PEDIATRIC SURGERY

VOLUME 2

PEDIATRIC SURGERY

Edited by

KENNETH J. WELCH, M.D.

Clinical Professor of Surgery, Harvard Medical School,
Senior Associate in Surgery, The Children's Hospital,
Boston, Massachusetts

JUDSON G. RANDOLPH, M.D.

Professor of Surgery and Child Health, George Washington University,
Surgeon-in-Chief, Children's Hospital National Medical Center,
Washington, D.C.

MARK M. RAVITCH, M.D.

Professor of Surgery, University of Pittsburgh,
Surgeon-in-Chief, Emeritus, Montefiore Hospital, Pittsburgh, Pennsylvania

JAMES A. O'NEILL, JR., M.D.

Professor of Pediatric Surgery, University of Pennsylvania School of Medicine,
Surgeon-in-Chief, The Children's Hospital of Philadelphia,
Philadelphia, Pennsylvania

MARC I. ROWE, M.D.

Professor of Pediatric Surgery, University of Pittsburgh School of Medicine,
Chief of Surgical Services, Children's Hospital of Pittsburgh,
Pittsburgh, Pennsylvania

FOURTH EDITION
Volume 2

YEAR BOOK MEDICAL PUBLISHERS, INC.
CHICAGO • LONDON • BOCA RATON

2 3 4 5 6 7 8 9 0 KC 89 88 87

Library of Congress Cataloging in Publication Data
Main entry under title:

Pediatric surgery:

   Includes bibliographies and index.
   1. Children—Surgery. I. Welch, Kenneth J.
[DNLM: 1. Surgery—in infancy & childhood. WO 925 P371]
RD137.P42 1986   617'.98   85-13775
ISBN 0-8151-9210-X

Notice

   Every effort has been made by the editors, the authors, and the publisher of this work to ensure that the procedures and treatment protocols presented herein were in accord with established practice at the time of publication. It should be noted, however, that procedures and treatment are subject to change and modification. In every case the reader is advised to check the latest publications on a given topic and to review recent drug product information to assure that changes have not been made, particularly in the recommended dosage of a drug or in contraindications for its administration.

Sponsoring Editor: Daniel J. Doody
Manager, Copyediting Services: Frances M. Perveiler
Copyeditor: Deborah Thorp
Production Project Managers: Carol Ennis Coghlan, R. Allen Reedtz
Proofroom Supervisor: Shirley E. Taylor

Preface to the First Edition

Pediatric surgery today is one of the most vigorously growing fields in surgery. The establishment of chairs, divisions, and departments of pediatric surgery in university centers attests to an increasing awareness of the special problems in this field. Several societies have been founded to promote knowledge in this area, and special sections exist in others. Two journals are devoted entirely to pediatric surgery, a third has a special department and others publish special issues concerned with its problems.

In June of 1959, an editorial board was formed to enroll the services of recognized authorities in writing a complete textbook of pediatric surgery that would reflect the best thoughts of men from representative institutions, covering a wide geographic area in the United States, Canada and England. As in any branch of surgery, during a period of rapid development and experimentation, much of the material is new, and much of it is as yet unpublished elsewhere in any form.

Our colleagues in many countries are contributing importantly to the growth of pediatric surgical knowledge. They will find repeated references to their published material. We regret that we could not enlist the services of many worthwhile contributors from Australia, Scandinavia and Continental Europe.

This project was conceived to meet the need for a comprehensive work on pediatric surgery presented from as broad a point of view as possible. There was agreement that all aspects of pediatric surgery would be covered, although, in order to limit the work to a reasonable size, it was necessary to restrict the space allotted to such specialty fields as ophthalmology, otolaryngology, orthopedics, and neurosurgery. The heaviest concentration is in the traditional fields of general, thoracic, and urologic surgery.

Particular emphasis has been laid on appropriate treatment of the physiologic, anatomic and embryologic aspects of specific surgical problems. Because we feel that the current state of knowledge is best understood in the light of its development, we have prefaced many subjects with an historical résumé.

Contributors have been urged to express their own feelings clearly on controversial points, to draw particularly on their own experience and, in addition, to evaluate and comment upon the work of others. To this end, we have encouraged extensive bibliographic lists, with annotations in the text. Particular attention has been paid to the illustrations and the publishers have been generous concerning the number included.

Our contributors have been cooperative, prompt, and patient with our editorial suggestions, and we are grateful to them. Some duplication of coverage will necessarily occur in a multiauthor textbook, and we think this not undesirable. Differences of opinion are expressed in some areas, and such differences will be found to exist. In details of treatment, and in other matters, in a variety of aspects of pediatric surgery, the editors do not hold uniform opinions—nor do the contributors. It was felt important only that an individual contribution present a valid and supportable point of view and a satisfactory method of treatment.

It is hoped that the various sections are developed in a manner systematic enough to make them useful to the student or house officer interested in the field of pediatric surgery, that the presentations are broad enough and sufficiently free from surgical minutiae to be useful to the pediatrician and yet detailed enough to convey to the informed general surgeon each author's assessment of current knowledge in his field and his own recommendations.

We have felt strongly that the value of this presentation would be increased in direct proportion to the briefness of time between the preparation of the manuscript and publication. In a multiauthor work, a good deal of time is necessarily expended in the transmission of manuscripts from authors to editors, in circulation among editors, and resubmission to authors for consideration of joint editorial suggestions. Six months were spent by the editorial board in organizing the form of the work, the division of subject matter, the matter of presentation, the division of editorial responsibilities and the assignment of subjects to the editors and contributors. The actual writing, editing, and publication have been accomplished in less than two years.

The editorial board has functioned in a coordinated effort. While the editors were individually responsible for given Parts, each contributed Sections to Parts for which others were editorially responsible. Every chapter has been reviewed by several members of the board. The distribution of a model chapter, prepared by Doctor Mustard, greatly simplified the problem of achieving uniformity. Doctor Welch served as chairman of the board and was editorially responsible for PART I: *General*, PART II: *Head and Neck*, and PART V: *Genitourinary System*. Doctors Mustard and Ravitch were responsible for PART III: *The Thorax*, Doctor Mustard for PART VI: *Integument and Musculoskeletal System*, and Doctor Ravitch for PART VII: *Nervous System*. Doctors Benson and Snyder prepared PART IV: *Abdomen*. The selection of contributors was a joint editorial effort. Mrs. Muriel McL. Miller was responsible for the uniform pen and ink illustration concept.

We wish to acknowledge our gratitude to our secretaries, Mrs. Ralph Conjour, Miss June Gerkens, Mrs. Grace Crabbe, Mrs. Josephine Dyer, and Miss Linda Morse, for their tolerance and patience, and their willingness to type and retype manuscripts at a rapid pace and make early publication a reality.

We are grateful also to the staff of Year Book Medical Publishers for their enthusiasm and cooperation. The many meetings of the editorial board have been made possible through their generous support.

THE EDITORS

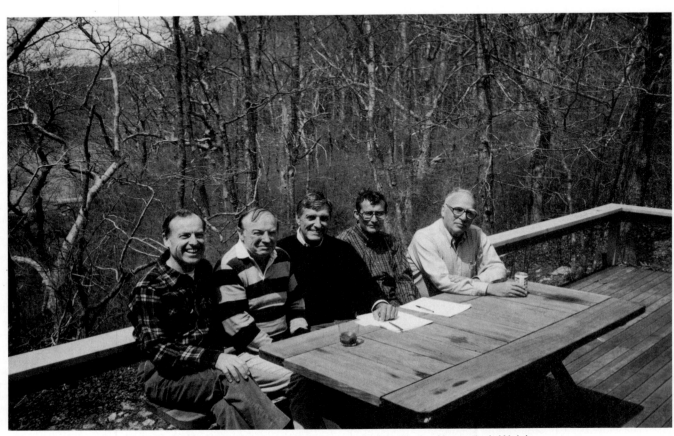

The Editors *(from left to right)*: James A. O'Neill, Jr., Kenneth J. Welch, Judson G. Randolph, Marc I. Rowe, and Mark M. Ravitch.

Preface to the Fourth Edition

This edition sees publication a quarter century after the appearance of the first.

With changes in organization and content and the roster of contributors, this edition is in many respects a new book. There are 33 new chapters representing either the presentation of new subjects (or phases of new subjects), or elevation of the status of a brief treatment offered previously. Discussions of the major malignant neoplasms of childhood have been collected in Part III rather than appearing in the various organ- or system-related sections of the book. Transplantation was considered to deserve its own section (Part IV) and an allocation of space that recognized the increasing importance of this exciting area.

Among the 33 new chapters and the subjects accorded expanded treatment are those on teratology, prenatal diagnosis, respiratory support, the immunocompromised child, newer imaging technologies, retinoblastoma, superior vena cava syndrome, esophageal rupture and perforation, gastrostomy, necrotizing enterocolitis, primary peritonitis, ileostomy and colostomy, non-Hodgkin's lymphoma, and six chapters on transplantation.

The increasing scope and complexity of what might be called general pediatric surgery led to the reluctant appreciation that not as much space could be devoted to the special fields as in previous editions. Most notably this has led to a sharp contraction and reorientation of the section that was devoted to cardiac surgery. That section, superbly organized and largely written by Dr. Mustard in the first two editions and brilliantly carried on by Dr. Aberdeen in the third, was in its own right a textbook of pediatric cardiac surgery. The sections on orthopedics and neurosurgery have also been reoriented.

Dr. Aberdeen has retired from the editorial board, as has Dr. Clifford Benson, one of the original editors, and a stalwart editor and contributor to the first three editions. We were delighted that he consented to contribute, once more, the chapter on pyloric stenosis. Drs. O'Neill and Rowe fill the places in the editorial board left by the retirement from it of Drs. Aberdeen and Benson.

The roster of 149 contributors includes 83 new names, recognizing the emergence of new authorities, new possessors of special knowledge. The contributors have been patient and cooperative in responding to the requirements of the book and we are grateful to them.

In the matter of editorial assignment to the various parts, Dr. Rowe took responsibility for PART I—*General,* PART IV—*Transplantation,* and PART IX—*Special Areas of Pediatric Surgery;* Dr. O'Neill, PART II—*Trauma,* and with Dr. Ravitch, PART VII—*The Abdomen;* Dr. Randolph, PART III—*Principal Malignant Tumors,* and with Dr. Ravitch, PART VI—*The Thorax;* Dr. Ravitch, PARTS VI and VII as noted, and PART X—*Skin, Soft Tissues, and Blood Vessels;* and Dr. Welch, PART V—*Head and Neck,* and PART VIII—*The Genitourinary System.*

Dr. Welch served as chairman of the board and Dr. Ravitch functioned as the "final common pathway" for all manuscripts and galleys. Our secretaries—Ruth Jacobson, Suzanne Danais, Katie Moran, Elizabeth Smith, and Norma Hackwelder—have been patient, tolerant, hardworking, and resourceful in typing and retyping manuscripts, tracking and routing contributions with persistence and good humor.

The informal portrait of the editors was taken in the final editorial work session, during a lunch break at which we discussed our hopes for the Fourth Edition and our desire that it prove helpful to pediatric surgeons and surgical residents the world over.

Once more Year Book Medical Publishers has been unstintingly cooperative and efficient and strongly endorsed and supported our efforts to make this essentially new book as complete, authoritative, and handsomely produced as the three preceding editions.

THE EDITORS

Contributors

ABERDEEN, EOIN, M.D.: Associate Professor, Department of Critical Care and Emergency Medicine, State University of New York, Emergency Room Physician, Upstate Medical Center, Syracuse, New York

ADKINS, JOHN C., M.D.: Clinical Assistant Professor of Pediatric Surgery, University of Pittsburgh, Attending Surgeon, Children's Hospital of Pittsburgh, Pittsburgh, Pennsylvania

ALTMAN, R. PETER, M.D.: Professor of Surgery and Pediatrics, Columbia University, College of Physicians and Surgeons, Director, Division of Pediatric Surgery, Babies Hospital, Columbia-Presbyterian Medical Center, New York, New York

AMOURY, RAYMOND A., M.D.: Katherine Berry Richardson Professor of Pediatric Surgery, University of Missouri–Kansas City School of Medicine, Surgeon-in-Chief, The Children's Mercy Hospital, Kansas City, Missouri

ANDERSON, KATHRYN D., M.D.: Professor of Surgery and Child Health Development, George Washington University, Senior Attending Surgeon, Children's Hospital National Medical Center, Washington, D.C.

ARENSMAN, ROBERT M., M.D.: Assistant Clinical Professor of Surgery, Louisiana State University Medical College, Chief, Division of Pediatric Surgery, Ochsner Medical Institutions, New Orleans, Louisiana

ASCHER, NANCY L., M.D., Ph.D.: Assistant Professor, Department of Surgery, University of Minnesota, Clinical Director, Liver Transplant Program, University of Minnesota Hospitals, Minneapolis, Minnesota

ASHCRAFT, KEITH W., M.D.: Clinical Professor, University of Missouri–Kansas City School of Medicine, Chief of Urology, Children's Mercy Hospital, Kansas City, Missouri

BARTLETT, ROBERT H., M.D.: Professor of Surgery, University of Michigan, Head, Section of General Surgery, Director, Surgical Intensive Care Unit, University of Michigan Medical Center, Ann Arbor, Michigan

BARTONE, FRANCIS F., M.D.: Professor of Surgery, Head, Section of Urology, Professor of Pediatrics, University of Nebraska, Omaha, Nebraska

BELMAN, A. BARRY, M.D., M.S.: Professor of Urology and Child Health and Development, George Washington University School of Medicine and Health Sciences, Chairman, Department of Urology, Children's Hospital National Medical Center, Washington, D.C.

BENSON, CLIFFORD D., M.D., F.A.C.S., F.A.A.P.: Professor of Clinical Surgery, Wayne State University School of Medicine, Emeritus Surgeon-in-Chief, Children's Hospital of Michigan, Consulting Surgeon, Bon Secours Hospital, Grosse Pointe, Michigan

BETTS, EUGENE K., M.D.: Assistant Professor of Anesthesia, The University of Pennsylvania, Senior Anesthesiologist and Director, Anesthesia Operating Room Service, The Children's Hospital of Philadelphia, Philadelphia, Pennsylvania

BISHOP, HARRY C., M.D.: Professor of Pediatric Surgery, University of Pennsylvania School of Medicine, Senior Surgeon, The Children's Hospital of Philadelphia, Philadelphia, Pennsylvania

BOIX-OCHOA, J., M.D.: Professor of Pediatric Surgery, Autonomous University, Chief, Department of Pediatric Surgery, Children's Hospital, Barcelona, Spain

BOLES, E. THOMAS, JR., M.D.: Professor and Director, Division of Pediatric Surgery, Ohio State University College of Medicine, Chief, Department of Pediatric Surgery, Children's Hospital, Columbus, Ohio

BOLEY, SCOTT J., M.D.: Professor of Surgery and Pediatrics, Chief, Pediatric Surgical Services, Albert Einstein College of Medicine, Chief of Pediatric Surgery, Montefiore Medical Center, New York, New York

BRUCE, DEREK A., M.B., Ch.B.: Associate Professor, Neurosurgery and Pediatrics, University of Pennsylvania School of Medicine, Associate Neurosurgeon, Children's Hospital of Philadelphia, Philadelphia, Pennsylvania

BUNTAIN, WILLIAM L., M.D.: Professor of Surgery, Director, Division of Pediatric Surgery, University of Tennessee Memorial Hospital, Knoxville, Tennessee

CALDAMONE, ANTHONY A., M.D., M.M.S.: Assistant Professor of Surgery (Urology), Case Western Reserve University School of Medicine, Head, Pediatric Urology, Rainbow Babies and Children's Hospital, Cleveland, Ohio

CAMPBELL, JOHN R., M.D.: Professor of Surgery and Pediatrics, Chief of Pediatric Surgery, Acting Chairman, Department of Surgery, Oregon Health Sciences University School of Medicine and University Hospitals, Portland, Oregon

CATLIN, FRANCIS I., M.D.: Professor of Otorhinolaryngology and Communicative Sciences, Baylor College of Medicine, Chief of Otolaryngology Services, St. Luke's Episcopal Texas Children's Hospitals, Houston, Texas

CHEW, EMILY Y., M.D.: Lecturer, University of Toronto, Staff Ophthalmologist, Toronto General Hospital and the Hospital for Sick Children, Toronto, Ontario

COLODNY, ARNOLD H., M.D.: Associate Professor of Surgery, Harvard Medical School, Senior Surgeon, Associate Director, Division of Urology, Children's Hospital, Boston, Massachusetts

CORAN, ARNOLD G., A.B., M.D.: Professor of Surgery, Head of the Section of Pediatric Surgery, University of Michigan Medical School, Surgeon-in-Chief, Mott Children's Hospital, Ann Arbor, Michigan, Chief of the Division of Pediatric Surgery, Henry Ford Hospital, Detroit, Michigan

CRAWFORD, JOHN D., M.D.: Professor of Pediatrics, Harvard Medical School, Chief, Pediatric Endocrinology-Metabolic Unit, Massachusetts General Hospital, Boston, Massachusetts

CRAWFORD, JOHN S., M.D., C.M., D.O.M.S. (Eng.), F.R.C.S.(C.): Emeritus Professor of Ophthalmology, University of Toronto, Former Ophthalmologist-in-Chief, Hospital for Sick Children, Toronto, Ontario

CROMIE, WILLIAM J., M.D.: Associate Professor of Surgery and Pediatrics, Head, Section of Pediatric and Reconstructive Urology, Albany Medical College of Union University, Albany, New York

D'ANGIO, GIULIO J., M.D.: Professor of Radiology, Professor of Radiation Therapy, Professor of Pediatric Oncology, University of Pennsylvania, Director, The Children's Cancer Research Center, The Children's Hospital of Philadelphia, Philadelphia, Pennsylvania

DAVIDSON, RICHARD S., M.D.: The Children's Hospital of Philadelphia, Philadelphia, Pennsylvania

DEAN, RICHARD H., M.D.: Professor of Surgery, Head, Division of Vascular Surgery, Vanderbilt University School of Medicine, Nashville, Tennessee

de LORIMIER, ALFRED A., M.D.: Professor of Surgery, School of

Medicine, University of California at San Francisco, Chief of Pediatric Surgery, University of California, San Francisco, Children's Hospital, San Francisco, California

de VRIES, PIETER A., M.D.: Professor of Surgery, Chief, Section of Pediatric Surgery, University of Kansas Medical Center, Kansas City, Kansas

DONAHOE, PATRICIA K., M.D.: Associate Professor of Surgery, Harvard Medical School, Chief of Pediatric Surgery, Director of Pediatric Surgical Research Laboratory, Massachusetts General Hospital, Boston, Massachusetts

DOWNES, JOHN J., M.D.: Professor of Anesthesia and Pediatrics, University of Pennsylvania, Anesthesiologist-in-Chief and Director, Department of Anesthesia and Critical Care, The Children's Hospital of Philadelphia, Philadelphia, Pennsylvania

DUCKETT, JOHN W., M.D.: Professor of Urology, University of Pennsylvania School of Medicine, Director, Division of Urology, The Children's Hospital of Philadelphia, Philadelphia, Pennsylvania

EATON, RICHARD G., M.D.: Associate Professor of Surgery, Columbia College of Physicians and Surgeons, Co-Chief, Hand Surgery Service, The Roosevelt Hospital, New York, New York

EDGERTON, MILTON T., M.D.: Chairman, Department of Plastic and Maxillofacial Surgery, University of Virginia Medical Center, Charlottesville, Virginia

EDHOLM, CURTIS D., M.D.: Associate Professor of Surgery (Orthopedic), Michigan State University College of Human Medicine, Project Director, Area Child Amputee Center, Mary Free Bed Hospital and Rehabilitation Center, Grand Rapids, Michigan

EICHELBERGER, MARTIN R., M.D.: Associate Professor of Surgery and Child Health, George Washington University, Director, Emergency Trauma Services, Children's Hospital National Medical Center, Washington, D.C.

EIN, SIGMUND H., M.D., C.M., F.R.C.S.(C.), F.A.C.S., F.A.A.P.: Assistant Professor, Department of Surgery, Faculty of Medicine, University of Toronto, Staff Surgeon, The Hospital for Sick Children, Consultant Staff, Division of Pediatrics, Women's College Hospital, Toronto, Ontario

EPSTEIN, MELVIN H., M.D.: Professor and Chairman, Department of Neurosurgery, Brown University, Providence, Rhode Island

FILLER, ROBERT M., M.D., F.A.A.P., F.R.C.S.(C.): Professor of Surgery and Pediatrics, University of Toronto, Surgeon-in-Chief, The Hospital for Sick Children, Toronto, Ontario

FILSTON, HOWARD C., M.D.: Professor of Pediatric Surgery and Pediatrics, Duke University School of Medicine, Chief of Pediatric Surgery Service, Duke University Medical Center, Durham, North Carolina

FIRLIT, CASIMIR F., M.D., Ph.D.: Professor of Urology, Northwestern University Medical School, Chairman, Division of Urology, Head, Renal Transplantation, Children's Memorial Hospital, Chicago, Illinois

FONKALSRUD, ERIC W., M.D.: Professor and Chief of Pediatric Surgery, Vice Chairman, Department of Surgery, UCLA School of Medicine, Los Angeles, California

GANS, STEPHEN L., M.D., F.A.C.S., F.A.A.P.: Clinical Professor of Surgery, UCLA School of Medicine, Attending Surgeon, Cedars-Sinai Medical Center, Los Angeles, California

GRIFFIN, PAUL P., M.D.: Professor of Orthopaedic Surgery, Harvard Medical School, Orthopaedic Surgeon-in-Chief, The Children's Hospital, Boston, Massachusetts

GRIFFITH, BARTLEY P., M.D.: Assistant Professor of Surgery, University of Pittsburgh School of Medicine, Pittsburgh, Pennsylvania

GROFF, DILLER B. III, M.D., F.A.C.S., F.A.A.P.: Professor of Pediatric Surgery, University of Louisville School of Medicine, Surgeon-in-Chief, Kosair Children's Hospital, Louisville, Kentucky

GROSFELD, JAY L., M.D.: Lafayette F. Page Professor and Chairman, Department of Surgery, Indiana University School of Medicine, Surgeon-in-Chief, James Whitcomb Riley Hospital for Children, Indianapolis, Indiana

GUZZETTA, PHILIP C., M.D.: Assistant Professor, Department of Child Health and Development, George Washington University,

Attending Surgeon, Children's Hospital National Medical Center, Washington, D.C.

HALLER, J. ALEX, JR., M.D.: Robert Garrett Professor of Pediatric Surgery, Professor of Emergency Medicine, Professor of Pediatrics, The Johns Hopkins University School of Medicine, Children's Surgeon-in-Charge, The Johns Hopkins Hospital, Baltimore, Maryland

HARDY, BRIAN E., M.B., Ch.B.: Associate Professor of Surgery, University of Southern California, Chief, Division of Urology, Children's Hospital of Los Angeles, Los Angeles, California

HARRISON, MICHAEL R., M.D.: Associate Professor of Surgery, University of California at San Francisco, Attending Pediatric Surgeon, USCF Children's Medical Center, San Francisco, California

HAYS, DANIEL M., M.D.: Professor of Surgery and Pediatrics, University of Southern California School of Medicine, Attending Surgeon, Children's Hospital of Los Angeles, Los Angeles, California

HELLER, RICHARD M., M.D.: Professor of Radiology and Radiological Sciences, Associate Professor of Pediatrics, Vanderbilt University School of Medicine, Nashville, Tennessee

HENDREN, W. HARDY, M.D., F.A.C.S.: Professor of Surgery, Harvard Medical School, Chief of Surgery, Children's Hospital Medical Center, Boston, Massachusetts

HERSH, STEPHEN P., M.D.: Co-Director, Medical Illness Counseling Center, Chevy Chase, Maryland

HILL, J. LAURANCE, M.D.: Professor of Surgery, University of Maryland, Baltimore, Maryland

HOLCOMB, GEORGE W., JR., M.D.: Clinical Professor of Pediatric Surgery, Vanderbilt University School of Medicine, Staff Pediatric Surgeon, Vanderbilt Children's Hospital, Nashville, Tennessee

HOLDER, THOMAS M., M.D.: Clinical Professor of Surgery, University of Missouri–Kansas City School of Medicine, Chief, Thoracic and Cardiovascular Surgery, Children's Mercy Hospital, Kansas City, Missouri

HOWELL, CHARLES G., M.D.: Associate Professor of Pediatric Surgery and Pediatrics, Medical College of Georgia, Augusta, Georgia

IWATSUKI, SHUNZABURO, M.D.: Associate Professor of Surgery, University of Pittsburgh School of Medicine, Pittsburgh, Pennsylvania

JAFFE, NORMAN, M.D.: Professor of Pediatrics, University of Texas, Chief, Division of Pediatrics, M. D. Anderson Hospital and Tumor Institute, Houston, Texas

JEFFS, ROBERT D., M.D.: Professor of Pediatric Urology, The Johns Hopkins University School of Medicine, Professor and Director, Division of Pediatric Urology, The Johns Hopkins Hospital, Baltimore, Maryland

JEWETT, THEODORE C., JR., M.D.: Professor of Surgery and Pediatrics, State University of New York at Buffalo, Associate Chairman, Department of Pediatric Surgery, The Children's Hospital of Buffalo, Buffalo, New York

JOHNSON, DALE G., M.D.: Professor of Surgery, Professor of Pediatrics, University of Utah College of Medicine, Chief of Surgery, Primary Children's Medical Center, Salt Lake City, Utah

JONES, PETER G., M.S. (Melb.), F.R.C.S., F.R.A.C.S., F.A.C.S., F.A.A.P. (Hon.): Fellow, Trinity College, Clinical Instructor, University of Melbourne, Surgeon, Royal Children's Hospital, Melbourne, Victoria, Australia

KABAN, LEONARD B., D.M.D., M.D., F.A.C.S.: Associate Professor, Oral and Maxillofacial Surgery, Harvard School of Dental Medicine, Associate in Surgery, Children's Hospital, Surgeon, Brigham and Women's Hospital, Boston, Massachusetts

KASS, EVAN J., M.D., F.A.A.P., F.A.C.S.: Chief, Pediatric Urology, William Beaumont Hospital, Royal Oak, Michigan

KEVY, SHERWIN V., M.D.: Associate Professor at Pediatrics, Harvard Medical School, Director of Transfusion Service, The Children's Hospital Medical Center, Boston, Massachusetts

KEYSER, JOHN J., M.D., F.A.C.S.: Clinical Instructor in Surgery, Columbia College of Physicians and Surgeons, Attending, Plastic, Reconstructive and Hand Surgery, St. Luke's Roosevelt Hospital Center, New York, New York, Chairman, Section of Plastic Surgery, Morristown Memorial Hospital, Morristown, New Jersey

KING, DENIS R., M.D.: Associate Professor of Surgery, Ohio State University College of Medicine, Children's Hospital, Columbus, Ohio

KING, LOWELL R., M.D.: Professor, Division of Urology, Department of Surgery, Department of Pediatrics, Duke University Medical Center, Durham, North Carolina

KOSLOSKE, ANN M., M.D.: Clinical Professor of Surgery and Pediatrics, University of New Mexico School of Medicine, Director of Pediatric Surgery, University of New Mexico Hospital, Albuquerque, New Mexico

KOTTMEIER, PETER K., M.D.: Professor of Surgery, State University of New York, Chief of Pediatric Surgery, Downstate Medical Center, Brooklyn, New York

LACKMAN, RICHARD D., M.D.: Assistant Clinical Professor and Chief, Musculoskeletal Tumor Service, Thomas Jefferson University, Philadelphia, Pennsylvania

LaROSSA, DONATO, M.D.: Associate Professor of Surgery, University of Pennsylvania School of Medicine, Director, Microsurgery Laboratory, Hospital of the University of Pennsylvania, Philadelphia, Pennsylvania

LEAPE, LUCIAN L., M.D.: Professor of Surgery, Tufts University School of Medicine, Chief, Pediatric Surgery, New England Medical Center, Boston, Massachusetts

LILLY, JOHN R., M.D.: Professor of Surgery, Department of Surgery, Chief of Pediatric Surgery, University of Colorado School of Medicine, Denver, Colorado

LINDSAY, WILLIAM K., M.D., B.Sc. (Med.), F.R.C.S. (C.), F.A.C.S.: Professor, Department of Surgery, Chairman, Interhospital Coordinating Committee for Plastic Surgery, Head, Division of Plastic Surgery, University of Toronto School of Medicine, The Hospital for Sick Children, Toronto, Ontario

LLOYD, DAVID A., M.D.: Associate Professor of Surgery, University of Pittsburgh School of Medicine, Pediatric Surgeon, Department of Surgery, Children's Hospital of Pittsburgh, Pittsburgh, Pennsylvania

LONG, DONLIN M., M.D., Ph.D.: Professor and Chairman, Department of Neurosurgery, The Johns Hopkins University School of Medicine, Baltimore, Maryland

MARTIN, LESTER W., M.D.: Professor of Surgery and Pediatrics, University of Cincinnati College of Medicine, Director of Pediatric Surgery, Children's Hospital Medical Center, Cincinnati, Ohio

MASTERSON, JOHN S.T., B.Sc., M.D., F.R.C.S.(C.): Clinical Instructor, University of British Columbia, Active Staff, Children's Hospital of British Columbia, Vancouver, British Columbia

MAUER, S. MICHAEL, M.D.: Professor of Pediatrics, Division of Nephrology, Department of Surgery, University of Minnesota, Minneapolis, Minnesota

MORGAN, RAYMOND F., M.D., D.M.D., F.A.C.S.: Associate Professor of Surgery, University of Virginia Medical Center, Charlottesville, Virginia

MULLIKEN, JOHN B., M.D., F.A.C.S.: Associate Professor in Surgery, Harvard Medical School, Surgeon, The Children's Hospital, Boston, Massachusetts

MURRAY, JOSEPH E., M.D.: Professor of Surgery, Harvard Medical School, Chief of Plastic Surgery, Children's Hospital and Brigham and Women's Hospital, Boston, Massachusetts

MYERS, NATHAN A., A.M., F.R.C.S., F.R.A.C.S.: Professorial Associate, University of Melbourne, Senior Surgeon, Royal Children's Hospital, Melbourne, Australia

NADLER, HENRY L., M.D.: Dean, School of Medicine, Professor of Pediatrics, Professor of Obstetrics, Wayne State University, Director, Genetic, Metabolic, and Developmental Disorders Clinic, Children's Hospital of Michigan, Detroit, Michigan

NAJARIAN, JOHN S., M.D.: Regents' Professor and Chairman, Department of Surgery, University of Minnesota Hospital, Minneapolis, Minnesota

O'NEILL, JAMES A., JR., M.D., F.A.C.S., F.A.A.P.: Professor of Pediatric Surgery, University of Pennsylvania School of Medicine, Surgeon-in-Chief, The Children's Hospital of Philadelphia, Philadelphia, Pennsylvania

OTHERSEN, H. BIEMANN, JR., M.D.: Professor of Surgery and Pediatrics, Medical University of South Carolina, Chief, Pediatric Surgery, Medical University Hospital, Charleston, South Carolina

PAE, WALTER E., JR., M.D.: Assistant Professor of Surgery, The Pennsylvania State University, Staff Surgeon, The Milton S. Hershey Medical Center, Hershey, Pennsylvania

PASHBY, ROBERT C., M.D.: Assistant Professor, Department of Ophthalmology, University of Toronto, Active Staff, The Hospital for Sick Children, Toronto, Ontario

PENA, ALBERTO, M.D.: Surgeon-in-Chief, National Institute of Pediatrics, Pre and Post Graduate Professor of Pediatric Surgery, Military Medical School and Faculty of Medicine of the University of Mexico, Mexico City, Mexico

PETTITT, BARBARA J., M.D.: Assistant Professor of Surgery and Pediatrics, Emory University School of Medicine, Attending Surgeon, Henrietta Egleston Hospital for Children, Grady Memorial Hospital, Atlanta, Georgia

PHILIPPART, ARVIN I., M.D.: Associate Professor of Surgery, Wayne State University School of Medicine, Chief of Pediatric General Surgery, Chairman of Surgical Services, Children's Hospital of Michigan, Detroit, Michigan

PRINGLE, KEVIN C., M.B., Ch.B., F.R.A.C.S.: Associate Professor, University of Iowa College of Medicine, Associate Professor of Surgery (Pediatrics), Department of Surgery, University of Iowa Hospitals and Clinics, Iowa City, Iowa

RANDOLPH, JUDSON G., M.D.: Professor of Surgery and Child Health, George Washington University, Surgeon-in-Chief, Children's Hospital National Medical Center, Washington, D.C.

RAPHAELY, RUSSELL C., M.D.: Associate Professor of Anesthesiology and Pediatrics, University of Pennsylvania School of Medicine, Director, Pediatric Intensive Care Complex, The Children's Hospital of Philadelphia, Philadelphia, Pennsylvania

RAVITCH, MARK M., M.D.: Professor of Surgery, University of Pittsburgh, Surgeon-in-Chief, Montefiore Hospital, Pittsburgh, Pennsylvania

REEMTSMA, KEITH, M.D., D.M.Sci.: Valentine Mott Professor of Surgery, Chairman, Department of Surgery, Columbia University College of Physicians and Surgeons, Director, Surgical Service, Presbyterian Hospital, New York, New York

RETIK, ALAN B., M.D.: Professor of Surgery (Urology), Harvard Medical School, Chief, Division of Urology, The Children's Hospital, Boston, Massachusetts

RODGERS, BRADLEY M., M.D.: Professor of Surgery and Pediatrics, University of Virginia Medical Center, Chief, Children's Surgery, University of Virginia Hospital, Charlottesville, Virginia

ROSEN, FRED S., M.D.: The James L. Gamble Professor of Pediatrics, Harvard Medical School, Chief, Division of Immunology and Renal Division, The Children's Hospital, Boston, Massachusetts

ROSENBAUM, KENNETH N., M.D.: Associate Professor of Child Health and Development, George Washington University, Director, Clinical Genetics and Genetics Laboratory, Children's Hospital Medical Center, Washington, D.C.

ROWE, MARC I., M.D.: Professor of Pediatric Surgery, University of Pittsburgh School of Medicine, Chief of Surgical Services, Children's Hospital of Pittsburgh, Pittsburgh, Pennsylvania

RUSH, BENJAMIN F., Jr., M.D., F.A.C.S.: Professor and Chairman, Department of Surgery, University of Medicine and Dentistry of New Jersey, New Jersey Medical School, Surgeon-in-Chief, University Hospital, Newark, New Jersey

SANTOS, GEORGE W., M.D.: Professor of Oncology and Medicine, The Johns Hopkins University School of Medicine, Active Staff in Medicine and Oncology, The Johns Hopkins Hospital, Baltimore, Maryland

SANTULLI, THOMAS V., M.D.: Professor Emeritus of Surgery, Special Lecturer in Surgery, Columbia University, Consultant in Surgery, Columbia-Presbyterian Medical Center, New York, New York

SCHNAUFER, LOUISE, M.D.: Associate Professor, Pediatric Surgery, University of Pennsylvania School of Medicine, Associate Surgeon, Children's Hospital of Philadelphia, Philadelphia, Pennsylvania

SCHULLINGER, JOHN N., M.D., F.A.C.S., F.A.A.P.: Associate Clinical Professor of Surgery, Columbia University College of Physicians and Surgeons, Associate Attending Surgeon, Columbia-Presbyterian Medical Center (Babies Hospital), New York, New York

SCHUSTER, SAMUEL R., M.D.: Associate Professor of Surgery, Harvard Medical School, Senior Associate Surgeon, Children's Hospital of Boston, Boston, Massachusetts

SEASHORE, JOHN H., M.D.: Professor of Surgery and Pediatrics, Yale University School of Medicine, Attending Physician, Yale-New Haven Hospital, New Haven, Connecticut

SHAW, ANTHONY, M.D.: Clinical Professor of Surgery, UCLA School of Medicine, Director, Pediatric Surgery, City of Hope National Medical Center, Attending Surgeon, UCLA Medical Center, Los Angeles, California

SHAW, BYERS W., JR. M.D.: Associate Professor of Surgery, Chief, Transplantation Section, Department of Surgery, University of Nebraska, Omaha, Nebraska

SIEBER, WILLIAM K., M.D.: Clinical Professor of Surgery, University of Pittsburgh, Senior Staff, Children's Hospital of Pittsburgh, Pittsburgh, Pennsylvania

SMITH, BRUCE M., M.D.: Assistant Clinical Professor of Surgery, Vanderbilt University Medical Center, Chief, Vascular Surgical Service, Nashville Veterans Administration Medical Center, Nashville, Tennessee

SMITH, E. IDE, M.D.: Professor of Surgery, University of Oklahoma College of Medicine, Chief, Pediatric Surgery Service, Oklahoma Children's Memorial Hospital, Oklahoma City, Oklahoma

SNYDER, HOWARD McC. III, M.D.: Assistant Professor of Surgery/ Urology, University of Pennsylvania School of Medicine, Associate Director, Division of Pediatric Urology, Children's Hospital of Philadelphia, Philadelphia, Pennsylvania

SOPER, ROBERT T., M.D.: Professor of Surgery, University of Iowa College of Medicine, Director of Pediatric Surgery Service, University of Iowa Hospitals and Clinics, Iowa City, Iowa

STARZL, THOMAS E., M.D., Ph.D.: Associate Professor of Surgery, University of Pittsburgh School of Medicine, Staff Surgeon, University-Presbyterian Hospital, Pittsburgh, Pennsylvania

STEPHENS, F. DOUGLAS, M.S. (Melb.), F.R.A.C.S.: Professor Emeritus of Surgery and Urology, Northwestern University Medical School, Pediatric Urologist, Children's Memorial Hospital, Chicago, Illinois

STONE, H. HARLAN, M.D.: Professor of Surgery and Chief, Division of General Surgery, University of Maryland School of Medicine, Chief of General Surgery, University of Maryland Hospital, Baltimore, Maryland

TELANDER, ROBERT L., M.D.: Head, Section of Pediatric Surgery, Professor of Surgery, Mayo Medical School, Consultant and Surgeon in Pediatric Surgery, St. Marys Hospital, Rochester, Minnesota

TEMPLETON, JOHN M., JR., M.D.: Assistant Professor of Pediatric Surgery, University of Pennsylvania School of Medicine, Associate Surgeon, The Children's Hospital of Philadelphia, Philadelphia, Pennsylvania

TERNBERG, JESSIE L., M.D., Ph.D.: Professor of Surgery and Pediatrics, Chief, Division of Pediatric Surgery, Washington University School of Medicine, Hospital Director, Division of Pediatric Surgery, Children's Hospital of the Washington University Medical Center, St. Louis, Missouri

THOMPSON, NORMAN W., M.D.: Henry King Ransom Professor of Surgery, University of Michigan School of Medicine, Chief, Division of Endocrine Surgery, University of Michigan Medical Center, Ann Arbor, Michigan

TOULOUKIAN, ROBERT J., M.D.: Professor of Surgery and Pediatrics, Yale University School of Medicine, Chief, Pediatric Surgery, Attending Surgeon, Yale-New Haven Hospital, New Haven, Connecticut

TUNELL, WILLIAM P., M.D.: Professor of Surgery, University of Oklahoma College of Medicine, Attending Surgeon, Oklahoma Children's Memorial Hospital, Oklahoma City, Oklahoma

UDVARHELYI, GEORGE B., M.D., F.A.C.S.: Professor Emeritus of Neurosurgery, Associate Professor Emeritus of Radiology (Neuroradiology), The Johns Hopkins University School of Medicine, Emeritus Staff Neurosurgeon, The Johns Hopkins Hospital, Baltimore, Maryland

VOTTELER, THEODORE P., M.D.: Clinical Associate Professor of Surgery, University of Texas Health Science Center, Director of Surgical Services, Children's Medical Center, Dallas Texas

WALDHAUSEN, JOHN A., M.D.: John W. Oswald Professor of Surgery, Chairman, Department of Surgery, The Pennsylvania State University, Chief of Surgery, The Milton S. Hershey Medical Center, Hershey, Pennsylvania

WATTS, HUGH G., M.D.: Professor of Orthopedic Surgery, University of Pennsylvania School of Medicine, Philadelphia, Pennsylvania

WEBER, COLLIN J., M.D., D.M.Sci.: Assistant Professor of Surgery, Director of Endocrine Transplant, Department of Surgery, Columbia College of Physicians and Surgeons, Assistant Attending Surgeon, The Presbyterian Hospital, New York, New York

WEBER, THOMAS R., M.D.: Associate Professor of Surgery, St. Louis University School of Medicine, Director, Department of Pediatric Surgery, Cardinal Glennon Children's Hospital, St. Louis, Missouri

WEINTRAUB, WILLIAM H., M.D.: Vice Chairman and Professor of Surgery, Temple University School of Medicine, Director, Department of Surgery, St. Christopher's Hospital for Children, Philadelphia, Pennsylvania

WEITZMAN, JORDAN J., M.D., F.A.C.S.: Associate Clinical Professor of Surgery, University of Southern California, Chairman, Section of Pediatric Surgery, Cedars-Sinai Medical Center, Los Angeles, California

WELCH, KENNETH J., M.D., F.A.C.S.: Clinical Professor of Surgery, Harvard Medical School, Senior Associate in Surgery, The Children's Hospital, Boston, Massachusetts

WHITAKER, LINTON A., M.D.: Professor of Surgery (Plastic), University of Pennsylvania School of Medicine, Chief of Plastic Surgery, Children's Hospital of Philadelphia, Philadelphia, Pennsylvania

WHITAKER, ROBERT H., M.Chir., F.R.C.S.: Associate Lecturer, Cambridge University, Consultant Paediatric Urologist, Addenbrooke's Hospital, Cambridge, England

WIENER, EUGENE S., M.D.: Clinical Assistant Professor of Pediatric Surgery, University of Pittsburgh, Attending Staff, Children's Hospital, Pittsburgh, Pennsylvania

WINFIELD, JEFFREY A., M.D., Ph.D.: Assistant Professor of Neurosurgery/Pediatrics, State University of New York, Upstate Medical Center, Syracuse, New York

WOOLLEY, MORTON M., M.D.: Professor of Surgery, University of Southern California School of Medicine, Surgeon-in-Chief and Head, Department of Surgery, Children's Hospital of Los Angeles, Los Angeles, California

ZIEGLER, MORITZ M., M.D.: Associate Professor of Pediatric Surgery, University of Pennsylvania School of Medicine, Associate Surgeon, The Children's Hospital of Philadelphia, Philadelphia, Pennsylvania

ZUKER, RONALD M., M.D., F.R.C.S.(C.), F.A.C.S.: Assistant Professor of Surgery, University of Toronto, Consultant in Plastic Surgery, The Hospital for Sick Children, Director of the Burn Unit, Toronto General Hospital, Toronto, Ontario

Contents

VOLUME 2

PART VII. ABDOMEN

SECTION TWO: STOMACH AND DUODENUM

SECTION THREE: THE SMALL INTESTINE

PART VIII. GENITOURINARY SYSTEM

SECTION ONE: KIDNEY AND URETER

PART IX. SPECIAL AREAS OF PEDIATRIC SURGERY

SECTION ONE: CARDIAC SURGERY

SECTION TWO: NEUROSURGERY

SECTION THREE: ORTHOPEDICS

PART X. SKIN, SOFT TISSUES, AND BLOOD VESSELS

Contents

PART II. TRAUMA

PART III. PRINCIPAL MALIGNANT TUMORS

PART IV. TRANSPLANTATION

PART V. HEAD AND NECK

PART VI. THORAX

SECTION ONE: THE THORACIC PARIETES

SECTION TWO: THE AIRWAY, LUNGS, AND PLEURA

Color Plates

PART VII

Abdomen

PLATE III

A. Omphalocele. This large defect measured 8 cm in diameter. The sac contained intestine, a large portion of the liver, and a portion of the heart, which protruded through an anterior defect in the pericardium and diaphragm. Congenital heart disease completed the "pentalogy of Ravitch and Cantrell." A Silon prosthesis was placed for initial coverage and gradual closure of the abdomen was accomplished successfully over a three-week period. Correction of the cardiac lesion, usually a tetralogy of Fallot, was left for a later stage.

B. Gastroschisis. This low–birth-weight infant was born with antenatal prolapse of most of the intestine through a relatively small opening at the right of the umbilicus. Staged closure of the abdomen with a Silon prosthesis was accomplished within ten days. Parenteral nutritional support was required for three weeks until full return of normal gastrointestinal function.

C. Patent omphalomesenteric duct, with complete eversion of proximal and distal loops of bowel. The Y-shaped mass presents a mucosal external surface. In this 23-day-old child, the fecal discharge came entirely from one arm of the "Y." The stem of the "Y" had room within it for a knuckle of bowel that was herniated up into the serosa-lined cavity. A small incision around the umbilicus allowed the bowel to be reduced, the omphalomesenteric persistence to be amputated, and the bowel to be closed. This is the most complete form of persistence of an omphalomesenteric duct. If only one end persists, it leaves a Meckel's diverticulum and, if the other, no more than a tuft of mucosa in the umbilicus.

D. Necrotizing enterocolitis. Vascular thromboses, marked distention, pneumatosis, and widespread necrosis are evident in this 3-day-old low–birth-weight infant with respiratory distress syndrome. Resection and high ileostomy permitted survival, but manifestations of "short bowel syndrome" required long-term parenteral nutrition, even following reanastomosis at 6 weeks of age.

E. Non-Hodgkin's lymphoma of small bowel. The tumor was easily palpable through the abdominal wall of this 4-year-old child who had vague symptoms. The U-shaped loop at the left is diffusely replaced by tumor, so that its lumen is a mere slit. There is obvious disproportion between the proximal dilated bowel *(left)* and the distal collapsed bowel *(lower center),* but the child had no obstructive symptoms. The involved segment of bowel was resected and multiagent chemotherapy initiated.

F. Intussusception. This 10-year-old child had Henoch-Schönlein purpura and developed signs and symptoms of intestinal obstruction confirmed on x-ray. Shown is a jejunal intussusception which was reduced operatively. Note the nodular areas of vasculitis.

PLATE III

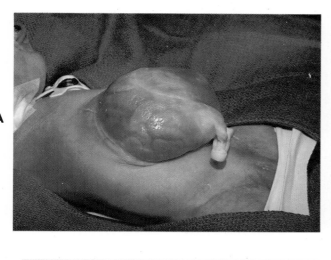

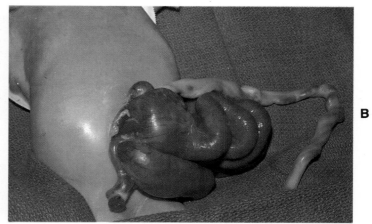

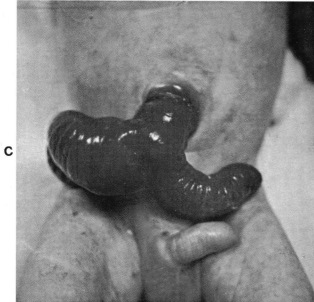

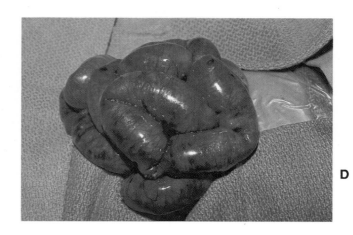

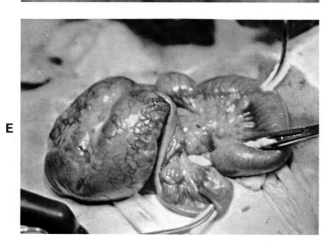

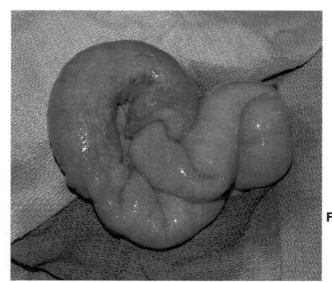

PLATE IV

A. Chylous cyst of the mesentery. A 4-year-old boy had abdominal colic with vomiting, as well as a lifelong history of intermittent attacks of a similar nature. There was dullness in the upper abdomen, but no palpable mass. The involved segment had twisted, producing a volvulus, and this twisting had probably occurred intermittently. The chylous cyst, filled with a creamy material, bulges its thin lobulations through the mesentery of the small bowel *(center)*, stretched out over the tumor. As in most mesenteric cysts, it was necessary to resect the bowel, together with the cyst, and perform an end-to-end anastomosis. Other cysts occasionally become manifest by the development of acute inflammation, suggesting appendicitis in their symptomatology.

B. Multiple jejunal atresias. Proximal jejunal atresias are shown in a newborn premature infant. A portion of the dilated proximal bowel and the atretic segment up to the distal patent bowel were resected, and end-to-back anastomosis performed as well as gastrostomy. Following one month of parenteral nutrition, it was possible to wean the baby to full oral feedings. Usually some form of tapering procedure would be performed on the residual dilated proximal bowel.

C. Hirschsprung's disease. Typical narrowing of the aganglionic rectosigmoid area with dilatation of the sigmoid were found at operation in a 3-week-old infant. A colostomy was performed in the sigmoid after frozen section determined the presence of normal ganglion cells. Resection of the aganglionic segment and endorectal pull-through were successfully accomplished when the child weighed 20 lb.

D. Hirschsprung's disease. Photomicrographs from a resected specimen in a child with a classic history of constipation and distention from birth and with typical operative findings. The left view, from the dilated hypertrophied proximal bowel, shows clearly the numerous large ganglion cells of the myenteric plexus of Auerbach and the inconspicuous nerve fibers. The right view, a section through the narrowed distal segment, shows a complete absence of ganglion cells and a great prominence of whorls of neurofibrillae. These are regular findings in the narrowed distal segment in Hirschsprung's disease. Distally, the aganglionic segment begins with the internal sphincter; and proximally it extends uninterruptedly until normal bowel is reached, usually in the sigmoid but occasionally in the more proximal areas of the colon, and, at times, well up into the small bowel. Occasionally the entire small intestine is involved, along with the colon. "Skip" areas are not reliably known to occur.

E. Intestinal duplication. A large enteric cyst near the ileocecal junction in a 12-day-old child who had great abdominal distention. Serosa-covered, muscle-walled, and mucosa-lined cysts of this kind, when localized, as in this instance, usually do not communicate with the bowel. A common muscular coat between the bowel and the cyst usually requires resection of the attached bowel, as was performed in this instance, with an end-to-end anastomosis. Long tubular duplications frequently communicate with the bowel; they are lined in whole, or in part, by gastric mucosa, so that junctional ulcers occur, presenting with massive hemorrhage. If resection of these duplications is precluded by the length of bowel involved, it is possible to strip the mucosal-submucosal lining from the duplication, leaving the innocuous muscle behind. Enteric cysts in the duodenum and other special locations require individual operative procedures.

F. Granulomatous ileitis. This 14-year-old boy required operation because of chronic pain, diarrhea, weight loss, and partial obstruction despite intensive supportive therapy. He improved remarkably after operation, but developed recurrent disease one year later, although he has not yet required reoperation. After the second operation, as after the first, there is a 50% to 60% likelihood of freedom from recurrence.

PLATE IV

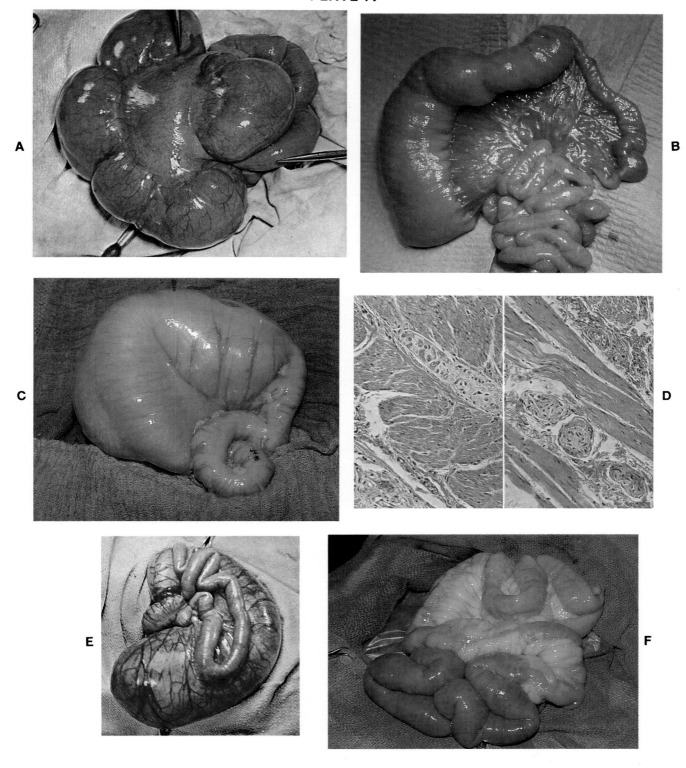

74 Anthony Shaw
Disorders of the Umbilicus

Clinical Embryology

ACCORDING TO traditional embryological doctrine,[13, 22] the anterior abdominal wall develops initially by a combination of lateral infolding and acute ventral flexion of the trilaminar disk-shaped embryo, beginning in the fourth week of life. The amniotic cavity, which initially occupies the dorsal position (Fig 74–1,A), is pulled around to surround the embryo, compressing and narrowing the ventral attachment of embryo to yolk sac (Fig 74–1,B). The coelomic cavity created by the curling of the embryo incorporates a portion of the yolk sac that differentiates into mid- and hindguts—the primitive alimentary canal.

The embryonic attachment to the chorion, the body stalk, contains the umbilical arteries and veins as well as the allantois, a slender projection of the yolk sac that opens into the portion of the hindgut that later becomes the bladder (Fig 74–1,B,C). With infolding of the embryonic disk and displacement of the yolk sac by the amniotic cavity, the attenuated connection between the extracoelomic yolk sac and midgut, known as the vitelline or omphalomesenteric duct, and its developing blood supply fuse with the structures of the body stalk into a cord-like structure. This cable, along with a matrix of primitive mesenchymal tissue (Wharton's jelly) and an outer covering of amnion, comprises the umbilical cord (Fig 74–1,D).

As the infolding continues, accompanied by the ventral migration of mesoderm that differentiates into fatty, muscular, and fascial tissues, the area of cord insertion, initially broad, contracts to a small fibromuscular ring that closes by the time of birth, assuring the integrity of the abdominal wall.

Klippel proposed a concept of embryogenesis in which the mathematics of vector analysis are applied to the developing embryo, which is considered a vector field.[20] According to this construct, development of the embryo proceeds not by an infolding process but outward from a fixed midpoint—a process comparable to the blowing of a bubble.

Umbilical Disease

Major signs of umbilical disease in infants and children are one or a combination of the following: drainage, mass, hernia.

Umbilical Drainage

Drainage from the umbilicus in the early weeks of life following separation of the umbilical cord may be due to the presence of vestigial embryonal structures derived from vitelline duct, urachus or umbilical vessels, umbilical sepsis (omphalitis), or a combination, i.e., infection of an embryonal vestige.

The *vitelline duct* has usually disappeared by the seventh fetal week, although the umbilical portion of the vitelline artery and vein may normally persist long beyond that time. Vestiges of duct and/or vessels include umbilical sinus, fistula, Meckel's diverticulum (see Chap. 87), cysts, polyps, and bands (Fig 74–2).

Unlike the vitelline duct, the *urachus* usually persists and is normally found as a cord-like structure from the dome of the bladder to the lower rim of the umbilical ring, flanked by the two umbilical ligaments (arteries). Dissections of adult cadavers have shown that all or part of the mucosa-lined urachal lumen persists throughout life, although normally collapsed or occluded by desquamated epithelial cells.[1] The urachus may be symptomatic if it communicates widely between bladder and umbilical skin as a urinary fistula, if cysts develop along its course, or if either its umbilical or bladder ends remain open, resulting in urachal sinus or bladder diverticulum, respectively (Fig 74–3).

Fistulae of vitelline (see Fig 74–2,C) or urachal (see Fig 74–3,A) ducts following separation of the umbilical cord and manifested by drainage of intestinal contents or urine, respectively, present little in the way of diagnostic difficulty but are rarely seen. Some degree of asymptomatic umbilical prolapse (intussusception) of the ileum through the umbilicus (Fig 74–4,A) is common with large patent vitelline ducts. Such prolapse rarely progresses to bowel obstruction or compromise of circulation of the prolapsed intestine. Urinary fistula may be suspected at birth when a "giant" umbilical cord is present. The enormous size of such a cord is due to swelling of Wharton's jelly as a result of absorption of the hypotonic fetal urine.[27] The connection of an umbilical fistula, intestinal or urinary, is easily confirmed by injection of contrast material (Fig 74–4,B). Lower urinary tract obstruction may be associated with urachal fistula and should be ruled out by appropriate radiographic and endoscopic studies before resection of the persistent urachus.

Umbilical drainage is much more likely to be due to vestigial sinuses (see Figs 74–2,B and 74–3,B) than to fistulae. Symptomatic drainage may appear at any age as a result of infection.

Purulent umbilical drainage, especially in the newborn, must always be considered a potential precursor of systemic sepsis, and the source of drainage must be rapidly identified and treated. A sinus opening may be hidden deep in the navel, especially in the presence of inflammation and edema. An otoscope serves well as an umbilicoscope to identify a recessed sinus opening and can permit visualization of the entire extent of relatively shallow tracts. Passage of a radiopaque catheter permits radiographic assessment of the extent and direction of deeper tracts, which may be helpful in differential diagnosis and in subsequent surgical management (Fig 74–5). In the absence of acute infection, injection of a drop or two of contrast solution may give additional useful information.

An infected *vestigial umbilical artery* (lateral umbilical ligament) was a common source of neonatal mortality in the early days of the century and is still a rare cause of purulent umbilical drainage in the newborn. A draining sinus that originates in the lateral inferior portion of the lower abdomen is more likely an infection of the vestigial umbilical artery (see Fig 74–5) than of the urachus, which is a midline structure.

Pilonidal sinuses with purulent drainage occur, rarely, in the umbilicus, perhaps caused by the drawing down of shed hairs into a deep umbilical recess by the "tugging action" of the urachus.[26] Gupta and Gupta recently reported such a case—a 17-year-old male with purulent umbilical drainage in whom a clump of hair was found impacted within an infected urachal sinus.[14]

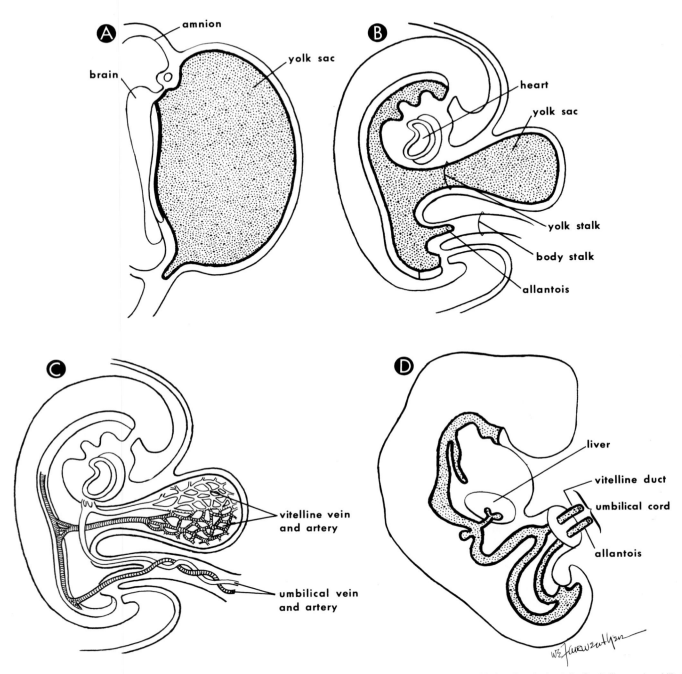

Fig 74–1.—Development of umbilical cord. **A,** embryonic disk. Yolk sac in contact with entire ventral surface. **B,** ventral attachment of yolk sac narrowed and lengthened as a result of folding of embryo. Intracoelomic portion of yolk sac forms gut. Allantois buds from hindgut into body stalk. **C,** vitelline and umbilical vessels develop in yolk and body stalks, respectively. **D,** yolk and body stalks fused into umbilical cord. Development of abdominal wall narrows umbilical ring.

Spontaneous intestinal umbilical fistula has been reported in adolescents with *Crohn's disease*.[17, 23]

In treating fistulae and sinuses of the umbilicus, control of local infection and treatment of generalized sepsis should precede efforts to eradicate the anatomic anomaly. Systemic and local measures include appropriate antibiotics, debridement, and promotion of drainage.

All umbilical sinuses and fistulae can be excised through an intraumbilical incision, circumscribing the cutaneous orifice and "coring out" the tract, preserving the umbilicus. Dissection along the serosal aspect of a vitelline fistula permits delivery of the entire tract and segment of bowel to which it is attached (see Fig 74–4,C). The fistula is excised and the ileal defect closed transversely. The fascia is closed; the intraumbilical skin defect can usually be closed. The resulting scar is inapparent (see Fig 74–4,D).

The lumen of the vitelline duct may be obliterated, leaving a cord running from the serosal surface of the distal ileum (or from

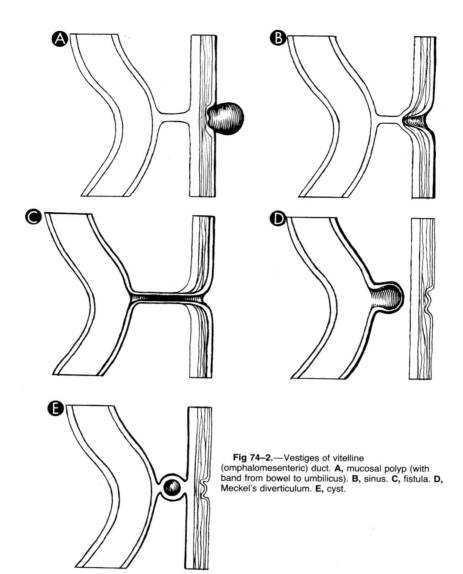

Fig 74–2.—Vestiges of vitelline (omphalomesenteric) duct. **A,** mucosal polyp (with band from bowel to umbilicus). **B,** sinus. **C,** fistula. **D,** Meckel's diverticulum. **E,** cyst.

the tip of a Meckel's diverticulum) to the umbilical ring (see Fig 74–2,*A* and *B*). (Such a cordlike structure may represent a vestige of vitelline vessels rather than of the duct itself.) Such cords provide a point of fixation to the abdominal wall about which a volvulus or internal hernia of small bowel may occur. Intra-abdominal cords should be identified and excised (along with a Meckel's diverticulum, if attached) in the coring out of an umbilicus sinus of vitelline origin.

Urachal fistulae and sinuses may also be excised through an intraumbilical incision. A short inferior extension may rarely be required to improve exposure of the vesicourachal junction. The urachal tract should be excised with a button of bladder wall and the bladder closed with absorbable sutures.

In excising an infected umbilical artery, the tract should be divided proximally, near its junction with the iliac artery.

While umbilical drainage due to local sepsis is commonly associated with a vestigial sinus in the older child and adolescent, umbilical sepsis in the infant may be associated with retained umbilical cord elements,[5, 16] or ectopic tissue;[25] most commonly, it represents poor hygienic practices and/or nosocomial infection.

Omphalitis may progress dramatically from minimal erythema of the umbilical area to florid cellulitis and sepsis in hours and therefore must be treated vigorously when its earliest manifestations are recognized (Fig 74–6). Omphalitis in newborn nurseries has been all but eliminated by scrupulous hand-washing on the part of professional personnel, isolation of infants with overt infections, asepsis in cord handling, and the use of antiseptics in the bathing of neonates. Routine culturing of the umbilical area may reveal colonization by pathogenic organisms in time to prevent infection.

Omphalitis associated with defective neutrophil mobility has been described in several newborns with delayed separation of the umbilical cord.[5, 16] Such infections may respond poorly to medical measures and may require excision of the cord remnant.

Umbilical Masses

Many of the masses, small and large, which appear in, under, or at the periphery of the umbilicus, are, like most umbilical sinuses and fistulae, manifestations of disease in remnants of the

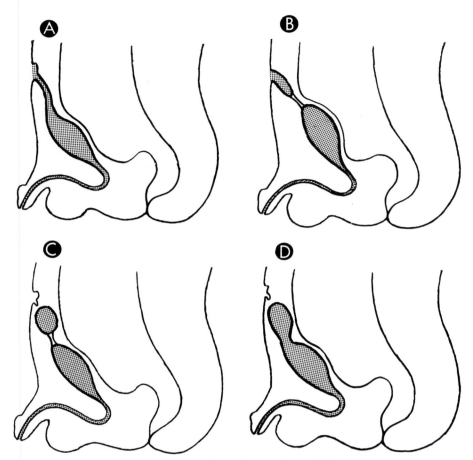

Fig 74–3.—Vestiges of urachus. **A**, fistula. **B**, sinus. **C**, cyst. **D**, bladder diverticulum.

vitelline duct or urachus or vestiges of other structures which, during embryonic life, were related to the umbilical cord or traversed the umbilical ring.

A friable pink excrescence persisting in the umbilical dimple following separation of the cord may enlarge into a mushroom of oozing granulation tissue—*umbilical granuloma*—often associated with persistent umbilical drainage and swelling and erythema of the surrounding skin. Small granulomas may be eradicated by one or two applications of silver nitrate. The larger ones may require excision, with cauterization of the base. Epithelialization will then take place, with complete healing. If cellulitis is present, local measures and antibiotics are indicated.

Umbilical polyp (see Fig 74–2,A) is a glistening cherry-red nodule that may be seen in the umbilical dimple after separation of the cord. This nodule, or umbilical polyp, a remnant of vitelline duct, usually consists of small-bowel mucosa but may rarely be gastric mucosa, the latter occasionally eroding the periumbilical skin. Umbilical polyps are often mistaken for granulomas. However, they do not yield to silver nitrate and must be excised. A central core of the umbilicus should be excised in continuity with the polyp in order to identify and remove contiguous intraabdominal vitelline duct vestiges.

Urachal cysts (see Fig 74–3,C) may occur anywhere along the urachal tract from the bladder to the umbilicus and may escape detection in infancy, causing symptoms in the older child or adult as an enlarging suprapubic or infraumbilical mass. Infection of urachal cysts with abscess formation results in an ovoid, painful, tender midline mass, accompanied by systemic signs of acute infection. Urachal abscess may drain through the umbilicus, rupture into the peritoneal cavity, causing peritonitis, or cause a spreading infection of the anterior abdominal wall or retroperitoneal tissues. Urachal abscess may occur in infancy but is more common in adolescents and young adults.

Urachal cysts should be excised in continuity with the rest of the urachal tract. Urachal abscess should be promptly drained. The infection may destroy the secretory cyst lining, preventing recurrence. However, Blichert-Toft and Nielsen reported recurrence in nine of twenty-nine abscesses treated by drainage alone.[3]

Much more rare than urachal cysts are *vitelline cysts* (see Fig 74–2,E) formed from mucosa-lined pockets along the course of the vitelline duct. Such cysts may be quite large at birth.

Although rare, *dermoid cysts* and *vascular malformations* have long been known to occur in the umbilicus.[10] Umbilical nodules of metastatic *adenocarcinoma* have been described both as accompanying obvious abdominal carcinomatosis[10] and as the first sign of visceral cancer in adults.[24]

Ectopic liver has appeared as an umbilical nodule, probably as a result of entrapment of the tip of the right lobe during closure of the umbilical ring.[25] *Adenocarcinoma of the urachus* may present as a subumbilical mass and has a very poor prognosis.[19] Over 70% occur in males, most of whom are middle-aged or elderly. The youngest reported patient with carcinoma of the urachus was a 15-year-old female who had a urachal abscess drained at age 13 and died of metastases to lungs and bone at age 22.[8]

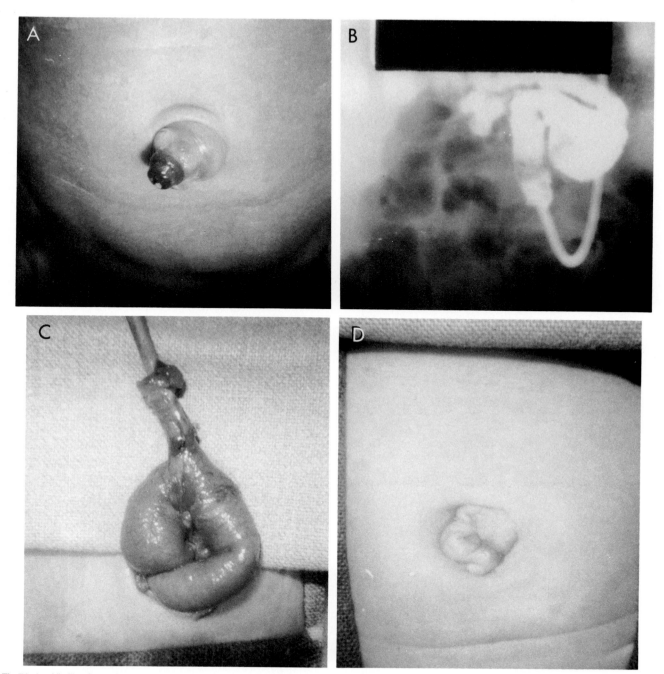

Fig 74–4.—Vitelline fistula (patent omphalomesenteric duct). **A,** ileostomy-like umbilical protrusion draining stool in 1-month-old girl. **B,** fistulogram showing filling of ileum via a Meckel's diverticulum. **C,** fistula, including Meckel's diverticulum and ileum delivered through umbilicus. **D,** appearance of umbilicus following closure of intraumbilical incision.

Umbilical Hernia

At birth, the contracted umbilical ring is normally reinforced by the round ligament (umbilical vein), urachus, lateral umbilical ligaments (vestigial umbilical arteries), and Richet's umbilical fascia (a subumbilical extension of transversalis fascia). Incomplete development, imperfect attachment, or weak areas in either ligamentous or fascial structures may predispose to herniation at the umbilicus. The defect is usually noticed within a few days or weeks following separation of the cord. A fine historical and anatomical review is provided by Woods.[29]

INCIDENCE.—Umbilical hernias are seen in many animal species as well as in man. There is a high familial incidence, but no genetic pattern of inheritance has been identified. The frequency of congenital umbilical hernias has been reported to be six to ten times higher in blacks than in whites, with the incidence in the former ranging from 25% to 50% in the early months of life.[9, 12] In contrast, a recent study of a large number of South African white and black children[4] found little difference in incidence between the two groups—a surprising finding, much at odds with reported observations in American pediatric populations. Umbilical hernia is commonly associated with a number of congenital

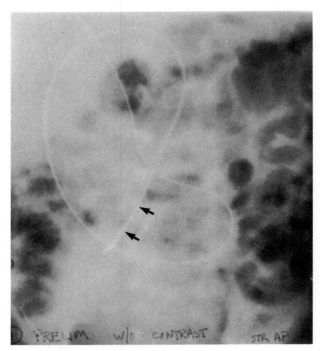

Fig 74–5.—Purulent umbilical drainage in newborn. Opaque catheter passed through sinus opening follows course of right umbilical artery *(arrows).*

malformations including thyroid dysgenesis, trisomy 18, trisomy 13, Beckwith syndrome, and Hurler syndrome.[2]

NATURAL HISTORY.—Unfortunately, there are no definitive longitudinal prospective studies of stable populations with umbilical hernia from birth to adulthood in whom hernia repair has been withheld. Thus, most of the statements in the literature about rates of spontaneous closure related to such factors as size of defect, age, sex, race, effectiveness of adhesive strapping, and so on, are of dubious validity. It is not even known whether most, or even many, adult umbilical hernias were present in childhood. Fewer than 10% of adults admitted for umbilical hernia repair in one study recalled having an umbilical hernia in childhood.[18] The voluminous but flawed umbilical literature *does* allow the following conclusions to be drawn: (1) most congenital umbilical hernias close spontaneously, and most of these in the first 3 years of life. (2) Small umbilical hernias close earlier than large umbilical hernias (size referring to ring diameter, not length of protrusion). (3) Many umbilical hernias still present at age 4–5 years close by puberty.

Claims that adhesive strapping helps cure umbilical hernia are not supported by the available data. Careless strapping may cause maceration of skin, and tight banding has caused death by asphyxia.[11]

Complications of umbilical hernia include incarceration and strangulation of intestine or omentum and perforation of umbilical skin with drainage (Fig 74–7) or evisceration, all very uncommon in childhood.

TREATMENT.—Perforation, incarceration, and pain clearly related to the hernia are compelling indications for surgical management of umbilical hernia. If it is true that incarceration carries with it a high mortality rate in later life,[15] especially in multiparous women, it seems reasonable to repair umbilical hernias before full maturity. On the other hand, because the likelihood of complication of umbilical hernia is low and the prospects of spontaneous closure excellent, there is rarely justification for correc-

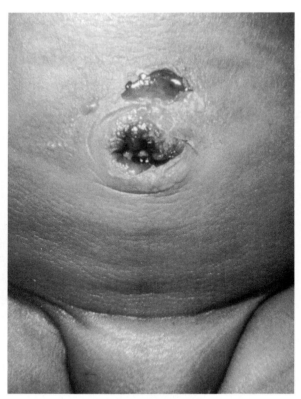

Fig 74–6.—Streptococcal sepsis originating in umbilicus in newborn nursery. Death occurred in less than 24 hours after diagnosis.

tion of an uncomplicated umbilical hernia in early childhood. Indeed, in the absence of symptoms, physical and psychological, with a known low incidence of complications, with the natural history disposing toward continuing closure, it seems reasonable to defer repair until adolescence. However many parents prefer repair at an earlier age, especially when the protrusion is large and the child self-conscious about it. In the absence of compli-

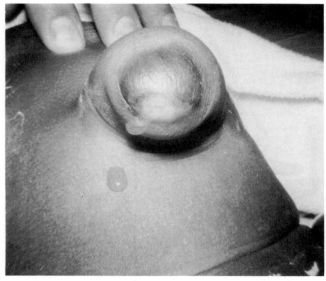

Fig 74–7.—Drainage from tiny spontaneous perforation of umbilical hernia. Sinogram showed free flow into peritoneal cavity.

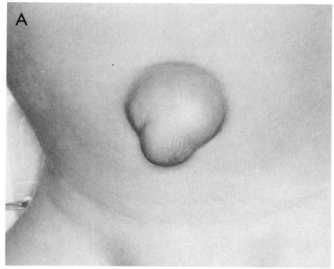

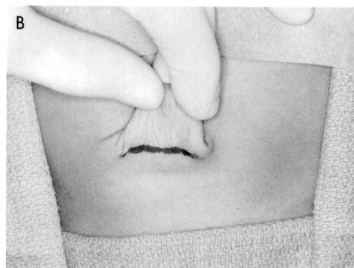

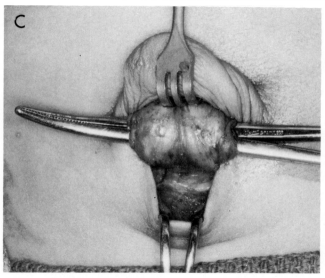

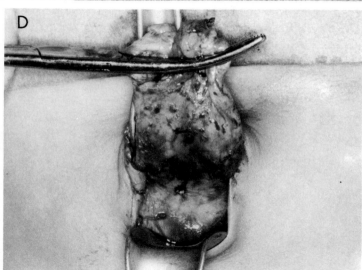

Fig 74–8.—Repair of umbilical hernia. **A,** typical umbilical hernia. **B,** site of incision within umbilical skin. **C,** dissection around base of sac completed. Sac still attached to umbilical skin. **D,** intact sac separated from umbilical skin. **(Continued)**

cations, I try to defer repair until school age at least. If incarceration occurs, it can usually be reduced manually with the aid of sedation and the hernia repaired electively.

TECHNIQUE.—The operation is performed under general anesthesia, usually without overnight admission. A transverse incision is made within a fold of the inferior aspect of the umbilicus and carried through the thin layer of subcutaneous fat and areolar tissue to the linea alba at the inferior rim of the umbilical ring (Fig 74–8,A and B). *The incision should not extend beyond the umbilicus.* By sharp and blunt dissection, the plane around the hernia ring at the level of the linea alba is defined and the sac is then sharply dissected away from the umbilical skin (Fig 74–8,C and D). In preference to transecting the sac, which often requires ligation of vessels in the preperitoneal fat and deepening of the anesthesia to prevent evisceration, I prefer to use the maneuver of Miller,[21] followed by transverse closure of the fascial ring (Fig 74–8,E and F). The underside of the umbilical skin is then tacked to the suture and to the skin line with a fine suture and the skin closed with three fine absorbable intracutaneous

sutures (Fig 74–8,G). A fluffed sponge or wad of cotton is compressed into the umbilical dimple and a pressure dressing is applied (Fig 74–8,H), which must remain in place for 3 or 4 days to prevent a wound hematoma, the most common and troublesome complication of umbilical hernia repair.

In a twenty-year experience of several thousand cases, neither Miller nor I are aware of any complications resulting from intraperitoneal invagination of the hernia sac. Wound hematoma has been rare and usually related to incorrect application or premature removal of the compression dressing. I have seen no recurrence with this technique. The cosmetic result is gratifying.

The Umbilicus as a Therapeutic Portal

The umbilical arteries continue to play vital monitoring and therapeutic roles in newborn intensive care, although the increasing reliability of transcutaneous blood gas monitoring is reducing the need for invasive techniques.

Concern about the complications of portal vein thrombosis and necrotizing colitis, coupled with the reduced need for exchange

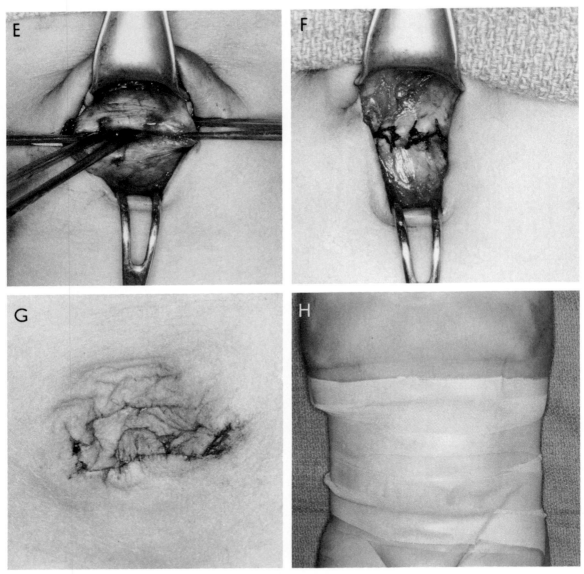

Fig 74–8 Cont.—E, Miller maneuver; sac invaginated. Inferior and superior edges of ring clearly seen. **F,** transverse closure. **G,** appearance at completion of operation. **H,** pressure dressing.

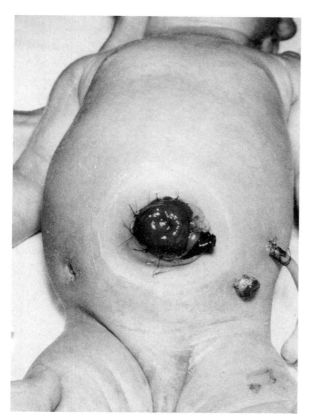

Fig 74–9.—Newborn with gastroschisis and ileal atresia; closure of abdominal defect with proximal ileostomy. Mucous fistula in left lower quadrant. Infant did well.

transfusions since the introduction of RhoGam and phototherapy, have in recent years decreased the use of the umbilical vein by neonatologists. The umbilical vein, however, remains the preferred route of access for exchange transfusions or when rapid lifesaving transfusion therapy is required in the newborn. Incidence of umbilical vein catheter complications is directly related to duration of cannulation.

The umbilicus has proved a good site for placement of end colostomy following abdominal perineal resection in adults.[28] Umbilical placement has been recommended for temporary colostomy and ileostomy in infants[7] and for permanent urinary stomas in children with myelodysplasia.[6] By suturing an end ileostomy into the umbilical defect of a newborn with gastroschisis and ileal atresia, I relieved the bowel obstruction while achieving a relaxed closure of the abdominal wall (Fig 74–9).

REFERENCES

1. Begg R.D.: The urachus: Its anatomy, histology and development. *J. Anat.* 64:170, 1930.
2. Bergsma D.: *Birth Defects: Atlas and Compendium.* Baltimore, Williams & Wilkins Co., 1973.
3. Blichert-Toft M., Nielsen C.W.: Congenital patent urachus and acquired variants. *Acta Chir. Scand.* 137:807, 1971.
4. Blumberg N.A.: Infantile umbilical hernia. *Surg. Gynecol. Obstet.* 150:187, 1980.
5. Bowen T., Ochs H.D., Wedgwood R.J.: Chemotaxis and umbilical separation. *Lancet* 2:302, 1979.
6. Braren V., Workman C.H., Johns O.T., et al.: Use of the umbilical area for placement of a urinary stoma. *Surg. Gynecol. Obstet.* 148:543, 1979.
7. Cameron G.S., Lau G.Y.P.: The umbilicus as a site for temporary colostomy in infants. *J. Pediatr. Surg.* 17:361, 1982.
8. Cornil C., Reynolds C.T., Kickham C.J.E.: Carcinoma of the urachus. *J. Urol.* 98:93, 1967.
9. Crump E.P.: Umbilical hernia: I. Occurrence of the infantile type in Negro infants and children. *J. Pediatr.* 40:214, 1952.
10. Cullen T.S.: *Embryology, Anatomy, and Diseases of the Umbilicus Together With Diseases of the Urachus.* Philadelphia, W.B. Saunders Co., 1916, pp. 351–372.
11. Emory J.L.: Infant deaths associated with tight umbilical binders. *Proc. R. Soc. Med.* 60:10, 1967.
12. Evans A.G.: The comparative incidence of umbilical hernias in colored and white infants. *J. Natl. Med. Assn.* 33:158, 1941.
13. Gasser R.F.: *Atlas of Human Embryos.* Hagerstown, Md., Harper & Row, 1975, pp. 25–44.
14. Gupta S., Gupta S.: Pilonidal sinus of the umbilicus with urachal adenoma. *Trop. Geogr. Med.* 33:393, 1981.
15. Haller J.A., et al.: Repair umbilical hernias in childhood to prevent adult incarceration. *Am. Surg.* 37:245, 1971.
16. Hayward A.R., Leonard J., Wood C.B.S., et al.: Delayed separation of the umbilical cord, widespread infections and defective neutrophil mobility. *Lancet* 1:1099, 1979.
17. Hiley P.C., Cohen N., Presant D.H.: Spontaneous umbilical fistula in granulomatous (Crohn's) disease of the bowel. *Gastroenterology* 60:103, 1971.
18. Jackson O.F., Muglen L.H.: Umbilical hernia: A retrospective study. *Calif. Med.* 113:8, 1970.
19. Jacobo E., Loening S., Schmidt J.D., et al.: Primary adenocarcinoma of the bladder: A retrospective study of 20 patients. *J. Urol.* 117:54, 1977.
20. Klippel C.H. Jr.: In El Shafie M., Klippel C.H. Jr. (eds.): *Associated Congenital Anomalies.* Baltimore, Williams & Wilkins Co., 1981, pp. 157–163.
21. Miller B.M.: Personal communication.
22. Moore K.L.: *The Developing Human: Clinically Oriented Embryology.* Philadelphia, W.B. Saunders Co., 1973. pp. 54–59.
23. Rentz T.W., Warden C.S., Garcia F.J., et al.: Crohn's disease with spontaneous ileoumbilical and ileovesical fistulae. *Dig. Dis. Sci.* 24:316, 1979.
24. Scarpa F.J., Dineen J.P., Boltax R.S.: Visceral neoplasia presenting at the umbilicus. *J. Surg. Oncol.* 11:351, 1979.
25. Shaw A., Pierog S.: "Ectopic" liver in the umbilicus. *Pediatrics* 44:448, 1969.
26. Steck W.D., Helwig E.B.: Umbilical granulomas, pilonidal disease and the urachus. *Surg. Gynecol. Obstet.* 120:1043, 1965.
27. Tsuchida Y., Ishida M.: Osmolar relationships between enlarged umbilical cord and patent urachus. *J. Ped. Surg.* 4:465, 1969.
28. Turnbull R.B.: The colostomies, in Maingot R. (ed.): *Abdominal Operations,* ed. 7. New York, Appleton-Century-Crofts, 1980, pp. 2319–2323.
29. Woods G.E.: Some observations on umbilical hernia in infants. *Arch. Dis. Child.* 28:450, 1953.

75 SAMUEL R. SCHUSTER

Omphalocele and Gastroschisis

OMPHALOCELE is a relatively rare condition that is estimated to occur once in 6,000 to once in 10,000 births. The embryology, terminology, and classification of congenital malformations of the anterior abdominal wall have been in an increasing state of confusion during the past 25 years. This confusion revolves around the more frequent description of a type of abdominal wall defect that has been termed "gastroschisis." There is no unanimity of opinion as to the definition of the term. A review of the literature[3, 5, 7, 9, 28, 31, 37, 38, 40, 48, 54, 55] suggests that this confusion may be based on differing understanding or interpretation of the embryology of the abdominal wall.

Embryology of the Abdominal Wall and Small Intestine

At the beginning of the third week of development, the primitive gut of the embryo is already demarcated into three regions: foregut, midgut, and hindgut. These primordia of the future intestinal tract are developmentally related to the embryologic folds that play an important role in the configuration of the abdominal wall. The cephalic, caudal, and lateral folds are each composed of somatic and splanchnic layers.

CEPHALIC FOLD.—This fold lies anteriorly and contains the foregut from which will develop the pharynx, the esophagus, and stomach. The splanchnic layer enfolds the heart and great vessels and will close the foregut in front, while the somatic layer forms the thoracic and epigastric wall as well as the septum transversum. Early failure of formation of the somatic layer of the cephalic fold causes an underlying epigastric abdominal wall defect or celosomia (persistence of extraembryonic coelom) that should be referred to as an "epigastric omphalocele." This type of omphalocele is frequently associated with lower thoracic wall malformations, diaphragmatic defects, and cardiac anomalies (Fig 75–1,A) (see also Chap. 57).

CAUDAL FOLD.—Posteriorly, in the smaller, caudal, fold, lies the hindgut with its ventral allantoic outgrowth; the hindgut gives rise to the colon and rectum. The splanchnic layer of this fold closes the hindgut in front, while the somatic layer, including the allantois, the forerunner of the urinary bladder, will form the hypogastric abdominal wall. Failure of normal formation of the caudal fold can affect both layers. Splanchnic layer deficiencies result in partial agenesis of the hindgut, while failure of normal formation of both layers leads to a lower abdominal wall defect or celosomia (extraembryonic coelom) that can be termed a "hypogastric omphalocele." This complex also includes agenesis of the hindgut (imperforate anus) with a fistula between the intestine and an open or exstrophied bladder (Fig 75–1,C). When there is isolated failure of the somatic layer, the anus is normal but the hypogastric wall in front of the allantois is absent. This absence leads to exstrophy of the urinary bladder combined with a lower abdominal or hypogastric omphalocele (see Chap. 76).

LATERAL FOLDS.—The lateral folds, comprised of somatic and splanchnic layers, enfold the midgut and form the lateral walls of the abdomen, ultimately helping to form the future umbilical ring. The somatic layers of these folds extend to the wall of the amniotic sac surrounding the embryo and form the abdominal wall. Failure of normal embryonic folding and fusion at the level of the lateral folds prevent the anterior abdominal wall from closing completely. In such cases, the umbilical ring remains widely open. This results in a middle celosomia or extraembryonic coelom communicating in varying degrees of magnitude with the intraembryonic coelom[5, 9, 18, 28, 54] (Fig 75–1,B). The ultimate diameter of this communication with the extraembryonic coelom will determine whether or not the persistent celosomia should be termed "omphalocele" or "hernia of the umbilical cord."

DEVELOPMENT AND ATTACHMENT OF THE MIDGUT.—During the third and fourth weeks of fetal life the embryo grows rapidly, whereas the yolk sac and the opening into the midgut do not. The opening in the midgut continues to decrease in size, and by the fifth week the connection with the yolk sac has no larger a diameter than that of the gut itself and is referred to as the vitelline duct, or the omphalomesenteric duct. At this time, the junction between the large and small intestine first becomes apparent as a ventral swelling just posterior to the yolk stalk, and for the first time elongation of the midgut proceeds faster than does elongation of the body of the embryo. The discrepancy in growth between the intestine and the fetal body, the abdominal cavity of which cannot contain the more rapidly enlarging gut, results in an extrusion of most of the midgut into the base of the umbilical cord, where it will normally reside in diminishing amounts from the fifth to the tenth weeks. A diagrammatic representation of this stage of development is seen in Figure 75–2. By the eleventh week of fetal life, all of the alimentary tract should normally have withdrawn into the abdomen, sufficient rotation having taken place so that the cecum lies in the epigastrium below the stomach. By the twelfth week, rotation of the colon should be complete, with the cecum in its final position in the right lower quadrant.

Rotation is not synonymous with fixation. Fixation of the bowel does not occur rapidly and may not even be completed during intrauterine life, continuing to take place from the twelfth week of gestation to well after birth. The final arrangement of the colon with fixation of the ascending and descending portions to the parietal peritoneum occurs over many months. Fixation may be arrested in various stages of completion. Failure of fixation, until birth or even thereafter, becomes important when we observe that a varying degree of malrotation with abnormal fixation is virtually always present in association with omphalocele, hernia of the umbilical cord, and even gastroschisis.[27, 33]

Definitions of Terms and Clinical Observations Related to Developmental Anatomy

Omphalocele (Exomphalos, Amniocele)

In 1949, Benson et al.[4] suggested two terms to emcompass those congenital defects in which the abdominal viscera remained herniated through the umbilical and supraumbilical portions of the abdominal wall into a sac covered by peritoneum and

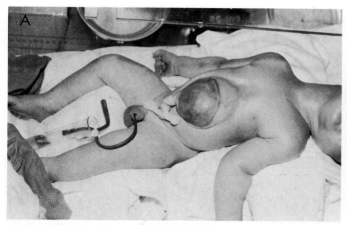

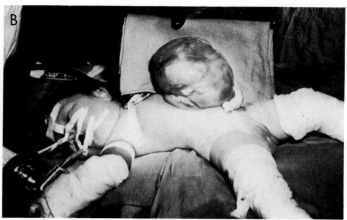

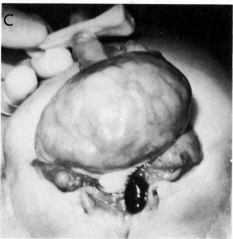

Fig 75–1.—Types of omphalocele. **A,** newborn with abdominal wall anomaly secondary to abnormal development of cephalic fold of the embryo. The typical epigastric omphalocele is associated with a lower thoracic wall malformation resulting in a cleft sternum, diaphragmatic defect, pericardial defect, and cardiac anomaly (see Cantrell's Pentalogy, Chap. 57). **B,** typical omphalocele from lateral fold developmental abnormality. The epigastric and hypogastric portions of the abdominal wall are normal. The defect lies between these areas and is greater than 4 cm in diameter. The overlying membrane is intact, and the muscular abdominal wall is normal. The umbilicus arises from an anterior position on the omphalocele. **C,** hypogastric omphalocele, the result of caudal fold abnormality. Associated defects include exstrophy of the bladder, imperforate anus, and, in this instance, a prolapsing rectovesical fistula (see Cloacal Exstrophy, Chap. 76).

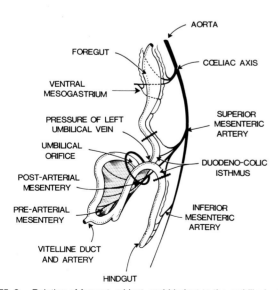

Fig 75–2.—Relation of foregut, midgut, and hindgut to the umbilical artery at the seventh to eighth week of fetal life. The elongation of the midgut is proceeding faster than the elongation of the body of the embryo, and the midgut has been extruded into the base of the umbilical cord, where it normally resides during the fifth to tenth weeks. Note the umbilical orifice and vitelline duct.

amniotic membrane. They arbitrarily chose to call those with an umbilical defect greater than 4 cm in diameter "omphalocele" or "amniocele," while those in which the defect had a diameter of less than 4 cm were termed "hernia of the umbilical cord."

The causative factors in the formation of an omphalocele have been the subject of considerable discussion, and many of the views held have been contradictory. In 1940, Gross and Blodgett[31] suggested that omphalocele is probably due to arrest of, or retardation in, the development of the abdominal cavity at the third month of fetal life. They proposed that the abdominal cavity itself was the primary culprit, since it did not develop rapidly enough and some of the abdominal viscera remained in the base of the umbilical cord because of insufficient space within the abdomen. Only one year later, Ladd and Gross,[37] in their classic textbook, suggested that an omphalocele occurred in the third month of fetal life because of the disparity between the size of the abdominal cavity and the viscera, resulting primarily from retarded development of the abdominal parietes, as opposed to the previously held view of Gross and Blodgett[31] that it was secondary to inadequate space within the abdomen. They may have actually meant the same thing.

A more significant interpretation of the etiology was proposed by Margulies,[38] who concluded that the structural defects ultimately resulting in the presence of an omphalocele occurred before the end of the third week of embryonal development, since the formation of the abdominal parietes should be virtually complete by that time under normal circumstances. Margulies therefore concluded that, once the abdominal wall had been formed normally, no herniation covered by an amnion could develop.

These observations, based on sound embryologic study, lend credence to the idea that abnormal development of the parietes before the third week of embryonal life somehow will prevent the later return of the midgut into the abdomen. This failure of midgut return results in a diminished stimulus to the increase of the space within the abdominal cavity, which therefore is inordinately small. Thus, not only has the gut lost its right of domicile, but other viscera, already residing in the intraembryonic coelom, may secondarily herniate through the persistent opening communicating with the extraembryonic coelom. The degree of closure or contraction of the umbilical ring determines which structures may later be found outside the abdomen.

Hernia of the Umbilical Cord

A hernia of the umbilical cord has been defined as an umbilical defect with a diameter of less than 4 cm and a sac that contains only loops of intestine[4] (Fig 75–3). This definition is consistent with the explanation by Margulies[38] that hernias into the umbilical cord result from failure of continuing closure or contracture of the umbilical ring during the eighth to the tenth weeks. By this time in fetal life, most of the midgut should normally have returned to the abdominal cavity. When all, or most, of the midgut returns to the intraembryonic coelom from the extraembryonic coelom, the abdominal cavity has developed sufficient volume to contain it. If all of the midgut does not return to the intraembryonic coelom, the extraembryonic coelom fails to disappear completely and an umbilical defect persists. This herniation usually involves only a small segment of the midgut. However, if a tear of the membrane covering a "hernia of the umbilical cord" occurs and there has been poor fixation of the gut, extensive herniation may occur and many loops of midgut may find their way out through the tear. Small hernias of the umbilical cord in which the membrane remains intact and gradually becomes epithelialized are referred to as "cutis navel."

In summary, abnormalities in the morphogenesis of the abdominal wall of the embryo lead to a general category of defects that can best be termed "celosomias" and are commonly referred to as "omphaloceles" or "exomphalos." Despite failure of absolutely normal morphogenesis, differentiation of the mesoderm continues. The abdominal wall muscles are normally formed in a

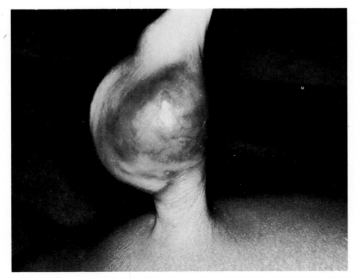

Fig 75–3.—Hernia of the umbilical cord. The umbilical ring is less than 4 cm in diameter; the hernia contains only small intestine. There is no deficiency of skin. An omphalomesenteric duct may be attached to the underside of the umbilicus.

newborn with omphalocele or gastroschisis. Since failure of return of the intestinal loops from the extraembryonic coelom seems to be related to failure of normal morphogenesis of the folds comprising the ventral wall, it is strongly suggested that completion of the closure of the ventral wall by the embryonic folds is a prerequisite for return of the extracoelomic intestine into the abdominal cavity. The mesoderm component, however, appears to develop normally, and normal abdominal wall muscles are present.

Gastroschisis

Divergent views are held as to the origin and definition of this term. In the nineteenth- and early 20th-century literature, the term was applied to the condition we now commonly call omphalocele. Ballantyne,[3] in 1904, designated by "gastroschisis" all somatic abdominal defects with the exception of the physiologic "hernia of the umbilical cord" and concluded: "And now at the beginning of the 20th century there are so many cases of 'gastroschisis' on record that the mere task of collecting all of the references is arduous."

In contrast to this, Moore and Stokes, in 1953,[39] found only five cases of gastroschisis in the literature. It is obvious that the term had been redefined. They defined the condition as one wherein the defect in the abdominal wall is in an extraumbilical location and without a membranous sac. Other features common to this group of patients were said to be a small peritoneal cavity and malrotation of the bowel. Such features hardly seem exclusive, since a poorly developed peritoneal cavity and malrotation of the bowel are commonly found in the patient with ordinary omphalocele.

In 1963, Moore[40] gathered 31 cases from the literature that he believed satisfied his criteria for the diagnosis of "gastroschisis." He further subclassified gastroschisis into antenatal and perinatal varieties, based on the consistency of the bowel and the adequacy of the peritoneal cavity. Patients with the antenatal type were those with thickly matted bowel covered with a gelatinous matrix and a relatively small peritoneal cavity. These patients were presumed to have had long-standing evisceration and exposure of the viscera to amniotic fluid in utero. In the perinatal type there was said to be minimal serosal reaction, and the peritoneal cavities of these patients were frequently able to accommodate this relatively normal bowel that occupies a smaller volume. Patients with this type were believed to have had evisceration close to the time of parturition. It has been demonstrated experimentally that prolonged exposure of the bowel to amniotic fluid causes serositis with apparent shortening of the bowel and increase in bulk of the eviscerated bowel. Long-term exposure of the bowel to amniotic fluid is probably a major cause of the discrepancy between the mass of the herniated bowel and the volume of the abdominal cavity in some patients with gastroschisis. The accepted embryogenesis of "omphalocele" and of "hernia of the umbilical cord" is based on known fetal observations. The developmental anatomy of gastroschisis is thus far based on speculation. Shaw[54] points out that embryologists have not given us any clinical evidence of gastroschisis existing in *early* human fetal specimens, i.e., abdominal wall defects without sacs, separated from a normally inserted umbilical cord by full thickness of abdominal wall.

There have been a number of attempts to describe the embryogenesis of gastroschisis as a separate event in development. Bill,[7] stating that gastroschisis was not yet explained embryologically, ascribed the origin to a failure of the lateral portion of the abdominal wall to join its upper and lower components, a little lateral to the umbilical remnants. If this were indeed the case, one might expect the defect to be farther from the umbilicus than it usually is. Duhamel[18] postulated that gastroschisis might be due to "a relatively early teratogenic action which may prevent the differentiation of the embryonic mesenchyme forming the framework of the somatopleure with subsequent resorption of the ectodermal layer of the somatopleure in the region of the lateral fold."

Gray and Skandalakis[28] indicated that "the defect lies in the failure of the musculature migrating from the dorsal myotomes completely to invade the splanchnopleure of the embryonic abdominal wall." If this were the case, one would expect greater abnormality in the differentiation and structure of the abdominal wall musculature. More specifically, one would expect the rectus muscles to have a much greater diastasis than is usually present in the patient with gastroschisis, and the rectus muscles would probably be deformed—which is not the case.

Bernstein[5] attempted to differentiate gastroschisis from a true umbilical hernia by stating that the latter is covered by a peritoneal sac, whereas in the former the extruded organs develop extracorporeally, immersed in the surrounding amniotic fluid containing vernix caseosa, debris, and meconium. His supposition therefore seemed to be that the eviscerated bowel in gastroschisis had never returned to the abdominal cavity and was never covered by a membrane. This theory is not consistent with the later thesis that gastroschisis occurs secondary to development of a paraumbilical abdominal wall defect through which the intra-abdominal viscera herniated after they had returned to the abdomen in the normal course of development.

Gastroschisis, as frequently described at present, must have most, if not all, of the following features: (1) the umbilical cord is to the left of the hernia defect and separated from it by a bridge of skin; (2) there is no sac; (3) small intestine is herniated, with extremely rare herniation of a portion of the liver; (4) the eviscerated loops of bowel are thickened, adherent, and covered by a confluent gelatinous layer; (5) the herniated bowel is more frequently infarcted or associated with atresia than in omphalocele; (6) other major congenital malformations are infrequent; (7) the abdominal cavity is more adequately developed than in cases of large omphalocele.

In a lucid analysis of the etiology of gastroschisis, Shaw[54] pointed out that the features commonly found in patients with gastroschisis are readily explained if it is postulated that this condition is simply a "hernia of the umbilical cord" in which rupture or tear of the membrane occurred after completion of the infolding of the somatic components of the anterior abdominal wall but before complete closure of the umbilical ring and complete fixation of the bowel in the peritoneal cavity. The amount of bowel herniating through this tear in the membrane depends on the degree of fixation of the midgut that had occurred before the tear took place. The condition of the eviscerated bowel depends on how long before birth the accidental rupture of the membrane took place. The longer the bowel was exposed to amniotic fluid, the more severe the changes in appearance and consistency of the bowel. Several previous observations are consistent with Shaw's theory.

Reed,[47] in 1913, illustrated a baby in whom the bowel was outside the abdomen, having passed through a tear in the wall of the umbilical cord several inches from the abdominal wall. This rupture of the cord, which presumably occurred just before birth, is most probably the initial event in gastroschisis. The interval between such an event and birth determines whether or not there has been time for disappearance of all or part of the membrane along the margin of the defect and also whether or not there has been sufficiently long exposure of the viscera to the amniotic fluid to produce matting, discoloration, thickening, and apparent foreshortening of the intestines. The "shortening" of the bowel noted in many patients with gastroschisis is proba-

bly more apparent than real and has been demonstrated to be reversible after the intestines have been successfully returned to the abdominal cavity (Fig 75–4). The small size of the umbilical ring in hernias of the umbilical cord, as in patients who have gastroschisis, is probably the major factor in compromising the blood supply of the herniated viscera. This results from compression at the ring margin, resulting in engorgement and even necrosis of the emerging loop of bowel. If the accident of herniation through a tear in a "hernia of the umbilical cord" occurred early enough in intrauterine life, then compression necrosis or compromise of the blood supply of the bowel by the small umbilical ring could result in an atretic segment of the bowel. It is well known that atresia is more frequently seen in patients with gastroschisis than in those with omphalocele. Prematurity is more common (about 60%) with gastroschisis.

Bremer[9] further substantiated the fact that gastroschisis is more likely to represent evisceration via a physiologic umbilical hernia, since the physiologic hernia contained only midgut and never the liver or other viscera, which are so often present in omphalocele but not in gastroschisis.

The defect in a patient with gastroschisis is always clearly between the medial borders of the rectus muscles and not through the substance of the muscle itself. The incidence of nongastrointestinal anomalies is low in patients with gastroschisis, consistent with the abdominal evisceration, being the result of a rupture of the umbilical membrane during a normal embryologic phase rather than the result of a teratologic insult.

The absence of a membrane along the margin of the defect has been claimed to differentiate gastroschisis from other forms of hernia or omphalocele. Shaw[54] theorizes that remnants of a sac would not cling for any significant length of time to the edge of a defect in the sac if this defect, or tear in the sac, had developed any significant time before birth, but would resorb on the side of the umbilical ring and become consolidated with the cord on the other. Rickham[48] tends to support this thesis. He reported his experience with the treatment of exomphalos and gastroschisis and observed that in some cases of the latter remnants of the sac are attached to part of the circumference of the abdominal opening. He had three such cases which were otherwise identical to those with no sac remnant and classically described as "gastroschisis."

Moore,[41] reviewing 258 reported cases of gastroschisis, observed that malformations of the small intestine were rare (1%) in patients with omphalocele, compared with patients with gastroschisis (14%). Two thirds of the jejunoileal malformations occurring with gastroschisis were either atresia or stenosis, which might well have resulted from ischemia and autoamputation, the strangulating effect of the small abdominal ring, further enhanced by the edema and swelling of the bowel, resulting from its exposure to amniotic fluid. The striking mobility of the bowel secondary to its lack of normal mesenteric attachment may also allow it to twist and undergo a secondary volvulus and strangulation. Meckel's diverticula are commonly seen with hernias of the umbilical cord, and prolonged tethering of the bowel by the omphalomesenteric duct attachment to the cord may be instrumental in preventing that part of the bowel from returning to the abdominal cavity. The distal ileum held out by this tethering mechanism becomes the most common site of atresia or strangulation.

One feature that has not been readily explained is the bridge of skin separating the umbilical cord from the defect through which the bowel herniated. Shaw[54] proposed a logical explanation: "It seems apparent that once the membrane of an omphalocele or Hernia of the Cord has ruptured in utero, skin grows in from the edge of the defect and, as in the so-called cutis navel, grows about the base of the cord. Such ingrowth of skin at the

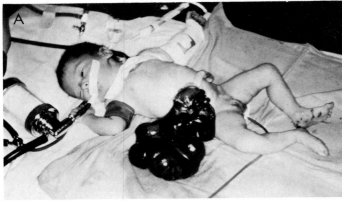

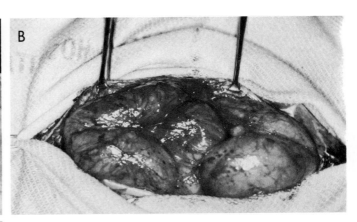

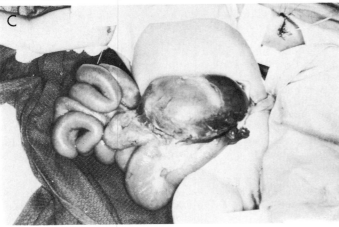

Fig 75–4.—Gastroschisis. **A,** newborn with a typical "foreshortened," confluent, matted, conglomerate mass of bowel commonly associated with the term "gastroschisis." This has herniated through a small defect in the abdominal wall between the rectus muscles. **B,** appearance of intestinal tract in the same patient just before completion of the final stage in repair of the abdominal wall. The infant had a superficial infection, resulting in separation of the prosthetic material, and was treated with open dressings of Mercurochrome. The ventral hernia was ultimately successfully closed with a staged technique using prosthetic materials. The membrane, which had been formed after the initial covering with polyethylene, allowed the bowel to recover, the heavy neonatal fibrinous deposit seen in **A** to be resorbed and the bowel to appear quite normal. It does not, in any way, resemble the original appearance in **A. C,** ruptured omphalocele, demonstrating a herniated liver. This is far more likely to occur in an antenatal rupture of an omphalocele than in a gastroschisis.

cord base results in a decrease of the size of the defect and also may result in the formation of a skin bridge, separating the defect from the umbilical cord which would then give the latter the appearance of normal insertion." However, the defect clearly remains medial to the rectus muscles which are intact. This again emphasizes the importance of the observation that the defect in gastroschisis lies between the recti and is not directly through the muscle.

The single finding most often used to identify gastroschisis as a separate developmental entity is that the defect is almost always to the right of the cord and therefore presumably due to a unique developmental abnormality. Shaw[54] explains this on the basis of normal embryologic anatomy, with the help of Max Brödel's illustrations (Fig 75–5). Whereas a 7-mm embryo has both a left and a right umbilical vein, in an 18-mm embryo the intestine has almost completely withdrawn from the cord and the right umbilical vein has disappeared. The remaining umbilical vein lies to the left. In the 12-cm embryo, the umbilical ring has been obliterated and the umbilical vein is attached to the left of a funnel-shaped depression. In the successive stages of development of a postnatal umbilical hernia, note that the umbilical vein is to the left of a weak area.

These observations are confirmable in infants with intact omphaloceles or "hernias of the umbilical cord," as well as at laparotomy or autopsy. The usual course of the umbilical vein from the left side of the umbilical ring is easily observed, and it appears that rupture would be easiest through the less well-supported and more vulnerable right side of the umbilical hernia sac. With rupture of the sac, the cord attachment appears to the left and slightly below the defect.

Based on the foregoing embryologic and clinical considerations, we should consider gastroschisis the result of an antenatal or perinatal tear or rupture through the membrane of a "hernia of the umbilical cord," with evisceration of intestine through this defect. At this stage of development, normal fixation of the bowel has not been completed, and the resultant mobility of the intestine can allow extensive evisceration.

This has more recently been confirmed by Glick et al.,[26] who demonstrated by serial antenatal ultrasonography the transformation of an antenatally ruptured "hernia of the umbilical cord" into a typical "gastroschisis" at birth.

Table 75–1 presents a classification of congenital abdominal wall defects based on the original developmental failure or event that produced them.

Associated Malformations

These occur more frequently with omphalocele than with gastroschisis or hernia of the umbilical cord. Some are part of three specific syndromes: (1) the lower midline syndrome with vesicointestinal fistula, imperforate anus, colonic agenesis, and bladder exstrophy (see Fig 75–2,*C*); (2) the upper midline syndrome described by Cantrell, Haller, and Ravitch[11] (see Chap. 57), which includes sternal diaphragmatic, pericardial, and cardiac defects (see Fig 75–2,*A*); (3) the Beckwith-Wiedemann syndrome with macroglossia and gigantism. This also occurs sporadically in association with trisomy D, and less often with trisomy E.

Cardiovascular malformations had been reported to occur in approximately 15–25% of infants with omphalocele. To determine the incidence more exactly, the diagnosis files at Children's

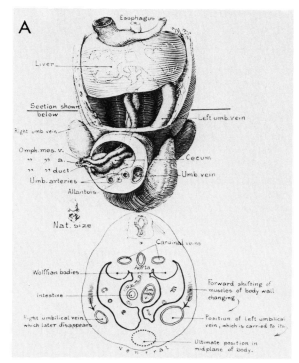

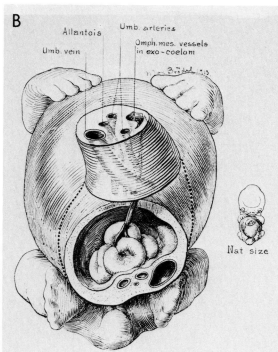

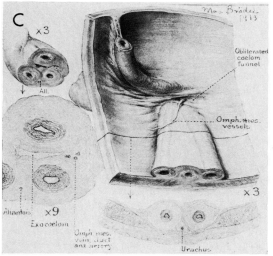

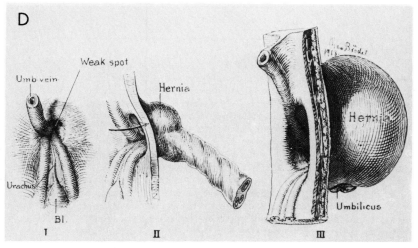

Fig 75–5.—Max Brödel drawings of the embryology of the umbilicus. **A,** 7-mm embryo showing left and right umbilical veins. **B,** in an 18-mm embryo, the intestine has almost withdrawn from the umbilical cord. The right umbilical vein has disappeared. The remaining umbilical vein lies to the left as it enters the abdominal wall. **C,** relations at the umbilical funiculus near birth. The umbilical ring has been obliterated and the umbilical vein is attached to the left of the funnel-shaped depression. **D,** successive stages of development of a postnatal umbilical hernia. The umbilical vein strengthens the left side of the umbilical ring, and rupture appears to be easier through the less well-supported and more vulnerable right side of the umbilical hernia defect. If the sac ruptured (as in gastroschisis), the cord attachment would appear to the left and slightly inferior to the defect.

(From Cullen T.S.: *The Umbilicus and Its Diseases.* Philadelphia, W.B. Saunders Co., 1916. Used by permission.)

Hospital, Boston, were searched and the records of all patients with omphalocele between 1947 and 1973 reviewed.[29] In addition, the files of the Regional Infant Cardiac Program (RICP) were searched for case reports of infants with an associated diagnosis of omphalocele seen between 1968 and 1972. The RICP registry includes nearly all the ill infants in the New England geographic area with significant congenital heart disease and therefore provides an accurate estimate of the incidence of omphalocele in a population of patients with serious congenital heart disease.

Patients with omphalocele were divided into subgroups shown in Tables 75–2 and 75–3. The category of isolated omphalocele comprised patients with no other major anomalies, except for a single patient with tracheosophageal fistula. Those with a specific recognizable syndrome (upper midline defect or lower midline defect) were placed in separate subgroups. The last category, multiple congenital anomalies, included patients with omphalocele plus two major additional extracardiac malformations (myelomeningocele, microcephaly).

Of 159 infants with omphalocele admitted to Children's Hos-

TABLE 75–1.—PROPOSED TERMINOLOGY FOR CONGENITAL
ABDOMINAL WALL DEFECTS RELATED TO ETIOLOGY
AND DEFINITIVE FEATURES

TERMINOLOGY	ETIOLOGY
Epigastric omphalocele	Cephalic fold abnormality ⎤ Diameter of
Omphalocele	Lateral fold abnormality ⎬ defect greater
Hypogastric omphalocele	Caudal fold abnormality ⎦ than 4 cm
Ruptured omphalocele	Ante- or perinatal rupture of the above
Hernia of the umbilical cord	Incomplete closure of umbilical ring (diameter of defect less than 4 cm; contains small bowel only)
Gastroschisis	Ante- or perinatal rupture of hernia of umbilical cord

TABLE 75–2.—SELECTED MALFORMATIONS ASSOCIATED WITH OMPHALOCELE,
CHILDREN'S HOSPITAL, BOSTON, 1947–1973*

MALFORMATIONS	TOTAL	WITHOUT CHD† NO.	%	WITH CHD NO.	%
Isolated	127	114	90	13	10
Specific syndromes	10	3	30	7	70
Diaphragmatic hernia and other upper midline defects	5	0	0	5	100
Exstrophy of the bladder and other lower midline defects	9	9	100	0	0
Multiple anomalies, malposition, ectopia cordis	8	2	25	6	75
Multiple anomalies	5	2	40	3	60
Malposition, ectopia cordis	3	0	0	3	100
Total no. of patients	159	128	80.5	31	19.5

*From Greenwood et al.[29]
†CHD = congenital heart disease.

pital, Boston, 31 (19.5%) had associated congenital heart disease (see Table 75–2). Clearly distinguishable syndromes were present in three of 128 infants with omphalocele without heart disease, and in seven of 31 with congenital heart disease. Additional multiple congenital anomalies not part of any recognizable syndrome were present in two of 128 infants without, and in three of 31 with, congenital heart disease. A low midline defect consisting of exstrophy of the bladder with or without imperforate anus, cloacal anomaly, or myelomeningocele was present in nine of 128 infants with omphalocele and no heart disease and in none of those with associated congenital heart disease. Upper midline defects, including a diaphragmatic hernia, always were associated with a congenital cardiac malformation. Of 1,566 infants with congenital heart disease registered in the RICP, 11 (0.6%) had an omphalocele.

Table 75–3 summarizes the types of congenital heart disease, associated anomalies, and prognosis of the group of 37 infants with omphalocele and congenital heart disease. The most common cardiac lesion was tetralogy of Fallot (33%); the next most common category was atrial septal defect (secundum 19%). Among the 15 infants with simple omphalocele and congenital heart disease, six had tetralogy of Fallot. Specific genetic syndromes were present in seven patients and included trisomies D, E, and 21 with Beckwith syndrome. Both infants with trisomy 21 had an endocardial cushion defect. In seven patients, omphalocele was associated with diaphragmatic hernia, and in five of these the cardiac lesion was tetralogy of Fallot. Six of the eight babies with multiple congenital anomalies or heterotaxia had complex cardiac lesions.

Congenital heart disease was not recognized until postmortem examination in nine of the 37 infants. These were relatively simple and less severe anomalies (ASD, 6; VSD, 2; coarctation, 1).

The mortality of the total group of infants with omphalocele and congenital heart disease was very high (81%); death was thought to be directly related to the heart lesion in only six of the 30 who expired (20%). Mortality among the 128 patients with omphalocele without heart disease was 31%. Almost all infants underwent operation of some form for the omphalocele, and in only a few was a cardiac procedure performed.

From this study,[29] it was determined that omphalocele and congenital heart disease coexist in 30 times greater frequency than would be predicted by chance alone. Congenital heart disease was encountered in 19.5% of patients with omphalocele. In over half of these patients, a specific syndrome appeared to be related, in part, to which of the four embryonic folds failed to converge during embryonic development. The most common cardiac lesion encountered was tetralogy of Fallot—12 of 37 infants with omphalocele.

Examination of Table 75–3 leads to a number of diagnostic implications. The newborn with specific syndromes should be clearly recognizable and generally exhibits the heart disease characteristic of the syndrome, i.e., atrioventricular canal in trisomy 21. Infants with diaphragmatic hernia, alone or in the midline defect syndrome, characteristically have tetralogy of Fallot. The infants with multiple anomalies or malposition of the viscera generally exhibit complex cardiovascular lesions.

Among infants with an otherwise isolated omphalocele and congenital heart disease, the most common form is again tetralogy of Fallot. A variety of other cardiac lesions may occur, such as left-to-right shunts, ventricular septal defects, or atrial septal defects. The prognosis of infants with omphalocele and congenital heart disease is poor. In them, the mortality rate in this series was approximately 80%, compared with 30% for infants without heart disease. Awareness that tetralogy of Fallot is the most common serious cardiac malformation associated with omphaloceles

TABLE 75–3.—Cardiovascular Malformations Associated with Omphalocele, Children's Hospital, Boston, 1947–1973 and Regional Infant Cardiac Program 1968–1972

OMPHALOCELE CATEGORY	NO. OF PATIENTS	MAJOR CARDIAC LESIONS				OUTCOME	
		ASD 2°	T/F	COMPLEX LESIONS*	MISCELLANEOUS LESIONS	DEAD	ALIVE
Isolated†	15	3	6		VSD (2), VSD and PS (1), CoAo (2), PDA (1)	10	5
Specific syndrome							
Trisomy 21	2				AVC (2)	2	0
Trisomy D	2	2				2	0
Trisomy E	1				VSD and ASD (1)	1	0
Beckwith	2	1	1			2	0
Diaphragmatic hernia							
Isolated	5		4		CoAo (1)	4	1
Midline defect syndrome	2		1	1		2	0
Multiple anomalies, malpositions, ectopia cordis	8	1		6	ASD 1° (1)	7	1
TOTALS	37	7	12	7	11	30	7

VSD = ventricular septal defect; ASD = atrial septal defect; 2° = secundum; 1° = primum. AVC = atrioventricular canal; T/F = tetralogy of Fallot; PS = pulmonic stenosis; CoAo = coarctation of aorta; PDA = patent ductus arteriosus.

*Includes one patient each with (1) aortic arch atresia; (2) ectopia cordis and left ventricular diverticulum; (3) ectopia cordis, tricuspid atresia and pulmonary stenosis; (4) total anomalous pulmonary venous return, ventricular septal defect, pulmonary atresia; (5) atrioventricular canal, coarctation, conjoined twins; (6) dextrocardia and situs inversus; (7) dextrocardia, ventricular septal defect and patent ductus arteriosus.

†Five of these had one additional anomaly: 4 were minor (2 hypoplastic lung, 1 Klippel-Feil anomaly, 1 talipes equinovarus) and 1 major (tracheoesophageal fistula).

From Greenwood et al.[29]

should lead to more aggressive early palliation or corrective cardiac operation in these patients.

Prenatal Management

There have been recent efforts to make an antenatal diagnosis of certain congenital malformations. Although there have not yet been any attempts to treat this lesion in the fetus, it appears beneficial to know if a child is going to be born with a large omphalocele or gastroschisis so that preparations to facilitate delivery and possible transport for treatment can be made well in advance. Nicolini et al.[42] report a case in which the antenatal diagnosis of an omphalocele containing a "large" amount of fluid was made by ultrasound. To facilitate delivery, the omphalocele was aspirated of 320 ml of clear yellow fluid 2 hours before cesarean section.

In another report of a prenatal diagnosis of a large omphalocele made by ultrasound, Dell'Agnola et al.[15] raise the question of antenatal intrauterine correction. They conclude that "fetal surgery for prenatal surgical correction of an omphalocele seems to be at present a dangerous procedure, until we have more experience and more accurate parameters of ultrasound fetal imaging." They go on to say that "at present, ultrasound diagnosis of fetal omphalocele in late pregnancy should be used only to alert us to avoid rupture of the sac or other complications during delivery, and to plan for correct perinatal management."

I have grave doubts from the surgical and moral points of view that antenatal surgical intervention for definitive treatment of either omphalocele or gastroschisis is, or ever will be, appropriate.

Treatment

The mortality rate of infants with a large omphalocele or gastroschisis has been reported to range from 34% to more than 80%. For many years, patients with antenatal rupture of the sac of a large omphalocele or gastroschisis had a mortality rate approaching 100%.

The severity of the condition and its poor prognosis were first described in the sixteenth century by Ambroise Paré.[44] The first successful surgical treatment was reported by Hey[33] in 1803. It was concluded that the condition was almost always fatal because of associated malformations or because the large size of the hernia prevented its reduction. A variety of methods of therapy, both operative and nonoperative, have been utilized with varying degrees of success.

Nonoperative (Conservative) Treatment

Successful treatment of a patient by alcohol dressing, without operation, was reported by Ahlfeld[1] in 1899 and by Cunningham[14] in 1956. In 1957, Grob[30] reported the treatment of omphalocele by application of 2% aqueous solution of Mercurochrome. Because of the danger of mercury intoxication, it is now recommended that Mercurochrome, if used at all,[58] be used as a 0.5% solution in 65% alcohol at hourly intervals for the first 48 hours.[20] The frequency of applications should then be reduced to once a day until a solid eschar forms. As epithelialization progresses from the periphery of the lesion, the eschar separates. Mercurochrome should not be applied to granulating surfaces, as excess absorption may result in mercury intoxication. Venugopal and associates[58] reported 15 infants treated in this manner with five deaths, a 33.3% mortality. Epithelialization of the sac may take as long as 10–19 weeks and in many instances, despite epithelialization of the sac, a large and persistent ventral hernia will require later therapy which, in a significant number of patients, will have to be a staged correction (Fig 75–6).

In 1977, Fagan et al.[20] reported a study of organ mercury levels in infants with omphaloceles treated with an organic mercurial antiseptic. Although they did not specify the strength or fre-

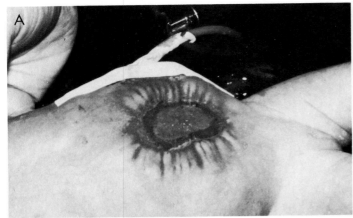

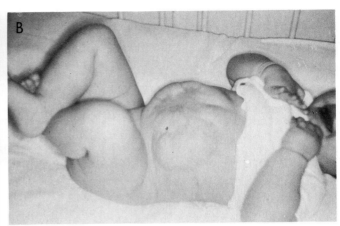

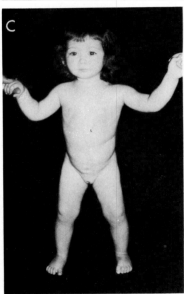

Fig 75–6.—Omphalocele: Mercurochrome treatment. **A,** during course of treatment by application of Mercurochrome. Note the eschar in center and the contracting rim of epithelium. **B,** same patient following complete spontaneous epithelialization of the anterior abdominal wall. A large ventral hernia remains. **C,** ultimate result after abdominal wall reconstruction.

quency of Merthiolate used in the study group, their results showed that thiomersal can induce blood and organ levels of organic mercury well in excess of the minimum toxic level in adults and fetuses. Because of the potential for mercury toxicity, it would probably be well to avoid its use completely, and, if need be, revert to simple 65% alcohol as an escharotic agent.

We have rarely used the Mercurochrome technique, although there do appear to be several indications for the use of a nonoperative method of treatment: (1) in the newborn with giant, intact membrane omphalocele who also has other life-threatening anomalies, the correction of which takes precedence over repair of the omphalocele; (2) in the patient with other anomalies that complicate repair of the omphalocele; (3) in the neonate with severe associated anomalies that may not be consistent with survival; (4) in the patient with a large omphalocele or gastroschisis who has been started on a program of multiple staged repairs using prosthetic materials but who has developed infection along the suture line, resulting in separation of the prosthetic material and its removal.

Operative Treatment

Primary operative repair of omphaloceles has been attempted since the first surgical treatment by Hey.[33] The ideal repair is complete primary closure without compromising the patient's respiratory state, venous return, or intestinal blood supply. Patients with small or medium-sized omphaloceles in whom the liver is not herniated can usually withstand a primary repair. Frequently, complete repair during the initial procedure can be accomplished in patients with gastroschisis; however, when the herniated mass is very large and, on the rare occasion when the liver makes up part of the herniated mass, primary complete repair may be dangerous despite manual stretching of the abdominal wall. Attempts at primary repair of very large omphaloceles or gastroschisis are often heroic, but brutal, efforts to squeeze more into a small abdominal cavity than it can contain (Fig 75–7). By force, the surgeon may be able to crowd intestines back into the abdomen and repair the musculofascial layers only to have death occur a few hours following operation secondary to severe respiratory distress and circulatory collapse. The respiratory problems are caused by marked elevation and immobilization of the diaphragm, while the circulatory collapse is secondary to compression of the inferior vena cava and decreased return of blood to the heart. Despite the availability of ventilatory support, the surgeon should avoid a compromising approach when a safe, staged, method for gradual enlargement of the abdominal cavity is available.

To obviate the above problems, Williams, in 1930,[60] first sug-

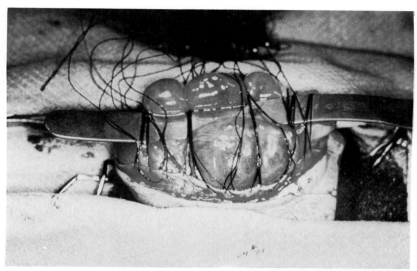

Fig 75–7.—Giant omphalocele: attempt at primary reconstruction. Note the virtual impossibility, even with brute force, of squeezing the viscera into the small abdominal cavity. If the sutures were to hold, the baby would be at great hazard of decreased return of blood to the heart from the vena cava compression and respiratory distress from elevation of the diaphragm.

gested a staged procedure; and Gross, in 1948,[32] described a technique of repairing the abdominal wall in two stages. The essential feature of the first stage was the preservation of the amniotic membrane, covering it with flaps of widely mobilized skin. No attempt was made to crowd the viscera back into the small abdominal cavity. Many such patients survived who would not have done so formerly. A few patients, even with this type of closure, required immediate release of the skin sutures to reverse the effects of the marked increase of abdominal pressure (Fig 75–8). Although Gross' staged technique[32] was a major step in improving survival in patients with large omphaloceles, it did not always subsequently result in the anticipated increase in size of the abdominal cavity. When these patients returned for the second procedure, i.e., correction of the large ventral hernia, many were found not to have had any increase in space within the abdomen. The herniated viscera had remained outside the abdomen lying on the surface of the abdominal wall. There had not been any stimulus within the abdomen to increase the size of the abdominal cavity (Figs 75–9, 75–10).

A useful technique for enlarging the abdominal space in such patients was popularized by Ravitch.[46] Goñi Moreno[27] in 1947 used progressive pneumoperitoneum in the repair of large hernias in adults. Ravitch proposed the use of this technique in patients, such as the one in Figure 75–10, left with large ventral hernias after initial treatment of an omphalocele by skin coverage with the Gross technique. The method involves the insertion of a polyethylene catheter under local anesthesia into the peritoneal cavity in one of the lower quadrants through an area of normal full-thickness abdominal wall. The proper free intraperitoneal position of the catheter is checked fluoroscopically by the injection of a few milliliters of radiopaque material. The catheter is fixed to the skin and attached to a stopcock. Thereafter, the abdomen is distended with air at least once a day to the point of tolerance. The potential complications include: (1) air embolism

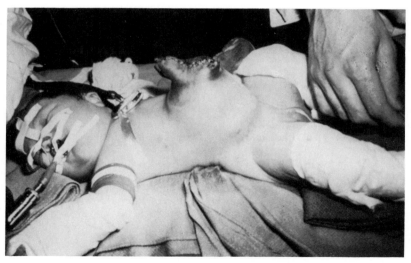

Fig 75–8.—Omphalocele. Attempted skin closure by extensive undermining, according to the technique of Gross. Despite the many advantages of this technique, even this kind of closure may not be successful, as this patient demonstrates. This child's abdomen had to be reopened because of poor viability of the skin and excessive intra-abdominal pressure, causing respiratory embarrassment.

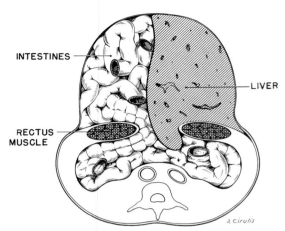

Fig 75–9.—Diagrammatic cross section of a patient with a persistent large ventral hernia following first-stage Gross repair. The herniated viscera and liver lie subcutaneously on the muscular abdominal wall and depress it. The abdominal cavity is small, and there is little space between the level of the ventral muscles and the vertebral column.

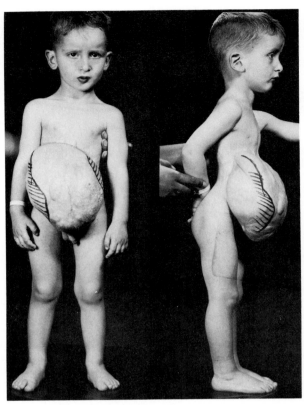

Fig 75–10.—Huge ventral hernia after Gross technique coverage of large omphalocele. The problem is that illustrated in the diagram in Figure 75–9. Most of the viscera, including the liver and spleen, are outside the abdomen, lying upon the abdominal muscles. Lateral view shows the very small size of the abdominal cavity.

if a catheter should be inserted directy into the liver; (2) insertion of too much air, resulting in respiratory difficulty, grunting, anorexia, and vomiting; (3) subcutaneous emphysema; (4) hepatic vein thrombosis secondary to attenuation of the hepatic vein; (5) perforation of a loop of bowel, resulting in peritoneal contamination. Ravitch recommended an initial operation to free up the liver when it is "riding forward on the shelves of the recti as the abdomen is distended with air." The recti can then be stretched over the liver without elongating the hepatic vein and inviting hepatic vein occlusion when ultimately the liver is replaced. The pneumoperitoneum is required for a variable period of time, and the longer it can be maintained the more adequate will be the size of the peritoneal cavity. We have not utilized this technique.

We generally adopt a staged operative approach to the treatment of giant omphaloceles and gastroschisis when they are not *reasonably* amenable to safe primary repair. A variety of operative methods have been proposed to facilitate complete primary closure of the abdominal wall, either by enlarging the abdominal cavity or by decreasing the volume of material to be returned. In 1956, Buchanan and Cain[10] resected the spleen and a large portion of the right lobe of the liver to close the skin during the first stage of a Gross repair. As recently as 1968, Kleinhaus et al.[35] performed a partial hepatectomy in the repair of an omphalocele to aid in closure of the abdominal wall. Sigmoidotomy with evacuation of the contents of the sigmoid colon has been recommended to decrease the volume of material to be returned to the abdomen.[16] Such interference with the viscera is to be deplored.

Transverse division of the rectus muscles[50, 51] was said to cause a greater relaxation of the abdominal wall fascia and skin and an increase in size of the abdominal cavity. The skin had been widely mobilized and used to cover the ventral surface of the abdomen.

In 1966, Dickey[17] suggested that surgical repair may not be successful in the massive omphalocele until the ratio of liver size to body cavity size is low. He pointed out that the change in body proportion and contour resulting in the loss of an infant potbelly is usually fairly well advanced by age 5 years, when replacement of an exteriorized liver and other viscera have a greater chance of success. The presumption was that the abdominal cavity would continue to grow despite the absence of the abdominal viscera within it. This is highly unlikely. Dickey also recommended that the boundaries of the right subdiaphragmatic

space be widened by cutting costal cartilages to allow exaggerated fan-like lateral and anterior expansion of the rib cage.

Croom and Thomas, in 1971,[13] proposed a unique closure of the abdominal wall utilizing skin and muscle flaps to repair a gastroschisis. Despite the magnitude of the operative procedure, they believed that it was justified since they obtained an immediate primary closure with autogenous tissue while avoiding the risk of excessive intra-abdominal pressure, compromise of cardiorespiratory function, and the danger of infection associated with the use of prosthetic materials. Köllermann and Schwarzer[36] utilized complex skin flaps to create a ventral hernia.

Ein and Shandling[19] used a polymer membrane in a neonate born with a giant omphalocele to promote the growth of granulation tissue over the eventrated viscera. These granulations became epithelialized within 4–6 weeks. As they stated, this method does not eliminate the need for a later repair of the resultant large ventral hernia. This later correction may or may not need to be done in stages with prosthetic materials. Their principal goal was to "eliminate the necessity for surgery in the newborn period." Although this technique may be useful in neonates with other complicating problems in whom one wishes to avoid operation, the otherwise uncomplicated giant omphalocele that cannot be safely repaired in a single operation can be treated more expeditiously with prosthetic materials in a series of staged procedures.

In 1959, we first used prosthetic materials to gradually enlarge the abdominal cavity with staged operative procedures. This was initially reported in 1964 and published in 1967.[52] Since that time, a number of techniques have been reported utilizing this basic principle of staged closure with prosthetic materials, but with various modifications.[2, 8, 23, 25, 34, 56, 57]

One of the more widely accepted modifications has been that proposed by Allen and Wrenn[2] in 1969. They termed their prosthetic sac attached to the abdominal wall a "silo" and initially sutured a single sheet of impermeable Silastic material around the circumference of the defect through which the viscera were herniated. Following the circumferential suturing around the defect, they used a running suture to close the sheet of Silon along its side and over the top. Postoperative management included dripping local antibiotics into the dressing continuously and reducing the size of the prosthetic sac at 1–3-day intervals by suturing or by simply squeezing it off and tying the sac to reduce its size.

With this technique, any delay in repair and removal of the Silon beyond 7–10 days often results in infection along the suture line and resultant loss of the prosthetic material. There can be no symphysis between the Silon and the patient's tissues. The subsequent operative stages remain totally dependent on the continuing integrity of the sutures holding the Silon in place. The sutures tend to pull out if infection occurs along the suture line. We prefer the method of staged repair with prosthetic materials shown in Figures 75–11 and 75–12.

Repair of Skin-Covered Omphalocele with Secondary Ventral Hernia (see Fig 75–11)

In these children, the problem is that the intestines, and often the liver, are under the widely dissected skin flaps overlying the muscles of the anterior abdominal wall and even the lower ribs, so that the growth of the viscera merely stretches the skin and does not enlarge the coelom.

The gastrointestinal tract is decompressed with nasogastric suction for 24–48 hours and the first stage undertaken under general anesthesia. A central venous line for hyperalimentation is placed at this time. All intravenous lines should be placed in the upper half of the body because increased abdominal pressure may interfere with the flow of fluid from lower-limb veins. The subcutaneous space is excluded from continuity with the coelom by suturing a sheet of knitted Teflon mesh on each side to the edge of the rectus. The viscera are protected from adhesion to the mesh by a thin sheet of nonreactive material tacked to the lateral gutter on either side. The very fine, medical-grade polyethylene, which we used initially, is no longer obtainable and we employ Dow Corning Silastic sheeting, 0.005–0.010 mm thick. The flaps of mesh are sutured together in the midline without any great degree of tension and the skin closed. The closure, which may at first seem snug, becomes slack with remarkable speed; and in a day or two, without anesthesia, the skin may be reopened and the Teflon mesh resutured to take up the slack, excising the redundant portion of mesh. The skin is closed again. To prevent infection, the entire surface of the repair, particularly the suture line, is coated with a heavy layer of Betadine ointment. The baby is then wrapped with a loose Curlex bandage, which is undisturbed until the next stage. Depending on the size of the initial hernia, completion of the procedure may require only two stages in some and four or five in others. The last stage, like the first, is performed under general anesthesia. The plastic liner is removed by simple traction, the last of the mesh excised, and the recti approximated in the midline. This may sometimes require near-and-far sutures.

Repair of Giant Omphalocele with Intact Membrane (see Fig 75–12)

As soon after birth as possible, with a nasogastric tube in place, an incision is made in the skin completely around the om-

phalocele sac and as close to the skin-sac junction as possible without opening into the sac. The retention of this very narrow strip of skin has caused no difficulty. The skin is dissected back only modestly. The repair is identical to that just discussed for giant ventral hernia, following employment of the Gross primary repair of omphalocele except that, since the intact sac membrane is available, there is no risk of bowel adhesion to the sheets of Teflon mesh and interposition of a sheet of Silastic is not required. Since the abdomen has not been opened, a gastrostomy tube is not inserted. We do not agree with the recommendation made by some that the omphalocele membrane be opened and the abdomen explored. This complicates the repair, and without it intestinal obstruction, for whatever reason, is relatively uncommon. The skin usually cannot be closed and is simply tacked as high on the mesh as it reaches comfortably. The routine employment of nasogastric drainage and central venous hyperalimentation permits decompression of the intestine and provision of adequate nutrition during the staged reconstruction of the abdominal wall. The mesh is excised in stages, the skin usually being closed at the second stage. After the abdominal wall has been repaired and has healed, laparotomy for correction of any intestinal problem can be more readily performed than it could have previously.

Figure 75–13 shows a patient with a large omphalocele and intact membrane during staged mesh repair. The retained membrane has prevented adhesion between the underlying bowel and the mesh. It also contains the visceral mass as a readily manipulated unit.

Repair of Ruptured Omphalocele and Gastroschisis

The bowel in children with ruptured omphalocele or gastroschisis has been herniated since well before birth, and the exposure to amniotic fluid has produced edema, fibrin deposition, and matting of the bowel into a conglomerate mass (Fig 75–14,A). It is generally best not to attempt to dissect and separate the loops of bowel. If intestinal perforations are created, they should be corrected and any suture line turned away from the overlying prosthetic material, burying it within the abdomen. The staged repair in other respects is identical to that already discussed for a giant skin-covered omphalocele with secondary ventral hernia. The gastrostomy is placed at the first operation and brought through the abdominal wall far laterally, removing Silastic for a small distance around the tube, so that the stomach can adhere to the parietal peritoneum.

Figure 75–15 shows the staged repair of a gastroschisis.

Helpful Adjuncts in Surgical Therapy

Several advances have improved the care and survival of newborns with giant omphalocele and/or gastroschisis.

For the recognition and management of the respiratory embarrassment that may be associated with repair of omphalocele, the degree of the baby's oxygenation is carefully monitored. Monitoring of tissue oxygenation by transcutaneous techniques has become increasingly useful (see Chap. 5) but may not be universally available. The umbilical arteries in these infants cannot be used for catheterization in the ordinary way. Filston and Izant[22] developed a fairly simple and useful technique for translocating the umbilical arteries to the lower abdomen for easy catheterization outside the operative field.

Prolonged intestinal dysfunction continues to be a major problem in the management of patients with gastroschisis and giant omphaloceles, despite surgical advances that have helped in the overall repair of these difficulties. In 1971, Filler et al.[21] described a method of maintaining nutrition in these patients by central venous infusion of fat-free amino acid–glucose solution.

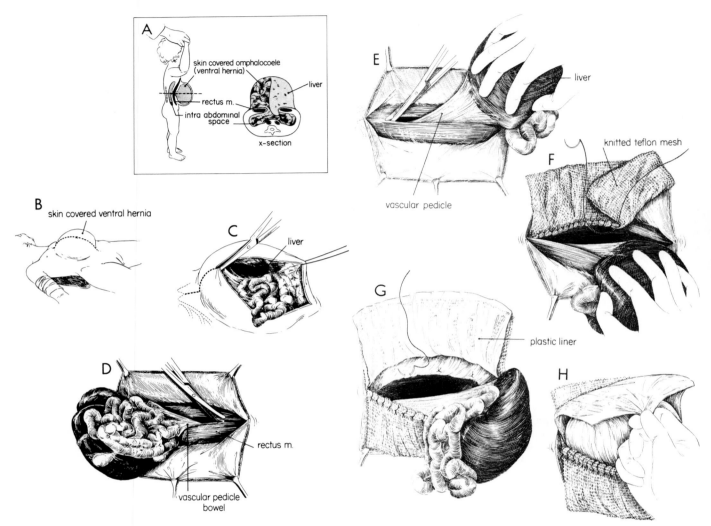

Fig 75–11.—Technique for repair of a previously skin-covered omphalocele (secondary ventral hernia). **A,** lateral view of the patient (sagittal section cutaway) and a cross-section to demonstrate the relation of the hernia to the layers of the abdominal wall. The intra-abdominal space is small and the recti are displaced posteriorly by the hernial mass. The herniated viscera spread, like the cap of a mushroom, subcutaneously over the abdominal wall, further depressing it posteriorly. If dissection of the skin flaps initially was carried up over the costal margin, the hernial mass may overlie the lower portion of the chest cage as well, compressing the lower ribs posteriorly and obliterating the subphrenic space that might normally accept the liver. Patients with liver herniation present the greatest problems. **B,** general anesthesia is used for the first stage, the patient supine, the *dotted line* representing the xiphoid-to-pubis midline incision. **C,** the skin has been opened and the peritoneal cavity entered. The intestines and liver are widely adherent to the overlying skin, and special care must be taken to avoid perforating bowel. **D,** the recti are separated inferiorly. One sees the nonrotated, unfixed bowel on its vascular pedicle. The anterior rectus sheath is preserved for later attachment of the prosthetic sheets. The midline is opened to the pubis. **E,** superiorly the midline is incised to the xiphoid process. This long incision produces a wide circumference for the Teflon-constrained enclosure and a larger opening through which the intestines can return, preventing compression and angulation of the bowel against the edges of a small abdominal wall defect. Angulation of the bowel can prevent its return to the abdomen, while compression

may be responsible for erosion and perforation. The liver, herniated out of the abdomen, is on a long pedicle and obstruction of venous return is easily produced. The assistant is responsible for maintaining the liver in midposition without traction or angulation of its pedicle. **F,** the abdominal opening extends from the xiphoid to the pubis; the medial edges of the recti are clearly defined. The anterior rectus fascia has been preserved. A folded edge of knitted Teflon mesh is being secured to the medial edges of the recti and fascia with heavy, interrupted, nonabsorbable sutures. Currently a long-lasting absorbable suture such as PDS is acceptable. The mesh is folded in this manner so that the narrow, outer edge may ultimately be secured on the anterior surface of the rectus sheath.[10] **G,** a second sheet of mesh has been similarly secured to the opposite rectus muscle. A sheet of very thin and soft synthetic material (Silastic, Dow Corning cat. no. 500-1 or 500-3) to serve as a lining membrane is sutured in the gutter on each side with a few interrupted sutures. A portion of the lining membrane will be excised from around the point of passage of the gastrostomy tube to permit adherence of the stomach to the abdominal wall. The gastrostomy is brought far laterally. A rigid lining material is to be avoided, lest it cause bowel erosion and fecal fistulae. **H,** the Silastic sheets from the two sides are overlapped (and do not need to be sutured together), preventing adherence of the viscera to the parietal peritoneum and to the Teflon mesh. Further, the Silastic sheets function as a sac, forcing the intestinal mass back into the abdominal cavity at subsequent stages, like a plastic-wrapped package. **(Continued)**

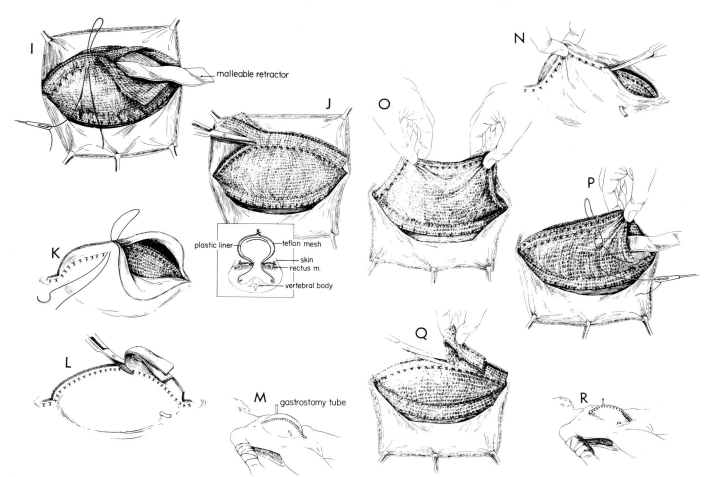

Fig 75–11 Cont.—I, the gut is pressed down by a malleable retractor as the sheets of netted Teflon mesh are secured to each other in the midline with horizontal mattress sutures, using an eyed probe with a blunt tip to make perforation of a loop of bowel less likely. The interstices of the mesh are large enough to receive the probe without difficulty. The outer fold of the Teflon is laid over the anterior rectus sheath and secured with just a few sutures to provide a broad area over which the mesh can "heal" to the underlying fascia. This area of symphysis helps avoid infection and prevents separation of the mesh and fascia during subsequent stages. A mesh material with large interstices has decided advantages over a single layer of impermeable material such as silicone, or even a very finely woven mesh. Finely woven material does not allow ready growth of tissue into its interstices. Premature separation of the prosthetic material is likely if infection involves the suture line (see Fig 75–16). **J,** closure of the mesh and removal of the excess. The surgeon must determine now if the patient has adequate spontaneous pulmonary exchange. If the closure appears to have been too tight, the suture line must be reopened and the sutures replaced farther out on the mesh, relieving the intra-abdominal tension. A cross-section shows what has been accomplished *(inset).* The bowel is entirely within the newly formed sac and does not overlie the muscular abdominal wall. **K** and **L,** the skin is closed and the excess excised. **M,** completion of the first stage, which has reduced the size of the hernia by only a modest degree. **N,** within 24–72 hours, the second stage can be carried out without anesthesia. The gastrostomy has been on suction in the interval. Note the striking laxity of the skin after this brief period. **O,** the looseness of the mesh is similarly apparent. **P,** the mesh is opened, the intestines depressed by a malleable retractor on the Silastic sheeting, and a new row of horizontal mattress sutures placed in the mesh behind the original row. The drawing suggests that the subcutaneous dissection is carried out beyond the attachment of mesh to the rectus sheath, but in fact it is important to avoid such a dissection to retain a firm and uninterrupted bond between skin, mesh, and fascia. **Q,** the excess mesh is resected after it has been determined that there is no significant compromise of ventilation. **R,** the skin is closed once more. The hernia is smaller. The number of stages required varies, depending on the size of the initial omphalocele. Only the first and last stages require anesthesia. **(Continued)**

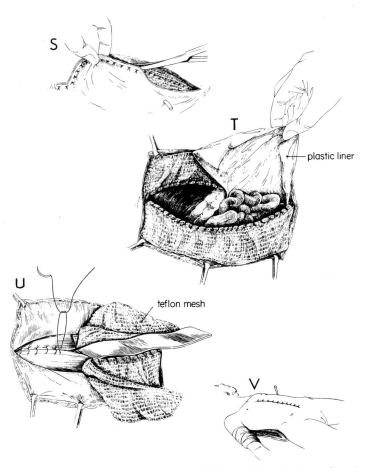

Fig 75–11 Cont.—S, at the last stage, the skin is reopened. **T,** the plastic liner is removed, simply by traction. **U,** the Teflon mesh is separated from the recti and entirely removed. The rectus edges are approximated with heavy absorbable monofilament sutures. Occasionally the tension is sufficient to require the use of "pulley stitches." **V,** completed procedure.

This has become a mandatory adjunct in the therapy of infants with giant omphaloceles, particularly those who have had antenatal rupture of omphalocele or gastroschisis. The intestines of these patients, as a result of prolonged exposure to amniotic fluid, have become thickened, edematous, and adherent and are subject to prolonged ileus and dysfunction that may last for weeks, if not months. Despite this, patients can be maintained in a virtually normal nutritional state by central venous hyperalimentation. Before this method of nutrition, there was frequently great concern about mechanical intestinal obstruction and the need for operative intervention to correct it. Premature and hazardous operative procedures were often undertaken in these patients to avoid the complications and mortality of prolonged starvation. More often than not, these efforts were not necessary, since the "obstruction" was more commonly intestinal dysfunction rather than a real mechanical obstruction. The central venous line for hyperalimentation placed during the first stage of the operative correction provides a margin of safety so that nutrition is maintained and there is time for complete repair and healing of the abdominal wall before any need for surgical intervention to correct a mechanical obstruction.

Prolonged intestinal decompression is obviously necessary in the face of prolonged intestinal dysfunction, and the establishment of a properly placed gastrostomy at the initial operative procedure provides for prolonged gastric suction without the use of a nasal or oral suction catheter. This combination of central venous hyperalimentation and gastric suction enables us to maintain normal nutrition until the abdominal wall has been completely reconstructed.

Complications and Their Management

RESPIRATORY DISTRESS.—When respiratory distress occurs immediately after operation, the surgeon must assume that the repair has been overly tight. It is because of this possibility that the staged repairs are done either without anesthesia or with light general anesthesia (first and last stages). This permits a more accurate determination of the patient's ability to ventilate. At each stage, the excess mesh should not be removed until the determination is made that the proposed closure is tolerated. If necessary, the suture line in the mesh can be moved more peripherally and the baby assessed again before the "excess" mesh is cut away.

Occasionally, patients, particularly prematures, after operation demonstrate inadequate ventilatory ability, as evidenced by abnormal blood gases. Such infants benefit from assisted ventilation, which is usually necessary for only a few hours or days and can overcome a serious temporary setback in their management. Gierup et al.[24] demonstrated its usefulness in the report of their experience with this problem.

INFECTION.—Infection has sometimes been a problem in association with the use of prosthetic material in the staged repair

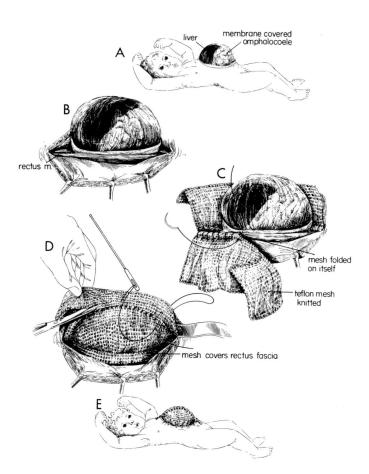

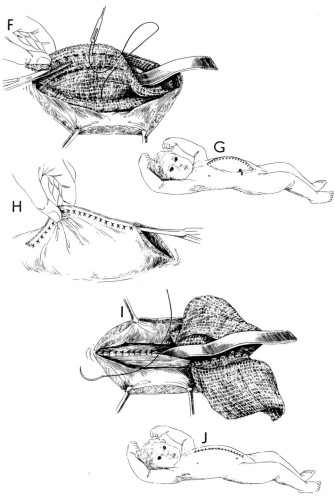

Fig 75–12.—Technique for repair of a giant omphalocele with an intact membrane. **A,** neonate with a typical large membrane-covered omphalocele. *Dotted line* around the omphalocele-skin junction indicates the line of incision, which will leave a very narrow margin of skin attached to the omphalocele, sufficient only to prevent opening into the peritoneal cavity. **B,** a skin flap has been elevated all around the omphalocele, not too widely lest the blood supply be compromised. It is not necessary to cover the omphalocele completely with skin in the first stage. **C,** the medial edges of the recti are identified and a folded sheet of Teflon mesh applied to each edge. **D,** the mesh has been additionally tacked to the edge of the rectus with another row of sutures, and now the two sheets of mesh are drawn together, sutured in the midline, and the excess cut away. Since the omphalocele membrane is intact, there is no need for a plastic lining. **E,** at the end of the first stage, there is usually not enough skin available to cover the entire

herniated mass, but the skin edge has been loosely sutured to the mesh as high as can be done easily without undue tension. The entire area of mesh and suture line is covered with Betadine ointment and sterile dressing. **F,** second stage, 24–72 hours later, is done without anesthesia. The suture line in the mesh is opened, a malleable retractor inserted over the intact omphalocele, and the sac containing the herniated viscera pressed into the abdomen. Another row of sutures is placed behind the ones originally placed in the mesh to maintain the reduction achieved. **G,** the skin can now be closed over the partially reduced omphalocele. The number of required stages depends entirely on the size of the initial omphalocele. **H,** final stage. The lax skin is reopened. **I,** the skin has been dissected off the mesh, which is completely removed. The recti are approximated and the skin closed. **J,** complete reconstruction of the abdominal wall after the final stage.

of omphaloceles or gastroschisis. Venugopal, Zachary, and Spitz[58] reported their experience in 1976. In a total of 91 patients treated by various methods, 17 were treated with a single nonpermeable prosthetic layer of Silastic sheeting, and in six of these there was separation from the abdominal wall. The mortality rate for this group was over 64%, most succumbing to infection and septicemia. Our own experience with infection has confirmed the fact that the use of Silon sheeting as a single prosthetic layer (an impermeable type of material) makes the patient much more prone to infection along the suture line. In the face of such infection, there is a great likelihood of separation of the Silon material and resultant delay in closure. Resuturing the material, in the presence of infection, is usually unsuccessful and the staged repair with prosthetic material has to be abandoned. This kind of problem is directly related to the nature of the material used.

The impermeable Silon sheeting, as the only layer in the repair, does not allow actual healing of the tissues to and through it. Integrity of the sutures is required to keep it in place. The sheeting acts as a foreign body being bathed continuously in a pool of serum. For all practical purposes, it creates a pocket of serum-filled dead space around itself, which is less resistant to infection than a closed and healing wound.

It has been our experience that, when infection of this type does occur, it usually does not extend intraperitoneally, although overwhelming sepsis may nevertheless occur. Further attempts at closure should not be made once infection has occurred. Instead, the prosthetic material should be removed and a nonoperative approach such as application of an escharotic agent, pursued. By the time the infection has produced separation of the prosthetic material, a "membrane" has formed over the her-

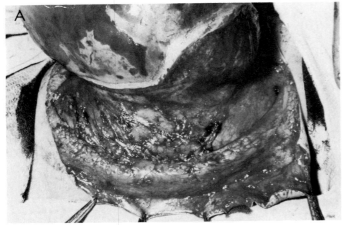

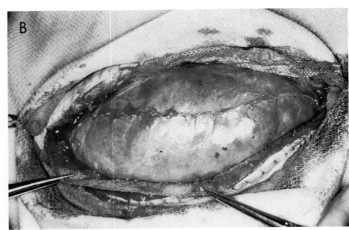

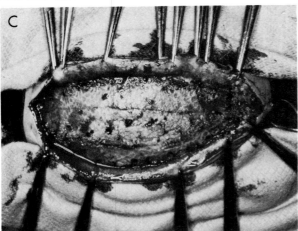

Fig 75–13.—Omphalocele with intact sac preserved during staged Teflon mesh repair. **A,** note the thin rim of skin attached to the sac, preserving its integrity. **B,** intermediate stage of repair. The natural membrane of the omphalocele has served to prevent adhesions between the underlying bowel and the mesh and to hold the visceral mass, which can be manipulated as a single contained unit. The omphalocele sac has not adhered to the Teflon, as can clearly be seen. The remaining edges of the Teflon will be sutured together. **C,** final stage. For the first time, the skin is dissected back to the rectus muscle beyond the mesh. The mesh has been so completely incorporated in the tissues that it is hard to recognize.

niated bowel in response to the overlying plastic material, providing a surface on which the chosen agent may be applied (Figs 75–15, 75–16).

Gierup et al.[24] analyzed their experience with 61 patients with abdominal wall defects (omphalocele 37, gastroschisis 24) over a 24-year period. They divided their patients into three different groups:

The first group, in the first 10 years, was principally babies with omphaloceles of small size, who did not require total parenteral nutrition (TPN) or assisted postoperative ventilation. They were treated with primary closure or painting with Mercurochrome.

The second group, in the next 5 years, was fairly evenly distributed between omphalocele and gastroschisis. TPN was given in 66% of cases and assisted ventilation was used in 20%. The repairs were with the staged Silo technique in approximately half the patients.

The third group, made up of the patients in the last 5-year period, was characterized by use of a "radical primary closure" with a concomitant increase in the use of assisted postoperative ventilation and TPN in 66%.

They concluded that the Silon pouch closure was not successful because of high incidence of sepsis. They tended to attribute the sepsis to the frequent use of central venous lines, although they provided no bacteriological evidence. Their experience, that sepsis occurs more frequently when a prosthetic impermeable membrane of Silastic is used as a *single* layer, was consistent with that of others.[49, 53] They further demonstrated that "radical primary closure" requires frequent need for postoperative ventilatory support because of elevation and immobilization of the diaphragm and circulatory collapse secondary to compression of the inferior vena cava. Despite this, they advocate the continued use of "radical primary closure" rather than a staged repair. They have failed to understand the basic principle of the staged repair and do not understand the *real* etiology of their problems.

Although a single-stage primary repair is desirable, the principal objective in the treatment of the neonate born with either a very large omphalocele or gastroschisis is to avoid any compromise of the patient's spontaneous ventilation. Despite the modern availability of mechanical ventilatory support, the surgeon should not include this as a routinely planned part of the postoperative care by insisting on "radical primary closure." The basic principle should be a gradual increase in the size of the abdominal cavity if primary closure cannot be carried out without compromising the patient's respiratory function. This is borne out by the fact that, despite ventilatory support, Gierup et al.[24] had several patients who died because of their inability to ventilate properly following "radical primary closure." Despite this, they have concluded that "From our positive experience has emerged a firm belief that [*almost*] all cases can be treated with radical primary repair."

During the past 13 years, our own experience has been quite different. There have not been any deaths related to the surgical repair or its complications. Patients who have died, with one

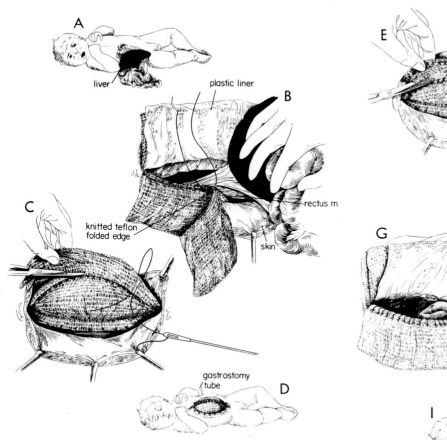

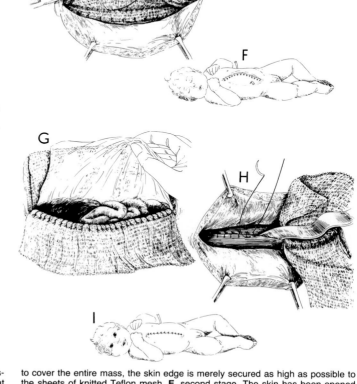

Fig 75–14.—Technique of staged repair of a ruptured omphalocele or gastroschisis not safely treatable by a single-stage procedure. **A,** newborn with what may either be antenatal rupture of an omphalocele or a gastroschisis. In this instance, because the liver is herniated outside the body cavity, it is almost certainly an omphalocele rather than a gastroschisis. **B,** the small opening through which the viscera have herniated has been enlarged, from xiphoid to symphysis. A folded edge of knitted Teflon mesh is secured to the medial edge of the rectus muscle with interrupted, nonabsorbable sutures or a long-lasting absorbable suture (PDS). The inner plastic lining material of thin Silastic film is secured in the posterolateral peritoneal gutter. Gastrostomy is placed as shown in Figure 75–11. **C,** the Silastic lining sheets are overlapped, covering the herniated mass of viscera, the knitted Teflon sheets sutured in the midline, and the excess resected. **D,** the patient following completion of the first stage. With insufficient skin to cover the entire mass, the skin edge is merely secured as high as possible to the sheets of knitted Teflon mesh. **E,** second stage. The skin has been opened (again, not dissected back as widely as the artist has shown), a few of the Teflon sutures removed, the Silastic-covered bowel depressed by the retractor, and a new row of sutures placed in the Teflon mesh behind those of the first stage. The excess mesh is resected after it has been determined that there has been no compromise of respiration. **F,** the patient following this stage. The skin edges have now been approximated in the midline. **G,** final stage. The plastic liners are removed. For the first time, the skin is dissected off the Teflon mesh to its edges on the anterior rectus sheath. **H,** the Teflon mesh is removed and the muscles closed in the midline. **I,** completed procedure, with reconstruction of the abdominal wall.

exception, have done so as a result of associated severe malformation or severe prematurity. One patient died as a result of a massive midgut volvulus.

Silon, as a single prosthetic layer material, is *not* acceptable in the staged repair for these infants. Theoretically, it has an advantage since it is a single material. If one could always assume that everything will proceed smoothly and the entire repair will be complete in 7–10 days *before* any infection has led to loss of the prosthetic material, Silon would be acceptable. However, delays occur and infection is always possible. A wide-mesh material such as the knitted Teflon we use is far more satisfactory. Since the mesh is actually incorporated into the tissues, there is no dead space between the prosthesis and the abdominal wall laterally when it is sutured, and this part of the mesh is exposed only at the initial operative procedure and at the final procedure when the mesh is removed. Our most recent results substantiate

this. Figure 75–13,*C* shows a patient just about to undergo the final stage, at which the prosthetic materials are going to be removed. The bonding has been so secure that one can hardly recognize the mesh incorporated in the tissues. On the underside there has been no adherence between the underlying bowel and the mesh because of the lining membrane of thin Silastic film.

ENTERIC FISTULAE.—From time to time there have been problems with the development of enterocutaneous fistulae beneath the prosthetic material. The cause is not entirely clear. In a patient in whom a heavy Silon material was used, the continuous friction of a firm fold of the material against the bowel wall apparently produced erosion and subsequent fistula.

Another site of fistula formation is at the point of egress of the bowel from the abdomen. In gastroschisis, the defect in the abdominal wall may be small. The bowel coming through the de-

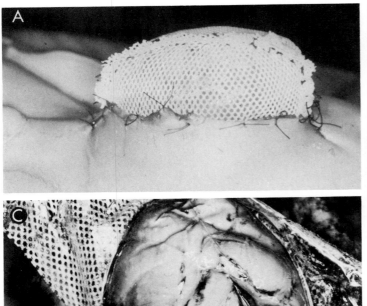

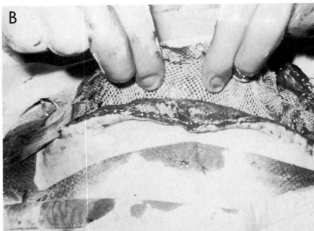

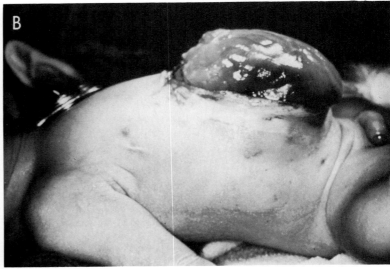

Fig 75–15.—Gastroschisis: staged repair. **A,** following the first stage. The lining membrane of Silastic is visible through the interstices of the overlying Teflon mesh. The skin has been loosely sutured to the mesh without placing undue tension on the flaps. **B,** interval stage. Note the laxity of the mesh held up between the thumb (not seen) and fingers of the two hands. The skin has not been separated from over the line of sutures securing the mesh to the rectus muscle. Avoiding such exposure of this suture line until the final stage allows firm adherence and healing between the mesh and the surrounding tissues and decreases the potential for infection around this suture line. **C,** at the final stage, the pseudomembrane over the herniated bowel has formed under the film of Silastic. Should infection necessitate removal of the prosthetic materials, this membrane will be a superb base for application of the escharotic agent.

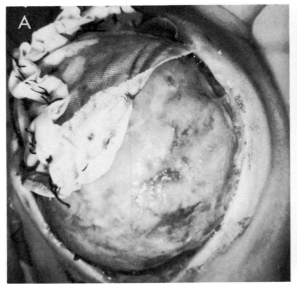

Fig 75–16.—The problem of infection of the suture line, resulting in separation of prosthetic materials. **A,** the prosthetic materials have partially separated. They were removed, leaving the good membrane resulting from the use of polyethylene. Mercurochrome was applied to bring about epithelialization over the her-

niated mass. **B,** infection in another patient, in whom Silon was used, resulted in separation of the prosthetic material. Once again, the membrane formed in response to the smooth plastic sheeting contains the visceral mass and provides a base for the application of Mercurochrome.

fect may angulate and become compressed against the firm margin of this defect, compromising the blood supply of the bowel and resulting in gangrene and perforation; or the bowel wall may erode at the point of compression. To prevent this, it is important to enlarge the opening into the intra-abdominal cavity at the initial operation. This also enhances the ease with which the bowel can re-enter the abdomen. Finally, excessive pressure on the bowel wall by overzealous tightening of the prosthetic material can conceivably cause erosion and vascular compromise with subsequent fistulization. The basic premise of these staged procedures is a *gradual* increase in pressure to *enlarge the abdominal cavity* without a marked increase in pressure at any one time.

INTESTINAL OBSTRUCTION.—Prolonged intestinal dysfunction is frequently seen in association with giant omphalocele and gastroschisis. In some instances, this is based on a very real mechanical obstruction. In many instances, it is related to the grossly evident changes in the bowel as a result of prolonged exposure to the amniotic fluid before birth. A few patients have a clearly evident atresia at the initial examination. The surgeon should not actively look for intestinal obstruction by removing the membrane of an omphalocele or dissecting out a conglomerate mass of bowel in a patient with gastroschisis.

The primary surgical concern is reconstruction and healing of the abdominal wall while the patient is kept on continuous gastric suction and nutrition is maintained by intravenous hyperalimentation. If intestinal obstruction is still evident after the abdominal wall has been reconstructed, diagnostic x-ray studies should be carried out and the required surgical treatment insti-

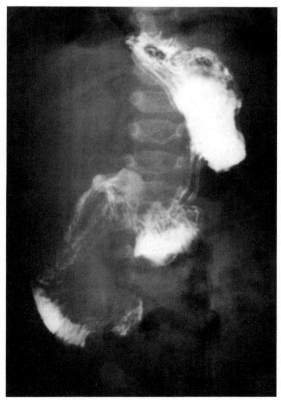

Fig 75–17.—Upper GI series in a patient who had repair of a massive omphalocele. The patient has gastric outlet obstruction. The liver is mainly on the right side of the abdomen but occupies a portion of the epigastrium. At laparotomy, the spleen and splenic pedicle were found anterior to the stomach, the splenic pedicle obstructing the outlet. Reorienting the viscera to their normal relative positions solved the problem. Splenectomy was not necessary.

tuted. One should bear in mind that, in patients with gastroschisis, nonmechanical dysfunction may last as long as 3 or 4 months following birth.

GASTRIC OUTLET OBSTRUCTION.—Kook et al.[43] reported a pyloroduodenal deformity that can occur as a result of the liver malformation associated with omphalocele.

We have seen two patients born with a large omphalocele who later presented with gastric outlet obstruction. Both were initially treated with nasogastric suction. The first patient responded well, with resolution of the obstructing mechanism, whereas the second patient had continued obstruction and required operation (Fig 75–17). The spleen was found in the midline, anterior to the stomach. The hilar splenic vessels and the pancreas were directly anterior to the stomach, obstructing the gastric outlet. The stomach appeared to have been displaced into a fossa behind these structures. The spleen, pancreas, and stomach were carefully mobilized and repositioned in their normal positions. The postoperative course was uncomplicated.

ANGULATION OF VENA CAVA.—An interesting observation has been made in three children who had cardiac catheterization following staged repair of a large omphalocele.[59] Angulation of the inferior vena cava–right atrial (IVC–RA) junction was noted in all three. The surgical procedure for repair of the omphalocele in each case was staged reduction. During cardiac catheterization, passing the catheter from the IVC to the RA was difficult in each case, and an abnormal insertion of the IVC into the RA was confirmed by angiography. The angiograms in Figure 75–18 compare a normal IVC–RA junction with that in two patients following repair of a large omphalocele. The angulation of the IVC–RA junction in such patients may be a congenital defect or secondary to the operation. Previous pathologic studies of omphaloceles have not described anomalies of systemic venous return, and review of our own autopsy material does not demonstrate deviation or angulation of the IVC–RA junction. However, the abnormality may not be obvious during postmortem manipulation.

Patients in whom the liver is part of the herniated visceral mass clearly have an attenuated and isolated hepatic vascular pedicle. It is reasonable, therefore, to assume that the abnormality of angulation of the IVC–RA junction is positional in origin, relating to settling or fixation of the IVC during repositioning of the liver. Since this was found in each of three patients who underwent cardiac catheterization, the venous abnormality may be relatively common in patients after omphalocele repair. There do not seem to be any symptoms related to this disorder. There is no reason for routine inferior venacavograms, since no therapy is indicated. However, pediatricians, cardiologists, and surgeons should be aware of this problem, since special care needs to be taken when inserting the IVC cannula for cardiopulmonary bypass or cardiac catheterization.

URETERAL NOTCHING.—In some patients after repair of a large omphalocele or gastroschisis there may be at least a transient element of obstruction of venous return from the lower part of the body with no outward evidence of vascular compromise. Cleveland et al.[12] have shown that some of these patients may develop sizable venous collaterals that may partially compress the ureters enough to produce a notched appearance (Fig 75–19).

RENAL MALPOSITION.—Pinckney et al.[45] described nine patients with omphalocele who were later found to have abnormally positioned kidneys. In eight of these, the kidneys were immediately subdiaphragmatic. In one patient, they were more

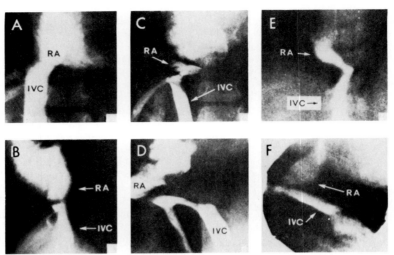

Fig 75–18.—Angulation of the inferior vena cava–right atrial junction after repair of omphalocele. Angiocardiograms: **top row,** anteroposterior views; **bottom row,** lateral views. **A** and **B,** normal infant; **C, D** and **E, F,** two patients after omphalocele repair. There is evident angulation of the junction of the inferior vena cava with the right atrium.

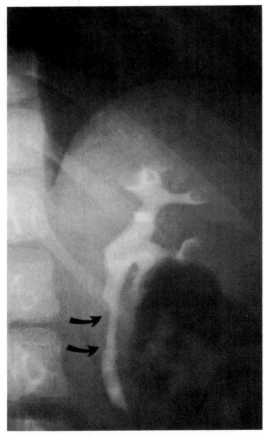

Fig 75–19.—Pyelogram in a patient who had repair of a giant omphalocele, showing close-up of the left kidney. *Arrows* mark vascular impressions, "notching," on the left ureter just below the ureteropelvic junction. These are from large venous collaterals presumably resulting from some element of obstruction of venous return from the lower half of the body during reconstruction of the abdominal wall. This film again shows how the upper border of the kidney has been displaced and actually touches the undersurface of the diaphragm.

caudal than normal. It is important to recognize that asymptomatic malposition of the kidneys in these patients does not require imaging procedures (Fig 75–20).

LIVER MALFORMATION AND MALPOSITION.—The patients born with an omphalocele or gastroschisis, the liver herniated out of the abdomen, present the greatest challenge to the surgeon. In most, the abdominal wall can be surgically repaired. Despite the normal postoperative appearance of the abdominal wall, the liver usually retains a globular shape and continues to reside high in the midline just below the xiphoid process. There is no functional abnormality. However, since the liver is not in its usual protected, subcostal position, it is more vulnerable to direct trauma. These patients should be cautioned to avoid body-contact sports. The patient and parents should be made aware of the fact that the liver in this position is often mistaken for an abnormal abdominal mass (see Fig 75–20).

INGUINAL HERNIA.—Inguinal hernia following complete repair of a large omphalocele or gastroschisis is a fairly frequent finding (Fig 75–21). It is most likely related to the increased pressure within the abdomen during the course of repair. The increased pressure undoubtedly has some effect on the internal inguinal ring and, if a patent processus vaginalis is present, there is a good likelihood that an inguinal hernia will develop, to be repaired in the usual manner.

Clinical Experience

This review of our experience begins in 1959 with the first use of the staged method utilizing prosthetic materials for abdominal wall defects. The series includes all patients admitted with the following diagnoses: (1) massive ventral hernia secondary to initial treatment of a large omphalocele by the Gross method of skin coverage; (2) hernia of the umbilical cord–fascial defect of less than 4 cm, with intact membrane and a herniated mass small enough for safe primary single-stage repair; (3) omphalocele with intact membrane; (4) ruptured omphalocele; (5) gastroschisis.

It is only during the past few years that serious attempts have been made at Children's Hospital, Boston, to differentiate between ruptured omphalocele and gastroschisis. Furthermore, the definition of these conditions undoubtedly varied, depending on

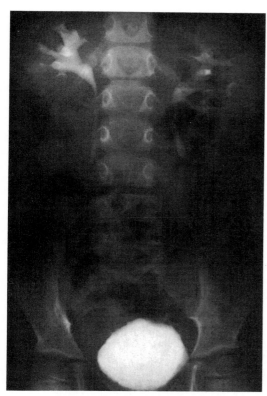

Fig 75–20.—Postoperative x-ray study of a patient who had repair of a massive omphalocele in which the liver was outside the abdomen. The kidneys are in an unusual position, having been elevated under the diaphragm. The renal pedicle on the right is at T11-12, and on the left at T-12/L-1. The liver can be seen as a midline epigastric mass. The indentations on the upper portion of the left ureter are from venous collaterals.

the views of the examining physician. In reviewing these patients, we have attempted, whenever possible, to redefine the initial anomaly based on information in the chart and our interpretation of the definition of these abdominal wall defects as described above. Despite these attempts to classify these patients clearly, there are undoubtedly some patients who have been in-

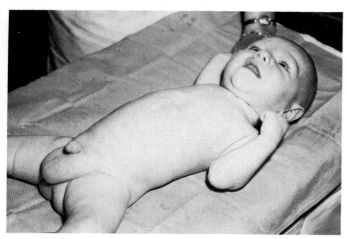

Fig 75–21.—Inguinal hernia in a patient who has had repair of a large omphalocele. This is a fairly frequent occurrence after repair of large omphaloceles, presumably due to the yielding of a patent processus vaginalis as a result of increased intra-abdominal pressure.

TABLE 75–4.—CONGENITAL
ABDOMINAL WALL DEFECTS,
1959–1983, CHILDREN'S
HOSPITAL, BOSTON

Secondary ventral hernia	19
Hernia of the umbilical cord	28
Omphalocele (intact membrane)	63
Omphalocele (ruptured)	40
Gastroschisis	36
TOTAL	186

TABLE 75–5.—METHODS OF TREATMENT
OF ABDOMINAL WALL DEFECTS, 1959–1983,
CHILDREN'S HOSPITAL, BOSTON

	NO. PATIENTS	DEATHS
Primary complete repair	87	11
Skin closure only	9	6
Staged repair		
"Preferred" method	54	13
Other method	26	11
Mercurochrome treatment	4	2
Other	1	. . .
No treatment	5	3
TOTAL	186	46

cluded as having ruptured omphaloceles who may well have had what we would today describe as "gastroschisis." The reverse may also be true. Despite these potential errors in classification, a review of this series of patients provides some very useful information.

In all, 186 patients were admitted with one of the foregoing diagnoses between January 1959 and January 1984. Table 75–4 gives the various diagnostic categories. Nineteen patients had a secondary ventral hernia following neonatal repair of an omphalocele using only skin coverage (17 at other hospitals and two at Children's Hospital). Twenty-eight patients had a hernia of the umbilical cord, and 63 patients had an intact omphalocele. A ruptured omphalocele was diagnosed in 40 patients, and 36 patients were considered to have a gastroschisis.

Table 75–5 shows the various methods of treatment, both operative and nonoperative. There were 87 patients who had a primary single-stage complete repair, nine patients initially treated only by skin coverage, and 80 patients treated in stages using prosthetic material. The latter group has been further subdivided into the group treated by what we consider the preferred method (54 patients), and a second group of 26 patients treated with other materials or methods that we presently do not consider optimal. Four patients were treated with Mercurochrome. One of these was treated elsewhere initially. One was managed with wet-to-dry dressing changes, and five patients did not receive any treatment.

Table 75–6 provides an analysis of the deaths. Group 1, patients who were managed without prosthetic materials, includes six patients who did not receive treatment but died of severe associated congenital anomalies. Group 2 is made up of patients treated in stages with prosthetic materials. Three patients in this group survived repair of the abdominal wall defects but died later of unrelated causes and are considered survivors in the statistics. One patient died following staged repair as a result of midgut volvulus with necrosis of the midgut, and is included as a surgical complication.

A relatively homogeneous group of infants could be identified who were, in general, of low birth weight, in most cases had no

Group 1: Treatment without prosthetic materials
(Total 81 patients)*

PRIMARY CAUSE OF DEATH	NO. PATIENTS
Inadequate perioperative resuscitation	1
Associated congenital anomalies	23
Surgical complications	3
TOTAL	22

Group 2: Treatment in stages with prosthetic materials
(Total 65 patients)

PRIMARY CAUSE OF DEATH	NO. PATIENTS
Inadequate perioperative resuscitation	7
Associated congenital anomalies	9
Surgical complications	10
TOTAL	24

*Includes 6 patients who were not treated and died of associated congenital anomalies.

associated life-threatening anomalies, sustained significant pre- and intraoperative stress and died at 24 to 96 hours secondary to a combination of renal and pulmonary failure with or without superimposed infection or CNS hemorrhage. The major factors contributing to this overwhelming stress in these fragile neonates were hypothermia, acidosis, hypotension and hypoxia. From review of the records, it is apparent that earlier in our series, insufficient attention was paid to perioperative resuscitation. The type of surgical management in this short-lived group is important only to the extent that operative trauma, or venous pooling caused by vena cava obstruction, contributes to the hypovolemia that leads to the vicious cycle of renal failure, fluid overload and pulmonary failure. Intelligent preoperative consideration and correction of these factors should prevent most of these deaths. It has become increasingly apparent that these patients need not be "rushed" directly to the operating room. A delay in operation is less dangerous than operating on a patient who has been inadequately prepared. We have not had such a death in the past six years.

The second category, associated congenital anomalies, includes all patients whose deaths were primarily related to associated life-threatening anomalies rather than to the abdominal wall defect itself. The most common associated anomalies were severe congenital heart defects, myelomeningoceles, with or without cloacal exstrophy, pulmonary hypoplasia and chromosomal anomalies such as trisomy D, trisomy E and in one case, D-D translocation.

The final category, surgical complications, includes those patients who die as a result of intestinal obstruction, fistula formation or infections related to the surgical procedures. It is of interest that in the past 11 years there have been only two deaths that might fall into this category. One of these two deaths occurred as a result of necrosis of a midgut volvulus. This was the only patient in the entire series who developed intestinal obstruction secondary to malrotation. The other death, during the course of staged repair, resulted from aspergillosis, with an aspergilloma that occluded the aorta. This patient also had serious congenital heart disease.

Of the total series of 186 patients, 81 were seen and treated during the most recent 11-year period. A staged method of closure using prosthetic materials was used in 35 of the patients in this group. This striking improvement in the results of therapy

was most likely related to the important lessons we have learned as follows:

1. Rapid completion of the stages. Initially, the goal was to cover the prosthetic material with skin at each stage and wait several weeks before the next stage to give maximal time for the abdominal wall to stretch. It became evident, however, that the incidence of wound infection increased with time and that the abdominal cavity could enlarge faster than originally anticipated. Removal of all prosthetic materials, and fascial closure, is now usually completed within 1–2 weeks.

2. Avoidance of surgical intervention for intestinal obstruction unless there is marked distention and/or evidence of bowel compromise. Resolution of what appears to be intestinal obstruction may take as long as 3–4 months in some patients after repair of gastroschisis or antenatal rupture of an omphalocele. When mechanical obstruction does indeed present, it is best to treat the patient by nonoperative bowel decompression until the abdominal wall problem has been resolved and all foreign material has been removed before embarking on operative correction. This, of course, assumes that there is no evidence that compromise of intestinal integrity has taken place.

3. Removal of all prosthetic material and employment of open techniques in the event of fistula formation or significant wound infection. The open technique we have used in the past included initial wet-to-dry dressings followed by 0.5% Mercurochrome applications. In the face of infection, a nonoperative approach is best calculated to result in a decrease in the incidence of systemic sepsis.

Among patients in whom prosthetic staging was employed, there were ten deaths due to primary surgical complications. Three of the deaths occurred early among the 54 patients in whom the preferred method of two-layer closure was used. Three deaths occurred among 20 patients in whom Silon was used as a one-layer closure, and three deaths among the six in whom other materials, or what we now consider to be nonstandard procedures, were used.

Growth, Development, and Late Morbidity

We have had a few patients who appear to have a period of abnormal intestinal behavior and possible malabsorption following correction of a particularly severe gastroschisis. Eventually, they have recovered and progressed to normal diets with good appetite and normal gastrointestinal behavior. We have not performed any metabolic studies on these patients. Berseth, et al,[6] carried out sophisticated metabolic studies on 22 survivors of gastroschisis and omphalocele. Although one third of the gastroschisis babies were small for gestational age at birth, no other predisposing factors for poor growth could be demonstrated. None of these children had intrinsic gastrointestinal or metabolic sequelae at three years of age as demonstrated by radiographic studies, fecal fat excretion, or serum chemistry screen. One third of those tested had IQs < 90; five had abnormal EEGs; one had impaired hearing. Intellectual impairment was related to length of hospitalization for nongastrointestinal causes. The authors felt that impairment of growth and intellectual outcome might be related to prematurity, small for gestation birth weight and nongastrointestinal neonatal complications.

It might be anticipated that these patients would be prime candidates for late intestinal obstruction. By virtue of the underlying anomaly they all have some degree of malrotation and malfixation. In addition, there are those born without a covering membrane or in whom the membrane was compromised, leading to the possibility of intra-abdominal adhesions. One might suppose that late intestinal obstruction would be a frequent complication. Surprisingly, this has not been the case. We have seen one patient who developed midgut volvulus with compromise of the bowel during the course of initial correction, but have not been confronted with intestinal obstruction as a late complication, although all patients and their families should be made aware of the potential for its development and also be aware of the presenting signs and symptoms of intestinal obstruction.

Wohl, et al,[61] recently studied the pulmonary function in a number of patients who had repair of a large omphalocele or gastroschisis as neonates. She was particularly interested in lung volume and flow. There were no abnormalities in lung volume or blood flow in these patients.

REFERENCES

1. Ahlfeld F.: Alkohol bei der Behandlung inoperabiler Brauchbruchen. *Monatsschr. Geburtshilfe Gynakol.* 10:124, 1899.
2. Allen R.G., Wrenn E.L.: Silon as a sac in the treatment of omphalocele and gastroschisis. *J. Pediatr. Surg.* 4:3, 1969.
3. Ballantyne J.W.: *Manual of Antenatal Pathology and Hygiene.* Edinburgh, 1904.
4. Benson C.D., Penherthy G.C., Hill E.J.: Hernia into the umbilical cord and omphalocele (amniocele) in the newborn. *Arch. Surg.* 58:833, 1949.
5. Bernstein P.: Gastroschisis, a rare teratological condition in the newborn. *Arch. Pediatr.* 57:505, 1940.
6. Berseth C.L., Malachowski N., Cohn R., et al.: Longitudinal growth and late morbidity of survivors of gastroschisis and omphalocele. *J. Pediatr. Gastro. Nutr.* 1:375, 1982.
7. Bill A.H.: Congenital defects of the umbilical region, in Preston F.W. (ed.): *General Surgery.* New York, Harper & Row, 1972.
8. Boles E.T.: Staged repair of huge ventral hernias. *J. Pediatr. Surg.* 6:618, 1971.
9. Bremer J.L.: *Congenital Anomalies of the Viscera.* Cambridge, Harvard University Press, 1957.
10. Buchanan R.W., Cain W.L.: A case of complete omphalocele. *Ann. Surg.* 143:552, 1956.
11. Cantrell J.R., Haller J.A., Ravitch M.M.: A syndrome of congenital defects involving the abdominal wall, sternum, diaphragm, pericardium and heart. *Surg. Gynecol. Obstet.* 107:602, 1958.
12. Cleveland R.H., Fellows K.E., Lebowitz R.L.: Notching of the ureter and renal pelvis in children. *Am. J. Roentgenol.* 129:837–844, 1977.
13. Croom R.D., Thomas C.G.: Repair of gastroschisis. *Surg. Gynecol. Obstet.* 132:689, 1971.
14. Cunningham A.A.: Exomphalos. *Arch. Dis. Child.* 31:144, 1956.
15. Dell'Agnola C.A., Baldrighi U., Agosti S.: After prenatal diagnosis of omphalocele, fetal surgery or postnatal correction? A case report. Personal communication, 1983.
16. Denes, J., Leb J., Lukacs F.V.: Gastroschisis. *Surgery* 63:701, 1968.
17. Dickey J.W.: Delayed repair of large omphalocele. *J. Fla. Med. Assoc.* 53:285, 1966.
18. Duhamel B.: Embryology of exomphalos and allied malformations. *Arch. Dis. Child.* 38:142, 1963.
19. Ein S.H., Shandling B.: A new non-operative treatment of large omphaloceles with a polymer membrane. *J. Pediatr. Surg.* 13:255–257, 1978.
20. Fagan D.G., Pritchard J.L., Clarkson T.W., et al.: Organ mercury levels in infants with omphaloceles treated with organic mercurial antiseptic. *Arch. Dis. Child.* 52:962–964, 1977.
21. Filler R.M., Eraklis A.J., Das J.B., et al.: Total intravenous nutrition, an adjunct to the management of infants with a ruptured omphalocele. *Am. J. Surg.* 121:454, 1971.
22. Filston H.C., Izant R.J.: Translocation of the umbilical artery to the lower abdomen: An adjunct to the postoperative monitoring of arterial blood gases in major abdominal wall defects. *J. Pediatr. Surg.* 10:225, 1975.
23. Geiger P.E.: Prenatally ruptured omphalocele. *Am. J. Surg.* 116:909, 1968.
24. Gierup J., Olsen K., Sundkirst K.: Aspects on the treatment of omphalocele and gastroschisis. Twenty years clinical experience. *Z. Kinderchirurgie* 35:3–6, 1982.
25. Gilbert M.G., Mencia L.F., Brown W.T., et al.: Staged surgical repair of large omphaloceles and gastroschisis. *J. Pediatr. Surg.* 3:702, 1968.
26. Glick L.G., Harrison M.R., Adzick N.S., et al.: The missing link in the pathogenesis of gastroschisis. *J. Pediatr. Surg.* (in press), 1985.
27. Goñi Moreno I.: Chronic eventrations and large hernias: Preoperative treatment by progressive pneumoperitoneum: Original procedure. *Surgery* 22:945, 1947.
28. Gray S.W., Skandalakis J.E.: *Embryology for Surgeons.* Philadelphia, W.B. Saunders Co., 1972.
29. Greenwood R.D., Rosenthal A., Nadas A.S.: Cardiovascular malformations associated with omphalocele. *J. Pediatr.* 85:818, 1974.
30. Grob M.: *Lehrbuch der Kinderchirurgie.* Stuttgart, Georg Thieme, 1957, p. 311.
31. Gross R.E., Blodgett J.B.: Omphalocele (umbilical eventration) in the newly born. *Surg. Gynecol. Obstet.* 71:520, 1940.
32. Gross R.E.: A new method for surgical treatment of large omphaloceles. *Surgery* 24:277, 1948.
33. Hey W.: *Practical Observations in Surgery.* London, Cadell & Davies, 1803, p. 266.
34. Hallabaugh R.S., Boles E.T.: The management of gastroschisis. *J. Pediatr. Surg.* 8:263, 1973.
35. Kleinhaus S., Kaufer N., Boley S.J.: Partial hepatectomy in omphalocele repair. *Surgery* 64:484, 1968.
36. Köllermann M.W., Schwarzer D.: Zum primären Verschluss grosser Bauchdeckendefekte bei Omphalocelen. *Chirurg.* 39:375, 1968.
37. Ladd W.E., Gross R.E.: *Abdominal Surgery of Infancy and Childhood.* Philadelphia, W.B. Saunders Co., 1941.
38. Margulies L.: Omphalocele (aminocele). *Am. J. Obstet. Gynecol.* 49:695, 1945.
39. Moore T.C., Stokes G.E.: Gastroschisis: Report of two cases treated by a modification of the Gross operation for omphalocele. *Surgery* 33:112, 1953.
40. Moore T.C.: Gastroschisis with antenatal evisceration of intestines and urinary bladder. *Ann. Surg.* 158:263, 1963.
41. Moore T.C.: Gastroschisis and omphalocele: Clinical difference. *Surgery* 82:561, 1977.
42. Nicolini V., Ferrazzi E., Bellotti M., et al.: Perinatal management of exomphalos diagnosed in late pregnancy. *Z. Kinderchirurgie, Hippokrates* 33:3, 1981.
43. Kook S.D., Strife J.L., Fischer K.C., et al.: Pyloroduodenal deformity due to liver malformation associated with omphalocele. *Am. J. Roentgenol.* 128:957–960, 1977.
44. Paré A.: *The Workes of That Famous Chiurgeon.* London: Th. Cotes and R. Young, 1634, book 24, p. 59.
45. Pinckney L.E., Moskowitz P.S., Lebowitz R.L., et al.: Renal malposition associated with omphalocele. *Radiology* 129:677–682, 1978.
46. Ravitch M.M.: Omphalocele: Secondary repair with the aid of pneumoperitoneum. *Arch. Surg.* 99–166, 1969.
47. Reed E.N.: Infant disemboweled at birth: Appendectomy successful. *JAMA* 61:199, 1913.
48. Rickham P.P.: Rupture of exomphalos and gastroschisis. *Arch. Dis. Child.* 38:138, 1963.
49. Rubin S.Z., Ein S.H.: Experience with 55 Silon pouches. *J. Pediatr. Surg.* 11:803–807, 1976 .
50. Safer D.J.: Rectus muscle transection for visceral replacement in gastroschisis. *Surgery* 63:988, 1968.
51. Savage J.P., Davey R.B.: The treatment of gastroschisis. *J. Pediatr. Surg.* 6:148, 1971.
52. Schuster S.R.: A new method for the staged repair of large omphaloceles. *Surg. Gynecol. Obstet.* 125:837, 1967.
53. Schuster S.R.: Omphalocele, hernia of the umbilical cord and gastroschisis, in *Pediatric Surgery*, ed. 3. Chicago, Year Book Medical Publishers, 1979, chap. 77.
54. Shaw A.: The myth of gastroschisis. *J. Pediatr. Surg.* 10:235, 1975.
55. Sherman J.J., Asch M.J., Isaacs H., et al.: Experimental gastroschisis in the fetal rabbit. *J. Pediatr. Surg.* 8:165, 1973.
56. Shermeta P.W., Haller J.A.: A new preformed transparent silo for the management of gastroschisis. *J. Pediatr. Surg.* 10:973, 1975.
57. Shin W.K.T.: Surgical treatment of gastroschisis. *Arch. Surg.* 102:524, 1971.
58. Venugopal S., Zachary R.B., Spitz L.: Exomphalos and gastroschisis: A 10-year review. *Br. J. Surg.* 63:523, 1976.
59. Waldman J.D., Fellows K.E., Paul M.H., et al.: Angulation of the inferior vena cava–right atrial junction in children with repaired omphalocele. *Pediatr. Radiol.* 5:142, 1977.
60. Williams C.: Congenital defects of the anterior abdominal wall. *Surg. Clin. North Am.* 10:805, 1930.
61. Wohl M.E.: Pulmonary function following repair of omphalocele and gastroschisis. Personal communication, 1983.

76 Moritz M. Ziegler / John W. Duckett / Charles G. Howell

Cloacal Exstrophy

History.—The first cases of cloacal exstrophy were described by Littre in 1709 and by Meckel in 1812.[19] By 1886, von Recklinghausen had collected 10 cases, and by 1901, Schwalbe had found 25 cases. By 1965, 53 cases had been reported; by 1968, 98 cases; and by 1976, the world's experience was 157 patients.[19] In the intervening 7 years, 18 more cases have been reported,[1, 4, 6, 9, 13] and the most recent report of our own 15 patients from Children's Hospital of Philadelphia[3] brings the current reported experience to 190 patients.

Before Rickham's report of successful surgical management in 1960 and his recommendation for staged total correction,[14] most children with cloacal exstrophy were allowed to die. Although Spencer, in 1965, supported the thesis of total correction,[16] others have suggested that the physical, emotional, and financial handicap was too great to warrant correction. This less aggressive attitude was supported by the very high mortality rates associated with correction; for example, only six of 23 patients from Boston Children's Hospital and only 17 of 34 patients in the period from 1968 to 1976 survived correction of this anomaly, as reported in the last edition of this book.[19] In our own series of 15 patients followed for an average of 9.5 years, 13 have survived following an aggressive regimen of sequential operation with vigorous perioperative support.[3] One must conclude today that a major effort should be made to salvage children with cloacal exstrophy.

Anatomy

Cloacal exstrophy, also termed vesicointestinal fissure, ileovesical fistula, or exstrophia splanchnica, is the most severe of the ventral abdominal wall defects. Classic cloacal exstrophy consists of an omphalocele superiorly, below which is an open plate of mucosa consisting of the two posterior walls of hemibladder on either side of a central strip of intestinal epithelium[8] (Figs 76–1, 76–2). In the latter central plate, prolapsed small bowel may be present superiorly (elephant-trunk deformity). The single or duplicated rectum, ending blindly, has an inferior orifice, and two duplicated appendiceal orifices may lie between these two intestinal lumens. Male genitalia usually are represented as a bifid penis on widely separated pubic bones; in the female, müllerian duct orifices may be exstrophied below the bladder mucosa, duplicate vaginas may end blindly, and a bifid clitoris may be present.

Of the vesical exstrophy complex of anomalies, 60% are classical exstrophy; 30% are epispadias (including balantic, penile, subsymphysial, and penopubic); and 10% comprise the cloacal exstrophies, superior vesical fissure, duplicate exstrophy or pseudoexstrophy.[5] Since the incidence of classic bladder exstrophy is 1 in 40,000 births, cloacal exstrophy and its variants would be expected in about 1 in 400,000. In the United States, we could anticipate 15 new cases per year.

Cloacal exstrophy variants are reported.[5] Embryologically, a covered cloacal exstrophy results from delayed mesenchymal migration after exstrophy of the bladder has already formed.[6] The umbilicus is situated low, adjacent to a thin scar over the anterior bladder wall. Epispadias may be present. We have seen two cases of "covered cloacal exstrophy" in which the external appearance was similar to covered bladder exstrophy, but inside, the posterior bladder was composed of ileocecal bowel. There was a short hindgut and imperforate anus. One of these cases had a duplicated distal bowel, as did two of our cloacal exstrophy patients.

Visceral sequestration is an entity also seen in the split symphysis variants. Segments of colon or ileum with mucosa on the exterior may be sequestered on the abdominal surface in association with exstrophy or epispadias in both males and females. Before such segments are discarded, consideration should be given to their possible use in urinary diversion or as vaginal substitutes.

Teratomatous lesions may also be present with visceral sequestration, or in association with split symphysis variants and exstrophy. This may represent a rudimentary attempt at twinning.

Embryogenesis

The exstrophic lesions represent abnormal embryogenesis (Fig 76–3) involving the cloacal membrane, rather than an arrest in development, since the normal embryo does not pass through such a phase. The cloacal membrane arises from a region adjacent to the original primitive streak. As the embryo and its tail elongate, this membrane rotates with the tail from a dorsal to ventral location; and in that new location the membrane forms the anterior wall of the primitive cloaca.[2, 15]

The Patten and Barry theory of embryologic maldevelopment suggests that the basic abnormality is a caudal displacement of the paired primordia of the genital tubercle, which permits persistence of a more cephalad cloacal membrane.[12] With no mesenchymal growth at the cephalic end of the cloacal membrane and with a simultaneous incomplete internal urorectal septal division, a disintegration of the cloacal membrane could establish both exstrophied bladder and bowel on the abdominal surface. The slightly dissimilar Marshall and Muecke theory states that the basic defect of cloacal exstrophy is in an abnormal overdevelopment of the cloacal membrane, which prevents migration of mesenchymal tissue between the endodermal and ectodermal layers.[11] With rupture of this unstable membrane at about the fifth week of embryonic life, before fusion of the genital tubercles and before the descent of the urorectal septum that separates cloaca into bladder and rectum, a midline infraumbilical defect results, exposing mucosa of the bladder and bowel and producing bifid external genitalia.

The developing structures of the abdominal wall are held apart by the wedge effect of the abnormally extensive cloacal membrane. This produces a separation of the pubic bones, varying degrees of a midline abdominal wall defect, and restricted fusion of the paired genital tubercles or the müllerian ducts. The precise form of the exstrophic lesion also depends on the timing of cloacal membrane dehiscence. If the rupture occurs after the urorectal septum begins to descend, the exstrophic gut may lie caudad to the bladder, an infrequent variant anomaly. If the rupture occurs as late as the seventh week, vesical exstrophy alone is the result.

Confusion exists regarding the embryology of cloacal exstrophy because none of these theories addresses the predilection for ileocecal intestinal prolapse, or the blind-ending colon with its associated imperforate anus. Johnston[8] suggests that the posterior wall of the cloaca moves forward, separating the ileum of the

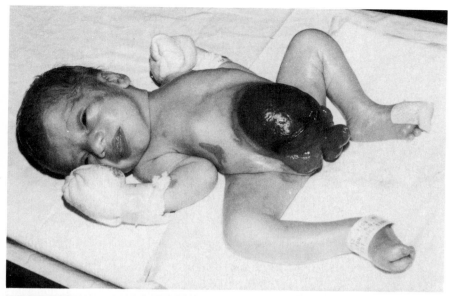

Fig 76–1.—Classic cloacal exstrophy characterized by a large omphalocele and a prolapsing terminal ileum ("elephant-trunk" deformity).

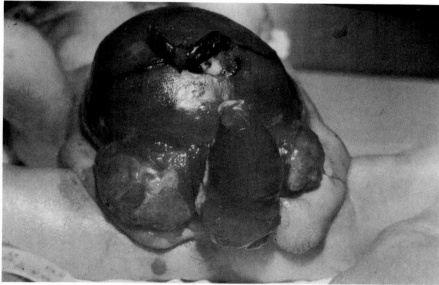

hindgut superiorly from the colonic orifice of the tailgut inferiorly, and involvement of the bowel in exstrophy greatly restricts its growth. Magnus[10] has suggested that a loop or loops of mid- or hindgut prolapses between the two bladder halves and becomes strangulated, a theory that potentially explains the multiple and variable intestinal plate orifices as well as the foreshortening of the intestine. This same confusion does not exist for the role that the cloacal membrane plays in the embryogenesis of cloacal exstrophy, since Muecke[11] has shown that surgical interference with membrane regression in the chick embryo produces an anatomical anomaly strikingly similar to human cloacal exstrophy.

Spectrum of Anomalies (Table 76–1)

In our series of 15 patients, there were 21 different anomalies in 11 of the patients.[3] Myelomeningocele occurred in seven patients—five lumbar, one sacral, and one thoracic—and there were associated vertebral anomalies. Scoliosis was present in six,

and bilateral clubfeet in an additional four children. One involved patient was one of a set of craniopagus conjoined twins, one had left facial paralysis, one had an atretic right upper lobe bronchus, and one had Factor VIII deficiency. The latter patient, who was genetically a male, had a gender conversion as a neonate because of an inadequate phallus. During this procedure, no problems with hemostasis were noted. At subsequent operation, the abnormal bleeding was encountered, and her "femaleness" delayed the appropriate diagnosis of Factor VIII deficiency.

All of our patients had omphaloceles, in two cases ruptured at the time of presentation.[3] An anteriorly placed anus was present in two children, and the rest all had imperforate anuses. Although colon length was variably foreshortened, none of our patients had congenitally short small bowel.

Thirteen of the 15 patients had the classic split bladder exstrophy with a hemibladder on either side of the exstrophied bowel.[3] Two single exstrophied bladders were also noted. Renal anomalies were seen in nine of the 15 children: one with bilateral

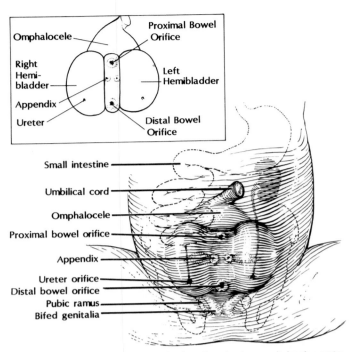

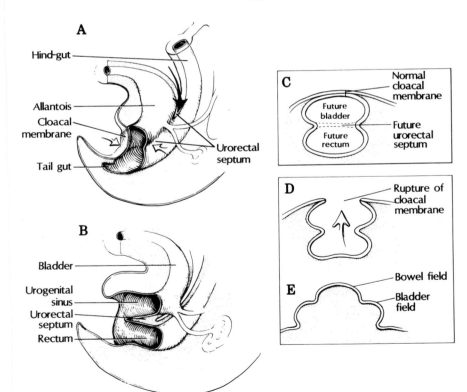

Fig 76–2.—Components of classic cloacal exstrophy: omphalocele; exstrophied bilateral hemibladders with ureteric or müllerian remnant orifices; central exstrophied ileocecal bowel plate with superior orifice of the terminal ileum, inferiorly, the colon, and centrally, the appendix; bifid rudimentary external genitalia; separated pubic rami.

renal agenesis, four with left renal agenesis, and four with crossed fused ectopia. One child had a hydronephrotic left kidney secondary to a severe left ureterovesical obstruction. Of the patients with ectopia, one had a solitary right kidney with a ureteral duplication and a hydroureteronephrosis of the lower pole to the right hemibladder with a crossed ectopia of the right upper pole to the left hemibladder. The other ectopia patient had a right double collecting system and hydronephrosis with the ureter ectopic to the vagina and the left upper pole ureter traversing to the opposite bladder.

Of the nine genetic males in our series, all had severe anomalies of the genitalia, including diminutive and separated corporal bodies, bifid scrota, and undescended testes.[3] Five of the six genetic females had bifid uteri, and one had a double vagina also. Three of the six had exstrophied vaginas and two, covered vaginal openings.

Treatment

Successful treatment of cloacal exstrophy (Fig 76–4) requires an aggressive multispecialty effort with a clear-cut captain of the ship who takes into account the total patient and who coordinates ancillary personnel including the stomal therapist, physical therapist, social worker, and family support network into the child's rehabilitation program. Accordingly, therapy must be directed sequentially and yet simultaneously for the abdominal wall defect with its omphalocele and the separated pubic bones, the exstrophied intestine with or without imperforate anus and bowel duplication, the exstrophied hemibladders, the malformed genitalia, and for the possible associated anomalies.[3, 5, 7] In the neonatal period, a reconstruction of considerable magnitude must be undertaken as the initial stage, a treatment plan which

Fig 76–3.—Embryologic basis for cloacal exstrophy in the 5-week human embryo. If the cloacal membrane ruptures before the urorectal septum descends, exstrophy of a central bowel field flanked by exposed mucosa of the hemibladders is the result. If cloacal separation begins by the downgrowth of the urorectal septum (6-week embryo) and then cloacal membrane disintegration occurs, the exstrophied gut may lie caudad to a single exstrophied bladder. Rupture of the cloacal membrane as late as the seventh week produces classic bladder exstrophy only.

TABLE 76–1.—SPECTRUM OF MULTIPLE ANOMALIES OF CLOACAL EXSTROPHY

1. Omphalocele and abdominal wall deficiency
2. Split symphysis anomaly
3. Bladder exstrophy (open plate of mucosa)
   a. 2 exstrophied hemibladders
   b. Interposed midline colonic segment
4. Ileocecal exstrophy
   a. Superior-orifice prolapsed ileum
   b. Single or duplicate inferior-orifice short blind-ending hindgut
   c. Usually duplicate appendiceal stumps in intermediate position
5. Imperforate anus
6. Bifid external genitalia
   a. Diminutive penis
   b. Bifid clitoris and labia
   c. Cryptorchidism
7. Duplex müllerian structures
   a. May be exstrophied vaginas at base of bladder mucosa
   b. May be atretic vaginas
8. Myelomeningocele
9. Other defects
   a. Talipes equinovarus
   b. Vertebral anomalies (scoliosis)
   c. Renal anomalies
      (1). Agenesis or multicystic
      (2). Megaureter
      (3). Hydronephrosis
      (4). Fusion anomalies, ectopia

should be managed by a pediatric surgeon and pediatric urologist who have had experience with this rare entity. There is ample time for transfer of these patients to major centers.

Abdominal Wall Defect

The preferred treatment of an omphalocele is neonatal primary closure, a procedure that becomes essential if the membrane is ruptured. From our recent experience with 17 newborn classical exstrophy reconstructions, neonatal approximation of the pubis is possible in the first 48 hours of life due to the flexibility of the bones and joints during the birth process. This bony approximation facilitates abdominal wall closure with or without application of a temporary prosthetic Silastic pouch. Of our 15 patients, 13 had primary fascial closures and two had staged closures following an initial application of such a Silastic pouch or silo.[3]

Intestinal Tract

Rickham, in 1960, presented four cases in which he learned by trial and error that preservation of the ileocecal segment was an important first step.[14] Unfortunately, this fact was not fully appreciated, and, even in the last edition of this text, establishment of an ileostomy was recommended.[19]

The primary goal of the intestinal surgery, re-emphasized in our report, is the preservation of a maximum length of bowel without discarding any colonic remnant, no matter how short or how "micro." Technically, the mucosal junction between bladder wall and colonic wall should be incised and the ileal and colonic

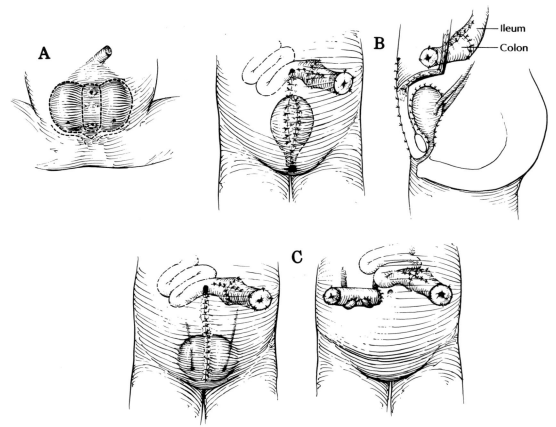

Fig 76–4.—Staged repair of cloacal exstrophy. The bowel and bladder mucosa are separated, and the ileocecal junction is tubularized and brought out as an end colostomy. The bladder halves are approximated only, or are turned in as a complete bladder exstrophy repair with approximation of the pubic rami; the omphalocele is also closed. Urinary diversion and genital reconstruction are deferred until later, although gender assignment is made in the neonatal period.

TABLE 76–2.—CLOACAL EXSTROPHY: CASE REPORTS

PATIENT	BIRTH DATE	AGE	SEX	GI ANOMALIES	GU ANOMALIES	GENITALIA ANOMALIES	OTHER ANOMALIES
MM	4/9/57	19 yrs died	M	Omphalocoele vesicointestinal fistula, short colon, imperforate anus (high)	Bladder exstrophy (split), 2 urethras, megaureters	Bifid scrotum, phallus and glans, severe chordee	Sacrococcygeal teratoma, myelomeningocoele, sacral anomalies
DS	9/18/61	21 yrs	F	Omphalocoele (rupture) vesicointestinal fistula, short colon, imperforate anus (high)	Bladder exstrophy (split)	Exstrophic vaginal opening, bifid clitoris, bifid uterus, 2 ovaries	Siamese twin (craniopagus, single lateral ventricle), myelomeningocoele, scoliosis
MKM	2/22/65	17 yrs	F	Omphalocoele, vesicointestinal fistula, short colon, imperforate anus (high)	Bladder exstrophy (split), megaureters	Laterally displaced vagina, bifid clitoris and uterus, 2 ovaries	Myelomeningocoele, scoliosis, sacral anomalies
JPO	7/29/68	14 yrs	M	Omphalocoele, vesicointestinal fistula, short colon, imperforate anus (high)	Bladder exstrophy (split), agenesis (L) kidney, crossed ectopia	Bifid scrotum, epispadias, (L) undescended testicle	Myelomeningocoele, patent ductus arteriosus, sacral anomalies
CI	4/1/68	14 yrs	F	Omphalocoele, vesicointestinal fistula, short colon, imperforate anus (high)	Bladder exstrophy (split), megaureters	Laterally displaced vagina, 2 ovaries, bifid uterus	Sacral anomalies
JD	7/29/71	10 yrs	M→F	Omphalocoele, vesicointestinal fistula, short colon, imperforate anus (high)	Bladder exstrophy (split), agenesis (L) kidney	Bifid scrotum, microphallus	Bilateral clubfeet, sacral anomalies
VJ	5/21/73	9 yrs	M→F	Omphalocoele, separate fecal fistula, low imperforate anus	Bladder exstrophy (split), agenesis (L) kidney, crossed ectopia, megaureters	1 corpora, no glans	Sacral anomalies
HY	9/16/75	6½ yrs	M→F	Omphalocoele, vesicointestinal fistula, short colon, imperforate anus (high)	Bladder exstrophy (split), crossed ectopia	Epispadias, bifid scrotum, bilateral undescended testicles	Myelomeningocoele, scoliosis, sacral anomalies
LL	5/25/77	5 yrs	F	Omphalocoele, vesicointestinal fistula, short colon, imperforate anus (high), malrotation	Bladder exstrophy (single), (R) double collecting system, ureter ectopic to vagina, crossed ectopia	Double vagina, bifid uterus, 2 ovaries	Sacral anomalies
CS	8/26/77	5 yrs	M→F	Omphalocoele, vesicointestinal fistula, imperforate anus (low), short colon	Bladder exstrophy (split), agenesis (L) kidney	Bifid scrotum and phallus, microphallus	Scoliosis, clubfeet
RM	5/5/78	4 yrs	M→F	Omphalocoele, vesicointestinal fistula, short colon, imperforate anus (high)	Bladder exstrophy (split)	Bifid scrotum and phallus, microphallus	Factor 8 deficiency, scoliosis, bilateral congenital hip dislocation
JB	6/30/79	3 yrs	M→F	Omphalocoele, vesicointestinal fistula, short colon, imperforate anus (high)	Bladder exstrophy (split), megaureters	Bifid scrotum, microphallus, bilateral undescended testicles	Myelomeningocoele (thoracic), atretic RUL bronchus, bilateral congenital hip dislocation
JT	8/21/79	2 days died	M	Omphalocoele, vesicointestinal fistula, short colon, imperforate anus (high), malrotation	Bladder exstrophy (split), bilateral renal agenesis	Bifid phallus and scrotum	Clubfeet
MC	9/4/79	2½ yrs	F	Omphalocoele, vesicointestinal fistula, short colon, imperforate anus (high)	Bladder exstrophy (split)	Exstrophy of vagina	Myelomeningocoele, clubfeet, (L) facial paralysis, twin
JF	4/11/81	1 yr	F	Omphalocoele, vesicointestinal fistula, duplicated colon (short), imperforate anus (high)	Bladder exstrophy (split), (L) ureterovesical obstruction, (L) cystic kidney	Bifid uterus, 2 ovaries, no vagina	Twin

TABLE 76–2.—CLOACAL EXSTROPHY: CASE REPORTS

MAJOR OPERATIONS (AGE—PROCEDURE)	CURRENT GU STATUS	STOMAS	MOTOR FUNCTION	INTELLIGENCE
2 days Closure omphalocoele, closure bladder, ileostomy, colon resection, excision sacrococcygeal teratoma, closure myelomeningocoele **1 year** Bil-Orchiopexy release chordee **2 years** Epispadias repair **6 years** Ileal loop diversion	Ileal conduit	Ileostomy, ileal conduit	Ambulatory	Normal
3 days Closure omphalocoele, ileocolonic anastomosis, colostomy **18 years** Ileal conduit, excision of bladder exstrophy, vagino and clitoroplasty	Ileal conduit	Colostomy, ileal conduit	Total paralysis of legs	Below normal
2 days Closure omphalocoele, ileostomy, colon resection **4 years** Ileal conduit **16 years** Vagino and clitoroplasty	Ileal conduit	Ileostomy, ileal conduit	Ambulatory with crutches	Normal
1 day Closure omphalocoele, ileocolonic anastomosis, colostomy, reapproximation hemibladders **3 months** Orchiopexy, herniorrhaphy **13 months** Ileal loop diversion, cystectomy **18 months** Epispadias repair	Ileal conduit	Colostomy, ileal conduit	Ambulatory	Normal
1 day Closure omphalocoele, ileocolonic anastomosis, colostomy, reapproximation hemibladders **22 months** Ileal loop diversion, cystectomy, vaginal reconstruction	Ileal conduit	Colostomy, ileal conduit	Ambulatory with leg splints	Normal
1 day Closure omphalocoele, ileocolonic anastomosis, colostomy, reapproximation hemibladders, gonadectomy, clitoroplasty **2½ years** Colon conduit, cystectomy, vaginoplasty	Colon conduit	Colostomy, colon conduit	Ambulatory	Normal
1 day Closure omphalocoele, closure bladder exstrophy, anoplasty **2½ years** Vesicostomy, RLP nephrectomy, bowel segment vaginoplasty	Closed bladder (CIC)		Normal	Normal
1 day Closure omphalocoele, ileocolonic anastomosis, colostomy, reapproximation hemibladders **9 months** Closure bladder exstrophy, penile lengthening **10 months** Orchiectomy, clitoroplasty **3 years** YDL	Closed bladder (CIC)	Colostomy	Ambulatory	Normal
1 day Closure omphalocoele, ileostomy, reapproximation hemibladders **4 months** Ileocolonic anastomosis, colostomy, (R) cutaneous ureterostomy, bladder closure	Closed bladder, incontinent	Colostomy	Ambulatory	Normal
1 day Closure omphalocoele, ileocolonic anastamosis, anoplasty **3 years** Excision bladder exstrophy, (R) cutaneous ureterostomy, vaginoplasty	Cutaneous ureterostomy	Cutaneous ureterostomy	Ambulatory	Below normal
1 day Closure omphalocoele, ileocolonic anastamosis, reapproximation hemibladders, gonadectomy, clitoroplasty, colostomy **6 months** Closure bladder exstrophy **4 years** Ileal conduit	Ileal conduit	Colostomy, ileal conduit	Ambulatory	Normal
1 day Closure omphalocoele (Silastic), ileocolonic anastomosis, colostomy, reapproximation hemibladders, gonadectomy, clitoroplasty **8 months** Repair myelomeningocoele	Ileal conduit	Colostomy, ileal conduit	Ambulatory with crutches	Normal
1 day Closure omphalocoele, ileocolonic anastomosis, reapproximation hemibladders, colostomy	Exstrophic bladder	Colostomy	Unknown	Unknown
1 day Closure omphalocoele (Silastic), ileocolonic anastomosis, reapproximation hemibladders, colostomy **3 months** Closure myelomeningocoele	Closed bladder, incontinent	Colostomy	Ambulatory	Normal
1 day Closure omphalocoele, ileostomy, (L) cutaneous pyelostomy **2 months** Closure ileostomy, ileocolonic anastomosis, colostomy and joining of 2 ends of duplicated colon, (R) cutaneous ureterostomy	(R) cutaneous ureterostomy, (L) pyelostomy	Ureterostomy, pyelostomy, colostomy	Ambulatory	Normal

plate should be folded into a tubular structure restoring the ileocecal junction and preserving *all* mucosa. No attempt should be made to "trim" the edges to make an end-to-end anastomosis. If a duplication of the colon is present, the duplicated segments should also be utilized, even antiperistaltically. The end colostomy should be placed well into the flank to avoid contamination of the abdominal closure. Relocation on the abdomen may be done later.

Two of our patients had intact colons with an anteriorly placed anus that required anoplasty only.[3] Two of our patients had colonic remnant resection with permanent end ileostomy done before transfer to our hospital. Nine patients had a primary reconstruction of the exstrophied ileocecal area with construction of an end colostomy. Two additional patients who were transferred following an initial ileostomy were re-explored because of malnutrition and high-output stomas. In one, the blind colon segment was found and converted to an end colostomy; the other had a short duplicated colon salvaged and anastomosed in continuity (one isoperistaltic, one with retrograde peristalsis) before bringing it out as an end colostomy. No patient had evidence of either congenital or iatrogenic short-bowel syndrome with inadequate small-bowel length. Only the two patients with ileostomies had long-term nutritional problems.

Infants with ileostomies are very difficult to manage. Their fluid losses are difficult to control and supplement, their weight gain is slow, and they are prone to develop mineral and trace element deficiencies and recurrent infections. In the past, these problems were attributed to "short-bowel syndrome," a condition that we believe may be functional but not anatomical.

Urinary Tract

The initial phase of management of the exstrophied bladder is the separation of the bowel from the bladder. If the two hemibladders are of adequate size and volume, they can be reapproximated and left exposed on the abdominal wall; or, after reapproximation both anteriorly and posteriorly, there can be a primary closure of the exstrophy, with no attempt to tighten the bladder neck. Taking advantage of the flexible bony pelvis in the first 48 hours of life, the surgeon can relocate the bladder into the pelvis and close the abdominal wall. As a primary procedure in our series, 13 patients had only an approximation of two hemibladders, while two recent patients had neonatal bladder closure.[3] In three patients a later bladder closure was effected, using iliac osteotomies. A continence procedure was provided with an ileal conduit diversion in seven patients. Four patients were managed by temporary cutaneous pyelostomy (three renal units) or ureterostomy (four units). Only one patient underwent nephrectomy, and one closed bladder was converted to a vesicostomy. Two patients remain incontinent following their bladder closure, one despite a Young-Dees-Leadbetter procedure, while a third can stay dry with intermittent catheterization. One recent patient has had only the initial reapproximation of hemibladders, the further management still pending.

Closure of the bladder, when attained, theoretically permits subsequent continence by clean intermittent catheterization. Intestinal augmentation of the bladder with the sacrifice of functional large bowel to serve as a urinary conduit should be deferred to see if the child has demonstrated an adequate intestinal length for the passage of formed stools (usually not the case). In one case we left a one-inch stoma of the colostomy and relocated the colon to the other side of the abdomen.[17] The solitary small ureter was connected to the stoma, onto which a collection device fits nicely and the patient is dry. An ileal conduit remains the first choice for long-term diversion, since the ileum is safer to sacrifice. Cutaneous ureterostomy utilizing a small cuff of bladder wall is also a reasonable permanent option. A Koch continent urinary reservoir may prove feasible in the future. If sequestrated bowel segments are present in the defect, every effort should be made to preserve these for use in attempts at reconstruction of the urinary tract to produce continence.

Genitalia

Although the majority of patients with cloacal exstrophy are genetic males, it has been recommended for more than a decade that males should be converted to females rather than attempt reconstruction of the inadequate genitalia into a functioning male phenotype[18] For psychodynamic reasons such gender-converting procedures should be done in the neonatal period. In our series, gender conversion was done five times in newborns and once in a 9-month-old. Corporal tissue is preserved for construction of an adequate clitoris. Of three reconstructed males, all were left with inadequate genitalia, a factor that may have contributed to the death of one by suicide.

In females, the bifid clitoris and labia may be reconstructed into a reasonably normal appearance at a later date. In the early stages, their dislocation should be of little concern. Depending on the severity of the lesion, there will most likely be a double vagina, uterus, and tubes, since the urorectal septum prevents fusion of the müllerian structures. Atresia of the vagina has been present in three of our cases associated with dysplastic uteri and tubes. The ovaries, however, were normal. We have seen several cases with exstrophy of the vagina just caudad to the bladder mucosa. This is very difficult to determine in the early phases. The lesion becomes apparent later, as late as puberty if the menstrual flow was obstructed by early reconstructive attempts. Recognition of the entity of vaginal exstrophy associated with cloacal exstrophy is important for appropriate staged reconstruction. Likewise, atresia of the distal müllerian structures is a possibility.

Myelodysplasia

About half of the children with cloacal exstrophy have a form of myelodysplasia—either a frank myelomeningocele (MMC) or a lipomeningocele. This must be repaired in accord with standard neurosurgical principles. If the open MMC is closed, a shunt for hydrocephalus is likely to be needed. There is recent evidence that a delay of several weeks in closing the MMC may not be detrimental. Certainly, delaying the therapy for the MMC facilitates early attack on the cloacal exstrophy.

Subsequent orthopedic splinting and prosthetics are integral parts of the rehabilitation of these children. Numerous orthopedic procedures are generally required as ambulation progresses. In addition, a network of support for the family is required from multidisciplinary clinics, stomal therapists, social service, and, most important, other parents.

Results (Table 76–2)

Until our report in 1983, the total of 175 patients with cloacal exstrophy included only 46 survivors, but in the period 1968–1976 survival approached 50%[19] In our own series, 13 of 15 (86%) children have survived following a protocol similar to that noted above.[3] Our two deaths included a neonate with renal agenesis and a 19-year-old who probably committed suicide. Ten of our 13 survivors have maintained an excellent nutritional status, while the two children treated by colectomy and permanent ileostomy have behaved like severe short-bowel syndrome patients with excessive stomal drainage and poor weight gain.

These results demand an informed and aggressive sequence of operations.[3, 5, 7] In the first stage in the newborn, the omphalocele should be closed, if possible. The ileocecal exstrophy plate should be separated from the hemibladders and the ileocecal region reconstructed, with preservation of all colonic bowel length forming an end colostomy stoma. The separated bladder halves should be reapproximated. It may be possible to close an adequate-sized bladder primarily, with simultaneous closure of the pubis. Surgery for urinary continence or permanent diversion can be delayed. At this same primary operation, except for a rare obvious phenotypic male with normal-appearing external genitalia, female gender assignment should be made; and subsequent appropriate reconstructive operations should be done in early life.

Whether the patient with cloacal exstrophy is permanently committed to two stomas or whether continence can be achieved by intermittent clean catheterization to eliminate one stomal appliance is speculative. Posterior sagittal anorectoplasty may isolate and identify pelvic floor muscular elements that potentially permit colonic pullthrough via the pelvic muscle complex, and this may possibly restore anorectal continence.

There is little speculation, however, that, with an aggressive, intelligent staged surgical approach, these unfortunate babies may be rehabilitated to happy contributing members of society— a little handicapped perhaps, but otherwise "normal."

REFERENCES

1. Allen R.G.: Omphalocele and gastroschisis, in Holder T.M., Ashcraft K.W. (eds.): *Pediatric Surgery.* Philadelphia, W.B. Saunders Co., 1980, pp. 572–588.
2. Ambrose S.S.: The anterior body wall, in Gray S.W., Skandalakis J.E. (eds.): *Embryology for Surgeons.* Philadelphia: W.B. Saunders Co., 1972, pp. 387–441.
3. Howell C., Caldamone A., Snyder H., et al.: Optimal management of cloacal exstrophy. *J. Pediatr. Surg.* 18:365–369, 1983.
4. Jeffs R.D.: Exstrophy and cloacal exstrophy. *Urol. Clin. North Am.* 5:127–140, 1978.
5. Johnston J.H.: The exstrophic anomalies, in Williams D.I., Johnston J.H. (eds.): *Paediatric Urology.* London: Butterworths, 1982, pp. 299–316.
6. Johnston J.H., Koff S.A.: Covered cloacal exstrophy: Another variation on the theme. *J. Urol.* 118:666–668, 1977.
7. Johnston J.H., Kogan S.J.: The exstrophic anomalies and their surgical reconstruction. *Curr. Prob. Surg.* August 1974, pp. 1–39.
8. Johnston T.B.: Extroversion of the bladder complicated by the presence of intestinal openings on the surface of the extroverted area. *J. Anat.* 48:89–106, 1913.
9. Koontz W.W., Joshi V.V., Ownby R.: Cloacal exstrophy with the potential for urinary control: An unusual presentation. *J. Urol.* 112:828–831, 1974.
10. Magnus R.V.: Ectopia cloacae—a misnomer. *J. Pediatr. Surg.* 4:511–519, 1969.
11. Muecke E.C.: The role of the cloacal membrane in exstrophy: The first successful experimental study. *J. Urol.* 92:659–667, 1964.
12. Patten B.M., Barry A.: The genesis of exstrophy of the bladder and epispadius. *Am. J. Anat.* 90:35–57, 1952.
13. Remigailo R.V., Woodard J.R., Andrews H.G., et al.: Cloacal exstrophy: 18-year survival of untreated case. *J. Urol.* 116:811–813, 1976.
14. Rickham P.P.: Vesico-intestinal fissure. *Arch. Dis. Child.* 35:97–102, 1960.
15. Ridley J.H.: The bladder and urethra, in Gray S.W., Skandalakis J.E. (eds.): *Embryology for Surgeons.* Philadelphia, W.B. Saunders Co., 1972, pp. 519–552.
16. Spencer R.: Exstrophia splanchnica (exstrophy of the cloaca). *Surgery* 57:751–766, 1965.
17. Sukarachana K., Sieber W.K.: Vesicointestinal fissure revisited. *J. Pediatr. Surg.* 13:713–719, 1978.
18. Tank E.S., Lindenauer S.M.: Principles of management of exstrophy of the cloaca. *Am. J. Surg.* 119:95–98, 1970.
19. Welch K.J.: Cloacal exstrophy (vesicointestinal fissure), in Ravitch M.M., Welch K.J., Benson C.D., et al. (eds.): *Pediatric Surgery.* Chicago: Year Book Medical Publishers, 1979, pp. 802–808.

77 THEODORE P. VOTTELER
Conjoined Twins

HISTORY.—Although a rare event, the birth of conjoined twins has always fascinated physician and layman alike. One of the first important medical books on the subject was written by Ambroise Paré, the most distinguished surgeon of the sixteenth century. In his work, *Of Monsters and Prodigies,*[42] he listed 11 generally accepted causes to explain the creation of all monsters, single or double. Most conjoined twins are stillborn, but up to the present more than 400 have survived, either remaining joined or surgically separated.

König[29] recorded the first successful separation of conjoined twins in 1689. In these twins, who were joined at the umbilicus, the division was accomplished by necrosing the band of tissue between the children with a constricting ligature. Kiesewetter[28] reviewed 24 attempts at surgical separation reported in the literature from 1689 to 1962. To 1984, over 85 successful separations, with survival of one or both twins, have been described in the English literature or lay press.

The inappropriate term "Siamese" twins was coined by P. T. Barnum, who promoted the exhibition of Chang and Eng Bunker, conjoined twins born in Siam in 1811.[25, 33] Their father was Chinese and their mother half Siamese and half Chinese. Both twins married; Eng's wife bore 12 children and Chang's wife 10. They died at age 63, Chang of pneumonia and Eng shortly after of hypovolemic shock. The term "Siamese twins" has persisted but has the unfortunate connotation of circus freaks. The term is inappropriate and should be avoided.[32]

Incidence

The birth of conjoined twins occurs in approximately 1 in 50,000 deliveries. Seventy percent are female, and in the past 60% are said to have been stillborn. Prenatal diagnosis of conjoined twinning by ultrasonography has led to increased cesarean section delivery and salvage of twins that would not have survived vaginal delivery.[22, 23] Although the incidence of reported cases in the literature and media seems to be increasing, it is doubtful that the true incidence has changed significantly. In a recent series,[18] 40% were stillborn, and an additional 35% survived only one day. Non-Caucasians may have a higher incidence than Caucasians.[9, 39] Maternal age is not significant, just as in monozygotic twinning.[47]

A significant number of these twins have congenital malformations not associated with the site of conjoining. At least 6% of conjoined twins were two of triplets, illustrating the high incidence of associated defects of morphogenesis rather than mere duplication. Perhaps 50% have an associated polyhydramnios.

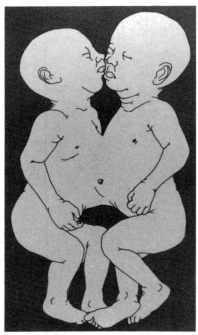

Fig 77–1.—Thoraco-omphalopagus twins. (From Votteler T.P.[57] Reprinted with permission.)

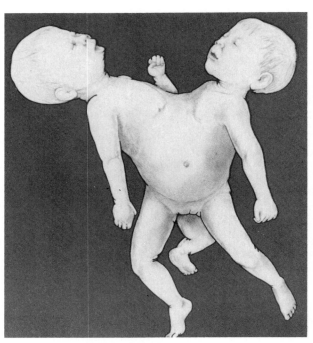

Fig 77–3.—Ischiopagus tripus twins. (From Votteler T.P.[57] Reprinted with permission.)

The etiology of conjoined twins is unknown, but the phenomenon occurs between the thirteenth and fifteenth day after fertilization with incomplete division of the zygote.[7, 8]

Classification

There are four basic types of conjoined twinning. The most common is thoracopagus-omphalopagus, representing 73% of cases reported. Pygopagus represents 19%, ischiopagus represents 6%, and the rarest, craniopagus, 2% (Figs 77–1 to 77–5).

Prenatal Diagnosis

Suspicion of conjoined twinning is raised in pregnancy complicated by polyhydramnios. Ultrasound technique with real-time scanning has established the diagnosis as early as the twelfth week of gestation.[48] Appropriate real-time and B-scan techniques avoid the need for invasive procedures such as amniocentesis.[13, 49, 62] Standard radiographs in the later stages of pregnancy may also lead to the suspicion of conjoined twinning but should be supplemented by appropriate sonography studies.[13, 22]

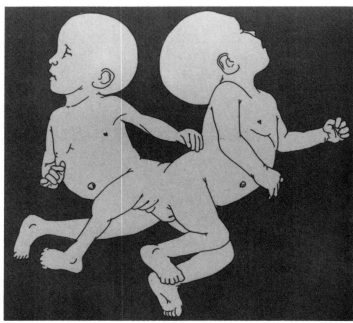

Fig 77–2.—Pygopagus twins. (From Votteler T.P.[57] Reprinted with permission.)

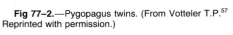

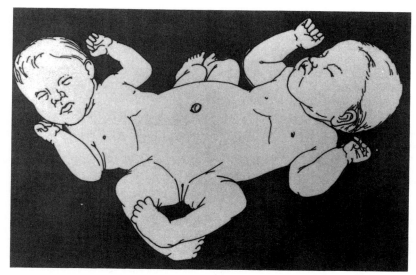

Fig 77–4.—Ischiopagus tetrapus twins. (From Votteler T.P.[57] Reprinted with permission.)

Antepartum Findings of Conjoined Twins

1. Bi-breech position by ultrasound and radiography
2. Single inseparable trunk by ultrasound with continuous external skin contour
3. Common heart sound by Doppler examination (thoracopagus)
4. Polyhydramnios by ultrasound
    50% conjoined twin pregnancies
    10% normal twin pregnancies
5. Bony fusion by radiography

6. En face position
7. Hyperextension of one or both cervical spines
8. Elongation of the fetal cranial vault
9. No change in relative position of twins on successive scans
10. Solitary large liver and heart
11. Solitary umbilical cord with over three vessels
12. Fetal body parts on the same level

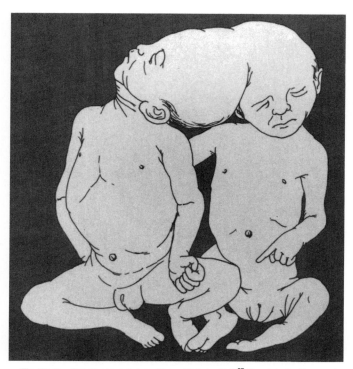

Fig 77–5.—Craniopagus twins. (From Votteler T.P.[57] Reprinted with permission.)

Ethics

The birth of conjoined twins raises serious ethical considerations.[43] The development of surgical separation techniques and anticipated long-term survival of one or both twins places parents and physicians in a unique and difficult situation from the moment of delivery.[32] Vying emphases on quality of life and sanctity of life place tremendous emotional burdens on all concerned. Decisions should be discussed in an atmosphere devoid of undue pressure from the media, the curious, or inexperienced physicians not possessing adequate knowledge of anticipated surgical results. Transfer of conjoined twins immediately after delivery to institutions with special interest in separation procedures is usually wise. Avoidance of publicity from the time of delivery is recommended to allow parents to receive and evaluate medical, religious, and ethical advice from knowledgeable consultants. The welfare of the conjoined twins should be paramount in discussions of future management.

Planned Surgical Separation

Subsequent to initial stabilization after delivery, it is preferable to complete all diagnostic studies required to delineate completely the extent of fusion of the twins. Creation of a team of surgeons, anesthesiologists, and nurses should be considered as soon as the diagnosis of conjoined twinning has been established and separation considered. Timing of the separation procedures depends on the anatomical findings as well as the ability of the twins to maintain normal growth and development. Indications for emergency separation procedures include: (1) one twin incapable of resuscitation or stillborn, (2) trauma to the connecting tissue during delivery, (3) an associated anomaly such as omphalocele, or (4) an unusual anomaly of one infant that cannot be readily corrected, i.e., severe cardiac defects.[20] Otherwise, efforts should be made to stabilize conjoined twins to allow a deliberately planned separation procedure. If possible, delay of separation procedures is wise for a period of time to allow growth and development. Excessive delay is usually unwise, however, and a planned separation procedure in the first year of life is recommended.

Anesthetic Management

Efficient planned anesthesia is required for successful separation (Fig 77–6). Keats et al.,[27] Jain,[26] Fournier et al.,[19] and Wong et al.[61] emphasized the unique aspects of the anesthetic management of these surgical procedures. Techniques vary with the experience and preference of involved anesthesiologists. Assignment of at least one member of the anesthetic team to each infant is wise, plus the addition of an overall anesthesia coordinator. Preoperative planning and rehearsal is beneficial for elective separation.[6] The extent of cross-circulation between infants is usually unpredictable, despite detailed preoperative studies. The effects of intravenous and inhalation agents may therefore be difficult to assess, and careful monitoring must be done. Hypothermia can be prevented by controlling operating suite temperature and by using warming devices, warm solutions and intravenous fluids, and heat-retaining skin coverage material on limbs and scalps. These measures permit prolonged operative procedures without significant temperature depression.

Difficulties in intubation are often encountered. Unusual changes in position to facilitate intubation should be minimized to prevent cardiovascular and respiratory alterations in the other twin. Orotracheal tubes should be replaced with nasotracheal tubes at the end of procedures to facilitate mechanical respiratory assistance in the postoperative period.

Blood loss is carefully monitored and replaced for each infant, realizing that transfusions for one infant may have a major effect on the other twin. If massive blood loss is anticipated, the use of autotransfusion equipment should be considered. Electrocautery is helpful to keep blood loss at a minimum. Extracellular fluid

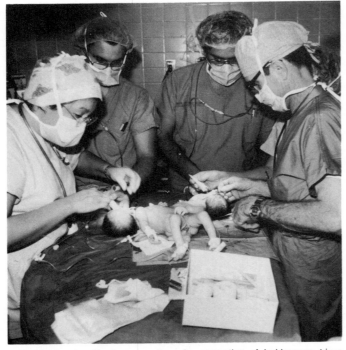

Fig 77–6.—Anesthesia preparations for separation of ischiopagus tripus twins. Surgical care shown in Figures 77–10 to 77–12. (From Votteler T.P.[57] Reprinted with permission.)

losses due to the exposure of large surfaces of viscera and soft tissue may, in themselves, require fluid volumes of 10 ml per kilogram per hour or greater. Steroid supplementation is rarely required. Monitoring techniques should include intra-arterial cannulas, central venous pressure lines, esophageal stethoscopes, frequent determination of arterial blood gases, and urinary bladder catheterization for renal output measurements in each infant.

The anesthesiologist should be aware of the ethical considerations created when decisions are made by the surgeon in favor of one twin to the detriment of the other.

Thoracopagus

These twins, who may be joined from the sternum to the umbilical region, constitute 73% of those reported. Seventy-five percent have varying degrees of cardiac fusion. Perhaps 90% have some degree of pericardial fusion. Although cardiac fusion usually precludes surgical separation, Synhorst, Matlak, et al.[53] separated such a pair with survival of one twin.

In utero ultrasonography diagnosis of cardiac fusion is possible but is not sufficiently accurate to be used as the only deciding factor in whether or not to recommend termination of pregnancy. Development of techniques to allow cardiac separation continues, and salvage of some of these infants may become possible. After delivery of thoracopagus-omphalopagus twins, evaluation of the cardiac status is of first importance. Studies to determine the degree of fusion should include two-dimensional echocardiography,[38] Doppler examination to determine flow patterns, as well as catheterization techniques. Nuclear cardiography may also be useful for complete evaluation. Magnetic resonance studies might delineate the extent of cross-circulation or organ fusion.

After this assessment, further investigations should establish the status of the gastrointestinal tracts, urinary systems, and liver-biliary organs.[34, 35] Liver scanning with an injection of ^{99m}Tc sulfur colloid into one twin can, at the same time, give useful information concerning the degree of cross-circulation and subsequent radioactivity of the other twin. Technetium DISIDA is useful to determine the status of the biliary tract. Arteriography by umbilical or other systemic arteries helps to determine thoracic and abdominal vascular patterns and suggests the extent of cross-circulation. Contrast material in the gastrointestinal tracts establishes the degree of fusion of the small intestine and colon.

In the absence of cardiac fusion to a degree which obviates it, separation of thoracopagus twins should be feasible. Pericardial substitutes may be utilized to prevent cardiac herniation and prosthetic material to reconstruct the chest wall. Sufficient skin mobilization usually is possible to close the operative defects. Secondary procedures for chest wall reconstruction may be left for later.

TABLE 77–1.—SURGICAL SEPARATIONS OF OMPHALOPAGUS TWINS WITH ASSOCIATED OMPHALOCELES

YEAR	SURGEON	SEX	SURVIVED	OMPHALOCELE
1963	Woolley[63]	M	One	Intact*
1964	Cywes[15]	F	One	Ruptured*
1965	Gans[20]	F	One	Ruptured*
1969	DeAngelis[16]	F	Both	Ruptured
1979	Messmer[36]	M	One	Intact
1980	Austin[3]	M	Both	Intact
1981	Votteler[57]	M	One	Ruptured*

*Imperforate anus.

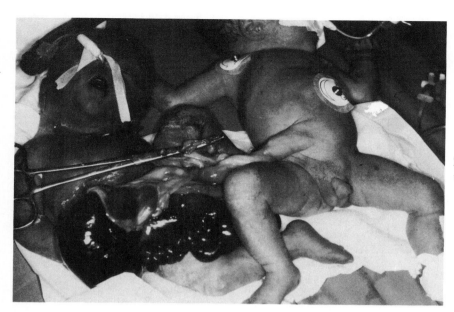

Fig 77–7.—Omphalopagus twins at birth with ruptured omphalocele and imperforate anus. Emergency separation. Twin on right survived with midileum enterostomy. (From Votteler T.P.[57] Reprinted with permission.)

Omphalopagus

Fusion of the liver must be anticipated when the junction of the twins includes the umbilical area. Compression techniques with individual vascular ligation can allow hepatic separation without excessive blood loss. Epigastric junction (omphalopagus) may be present without chest wall involvement. Such twins usually have a bridge of connecting liver tissue as well as a peritoneal communication. Separation should not present unusual technical problems. An omphalocele may complicate the repair as well as dictate an immediate separation procedure, particularly if it has ruptured during delivery. An unusual association has been the presence of imperforate anus in four of the seven omphalopagus twins successfully separated (Table 77–1) (Fig 77–7).

The majority of successful separations described in the literature and media have been of the thoracopagus-omphalopagus type. At least 46 have been discovered upon review of available descriptions in the English literature.

Pygopagus

Attachment at the buttocks area represents 19% of conjoined twins. Long-term survival is possible, but separation is feasible, as shown in Table 77–2.[58] Often the urinary tract and rectum are complete in each twin. Degrees of fusion may require separation procedures that leave one of the infants with a colostomy (Fig

77–8). Although the vertebral columns are usually in continuity, the spinal cords are usually separate. Metrizimide myelography, with CT scanning and ultrasound, are needed to establish the status of the spinal cords. If joined, they may still be separated without major neurologic deficit, utilizing urodynamic studies to preserve sacral nerve roots for each infant[57] (Fig 77–9). Skin or myocutaneous flaps can easily be constructed from adjacent glu-

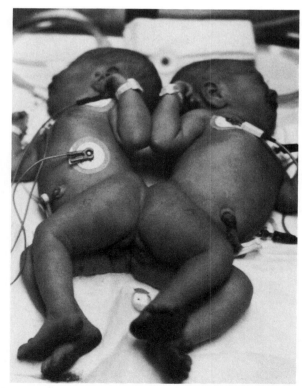

Fig 77–8.—Pygopagus twins at delivery. Separate vaginal and urethral orifices and common rectal opening. Twin on left developed necrotizing enterocolitis requiring colectomy. Separated at 14 months without rectal or bladder dysfunction. (From Votteler T.P.[57] Reprinted with permission.)

TABLE 77–2.—SURGICAL SEPARATIONS OF PYGOPAGUS TWINS

YEAR	SURGEON	SEX	SURVIVED
1953	Oschsner[59]	F	Both
1957	Koop[30]	F	Both
1962	Aird[2]	F	One
1965	Solerio[50]	F	Both
1971	Able[1]	M	Both
1974	Roy[14]	F	Both
1980	Goodwin[21]	F	One
1981	Votteler[58]	F	Both

From Votteler T.P.[58]

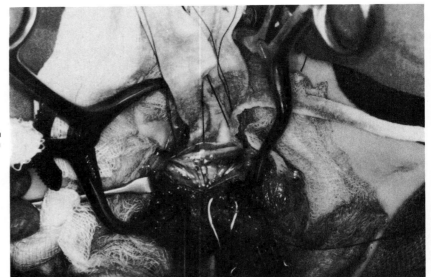

Fig 77–9.—Pygopagus twins. Spinal cords in continuity with common dura. No neurologic function loss after division. (From Votteler T.P.[57] Reprinted with permission.)

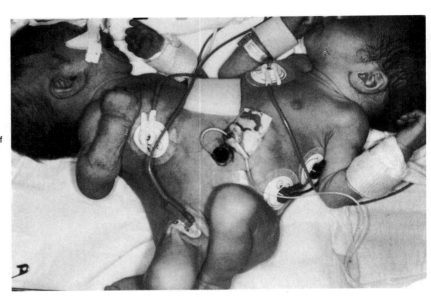

Fig 77–10.—Ischiopagus tripus twins 21 days old at time of separation. Twin on left died of multiple anomalies 8 hours after separation. (From Votteler T.P.[57] Reprinted with permission.)

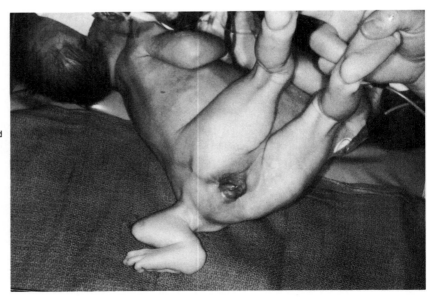

Fig 77–11.—Ischiopagus tripus twins showing perineal and lower limb anatomy. Common opening for urethra. Three vaginas and single rectum. (From Votteler T.P.[57] Reprinted with permission.)

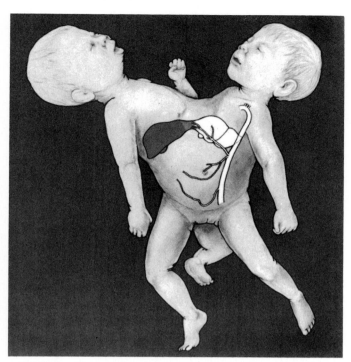

Fig 77–12.—Diagram of umbilical artery injection showing abdominal vascular patterns of ischiopagus twins in Figure 77–10. (From Votteler T.P.[57] Reprinted with permission.)

Ischiopagus

Approximately 6% of fusions extend from the umbilical area to include the lower trunk and pelvis with three limbs (tripus) or four limbs (tetrapus). These present challenging surgical problems and require careful preoperative planning (Figs 77–10, 77–11, 77–12). The gastrointestinal tract is often fused from the level of a Meckel's diverticulum. Various degrees of fusion of the bladder, vagina, and colon are to be anticipated, and often one twin requires at least temporary drainage of either the gastrointestinal or urinary tract. Successful separations of ischiopagus tripus twins are listed in Table 77–3. Separation of ischiopagus tetrapus twins with survival of one or both is listed in Table 77–4. Successfully separated ischiopagus twins require long-term rehabilitation—particularly orthopedic, gynecologic, and urologic. Satisfactory quality of life can be achieved, however (Fig 77–13), and pessimism initially evident when these infants are delivered should be tempered by extensive investigation to establish the maximum rehabilitation that can be achieved.

Craniopagus

Craniopagus, the rarest form, occurs once in 2,500,000 deliveries. A classification into partial or total forms, having a junction at either brow, vertex, or parietal bone,[41] has been devised. Partial forms have brain separation by bone or dura; each brain should have separate leptomeninges. The total form has an extensive connection of brain tissue or separation only by arachnoid layer. Separation of the latter type is most difficult. Feasibility of separation may depend on the presence of a superior sagittal

teal tissues to cover the operative defects. Preliminary colostomy is usually performed to prevent fecal contamination and subsequent infection of the flaps devised for coverage.

It is important to establish the optimum position of the patients for the neurosurgical procedure of separation of the spinal cord and dura. Indeed, in our separation in 1980,[57] the preoperative phases were done in the supine position, the infants being turned to the prone position to facilitate exposure of the spinal cord. Separation with the infants supine would not have been feasible.[54]

TABLE 77–3.—SURGICAL SEPARATIONS OF ISCHIOPAGUS TRIPUS TWINS

YEAR	SURGEON	SEX	SURVIVED
1968	Mestel[37]	F	Both
1971	Bissett[11]	?	One
1978	Votteler[57]	F	One
1979	Chao[12]	M	Both
1981	Bishop[10]	F	One
1981	Rector[45]	F	Both
1981	Raffensperger[44]	M	Both

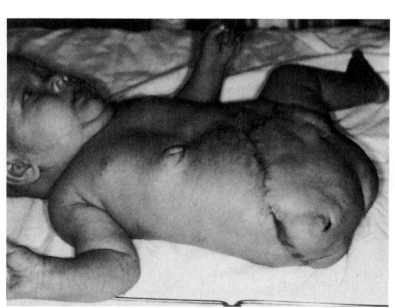

Fig 77–13.—Ischiopagus tripus twin survivor at 9 months of age. Skin and muscle coverage of pelvis and abdomen was achieved by utilizing tissues from the conjoined leg. Continence of urine and satisfactory bowel control at 6 years of age after abdominoperineal reconstruction at 9 months. Three vaginas left undisturbed. (From Votteler T.P.[57] Reprinted with permission.)

TABLE 77–4.—SURGICAL
SEPARATIONS OF ISCHIOPAGUS
TETRAPUS TWINS

YEAR	SURGEON	SEX	SURVIVED
1955	Spencer[51]	F	One
1965	Eades[17]	F	Both
1969	Hendren[31]	?	Both
1969	Louhimo[31]	?	One
1974	Koop[31]	F	Both

TABLE 77–5.—SURGICAL SEPARATION
OF CRANIOPAGUS TWINS

YEAR	SURGEON	SEX	CLASSIFICATION	SURVIVED
1952	Grossman[24]	M	Partial	One
1954	Murphey[59]	F	Total	One
1955	Voris[56]	F	Partial	Both
1956	Baldwin[4]	F	Partial	Both
1959	O'Connell[40]	M	Total	One
1961	O'Connell[40]	F	Total	One
1964	O'Connell[41]	F	Total	One
1968	Wolfowitz[60]	F	Partial	Both
1979	Roberts[46]	F	Total	Both
1981	Villarejo[55]	F	Total	One
1983	Anderson[52]	F	Partial	One

sinus for each brain, as venous drainage may be the critical parameter to allow successful separation. Closure of the resulting dural, bone, and scalp defects may tax the ingenuity of the neurosurgeon or plastic surgeon.

Preoperative studies should include computed tomography with or without contrast material, cerebral angiography, and, now, nuclear magnetic resonance studies.[5, 52] Metrizamide contrast studies may be useful if ventricular communication is suspected. Successfully separated craniopagus twins are listed in Table 77–5.

REFERENCES

1. Able L.W.: Personal communication.
2. Aird I.: The conjoined twins of Kano. *Br. Med. J.* 1:831, 1954.
3. Austin E., Schifrin B.S., Pomerance J.J., et al.: The antepartum diagnosis of conjoined twins. *J. Pediatr. Surg.* 15:332–334, 1980.
4. Baldwin M., Dekaban A.: The surgical separation of Siamese twins conjoined by the heads (cephalopagus frontalis) followed by normal development. *Am. J. Neurol. Neurosurg. Psych.* 21:195–202, 1958.
5. Bancovsky I., Bianco E., Moreira F.A.: Computed tomography in craniopagus occipitalis twins. *J. Comput. Assist. Tomogr.* 3:836–837, 1979.
6. Bell A.N.: Separating conjoined twins: A care plan. *AORN J.* 35:47–57, 1982.
7. Benirschke K., Chung K.K.: Multiple pregnancy. *N. Engl. J. Med.* 188:1329, 1973.
8. Benirschke K., Temple W.W., Bloor C.: Conjoined twins: Nosology and congenital malformations. *Birth Defects* 16:179–192, 1978.
9. Bhettay E., Nelson M.D., Beighton P.: Epidemic of conjoined twins in southern Africa. *Lancet* 2:741–743, 1975.
10. Bishop H.: Personal communication.
11. Borde J., Mitrofanoff P., Wallon P., et al.: A case of asymmetrical ischiopagus symelius conjoined twins, in *Progress in Pediatric Surgery*. Baltimore, University Park Press, 1974, p. 27.
12. Chao C.C., Susetio L., Luu K.W., et al.: Anaesthetic management for successful separation of tripus ischiopagal conjoined male twins. *Can. Anaesth. Soc. J.* 27:565–571, 1980.
13. Chen H.Y., Hsieh F.J., Huang L.H.: Prenatal diagnosis of conjoined twins by real-time sonography: A case report. *J.C.U.* 11:94–96, 1983.
14. Cloutier R., Levassiur L., Copty M., et al.: The surgical separation of pygopagus twins. *J. Pediatr. Surg.* 14:554–556, 1979.
15. Cywes S., Davies M.R., Rode H.: Conjoined twins—the Red Cross War Memorial Children's Hospital experience. *S. Afr. J. Surg.* 20:105–118, 1982.
16. DeAngelis R.R., Dursi J.F., Ibach J.R.: Successful separation of xiphopagus conjoined twins. *Ann. Surg.* 172:302, 1970.
17. Eades J.W., Thomas C.G.: Successful separation of ischiopagus tetrapus-conjoined twins. *Ann. Surg.* 164:1059–1072, 1966.
18. Edmonds L.D., Layde P.M.: Conjoined twins in the United States, 1970–1977. *Teratology* 25:301–308, 1982.
19. Fournier L., Goulet C., Waugh R., et al.: Anaesthesia for separation of conjoined twins. *Can. Anaesth. Soc. J.* 23:425–431, 1976.
20. Gans S.L., Morgenstern L., Gettelman E., et al.: Separation of conjoined twins in the newborn period. *J. Pediatr. Surg.* 3:565–574, 1968.
21. Goodwin C.: Personal communication.
22. Gore R.M., Filly R.A., Parer J.T.: Sonographic antepartum diagnosis of conjoined twins: Its impact on obstetric management. *JAMA* 247:3351–3353, 1982.
23. Greening D.G.: Vaginal delivery of conjoined twins. *Med. J. Aust.* 2:356–360, 1981.
24. Grossman H.J., Sugar O., Greeley P.W., et al.: Surgical separation in craniopagus. *JAMA* 153:201, 1953.
25. Guttmacher A.F., Nichols B.L.: Teratology of conjoined twins. *Birth Defects* 3:10–17, 1967.
26. Jain M.K.: Case of the month: Conjoined twins—craniopagus. *Indian Pediatr.* 16:727–728, 1979.
27. Keats A.S., Cave P.E., Slataper E.L., et al.: Conjoined twins—a review of anesthetic management for separating operations. *Birth Defects* 3:80–88, 1967.
28. Kiesewetter W.B.: Surgery on conjoined (Siamese) twins. *Surgery* 59:860, 1966.
29. König G.: Sibi invicem adnati feliciter separati. *Ephemerid Natur. Curios* 2:145, 1689.
30. Koop C.E.: The successful separation of pygopagus twins. *Surgery* 49:271, 1961.
31. Koop C.E., *Medical World News*, November 1974, pp. 90–99.
32. Lipsky K.: Conjoined twins: Psychosocial aspects. *AORN J.* 35:58–61, 1982.
33. Luckhardt A.B.: Report of the autopsy of the Siamese twins together with other interesting information covering their life, a sketch of the life of Chang and Eng. *Surg. Gynecol. Obstet.* 72:116–125, 1941.
34. Mann M.D., Coutts J.P., Kaschula R.O., et al.: The use of radionuclides in the investigation of conjoined twins. *J. Nucl. Med.* 24:479–484, 1983.
35. Margouleff D., Harper R.G., Kenigsberg K., et al.: Sequential scintiangiography of the hepato-splenic system of xiphopagus conjoined twins. *J. Nucl. Med.* 21:246–247, 1980.
36. Messmer B.J., Hornchen H., Kosters C., et al.: Surgical separation of conjoined (Siamese) xiphopagus twins. *Surgery* 89:622–625, 1981.
37. Mestel A.L., Golinko R.J., Wax S.H., et al.: Ischiopagus tripus conjoined twins: Case report of a successful separation. *Surgery* 69:75–83, 1971.
38. Miller D., Colombani P., Buck J.R., et al.: New techniques in the diagnosis and operative management of Siamese twins. *J. Pediatr. Surg.* 18:373–376, 1983.
39. Nelson M.M., Bhettay E., Beighton P.: Excessive Siamese twinning in southern Africa. *Afr. Med. J.* 50:697–698, 1976.
40. O'Connell J.E.A.: Craniopagus twins. *Br. Med. J.* 1:1333–1336, 1964.
41. O'Connell J.E.A.: Craniopagus twins: Surgical anatomy and embryology and their implications. *J. Neurol. Neurosurg. Psych.* 39:1–22, 1976.
42. Paré A.: Complete works, Johnson T. (trans.), 1678.
43. Pepper C.K.: Ethical and moral considerations in the separation of conjoined twins: Summary of two dialogues between physicians and clergymen. *Birth Defects* 3:128, 1967.
44. Raffensperger J.: Personal communication.
45. Rector J.: Personal communication.
46. Roberts T.: Personal communication.
47. Schinzel A.A., Smith D.W., Miller J.R.: Monozygotic twinning and structural defects. *J. Pediatr.* 95:921–930, 1979.
48. Schmidt W., Heberling D., Kubli F.: Antepartum ultrasonographic diagnosis of conjoined twins in early pregnancy. *Am. J. Obstet. Gynecol.* 139:961–963, 1981.
49. Siegfried M.S., Koptik G.F.: Prenatal sonographic diagnosis of conjoined twins. *Postgrad. Med.* 73:317–319, 1983.
50. Solerio L.: Separation of pygopagus twins. *Munich Med. Wochenschr.* 107:1549–1551, 1965.
51. Spencer R.: Surgical separation of Siamese twins: Case report. *Surgery* 39:827, 1956.
52. Stanley P., Anderson F.M., Seagall H.D.: Radiologic investigation of craniopagus twins (partial type). *AJNR* 4:206–208, 1983.

53. Synhorst D., Matlak M., Roan Y., et al.: Separation of conjoined thoracopagus twins joined at the right atria. *Am. J. Cardiol.* 43:662–665, 1979.
54. Venes J.: Personal communication.
55. Villarejo F., Soto M., Amaya C., et al.: Total craniopagus twins. *Child's Brain* 8:149–155, 1981.
56. Voris H., Slaughter W., Christian J., et al.: Successful separation of craniopagus twins. *J. Neurosurg.* 14:548–560, 1957.
57. Votteler T.P.: Surgical separation of conjoined twins. *AORN J.* 35:35–46, 1982.
58. Votteler T.P.: Necrotizing enterocolitis in a pygopagus conjoined twin. *J. Pediatr. Surg.* 17:555–557, 1982.
59. Wilson H., Storer E.: Surgery in Siamese twins: A report of three sets of conjoined twins treated surgically. *Ann. Surg.* 145:718, 1957.
60. Wolfowitz J., Kerr E.M., Levin S.E., et al.: Separation of craniopagus twins. *S. Afr. Med. J.* 42:412–424, 1968.
61. Wong K.C., Ohmura A., Roberts T.H., et al.: Anesthetic management for separation of craniopagus twins. *Anesth. Analg.* 59:883–886, 1980.
62. Wood M.J., Thompson H.E., Roberson F.M.: Real-time ultrasound diagnosis of conjoined twins. *J.C.U.* 9:195–197, 1981.
63. Woolley M., Joergenson E.: Xiphopagus conjoined twins. *Am. J. Surg.* 108:277, 1964.

78 Marc I. Rowe / David A. Lloyd
Inguinal Hernia

History.—In 176 A.D., Galen[82] wrote, "The duct descending to the testicle is a small offshoot [processus vaginalis peritonei] of the great peritoneal sac in the lower abdomen," an observation which established the pathogenesis of indirect inguinal hernia. As early as 1552 B.C., the Egyptians described inguinal hernias treated by external pressure.[59] The earliest record of surgical therapy for hernia was by Susruta[59] in the fifth century A.D.

During the early part of the nineteenth century, the anatomy of the inguinal canal was accurately described by Camper,[10] Cooper,[15] Hesselbach,[31] and Scarpa.[75] Lister's antisepsis[44] made feasible the deliberate reconstruction of the inguinal structures, and, in 1887, Bassini[4] and, in 1889, Halsted[29] reported the successful use of the now basic techniques of inguinal herniorrhaphy. Although Banks[3] recommended in 1884 that hernias be definitively treated by well-fitting trusses, he did condescend to operate on a few patients when the truss failed. He described complete removal of the hernia sac through the external ring, and this operation is now associated with his name. In 1899, Ferguson[22] described high ligation of the sac and reconstruction without altering the relation of the cord structures to the anatomical layers of the inguinal canal. He incised the external oblique aponeurosis to facilitate the dissection. MacLennan[50] in 1914 emphasized the desirability of elective operation as a definitive cure for inguinal hernia and influenced the transition from the use of trusses to definitive operation. He was a protagonist of early discharge of the child patient. Potts, Riker, and Lewis[62] supported the principle of simple high ligation and removal of the hernia sac for routine hernia repair in the child patient. This philosophy began a trend that has resulted in the current surgical management of infants and children with inguinal hernia. Under ideal circumstances, the recommended age for repairing an inguinal hernia is at the time of diagnosis. The generally accepted procedure is suture ligation of the sac at the internal ring. With certain exceptions, elective operation is now done in the outpatient surgical unit.[60]

Embryogenesis and Pathogenesis

Continued patency of the processus vaginalis is the principal factor in the development of congenital hernia and hydrocele. The patent processus vaginalis is a *potential* hernia and only when it contains some part of the abdominal viscera does it become an actual hernia. The difference between a congenital hernia and a congenital hydrocele is the diameter of the processus and the content of the sac; the former contains an intra-abdominal structure, while the latter contains peritoneal fluid alone.

The processus vaginalis develops during the third month of gestation as an outpouching of the peritoneal cavity through the internal inguinal ring.[80] At this time, the developing testis lies within the abdominal cavity. Descent of the testis commences after the seventh month of intrauterine life and is associated with extension of the processus vaginalis into the scrotum. The processus vaginalis appears to play an integral role in testicular descent, probably by providing the necessary hydraulic force that drives the testis into the scrotum.[55] That hormonal factors, notably testosterone, influence the descent of the testis has been established since 1931,[76] but the precise mechanisms remain unknown.

The processus vaginalis obliterates spontaneously from the internal inguinal ring to the testis after testicular descent has been completed. The distal processus persists as the tunica vaginalis. Incomplete obliteration of the processus predisposes to various patterns of fluid accumulation (hydrocele) and hernia (Fig 78–1). The time of normal postnatal closure of the processus vaginalis is not known. Some claim that closure occurs immediately after birth; others state that a high percentage remain open for several years. In 1969, Snyder et al.,[85] from a review of six published studies, concluded that, at birth, the processus vaginalis remains in communication with the peritoneal cavity in 80–94% of examined bodies. He further quoted Sachs[73] as finding that the processus vaginalis was completely open in 57% of the bodies of infants between the ages of 4 months and 1 year. Although Snyder's figures have been quoted by subsequent authors, they are difficult to interpret for several reasons. First, the data are derived from autopsy studies done between 1785 and 1885. Second, the definition of a "partially" or "completely" open processus vaginalis, descriptions used by several authors, is not clarified. Third, the data on patent processus vaginalis are further confusing because in some series whole bodies are referred to and in others, body halves. Recent information on the postnatal obliteration of the processus has been derived from contralateral exploration when a clinically apparent unilateral hernia was present. It is misleading to draw conclusions from these figures, since the patients all had hernias, demonstrating an inherent abnormality of the processus vaginalis, at least on one side.

Although the above studies give us no firm figures as to the frequency at any age of a processus vaginalis, they do indicate a relatively high incidence of patency of the processus vaginalis in normal infants for several months after birth. Data from adult

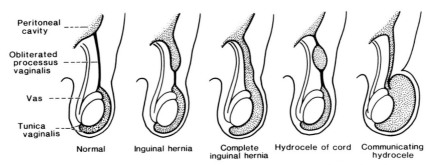

Fig 78–1.—Different forms of inguinal hernia and hydrocele arising from failure of the processus vaginalis to obliterate completely.

autopsy studies lend support to this impression. A postmortem study of adults dying without clinically apparent inguinal hernias demonstrated a patent processus vaginalis in 20% of groins examined.[56] The incidence of patent processus vaginalis in other autopsy studies varies from 15% to 37%. It appears that, in apparently normal individuals, not only does the processus vaginalis remain patent for several months after birth, but in some 20% patency persists throughout life.

A hernia is not inevitable when the processus vaginalis remains patent, and, from the adult autopsy studies quoted above, it is clear that patency of the processus may persist undetected throughout life. Therefore, factors other than simple patency of the processus are involved in the development of a clinically apparent inguinal hernia. The only factor positively identified is excess fluid in the peritoneal cavity. Whether this is due to the physical presence of the fluid, or is secondary to increased intra-abdominal pressure, is not known. There are several reports of indirect inguinal hernias developing in patients with ascites, with ventriculoperitoneal shunts, or undergoing peritoneal dialysis. Alexander and Tank[1] reported a 6-year-old boy who had a clinically apparent inguinal hernia on the left side confirmed by peritoneography and repaired at the time of placement of a peritoneal dialysis catheter. A small patent processus vaginalis seen on the opposite side was not operated on because of its small size. Following peritoneal dialysis, a symptomatic hernia promptly developed on the second side and required repair. Similarly, Grosfeld and Cooney[28] reported two patients, aged 5 and 7 years, without clinical evidence of an inguinal hernia who previously had ventriculoatrial shunts that were converted to ventriculoperitoneal shunts. These patients developed clinically apparent indirect inguinal hernias 1 month and 3 months, respectively, after placement of the ventriculoperitoneal shunts.

Incidence

Inguinal hernia repair is the most frequent general surgical operation performed by pediatric surgeons. In 1983, at Children's Hospital of Pittsburgh, out of a total of 2,281 general surgical operations, there were 852 inguinal hernia repairs (37%). The incidence of inguinal hernia in children ranges from 0.8% to 4.4%.[6] In premature infants the incidence rises to 30%, depending on the gestational age.[30]

AGE.—The incidence of inguinal hernia is highest during the first year of life, with a peak during the first month.[6] Approximately one third of children with hernia are less than 6 months of age at operation.[6, 32]

SEX.—Boys are affected approximately six times more often than girls;[32] reported sex ratios range from 3:1 to 10:1 in favor of males.[6, 32, 41, 51, 52, 70, 74, 94] Among newborn infants, particularly

prematures, the relative incidence of inguinal hernia in females is higher than in older children.[6, 30]

SIDE.—The predominance of right-sided hernias is well established. In boys, 60% of hernias occur on the right side, 30% on the left, and 10% are bilateral.[70] The incidence is similar in girls (right side 60%, left side 32%, bilateral 8%). In the figures quoted, a hernia was designated bilateral only if the diagnosis was made preoperatively; a simple patent processus vaginalis found on contralateral exploration was not considered a hernia.

FAMILY HISTORY.—An increased incidence of congenital inguinal hernia has been documented in twins and in individual families of patients with inguinal hernia.[6, 17] There is a history of another inguinal hernia in the family in 11.5% of patients.[46]

Clinical Features

An inguinal hernia appears as a bulge in the groin that extends toward, and often into, the scrotum with crying and straining. It may be present at birth or may not appear until weeks, months, or years later. The clinical signs of an inguinal hernia are a smooth, firm mass that emerges through the external inguinal ring lateral to the pubic tubercle and enlarges with increased intra-abdominal pressure. When the patient relaxes, the hernia either reduces spontaneously or can be reduced by gentle pressure upward and posteriorly, when it will suddenly slip back. The position of the testis must be ascertained, because a retractile testis lying outside the external inguinal ring appears as a groin swelling and is easily confused with an inguinal hernia. The distinction is made by manipulating the retracted testes into the scrotum and then examining the groin. An undescended testis may coexist with a hernia and must be identified, since orchiopexy will be required in addition to hernia repair.

Typically the patient is referred to a surgeon after a hernia has been seen by the parents or a pediatrician. Although the history may be characteristic, it is necessary to confirm the presence of the hernia by identifying the inguinal swelling. A quiet infant can be made to strain his abdominal muscles by stretching him out supine on the bed with legs extended and arms held straight above the head. Most infants will struggle to get free, increasing intra-abdominal pressure; this is reinforced by stimulating the infant to cry. Older children can be asked to blow up a balloon, perform the Valsalva maneuver, or cough, preferably while standing. Detecting thickening and silkiness on palpating the spermatic cord as it crosses the pubic tubercle (silk-glove sign) may be a useful diagnostic aid in patients in whom an inguinal hernia is suspected clinically.[6, 26] When the hernia cannot be demonstrated but has previously been identified by a pediatrician, most surgeons (65%) accept the diagnosis and operate.[72] The remainder reevaluate the patient at a second visit. If the hernia has been seen only by the parents, 55% of surgeons re-evaluate the patient at a second visit. When we are unable to demonstrate a hernia, we prefer to reevaluate the patient before undertaking an operation. A second inconclusive examination is a reasonable indication for a herniogram.

Management

An inguinal hernia will not resolve spontaneously and must be repaired because of the high risk of incarceration, particularly during the first months of life. Sixty-nine percent of incarcerated hernias occur below the age of 1 year, and in these younger patients the hernia tends to be irreducible: Rowe and Clatworthy[69] found that 71% of incarcerated hernias requiring operative reduction occurred in infants less than 11 months of age.

In most patients, elective inguinal hernia repair is safely done in the outpatient surgical unit. Exceptions are high-risk newborn infants (discussed later) and older children with cardiac, respiratory, or other disorders that increase the risk of anesthesia. These patients may be admitted either on the night before or on the morning of operation and are kept in hospital overnight for observation and monitoring.

In infants, endotracheal anesthesia, with its greater control over ventilation, is preferred. For older children, mask anesthesia is adequate. In all patients, venous access is obtained for administration of fluids and drugs. Regional anesthesia, by ilioin-guinal and iliohypogastric nerve block, has been suggested to minimize postoperative discomfort.[78, 84] In our experience, infants and young children appear to have minimal postoperative pain; analgesia is seldom required, and they are usually fully active within 24 hours.

Surgical Technique

The principal objective in correcting a pediatric inguinal hernia is high ligation of the hernia sac at the internal inguinal ring (Fig 78–2). A useful landmark is the pubic tubercle (Fig 78–2,*A*), immediately lateral to which lies the external inguinal ring. In the newborn, the internal ring lies almost directly beneath the external ring (Fig 78–2,*B*) and can be comfortably approached through the external ring without incising the external oblique aponeurosis.[3] With increasing age, the two inguinal rings become progressively farther apart as the inguinal canal lengthens, and the internal ring is approached by incising the overlying external oblique aponeurosis.

A transverse skin crease incision is made, the medial end of the incision above and lateral to the pubic tubercle (Fig 78–2,*A*). The precise situation of the incision depends on the age of the patient. The older child requires a more laterally placed incision to gain optimal exposure of the internal ring. The incision should be long enough to provide adequate exposure of the cord structures; a difficult and traumatic dissection can usually be attrib-

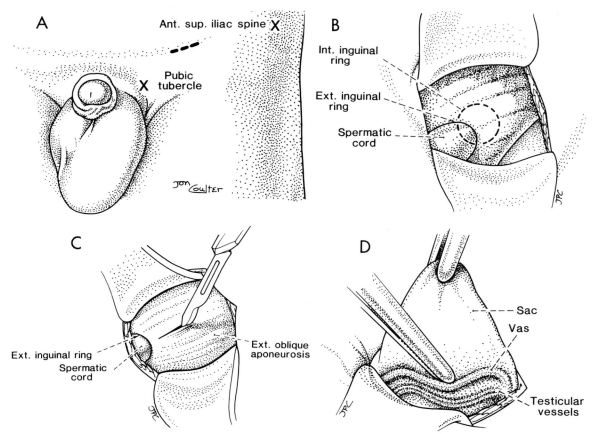

Fig 78–2.—Inguinal hernia repair in the male child. **A,** the incision is made in the skin crease above and lateral to the pubic tubercle, over the internal inguinal ring. **B,** in the infant up to about 1 year of age, the inguinal canal is short, and the internal inguinal ring can be approached through the external inguinal ring without incising the external oblique aponeurosis. The subcutaneous fat and Scarpa's fascia are divided, and the external oblique aponeurosis is cleared of overlying fat and connective tissue to expose the external inguinal ring. **C,** in the child 1 year of age or older, the incision in the external oblique aponeurosis is made lateral to the external inguinal ring, over the internal ring. **D,** the fibers of the cremasteric fascia are separated. The shiny white hernia sac is identified and lifted with blunt forceps. The vas deferens and testicular vessels are never held with forceps and are dissected off the hernia sac with the overlying areolar tissue. (Continued)

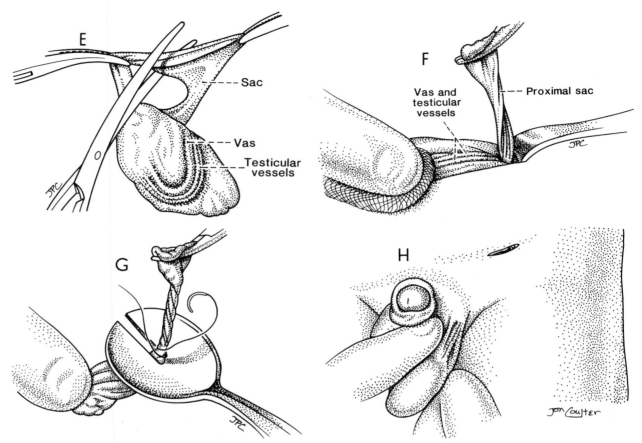

Fig 78–2 Cont.—E, the isolated sac is inspected to ensure that it is empty and is then divided. The distal portion of the sac is ignored. **F,** the proximal part of the sac is dissected into the internal inguinal ring until the preperitoneal fat is identified. The assistant applies gentle digital traction to the vas and testicular vessels to facilitate dissection. **G,** after twisting the sac two or three times, high ligation is performed using a transfixion suture. The grooved teaspoon is used to protect the cord structures during suture ligation. **H,** the testis is pulled well down into the scrotum, bringing the testicular vessels and the vas back to their normal positions in the inguinal canal. Fluid is expressed from the distal sac, which is neither ligated nor removed. The wound is closed in layers with absorbable sutures, including subcuticular sutures to the skin.

uted to inadequate exposure. The viability of the testis and the safe handling of the spermatic vasculature and vas deferens should never be jeopardized for the sake of a short incision.

The subcutaneous fat is separated to expose Scarpa's fascia, which in children is well developed and easily confused with the external oblique aponeurosis. Scarpa's fascia is picked up with fine hemostats and incised in the line of the skin incision, revealing a further layer of fatty tissue. This is cleared from the underlying external oblique aponeurosis. The external inguinal ring is identified lateral to the pubic tubercle, and the inguinal ligament and the fibers of the external oblique aponeurosis overlying the inguinal canal are delineated.

A short incision is made in the external oblique in the line of its fibers, lateral to the external ring (Fig 78–2,C). The incised edges of the external oblique fascia are elevated, taking care to identify and protect the underlying ilioinguinal nerve. The opening may be extended into the external ring, depending on the preference of the surgeon. Dissection under the inferior flap of the external oblique aponeurosis exposes the spermatic cord and the inguinal ligament. Using a hemostat or smooth forceps, the fibers of the cremasteric fascia are separated to expose the cord structures and the hernia sac. It is neither necessary nor desirable to free up the entire spermatic cord and lift it into the wound, as this may damage the underlying transversalis fascia and destroy the integrity of the posterior wall of the inguinal

canal. Using a pair of blunt forceps, the sac is lifted and the fine layer of connective tissue overlying the sac is dissected off it (Fig 78–2,D). Blunt dissection continues on the inferolateral aspect of the sac, usually revealing deep golden fat overlying the testicular vessels. The vas deferens, in turn, is usually situated below the testicular vessels. To avoid damaging the vessels and the vas, they must never be held with forceps. The vas and vessels can be safely dissected off the sac by grasping the areolar tissue immediately adjacent to them with forceps and "stripping" this tissue off the sac, taking with it these vulnerable structures. Should the sac tear, a pair of hemostats is used to appose the edges of the tear to prevent it extending through the internal inguinal ring into the peritoneal cavity.

After the cord structures have been separated from the sac at the point of dissection, the sac is inspected to insure that no abdominal viscera are trapped within it and then divided between hemostats (Fig 78–2,E). The proximal end of the sac is elevated and the cord structures, held under gentle traction by the assistant, are dissected from it (Fig 78–2,F). The dissection of the sac continues into the internal ring until the preperitoneal fat is identified. Having once again ascertained that the sac is empty, the surgeon twists it three or four times and ligates it at the level of the internal ring (Fig 78–2,G). It is helpful to use a grooved teaspoon to keep the adjacent cord structures from being caught up in the transfixion suture. A dilated internal ring

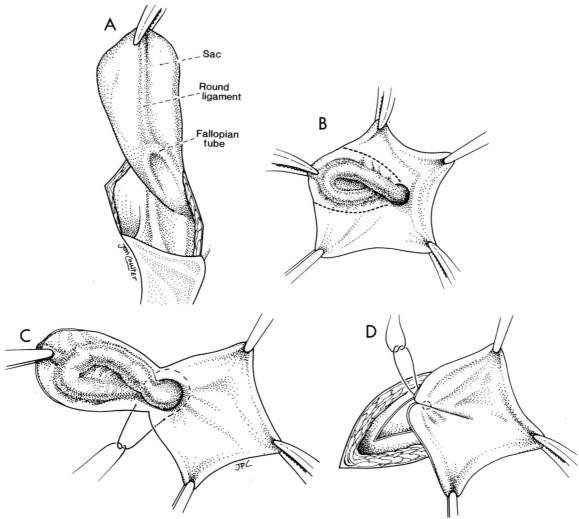

Fig 78–3.—Inguinal hernia repair in the female child. **A,** skin incision and exposure of the hernia sac are similar to that in the male child. After mobilizing the sac, the round ligament, which lies in the wall of the sac, is ligated and divided distally. The Fallopian tube may be seen in the wall of the sac as a sliding hernia. **B,** the hernia sac is opened and the Fallopian tube is searched for before the sac is ligated. If the Fallopian tube is not visible, it can be brought into view by traction on the round ligament. When the tube is present as a sliding hernia, it is immobilized by traction with a hemostat placed on the stump of the round ligament. An incision is made in the sac on either side of the Fallopian tube. **C,** a purse-string suture is placed around the neck of the sac at the level of the internal ring. **D,** the flap of hernia sac with the Fallopian tube is inverted through the internal inguinal ring into the peritoneal cavity. The purse-string suture is tied. The internal ring and the external ring may be closed with interrupted sutures. The wound is closed as in the male patient.

may be found when a large hernia is present and occasionally needs to be narrowed by placing one or two sutures in the edges of the transversalis fascia at the inferior aspect of the ring.

It is not necessary to remove the distal part of the hernia sac, which is simply left open. Attempts to remove a large adherent sac usually result in bleeding and hematoma and may injure the vas. Gentle traction on the testis returns the cord structures to the inguinal canal and the testis to the scrotum (Fig 78–2,*H*). If the testis is mobile and unattached to the scrotum, it is anchored to the scrotum by a suture tied over a dental roll, or by placing it in a dartos pouch. The external oblique aponeurosis and Scarpa's fascia are closed with interrupted sutures, and the skin with fine subcuticular chromic catgut sutures. The skin closure is reinforced with adhesive strips or a layer of collodion. At the end of the operation, the testis is again pulled well down into the scrotum to prevent its becoming adherent in a retracted position.

Inguinal Hernia in Girls

The skin incision and exposure of the inguinal canal are identical to those in the male. The hernia sac and round ligament are dissected up to the internal ring and the round ligament is divided and ligated. In 21% of cases,[27] the Fallopian tube, occasionally with the ovary or uterus, lies in the wall of the hernia sac as a sliding hernia and will not reduce into the peritoneal cavity (Fig 78–3,*A*). For this reason, we routinely open the sac and examine the interior. If the Fallopian tube is not easily visible, traction on the round ligament brings it into view so that its exact position can be determined. A high ligation is performed if a sliding hernia is not present.

In the presence of a sliding hernia, no attempt should be made to dissect the Fallopian tube off the inner wall of the sac, as this may lead to traumatic or ischemic stenosis of the tube. The technique described by Goldstein and Potts[27] entails making an incision in the wall of the open sac on either side of the Fallopian tube (Fig 78–3,*B*). A purse-string suture is placed around the neck of the sac (Fig 78–3,*C*), the flap of the hernia sac wall with the attached Fallopian tube is turned into the peritoneal cavity, and the suture tied (Fig 78–3,*D*). The internal ring may be closed with one or two interrupted sutures placed through edges of the transversalis fascia. An alternate method has been described by Woolley:[94] the hernia sac is ligated distal to the Fallopian tube and divided; the proximal sac is then invaginated into the peritoneal cavity through the internal ring, which is closed with sutures placed through the transversalis fascia. The external inguinal ring may also be closed. The external oblique aponeurosis, Scarpa's fascia, and the skin are closed as in the male.

Complications

Recurrent hernias, spermatic cord injuries, and testicular complications are discussed in the sections on contralateral exploration and incarcerated hernia.

IATROGENIC CRYPTORCHIDISM (TRAPPED TESTICLE).—Kiesewetter[39] reported two cases of iatrogenic cryptorchidism after inguinal herniorrhaphy in a series of 248 patients. In large series reported by Holder and Ashcraft,[32] McGregor et al.,[51] and Lynn and Johnson,[48] there were no instances of cryptorchidism on follow-up. Except in patients with congenital undescended testis, this abnormality occurs as a result of failure to pull the testis down to its normal position in the scrotum at the conclusion of hernia repair and to maintain it there.[37]

POSTOPERATIVE SCROTAL SWELLING.—Following hernia repair, fluid may accumulate in the distal sac, forming a recurrent hydrocele. Usually this resolves spontaneously; rarely, aspiration may be necessary. Scrotal hematoma may follow excision of the distal sac.

Contralateral Exploration

In 1955, Rothenberg and Barnett[68] reported contralateral groin explorations in 50 infants and children with unilateral inguinal hernias. They found that 100% of infants under 1 year of age and 65.8% of children over 1 year had "bilateral inguinal hernias." They concluded that, when a hernia defect is demonstrated on one side, it could be presumed to exist on the opposite side in three out of four patients and that routine groin exploration in all children with a unilateral clinically apparent inguinal hernia was indicated. Their study initiated a debate over the management of the opposite groin of a child with a unilateral inguinal hernia that has persisted for 30 years. Many reports followed, supporting or contesting Rothenberg and Barnett's findings and recommendations. McLaughlin and Kleager[52] and Mueller and Rader[57] found a high incidence of open processus vaginalis on the side opposite a clinically apparent inguinal hernia and recommended exploration. Fischer and Mumenthaler[23] reported a low incidence of patent processus on the contralateral side and raised the possibility of damage to the testicle during the course of the exploration. A comprehensive study published in 1958 by Clausen, Jake, and Binkley[13] examined some of the controversial aspects of the problem. They concluded that, although routine exploration could not be recommended, the mortality and morbidity of herniorrhaphy would not be increased by contralateral exploration in properly selected infants if the surgeon was skillful. Kiesewetter and Parenzan[41] recommended contralateral exploration in all children under 2 years of age. Gilbert and Clatworthy[26] reported their experience with routine contralateral exploration. They found a high incidence of patent processus vaginalis (60%) on the side opposite a clinically apparent inguinal hernia. They also noted that palpation of the cord on the side

opposite a clinically apparent inguinal hernia was relatively useless in predicting the presence of an occult hernia. They concluded that it was justifiable to perform "bilateral herniotomy" on an otherwise healthy infant or child with a unilateral clinically apparent hernia or hydrocele irrespective of age, sex, family history of hernia, history of prematurity, or side involved.

Sparkman[86] published an extensive review of the subject in 1962. The advantages of routine contralateral exploration were: (1) contralateral hernias were found in a high percentage of cases, (2) the cost of a second hospitalization was avoided, (3) the child was spared psychological trauma and the risk of a second anesthetic and operation, (4) the parents were spared the anxiety of second operation, and (5) the surgeon was spared the embarrassment occasioned by appearance of a second hernia. The drawbacks to contralateral exploration were: (1) many unnecessary operations were performed when routine exploration was done, (2) there was a possibility of technical mishaps, (3) the incidence of a patent processus vaginalis disclosed by blind contralateral operation appeared to be disproportionate to the incidence of hernias later developing in patients who had a unilateral repair. Sparkman[86] reviewed reports of 918 contralateral explorations published between 1952 and 1960. The overall incidence of contralateral open patent processus vaginalis was 57%. There was a higher incidence of positive explorations in younger children, decreasing with age. In 1,944 patients who had unilateral hernia repairs and who were followed for periods of 18 months to 37 years, contralateral hernias developed subsequently in 15.8% of patients, with a range of 4% to 34%. He summarized his findings as follows: (1) if routine bilateral exploration is performed on all infants and children, a contralateral patent processus vaginalis will be found in 50–60% of the entire group; (2) if a unilateral hernia repair is performed, the subsequent development of a contralateral hernia within the childhood years can be anticipated in at least 15–20% of the entire group.

In 1969, Rowe et al.[71] reviewed a series of 2,764 infants and children with inguinal hernias. This study was unique because of the large number of patients operated on in a single institution by a small group of surgeons who used the same criteria for determining patency of the processus and employed similar operative techniques for hernia repair and contralateral exploration. The focus of this study was on 1,965 patients who had a clinically apparent unilateral inguinal hernia and underwent exploration of the contralateral side in search of a patent processus vaginalis. A significant patent processus vaginalis was discovered in 946 (48%) patients. The definition of a significant processus was that it was at least 2 cm long and was patent as demonstrated by an obvious lumen or by passage of a probe or injection of fluid or air. The highest incidence of patency (63%) was in the first 2 months of life. After this, there was a steady fall in incidence until 2 years of age, when a leveling off occurred. From 2 years of age to 16, the incidence of patency was 41%. They reanalyzed their data in 1971[70] and concluded that it is reasonable to perform contralateral groin explorations but that the following criteria must be met: (1) the surgeon is skilled and experienced, (2) the anesthesiologist is an expert in administering anesthesia to infants and children and has the proper equipment, (3) the patient does not have a serious condition that will increase the risk of operation, (4) the operative procedure progresses smoothly and repair of the primary hernia takes less than 1 hour of anesthesia time. More recently, Holder and Ashcraft[32] reviewed their personal series of 1,000 consecutive patients with inguinal hernia. A total of 384 patients with unilateral inguinal hernia had contralateral exploration, with significant patent processus vaginalis found in 46% of cases. They also recommended bilateral operation.

Although the studies of the incidence of positive and negative findings after contralateral exploration are interesting and give information on the natural history of the processus vaginalis, they do not answer the most important question: How many patients who have operative repair of a unilateral clinically apparent inguinal hernia without contralateral exploration subsequently develop a clinically apparent inguinal hernia on the opposite side? Is the incidence of "open sacs" found at contralateral exploration the same as the incidence of contralateral hernias developing after unilateral hernia repair? Sparkman,[86] in an attempt to answer this question, analyzed the data from seven studies reported during the 1950s and 1960s from the American and foreign literature. A total of 1,944 patients were followed for periods ranging from 18 months to 37 years. The overall incidence of subsequent contralateral hernias was 15.8%; the lowest incidence was 4%, and the highest 34%. Most authors conceded that further extension of the period of follow-up would lead to an increase in the rate of development of contralateral hernias. In 1970, Bock and Sobye[5] reviewed 174 patients who had had unilateral inguinal hernia repair and were followed for 27–36 years. Their figure of 14.9% developing hernia on the opposite side is almost identical to the collective incidence found by Sparkman, 15.8%. More recently, McGregor et al.[51] reviewed 148 children who had unilateral hernia repair and then were followed for 10–20 years. Twenty-two percent of the patients eventually required repair of a hernia in the opposite groin.

It is obvious that the 15–22% incidence of hernias developing after unilateral hernia repairs is much lower than the 48–60% incidence of patent processus found at contralateral exploration. The discrepancy between the frequency of contralateral hernia and patent processus vaginalis was explained by Rowe et al.[71] as a natural consequence of obliteration of the processus vaginalis. They postulated that the contralateral processus vaginalis in infants with a unilateral inguinal hernia obliterates just before birth or in the first few months of life in about 40% of cases, leaving 60% still with a patent processus vaginalis. In another 20%, the processus obliterates over the next 2 years. After 2 years of age, about 40% of the children still have a patent processus vaginalis and no further obliteration takes place. Half of these children (20%) will develop an inguinal hernia sometime in their lives. The other half (20%) will live out their lifetimes with a patent processus vaginalis but never develop a clinically apparent inguinal hernia.

There are several treatment options in managing an infant or child with a unilateral inguinal hernia and no evidence of hernia on the opposite groin: (1) routine unilateral hernia repair and contralateral exploration, (2) unilateral hernia repair and contralateral exploration in selected cases, (3) unilateral inguinal hernia repair without contralateral exploration, (4) unilateral operation and employment of an intraoperative diagnostic procedure to determine patency of the contralateral processus vaginalis. If a processus is detected, bilateral operation is performed; (5) preoperative herniogram, with bilateral operation, if positive on the second side, and unilateral operation if negative.

Routine Bilateral Exploration

In 1958, Clausen et al.[13] surveyed the surgical staffs of 10 large children's hospitals and found that 40% of the surgeons routinely explored the side opposite a clinically apparent inguinal hernia. A year later, Gilbert and Clatworthy[26] surveyed 46 surgeons who were members of the Surgical Section of the American Academy of Pediatrics and found that 37% would routinely explore the opposite side. In 1981, Rowe and Marchildon[72] questioned 40 senior pediatric surgeons with an average of 17 years of clinical practice. Eighty percent routinely explored the opposite side in boys, and 90% the opposite side in girls. Their survey pointed out the fact that, in spite of the many articles that have been written about the controversy of the routine exploration of the contralateral side and the possible dangers attendant upon it, a large number of experienced pediatric surgeons routinely explore the opposite side.

The major advantage of contralateral exploration is that it allows the discovery and elimination of a patent processus vaginalis, and without a patent processus an indirect inguinal hernia cannot develop. The mortality and the common postoperative complications do not appear to be increased by extending the operation to include contralateral exploration. A major objection voiced by many is that contralateral exploration in the majority of instances is "unnecessary." In support of this contention, the available data indicate that no matter how many vaginal processes are discovered with contralateral explorations, a clinically apparent hernia develops after unilateral operation in only one out of every six.

Several authors have raised the serious question as to whether contralateral exploration unnecessarily exposes the vas, the epididymis, and the testicle to injury, resulting in the later development of infertility. Testicular atrophy has been documented as a complication following inguinal hernia repair but its incidence following contralateral exploration has never been reported. The reported percentages of testicular atrophy following unilateral inguinal hernia repair vary widely. Fischer and Mumenthaler in 1957[23] examined 587 patients following previous inguinal hernia repairs done by many surgeons from several hospitals in Switzerland. One percent of the patients on follow-up examination had frank testicular atrophy and another 2.7%, a testicle of reduced size. The method of repair was not described, nor was the incidence of incarcerated hernia. Fahlstrom et al.,[21] in a widely quoted study in 1963, found that 1% of all patients who had an inguinal hernia repair and 15% who had a hydrocele operation had testicular atrophy. It is doubtful if this information is relevant to hernia and hydrocele operations as they are presently done. Only 33 hernia repairs and 19 hydrocele operations were performed per year, a small experience. Two thirds of patients had their inguinal hernia treated by high ligation, but the majority had the distal sac totally excised. Of particular significance was the fact that the operation for correction of hydrocele involved inverting the processus vaginalis around the testicle. The incidence of incarcerated hernias was not reported. We believe that the data from both these reports do not indicate what the incidence of testicular atrophy may be when an exploration rather than a hernia repair is performed by experienced surgeons and when a simple high ligation is utilized to obliterate the open sac.

Inadvertent injury to the vas deferens resulting in later development of infertility is an operative injury that may occur during contralateral exploration and go unrecognized for many years. This injury was emphasized by Sparkman,[86] and figures from his review have been widely quoted. He stated that tissue examination of 313 hernia sacs from children who had undergone inguinal hernia repair revealed in five instances "segments of the vas deferens" and concluded that there was, therefore, an incidence of "proven injury" to the vas deferens of 1.6%. He then stated that "one can only speculate as to the frequency with which other vasa deferentia were transected or crushed without actual removal of identifiable segments." Because the implications of his data are so far-reaching, they bear careful scrutiny. His information relating to the vas came from patients operated on in three Dallas hospitals. The reference for this data is a personal communication to Sparkman by Wiener, the pathologist, and was listed as "unpublished data." To the best of our knowledge, the data have never been published in detail. We do not have a description of the histologic findings of the "vas," the incidence of incarcerated hernias, type of hernia repair used, or the experience of the surgeons. Walker and Mills[91] in 1983 presented pathologic information on inguinal hernia sacs that cast further doubt on Sparkman's statistics. These authors found that small glandular inclusions were present in approximately 6% of hernia sacs from prepubertal males. They believed that these structures were remnants of müllerian ducts and that, regardless of their cell origin, the inclusions were common findings in hernia sacs and spermatic cord tissue and were not segments of the vas deferens. They emphasized that these structures were of no clinical importance, except for the potential confusion with functional reproductive structures. Perhaps the "vas" segments identified by Wiener may have been these glandular structures.

More objective but indirect evidence on the vulnerability of the vas during hernia repair and exploration has recently been reported by Shandling and Janik.[35, 77] In their experimental studies, the vas deferens of rats was grasped with fingers, nontoothed Adson forceps, bulldog vascular clamps, and mosquito hemostats. Serial studies of the vas were done for 6 months. Damage was found with all manipulations except digital handling.

We performed a computer search of the recent literature on male infertility and found two articles published in 1979 dealing with inguinal herniorrhaphy and infertile men. Homonnai et al.,[34] over a 15-year period, studied 131 men who were referred to the fertility clinic at Tel Aviv and had undergone inguinal hernia repair between the ages of 2 and 35 years. Fourteen percent had slightly smaller testicles on the side of operation, and 85% had normal testicles. Various degrees of pathology in the semen accounted for infertility in the 112 men with normal-sized testicles. These semen findings were thought not to be related to the hernia operation. However, in the 19 men who had decreased testicular size, five had spermatic findings thought to be the result of operative injury. The authors concluded that, although 131 men had had inguinal hernia repairs and were infertile, only 14% of them had testicular atrophy or sperm findings that could be related to the hernia operation. The incidence of incarceration, the experience of the surgeon, and the type of hernia repair performed were not reported.

Friberg and Fritjofsson[25] studied sperm-agglutinating antibodies in infertile men who had undergone inguinal hernia repair. The antigenic properties of sperm had been first described in 1899. Later, it was found that spontaneously occurring agglutinating antibodies could be demonstrated in men and that these antibodies may be an important mechanism in male infertility. Operative injury to the vas deferens during inguinal hernia repair may result in obstruction to the efferent sperm transport pathways and cause the induction of spermatic auto-agglutinating antibodies. In a large series of patients studied for infertility, 76 men were found to have sperm agglutinating antibodies. A unilateral inguinal herniorrhaphy had been performed during childhood on 12 of these (16%). In 10 of the 12 men, the site of the previous herniorrhaphy was explored to ascertain the patency of the vas deferens and to find out if there had been an operative injury. In five of the 10 patients, an obstruction of the vas deferens was found in the area of the previous herniorrhaphy. The authors concluded that, during inguinal herniorrhaphy in a child, accidental transection or ligation of the tiny vas deferens can occur and may be a likely explanation of infertility in men who have had herniorrhaphy before puberty.

These two reports do not shed light on the incidence of infertility in men who have undergone either unilateral or bilateral inguinal operations as children but confirm that an association with herniorrhaphy does exist. It would appear that, if a childhood herniorrhaphy was a common cause of male infertility, more than two articles over the past 10 years would have been published in the infertility literature.

Unilateral Repair and Selected Contralateral Exploration

In order to reduce the number of unnecessary explorations and the danger of operative injury, factors such as age, sex, and side of the clinically apparent inguinal hernia have been used to select patients for exploration. It has been well established that there is a higher incidence of patent processus vaginalis on the side opposite a clinically apparent inguinal hernia in the first year of life, leading many surgeons to limit contralateral exploration to infants. Clausen et al.[13] observed that under 6 months of age a contralateral patent processus vaginalis was found in 73% of patients as compared with 37.3% of patients over 2 years of age. Rowe et al.[71] found that 63% of positive explorations were in the first 2 months of life and that there was a steady fall in patency until after 2 years of age when there was a leveling off at 41% positive explorations. Of greater significance is the parallel increased incidence of development of a contralateral inguinal hernia when the patient presents with a unilateral inguinal hernia in the first year of life. Kiesewetter and Parenzan[41] found that 42% of the patients who had their primary operation before 1 year of age subsequently developed a contralateral hernia, in contrast to 35% of children who had a repair between 1 and 2 years of age. Even more striking was the report of Bock and Sobye,[5] who found that 47.3% of patients who had their primary hernia before the age of one year developed a contralateral hernia, compared with only 11% of those whose primary hernia presented after the first year of life. These data suggest that infants who present with a unilateral inguinal hernia in the first year of life have a two to four times greater chance of subsequently developing a contralateral inguinal hernia than do children whose hernia presents after 1 year of age. Therefore, contralateral exploration during the first year of life prevents the development of a significant number of contralateral hernias; this is not true in older infants and children.

The side of the clinically apparent inguinal hernia is the second factor used to determine whether contralateral exploration is indicated. A review of five series[5, 13, 23, 41, 51] suggests that there is a slight increase in positive contralateral explorations if the patient presents with a unilateral clinically apparent left inguinal hernia. Approximately 62% of right explorations will be positive if there is a left inguinal hernia present, while 56% of left explorations will be positive if there is a right inguinal hernia. These figures do not strongly support the contention that there is a much higher yield when exploration is done in the presence of a left inguinal hernia. Nor is there a great difference in occurrence of a subsequent inguinal hernia whether a left inguinal hernia or a right inguinal hernia is present. Of the five studies analyzed,[5, 13, 23, 41, 51] three showed an increased incidence of right contralateral hernia following unilateral left inguinal hernia repair. In Bock and Sobye's series,[5] the incidence of right contralateral hernia was 20%, compared with 12.8% of left contralateral hernia. In the series of Claussen et al.,[13] the incidence of right contralateral hernia developing after contralateral exploration was 23%, compared with 13% on the left, and in McGregor and associates'[51] series the incidences were 41% and 14%, respectively. This is disputed by the studies of Kiesewetter and Parenzan[41] and of Fischer and Mumenthaler.[23] In the former series, 28% right contralateral hernias and 32% left contralateral hernias developed, while in the latter series there was an 11% incidence of contralateral hernias on each side.

Many surgeons believe that exploration should always be done when a girl has a unilateral inguinal hernia. The incidence of positive explorations in 359 girls with unilateral inguinal hernia was 57%. In Holder and Ashcraft's[32] series of 111 girls with unilateral inguinal hernia and contralateral exploration, 54% had a positive exploration. More recently, Wright[95] explored the opposite side in 100 girls with unilateral clinically apparent inguinal hernia; a significant processus vaginalis was found in 40% of the cases, and the ovary or tube was seen on the side of the patent processus vaginalis in only 5% of these cases. He therefore concluded that the risk of injury to the tube or ovary in a contralateral exploration was quite low, and that contralateral exploration should be done. There is only one study, that of Bock[5], recording the follow-up of girls with unilateral inguinal hernia who subsequently developed a contralateral hernia. The incidence was 8%, but only 25 patients were studied. Since the incidence of a positive patent processus vaginalis on the side opposite an inguinal hernia does not appear to be significantly higher in girls than in boys and the data on development of contralateral inguinal hernia are too small to be able to make any definite conclusions, the major reason for exploring the opposite side in a girl versus a boy would be the relative rarity of encountering reproductive structures that could be damaged within the operative field.

Unilateral Inguinal Hernia Repair Without Contralateral Exploration

Since approximately 20% of patients with unilateral clinically apparent hernia develop a contralateral hernia if only a unilateral operation is done, adding exploration of the groin to the operative procedure is unnecessary in 80% of cases. By performing only a unilateral operation, the danger of injuring the structures of the spermatic cord during contralateral exploration is eliminated. The major disadvantage of a unilateral repair is the necessity, if a contralateral hernia develops, for the patient to be brought back to hospital and subjected to a second operation and anesthetic, with the attendant psychic trauma and physical risk. At the time that many of the reports advocating contralateral inguinal explorations were written in the late 1950s and 1960s, the average hospital stay for a patient with an inguinal hernia repair was 3.3 days. It is now common practice to perform pediatric inguinal hernia repair in a day care unit. The patient is operated on in the morning and released by early afternoon. There is minimal separation from parents and the cost certainly, and psychic trauma probably, are reduced. In the 1980s, the development of pediatric anesthesia has reached the point where repetitive general anesthesia does not carry a high risk.

A common argument used to justify contralateral exploration rather than the unilateral operation has been that, by eliminating the processus vaginalis, one would prevent the development of a subsequent inguinal hernia and therefore eliminate the danger of a possible incarcerated hernia. In our review of published reports of incarcerated hernia, we were unable to find a single patient who developed a contralateral incarcerated hernia after a unilateral inguinal hernia repair. For several reasons, it appears that, if a child has had a unilateral inguinal hernia, a subsequent contralateral hernia will be diagnosed and operated on before incarceration. Several authors have noted the rapid development of a contralateral hernia after a unilateral inguinal hernia repair. Bock[5] found 27% of patients developing a contralateral hernia did so within 1 year and 50% within 3 years. McGregor et al.[52] found that, of the hernias that developed after unilateral hernia repair over a 10–30-year follow-up, 48% developed in the first year and 65% by the second. This information suggests that, if a surgeon elects to do a unilateral inguinal hernia repair, the majority of hernias that will subsequently develop on the opposite side will do so within a few years, still during childhood, and can be detected by routine follow-up by either the surgeon or the pediatrician. In addition, the chances of promptly detecting an inguinal hernia should be increased because the parents have already had recent experience with the clinical characteristics of an inguinal hernia.

Intraoperative Diagnosis of a Patent Processus Vaginalis

The fourth approach to the problem is to attempt, during an inguinal hernia repair, an intraoperative diagnostic maneuver to prove or disprove the presence of a contralateral patent processus vaginalis. Kramer and Davis[42] and Brown[7] described a method of detecting a contralateral patent processus vaginalis intraoperatively by inserting a Bakes choledochal dilator through the open neck of the hernia sac and attempting to slide it transperitoneally into a possible processus vaginalis on the opposite side. Kiesewetter[40] tested this procedure in 100 patients by passing the probe and then exploring the opposite side. He found that there were false abnormal and false normal findings in 13% of cases. Twenty-three percent of cases had equivocal findings. He concluded that, in nearly one third of cases, the dilator technique was not reliable in deciding whether or not to explore the opposite side. He also found that the technique was not applicable in several cases because the neck of the hernia sac was too small and precluded the insertion of the dilator.

The second intraoperative method of diagnosing a patent processus vaginalis or inguinal hernia on the side opposite the clinically apparent inguinal hernia is by intraoperative pneumoperitoneum, first reported by Skeie.[83] In 1970, Bulow[8] reported using artificial pneumoperitoneum in 117 patients as a method of perioperative demonstration of contralateral patent processus vaginalis. There were 93 boys and 24 girls, aged between 1 and 14 years. The hernia sac was isolated and opened and a cannula passed into the peritoneal cavity. The child was then placed in the Trendelenburg position and 500 to 3,000 ml of oxygen insufflated into the abdomen. A patent contralateral processus vaginalis frequently became visible, or crepitus was palpated over the groin. They reported 10% positive tests. One patient with a negative pneumoperitoneum study was subsequently admitted for a clinically apparent contralateral inguinal hernia. There were no air emboli or anesthetic complications. Mild subcutaneous emphysema in the inguinal area developed in one patient following rupture of the sac by the air insufflation.

Recently, Powell[63] reported a series of 256 patients who had intraoperative pneumoperitoneum. They had 61 positive tests, an incidence of 24%. This is well below the average finding of a contralateral process by exploration, which ranges between 45% and 48%, and by positive herniograms, which register between 30% and 60%, and suggests an incidence of false negatives of approximately 20%. The patients in the study did not have routine contralateral exploration, so the true incidence of false negative tests was not determined. During a follow-up period of 6 months to 4 years, three patients with negative tests returned with either a hernia or communicating hydrocele. There were no complications directly related to the procedure.

Preoperative Herniography

Herniography, first described by Ducharme et al.[18] in 1967, has been recommended as a safe and accurate preoperative method of identifying or excluding a patent processus vaginalis in patients with a unilateral inguinal hernia. Only if the examination is positive is contralateral exploration performed. Unnecessary explorations with the inherent risk of operative injury are avoided.

Herniography involves injection of radiopaque contrast medium through the anterior abdominal wall into the peritoneal cavity. With the patient prone and in a head-up position, radiographs will demonstrate filling of a patent processus vaginalis by the contrast medium with an accuracy of approximately 90–95%.[36, 93] In Jewett and associates'[36] large series, herniography identified a contralateral patent processus vaginalis in approximately 60% of infants under 6 months of age and in 30–40% of children older than 2 years, an incidence almost identical to that found by routine contralateral exploration.

In spite of favorable reports from those who have used it, herniography has not found wide acceptance. The procedure is painful; and complications, although uncommon, include abdominal wall hematoma with or without cellulitis, penetration of the intestine or bladder, and adverse reaction to the contrast medium.[20] Although those who have experience with herniography claim that none of these complications are serious,[14, 36] Ducharme himself has recently reported two patients with complications of herniography considered to be potentially life-threatening, namely hematoma of the bowel causing intestinal obstruction and cellulitis of the abdominal wall with septicemia.[19] In both cases, technical factors could be identified that led to these complications; nevertheless, Ducharme concluded that herniography should not be used simply to rule out a hernia or detect a contralateral sac or confirm a communicating hydrocele. He recommends that its uses should be restricted to clarifying the occasional difficult diagnosis of recurrent hernia or recurrent hydrocele.

In patients under 1 year of age with a unilateral hernia, the incidence of finding a patent processus vaginalis on the opposite side by herniography and by operative exploration is approximately 60%—so that the number of patients who would be excluded from exploration on the basis of a negative herniogram is about 40%. Over the age of 2 years, the likelihood of demonstrating a patent processus vaginalis on the opposite side by herniography is 26–40%, so that at least 60% of patients would be spared unnecessary exploration. Herniography therefore provides an effective alternative to routine contralateral exploration.

Comment

After analyzing our own experience and reviewing the literature, we have revised our policy and no longer routinely perform contralateral exploration when a unilateral hernia is present. Instead, we explore the contralateral groin in male infants less than 1 year of age, girls at all ages, and infants and children who have excess peritoneal fluid as a result of ventriculoperitoneal shunts, peritoneal dialysis, or ascites. These patients all have a high incidence of developing contralateral clinically apparent inguinal hernias. This selective policy avoids a large number of unnecessary explorations with the inherent risk of injury to the vas and testicular vessels. We reserve herniography for the following: (1) patients of any age in whom the diagnosis of inguinal hernia cannot be accurately determined clinically after repeated examination, (2) patients with suspected recurrent inguinal hernias not clearly demonstrated by clinical examination, and (3) patients undergoing placement of catheters for chronic ambulatory peritoneal dialysis. In these patients, the herniogram is done intraoperatively after placement of the catheter. If a patent processus vaginalis is demonstrated, it is repaired.

Irreducible Hernia (Incarceration and Strangulation)

An *incarcerated hernia* is one in which the contents of the sac cannot easily be reduced into the abdominal cavity. Incarceration does not refer to changes in the blood supply of the retained part nor to the intestinal obstruction usually produced. A *strangulated hernia* is one that is tightly constricted in its passage through the inguinal canal and has become or is likely to become gangrenous. Whereas in adults incarceration may be tolerated for years, most nonreducible inguinal hernias in children, unless

treated, rapidly progress to strangulation with infarction of the hernia contents. Initially, there is pressure on the herniated viscera as they pass through the internal ring, inguinal canal, and external ring, leading to impaired lymphatic and venous drainage. This in turn results in swelling of the herniated organ, which further increases the compression in the inguinal canal, ultimately resulting in total occlusion of the arterial supply. Progressive ischemic changes take place, culminating in gangrene and perforation of the herniated viscus. In girls, the herniated ovary may become strangulated.

In the 2,764 patients reported by Rowe and Clatworthy,[69] 351 (12%) of the hernias were incarcerated or strangulated on admission. Eighty-two percent of the incarcerated hernias were on the right side and 18% on the left. Eighty-three percent of the incarcerated hernias were found in boys and 17% in girls. Of 359 hernias in girls, 61 (17%) presented with incarceration, whereas, of 2,405 hernias in boys, 290 (12%) presented with incarceration, suggesting a slightly higher incidence of incarceration in girls than in boys. Of significance is the fact that, once incarcerated, 29% of hernias in females require surgical reduction, compared with 17% in boys.

The incidence of incarceration is highest in the first months of life (Fig 78–4). Of all incarcerated inguinal hernias in children, 69% occurred during the first year of life. The remaining 31% occurred between the ages of 1 and 15 years.

Diagnosis

The symptoms of an incarcerated hernia are irritability, abdominal pain, and, possibly, vomiting. A somewhat tense, fluctuant mass is present in the inguinal region and may extend down into the scrotum. The mass is well defined, usually nontender, and does not reduce. Occasionally, it may be transilluminated and must then be distinguished from a tense hydrocele.

With the onset of ischemic changes, the pain intensifies and the vomiting becomes bilious or feculent. Blood may be noted in the stools. The mass becomes tender, and often there is edema and reddening of the overlying skin, with increasing fever and progressive evidence of intestinal obstruction. The testes are usually normal, but in some patients with prolonged strangulation, the testis may be swollen and hard on the affected side, due to venous congestion resulting from compression of the spermatic veins and lymph channels at the inguinal ring by the tightly strangulated hernia mass.[12] On rectal examination the in-

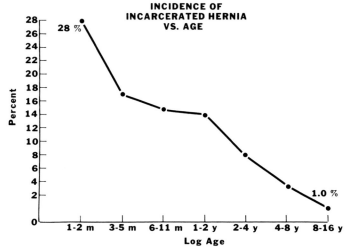

Fig 78–4.—Age-related incidence of incarcerated hernia in 351 infants and children. Newborn infants are at greatest risk for incarceration.

carcerated hernia can be palpated as it enters the internal inguinal ring. Abdominal radiographs demonstrate features of partial or complete intestinal obstruction. Gas may be seen in the scrotum, representing gas within the incarcerated bowel segments.

Differential Diagnosis

TORSION OF THE TESTICLE.—This may occur acutely without previous history of hernia, but there may be a history of undescended testis. With torsion, the testis may be pulled upward. There is acute, severe pain with nausea and vomiting. Local examination reveals a smooth, exquisitely tender mass in the inguinoscrotal region. The swelling does not extend through the external ring into the inguinal canal.

HYDROCELE OF THE CORD OR OF THE CANAL OF NUCK.—There is usually a previous history of swelling in the region of the inguinal canal. There are no associated symptoms, and the swelling is translucent, smooth, movable, and usually nontender. The external ring can be felt, and there is a definite upper limit to the swelling. On rectal examination, no abnormal thickening is palpated in the region of the internal ring. Occasionally, an acute hydrocele of the cord cannot be differentiated clinically from an incarcerated hernia, and operation is required.

INGUINAL OR FEMORAL LYMPHADENITIS.—There is usually evidence of recent infection in the area of lymphatic drainage covered by these lymph nodes, which manifest as tender, fixed nodules. The inguinal canal and spermatic cord are usually normal, as is rectal examination.

TORSION OF THE APPENDIX TESTIS.—This usually presents with acute pain in the scrotum. On examination, there is no evidence of an inguinal hernia in the inguinal canal or scrotum. Once the patient's apprehension has been overcome, it is usually possible to determine that the testis itself is not tender but that there is an extremely tender nodule at the upper pole of the testis.

Management

NONOPERATIVE.—An incarcerated, irreducible inguinal hernia, without evidence of strangulation, should initially be managed nonoperatively.[64, 69] One hundred percent of surveyed pediatric surgeons attempt nonoperative reduction of an incarcerated inguinal hernia in a clinically stable patient without evidence of strangulation. Seventy-five percent of surgeons employ some form of sedation, while 55% utilize some form of elevation. The principle of management is to obtain complete relaxation of the abdominal wall muscles by sedating the infant, relieving the pressure on the neck of the hernia sac. The Trendelenburg position allows the viscera to move cephalad, creating mild traction on the hernia contents. The foot of the crib is elevated to produce an incline of 30–40 degrees; different methods of wrapping the baby are used to maintain this position and prevent the child from slipping down the incline.

The sedated, elevated infant is observed for a period not exceeding 1½–2 hours. If, by this time, spontaneous reduction has not been achieved, most surgeons attempt gentle manual reduction. If this is not successful, immediate operation is performed. Under no circumstances should reduction be attempted under general anesthesia. Approximately 81% of incarcerated hernias reduce without operation. Elective repair is performed 48 hours later, by which time there is less edema, handling of the sac is easier, and the risk of complications is reduced.

OPERATIVE.—When the hernia cannot be reduced or is strangulated, operation is indicated. If there are signs of intestinal obstruction or strangulation, initial management consists of nasogastric intubation and broad-spectrum antimicrobial therapy. Fluid and electrolyte imbalance are corrected by intravenous infusions. When the child's condition is satisfactory, urgent inguinal exploration is undertaken. Should an apparently irreducible hernia spontaneously reduce after the child has been anesthetized, but before the incision is made, most surgeons (95%) proceed with hernia repair and do not attempt to identify the previously incarcerated viscus to ascertain its viability.[72] Nonviable bowel is extremely unlikely to be reduced in this way.

The skin incision is somewhat longer than for elective hernia repair, and the external oblique aponeurosis is opened into the external inguinal ring. The hernia sac is exposed. At this stage, several possible situations may develop:

1. The incarcerated intestine reduces before the sac is opened. If this occurs, the sac should be opened and inspected. If there is no evidence of intestinal ischemia, i.e., no blood-stained or foul-smelling fluid, most surgeons (82%) proceed with hernia repair without attempting to visualize the previously incarcerated bowel.[72] However, when there is evidence of intestinal ischemia, an attempt should be made to locate the previously incarcerated bowel through the sac in order to ascertain its viability. Should this not be successful, we recommend exploration through an abdominal incision in the right lower quadrant. If nonviable bowel is identified, it is resected.

2. If the bowel does not reduce spontaneously and, on opening the sac, is found to be viable, it is reduced and the hernia sac is repaired. Difficulty may be encountered at the internal ring in reducing the bowel. An attempt is made to dilate the internal ring with a small right-angle retractor; should this be inadequate, an incision made superiorly into the arching fibers of the internal oblique muscle permits reduction of the hernia contents.

3. If the hernia does not reduce spontaneously and the viability of the incarcerated intestine is in doubt, the hernia sac is opened and the incarcerated bowel is lifted out for inspection, taking care not to allow it to slip back into the peritoneal cavity. The internal ring is dilated or incised to allow the incarcerated bowel to be withdrawn into the wound until normal intestine is seen proximally and distally. The intestine is covered with a sponge moistened with warm saline for a period of not less than 5 minutes, timed by the clock. The intestine is again inspected for viability, notably mesenteric arterial pulsation, evidence of peristalsis, and color commensurate with adequate perfusion. If it is adjudged viable, it is reduced and the hernia is repaired. If, on the other hand, the intestine appears to be nonviable, resection and end-to-end anastomosis are performed. This may be done through the hernia incision, provided there is adequate exposure and the anastomosis can be easily reduced. Alternatively, a separate abdominal incision can be made to facilitate resection.

Operation for incarcerated hernia in the infant is particularly difficult because the sac is edematous and readily torn, rendering the testicular vessels and the vas vulnerable to trauma. Where possible, the sac is repaired by transfixion and ligation; however, for an edematous, friable sac, continuous or interrupted sutures may be more appropriate. The remainder of the incision is closed in the usual way.

Complications

The overall complication rate after elective hernia repair is approximately 2%; this rises to 19% following operation for incarcerated hernia.[69]

MORTALITY.—In 1939, Thorndike and Ferguson[88] reported an overall mortality of 2.8% for incarcerated hernias treated between 1927 and 1936. In 1954, Clatworthy and Thompson[12] reported one death in 135 patients treated for incarcerated hernia

(0.9%); at the same institution, a survey in 1970 revealed a 0% mortality for 351 patients treated with incarcerated hernia.[69] Since then, there have been several series of incarcerated hernia without mortality.[43, 58, 61]

INTESTINAL INJURY.—The incidence of intestinal infarction is extremely low. Between 1960 and 1965, the incidence of intestinal resection among 351 patients with incarcerated hernia was 1.4%.[69] A review of three series published since 1978 indicates no resections in 221 patients with incarcerated hernia.[43, 58, 61]

TESTICULAR COMPLICATIONS.—The blood supply to the testis may be impaired by compression of the testicular vessels by the incarcerated viscus. The incidence of testicular compromise in association with incarcerated inguinal hernia ranges from 2.6% to 5%.[58, 61, 69] The finding of a cyanotic testicle at emergency operation is common, approximately 11% to 29%. However, the actual incidence of testicular atrophy as indicated by histological examination or diminished size at follow-up is much lower, varying from 0% to a maximum of 19%.[43, 58, 61, 69] Unfortunately, reported series of patients treated by emergency operation consist of small numbers of patients, and the length of follow-up and the criteria for evaluation of the testis vary considerably. Recently, Puri et al.,[64] in an analysis of 87 boys with incarcerated hernia treated by nonoperative reduction, found unilateral testicular atrophy in two patients (2.3%). From the available data, we conclude that vascular compromise of the testis is common, but the risk of actual infarction is low. Unless the testis is frankly necrotic, it should not be removed. The herniated ovary and Fallopian tubes are also susceptible to vascular compromise and infarction.

RECURRENCE.—It is difficult to arrive at a precise incidence of recurrence after repair of an indirect inguinal hernia because factors such as sex and incarceration are not clearly defined in reported series. In general, the reported recurrence rate for uncomplicated hernias is 0% to 0.8%.[32, 39, 51, 70]

Certain factors said to predispose to recurrence include ventriculoperitoneal shunts, sliding hernia, and incarceration. Grosfeld and Cooney,[28] in a series of 25 patients with ventricular peritoneal shunts, identified three recurrent inguinal hernias (12%). In a series of 44 sliding hernias in girls reported by Goldstein and Potts,[27] there was one recurrence, an incidence of 2.3%. Patients operated on for irreducible or strangulated inguinal hernia who require emergency operation are also thought to have a higher recurrence rate. At Columbus (Ohio) Children's Hospital between 1946 and 1952, four of 69 (6%) patients operated on for incarcerated inguinal hernia developed a recurrence.[12] However, at the same institution between 1960 and 1965, 67 patients required emergency operation for incarcerated inguinal hernia, and no recurrences were recorded.[70]

In the series quoted above, with the exception of McGregor's, no attempts were made to contact patients for review. Therefore, the true incidence of recurrence is not known and is probably higher than given because patients who developed recurrences may have sought treatment at other institutions. Other series of patients with incarcerated inguinal hernias do not comment on recurrence in relation to sex, or whether management was operative or nonoperative.

Recurrent inguinal hernias may be indirect or direct. The majority are indirect and probably result from tearing a friable sac, a slipped ligature at the neck of the sac, or failure to ligate the sac high at the internal ring. Less frequently, recurrences present as direct hernias. In Fonkalsrud's[24] series of 14 direct inguinal hernias, four followed previous repair of an indirect hernia (31%). The likely genesis of the direct hernia is injury to the posterior wall of the inguinal canal during dissection of the sac and while mobilizing the structures of the spermatic cord.

Special Considerations

THE PREMATURE INFANT.—There is an increased incidence of inguinal hernia in premature infants. Walsh,[92] in a review of 82 infants weighing less than 2,000 gm, found a 13% incidence of inguinal hernia. Among 28 infants weighing less than 1,500 gm, seven (25%) had an inguinal hernia, compared with four (7%) among infants exceeding 1,500 gm. Rescoria and Grosfeld[65] recently reviewed 100 infants under 2 months of age who required inguinal hernia repair; 30% of these infants were prematures. In a small series reported by Harper et al.[30] of 37 premature infants weighing less than 1,000 gm, the incidence of inguinal hernia was 30%; two of these 11 infants had incarcerated hernias (18%). Although the incidence of incarceration in premature infants is difficult to determine from a review of reported series, Harper's data and our own impressions suggest that in them the risk of incarceration is increased.

There is strong evidence of an increased risk of life-threatening apnea following repair of an inguinal hernia in premature infants. In 1982, Steward[87] reviewed 71 infants undergoing operation for inguinal hernia. Intraoperative and postoperative respiratory complications occurred in 13 of 33 prematures (39%); six had apnea and required manual stimulation and/or mask ventilation. Among the 38 full-term infants, only one developed respiratory complications. Liu et al.[45] reviewed 41 premature infants anesthetized for a variety of reasons; seven of 41 infants who had not required ventilation before operation required postoperative ventilatory support because of apnea. A history of apnea in infants of less than 41 weeks of age from conception was associated with a 50% chance of requiring postoperative ventilation.[45] Apnea is not confined to patients with a positive history of respiratory distress syndrome. In Steward's[87] series, premature infants who experienced apnea were all under 10 weeks' postnatal age and weighed less than 3,000 gm at operation. Only two of six patients who developed apnea had a history of apnea, and nine other infants with a positive history of apnea did not develop postoperative respiratory difficulties.

The cause of postoperative apnea is not known. It may result from a combination of several factors. Immaturity of the diaphragm and intercostal muscles resulting in an increased tendency to fatigue has been documented,[38] probably because of the small number of fatigue-resistant muscle fibers in the ventilatory muscles of premature infants. Further, infants with apnea have alveolar hypoventilation during sleep, and abnormal responses to hypoxia and hypercapnia have been demonstrated. Anesthetic agents, particularly halogenated hydrocarbons, depress the brain-stem ventilatory control mechanisms, decrease the peripheral chemoreceptor response to hypoxia, and may impair the power and endurance of the respiratory muscles.

Admission and careful monitoring of these high-risk infants for 24 hours following operation is recommended. Rescoria and Grosfeld[65] offer the following guidelines for preterm and seriously ill newborn infants: (1) Infants with a reducible inguinal hernia who are already in the hospital are closely observed for irreducibility. The hernia is repaired before discharge, the precise timing of operation depending on the associated disease and the child's general status. (2) For premature infants who develop a reducible inguinal hernia while at home, early operation is recommended because of the high risk of incarceration. Following operation, the patient is admitted to the hospital for a 24-hour period of observation.

VENTRICULAR PERITONEAL SHUNTS AND PERITONEAL DIALYSIS.—In patients with patency of the processus vaginalis, procedures that introduce fluid into the peritoneal cavity may precipitate a hydrocele or hernia. Grosfeld and Cooney[28] found a high incidence of inguinal hernia (14%) following insertion of ventricular peritoneal shunts. Complications were common; 20% developed an incarceration and the hernia recurred in 16%. Based on this study, Grosfeld and Cooney made the following recommendations: (1) after ventriculoperitoneal shunt procedures, infants should be closely observed for the development of a clinical inguinal hernia; (2) operation should be done promptly after diagnosis because of the increased risk of incarceration; (3) the contralateral groin should be explored in the case of a clinical unilateral inguinal hernia.

There is a risk of inguinal hernia developing in patients on chronic ambulatory peritoneal dialysis. Intraoperative herniography is recommended at the time of insertion of the dialysis catheter, and hernia repair is performed if a patent processus vaginalis is demonstrated.[1]

SLIDING INDIRECT HERNIA.—The *Fallopian tube* is frequently found in the wall of the sac. This has been discussed above.

The *appendix* may be partly found in the wall of the sac, forming a sliding hernia. Appendectomy, if it can be done safely, allows high ligation of the hernia sac in the usual way.[66]

In the infant, the *bladder* may lie beneath the internal inguinal ring and may be pulled up with the hernia sac during dissection. High ligation of the hernia sac may include the bladder wall leading to hematuria and possible necrosis of the bladder and extravasation of urine. This is avoided by careful inspection of the neck of the sac at the time of transfixion. Occasionally, the bladder may extend high onto the medial wall of the sac as a true sliding hernia. Shaw and Santulli[79] recommend a flap operation, as in the Goldstein-Potts repair in the female.[27]

DIRECT INGUINAL HERNIA.—Direct inguinal hernia is rarely encountered in children and usually presents as a recurrent hernia after repair of a congenital indirect hernia.[90] At operation, a defect is found medial to the deep epigastric vessels. Fonkalsrud[24] recommends repairing the transversalis fascia; an alternative procedure, which we favor, is the Cooper ligament repair.

FEMORAL HERNIA.—Femoral hernias are rare in children. Fonkalsrud[24] reviewed 5,452 patients with groin hernias, and Burke,[9] 4,567 patients with groin hernias, a total of 10,019 infants and children. There were 21 patients with femoral hernia (0.2%). The ages ranged between 6 weeks and 13 years, and there were 18 females and 10 males, a ratio of almost 2:1. The correct preoperative diagnosis was made in eight of the 21 patients (38%). Four patients had bilateral femoral hernias, and in five patients the hernias were incarcerated. A Cooper ligament repair is recommended.

INHERITED DISORDERS OF CONNECTIVE TISSUE.—Patients with Hurler-Hunter or Ehlers-Danlos syndrome frequently have inguinal hernias and are prone to recurrence unless an inguinal floor repair is added to the usual high ligation of the sac. Coran and Eraklis[16] found that 36% of 50 patients with Hurler-Hunter syndrome followed at Children's Hospital Medical Center in Boston developed inguinal hernias. The recurrence rate was 56%, and formal herniorrhaphy, rather than a simple high ligation of the sac, was recommended.

CYSTIC FIBROSIS.—The incidence of absent vas deferens in the general population is 0.5–1%, based on vasectomy studies.[53, 96] In cystic fibrosis, abnormalities of the vas deferens ranging from obstruction to complete absence are found in 100% of patients.[89] The abnormality is usually bilateral. The incidence of inguinal hernia in cystic fibrosis is increased to between 6 and 15%.[33, 47] Failure to identify the vas deferens at operation should, therefore, lead to a sweat test. Since agenesis of the vas deferens is also found in association with renal dysgenesis in patients who do not have cystic fibrosis, if the sweat test is normal, evaluation of the upper urinary tract is recommended.

INTERSEX.—Rarely, a "girl" with a palpable gonad in the labia may actually be a male with testicular feminization syndrome, or a true hermaphrodite.[11] If an "ovary" is encountered in the hernia sac of a female patient, it should be carefully examined for evidence of testicular tissue. Males with testicular feminization syndrome do not have Fallopian tubes and uterus, but have a small testis. Hermaphrodites, on the other hand, may have a Fallopian tube in the hernia sac and examination of the gonad reveals an asymmetric ova-testis. In both situations, if an abnormal gonad is encountered, it should not be removed. Small wedge biopsy specimens are taken, the gonad is replaced, and the hernia repaired. The patient is further evaluated as discussed in Chapter 139.

SPLENOGONADAL FUSION.—Splenic tissue may be fused to an otherwise normal testis (splenotesticular fusion).[81] Presentation is with a scrotal mass, and the usual preoperative diagnosis is a testicular tumor. Orchidectomy is not necessary; intraoperative frozen section provides the diagnosis and allows preservation of the testis. Spleno-ovarian fusion may also be encountered.

ADRENAL REST.—Ectopic adrenal tissue appearing as a small mass of yellowish tissue in the apex of the hernia sac is not rare and was found in 10 of 385 operations for inguinal hernia (2.6%),[54] an incidental finding in each case.

Congenital Hydrocele

Hydrocele, commonest in infancy, is usually noted to have been present since birth, and often bilateral. Less commonly, a hydrocele does not become apparent until the child is several years of age. A typical hydrocele presents as a swelling of the scrotum that surrounds the testis and fluctuates in size, becoming smaller at night when the infant is asleep. Occasionally, it is tense and may lie above the testis (encysted hydrocele) (see Fig 79–1). At the external ring, the neck (funicular part) of the processus vaginalis narrows, and careful palpation determines that the hydrocele does not extend into the inguinal canal, thus differentiating it from a hernia. This can be difficult to determine in newborns. Attempts to "reduce" the tense hydrocele push it across and above the external ring, giving the impression of an incarcerated hernia, but the hydrocele is more mobile than a hernia and is not tender. The hallmark of a hydrocele is its brilliant transillumination. Occasionally, an incarcerated inguinal hernia containing gas-filled bowel is transilluminated, and diagnostic aspiration should therefore never be attempted.

In most children with congenital hydrocele, the processus vaginalis closes and the hydrocele resolves during the first 12–18 months of life. There is no evidence that a hydrocele will become a hernia, although in theory a hydrocele is a potential hernia.

The recommended management of a hydrocele, therefore, is not to operate during the first 2 years of life unless a hernia cannot be excluded with certainty. We do not distinguish between "communicating" and "noncommunicating" hydroceles, since most, if not all, hydroceles of childhood communicate with the peritoneal cavity to a greater or lesser degree. After age 2 years, we operate if the hydrocele shows no signs of resolution, or if it arises de novo, because in older children a hydrocele is not likely to resolve.

The operation for hydrocele is high ligation of the processus vaginalis, as for inguinal hernia. The distal part of the hydrocele sac is left open, and no attempt is made to remove it. Reaccumulation of fluid in the distal sac is rare and usually resolves spontaneously.

REFERENCES

1. Alexander S.R., Tank E.S.: Surgical aspects of continuous ambulatory peritoneal dialysis in infants, children and adolescents. *J. Urol.* 127:501, 1981.
2. Bakwin H.: Indirect inguinal hernia in twins. *J. Pediatr. Surg.* 6:165, 1971.
3. Banks W.M.: *Notes on Radical Cure of Hernia.* London, Harrison & Sons, 1884.
4. Bassini E.: Nuovo metodo per la cura radicale dellernia. Atti Congr. Ass. Med. Ital. (1887) *Pavia* 2:179, 1889.
5. Bock J.E., Sobye J.V.: Frequency of contralateral inguinal hernia in children. *Acta Chir. Scand.* 136:707, 1970.
6. Bronsther B., Abrams M.W., Elboim C.: Inguinal hernias in children—a study of 1,000 cases and a review of the literature. *JAMWA* 27:524, 1972.
7. Brown R.K.: Hernia diagnosis by transperitoneal probing of the contralateral groin. *Surg. Gynecol. Obstet.* 118:123, 1964.
8. Bulow S.: Artificial pneumoperitoneum during inguinal herniotomy in children. *Acta Chir. Scand.* 140:127, 1974.
9. Burke J.: Femoral hernia in childhood. *Ann. Surg.* 166:287, 1967.
10. Camper P.: *Icones Herniarum.* Frankfurt am Main, Varrentrapp & Wenner, 1801.
11. Carmichael D.H., Vorse H.B.: Female inguinal hernias and testicular feminization. *S. Med. J.* 74:772, 1981.
12. Clatworthy H.W. Jr., Thompson A.G.: Incarcerated and strangulated inguinal hernia in infants: A preventable risk. *JAMA* 154:123, 1954.
13. Clausen E.G., Jake R.J., Binkley F.M.: Contralateral inguinal exploration of unilateral hernia in infants and children. *Surgery* 44:735, 1958.
14. Cooney D.R., Dokler M.: Personal communication, 1984.
15. Cooper A.P.: *The Anatomy and Surgical Treatment of Abdominal Hernia.* London, Longman & Co., 1804–1807.
16. Coran A.G., Eraklis A.J.: Inguinal hernia in the Hurler-Hunter syndrome. *Surgery* 61:302, 1967.
17. Czeizel A., Gardonyi J.: A family study of congenital inguinal hernia. *Am. J. Med. Genet.* 4:247, 1979.
18. Ducharme J.C., Bertrand R., Chacar R.: Is it possible to diagnose inguinal hernia by x-ray? *J. Can. Radiol. Assoc.* 18:488–490, 1967.
19. Ducharme J.C., Guttman F.M., Poljicak M.: Hematoma of bowel and cellulitis of the abdominal wall complicating herniography. *J. Pediatr. Surg.* 15:318, 1980.
20. Ekberg O.: Complications after herniography in adults. *Am. J. Radiol.* 140:491, 1983.
21. Fahlstrom G., Holmberg L., Johansson H.: Atrophy of the testis following operations upon the inguinal region in infants and children. *Acta Chir. Scand.* 126:221, 1963.
22. Ferguson A.H.: Oblique inguinal hernia: Typical operation for its radical cure. *JAMA* 33:6, 1899.
23. Fischer V.R., Mumenthaler A.: Ist bilaterale Herniotomie bei Sauglingen und Kleinkindern mit einseitiger Leistenhernie angezeigt? *Helvet. Chir. Acta* 4:346, 1957.
24. Fonkalsrud E.W., deLorimier A.A., Clatworthy H.W. Jr.: Femoral and direct inguinal hernias in infants and children. *JAMA* 192:101, 1965.
25. Friberg J., Fritjofsson A.: Inguinal herniorrhaphy and sperm-agglutinating antibodies in infertile men. *Arch. Androl.* 2:317, 1979.
26. Gilbert M., Clatworthy H.W.: Bilateral operations for inguinal hernia and hydrocele in infancy and childhood. *Am. J. Surg.* 97:255, 1959.
27. Goldstein I.R., Potts W.J.: Inguinal hernia in female infants and children. *Ann. Surg.* 148:819, 1958.
28. Grosfeld J.L., Cooney D.R.: Inguinal hernia after ventriculoperitoneal shunt for hydrocephalus. *J. Pediatr. Surg.* 9:311, 1974.
29. Halsted W.S.: The radical cure of hernia. *Johns Hopkins Hosp. Bull.* 1:12, 1889.
30. Harper R.G., Garcia A., Sia C.: Inguinal hernia: A common problem of premature infants weighing 1,000 grams or less at birth. *Pediatrics* 56:112, 1975.
31. Hesselbach F.K.: *Neueste anatomisch-pathologische Untersuchungen uber den Ursprung und das Fortschreiten der Leisten- und Schenkelbruche.* Wurzburg, Baumgartner, 1814.
32. Holder T.M., Ashcraft K.W.: Groin hernias and hydroceles, in *Textbook of Pediatric Surgery.* Philadelphia, W.B. Saunders Co., 1980, p. 594.
33. Holsclaw D.S.: Increased incidence of inguinal hernia, hydrocele, and undescended testis in males with cystic fibrosis. *Pediatrics* 48:442, 1971.
34. Homonnai Z.T., Fainman N., Paz G.F., et al.: Testicular function after herniotomy. *Andrologia* 12:115, 1980.

35. Janik J.S., Shandling B.: The vulnerability of the vas deferens. II. The case against routine bilateral inguinal exploration. *J. Pediatr. Surg.* 17:585, 1982.
36. Jewett T.C. Jr., Kuhn J.P., Allen J.E.: Herniography in children. *J. Pediatr. Surg.* 11:451, 1976.
37. Kaplan G.W.: Iatrogenic cryptorchidism resulting from hernia repair. *Surg. Gynecol. Obstet.* 142:671, 1976.
38. Keens T.G., Bryan A.C., Levison H., et al.: Developmental pattern of muscle fibers in human ventilatory muscles. *J. Appl. Physiol.* 44:909–913, 1978.
39. Kiesewetter W.B.: Early surgical correction of inguinal hernias in infancy and childhood. *Am. J. Dis. Child.* 96:362, 1958.
40. Kiesewetter W.B.: Unilateral inguinal hernias in children. *Arch. Surg.* 115:1443, 1980.
41. Kiesewetter W.B., Parenzan L.: When should hernia in the infant be treated bilaterally? *JAMA* 171:287, 1959.
42. Kramer S.G., Davis S.E.: Transperitoneal detection of occult inguinal hernias. *Milit. Med.* 132:512–514, 1967.
43. LeCoultre C., Cuendet A., Richon J.: Frequency of testicular atrophy following incarcerated hernia. *Kinderchirurgie,* 39–41, 1983.
44. Lister J.: On a new method of treating compound fracture, abscess, etc. with observations on the conditions of suppuration. *Lancet* 1:326, 357, 387, 507, 2:95, 1867.
45. Liu L.M.P., Cote C.J., Goudsouzian N.G., et al.: Life-threatening apnea in infants recovering from anesthesia. *Anesthesiology* 59:506, 1983.
46. Loutfi A.H.: Inguinal hernia in infancy and childhood. *J. Egypt. Med. Assoc.* 50:655, 1967.
47. Lukash F., Zwiren G.T., Andrews H.G.: Significance of absent vas deferens at hernia repair in infants and children. *J. Pediatr. Surg.* 10:765, 1975.
48. Lynn H.B., Johnson W.W.: Inguinal herniorrhaphy in children. A critical analysis of 1000 cases. *Arch. Surg.* 83:573, 1961.
49. MacLennan A.: The simplified operation for the cure of hernia in infants. *Clin. J.* 43:29, 1914.
50. MacLennan A.: The radical cure of inguinal hernia in children with special reference to the embryonic rests found associated with the sacs. *Br. J. Surg.* 9:445, 1922.
51. McGregor D.B., Halverson K., McVay C.B.: The unilateral pediatric inguinal hernia: Should the contralateral side be explored? *J. Pediatr. Surg.* 15:313, 1980.
52. McLaughlin C.W. Jr., Kleager C.: The management of inguinal hernia in infancy and early childhood. *Am. J. Dis. Child.* 92:266, 1956.
53. Michelson L.: Congenital anomalies of the ductus deferens and epididymis. *J. Urol.* 61:384, 1949.
54. Michowitz M., Schujman E., Solowiejczyk M.: Aberrant adrenal tissue in the wall of a hernia sac. *Am. Surg.* 45:67, 1979.
55. Mickel R.E.: The external descent of the testes—a mechanical hypothesis revived. *S. Afr. J. Surg.* 20:289, 1982.
56. Morgan E.H., Anson B.J.: Anatomy of region of inguinal hernia. IV. The internal surface of the parietal layers. *Q. Bull. Northwestern Univ. Med. School* 16:20, 1942.
57. Mueller C.B., Rader G.: Inguinal hernia in children. *Arch. Surg.* 73:595, 1956.
58. Murdoch R.W.G.: Testicular strangulation from incarcerated inguinal hernia in infants. *J. R. Coll. Surg. Edinb.* 24:95, 1979.
59. Nyhus L.M., Harkins H.N.: *Hernia.* Philadelphia, J.B. Lippincott Co., 1964.
60. Othersen H.B. Jr., Clatworthy H.W.: Outpatient herniorrhaphy for infants. *Am. J. Dis. Child.* 116:78, 1968.
61. Palmer B.V.: Incarcerated inguinal hernia in children. *Ann. R. Coll. of Surg. Eng.* 60:121, 1978.
62. Potts W.J., Riker W.L., Lewis J.E.: The treatment of inguinal hernia in infants and children. *Ann. Surg.* 132:566, 1950.
63. Powell R.W.: Intraoperative diagnostic pneumoperitoneum (Goldstein test) in pediatric patients with unilateral inguinal hernias, personal communication.
64. Puri P., Guiney E.J., O'Donnell B.: Inguinal hernia in infants: The fate of the testis following incarceration. *J. Pediatr. Surg.* 19:44, 1984.
65. Rescoria F.J., Grosfeld J.L.: Inguinal hernia repair in the perinatal period and early infancy: Clinical considerations. *J. Pediatr. Surg.* 19:832, 1984.
66. Rose E., Santulli T.V.: Sliding appendiceal inguinal hernia. *Surg. Gynecol. Obstet.* 146:626, 1978.
67. Ross L.S., Gallo D.A., Prinz L.M., et al.: Testicular infarction due to strangulated inguinal hernias in infants. *J. Urol.* 102:644, 1969.
68. Rothenberg R.E., Barnett T.: Bilateral herniotomy in infants and children. *Surgery* 37:949, 1955.
69. Rowe M.I., Clatworthy H.W.: Incarcerated and strangulated hernias in children. *Arch. Surg.* 101:136, 1970.

70. Rowe M.I., Clatworthy H.W.: The other side of the pediatric inguinal hernia. *Surg. Clin. North Am.* 51:1371, 1971.
71. Rowe M.I., Copelson L.W., Clatworthy H.W.: The patent processus vaginalis and the inguinal hernia. *J. Pediatr. Surg.* 4:102, 1969.
72. Rowe M.I., Marchildon M.B.: Inguinal hernia and hydrocele in infants and children. *Surg. Clin. North Am.* 61:1137, 1981.
73. Sachs H.: Untersuchungen uber den Processus Vaginalis peritonei als Prädisponirendes. Moment fur die aussere Leistenhernie, Inaugural Dissertation, Dorpat, H. Laakman, 1885.
74. Santulli T.V., Shaw A.: Inguinal hernia: Infancy and childhood. *JAMA* 176:112, 1961.
75. Scarpa A.: *Sull'ernia del perineo* (Pavia: P. Bizzoni, 1821).
76. Schapiro B.: Ist der Kryptorchismus hormonell oder chirurgisch zu behandeln? *Dtsch. Med. Wochenschr.* 38:38, 1931.
77. Shandling B., Janik J.S.: The vulnerability of the vas deferens. *J. Pediatr. Surg.* 16:461, 1981.
78. Shandling B., Steward D.J.: Regional analgesia for postoperative pain in pediatric outpatient surgery. *J. Pediatr. Surg.* 15:477, 1980.
79. Shaw A., Santulli T.V.: Management of sliding hernias of the urinary bladder in infants. *Surg. Gynecol. Obstet.* 124:1314, 1967.
80. Shrock P.: The processus vaginalis and gubernaculum. *Surg. Clin. North Am.* 51:1263, 1971.
81. Sieber W.K.: Splenotesticular cord (splenogonadal fusion) associated with inguinal hernia. *J. Pediatr. Surg.* 4:208, 1969.
82. Singer C.: *Galen on Anatomical Procedures.* London, Oxford University Press, 1956.
83. Skeie E., Kongresreferat, Nordisk kirurgisk forchings 35. Kongres, Reykjavik, 1971.
84. Smith B.A.C., Jones S.E.F.: Analgesia after herniotomy in a paediatric day unit. *Br. Med. J.* 285, 1466, 1981.
85. Snyder W.H. Jr., Greaney E.M. Jr.: Inguinal hernia, in *Pediatric Surgery*, ed. 2. Chicago, Year Book Medical Publishers, 1969, p. 692.
86. Sparkman R.S.: Bilateral exploration in inguinal hernia in juvenile patients. *Surgery* 51:393, 1962.
87. Steward D.J.: Preterm infants are more prone to complications following minor surgery than are term infants. *Anesthesiology* 56:304, 1982.
88. Thorndike A. Jr., Ferguson C.F.: Incarcerated inguinal hernia in infancy and childhood. *Am. J. Surg.* 39:429, 1938.
89. Valman H.B., France N.E.: The vas deferens in cystic fibrosis. *Lancet* 2:566, 1969.
90. Viidik T., Marshall D.G.: Direct inguinal hernias in infancy and early childhood. *J. Pediatr. Surg.* 15:646, 1980.
91. Walker A.N., Mills S.E.: Glandular inclusions in inguinal hernial sacs and spermatic cords. *Am. J. Clin. Pathol.* 82:85, 1984.
92. Walsh S.Z.: The incidence of external hernias in premature infants. *Acta Paediatr.* 51:161, 1962.
93. White J.J., Haller J.A. Jr., Dorst J.P.: Congenital inguinal hernia and inguinal herniography. *Surg. Clin. North Am.* 50, 823, 1970.
94. Woolley M.M.: Inguinal hernia, in *Pediatric Surgery*, ed. 3. Chicago, Year Book Medical Publishers, 1979, p. 815.
95. Wright J.E.: Inguinal hernia in girls: Desirability and dangers of bilateral exploration. *Aust. Paediatr. J.* 18:55, 1982.
96. Young D.: Bilateral aplasia of the vas deferens. *Br. J. Surg.* 36:417, 1949.

79 Eric W. Fonkalsrud

Undescended Testes

HISTORY.—The earliest study of testicular descent was published in 1786 by John Hunter,[54] who found the testis still in the fetal abdomen during the seventh month and in the scrotum in the ninth. He believed that the descent of the testis was directed by a cord or ligament that he termed "the gubernaculum," although he surmised that the fault of maldescent originated in the testicles themselves.

Embryology

The urogenital ridge arises by the fourth gestational week as an invagination of the posterior wall of the coelomic cavity after degeneration of the pronephros. The urogenital ridge divides into the genital fold medially and into the mesonephric fold laterally by the sixth gestational week. A multilayered strip of epithelium covers the genital fold and represents the gonadal precursor, extending caudad from the diaphragm. Because the body trunk elongates cephalad more rapidly than the slower-growing genital fold, there is a gradual caudal shift of the maturing gonadal tissue until it lies approximately ten segments below its level of origin.[5] By the tenth gestational week, the caudal end of the enlarging gonad has developed a mesorchium and lies at the boundary between the abdomen and pelvis.

The embryonic development of the testis may be divided into three phases: intra-abdominal (1–7 months), canalicular (7–8 months), and scrotal (8–9 months). As the anterior abdominal wall develops, the gonad becomes attached at the site of the future inguinal canal by fibers of the developing corda gubernaculum.[17] The contractile nonstriated muscle fibers, and perhaps other components of the gubernaculum, are believed to cause the testicle to migrate through the inguinal canal by the seventh fetal month. The gubernaculum is attached superiorly to the proximal tip of the vas deferens and is believed to divide distally into several tails extending to the dartos muscle in the scrotum, Colles' fascia in the perineum, the pubic tubercle and crest, the inguinal ligament, and the fascia lata in the femoral triangle.[70] Although the testis normally follows the course of the scrotal extension, occasionally it may follow one of the other gubernacular tails to an ectopic location in the perineal, suprapubic, or femoral areas. The descent of the testis is attributed to the three combined forces of intra-abdominal pressure, intramuscular pressure due to the contraction of the muscles draped around the canal, and the guidance and active contraction of the gubernaculum.[104]

The left testis is believed slightly to precede the right in its descent, which possibly accounts for the fact that unilateral undescent is more frequent on the right.[106] The testis and gubernaculum are covered by peritoneum before the descent begins along the inguinal canal, dorsal to the peritoneal cavity. Before and during descent, the testis and spermatic cord enlarge and the vessels of the cord lengthen and become tortuous, increasing the mobility of the testis. The testis then progresses through the inguinal canal, and both the cremaster muscle and the internal spermatic fascia accumulate fibers.

During its descent into the scrotum, the testis carries with it an extension of the peritoneal cavity, the processus vaginalis. Later, the testis becomes covered by a reflected fold of the processus, although it lies entirely outside the peritoneal cavity. After the gonad reaches the scrotum, the gubernaculum becomes indistinct as an identifiable structure. Many aspects of the embryologic and morphologic development of the testicle remain undefined.

Hormonal Influences

Orchiectomy in the rabbit fetus before differentiation of the male urogenital tract has been shown to cause subsequent feminization of both the internal and external genitalia.[39, 60] The Sertoli cells of the testis produce a locally acting substance (müllerian inhibiting substance) responsible for regression of the paramesonephric (müllerian) duct.[12] The Leydig cells produce locally acting testosterone responsible for differentiating the mesonephric duct into wölffian structures.[59] Testicular secretion of testosterone into the general circulation and its peripheral conversion to dihydrotestosterone are responsible for masculinizing the external genitalia.[55] Defects in any of these testicular functions can result in conditions of male pseudohermaphroditism, with or without cryptorchidism.

Crowe, Cushing, and Homans[26] demonstrated the relation of the pituitary to the developing gonad, observing that hypophysectomy caused gonadal atrophy in dogs. Zondek[117] and Aschheim[8] described the presence of gonad-stimulating hormones in the human hypophysis. They[9] also presented evidence that the urine of pregnant women contains a male gonad-stimulating factor different from that found in the urine of postmenopausal women. Jost[60] showed that a sufficiently large amount of circulating male hormone in the fetus may cause testicular descent. Zondek[117] noted that high levels of gonadotropic hormones are present in the human maternal circulation until the third trimester, when they begin to drop. Nelson[86] demonstrated that maternal gonadotropic hormones stimulate production of androgenic hormones from the fetal testis. Deming[29] showed in the immature rhesus monkey that the testis increased 50% in size after injection of gonadotropin because of testicular and interstitial cell enlargement, as well as epididymal tubular enlargement. High levels of gonadotropin are present in the circulation during the last eight weeks of fetal development, and then are almost absent from birth until about 10–12 years of age, when the levels rise again.[113]

Technological advances in the development of highly purified gonadotropins and the application of radioimmunoassay methods have led to a new understanding of the role of hormones in reproductive physiology. Testicular descent is believed to be greatly influenced by the presence of these demonstrable hormones during fetal development; however, there is no clear evidence that true cryptorchid testes with mechanical obstruction will descend further in response to exogenous or endogenous hormones after the first three months of life.[84, 108] Failure of the testicle to descend during the third trimester may be related either to the inadequacy of the hormones, or to the failure of the testis to respond to them. Normal testicular volume is less than 2 ml up to the age of 11 years. At age 12 years, the volume ranges from 2 to 5 ml; at age 13 years from 5 to 10 ml, and at 15 years from 12 to 14 ml.[115]

The gonadotropin deficiency in cryptorchid boys stops the transformation from A to B spermatogonia, so influencing multiplication of the germ cells to a certain extent. In the iatrogenic cryptorchid testis, in the same maldescended position as the true cryptorchid testis, transformation from A to B spermatogonia occurs, even after years of being in an unfavorable position. The Leydig cells develop normally, but secondary changes, such as a significant diminution of the number of germ cells and a thickening of the collagen in the peritubular connective tissue, are discernible, owing to the unfavorable position. When the histologic findings are compared with the luetinizing hormone (LH) and follicle-stimulating hormone (FSH) plasma values, 80% of cryptorchid boys are found to have an impaired hypothalamic-pituitary-gonadal axis. The inability of most prepubertal cryptorchid boys to raise their FSH level, because they have severely damaged testes, underlines their hypogonadotropic state. In only 20% of cryptorchid boys studied has a rise in FSH plasma values occurred, usually in those with better testicular history.

Types of Undescended Testes

Retractile Testes

An extensive study of human inguinal anatomy by Browne[15] indicated that more than three fourths of the testes not located in the scrotum of children were held in a higher position by an "overactive" cremaster muscle. Retractile testes are believed to ascend from the scrotum because of an overactive cremasteric reflex and failure of complete attachment of the lower pole of the testicle to the scrotum by the gubernaculum. By this normal muscular action, the testes are spontaneously held high during periods of stimulation. Such testes usually descend into the scrotum spontaneously when the child is asleep or relaxes, as in a warm bath.

Retractile testes are usually bilateral, in contrast to true undescended testes. At puberty, the testicle becomes larger than the external ring. The cremaster muscle becomes less active, and the retractile testis usually remains in the scrotum. If at any time the testis is seen in the scrotum or can be manipulated into the scrotum, the patient has a retractile testis. Parents can be reassured that the testes will eventually reside in the normal scrotal position, usually well before puberty. In a review of 43 adults who as children were diagnosed as having bilateral retractile testes, Puri and Nixon[89] found the testicular volume normal for age in each; moreover, 74% of the married patients had children, a figure similar to that for the normal adult population of the same age.

Ectopic Testes

Cryptorchidism, a word derived from the Greek *cryptos* (hidden) and *orchis* (testis), correctly defines the position of abdominal undescended testes, although it is now applied to all forms of imperfectly descended testes. The true cryptorchid testis should be distinguished from an ectopic testis that has progressed normally through the inguinal canal and emerged from the external ring but has been directed away from the scrotum into the thigh, the suprapubic area, or the perineum. Transverse ectopia to the contralateral groin has been reported. Although it has been suggested that more than 75% of ectopic testes are located in the superficial inguinal pouch, Scorer[95] and others have indicated that such testes should be considered truly undescended rather than ectopic (Fig 79–1). The rarity of true ectopia is evidenced by the fact that in a review of more than 3,600 newborn males of whom 153 had testicular undescent, Scorer[95] found no infants with true ectopia. Approximately 80% of reported cases of ectopic testes are unilateral, usually normal in size, with normal spermatogenic and androgenic function. Regardless of location, they should be placed into the scrotum surgically because the spermatic cord will be sufficiently long. Attempts to move ectopic testes into the scrotum with hormone therapy have been ineffective.[58]

Anorchia

Normal male (wölffian) ductal development depends on fetal androgenic stimulation from the differentiated testis. With the complete absence of testicular tissue, female (müllerian) ductal development differentiates into the feminine configuration. Rarely, one testis may fail to develop, more commonly on the

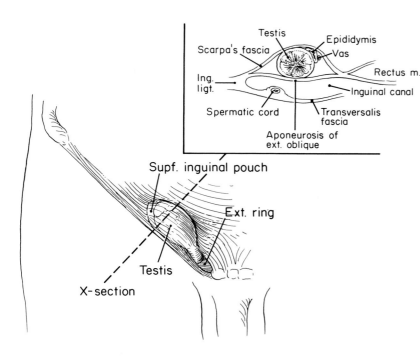

Fig 79–1.—Superficial inguinal pouch into which a retractile testis often ascends and in which a true cryptorchid testis frequently is located. Cross-section shows the location of the testis within the pouch, bounded anteriorly by Scarpa's fascia and posteriorly by the external oblique aponeurosis. The inguinal canal lies deep to the external oblique layer and superficial to the transversalis fascia. (Reprinted by permission from Fonkalsrud E.W.[37])

right and occasionally associated with ipsilateral agenesis of the kidney and ureter.[41] The vas deferens in these patients is usually hypoplastic and ends blindly at the internal inguinal ring. The ipsilateral scrotum is often underdeveloped.

Anorchia has been reported to occur in from 3.3% to 5.2% of boys operated on for cryptorchidism.[1, 42, 58] Anorchia is unilateral in approximately 80% of cases. The surgeon should be encouraged to seek a nonpalpable, high undescended testis inasmuch as total absence is unlikely.

On rare occasions, no viable testicular tissue on either side is evident, although the external genitalia are fully differentiated in masculine configuration at birth and a vestigial vas deferens terminates blindly in the abdomen. Since these patients are both genotypic and fully masculinized, phenotypic males, it is believed that the testes must have been present during early fetal development. Torsion or obstruction to testicular blood supply is believed to play a role in this "vanishing testis syndrome." Puberty is delayed, characterized by persistent elevation of plasma FSH and LH levels and low plasma testosterone levels.

Rivarola and associates[93] recommend giving a course of human chorionic gonadotropin (HCG) to males with bilateral nonpalpable testes to determine whether or not they are anorchic. If high undescended testes are present, the plasma testosterone levels increase significantly, but if the patient is anorchic, the testosterone level does not change. Although abdominal ultrasound and computer-assisted tomography (CAT) may be of some help in identifying intra-abdominal testes, surgical exploration is necessary to establish the diagnosis. Exogenously administered testosterone in early adolescence produces a gratifying response of male sexual maturation. Testicular prostheses can be inserted after testosterone therapy has enlarged the scrotum.

True Undescended Testes

Incidence

The frequency of undescended testes is higher in prematurely born than in term infants. Most undescended testes descend by the end of the first year. Unless there is an associated trouble-some hernia, no therapy is required during the first 2 years of life.

In a combined series reported by Benson and Lotfi,[11] the incidence of nondescent in the prematurely born infant averaged 26.5% and in the full-term infant 3.2%. At the end of the first year of life, approximately 5.4% of premature infants and 0.5% of full-term infants have undescended testes. Extensive statistics derived from a total of over 12 million military recruits over the past one-and-a-half centuries yield an average of 0.28% undescended testes.[114]

Scorer[97] noted that two thirds of the testes remaining undescended in full-term males at birth eventually descend into a normal position in the scrotum by 6 weeks of age (3 months for premature infants). If descent did not occur by this time, the testis never descended completely into the scrotum, remaining smaller than the contralaterally descended gonad. Scorer[95] found that only 28 of 3,612 boys examined at the age of 1 year still had one or both testes undescended, an incidence of 0.8%, probably representing the true incidence of undescended testes in boyhood. In almost half of these boys, the testicle was located in a high scrotal position, a condition that many other authors may not have classified as a cryptorchid testis, thus making the actual incidence of complete undescent approximatelty 0.4%. Scorer[96] further emphasized that the testis must reside in, or be capable of manipulation into, a position more than 8 cm below the pubic crest in order to be considered normally descended. Gonads that cannot be manipulated lower than 4–7 cm below the pubic crest have been classified as "incompletely descended" even though they eventually reside in the high scrotum; they are usually smaller than the normal descended testes of a male of the same age. In the most recent comprehensive statistical review of the subject, Campbell,[19] in 1959, reported that cryptorchidism occurred in 0.44% of adult males, based on 2.8 million U.S. Selective Service physical examinations between 1940 and 1944.

Approximately 14% of boys with cryptorchidism come from families in which other members have had the same condition. The mode of transmission is not known. Cryptorchidism appears frequently in anencephalic fetuses and is present in 44% of boys with a variety of cerebral lesions.[44]

Many physicians believe that in many cases cryptorchid testes will descend spontaneously when a boy passes through puberty to adolescence. Johnson[56] reported in 1939 that 544 cases of undescended testes were found in 31,609 boys (1.7%). Of the 544, 217 were lost to follow-up, 14 were operated on, and spontaneous descent occurred in 313. A similar incidence of spontaneous descent was noted by Ward and Hunter,[110] based on annual school examinations of 19,000 boys in Nottingham, England. Unfortunately, no definition was provided to indicate what constituted an undescended testis, and the examinations were performed by many doctors. Scorer[95] suggested that this series probably included many children with retractile testes, since almost half were reported to have bilateral undescent. It is also likely that many who were classified as having spontaneous descent at puberty had incompletely descended testes that came to lie in the upper scrotum. No clear evidence exists that the hormonal influences occurring at puberty that enlarge the testes and external genitalia, and decrease the muscular pull of the cremaster, have any effect on the embryologic migration of the true cryptorchid gonad from the abdomen or inguinal canal. Thus, contrary to some previous recommendations, there is no valid reason to defer the surgical management of true undescended testes until puberty.

The incidence of bilateral undescent has been reported from 10% to 25%.[42, 105] The right side is undescended slightly more often (53–58%) than the left (42–47%).

Causes of Undescent

The true cryptorchid testis may not descend because of an anatomical abnormality, a primary endocrine disorder, or other undetermined factors. In the majority of cryptorchid patients, there is no evidence of endocrine disorder, and there is evidence of normal secretion of pituitary gonadotropins stimulating the interstitial cells because, even when the testes remain within the abdomen, virilization occurs at puberty and normal levels of plasma testosterone and urinary 17-ketosteroids are usually found. Nonetheless, studies in mice by Hadziselimovic and Herzog[46] indicate that Leydig cells play a decisive role in normal testicular descent. Estrogens administered to the mother during the last trimester cause bilateral undescent; however, simultaneous administration of chorionic gonadotropin permits normal testicular descent. These observations have suggested that exogenous HCG might be efficacious for treating cryptorchid males up to the age of 6 months.

Mechanical failure of testicular descent is believed to stem from improper function of the gubernaculum, a shortened spermatic artery, a tight inguinal ring or canal, abnormal adhesions between the fetal testis and retroperitoneal tissues, cremaster muscle hyperactivity, or some other anatomical abnormality.[30] The gubernaculum is believed to be unimportant, except in guiding the descent of the testes, hence unlikely to be the source of undescent.[112] Abnormality of the abdominal musculature causing a true mechanical barrier is rarely observed during the surgical repair of undescended testes.

Shortening of the spermatic artery is typically the limiting factor preventing complete descent of a high cryptorchid testis and forms the basis for the standard orchiopexy.[36] The artery usually has a normal diameter and presumably carries a normal blood flow, although there is little information to substantiate this view; it is likely that alterations in testicular blood flow correlate with morphologic abnormalities and diminished spermatogenic function. The reason for arterial shortening is not known. Gonadotropic hormones may increase testicular blood flow and arterial diameter, together with testicular enlargement; however, a disproportionate lengthening of the spermatic artery due to hormones has not been reported. The vas deferens is rarely shortened in patients with undescended testes.

Bilateral cryptorchidism is present in almost all patients with certain anomalies of the abdominal wall such as bladder exstrophy, the prune-belly syndrome, and in many infants with gastroschisis and omphalocele. Hypospadias occasionally is associated with cryptorchidism, and in severe cases it may be difficult to differentiate such patients from those with intersex anomalies. More than 6% of boys with bilateral undescent have endocrine disorders causing hypogonadism, such as pituitary deficiency or primary testicular defects which, unless corrected, may adversely affect gonadal function regardless of whether orchiopexy is performed. Klinefelter syndrome, hypogonadism, and germinal wall aplasia have been reported in boys with bilateral undescent.[53]

Various intersex anomalies can be confused with bilateral cryptorchidism. Chromosome analysis; plasma and urine hormone determinations for 17-alpha-hydroxyprogesterone, 17-ketosteroids, pregnanetriol; as well as pelvic ultrasonography and genitourography are helpful procedures in identifying these patients.

Iatrogenic cryptorchidism occasionally follows inguinal herniorrhaphy, particularly in young patients, owing to infection or to attachment of the cremaster muscle or fascia to the abdominal wall during hernia repair.[61] This problem is more frequent in boys with an undeveloped scrotum. The testis should be returned to the scrotum as soon as feasible by operation to prevent testicular injury and degenerative changes.

Complications of Cryptorchidism

Decreased Spermatogenic Function

Failure of normal testicular descent causes the testis to be left at the higher temperature of the body long enough that, unless corrected, normal maturation may be severely retarded. The scrotal temperature ranges between 1.5 and 2.5 C lower than that of the abdomen. Placement of scrotal testes into the abdomen of experimental animals causes degeneration of the germinal epithelium; however, normal germinal maturation may again occur within 3–6 months after return of the testes to the scrotum.[83] Kiesewetter and associates[64] have shown that a maturing puppy testis placed into the abdomen or inguinal position loses weight and develops markedly altered tubular architecture. It is generally accepted that the scrotum and cremaster mechanism act as a servo regulator for the testis and that the degeneration of seminiferous tubules apparent in cryptorchid gonads is, in part, due to their location in a region of higher temperature. This concept has provided a rationale for therapeutic placement of the undescended testis into the scrotum, although it fails to explain why the contralateral, descended testis often has abnormal morphology.

For many years it was believed that the human male gonad remained in a resting stage from birth until approximately the fifth year of life. This opinion has been modified by studies of Städtler and Hartmann[107] showing that continuous testicular growth begins immediately after birth, as indicated by an increase in testicular size, tubular diameter, and the number of spermatogonia. Spermatogonia content, apart from tubular maturation, may be the crucial parameter when assessing the impairment of function of the undescended testis.[81] In a comprehensive study of testicular biopsy specimens, Mengel and associates[81] examined tissue from 515 undescended and 237 unilaterally descended testes. They found that the majority of unilateral cryptorchid testes have normal morphology and spermatogonia content during the first 2 years of life. However, gonads that remain out of the scrotum evidence, by the beginning of the third year, a statistically significant decrease in spermatogonia content and tubular growth. Hadziselimovic and associates[47] similarly observed no ultrastructural differences in the seminiferous tubules between scrotal and undescended testes up to the age of 1 year, but after that time significant differences were noted. Further studies demonstrated that the number of cells involved in DNA synthesis in cryptorchid testes and the rate of DNA production are markedly inferior to those in the contralateral, descended gonad.[75]

The most significant complication of cryptorchidism is the failure of the seminiferous tubules to mature normally, with resultant inability of the gonads to produce normal, mature sperm. Some authors indicate that the undescended testis is abnormal at birth or becomes so shortly thereafter,[74] whereas others maintain that the cryptorchid testis does not show degenerative changes until shortly before adolescence.[4, 101] Most recent studies, however, claim that, although slight histologic differences may be found between the normal and cryptorchid testis during the first 2 years of life, there is progressive, severe degenerative change in the nonscrotal testis during the ages of 2–5 years.[22, 87, 94] The difficulty in interpreting the disparate observations occurs partly because many authors have failed to indicate the degree of undescent of the testis, as defined by Scorer,[95] and because the studies have usually represented a wide age range.[71] The tubular fertility index (percentage of testicular tubules seen to contain spermatogonia, TFI) compares the germinal cell content of testes from different patients and is more reliable than comparison of the mean diameter of the tubules.[70] Testes of normal males have a TFI of 100% by the age of 15 years, but the level in cryptorchid testes remains at approximately 25%, without increase in late adolescence.[33] The TFI appears to correlate closely with the degree of descent of the testis;[33] gonads at the scrotal neck have a TFI of 42.4%, whereas those in the midinguinal canal have a TFI of 19.1%. The unilaterally descended testis in many males commences and completes spermatogenesis at an earlier age than does the normal testis, indicating a degree of hyperplasia. Approximately 4% of unilaterally descended testes show tubular dysgenesis. The remainder appear to have the capability of normal spermatogenesis at puberty.[33] Hecker and Hienz[51] found, in reviewing biopsies of both testes from 125 patients with unilateral cryptorchidism, that, although dystopic testes never matured beyond stage II, the contralaterally descended testes mature normally in only 40% of patients. In 6% of patients, the degenerative changes were even more pronounced in the scrotal than in the undescended testis. In summarizing six published reports, Hecker and Hienz[51] observed that, among 346 patients with uncorrected unilateral dystopia, the sperm counts of only 35% were sufficient to produce fertility. The study does not, however, take into account the wide age range in the patients and varying degrees of sexual activity. Hecker[50] has further suggested that a cryptorchid testis may adversely affect the contralaterally descended testis, and that, in patients older than 5 years, orchiectomy rather than orchiopexy should be performed. Studies by Mengel and Zimmermann[82] suggest that autoantibodies may be produced by an undescended testis, which can cause degenerative changes in the contralateral descended gonad.

Although the salutary effects of repositioning a cryptorchid testis into the scrotum have been reported by many authors, controversy persists concerning the optimal time for performing orchiopexy. It has been suggested that the longer the testis is maintained in the abdominal position before being placed into the scrotum, both experimentally and clinically, the more severe and permanent is the maturational arrest.[2] There is general agreement that placement of the cryptorchid testis into the scro-

tum after puberty does not influence spermatogenesis, and that atrophy of the spermatic tubules is irreversible by then.[2, 50] Karcher[62] reported that 100% of his patients with unilateral undescent who underwent surgical correction before the age of 10 years were normally fertile, whereas only 60% who had orchiopexy between 10 and 14 years of age were fertile, and only 35% who had repair after age 14 were fertile. This study corroborates the observations of Cywes and associates[28] that a satisfactory histologic result can be obtained in two thirds of boys who undergo orchiopexy before the age of 8 years, most of whom will have the possibility of parenthood, based on sperm counts.

If orchiopexy is performed without gentle cord lengthening, preventing tension or partial obstruction of the arterial or venous circulation to the gonad, even further damage may occur in a marginally functional testis.[14, 32] Evaluation of fertility subsequent to orchiopexy is complicated by the fact that the operative repair has not been standardized among different authors. Follow-up fertility studies subsequent to orchiopexy by Gross and Jewett,[42] McCallum,[80] Brunet and associates,[16] and Barcat[10] report a 70–80% fertility rate in males who underwent operation for bilateral cryptorchidism between 8 and 10 years of age. Bramble and associates[14] recorded an overall fertility rate of 48% in 21 males who underwent bilateral orchiopexy at an average of 11.5 years, using MacLeod's criteria[73] for seminal analysis. Studies by Cywes and associates[28] indicate that 68% of boys with unilateral undescent who undergo repair before age 8 have more than 200 million spermatozoa per milliliter and are fertile. Only 34% of boys who underwent repair of bilateral cryptorchidism before puberty had spermatozoa counts of more than 20 million. Most authors agree that the standard for fertility should be at least 20 million spermatozoa per milliliter, coupled with good motility and morphology.

Current evidence suggests that the optimal time for performing orchiopexy is before the age of 5 and possibly as early as 2 years. Most pediatric surgeons perform elective orchiopexy on boys younger than 4 years. Nonetheless, conclusive fertility studies involving sperm analyses and hormone assays to document the efficacy of this approach have not been reported.

Lee and associates[69] found that values for LH and FSH were elevated in bilaterally anorchic males. They concluded that elevated FSH levels correlate with compromised testicular function, whereas elevated LH levels indicate atrophic gonadal tissue, even in the young boy. Bramble and associates[14] suggest that the inverse relation of FSH hormone concentrations to sperm count indicates that secretion is controlled, at least partly, by some nonandrogenic factor produced in the testis and is associated with spermatogenesis.

Contrary to previous views, several reports state that androgen output by a cryptorchid testis may be reduced.[31, 90] Mancini and associates[74] noted impaired function of Sertoli cells in cryptorchid testes. It is uncommon for cryptorchid males to have abnormal Leydig cell function, but, when this occurs, LH levels become elevated, presumably as a result of decreased feedback of testosterone or its metabolites. Normal testosterone levels were recorded in 20 of 21 adults subsequent to bilateral orchiopexy in childhood, confirming the usual clinical observation that it is rare for a male with unilateral or bilateral undescent to have less androgen production or to show failure of virilization unless severe atrophy of both gonads is present.[7] Libido and potency are rarely impaired.

Hernia

The peritoneum from the lower abdomen normally descends with the testis through the inguinal canal and into the scrotum to form the eventual tunica vaginalis. The narrow processus vaginalis communicating between the tunica and the peritoneal cavity usually stretches and becomes compressed by the abdominal wall musculature in the inguinal canal, causing its obliteration within the first few weeks of life in normal males. When the testis is arrested in its normal descent, the factors usually causing closure of the patent processus do not become effective, resulting in persistence of the processus, which in most patients is sufficiently large to be classified as a hernia. Most authors indicate an incidence of accompanying hernia greater than 65%.[20, 42, 63, 105] Hernias may become symptomatic during the first several months of life so that repair is necessary despite the delicacy of the spermatic cord, which makes this a suboptimal time for orchiopexy. The trend to perform elective orchiopexy early, around the age of 2 years, has been reflected in the fact that surgeons generally repair nearly all clinically symptomatic hernias in cryptorchid males when they are diagnosed, regardless of age. Although cryptorchidism is usually asymptomatic, the presence of an associated hernia may produce inguinal pain. If a cryptorchid male undergoes repair of a symptomatic hernia, the testis should be simultaneously placed into the scrotum, because later reoperation in a scarred wound may risk serious injury to the testicular blood supply.

Torsion of the Undescended Testis

The true relation of torsion to testicular undescent is unknown, since almost all involved gonads are located within the scrotum. Additionally, it is rarely necessary to perform a concomitant orchiopexy to lengthen the spermatic cord sufficiently to permit placing the gonad into the lower scrotum. Hand[49] reported only three cases of torsion among 153 cryptorchid patients who were followed up to 33 years. When torsion is present in a cryptorchid testis, a nonviable gonad is more likely to result than if torsion occurs in a noncryptorchid testis.[68] Torsion may occur in an undescended testis that has undergone malignant degeneration. Of the adult cryptorchid testes involved in torsion, 65% were found to be malignant.[92]

Trauma

A cryptorchid testis residing in the inguinal canal is more vulnerable to trauma than is the normally descended gonad because of the relatively rigid posterior wall of the canal. Contraction of the abdominal musculature subjects the cryptorchid testis lodged in the inguinal canal to repeated alterations in pressure which, under certain circumstances, may be traumatic and painful. Testes lying in the superficial inguinal pouch are often exposed to direct and recurrent trauma.

Psychological Factors

An empty scrotum may cause considerable anxiety and embarrassment, often causing feelings of physical inferiority and concern about virility.[43] Anxiety is expressed by patients and parents regarding the possibility of sterility. Assurance from the physician about the likelihood of eventual fertility in most patients with unilateral undescent, and of virility in the majority of those with bilateral undescent, after proper management, alleviates many such concerns.

Development of Malignancy

A wide diversity of opinion exists regarding the role that cryptorchidism plays in testicular tumorogenesis. Various reports have shown that from 3.5% to 11.6% of testicular tumors arise in cryptorchid testes.[37] Gilbert and Hamilton[40] reported a collected series of over 7,000 cases of testicular malignancies, of which 840 were situated in an undescended testis (12% incidence). They indicated that cryptorchid males are approximately 48 times more likely to develop a testicular malignancy than those with normally descended testes. Since the average age of patients who develop testicular tumors is 35 years,[23] it is not surprising that numerous reported series of children who have undergone surgical repair of cryptorchidism fail to list any cases of malignancy.[69, 90] In a collective review of the literature, Martin and Menck[79] found 166 cases of germinal tumors in testes subsequent to orchiopexy. The age at which orchiopexy is performed appears to be a critical factor, inasmuch as they could find only five cases of tumor in boys who had undergone orchiopexy younger than 10 years.[103]

Inasmuch as most tumors reported to occur in cryptorchid males are germinal in origin, it is quite likely that a direct correlation exists between the degree of dysgenesis of the seminiferous tubules and the development of malignancy.[101] Indeed, the higher incidence of dysgenetic tissue in cryptorchid testes may account for the relative vulnerability to malignant degeneration.[102] The contralateral, descended testis occasionally shows evidence of varying degrees of dysgenesis; it is not surprising, therefore, that several authors note an increased incidence of neoplasia in the contralateral, descended testis in patients with unilateral undescent.[3] Approximately one of five testicular tumors reported in patients with cryptorchidism has developed in the scrotal testis.[57] Seminoma constitutes 30–40% of tumors in scrotal testes but 60% in undescended testes.[102] An abdominal cryptorchid testis is five times more likely to develop a malignancy than is an inguinal testis.[79] In a survey of 15 reports, Campbell[18] found that, although only 14.3% of undescended testes were intra-abdominal, such testes accounted for 48.5% of all tumors in cryptorchid testes. Symptomatic intra-abdominal testes frequently develop malignancy. When a testis cannot be identified at the time of inguinal exploration, intraperitoneal exploration is necessary to rule out a high abdominal testis. If an atrophic intra-abdominal gonad is found, it is wise to remove this testis rather than attempt to place it into the scrotum because the risk of developing malignancy outweighs the likelihood of achieving significant spermatogenic function. Following this same reasoning, several authors have suggested that orchiectomy be performed for unilateral undescent when the gonad has not been placed in the scrotum by the ages of 12 and 15 years.[27] Patients who undergo orchiopexy, and their families, must be advised of the risk of subsequent malignant degeneration.

Krabbe and associates[65] performed testicular biopsies in 50 men previously treated for undescended testes, three of whom had a pattern of carcinoma in situ. A characteristic abnormality of the seminiferous epithelium is present in this lesion. It is rare that carcinoma in situ is identified earlier than the age of 18 years,[100] although several reports suggest that malignant changes occur well in advance of overt tumors. It is possible that early orchiopexy, by age 2 years, might alter the incidence of this lesion.[77]

Any undescended testis which, when exposed surgically, shows considerable variation in size or configuration from what is normal for that age should have a biopsy and be observed closely during the ensuing years, or even removed. Dysplastic gonads occurring in males aged 8–10 years should be removed.

Seminoma accounts for approximately 60% of the germinal cell tumors found in cryptorchid testes.[103] Teratocarcinomas, embryonal carcinomas, and occasional adult teratomas are the other malignancies typically reported. Because of the surgical alteration in lymphatic drainage of the testis after inguinal or scrotal operation, it has been recommended that the inguinal lymph nodes be included in the therapeutic program, either by groin dissection or with irradiation as considered appropriate.[52, 76, 77]

The factors responsible for the association of germinal neoplasms of the testis in cryptorchidism have not been established; an altered environment, germinal atrophy, ischemia, hormonal imbalance, occurring separately or in various combinations, have been implicated. Although clinically these factors may suggest a cause-and-effect relation, there has been no laboratory substantiation of this view. Testicular tumors have not been produced experimentally.

Associated Anomalies

In addition to the major anomalies of the abdominal wall, endocrine disorders, and intersex malformations often occurring in males who have bilateral cryptorchidism, certain other developmental defects frequently are seen in patients with bilateral, and less frequently with unilateral, undescent.

URINARY TRACT ANOMALIES.—Approximately 9% of patients admitted for orchiopexy alone have major renal anomalies and another 9% have minor anomalies.[24] The most common major renal anomalies are renal hypoplasia, renal agenesis, ureteropelvic obstruction, and horseshoe kidney. It has been recommended that any male with urinary tract symptoms and unilateral undescent, as well as all those with bilateral cryptorchidism, undergo an intravenous pyelogram during the first year of life.[111] Others have found that the incidence of major renal anomalies is approximately 3% and that they are rarely associated with unilaterally cryptorchid testes. Therefore, routine urography in the asymptomatic child is not necessary.[109] Hypospadias occurs in approximately 3% of boys with bilateral undescent.

ANOMALIES OF THE EPIDIDYMIS AND VAS DEFERENS.—Abnormalities of the epididymis and vas deferens are common in cryptorchid testes, and the surgeon should inspect the testis closely at orchiopexy to note any unusual appearance. Many of these anomalies can limit the flow of spermatozoa and thus become a source of infertility.[96]

CHROMOSOMAL ABNORMALITIES.—Although occasional patients are reported to have chromosomal abnormalities in association with cryptorchidism, it has been our experience that changes in the chromosomal pattern are found mainly in those with bilateral cryptorchidism, in whom intersex anomalies are more frequent, and that chromosomal evaluation is justified in many cases of bilateral undescent.

Diagnosis

In over 85% of boys with an empty scrotum, the gonad may be palpated in the inguinal canal, superficial inguinal pouch, or in an ectopic location. An undeveloped scrotum is rare and usually occurs in association with a high inguinal or abdominal testis, or with atrophic or absent gonads. Careful examination with warm hands, and with the patient relaxed in a recumbent position, usually permits identification of retractile testes, which do not require specific treatment. When the gonad is identified in a suprascrotal position, notation should be made of the size compared with the contralateral gonad and to males of the same age, and also with regard to the shape and consistency of the testis. After palpation, the fingers of the examining hand are pressed flat against the patient's lower abdomen just above the gonad and then slowly brought down over the external inguinal ring with a sweeping motion in an attempt to manipulate the testis downward into the scrotum. The fingers of the other hand may assist by grasping the testis when it passes the scrotal neck, directing it into the scrotum as far as possible. After repeating this maneuver several times, the lowermost location in which the testis can be positioned should be noted, e.g., inguinal canal, superficial inguinal pouch, high scrotum, or low scrotum (normal).[95] If the

gonad cannot be manipulated into the scrotum, further examination in the standing or sitting position with legs crossed may cause the testis to descend slightly lower. Occasionally, mild sedation may be necessary to facilitate an optimal examination in a hyperactive child. If after several examinations the physician is unable to palpate a testicle, it is probably located within the abdomen, atrophic, or absent. Dogmatic statements regarding absence of a testis should not be made after a single examination.

When the testes cannot be palpated, a diagnostic course of HCG with plasma testosterone determination before and after the injection indicates the presence of Leydig cells, if the testosterone levels become elevated. Diagnostic ultrasound and/or CT scan may be helpful in identifying abdominal testes noninvasively. Selective arteriography, venography, and retroperitoneal pneumography can assist in locating abdominal testes; however, the indications for performing these extensive studies are minimal, since nearly all patients with nonpalpable gonads require surgical exploration.

Treatment

A testicle that fails to descend spontaneously, or that cannot be manipulated into a low scrotal position after the age of 12 months, should be considered cryptorchid and requires treatment. There is considerable disagreement regarding what constitutes optimal therapy and at what age it should be provided.

Hormone Therapy

Exogenously administered HCG may help to cause descent in occasional patients with bilateral cryptorchidism and can be helpful in causing descent of gonads that have no mechanical factor limiting descent. Nevertheless, there is no clear evidence in the United States that HCG enables the typical inguinal or abdominal undescended testes with short spermatic arteries to descend and remain permanently in the scrotum. There is also no clear evidence that hormone therapy improves testicular structure or fertility in cryptorchid males beyond that which would have occurred spontaneously at puberty. Nonetheless, recent studies in which HCG has been given during the first four years of life suggest that subsequent function of the gonad may be better than if hormones were not used. There also is no clear indication that hormone therapy will in any way benefit closure of the commonly accompanying hernia. Because of the occasional adverse effects accompanying injudicious administration of gonadotropins, this treatment should be used cautiously, with a definite protocol, in appropriately selected patients. Treatment consists of 10,000 units of HCG given over a short course of 1½–2 weeks by intramuscular injection in five to six doses. Lattimer and associates[66] believe that HCG could be helpful in enlarging the severely underdeveloped scrotum before orchiopexy. Others suggest a trial of HCG for almost all patients with bilateral undescent and for those with unilateral undescent in whom mechanical factors are not believed to be present. Most conclude that gonadotropins cause descent of only those testes that ultimately would have descended without treatment. Hormone administration is therefore recommended as a method of distinguishing testes destined to descend spontaneously from those requiring orchiopexy. Gonadotropin administration, even when it fails to cause descent, enlarges the testis and thus facilitates the subsequent operation. Early epiphyseal closure is an untoward effect that may occasionally be precipitated by hormone stimulation. Injudicious hormone treatment also is attended by the risk of seminiferous tubular degeneration and even atrophy of the retained undescended testis, particularly if high doses are given.[10, 85]

Testosterone administration has been reported to induce descent of cryptorchid testes in approximately one-fourth of the patients in whom it has been used.[48] The results achieved with androgen therapy have been far less convincing than those obtained with HCG and the reported clinical experience is sparse.

The isolation of luteinizing hormone-releasing hormone (LH-RH) has introduced new concepts in the treatment of cryptorchidism. Hadziselimovic[45] reports that 17 of 30 boys with cryptorchidism treated by intranasally administered LH-RH responded by having the testes descend into the scrotum. The results with LH-RH therapy have reportedly been superior to those obtained with the use of HCG. FSH levels have reportedly decreased significantly after 4 weeks of LH-RH therapy. No alterations in testosterone concentrations have been noted during treatment. The puberty-like side effects often observed with HCG therapy are absent with LH-RH. The success rate with LH-RH intranasal therapy is approximately 50%. Good results have been obtained with testes in the low inguinal canal, and this form of therapy has been recommended for both unilateral and bilateral cryptorchidism. The duration of treatment is usually one month, the dose 1.2 mg per day. The most noticeable descent is seen during the first 2 weeks. A slightly improved result has been noted with combined treatment using LH-RH followed by HCG therapy.[45] We currently use intramuscular HCG preoperatively in boys with unilateral undescent who have a small testis or in whom the gonad is located high in the inguinal canal or in the retroperitoneal space. We give between 7,000 and 10,000 IU of HCG, depending on the age of the patient, giving 1,500 IU every 2–3 days. We also use HCG in the same dosage level for boys with bilateral undescent who do not have a true mechanical cause for undescent, i.e., exstrophy of the bladder, omphalocele, prune-belly syndrome, etc.

The higher the cryptorchid testis resides above the scrotum, the more dysgenetic the morphology is likely to be. High testes rarely descend into the scrotum with HCG or LH-RH and

should usually be treated by orchiopexy by the age of 2–3 years. The undescended testis does not mature normally after the age of 2 years and may produce adverse effects on the contralateral descended testis, possibly by an autoimmune mechanism. A course of HCG for boys with low-lying undescended testes, both unilateral and bilateral, may produce descent in as many as 15% of patients, and may make the technical aspects of orchiopexy easier in those who do not respond. Unilateral cryptorchid testes that are dysplastic or located high should generally be removed before late adolescence.

Orchiopexy

The technique of orchiopexy currently in general use has been described and illustrated by several authors.[42, 67, 88, 106] The objective of the repair is to alter the course of the spermatic artery from the renal pedicle, to the internal inguinal ring, to the external inguinal ring, and to create in its place a direct line from the renal pedicle to the scrotum (Fig 79–2). An incision approximately 3–4 cm long is made through the lowermost abdominal skin crease (Fig 79–3). The external oblique aponeurosis is opened in the direction of its fibers through the external ring. An occasional patient with a high-lying testis has an unusually small external ring. The testicle is usually found protruding through the external ring inferior to the internal oblique muscle, with attachments to the pubis. The testis with its surrounding tunica vaginalis is mobilized from the gubernaculum and often tenacious surrounding attachments, permitting it to be elevated with gentle traction (Fig 79–4). The cremaster muscle is mobilized gently from the spermatic vessels and the vas deferens up to the level of the internal inguinal ring. The internal oblique muscle is divided laterally to the internal ring for approximately 1 cm to obtain better exposure (Fig 79–5). The inferior epigastric artery and veins are divided, and the transversalis fascia is

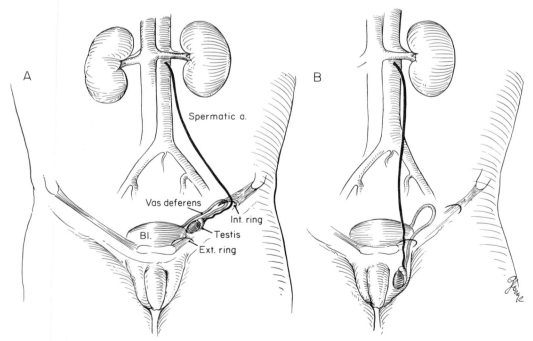

Fig 79–2.—Shortening the distance the spermatic artery must traverse. **A,** lengthy course of the spermatic artery descending from the aorta through the internal inguinal ring to the undescended testis in the inguinal canal. **B,** by transposing the internal inguinal ring medially to the pubis, the spermatic artery may be lengthened effectively to permit the testis to be placed into the scrotum, the basis of the standard orchiopexy. (Reprinted by permission from Fonkalsrud E.W.[37])

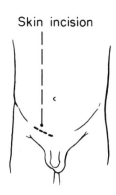

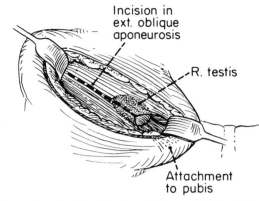

Fig 79–3.—Cutaneous incision for orchiopexy, made through the lower abdominal skin crease. The external oblique aponeurosis is incised, exposing the testis in its tunica vaginalis, usually lying just beneath the external ring or in the superficial inguinal pouch. (Reprinted by permission from Fonkalsrud E.W.[37])

opened widely through the internal ring to permit wide exposure of the retroperitoneal space (Fig 79–6). The accompanying hernia sac is separated from the spermatic vessels and the vas, often a delicate maneuver because the structures are tenaciously adherent and the sac tears easily. This maneuver can be facilitated by injecting a small amount of saline through a small-gauge needle between the hernia sac and the cord structures and then gently developing a plane by blunt dissection with a fine clamp (Fig 79–7). High ligation of the hernia sac is performed with a fine transfixion suture. The gonad is inspected to note its size, consistency, and any abnormal features. Biopsy is not routinely recommended because of the risk of further injury to the delicate organ, especially in the young child, unless any unusual features are apparent or if the child is older than 12. A thin wedge biopsy running longitudinally on the side opposite the epididymis is preferred, closing the wound with fine sutures. The testicle is then replaced into the tunica, the proximal end of which is closed loosely to prevent dislodgment outside the sac (Fig 79–8). The dissection is continued into the retroperitoneal space by elevating the peritoneum, sharply dividing the lateral spermatic fascia and bluntly mobilizing the spermatic vessels up to the lower pole of the kidney and the vas over to the bladder (Fig 79–9). The scrotum is then forcibly stretched by inserting a finger through the wound to the lowermost portion of the sac. A

small incision is made through the scrotal skin at this point and a space sufficiently large to accommodate the testis is developed between the dartos muscle and the scrotal skin by blunt dissection (Fig 79–10). A small opening is then placed in the dartos fascia and muscle layer through which a clamp is passed superiorly to direct the testicle downward through the scrotum (Fig 79–11). Twisting of the spermatic vessels must be avoided. The upper edge of the tunica is stitched to the dartos layer circumferentially to prevent upward displacement or subsequent torsion, and the testis placed subcutaneously. The scrotal skin is closed loosely with fine sutures of absorbable material (Fig 79–12). The transversalis fascia is then closed with nonabsorba-

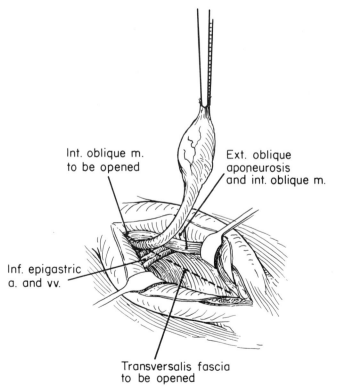

Fig 79–4.—The tunica vaginalis and enclosed testicle are mobilized from the gubernacular and fascial attachments to the pubis and adjacent soft tissues. (Reprinted by permission from Fonkalsrud E.W.[37])

Fig 79–5.—The cremaster muscle is teased free from the spermatic vessels and vas up to the internal inguinal ring. The internal oblique muscle is divided superior and lateral to the internal ring over a distance of 1 cm. (Reprinted by permission from Fonkalsrud E.W.[37])

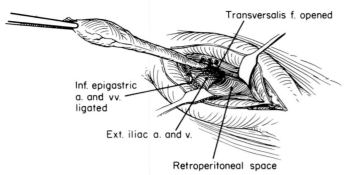

Fig 79–6.—The inferior epigastric artery and veins are divided, and the transversalis fascia is incised from the internal ring medially to the pubis to provide wide exposure of the retroperitoneal space. (Reprinted by permission from Fonkalsrud E.W.[37])

ble sutures, leaving a small opening just lateral to the pubis to function as the new internal inguinal ring (Fig 79–13). The internal oblique muscle is sutured to the shelving edge of the inguinal ligament, again leaving a small opening medially for the new internal ring. The external oblique aponeurosis is reapproximated. The skin closure is the same as that used for herniorrhaphy wounds. In children under 10 years of age, the operation is usually performed as an outpatient procedure. Despite the arrangement of the external ring almost directly over the new internal ring, which appears conducive to developing a direct hernia, this complication is extremely rare.

Correction of the High Cryptorchid Testis

The operative technique described for the standard orchiopexy should be used for almost all cryptorchid testes; deletion of any

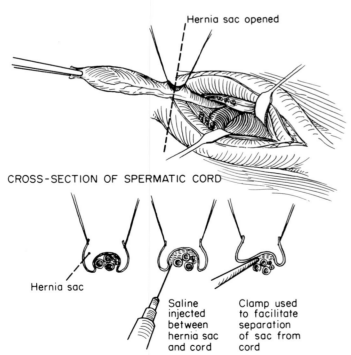

Fig 79–7.—The hernia sac is dissected free from the spermatic vessels and vas. Cross-section shows saline injection technique that occasionally is useful in separating a delicate but tenaciously adherent hernia sac from the spermatic vessels and vas. (Reprinted by permission from Fonkalsrud E.W.[37])

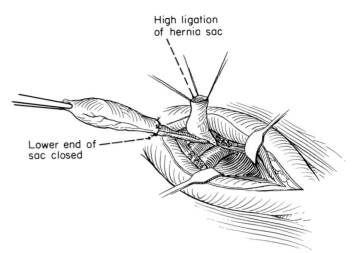

Fig 79–8.—The testicle is inspected for abnormalities and replaced into the tunica. The testicular end of the hernia sac is sutured closed to prevent dislodgment of the testicle outside the tunica. The proximal end of the hernia sac is ligated. (Reprinted by permission from Fonkalsrud E.W.[37])

of the steps is likely to result in a less than desirable outcome in which the spermatic vessels are subjected to undue tension with increased risk of vascular compromise and testicular retraction from the low scrotum. For high-lying testes that cannot be brought into the low scrotum by the standard orchiopexy (ap-

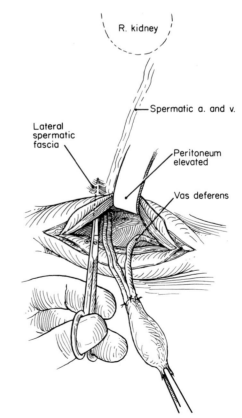

Fig 79–9.—The lateral spermatic fascia is divided, and the spermatic vessels dissected bluntly from the posterior surface of the peritoneum and retroperitoneal tissues up to the lower pole of the kidney. (Reprinted by permission from Fonkalsrud E.W.[37])

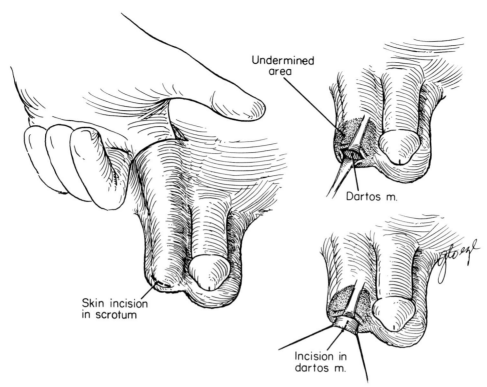

Undermined
area

Dartos m.

Incision in
dartos m.

Skin incision
in scrotum

Fig 79–10.—The scrotum is distended by the surgeon's index finger, and a small incision is made through the most dependent portion of the scrotal skin.

The dartos muscle and fascia are dissected free from the scrotal skin to form a subcutaneous pouch. (Reprinted by permission from Fonkalsrud E.W.[37])

proximately 5%), two-stage repair is preferred to placing great downward traction on the gonad.[34, 91] The lower pole of the tunica may be attached to the pubis or adjacent muscle, or it may be attached to an external cottonoid pledget by means of a pullout stitch of nylon. An interval of approximately one year is recommended before the second-stage operation is performed. Zer and associates[116] were able to position the testis satisfactorily in the low scrotum in 90% of their 62 patients on whom staged orchiorrhaphy was performed. Corkery[25] recommended placing the testis and spermatic cord in a Silastic envelope at the first operation in order to reduce the extensive adhesions between the testis and the inguinal tissues that usually make the second operation more tedious and bloody. Caution should be taken to avoid injury to the vessels of the gonad during the second operation because subsequent testicular atrophy is not uncommon, while the additional benefits of the second operation have not been clearly documented.

Fowler and Stephens[38] developed the "long-loop vas" orchiopexy, a technique for correcting the high undescended testis. The spermatic artery and veins are divided high up, which permits sufficient mobility to place the gonad into the scrotum in one operation. The testis then derives its blood supply entirely from a secondary vascular loop from the vessels of the vas deferens, collaterals from the deep epigastric vessels, and myriad branches entering the posterior wall of the processus vaginalis from the area of the gubernaculum (Fig 79–14). It has been stressed that the success of this operation depends on the fact that no dissection is performed within the substance of the cord, and that division of the spermatic vessels should be as high above the testicle as feasible to assure optimal vascularity. Adequacy of collateral circulation may be assessed by incising the tunica albuginea of the testis, then transiently occluding the spermatic

artery and examining for continued bleeding. This technique did not gain popularity until 1972 when Clatworthy and associates[21] reported 24 good results following 32 operations, three fourths of which were for intra-abdominal testes. Inasmuch as most authors have reported occasional atrophic testes following division of the spermatic artery, this procedure should be used cautiously and only when other techniques do not appear feasible.

Flinn and King[35] described a midline transabdominal approach, especially useful for patients with bilateral high cryptorchidism in whom both testes can be brought down through a single incision. This operation is particularly suitable for patients whose inguinal structures have been distorted from previous operations, as well as those with suspected testicular agenesis or intersex malformations. They noted uniformly good results in each of the 25 patients on whom the operation was performed. The preperitoneal approach also has been recommended for mobilizing the testis and spermatic cord.[13]

Microsurgical techniques for anastomosis of the spermatic vessels to the vessels of the thigh or branches of the inferior epigastric vessels have been reported with some success in the management of the high undescended testis. Silber and Kelly[99] reported the first successful case of microvascular reconstruction in 1976.

Abdominal Exploration

When the testicle cannot be located after extensive exploration of the retroperitoneal space, it has been our experience that transperitoneal exploration through the same inguinal incision slightly extended (LaRoque maneuver) is necessary to completely exclude the possible presence of a gonad. The intra-abdominal testis may be missed easily during the retroperitoneal

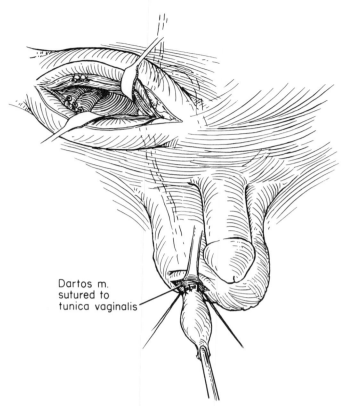

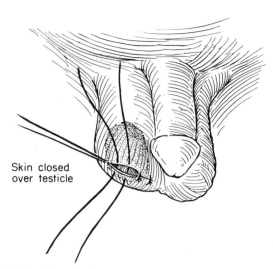

Fig 79–11.—The testicle is brought down through an opening in the dartos muscle and placed into the subcutaneous scrotal pouch. The dartos muscle is sutured to the upper end of the tunica circumferentially. (Reprinted by permission from Fonkalsrud E.W.[37])

Dartos m. sutured to tunica vaginalis

Skin closed over testicle

Fig 79–12.—The scrotal skin is closed over the testis with absorbable stitches. (Reprinted by permission from Fonkalsrud E.W.[37])

dissection since it is suspended in the peritoneal cavity by the mesorchium, as is the normal ovary. Two of our patients who previously underwent extensive retroperitoneal exploration and insertion of scrotal prostheses after failure to identify a gonad, when later explored abdominally were found to have intra-abdominal testes. Martin[78] has seen two patients who developed malignant tumors in intra-abdominal undescended testes that were not identified during previous retroperitoneal exploration.

The high incidence of malignant tumors in untreated undescended testes has led Martin and Menck[79] and others to focus on the appropriate treatment of the patient first seen after puberty. Comparing the risk of death due to malignancy with the risk after orchiectomy, they concluded that between the ages of

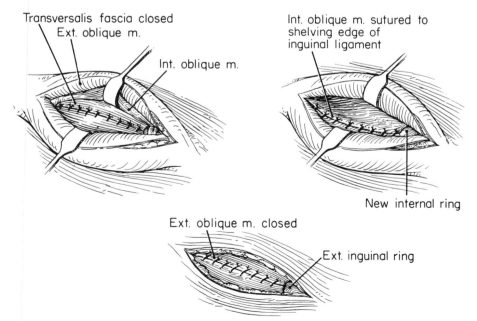

Transversalis fascia closed
Ext. oblique m.
Int. oblique m.

Int. oblique m. sutured to shelving edge of inguinal ligament

New internal ring

Ext. oblique m. closed
Ext. inguinal ring

Fig 79–13.—The transversalis fascia is reapproximated, leaving a small opening just lateral to the pubis to serve as the new internal inguinal ring. The internal oblique muscle is approximated to the shelving edge of the inguinal ligament, again leaving an opening for the spermatic cord medially. The external oblique aponeurosis is approximated. (Reprinted by permission from Fonkalsrud E.W.[37])

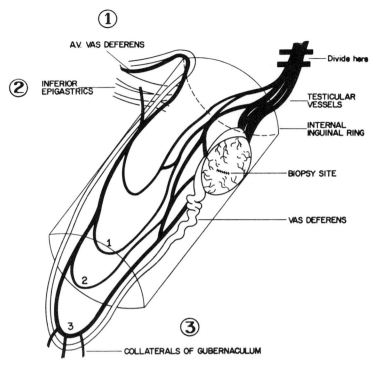

① A.V. VAS DEFERENS
② INFERIOR EPIGASTRICS

Divide here

TESTICULAR VESSELS

INTERNAL INGUINAL RING

BIOPSY SITE

VAS DEFERENS

③

1
2
3

COLLATERALS OF GUBERNACULUM

Fig 79–14.—Rationale for the "long-loop vas" orchiopexy. The three significant collateral vascular pathways (the artery and vein of the vas deferens, the inferior epigastric vessels, and the vessels of the gubernaculum) provide circulation to the testis when the major vascular pedicle is divided well above the gonad itself. Several arcades *(1, 2, 3)* across the bottom of the major long loop of the vas deferens can usually be spared and adequate length achieved. Free bleeding from the biopsy site confirms adequacy of the arterial blood supply. (Reprinted by permission from Clatworthy H.W. Jr. et al.[21])

15 and 50, all unilateral undescended inguinal, as well as all intra-abdominal testes, should be removed.

When anorchia is present, or when the testicle is removed, in most patients, regardless of age, a soft Silastic testicular prosthesis should be placed into the scrotum through the inguinal incision and secured in place. If the patient is a young boy, a larger prosthesis may be necessary after he achieves puberty.

Complications

Following orchiopexy, complications severe enough to jeopardize function of the gonad occur in less than 5% of operations performed by experienced surgeons. The most serious concerns are obstruction of the delicate vascular supply to the testis by direct injury, compression from twisting the vascular pedicle or closing the abdominal musculature too tightly, or from narrowing the vessels by placing them under significant tension as the testis is placed into the scrotum. Since the function of the cryptorchid testis in many instances is less than optimal, there is sufficient indication that the additional insult of vascular injury may worsen the prognosis for function even after the testis is placed into the scrotum. Severe vascular obstruction usually causes testicular atrophy within a few weeks. Transient testicular swelling due to partial obstruction of lymphatic and venous drainage is common, usually subsiding within 2–4 weeks. Injury to the vas is believed to be relatively rare. Retraction of the testis up to the external inguinal ring or higher has been uncommon since we adopted the dartos pouch technique of anchoring the testis as standard. Recurrent direct hernia and scrotal hematoma are rare after orchiopexy.

Results

During recent years, there has been a steady trend toward treatment of undescended testes at an early age. Morphologic and clinical evidence has increased to support the view that mat-uration of the cryptorchid testis is retarded after the age of 2–3 years and that placement of the testis into the scrotum improves the potential of further maturation and fertility if the spermatic vessels or the gonad itself are not injured in the process.[6, 47, 81, 107] The 35% incidence of fertility reported in a collected series of 346 patients with uncorrected unilateral undescent[51] sharply disagrees with the 80% fertility reported by Gross and Replogle[43] in patients with unilateral undescent who underwent orchiopexy before puberty, and the nearly 100% fertility reported by Karcher[62] in boys who underwent repair before the age of 10. Patients with bilateral cryptorchidism are sterile; however, those with bilateral undescent who have been treated by orchiopexy beween the ages of 3 and 10 years have a fertility rate of 37%, based on semen analysis.[98] There is strong evidence, therefore, that orchiopexy improves the likelihood of fertility. When orchiopexy for bilateral undescent is performed before the age of 5 years, more than 50% of patients will be fertile and 31% will be normospermatic,[53] further supporting the practice of early operation. Moreover, Martin and Menck[79] pointed out the rare occurrence of late malignant change in testes that have been brought down early as being a strong argument in favor of early treatment.

REFERENCES

1. Abeyratne M.R., Aherne W.A., Scott J.E.S.: The vanishing testis. *Lancet* 2:822, 1969.
2. Alojzy M.: Significance of biopsy research in cryptorchidism in children. *Arch. Dis. Child.* 38:170, 1963.
3. Altman B.L., Malament M.: Carcinoma of the testis following orchiopexy. *J. Urol.* 97:498, 1967.
4. Anderson H.: Biopsy studies in cryptorchidism. *Acta Endocrinol.* 18:567, 1955.
5. Arey L.B.: *Developmental Anatomy.* Philadelphia, W.B. Saunders Co., 1940, p. 301.
6. Atkinson P.M.: A followup study of surgically treated cryptorchid patients. *J. Pediatr. Surg.* 10:115, 1975.
7. Atkinson P.M., Epstein M.T., Rippon A.E.: Plasma gonadotropins

and androgens in surgically treated cryptorchid patients. *J. Pediatr. Surg.* 10:27, 1975.
8. Aschheim S.: Über die funcktion des Ovariums. *Z. Geburtsh. Gynak.* 90:387, 1926.
9. Aschheim S., Zondek B.: The hormone of the anterior lobe of the hypophysis and the ovarian hormone in the urine of pregnant women. *Clin. Wochenschr.* 6:1322, 1927.
10. Barcat J.: L'ectopie testiculaire: Statistique clinique et operatoire des services de chirurgie infantile des enfants—malades de 1914 à 1950. *Mem. Acad. Chir.* 83:909, 1957.
11. Benson D.C., Lotfi M.W.: The pouch technique in the surgical correction of cryptorchidism in infants and children. *Surgery* 62:967, 1967.
12. Blanchard M.G., Josso N.: Source of the anti-Müllerian hormone synthesized by the fetal testis: Müllerian-inhibiting activity of fetal bovine Sertoli cells in tissue culture. *Pediatr. Res.* 8:968, 1974.
13. Boley S.J., Kleinhaus S.A.: A place for the Cheatle-Henry approach in pediatric surgery. *J. Pediatr. Surg.* 1:394, 1966.
14. Bramble F.J., Houghton A.L., Eccles S.: Reproductive and endocrine function after surgical treatment of bilateral cryptorchidism. *Lancet* 2:311, 1974.
15. Browne D.: Some anatomical points in operation for undescended testicle. *Lancet* 1:460, 1933.
16. Brunet J., DeMowbray R.R., Bishop P.M.F.: Management of the undescended testis. *Br. Med. J.* 5084:1367, 1958.
17. Burton C.C.: The embryologic development and descent of the testis in relation to congenital hernia. *Surg. Gynecol. Obstet.* 2:284, 1958.
18. Campbell H.E.: Incidence of malignant growth of the undescended testicle. *Arch. Surg.* 44:353, 1942.
19. Campbell H.E.: The incidence of malignant growth of the undescended testicle: A reply and re-evaluation. *J. Urol.* 81:663, 1959.
20. Clatworthy H.W. Jr., Gilbert M., Clement A.: The inguinal hernia, hydrocele and undescended testicle problem in infants and children. *Postgrad. Med. J.* 22:122, 1957.
21. Clatworthy H.W. Jr., Hollabaugh R.S., Grosfeld J.L.: The "long loop" vas orchiopexy for the high undescended testis. *Am. Surg.* 38:69, 1972.
22. Cohn B.D.: Histology of the cryptorchid testis. *Surgery* 62:536, 1967.
23. Colby F.H.: *Essential Urology.* Baltimore, Williams & Wilkins Co., 1956.
24. Cook G.T., Marshall V.F.: The association of undescended testes and renal abnormalities. Presented at the Annual Meeting of the American Academy of Pediatrics, Washington, D.C., November 1968.
25. Corkery J.J.: Staged orchiopexy: A new technique. *J. Pediatr. Surg.* 10:515, 1975.
26. Crowe S.J., Cushing H., Homans J.: Experimental hypophysectomy. *Bull. Johns Hopkins Hosp.* 21:127, 1910.
27. Cunningham J.H.: New growth developing in undescended testicles. *J. Urol.* 5:471, 1921.
28. Cywes S., Retief P.J.M., Louw J.H.: Results following orchiopexy, in Fonkalsrud E.W., Mengel W. (eds.): *The Undescended Testis.* Chicago, Year Book Medical Publishers, 1981.
29. Deming C.L.: Hormonal bases for the treatment of the undescended testis. *Am. J. Surg.* 38:186, 1937.
30. Eccles W.M.: The anatomy, physiology and pathology of the imperfectly descended testis. *Lancet* 1:569, 1902.
31. Engberg H.: Investigations on the endocrine function of the testicle in cryptorchidism. *Proc. R. Soc. Med.* 42:652, 1949.
32. Fahlstrom G., Holmberg L., Johannson H.: Atrophy of testis following operation on the inguinal region in infants and children. *Acta Chir. Scand.* 126:221, 1963.
33. Farrington G.H.: Histologic observations in cryptorchidism: The congenital germinal-cell deficiency of the undescended testis. *J. Pediatr. Surg.* 4:606, 1969.
34. Firor H.V.: Two-stage orchiopexy. *Arch. Surg.* 102:598, 1971.
35. Flinn R.A., King L.R.: Experiences with the midline transabdominal approach in orchiopexy. *Surg. Gynecol. Obstet.* 131:285, 1971.
36. Fonkalsrud E.W.: Current concepts in the management of the undescended testis. *Surg. Clin. North Am.* 50:847, 1970.
37. Fonkalsrud E.W.: The undescended testis. *Curr. Prob. Surg.* 15:5, 1978.
38. Fowler R., Stephens F.D.: The role of testicular vascular anatomy in the salvage of high undescended testis. *Aust. N.Z. J. Surg.* 29:92, 1959.
39. Gaspar M.R., Kimber J.H., Berkaw K.A.: Children with hernias, testes and female external genitalia. *Am. J. Dis. Child.* 91:542, 1956.
40. Gilbert J.B., Hamilton J.B.: Incidence and nature of tumors in ectopic testes. *Surg. Gynecol. Obstet.* 71:731, 1940.
41. Glenn J.F.: The prostate, seminal vesicles, penis and testes, in Sabiston D.C. Jr. (ed.): *Davis-Christopher Textbook of Surgery.* Philadelphia, W.B. Saunders Co., 1972, p. 1562.
42. Gross R.E., Jewett T.C. Jr.: Surgical experiences from 1222 operations for undescended testes. *JAMA* 160:634, 1956.
43. Gross R.E., Replogle R.L.: Treatment of the undescended testis. *Postgrad. Med. J.* 34:266, 1963.
44. Hadziselimovic F.: Current treatment of cryptorchidism. *Dial. Ped. Surg.* 6:2, 1983.
45. Hadziselimovic F.: Treatment of cryptorchidism with GNRH. *Urol. Clin. North Am.* 9:413, 1982.
46. Hadziselimovic F., Herzog B.: The meaning of the Leydig cell in relation to the etiology of cryptorchidism: An experimental and electron-microscopic study. *J. Pediatr. Surg.* 11:1, 1976.
47. Hadziselimovic F., Herzog B., Seguchi H.: Surgical correction of cryptorchidism at 2 years: Electron microscopic and morphologic investigation. *J. Pediatr. Surg.* 10:19, 1975.
48. Hamilton J.B., Hubert G.: Effect of synthetic male hormone substance on descent of testicles in human cryptorchidism. *Proc. Soc. Exp. Biol. Med.* 39:4, 1938.
49. Hand J.R.: Treatment of undescended testis and its complications. *JAMA* 164:1185, 1957.
50. Hecker W.C.: Neuere Gesichtspunkte zum Kryptorchismus Problem. *Munch. Med. Wochenschr.* 113:1125, 1971.
51. Hecker W., Hienz H.A.: Cryptorchidism and fertility. *J. Pediatr. Surg.* 2:513, 1967.
52. Herr H.W., Silbert I., Martin D.C.: Management of inguinal lymph nodes in patients with testicular tumors following orchiopexy, inguinal or scrotal operations. *J. Urol.* 110:223, 1973.
53. Hortling H., Chappelle A., Johansson C.J., et al.: An endocrinological followup study of operated cases of cryptorchidism. *J. Clin. Endocrinol. Metab.* 27:120, 1967.
54. Hunter J.: *Observations on Certain Parts of the Animal Economy.* London, Longmans, Greene & Co., 1786.
55. Imperato-McGinley J., et al.: Steroid 5-alpha reductase deficiency in man: An inherited form of male pseudohermaphroditism. *Science* 186:1213, 1974.
56. Johnson W.W.: Cryptorchidism. *JAMA* 113:25, 1939.
57. Johnson D.E., Woodhead D.M., Pohl D.R., et al.: Cryptorchidism and testicular tumorigenesis. *Surgery* 63:919, 1968.
58. Jones P.G.: Undescended testes. *Aust. Paediatr. J.* 2:36, 1966.
59. Jost A.: A new look at the mechanisms controlling sex differentiation in mammals. *Johns Hopkins Med. J.* 130:38, 1972.
60. Jost A.: Sur le rôle des gonads foetales dans la differentiation sexuelle somatique de l'embryon du lapin. *Cr. Assoc. Anat.* 34:255, 1947.
61. Kaplan G.W.: Iatrogenic cryptorchidism resulting from hernia repair. *Surg. Gynecol. Obstet.* 142:671, 1976.
62. Karcher G.: Die Fertilitaet des behandelten pathologischen Hodenhochstandes unter besonderer Beruecksichtigung des Zeitpunktes der hormonellen bzw. operativen Therapie, *Arch. Clin. Chir.* 317:288, 1967.
63. Kiesewetter W.B.: Undescended testes. *W. Va. Med. J.* 52:235, 1956.
64. Kiesewetter W.B., Kalayoglu M., Sachs B.: The effect of abnormal position, scrotal repositioning and human gonadotropic hormone on the developing puppy testis. *J. Pediatr. Surg.* 8:739, 1973.
65. Krabbe S., Skakkebaek N.E., Berthelsen J.G., et al.: High incidence of undetected neoplasia in maldescended testes. *Lancet* 1:999, 1979.
66. Lattimer J.K., Smith A.M., Dougherty L.J., et al.: The optimum time to operate for cryptorchidism. *Pediatrics* 53:96, 1974.
67. Laughlin V.C.: Orchidofunicolysis. *J. Urol.* 77:39, 1957.
68. Leape L.: Torsion of the testis: Invitation to error. *JAMA* 200:669, 1967.
69. Lee P.A., Hoffman W.H., White J.J., et al.: Serum gonadotropins in cryptorchidism. *Am. J. Dis. Child.* 127:530, 1974.
70. Lemeh C.N.: A study of the development and structural relationships of the testis and gubernaculum. *Surg. Gynecol. Obstet.* 40:535, 1925.
71. Levin A., Sherman J.O.: The undescended testis. *Surg. Gynecol. Obstet.* 136:473, 1973.
72. Mack W.S., Scott L.S., Ferguson-Smith M.A., et al.: Ectopic testis and true undescended testis: A histological comparison. *J. Pathol.* 82:439, 1961.
73. MacLeod J.: Semen quality in 1000 men of known fertility and in 800 cases of infertile marriage. *Fertil. Steril.* 2:115, 1951.
74. Mancini R.E., Rosenberg E., Cullen M., et al.: Cryptorchid and scrotal human testes. I. Cytological, cytochemical and quantitative studies. *J. Clin. Endocrinol. Metab.* 25:927, 1965.
75. Markewitz M., Lattimer J.K., Veenema R.J.: A comparative study of germ cell kinetics in the testis of children with unilateral cryptorchidism: A preliminary report. *Fertil. Steril.* 21:806, 1970.

76. Martin D.C.: Malignancy in the cryptorchid testis. *Urol. Clin. North Am.* 9:731, 1982.
77. Martin D.C.: Malignancy and the undescended testis, in Fonkalsrud E.W., Mengel W. (eds.): *The Undescended Testis.* Chicago, Year Book Medical Publishers, 1982.
78. Martin D.C.: Personal communication.
79. Martin D.C., Menck H.R.: The undescended testis: Management after puberty. *J. Urol.* 114:77, 1975.
80. McCallum D.W.: Clinical study of the spermatogenesis of undescended testes. *Arch. Surg.* 31:290, 1935.
81. Mengel W., Hienz H.A., Sippe W.G., et al.: Studies on cryptorchidism: A comparison of histological findings in the germinative epithelium before and after the second year of life. *J. Pediatr. Surg.* 9:445, 1974.
82. Mengel W., Zimmermann F.A.: Immunologic aspects of cryptorchidism, in Fonkalsrud E.W., Mengel W. (eds.): *The Undescended Testis.* Chicago, Year Book Medical Publishers, 1981.
83. Moore C.R.: The biology of mammalian testis and scrotum. *Q. Rev. Biol.* 1:4, 1926.
84. Moore N.S., Tapper S.M.: Cryptorchidism: A theory to explain its etiology. *J. Urol.* 43:204, 1940.
85. Myers R.P., Kelalis P.P.: Cryptorchidism reassessed: Is there an optimal time for surgical correction? *Mayo Clin. Proc.* 48:94, 1973.
86. Nelson W.O.: Effect of gonadotropic hormone injections upon the hypophysis and sex accessories of experimental cryptorchid rats. *Proc. Soc. Exp. Biol. Med.* 31:1192, 1933.
87. Nelson W.O.: Mammalian spermatogenesis. *Rec. Prog. Horm. Res.* 6:29, 1951.
88. Prentiss R.J., Mullenix R.B., Whisenand J.M.: Medical and surgical treatment of cryptorchidism. *Arch. Surg.* 70:283, 1955.
89. Puri P., Nixon H.H.: Bilateral retractile testes—subsequent effects on fertility. *J. Pediatr. Surg.* 12:563, 1977.
90. Raboch J., Starka L.: Plasmatic testosterone in bilateral cryptorchids in adult age. *Andrologia* 4:107, 1972.
91. Redman J.F.: The staged orchiopexy: A critical review of the literature. *J. Urol.* 117:113, 1977.
92. Riegler H.C.: Torsion of intra-abdominal testis. *Surg. Clin. North Am.* 52:371, 1972.
93. Rivarola M.A., Bergada C., Cullen M.: HCG stimulation test in prepubertal boys with cryptorchidism in bilateral anorchia and in male pseudohermaphroditism. *J. Clin. Endocrinol. Metab.* 31:526, 1970.
94. Robinson J.N., Engle E.T.: Some observations on the cryptorchid testis. *J. Urol.* 71:726, 1954.
95. Scorer C.G.: The descent of the testis. *Arch. Dis. Child.* 39:605, 1964.
96. Scorer C.G.: Descent of the testes in the first year of life. *Br. J. Surg.* 27:374, 1955.
97. Scorer C.G.: The incidence of incomplete descent of the testicle at birth. *Arch. Dis. Child.* 31:198, 1956.
98. Scott L.S.: Delayed treatment of cryptorchidism with subsequent infertility. *Fertil. Steril.* 18:782, 1967.
99. Silber S.J., Kelly J.: Successful autotransplantation of an intra-abdominal testis to the scrotum by microvascular technique. *J. Urol.* 115:452, 1976.
100. Skakkebaek N.E., Berthelsen J.G., Muller J.: Carcinoma-in-situ of the undescended testis. *Urol. Clin. North Am.* 9:377, 1982.
101. Sohval A.R.: Histopathology of cryptorchidism. *Am. J. Med.* 16:346, 1954.
102. Sohval A.R.: Testicular dysgenesis as an etiologic factor in cryptorchidism. *J. Urol.* 72:693, 1954.
103. Sohval A.R.: Testicular dysgenesis in relation to neoplasm of the testicle. *J. Urol.* 75:285, 1975.
104. Sonneland S.G.: Undescended testicle. *Surg. Gynecol. Obstet.* 40:535, 1925.
105. Snyder W.H. Jr., Chaffin L.: Surgical management of undescended testes. *JAMA* 157:129, 1955.
106. Snyder W.H. Jr., Greaney E.M. Jr.: Cryptorchidism, in Mustard W., Ravitch M.M., Snyder W.H. Jr., et al. (eds.): *Pediatric Surgery.* Chicago, Year Book Medical Publishers, 1969.
107. Städtler F., Hartmann R.: Histologic and morphological studies of prepubertal testicular development in normal and in cerebrally damaged boys. *Dtsch. Med. Wochenschr.* 97:104, 1972.
108. Thompson W.O., Heckel N.J.: Undescended testes: Present status of glandular treatment. *JAMA* 112:397, 1939.
109. Tvetter K.J., Fjaerli J.: Roentgenologic findings in cryptorchidism. *Scand. J. Urol. Nephrol.* 9:171, 1975.
110. Ward B., Hunter W.M.: The absent testicle: A report on a survey carried out among schoolboys in Nottingham. *Br. Med. J.* 5179:1110, 1960.
111. Watson R.A., Lennox K.W., Gangai M.P.: Simple cryptorchidism: The value of the excretory urogram as a screening method. *J. Urol.* 11:789, 1974.
112. Wells L.J., State D.: Misconception of the gubernaculum testis. *Surgery* 22:502, 1947.
113. Womack E.B., Koch F.C.: Undescended testis. *Endocrinology* 16:267, 1932.
114. Woolley M.M.: Cryptorchidism, in Ravitch M.M., Welch K.J., Benson C.D., et al. (eds.): *Pediatric Surgery.* Chicago, Year Book Medical Publishers, 1979.
115. Zachman M., Prader A., Kind H.P., et al.: Testicular volume during adolescence, cross-sectional and longitudinal studies. *Helv. Paediatr. Acta* 29:61, 1974.
116. Zer M., Wolloch Y., Dinstman M.: Staged orchiorrhaphy. *Arch. Surg.* 110:387, 1975.
117. Zondek B.: Über die Funcktion des Ovariums. *Ztschr. Geburtsh. Gynak.* 90:372, 1926.

80 Bradley M. Rodgers

Gastrostomy: Indications and Technique

History.—The use of a gastrostomy was first suggested in 1837 by Egeberg, a Norwegian Army surgeon, as a method of feeding patients with carcinoma of the esophagus.[5] Watson of New York appears to have made the first similar suggestion in the American literature in 1844.[19] After experimenting with gastrostomies in dogs, Sédillot, of Strasbourg, performed the first gastrostomy in a human in 1849.[15] This patient died 10 days after the gastrostomy from peritonitis caused by leakage about the tube. The first successful use of a gastrostomy is attributed to Jones, a surgeon from London, in 1875.[12] The first suggestion for the use of a gastrostomy for decompression of the gastrointestinal tract was made by Horsley in 1939, but the merits of this technique were not widely recognized until the reports of Farris and Smith in 1956.[6] The importance of the use of gastrostomy for feeding purposes in pediatric surgery was recognized by the pioneering efforts of Leven in 1941 in the staged correction of infants with esophageal atresia.[13]

Gastrostomy, the creation of a fistula between the lumen of the stomach and the abdominal wall, is one of the most commonly employed techniques in pediatric surgery. While procedures for performing "temporary" gastrostomies, with a serous lining of the tract, and "permanent" gastrostomies, with a full mucosal lining of the fistula, have been described, gastrostomies employed in children are nearly all of the "temporary" type. These gastrostomies are simpler to perform, less likely to leak gastric juice onto the skin, and close spontaneously when the tube is removed. The disadvantage of this technique over the "permanent" type of gastrostomy is that to keep the tract open the catheter must remain continuously in the fistula into the stomach. The use of gastrostomy is so widespread in infants and children because of the inherent disadvantages of nasogastric tubes. The tubes used for small patients are of limited caliber and tend to occlude, and a tube through the oropharynx increases oral secretions and induces aerophagia, both contributing to gastrointestinal distention if the tubes become obstructed.[17] Nasal obstruction caused by these tubes may precipitate respiratory distress in the small infant, an obligatory nasal breather. The use of a gastrostomy tube avoids the trauma to the upper airway and lower esophagus caused by nasogastric tubes. A gastrostomy tube allows for more efficient gastrointestinal decompression and facilitates the feeding and mobility of the patient.

The principal indications for gastrostomy in pediatric surgery are for feeding, for gastrointestinal decompression, and for retrograde esophageal dilation. In most series, approximately 20% of the gastrostomies performed are used exclusively for feeding purposes.[11] These may be in patients with anatomic or neurologic abnormalities precluding normal feeding. Approximately 55% of gastrostomies in children are employed primarily for decompression of the gastrointestinal tract, most commonly in newborns with intestinal abnormalities requiring anastomosis. Occasionally, gastrostomy may be employed in patients with significant abdominal trauma or peritonitis who are expected to have prolonged postoperative ileus. Approximately 25% of the gastrostomies in children are performed to facilitate esophageal dilatation. These are in patients with anastomotic stricture following repair of esophageal atresia, or children with stricture secondary to ingestion of caustics. Passage of a string through the mouth and esophagus and out the gastrostomy allows the Tucker dilators to be pulled through the lumen either retrograde or antegrade.

There are few contraindications to gastrostomy in children. If one contemplates the construction of a reverse gastric tube for esophageal replacement, the use of a gastrostomy may be contraindicated, but even in this situation, if the stomach is of sufficient size, a carefully placed gastrostomy may be employed, preserving the stomach along the greater curvature for the creation of the gastric tube. The use of a gastrostomy alone for feeding purposes in patients with significant gastroesophageal reflux will often precipitate reflux of tube feedings and aspiration, but gastrostomy may be an important adjunct to the Nissen fundoplication in these patients.

Technique

The technique used for creation of a temporary gastrostomy in children is a modification of the procedure originally described by Stamm in 1894.[18] Although the operation may be performed under general or local anesthesia, for children most surgeons prefer the use of general anesthesia, reserving local anesthesia for older patients or those with significantly impaired central nervous system function. When performed as a primary procedure, a small transverse left upper quadrant incision is made overlying the left rectus muscle (Fig 80–1). The muscle itself may be divided transversely or split vertically and the peritoneum entered. The stomach is identified by its pale color and the characteristic vasculature along the greater curvature. A site on the anterior wall of the stomach at the junction of the upper and middle third, along the greater curvature, is usually chosen for insertion of the gastrostomy tube. The gastrostomy site must reach the abdominal wall without tension and should be well away from the pylorus to minimize the possibility of the gastrostomy tube prolapsing into the duodenum. A purse-string suture of 3-0 or 4-0 silk is placed in the gastric wall, and an opening is made into the lumen of the stomach with the electrocautery. Meticulous hemostasis must be achieved in the vascular submucosa of the stomach. The opening is dilated with a hemostat and a dePezzer catheter placed into the stomach. An 18- or 20-F catheter is usually employed, although a 16-F may be used in the premature infant. The catheter is prepared by excising the distal end, creating a single-hole, flanged catheter. The purse-string suture is tied, preserving the needle for later suture of the stomach to the abdominal wall. A second inverting purse-string suture is then placed, approximately 5 mm outside the first. This suture is placed so that the knot will be opposite the first, and the needle is also preserved. The spot for exit of the gastrostomy tube is selected in the left upper quadrant. This should be separate from the primary surgical incision to minimize wound contamination and should be at least a centimeter away from the costal arch, to avoid perichondritis. A stab incision is made at the site selected and a clamp passed into the abdominal cavity. The gastrostomy catheter is grasped and pulled through the abdominal wall. This tract and skin incision should be tight about the tube to minimize the possibility of a leak of gastric contents.

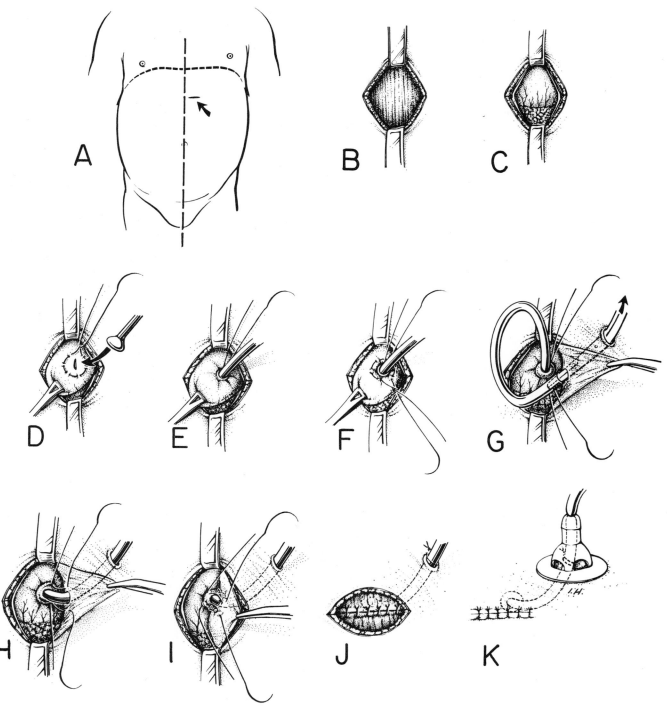

Fig 80–1.—Operative technique for temporary gastrostomy. **A,** small incision is made in a natural skin fold in the left upper quadrant. **B,** rectus muscle is divided or its fibers split, and the peritoneum opened to expose **(C)** the greater curvature of the stomach. **D,** silk purse-string suture is placed in the body of the stomach, along the greater curvature, and a modified dePezzer catheter is inserted through a gastrotomy. **E,** first purse-string is secured, and a second is placed **(F)** so that the knots of the two will be on opposite sides of the gastrostomy tube. **G,** a site for the emergence of the tube is selected, away from the primary incision and the costal margin. A clamp is inserted through a stab wound and the tube pulled through the abdominal wall. **H,** the two purse-string sutures are secured to the parietal peritoneum behind the gastrostomy tube. **I,** additional sutures secure the stomach to the abdominal wall anterior to the tube. **J,** wound is closed in layers and the gastrostomy tube secured to the skin with a nylon suture. **K,** tube is placed through a nipple to maintain slight tension and to keep the tube from rotating and eroding the abdominal wall skin. (Modified from Holder and Gross[10] and Meeker and Snyder.[14])

The stomach is then carefully fixed to the abdominal peritoneum by first anchoring the two purse-string sutures posterior to the gastrostomy catheter and then placing several additional seromusculature sutures anteriorly. This is a most important step in minimizing complications, and care must be taken to be certain that the stomach is securely fastened to the abdominal wall completely around the gastrostomy exit. The gastrostomy tube is then secured to the skin with a 3-0 nylon suture, and gentle traction is maintained on the tube by passing it through a sterile nipple, which grips it firmly and is pressed down upon the skin. The primary incision is closed in layers with absorbable sutures, and the gastrostomy is left to gravity drainage for 48–72 hours before it is elevated and used for feeding purposes. When used for early postoperative decompression, the gastrostomy tube should be irrigated frequently with 3 cc of sterile saline or air in order to maintain its patency.

A technique for the endoscopic-percutaneous insertion of a gastrostomy has been described by Gauderer and associates.[8] This technique may be useful for placement of feeding gastrostomies, particularly in children with neurologic impairment.

Complications

The greatest deterrent to widespread acceptance of the use of gastrostomy tubes has been the incidence of complications and the occasional mortality attributed to this procedure. The deaths reported are almost all due to leakage of gastric contents into the peritoneal cavity from disruption of the union between the stomach and abdominal wall. It appears clear that increasing experience with the technique of gastrostomy and meticulous attention to the operative details of this procedure have virtually eliminated the fatalities from gastrostomy and have minimized the complications. Conner and Sealy, in 1956, reported a 30.7% fatality rate from gastrostomies performed in the neonatal period.[3] By 1966, Haws and associates were able to report only a 16% morbidity rate, 6% major and 10% minor, in 240 children undergoing gastrostomy.[9] That series had a 4% mortality, most of the deaths occurring in neonates. Holder et al., in 1972, had a single fatality in 280 gastrostomies (0.4%) and only a 2.5% incidence of major morbidity.[11] Gallagher et al., in 1973, reported a 2% major morbidity and 7% minor morbidity, with a single death from intra-abdominal leak in a neonate.[7] Campbell, in 1974, reported 8% minor and 7% major complications from gastrostomies in children, without a single death.[2] In all series, the mortality from gastrostomy occurs primarily in neonates, emphasizing the meticulous attention that must be paid to technique in managing these infants.

The most serious complication of the gastrostomy procedure is separation of the stomach from the abdominal wall. This may occur because of inadequate fixation of the serosa of the stomach to the parietal peritoneum, or from early dislodgment of the gastrostomy tube before a fibrinous seal around the gastrostomy has developed. Careful fixation of the gastric wall to the abdominal peritoneum is essential. In small children and uncooperative older patients, loose arm restraints should be used so that the patient cannot pull at the gastrostomy tube. Dislodgment of the gastrostomy tube in the first 72 hours is a major complication. Blind reinsertion of another tube may push the stomach away from the abdominal wall and create a fatal peritoneal leak. The tube should be reinserted either under direct operative control or with gentle manipulation under fluoroscopy to be certain that it passes directly into the gastric lumen. Passage of the tube outside the stomach and injection of feedings into the peritoneal cavity is not unknown. A Foley catheter should be employed for this purpose and the balloon inflated to hold the stomach against the abdominal wall until further healing.

Leakage of gastric contents around the tube onto the abdominal wall is the most common complication following gastrostomy.[16] Usually, this complication indicates that the flange of the gastrostomy tube has slipped into the gastric lumen, allowing for passage of the gastric contents externally (Fig 80–2). Gentle traction on the tube and impaction of the flange against the inner surface of the fistula usually eliminates this problem. Allowed to persist, the inflammation caused by this leakage erodes the skin and fistula tract, creating a large hole in the abdominal wall. Occasionally it may be necessary to remove the tube and control the fistula with a bulky elastic dressing for several days to allow the hole to close partially before a smaller tube is inserted.

Migration of the gastrostomy tube, either through the pylorus into the duodenum or retrograde into the esophagus, may cause serious complications. Any patient with a gastrostomy who begins to vomit should be suspected of having an obstruction caused by such migration. Contrast roentgenograms may be helpful to define the position of the tube in these patients. If there is any question, the tube should be removed and a new one inserted.

Persistence of the gastrocutaneous fistula after removal of the gastrostomy tube occurs in 10–18% of patients with long-stand-

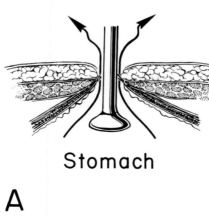

Stomach

A

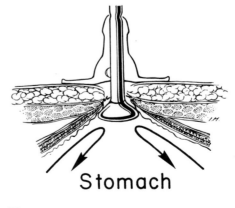

Stomach

B

Fig 80–2.—Leakage from gastrostomy. **A,** the most common cause for leakage about the gastrostomy tube is advancement of the flange of the tube into the gastric lumen. **B,** impingement of the flange against the gastric wall seals the gastrostomy and prevents leakage. The tube may be held in this position by the rubber nursing nipple at the skin level.

ing gastrostomies. In most cases, this persistence is caused by growth of gastric mucosa along the fistula. Usually, cautery of this tract with silver nitrate or the electrocautery is sufficient to allow closure. Occasionally, a more formal operative technique, such as excision of the epithelial lining and temporary reinsertion of a smaller gastrostomy tube or excision of the lining and a layered closure of the abdominal wall, may be necessary.[1, 4]

REFERENCES

1. Bishop H.C.: Simplified closure of the long-standing gastrostomy. *J. Pediatr. Surg.* 16:571, 1981.
2. Campbell J.R., Sasaki T.M.: Gastrostomy in infants and children: An analysis of complications and techniques. *Am. Surg.* 9:505, 1974.
3. Conner R.G., Sealy W.C.: Gastrostomy and its complications. *Ann. Surg.* 143:245, 1956.
4. Ducharme J.C., Youssef S., Tilkin F.: Gastrostomy closure: A quick, easy, and safe method. *J. Pediatr. Surg.* 12:729, 1977.
5. Egeberg C.A.: Om Behandlingen af impenetrable Stricturer i Madroret (Oesophagus). *Norsk Magazin Laegevidenskaben* 2:97, 1841.
6. Farris J.M., Smith G.K.: An evaluation of temporary gastrostomy—a substitute for nasogastric suction. *Ann. Surg.* 144:475, 1956.
7. Gallagher M.W., Tyson K.R.T., Ashcraft K.W.: Gastrostomy in pediatric patients: An analysis of complications and techniques. *Surgery* 74:556, 1973.
8. Gauderer M.W.L., Ponsky J.L., Izant R.J. Jr.: Gastrostomy without laparotomy: A percutaneous endoscopic technique. *J. Pediatr. Surg.* 15:872, 1980.
9. Haws E.B., Sieber W.K., Kiesewetter W.B.: Complications of tube gastrostomy in infants and children. *Ann. Surg.* 164:284, 1966.
10. Holder T.M., Gross R.E.: Temporary gastrostomy in pediatric surgery: Experience with 187 cases. *Pediatrics* 26:36, 1960.
11. Holder T.M., Leape L.L., Ashcraft K.W.: Gastrostomy: Its use and dangers in pediatric patients. *N. Engl. J. Med.* 286:1345, 1972.
12. Jones S.: Gastrostomy for stricture (cancerous?) of esophagus. Death from bronchitis forty days after operation. *Lancet* 1:678, 1875.
13. Leven N.L.: Congenital atresia of the esophagus with tracheoesophageal fistula. *J. Thorac. Surg.* 10:648, 1941.
14. Meeker I.A., Snyder W.H.: Gastrostomy for the newborn surgical patient: A report of 140 cases. *Arch. Dis. Child.* 37:159, 1962.
15. Sédillot, C.E.: Opération de gastro-stomie pratiquée pour la première fois le 13 Novembre 1849. *Gaz. Méd. Strasbourg* 9:366, 1849.
16. Shackelford R.T., Zuidema G.D.: Gastrostomy, in *Surgery of the Alimentary Tract*. Philadelphia, W.B. Saunders Co., 1981, p. 332.
17. Smith G.K., Farris J.M.: Re-evaluation of temporary gastrostomy as a substitute for nasogastric suction. *Am. J. Surg.* 102:168, 1961.
18. Stamm M.: Gastrostomy by a new method. *Medical News* 65:324, 1894.
19. Watson J.: Practical observations on organic obstructions of the esophagus; preceded by a case which called for esophagotomy and subsequent opening of the trachea; with accompanying illustrations. *Am. J. Med. Sci.* 8NS:309, 1844.

81 Clifford D. Benson

Infantile Hypertrophic Pyloric Stenosis

History.—In the United States, Hezekiah Beardsley, in 1788, reported one of the first cases of congenital pyloric stenosis.[10] The child died at the age of 5 years, and necropsy revealed an obstructing scirrhosity at the pylorus. In 1877, Hirschsprung[17] presented two cases and provided an accurate description that established the condition as a distinct clinical entity. In 1907, Pierre Fredet[12] suggested that the pyloric muscle be split, leaving the mucosa intact, the muscle being closed transversely. Rammstedt,[26] in 1912, described an operative procedure similar to Fredet's but did not suture the circular muscle over the gaping submucosa. His is the operation that has proved to be curative and is accepted the world over as the procedure for congenital pyloric stenosis. Before 1907, gastroenterostomy was advocated and was attended by a mortality rate of approximately 50%. Subsequently, it was found that the pyloric muscle tumor persisted after gastroenterostomy, but after the Rammstedt operation, the tumor disappeared within 10–14 days.[34] Mack[21] and Ravitch[27] have published historical accounts of the development of the surgical treatment of pyloric stenosis.

Etiology and Pathology

The exact cause of pyloric stenosis is still obscure. Belding and Kernohan[1] found a decreased number of ganglion cells and nerve fibers in the pylorus, which they ascribed to degenerative changes. Friesen et al.[13] observed that the ganglion cells are not greatly diminished in number, but that they are not mature, and stated that failure of ganglion cell development rather than degeneration led to pyloric stenosis. Zuelzer[35] failed to see any significant changes in ganglion cells.

Heredity and family predisposition have been implicated. There is a 6.9% incidence of pyloric stenosis in children of affected parents. The female parent who had pyloric stenosis as an infant has a four times greater chance of having affected offspring than does a similarly affected male parent.[23] Berglund and Rabo[6] found that 4.5% of close relatives, and one of 11 brothers of affected patients, had had pyloric stenosis. Pollock et al.[24] found an incidence of 1 in 300 live births in the Los Angeles area, and Laron and Horne[19] found the incidence to be 1 in 913 live births in the Pittsburgh area. They also found an incidence in white infants of 1 in 830, compared with an incidence in black infants of 1 in 2073.

Male infants are affected more often than females, in a ratio of 4:1. According to most authors, the firstborn is most often affected.

Lynn[20] proposed a simple physiologic explanation that milk curds propelled by the gastric musculature against a pyloric canal in spasm produce edema of the pyloric mucosa and submucosa that narrows the pyloric canal. He postulated a concomitant response of work hypertrophy of the pyloric and gastric musculature, setting up a vicious cycle that progresses to a high-grade obstruction of the pyloric canal. Hypergastrinemia was found by Spitz and Zail[33] in affected infants, and they suggested an etiologic role for gastrin. Rogers et al.[29] failed to confirm this finding but demonstrated hyperacidity in infants with pyloric stenosis.

Symptoms and Signs

Rarely, the onset of symptoms may occur at birth.[24] Occasionally, the diagnosis has been made as early as the fourth or fifth day, and in one instance as late as 5 months.[28] In our experience, the average clinical onset occurs at 3 weeks. Vomiting is the initial sign, and the vomitus is almost always free of bile. Initially, the baby may vomit once or twice a day, but, as the obstruction increases, the vomiting becomes more constant and more forceful. Occasionally, the fluid vomited may be brownish or frankly blood-streaked due to bleeding from capillaries in the gastric mucosa ruptured by the frequent vomiting. As the vomiting continues, dehydration appears, followed by weight loss and dramatic failure to grow. Marked alkalosis develops as a consequence of chloride loss in the vomitus.

Gastric peristalsis can often be seen as an impressive wave passing from the left upper quadrant across to the right in infants with well-established clinical pyloric stenosis. While these waves can be seen in other conditions, such as severe pylorospasm or gastric duplication, they are highly suggestive of pyloric stenosis. A firm, small, movable mass, most often described as the size and shape of an olive, is found in the right upper quadrant. This mass is pathognomonic and, depending on the experience and the patience of the examiner, can be felt in 70–90% of infants with hypertrophic pyloric stenosis.

X-ray examination following a barium meal is helpful in the diagnosis when a tumor cannot be palpated. A thin mixture of barium is used to aid in outlining the narrowed and elongated pyloric canal (Fig 81–1). A careful roentgen examination should include study of the esophagus to rule out gastroesophageal reflux. Reflux may closely simulate pyloric stenosis because vomiting is the main symptom and weight loss often occurs. Gastric retention of barium is not definitive, since other conditions such as pylorospasm and central nervous system lesions may impede gastric emptying. However, rapid gastric emptying of barium excludes the diagnosis of pyloric stenosis. If a barium study is necessary to confirm the diagnosis of pyloric stenosis, excess barium should be lavaged from the infant's stomach with a large-bore catheter introduced orally before the induction of anesthesia for pyloromyotomy.

In the past several years, abdominal sonography has been used as a diagnostic aid in pyloric stenosis.[7] This technique has a false negative rate of 5–10% and does not exclude other diagnoses such as chalasia and malrotation with duodenal bands. Radiation exposure is not a factor in single gastrointestinal series in infants,

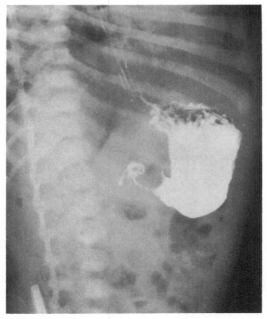

Fig 81–1.—Pyloric stenosis. Roentgenogram demonstrating an elongated and narrowed pyloric canal. The pathognomonic pyloric tumor should be palpable in 85–90% of cases, in whom x-ray or sonography (less reliable) is not necessary.

and in our department barium swallow has an accuracy rate of 95%.

ASSOCIATED JAUNDICE.—Jaundice occurs in association with pyloric stenosis in 1–2% of infants. The cause is not known but is thought to be related to acute starvation with an immature liver. In our experience, the bilirubin level is mainly in the indirect fraction. In the usual case of pyloric stenosis, the jaundice disappears 5–10 days after the Rammstedt procedure. Twenty infants in our series of 1,872 patients had associated jaundice with elevated indirect bilirubin values. In all, the jaundice cleared promptly after the Rammstedt procedure.

Operative Treatment

PREPARATION.—Since the diagnosis is being made progressively earlier, fewer infants are being seen in an advanced state of severe dehydration, malnutrition, and alkalosis with hypochloremia and hypokalemia. The aim in preparing these infants for operation is to restore sodium, chloride, potassium, and water losses as quickly as possible and to ensure sufficient hemoglobin and protein levels in the rare instance when these factors are depressed. As a rule, most babies with pyloric stenosis can be operated on within 24 hours after admission to the hospital. Occasionally, a severely depleted infant requires a longer period of preparation. With improved understanding of fluid and electrolyte management of neonates, morbidity and mortality have been steadily reduced. In the past two decades, an infant operated on for pyloric stenosis has rarely been lost.

From a practical point of view, infants with pyloric stenosis can be divided into three main groups: those with mild, moderate, and severe symptoms.[2] In the mild cases, the infant is not dehydrated, or only mildly so, and has only slight metabolic alkalosis with carbon dioxide content of 25 mEq/L or less. In moderate cases, the carbon dioxide content is 26–35 mEq/L with correspondingly more impressive dehydration and weight loss. In the severe category, there is malnutrition, alkalosis with CO_2 content above 35 mEq/L, hypokalemia, or even tetanic convulsions. Kumar and Bailey[18] found that serum chloride, carbon dioxide content, and hemoglobin are often unreliable indices of the extent of fluid and electrolyte disturbances in pyloric stenosis. Similarly, total body potassium may be markedly depleted before serum samples reflect hypokalemia. Patients in the mild and moderate groups can be managed by a variety of regimens, and, as long as appropriate amounts of parenteral fluids and proper aliquots of salt are administered, if renal function is good, these infants do well. Severely depleted infants tax the judgment and ability of the physician to prepare them properly for operation. The greatest error is to rush a poorly prepared infant to operation. When long-standing vomiting has led to acute starvation, severe alkalosis, and dehydration, careful preparation over a 3–5 day course may be wise.

With minimal dehydration and no significant electrolyte disturbance, we offer oral feedings consisting of 60 ml of balanced electrolyte solution every 3 hours up to 4 hours before operation. In some cases, it is necessary first to lavage the stomach with normal saline to remove obstructing milk curd and barium. Two to three mEq of potassium chloride may be added to each feeding after satisfactory renal function has been assured. If vomiting persists, or if the level of dehydration suggests the need for intravenous fluids, oral feedings are withheld and 5% dextrose in 0.33% saline is administered intravenously in amounts of 50–70 ml/lb/24 hr, depending on the amount of hydration needed. After the infant has voided, 5–10 mEq of potassium chloride is added to each 250-ml intravenous bottle. It is recommended that the total amount of potassium chloride administered not exceed 40 mEq in 24 hours.

Moderate and severe fluid and electrolyte disturbances must be corrected with intravenous therapy. In addition to serum electrolyte levels as an indication of the severity of derangement, we use known weight loss as an aid in estimating the water deficit. Each pound of weight loss approximates 450 ml of water deficit. We have found that, for each pound of weight loss, one day is required for correcting water and electrolyte deficits. The malnourished, hypoproteinemic infant is given 5 ml/lb/day of plasma or colloid, and hemoglobin deficiencies are corrected with 5–10 ml/lb of packed red cells.

Moderately severe electrolyte derangements are corrected by giving the first half of the calculated replacement as 5–10% dextrose in 0.45% normal saline. Potassium chloride, 20–40 mEq in each liter of intravenous fluids, is added after the infant has voided. Infants with severe electrolyte disturbances receive their initial calculated replacement as one part 5% dextrose in 0.45% normal saline, one part normal saline, and the remainder, including maintenance fluids, as 5% dextrose in 0.33% normal saline. Potassium chloride is added as calculated above after satisfactory renal function has been assured. Serum electrolytes are measured after every 12–24 hours of therapy, and operation is deferred as long as necessary until the constituents of serum, plasma, and blood have reached satisfactory levels and total body water is judged to be sufficient.

Once the stomach has been emptied, most of these infants stop vomiting. A few, however, persist, and a nasogastric tube is then introduced and attached to a low-pressure suction device. The stomach is again emptied just before induction of anesthesia.

ANESTHESIA.—Local anesthesia was used frequently in many clinics here and abroad before 1945. General anesthesia is now standard practice because the infant's preoperative status is generally strong and there has been such progress in pediatric anesthesia.

OPERATION.—The Rammstedt pyloromyotomy is universally accepted. The abdomen is opened through a right transverse skin incision well above the liver edge; the rectus muscle is then split vertically. We discontinued use of the vertical skin incision because it lengthened with growth, yielding a poor cosmetic result. The transverse skin incision remains small and inconspicuous. Many surgeons prefer transverse division of the rectus muscle, and some still prefer the gridiron incision that was so important to healing in depleted subjects when first advocated in 1940 by Robertson.[30]

The tumor is delivered into the wound and often is retained there by the wound edges. The prepyloric area is grasped with moist gauze and rotated inferiorly to expose the anterosuperior border of the hypertrophied pylorus. An incision is made through the serosa and extended through the circular muscle, the length of the tumor (Fig 81–2,A). Care is taken to start the incision just proximal to the white line that denotes the junction of the pylorus and duodenum. The circular muscle is then spread bluntly. Some surgeons use the back end of the knife handle to accomplish this important maneuver; others use the jaws of the curved hemostat. For many years, we have successfully used a pyloric spreader (Fig 81–3), which was developed specifically for the Rammstedt operation to ensure that all muscle fibers are thoroughly, yet safely, ruptured. With completion of this step, the gastric submucosa pouts up into the cleft, indicating release of the obstructive process.

On the duodenal side, it is important to spread gently under the white line to divide all fibers at this end of the pyloric incision without tearing the thin, vulnerable duodenal mucosa. Most perforations occur at this location, but this complication can be avoided if the original incision stops just short of the white line that demarcates the true junction of the stomach and duodenum. If the duodenum is opened, the perforation must not go unrecognized. Many surgeons routinely milk the duodenum toward

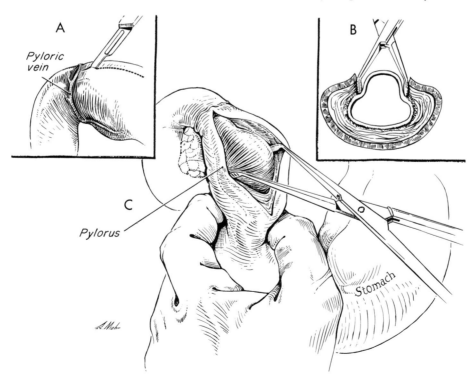

Fig 81–2.—Pyloric stenosis: operative technique of pyloromyotomy. **A,** incision made on anterosuperior surface through avascular area.
B, cross-section of hypertrophied pylorus after operation has been completed.
C, circular muscle is separated, allowing submucosa to bulge.

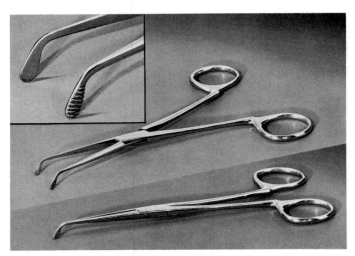

Fig 81–3.—Author's pylorus spreader.

the pylorus to search for bile-stained fluid that will be expressed through a mucosal rent. Disruption of the duodenum is best repaired with nonabsorbable sutures and a tag of omentum. In rare instances, secure closure of the ruptured duodenum compromises the pyloromyotomy. In such circumstances, the pylorus should be rotated 45 degrees and a fresh pyloric incision made, repeating all steps of the Rammstedt procedure. Before the pylorus is returned to the abdomen, a search should be made for bleeding, which may require cautery or suture ligation for control. At the conclusion of the operation, the peritoneum and posterior rectus sheath are closed by a running suture of 3-0 chromic catgut, and the anterior rectus sheath is closed with interrupted 4-0 silk sutures. The skin edges are meticulously approximated.

POSTOPERATIVE CARE.—The gastric tube is removed as soon as the infant recovers from the anesthesia. When a duodenal perforation has occurred, the gastric tube is left in place for 48 hours to assure gastric decompression.

Parenteral fluids in the form of 5% glucose in 0.33% normal saline are given to maintain a fluid intake of 50 ml/lb/day until oral fluid intake is sufficient.

Oral feedings are begun 8 hours after operation, provided the infant is alert and has a good sucking reflex. Scharli and Leditschke[31] have confirmed by manometric and roentgenologic studies that gastric peristalsis is depressed for 12–18 hours after the Rammstedt operation. Commencement of oral feedings early in the postoperative period is thus unwise, as more vomiting often occurs; vomiting in the postoperative period is markedly reduced if oral fluids are withheld for the first 8 hours. A number of different postoperative feeding routines are popular. Ours utilizes 10% dextrose, alternated with half-strength formula every 2 hours, beginning with 10 ml and increasing by 10 ml every 4 hours until 60 ml (2 oz) is taken and retained at one feeding. The formula is then increased to full strength. Some regurgitation of a portion of the feedings occurs in about one third of the infants in the early postoperative period but is not a serious problem. If vomiting occurs frequently in the first 24 hours after operation, the stomach is washed out to remove excess mucus, and the feeding routine recommenced at the beginning, after which vomiting usually ceases.

COMPLICATIONS.—Incomplete pyloromyotomy, recognized by unrelieved projectile vomiting, is a rare problem in experienced hands. In this circumstance, x-ray studies are not helpful, since it is difficult to show an open pylorus postoperatively.

Perforation of the duodenum or stomach during the Rammstedt procedure is or should be a rare occurrence. I have experienced this only once, when perforation occurred on the gastric side in a premature infant in the initial muscle separation. In our total experience of 1,872 Rammstedt operations, the incidence of perforation was 2.3%; this includes all operations performed by the attending and resident staffs. All perforations but one were recognized and closed. The patient with unrecognized perforation died of peritonitis. Two wound disruptions occurred in the 1,872 patients, and secondary repair was successful in both.

LENGTH OF HOSPITALIZATION.—During the past four decades at our institution, the average preoperative hospital stay has been reduced from 3½ days to 1 day and the average postoperative stay reduced from 13.5 to 2 days.

MORTALITY.—The mortality rate is low, 0.3%, in this series of 1,872 patients. There have been no deaths in the last 1,155 babies undergoing pyloromyotomy. Four of our patients had tracheoesophageal fistula complicated by pyloric stenosis. The Rammstedt procedure was successfully performed at 3–4 weeks in each patient. Two other patients had associated mediastinal neuroblastoma excised successfully 3 weeks after the pyloromyotomy, and both are well 14 years postoperatively.[4] Two other patients had associated complicating congenital cardiac problems: one premature infant required ligation of a patent ductus at 3 days of age. Three weeks later, a Rammstedt operation was successfully performed. The second had ventricular and atrial septal defects; pyloromyotomy was uneventfully performed, but the infant died of cardiac failure several weeks after discharge. A male infant had an associated sacral teratoma excised at 3 days of age and a Rammstedt operation performed at 3 weeks of age with an uneventful recovery from both operations. Mortality in other reported series has been: Gross,[15] 928 cases with nine deaths, no deaths in 188 cases, 1964–1966; Donovan,[10] 350 cases with one death; Potts,[25] 750 cases with one death; Scharli et al.,[32] two deaths in the last 377 infants operated on; Donnellan,[9] no deaths related to the condition in 215 patients. These figures attest to the extremely low mortality rates in the large pediatric centers in North America.

Nonoperative Treatment

Nonoperative treatment of pyloric stenosis has been reported from England and Scandinavia[22] but has never gained favor in the Americas. Berglund and Rabo,[5] in following these patients, found a significant correlation between weight loss and duration of the inanition accompanying medical management and the eventual adult height. Satisfactory results may ultimately be obtained by medical management, but medical treatment takes considerably longer, necessitates a prolonged hospital stay, and requires daily effort to assure adequate nutrition. In contrast, most babies operated on are sent home on the third postoperative day. In view of the prolonged hospitalization required and the potential morbidity, medical management of pyloric stenosis should be reserved for isolated instances when operation is contraindicated because of coexisting disease.

REFERENCES

1. Belding H.D., Kernohan J.W.: A morphologic study of the myenteric plexus and musculature of the pylorus with special reference to the changes in hypertrophic pyloric stenosis. *Surg. Gynecol. Obstet.* 97:322, 1953.
2. Benson C.D., Alpern E.B.: Preoperative and post-operative care of congenital pyloric stenosis. *Arch. Surg.* 75:877, 1957.
3. Benson C.D., Lloyd J.R.: Infantile pyloric stenosis. *Am. J. Surg.* 107:429, 1964.
4. Benson C.D.: Infantile pyloric stenosis. *Prog. Pediatr. Surg.* 1:63, 1969.

5. Berglund G., Rabo E.: A long-term follow-up investigation of patients with hypertrophic pyloric stenosis—with special reference to the physical and mental development. *Acta Paediatr. Scand.* 62:125, 1973.
6. Berglund G., Rabo E.: A long-term follow-up of patients with pyloric stenosis—with special reference to heredity and later morbidity. *Acta Paediatr. Scand.* 62:130, 1972.
7. Blumhagen J.D., Noble H.G.S.: Muscle thickness in hypertrophic pyloric stenosis: Sonographic determination. *AJR* 140:221, 1983.
8. Corner B.D.: Hypertrophic pyloric stenosis in infancy treated with methyl scopolamine nitrate. *Arch. Dis. Child.* 30:377, 1955.
9. Donnellan W.: Cited in Maingot R.: *Abdominal Operations*, ed. 5. New York, Appleton-Century-Crofts, 1969, vol. 1.
10. Donovan E.J.: Hezekiah Beardsley, congenital hypertrophic stenosis of the pylorus. *Arch. Pediatr.* 75:359, 1958.
11. Donovan E.J.: In discussion of Robertson.[30]
12. Dufour H., Fredet P.: La Sténose hypertrophique du pylore chez le nourisson et son traitement chirurgical. *Rev. Chir.* 37:208, 1908.
13. Friesen S.R., Boley J.O., Miller D.R.: The myenteric plexus of the pylorus: Its early normal development and its changes in hypertrophic pyloric stenosis. *Surgery* 39:21, 1956.
14. Gordon H.E., Pollack W.F., Norris W.J., et al.: Hypertrophic pyloric stenosis: Experience with 1,573 cases at Los Angeles Children's Hospital. *West. J. Surg.* 67:139, 1959.
15. Gross R.E.: Cited in Maingot R.: *Abdominal Operations*, ed. 5. New York, Appleton-Century-Crofts, 1969, vol. 1.
16. Hight E.W., Benson C.D., Philippart A.I., et al.: Management of mucosal perforation during pyloromyotomy for infantile pyloric stenosis. *Surgery* 90:85–86, 1981.
17. Hirschsprung H.: Fälle von angeborener Pylorusstenose: Beobachtungen bei Sauglingen. *Jahrb. Kinderhlk.* 28:61, 1888.
18. Kumar V., Bailey W.C.: Electrolyte and acid base problems in hypertrophic pyloric stenosis in infancy. *Indian Pediatr.* 12:839, 1975.
19. Laron Z., Horne L.M.: The incidence of infantile pyloric stenosis. *Am. J. Dis. Child.* 94:151, 1957.
20. Lynn H.: The mechanism of pyloric stenosis and its relationship to preoperative preparation. *Arch. Surg.* 81:453, 1960.
21. Mack H.C.: A history of hypertrophic pyloric stenosis and its treatment. *Bull. Hist. Med.* 12:465, 595, 666, 1942.
22. Malmberg N.: Hypertrophic pyloric stenosis: A survey of 136 successive cases with special references to treatment with Scopyl. *Acta Pediatr.* 38:472, 1949.
23. McKeown T., MacMahon B.: Infantile hypertrophic pyloric stenosis in parent and child. *Arch. Dis. Child.* 30:497, 1955.
24. Pollock W.F., Norris W.J., Gordon H.E.: The management of hypertrophic pyloric stenosis at the Los Angeles Children's Hospital (a review of 1,422 cases). *Am. J. Surg.* 94:335, 1957.
25. Potts W.E.: *The Surgeon and the Child.* Philadelphia, W.B. Saunders Co., 1959.
26. Rammstedt C.: Zur Operation der angeborenen Pylorus-stenose. *Med. Klin.* 8:1702, 1912.
27. Ravitch M.M.: The story of pyloric stenosis. *Surgery* 48:1117, 1960.
28. Rendle-Short J., Zachary R.B.: Congenital pyloric stenosis in older babies. *Arch. Dis. Child.* 30:70, 1955.
29. Rogers I.M., Drainer I.K., Moore M.R., et al.: Plasma gastrin in congenital hypertrophic pyloric stenosis. *Arch. Dis. Child.* 50:467, 1975.
30. Robertson D.E.: Congenital pyloric stenosis. *Ann. Surg.* 112:786, 1940.
31. Scharli A.F., Leditschke J.F.: Gastric motility after pyloromyotomy in infants: A reappraisal of postoperative feeding. *Surgery* 64:113, 1968.
32. Scharli A., Sieber W.K., Kiesewetter W.B.: Hypertrophic pyloric stenosis at the Children's Hospital of Pittsburgh from 1912 to 1967. *J. Pediatr. Surg.* 4:108, 1969.
33. Spitz L., Zail S.S.: Serum gastrin levels in congenital hypertrophic pyloric stenosis. *J. Pediatr. Surg.* 11:33, 1976.
34. Wollstein M.: Healing of hypertrophic pyloric stenosis after the Fredet-Ramstedt operation. *Am. J. Dis. Child.* 23:511, 1922.
35. Zuelzer W.: Personal communication.

82 JESSIE L. TERNBERG

Peptic Ulcer—Acute and Chronic

PEPTIC ULCER DISEASE is caused by the digestive action of pepsin in the presence of acid on gastrointestinal mucosa, producing a penetrating lesion. The erosion or ulcer produced is located primarily in the stomach or duodenum but can also be in the esophagus, or in a segment of bowel that has been anastomosed to the stomach or duodenum. In addition, ulcers can arise in gastrointestinal mucosa adjacent to functional ectopic gastric mucosa, in an intestinal duplication, or in a Meckel's diverticulum. The history of peptic ulcer disease in infants and children dates back to 1826 with the description by von Siebold[63] of a perforated gastric ulcer in a 2-day-old infant. A collective review of the literature on peptic ulcers in children covering 243 patients was published by Bird et al. in 1941.[6] The introductory paragraph of this paper states that peptic ulcer of the stomach and duodenum in infants and children, although considered a rare lesion, is not an uncommon disease. Reports of other series have continued to suggest peptic ulcer occurs more frequently in childhood than has been reported and should be given more clinical consideration in pediatric practice.[4, 18, 40, 59] Despite these early papers, the general impression of peptic ulcer disease as an uncommon problem in childhood lingers. This is demonstrated by the almost ubiquitous statement in subsequent reports that peptic ulcer disease, once considered rare in infants and children, is being recognized with increasing frequency.[13, 15, 66]

The collected series by Bird et al.[6] included 119 patients who had been operated on for their peptic ulcer disease. Ulcers in infants aged 1–15 days characteristically had presented precipitously with hemorrhage or perforation. There were no premonitory signs or symptoms. No other preceding or associated problem, such as sepsis, shock, or intracranial hemorrhage, was noted. The ulcers in these neonates were primarily in the duodenum or pylorus and were described as acute, without cellular reaction or bacterial invasion. Preschool children, on the other hand, frequently had an illness before the onset of the graver symptoms of an ulcer catastrophe, such as hemorrhage or perforation. The possible heterogeneity of the etiology of the ulcers was apparently not recognized. The differences noted were ascribed to age.

The useful classification of peptic ulcers into primary and secondary was presented by Schuster and Gross[56] in 1963. Primary ulcers were defined as those in which the ulcer was the principal clinical and pathological entity. Secondary ulcers were the result of other underlying disease. This separation is useful in discussing etiology, diagnosis, and treatment.

Secondary Peptic Ulcer Disease

Secondary ulcers, also referred to as stress ulcers, are acute ulcers in children. In the adult, stress ulcers are multiple superficial mucosal erosions found primarily in the fundus of the stomach and associated with major physical or thermal trauma, sepsis, shock, or similar serious medical problem. These ulcers should be considered separately from ulcers that result from ingestion of drugs or chemicals and perhaps also from ulcers associated with intracranial problems (Cushing's ulcer). Drug and chemical-induced ulcers resemble stress ulcers in their appearance and in their distribution. The ulcer that occurs with intracranial problems, such as tumors or head injuries, however, is usually a single, deep ulcer, prone to perforation. Studies in adults indicate gastric hypersecretion is not associated either with stress ulcers or with ulcers resulting from drug ingestion.[33, 41] Cushing's ulcers, on the other hand, have been shown to be associated with an increased acid output.[25, 47] Secondary ulcers in children are frequently single and deep, similar to the Cushing ulcer, instead of the usual multiple superficial ulcerations seen secondary to stress in the adult. No studies, however, have been done to determine whether gastric hypersecretion is present in the child with a stress ulcer.

A wide range of clinical and laboratory studies have been undertaken to clarify the pathogenesis of stress peptic ulcers. Acid is considered requisite, even though hypersecretion is usually not present except with Cushing's ulcer. It appears that most of the factors contributing to the development of stress ulcers do so by reducing the ability of the stomach to protect itself against acid injury rather than by increasing the amount of acid secretion.[58] All investigators agree that mucosal ischemia is basic to the pathogenesis of stress ulcers.[10] Normally, small amounts of hydrogen ion diffuse into the mucosa but are rapidly cleared or neutralized if there is adequate mucosal blood flow. Ischemia reduces the capacity for neutralization of the acid entering the tissue, leading to an accumulation of hydrogen ions within the tissue and subsequent mucosal ulceration. It appears that the adverse effect of ischemia on energy metabolism is an additional factor, reducing the ability of the mucosa to defend itself against injury.[36] Intravenous infusions of sodium bicarbonate given during the experimental production of mucosal injury by hemorrhagic shock have had a protective effect. This suggests that the pH of arterial blood perfusing the stomach also may be important in determining the ability of the gastric mucosa to protect itself against acid injury.[11] It appears, then, that ischemia, energy deficits, and systemic acidosis are all important factors in the pathogenesis of stress ulcers.

In drug-induced ulcers, the drug has disrupted the mucosal permeability barrier.[42] The gastric mucosa cannot contain the hydrogen ion within the lumen, and the ulcer results from an excessive back diffusion of hydrogen ion into the mucosal cells.

Prostaglandins have a protective effect in the prevention of experimentally induced stress ulcers.[39] The mechanism of the protective effect is uncertain. It is known that prostaglandins stimulate chloride ion transport out of the cell, exchanging it for bicarbonate ion. Available bicarbonate is increased within the cell, increasing the ability of the cell to buffer acid entering it.[20] Endogenous prostaglandins also have a role in maintaining adequate blood flow to the gastric mucosa, and this may affect the ability of the mucosa to withstand formation of stress ulcers.[54]

In general, stress ulcers in children resemble Cushing's ulcer in adults, being duodenal, single, and deeply penetrating, compared with the multiple superficial ulcerations in the adult with stress ulceration. Notable exceptions to the isolated duodenal ulcer were reported by Morden et al.[44] In this series of 10 patients with severe complicated medical illnesses, all patients had multiple gastric ulcers, and hemorrhage was the most common presentation.

Williams et al.[65] reported the largest series of stress ulcers in children. The 194 cases consisted primarily of Curling's ulcers, the stress ulcer that arises secondary to burn trauma. One hundred of these ulcers were diagnosed clinically; the rest were found at autopsy. The ulcer was located in the duodenum in 43 of the 63 cases in which a site was identified. The only significant gastric ulcers in the series were diagnosed after perforation. In 18 patients, the data were considered sufficient for estimation of the rate of bleeding. Expressed as a percentage of the total blood volume for 24 hours, if the rate of bleeding was over 60%, no patient lived who was not operated on. Of the bleeding patients operated on, 60% died. These were all patients with duodenal ulcers. If the percentage of blood volume lost per 24 hours was less than 60%, all patients lived without an operation, the bleeding stopping spontaneously. There were no documented cases of severe, persistent gastric bleeding, nor were there any deaths from gastric hemorrhage. In another series reported by Grosfeld et al.,[22] of 29 patients, two secondary to burns and none secondary to intracranial lesions, the distribution of duodenal to gastric lesions was almost equal. All these ulcers were solitary, except in one child in whom multiple ulcers were found at autopsy. In another series of 25 patients with secondary ulcers, the lesions were almost equally distributed between the duodenum and the stomach.[15] The single gastric ulcers in these studies were usually prepyloric and therefore similar in most respects to duodenal ulcers.

Diagnosis

The secondary ulcer is an acute ulcer. Although the reported ages of patients with secondary ulcers have ranged from 1 day to 18 years, the greatest number of patients are less than 6 years old. Diagnosis is therefore more difficult and usually made when a catastrophe, such as hemorrhage and/or perforation, occurs. Typical peptic ulcer pain is absent in children less than 6 years of age and only occurs in 8% of patients over 6. Atypical pain occurs in 8% of patients less than 6 years of age and in 39% of patients over 6 years of age. Vomiting, a very common sign, occurs in 92% of secondary ulcer cases in children less than 6 years of age. Vomiting is also fairly common in the child over 6 years of age with secondary ulcer—54% of reported cases. Gastrointestinal bleeding, the predominant presentation of secondary ulcers, occurs in 92% of patients less than 6 years old and in 77% of those over 6 years of age. A significant percentage of patients in all series presented with perforation, although it appears gastrointestinal bleeding preceded or was closely associated with perforation in many cases.[5]

The diagnosis of secondary ulcer has been made by contrast radiological studies, endoscopy, angiography, laparotomy, and autopsy. The known occurrence of secondary ulcers in association with physiological stress should lead to diagnosis before signs and symptoms become catastrophic. Radiological diagnosis can be difficult in the presence of hemorrhage, as blood clots can mask the ulcer. Endoscopy has been used with increasing frequency. The availability of modern fiberoptic endoscopic equipment has contributed to the improved diagnostic capability of endoscopy. In one report, 85% of children with upper GI bleeding were diagnosed with endoscopy, compared with 62% by radiological studies.[60] Angiography can be useful in locating a bleeding ulcer if the rate of bleeding is at least 0.5 ml/min.[19, 61]

Treatment

Prevention is the preferred treatment goal for stress ulcers. It has been shown experimentally that, under simulated clinical conditions, development of stress ulcers requires a low gastric juice pH. The use of antacids prophylactically to maintain gastric intraluminal pH at 6.0 or greater may contribute to a decrease in incidence. Supportive care with improved ventilatory support, maintenance of vascular volume, correction of acid-base imbalances, and nutritional support also may contribute to the ability of the gastric mucosa to withstand acid pepsin injury.

The effectiveness of histamine H_2 receptor antagonists in the prevention of stress ulcers is disputed. A histamine H_2 antagonist is probably indicated in the prevention and treatment of Cushing's ulcers because of the known association with hypersecretion of acid. Although there is no experimental evidence to indicate hypersecretion of acid in association with Curling's ulcers, the clinical similarity of these ulcers to Cushing's ulcers in children suggests that a histamine H_2 antagonist might be beneficial.

When a secondary ulcer presents with bleeding, immediate supportive treatment with balanced salt solution and blood transfusion is frequently adequate. If massive hemorrhage occurs, op-

eration is indicated. Massive hemorrhage has been defined as blood loss in 24 hours equal to the total estimated blood volume in infants less than 2 years of age, and half of the estimated blood volume in older children. This correlates with the report of Williams et al.[65] that no child recovered without an operation if the rate of blood loss was over 60% of the estimated blood volume for 24 hours. The successful use of selective intra-arterial vasopressin to manage bleeding stress ulcer in a child has been reported.[32] There are also reports of several unsuccessful attempts to control bleeding stress ulcers with vasopressin.[22, 44] Although bleeding often precedes perforation of a secondary ulcer, perforation can be the initial presentation of a secondary ulcer and demands operation.

The operative procedures used in the treatment of stress ulcers have ranged from simple closure of a perforation, to oversewing of the base of a bleeding ulcer, to gastrectomy (Table 82–1). As a general rule, these ulcers are not associated with an ulcer diathesis, and therefore they should respond to the sim-

TABLE 82–1.—SURGICAL TREATMENT OF STRESS (SECONDARY) PEPTIC ULCERS*

PRIMARY DISEASE	PATIENT AGE	LOCATION	PRESENTATION	TREATMENT	RESULT	SUMMARY
Acute encephalopathy	9 yr	Stomach	Perforation	Closure only	Survived	
Arteriovenous malformation with subarachnoid and intraventricular hemorrhage	8 yr	Duodenum	Perforation	Vagotomy, antrectomy, Bilroth I	Survived	4 cases of Cushing's ulcer: 3 with perforation, 1 with bleeding
Cerebral tumor	8 yr	Duodenum	Perforation	Vagotomy and pyloroplasty	Died on 17th postop day of primary disease	Vagotomy and pyloroplasty or vagotomy and antrectomy used to treat 3 cases with unresolved neurologic problems. No recurrence of ulcer disease
Pineal area tumor	1 yr	Duodenum	Massive GI hemorrhage	Vagotomy and pyloroplasty	Survived	No death from ulcer disease
20% full and deep partial-thickness burn	1½ yr	Duodenum	Perforation	Vagotomy and pyloroplasty	Survived	1 case of Curling's ulcer; burns healed 6 weeks after vagotomy and pyloroplasty
Open-heart operation	6 yr	Duodenum	Massive GI hemorrhage	Vagotomy and pyloroplasty	Survived	4 cases massive GI bleeding; 1 rebled after 90% gastrectomy
Sepsis, paraplegia	14 yr	Duodenum	Massive GI hemorrhage	Vagotomy and pyloroplasty	Survived	
Sepsis	6 mo	Duodenum	Massive GI hemorrhage	Closure	Survived	
Sepsis, thrombocytopenia	6 yr	Stomach	Massive GI hemorrhage	90% gastrectomy	Rebled, died	
Sepsis, neurologic damage	5 wk	Stomach	Perforation	Closure	Died 2 wk postop	
Reflux, aspiration, neurologic damage	2 mo	Duodenum	Perforation	Closure	Survived	10 cases of perforation, all 6 months or less of age. Closure of perforation with 5 surviving patients
Disseminated varicella	2 mo	Duodenum	Perforation	Jejunal patch	Died 1 day postop	
Vomiting, diarrhea	6 mo	Duodenum	Perforation	Excision and gastrojejunostomy	Died 2 days postop	
Failure to thrive, cardiorespiratory arrest at home	5 wk	Duodenum	Perforation	Closure	Survived	
Inborn error of metabolism, acute hepatic necrosis	2 mo	Duodenum	Perforation	Closure	Died 4 days postop	
Congestive heart failure	6 mo	Duodenum	Perforation	Closure	Survived	
Inborn error of metabolism, hepatic failure	9 wk	Duodenum	Perforation	Closure	Died 9 days postop	
Sepsis, multiple congenital anomalies	6 wk	Duodenum	Perforation	Closure	Survived	
Cystic fibrosis, sepsis	2 mo	Duodenum	Perforation	Closure	Survived	

*10-year experience, St. Louis (Mo.) Children's Hospital.

plest operative procedure that effectively treats the presenting problem. Since stress ulcers are secondary to an underlying disease, recurrence of the ulcer is possible if the underlying problem is unresolved, and this must be considered when deciding on the appropriate operation. The simplest procedure, plication and/or oversewing of the bleeding point, has been demonstrated to be effective. On the other hand, when it is apparent that the underlying problem will remain unresolved for an extended period of time, it may be appropriate to perform a more definitive ulcer procedure. Vagotomy with pyloroplasty is recommended most frequently. Vagotomy with antrectomy may be necessary to control the problem in burn patients and patients with intra-cranial problems.[48] Antrectomy may also be necessary for very large perforations that cannot be closed by a pyloroplasty, although the possibility of serosal patching to close such large defects should be kept in mind. In adults, even total gastrectomy has been recommended, although not by many, to treat multiple gastric ulcers. Such a procedure is rarely indicated in the child. The surgeon who operates on a child for ulcer disease must remember that the patient must continue to grow and develop; therefore, the simplest, least disruptive procedure must be selected. Follow-up studies of infants and children who have had partial gastrectomies suggest that the operation does not have a detrimental effect.[43] Other evidence, however, suggests that these children indeed have problems—for example, low hemoglobin levels.[62] Experimental evidence comparing the effects of gastrectomy and of vagotomy with pyloroplasty on the growth and development of puppies[8] and miniature swine[49] suggests that vagotomy with pyloroplasty produces less disturbance of growth patterns than gastrectomy. Follow-up information on children who have had vagotomy with pyloroplasty indicates that the treatment has been effective, without producing subsequent problems.[29] In view of the late reports of osteoporosis and iron deficiency developing in adults who have had various operations for peptic ulcer disease,[34, 45] some reservations must be retained concerning possible future problems in the child who has had an ulcer operation.

Drugs can cause secondary ulcers by damaging the mucosa, allowing acid pepsin digestion to occur. Aspirin is a common agent producing drug-induced secondary ulcers. Overdosage of another commonly available medication, ferrous sulfate, has also been implicated as a cause of ulcers in children. The causal relation of steroid therapy to development of secondary ulcers remains the subject of debate. Evidence exists to indicate that steroids are not a contributory factor,[14] as well as to indicate that they are.[46] In general, drug-induced ulcers should respond to conservative supportive treatment.

Primary Peptic Ulcer Disease

Primary peptic ulcer disease is not known to be the result of underlying illness or trauma. These peptic ulcers are most frequently duodenal or prepyloric. Duodenal and prepyloric ulcers are similar in that they are usually associated with higher levels of acid secretion and the patients, both adults and children, are predominantly of blood group O. The adult duodenal peptic ulcer patient is also more likely to be a nonsecretor of ABH blood group substances. This excess of nonsecretors has not been noted in children with peptic ulcer disease.[26, 31]

Gastric ulcers other than prepyloric occur primarily in younger patients who generally have hyposecretion of acid, but not achlorhydria, and are most frequently of blood group A. The ulcer is usually in the area of the junction of parietal cells with the pyloric mucosa.[28]

The true incidence of primary peptic ulcer disease is difficult to assess. An epidemiological study done in Erie County, N.Y.,

found the incidence to be 0.5 in 100,000 children during 1947–1949 and 3.9 in 100,000 children during 1956–1958.[59] Another survey in the same area indicated 1.7% of private-practice pediatric patients had peptic ulcer disease. Primary peptic ulcers occur most frequently after the age of 6 years with the incidence increasing progressively into the teen years. A 1.3:1 ratio of males to females is present up to 14 years of age, increasing to 2.8:1 for 15–19-year-old patients.

The question has been raised whether childhood peptic ulcer disease is the same as that seen in adults. A strong familial tendency has been noted. From 33–56% of children with ulcer disease have first- and second-degree relatives with peptic ulcer disease.[7, 23, 53] The incidence of peptic ulcers is also higher in monozygous than in dyzygous twins. Heritability of peptic ulcer disease has been calculated at 0.91 for children by Jackson,[26] considerably higher than the heritability calculation of 0.37 derived for adults by Fällström.[18] A family history positive for peptic ulcer disease is considered an important characteristic of ulcer disease in children.

Studies on acid and pepsinogen secretion have been done in infants and children. Acid secretion has been identified in the fetal stomach as early as the 19th week and pepsin secretion by the 34th week.[64] Term babies are able to secrete acid and pepsin. The premature infant can also secrete acid and pepsin, but not as much as the term infant. In neonates, the parietal cell mass per unit area is two to three times that found in adults.[50] A relatively high acid secretion by infants has been noted during the first week to 10 days of life.[38] Maternal gastrin may be responsible for both the increased parietal cell mass and the high acid secretion. Acid secretion rapidly decreases after about 10 days of age.[2] During the next 4 months, acid and pepsin secretion increase, paralleling weight instead of age. The increase continues gradually throughout childhood.

Elevated levels of acid secretion have been reported in children with peptic ulcer disease. As in the data from adult studies, elevated acid secretion does not seem to be great or consistent enough to be useful in identifying the child with peptic ulcer disease (Table 82–2). For example, Ghai et al.[21] used the augmented histamine test to study 18 children with ulcer disease and 16 control children (no ulcer disease). They found no significant increase in basal output of acid in the ulcer patients. There was an increase in the mean maximal and peak acid output, but the two groups overlapped, the maximal and peak values increasing with the patient's age and weight. A similar relation of age, weight, and acid secretion was noted by Robb et al., although no difference was noted between the acid secretion of 49 children with duodenal ulcers and 30 children with dyspepsia and no ulcer.[53]

Diagnosis

The clinical features of peptic ulcer disease in children can easily be confused with many other disorders, and this is basic to the problem of determining the incidence of ulcer disease in children. Signs in the infant include refusal of feedings, persistent crying, and vomiting.[27] The diagnosis is usually made when one of the more dramatic presentations, such as perforation and/or bleeding, occurs.

Vomiting is the predominant sign of ulcer disease in the preschool child. Abdominal pain is also common and is recognized with increasing frequency as the child becomes older. The pain is vague and difficult to describe, even for the older child.[15, 57] It does not have the relation to meals and relief produced by eating observed in the adult patient. Intermittent pain, however, is characteristic, with relief lasting days to weeks followed by recurrence, and should suggest the possibility of an ulcer. Noctur-

TABLE 82–2.—Surgical Treatment of Primary Peptic Ulcers*

INDICATION FOR OPERATION	PATIENT AGE	LOCATION	PROCEDURE	RESULT	SUMMARY
Perforation	16 yr	Duodenum	Omental plication	No recurrence, 4-yr follow-up	
Massive bleeding	16 yr	Duodenum	Vagotomy and pyloroplasty	No recurrence, 9-yr follow-up	
Massive bleeding	6 yr	Duodenum	Vagotomy and pyloroplasty	No recurrence, 10-yr follow-up	11 cases operated on for primary peptic ulcer disease:
Massive bleeding	13 yr	Duodenum	Vagotomy and pyloroplasty	No recurrence, 6-yr follow-up	1, perforation
Massive bleeding	13 yr	Gastric antrum	Ulcer oversewn	Recurrent bleeding after 1 yr, no operation. No recurrence, 4 yr	5, massive bleeding 2, obstruction 3, intractable symptoms
Massive bleeding	16 yr	Duodenum	Vagotomy and pyloroplasty	Recurrent ulcer symptoms 5 yr after operation	1 with recurrent bleed after ulcer oversewn;
Obstruction	8 yr	Duodenum	Vagotomy and pyloroplasty	No recurrence, 10 yr	1 with recurrent symptoms after vagotomy and
Obstruction	22 mo	Gastric antrum	Vagotomy and pyloroplasty	No recurrence, 7 yr	pyloroplasty; 1 with dumping after vagotomy and antrectomy
Intractable symptoms	17 yr	Duodenum	Selective vagotomy	No recurrence, 1 yr	
Intractable symptoms	16 yr	Duodenum	Parietal vagotomy	No recurrence, 7 yr	
Intractable symptoms following vagotomy and gastrojejunostomy done for peptic ulcer disease elsewhere	9 yr	Jejunum	Takedown of gastrojejunostomy, antrectomy, and gastroduodenostomy	"Dumping" problems developed in 7 mo	

*10-year experience, St. Louis (Mo.) Children's Hospital.

nal pain is also somewhat characteristic, and when it recurs should suggest peptic ulcer.

The diagnosis of peptic ulcer disease is made primarily by radiological examination or by endoscopy unless the ulcer presents with perforation, obstruction, or severe bleeding. Gastric analysis is not a useful diagnostic test.

Treatment

The treatment of peptic ulcer disease in children parallels that for adults. Antacids and histamine H_2 receptor antagonists (e.g., cimetidine) are the mainstays of medical therapy. There have been few studies of the pharmacokinetics of cimetidine in infants and children.[12] The current recommended dose is 20–40 mg/kg/24 hr. In infants, the lower dose appears to be adequate and safer.[9]

Surgical treatment has been reserved for ulcer complications such as perforation, bleeding, obstruction, and intractable pain (see Tables 82–1 to 82–3). Follow-up studies of children with ulcer disease treated medically show a high rate of recurrence throughout childhood and into adult life.[37, 51] Increasing numbers of these patients eventually require surgical treatment. Because of the prolonged morbidity reported for these patients, earlier surgical treatment has been recommended.[52] Vagotomy with py-

loroplasty is recommended as effective treatment, with a minimal effect on subsequent growth and development.[29] In the last decade, highly selective or parietal cell vagotomy has been used extensively in several centers to treat adult disease. There is no reported experience of this procedure for children. It appears to be a useful procedure in the child, with fewer side effects. The anticipated increased rate of ulcer recurrence, as compared with that from a truncal vagotomy demonstrated in adults, has been deemed acceptable in children in the context of producing a minimal disturbance of growth and development while providing a reasonable long-term result.[24]

There are some notable exceptions to this discussion of primary ulcers that should be briefly discussed for clarification. The bleeding or perforated ulcer occurring in the first 1–2 weeks of life and unassociated with other illness or stress appears to be an acute ulcer and may result from hypersecretion of acid caused by maternal gastrin. These ulcers most commonly bleed and respond to nasogastric decompression, with careful lavage to keep clots evacuated from the stomach, and supportive treatment to cover the blood losses. Perforation can also occur and should have prompt operation using the simplest method that will safely close the defect. This can be suture or pyloroplasty. If the operation is for hemorrhage, simple oversewing of the ulcer bed should suffice. There is no evidence that these ulcers recur.

TABLE 82–3.—Surgical Treatment of Neonatal Peptic Ulcers*

PATIENT AGE	LOCATION	PRESENTATION	PROCEDURE RESULT	
3 days	Duodenum	Perforation	Closed by Finney pyloroplasty	No recurrence, 10 yr
3 days	Duodenum	Massive hemorrhage	Ulcer oversewn	No recurrence, 9 yr

*10-year experience, St. Louis (Mo.) Children's Hospital. 78 newborn infants (2.8% of admissions) were observed for hematemesis in the neonatal intensive care unit within a 5-year period. Treatment consisted of gastric decompression and transfusions as indicated. None required operation.

Chronic partial obstruction secondary to a congenital problem, such as a duodenal web,[3, 30] or to hypertrophic pyloric stenosis[35] can also result in peptic ulcers in infants and children. It is important to identify the cause in this situation, as the ulcer can be completely relieved by treatment of the obstruction.

The Zollinger-Ellison (Z-E) syndrome is extremely rare in children.[55] The registry for Z-E patients includes 28 children followed up to 21 years.[67] The diagnosis may be suggested by large rugal stomach folds, duodenal dilatation, and edema of the small-bowel mucosa and confirmed by an elevated serum gastrin level. In adults, a calcium infusion test has been used to help identify the Z-E patient. The calcium markedly elevates serum gastrin levels in such patients. This infusion test has also been demonstrated to be reliable in a child.[1] Treatment traditionally has been total gastrectomy unless the pancreatic tumor can be completely resected. A histamine H_2 antagonist has been reported to eliminate the need for gastrectomy in a child.[17] Longer follow-up and experience with more patients using a histamine H_2 antagonist will be necessary before reliable conclusions can be drawn.

REFERENCES

1. Abe K., Nukawa N., Sasaki H.: Zollinger-Ellison syndrome with Marden-Walker syndrome. *Am. J. Dis. Child.* 133:735, 1979.
2. Agunod M., Yamaguchi N., Lopez R., et al.: Correlative study of hydrochloric acid, pepsin and intrinsic factor secretion in newborns and infants. *Am. J. Dig. Dis.* 14:400, 1969.
3. Airan B., Yadav K., Yadov R.V.S.: Congenital incomplete duodenal diaphragm with prediaphragmatic duodenal ulcer. *Am. J. Gastroenterol.* 72:426, 1979.
4. Alexander F.K.: Duodenal ulcer in children. *Radiology* 56:799, 1951.
5. Bell M.J., Keating J.P., Ternberg J.L., et al.: Perforated stress ulcers in infants. *J. Pediatr. Surg.* 16:998, 1981.
6. Bird C.E., Limper M.A., Mayer J.M.: Surgery in peptic ulceration of stomach and duodenum in infants and children. *Ann. Surg.* 114:526, 1941.
7. Blodgett M.D., Morris N., Lurie H.J.: Children with peptic ulcers and their families. *J. Pediatr.* 62:280, 1963.
8. Boley S.J., Krieger H., Schwartz S., et al.: The effect of operations for peptic ulcer on growth and nutrition of puppies. *Surgery* 57:441, 1965.
9. Chattriwalla Y., Colon A.R., Scanlon J.W.: The use of cimetidine in the newborn. *Pediatrics* 65:301, 1980.
10. Cheung L.Y., Chang N.: The role of gastric mucosal blood flow and H^+ back-diffusion in the pathogenesis of acute gastric erosions. *J. Surg. Res.* 22:357, 1977.
11. Cheung L.Y., Porterfield G.: Protection of gastric mucosa against acute ulceration by intravenous infusion of sodium bicarbonate. *Am. J. Surg.* 137:106, 1979.
12. Chin T.W.F., MacLeod S.M., Fenje P., et al.: Pharmacokinetics of cimetidine in critically ill children. *Pediatr. Pharmacol.* 2:285, 1982.
13. Christie D.L., Ament M.E.: Diagnosis and treatment of duodenal ulcer in infancy and childhood. *Pediatr. Ann.* 5:673, 1976.
14. Conn H.O., Blitzer B.L.: Nonassociation of adrenocortico-steroid therapy and peptic ulcer. *N. Engl. J. Med.* 294:473, 1976.
15. Deckelbaum R.J., Roy C.C., Lussier-Lazaroff J., et al.: Peptic ulcer disease: A clinical study in 73 children. *CMA J.* 111:225, 1974.
16. Donovan E.J., Santulli R.V.: Gastric and duodenal ulcers in infancy and in childhood. *Am. J. Dis. Child.* 69:176, 1945.
17. Drake D.P., MacIver A.G., Atwell J.D.: Zollinger-Ellison syndrome in a child: Medical treatment with cimetidine. *Arch. Dis. Child.* 55:226, 1980.
18. Fällström S.P., Reinard T.: Peptic ulcer in children. *Acta Paediatr.* 50:431, 1961.
19. Fliegel C.P., Herzog B., Signer E., et al.: Bleeding gastric ulcer in a newborn infant diagnosed by transumbilical aortography. *J. Pediatr. Surg.* 12:589, 1977.
20. Garner A., Flemstrom G., Heylings J.R.: Effects of antiinflammatory agents on acid and bicarbonate secretions in the amphibian—isolated gastric mucosa. *Gastroenterology* 77:451, 1979.
21. Ghai O.P., Singh M., Walia B.N.S., et al.: An assessment of gastric acid secretory response with "maximal" augmented histamine stimulation in children with peptic ulcer. *Arch. Dis. Child.* 40:77, 1965.
22. Grosfeld J.L., Shipley F., Fitzgerald J.F., et al.: Acute peptic ulcer in infancy and childhood. *Am. Surg.* 44:13, 1978.
23. Habbick B.F., Melrose A.G., Grant J.C.: Duodenal ulcer in childhood: A study of predisposing factors. *Arch. Dis. Child.* 43:23, 1968.
24. Harmon J.W., Jordan P.H. Jr.: Verdict on vagotomy. *Gastroenterology* 81:809, 1981.
25. Idjadi F., Robbins R., Stahl W.M., et al.: Prospective study of gastric secretion in stress patients. *J. Trauma* 11:681, 1971.
26. Jackson R.H.: Genetic studies in peptic ulcer in childhood. *Acta Paediatr.* 61:493, 1971.
27. Johnson D., L'Heureux P., Thompson T.: Peptic ulcer disease in early infancy: Clinical presentation and roentgenographic features. *Acta Paediatr. Scand.* 69:753, 1980.
28. Johnson H.D., Love A.H.G., Rogers N.H., et al.: Gastric ulcers, blood groups and acid secretion. *Gut* 5:402, 1964.
29. Johnston P.W., Snyder W.H.: Survey of vagotomy and pyloroplasty in infants and children. *Am. J. Surg.* 120:173, 1970.
30. Keramides D.C., Voyatzis N.: Duodenal ulcer associated with incomplete duodenal diaphragm. *J. Pediatr. Surg.* 10:837, 1975.
31. Langman M.S., Doll R.: ABO blood groups and secretor status in relation to clinical characteristics of peptic ulcers. *Gut* 6:270, 1965.
32. Lerner A.G., Meng C.H., Schneider K.M.: Selective intra-arterial vasopressin in the management of stress ulcers in childhood. *Pediatrics* 51:126, 1973.
33. Lucas C.E., Sugawa C., Riddle J.: Natural history and surgical dilemma of "stress" gastric bleeding. *Arch. Surg.* 102:266, 1971.
34. Magnusson B., Hallberg L., Arvidsson B.: Iron absorption from food and from ferrous ascorbate. *Scand. J. Haem.* (suppl.) 26:69, 1976.
35. Mendl K., Jenkins R.T., Penlington E.F.: Gastric ulcer in the newborn and its association with antral spasm resulting in hypertrophic pyloric stenosis. *Br. J. Radiol.* 35:831, 1962.
36. Menguy R.: Role of gastric mucosal energy metabolism in the etiology of stress ulceration. *World J. Surg.* 5:175, 1981.
37. Michener W.M., Kennedy R.L.J., Du Shane J.W.: Duodenal ulcer in childhood. *Am. J. Dis. Child.* 100:814, 1960.
38. Miller R.A.: Observations on the gastric acidity during the first month of life. *Arch. Dis. Child.* 15:22, 1941.
39. Miller T.A., Jacobson E.D.: Gastrointestinal cytoprotection by prostaglandins. *Gut* 20:75, 1979.
40. Millikan J.C.: Duodenal ulceration in children. *Gut* 6:25, 1965.
41. Moody F.G., Cheung L.Y.: Stress ulcers: Their pathogenesis, diagnosis, and treatment. *Surg. Clin. North Am.* 56:1469, 1976.
42. Moody F.G., Zalewsky C.A., Larsen K.R.: Cytoprotection of the gastric epithelium. *World J. Surg.* 5:153, 1981.
43. Moore T.C.: Gastrectomy in infancy and childhood. *Ann. Surg.* 162:91, 1965.
44. Morden R.S., Schullinger J.N., Mollitt D.L., et al.: Operative management of stress ulcers in children. *Ann. Surg.* 196:18, 1982.
45. Morgan D.B., Hunt G., Peterson C.R.: The osteomalacia syndrome after stomach operations. *Am. J. Med.* 155:395, 1970.
46. Nesser J., Reitman D., Sacks H.S., et al.: Association of adrenocorticosteroid therapy and peptic ulcer disease. *N. Engl. J. Med.* 309:21, 1983.
47. Norton L., Greer J., Eiseman B.: Gastric secretory response to head injury. *Arch. Surg.* 101:200, 1970.
48. O'Neill J.A. Jr., Pruitt B.A. Jr., Moncrief J.A.: Surgical treatment of Curling's ulcer. *Surg. Gynecol. Obstet.* 126:40, 1968.
49. Othersen B.H. Jr., Garcia R., Doering E.J.: The effect of gastric resections and denervation upon growth in miniature swine. *J. Pediatr. Surg.* 8:159, 1973.
50. Polacek M.A., Ellison E.H.: Gastric acid secretion and parietal cell mass in the stomach of a newborn infant. *Am. J. Surg.* 111:777, 1966.
51. Puri P., Boyd E., Blake N., et al.: Duodenal ulcer in childhood: A continuing disease in adult life. *J. Pediatr. Surg.* 13:525, 1978.
52. Ravitch M.M., Duremdes G.D.: Operative treatment of chronic duodenal ulcer in childhood. *Ann. Surg.* 171:641, 1970.
53. Robb J.D.A., Thomas P.S., Orszulok J., et al.: Duodenal ulcer in children. *Arch. Dis. Child.* 47:688, 1972.
54. Robert A., Lancoster C., Huncher A.J., et al.: Mild irritants prevent gastric necrosis thru prostaglandin formation. *Gastroenterology* 74:1086, 1978.
55. Rosenlund M.L.: The Zollinger-Ellison syndrome in children: A review. *Pediatrics* 141:884, 1967.
56. Schuster S.R., Gross R.E.: Peptic ulcer disease in childhood. *Am. J. Surg.* 105:324, 1963.
57. Seagram C.G.F., Stephens C.A., Cumming W.A.: Peptic ulceration at the Hospital for Sick Children, Toronto, during the 20-year period 1949–1969. *J. Pediatr. Surg.* 8:407, 1973.
58. Skillman J.J., Silen W.: Stress ulcers. *Lancet* 2:1303, 1972.
59. Sultz H.A., Schlesinger E.R., Feldman J.G., et al.: The epidemiology of peptic ulcer in childhood. *Am. J. Pub. Health* 60:492, 1970.
60. Tedesco F.J., Goldstein P.D., Gleason W.A., et al.: Upper gastroin-

testinal endoscopy in the pediatric patient. *Gastroenterology* 70:492, 1976.
61. Ternberg J.L., Koehler P.R.: The use of arteriography in the diagnosis of the origin of acute gastrointestinal hemorrhage in children. *Surgery* 63:686, 1968.
62. Tsuchida Y., Makino S., Ishida M.: A follow-up study of subtotal gastrectomy in infancy and early childhood. *J. Pediatr. Surg.* 9:499, 1974.
63. von Siebold A.E.: Brand in der kleinen Kurvatier des Magens eines atrophischen Kindes. *J. Geburtsh. Frauenzimmer. Kinderkr.* 5:3, 1826.
64. Wagner H.: The development to full functional maturity of the gastric mucosa and the kidneys in the fetus and newborn. *Biol. Neonat.* 3:257, 1961.
65. Williams J.W., Pannell W.P., Sherman R.T.: Curling's ulcer in children. *J. Trauma* 16:639, 1976.
66. Williams R.S., Ahmed S.: Peptic ulcer in childhood. *Aust. Paediatr. J.* 13:299, 1977.
67. Wilson S.D.: The role of surgery in children with the Zollinger-Ellison syndrome. *Surgery* 92:682, 1982.

---

83 John R. Campbell
Other Conditions of the Stomach

Congenital Gastric Outlet Obstruction

HISTORY.—Congenital gastric outlet obstruction, not common in the newborn period, has been recognized only in comparatively recent years. In 1937, Bennett[2] reported a 4-day-old infant who died 36 hours after operation for "pyloric stenosis." Autopsy revealed the cause of obstruction to be a complete prepyloric diaphragm. In 1940, Touroff and Sussman[31] successfully removed a complete prepyloric diaphragm in a 1-day-old infant. Metz et al.,[21] in 1951, reported a 3-day-old infant who had a double diaphragm that caused a cyst-like structure between two membranes. Incision of the diaphragms resulted in recovery. In 1951, Benson and Coury[3] reported the third successful operation, and in 1959, Brown and Hertzler[6] reported successful treatment of two premature infants. There are at least six reports of familial occurrence, and there is some suggestion of an autosomal recessive mode of inheritance.[1, 3, 5, 18, 23, 30]

Etiology and Pathology

When these lesions are discovered in an infant, there is no question of their congenital origin. Identical lesions are seen in adults, frequently with little history to suggest a congenital origin, and it has been argued that they might be acquired.[7, 12, 24, 28] Most believe that they arise following an in utero vascular accident, as with other small and large intestinal atresias, although others think that failure of recanalization may be the cause. Maternal hydramnios occurs in about half of the cases.[20] Gerber and Aberdeen,[14] in an extensive review, proposed the following classification:
I. Pyloric
  A. Membrane
  B. Atresia
II. Antral (1 cm or more proximal to pylorus)
  A. Membrane
  B. Atresia

Atresias can usually be recognized at operation, and occasionally a fibrous cord may join two blind ends (Fig 83–1). Gastrotomy and passage of catheters may be required to detect membranous obstructions (Fig 83–2).

The infant with complete gastric outlet obstruction, proximal to the entry of the common bile duct, vomits nonbile-stained material.[11, 26, 27] Frequently the diaphragm, although perforate, produces essentially complete obstruction. Respiratory problems are common, and dyspnea, tachypnea, cyanosis, and excessive salivation may be mistaken for esophageal atresia. The abdomen is scaphoid unless the stomach is distended. If diagnosis is delayed, the stomach may perforate. The passage of a meconium stool may mislead the casual observer.

Diagnosis

Roentgen examinations confirm the clinical diagnosis (Fig 83–3). It may be necessary to aspirate the stomach of liquid contents and reinstill a similar volume of air. Injections of opaque material are unnecessary. Films taken in various positions may be needed to establish the correct diagnosis.

Talwalker[29] emphasized the difficulty in diagnosing pyloric atresia at laparotomy, and recommended generous proximal gastrotomy. Haller and Cahill[16] warn against missing a pyloric web in association with a duodenal atresia. Conversely, a wide gastrotomy and distal passage of a catheter after excision of the prepyloric diaphragm discloses any duodenal diaphragm.

Treatment

Excision of a complete or perforate diaphragm with Heineke-Mikulicz pyloroplasty is the most straightforward correction. In the presence of atresia with a gap, gastroduodenostomy will be necessary. A temporary tube gastrostomy is useful.

Prognosis

With early diagnosis and operation, and with current neonatal supportive care, survival should be anticipated. Mortality has been associated with delayed diagnosis[1, 18, 23] and with associated conditions.[25] Fifty-nine cases of congenital pyloric atresia have been reported, with a familial occurrence described in 13 infants in six families, with a high and unexplained mortality in this familial group.

Incomplete Pyloric-Prepyloric Diaphragm in Infants and Children

Fiberoptic panendoscopy has, as yet, been carried out infrequently in cases of this lesion but may clarify roentgenographic findings. Dilute barium may be required in diagnosis of these incomplete lesions (Fig 83–4), which are being reported with increasing frequency, especially in adults.[1, 4, 5, 8, 9, 13, 15, 17, 19, 23, 32] The prognosis should be excellent

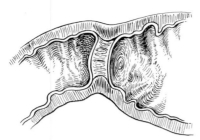

Fig 83–1.—Pyloric atresia. Note that the seromuscular layers are uninterrupted. The tissue between the gastric and duodenal mucosae was of two types, fibrous and areolar.

after excision of the diaphragm and either end-to-end anastomosis or pyloroplasty. Meconium peritonitis has been reported in association with a prepyloric mucosal diaphragm.[10]

REFERENCES

1. Bar-Maor J.A., Nissan S., Nevo S.: Pyloric atresia: A hereditary congenital anomaly with autosomal recessive transmission. *J. Med. Genet.* 9:70, 1972.
2. Bennett R.J. Jr.: Atresia of pylorus. *Am. J. Dig. Dis.* 4:44, 1937.
3. Benson C.D., Coury J.J.: Congenital intrinsic obstruction of stomach and duodenum in the newborn. *Arch. Surg.* 62:856, 1951.
4. Berman J.K., Ballenger F.: Prepyloric membranous obstruction. *Q. Bull. Ind. Univ. Med. Center* 4:14, 1948.
5. Bronsther B., Nadeau M.R., Abrams M.W.: Congenital pyloric atresia: A report of three cases and a review of the literature. *Surgery* 69:130, 1971.
6. Brown R.P., Hertzler J.H.: Congenital prepyloric gastric atresia. *Am. J. Dis. Child.* 97:857, 1959.
7. Creedon F.: The adult pyloric mucosal diaphragm. *Br. J. Surg.* 55:818, 1968.
8. Cremin B.J.: Neonatal prepyloric membrane. *S. Afr. Med. J.* 41:1076, 1967.
9. Cremin B.J.: Congenital pyloric antral membranes in infancy. *Radiology* 92:509, 1969.
10. DeSpirito A.J., Guthorn P.J.: Recovery from meconium peritonitis associated with diaphragm-like obstruction of the prepyloric mucosa. *J. Pediatr.* 50:599, 1957.
11. Ducharme J.C., Bensoussan A.L.: Pyloric atresia. *J. Pediatr. Surg.* 10:149, 1975.
12. Felson B., Berkmen Y.M., Hoyumpa A.M.: Gastric mucosal diaphragm. *Radiology* 92:513, 1969.

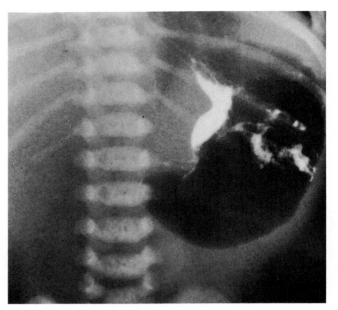

Fig 83–3.—Pyloric atresia in a newborn. Air provides excellent contrast. No air beyond the pylorus. This child was readmitted to the hospital dehydrated and with hypochloremic, hypokalemic alkalosis after early postnatal discharge. End-to-end gastroduodenostomy was successful.

13. Fujioka M., Fisher S., Young L.W.: Pseudoweb of the gastric antrum in infants. *Pediatr. Radiol.* 9:73, 1980.
14. Gerber B.C., Aberdeen S.D.: Prepyloric diaphragm: An unusual abnormality. *Arch. Surg.* 90:472, 1965.
15. Hait G., Esselstyn C.B., Rank G.B.: Prepyloric mucosal diaphragm (antral web): Report of a case and review of the literature. *Arch. Surg.* 105:486, 1972.
16. Haller J.A., Cahill J.L.: Combined congenital gastric and duodenal obstruction. *Surgery* 63:503, 1968.
17. Jinkins J.R., Ball T.I., Clements J.L. Jr., et al.: Antral mucosal diaphragms in infants and children. *Pediatr. Radiol.* 9:69, 1980.
18. Keramidas D.C., Voyatzis N.: Pyloric atresia: Report of a second occurrence in the same family. *J. Pediatr. Surg.* 7:445, 1972.
19. Liechti R.E., Mikkelson W.P., Snyder W.H. Jr.: Prepyloric stenosis caused by congenital squamous epithelial diaphragm-resultant infantilism. *Surgery* 53:670, 1963.
20. Lloyd J.R., Clatworthy H.W. Jr.: Hydramnios as an aid to the early diagnosis of congenital obstruction of the alimentary tract: A study of the maternal and fetal factors. *Pediatrics* 21:903, 1958.
21. Metz A.R., Householder R., DePree J.F.: Obstruction of the stomach due to congenital double septum with cyst formation. *Trans. West. Surg. Assoc.* 50:242, 1951.
22. Nanagas V., Hartley-Smith E.: Incomplete pyloric diaphragm. *J. Pediatr. Surg.* 9:551, 1974.
23. Olson L., Grotte G.: Congenital pyloric atresia: Report of a familial occurrence. *J. Pediatr. Surg.* 11:181, 1976.
24. Parrish R.A. Jr., Sherman H.S., Moretz W.H.: Congenital antral membrane. *Surgery* 59:681, 1966.
25. Peltier F.A., Tschen E.H., Raimer S.S., et al.: Epidermolysis bullosa lethalis associated with congenital pyloric atresia. *Arch. Dermatol.* 117:728, 1981.
26. Salzberg A.M., Collins R.E.: Congenital pyloric atresia. *Arch. Surg.* 80:501, 1960.
27. Saw E.C., Arbegast N.R., Comer T.: Pyloric atresia: A case report. *Pediatrics* 51:574, 1973.
28. Shartsis J.M., Fox T.A.: Pyloric diaphragm in an adult. *Gastroenterology* 56:580, 1969.
29. Talwalker V.C.: Pyloric atresia: A case report. *J. Pediatr. Surg.* 2:458, 1967.
30. Thompson N.W., Parker W., Schwartz S., et al.: Congenital pyloric atresia. *Arch. Surg.* 97:792, 1968.
31. Touroff A.S.W., Sussman R.M.: Congenital prepyloric membranous obstruction in a premature infant. *Surgery* 8:739, 1940.
32. Wutenberger H.: Gastric atresia. *Arch. Dis. Child.* 36:161, 1961.

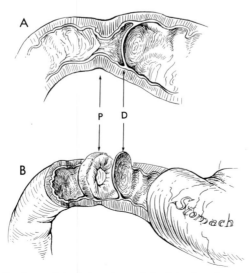

Fig 83–2.—Congenital pyloric and prepyloric obstruction. **A,** prepyloric membrane, **B,** antral diaphragm. *P* = pylorus; *D* = diaphragm.

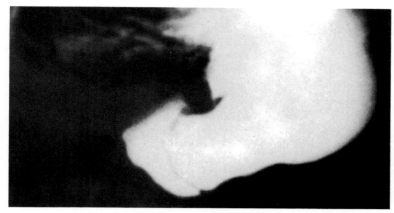

Fig 83–4.—Incomplete antral diaphragm in a newborn. This infant had non-bile-stained vomitus shortly after birth. A swallow of dilute barium made the diagnosis in this incomplete obstruction. Heineke-Mikulicz pyloroplasty and excision of the web were successful.

Volvulus of the Stomach

HISTORY.—General descriptions of gastric volvulus have appeared in the literature since the first description by Berti in 1866.[1] Borchardt,[2] in 1904, described the classic triad of observations: (1) acute or localized distention of the epigastrium associated with pain, (2) inability to pass a nasogastric tube, and (3) nonproductive attempts at vomiting. It was not until 1923 that the characteristic roentgen findings of acute gastric volvulus were described. Since then, numerous case reports have appeared of adults and of children, including a review of the world literature by Cole and Dickinson.[5] Acute gastric volvulus in children is a rare condition, representing 44 of 250 cases reported in their review. Chronic gastric volvulus is encountered more frequently than the acute form, and in adults is often seen with paraesophageal hiatus hernia. Acute gastric volvulus, on the other hand, is a true surgical emergency.

Description and Classification

Gastric volvulus is rare, since the stomach is held securely in place by the gastrophrenic ligaments and the esophageal hiatus, the retroperitoneal fixation of the duodenum, the short gastric vessels, and the gastrocolic ligament. It occurs, therefore, only when there is laxity or absence of these attachments. It is occasionally associated with eventration of the diaphragm, diaphragmatic hernia, congenital bands, elongated gastric attachments, or absence of the gastrocolic ligament. Disorders of rotation are the suspected cause. Mental retardation has been noted in association, and asplenia or a mobile spleen are common.[7] It is commoner in males than females.[3, 5, 9]

Diagnosis of acute gastric volvulus associated with diaphragmatic hernia is usually made at operation. When it occurs alone, the symptoms will be those of high intestinal obstruction or, if vascular compromise has occurred, the local and systemic manifestations of gangrene. Occasionally, the distended stomach causes an epigastric fullness or mass.

Gastric volvulus is classified according to the plane of rotation (Fig 83–5). In organoaxial volvulus, the stomach rotates on its long axis; the greater curvature passes anteriorly but may be displaced posteriorly. In the less common mesenterioaxial volvulus, rotation is on an axis from greater to lesser curvature, the pylorus or cardia commonly rotating anteriorly. The opposite rotation may occur. The torsion may be total, involving the entire stomach, or partial and limited to the pyloric end. The rotating section most often passes anteriorly.

Radiologic Features

Roentgenographic examination (Fig 83–6) often provides a definitive diagnosis. de Lorimier and Penn[6] specified the roentgenologic features of acute volvulus of the stomach: (1) localized massive distention of the upper abdomen; (2) visualization of the outline of a "hairpin" loop with incisura toward the right upper quadrant; (3) fixation of the loop regardless of the position of the patient; (4) delimitation of ingested barium at the tapered extremity of the esophagus, the so-called bird's beak; (5) possible evidence of a hiatal sacculation or other diaphragmatic herniation; and (6) deviation of the position of the spleen.

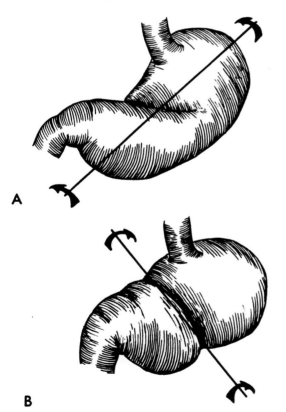

A

B

Fig 83–5.—Gastric volvulus. **A,** organoaxial. The greater curvature usually passes forward, as depicted, but may rotate posteriorly. **B,** mesenteroaxial. The pylorus or the cardia commonly rotates anteriorly, but the opposite may occur. (From Cole and Dickinson: *Surgery* 70:707, 1971; used by permission.)

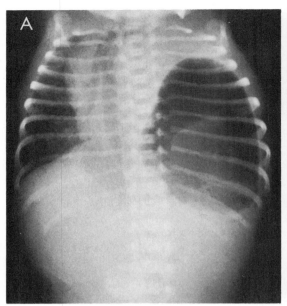
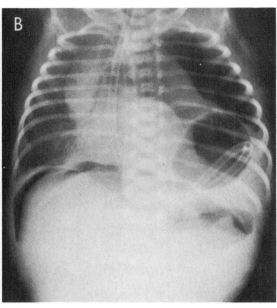

Fig 83–6.—Acute gastric volvulus in a 1,060-gm newborn with diaphragmatic hernia. **A,** acutely ill premature infant seized with respiratory distress at 12 hours. **B,** at 24 hours, on transfer to the surgical service in desperate condition, pneu- moperitoneum and a left pneumothorax are seen. The gangrenous portion of the stomach was resected—after reduction of the volvulus—and the diaphragm re- paired. The child survived.

Treatment

This is one of the true acute emergencies in pediatric surgery, and operation should be undertaken before vascular compromise occurs. There is no place for simple decompression with a naso- gastric tube. At operation, gastric decompression by needle tro- car or gastrotomy facilitates reduction. The puncture or gas- trotomy should be closed before reduction, since the site may not be accessible after reduction. Gastrostomy or anterior gastro- pexy is then performed. Recurrence in spite of fixation has been reported.[8]

REFERENCES

1. Berti A.: Singolare attortigliamento dell' esofago col duodeno sequito da rapida morte. *Gass. Med. Ital.* 9:139, 1866.
2. Borchardt M.: Zur Pathologie und Therapie des Magenvolvulus. *Arch. Klin. Chir.* 74:243, 1904.
3. Campbell J.B.: Neonatal gastric volvulus. *AJR* 132:723, 1979.
4. Carter R., Brewer L.A. III, Hinshaw D.B.: Acute gastric volvulus: A study of 25 cases. *Am. J. Surg.* 140:99, 1980.
5. Cole B.C., Dickinson S.J.: Acute volvulus of the stomach in infants and children. *Surgery* 70:707, 1971.
6. DeLorimier A.A., Penn L.: Acute volvulus of the stomach, empha- sizing management hazards. *Am. J. Roentgenol.* 77:627, 1957.
7. Singleton A.C.: Chronic gastric volvulus. *Radiology* 34:53, 1940.
8. Tanner N.C.: Chronic and recurrent volvulus of the stomach with late results of "colonic displacement." *Am. J. Surg.* 115:505, 1968.
9. Ziprkowski M.D., Teele R.L.: Gastric volvulus in childhood. *AJR* 132:921, 1979.

Gastrointestinal Perforations in the Newborn

HISTORY.—Perforation of the gastrointestinal tract of the newborn without demonstrable cause was first reported by Siebold.[24] Such lesions eventually acquired the label of "spontaneous perforations." Stern et al.,[26] in 1929, reported one of the earliest attempts at operative interven- tion, but it was not until 1943 that a neonatal gastrointestinal perforation was closed successfully.[1] With rare exception,[27] perforations in stomach, duodenum, small intestine, or colon were considered different entities. In 1964, Lloyd et al.[17] reported 61 cases of so-called spontaneous perfo- ration of the gastrointestinal tract of the newborn and called attention to the fact that these lesions were the result of ischemic necrosis, regardless of location. The undesirable side effects of an asphyxial defense mecha- nism, known as selective circulatory ischemia, activated by perinatal stress, hypoxia, or shock, were implicated as the principal factors causing these lesions.[2, 3, 12, 28] In 1969, Lloyd[16] reviewed the world literature and found 315 cases of gastrointestinal perforation in neonates qualifying as ischemic lesions. Additional reports, although categorized variously as spontaneous gastric perforations or necrotizing enterocolitis, bring the total of reported cases into the thousands.

Etiology and Pathology

Ischemic necrosis with perforation of the gastrointestinal tract is a unique surgical disease of the newborn because, in contrast to other disorders in this chapter, it is an acquired lesion. Al- though the same etiologic process leads to necrotizing enterocol- itis without perforation, the latter will be discussed separately (see Chap. 100). In this condition, we exclude perforations with such obvious causes as intubation, obstruction distal to the per- foration, and accidental gastric overinsufflation. However, Hol- gersen,[10] in a recent re-evaluation, compared 28 cases of spon- taneous gastric perforation to 10 experimental mechanical gastric disruptions in animals and thought there was sufficient evidence to support the thesis that neonatal gastric perforation is due to overdistention. Explanations considered in the past and now dis- carded are congenital muscular defects,[9] increased gastric acid- ity,[18] and compression of a fluid-filled stomach during birth.[23, 25] Although ischemia may be the common denominator, a multifac- torial etiology is likely, including bacterial colonization of the gut with pathogenic organisms[14] and the presence of a hyperosmolar luminal substrate such as carbohydrate. Kiesewetter[13] suggested that a hypothalamic-pituitary-adrenal mechanism activated by perinatal stress, including anoxia, could result in gastromalacia and subsequent perforation of the stomach. Gregory et al.[6] doc- umented perinatal stress in 39 of 42 infants with ischemic necro- sis of the gut. The actual mechanisms by which these ischemic changes are induced remain uncertain. It is believed that blood is shunted to the heart and the brain at the expense of the pe- ripheral, renal, and mesenteric vascular beds. The reader is re- ferred to the works of Scholander[21, 22] and Elsner et al.[3] for the details of this "diving reflex" in mammals and in man. Asphyxia

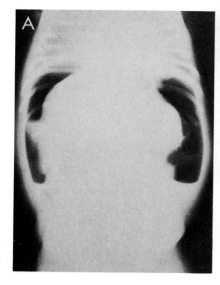
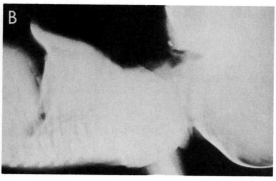

Fig 83–7.—Spontaneous perforation of the stomach. Plain upright posteroanterior **(A)** and lateral **(B)** films of the abdomen, showing massive pneumoperitoneum.

at birth in infants with low Apgar scores is particularly likely to lead to intestinal perforation. Redistribution of blood flow during hypoxia and/or hypovolemia or other stress states,[29] with shunting away from mesenteric vascular beds, is thought to result in microvascular injury[7, 8] and subsequent loss of mucosal integrity.[11] Persistence of the ischemic insult, allowing extension of microvascular thrombosis, leads to the transmural necrosis seen in intestinal perforation. The periods of stress and potential mesenteric ischemia may be temporally remote from the recognition of perforation. Indomethacin therapy in low birth weight infants has been implicated in gastrointestinal perforations.[5, 19] One can speculate as to whether the cause is indomethacin or the low birth weight.

Signs and Symptoms

The first indication of perforation usually occurs at 4–5 days of life. Abdominal distention is frequently abrupt and rapidly progressive. Signs of hypovolemia and decreased perfusion are usually present. Respiratory difficulty from massive pneumoperitoneum may be the first indication. Early radiographs may not reveal pneumoperitoneum, which becomes obvious with time (Fig 83–7).

Infants born of pregnancies characterized by abruptio placentae, placenta previa, amnionitis, and infants delivered by emergency cesarean section are at increased risk and should be carefully observed for 4–5 days. Pressure from utilization review bodies should be resisted, and early discharge from the hospital of infants at risk of gastric perforation is to be avoided.

The infant who seems to be progressing satisfactorily and suddenly refuses feedings, or who is listless and apathetic, and in whom a septic work-up is undertaken should have feedings discontinued. Serial abdominal radiographs should be obtained until the cause of the problem is elucidated.

The incidence and sex distribution in the population as a whole is unknown. An excellent review by Rosser et al.[20] provides information relative to the incidence among the black population, an incidence of 1 in 2,900 live births. In this series, four times more males than females were afflicted.

Treatment

Preoperative Preparation.—The infant with gastrointestinal perforation deteriorates rapidly, and early recognition and prompt treatment are essential for a favorable outcome. Linkner and Benson[15] stressed rapid resuscitation—fluid and colloid administration, blood transfusion, correction of acidosis, antibiotics, nasogastric suction, and only essential diagnostic studies—with attention to the prevention or correction of hypothermia. Aspiration of the pneumoperitoneum with a blunt needle or plastic catheter may relieve life-threatening respiratory distress. Some of these infants will require immediate respiratory support. If transportation to a tertiary care nursery is indicated, resuscitation should begin before transport, and the infant should be transported by experienced personnel who can continue the resuscitation en route.

Operation.—A transverse right supraumbilical incision can be extended into a full upper abdominal transverse incision to approach any site of perforation. Systematic exploration of the abdomen should be carried out, directed by the location of the greatest peritoneal soilage. Perforation sites may be occult and, after careful examination of the bowel from the esophageal hiatus to the pelvic floor, exploration of the lesser omental space may be necessary. Looking for bubbles when the abdomen is filled with warm saline has been suggested. Failure to demonstrate the actual site of perforation occurs in about 10% of cases, and in the majority of such instances the perforation may be sealed. The decision to take down adhesions and to look for the site is a difficult one. If it can be determined that there is no continued soilage, and there is no distal obstruction, the bowel may best be left undisturbed. If the site of perforation is discrete and the adjacent bowel healthy, the perforation may be closed in layers with nonabsorbable sutures. If there is massive necrosis, resection may be necessary. Whether to perform an anastomosis or a double-barreled enterostomy depends on the level of the perforation. Infants tolerate high intestinal fistulae poorly and there is a tendency toward more frequent primary anastomoses, although the sick infant's best chance for survival may depend on a short operative procedure with exteriorization of the perforation. Resection at times may need to be massive, and resections approaching total gastrectomy are sometimes necessary.[4] It is an error to finish an operation without finding some explanation of the cause. Hirschsprung's disease and colonic atresia have presented in just this manner, as intestinal perforation "without explanation." Aerobic and anaerobic cultures should always be obtained.

Certain infants with respiratory distress syndrome, on high-pressure ventilatory support, develop pneumoperitoneum.[30] These are patients at greatest risk of ischemic gut necrosis. However, pulmonary alveolar rupture may occur, and air may dissect down the bronchial sheath into the mediastinum and into the abdomen, producing a picture identical to that of gastrointestinal perforation. It is important to avoid an unnecessary operation in these critically ill infants. The recognition of pneumomediastinum or pneumopericardium may allow the surgeon to observe these infants. If one cannot exclude ischemic gut necrosis as the cause, abdominal exploration should be undertaken.

POSTOPERATIVE MANAGEMENT.—Most of these sick infants return to the intensive care nursery with their tracheas intubated. Extubation, adjustments in fluid and colloid administration, removal of nasogastric tubes, and institution of oral feedings must be individualized. Loss of fluid from the intravascular space into the peritoneum may be massive, and appropriate replacement requires careful monitoring of urinary output, pulmonary and cardiac status, and intestinal function.

PROGNOSIS.—Except for the isolated gastric perforation, the survival rate of these infants continues to be discouraging; the prognosis is determined by the maturity of the infant, associated conditions, the duration between perforation and resuscitation, the exactness of the surgical procedure, and the aggressiveness of the postoperative care. Early series[16] reported survival of approximately 30%. More recent series suggest greater than double that survival.

REFERENCES

1. Agerty H.A., Ziserman A.J., Schollenberger C.L.: A case of perforation of the ileum in a newborn infant with operation and recovery. *J. Pediatr.* 22:223, 1943.
2. Barlow B., Santulli T.V.: Importance of multiple episodes of hypoxia or cold stress on the development of enterocolitis in an animal model. *Surgery* 77:687, 1975.
3. Elsner R., Franklin R.L., Van Citters R.L., et al.: Cardiovascular defense against asphyxia. *Science* 153:941, 1966.
4. Graivier L., Rundell K., McWilliams N., et al.: Neonatal gastric perforation and necrosis: Gastrectomy and colonic interposition with survival. *Ann. Surg.* 177:428, 1973.
5. Gray P.H., Pemberton P.J.: Gastric perforation associated with indomethacin therapy in a pre-term infant. *Aust. Paediatr. J.* 16:65, 1980.
6. Gregory J.R., Campbell J.R., Harrison M.W., et al.: Necrotizing enterocolitis. *Am. J. Surg.* 141:562, 1981.
7. Harrison M.W., Connell R.S., Campbell J.R., et al.: Microcirculatory changes in the gastrointestinal tract of the hypoxic puppy: An electron microscope study. *J. Pediatr. Surg.* 10:599, 1975.
8. Harrison M.W., Connell R.S., Campbell J.R., et al.: Fine structural changes in the gastrointestinal tract of the hypoxic puppy: A study of the natural history. *J. Pediatr. Surg.* 12:403, 1977.
9. Herbut P.A.: Congenital defect in the musculature of the stomach with rupture in a newborn infant. *Arch. Pathol.* 36:91, 1943.
10. Holgersen L.O.: The etiology of spontaneous gastric perforation of the newborn: a reevaluation. *J. Pediatr. Surg.* 16:608, 1981.
11. Hopkins G.B., Gould V.E., Stevenson J.K., et al.: Necrotizing enterocolitis in premature infants. *Am. J. Dis. Child.* 120:229, 1970.
12. James L.S.: Biochemical aspects of asphyxia at birth, in *Adaptation to Extrauterine Life.* 31st Ross Conference on Pediatric Research. Columbus, Ohio, Ross Laboratories, 1959, p. 66.
13. Kiesewetter W.B.: Spontaneous rupture of the stomach in the newborn. *Am. J. Dis. Child.* 91:162, 1956.
14. Kosloske A.M.: Necrotizing enterocolitis in the neonate. *Surg. Gynecol. Obstet.* 148:259, 1979.
15. Linkner L., Benson C.: Spontaneous perforation of the stomach in the newborn. *Ann. Surg.* 149:525, 1959.
16. Lloyd J.R.: The etiology of gastrointestinal perforations in the newborn. *J. Pediatr. Surg.* 4:77, 1969.
17. Lloyd J.R., Espiasse E., Bernstein J.: Etiology of gastrointestinal perforations in the newborn. *Harper Hosp. Bull.* (Detroit) 22:224, 1964.
18. Miller R.A.: Gastric acidity during the first year of life. *Arch. Dis. Child.* 17:198, 1942.
19. Nagaraj H.S., Sandhu A.S., Cook L.N., et al.: Gastrointestinal perforation following indomethacin therapy in very low birth weight infants. *J. Pediatr. Surg.* 16:1003, 1981.
20. Rosser S.B., Clark C.H., Elechi E.N.: Spontaneous neonatal gastric perforation. *J. Pediatr. Surg.* 17:390, 1982.
21. Scholander P.F.: The master switch of life. *Sci. Am.* 209:92, 1963.
22. Scholander P.F.: Circulatory adjustment in pearl divers. *J. Appl. Physiol.* 17:184, 1962.
23. Shaw A., Blank W.A., Santulli T.V., et al.: Spontaneous rupture of the stomach in the newborn, a clinical and experimental study. *Surgery* 58:561, 1965.
24. Siebold A.E.: Brand in der Kleinen Kurvatier des Magens eines atrophischen Kindes. *J. Geburtsch. Frauenzimmer. Kinderkr.* 5:3, 1826.
25. Silbergleit A., Berkas E.M.: Neonatal gastric rupture. *Minn. Med.* 49:65, 1966.
26. Stern M.A., Perkins E.L., Nessa N.J.: Perforated gastric ulcer in a 2-day-old infant. *Journal Lancet* 49:492, 1929.
27. Thelander H.E.: Perforation of the gastrointestinal tract of the newborn infant. *Am. J. Dis. Child.* 58:371, 1939.
28. Touloukian R.J.: Gastric ischemia: The primary factor in neonatal perforation. *Clin. Pediatr.* 12:219, 1973.
29. Touloukian R.J., Posch J.N., Spencer R.: The pathogenesis of ischemic gastroenterocolitis of the neonate: Selective gut mucosal ischemia in asphyxiated neonatal piglets. *J. Pediatr. Surg.* 7:194, 1972.
30. Zerella J.T., McCullough J.Y.: Pneumoperitoneum in infants without gastrointestinal perforation. *Surgery* 89:163, 1981.

Lactobezoar

HISTORY.—Inspissated formula causing intestinal obstruction in the premature infant was first reported in 1969.[2] Although it had undoubtedly occurred much earlier, the increasing survival of premature infants, in whom this condition usually occurs, made its recognition more common. The advent of total parenteral nutrition and the tendency toward cautious feeding of the premature have undoubtedly reduced the incidence in today's intensive care nurseries.

Etiology and Pathology

The immediate and early undiluted breast milk feeding of infants has long been known to reduce the serum bilirubin and prevent symptomatic hypoglycemia. This tendency toward early feeding when applied to the premature infant can result in the formation of lactobezoars that temporarily cause gastric obstruction (Fig 83–8,A). The typical age at presentation is 5–14 days,[2] although a 4½-month-old infant was readmitted to the hospital with a lactobezoar obstructing the stomach after powdered milk was substituted for evaporated milk and water.[4] Bennett and Herman[1] reported a 2-year-8-month-old boy who developed a milk curd cast after a whooping-cough type of illness of 1 month's duration. Powdered formulas have most often been incriminated. Majd and LoPresti[4] postulated that concentrated formulas produce diarrhea with subsequent dehydration. To reconstitute the depleted extracellular volume, water is absorbed from the gastrointestinal tract, including the stomach. A lactobezoar is thus formed, causing mechanical obstruction of the stomach and vomiting.

Treatment

Most infants and children respond to nonoperative treatment (Fig 83–8,B). Feedings are discontinued, a nasogastric tube is used to empty the stomach, and dehydration, if present, is corrected. Total parenteral nutrition in the fragile premature allows delay, and cautious resumption of oral feedings. If the correct diagnosis is made, operation can be avoided.[3, 5]

REFERENCES

1. Bennett P., Herman S.: Curious curd. *Lancet* 1:1430, 1975.
2. Editorial: New hazards for the newborn. *Br. Med. J.* 4:633, 1969.
3. Erenberg A., Shaw R.D., Yousefzadeh D.: Lactobezoar in the low-birth-weight-infant. *Pediatrics* 63:642, 1979.
4. Majd M., LoPresti J.M.: Lactobezoar. *Am. J. Roentgenol.* 116:575, 1972.

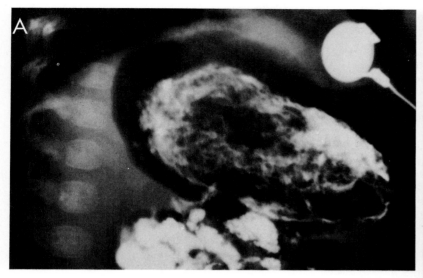

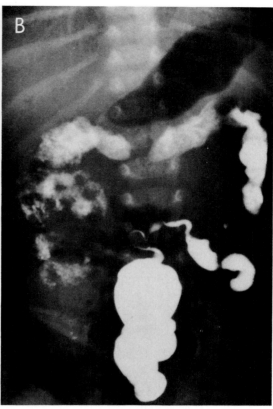

Fig 83–8.—Lactobezoar in a premature infant. **A,** barium-impregnated milk curd cast of stomach. **B,** lactobezoar now gone from the stomach 17 hours after barium was ingested and formula feedings were discontinued.

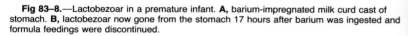

5. Schreiner R.L., Brady M.S., Franken E.A., et al.: Increased incidence of lactobezoars in low birth weight infants. *Am. J. Dis. Child.* 133:936, 1979.

Congenital Microgastria

HISTORY.—Dide,[4] in 1894, performed a necropsy on a feeble-minded and epileptic woman whose stomach was abnormally small and abnormally oriented. Caffey,[3] who cited Dide's report, described the clinical and radiographic findings in a 6-month-old infant who had congenital microgastria and failure of rotation. Blank and Chisholm[2] reported an example seen in 1947 but not reported until 1973. Increasing regionalization of the care of infants and children in hospitals for children has resulted in increased recognition of this condition.[1, 6, 10]

Etiology and Pathology

This is a rare congenital anomaly of the caudal part of the embryological foregut, characterized by a small, tubular stomach, megaesophagus, and incomplete gastric rotation. The esophageal, gastric, small, and large intestinal mucosae are normal. There are many associated conditions of the gastrointestinal tract. Nonrotation of the midgut may occur. One of our patients had duodenal obstruction secondary to nonrotation of the midgut, and duodenal bands and ileal duplication leading to a localized volvulus. At a second operation, when the duodenum remained obstructed, a duodenal mucosal diaphragm was excised. In the postoperative period, hiatal hernia and gastroesophageal reflux were observed. A transverse liver was noted at operation. Multiple thoracic hemivertebrae were present. Absence of the gallbladder has been reported.[9] Massive and persistent reflux into the biliary tract may occur (Fig 83–9). One of our patients had a single atrium, a single ventricle, and total anomalous pulmonary venous return into the portal vein. This child's mother took diphenylhydantoin during her pregnancy. Situs inversus and asplenia have been reported.[7] Skeletal anomalies are common and include micrognathia, radial and ulnar hypoplasia, oligodactyly, and hypoplastic nails. Anophthalmia has been reported.

Clinical Presentation and Pathophysiology

The most frequent signs are vomiting and failure to thrive. Malnutrition and developmental delay may result. Diarrhea is common. One of our patients, although proved not to have cystic fibrosis, was improved by taking pancreatic enzymes. Aspiration pneumonia is common in these infants. An incompetent lower esophageal sphincter has been demonstrated.[11] When coupled with reduced gastric capacity and a dilated esophagus, vomiting, esophageal erosion, and aspiration are common. Although not well studied, it is postulated that malnutrition and diarrhea may result from a small gastric capacity with rapid emptying and a dumping syndrome. Bacterial overgrowth and a blind loop-like syndrome have been suggested to explain the diarrhea and malnutrition, but the Shilling test has been normal in those patients studied.[11]

Investigation

Examination of the gastrointestinal tract with barium is usually the first study and demonstrates the features mentioned above. Imaging techniques augment the radiographs. Endoscopy has proved difficult and confusing. Appropriate cardiac studies will be dictated by the specific findings, and asplenia may be demonstrated by examination of the peripheral blood and by nuclear imaging. If gastroesophageal reflux is a clinical feature, manometry and esophageal pH studies may be appropriate. In pa-

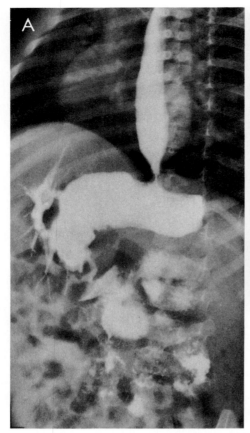

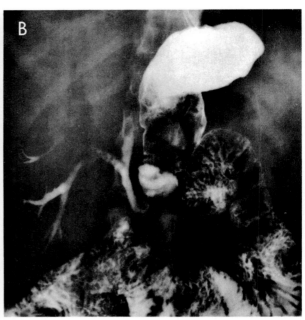

Fig 83–9.—Microgastria. **A,** chest and abdomen in oblique view. Early in the examination, the stomach is filled with barium; the long axis is in an oblique plane. The duodenal bulb is not identifiable, and the duodenum lacks the normal curves. The proximal loops of jejunum are in the normal location in the left upper quadrant. Barium has refluxed into the bile ducts. The esophagus is not dilated. **B,** upper gastrointestinal examination was repeated when the patient was 27 years old. The stomach has grown, but it remains smaller than normal and has not differentiated into its normal parts. Barium again has refluxed into the bile ducts. The loop of small bowel closest to the left side of the stomach is presum- ably the loop of jejunum anastomosed 26 years earlier. This patient presented at 1 year of age with fever and bile-stained vomitus and a history of regurgitation of feedings since birth. Division of duodenal bands and a Ladd procedure failed to completely relieve her symptoms, and a gastrojejunostomy was performed. Thirty-six years later she eats small amounts of food frequently because she fills up quickly. She has no symptoms of "dumping." She is currently employed, has borne three children, weighs 47.3 kg, and is 156.2 cm tall. (From Blank E., Chis- holm A.J.: *Pediatrics* 51:1037, 1973; used by permission.)

tients with diarrhea, malnutrition, or growth retardation, intestinal absorption studies may elucidate the cause.

Treatment

Medical treatment should be tried first. Constant nasogastric feedings may allow a patient to grow and the stomach to enlarge, so that the patient can then tolerate normal feedings. Total parenteral nutrition and other supportive care may be helpful. The longest reported survivor (see Fig 83–9) was treated by gastrojejunostomy. She eats small amounts of food frequently because she fills up quickly. She has no symptom of "dumping." She is currently employed, has borne three children, weighs 42.3 kg, and is 156.2 cm tall, 36 years later. Construction of a jejunal reservoir has been recommended by several authors,[5, 8] and the early follow-up is encouraging. When gastroesophageal reflux cannot be managed medically, fundoplication should be considered, although this may further reduce gastric capacity. The use of antiperistaltic segments and vagotomy are still considered experimental.

REFERENCES

1. Anderson K.D., Guzzetta P.C.: Treatment of congenital microgastria and dumping syndrome. *J. Pediatr. Surg.* 18:747, 1983.
2. Blank E., Chisholm A.J.: Congenital microgastria, a case report with a 26-year follow-up. *Pediatrics* 51:1037, 1973.
3. Caffey J.: *Pediatric X-Ray Diagnosis: A Textbook for Students and Practitioners of Pediatrics, Surgery and Radiology,* ed. 3. Chicago, Year Book Medical Publishers, 1956, p. 496.
4. Dide M.: Sur un estomac d'adulte à type foetal. *Bull. Soc. Anat. Paris* 69:669, 1894.
5. Gerbeaux J., Couvreur J., Vialas M., et al.: Absence congénitale d'estomac. *Ann. Pédiatr.* 18:349, 1971.
6. Hochberger O., Swoboder W.: Congenital microgastria: A follow-up observation over six years. *Pediatr. Radiol.* 2:207, 1974.
7. Kessler H., Smulevicz J.J.: Microgastria associated with agenesis of the spleen. *Radiology* 107:393, 1973.
8. Neifeld J.P., Berman W.F., Lawrence W., et al.: Management of congenital microgastria with a jejunal reservoir pouch. *J. Pediatr. Surg.* 15:882, 1980.
9. Schulz R.D., Niemann F.: Kongenitale Mikrogastrie in verbindung mit Skelettmissbildungen-ein neues Syndrom. *Helv. Paediat. Acta* 26:185, 1971.
10. Shackelford G.D., McAlister W.H., Brodeur A.E., et al.: Congenital microgastria. *Am. J. Roentgenol.* 118:72, 1973.
11. Welch K.J.: Personal communication.

84 Louise Schnaufer

Duodenal Atresia, Stenosis and Annular Pancreas

HISTORY.—In 1733, Calder[1] described two children born with "preternatural conformation of the guts," the first reported cases of duodenal atresia. Few additional cases were reported until 1877, when Theremin[16] reported having seen two cases over an 11-year period among 111,451 children admitted to the Foundling Hospital in Vienna and nine cases in 150,000 admissions to a similar hospital in St. Petersburg. In 1901, Cordes[2] found 56 cases in the literature, added one of his own, and described the clinical manifestations of the anomaly. Although 73 enterostomies and nine anastomoses had been performed before 1911, there were no survivors and many believed that technically this anomaly could not be repaired.[17] Ernst,[4] of Copenhagen, is credited as being the first, in 1914, to operate successfully on a child with duodenal atresia. A follow-up of the patient in 1975 found him to be in good health at age 61.[13] In 1929, Kaldor[8] had found 250 cases of duodenal atresia reported in the literature. Yet by 1931, there were only nine survivors located by Webb and Wangensteen.[17] They realized that the heavy catgut sutures produced large holes in the thin duodenal wall and found that the use of fine black silk sutures prevented leaks. They also initiated the technique of inflating the distal duodenal segment with air for an easier anastomosis. Finally, in 1941, Ladd and Gross refined the techniques that are in use today.[9]

Embryology and Pathogenesis

In 1902, Tandler[15] proposed his theory that failure of recanalization of the duodenal lumen produces stenosis, atresia, or formation of a mucosal web. During the second month of intrauterine life, there is exuberant growth of the epithelial lining before the size of the gut has increased sufficiently to accommodate it, obliterating the lumen. This is particularly true in the esophagus, duodenum, and rectum. As the gut grows, vacuolization of the solid core of cells begins, and the lumen is recanalized by the end of the eighth to the tenth week. Failure of coalescent vacuolization is thought to produce obstruction of the duodenum in the newborn. At the same time, there may be anomalies of the pancreas and extrahepatic ductal system. The error of recanalization seems to occur most often at the site of the papilla of Vater, and frequently the common duct is found opening at an intraluminal web

The pancreas develops from two primordia, the dorsal and ventral pancreatic buds. The dorsal pancreas arises from the dorsal wall of the duodenum, and the ventral pancreas arises to the right of the midline in an angle between the duodenum and the hepatic diverticulum. As rotation of the gut continues, the ventral pancreas begins to grow around the right side of the duodenum until it meets the dorsal bud, with which it merges, and fuses with the duct of the dorsal pancreas to form Wirsung's duct. The most commonly held theory on the formation of annular pancreas is Lecco's[10] suggestion that the tip of the ventral pancreas becomes fixed to the duodenal wall and, as rotation occurs, is drawn around the right side of the duodenum to fuse with the dorsal pancreas.

Pathology

Obstruction of the lumen of the duodenum may take several forms and may be partial or complete.

Stenosis

Stenosis, a narrowing of the intestinal lumen, is usually associated with extrinsic indentation of the duodenal wall. Partial obstruction may be caused by mesenteric bands associated with malrotation of the colon by an anterior (i.e., preduodenal) portal vein, by aberrant pancreatic tissue in the duodenal wall, or by an annular pancreas. The degree of obstruction varies, and often the patient may not become symptomatic until later in life.

Partial obstruction may be caused by a mucosal web, leaving a crescentic opening of variable size, or by an all but complete diaphragm with a central opening. It is postulated that the perforation may have developed in formation of the diaphragm or secondarily, as a result of intraluminal pressure during fetal growth. Incomplete webs and perforated diaphragms may cause neonatal obstruction or a degree of obstruction that does not attract attention until later in childhood.

Atresia

As described by Gray and Skandalakis[6] and by others, three types of atresia occur:

TYPE 1.—The atresia is produced by an intact diaphragm or membrane which is formed of mucosa and submucosa. The muscularis is intact. Externally there is no evidence of the site of the membrane other than the discrepancy in size between the proximal and distal segments. An interesting variation of the intact membrane is the wind-sock anomaly, caused by elongation of the membrane due to peristalsis and high proximal intraluminal pressure (Fig 84–1,E). The actual site of the origin of the wind sock may be several centimeters proximal to the level of obstruction distally. Pressure on the wind sock by an intraluminal catheter produces an indentation in the bowel wall at the origin of the diaphragm.

TYPE 2.—The two blind ends of the duodenum are connected by a short fibrous cord along the edge of the intact mesentery (Fig 84–1,B).

TYPE 3.—There is no connecting fibrous cord between the blind ends, which are separated by some distance; and the mesentery is absent, in a V-shaped defect (Fig 84–1,C).

Annular pancreas may be associated with duodenal atresia and may not itself necessarily be the cause of the obstruction.

The gross anatomical findings in infants with congenital duodenal obstruction are a greatly dilated duodenum with hypertrophied walls and a dilated pylorus and stomach. The duodenum distal to the obstruction, since it has been unused, is small and thin-walled (Fig 84–1,A).

Annular Pancreas

Perhaps the most common form of external compression on the second part of the duodenum is annular pancreas. Thin, flat

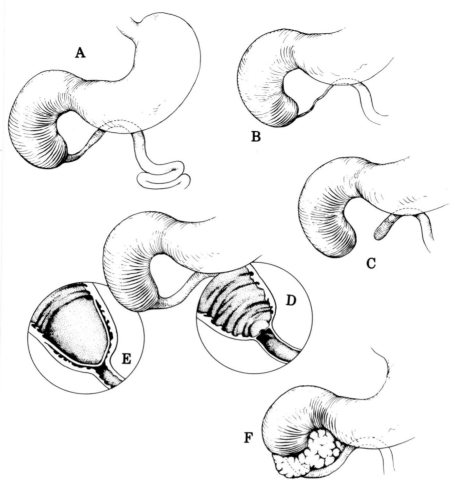

Fig 84–1.—Various types of anomalies causing duodenal obstruction. **A,** type 1 atresia with intact membrane producing marked discrepancy in size between proximal and distal segments. **B,** blind ends of duodenum connected by a fibrous cord. **C,** blind ends are separated, and the mesentery is absent at the separation. **D,** intraluminal membrane with a perforation. **E,** wind-sock anomaly. Note that an incision in the distal portion of the dilated segment would still be beyond the obstruction. **F,** annular pancreas.

segments of pancreatic tissue either completely or partially surround the duodenum and may cause partial or complete obstruction (Fig 84–1,*F*). The ring of pancreatic tissue is thought to be due to the persistent ventral primordium of the pancreas, which normally rotates around the duodenum to join the dorsal bud to become the head of the pancreas. In addition to the annular pancreas, there is commonly either stenosis or atresia of the duodenum at the same level (Fig 84–2).[3] Some cases of annular pancreas are found only incidentally at laparotomy.

Another form of extrinsic pressure on the duodenum may be from Ladd's bands, associated with rotation and fixation anomalies of the midgut.

Location and Incidence

Stenosis or atresia of the duodenum is usually limited to the first and second parts of the duodenum. It is relatively uncommon proximal to the ampulla of Vater, the most common site being just at the ampulla. Frequently, the end of the common duct is incorporated in the intraluminal membrane. Multiple atresias of the duodenum are quite rare.

Louw[12] classified 138 cases of intestinal stenosis and atresia both by type and by location. Seventy-five percent of stenoses occurred in the duodenum, 20% in the ileum, and 5% in the jejunum. Forty percent of atresias occurred in the duodenum, 35% in the ileum, and 25% in the jejunum.

The reported incidence of congenital duodenal obstruction varies from 1 in 20,000 births to 1 in 40,000 births. Rickham and Johnston[14] believe these estimates are too low. During a 12-year period, 68 infants with intrinsic duodenal obstruction were seen at the Liverpool Neonatal Surgical Center, and this number corresponded to an incidence of roughly 1 in 10,000 births. In this series, 60% of the infants with duodenal obstruction were born prematurely.

Associated Anomalies

Roughly 30% of babies with congenital duodenal obstruction also have Down syndrome. In a 1968 study of 503 cases of duodenal obstruction surveyed by the Surgical Section of the American Academy of Pediatrics, Down syndrome occurred in approximately one-third of the series, followed in frequency by associated malrotation anomalies and congenital heart disease. In several series, 70% of babies with annular pancreas had other anomalies.[5, 18]

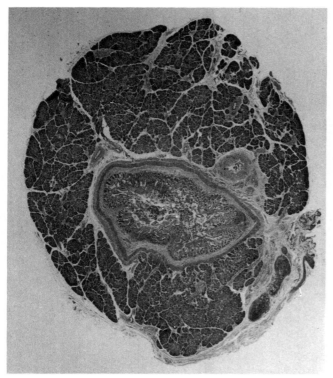

Fig 84–2.—Microscopic cross-section of duodenum showing annular pancreas and stenotic lumen. Duodenal atresia is often associated with annular pancreas.

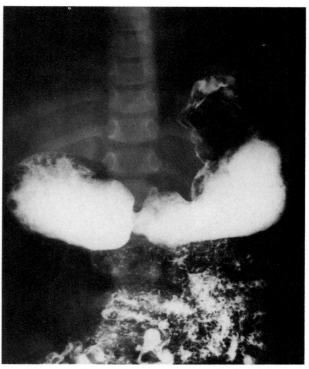

Fig 84–3.—Duodenal obstruction due to annular pancreas. Five-year-old boy with Down syndrome who had been vomiting intermittently for 3 years and was poorly nourished. Gastrointestinal series showed a huge duodenal bulb half the size of the stomach. In the second portion of the duodenum, there was a pronounced narrowing. Distal to this, the duodenum was normal. At operation, an annular pancreas was found causing the stenosis and partial obstruction. Duodenojejunostomy solved the problem.

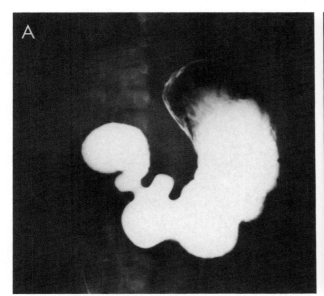

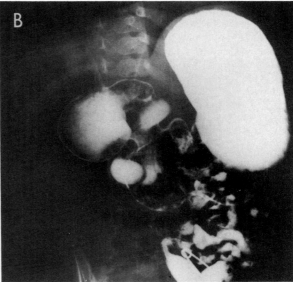

Fig 84–4.—Duodenal web with central perforation. Two-month-old female with such intense vomiting, of 1 month's duration, that she was back to her birth weight. **A,** barium meal shows a dilated proximal duodenum. **B,** distal to this, a narrow column of barium enters the distal duodenum through a pinpoint opening.

This indicates an intraluminal web with a central opening. At operation, the web was excised and a duodenoplasty performed, resulting in good emptying of the proximal duodenum.

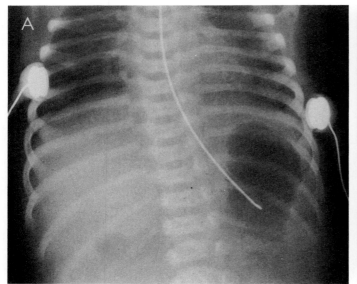

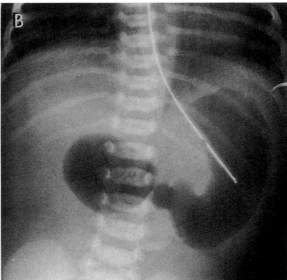

Fig 84–5.—Duodenal atresia; 3-day-old baby with bilious vomiting and absence of meconium stools. **A,** plain film of abdomen suggests a double-bubble sign. No gas is seen in lower abdomen. **B,** instillation of 60 cc of air through a nasogastric tube shows a typical double-bubble sign, indicating obstruction of the duodenum. At operation, duodenal atresia was found and corrected by duodenoduodenostomy.

Clinical Picture

The association between the maternal history of polyhydramnios and high intestinal obstruction in the newborn is well known, and most researchers find that it occurs in approximately 50% of cases. It is less common in infants born with atresia of the lower small intestine or colon. Amniotic fluid swallowed by the fetus is normally absorbed in the distal small intestine, so that an obstruction high in the duodenum results in an abnormal accumulation of amniotic fluid.[11]

Vomiting of bile-stained material, often within a few hours of birth, is the most common and often the earliest sign in the infant with duodenal obstruction. High intestinal obstruction should be suspected if the gastric aspirate in a neonate who has not vomited exceeds 30 cc of bile-stained fluid. Rarely does a duodenal obstruction occur above the level of the ampulla of Vater, when the vomitus would be colorless, perhaps delaying the diagnosis. Continual vomiting may lead to gastritis and blood-stained vomitus.

Abdominal distention is not the common finding in these infants that it is in those with lower intestinal obstruction. A fullness in the epigastrium due to the dilated stomach may be visible, or the abdomen may be quite scaphoid because of the absence of gas in the intestine.

Absence of meconium stools is a dependable sign of complete intestinal obstruction in the newborn. A few babies with duodenal obstruction may pass one or two small meconium stools shortly after birth, and those with a perforated duodenal web pass meconium and then bile-stained stools.

The diagnosis of duodenal obstruction is not always made during the neonatal period. Depending on the severity of the obstruction, the symptoms may mimic a feeding problem or pyloric

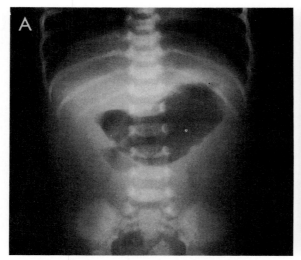

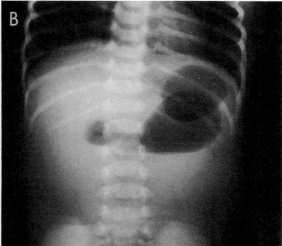

Fig 84–6.—Malrotation and volvulus. This 1-day-old baby had been vomiting bilious material. Supine **(A)** and upright **(B)** films show a dilated stomach and moderate dilatation of the third part of the duodenum where the air stops abruptly. At operation, a volvulus of the small intestine at the fourth part of the duodenum was found and reduced. Since atresias and webs are rarely found in the distal duodenum, volvulus or malrotation should be suspected.

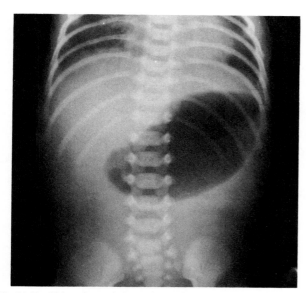

Fig 84–7.—Malrotation and obstruction by Ladd's bands. This 2-day-old girl had bilious vomiting and abdominal distention. Plain film of the abdomen shows a large, dilated stomach and a small amount of air in the first part of the duodenum. Operation disclosed malrotation with duodenal bands. Division of the bands and a Ladd procedure relieved the obstruction. The duodenum in this anomaly is generally not as dilated as in duodenal atresia or intraluminal web.

stenosis, and some children with duodenal stenosis or a perforated web may not present compelling symptoms until late childhood (Figs 84–3 and 84–4).

Diagnosis

The diagnosis of duodenal obstruction is made by a simple upright film of the abdomen. A large, air-distended stomach with a fluid level, a markedly distended first portion of the duodenum with a fluid level, and no evidence of air in the remaining GI tract, are diagnostic and known as the "double-bubble" sign. These findings may be obscured if there is considerable fluid in the stomach and duodenum. If the stomach is aspirated and approximately 60 cc of air instilled by nasogastric tube, a spectac-

ular double-bubble sign will be seen (Fig 84–5). A barium study is not necessary and provides no additional information.

Atresia is not difficult to diagnose radiologically. In cases of partial duodenal obstruction, the possibility of malrotation and volvulus or duodenal bands must be considered. Peritoneal bands, across the second portion of the duodenum from the abnormally positioned cecum, may produce a partial obstruction so that the proximal duodenum is only modestly dilated (Figs 84–6 and 84–7). There may also be scattered bubbles of air throughout the intestinal tract, and this may be confused with duodenal stenosis or a perforated web. Correction of the anomaly becomes more urgent if malrotation is present, confirmed by an upper GI study demonstrating presence or absence of the C-loop of the duodenum and the ligament of Treitz.

Prenatal diagnosis of duodenal atresia has become common with the routine use of maternal ultrasonography[7] for complications such as polyhydramnios in the third trimester of pregnancy. The obstructed stomach and first part of the duodenum of the fetus can easily be seen as large, fluid-filled, cystic masses (Fig 84–8).

Management

Preoperative Treatment

Neonates with high intestinal obstruction are usually admitted to the neonatal surgical unit in the first 24 hours of life because of the prenatal diagnosis by ultrasonography, the suspicion of a problem because of maternal polyhydramnios, or the early onset of symptoms. Correction of the anomaly is not an extreme emergency. If the child is in good condition and has no other life-threatening anomalies, surgical correction may be undertaken immediately. If volvulus has been excluded, operation may be postponed as long as necessary to evaluate an infant with a severe cardiac anomaly, severe metabolic imbalance, or respiratory distress syndrome. Some infants may require prolonged resuscitation and may be managed for several weeks by continuous gastrointestinal decompression and total parenteral nutrition.

Operation

The area of obstruction in the duodenum is easily approached through a supraumbilical right transverse abdominal incision.

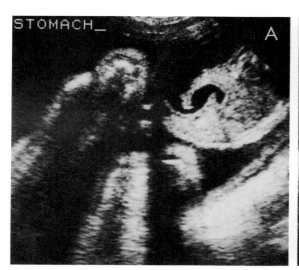

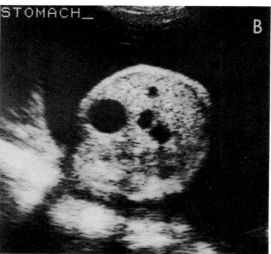

Fig 84–8.—Ultrasound study of fetus of 37 weeks' gestation performed because of maternal polyhydramnios. **A,** coronal view of fetus showing dilated stomach and duodenum. **B,** transverse view of fetus showing stomach bubble and two loops of duodenum. The baby was delivered by cesarean section at night because of fetal distress, transferred, and operated on at 14 hours of age. A complete duodenal web was found and excised.

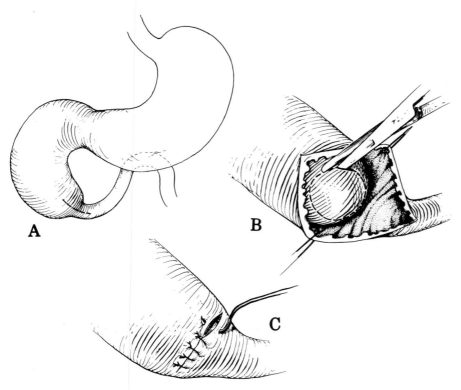

Fig 84–9.—Excision of duodenal web. **A,** a vertical incision is made at site of obstruction. **B,** web is excised carefully to avoid damage to ampulla of Vater. **C,** incision is closed transversely.

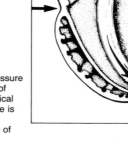

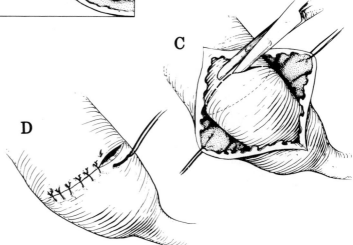

N G tube

Fig 84–10.—Excision of wind-sock membrane. **A,** pressure of catheter at bottom of wind sock produces indentation of wall, indicating point of attachment of membrane. **B,** vertical incision made at indentation site. **C,** wind-sock membrane is excised. **D,** incision is closed transversely. Note that a duodenojejunostomy made from the distal dilated portion of the duodenum would have been below the obstructing diaphragm, which can be missed.

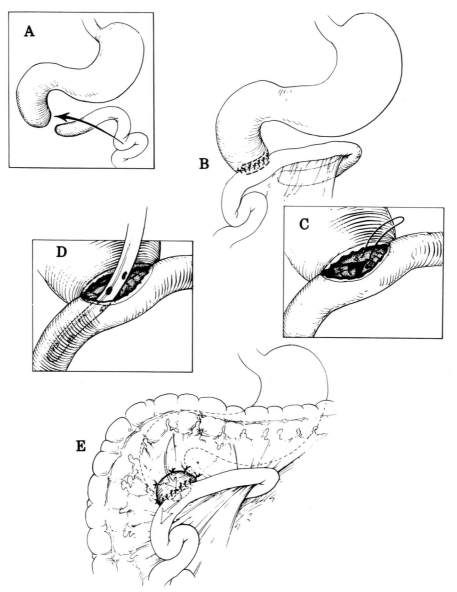

Fig 84–11.—Duodenojejunostomy for duodenal atresia. **A, B, C,** a loop of proximal jejunum is brought through an opening in the transverse mesocolon and anastomosed to the most dependent portion of the obstructed duodenum. **D,** before the anastomosis is completed, a catheter is inserted and the distal small bowel irrigated with saline to rule out additional sites of obstruction. **E,** the duodenum is sutured to the mesocolon to prevent herniation of the jejunum through the mesocolon.

The lesser omental sac is opened, the entire duodenum inspected, and the point of obstruction determined. The choice of operation depends on the type of anomaly encountered.

A simple duodenal web or diaphragm may be easily excised through a longitudinal incision across the area of obstruction (Fig 84–9). Care must be taken in excising the web because the opening of the ampulla of Vater is frequently in the web itself. Cautery or suturing of the mucosa of the web in this area is contraindicated because of possible damage to the entrance of the bile duct. The vertical incision is closed transversely, enlarging the lumen and preventing stricture, with 5-0 or 6-0 silk sutures. If one suspects a wind-sock anomaly, in which the elongated web may produce distention of the duodenum several centimeters beyond the attachment of the diaphragm to the duodenal wall, an intraluminal nasogastric tube may be used to find this point. Pressure on the tube at the bottom of the web produces an in-

dentation in the duodenal wall, indicating the point of attachment, and the incision should be placed at that point (Fig 84–10).

The standard bypass procedure for duodenal atresia or annular pancreas has long been a retrocolic duodenojejunostomy. A loop of jejunum is brought through an opening in the right transverse mesocolon and anastomosed to the most dependent portion of the dilated duodenum, using a two-layer anastomosis of 5-0 chromic catgut in the mucosal layer and 5-0 black silk sutures in the seromuscular layer. The anastomosis is then pulled through the opening in the mesocolon and the duodenal wall sutured to the mesocolon to avoid constriction of the jejunal limbs by the mesocolic ring (Fig 84–11). The temptation to divide the pancreatic ring must be resisted because (1) there is often an intrinsic duodenal obstruction, (2) some of the pancreatic tissue may be intramural, and (3) pancreatitis or a pancreatic fistula may result.

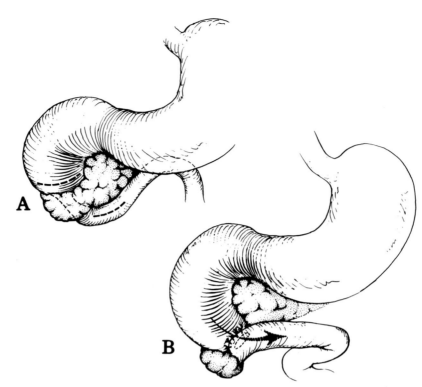

Fig 84–12.—Duodenoduodenostomy for annular pancreas. The temptation to divide the pancreas must be resisted because (1) there may be duodenal atresia, (2) some of the pancreatic tissue is intramural, (3) pancreatitis may result.

Duodenoduodenostomy, a more physiologic bypass procedure for intrinsic duodenal obstruction, requires considerably more dissection, with reflection of the right colon to mobilize a greater length of duodenum by the Kocher maneuver. A transverse incision is made in the lowest portion of the proximal duodenum and a vertical incision in the smaller distal segment. Since the posterior walls of both portions of the duodenum remain intact, an anterior closure is done with inverting single-layer sutures of fine silk (Fig 84–12).

Multiple atresias or webs are uncommon; but, before completing any of these anastomoses, one must nevertheless rule out additional sites of obstruction. A small catheter should be threaded into the distal small intestine and saline injected until it reaches the colon, thus confirming patency (see Fig 84–11,*D*).

Gastrojejunostomy as a means of bypassing a duodenal obstruction should never be done because of long-term problems with marginal ulceration, bleeding, and stricturing of the anastomosis.

The use of gastrostomy for postoperative drainage is argued. Some surgeons believe it is an absolute necessity in premature infants, and others find that nasogastric drainage is adequate. If the proximal duodenum is very large and dilated, the postoperative stasis may be prolonged and the anastomosis slow to function. Very soft mercury-tipped Silastic jejunal feeding tubes allow transanastomotic or separate jejunal intubation for early postoperative feeding. However, insertion of these tubes can be difficult and time-consuming, and they frequently become coiled, kinked, or displaced. Peripheral or central hyperalimentation is a more reliable means of nutrition and, once the amount of gastric aspirate decreases, indicating a functioning anastomosis, the infant can be started on oral feedings.

Results

Forty-four patients with duodenal obstruction were treated at the Children's Hospital of Philadelphia during 1977–1983. Four patients died postoperatively, one with Down syndrome and three with Vater syndrome, a mortality rate of 9%. Ten children, or 23%, had Down syndrome, and six of the ten had annular pancreas. Thirteen other children had multiple severe anomalies, but there were no deaths in this group.

REFERENCES

1. Calder J.: Two examples of children born with preternatural conformation of the guts. *Med. Essays* (Edinburgh) 1:203, 1733.
2. Cordes L.: Congenital occlusion of the duodenum. *Arch. Pediatr.* 18:401, 1901.
3. Elliott M.B., Kliman M.R., Elliott K.A.: Pancreatic annulus: A sign or cause of duodenal obstruction? *Can. J. Surg.* 11:357, 1968.
4. Ernst N.P.: A case of congenital atresia of the duodenum treated successfully by operation. *Br. Med. J.* 1:1644, 1916.
5. Free E.A., Gerald B.: Duodenal obstruction in the newborn due to annular pancreas. *Am. J. Roentgenol.* 103:321, 1968.
6. Gray S.W., Skandalakis J.E.: *Embryology for Surgeons.* Philadelphia, W.B. Saunders Co., 1972.
7. Hayden C.K., Schwartz M.Z., Davis M., et al.: Combined esophageal and duodenal atresia: Sonographic findings. *Am. J. Radiol.* 140:225, 1983.
8. Kaldor J.: Atresia of the duodenum and duodenal diverticula. *Ann. Surg.* 89:6, 1929.
9. Ladd W.E., Gross R.E.: *Abdominal Surgery of Infancy and Childhood.* Philadelphia, W.B. Saunders Co., 1941.
10. Lecco T.M.: Zur Morphologie des Pankreas annulare. *Sitzungsb. Akad. Wissensch. Cl.* 119:391, 1910.
11. Lloyd J.R., Clatworthy H.W.: Hydramnios as an aid to the early diagnosis of congenital obstruction of the alimentary tract. *Pediatrics* 21:903, 1958.
12. Louw J.H.: Investigations into the etiology of congenital atresia of the colon. *Dis. Colon Rectum* 7:471, 1964.

13. Madsen C.M.: Duodenal atresia—60 years of follow-up (case report). *Prog. Pediatr. Surg.* 10:61, 1977.
14. Rickham P.P., Johnston J.H.: *Neonatal Surgery.* New York, Appleton-Century-Crofts, 1969.
15. Tandler J.: Zur Entwicklungsgeschichte des menschlichen Duodenums. *Morphol. Jb.* 29:187, 1902.
16. Theremin E.: Ueber kongenitale Occlusionen des Duenndarms. *Deutsche Ztschr. Chir.* 8:34, 1877.
17. Webb C.H., Wangensteen O.H.: Congenital intestinal atresia. *Am. J. Dis. Child.* 41:262, 1931.
18. Whelan T.J. Jr., Hamilton G.B.: Annular pancreas. *Ann. Surg.* 146:252, 1957.

85   Jay L. Grosfeld

Jejunoileal Atresia and Stenosis

HISTORY.—Goeller is credited with the first description of ileal atresia in 1684.[24] Other early observations concerning intestinal atresia were recorded by Calder (1773)[81] and Osiander (1779).[28] Voisin performed an enterostomy for intestinal atresia in 1804, and Meckel published a review of the topic and speculated on its etiology in 1812. In 1889, Bland-Sutton[9] proposed a classification of the types of atresia and postulated that intestinal atresia occurred at the sites of "obliterative embryological events," such as atrophy of the vitelline duct. In 1894, Wanitschek unsuccessfully attempted the first resection and anastomosis for intestinal atresia.[28] In 1900, Tandler[73] proposed the theory that atresia was related to failure of recanalization (vacuolization) of the solid-cord stage of bowel development. These observations were confirmed by Johnson in 1910.[38] In 1911, Fockens[25] performed the first successful anastomosis for intestinal atresia. In 1912, Spriggs[71] suggested that mechanical accidents, including vascular occlusions, might be responsible for these occurrences. This concept was supported by clinical observations on atresia by Davis and Poynter (1922)[19] and Webb and Wangensteen (1931).[81] Evans'[24] extensive review (1951) concerning 1,498 instances of gastrointestinal atresia documented a successful result in only 139 infants. The classic experimental observations of Louw and Barnard[45] (1955) confirming the role of late intrauterine mesenteric vascular accidents as the cause of most jejunoileal atresias laid the foundations for the modern-day understanding and care of these interesting anomalies.

Incidence

Jejunoileal atresia and stenosis is a significant cause of neonatal intestinal obstruction. "Atresia" refers to a congenital obstruction due to complete occlusion of the intestinal lumen and accounts for 95% of cases. "Stenosis" is defined as a partial intraluminal occlusion, resulting in an incomplete intestinal obstruction, and accounts for 5% of jejunoileal obstructions. During the past two decades, a better understanding of etiologic factors and impaired intestinal function, as well as refinements in operative technique and pre- and postoperative care (especially in the area of nutritional support), have led to a significant improvement in survival in these cases.

The incidence of jejunoileal atresia has been reported from as high as 1 in 330 (United States) and 1 in 400 (Denmark) live births[35] to 1 in 1,500 live births.[24] Of 118 cases of intestinal atresia and stenosis treated at the James Whitcomb Riley Hospital for Children, Indianapolis, from 1973 to 1983, 55 were jejunoileal, 53 duodenal, and 10 colonic. Nixon and Tawes,[56] however, noted a 2:1 ratio in the frequency of jejunoileal to duodenal atresias. In a review of 619 cases of jejunoileal atresia and stenosis from the experience of members of the Surgical Section of the American Academy of Pediatrics, de Lorimier et al.[20] noted that boys and girls were equally affected. Although the mean birth weight in this relatively large group of babies was 2.7 kg (range, 0.9–4.8 kg), one third of the infants with jejunal atresia, one fourth of those with ileal atresia, and more than one half of those with multiple atresias were of low birth weight. Whereas 30% of infants with duodenal atresia or stenosis have Down syndrome, mongolism is relatively uncommon in patients with jejunoileal atresia. Nixon and Tawes[56] noted only two cases of mongolism among 127 cases, and de Lorimier et al.,[20] only five among 619 cases. The only one of 49 infants with jejunoileal atresia at our institution who had Down syndrome had coexisting duodenal atresia.

Etiology

The early concepts concerning the etiology of jejunoileal atresia were briefly considered in the historical sketch. In 1900, Tandler[73] theorized that intestinal atresia was related to a lack of revacuolization of the solid-cord stage of intestinal development. In 1959, Lynn and Espinas[46] confirmed some of Tandler's observations concerning epithelial plugging. Although mucosal atresia was frequently noted in instances of duodenal atresia, jejunoileal atresia as a result of epithelial plugging was uncommon. Most jejunoileal atresias are separated by a cord-like segment or a V-shaped mesenteric gap defect. Clinical observations by Louw and Barnard,[45] Santulli and Blanc,[68] and Nixon[54] that bile pigments, squames, and lanugo hairs often found distal to atretic segments strongly suggested that some factor other than epithelial plugging was involved. Fetal bile secretion and the swallowing of amniotic fluid begin in the 11th and 12th weeks of intrauterine life, respectively—well after revacuolization of the solid-cord stage.[35] Postmortem observations of vascular abnormalities, such as deficiency in arteriomesenteric arcades, added strength to suspicions that other etiologic factors were involved.

In 1955, Louw and Barnard[45] subjected dog fetuses to ligation of mesenteric vessels and strangulation obstruction late in the course of gestation. Ten to 14 days later, examination of affected fetal intestine demonstrated a variety of atretic conditions similar to those observed clinically in human neonates. These findings strongly suggested that most jejunoileal atresias are a result of a late intrauterine mesenteric vascular catastrophe. Courtois[18] (1959) demonstrated that, after fetal operations in rabbits, intrauterine intestinal perforation can heal without a trace (with or without evidence of meconium peritonitis) or result in stenosis or atresia. He further observed that, if an intestinal loop was isolated, resorption of the loop occurred if its blood supply was poor. Santulli and Blanc (1961),[68] Abrams (1968),[1] and Koga et al. (1975)[39] confirmed these findings in experimental studies performed on fetal rabbits, sheep, and dogs respectively.

Frequent clinical instances of intestinal atresia as a result of late intrauterine mesenteric vascular insults such as volvulus, intussusception, internal hernia, and constriction of the mesentery in a tight gastroschisis or omphalocele defect have been observed. de Lorimier et al.[20] noted evidence of bowel infarction in 42% of 619 cases. Nixon and Tawes[56] noted macroscopic or microscopic intrauterine peritonitis in 61 of 127 patients, with an obvious volvulus in 44. Murphy[52] noted that 5% of atresias were related to fetal internal hernia. Reports by Santulli and Blanc,[68] Nixon and Tawes,[56] and Okmian and Kovamees[58] document atresia related to bowel incarceration in an omphalocele. Iatrogenic postpartum ileal atresia due to umbilical clamping of an occult omphalocele was reported by Vassy and Boles[79] and by Landor et al.[40] Grosfeld and Clatworthy[30] observed the occurrence of jejunal atresia with infarction of the entire midgut in a tight gastroschisis defect. In the American Academy of Pediatrics Survey, atresia associated with gastroschisis was observed in 2% of patients.[20] Intrauterine intussusception is an infrequently reported

TABLE 85–1.—JEJUNOILEAL ATRESIA:
CLINICAL PRESENTATION

FINDING	IN JEJUNAL ATRESIA (%)	IN ILEAL ATRESIA (%)
Polyhydramnios	38	15
Bilious vomiting	84	81
Abdominal distention	78	98
Failure to pass meconium	65	71
Jaundice	32	20

cause of atresia. Evans'[24] review of 1,498 cases recognized only nine examples of atresia associated with intussusception. Like that of intussusception after birth, the etiology of intrauterine intussusception is unknown. Most of these infants are full-term without associated malformations and have a single cord or gap type of atresia that is not associated with cystic fibrosis.[31, 60, 62, 70, 76] In the 55 patients with jejunoileal atresia or stenosis at James Whitcomb Riley Hospital for Children in Indianapolis, volvulus was detected in 21, intussusception in two, internal hernia in one, gastroschisis with antenatal peritonitis in 10, and evidence of meconium peritonitis in 10. The late occurrence of such events accounts for the relatively low incidence (7%) of associated extraintestinal anomalies.[20] In rare instances, jejunoileal atresia has been observed to coexist with biliary atresia, duodenal atresia, colon atresia, gastric atresia, and in mothers with migraine headaches receiving Cafergot during pregnancy.[27, 32, 33, 34, 41] Fortunately, most infants with jejunoileal atresia have only this single abnormality and are otherwise normal.

Diagnosis

Clinical Presentations

The pertinent signs of jejunoileal atresia include maternal polyhydramnios, bilious vomiting, abdominal distention, jaundice, and failure to pass meconium on the first day of life (Table 85–1).[20, 29, 43, 52, 80] Polyhydramnios is observed in 24% of cases and is more commonly noted in instances of proximal jejunal atresia (38%).[20] Prenatal ultrasonography in mothers with polyhydramnios has identified small-bowel obstruction associated with atresia, volvulus, and meconium peritonitis.[2, 42, 47] These observations suggest that ultrasonography should be routinely performed in the presence of polyhydramnios. Bilious vomiting is slightly more common in jejunal atresia (84%), while abdominal distention is more frequently noted in cases of ileal atresia (98%).[29] Jaundice occurs in 32% of infants with jejunal atresia and 20% of those with ileal atresia.[20] Jaundice in these cases of small-bowel obstruction is characteristically associated with an elevation of indirect bilirubin.[11, 57] Although most infants fail to pass meconium, occasionally meconium and necrotic tissue may be passed per rectum.[29, 31, 56, 76] Abdominal distention is a frequent clinical feature in instances of jejunoileal atresia. Proximal jejunal atresia may be associated with upper abdominal distention. More generalized distention usually denotes a low obstruction (e.g., distal small bowel or colon) in which many loops of bowel are filled with air proximal to the level of obstruction. Severe distention may be associated with respiratory distress due to elevation of the diaphragm, easily visible veins, and "intestinal patterning" characterized by visible loops of bowel (occasionally with peristaltic waves) on the abdominal wall. While distention usually develops 12–24 hours after birth, abdominal distention noted immediately at birth suggests the presence of giant cystic meconium peritonitis.[13]

X-Ray Findings

The diagnosis of jejunoileal atresia usually is confirmed by roentgen examination of the abdomen. Erect and recumbent abdominal films are obtained in each case. Thumb-sized intestinal loops ("rule of thumb") and air-fluid levels are highly suggestive of intestinal obstruction in the newly born.[15] High jejunal atresia may present with a few air-fluid levels and no further gas beyond that point (Fig 85–1). The lower the atresia, the more apparent the clinical distention and the greater the number of distended intestinal loops and air-fluid levels observed on x-ray. The site of atresia may appear as a larger loop with a significant air-fluid level (Fig 85–2). Peritoneal calcification is seen in 12% of cases on plain films and signifies the presence of meconium peritonitis, a sign of intrauterine bowel perforation (Fig 85–3). In addition, instances of intraluminal calcification ("mummification") may be observed, indicating an antenatal volvulus.[6, 36] In instances of giant cystic meconium peritonitis, plain films of the abdomen may demonstrate a very large air-fluid level in a meconium pseudocyst.[13] This type of occurrence is related to a late intrauterine perforation, resulting in an encapsulated mass of perforated bowel and meconium.[29]

The newborn rarely demonstrates colonic haustral markings on a plain abdominal radiograph, which may simply show dilated loops of bowel without actually differentiating between the small and large bowel. A barium enema should be performed in each instance of suspected neonatal intestinal obstruction. The first enema the baby receives should be the barium enema, which, when performed by trained radiologists with experience in obstructive cases in neonates and infants, usually involves minimal risk. The barium enema serves three purposes: (1) to distinguish between small- and large-bowel distention, (2) to determine if the colon is used or unused (microcolon), and (3) to locate the position of the cecum in regard to intestinal rotation and fixation.[29] The great majority of infants with jejunoileal atresia demonstrate a microcolon, an observation that usually limits the obstruction to the distal small intestine (see Fig 85–3). Microcolon is directly related to the fact that little succus entericus has passed the area of obstruction in the distal fetal small bowel and the unused colon does not distend.[6] Rarely, however, the colon may appear of normal caliber if the intrauterine vascular catastrophe leading to atresia occurred extremely late in gestation (Fig 85–4). This is particularly true in instances of atresia related to intrauterine intussusception.[31, 62, 76] Malrotation may be observed in approximately 10% of patients with jejunoileal atresia.[20, 56]

There is usually no indication to perform upper gastrointestinal contrast studies in instances of complete obstruction. In cases of intestinal stenosis (with an incomplete obstruction), this study may prove quite useful. A small-bowel contrast enteroclysis study has a higher diagnostic yield than the routine small-bowel series.

Differential Diagnosis

Newborn infants with intestinal obstruction from other causes may present with a clinical picture quite similar to that of infants with jejunoileal atresia. These causes include malrotation with or without volvulus, meconium ileus, bowel duplication, internal hernia, colonic atresia, adynamic ileus due to sepsis, and total colonic aganglionosis.[12, 35, 44] The contrast barium enema often yields valuable information that frequently rules out certain causes of obstruction, particularly colonic atresia and aganglionosis. Jejunoileal atresia may coexist with malrotation (9%), meconium peritonitis (12%), meconium ileus (9–10%) and rarely aganglionosis, so that a clear differentiation is not always possi-

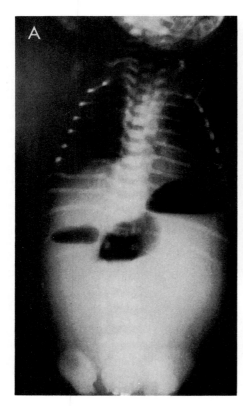

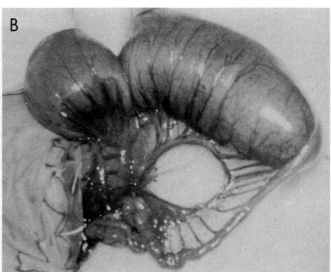

Fig 85–1.—High jejunal atresia. **A,** plain abdominal x-ray film. Note the three gas bubbles, suggesting the obstruction is just beyond the duodenum. **B,** at laparotomy a type I mucosal atresia of the proximal jejunum was observed. (From Grosfeld.[29])

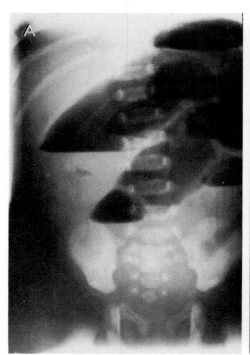

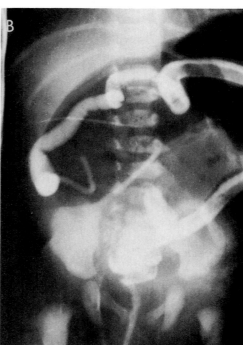

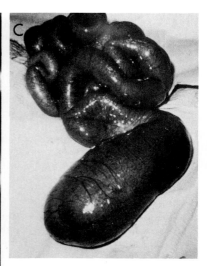

Fig 85–2.—Ileal atresia. **A,** erect abdominal x-ray film, showing distended intestinal loops with air-fluid levels. **B,** contrast enema demonstrates a microcolon (unused) suggestive of small bowel obstruction. **C,** atresia of the ileum (type IIIa) at laparotomy. (From Grosfeld.[29])

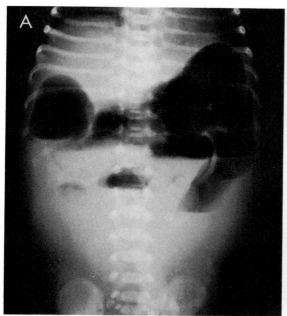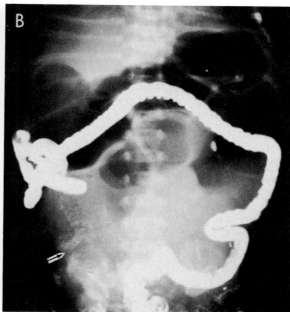

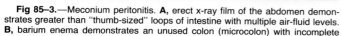

Fig 85–3.—Meconium peritonitis. **A,** erect x-ray film of the abdomen demonstrates greater than "thumb-sized" loops of intestine with multiple air-fluid levels. **B,** barium enema demonstrates an unused colon (microcolon) with incomplete rotation (cecum in right upper quadrant) and calcification in the right lower quadrant *(arrow)* indicative of meconium peritonitis. (From Grosfeld.[29])

ble.[13, 20, 29, 44, 56, 59] A careful family history regarding cystic fibrosis may permit preoperative identification of infants with meconium ileus. Infants with uncomplicated meconium ileus often have significant dilatation of loops of varying sizes and few, if any, air-fluid levels. This latter observation is related to the fact that meconium in these patients is extremely viscid and fails to layer out as an air-fluid interface until the infant is kept upright for 10–15 minutes.[29] A "ground-glass" appearance (Neuhauser's sign)[53] or the "soap-bubble sign" of Singleton[69] may be observed in the right lower quadrant and represents the viscid meconium mixed with air. Careful evaluation of these patients may avoid an unnecessary operation, as at least half of these uncomplicated cases of meconium ileus respond to nonoperative therapy in the form of a Gastrografin enema (see Chap. 86). Instances of meconium ileus complicated by atresia, volvulus, or gangrenous bowel require operative intervention, and the appropriate diagnosis in such obstructed patients will be made at the time of laparotomy.

Pathologic Findings

Atresias of the small intestine are equally distributed between the jejunum (51%) and the ileum (49%). The proximal jejunum is the site of atresia in 31% of cases, distal jejunum 20%, proximal ileum 13%, and distal ileum 36%.[20] The atresia is usually single (>90%) but may be multiple in 6–20% of cases.[19, 20, 29, 32]

The classification of jejunoileal atresia has changed only slightly since the early observations of Bland-Sutton[9] and Spriggs.[71] Louw[44] recognized three types of jejunoileal atresia. Type I refers to a mucosal (septal) atresia with an intact bowel wall and mesentery. Type II has two atretic blind ends connected by a band of fibrous tissue (cord) and an intact mesentery, and type III has the two ends of atretic bowel separated by a gap (V-shaped defect) in the mesentery (Fig 85–5). This has been the classification used most extensively throughout the literature, particularly in the large reviews.[20, 56] In evaluating 559 cases of jejunoileal atresia, de Lorimier et al.[20] noted 19% were type I,

31% type II, and 46% type III. Nixon and Tawes[56] similarly found type III cases to be the most common variant. While many type III cases are associated with shorter bowel length due to intrauterine resorption of fetal gut subjected to a vascular insult, most type I and II cases have reasonably normal length of remaining intestine. Foglia et al. reported an unusual type I case in which a 40-cm segment of bowel had an occluded lumen.[26]

Little attention has been given to cases of multiple atresias and foreshortened bowel associated with prematurity and a high mortality. At operation, there is a "string-of-beads" or "string-of-sausages" appearance (see Fig 85–5).[35] Rittenhouse et al.[65] reported that multiple atresias occurred in 14% of cases and noted one infant with 25 separate atresias. An intrauterine inflammation was considered a possible cause. Guttman et al.[34] reported a family pattern of multiple atresias affecting the stomach, duodenum, small bowel, and colon occurring in French Canadians near the St. John River in Quebec. Because of the high degree of consanguinity observed in this group, these authors, as well as Teja et al.,[74] proposed that extensive multiple atresias occur most likely as an expression of a rare autosomal recessive gene. Mishalany and Najjar[50] reported three cases of jejunal atresia in one family.

Another unusual group of patients are those with "apple-peel" atresia or "Christmas-tree" deformity. They present with jejunal atresia near the ligament of Treitz, foreshortened bowel, a large mesenteric gap, and the bowel distal to the atresia precariously supplied in retrograde fashion by anastomotic arcades from the ileocolic, right colic, or inferior mesenteric artery.[28, 83, 86, 87] Ros Mar et al. observed 12 cases of apple-peel deformity among 37 cases of jejunoileal atresia (32.4%).[67] Zerella and Martin, however, observed the "apple-peel" variant of atresia in 7 of 59 cases (11%) of jejunoileal atresia.[86] Patients with this distinct variation of atresia appear to have a familial pattern, are often of low birth weight and have an increased number of associated anomalies.[10]

Martin and Zerella[49] proposed a new classification to include instances of multiple atresia and "apple-peel" atresia. We have

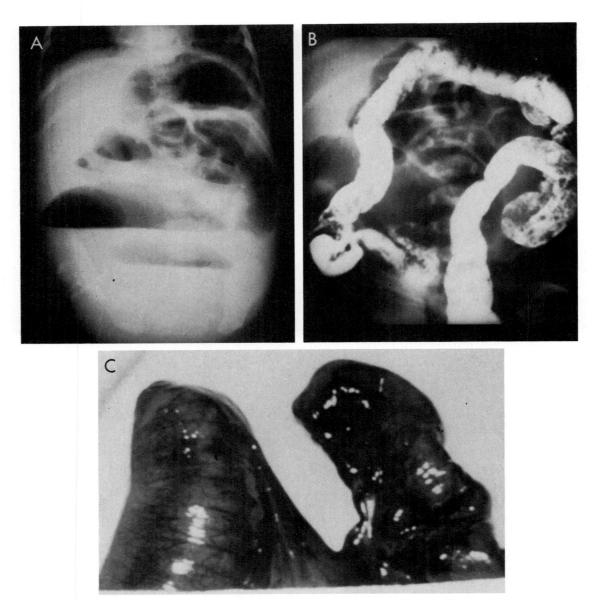

Fig 85–4.—Ileal atresia. **A,** upright x-ray film of abdomen, showing distended loops of intestine with air-fluid levels. **B,** contrast enema showing normal-caliber colon filled with debris. **C,** at laparotomy, ileal atresia with a V-shaped defect in the mesentery (type IIIa) and evidences of an intrauterine intussusception were found. (From Grosfeld.[29])

modified this classification somewhat to retain the previous nomenclature of Louw, add "apple-peel" atresia as a special form of type III (IIIb), and consider multiple atresias as type IV (see Fig 85–5). Of 49 patients with atresia at James Whitcomb Riley Hospital for Children, 31 had jejunal and 18, ileal atresia. There were nine cases of type I atresia, 14 type II, 17 type IIIa, two type IIIb, and nine type IV.

Treatment

Preoperative Management

During initial evaluation, the infant is maintained in a warm humidified environment (either in an Isolette or under an overhead warmer) to avoid hypothermia. An orogastric tube (no. 10) is passed and taped to the cheek. The stomach contents are as-

pirated and presence of bile noted. The tube is placed on intermittent suction to decompress the stomach and to prevent vomiting and further gaseous distention of the obstructed bowel from swallowed air. This is a key prerequisite if the infant is to be transferred from a community or general hospital to a neonatal intensive care facility. These precautions should also be in effect before the infant is evaluated in the x-ray department, as aspiration during transportation is a significant complication and should be carefully avoided. The infant should always be attended by experienced personnel.

The infant's weight is determined and baseline laboratory data including complete blood count, platelet count, blood urea nitrogen, bilirubin, glucose, calcium, pH and blood gas tensions, serum electrolytes, and type and crossmatch are obtained by microtechniques. Urinary volume, specific gravity, and osmolality are also measured. The extent of the preoperative preparation

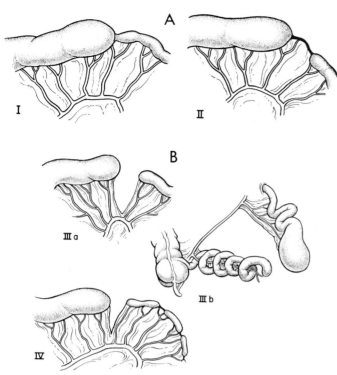

Fig 85–5.—Classification of intestinal atresia. *Type I,* mucosal (membranous) atresia with intact bowel wall and mesentery. *Type II,* blind ends are separated by a fibrous cord. *Type IIIa,* blind ends are separated by a V-shaped *(gap)* mesenteric defect. *Type IIIb,* "apple-peel" atresia. *Type IV,* multiple atresias ("string of sausages").

depends primarily on the delay in diagnosis, the degree of fluid and electrolyte imbalance, and the presence of peritonitis. An adequate intravenous route is established by percutaneous insertion of a short 22-gauge Teflon or silicone catheter in the scalp, or dorsum of the foot or hand. We avoid "cutdowns," as they are rarely necessary unless total parenteral nutrition is required. Routine catheterization of the umbilical vein is avoided because of the increased risk of sepsis; it is used occasionally, however, for exchange transfusion in this group of patients with an increased incidence of hyperbilirubinemia. If the infant has associated respiratory distress related to aspiration of vomitus or severe distention, a percutaneous arterial catheter is inserted into the right radial artery for more accurate PaO_2 monitoring above the level of neonatal right-to-left shunts through the patent ductus and foramen ovale.

The infant's fluid deficits are evaluated and replacement therapy initiated. Bilious drainage from the nasogastric tube is replaced milliliter for milliliter with lactated Ringer's solution. In instances of peritonitis and/or severe distention, Plasmanate or lactated Ringer's solution is administered at a rate of 20 ml/kg over a 30-minute period, and, in instances of obstruction without perforation, an empirical infusion of 10 ml/kg is employed to correct hypovolemia related to third-space losses sequestered in the peritoneal cavity or the obstructed proximal bowel. Additional fluids (Plasmanate or lactated Ringer's solution) may be necessary to maintain the infant's blood pressure above 50 mm Hg and establish appropriate urine flow (1–2 ml/kg/hr). A 10% dextrose in 0.25% normal saline solution is employed for maintenance.

Vitamin K, oxide (Aquamephyton, 1 mg intramuscularly) is routinely given. Intravenous antibiotics are usually employed (ampicillin, 100 mg/kg/day, and gentamicin, 5 mg/kg/day).

Preoperative preparation may take from 1 to 4 hours, according to the severity of the infant's condition and the degree of hypovolemia.

Operating Room Care

Following appropriate preparation, the infant is taken to the operating room, and similar precautions concerning transportation and preservation of an appropriate thermal environment are observed. The operating room temperature is kept between 75 and 80 F. The patient is placed under a heat lamp on a protected warming blanket, and limbs are wrapped with Webril gauze. The umbilicus is prepared with a warm iodophor solution and suture-ligated following resection of the clamped cord. The obstructed patient should be intubated while awake to avoid aspiration, and the location of the endotracheal tube should be evaluated by careful auscultation. Monitoring of blood pressure (Doppler), electrocardiogram, pulse, and temperature (skin or axillary probe) is routine in each case. Arterial pH and blood gas tensions are acquired as necessary. Nonexplosive inhalation anesthesia (usually halothane) is employed. The gases are warm and humidified to prevent heat loss and drying of the tracheobronchial tree. Dry anesthetic gases may cause destruction of cilia, desquamation of cells into the lumen, and a decrease in mucus production.[14, 48] These changes result in an increased incidence of postoperative pulmonary complications related to delayed endobronchial clearance and plugging. The abdomen is gently prepared (painted rather than scrubbed) with a warm iodophor (Betadine) solution. Four towels are used to drape the abdomen and are held in place with a sterile transparent adhesive plastic drape, which is applied over the operative field. This drape is then covered by a pediatric laparotomy sheet with an aperture through which the procedure is carried out.

A right supraumbilical transverse incision allows excellent access to all areas of the peritoneum. We routinely employ a fine-tipped infant electrocoagulator with a pencil-like fingertip control to achieve hemostasis. This avoids blood loss and obviates the need for time-consuming clamping and tying techniques. Fluid administration during operation usually consists of an infusion of 5–10 ml/kg/hr of 5% dextrose in lactated Ringer's solution to replace sequestered tissue fluid losses related to dissection. Equal volumes of lactated Ringer's solution are administered to replace intraoperative losses from the nasogastric tube and any bowel content aspirated during the procedure. Warmed whole blood is transfused if losses are greater than 10% of the estimated blood volume (80 ml/kg of body weight). Small-volume aspiration-collecting systems and close monitoring of sponge weights facilitate these estimates. Blood loss up to 10% of the estimated blood volume is replaced by infusion of 5% dextrose in lactated Ringer's solution.

Operative Techniques

The operation of choice in jejunoileal atresia and stenosis is related to the pathologic findings and the specific set of circumstances encountered in each individual case.[32] The actual decision as to the most appropriate procedure depends on the pathologic type of obstruction (e.g., stenosis or atresias types I, II, IIIa, IIIb, or IV) and the presence of malrotation, volvulus, meconium ileus, or variants of meconium peritonitis. An additional set of complicated circumstances occurs in infants with atresia or stenosis associated with gastroschisis or omphalocele, where primary closure of the abdominal wall may present a problem.

Appropriate credit should be given to Louw,[44] Nixon,[55, 56] and Benson,[5] on whose experience much of the current trend in operative therapy is based. They independently became aware that retention and use of the dilated blind proximal atretic segment of intestine in any type of anastomosis led to a high incidence of delayed function of the anastomosis, manifested by obstruction. Although the side-to-side anastomosis was commonly used in the early attempts at surgical correction of jejunoileal atresia, functional obstruction and subsequent development of the blind loop syndrome frequently complicated this operation.[5, 44, 55] Nixon[55, 56] noted that the change in the dilated proximal atretic segment consisted of smooth muscle hypertrophy and enlargement of the bowel diameter. He suggested this segment of bowel had ineffective peristalsis and failed to function at lower pressures after operation. de Lorimier et al.[21] and Cloutier[16] suggested that hyperplasia is the main change occurring in intestinal smooth muscle above a chronic obstruction. In instances of a chronic complete obstruction, such as jejunal atresia, hyperplasia may be so extreme that a state of decompensation is reached in which even strong contractions never close the intestinal lumen sufficiently to increase in pressure or to allow efficient propulsion at the normal inlet pressure.[16] Experience has shown that, in cases of proximal jejunal atresia (with adequate length of intestine), resection of the dilated atretic segment at the ligament of Treitz (as advocated by Nixon,[55] Benson,[5] and Louw[44]) followed by an end-to-oblique anastomosis obviates these complications and usually results in a successful outcome. When there is a limited length of remaining bowel (e.g., short gut), a reduction tapering antimesenteric jejunoplasty, as suggested by Thomas, has proved useful.[75] Reports by Howard and Othersen[37] and by Weber et al.[82] confirm the applicability of tapering enteroplasty in selected cases. de Lorimier and Harrison reported that intestinal imbrication also effectively reduced the caliber of distended bowel and restored function.[22] Wide proximal resection and anastomosis is also utilized for instances of single or multiple atresias of the middle small bowel or distal ileum. Benson and associates[5] suggested that an end-to-side ileo-ascending colonic anastomosis is a reasonable alternative in instances of distal ileal atresia. The major disadvantage of this procedure is bypassing the ileocecal valve.

At operation, the bowel is inspected and the proximal and distal ends of the atresia identified. Gentle evisceration often facilitates this inspection. Malrotation, volvulus, and/or segments of partially resorbed fetal intestine that may be involved in an intrauterine volvulus may be observed. The twisted bowel is carefully reduced so that a complete evaluation of the pathologic anatomy is possible. A pursestring suture is placed in the distal atretic end of bowel, and saline is injected through a 25-gauge needle to rule out an unsuspected distal atretic mucosal membrane or web. If bowel length is adequate, the proximal dilated atretic segment is resected back to the level where the bowel diameter approaches 1.0–1.5 cm (in instances of ileal atresia) or to the ligament of Treitz in instances of proximal jejunal atresia. A Bainbridge infant bowel clamp is applied at a 90-degree angle on the proximal bowel. A short segment of the distal atretic segment is resected at a 45-degree angle more distal on the antimesenteric side, and an additional Bainbridge clamp is used (Fig 85–6,A). If there is still a discrepancy in the size of the two lumina, a short antimesenteric incision in the distal atretic bowel alleviates this difference. A two-layer interrupted 5-0 silk end-to-oblique anastomosis is then performed (Fig 85–6,B). All of the posterior outer layer seromuscular sutures are inserted (usually no more than five) before being tied. The clamps are removed, and the crushed tissue trimmed. The posterior inner layer is inserted and is brought around anteriorly as an interrupted inverting Connell suture (in-out, out-in) with the knots on the inside. The anastomosis is completed with an outer anterior seromuscular interrupted 5-0 silk Lembert closure. The mesenteric defect is carefully approximated, tucking the longer proximal mesentery to prevent a kink at the anastomosis.[56]

In cases of jejunal atresia with significantly foreshortened bowel, a tapering antimesenteric reduction jejunoplasty is accomplished with the GIA autostapling device (Fig 85–6,C). The most bulbous distal portion of the proximal atretic segment is resected and a 22–24-F catheter is inserted into the lumen along the mesenteric side. The antimesenteric border of the bowel is then resected between two rows of autostaples up to the ligament of Treitz. The remaining staple line is oversewn with interrupted 5-0 silk sutures and the procedure completed by an end-to-oblique anastomosis, as previously noted. The dissection and anastomosis are presently performed with the aid of magnifying

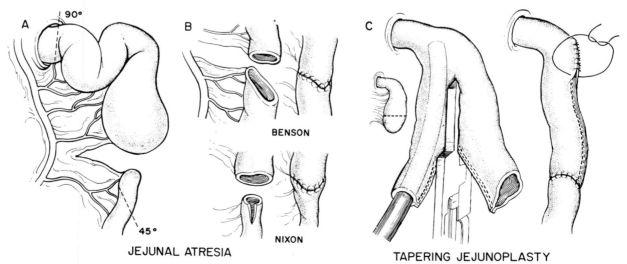

JEJUNAL ATRESIA   TAPERING JEJUNOPLASTY

Fig 85–6.—Jejunal atresia: techniques of anastomosis. **A,** the proximal jejunal atretic segment is resected at the ligament of Treitz at a 90-degree angle and the distal segment at a 45-degree angle. **B,** end-to-oblique anastomosis is carried out by the techniques of Benson (one-layer) or Nixon (two-layer) with fine interrupted silk sutures. **C,** tapering proximal jejunoplasty: the bulbous distal portion of the atresia is resected and a tube is placed in the mesenteric side of the lumen; antimesenteric resection with the GIA autostapler is carried out up to the ligament of Treitz. End-to-end anastomosis completes the procedure. Note that the staple line is also oversewn with interrupted 5-0 silk sutures.

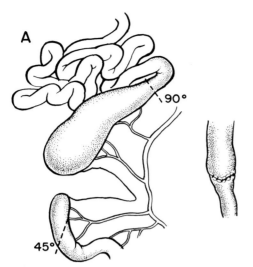

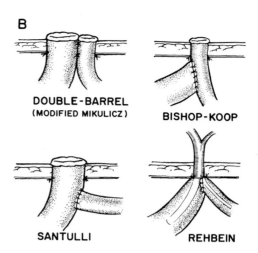

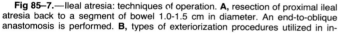

Fig 85–7.—Ileal atresia: techniques of operation. **A,** resection of proximal ileal atresia back to a segment of bowel 1.0-1.5 cm in diameter. An end-to-oblique anastomosis is performed. **B,** types of exteriorization procedures utilized in in-

stances of severe peritonitis, questionable bowel viability, and meconium ileus. The double-barrel side-by-side (modified Mikulicz) enterostomy is preferred.

loupes of 2½–3× power. These loupes allow a much more precise placement of the anastomotic sutures and greatly facilitate the operative procedure.

A primary anastomosis is not attempted in instances of ileal atresia associated with volvulus when the vascular integrity of the intestine is in question, in severe meconium peritonitis, or with obvious meconium ileus. In these cases, resection of the atretic ileal segments and exteriorization are carried out. The most expeditious procedure is a side-by-side (modified Mikulicz)[3, 7, 63, 66] double-barrel enterostomy brought out through the wound and fixed to the abdominal wall layers with a few 5-0 interrupted silk sutures (Fig 85–7). The Bishop-Koop (distal stoma),[8] Santulli (proximal stoma),[68] and Rehbein (tube)[64] anastomotic enterostomies are probably equally acceptable procedures in this regard. We use the double-barrel enterostomy, as it is rapidly performed, avoids an intraperitoneal anastomosis, and allows the stomas to be easily evaluated for intestinal viability in the postoperative period. Although this does create an end-ileostomy stoma, appropriate stomal and skin care and parenteral nutrition by either a central or peripheral route usually obviate any problems. Reoperation at a later date requires a limited "target" laparotomy to restore intestinal continuity by end-to-end anastomosis and has not been a problem in our hands. We have neither employed transanastomotic Silastic decompression catheters in instances of proximal jejunal anastomosis,[35, 56] nor used an appendicostomy catheter (as suggested by Suruga[72]) in distal ileal anastomoses.

A Stamm gastrostomy is usually performed as an adjunct to these intestinal procedures (see Chap. 80). The tube (no. 14 or 16 Pezzer catheter) is brought out of a stab wound in the left upper quadrant. This is a useful method of decompressing the stomach and has the advantage of avoiding long-term orogastric intubation in patients with prolonged ileus or anastomosis dysfunction in the postoperative period. The abdominal wall is closed in layers; continuous 4-0 chromic catgut is used on the peritoneum and interrupted inverting 4-0 polypropylene sutures on the fascial layers. Skin edges are approximated with Steri-Strips.

At the James Whitcomb Riley Hospital for Children, 31 patients were treated for jejunal atresia. Nine were managed by wide proximal resection back to the ligament of Treitz, and 10

had a tapering jejunoplasty followed by end-to-oblique anastomosis. Five infants had minimal resection of the proximal atretic segment and a temporary double-barrel enterostomy. Successful anastomosis was accomplished at a second procedure. One patient with gastroschisis had an end jejunostomy. Six patients were transferred following initial procedures done at other institutions. Five required reoperation due to anastomotic obstruction in three and atonic dilated proximal jejunum that had not been initially resected or tapered in two. Of 18 patients with ileal atresia, 10 were treated by exteriorization procedures and eight by wide proximal resection and end-to-oblique anastomosis, including three with tapering enteroplasty. Six patients with intestinal stenosis were managed by resection and anastomosis in five and transverse jejunoplasty in one.

Ten of 55 patients with jejunoileal obstruction had gastroschisis. Eight patients had bowel atresia and two, intestinal stenosis. Six patients with bowel atresia were managed by initial enterostomy and two by minimal resection and anastomosis. One patient had an associated colon atresia. In three, staged abdominal wall closure using Dacron-reinforced Silastic was necessary because of a small abdominal cavity. The two infants with stenosis were treated by resection and primary anastomosis in one and a transverse jejunostomy in the other. Both required temporary Silastic closure for 7–12 days. Primary bowel anastomosis and enterostomy are well tolerated even in the presence of prosthetic materials. No instance of infection related to the enterostomy or anastomotic leak was encountered. Subsequent end-to-end anastomosis was accomplished in each of the three atresia patients.

Postoperative Care

After a brief period of close observation in the recovery room, the infant is returned to the newborn intensive care unit and placed in a warm, humid, well-monitored environment. The gastrostomy tube is placed on straight drainage and the head of the Isolette is elevated at 30 degrees. Maintenance fluids are administered at 80–100 ml/kg/day; a solution containing 10% dextrose in 0.25% normal saline (delivering approximately 40 mEq/L of sodium chloride) is used. Potassium chloride (2–3 mEq/kg/day) is also infused, not in excess of 40 mEq/L. Losses related to gastric drainage are replaced milliliter for milliliter with 0.45% normal saline in 5% dextrose and water if the drainage fluid is clear (gastric juice) and by 5% dextrose and water in lactated Ringer's solution if it is green (intestinal drainage). Infusions should contain vitamins B and C, required for wound healing. Occasionally, an additional fluid bolus to counteract excessive third-space losses may be required. A urine output of 40–50 ml/kg/day, specific gravity of 1.005–1.015, and weight stability usually indicate appropriate hydration. The infant's Dextrostix, acid-base balance, and bilirubin levels are closely monitored to avoid hypoglycemia, acidosis, and kernicterus. If the bilirubin level exceeds 8 mg/100 ml, the infant is placed under Bililite phototherapy, as kernicterus may occur at unusually low levels in seriously ill neonates, particularly in the premature and in babies small for their gestational age. Exchange transfusion is undertaken when the bilirubin level exceeds 3.75 times the total protein as measured on a refractometer. Serum electrolyte values are obtained daily for the first few postoperative days. When the infant has spontaneous bowel motions and the gastric drainage fluid is clear and of minimal volume, the gastrostomy tube is elevated as a "burp tube." If no excessive gastric or intestinal reflux occurs, clear liquids are initiated (Pedialyte) at ½ oz every 3 hours and advanced in volume, and then a half-strength and finally a full-strength low osmolar small-curd formula (Isomil or Nutramigen) is given. The newborn infant requires 120 calories/kg/day to grow appropriately. Lactose intolerance is a frequent problem following major bowel resection, and milk-curd obstruction of the small intestinal anastomosis may occur if a large-curd formula (Similac or Enfamil) is used initially.[17] Malabsorption and diarrhea may be significant in infants with short bowel, those in whom the ileocecal valve has been resected, and in infants with multiple atresias or "apple-peel" atresia.[29, 32, 35, 49] Formulas that contain long-chain fats should be avoided in these patients. Instead, a medium-chain triglyceride and/or casein hydrolysate diet (Portagen or Pregestimil) is offered. Occasionally, a carbohydrate-free or an easily absorbable elemental diet such as nonflavored Vivonex may also be useful. If these formulas are not tolerated, total parenteral nutrition with a high-calorie (25% glucose, 2½% Freamine) infusion is delivered via a centrally placed Silastic (Broviac) catheter tunneled from the chest wall to a venotomy in the external or internal jugular vein or cephalic vein and advanced to the superior vena cava. This solution delivers 1 calorie per milliliter of infusate. In addition, a 10% intravenous fat solution (Intralipid) may be given through a peripheral vein. This material is isosmolar, supplies free fatty acids, and delivers an additional 1.1 calorie per milliliter. This may be infused up to 4 gm/kg/day. These vital adjunctive measures of therapy prevent inanition due to protein-calorie malnutrition (so commonly seen in past years) in cases of prolonged gastrointestinal tract malfunctions and allow time for bowel adaptation to occur. Twenty-seven of 49 infants with jejunoileal atresia at James Whitcomb Riley Hospital for Children received total parenteral nutrition. During the postoperative period, all infants with jejunoileal atresia undergo a sweat test to rule out cystic fibrosis, which occurred in six of 49 cases (12.2%).

Morbidity and Mortality

The most common cause of death in infants with jejunoileal atresia is infection related to pneumonia, peritonitis, or sepsis.[20] The most significant postoperative complications include functional intestinal obstruction at the site of anastomosis and anastomotic leak.[20, 56] Other contributing factors affecting morbidity and mortality include respiratory distress, prematurity, short-bowel syndrome, and postoperative volvulus with bowel infarction.[20] Nixon and Tawes[56] found that the most common primary

cause of death was an anastomotic leak or dysfunction, which occurred in 15% of cases.

A relatively low survival rate (58%) has been observed in instances of jejunal atresia.[20] The prognosis improves with more distal obstructions, with a 75% survival rate noted in instances of ileal atresia. An increased mortality is observed in multiple atresias (57%), apple-peel atresias (71%), and when atresia is associated with meconium ileus (65%), meconium peritonitis (50%), and gastroschisis (66%).[20, 29, 49] Nixon and Tawes[56] suggested the use of "risk" and "treatment" groups for critical evaluation of survival and mortality data in intestinal atresia. Infants were placed into three "risk" groups: group A patients are infants weighing more than 5½ lb with no other significant abnormalities; group B infants weigh 4–5½ lb or have a moderately severe associated abnormality; group C infants weigh less than 4 lb and/or have associated severe abnormalities. As expected, infants in group C had the worst survival data (32%), while infants in group A or B had an 81% survival rate. "Treatment" groups were divided into groups with high jejunal, middle small bowel, and terminal ileal atresias. Patients with high jejunal atresia in group A or B had a 60% survival, while all eight patients in group C died. Survival occurred in 82% of middle small-bowel atresias in group A or B, but was only 32% in group C. Survival for atresias involving the terminal ileum in infants in group A or B was 100%, but dropped to 50% for infants in group C. de Lorimier et al.[20] evaluated the effect of wide proximal resection and end-to-end anastomosis on survival. Resection improved survival in jejunal atresia from 39% to 66% but had little effect on the overall survival in instances of ileal atresia. Louw[44] reported a 94% survival rate following wide proximal resection and end-to-oblique one-layer anastomosis in 33 infants with jejunoileal atresia. There were two anastomotic leaks. The only two deaths in this series occurred in infants categorized as group C patients. Martin and Zerella[49] reported a 100% survival rate in 23 patients with jejunoileal atresia treated since 1968. All data on survival rates are summarized in Table 85–2.

Fifty of 55 infants with jejunoileal atresia or stenosis treated at James Whitcomb Riley Hospital for Children (1974–1983) survived (91%). One infant with high jejunal atresia had short bowel (16 cm of proximal dilated jejunum anastomosed to transverse colon) and died of sepsis after 3 months of hyperalimentation. A second death occurred in a group C patient who weighed 3 lb 2 oz and had gastroschisis associated with ileal atresia. This patient's demise was related to respiratory insufficiency and bronchopulmonary dysplasia. One anastomotic leak occurred in an infant with ileal atresia and volvulus. Reoperation with exteriorization was followed by survival. Five infants initially treated without proximal resection required subsequent reoperation for obstruction. All responded to resection and anastomosis. All nine patients with multiple atresias, both infants with apple-peel atresia, eight of 10 infants with gastroschisis, nine of 10 with meco-

TABLE 85–2.—PERCENT SURVIVAL IN JEJUNOILEAL ATRESIA

	JEJUNAL	MIDBOWEL	ILEAL	ALL CASES
de Lorimier et al.[20] (1969)	58	—	75	68
Nixon and Tawes[56] (1971)	33	65	77	62
Louw[44] (1967)	Locations not specified			94
Grosfeld, Riley Hospital (1976)	92	—	92	92
Martin and Zerella[49] (1976)	Locations not specified (since 1968)			100

nium peritonitis, and eight of 10 patients with short bowel following extensive bowel resection survived. Improved survival in these patients was related to appropriate resection or tapering enteroplasty and end-to-oblique anastomosis, or exteriorization with a late anastomosis in selected cases. The aggressive use of total parenteral nutrition as an adjunctive method of therapy has significantly improved the overall outlook of infants with jejunoileal atresia. Intravenous hyperalimentation avoids protein-calorie malnutrition, establishes positive nitrogen balance, and allows for a relatively safe "waiting period" in instances of jejunoileal atresia associated with anastomotic dysfunction or gastroschisis. This has also been extremely useful in instances of short-bowel syndrome and in infants with temporary exteriorization procedures who have enterostomy dysfunction. After massive bowel resection, parenteral hyperalimentation maintains the nutritional needs of the infants while allowing appropriate healing and time for adaptive mechanisms eventually to become effective. Adaptation is characterized by villus hypertrophy, mucosal cell hyperplasia, and increased bowel wall thickness and circumference. Unfortunately, total parenteral nutrition may be associated with severe cholestasis resulting in progressive liver disease and subsequent hepatic failure. Two deaths in the current series were related to liver failure associated with total parenteral nutrition.

Infants with middle small-bowel resection have a better prognosis than those in whom the ileocecal valve has been resected. Wilmore's review[85] of 50 infants with significant small-bowel resection suggests that most infants with more than 35 cm of intestine following middle small-bowel resection and with intact ileocecal valves survive. Survival drops to 50% if only 15–25 cm of the bowel remains and decreases to 0 in infants with less than 15 cm of remaining small bowel and an intact ileocecal valve or less than 40 cm of proximal bowel if the ileocecal valve has been resected. We believe that hyperalimentation and special elemental diets have changed these observations somewhat, as we have treated two infants with 20 cm and 30 cm of remaining small bowel, respectively, with excision of the ileocecal valve who have survived. There is good evidence to suggest that the infant's bowel lengthens in the first year of life, which may play a role in these observations.[35, 78, 84]

While most infants with a 50% middle small-bowel resection will have a normal growth and developmental pattern, others with more extensive resections may not. Infants with more distal resections, particularly those in whom the ileocecal valve is excised, are more subject to malabsorption (fat, bile salts, vitamin B$_{12}$, calcium, magnesium), diarrhea (steatorrhea), and increased bacterial proliferation in the small bowel.[4, 84, 85] Although infants with short bowel survive, they may continue to have significant problems that must be closely monitored. Long-term follow-up with regard to growth and development is essential. The care of many of these infants is exacting and demanding and should take place in a well-equipped neonatal and pediatric center with personnel skilled in the management of these unusual problems.

REFERENCES

1. Abrams J.S.: Experimental intestinal atresia. *Surgery* 64:185, 1968.
2. Baxi L.V., Yeh M.N., Blanc W.A., et al.: Antepartum diagnosis and management of in-utero intestinal volvulus with perforation. *N. Engl. J. Med.* 308:1519, 1983.
3. Bell R.H., Johnson F.E., Lilly J.R.: Intestinal anastomosis in neonatal surgery. *Ann. Surg.* 183:276, 1976.
4. Benson C.D., Lloyd J.R., Krabbenhoft K.: The surgical and metabolic aspects of massive small bowel resection in the newborn. *J. Pediatr. Surg.* 2:227, 1967.
5. Benson C.D., Lloyd J.R., Smith J.D.: Resection and primary anastomosis in the management of stenosis and atresia of the jejunum and ileum. *Pediatrics* 26:265, 1960.
6. Berdon W.E., Baker D.H., Santulli T.V., et al.: Microcolon in newborn infants with intestinal obstruction: Its correlation with the level and time of onset of obstruction. *Radiology* 90:878, 1968.
7. Birtch A.G., Coran A.G., Gross R.E.: Neonatal peritonitis. *Surgery* 61:305, 1967.
8. Bishop H.C., Koop C.E.: Management of meconium ileus. *Ann. Surg.* 145:410, 1957.
9. Bland-Sutton J.: Imperforate ileum. *Am. J. Med. Sci.* 98:457, 1889.
10. Blyth H., Dickson J.A.S.: Apple-peel syndrome (congenital intestinal atresia): A family study of 7 index patients. *J. Med. Genet.* 6:275, 1969.
11. Boggs T.R., Bishop H.: Neonatal hyperbilirubinemia associated with high obstruction of the small bowel. *J. Pediatr.* 66:349, 1965.
12. Careskey J., Weber T.R., Grosfeld J.L.: Total colonic aganglionosis: Analysis of 16 cases. *Am. J. Surg.* 143:160, 1982.
13. Careskey J., Grosfeld J.L., Weber T.R., et al.: Giant cystic meconium peritonitis (GCMP): Improved survival based on clinical and laboratory observations. *J. Pediatr. Surg.* 17:482, 1982.
14. Chalon J., Loew D.A., Malebranche J.: Effects of dry anesthetic gases on tracheobronchial ciliated epithelium. *Anesthesiology* 37:338, 1972.
15. Clatworthy H.W. Jr.: Personal communications.
16. Cloutier R.: Intestinal smooth muscle response to chronic obstruction: Possible application in jejunoileal atresia. *J. Pediatr. Surg.* 10:3, 1975.
17. Cook R.C.M., Rickham P.P.: Neonatal intestinal obstruction due to milk curds. *J. Pediatr. Surg.* 4:599, 1969.
18. Courtois B.: Les origines foetales des occlusions congenitales du grele dites par atresia. *J. Chir.* 78:405, 1959.
19. Davis D.L., Poynter C.W.M.: Congenital occlusions of intestines with report of a case of multiple atresias of jejunum. *Surg. Gynecol. Obstet.* 34:35, 1922.
20. de Lorimier A.A., Fonkalsrud E.W., Hays D.M.: Congenital atresia and stenosis of the jejunum and ileum. *Surgery* 65:819, 1969.
21. de Lorimier A.A., Norman D.A., Gooding C.A., et al.: A model for the cinefluoroscopic and manometric study of chronic intestinal obstruction. *J. Pediatr. Surg.* 8:785, 1973.
22. de Lorimier A.A., Harrison M.R.: Intestinal imbrication for atresia and pseudo-obstruction. *J. Pediatr. Surg.* 18:734, 1983.
23. Dickson J.A.S.: Apple-peel small bowel: An uncommon variant of duodenal and jejunal atresia. *J. Pediatr. Surg.* 5:595, 1970.
24. Evans C.H.: Atresias of the gastrointestinal tract. *Surg. Gynecol. Obstet.* 92:1, 1951.
25. Fockens P.: Ein operativ geheilter Fall von Kongenitaler Duenndarm Atresie. *Zentralbl. Chir.* 38:532, 1911.
26. Foglia R.P., Jobst S., Fonkalsrud E.W., et al.: An unusual variant of a jejuno-ileal atresia. *J. Pediatr. Surg.* 18:182, 1983.
27. Graham J.N., Marin-Padilla M., Hoefnagel D.: Jejunal atresia associated with Cafergot ingestion during pregnancy. *Clin. Pediatr.* 22:226, 1983.
28. Gray S.W., Skandalakis J.E.: *Embryology for Surgeons.* Philadelphia, W.B. Saunders Co., 1972, p. 151.
29. Grosfeld J.L.: Alimentary tract obstruction in the newborn. *Curr. Prob. Pediatr.*, January 1975.
30. Grosfeld J.L., Clatworthy H.W. Jr.: Intrauterine midgut strangulation in a gastroschisis defect. *Surgery* 67:519, 1970.
31. Grosfeld J.L., Clatworthy H.W. Jr.: The nature of ileal atresia due to intrauterine intussusception. *Arch. Surg.* 100:714, 1970.
32. Grosfeld J.L., Ballantine T.V.N., Shoemaker R.: Operative management of intestinal atresia and stenosis based on pathologic findings. *J. Pediatr. Surg.* 14:368, 1979.
33. Grosfeld J.L., Dawes L., Weber T.R.: Current management of abdominal wall defects: Gastroschisis and omphalocele. *Surg. Clin. North Am.* 61:1037, 1981.
34. Guttman F.N., Braun P., Garance P.H., et al.: Multiple atresias and a new syndrome of hereditary multiple atresias involving the gastrointestinal tract from stomach to rectum. *J. Pediatr. Surg.* 8:633, 1974.
35. Hays D.M.: Intestinal atresia and stenosis. *Curr. Prob. Surg.* October 1969.
36. Houston C.S., Wittenborg M.H.: Roentgen evaluation of anomalies of rotation and fixation of the bowel in children. *Radiology* 84:1, 1965.
37. Howard E.R., Othersen, H.B.: Proximal jejunoplasty in the treatment of jejunal atresia. *J. Pediatr. Surg.* 8:685, 1973.
38. Johnson F.P.: The development of the mucous membrane of the esophagus, stomach, and small intestine in the human embryo. *Am. J. Anat.* 10:521, 1910.
39. Koga Y., Hayashida Y., Ikeda K., et al.: Intestinal atresia in fetal dogs produced by localized ligation of mesenteric vessels. *J. Pediatr. Surg.* 10:949, 1975.

40. Landor J.H., Armstrong J.H., Dickson O.B., et al.: Neonatal obstruction of bowel caused by accidental clamping of small omphalocele: Report of two cases. *South. Med. J.* 56:1236, 1963.

41. LeCoultre C., Fete R., Cuendet A., et al.: An unusual association of small bowel atresia and biliary atresia: A case report. *J. Pediatr. Surg.* 18:136, 1983.

42. Lituania M., Cordone M.S.: Prenatal diagnosis of jejunal atresia by ultrasound (apple-peel syndrome). *Gaslini.* 12:197, 1980.

43. Lloyd J.R., Clatworthy H.W. Jr.: Hydramnios as an aid to the early diagnosis of congenital obstruction of the alimentary tract: A study of maternal and fetal factors. *Pediatrics* 21:903, 1958.

44. Louw J.H.: Resection and end-to-end anastomosis in the management of atresia and stenosis of the small bowel. *Surgery,* 62:940, 1967.

45. Louw J.H., Barnard C.N.: Congenital intestinal atresia: Observations on its origin. *Lancet* 2:1065, 1955.

46. Lynn H.B., Espinas E.E.: Intestinal atresia. *Arch. Surg.* 79:357, 1959.

47. Magliner B.M., Apelman Z., Lancet M., et al.: Antenatal diagnosis of fetal intestinal obstruction by ultrasonography. *Harefuah* 101:5, 1981.

48. Marfitia S., Donahoe P.K., Hendren W.H.: Effect of dry and humidified gases on the respiratory epithelium in rabbits. *J. Pediatr. Surg.* 10:593, 1975.

49. Martin L.W., Zerella J.T.: Jejunoileal atresia: Proposed classification. *J. Pediatr. Surg.* 11:399, 1976.

50. Mishalany H.G., Najjar F.: Familial jejunal atresia: Three cases in one family. *J. Pediatr. Surg.* 73:753, 1968.

51. Moya F., Apgar V., James L.S., et al.: Hydramnios and congenital anomalies: Study of a series of 74 patients. *J.A.M.A.* 173:1552, 1960.

52. Murphy D.A.: Internal hernias in infancy and childhood. *Surgery* 55:311, 1964.

53. Neuhauser E.B.: Roentgen changes associated with pancreatic insufficiency in early life. *Radiology* 46:319, 1946.

54. Nixon H.H.: Intestinal obstruction in the newborn. *Arch. Dis. Child.* 30:13, 1955.

55. Nixon H.H.: An experimental study of propulsion in isolated small intestine and applications to surgery in the newborn. *Ann. R. Coll. Surg. Engl.* 27:105, 1960.

56. Nixon H.H., Tawes R.: Etiology and treatment of small intestinal atresia: Analysis of a series of 127 jejunoileal atresias and comparison with 62 duodenal atresias. *Surgery* 69:41, 1971.

57. Odell G.B.: Physiologic hyperbilirubinemia in the neonatal period. *N. Engl. J. Med.* 277:193, 1967.

58. Okmian L.G., Kovamees A.: Jejunal atresia with intestinal aplasia: Strangulation of the intestine in the extraembryonic coelom of the bellystalk. *Acta Paediatr. Scand.* 53:65, 1964.

59. Olsen M.M., Luck S.R., Lloyd-Still J., et al.: The spectrum of meconium disease in infancy. *J. Pediatr. Surg.* 17:479, 1982.

60. Parkkulainen K.U.: Intrauterine intussusception as a cause of intestinal atresia. *Surgery* 44:1106, 1958.

61. Pokorny W.J., Harberg F.J., McGill C.W.: Gastroschisis complicated by intestinal atresia. *J. Pediatr. Surg.* 16:261, 1981.

62. Rachelson M.H., Jernigan J.R., Jackson W.F.: Intussusceptum in the newborn infant with spontaneous expulsion of the intussusception: Case report and review of the literature. *J. Pediatr.* 47:87, 1955.

63. Randolph J.G., Zollinger R.M. Jr., Gross R.E.: Mikulicz resection in infants and children: A 20-year survey of 196 patients. *Ann. Surg.* 158:481, 1963.

64. Rehbein F., Halsband H.: A double tube technique for the treatment of meconium ileus and small bowel atresia. *J. Pediatr. Surg.* 3:723, 1968.

65. Rittenhouse E.A., Beckwith J.B., Chappell J.S., et al.: Multiple septa of the small bowel: Description of an unusual case with review of the literature and consideration of etiology. *Surgery* 71:371, 1972.

66. Rosenmann J.E., Kosloske A.M.: A reappraisal of the Mikulicz enterostomy in infants and children. *Surgery* 91:34, 1982.

67. Ros Mar Z., Diez-Pardo J.A., Rosmiguel M., et al.: Apple-peel small bowel: A review of 12 cases. *Z. Kinderchir. Grenzgeb.* 29:313, 1980.

68. Santulli T.V., Blanc W.A.: Congenital atresia of the intestine: Pathogenesis and treatment. *Ann. Surg.* 154:939, 1961.

69. Singleton E.B.: Radiologic evaluation of intestinal obstruction in the newborn. *Radiol. Clin. North Am.* 1:571, 1963.

70. Spencer R.: The various patterns of intestinal atresia. *Surgery* 64:661, 1968.

71. Spriggs N.I.: Congenital intestinal occlusion. *Guys Hosp. Rep.* 66:143, 1912.

72. Suruga K., Tsunoda A., Masuda H., et al.: Some problems of congenital intestinal atresia. *Z. Kinderchir.* 3:29, 1966.

73. Tandler J.: Zur Entwicklungsgeschichte des menschlichen Duodenum in fruhen Embryonalstadien. *Morphol. Jahrb.* 29:187, 1900.

74. Teja K., Schnatterly P., Shaw A.: Multiple intestinal atresia: Pathology and pathogenesis. *J. Pediatr. Surg.* 16:194, 1981.

75. Thomas C.G. Jr.: Jejunoplasty for correction of jejunal atresia. *Surg. Gynecol. Obstet.* 129:545, 1969.

76. Todani T., Tabuchi K., Tanaka S., et al.: Intestinal atresia due to intrauterine intussusception: Analysis of 24 cases in Japan. *J. Pediatr. Surg.* 10:445, 1975.

77. Touloukian R.J.: Intestinal atresia and stenosis, in Holder T.M., Ashcraft K.W. (eds.): *Pediatric Surgery.* Philadelphia, W.B. Saunders Co., 1980, pp. 331–345.

78. Touloukian R.J., Walker G.J.: Normal intestinal length in preterm infants: An autopsy study. *J. Pediatr. Surg.* 18:720, 1983.

79. Vassy L.E., Boles E.T.: Iatrogenic ileal atresia secondary to clamping of an occult omphalocele. *J. Pediatr. Surg.* 10:799, 1975.

80. Wagner M.L., Rudolph A.J., Singleton E.B.: Neonatal defects associated with abnormalities of the amnion and amniotic fluid. *Radiol. Clin. North Am.* 6:279, 1968.

81. Webb C.H., Wangensteen O.H.: Congenital intestinal atresia. *Am. J. Dis. Child.* 41:262, 1931.

82. Weber T.R., Vane D.W., Grosfeld J.L.: Tapering enteroplasty in infants with bowel atresia and short gut. *Arch. Surg.* 117:684, 1982.

83. Weitzman J.J., Vanderhoof R.S.: Jejunal atresia with agenesis of the dorsal mesentery with "Christmas tree" deformity of the small intestine. *Am. J. Surg.* 111:443, 1966.

84. Wilkinson A.W.: Some effects of extensive intestinal resection in childhood: Symposium on intestinal absorption and malabsorption, Zürich, 1967. *Mod. Prob. Paediatr.* 11:191, 1968.

85. Wilmore D.W.: Factors correlating with a successful outcome following extensive intestinal resection in the newborn infant. *J. Pediatr.* 80:88, 1972.

86. Zerella J.T., Martin L.W.: Jejunal atresia with absent mesentery and a helical ileum. *Surgery* 80:550, 1976.

87. Zwiren G.T., Andrews H.G., Ahmann P.: Jejunal atresia with agenesis of the dorsal mesentery ("apple-peel small bowel"). *J. Pediatr. Surg.* 7:414, 1972.

Meconium Ileus

HISTORY.—In 1905, Landsteiner[50] described the association of intestinal obstruction, due to inspissated meconium in the newborn, with pathologic changes in the pancreas. Later, Kornblith and Otani[48] and Hurwitt and Arnheim[43] reported patients with meconium ileus and congenital stenosis of the pancreatic ducts. Fanconi et al.[24] coined the term "cystic fibrosis of the pancreas" for the combination of pancreatic insufficiency and chronic pulmonary disease in infancy.

In 1938, Andersen[1] described meconium ileus as an early manifestation of cystic fibrosis, noting the histologic similarity between the pancreatic lesions in both conditions. Farber,[25] in 1944, contended that, in meconium ileus, the abnormality of meconium was a consequence of pancreatic achylia, a theory supported by Andersen. In 1952, Bodian[7] ascribed the viscid nature of the meconium to abnormal mucus secreted by the intestine in infants with cystic fibrosis. The surgical treatment of meconium ileus resulted in early postoperative death until 1948, when Hiatt and Wilson[38] described the successful management by intraoperative removal of the impacted meconium with saline irrigations through an ileotomy. Since then, different surgical techniques have been described: notably, Mikulicz resection and ileostomy by Gross,[37] resection with primary anastomosis by Swenson,[90] distal chimney enterostomy by Bishop and Koop,[6] and proximal chimney enterostomy by Santulli.[81] At the same time, a variety of solutions, including saline, pancreatic enzymes, hydrogen peroxide, N-acetylcysteine and polysorbate-80 were used to liquefy the abnormal meconium. Rectal irrigation with these fluids was also reported to produce successful results in a small number of cases. In 1969, Noblett[66] reported relief of the obstruction in four consecutive infants with meconium ileus, using a hyperosmolar Gastrografin enema. This method is now the preferred technique for managing uncomplicated meconium ileus. Before 1964, the results of operative treatment were uniformly poor. The operative mortality was approximately 70%, and the survival rate at 1 year was 10%.[28] Since then, the operative mortality has decreased to 20%, with long-term survival of 75%.[80] These improved results can be attributed to advances in the management of newborn infants undergoing operation and to improved surgical technique. In addition, the modern sweat test[29] has made possible the early diagnosis and management of the underlying cystic fibrosis.

Pathogenesis

Cystic fibrosis is transmitted as an autosomal recessive trait. Neither parent is affected, but both are heterozygotes carrying the abnormal gene. Consequently, there is a 1-in-4 chance of the condition occurring with each conception. The estimated incidence of heterozygotes is 1 in 20, making this the commonest genetically determined potentially lethal disease in the Caucasian population. There is, at present, no reliable test for identifying heterozygotes or for detecting cystic fibrosis in utero. Meconium peritonitis in an unborn infant has been detected by sonography.[26]

Cystic fibrosis results from an abnormality of exocrine gland secretions throughout the body. Despite extensive investigations, the basic cause of the abnormality remains unknown.[18] The clinical manifestations of cystic fibrosis are due to the hyperviscous mucous secretions that obstruct organ passages, and chemically abnormal secretions from the serous glands. The organs principally involved are the pancreas, lungs, sweat glands, and intestine; also affected are the liver, salivary glands, reproductive organs, and nasal mucous membranes.

The lungs are normal at birth; subsequently, after months or years, progressive diffuse pulmonary disease develops as a result of mucous plugging of the small airways, with secondary infection. The exocrine pancreas is affected during fetal life. The abnormal secretions obstruct the pancreatic duct system, leading to retention of pancreatic secretions, progressive flattening and atrophy of the acinar cells, and, ultimately, replacement of the exocrine tissue by fatty tissue and fibrosis.[2, 7] Approximately 85%–90% of patients with cystic fibrosis have an advanced pancreatic lesion by early infancy and absence of pancreatic enzymes in the duodenal content.[7, 88]

The intestinal abnormalities also manifest during fetal life. Meconium ileus is uncommon in premature infants, suggesting that the gross pathologic changes take place during the last few weeks of fetal life. The small-intestinal mucous glands produce a hyperviscous secretion. The meconium formed in utero is abnormally sticky, with a low water content,[18, 22] and adheres firmly to the mucosa of the small intestine, producing intraluminal obstruction. Glanzmann and Berger[30] found in the meconium from a patient with meconium ileus a protein which, in the presence of water, combined with fat to produce a very firm jelly. This protein was not present in normal meconium. In 1952, Buchanan and Rapoport[10] showed that meconium from patients with meconium ileus contained less carbohydrate and more protein than normal meconium and suggested that the increased viscosity of the abnormal meconium was due to mucoproteins. Green, Clarke, and Shwachman[35] found the major protein constituents in extracts of meconium from patients with meconium ileus to be albumin. This has been confirmed by others, including Stephan[89] in 1975, who notes that albumin has also been found in the meconium of infants with ileal atresia and melena neonatorum. The detection of albumin in meconium has been used as a screening test for cystic fibrosis.[36]

Contrary to the original concepts of the pathogenesis of meconium ileus,[1, 25] deficiency of pancreatic enzymes is probably not the major cause of the abnormal meconium in meconium ileus. Several studies have shown that there is not a consistent correlation between meconium ileus and the severity of the pancreatic disease.[7, 30, 70, 91] Further, patients with severe pancreatic involvement due to cystic fibrosis and patients with pancreatic achylia unrelated to cystic fibrosis have a low incidence of meconium ileus.[5, 86] Meconium ileus thus appears to be mainly the result of abnormal intestinal secretions; the pancreatic lesion seems to play only a secondary role.[91]

Sodium, chloride, and (to a lesser extent) potassium levels in the sweat are elevated from birth and are unrelated to the severity or distribution of organ involvement. The sweat electrolyte defect is explained by the impermeability of cystic fibrosis epithelia to chloride ions. As sodium is actively pumped out of luminal fluids, chloride ions cannot follow; this tends to hold sodium back in the lumen.[74] This defect is also present in respiratory epithelia.[46] Severe salt depletion and cardiovascular collapse may occur as a result of the loss of electrolytes. The sweat test, based on the increased sodium and chloride content of sweat, is the cardinal laboratory determination for the diagnosis of cystic fibrosis but must correspond to the clinical picture.

Incidence

In Caucasian communities, the incidence of cystic fibrosis ranges from 1 in 1,150 to 1 in 2,500 live births.[14, 49, 89] The disease is rare in American Negroes and is virtually unknown in native African Negroes and in Mongolian and Asian peoples.[3] The reported incidence of meconium ileus in cystic fibrosis ranges from 7% to 25%; the mean incidence is approximately 15%.[4, 20, 41, 57, 59, 70] There is no significant difference in the sex incidence of meconium ileus.[20, 41, 57] Meconium ileus accounts for 9–33% of neonatal small intestinal obstructions.[16, 17]

Pathology

Meconium ileus may be simple (uncomplicated) or complicated. The two forms occur with approximately equal frequency, the reported incidence of simple meconium ileus ranging from 41% to 67%.[20, 41, 58, 65, 69, 80]

Simple Meconium Ileus

The pathologic features of simple meconium ileus are characteristic. The obstruction occurs in the midileum, which is markedly dilated, reaching a diameter of several centimeters,[80] and is

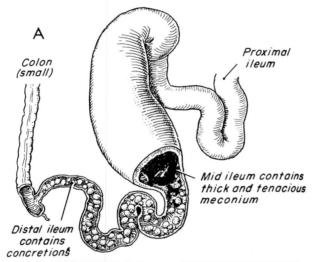

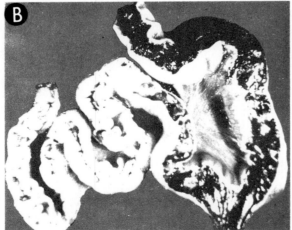

Fig 86–1.—Morphologic features of meconium ileus. Hyperperistalsis secondary to the meconium obstruction produces hypertrophy of the dilated proximal ileum. The distal ileum contains "rabbit-pellet" meconium concretions. The narrow colon is empty.

filled with thick, tenacious, dark green, tarry meconium (Fig 86–1). The intestinal wall is congested and hypertrophied. Proximally, the small intestine becomes progressively less distended and the contents change to a relatively normal semifluid consistency. Distal to the obstruction, the ileum is narrow and contains pellets of gray, inspissated meconium with the consistency of putty (rabbit pellets), giving the bowel a beaded appearance. The colon is narrow and empty, the so-called microcolon.

Complicated Meconium Ileus

The complications associated with meconium ileus include intestinal volvulus, atresia, necrosis, perforation, meconium peritonitis, and pseudocyst (Fig 86–2). All are mechanical complications of the primary disorder. The large meconium bolus, increasingly impacted further into the ileum by peristalsis, produces ischemic necrosis and perforation of the intestinal wall. This may occur before birth, leading to aseptic meconium peritonitis. In 30%–62% of patients, the heavy, meconium-filled segment of bowel has twisted as a result of the hyperperistalsis in response to obstruction, producing volvulus.[39, 41, 69] The ischemic bowel at the base of the volvulus may perforate or may heal forming a stricture or complete atresia. Ischemic necrosis of the entire volvulus, with extravasation and liquefaction of meconium, results in a pseudocyst (giant cystic meconium peritonitis).[63] Rarely, the extravasated meconium causes diffuse meconium ascites. Postnatal volvulus and perforation causes bacterial peritonitis. Perforation of the colon distal to the small-intestinal obstruction has been noted in several reports; some patients had had enemas—in others the cause remains unknown. A possible explanation is stercoral ulceration of impacted, hard, inspissated meconium pellets in the colon.[20, 23, 101]

Histology

The histologic feature of the intestinal mucosa in patients with meconium ileus is distention of the goblet cells and mucous glands, which are filled with homogeneous eosinophilic material. This merges with the intraluminal meconium, forming a cast of the crypts and villi. The intestinal muscle layers are hypertrophied as a result of the thwarted intrauterine peristalsis.

Clinical Features

A family history of cystic fibrosis, a valuable diagnostic feature, is present in 10%–33% of patients.[51, 58, 65, 69, 80] In Donnison's review, 19 of 148 families had more than one child with cystic fibrosis.[20] A maternal history of hydramnios, recorded in up to 19% of patients,[40, 44] is more common in the complicated form of meconium ileus.[51, 65, 80]

Meconium ileus is uncommon in premature infants.[41, 44, 57, 59, 65, 80] In Noblett's series, 12 of 89 patients with meconium ileus weighed less than 2.5 kg; most were small for gestational age and not premature infants.[65] O'Neill reported an unusually high incidence of premature patients (33%); however, no further information was given about these infants.[69] Associated congenital anomalies are rare.[20, 41, 44, 59, 65]

With simple meconium ileus, the presentation resembles distal ileal obstruction and manifests itself 24–48 hours after birth.[44, 65] There is increasing generalized abdominal distention and bilious vomiting. Usually, no stools are passed. If the abdomen is not grossly distended, dilated loops of bowel are visible. The impacted intraluminal meconium is palpable as a doughy, rubbery substance, mainly on the right side. Typically the anus and rectum are narrow, and this may be misinterpreted as anal stenosis. A small amount of dry or sticky gray meconium may be present in the anus.

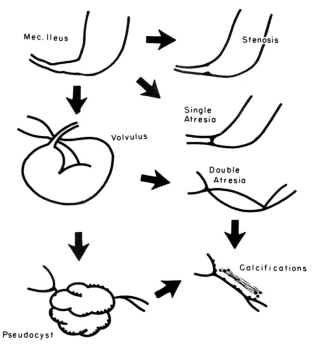

Fig 86–2.—Intestinal complications of meconium ileus. A localized area of ischemia may heal with stenosis or atresia. Volvulus occurs when hyperperistalsis leads to rotation of the heavy, meconium-filled, obstructed segment. A pseudocyst results from necrosis and liquefaction of the twisted segment and its contained meconium. The affected segment may reabsorb, leaving a long atretic segment and calcified remnants.

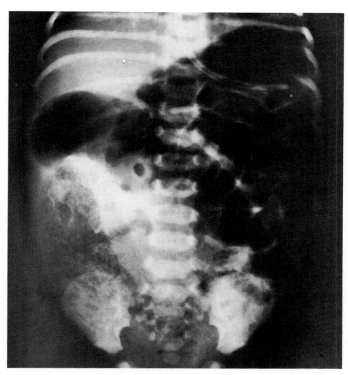

Fig 86–3.—Simple meconium ileus. This abdominal radiograph of a newborn infant with uncomplicated meconium ileus demonstrates, in the right iliac fossa, the soap-bubble appearance of the impacted meconium. Proximal to this are varying degrees of gaseous distention of the small intestine.

Complicated meconium ileus has a more acute onset, usually within 24 hours of birth. There is severe and progressive abdominal distention, which may lead to respiratory distress, particularly if there is postnatal intestinal perforation and pneumoperitoneum. The veins of the abdominal wall may be prominent. Edema and red discoloration of the abdominal wall usually indicate an underlying pseudocyst or peritonitis. A mass, representing a pseudocyst or matted loops of meconium-filled bowel, may be palpated.[65, 80] Rectal prolapse has been seen in an infant 7 hours after birth.[58] Infants with complications may be significantly hypovolemic.[58]

Radiologic Features

With simple meconium ileus, abdominal radiographs demonstrate distended, gas-filled intestinal loops. The degree of distention is uneven, some loops being considerably more dilated than others (Fig 86–3). Usually, it is not possible to differentiate between small and large bowel loops on the plain radiographs. In a patient with a positive family history of cystic fibrosis, this plain radiographic pattern is diagnostic of meconium ileus.[51] In some patients, the intestinal dilatation and air-fluid levels resemble ileal atresia. In others, there is no abrupt termination of the visualized gas to indicate a point of obstruction. Instead, minute bubbles of gas can be seen scattered through the distal ileum due to a mixture of air with the tenacious meconium[64] (Fig 86–3). This coarse, granular "soap-bubble" appearance depends on the viscosity of the meconium. It is not a constant feature and was seen by Herson in 12 of 17 patients (70%) with meconium ileus.[42] A similar bubbly appearance has also been noted in patients with colon obstruction associated with imperforate anus, Hirschsprung's disease, meconium plug syndrome, and atresia of the small intestine.[51]

An absence or paucity of air-fluid levels in meconium ileus was described by Zimmer[102] in 1948 and subsequently by White[97] in 1956. This, too, is due to the viscosity of the meconium. It is not a constant finding, and in two series the absence of air-fluid levels was noted in only 25% of uncomplicated cases.[42, 51] A few fluid levels may be present in the proximal small intestine, where the contents are more liquid. Air-fluid levels may be absent in other forms of intestinal obstruction if the intraluminal fluid and gas have been removed by intestinal suction before the radiologic examination, leading to an incorrect diagnosis of meconium ileus. The "typical" radiologic signs of meconium ileus are also seen in patients with inspissated meconium obstructing the terminal ileum who are subsequently proved not to have cystic fibrosis.[51]

With complicated meconium ileus a variety of radiologic features present, depending on the nature of the complication. Calcification on the abdominal films usually indicates meconium peritonitis resulting from intrauterine intestinal perforation (Fig 86–4); rarely, the inspissated intraluminal meconium will calcify. In the absence of calcification, the radiologic features on plain films are often not diagnostic (Fig 86–5). One third of the complicated cases reviewed by Leonidas[51] had no radiologic features that suggested complication. When there is associated proximal intestinal obstruction, such as intestinal atresia, prominent air-fluid levels may be visible. White[97] suggested that air-fluid levels on plain radiographs indicate the complicated form of meconium ileus. Because of the thick meconium in the intestine, volvulus may occur without air-fluid levels, the appearance being that of uncomplicated meconium ileus. A pseudocyst (Fig 86–6) may appear as a large dense mass with a rim of calcification and proximal intestinal obstruction.

Barium enema examination demonstrates the colon and distal

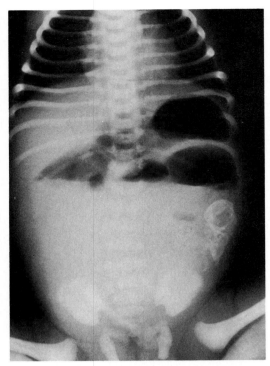

Fig 86–4.—Complicated meconium ileus. The erect abdominal radiograph shows intraperitoneal calcification in the left lower quadrant. Multiple air-filled levels are present in several dilated intestinal loops. The patient had meconium ileus with meconium peritonitis and ileal atresia.

ileum, which cannot be reliably identified on plain radiographs. The colon is characteristically of normal length and small caliber and is empty (microcolon, unused colon). Hypertonic water-soluble contrast materials should not be used for diagnosis of intestinal obstruction, especially Hirschsprung's disease,[73] since rapid fluid loss into the intestinal lumen and absorption of contrast medium lead to hypovolemia and hypertonicity,[78, 79] particularly if the hypertonic material is retained proximal to the obstruction.

Diagnosis of Cystic Fibrosis

Diagnostic tests for cystic fibrosis should be done as soon as possible. Usually this is not practical before operation.

Sweat Test

The sweat test is the most accurate method of diagnosing cystic fibrosis and can be done in the newborn infant. The pilocarpine iontophoresis method[29] provides a quantitative estimate of sodium and chloride on an accurately collected amount of uncontaminated sweat from the forearm, leg, or back. Pilocarpine is a cholinergic drug that stimulates sweat production.[71] The drug is placed on the skin, into which it is driven by application of a small (3–4 ma) electrical current for 5 minutes. Sweat is then collected for the next hour on filter paper secured to the area with an airtight binder to prevent evaporation. The sweat is eluted from the filter paper, and the sodium and chloride concentrations are measured. Concentrations of sodium and chloride above 60 mEq/L are diagnostic if at least 100 mg of sweat is collected. Although Donnison[20] reports a 90% success rate for sweat tests done during the first few days of life, at that age it may be impossible to obtain sufficient sweat for an accurate test.[21] In addition, the sweat electrolyte levels of normal infants

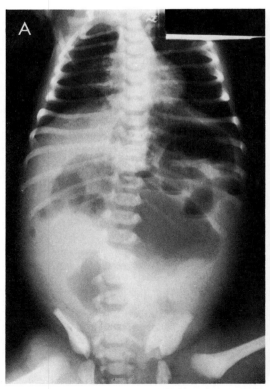

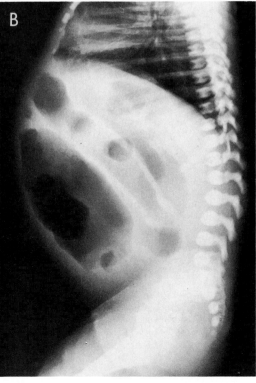

Fig 86–5.—Complicated meconium ileus. **A,** erect abdominal radiograph. Fluid levels are seen in the left upper quadrant but not in the extremely distended central loop. **B,** lateral abdominal radiograph demonstrates varying degrees of gaseous intestinal distention, with the most distended loop lying in an anterior position. At operation, this patient had meconium ileus with ileal volvulus and atresia.

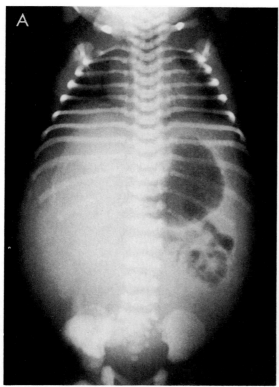 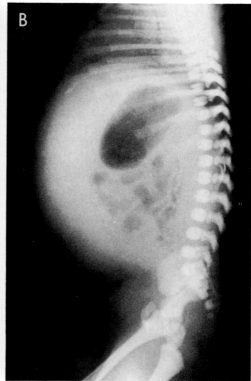

Fig 86–6.—Complicated meconium ileus. **A,** supine abdominal radiograph demonstrates a large opaque area on the right with diffuse and linear calcifications in the upper abdomen. Small, gas-filled loops of jejunum are displaced to the left. There is edema of the abdominal wall. **B,** lateral abdominal radiograph shows gross abdominal distention. No dilated loops of intestine are visible, and calcification is not seen on this view. Findings at operation were meconium ileus with a pseudocyst, meconium peritonitis, and jejunal atresia.

may be high during the first few days of life.[2, 21] Therefore, it is advisable to repeat the study after 4–6 weeks. There is no justification for delaying for months before attempting the definitive test.

Meconium Paper Strip Test

The Boehringer-Mannheim (BM) paper strip test, which is now used in some nurseries as a screening test for cystic fibrosis, is not diagnostic of meconium ileus. The test depends on the demonstration of excess albumin in the initial meconium, using a simple dipstick technique. The test strip is an intense blue when albumin is present at concentrations over 20 mg/gm of meconium. Meconium from normal infants seldom contains more than 3 mg/gm; that of infants with cystic fibrosis may contain up to 80 mg/gm. False positive results have been obtained in premature infants, in melena neonatorum, and in other forms of intestinal obstruction, such as ileal atresia. Thus, while a positive BM test result is suggestive, it is not absolutely indicative of cystic fibrosis in an infant with intestinal obstruction.

Tryptic Activity

Laboratory tests for the presence of tryptic activity in the duodenal aspirate or initial meconium are not reliable.[75, 88]

Immunoreactive Trypsin (IRT) Assay

This blood spot test identifies elevated concentrations of IRT in newborn infants with cystic fibrosis. Use of the assay in a statewide screening test was reported by Wilcken et al. in Aus-

tralia.[98] The test was very sensitive but was less specific in newborn than in older infants. Further evaluation of this assay is needed[96] and is currently under way.

Differential Diagnosis

A positive diagnosis can usually be made after evaluating the clinical and radiologic features. In an infant with obstruction of the small intestine, a positive family history of cystic fibrosis is usually diagnostic. In the absence of a family history, simple meconium ileus must be distinguished from other forms of distal intestinal obstruction. On a plain radiograph showing multiple dilated loops of intestine, small bowel cannot be distinguished from large bowel. Barium enema examination demonstrates the narrow "microcolon" and excludes the different causes of large-bowel obstruction, including meconium plug syndrome,[12] Hirschsprung's disease, small left-colon syndrome,[15] functional immaturity of the intestine,[53, 93] and colonic atresia. Patients with meconium plug (anorectal plug) syndrome should be evaluated for cystic fibrosis. In two recent reports, the disease was identified in 14%–25% of infants with meconium plug syndrome.[67, 77]

With the finding of an unused colon of small caliber, total colonic aganglionosis and ileal atresia must be excluded. In the latter case, barium refluxing into the terminal ileum will be impeded by the atresia and will not enter the proximal dilated bowel. In both total colonic aganglionosis and meconium ileus, barium refluxing into the terminal ileum ultimately enters dilated small intestine. With meconium ileus, the bolus of impacted meconium is outlined as a large filling defect, whereas in Hirschsprung's disease, the bowel contents are more liquid and air-fluid levels are visible in the dilated small bowel on a radiograph taken with the baby erect.[9, 45] The diagnosis of Hirschsprung's disease is confirmed by rectal biopsy.

"Meconium ileus" may occur in patients who do not have cystic fibrosis.[51] Emery[23] described three infants with a meconium plug obstruction of the ileum: two had passed meconium before manifesting intestinal obstruction. Rickham and Boeckman[76] reported seven patients with what they termed "meconium disease." One had a meconium plug obstructing the jejunum; the others had obstruction of the distal ileum and colon by sticky, inspissated meconium, which in some was yellow-white. Similar findings were reported in siblings by Dolan and Touloukian.[19] Vinograd[94] described seven very low birth weight premature infants with meconium disease, successfully treated by enemas. None of these patients had cystic fibrosis, and all appeared to have normal pancreatic function, although Rickham and Boeckman[76] found an abnormal glucose tolerance curve in three of five long-term survivors. Rarely, meconium ileus has occurred in infants with pancreatic achylia due to pancreatic duct stenosis, in the absence of cystic fibrosis.

With complicated meconium ileus, the features of the complication—for example, intestinal atresia or volvulus—may predominate and meconium ileus may not be suspected until operation or until pathologic study of the resected surgical specimen. Patients with unusual forms of obstruction, such as volvulus of the small intestine without malrotation, or neonatal intussusception, should have a sweat test after operation to exclude cystic fibrosis.

Management

Nonoperative Management

Nonoperative management applies only to patients with simple, uncomplicated meconium ileus. Until 1969, most patients with simple meconium ileus were treated by operative removal of the impacted meconium. Some patients with mild or incomplete intestinal obstruction were successfully treated by enema, using different solutions including saline, pancreatine solution,[20] polysorbate-80 (Tween-80),[8, 17] and N-acetylcysteine (Mucomist).[62, 83, 84] Hydrogen peroxide has also been used successfully,[67] but adverse effects due to gas embolism preclude its further use.[13, 85]

In 1969, Noblett[66] reported four infants with uncomplicated meconium ileus in whom obstruction was relieved following high hyperosmolar enema. Subsequent experience has confirmed the efficacy of this technique, which has now become the preferred method of treatment of simple meconium ileus.[65, 95] Noblett used Gastrografin, a hyperosmolar water-soluble radiopaque solution of meglumine diatrizoate with 0.1% polysorbate-80 (Tween-80), a wetting agent, and 37% organically bound iodine. The success of Gastrografin in relieving the obstruction in meconium ileus is due to its high osmolarity (1,900 mOsm/L), which draws fluid into the intestinal lumen, disimpacting the mass of meconium and softening it. The polysorbate was thought to contribute to the disimpaction, but sodium diatrizoate (Hypaque 40%), a hyperosmolar solution that does not contain the wetting agent, has also proved effective in relieving uncomplicated meconium ileus, suggesting that it is the fluid flux that relieves the obstruction.[27] Studies on rats by Lutzger and Factor[56] suggested a possible damaging effect of polysorbate-80 on the intestinal mucosa. Although this was not confirmed by Wood et al.,[100] who observed no deleterious effects on rat colon using a 10% solution of polysorbate-80, diatrizoate solutions (including Gastrografin and Gastroview) are now supplied without the wetting agent. Hyperosmolar contrast agents are reserved for the *therapeutic*

management of simple meconium ileus; for reasons already discussed, barium should be used for all *diagnostic* enemas in the newborn.

Noblett[66] defined the following requirements that must be fulfilled before a hyperosmolar enema is used in the management of simple meconium ileus: (1) a diagnostic barium enema must have excluded other causes of distal intestinal obstruction; (2) there should be no clinical or radiologic evidence of complications such as volvulus, atresia, perforation, or peritonitis; (3) the patient should have been fully prepared as if for operation, including correction of fluid and electrolyte abnormalities and hypothermia; (4) prophylactic antimicrobials should have been given; (5) the patient must be evaluated by a surgeon, who will decide whether to treat the patient with hyperosmolar enema or by operation, and who will follow the patient; (6) the contrast enema must be done under fluoroscopic control.

TECHNIQUE FOR HYPEROSMOLAR ENEMA.—Before commencing the study, an intravenous infusion of 5% dextrose and 0.2% normal saline is begun, at a rate equal to twice the maintenance requirement of the child. This infusion is continued for six hours while the urine output, serum and urine osmolality, hematocrit, and serum electrolytes are monitored and used to adjust the rate of intravenous fluid administration.[78, 79]

Under fluoroscopic control, a 50% solution of Gastrografin in water is infused into the rectum and colon through a catheter firmly taped to the buttocks to prevent contrast leaking through the anus. To minimize the risk of perforation, balloon catheters are not inflated, and the Gastrografin is infused slowly at a low hydrostatic pressure or carefully injected by syringe. Injection by syringe produces variable and uncontrolled pressures. When the Gastrografin enters the dilated, gas-filled ileum, the catheter is removed and an abdominal film taken to ensure that intestinal perforation has not occurred (Fig 86–7). Usually, there is rapid passage of semiliquid meconium, which continues during the ensuing 24–48 hours. Radiographs are taken at 12 and 24 hours to evaluate progress and exclude late perforation. A second enema may be required if evacuation is incomplete.[65, 94] The second procedure should be done cautiously, as complications are more likely to occur after repeated enemas.[65] Failure to pass meconium within a few hours of a technically successful enema, or progressive distention, are indications for operation, not for repetition of the enema. Following relief of the obstruction by enema, acetylcysteine is given by nasogastric tube. Feeding is begun when signs of obstruction have subsided, usually within 48 hours. Palpable loops of intestine may be evident for several days.

Despite widespread use of hypertonic enemas, there are few reported series of patients treated in this way. Noblett[65] reported 18 patients managed by Gastrografin enema, in 14 (63%) of whom the obstruction was successfully relieved. Four patients required operation: two for intestinal perforation, and two because the Gastrografin did not reflux into the ileum. In Wagget's[95] series of seven patients, five were disimpacted by Gastrografin enema, and two required operation for intestinal perforation. In the six patients reported by Lillie and Chrispin,[55] Gastrografin enema was successful in five, and one was operated on for a late intestinal perforation. A major advantage of nonoperative therapy is the near-absence of pulmonary problems, a major cause of morbidity following operation.[95] A further advantage is the reduced hospital stay; in Noblett's series, the mean hospital stay for patients treated nonoperatively was 3.5 weeks, compared with 8 weeks for patients who required operation.[65]

COMPLICATIONS OF HYPEROSMOLAR ENEMA THERAPY.—Hypovolemic shock is a potentially fatal complication[78, 94] caused by

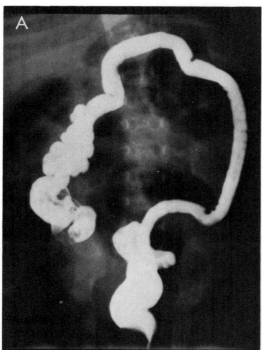
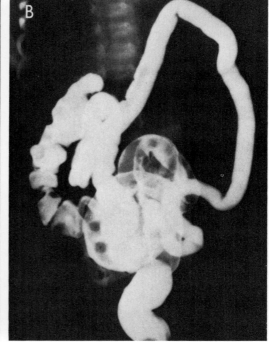

Fig 86–7.—Simple meconium ileus. Therapeutic Gastrografin enema. **A,** narrow, empty microcolon and appendix are filled with Gastrografin. **B,** Gastrografin has refluxed into the distal ileum, outlining the "rabbit-pellet" meconium concretions.

fluid loss into the intestinal lumen and aggravated by hypertonicity and osmotic diuresis. This can be avoided by concurrent intravenous fluid therapy and slow infusion of contrast.

A major complication associated with therapeutic hyperosmolar enema is intestinal perforation. Early perforation during administration of the contrast agent is immediately recognized fluoroscopically and is more likely to occur with repeated enemas.[58, 65] Wagget[95] reported rupture of the sigmoid colon attributed to distention of the balloon of the rectal catheter in the unused colon; despite immediate operation, the patient succumbed to respiratory complications.

Late intestinal perforation of the ileum or cecum may occur 12 hours to 2 days after therapeutic enema.[65] Possible factors leading to perforation are severe intestinal distention by fluid drawn into the intestinal lumen and injury to the bowel wall by the contrast medium. Studies in rats by Lutzger and Factor[56] showed extensive acute inflammatory reaction in the colon following Gastrografin enema, reaching a maximum 48–96 hours after the enema. The reaction was worse from solutions containing polysorbate-80 (Tween-80) than from Hypaque-25 alone. Wood et al.[100] studied the effects of diatrizoate solutions with and without polysorbate-80 in rats. Twenty-four hours after the enema, there were no pathologic changes in the colon unless there was associated colonic distention. Leonidas et al.[52] reported two newborn infants who died within 72 hours after Gastrografin enemas with bowel necrosis, perforation, and peritonitis. An infant with uncomplicated meconium ileus who was successfully disimpacted by a therapeutic hyperosmolar enema using Renografin-76 was reported by Grantmyre et al.[34] to develop septicemia and intestinal perforation 60 hours later as a result of extensive necrotizing enterocolitis, which proved fatal.

The likely pathogenesis of intestinal perforation or necrotizing enterocolitis following hyperosmolar enema is ischemia produced by intestinal distention.[99, 100] For this reason, diluted hyperosmolar agents should be used to modify the fluid flux, and the contrast should be infused slowly to avoid overdistention. Wood et al.[100] found that 10% polysorbate-80 did not cause a mucosal reaction in rats and successfully used a solution of 1–2% polysorbate-80 with isotonic Gastrografin diluted in water to give a final osmolality of 320–340 mOsm/L in two patients with meconium ileus and three others with meconium or fecal impaction.

Operative Management

Operation is indicated if the hyperosmolar enema fails to relieve the obstruction, in patients with complicated meconium ileus, and when the diagnosis is in doubt. Operation is not undertaken until fluid and electrolyte deficits have been corrected, and vitamin K and antibiotics have been administered.

SIMPLE MECONIUM ILEUS.—The object of operative management, when it becomes necessary, is complete evacuation of meconium from the small intestine proximal and distal to the level of obstruction. This is accomplished by irrigating the intestine through an enterotomy placed in the dilated hypertrophic ileum. Intestinal resection may also be necessary.

The abdomen is entered through a supraumbilical transverse incision. The typical features of meconium ileus (see Fig 86–1) are identified. The distal ileum may have been evacuated by the preoperative hyperosmolar enema. An incision is made into the dilated obstructed ileum. Meconium in the proximal small intestine, and residual meconium in the distal intestine are slowly evacuated by irrigation through the enterotomy using warm saline, 2% or 4% N-acetylcysteine, or a 50% diatrizoate solution. The enterotomy is then closed. Undiluted Gastrografin used for operative irrigation has caused acute hypovolemia.[61] Pancreatic enzymes or hydrogen peroxide are not recommended. If the obstruction is not completely relieved, or if the intestine has been injured, the dilated segment of ileum is resected. The length of the resected bowel should be minimized to avoid aggravating the malabsorption encountered with cystic fibrosis.

There are a number of techniques for reconstruction after intestinal resection:

1. Primary end-to-end anastomosis was recommended by Swenson.[90] Santulli[80] stated that this procedure is associated with a high incidence of postoperative obstruction from adhesions and leakage from the anastomotic site, because of excessive manipulation during disimpaction of the intestine, and reported three survivors out of 10 patients. Recently, Chappell[11] used resection and primary anastomosis successfully in seven patients, and Mabogunje et al.[58] report primary anastomosis in 18 patients with only one death. They emphasize that the resection should be adequate, the ends of the anastomosed bowel must have a good blood supply and must not have been traumatized, and the intestine must be cleared of meconium.

2. Distal chimney enterostomy, described by Bishop and Koop,[6] consists of a Roux-en-Y anastomosis between the end of the proximal segment and the side of the distal segment, approximately 4 cm from the open end. The open limb of the distal segment is brought out as an ileostomy. This technique allows normal gastrointestinal transit while providing a safety valve through the ileostomy in the event of a distal obstruction. The technique has been slightly modified by angulating the proximal segment onto the distal segment so that the proximal segment enters the distal limb obliquely, directing the intestinal content distally away from the ileostomy stoma.[75]

3. Proximal chimney enterostomy, described in 1961 by Santulli,[81] is the reverse of the Bishop-Koop anastomosis. The end of the distal limb is anastomosed to the side of the proximal limb, the end of which is brought out through the abdominal wall as an enterostomy. This method facilitates irrigation and decompression of the proximal small intestine. A catheter is placed in the distal intestine at the time of operation and is brought out through the stoma; drainage from the enterostomy is collected and instilled into the distal bowel through this catheter. Intestinal transit is assessed by intermittently clamping the enterostomy.

4. A Mikulicz double-barreled enterostomy was recommended by Gross[37] and has the advantage of being quick, since it is not necessary to clear the meconium from the intestine at the time of operation.[20] Further, it avoids an intra-abdominal anastomosis when there is doubt about the safety of such a procedure. A spur-crushing clamp is later applied. At Children's Hospital in Melbourne, double enterostomy without resection was the most frequently used procedure.[65] Resection was performed only when the bowel was not viable, and trauma to the congested bowel was minimized by not attempting to remove all the meconium at operation. Acetylcysteine was administered by nasogastric tube after operation. On the third or fourth postoperative day, Gastrografin was used to wash out any remaining meconium and demonstrate patency of the distal intestine. The enterostomy was closed five to seven days after operation by intraperitoneal end-to-end anastomosis.

Comment.—Primary end-to-end anastomosis is the method of choice, provided the intestine is healthy and well cleaned out proximally and distally as far as the anus. As an alternative, we prefer the Bishop-Koop anastomosis with distal ileostomy. The ileostomy output diminishes when normal gastrointestinal function returns, and there is no urgency to close the stoma. An advantage of the Santulli and Mikulicz procedures is that it is not necessary to evacuate the intestine at operation; however, early closure of the stoma may be necessary to prevent excessive fluid losses from the proximal stoma.

COMPLICATED MECONIUM ILEUS.—The treatment is always operative when there are complications. The actual procedure depends on the findings at operation. Nonviable, atretic, or severely distended intestine is resected and adhesions are lysed. A Bishop-Koop procedure is preferred; alternatively a Mikulicz procedure may be used. The enterostomy is closed when normal gastrointestinal function has returned, after barium enema has demonstrated patency of the distal intestine. Primary end-to-end anastomosis is not recommended unless the remaining intestine appears completely normal.

Postoperative Management

Following operation, 10% acetylcysteine by nasogastric tube or by mouth may aid the passage of meconium. Oral feedings, usually Pregestimil, are begun when gastrointestinal function has been established. A pancreatic enzyme preparation (Cotazym-S or Pancrease) is given with each feeding. Vitamin and salt supplements are provided. Failure to thrive due to impaired intestinal absorption or because of extensive small-bowel resection may necessitate a modified diet, including medium-chain triglycerides.

Prophylactic pulmonary therapy is begun immediately after operation. This includes chest percussion or vibration and postural drainage. Antibiotic therapy is begun before operation and modified on the basis of cultures from the upper respiratory tract and sputum.

Postoperative Complications

Gastrointestinal

Early gastrointestinal complications include persistent or recurrent obstruction due to inspissated meconium, anastomotic dehiscence, and secondary obstruction due to adhesions or volvulus around the fixed point of the ileostomy stoma. In the event of early postoperative obstruction, Gastrografin contrast studies by nasogastric tube, by enema, or by instillation through the ileostomy stoma demonstrate the obstruction and are usually effective in clearing residual inspissated meconium. If this is not successful or if the obstruction is mechanical, reoperation is required.

Late gastrointestinal complications include malabsorption and recurrent episodes of meconium obstruction (meconium ileus equivalent, see below). Malabsorption may be due to impaired intestinal absorption or extensive small-intestinal resection. Rectal prolapse and intussusception occur in infants with cystic fibrosis[33, 65, 86] but are less common in patients receiving enzyme replacement. Disaccharide intolerance affects up to 20% of patients with meconium ileus, usually following meconium peritonitis and atresia. Prolonged jaundice may result from accumulation of thick bile in the biliary system. Fifty percent of patients with jaundice and cystic fibrosis have meconium ileus.[92]

Pulmonary

These were a major cause of postoperative morbidity and mortality in early series.[20, 40] With early prophylactic therapy, the outcome has considerably improved.[28, 65] Nonoperative treatment, with hyperosmolar enemas, has reduced the incidence of severe pulmonary complications. Pulmonary infection requires aggressive therapy with systemic antibiotics, and physical therapy with postural drainage. Late pulmonary complications are the result of progressive primary disease.

Operative Results

Major developments in the surgical management of meconium ileus took place during the early 1960s. Before this, the mortality rates following operation ranged from 50% to 91%,[17, 20, 28, 40, 41, 44, 57, 58, 59, 69, 82] and the survival rate at 1 year ranged from 0% to 30%. Subsequently, improved operative mortality rates of 11%–30% have been reported,[28, 57, 58, 65, 80, 82] with survival rates at 1 year of 60%–71%. In recent small series by Chappel[11] and MacManus,[60] there were no operative deaths. The operative mortalities for simple and complicated meconium ileus do not differ significantly.[58, 65, 80]

Prognosis

After recovery from neonatal meconium ileus, the long-term outlook depends on the severity and rate of progression of the pulmonary disease. Life tables of patients with cystic fibrosis[29] show improved survival of patients with and without meconium ileus, due largely to early diagnosis and treatment. Shwachman[87] reported ten patients aged 28 to 35 years of age who, as newborns, had meconium ileus. Five were managed by rectal irrigation, and five were operated on. Intestinal impaction occurred in four patients in their late teens: two continue to have gastrointestinal symptoms. All have pulmonary disease: five are in fair to excellent condition, two have significantly compromised respiratory disease, and three have died as a result of progressive lung disease.

Meconium Ileus Equivalent

Meconium ileus equivalent is an uncommon complication of cystic fibrosis affecting approximately 10% of older children.[71] The intestinal contents remain abnormal through life, and at any age beyond the newborn period the thick, putty-like fecal matter may impact in the intestine, producing symptoms and signs of intestinal obstruction. In most patients, the reason for the obstruction is inadequate dosage, omission of pancreatic enzyme therapy, or dietary indiscretion (e.g., a birthday party). There is no relation to the severity of abnormalities in other organs. Dehydration following upper respiratory infection with fever, or following operation, may be a precipitating factor, and obstruction has followed upper gastrointestinal barium examination.[31]

The clinical picture is of intestinal obstruction. Dilated loops of bowel are visible, and firm, rubbery masses of inspissated intestinal content may be palpated. The differential diagnosis includes inspissated milk syndrome, intussusception, and appendiceal abscess. Intussusception of the appendix may coexist with meconium ileus equivalent.[80]

Radiographs show proximal small-bowel distention with air-fluid levels and a mottled, soap-bubble appearance representing the fecal mass, usually in the right iliac fossa. Barium enema examination outlines the fecal masses and excludes intussusception. In cystic fibrosis, the colonic mucosa has a characteristic cobblestone appearance.[31, 72] Barium follow-through studies are contraindicated.

In most cases the obstruction can be relieved by hyperosmolar enemas with Gastrografin, as described for meconium ileus.[57] Hypaque and acetylcysteine enemas have also been used with success. The proximal intestine is decompressed by nasogastric tube. Pancreatic enzymes or acetylcysteine administered through the gastric tube may help soften the inspissated intestinal content. Operation is necessary for the rare refractory case. Patients with abdominal pain without established intestinal obstruction may have relief of symptoms with oral *N*-acetylcysteine.[32, 54] Pancreatitis and duodenal ulcer must be excluded.[47, 88]

REFERENCES

1. Andersen D.H.: Cystic fibrosis of the pancreas and its relation to celiac disease. *Am. J. Dis. Child.* 56:344, 1938.
2. Andersen D.H.: Cystic fibrosis of the pancreas. *J. Chron. Dis.* 7:58, 1958.
3. Anderson C.M., Goodchild M.C.: *Cystic Fibrosis: Manual of Diagnosis and Management.* Boston, Blackwell Scientific Publications, 1976.
4. Allan D.L., Robbie M., Phelan P.D., et al.: Familial occurrence of meconium ileus. *Eur. J. Pediatr.* 135:291, 1981.
5. Auburn R.P., Feldman S.A., Gadacz T.R., et al.: Meconium ileus secondary to partial aplasia of the pancreas: Report of a case. *Surgery* 65:689, 1969.
6. Bishop H.C., Koop C.E.: Management of meconium ileus: Resection, Roux-en-Y anastomosis and ileostomy irrigation with pancreatic enzymes. *Ann. Surg.* 145:410, 1957.
7. Bodian M.: *Fibrocystic Disease of the Pancreas.* New York, Grune & Stratton, 1953.
8. Bowring A.C., Jones R.F.C., Kern I.B.: The use of solvents in the intestinal manifestations of mucoviscidosis. *J. Pediatr. Surg.* 5:338, 1970.
9. Bryk D.: Meconium ileus: Demonstration of the meconium mass on barium enema study. *Am. J. Roentgenol.* 95:214, 1965.
10. Buchanan D.J., Rapoport S.: Chemical comparison of normal meconium and meconium from a patient with meconium ileus. *Pediatrics* 9:304, 1952.
11. Chappell J.S.: Management of meconium ileus by resection and end-to-end anastomosis. *S. Afr. Med. J.* 52:1093, 1977.
12. Clatworthy H.W., Howard W.H.R., Lloyd J.: The meconium plug syndrome. *Surgery* 39:131, 1956.
13. Danis R.K., Brodeur A.E., Shields J.: The danger of hydrogen peroxide as a colonic irrigating solution. *J. Pediatr. Surg.* 2:131, 1967.
14. Danks D.M., Allan J., Anderson C.M.: A genetic study of fibrocystic disease of the pancreas. *Ann. Hum. Genet.* 28:323, 1965.
15. Davis W.S., Allen R.P., Favara B.E., et al.: Neonatal small left colon syndrome. *Am. J. Roentgenol.* 120:322, 1974.
16. de Lorimier A.A., Fonkalsrud E.W., Hays D.M.: Congenital atresia and stenosis of the jejunum and ileum. *Surgery* 65:819, 1969.
17. Dey D.L.: The surgical treatment of meconium ileus. *Med. J. Aust.* 50:179, 1963.
18. Di Sant'Agnese P.A., Davis P.B.: Research in cystic fibrosis. *N. Engl. J. Med.* 295:481, 1976.
19. Dolan T.F. Jr., Touloukian R.J.: Familial meconium ileus not associated with cystic fibrosis. *J. Pediatr. Surg.* 9:821, 1974.
20. Donnison A.B., Shwachman H., Gross R.E.: Review of 164 children with meconium ileus seen at the Children's Hospital Medical Center, Boston. *Pediatrics* 37:833, 1966.
21. Elian E., Shwachman H., Hendren W.H.: Intestinal obstruction of the newborn infant. *N. Engl. J. Med.* 264:13, 1961.
22. Emery J.L.: Laboratory observations on the viscidity of meconium. *Arch. Dis. Child.* 29:34, 1954.
23. Emery J.L.: Abnormalities in meconium of the foetus and newborn. *Arch. Dis. Child.* 32:17, 1957.
24. Fanconi G., Uehlinger E., Knauer C.: Das Coeliakiesyndrom bei angeborener zystischer Pancreasfibromatose und Bronchiektasien. *Wien. Med. Wochenschr.* 27/28:753, 1936.
25. Farber S.J.: The relation of pancreatic achylia to meconium ileus. *J. Pediatr.* 24:387, 1944.
26. Fleischer A.C., Davis R.J., Campbell L.: Sonographic detection of a meconium-containing mass in a fetus: A case report. *J. Clin. Ultrasound* 11:103, 1983.
27. Frech R.S., McAlister W.H., Ternberg J., et al.: Meconium ileus relieved by 40 per cent water-soluble contrast enemas. *Radiology* 94:341, 1970.
28. George L., Norman A.P.: Life tables for cystic fibrosis. *Arch. Dis. Child.* 46:139, 1971.
29. Gibson L.E., Cooke R.E.: A test for concentration of electrolytes in sweat in cystic fibrosis of the pancreas utilizing pilocarpine by iontophoresis. *Pediatrics* 23:545, 1959.
30. Glanzmann V.E., Berger H.: Uber mekoniumileus. *Ann. Paediatr.* 175:33, 1950.
31. Glick S.K., Kressel H.Y., Laufer I., et al.: Meconium ileus equivalent: Treatment with hypaque enema. *Diagn. Imaging* 49:149, 1980.
32. Gracey M., Burke V., Anderson C.M.: Treatment of abdominal pain in cystic fibrosis by oral administration of N-acetylcysteine. *Arch. Dis. Child.* 44:404, 1969.
33. Graham W.P., Halden A., Jaffe B.F.: Surgical treatment of patients with cystic fibrosis. *Surg. Gynecol. Obstet.* 122:373, 1966.
34. Grantmyre E.B., Butler G.J., Gillis D.A.: Necrotizing enterocolitis

after Renografin-76 treatment of meconium ileus. *Am. J. Radiol.* 136:990, 1981.

35. Green M.N., Clarke J.T., Shwachman H.: Studies in cystic fibrosis of the pancreas: Protein pattern in meconium ileus. *Pediatrics* 21:635, 1958.
36. Green M.N., Shwachman H.: Presumptive tests for cystic fibrosis based on serum protein in meconium. *Pediatrics* 41:989, 1968.
37. Gross R.E.: *The Surgery of Infancy and Childhood.* Philadelphia, W.B. Saunders Co., 1953.
38. Hiatt R.B., Wilson P.E.: Celiac syndrome. Therapy of meconium ileus: Report of eight cases with a review of the literature. *Surg. Gynecol. Obstet.* 87:317, 1948.
39. Hill J.T., Snyder W.H., Pollock W.F.: Uncomplicated meconium ileus. *Arch. Surg.* 88:522, 1964.
40. Hill J.T., Snyder W.H., Pollock W.F.: Management of complicated meconium ileus. *Am. J. Surg.* 108:233, 1964.
41. Holsclaw D.S., Eckstein H.B., Nixon H.H.: Meconium ileus: A 20-year review of 109 cases. *Am. J. Dis. Child.* 109:101, 1965.
42. Herson R.E.: Meconium ileus. *Radiology* 68:568, 1957.
43. Hurwitt E.S., Arnheim E.E.: Meconium ileus associated with stenosis of the pancreatic ducts. *Am. J. Dis. Child.* 64:443, 1942.
44. Kalayoglu M., Sieber W.K., Rodnan J.B., et al.: Meconium ileus: A critical review of treatment and eventual prognosis. *J. Pediatr. Surg.* 6:290, 1971.
45. Keats T.E., Smith T.H.: Meconium ileus: A demonstration of the ileal meconium mass by barium enema examination. *Radiology* 89:1073, 1967.
46. Knowles M., Gatzy J., Boucher R.: Relative ion permeability of normal and cystic fibrosis nasal epithelium. *J. Clin. Invest.* 71:1410, 1983.
47. Kopel F.B.: Gastrointestinal manifestations of cystic fibrosis. *Gastroenterology* 62:483, 1972.
48. Kornblith B.A., Otani S.: Meconium ileus with congenital stenosis of the main pancreatic duct. *Am. J. Pathol.* 5:249, 1929.
49. Kramm E.R., Crane M.M., Sirken M.G., et al.: A cystic fibrosis pilot survey in three New England states. *Am. J. Public Health* 52:2041, 1962.
50. Landsteiner K.: Darmverschluss durch eingedictes Meconium Pankreatitis. *Zentralbl. Allg. Pathol.* 16:903, 1905.
51. Leonidas J.C., Berdon W.E., Baker D.H., et al.: Meconium ileus and its complications: A reappraisal of plain film roentgen diagnostic criteria. *Am. J. Roentgenol.* 109:598, 1970.
52. Leonidas J.C., Burry V.F., Fellows R.A., et al.: Possible adverse effect of methylglucamine diatrizoate compounds on the bowel of newborn infants with meconium ileus. *Radiology* 121:693, 1976.
53. Le Quesne G.W., Reilly B.J.: Functional immaturity of the large bowel in the newborn infant. *Radiol. Clin. North Am.* 13:331, 1975.
54. Lillibridge C.B., Docter J.M., Eidelman S.: Oral administration of N-acetylcysteine in the prophylaxis of "meconium ileus equivalent." *J. Pediatr.* 71:887, 1967.
55. Lillie J.G., Chrispin A.R.: Investigation and management of neonatal obstruction by Gastrografin enema. *Ann. Radiol.* 15:237, 1972.
56. Lutzger L.G., Factor S.M.: Effects of some water-soluble contrast media on the colonic mucosa. *Radiology* 118:545, 1976.
57. McPartlin J.F., Dickson J.A.S., Swain V.A.J.: Meconium ileus: Immediate and long-term survival. *Arch. Dis. Child.* 47:207, 1972.
58. Mabogunje O.A., Wang C.I., Mahour G.H.: Improved survival of neonates with meconium ileus. *Arch. Surg.* 117:37, 1982.
59. MacDonald J.A., Trusler G.A.: Meconium ileus: An eleven-year review at the Hospital for Sick Children, Toronto. *Can. Med. Assoc. J.* 83:881, 1960.
60. MacManus L.E., Rongaus V.A., Klein R.L.: Meconium ileus with cystic fibrosis. *J. Am. Osteopath. Assoc.* 81:616, 1982.
61. Maneksha F.R., Betta J., Zawin M., et al.: Intraoperative hypoxia and hypotension caused by Gastrografin-induced hypovolemia. *Anesthesiology* 61:454, 1984.
62. Meeker I.A., Kincannon W.N.: Acetylcysteine used to liquefy inspissated meconium causing intestinal obstruction in the newborn. *Surgery* 56:419, 1964.
63. Moore T.C.: Giant cystic meconium peritonitis. *Ann. Surg.* 157:566, 1963.
64. Neuhauser E.B.D.: Roentgen changes associated with pancreatic insufficiency in early life. *Radiology* 46:319, 1946.
65. Noblett H.: Meconium ileus, in Ravitch M.M., Welch K.J., Benson C.D., et al. (eds.): *Pediatric Surgery,* ed. 3. Chicago, Year Book Medical Publishers, 1979.
66. Noblett H.R.: Treatment of uncomplicated meconium ileus by Gastrografin enema: A preliminary report. *J. Pediatr. Surg.* 4:190, 1969.

67. Olim C.B., Ciuti A.: Meconium ileus: A new method of relieving obstruction. *Ann. Surg.* 140:736, 1954.
68. Olsen M.M., Luck S.R., Lloyd-Still J., et al.: The spectrum of meconium disease in infancy. *J. Pediatr. Surg.* 17:479, 1982.
69. O'Neill J.A., Grosfeld J.L., Boles E.T., et al.: Surgical treatment of meconium ileus. *Am. J. Surg.* 119:99, 1970.
70. Oppenheimer E.H., Esterly J.R.: Pathological evidence of cystic fibrosis patients with meconium ileus. *Pediatr. Res.* 7:339, 1973.
71. Orenstein D.M.: Diagnosis of cystic fibrosis. *Semin. Resp. Med.,* in press.
72. Pilling D.W., Steiner G.M.: The radiology of meconium ileus equivalent. *Br. J. Radiol.* 54:562, 1981.
73. Poole C.A., Rowe M.I.: Distal neonatal intestinal obstruction: The choice of contrast material. *J. Pediatr. Surg.* 11:1011, 1976.
74. Quinton P.M., Bijman J.: Higher bioelectric potentials due to decreased chloride absorption in the sweat glands of patients with cystic fibrosis. *N. Engl. J. Med.* 308:1185, 1983.
75. Rickham P.P.: Intraluminal intestinal obstruction. *Prog. Pediatr. Surg.* 2:73, 1971.
76. Rickham P.P., Boeckman C.R.: Neonatal meconium obstruction in the absence of mucoviscidosis. *Am. J. Surg.* 109:173, 1965.
77. Rosenstein B.J., Langbaum T.S.: Incidence of meconium abnormalities in newborn infants with cystic fibrosis. *Am. J. Dis. Child.* 134:72, 1980.
78. Rowe M.I., Furst A.J., Altman D.H., et al.: The neonatal response to Gastrografin enema. *Pediatrics* 48:29, 1971.
79. Rowe M.I., Seagram G., Weinberger M.: Gastrografin-induced hypertonicity. *Am. J. Surg.* 125:185, 1973.
80. Santulli T.V.: Meconium ileus, in Holder T.M., Ashcraft K.W. (eds.): *Pediatric Surgery.* Philadelphia, W.B. Saunders Co., 1980.
81. Santulli T.V., Blanc W.A.: Congenital atresia of the intestine: Pathogenesis and treatment. *Ann. Surg.* 154:939, 1961.
82. Schennach W., Menardi G., Stauffer U.G.: Zur Prognose des Mekoniumileus. *Z. Kinderchir.* 18:161, 1976.
83. Schiller M., Grosfeld J.L., Morse T.S.: Nonoperative treatment of meconium ileus: An experimental study in rats. *Am. J. Surg.* 122:22, 1971.
84. Shaw A.: Safety of N-acetylcysteine in treatment of meconium obstruction of the newborn. *J. Pediatr. Surg.* 4:119, 1969.
85. Shaw A., Cooperman A., Fusco J.: Gas embolism produced by hydrogen peroxide. *N. Engl. J. Med.* 277:238, 1967.
86. Shwachman H.: Gastrointestinal manifestations of cystic fibrosis. *Pediatr. Clin. North Am.* 22:787, 1975.
87. Shwachman H.: Meconium ileus: Ten patients over 28 years of age. *J. Pediatr. Surg.* 18:570, 1983.
88. Shwachman H., Lebenthal E., Khaw K.T.: Recurrent acute pancreatitis in patients with cystic fibrosis with normal pancreatic enzymes. *Pediatrics* 55:86, 1975.
89. Stephan U., Busch E.W., Kollberg H., et al.: Cystic fibrosis detection by means of a test-strip. *Pediatrics* 55:35, 1975.
90. Swenson O.: *Pediatric Surgery,* ed. 2. New York, Appleton-Century-Crofts, 1962.
91. Thomaidis T.S., Arey J.B.: The intestinal lesions in cystic fibrosis of the pancreas. *J. Pediatr.* 63:444, 1963.
92. Valman H.B., France N.E., Wallis P.G.: Prolonged neonatal jaundice in cystic fibrosis. *Arch. Dis. Child.* 46:805, 1971.
93. Vanhoutte J.J., Katzman D.: Roentgenographic manifestations of immaturity of the intestinal neural plexus in premature infants. *Radiology* 106:363, 1973.
94. Vinograd I., Mogle P., Peleg O., et al.: Meconium disease in premature infants with very low birth weight. *J. Pediatr.* 103:963, 1983.
95. Wagget J., Bishop H.C., Koop C.E.: Experience with Gastrografin enema in the treatment of meconium ileus. *J. Pediatr. Surg.* 5:649, 1970.
96. Warwick W.J.: Cystic fibrosis and meconium ileus. *J. Pediatr.* 103:1008, 1983.
97. White H.: Meconium ileus: A new roentgen sign. *Radiology* 66:567, 1956.
98. Wilcken B., Brown A.R.D., Urwin R., et al.: Cystic fibrosis screening by dried blood spot trypsin assay: Results in 75,000 newborn infants. *J. Pediatr.* 102:383, 1983.
99. Wood B.P., Katzberg R.W.: Tween-80/diatrizoate enemas in bowel obstruction. *Am. J. Roentgenol.* 130:747, 1978.
100. Wood B.P., Katzberg R.W., Ryan D.H., et al.: Diatrizoate enemas: Facts and fallacies of colonic toxicity. *Radiology* 126:441, 1978.
101. Zachary R.B.: Meconium and faecal plugs in the newborn. *Arch. Dis. Child.* 32:22, 1957.
102. Zimmer J.: Microcolon: With report of two cases. *Acta Radiol.* 29:228, 1948.

Meckel's Diverticulum

HISTORY.—In 1809, Johann Friedrich Meckel the Younger detailed in human development that persistence of the yolk sac duct can result in a vestigial structure connected with the intestine. He described this structure as the diverticulum which now bears his name.[11] Fredericus Ruysch had pictured such an ileal diverticulum a century earlier.[16]

Incidence

Meckel's diverticulum occurs in approximately 2% of the population.[1, 7, 10, 20, 21] It may be asymptomatic and unsuspected throughout the life of most individuals until found at autopsy, may be an incidental finding during celiotomy, or a complication may make it manifest clinically.

Embryology

The yolk sac is connected to the primitive gut by the yolk stalk or vitelline (omphalomesenteric) duct. This attenuates, involutes, and separates from the intestine between the fifth and seventh weeks of gestation.[7] Failure of the yolk stalk to disappear completely results in persistence of vitelline (omphalomesenteric) duct remnants, whose anatomy is determined by the stage at which arrest of involution occurs. The derivation and spectrum of such anomalies has been amply described[7, 19, 20] and can be depicted graphically (Fig 87–1; see also Fig 87–5).

Anatomy and Histology

Based on the classical monograph of Söderlund[20] and the work of earlier authors,[19, 22] these anomalies can be tabulated into six major groups. Meckel's diverticulum is by far the most common (Table 87–1). In 74%, the tip of the diverticulum is free.[20]

The blood supply of Meckel's diverticulum is derived from the vitelline vessels and usually terminates in the diverticulum, but may continue to the abdominal wall, and occasionally remains attached to the umbilicus even after involution of the diverticulum[7] (Fig 87–1,A and F).

Meckel's diverticulum arises from the antimesenteric aspect of the ileum, 40–100 cm proximal to the ileocecal valve. It is a true diverticulum containing all layers of the intestinal wall (Fig 87–1,E). Söderlund[20] employed serial sections in a study of 88 cases of symptomatic and nonsymptomatic Meckel's diverticula and found heterotopic gastric mucosa in 39 cases (44%). Gastric mucosa was found in 35% of asymptomatic diverticula and in 75% of those producing symptoms. Fundic glands presumed capable of producing hydrochloric acid were found in 38 of the 39 specimens, and accompanying pyloric glands in 29 of the cases. Söderlund[20] also correlated an increased measured area of gastric mucosa (1.2 cm^2 or greater) with a high incidence of peptic ulceration in the diverticula examined. Pancreatic tissue has been found in about 5% of excised Meckel's diverticula with or without gastric mucosa in the diverticulum.

Natural History of Meckel's Diverticulum

While Meckel's diverticulum is generally a silent lesion, in two series disease was found in 27% of 190 cases[5] and 34% of 413 cases.[20] These figures are high. A more realistic figure was de-

rived by Soltero and Bill,[21] who calculated a 4.2% risk of disease, diminishing with advancing age. This is consistent with observations that 45% of patients with symptomatic diverticula present at under 2 years of age.[1, 8]

The frequency of specific complications of Meckel's diverticulum varies, but an approximation was derived from six series totaling 830 cases of complicated Meckel's diverticulum[1, 8, 10, 17, 20, 21] as follows: (1) bleeding, 32%; (2) intestinal obstruction, 35%; (3) diverticulitis (with or without perforation), 22%; (4) umbilical fistula, 10%; (5) other umbilical lesions, hernias, tumors, miscellaneous, 1%. Except for a higher incidence of hernia and a lower incidence of umbilical fistula anomalies, these results are in approximate concordance with the analysis of 1,605 cases collected by Moses[12] in 1947.

There is a variable male predominance in patients with symptomatic diverticula. Hemorrhage and obstruction are more common in infants and young children, and diverticulitis in older children.[1]

Hemorrhage—Clinical Presentation and Diagnosis

Bleeding from a Meckel's diverticulum is usually painless and is most often seen in children under 5 years of age.[1, 8] It originates from a peptic ulceration of ileum adjacent to ectopic gastric mucosa, whether this junction is within the diverticulum or in the ileum adjacent to its base.[20] Bleeding varies from minimal, recurrent episodes of hematochezia to massive, shock-producing hemorrhage. The appearance of the material passed by rectum can usually be correlated with the rate of bleeding, the volume of blood, and the level of peristaltic activity. In general, the more brisk the hemorrhage, the brighter red the blood expelled. At first the stools are frequently brick-red and bulky with "currant-jelly" stools associated with persistent bleeding. Tarry stools originating from a Meckel's diverticulum or another site in the lower intestine suggest minor bleeding with slow intestinal trans-

TABLE 87–1.—RELATIVE FREQUENCY OF VITELLINE DUCT REMNANTS (413 CASES)*

ABNORMALITY		FREQUENCY (%)
Meckel's diverticulum and related abnormalities		
Meckel's diverticulum (399 cases)		97
Tip attached to body wall (22 cases)	5.3 ⎫	(23)
or other structure (72 cases)	17.4 ⎭	
Tip unattached (305 cases)		74
Remnant of vitelline vessels attached to umbilicus		—
Solid cord from ileum to umbilicus		—
Umbilical abnormalities		
Umbilical cord cyst, umbilical mucosal remnant ("polyp"), umbilical sinus (5 cases)		1.2
Cystic remnant of vitelline duct		
In body wall		
In abdominal cavity (1 case)		0.24
Omphaloileal fistula (10 cases)		2.4

*From Söderlund.[20]

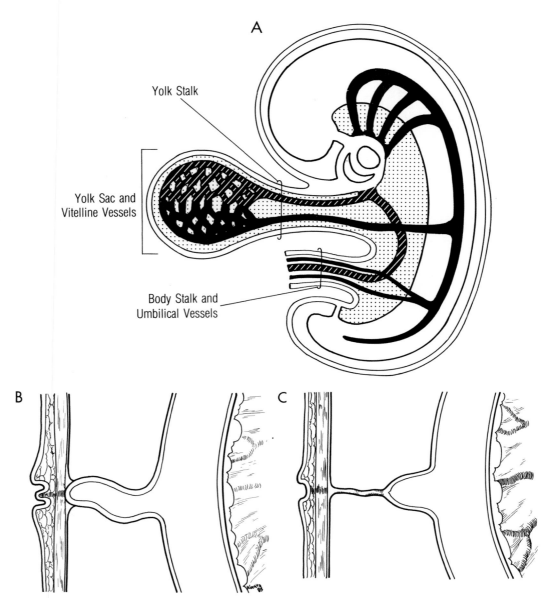

Fig 87–1.—Derivation of persistent vitelline (omphalomesenteric) duct remnants and spectrum of anomalies. Those illustrated are intraperitoneal and can produce important clinical manifestations. **A,** embryo before the fifth week of fetal life, showing pertinent structures before involution. The communication between the yolk sac and the intestinal primordium narrows and elongates to become the yolk stalk or vitelline (omphalomesenteric) duct, which joins the fetal intestine at the midgut. The developing vitelline vessels ramify over the yolk sac, which serves as the main source of nourishment for the embryo. As utilization of the yolk sac proceeds to completion, the vitelline duct fuses with the body stalk to form the umbilical cord. Thereafter umbilical vessels transport nutrients from the functioning placenta to the fetus. **B,** Meckel's diverticulum is the most common of the vitelline (omphalomesenteric) duct remnants. It can persist in its entirety and remain attached to the body wall. **C,** it can remain attached to the body wall by an intervening fibrous cord which results from involution and obliteration of the distal portion of the vitelline duct leaving the more proximal diverticulum in continuity with the ileum. **(Continued.)**

port and consequent alteration of the blood passed. This is in contrast to the tarry stools seen in patients with gastric bleeding. Meckel's diverticulum can be eliminated as a significant diagnostic possibility in such patients, as tarry stools are far more likely due to bleeding from a proximal site in the gastrointestinal tract. Chronic rectal bleeding from a Meckel's diverticulum occasionally produces significant anemia, as do other causes of lower intestinal bleeding. The latter include polyps, blood dyscrasia, intestinal hemangiomas, and arteriovenous malformations. In the absence of an episode of massive rectal bleeding, appropriate hematologic studies, endoscopy, and barium contrast studies should be done to rule out such sources of bleeding. Barium

studies are of little value where Meckel's diverticulum is suspected, as the overlay of contrast-containing loops of intestine hide the diverticulum.

The most helpful study in confirming a diagnosis of Meckel's diverticulum is the "Meckel's scan." In 1970, Jewett, Duszynski and Allen[9] first described this technique, based on the affinity of the isotope ^{99m}Tc pertechnetate for gastric mucosa and the resultant imaging of a Meckel's diverticulum that contains parietal cells. There is a significant incidence of false negative studies.[3, 15] Berquist et al.[3] reviewed the specificity of scintigraphic findings in 100 cases of suspected Meckel's diverticulum in adults and children. Eight patients proved to have Meckel's diverticula.

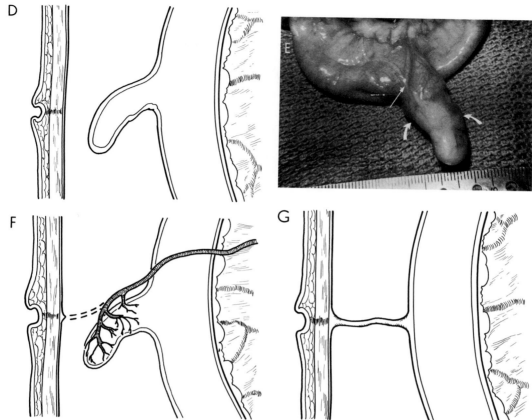

Fig 87–1 Cont.—D, Meckel's diverticulum remains unattached in the majority (74%) of cases.[20] **E,** typical appearance of Meckel's diverticulum at celiotomy. It arises from the antimesenteric border of the ileum, usually within 100 cm of the ileocecal junction, and is of approximately the same caliber as the ileum. The majority of symptomatic Meckel's diverticula (75%) contain heterotopic elements (most commonly gastric mucosa) that can often be seen and palpated on external examination, as in this case. The pale appearance (distal to curved arrows) represents heterotopic gastric mucosa within the diverticulum. Ease of palpability can be correlated with an increased measured area of gastric mucosa in the diverticulum.[20] The blood supply is seen continuing from beneath the ileal serosa into the body of the diverticulum *(straight arrow)*. **F,** the blood supply is derived from the paired vitelline (omphalomesenteric) arteries that pass on either side of the mesentery to ramify over the yolk sac. The left vitelline artery normally disappears, while the proximal part of the right vessel becomes the superior mesenteric artery. Its distal segment persists as an end artery of this parent vessel and supplies remnants of the vitelline duct. The vitelline (omphalomesenteric) vessels usually terminate in the diverticulum but can continue to the abdominal wall *(dotted line)*. **G,** in the latter instance, the vitelline vessels may also persist as a fibrous cord connecting ileum to the umbilicus after complete involution of the diverticulum. This can set the stage for intestinal obstruction.

One was false negative, and two were false positive examinations. False positive scans have been reported in patients with other abnormalities, such as intussusception, hydronephrosis, and arteriovenous malformations; however, when Berquist and associates[3] scanned patients with these lesions, they found them all to be negative. Similar results were found in an exclusively pediatric series.[15] Positive scans have nevertheless been seen in children with intestinal bleeding from unusual sources other than Meckel's diverticulum. These have included ectopic gastric mucosa in the ileum, and papillary lymphoid hyperplasia of the ileum.[18] Use of cimetidine[13] and pentagastrin[23] to enhance gastric mucosal imaging improves results. Angiography has been used to visualize a bleeding Meckel's diverticulum[6] but is more appropriate for evaluating arteriovenous malformations.

An illustrative case of bleeding Meckel's diverticulum is shown, with correlation of a diagnostic scan, operative findings and surgical pathology, in Figure 87–2.

Management

Massive hemorrhage from Meckel's diverticulum is episodic, and spontaneous cessation is the rule. In view of this, blood is replaced rapidly and an elective operation is planned when the patient's condition is stable. If the technetium scan is negative, the patient may be observed, but a repeat episode of serious bleeding is an indication for operation to search for a Meckel's diverticulum, duplication, hemangioma, or arteriovenous malformation.

Procedure

A transverse right lower quadrant incision may be used and the diverticulum located by tracing the ileum proximal from its junction with the cecum. This segment of intestine is downstream from the diverticulum and may appear dark due to intraluminal blood. The feeding artery on the surface of the ileum should be ligated. Diverticulectomy without segmental ileal resection can usually be carried out when bleeding is the indication for operation. The ileum at the base of the diverticulum can be amputated obliquely and closed over a clamp. Alternatively, seromuscular sutures can be placed at the junction of diverticulum and ileum and a wedge excision performed, especially if an ileal ulceration is suspected. The open two-layered closure of the ileum is transverse to its long axis. Safe closure of healthy intestine is anticipated using either method or a stapling device. Occasionally, the base of the diverticulum is so broad that an ileal resection is required. The results of operation for bleeding Meckel's diverticulum are excellent.

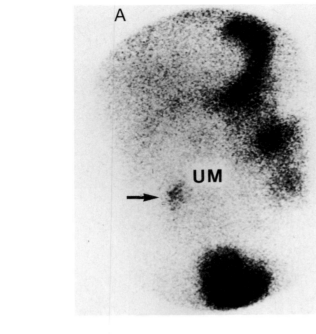

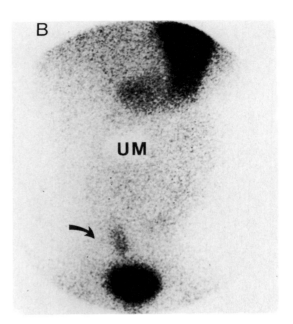

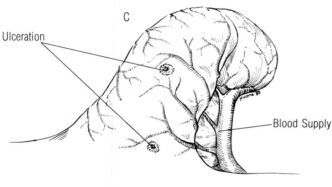

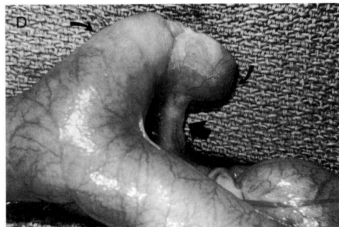

Fig 87–2.—Meckel's diverticulum and hemorrhage. **A,** Meckel's scan. Technetium-99m pertechnetate selectivity concentrates in gastric mucosa whether in stomach or in a Meckel's diverticulum. It is presumably excreted and can thereafter be followed into the upper intestine. Some of the isotope, excreted in the urine, collects in the bladder. Sites of isotope accumulation appear as the darkest areas on the scan. In this case, isotope outlines stomach, proximal intestine, and a Meckel's diverticulum *(arrow)* to the right of the umbilical marker *(UM)*. The urinary bladder is distended. **B,** patient has voided. With contraction of the bladder, the ileum and diverticulum have moved downward *(curved arrow)*. This is an interesting demonstration of the natural mobility of Meckel's diverticulum. (Courtesy of Dr. Donald R. Germann, St. Luke's Hospital of Kansas City, Mo.) **C,** diagram drawn from operative findings in this case illustrates two possible sites of peptic ulceration in Meckel's diverticulum. Ulcerations (exaggerated in size) are generally single and found at junction of heterotopic gastric mucosa and ileal mucosa within the diverticulum, usually at its neck—in other cases in the ileum near its junction with the diverticulum. This location is generally related to extension of heterotopic gastric mucosa to the base of the diverticulum. Note blood supply entering and "tethering" the diverticulum. **D,** diverticulum at operation 1 day following the diagnostic scan. As in the diagram, it has a somewhat different form compared with the more nearly typical Meckel's diverticulum in Figure 88–1,*E.* Heterotopic tissue could be suspected from external inspection of the diverticulum. It had a whitish appearance, was easily palpable (shown bounded by *small arrows*). As in the diagram, the blood supply *(large arrow)* enters the diverticulum along a broad expanse from its course in the mesentery, proceeds almost to the tip of the diverticulum, and "tethers" or curves back toward its junction with the ileum. As in most cases the blood supply was discrete and could be precisely secured for division and ligation. **(Continued.)**

Intestinal Obstruction

Meckel's diverticulum can cause intestinal obstruction in a number of ways (Fig 87–3); the principal mechanisms are: intussusception (Fig 87–3,*A*) or herniation, kinking, or volvulus in relation to a persistent remnant of the vitelline duct (Fig 87–3,*B* and *C*). In three series totaling 182 cases,[8, 17, 20] intussusception was the cause of intestinal obstruction in 47% of cases and herniation, bands, kinking, and volvulus in 53%. Except for Meckel's diverticulum incarcerated in an inguinal hernia (Meckel's hernia, Littre's hernia)[2] (Fig 87–3,*G*), the clinical presentation is that of intestinal obstruction of uncertain etiology. The Meckel's diverticulum is seldom diagnosed preoperatively.

Intussusception

When Meckel's diverticulum inverts into the ileum, it initially acts as a lead point of an ileoileal intussusception (Fig 87–3,*A1* and *A2*). Rapid progression of the intussusception to the ileoileal-ileocolic variety can lead to early vomiting, a palpable abdominal mass, and vascular compromise. Barium enema can be used to confirm intussusception as the mechanism of intestinal obstruc-

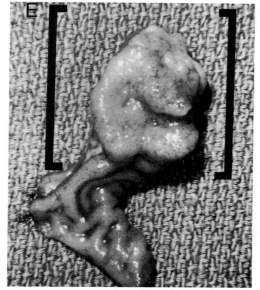

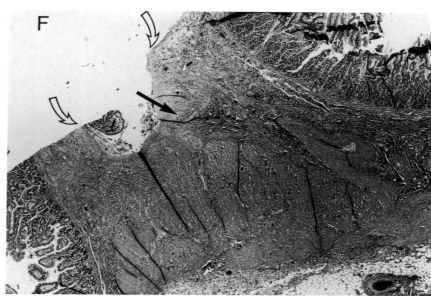

Fig 87–2 Cont.—E, opened specimen clearly shows the rugated appearance of heterotopic gastric mucosa *(brackets)*. Normal ileal mucosa is seen below. *Ink lines* indicate original relationship of ileal mucosa to linear ileum. Fundic glands, presumed capable of producing hydrochloric acid, are found in almost all serially sectioned diverticula containing gastric mucosa.[20] A tiny peptic ulcer (not visible) was seen on close inspection beneath an overhanging gastric mucosal fold. **F,** photomicrograph of the specimen (×16, hematoxylin and eosin stain), showing the peptic ulceration. Boundaries of crater are indicated by *curved arrows.* The ulcer occurred at junction of gastric mucosa (upper right) and ileal mucosa (lower left). The presumed source of hemorrhage was the small muscular artery *(straight arrow)* with partial necrosis of its wall adjacent to the ulcer crater. (Courtesy of Dr. Eugene C. Beatty and Ms. Carolyn Finley, Children's Mercy Hospital, Kansas City, Mo.)

tion when the ileoileal component has entered the colon, and to attempt its hydrostatic reduction. Failure to produce reflux of contrast into the terminal ileum or persistence of symptoms after apparent reduction indicates exploration to rule out ileoileal intussusception. If this complex lesion can be reduced, the diverticulum can be resected as in diverticulectomy for hemorrhage. Occasionally, reduction may be so traumatic as to damage the intestine and make resection and enteroenterostomy the safest procedure. When the intussusception is irreducible, the diverticulum is in the intussusception and will be part of the resected specimen (see Chap. 88).

Intestinal Obstruction Related to Persistent Remnants of the Vitelline Duct

Persistent remnants of the vitelline duct may extend as fibrous cords to the abdominal wall (behind the umbilicus) from a Meckel's diverticulum (see Figs 87–1,*B* and *C*; 87–3,*B*); from the base of the mesentery where the vitelline vessels have persisted as a cord (Fig 87–1,*F*); or from a segment of intestine, the diverticulum having completely involuted (see Figs 87–1,*G* and 87–3,*C*). The mechanisms of intestinal obstruction are (1) kinking or herniation of a loop of intestine in relation to one of the above types of fibrous cords (see Figs 87–1,*B,C,F,G* and 87–3,*B*) or (2) an intestinal volvulus based on a vitelline remnant that serves as a fixed point around which the volvulus occurs (see Fig 87–3,*C*). Other less common mechanisms of obstruction are shown in Figure 87–3,*D-G.*

Management of Intestinal Obstruction Related to Persistent Vitelline Duct Remnants

The preoperative management is that of any patient with intestinal obstruction—nasogastric suction, intravenous fluids, and parenteral antibiotics whenever there is suspected strangulation. Operative intervention within an hour or two is indicated in patients who are easily stabilized. In profoundly sick children, op-

eration is undertaken after resuscitation or when no further improvement is anticipated—in any case within four or five hours. A transverse incision above the umbilicus is recommended for adequate exposure. The mechanism of obstruction is identified and relieved (see Fig 87–3). This generally involves division of a causative band and unkinking of the intestine with excision of the Meckel's diverticulum (see Fig 87–3,*B*); derotation of a nonstrangulated volvulus (see Fig 87–3,*C*); resection of a twisted diverticulum[8] (see Fig 87–3,*D*); resection of a long Meckel's diverticulum and a "knotted" loop of intestine[25] (see Fig 87–3,*E*); dividing a mesodiverticular band[14] (see Fig 87–3,*F*); and reducing and repairing a Meckel's or Littre's hernia through an inguinal approach with concomitant or later diverticulectomy[2] (see Fig 87–3,*G*). Resection is obviously indicated for intestinal infarction, whatever the mechanism. Giant Meckel's diverticulum is an unusual cause of intestinal obstruction that presents as an abdominal mass in the newborn and requires prompt resection.[24]

Meckel's Diverticulitis

Meckel's diverticulum may be the site of inflammation producing a clinical picture indistinguishable from acute appendicitis. Early in the course, pain is periumbilical. Physical findings may be anywhere in the lower abdomen due to the motility of the ileum. A diagnosis of acute appendicitis is almost always made, and, when a normal appendix is found at laparotomy, a Meckel's diverticulum is searched for by examining the distal ileum for up to 3–4 ft.

Analysis of three series, consisting of 126 cases,[1, 17, 21] indicates that approximately one third (36%) of cases of Meckel's diverticulitis are complicated by perforation. As in acute appendicitis, the prognosis in Meckel's diverticulitis depends on whether or not perforation has occurred, although the mechanism may be different. In some cases, it is presumed that the ectopic gastric mucosa produces peptic ulceration of the adjacent ileal mucosa in the diverticulum, followed by bacterial invasion, necrosis, and perforation.[1, 20] An abscess can be formed or spreading peritoni-

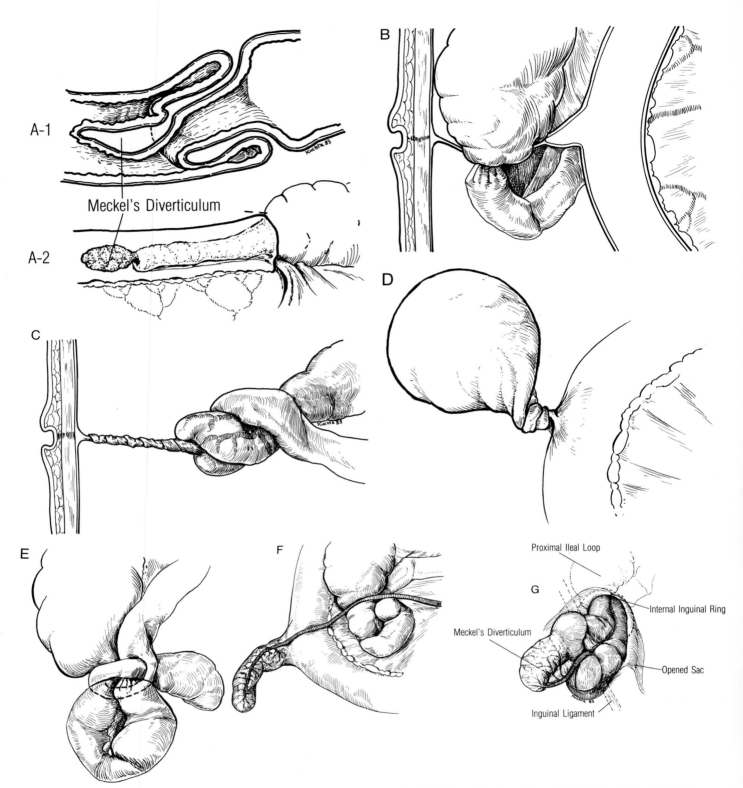

Fig 87–3.—Meckel's diverticulum and possible mechanisms of intestinal obstruction. Intussusception **(A)** and obstruction related to cord-like remnants of the vitelline duct **(B** and **C)** are the most common mechanisms. Remaining mechanisms **(D** to **G)** are seldom encountered. **A-1,** intussusception. Meckel's diverticulum inverted into the ileum as a lead point in an ileoileal intussusception. The diverticulum itself may not be turned inside out. **A-2,** diverticulum has intussuscepted further and can progress into the ascending colon as an ileoileal-ileocolic intussusception. **B,** kinking of a loop of small bowel on a cord-like vitelline duct remnant between Meckel's diverticulum and the umbilicus. **C,** volvulus caused by torsion of loops of small intestine around the fixed point of a fibrous cord remnant of the vitelline duct. **D,** twisting of Meckel's diverticulum at its base, causing diverticular obstruction with possible infarction. **E,** "knotting" or "lassoing" of linear ileum by a long Meckel's diverticulum that has formed a knot by looping around itself. It can obstruct both the ileum and itself. **F,** mesodiverticular band containing the vitelline vessels passes across the ileum to the diverticulum. It is separated from the mesentery and forms a band under which a loop of small intestine has herniated and become obstructed. **G,** Littre's hernia consists of a loop of ileum with a Meckel's diverticulum in an inguinal hernia sac. Shown here is an indirect hernia containing intestine and diverticulum. The hernia sac has been opened before reduction and inguinal herniorrhapy. The proximal limb of intestine is dilated due to obstruction by the constricting internal inguinal ring, while the distal limb has emptied beyond the obstruction.

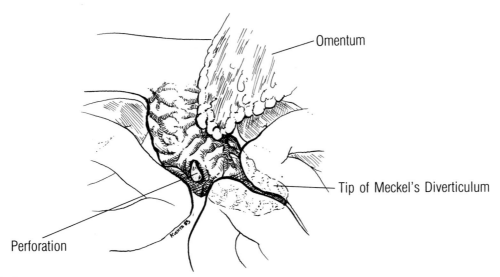

Fig 87–4.—Meckel's diverticulum and inflammation. As in appendicitis, perforation can occur as a consequence of Meckel's diverticulitis. Spreading peritonitis is more likely to occur than in appendicitis because the diverticulum lies free in the peritoneal cavity. Some anatomical limitations in the "walling off" process are shown here, with a perforated Meckel's diverticulum only partly surrounded by loops of adjacent small intestine and a short, filmy omentum.

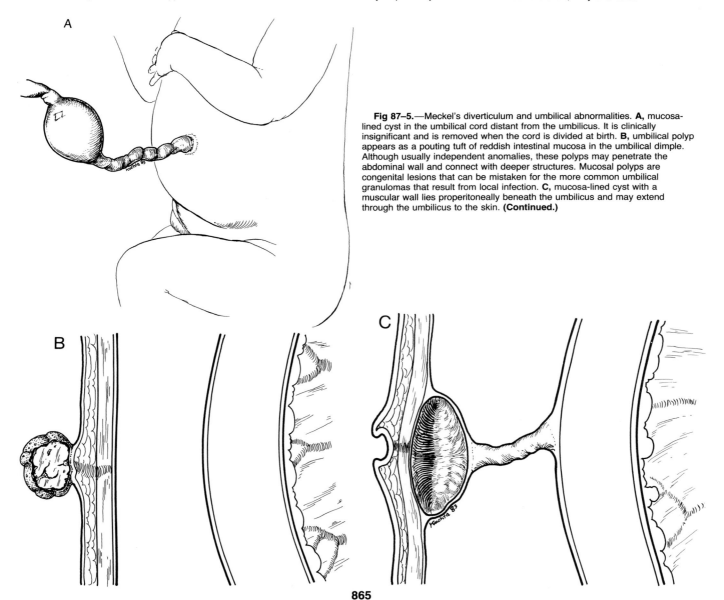

Fig 87–5.—Meckel's diverticulum and umbilical abnormalities. **A,** mucosa-lined cyst in the umbilical cord distant from the umbilicus. It is clinically insignificant and is removed when the cord is divided at birth. **B,** umbilical polyp appears as a pouting tuft of reddish intestinal mucosa in the umbilical dimple. Although usually independent anomalies, these polyps may penetrate the abdominal wall and connect with deeper structures. Mucosal polyps are congenital lesions that can be mistaken for the more common umbilical granulomas that result from local infection. **C,** mucosa-lined cyst with a muscular wall lies properitoneally beneath the umbilicus and may extend through the umbilicus to the skin. **(Continued.)**

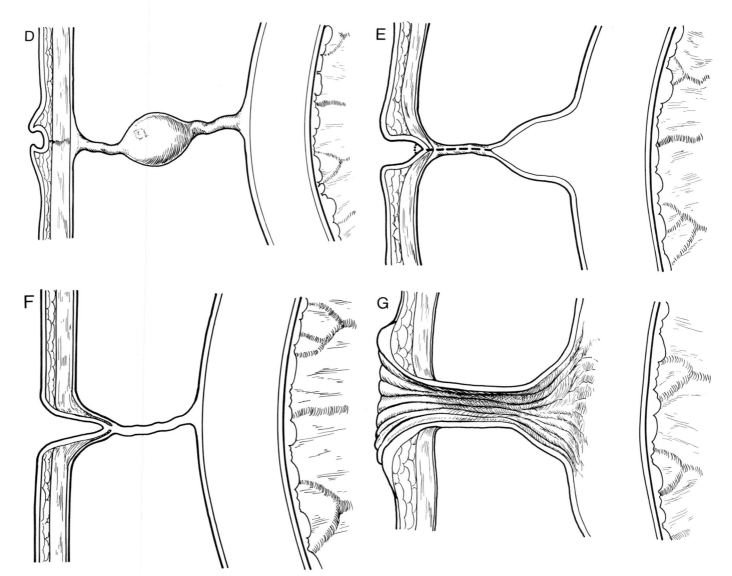

Fig 87–5 Cont.—D, mucosa-lined cyst with smooth muscle wall may persist in the midportion of an otherwise obliterated vitelline duct. **E,** umbilical sinus represents an external vestige of the vitelline duct. It can be a source of infection with purulent drainage. The sinus shown here can be connected to Meckel's diverticulum by an obliterated internal portion of the vitelline duct or by a patent continuation of the duct from the floor of the sinus *(dotted lines).* **F,** another anatomical variant of umbilical sinus. The floor of the sinus is connected directly to the ileum by an obliterated cordlike remnant of the vitelline duct without an intervening Meckel's diverticulum. As in Figures 87–1,*C* and 87–3,*B* and *C,* this may cause intestinal obstruction as well as infection and drainage from the umbilical sinus. **G,** omphaloileal (umbilical-intestinal) fistula resulting from persistent patency of vitelline duct with the fetal intestine. Note the intestinal folds extending from the ileal lumen to the skin. In some cases, this lining contains gastric mucosa. Treatment requires circumscribing the umbilical opening and tracing the duct to the ileum, where it is amputated and the ileum closed. A separate subumbilical incision may be required, or used primarily to approach this anomaly.

tis can occur rapidly, since the diverticulum lies free in the peritoneal cavity (Fig 87–4). This lack of localization is especially dangerous in the infant and requires prompt resection with primary anastomosis. Exteriorization should be considered for critically ill patients.[4]

Umbilical Abnormalities

Approximately 2–10% of patients with Meckel's diverticulum present with abnormalities related to the umbilicus.[1, 8, 10, 17, 20] There may be an external, mucosa-lined cyst of the umbilical cord[1] (Fig 87–5,*A*). The umbilicus may be covered by a polypoid tuft of recognizable intestinal mucosa. These umbilical mucosal remnants are usually independent anomalies with no connection to deeper structures such as Meckel's diverticulum or ileum (Fig 87–5,*B*). They are sometimes mistaken for umbilical granulomas. A mucosal "polyp" should be suspected if it persists after one or two applications of silver nitrate, and the "granulations" may in fact be ileal mucosa. Mucosal "polyps" require excision. Other surgical lesions are vitelline duct cysts that may be in the abdominal wall beneath the umbilicus (Fig 87–5,*C*) or within the abdomen (Fig 87–5,*D*). They should be excised when encountered.

Discharge at the umbilicus is another obvious manifestation and requires elucidation by probe and/or injection of radiopaque contrast material. An umbilical sinus may be isolated, connected with a Meckel's diverticulum (Fig 87–5,*E*), or may communicate directly with the ileum without an intervening diverticulum (Fig 87–5,*F*). If a tract is present, it should be examined for mucosa and its extent delineated by injecting radiopaque contrast into a catheter positioned in the sinus lumen. Radiographs may show the tract extending only a few millimeters or several centimeters. In some cases, a communication with the small bowel will be demonstrated and a diagnosis of omphaloileal fistula made.

In patients with an obvious omphaloileal fistula, the vitelline duct has remained patent (Fig 87–5,*G*), and the external appearance may vary from a rosette of mucosa resembling an ileostomy to a striking degree of ileal prolapse, which may result in intestinal obstruction and compromise of the blood supply. If discharged contents are clearly ileal, further work-up is unnecessary. If there is any question regarding the termination of an umbilical fistula, a catheter can be passed and contrast injected to delineate the tract and any communication with the intestine, urinary bladder (via a patent urachus), or both. Dissection is facilitated by a catheter in the fistula.

Surgical management of these umbilical sinus or fistula anomalies (Fig 87–5,*E-G*) consists of an intraumbilical incision that circumscribes the sinus opening and traces any underlying tract to its full extent, with excision of any deeper anomalous structures. A subumbilical incision can also be used and the umbilical end of the tract transected or circumscribed, detached, and removed in continuity with any persistent abnormal structures. Any connections to the intestine should be dismantled carefully.

Meckel's Diverticulum and Neoplasms

Neoplasms are seldom encountered in Meckel's diverticulum. The benign tumors (e.g., lipoma, myoma, fibroma, neurofibroma, angioma) may cause intussusception. Carcinoids, sarcomas, and carcinomas have been seen, the adenocarcinomas probably arising from heterotopic gastric mucosa.[20]

Management of Meckel's Diverticulum Found Incidentally

The management of Meckel's diverticulum found incidentally during an abdominal procedure is somewhat controversial. The concept of excision in virtually all cases[1, 20] has been tempered by a realization that there is only a small chance of a truly asymptomatic diverticulum causing disease during life.[21] Diverticulectomy is indicated when Meckel's diverticulum is found with persistent vitelline duct remnants that predispose to intestinal obstruction. Diverticula containing palpable heterotopic tissue or tumors should also be excised. Diverticulectomy is also warranted, even if an apparently normal diverticulum is found at laparotomy, for abdominal pain of unknown etiology. Excision of a Meckel's diverticulum found during operative closure of gastroschisis is contraindicated, as the suture line will almost always disrupt.

REFERENCES

1. Benson C.D.: Surgical implications of Meckel's diverticulum, in Ravitch M.M., Welch K.J., Benson C.D., et al. (eds.): *Pediatric Surgery*, ed. 3. Chicago, Year Book Medical Publishers, 1979, pp. 955–960.
2. Baillie R.C.: Incarceration of a Meckel's inguinal hernia in an infant. *Br. J. Surg.* 46:459–461, 1959.
3. Berquist T.H., Nolan N.G., Stephens D.H., et al.: Specificity of 99m Tc-pertechnetate in scintigraphic diagnosis of Meckel's diverticulum: Review of 100 cases. *J. Nucl. Med.* 17:465–469, 1976.
4. Canty T., Meguid M.M., Eraklis A.J.: Perforation of Meckel's diverticulum in infancy. *J. Pediatr. Surg.* 10:189–193, 1975.
5. DeBartolo H.M. Jr., van Heerden J.A.: Meckel's diverticulum. *Ann. Surg.* 183:30–33, 1976.
6. Faris J.C., Whitley J.E.: Angiographic demonstration of Meckel's diverticulum. *Radiology* 108:285–286, 1973.
7. Gray S.W., Skandalakis J.E.: *Embryology For Surgeons*. Philadelphia, W.B. Saunders Co., 1972, pp. 156–167.
8. Gross R.E.: *The Surgery of Infancy and Childhood*. Philadelphia, W.B. Saunders Co., 1953, pp. 212–220.
9. Jewett T.C. Jr., Duszynski D.O., Allen J.E.: The visualization of Meckel's diverticulum with 99m Tc-pertechnetate. *Surgery* 68:567–570, 1970.
10. McParland F.A., Kiesewetter W.B.: Meckel's diverticulum in childhood. *Surg. Gynecol. Obstet.* 106:11–14, 1958.
11. Meckel J.F.: Ueber die Divertikel am Darmkanal. *Arch. Physiol.* 9:421–453, 1809.
12. Moses W.R.: Meckel's diverticulum. *N. Engl. J. Med.* 237:118–122, 1947.
13. Petrokubi R.J., Baum S., Rohrer G.V.: Cimetidine administration resulting in improved pertechnetate imaging of Meckel's diverticulum. *Clin. Nucl. Med.* 3:385–388, 1978.
14. Raffensperger J.G. Meckel's diverticulum, in *Swenson's Pediatric Surgery*, ed. 4. New York, Appleton-Century-Crofts, 1980, pp. 452-455.
15. Rosenthall L., Henry J.N., Murphy D.A., et al.: Radiopertechnetate imaging of the Meckel's diverticulum. *Radiology* 105:371–373, 1972.
16. Ruysch F.: *Opera Omnia*. Amsterdam, Jansson-Waesberg, 1757.
17. Seagram C.G.F., Louch R.E., Stephens C.A., et al.: Meckel's diverticulum: A 10-year review of 218 cases. *Can. J. Surg.* 11:369–373, 1968.
18. Shigemoto H., Fujita W., Nishimoto T., et al.: Scintigraphic detection of intestinal bleeding in infants and children, in Raynaud C. (ed.): *Nuclear Medicine and Biology Advances*. New York, Pergamon Press, 1983, pp. 979–982.
19. Sibley W.L.: Meckel's diverticulum: Dyspepsia Meckeli from heterotopic gastric mucosa. *Arch. Surg.* 49:156–166, 1944.
20. Söderlund S.: Meckel's diverticulum, a clinical and histologic study. *Acta Chir. Scand.* (suppl.), 248:13–233, 1959.
21. Soltero M.J., Bill A.H.: The natural history of Meckel's diverticulum and its relation to incidental removal. *Am. J. Surg.* 132:168–173, 1976.
22. Thompson J.E.: Perforated peptic ulcer in Meckel's diverticulum. *Ann. Surg.* 105:44–55, 1937.
23. Treves S., Grand R.J., Eraklis A.J.: Pentagastrin stimulation of technetium-99m uptake by ectopic gastric mucosa in Meckel's diverticulum. *Radiology* 128:711–712, 1978.
24. Tunell W.P.: Meckel's diverticulum, in Holder T.M., Ashcraft K.W. (eds.): *Pediatric Surgery*. Philadelphia, W.B. Saunders Co., 1980, pp. 457–464.
25. Walsh A.: Knot in Meckel's diverticulum causing acute intestinal obstruction. *Br. J. Surg.* 37:475–476, 1950.

88 Mark M. Ravitch

Intussusception

HISTORY.—Intussusception has been differentiated from other forms of intestinal obstruction for less than 300 years. In the mid-seventeenth century, Paul Barbette[4] of Amsterdam clearly described intestinal invagination and suggested operative reduction. John Hunter[54] described intussusception accurately and discussed a postmortem specimen. Reduction from below by means of enemas, injection of air or gas, or manipulation with a wand were all attempted.[98] In the mid-nineteenth century, the disease was almost universally fatal but occasionally responded to inflation of the bowel with a bellows or to enemas.[75] The first successful operation for intussusception in an infant was performed by Jonathan Hutchinson[55] in 1871. Hirschsprung[48] of Copenhagen in 1876 published the first of a series of reports dealing with the systematic reduction of intussusception by hydrostatic pressure. His results were superior to those achieved by primary operative treatment for the next 70 years. In 1913, Ladd[67] published the first reproduction of a radiograph of a contrast enema in intussusception. He considered that the diagnosis might be so made in obscure cases, but that it would not be a therapeutically useful maneuver. Hipsley,[47] of Australia, achieved great success with hydrostatic (saline) pressure reduction. In 1927, in the United States, Retan[103] and Stephens[115] independently described the use of contrast enema reduction of intussusception; and Pouliquen[92] in France and Olsson and Pallin[81] in Scandinavia reported their experiences with the method. Our experience with barium enema began in 1939, and our first paper on the barium enema reduction of intussusception appeared in 1948.[101] Unreported experience with barium enema reduction must have antedated these reports. McArthur, in Chicago, in 1920, in discussion at a meeting, described its use.[99]

The first successful resection of an intussusception in a child was by Clubbe,[11] of Australia, in 1897. In 1831, in Tennessee, J.R. Wilson reduced an intussusception in a Negro slave by operation,[122] but the first successful resection of an intussusception in a child in this country was reported by Peterson[89] in 1908.

Intussusception, the invagination of a portion of the intestine into itself, is one of the classic subjects of pediatric surgery. The characteristic case of intussusception occurs in a well-nourished male child of 8 months awakened from sleep with what appears to be violent abdominal pain. The child cries out in sudden pain and vomits. Soon thereafter he passes a normal stool. Almost at once he seems well, playful, and may eat until stricken by another bout of colicky pain. With each bout he turns pale, may sweat, and becomes markedly apathetic, a sign long recognized and now rediscovered.[9, 112, 124] Thereafter he vomits repeatedly, has obvious bouts of recurrent peristaltic pain, and begins to pass bloody mucus per rectum. Presently, persistent apathy, pallor, and evidences of dehydration appear. The intestinal obstruction, which has in fact existed from the onset, does not become clinically manifest for many hours. The condition is likely to be fatal in 2–4 or 5 days if not interrupted. The invagination begins at or near the ileocecal valve, and examination of the bowel shows no obvious local anatomical cause for intussusception.

This is the classic picture, and it is so typical that the diagnosis may frequently be made over the telephone. The variations of the picture, however, are of interest and are of great importance in facilitating the diagnosis of the less typical cases, which are the only ones in which a fatal issue is at all likely today.[96]

Incidence

Intussusception is seen with striking variation in frequency in several parts of the world. At the Harriet Lane Home of the Johns Hopkins Hospital, with a very large outpatient department

and a special interest in intussusception, we saw no more than six to eight instances a year, and it appears that other clinics in the country do not see appreciably more. Denver Children's Hospital[82] saw about five cases per year; Los Angeles Children's Hospital[114] 14 per year; Charity Hospital in New Orleans[58] five per year; Boston Children's Hospital[42] almost 20 per year; Children's Hospital in Cincinnati[70] six per year; Babies Hospital in New York[108] about eight per year; Children's Memorial Hospital in Chicago[31] ten per year, and St. Louis Children's Hospital[123] about seven per year. In contrast with this American experience, the Hospital for Sick Children, Toronto,[25] reports 354 cases in ten years. In that very large hospital, this may not mean a higher incidence rate. Royal Children's Hospital, Melbourne, in 1970 reported 203 cases in seven years,[2] and in 1975–1978, 120 cases,[77] still 30 cases per year. Strang,[117] from the Royal Hospital for Sick Children in Glasgow, reported an experience of 400 cases from 1946 to 1957, the number per year varying from 25 to 59. In 1970, from the same hospital, Dennison and Shaker[18] reported 288 cases seen from 1959 to 1968. They stated that there had been a sharp decrease in the frequency with which cases were seen, the first report from their hospital being from one of the two surgical services and the second from both. Also from Scotland, Pollet and Hems report a one-third decrease in incidence of intussusception in Aberdeen and two surrounding counties in 1967–1976 compared with 1950–1959, particularly in rural areas.[91] Hellmer,[46] from the University of Lund in Sweden, reported 54 cases per year, and Nordentoft,[78] in Copenhagen, collected 63 cases per year. In Nigeria,[12, 28, 57] intussusception is a common disease in children over 5 years and tends to be subacute or chronic. The same is true in Taiwan and in mainland China.

Studies of absolute incidence of intussusception in this country are not available; but, in Birmingham, England, MacMahon[72] reported an incidence of 1.9 per 1,000 live births, and Newcastle-on-Tyne[13] has over 4 per 1,000 births. Smith[113] from Edinburgh reported a figure of 1.57 per 1,000 live births, like that in Birmingham. In all three cities, the incidence of pyloric stenosis is uniform. The differences in the incidence of intussusception, although not understood, are of an order to be significant. There has been some thought that the incidence of intussusception has fallen in this country, but this is not apparent from the experience in the hospitals of the editors of these volumes.

SEX INCIDENCE.—All series report a strong male preponderance, usually in the order of 3:2. The male preponderance is more striking in the latter months of infancy.

RACIAL INCIDENCE.—Intussusception may be more common in white children than in black children, but the difference in hospitals in this country, seeing large numbers of children of both races, is at most not great.

AGE INCIDENCE.—Intussusception occurs largely in the first year of life and most commonly from the fifth to the ninth month. Sixty to 65% of the children are less than 1 year of age (Fig 88–1).

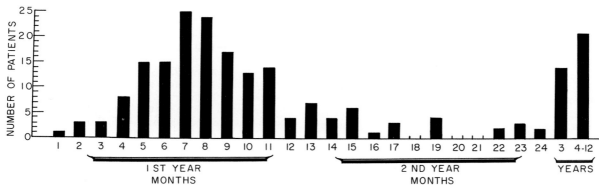

Fig 88–1.—Intussusception: age of incidence in 205 cases at The Johns Hopkins Hospital, 1893–1960. The peak of incidence is from the fifth through the ninth month (45% of all cases), 62% occurring from the fourth through the 12th month. More than 80% of the children were under 2 years of age.

Intussusception in the fetus, with gangrene and absorption of the intussuscepted portion, has been found to be a cause of intestinal atresia.[52, 85] Intussusception at times occurs in the newborn,[40, 86, 94, 118, 126] and about 0.3% of cases occur in the first month of life. The newborn infants who have had intussusception have been, for the most part, mature, full-term infants in good vigor, and the symptoms of their intussusceptions were in no wise unusual.

SEASONAL INCIDENCE.—No general agreement prevails regarding a seasonal variation in the incidence of intussusception. In our experience,[102] there seemed to be two peaks of incidence, one in spring and summer, possibly the season of enteritis, and another in midwinter, during the time of maximal incidence of respiratory infections (Fig 88–2). Strang[117] found a suggestion of similar peaks in his Glasgow experience. There is so much variation in the reported series that this probably has no significance. Mulcahy,[77] from the Royal Alexandria Hospital in Sydney, makes the point that their seasonal variation in incidence of intussusception is not great and shows no correspondence to the seasonal incidence of gastroenteritis.

Nutrition and Previous Health

Intussusception tends to occur in sturdy, well-nourished infants, and it is relatively uncommon to see it in malnourished children. In our experience, perhaps one child in 10 had diarrhea before the onset of what was obviously intussusception, and

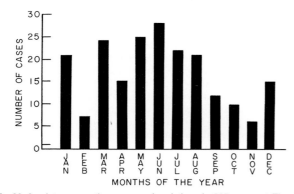

Fig 88–2.—Intussusception: seasonal variations in 205 cases at The Johns Hopkins Hospital, 1893–1960. There is an apparent peak in midsummer and another in midwinter, conceivably reflecting periods of maximal incidence of enteritis and respiratory infections. On the whole, it is difficult to sustain the case for sharp seasonal variation on the basis of these or other figures.[77]

an occasional child had received cathartics for constipation just before the onset of symptoms, or had been severely constipated. A good many of the children had upper respiratory infection at the time of the intussusception. Dennison[17] in particular found a much more constant correlation with upper respiratory infection than with seasonal diarrhea.

It is frequently stated that the high incidence of intussusception in some European countries is associated with the fact that children there are frequently breast fed and that the subsequent change from breast milk to cow's milk plays a part in the occurrence of intussusception. This theory has never been subjected to epidemiologic analysis.

Previous Attacks; Spontaneous Reduction

About 7% of our patients had had an entirely similar attack at intervals of ten days to six months before the attack of intussusception that brought them to the hospital. Our experience suggests that, in children with such histories, operation and the search for polyps or other causative lesions will be more fruitful than in other children. Others have reported an incidence of 5% or 6% for spontaneous and complete reduction of intussusception between the time of diagnosis and the time of laparotomy in patients undergoing primary operation.[19, 38]

The fact that repeated attacks of intussusception may occur before the attack that is brought under treatment suggests the possibility that further attacks may ensue at some period after the operative or hydrostatic-pressure reduction of the intussusception. In fact, recurrence rates of 4–6% have been recorded without regard to the method of treatment.[19]

SPONTANEOUS SLOUGHING OF THE INTUSSUSCEPTUM.—The spontaneous reductions cited above are instances of restitution to the normal state. From the earliest days of our knowledge of intussusception, it has also been known that in some instances the intussusception becomes gangrenous and sloughs, the bowel fusing at the neck of the intussusception, preserving its continuity, while the sphacelated intussusceptum is passed by rectum, with recovery. This requires the rapid production of gangrene and slough before the patient succumbs to intestinal obstruction, and requires adherence of the proximal and distal bowel at the neck of the intussusception. Recovery after such an accident may be permanent, but progressive cicatricial constriction may ultimately produce intestinal obstruction. Such instances, which are today rare and evidences of neglect, at an earlier date represented almost the only hope for survival. The bowel sloughs required 11–21 days to develop and occurred chiefly in older children.[59, 69, 102, 104]

Signs and Symptoms

The many analyses from various countries show close correspondence in the clinical picture the world over.

The chief complaint in 44% of our cases was vomiting and, in almost the same number, passage of blood per rectum.[102] The patients being largely infants, in only about one of four did the mothers consider abdominal pain to be the chief complaint.

The symptoms of onset tend to differ somewhat from the symptoms that predominate when the infants are seen. In almost half the babies, abdominal pain is the first symptom to attract attention; in only about a third is vomiting the initial sign. Blood per rectum as the first sign was seen in little more than 10%. For obvious reasons, pain is increasingly the first symptom in the older age groups, whereas blood in the stool is the first recognized sign almost solely in infants in the first 2 years of life, when the less dramatic symptoms may not command the mother's attention.

PAIN.—The characteristic pain is colicky, intermittent, and, obviously, extremely severe. Colicky pain at some point in the course of the disease is almost invariably recognized in children older than 2 years, and somewhat less commonly in smaller infants.

VOMITING.—Almost all infants vomit in the course of the illness and more than 80% of older children. In infants, vomiting tends to begin earlier. The early vomiting is reflex. The vomiting of intestinal obstruction is a late sign and should never be seen in a properly handled case of intussusception.

BLEEDING.—Blood in the rectal discharge is seen in 95% of the infants and 65% of the older children. A bloody rectal discharge may appear within the first 2 or 3 hours of the onset or may not appear for a day. In most cases, the blood is prominently mixed with mucus, producing characteristic currant-jelly stools. At times, the production of mucus is very great and only traces of blood are seen; in other instances, there is copious passage of a thin, mahogany-colored fluid or what appears to be clotted blood. In many patients, the first evidence of blood is seen when the examining finger is withdrawn from the rectum. The amount of blood lost externally, while rarely great, when added to the fluid lost in the bowel wall and lumen and by vomiting, contributes to collapse.

DEFECATION.—In most cases of intussusception, once the baby has evacuated the bowel content that was distal to the intussusceptum, feces and flatus are not passed and intestinal obstruction is complete. In an occasional instance of chronic nonobstructing intussusception, stools continue to be passed. What is apt to be more confusing is the occurrence of diarrhea after the onset of intussusception, seen in almost 7% of our patients. This creates the danger of a misdiagnosis of dysentery and resultant catastrophic delay. Prolapse of the intussusception through the anus occurred in about 3% of children in the Johns Hopkins series.

Examination of the Patient

The children characteristically lie quietly on the examining table, are frequently apathetic and often quite strikingly prostrated, to the point of being cold, sweaty, and unresponsive. In almost half our patients, prostration has been evident, and in the days when patients died of intussusception, severe prostration was a grave prognostic sign. From time to time, the children become restless and fretful, or scream out, drawing up their legs with obvious pain; and at such times the abdomen, usually flat and flaccid, remains so, but the violent peristaltic effort may

make the mass of the intussusceptum more readily felt. We have been able to feel a mass in some 85% of our patients, either abdominally or rectally, and others report a palpable mass in as many as 95%. In most cases, if a rectal mass is palpable, the intussusceptum is so long that an abdominal mass can be felt as well. In an occasional case, a mass is felt only per rectum, and at times only by bimanual examination. Palpation of the mass is likely to be pathognomonic in children in whom the question of intussusception has been raised. Early, the abdomen is flat or actually scaphoid, although very rarely the intussusception presents a visible protuberance. The abdomen typically is soft and not tender. The intussusception itself may be tender when palpated, and there may be a little muscular resistance over it. Early in the progress of a characteristic intussusception, the mass passes into the hepatic flexure behind the right costal margin and under the right lobe of the liver, and at such times it may be difficult or impossible to feel. As time passes, the picture is confused by the superimposition of nonspecific signs of intestinal obstruction—distention and intestinal patterns that may obscure the mass. The typical mass is sausage-shaped or cylindric. The pull of the mesentery on the intussuscepted bowel, between the layers of which it has been drawn, constrains the tumor to arch in a curve, imparting the characteristic sausage shape.

Fever is common, and is highest and commonest in younger children. Again, in the days when death from intussusception occurred, high fever was of grave prognostic significance. The pulse does not rise with intussusception except during the episodes of colic, or later when severe dehydration or the shock attendant upon gangrene of the bowel produces general deterioration. Leukocytosis is common but of no diagnostic or prognostic significance.

A barium enema is undertaken for diagnosis if *any* suspicion is raised about the possibility of the diagnosis, and in all such cases, the patient is formally posted for immediate operation. In adults[20, 51, 84, 125] and in children,[65] positive diagnosis of intussusception has been made by sonography and even by computed tomography. How sensitive and how accurate sonography may be, and hence its utility as a screening method, remains to be seen. Barium enema is 100% accurate in the diagnosis of intussusception, and diagnosis merges into treatment.

Pathogenesis of the Disease and of its Symptomatology

The reasons for the occurrence of intussusception in infants are uncertain. It has been suggested that there is a greater disproportion between the size of the ileum and the ileocecal valve in infants than in older children. Use of the terms "ileocolic," "ileocecolic" and other compound designations is not helpful and tends to obscure the fact that the great majority of intussusceptions—95% or more—begin at or near the ileocecal valve. A few intussusceptions occur well up in the small bowel and produce even more violent symptoms. An occasional intussusception begins in the colon and is likely to have less striking manifestations.[8, 16, 56] In a few intussusceptions (2%–8% of all), the leading point of the intussusception is a recognizable lesion of the bowel wall such as a polyp, Meckel's diverticulum, a nodule of ectopic pancreas, a very small enterogenous cyst or an enormously hypertrophied lymphoid patch. We[101] have observed in experimental intussusception in dogs that, once the intussusception has developed, the intense local edema produces substantial enlargement of the adjacent lymph nodes. Caution must therefore be exercised in the deduction that, since large lymph nodes are found adjacent to an intussusception, enlargement of lymphoid tissue must have played a part in the production of the intussusception. Nevertheless, at times a clearly demarcated, almost intraluminal mass of lymphoid tissue has been seen, and the richness of the lymphoid tissue of the bowel in infants is one of the clear differences between them and older patients and one of the more likely of the possible pathogenic factors.[15, 109] The association of enlargement of the lymph nodes with respiratory infections is accepted, and some 21% of our patients had either otitis media or an upper respiratory infection or both at the time of admission. Dennison[17] was particularly impressed with a similar association in his series in Glasgow. In Strang's[117] analysis of 400 cases from the same clinic, the mesenteric nodes, commented on in 318 cases, were grossly enlarged in 35%, moderately enlarged in 16%, and mildly enlarged in 27%.

A good deal of interest has centered on the culture of stools and intestinal lymph nodes for viruses, and several groups have reported much higher recovery of adenoviruses from children with intussusception and with mesenteric adenitis than from controls who were simultaneously in the hospital.[7, 35, 107]

The human reovirus-like agent (HRVL, reovirus, rotavirus infantile gastroenteritis virus) is a cause of gastroenteritis in children.[23, 60] Konno et al., in a study of 30 infants with clinical enteritis and intussusception, found rotavirus in the stools of 11 by electron microscopy and significant titer of antibodies in the blood of five of seven children studied.[63, 64]

Thomas and Zachary,[119] reporting on identical twins, both of whom had intussusception within 24 hours, corrected our previous statement that siblings are at no increased risk. They pointed out that both twins had adenovirus in appendix and lymph node, large lymph nodes, and Peyer's patches. Reports from Tel-Aviv,[111] Tenerife,[39] and Adelaide[120] record sibling cases and father-and-son cases. We have treated two brothers within 24 hours, operating on the second who had hypertrophied Peyer's patches of almost tumor-like proportions.

In 205 cases of intussusception, of which 63 were not operated on, we encountered two small enteric cysts, six Meckel's diverticula, five polyps, one ectopic focus of pancreatic tissue, and two instances of unusually large and discrete patches of ileal lymphoid tissue. The total is thus 16 of 205 cases, or 7.8%. Eleven of the 16 patients were over 1 year of age. In Strang's 400 cases, all operated on, there were only eight (2%) obvious lesions. Two of these patients had Henoch-Schönlein purpura, a circumstance reported by others.[6, 29, 87] The abdominal pain of this illness may, more often than is recognized, represent transient intussusception. This probably represents one of a series of conditions in which localized edema or hemorrhage appears to incite intussusception. Thus, intussusception has been seen also in hemophiliacs,[33] in children with abdominal trauma, in leukemics, with and without chemotherapy.[3, 22, 71, 121]

The suggestion, then, is that specific causative lesions requiring resection are uncommon, and particularly uncommon in the infants who have the major proportion of intussusceptions. Lymphosarcoma is the occasional cause of a type of chronic nonstrangulating intussusception in older children.[41, 62] The vermiform appendix may participate in or initiate an intussusception in one of a number of ways,[66] but ordinarily it is merely drawn into the space between the intussusceptum and the intussuscipiens and there compressed. Children with cystic fibrosis are at special risk. Shwachman's[50] series, from Children's Hospital, Boston, had, by 1971, accounted for 22 intussusceptions in 19 patients with cystic fibrosis. All were over 4 years of age and averaged 9¾ years.

Intussusception after abdominal operative manipulations, especially renal, is a familiar event in the animal laboratory.[98] It has become apparent that intussusception in the postoperative period in infants and children occurs more often than would be expected by chance.[10, 19, 74, 76, 110, 116] It has occurred after resection of coarctation of the aorta, reduction of strangulated umbil-

ical hernia, resection of Wilms tumor, biopsy of neuroblastoma, operations for Hirschsprung's disease, imperforate anus, and right hepatectomy. It is obvious that many of the instances do not involve operations on the small bowel itself, and some do not even involve manipulation of the bowel to any significant degree. The diagnosis is arrived at slowly. The initial diagnosis is usually ileus due to adhesions, and symptoms are present for several days before operation is undertaken. Because of the recent abdominal incision and frequent distention, the mass of the intussusception is almost never felt. Furthermore, the intussusception is almost entirely in the small bowel, and such intussusception masses are often not palpable. Barium enema has rarely been helpful in making the diagnosis, since the intussusception is above the ileocecal valve. Awareness of the occurrence of intussusception in the postoperative period in children operated on for any lesion, realization that intestinal obstruction from adhesions ordinarily comes on later than the two to four days after operation in which intussusception is likely to appear, and unwillingness to rely on gastrointestinal suction for the treatment of mechanical intestinal obstruction are required if one is to treat these children with the same promptness with which one treats the usual intussusception. The treatment is operative reduction. Although recurrence after operative reduction of the usual ileocecal intussusception is not rare (and some postoperative intussusceptions have occurred high in the small bowel in patients who have had recent laparotomy for the classic intussusception at the ileocecal junction), a second postoperative intussusception after reduction of the first has not been reported, even though the postoperative intussusception itself is at times multiple.

Occasionally, a long indwelling tube causes intussusceptions in the small bowel, with a confusing picture of cramps and intermittent intestinal obstruction. We have seen one child with two such episodes, each relieved by operation, at one of which multiple intussusceptions were found.

It is important to realize that, from the first moment of invagination, the mesentery of the invaginated bowel is compressed between the layers of the intussusceptum. Figure 88–3 shows the sharp U-shaped turn taken by the bowel at the two ends of the intussusceptum, so that the outer layer of the intussusceptum is trapped between these two bends and its blood supply acutely angulated at these points as well as compressed in the entire segment that lies between these points. The result is almost immediate venous compression, venous stasis, and edema. The process rapidly leads to swelling of the tissues and still more venous obstruction. Histologically, it is reflected by enormous distention of the vessels of the bowel and by a filling of the mucosal cells of the intussuscepted bowel with mucus, so that the mucosa seems to be composed almost entirely of goblet cells. The goblet cells discharge mucus into the bowel, where it mixes with the blood that seeps from the engorged intestine to form characteristic currant-jelly stools. As venous obstruction and edema increase while arterial inflow continues, the tissues become engorged to the point at which the tissue pressure finally exceeds the arterial pressure, circulation ceases, and gangrene ensues. We have demonstrated[100] experimentally that, when necrosis begins in intussusception, it begins at the distal end of the outer or returning layer of the intussusceptum and then extends proximally. The innermost layer of the intussusceptum becomes gangrenous much later. The outermost layer, the intussuscipiens, rarely, if ever, suffers.

In animals, when viable intussusceptions are reduced operatively under sterile conditions and cultures are taken from the apparently intact serosal surface, pathogenic bacteria are frequently recovered.[98] This *durchwanderung* was postulated in 1897 by D'Arcy Power[93] and is the undoubted explanation for

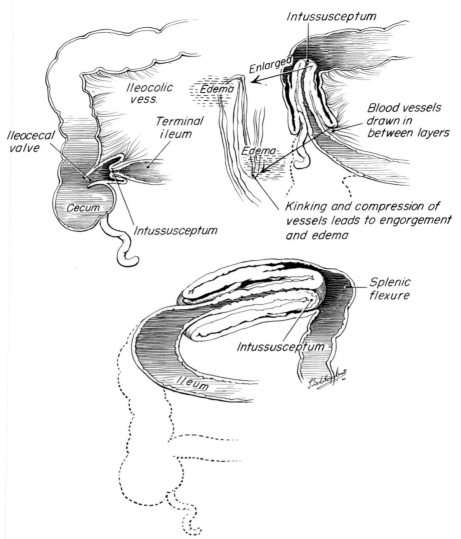

Fig 88–3.—The development of an intussusception. The great majority of intussusceptions in infants and children are of the kind shown here. The intussusception begins at or near the ileocecal valve without obvious local anatomical lesion to cause it. From the first moment, there is simultaneous interference with patency of the alimentary canal and with the vascular supply of the intussusceptum. The drawings indicate the manner in which the mesenteric vessels are drawn between the layers of the intussusception and compressed. The slight interference with lymphatic and venous drainage, which occurs almost at once, results in edema and an increase of tissue pressure. This further increases resistance to the return of venous blood. Venules and capillaries become enormously engorged, and bloody edema fluid drips into the lumen. The mucosal cells swell into goblet cells and discharge mucus, which, mixing in the lumen with the bloody transudate, forms the currant-jelly stool. Edema increases until venous inflow is completely obstructed. As arterial blood continues to pump in, tissue pressure rises until it is higher than arterial pressure, and gangrene ensues. The drawings indicate the sharp U-shaped turns of the bowel and mesenteric vessels at either end of the intussusceptum. The outer coat of the intussusceptum (middle layer of the intussusception) is isolated between the two sharp bends and understandably is the first to become gangrenous. Gangrene appears in this coat near the tip of the intussusception and progresses back toward the neck of the intussusceptum. Rarely, the intussuscipiens is damaged. (From Ravitch.[98])

the frequent wound infections in the preantibiotic era and for the common occurrence of high fever after the reduction of intussusception.

Treatment

Operative

The standard treatment of intussusception in the British Isles, in the United States, and in most of Europe was formerly immediate operative reduction. Stress was laid on the necessity for spectacular haste in moving such patients to the operating room. It is now generally accepted that the immediate need of a child with intussusception is for intravenous fluids or blood; for gastric aspiration, as in any type of intestinal obstruction; and for the administration of antibiotics, as in any other situation where the vascular supply of the bowel may be jeopardized.

These things having been attended to, if primary operative therapy is to be employed, the abdomen is entered through a low midline incision to allow access to the intussusception throughout its reduction around the colon. The intussusception is milked back by progressive compression of the bowel just distal to the intussusception, driving it proximally (Fig 88–4). If the bowel reduces easily and rapidly, there is no need to deliver the intussusception or to question the viability of the bowel. If the bowel stubbornly resists reduction, it is preferable to resect it at once rather than to use excessive force and risk rupturing the bowel and contaminating the wound and peritoneal cavity. Min-

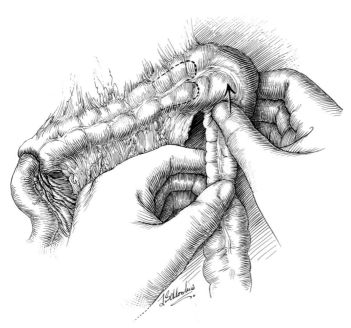

Fig 88–4.—Intussusception: manual reduction. If barium enema fails or intussusception is met with during laparotomy for intestinal obstruction, manual reduction is required. The bowel is occluded immediately distal to the intussusception with the fingers of one hand and stripped proximally with the fingers of the other. In effect, this increases intraluminal pressure just as enema does. The bowel should not be pulled upon. Saline solution or mineral oil injected between the coats may help. If reduction is not readily achieved, resection and anastomosis should be performed.

eral oil may be gently injected between the coats of the intussusception to aid in the reduction, but attempts to stretch the neck of the intussusception with instruments result in disaster, and incision of the neck of the intussusception invites contamination of the operative field. In any case, it is seldom that an intussusception so difficult to reduce as to require these strenuous methods will prove not to require resection because of gangrene or doubtful viability. The reduced bowel is frequently beefy red or blue-black in color, and yet, after several minutes of observation, it will be seen to have a good tone and to be capable of peristalsis. As in any other form of mechanical intestinal obstruction, bowel of questionable viability is safest resected.

A variety of methods have been proposed for dealing with gangrenous or nonreducible intussusception. The unsatisfactory experiences of an earlier day with primary resection and anastomosis in these sick infants with edematous, obstructed bowel led a number of clinics to adopt staged operations of various kinds. Gross[42] described his "aseptic" Mikulicz procedure. As is true in a number of other fields of pediatric surgery, the more exacting demands of conditions in tiny patients at first retarded the adoption of bold primary procedures to replace the older, complicated staged procedures.

The current experience with direct resection and primary anastomosis yields recovery rates as high as with the less attractive staged procedures, and this more straightforward and definitive procedure is now the one most frequently advocated and performed.

Nonoperative

The hydrostatic-pressure reduction of intussusception, which had been in fairly common but sporadic and unsystematic use for years, was systematized by Hirschsprung[48] of Copenhagen. He

reported his first experience with this treatment in 1876. By 1905,[49] he was able to report on 107 personal cases of intussusception with results so superior to any previously reported that his contemporaries seem to have doubted his conclusions. In self-defense, he published a concise account of each of his 107 cases, with a 35% mortality, in contrast to the usual 80% mortality from operation. It was not until the period 1925–1930 that reports of mortality rates lower than his began to appear from clinics primarily employing operation. Hirschsprung's successors in Copenhagen attempted to add manual disinvagination of the intussusception through the intact abdominal wall but abandoned the method because of increased morbidity. Hipsley, of Sydney, Australia, dissatisfied with a mortality of 8% for the operative treatment of intussusception (remarkable enough for the time), began the regular treatment of intussusception by hydrostatic pressure with normal saline solution, and in 1926 reported on 100 patients so treated, with a mortality of 5%, which, for the time, was spectacularly low.[47] The introduction of the barium enema in controlled hydrostatic pressure in 1927[92, 103] led to the popular use of this method in Scandinavia and South America.

Our experience with hydrostatic pressure began at The Johns Hopkins Hospital in 1939 and was limited to barium enema reduction.[100] From 1939 to 1946, barium enema became increasingly the method of choice for the treatment of intussusception at that hospital and, since 1946, has been universally the method of choice. The demonstration[100] that during the period 1939–1947 there were 21 primary operative reductions with five deaths, a mortality of 24%, and 27 primary enema reductions with no deaths had a good deal to do with influencing the practice of the surgical service. The Johns Hopkins series consisted of 101 cases of intussusception in infants and children treated primarily by barium enema from 1939 to January 1, 1966. There were two deaths in the series (see Fig 88–9).

To achieve success with barium enema reduction, the principles outlined in Table 88–1 must be rigorously observed. Numerous reports testify to the general shift toward barium enema reduction—Ireland,[14] United States,[53] France,[21] Scotland,[91] Nigeria,[80] Scandinavia,[26, 46, 73, 78, 79] Russia,[61] Japan,[44] and many others. Reports from some areas[95] suggest patients are seen so late that barium enema reduction should not be tried, and others[27, 90] have such low success rates as to be unenthusiastic. In most of the Western world, the question today is principally whether to start with barium enema reduction in all cases, or only in those who show "no intestinal obstruction."[36, 106] Nevertheless, there are those, notably in France,[1, 88] who refuse to accept the massive evidence for the advantages of hydrostatic-pressure reduction.

TECHNIQUE OF BARIUM ENEMA REDUCTION.—Once the diagnosis of intussusception is entertained, the operating room is no-

TABLE 88–1.—PRINCIPLES OF BARIUM ENEMA REDUCTION

1. Call operating room and schedule operation.
2. Perform nasogastric suction; administer IV fluids or blood, and antibiotics.
3. Insert ungreased Foley catheter in rectum, distend balloon, and pull down against levators. Strap in place.
4. Wrap legs.
5. Let barium run from height of 3 ft 6 in. above table.
6. Fluoroscope intermittently.
7. Abandon if barium column is stationary, and its outline unchanging, for 10 minutes.
8. Reduction is marked by
   a) *free flow of barium well into small bowel.*
   b) expulsion of feces and flatus with the barium.
   c) disappearance of mass.
   d) response of child.

tified and the patient formally posted for operation. In most cases, the intussusception will have been reduced before the operating room has had time to send for the patient. Intravenous fluid administration is begun at once. In more severely shocked children, blood is matched and transfusion begun in the fluoroscopy room. As with any type of intestinal obstruction, the stomach is emptied and a nasogastric tube left in place. The advent of fluoroscopic screen intensification with observation of the video image in a lighted room eliminated the risk of unobserved vomiting and aspiration in the dark fluoroscopic room. An ungreased 45-ml Foley bag catheter is inserted into the rectum, the balloon inflated fully, pulled down against the levators, and the buttocks strapped tightly together with adhesive. It is remark-

able to see how large a balloon a tiny infant can expel if it struggles.[37] Wrapping the baby is helpful.[37] The catheter is connected to an ample reservoir of barium 3 feet to 3 feet 6 inches above the table. We do not employ anesthesia or sedation. The barium is permitted to run into the rectum uninterruptedly, although the flow may be momentarily halted while spot films are exposed. The barium usually will be seen to run rapidly into the rectum and colon until the head of the barium column meets the intussusception. At this point, the rounded head of the advancing barium column suddenly becomes concave, forming a meniscus around the head of the intussusception, much as a column of barium in the vagina would outline the cervix (Figs 88–5 to 88–7). For purposes of documentation, a film is generally exposed

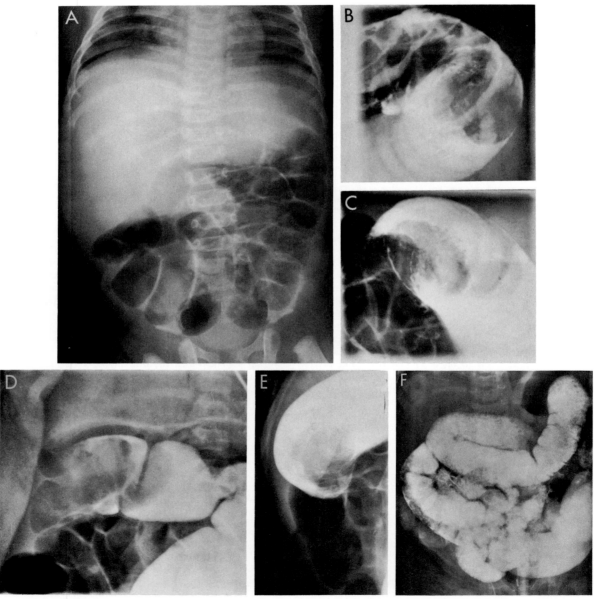

Fig 88–5.—Intussusception: barium enema reduction. A 3-month-old infant with symptoms for 24 hours was moderately prostrated and received intravenous fluids during the reduction, which required 15 minutes. The child was discharged from hospital on the third day. **A,** plain film shows numerous distended loops and a nonspecific picture of intestinal obstruction. **B,** the intussusceptum is met just distal to the splenic flexure; the sharply concave filling defect is plainly seen. A little barium has seeped around the intussusceptum. **C,** the intussusceptum is being displaced proximally. **D,** the intussusceptum is now in midtransverse colon. Here the intussuscipiens grips it less closely and more barium seeps between the two, producing a long U-shaped defect in the barium. **E,** the filling defect shows in the hepatic flexure. **F,** the intussusception rapidly gives way, and the filling of numerous loops of small bowel gives evidence of complete reduction.

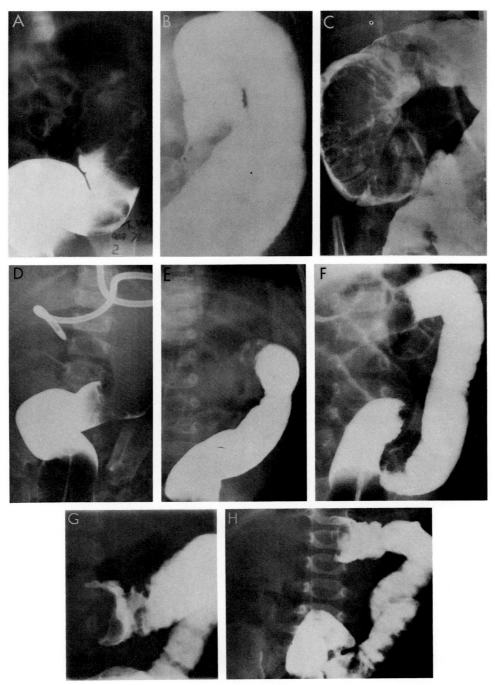

Fig 88–6.—Intussusception: barium enema reduction. Appearance of intussusception *when first observed* in eight infants. In most cases, the intussusception reduced substantially between the time of recognition and the time the first film was exposed. In **D,** for instance, the intussusception protruded from the anus and had to be replaced manually to allow introduction of the catheter. In all eight infants, the intussusception was completely reduced by barium enema. **A,** intussusception first met in the rectum. **B,** intussusception in the left transverse colon.

C, intussusception in midtransverse colon. The intussusception fits loosely in the right colon, and barium between the coats of the intussusception gives a semblance of the coiled-spring sign. **D,** intussusception originally prolapsed through anus. Note gastric tube for emptying stomach. **E,** intussusception at splenic flexure. **F,** intussusception in left transverse colon. **G** and **H,** intussusceptions in midtransverse colon.

to show the intussusception when first encountered, and at least one more, after evacuation, to show complete reduction. As the hydrostatic pressure of the column of barium is maintained, the meniscus lengthens, the horns extending proximally along the intussusceptum until suddenly the intussusceptum is displaced

and the meniscus flattens out again. This process is repeated, sometimes with extreme rapidity, until the intussusceptum is reduced to the cecum and through the ileocecal valve. In the transverse and ascending colon, the intussusceptum frequently fits loosely enough in the larger-caliber intussuscipiens, so that

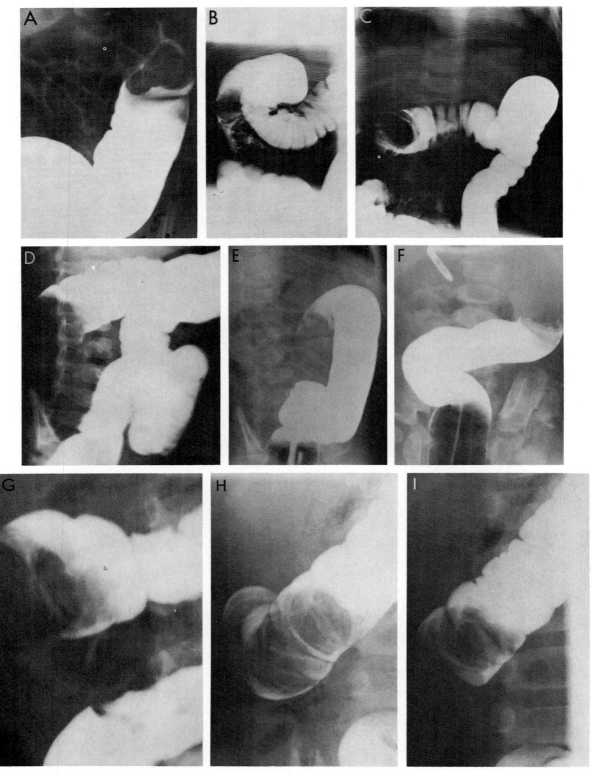

Fig 88–7.—Intussusception: barium enema reduction. Appearance at various stages of reduction in a number of patients. **B** and **C** are of the same patient, and **H** and **I** of another patient. The others are all of individual patients.

barium seeps between the intussusceptum and the intussuscipiens, producing the coiled-spring appearance, even in acute intussusceptions. One should take care to see that the barium flows freely into the ileum. If the ileum does not fill freely (Fig 88–8), one should operate at once, even though the intussusception has apparently been reduced through the ileocecal valve and the cecum fills without any defect. Little harm is done by a McBurney incision, which discloses that the intussusception had been, in fact, completely reduced; real harm may result if the reduction is incorrectly assumed to be complete. At times, when the intussusception rests entirely within the small bowel, it can be demonstrated by barium refluxing through the ileocecal valve up to the intussusceptum. This is not dependable, and in any case, at this level one makes no attempt to reduce an intussusception by barium enema. Intussusceptions entirely limited to the small bowel usually present the picture of intestinal obstruc-

tion. In such patients, if the barium enema shows no intussusception in the colon, operation for the intestinal obstruction should be undertaken at once.

There is great variation in the speed with which reduction can be achieved. In one newborn with an intussusception of the transverse colon, fluorographic motion pictures were taken of the entire reduction. The continuous film strip covers a period of less than 5 seconds. At other times, reduction may be extremely stubborn. Not rarely, there is a momentary pause when the intussusception is encountered, then steady reduction to the splenic flexure. Delay at the splenic flexure may be followed by rapid reduction to the hepatic flexure, when there may again be some delay. Filling of the cecum is often slow, and the cecum may distend quite markedly before a sudden rush of barium into the small bowel denotes complete reduction. In 1977, Fisher and Germann, of Kansas City,[30] described their success with gluca-

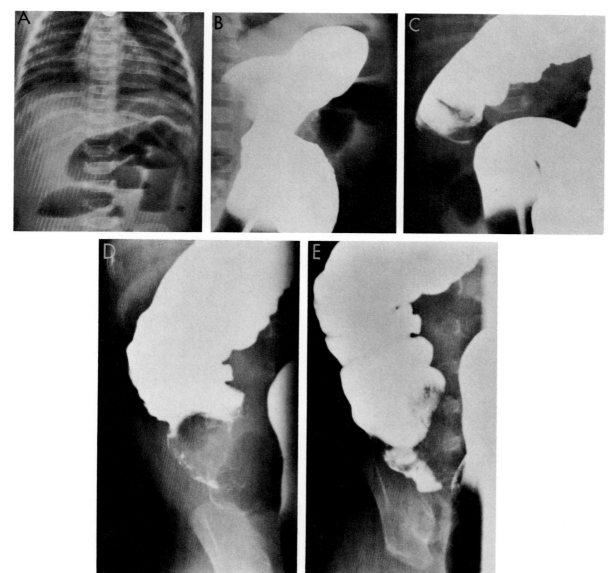

Fig 88–8.—Intussusception: incomplete reduction. A 6-month-old infant had vomited for 36 hours. A mass was felt on rectal examination and the intussusception was readily reduced to the cecum. At operation, undertaken at once, a small residual intussusception in the terminal ileum was readily reduced. A cigar-shaped area of lymphoid hyperplasia was found. **A,** plain film shows dilated loops and fluid levels. **B,** the intussusception reduced so rapidly from the rectum that the first film taken shows it in the left transverse colon. **C,** the intussusception is now at the hepatic flexure. **D,** the cecum fills incompletely. **E,** the cecum is almost completely filled and some barium is in the ileum. No further progress was made, and after 10 minutes the reduction was completed by operation.

gon in completing a stalled barium enema reduction in two infants. Eleven months later, Boles[53] published an optimistic report of experience with glucagon, successfully reducing 84% of 25 intussusceptions. Haase and Boles[43] put this to experimental test in puppies and thought reduction was easier, but no more certain, when glucagon was used. Lanocita and Castiglioni[68] thought that, with the use of glucagon, they had converted an apparent failure to a successful reduction. A cooperative double-blind study of 31 children with intussusception in five university centers "failed to show any therapeutic value of glucagon in hydrostatic reduction of intussusception."[32]

We have no hesitation in continuing the reduction for as long as 45 minutes or an hour, *so long as steady progress is being made.* The children are receiving intravenous fluids or blood as needed during the procedure, and the roentgen exposure is only fractional and intermittent. Once it is obvious that there has been an absolute arrest of the barium column for 10 minutes or so, nothing is to be gained by persisting, and operation should be undertaken. Presently, we rely, in general, on one continuous sustained injection. The intussusception, if not completely reduced, is almost invariably reduced to the cecum, although in a few instances it has returned no farther than the ascending colon. It is of the utmost importance to be certain that there is free filling with barium of many loops of small bowel.

The distended cecum and the sigmoid may overlap and, between them, fill the field, obscuring the ileum. In no circumstance do we manipulate the abdomen, however great the temptation. In no circumstance do we raise the cannister of barium higher than 3 feet 6 inches above the table. Neglect of these precautions invites rupture of the bowel or reduction of gangrenous bowel. If the colon becomes so distended with barium that it is difficult or impossible to be certain that the loops of small bowel have filled, the catheter is removed, the child allowed to evacuate and then fluoroscoped once more. The loops of small bowel filled with barium are usually seen framed by the colon. Immediately after completion of the reduction, powdered charcoal is deposited in the patient's stomach through the tube already in place. Six hours later, an enema is administered to recover the charcoal and prove beyond doubt the relief of the obstruction. This method, introduced by Hipsley, assures one that the obstruction has been relieved but does not necessarily demonstrate that the intussusception has been totally reduced.

The successful reduction of an intussusception by barium enema is indicated by the following:

1. The free flow of barium well into the the small bowel. This is the sine qua non of complete reduction and must be insisted upon in all patients who are not to have an immediate operation. The remaining criteria are merely confirmatory.

2. Return of feces or flatus with the barium.

3. Disappearance of the mass. At times, a mass may persist, even in the face of adequate and clear radiologic evidence of complete reduction of the intussusception. The mass, in such cases, is the swollen edematous bowel previously involved in the intussusception.

4. Clinical improvement of the patient, who may fall into a natural sleep.

5. Subsequent recovery in the stool of the charcoal given by stomach tube.

RESULTS.—Of 101 intussusceptions treated primarily by barium enema, 65 were reduced by the barium enema alone, an incidence of 65% (Fig 88–9). Of 36 patients who were operated on, reduction had been achieved by barium enema in eight, so that the operation was merely confirmatory. The barium enema therefore completely reduced the intussusception in 73 of the 101 cases. There were three recurrences in the 101 cases, an

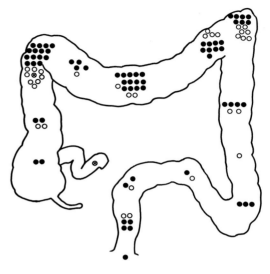

INTUSSUSCEPTION   1939–1966

Reduced by

◉ Barium Enema Alone 65/101

◎ Barium Enema and Operation 36/101
Operative Confirmation 8/101
Operative Reduction 28/101

(⊗ Deaths 2/101)

Fig 88–9.—Intussusception: results of treatment of 101 patients at The Johns Hopkins Hospital, 1939–1966. Sixty-five were reduced by barium enema alone; eight were found at operation to have been reduced by the barium enema; 28 were reduced at operation and in almost every one, the barium had reduced the intussusception to the cecum or right colon. The two deaths were not related to the barium enema (see text): one was of a child with intussusception above the cecum, operated on at once, and the other, of a child in hospital with pulmonary complications of mucoviscidosis from which he died.

incidence no higher than that reported for primary operative reduction of intussusception. There were two deaths in the series. The first was of a 10-month-old infant shown by barium enema to have, well up in the small bowel, an intussusception that had never reached the colon (Fig 88–10). Immediate operation disclosed a gangrenous intussusception. The baby died 2 weeks later of a Pseudomonas wound infection, peritonitis, and septicemia. The second death was in an older boy admitted to the hospital for pulmonary complications of cystic fibrosis of the pancreas. Intussusception developed, was promptly recognized, and was reduced by barium enema. The next day his abdomen was flat, but there was blood in his stools and a mass was felt in the right lower quadrant. Operation was undertaken without barium enema and, as might have been anticipated, all that was found was the edematous bowel, which is not rare 24 hours after reduction. The boy died of the respiratory disease during this hospitalization. The bowel had remained viable and functioning.

DISCUSSION.—In my opinion, the barium enema can and should be administered to every child with intussusception, regardless of the duration of the disease or the child's condition. Present and previous clinical experience supported by experimental studies, together with the great mass of reported material, convince me that, if manual pressure is avoided and if the barium cannister is no higher than 3 feet 6 inches above the operating table, gangrenous bowel will not be reduced and perforation of the intestine will not occur. We have seen infants brought in in such a degree of collapse that it seems almost certain that the bowel must be gangrenous, who have yet had in-

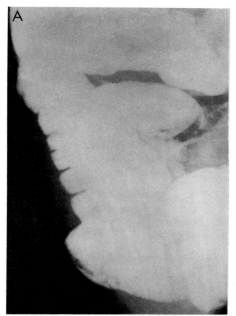
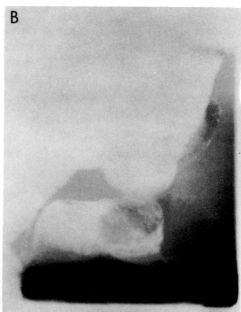

Fig 88–10.—Ileoileal intussusception not reduced by barium enema. The filling defect in this 10-month-old infant was first encountered in the small bowel. Enema reduction is not attempted in such patients. At immediate operation, a gangrenous irreducible intussusception was found 20 cm proximal to the ileoce- cal valve. Resection and anastomosis were performed. The child ultimately died of septicemia and generalized moniliasis, the first death (March 20, 1959) in The Johns Hopkins series since 1946.

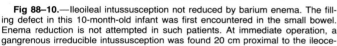

tussusceptions reduced while blood was being administered and have not required operation. It is scarcely possible to make an absolute diagnosis of gangrene of an intussusception without operation. No time is lost by use of the barium enema, since the operating room is being readied and the child is having gastric aspiration, supportive intravenous fluid therapy or transfusion, and antibiotics at the same time. Furthermore, even if the intussusception should prove to be incompletely reduced by the barium enema, the more of the intussusception that is reduced by the enema, the less remains to be done in the operating room. The problem of reducing an intussusception found at operation to be in the right colon or the cecum is quite another from that of reducing an intussusception in the rectum or the sigmoid. Reports from Colorado,[83] New Orleans,[59] St. Louis,[123] and California[45] all list a number of patients with mechanical intestinal obstruction due to adhesive bands, occurring from 2 months to 3½ years after operation for intussusception. We[102] reported 12 such cases, three of them fatal, developing weeks, months, or years after operative reduction in the early series at Johns Hopkins Hospital. With barium enema, some 65%–75% of patients are spared the need for anesthesia and incision. It is also of interest that the incidence of resection is much lower in patients treated primarily by barium enema. Presumably, this indicates that a number of the resections that are otherwise performed are made necessary by operative trauma to the bowel during the reduction or represent resections of bowel mistakenly thought to be nonviable.

When the Johns Hopkins series was begun, the difference in the reported mortalities from the clinics treating intussusception primarily by hydrostatic pressure and those from clinics resorting primarily to operation was striking, and entirely in favor of the former. Today, there is essentially no mortality from intussusception treated in the best pediatric surgical clinics, except in children already irretrievably moribund at admission, or in those with complicating disease. A comparative study of current mortality statistics is therefore of little value. The advantage of hy- drostatic pressure today lies in the avoidance of an anesthetic and laparotomy in over 70% of patients.

Objections commonly raised to the barium enema treatment[127] are these:

1. The original diagnosis may be uncertain.

2. It is difficult to be sure of reduction.

3. Will not the recurrence rate be higher?

4. Polyps and other tumors cause many intussusceptions and will not be found.

5. In unsuccessful cases, a dangerous delay will have been caused.

6. The bowel may rupture.

7. Nonviable bowel may be reduced.

These objections may be answered as follows:

1. Diagnosis by fluoroscopy is simple and accurate and, as a matter of fact, offers a distinct advantage. Not only have many intussusceptions been reduced inadvertently by radiologists in the course of examinations intended to be diagnostic, but, human nature being what it is, pediatricians are much more likely to make a tentative diagnosis of intussusception before they are absolutely certain of it, if to do this commits them and their little patients merely to an enema rather than to an operation. The result is substantially earlier definitive treatment.

2. Accuracy of diagnosis of complete reduction is high. We have made an erroneous diagnosis twice, the last time over 35 years ago. Since we made it an iron-clad policy to operate in every case in which there is not free filling of many loops of small bowel, we have had no fear of mistaken diagnosis of complete reduction. On the contrary, we have had eight instances in which operation disclosed the fact that reduction by the enema actually had been complete.

3. Rate of recurrence is no higher than that in series of patients treated primarily by operation.

4. The actual incidence of specific causative lesions in the Johns Hopkins series was 6.5%, in others even lower; these were practically all in children over 2 years of age.[97] The tumors that

cause intussusception are rarely dangerous of themselves. Polyps may be cause intussusceptions or anemia from bleeding but are not dangerous if not discovered at once. Meckel's diverticula occur in at least 1% of the population anyway. Large lymphoid patches usually cause no other trouble, and such rare lesions as the occasional small enteric cyst and focus of ectopic pancreatic tissue are of little consequence except as they cause intussusception. Lymphosarcomas that cause chronic intussusception with persistent filling defects are not likely to be missed.

5. Usually, less than half an hour is required from start to finish to reduce an intussusception by enema. It is our practice to call the operating room as soon as the diagnosis is entertained, and we have usually finished the reduction in time to cancel the procedure before preparations in the operating room have been completed. This time, in any case, is employed for lavage of the stomach, administration of blood or intravenous fluids, and antibiotics.

6. The bowel can rupture with hydrostatic pressure, of course, as well as with manual reduction during operation, but rupture is much less likely to occur with the enema, since less force is employed and that force is diffusely distributed. We have never ruptured the bowel with barium enema.

However, the Toronto-Ottawa collective report[24] lists seven bowel perforations in 25 years, six of these since 1974. All the infants had been sick, five of the intussusceptions were of at least 72 hours' duration, and all had obvious intestinal obstruction. Their high success rate (85%) raises the question of excessive zeal in attempted reduction.

7. As for reducing nonviable bowel, it appears from our experimental work and the clinical evidence that, with barium at a height of 3 feet 6 inches, one does not reduce gangrenous bowel. Irreducibility of an intussusception is determined by adhesions between the sheaths and by the degree of edema. Both factors increase with time and become more effective in preventing reduction as the damage to bowel increases. By the time constriction is so severe as to have produced gangrene, the moderate hydrostatic pressure employed will not reduce the bowel. It is important to note that the stress of this pressure is borne by the outer sheath, the intussuscipiens, which usually remains viable to the end.

It is to be re-emphasized that the method is not a substitute for operation nor an escape from operation. It is as much a surgical procedure as is the reduction of a fracture by traction. The surgeon should be as ready to perform a laparotomy if it proves necessary as the orthopedist is to perform an open reduction. *The treatment should be carried out by a surgeon and in a hospital.* It is not an office procedure or a kitchen-table remedy nor a radiological procedure undertaken in the absence of the surgeon. A survey of the literature indicates an increasing interest in the United States[5, 34, 45, 59, 83, 105, 108] and in some clinics in England[127] and Ireland[14] in hydrostatic pressure reduction with the barium enema, with essential confirmation of the results of earlier investigators.

REFERENCES

1. Aubrespy P., Derlon S., Alessandrini P., et al.: Invagination intestinale aiguë du nourrisson et de l'enfant. *Chir. Pediatr.* 24:392, 1983.
2. Auldist A.W.: Intussusception in a children's hospital: A review of 203 cases in seven years. *Aust. N.Z. J. Surg.* 40:136, 1970.
3. Badertscher V.A.: Traumatic triple intussusception of the ileum in a child. *J.A.M.A.* 112:422, 1939.
4. Barbette P.: *Oeuvres chirurgiques et anatomiques.* Geneva, François Miege, 1674, p. 522.
5. Bass L.W., Sieber W.K., Girdany B.R.: The treatment of ileocolic intussusception. *J. Pediatr.* 55:51, 1959.
6. Beck A.R., Leichtling J.J.: Intussusception in Henoch-Schoenlein's purpura. *Mt. Sinai J. Med.* 39:397, 1972.
7. Bell T.M., Steyn J.H.: Viruses in lymph nodes of children with mesenteric adenitis and intussusception. *Br. Med. J.* 2:700, 1962.
8. Bower R.J., Kiesewetter W.B.: Colo-colic intussusception due to a hemangioma. *J. Pediatr. Surg.* 12:777, 1977.
9. Braun P., Germann-Nicod I.: Altered consciousness as a precocious manifestation of intussusception in infants. *Z. Kinderchir.* 33:307, 1981.
10. Brown P.M., Thronfeldt R.: Intussusception in the early postoperative period. *Am. J. Dis. Child.* 107:297, 1964.
11. Clubbe C.P.B.: *The Diagnosis and Treatment of Intussusception,* ed. 2. London, Hodder & Stoughton, 1921.
12. Cole G.J.: Caecocolic intussusception in Ibadan. *Br. J. Surg.* 53:415, 1966.
13. Court D., Knox G.: Incidence of intussusception in Newcastle children. *Br. Med. J.* 2:408, 1959.
14. Courtney D.F., Kelleher J., O'Donnell B.: Intussusception—a change in policy where management has been satisfactory. *Ir. J. Med. Sci.* 150:69, 1981.
15. Danis R.K.: Lymphoid hyperplasia of the ileum—always a benign disease? *Am. J. Dis. Child.* 127:656, 1974.
16. Davies M.R.Q., Cywes S.: Colonic intussusceptions in children. *S. Afr. Med. J.* 54:517, 1978.
17. Dennison W.M.: Acute intussusception in infancy and childhood. *Glasgow Med. J.* 29:71, 1948.
18. Dennison W.M., Shaker M.: Intussusception in infancy and childhood. *Br. J. Surg.* 57:679, 1970.
19. Dodrill F.D., Benson C.D.: Coarctation of the aorta with both subclavian arteries arising from the distal segment complicated by postoperative intussusception. *Surgery* 51:809, 1962.
20. Donovan A.T., Goldman S.M.: Computed tomography of ileocecal intussusception: Mechanism and appearance. *J. Comput. Assist. Tomogr.* 6:630, 1982.
21. Ducharme J.C., Perreault G., Cyr R., et al.: L'invagination intestinale: 188 malades traités au cours d'une periode de 22 ans. *Chir. Pédiatr.* 23:23, 1982.
22. Dudgeon D.L., Hays D.M.: Intussusception complicating the treatment of malignancy in childhood. *Arch. Surg.* 105:52, 1972.
23. Editorial: Virus of infantile gastroenteritis. *Br. Med. J.* 3:555, 1975.
24. Ein S.H., Mercer S., Humphry A., et al.: Colon perforation during attempted barium enema reduction of intussusception. *J. Pediatr. Surg.* 16:313, 1981.
25. Ein S.H., Stephens C.A.: Intussusception: 354 cases in 10 years. *J. Pediatr. Surg.* 6:16, 1971.
26. Eklöf O.A., Johanson L., Löhr G.: Childhood intussusception: Hydrostatic reducibility and incidence of leading points in different age groups. *Pediatr. Radiol.* 10:83, 1980.
27. El-Barbari M., Bashir A.Y., Ibrahim A.H.: Intussusception in infancy and childhood in Egypt. *J. Egypt. Med. Assoc.* 61:23, 1978.
28. Elebute E.A., Adesola A.O.: Intussusception in western Nigeria. *Br. J. Surg.* 51:440, 1964.
29. Emanuel B., Lieberman A.D., Rosen S.: Intussusception due to Henoch-Schönlein purpura. *Ill. Med. J.* 122:162, 1962.
30. Fisher J.K., Germann D.R.: Glucagon-aided reduction of intussusception. *Radiology* 122:197, 1977.
31. Fox P.F.: Intussusception: Surgical treatment. *Surg. Clin. North Am.* 36:1501, 1956.
32. Franken E.A. Jr., Smith W.L., Chernish S.M., et al.: The use of glucagon in hydrostatic reduction of intussusception: A double-blind study of 30 patients. *Radiology* 146:687, 1983.
33. Fripp R.R., Karabus C.D.: Intussusception in haemophilia. *S. Afr. Med. J.* 52:617, 1977.
34. Frye T.R., Howard W.H.R.: The handling of ileocolic intussusception in a pediatric medical center. *Radiology* 97:187, 1970.
35. Gardner P.S., Knox E.G., Court S.D.M., et al.: Virus infection and intussusception in childhood. *Br. Med. J.* 2:697, 1962.
36. Gelov N.: Experience with the treatment of acute intestinal invagination in infancy. *Khirurgiia* 3:513, 1978.
37. Girdany B.R., Bass L.W., Sieber W.K.: Roentgenologic aspects of hydrostatic reduction of ileocolic intussusception. *Am. J. Roentgenol.* 82:455, 1959.
38. Goldman L., Elman R.: Spontaneous reduction of acute intussusception in children. *Am. J. Surg.* 49:259, 1940.
39. Gonzalez Bethencourt J.V., Cruz Diaz M.M.: Invaginación intestinal en gemelas lactantes. *Rev. Esp. Enf. Ap. Digest.* 60:615, 1981.
40. Goodhead B.: Intussusception in the newborn. *Br. J. Surg.* 53:626, 1966.
41. Götz M., Weissenbacher G.: Ileocócales Lymphosarkom unter dem Bild einer chronisch rezidivierenden Invagination. *Monatschr. Kinderh.* 121:72, 1973.
42. Gross R.E., Ware P.F.: Intussusception in childhood: Experiences from 610 cases. *N. Engl. J. Med.* 239:645, 1948.
43. Haase G.M., Boles E.T. Jr.: Glucagon in experimental intussusception. *J. Pediatr. Surg.* 14:664, 1979.
44. Hashimoto S.: A new simplified technique of hydrostatic reduction

of intussusception minimizing x-ray exposure. *Nippon Igaku Hoshawen Gakkai Zasshi* 39:17, 1979.

45. Hays D.M., Gwinn J.L.: The changing face of intussusception. *J.A.M.A.* 195:817, 1966.
46. Hellmer H.: Intussusception in children: Diagnosis and therapy with barium enema. *Acta Radiol.* (suppl. 65), 1948.
47. Hipsley P.L.: Intussusception and its treatment by hydrostatic pressure: Based on an analysis of one hundred consecutive cases so treated. *Med. J. Aust.* 2:201, 1926.
48. Hirschsprung H.: Et Tilfaelde af subakut Tarminvagination. *Hospitals-Tidende* 3:321, 1876.
49. Hirschsprung H.: 107 Fälle von Darminvagination bei Kindern, behandelt im Königin Louisen-Kinderhospital in Kopenhagen während der Jahre 1871–1904. *Mitt. Grenzgeb. Med. Chir.* 14:555, 1905.
50. Holsclaw D.S., Rocmans C., Shwachman H.: Intussusception in patients with cystic fibrosis. *Pediatrics* 48:51, 1971.
51. Holt S., Samuel E.: Multiple concentric ring sign in the ultrasonographic diagnosis of intussusception. *Gastrointest. Radiol.* 3:307, 1978.
52. Hopfgartner L., Wurnig P.: Ein Fall von pränataler Invagination: Ein Beitrag zur Genese der Dunndarmatresien: A Case of Pre-natal Intussusception. *Z. Kinderchir.* 13:328, 1973.
53. Hoy G.R., Dunbar D., Boles E.T. Jr.: The use of glucagon in the diagnosis and management of ileocolic intussusception. *J. Pediatr. Surg.* 12:939, 1977.
54. Hunter J.: On introsusception. *Trans. Soc. Improvement of Medical and Chirurgical Knowledge* 1:103, 1793.
55. Hutchinson J.: A successful case of abdominal section for intussusception. *Proc. R. Med. Chir. Soc.* 7:195, 1873.
56. Ippolito R.J., Touloukian R.J.: Colocolic intussusception in an older child. *Clin. Pediatr.* 17:720, 1978.
57. Joly B.M., Thomas H.O.: Non-infantile idiopathic intussusception in western Nigeria. *W. Afr. Med. J.* March 1954, p. 3.
58. Kahle H.R.: Intussusception in children under two years of age. *Surgery* 29:182, 1951.
59. Kahle H.R., Thompson C.T.: Diagnostic and therapeutic considerations of intussusception. *Surg. Gynecol. Obstet.* 97:693, 1953.
60. Kapikian A.Z., Kim H.W., Wyatt R.G., et al.: Recent advances in the aetiology of viral gastroenteritis. *Ciba Found. Symp.* 42:273, 1976.
61. Khristich A.D., Portnoy V.M.: Treatment of intestinal invagination in children. *Klin. Khir.* 6:9, 1977.
62. Kobayashi A., Akiyama H., Kawai S., et al.: Chronic intussusception associated with ileocecal lymphosarcoma. *Helv. Paediatr. Acta* 30:315, 1975.
63. Konno T., Suzuki H., Kutsuzawa T., et al.: Human rotavirus and intussusception. *N. Engl. J. Med.* 297:945, 1977.
64. Konno T., Suzuki H., Kutsuzawa T., et al.: Human rotavirus infection in infants and young children with intussusception. *J. Med. Virol.* 2:265, 1978.
65. Kozarek J.A., Starshak R.J.: Ultrasonic ring sign. *Wisconsin Med. J.* 79:26, 1980.
66. Krasna I.H., Beardmore H.E.: Appendicocecal intussusception: A case report. *Can. J. Surg.* 12:229, 1969.
67. Ladd W.E.: Progress in the diagnosis and treatment of intussusception. *Boston M. & S. J.* 168:542, 1913.
68. Lanocita M., Castiglioni G.: Impiego del glucagone nella riduzione dell'invaginazione intestinale. *La Radiologi Medica* 66:513, 1980.
69. Leichtenstern O.: Intussusception, Invagination und Darmeinschiebung, in *Ziemssen's Cyclopaedia of the Practice of Medicine*, 1877, vol. 7, p. 610.
70. Ling J.T.: Intussusception in infants and children. *Radiology* 62:505, 1954.
71. Lyon D.C.: Intussusception complicating anticoagulant therapy. *Br. Med. J.* 2:345, 1968.
72. MacMahon B.: Data on the etiology of acute intussusception in childhood. *Am. J. Hum. Genet.* 7:430, 1955.
73. Madsen C.M.: Personal communication, March 9, 1978.
74. McGovern J.B., Gross R.E.: Intussusception as a postoperative complication. *Surgery* 63:507, 1968.
75. Mitchell S.: Intussusception in children. *Lancet* 1:904, 1837-38.
76. Mollitt D.L., Ballantine T.V.N., Grosfeld J.L.: Postoperative intussusception in infancy and childhood: Analysis of 119 cases. *Surgery* 86:402, 1979.
77. Mulcahy D.L., Kamath K.R., de Silva L.M., et al.: A two-part study of the aetiological role of rotavirus in intussusception. *J. Med. Virol.* 9:51, 1982.
78. Nordentoft J.M.: The value of the barium enema in the diagnosis and treatment of intussusception in children, illustrated by about 500 Danish cases. *Acta Radiol.* 24:484, 1943.
79. Nordshus T., Swensen T.: Barium enema in pediatric intussusception. *Fortschr. Rontgenstr.* 131:42, 1979.

80. Odita J.C., Piserchia N.E., Diakporomre M.A.: Childhood intussusception in Benin City, Nigeria. *Trop. Geogr. Med.* 33:317, 1981.
81. Olsson Y., Pallin G.: Über das Bild der akuten Darminvagination bei Röntgenuntersuchung und über Desinvagination mit Hilfe von Kontrastlavements. *Acta Chir. Scand.* 61:371, 1927.
82. Packard G.B., Allen R.P.: Results in the treatment of intussusception in infants and children. *Surgery* 41:567, 1957.
83. Packard G.B., Allen R.P.: Intussusception. *Surgery* 45:496, 1959.
84. Parienty R.A., Lepreux J.F., Gruson B.: Sonographic and CT features of ileocolic intussusception. *A.J.R.* 136:608, 1981.
85. Parkkulainen K.V.: Intrauterine intussusception as a cause of intestinal atresia. *Surgery* 44:1106, 1958.
86. Patriquin H.B., Afshani E., Effman E., et al.: Neonatal intussusception. *Radiology* 125:463, 1977.
87. Pellerin D.: Les manifestations chirurgicales du purpura rhumatoide. *Ann. Chir. Infant.* 6:289, 1965.
88. Pellerin D.: Traitément de l'invagination intestinale aiguë du nourrisson. *Chirurgie* 107:398, 1981.
89. Peterson E.W.: Remarks on acute intestinal obstruction with especial reference to intussusception. *Medical Record* 74:438, 1908.
90. Petrović, S., Jovanović, D., Stojanović, S., et al.: Akutne crevne invaginacije u dece. *Acta Chir. Iugosl.* 25:31, 1978.
91. Pollet J.E., Hems G.: The decline in incidence of acute intussusception in childhood in north-east Scotland. *J. Epidemiol Community Health* 34:42, 1980.
92. Pouliquen M., de la Marnierre: Indication du lavement bismuthé dans certaines formes d'invaginations intestinales. *Bull Mém. Soc. Nat. Chir.* 53:1016, 1927.
93. Power D.: The Hunterian lectures on the pathology and surgery of intussusception. *Br. Med. J.* 1:381–388, 453–456, 514–516, 1897.
94. Rachelson M.H., Jernigan J.P., Jackson W.F.: Intussusception in newborn infant. *J. Pediatr.* 47:87, 1955.
95. Rao P.L.N.G., Prsaad C.N., Mitra S.K., et al.: Intussusception in infancy and childhood. *Indian J. Pediatr.* 46:126, 1979.
96. Ravitch M.M.: Consideration of errors in the diagnosis of intussusception. *Am. J. Dis. Child.* 84:17, 1952.
97. Ravitch M.M.: Intussusception in infancy and childhood. *N. Engl. J. Med.* 259:1058, 1958.
98. Ravitch M.M.: *Intussusception in Infants and Children.* Springfield, Ill., Charles C Thomas, Publisher, 1959.
99. Ravitch M.M.: In *A Century of Surgery.* Philadelphia J.B. Lippincott Co., 1981, p. 566
100. Ravitch M.M., McCune R.M. Jr.: Reduction of intussusception by barium enema: A clinical and experimental study. *Ann. Surg.* 128:904, 1948.
101. Ravitch M.M., McCune R.M. Jr.: Reduction of intussusception by hydrostatic pressure: An experimental study. *Bull. Johns Hopkins Hosp.* 82:550, 1948.
102. Ravitch M.M., McCune R.M. Jr.: Intussusception in infants and children. *J. Pediatr.* 37:153, 1950.
103. Retan G.M.: Nonoperative treatment of intussusception. *Am. J. Dis. Child.* 33:765, 1927.
104. Robb W.A.T., Souter W.: Spontaneous sloughing and healing of intussusception: Historical review and report of a case. *Br. J. Surg.* 49:542, 1962.
105. Robins M.M., Plenk H.P.: Intussusception in childhood. *Pediatrics* 25:592, 1960.
106. Rosenkrantz J.G., Cox J.A., Silverman F.N., et al.: Intussusception in the 1970s: Indications for operation. *J. Pediatr. Surg.* 12:367, 1977.
107. Ross J.G., Potter C.W., Zachary R.B.: Adenovirus infection in association with intussusception in infancy. *Lancet* 2:221, 1962.
108. Santulli T.V., Ferrer J.M. Jr.: Intussusception: An appraisal of present treatment. *Ann. Surg.* 143:8, 1956.
109. Schenken J.R., Kruger R.L., Schultz L.: Papillary lymphoid hyperplasia of the terminal ileum: An unusual cause of intussusception and gastrointestinal bleeding in childhood. *J. Pediatr. Surg.* 10:259, 1975.
110. Shaw A., Francois E.: An unusual case of postoperative intussusception. *Surgery* 59:455, 1966.
111. Siegal B., Gindin J.: Familial intussusception. *Harefuah* 95:390, 1978.
112. Singer J.: Altered consciousness as an early manifestation of intussusception. *Pediatrics* 64:93, 1979.
113. Smith I.M.: Incidence of intussusception and congenital hypertrophic pyloric stenosis in Edinburgh children. *Br. Med. J.* 1:551, 1960.
114. Snyder W.H. Jr., Kraus A.R., Chaffin L.: Intussusception in infants and children: A report of 143 consecutive cases. *Ann. Surg.* 130:200, 1949.
115. Stephens V.R.: Ileocaecal intussusception in infants with special reference to fluoroscopic findings. *Surg. Gynecol. Obstet.* 45:698, 1927.

116. Stevenson E.O.S., Hays D.M., Snyder W.H. Jr.: Postoperative intussusception in infants and children. *Am. J. Surg.* 113:562, 1967.
117. Strang R.: Intussusception in infancy and childhood. *Br. J. Surg.* 46:484, 1959.
118. Talwalker V.C.: Intussusception in the newborn. *Arch. Dis. Child.* 37:203, 1962.
119. Thomas G.G., Zachary R.B.: Intussusception in twins. *Pediatrics* 58:754, 1976.
120. Thomas M.P., McKay D.G.: Idiopathic intussusception occurring in father and son, with a post-operative intussusception in the son. *Aust. Paediatr. J.* 15:281, 1979.
121. Thompson J.H., Posel M.M.: A case of intussusception in acute lymphatic leukaemia. *Lancet* 218:1180, 1930.
122. Thompson W.W.: A case of introsusception in which an operation

was successfully resorted to by John R. Wilson, M.D. *Transylvania J. Med.* 8:486, 1835.
123. Thurston D.L., Holowach J., McCoy E.E.: Acute intussusception: Analysis of one hundred sixteen cases at St. Louis Children's Hospital. *Arch. Surg.* 67:68, 1953.
124. Thurston D.L., Thurston J.H., McCoy E.E.: "Knocked out"—an early sign of intussusception. *Pediatrics* 65:1057, 1980.
125. Uhland H., Parshley P.F.: Obscure intussusception diagnosed by ultrasonography. *JAMA* 239:224, 1978.
126. Yoo R.P., Touloukian R.J.: Intussusception in the newborn: A unique clinical entity. *J. Pediatr. Surg.* 9:495, 1974.
127. Zachary R.B.: Acute intussusception in childhood. *Arch. Dis. Child.* 30:32, 1955.

89 E. IDE SMITH

Malrotation of the Intestine

HISTORY.—The development of knowledge concerning the failure of rotation and fixation of the intestinal tract has had a number of milestones. Up until the turn of the century, many articles described individual situations found at operation or at autopsy. These could not be placed in context until the embryology was understood. Each clinical case of malrotation represents a failure at some point of this embryologic process.

The first good description of the embryology was written in 1898 by Franklin P. Mall,[27] Professor of Anatomy at Johns Hopkins, who had studied in Germany with the celebrated embryologist His. Mall described the process of rotation and then fixation of the bowel, based on studies of embryos by His and on reconstructions of embryos in his own department, and described the continuing process as the embryo developed.

Fraser and Robbins,[14] of St. Mary's Hospital at the University of London, expanded the observations of Mall from their own studies of a large group of embryos.

In 1923, in the *British Journal of Surgery*, there appeared an article entitled "Anomalies of intestinal rotation: Their embryology and surgical aspects," by Norman N. Dott of Edinburgh.[10] This was the first clear correlation between the embryologist's observations and the problems seen clinically. The simplified embryologic drawings, by Dott himself, have served as models for most succeeding authors. He correlated the findings in two of his own cases and 40 collected from the literature with various failures of development.

Since then, many articles have described clinical cases in relation to the stage of embryologic failure. Waugh,[36] in 1928, described two cases of volvulus due to nonrotation. Haymond and Dragstedt,[17] in 1931, described the findings and the embryology of one of the types of internal hernia. Gardner and Hart[15] described two cases of their own, and classified 104 cases new in the literature since Dott's article. Wakefield and C. Mayo[34] described 13 cases, and McIntosh and Donovan[28] described 20. William E. Ladd, in 1936, wrote the classic article on treatment of this condition, describing 21 cases.[24] He had, in 1932,[23] described ten cases of malrotation and volvulus and their treatment by counterclockwise detorsion. In the 1936 article, he emphasized the importance of dividing the bands over the duodenum, and then placing the cecum in the left upper quadrant. Close reading of this article shows that his attention had been directed to the rarely found bands that go to the *right* of the duodenum, while he did not identify the more frequently encountered bands that enclose the duodenum and cecum. His plan of releasing the duodenum and putting the cecum in the left upper quadrant remains the cornerstone of surgical treatment for nonrotation with midgut volvulus. It has recently been advocated that this positioning be fixed by sutures.[6, 7] In 1953, R.E. Gross[16] published a review of 156 cases.

In 1954 appeared the clear and most useful presentation by William Snyder, one of the original editors of these volumes, and Lawrence Chaffin.[31] The embryology of malrotation was compared to the twisting of a loop of rope around a central band representing the superior mesenteric

vessels. This simple means of demonstrating the process has done much for its understanding by succeeding generations of surgeons.

Embryology

The section on embryology that follows was written by William Snyder and Lawrence Chaffin for previous editions of this book. Their description is retained because of its clarity.

Normal Rotation

Terminology

Rotation will be described as it affects the two ends of the intestinal tract, that is, the proximal *duodenojejunal loop* and the distal *cecocolic loop*, and the simultaneous rotation of these two components will be indicated. Most authorities have referred to the process as involving the midgut,[16, 25] but we prefer to include the entire intestinal tract in the process.

DUODENOJEJUNAL LOOP.—Everyone is familiar with the normal adult position of the stomach, duodenum, and first part of the jejunum. Starting at this *upper end* of the adult intestinal tube and describing its fixed relation to the superior mesenteric artery, it is clear that the stomach is above or anterior to the artery, the second portion of the duodenum is to the right of the artery, the third portion of the duodenum lies beneath the artery, and the fourth portion (the distal duodenum and first part of the jejunum) is to the left of the artery. If, then, the embryologic fact is remembered that this whole section of the intestinal tract—that is, *duodenojejunal loop*—starts in the embryo in the same position as that of the stomach (Fig 89–1) in the adult, and if the other components of the loop eventually take the position described above, it is perfectly clear that the duodenojejunal loop has rotated around the superior mesenteric artery from above (see Fig 89–1), to the right 90 degrees (Fig 89–2), to beneath another 90 degrees, or a total thus far of 180 degrees (Fig 89–3), to its final place to the left of the artery, for an additional swing of another 90 degrees, or a total arc of 270 degrees (Fig 89–4).

The direction of the swing is obvious, for it is determined by

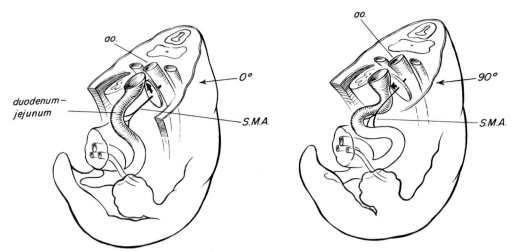

Fig 89–1 (left).—Schematic ventrolateral view of a 5-mm embryo. The intestinal tract forms a slight curve forward. The superior mesenteric artery *(SMA)* passes at right angles from the aorta *(ao)* to the curve of the intestine. A disk has been drawn around the SMA at its base; *arrow* points superiorly to the starting position, or 0-degree rotation, of the duodenojejunal loop. Rotation proceeds around the artery as an axis.

Fig 89–2 (right).—Schematic ventrolateral view of a 10-mm embryo. The duodenojejunal loop has passed from a position above the superior mesenteric artery *(SMA)* to the right of the artery and thus has rotated through an arc of 90 degrees from its starting position, as indicated by the arrow in the disk. This is considered to be the first stage of rotation.

the normal final position of the stomach and the first, second, third, and fourth portions of the duodenum in the adult.

ORIENTATION FOR SIDE AND DIRECTION OF ROTATION.—In the above description, the right side is obviously the patient's right, not the right side for the observer who, standing at the patient's side, facing the patient's head, looks down upon the patient. But, when the description of the *direction* of the rotation is given according to the motion of the hands of a clock, the direction is indicated from the viewpoint of the observer. An imaginary clock is placed face up on the posterior wall of the embryo or baby. The pivot point of the hands, that is, the axis of their rotation, is the superior mesenteric artery. The duodenojejunal loop moves in a direction opposite to the hands of the clock. The rotation is counterclockwise.

CECOCOLIC LOOP.—In the adult, the terminal ileum, cecum, and right colon lie on the right side of the abdomen to the right

of the superior mesenteric artery. In the embryo, they lie beneath the artery. This cecocolic loop, like the duodenojejunal loop, passes counterclockwise from its starting point beneath the artery (Fig 89–5), to the left of the artery 90 degrees (Fig 89–6), above to 180 degrees (Fig 89–7), and to the right of the artery, through a total arc of 270 degrees (Fig 89–8). In this manner, the cecocolic loop normally achieves its adult position.

SIMULTANEOUS ROTATION OF BOTH ENDS AND OF THE ENTIRE INTESTINAL TRACT.—The rotation is best visualized by attaching a loop of rope (Fig 89–9) above and below the metal spoke (wire) on a piece of wood. Now, grasp the loop in the left hand and turn it through three quarters of a turn to the left. Watch the proximal portion of the upper limb of the rope. It turns from its initial position above the wire, to the right of it, beneath it, and to the left of it. At the same time, the lower limb of the rope lies beneath the wire at the start of the turn, then it goes to the left,

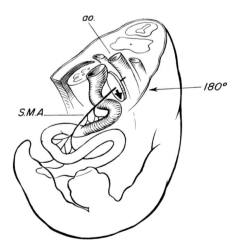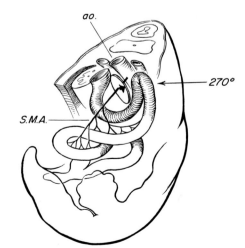

Fig 89–3 (left).—Schematic ventrolateral view of a 25-mm embryo, indicating further rotation of the duodenojejunal loop to a position below the superior mesenteric artery *(SMA)*, through an arc of 180 degrees. Extension of the remainder of the intestines into the cord is not shown.

Fig 88–4 (right).—Schematic ventrolateral view of a 40-mm embryo, indicat-

ing final rotation of the duodenojejunal loop to a position immediately on the left of the superior mesenteric artery *(SMA)*, this loop having passed from a position superior, to the right beneath and to the left, or through an arc of 270 degrees in counterclockwise direction. This final rotation of the duodenojejunal loop takes place as the intestines return from the cord.

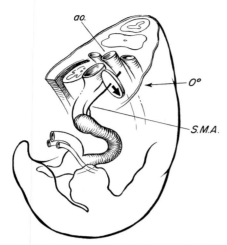

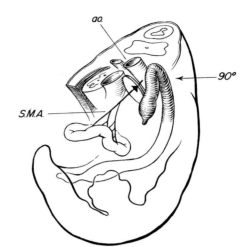

Fig 89–5 (left).—Schematic ventrolateral view of a 5-mm embryo, indicating the forward bend of the intestinal tract. The cecocolic loop is emphasized as it lies inferior to the superior mesenteric artery *(SMA)*, or in a position of a 0-degree rotation, indicated on the disk around the base of the SMA. The 0-degree rotation position for this loop is inferior to the SMA, whereas that for the duodenojejunal loop is superior.

Fig 89–6 (right).—Schematic ventrolateral view of a 40-mm embryo, showing position of the cecocolic loop at the left of the superior mesenteric artery *(SMA)*, the loop having rotated through an arc of 90 degrees from its starting position inferior to the artery (see disk at base of SMA). This phase of rotation is maintained while the intestines are in the cord and at the moment they drop back into the abdomen.

then above and finally to the right of the wire. If the upper limb is considered to represent the duodenojejunal loop, the wire, the superior mesenteric artery, and the lower limb the cecocolic loop, the position of these structures in their process of rotation will have been made clear. Of course, the entire process can be studied in minute detail with a dissecting microscope and a large series of embryos ranging in age from 1 to 3 months. At about 1 month of fetal life, or when the embryo has reached the 5-mm stage, the intestinal tract represents almost a straight tube with a slight anterior bulge in the central portion. The superior mesenteric artery comes forward from the posterior wall to the center of the bulge (see Figs 89–1 to 89–5). Changes take place rapidly as the intestines form within an extension of the abdomen into the cord. The stomach remains in its original position anterior and above the superior mesenteric artery. As the days pass, however, the duodenum begins to curve downward and to the

right of the artery. The jejunum and small intestine extend into the cord along with the cecum, right colon, and part of the transverse colon. Both loops have thus passed from a position in front of the artery to the side of the artery (see Figs 89–2 and 89–6). It was taught previously that both loops remained in this relation until the intestines returned from the cord, back into the abdomen.[10, 14] It has been demonstrated, however,[27] and verified by Snyder and Chaffin,[31] that rotation of the duodenojejunum continues during the extracoelomic phase of intestinal development and, at about the eighth week, or when the embryo is about 25 mm long, the third portion of the duodenum comes to lie beneath the artery (see Fig 89–3), which increases the rotation of this segment to 180 degrees. Finally at about 10 weeks, or when the embryo is about 40 mm long, the intestines return to the abdomen. This must be a fairly rapid process, as not many specimens of this stage of development have been described. When

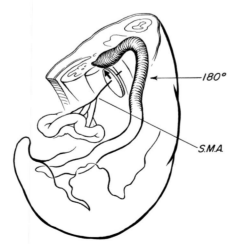

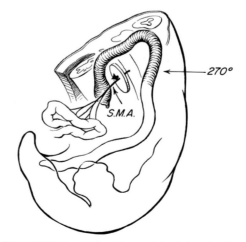

Fig 89–7 (left).—Schematic ventrolateral view of a 40-mm embryo, indicating rotation of the cecocolic loop to a position superior to the superior mesenteric artery *(SMA)*, or rotation through an arc of 180 degrees, from the starting position inferior to the SMA. This phase takes place immediately after return of the intestines from the cord into the abdomen.

Fig 89–8 (right).—Schematic ventrolateral view of a 40-mm embryo, showing final position of the cecocolic loop to the right of the superior mesenteric artery *(SMA)*, this loop having passed from a position beneath, to the left, superior, and finally to the right, or through an arc of 270 degrees, in a counterclockwise direction.

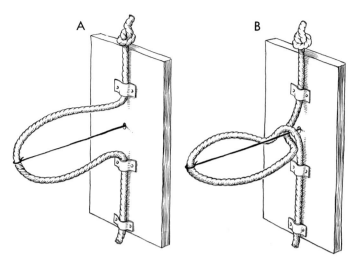

Fig 89–9.—Mechanical demonstration of intestinal rotation. A rope is attached to a board at both ends, with a wire extending at right angles from the board to the base of the loop. In **A,** the top limb of the rope corresponds to the duodenojejunal loop, the wire to the superior mesenteric artery, and the bottom limb to the cecocolic segment. In **B,** the rope loop has been grasped by the hand and rotated through an arc of 270 degrees, or three fourths of a complete turn around the wire as the axis, in a counterclockwise direction. Thus, in **B** the top limb has become the bottom one, and the bottom limb the top. By following the movements of the two limbs around the wire close to the board, one can visualize the process of rotation of the intestine in the embryo.

the intestines return, the small bowel does so first, and it pushes the fourth portion of the duodenum and jejunum to the left of the superior mesenteric artery; this completes the rotation of this segment of the bowel (see Fig 89–4). The cecum and right colon return to the abdomen last and on the left side (see Fig 89–6). This loop then passes anterior or above the artery (see Fig 89–7) and finally to its adult position on the right side of the artery (see Fig 89–8).

With a hand on the top of the steering wheel, a three-quarter turn to the left will execute the process of rotation of the duodenojejunal loop around the steering post (superior mesenteric artery). With a hand on the bottom of the steering wheel, a three-quarter turn to the left will execute the process of rotation of the cecocolic loop.

This is the process of normal rotation with the sequence of events postulated from bits of evidence contributed by many observers. It does not lend itself to a breakdown into stage I, II, and III, as previously described[14] because it is a continuing process and is better understood and remembered by comparing it with the swing of a twisted rope or the turn of a steering wheel. This description may be an oversimplification, but it offers the advantage of being easily remembered and reconstructed in one's mind at the operating table.

Classification of the Abnormalities of Intestinal Rotation

The surgical problems resulting from the abnormalities of rotation are classified by the stage at which the error occurs in the mid-gut loop. It should be clear that the abnormalities of intestinal rotation (Fig 89–10) represent a spectrum with a multitude of intermediate stages.[3] The three defined stages are arbitrary groupings. Although the upper (prearterial or duodenojejunal) limb usually is thought to complete its rotation before the lower (postarterial or cecocolic) limb, all of the combinations of failure of, or incomplete rotation of, either limb are possible. There may also be a reversal of rotation. The organs of the peritoneum may

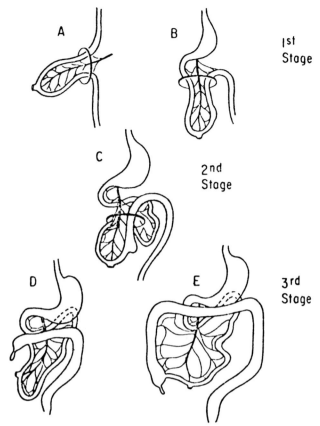

Fig 89–10.—Normal intestinal rotation. **A,** 6 weeks gestational age, nonrotation. **B,** 8 weeks gestational age, incomplete rotation. **C,** 9 weeks gestational age, incomplete rotation. **D,** 11 weeks gestational age. **E,** 12 weeks gestational age. (From Filston and Kirks,[12] modified from Snyder and Chaffin,[31] by permission.)

also be involved in situs inversus. The potential clinical problems associated with each of the stages are shown in Table 89–1.

Terminology

Clinically, although objections can justifiably be raised to the term "malrotation,"[11] it has been used and accepted beyond the point of recall for abnormalities of the process of intestinal rotation and attachment. The term "nonrotation" is used for the first stage (see Fig 89–10), while "incomplete rotation" or "mixed rotation" is used for abnormalities of the second stage.

Associated Abnormalities Seen With Malrotation

Malrotation is an integral part of congenital diaphragmatic hernia and of abnormalities of the abdominal wall—omphalocele and gastroschisis. In gastroschisis, the midgut is nonrotated, while in the other two conditions there may be nonrotation or incomplete rotation.

Associated abnormalities are seen in 30%–62% of reported series of malrotation.[12, 22, 33] Fifty percent of patients with duodenal atresia and one third of those with jejunoileal atresia have associated malrotation. Association of malrotation with Hirschsprung's disease has also been noted. Mesenteric cysts have been found in malrotation. Whether this is a factor that plays a role in the development of malrotation or results from the lymphatic obstruction in chronic volvulus is not clear.[4]

TABLE 89–1.—Classification of Abnormalities of Intestinal
Rotation and Fixation

STAGE	EMBRYOLOGICAL	CLINICAL
I. Nonrotation	Midgut lengthens on superior mesenteric artery	Midgut volvulus
II. Incomplete rotation	Return prearterial and postarterial loops and rotation	Midgut volvulus; duodenal obstruction; reverse rotation (internal hernia)
III. Incomplete fixation	Descent of cecum; fixation of mesenteries	Internal hernia; cecal volvulus

Clinical Manifestations

Malrotation leads to three clinical problems: (1) volvulus, acute and chronic; (2) duodenal obstruction, acute and chronic; (3) internal herniation.

Volvulus of the Midgut

With normal rotation and fixation, the mesentery is broad-based (Fig 89–11). Because of the narrow pedicle formed by the base of the mesentery in malrotation, volvulus of the midgut may occur (Fig 89–12). Other predisposing causes are an undue length of the mesentery and a point of adhesion at the convexity of the loop that acts as an axis for rotation.[10] Dott cites as exciting causes (1) unusual effort or accidental movement of the body, (2) abnormal peristaltic motility of the intestine, and (3) undue distention of the intestine.[10] It seems reasonable to speculate that distention and abnormal movement may be the factors that initiate a torsion of the intestine leading to clinical midgut volvulus.

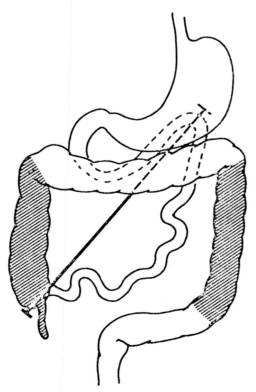

Fig 89–11.—Normal fixation of the mesentery of the midgut. The normal broad base extends from the ligament of Treitz to the ileocecal junction and prevents twisting of the intestine. Both ascending and descending colon are fixed retroperitoneally. (From Filston and Kirks,[12] modified from Snyder and Chaffin,[31] by permission.)

Asymptomatic malrotation in an adult suggests that malrotation does not inevitably lead to volvulus.

Acute Midgut Volvulus

The majority of patients with midgut volvulus present in the first year of life. In a group of 74 patients, 23 were seen in the first 7 days of life; 16 from 7 to 30 days of life, and 24 from 1 to 12 months. Only 11 were over 1 year of age.[2]

Signs and Symptoms.—The primary presenting sign is the sudden onset of bilious vomiting. Abdominal distention and a mass are common. With the onset of the acute obstruction, the distal colon empties. As vascular compromise increases, intraluminal bleeding may occur. Blood is often passed per rectum, and at times there is hematemesis. The patient develops a firm distended abdomen, hypovolemia, and shock. Abdominal distention in an infant with a gasless abdomen on plain roentgenograms should always raise the suspicion of midgut volvulus. Midgut volvulus is one of the most serious emergencies seen in the neonate or infant.

The infant with midgut volvulus appears in acute pain, is clearly in acute distress, has grunting respirations, and may be pale. Abdominal tenderness varies with the degree of vascular compromise. Abdominal guarding usually precludes palpation of thickened intestinal loops. On rectal examination, stool is usually absent, but, if present, is guaiac-positive or shows gross blood.

Suspicion of volvulus is raised by the history and a plain film of the abdomen, although definitive diagnosis requires contrast studies. With shock or a clear indication for exploration, contrast studies may be dispensed with. Intestinal obstruction in the newborn requires urgent relief. The possibility of volvulus accentuates that urgency, since a few hours may be the difference between a totally reversible condition on the one hand and loss of most of the intestine on the other.

Chronic Midgut Volvulus

Although less frequent than acute volvulus of the midgut, intermittent or partial volvulus occurs.[13, 19, 20] Intermittent or partial twisting results in lymphatic and venous obstruction with a significant enlargement of the associated mesenteric lymph nodes. Mild to severe protein calorie malnutrition has been reported in children with incomplete rotation.[19] Both absorption and transport are impaired by the venous and lymphatic stasis. An increased predisposition to infection is also present.[19]

Signs and Symptoms.—Recurrent abdominal pain and a malabsorption picture are the two primary presentations of chronic midgut volvulus. Janik and Ein[20] emphasized that bilious vomiting with chronic abdominal pain in infancy or childhood should be considered a mechanical problem until proved otherwise. Patients may have nonbilious vomiting as well from reflex irritation from gastroduodenal distention.

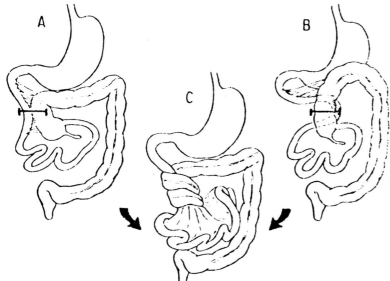

Fig 89–12.—Pathophysiology of midgut volvulus with malrotation. The narrow mesenteric attachment in nonrotation **(A)** or incomplete rotation **(B)** predisposes to midgut volvulus **(C).** (From Filston and Kirks,[12] modified from Snyder and Chaffin,[31] by permission.)

Malrotation in the Asymptomatic or Minimally Symptomatic Patient

The finding of malrotation either by x-ray films or at operation in a patient with nonrelated disease poses a problem. How dangerous is the incompletely rotated gut to the patient? Although variations in rotation are seen in adults, these may represent a potential hazard at any age. Of 50 adult patients reported with abnormalities of rotation by Wang and Welch,[35] 26 patients had symptoms referable to the abnormality. Filston and Kirks[12] advise exploration of the asymptomatic infant under 2 in whom definite malrotation is demonstrated. Firor and Steiger[13] believe that operative correction is indicated in all patients in whom a rotational abnormality could be complicated by midgut volvulus. There appears to be general acceptance that, in the patient with acute or chronic abdominal symptoms, particularly pain and/or vomiting, exploration of a proved malrotation is indicated.[9]

Duodenal Obstruction

Duodenal obstruction may be acute or chronic. It is usually present with acute volvulus but can occur independently.

Acute Duodenal Obstruction

Acute duodenal obstruction is usually caused by compression of the third portion of the duodenum by peritoneal bands (Ladd's bands) or by kinking of the bowel as a result of the bands[24] (see Fig 89–21,*D*). Duodenal obstruction is more common in the newborn or infant but can occur later in life.

SIGNS AND SYMPTOMS.—The infant or newborn usually presents with forceful, bilious vomiting. Abdominal distention may or may not be present, depending on the degree of gastroduodenal decompensation achieved by vomiting. Gastric waves may be present.[28] The obstruction may be complete or incomplete, so that a newborn may have passed meconium or the infant may have passed a stool. Jaundice may be present.[29] Malrotation is often accompanied by intrinsic duodenal obstruction. "Double-bubble" duodenal enlargement is seen on the plain abdominal x-ray film. A contrast study of the colon may suggest a rotational abnormality. Contrast study of the duodenum is diagnostic.

Chronic Duodenal Obstruction

Chronic, recurrent, or subacute obstruction of the duodenum is produced when the prearterial limb does not complete its normal rotation and is fixed by adhesions and peritoneal bands that may twist, angulate, or kink the duodenum, causing partial obstruction.[26] Some degree of volvulus may pull on the bands and contribute to the kinking. The obstruction is usually in the third, not the second, portion of the duodenum.

SIGNS AND SYMPTOMS.—Vomiting, usually bilious, is the chief symptom. Failure to gain weight and intermittent colicky ab-

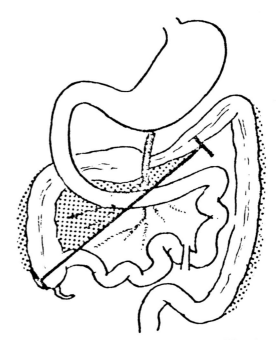

Fig 89–13.—Reverse rotation of duodenum and colon. When the colon rotates beneath the superior mesenteric artery, partial obstruction of the midtransverse colon may occur. This is caused by pressure of the vessels and by bands from the mesentery to the small bowel.

dominal pain are common. The usual age at diagnosis ranges from infancy to the preschool period. Transient dilatation of the duodenum without reflux can reflexly stimulate gastric regurgitation. Contrast studies, although diagnostic, must be carefully performed because the changes from the normal may be subtle.

Reverse Rotation With Colonic Obstruction

In this rare abnormality (Fig 89–13), the duodenum and jejunum lie anterior to the superior mesenteric vessels, which obstruct the posteriorly lying transverse colon. The transverse colon must pass through a tunnel beneath the mesentery, and this produces a chronic or complete obstruction of the colon. The condition is usually seen in adults and is rarely reported in children.[35]

Internal Herniation

Lack of fixation of the mesentery of the right and left colon, and of the duodenum, results in the formation of potential her-

nial pouches. Internal hernias cause recurrent entrapment of bowel with partial obstruction, which may progress to complete obstruction and strangulation. The most commonly seen internal hernias are the right and left mesocolic hernias, as described by Willwerth et al.[37] The term "mesocolic" is preferred to "paraduodenal." The right mesocolic hernia is produced when the prearterial limb fails to rotate around the superior mesenteric artery and the loops are entrapped by the mesentery of the cecum and colon (Fig 89–14,A). A left mesocolic hernia is produced when the unsupported area of the descending mesocolon between the inferior mesenteric vein and the posterior parietal attachment is ballooned out by the small intestine as it migrates to the left superior portion of the abdominal cavity. The cecum has completely rotated and lies in a normal position in the right lower quadrant. The ileum exits from the sac, but at a variable distance from the ileocecal valve (Fig 89–14,B and C).

SIGNS AND SYMPTOMS.—There is recurrent and intermittent intestinal obstruction. The patient has recurrent bouts of colic,

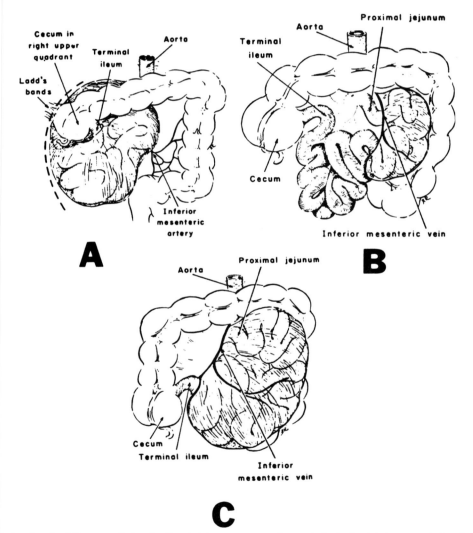

Fig 89–14.—Mesocolic hernias. **A,** right mesocolic hernia. Prearterial segment of the midgut has failed to rotate. Postarterial segment does not rotate, trapping most of the small bowel behind the right mesocolon. *Hatched line* indicates the surgical incision used to reduce the hernia. **B,** left mesocolic hernia. Initial rotation of the small intestine is normal. During migration to the left superior portion of the abdomen, the bowel invaginates an avascular portion of the left mesocolon posterior to the interior mesenteric vein. **C,** left mesocolic hernia. Small intestine, except for portions of the distal ileum, is trapped beneath the left mesocolon. Note that the inferior mesenteric vein delineates the right margin of the sac and is an integral part of the neck of the sac. (From Willwerth et al.[37] Used with permission. **B** and **C** based on Callander C.L., et al.: *Surg. Gynecol. Obstet.* 60:1052, 1935.)

which may lead to constant abdominal pain, vomiting, and sometimes constipation. The symptoms are often considered psychological. Roentgenograms taken during an attack may suggest small-intestinal obstruction and an abnormal appearance of the cecum and right colon.

Volvulus of the Cecum

With lack of fixation of the cecum, terminal ileum, and proximal ascending colon, twisting of this segment is possible, seen more frequently in the older patient. The symptoms are acute severe abdominal pain, nausea, and vomiting. Complete obstruction may develop. Distention may be right-sided. The pathognomonic abdominal x-ray film shows a large air-filled loop of colon occupying the left upper quadrant, with its convex surface facing the left lower quadrant, and the picture of small-bowel obstruction may be present.[1]

Radiological Diagnosis of Abnormalities of Rotation

Diagnostic radiologic study is the basis of the clinical evaluation of problems of intestinal rotation. The normal relations of the stomach, duodenum, ligament of Treitz, and the ileocecal region are shown in Figure 89–11. *The mesentery is the key to abnormalities of rotation.*[5, 18] The plain abdominal x-ray film may suggest malrotation if no clearly demonstrable colonic gas is seen on the baby's right. Differentiation of gas-filled small or large intestine in the newborn and infant is very difficult. Volvulus of the midgut is often characterized by the absence of gas in the abdomen, but infants with volvulus may show a radiographic pattern ranging from the gasless abdomen (Fig 89–15,A) to one simulating low intestinal obstruction (Fig 89–16).[21] A nasogastric tube, passing into a nonrotated duodenum, may be a giveaway

(Fig 89–17). The intestine may also appear thickened and edematous (see Fig 89–16).

Obstruction of the duodenum is evident with distention of the gastroduodenal segment—"double-bubble sign" (see Fig 89–15,A).

Barium is preferred for contrast studies from below or above. Barium enema demonstrates a high or abnormally mobile cecum, which suggests shortening of the mesenteric attachment (Fig 89–18). The cecum may be directed transversely or have a fixed position. With volvulus, there should be obstruction in the transverse colon. Simpson et al.[30] have commented that complete obstruction to the retrograde flow of contrast media is rare in malrotation with volvulus.

Examination of the upper gastrointestinal tract provides more specific diagnostic clues. One looks for an abnormal position of the ligament of Treitz, obstruction of the duodenum (often with a spiral or corkscrew appearance), and the presence of the jejunum on the right side (see Figs 89–18, 89–19). The duodenum, in malrotation, lies to the left of the spine and ascends to a point halfway between the lesser and greater curvatures of the stomach. In chronic obstruction and volvulus, there is thickening of the mucous membrane of the small intestine, as seen in malabsorption syndromes.[11] Chronic duodenal obstruction often requires very careful and skillful examination[3] (Fig 89–19). With a right mesocolic hernia the relation of ascending and transverse colon may be abnormal. Contrast studies show entrapment of small intestine (Fig 89–20).

Treatment

Preoperative Management

Preparation of the bowel is usually not necessary in the elective case and not feasible in the emergency one. The correction

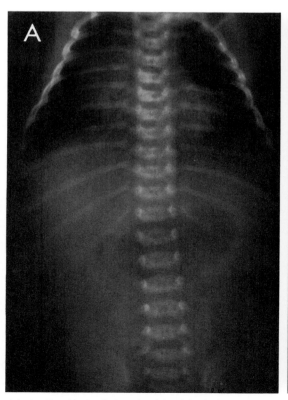
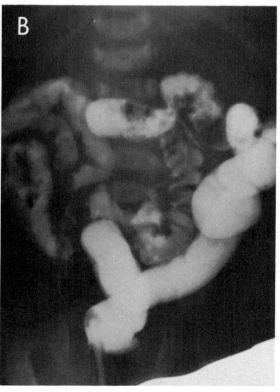

Fig 89–15.—Infant with midgut volvulus. **A,** plain abdominal examination shows absent air pattern except for dilatation of stomach and duodenum, indicative of duodenal obstruction. **B,** barium enema shows entire colon on left of abdomen in abnormal position with some reflux of barium into ileum.

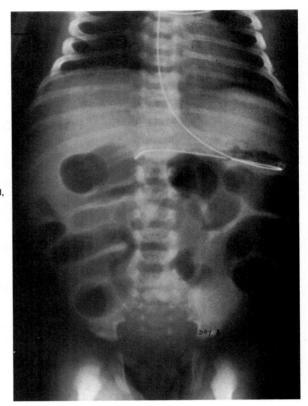

Fig 89–16.—Eight-day-old infant with midgut volvulus. A number of loops are distended, suggesting low intestinal obstruction but with centrally based intestinal loops that are thickened and edematous. With simple obstruction, there would be less space between loops.

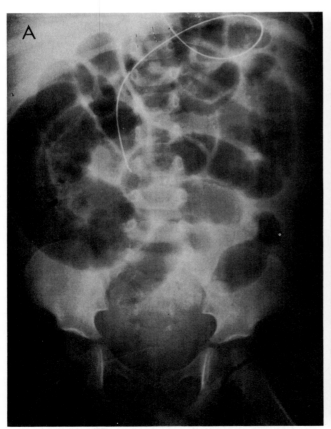

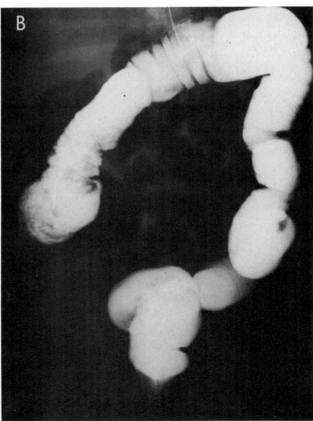

Fig 89–17.—Four-year-old male with malrotation and volvulus. **A,** plain abdominal examination shows downward course of nasogastric tube, suggesting incomplete rotation but with dilated loops of small intestine. **B,** barium enema demonstrates abnormal location of cecum and mobility of the right colon, suggesting malrotation.

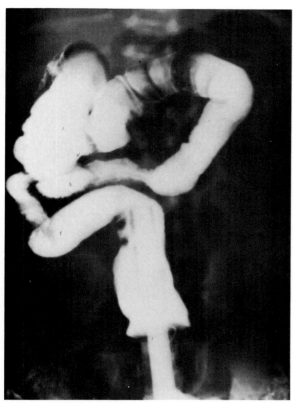

Fig 89–18.—Seven-day-old infant with malrotation and volvulus. Barium enema demonstrates abnormal positioning of the cecum and ascending colon with paralleling of ascending and transverse colon.

of metabolic abnormalities is begun, but the infant with midgut volvulus can be resuscitated or corrected only to a point. Additional time lost in efforts at total correction or precise diagnosis may mean the difference between a normal child and one with short-gut syndrome. With a nasogastric tube for decompression, adequate intravenous access, preoperative antibiotics parenterally, operation is undertaken as quickly as possible in the emergency case.

Operative Technique

Recognition of Abnormalities of Rotation

The peritoneal cavity is entered through an upper transverse muscle-dividing incision slightly skewed to the right. Recognizing a rotation abnormality is not easy, even when it is suspected, and less easy when it is encountered as an incidental finding. The two most constant anatomical points in the abdomen are the position of the pylorus and of the splenic flexure. A seemingly normal position of the cecum in the right middle or lower quadrant and an apparent leftward course of the duodenum are not positive proof of normal rotation, nor do they rule out malrotation. Several signs suggest a rotational abnormality: (1) abnormal peritoneal bands from the ileum or right colon to the parietal peritoneum or to the duodenum; (2) fixation of the duodenum and/or upper jejunum to the cecum or right colon; (3) visualization of the entire duodenum, particularly the third and fourth portions at the base of the mesentery of the transverse colon; (4) abnormal position and mobility of the cecum or of the duodenum along the right gutter.

We have found it helpful in the identification of malrotation to locate the ileocecal region, and to attempt to orient the ileal mesentery so that it lies flat on the surgeon's palm. If normal, the cecum then lies on the patient's right and the ileum to the left. Often there remains some question as to how the mesentery

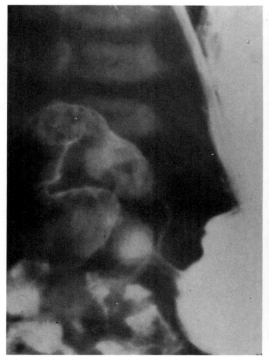
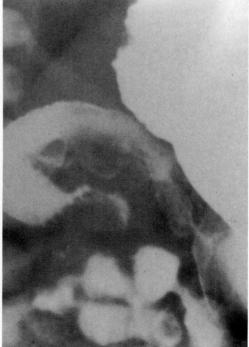

Fig 89–19.—One-day-old girl with acute duodenal obstruction due to twisting of the duodenum. Contrast study on left shows corkscrew appearance of the duodenum, with mild dilatation visible on both views.

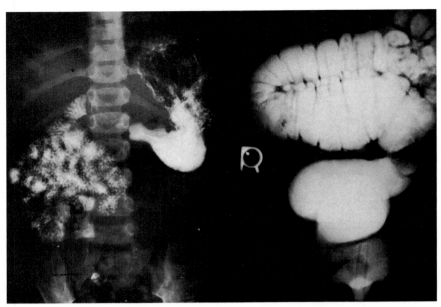

Fig 89–20.—Four-year-old boy with right mesocolic hernia. **Left,** upper gastrointestinal contrast study showing fixation of small intestines on the right. **Right,** barium enema showing displacement of the cecum with near superimposition of the ascending and transverse colon.

really lies. Narrowness of the mesenteric attachment is usually apparent. Sometimes it is only after separation of the cecum and right colon at the duodenocolic isthmus that malrotation is clearly evident.

Reduction of Volvulus

After the peritoneum has been opened, midgut volvulus can often be diagnosed by the appearance of the compromised small intestine (Fig 89–21,*A*). The entire mass of small and large intestine must be delivered through the incision and out of the peritoneal cavity, avoiding strong traction on the bowel or mesentery. With this maneuver, the twist at the base of the mesentery is visualized (Fig 89–21,*B*). Reduction of the bowel is carried out in a counterclockwise motion (Fig 89–21,*C*). One or more turns are required to reduce the volvulus and to bring the transverse colon and cecum into view anterior to the mesenteric pedicle (Fig 89–21,*D*). Improvement in the color of the intestine usually accompanies the reduction unless the bowel is already severely compromised or necrotic.

With the advent of total parenteral nutrition, the management of midgut volvulus has changed. It is possible to sustain infants with massive loss of intestine until adjustment and growth allow the child to grow on oral intake. It is also possible to have an infant who is totally dependent on parenteral nutrition.

While the management of these patients must be individualized, three principles can be followed: (1) preservation of maximal length of intestine has the highest priority, and one should err on the side of leaving intestine; (2) anastomoses between questionable ends of intestine are avoided except in rarest instances where that extra length lost with the subsequent closure of an enterostomy may be significant; (3) with extremely short lengths of viable intestine, the clinical decision is an individual one for the operator.

When the intestine appears viable, simple enterolysis and a Ladd procedure suffice. When the bowel is questionable throughout, but probably viable, a Ladd procedure plus gastrostomy is done. A localized gangrenous segment, with ample remaining bowel of good appearance, may be resected and a primary anastomosis performed. When there is gangrene, and a question of viability at the ends, or with skip areas, an enterostomy can be performed in order that the ends may be observed.

A second look operation is usually performed when there are multiple areas of very questionable viability, or when the entire midgut appears nonviable, or when clinical signs and symptoms suggest additional loss of bowel. At 12–24 hours, it may be obvious that there has been no recovery and that the situation is irredeemable, or bowel previously thought probably nonviable has pinked up, permitting a resection only of surely compromised bowel.

Our own experience with midgut volvulus and duodenal obstruction without other abnormalities such as omphalocele, atresia, etc., is shown in Table 89–2.

Relief of Duodenal Obstruction; Division of Ladd's Bands

Following the reduction of the volvulus, any duodenal bands causing obstruction are identified; dissection is begun either at the pyloric end or the duodenojejunal end (see Fig 89–21,*D*). The bands usually attach closely to the cecum or right colon close to the superior mesenteric vessels, the so-called duodenocolic isthmus. Dissection is carried out very close to the serosa of the duodenum, with careful attention to the superior mesenteric vessels and to the hepatic triad superiorly and medially. Sharp dissection is usually employed, but at times the thin peritoneal reflections can be pushed away bluntly. Many times, a plane can be developed with a right-angle clamp. There are sometimes medial attachments, particularly in the chronic duodenal obstructions.

In all cases, it is imperative to prove that there is no intrinsic obstruction. This is accomplished by passage through the duodenum of a nasogastric tube of adequate size or by the passage of a Foley catheter via nasopharynx or gastrotomy (Fig 89–21,*E*). The demonstration that air passes through the duodenum is not sufficient. The obstructive bands may also involve the ileum or progress down onto the jejunum. Houston and Wittenborg[18] pointed out that bands may also run to the gallbladder and the liver.

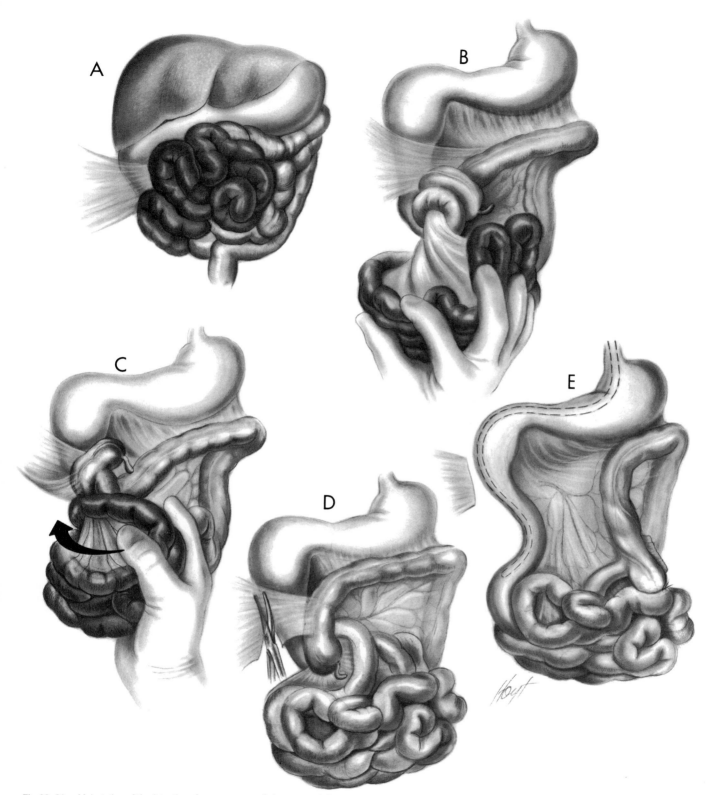

Fig 89–21.—Malrotation of the intestine. **A,** appearance of viscera as abdominal cavity is opened. The small intestines are seen at once, and appear to hide the colon. Vascular compromise of intestine may be obvious. **B,** entire intestinal mass is delivered out of the wound and drawn downward, showing the base of the mesentery. Coils of intestine or ascending colon are wrapped around the root of an incompletely anchored mesentery. The volvulus has taken place in a clockwise direction. The descending duodenum is dilated because of extrinsic pressure from Ladd's bands or peritoneal folds that cross it. **C,** volvulus is reduced by taking the entire intestinal mass in the hand and rotating it, counterclockwise (in most cases). **D,** with reduction of the volvulus, the cecum lies in the right paravertebral gutter. The peritoneal folds from the cecum obstruct the duodenum. The folds are incised close to the lateral serosal border of the duodenum. The underlying superior mesenteric pedicle is identified and carefully preserved. **E,** appearance of the intestines and ascending colon at the end of the operation. The duodenum descends along the right gutter. The small intestines lie on the right side of the abdomen, while the cecum and ascending colon are in the midline or left side of the abdomen. The superior mesenteric artery and its branches are left exposed as shown. A nasogastric tube has been passed into the jejunum to rule out intrinsic obstruction. (Modified from Ladd and Gross,[25] by permission.)

TABLE 89–2.—MIDGUT VOLVULUS AND EXTRINSIC DUODENAL
OBSTRUCTION WITHOUT OTHER ABNORMALITY, OKLAHOMA
CHILDREN'S MEMORIAL HOSPITAL, 1970–1983

	PROCEDURE		
DISORDER	LADD ONLY	LADD, RESECTION, AND ANASTOMOSIS	LADD AND ENTEROSTOMY
Midgut volvulus			
Acute	4 (2)*	2	5†
Chronic	—	—	—
Duodenal obstruction			
Acute	12	—	—
Chronic	7	—	—

*Two patients had second procedures. Number in parentheses indicates deaths.
†One patient had a second procedure.

Gastrostomy is advised when there is evidence of prolonged gastroduodenal distention that may be slow to resolve, and in patients with significant loss of intestine in whom short-gut syndrome is likely.[2] An appendectomy is also usually performed. Often, dissection of the cecal segment has resulted in sacrifice of the appendiceal vessels.

Treatment of Colonic Obstruction Secondary to Reversed Rotation

In the past, various procedures were recommended, which involved division of the colon with anastomosis anterior to the duodenum.[35] Currently, it is recognized that reflection of the colon and reversal of the rotation can free the colon satisfactorily.

Operative Repair of Mesocolic (Paraduodenal) Hernia

Willwerth et al.[37] suggest that right mesocolic hernia is best treated by freeing the small intestine by incising the lateral peritoneal margin of the right colon and reflecting the colon to the left.

Treatment of the left mesocolic hernia can be more difficult. Sometimes the small intestine can be reduced through the neck of the sac. The key to the repair and reduction is the mobilization of the inferior mesenteric vein, which runs along the anterior margin of the neck of the sac (see Fig 89–14,*B* and *C*) and must be spared. An incision is made to the right of the vein, allowing reduction of the bowel. The peritoneum adjacent to the vein is sutured to the posterior peritoneum to close the neck of the sac.

Cecal Volvulus

Reduction of the volvulus is followed by fixation or by cecostomy where the bowel is viable. Where the bowel is compromised, resection is advised.

Fixation of the Mesentery

Because of the dangers of recurrent volvulus, Brennom and Bill[7] advised a stabilization of the mesentery by fixation of the duodenum and of the colon. The initial report showed superiority of fixation over nonfixation.[6] Subsequently, Stauffer and Herrmann[32] presented data that suggest no advantage of fixation. The majority consensus appears to concur with the recommendations of Stauffer.[2, 22, 33] The fixation base of the mesentery may actually be improved by separating the colonic portion of the isthmus from the duodenum.

Malrotation Discovered in the Course of an Unrelated Operation

Dott[10] pointed out the dangers of malrotation unrecognized in an abdominal operation, citing a gastroileostomy being performed instead of a gastrojejunostomy. Recognizing abnormalities of rotation is important in all procedures where small intestine is used, as for example, in Roux-en-Y loops, urinary conduits, and the like. Antiperistaltic loops may be created, torsion may occur in the reanastomosis, and twisting of the mesentery with intestinal obstruction may occur if the true anatomy is not recognized.

Locating an acutely inflamed appendix in a patient with malrotation is difficult but may be anticipated by the absence of a cecal shadow in the right lower quadrant. In Collins' study of 71,000 human appendix specimens, 2,849 were in an abnormal position within the abdomen due to incomplete rotation of the large bowel: 2,781 of these were in the right upper quadrant, only 40 (0.05%) in the left upper quadrant, and 28 (0.03%) in the left lower quadrant.[8]

Postoperative Management and Complications

Return of intestinal function depends on the duration and extent of the obstruction. Marginally viable bowel with mucosal injury and the short-gut syndrome are special problems. In an uncomplicated external obstruction due to duodenal bands, duodenal function returns in 3–5 days. Small initial feedings, such as those used in pyloric stenosis, have been advised.[22] In the absence of intrinsic congenital obstruction, return of gastroduodenal function should be relatively prompt.

The complications are those of general intestinal pediatric surgery—superficial wound infections, postoperative obstruction due to adhesive bands, or postoperative intussusception.

Mortality is primarily associated with extensive intestinal necrosis in midgut volvulus.[2]

Results

Recurrence of the volvulus is infrequent. Ten percent of patients in Stauffer's[32] series required reoperation for obstruction or volvulus. In the Boston Children's series of 441, only two patients had recurrent obstruction, and in the Los Angeles series there were no recurrences.[2] Morbidity of recurrent abdominal symptoms or pain in patients with chronic volvulus or obstruction is more significant: 20% in Stauffer's report.[32] The overall results in correction of malrotation in older children with abdominal pain, vomiting, or malabsorption are anecdotal,[13, 20] but appear quite satisfactory.

REFERENCES

1. Anderson A., Bergdahl L. Van der Linden W.: Volvulus of the cecum. *Ann. Surg.* 181:876–880, 1975.
2. Andrassy R.J., Mahour G.H.: Malrotation of the midgut in infants and children. *Arch. Surg.* 116:158–160, 1981.
3. Balthazar E.J.: Intestinal malrotation in adults: Roentgenographic assessment with emphasis on isolated complete and partial nonrotations. *Am. J. Roentgenol.* 126:358–367, 1976.
4. Bentley J.F.R.: Mesenteric cysts with malrotated intestine. *Br. Med. J.* 2:223–225, 1959.
5. Berdon W.E., Baker D.H., Bull S., et al.: Midgut malrotation and volvulus. *Radiology* 96:365–383, 1970.
6. Bill A.H., Grauman D.: Rationale and technic for stabilization of the mesentery in cases of nonrotation of the midgut. *J. Pediatr. Surg.* 1:127–135, 1966.
7. Brennom W.S., Bill A.H.: Prophylactic fixation of the intestine for midgut nonrotation. *Surg. Gynecol. Obstet.* 138:181–184, 1974.
8. Collins D.C.: 71,000 human appendix specimens: A final report, summarizing forty years' study. *Am. J. Proctol.* 14:365–381, 1963.

9. Devlin H.B.: Midgut malrotation causing intestinal obstruction in adult patients. *Ann. R. Coll. Surg. Engl.* 48:227–237, 1971.
10. Dott N.M.: Anomalies of intestinal rotation: Their embryology and surgical aspects, with report of 5 cases. *Br. J. Surg.* 11:251–286, 1923.
11. Estrada R.L.: *Anomalies of Intestinal Rotation and Fixation.* Springfield, Ill., Charles C Thomas, Publisher, 1958.
12. Filston H.C., Kirks D.R.: Malrotation—the ubiquitous anomaly. *J. Pediatr. Surg.* 16:614–620, 1981.
13. Firor H.V., Steiger E.: Morbidity of rotational abnormalities of the gut beyond infancy. *Cleve. Clin. Q.* 50:303–309, 1983.
14. Fraser J.E., Robbins R.H.: On the factors concerned in causing rotation of the intestine in man. *J. Anat. Physiol.* 50:75–110, 1915.
15. Gardner C.E., Hart D.: Anomalies of intestinal rotation as a cause of intestinal obstruction. *Arch. Surg.* 29:942–981, 1934.
16. Gross R.E.: *The Surgery of Infancy and Childhood.* Philadelphia, W.B. Saunders Co., 1953.
17. Haymond H.E., Dragstedt L.R.: Anomalies of intestinal rotation. *Surg. Gynecol. Obstet.* 53:316–329, 1931.
18. Houston C.S., Wittenborg M.H.: Roentgen evaluation of anomalies of rotation and fixation of the bowel in children. *Radiology* 84:1–18, 1965.
19. Howell C.G., Vozza F., Shaw S., et al.: Malrotation, malnutrition and ischemic bowel disease. *J. Pediatr. Surg.* 17:469–473, 1982.
20. Janik J.S., Ein S.H.: Normal intestinal rotation with nonfixation: A cause of chronic abdominal pain. *J. Pediatr. Surg.* 14:670–674, 1979.
21. Kassner E.G., Kottmeier P.K.: Absence and retention of small bowel gas in infants with midgut volvulus: Mechanisms and significance. *Pediat. Radiol.* 4:28–30, 1975.
22. Kiesewetter W.B., Smith J.W.: Malrotation of the midgut in infancy and childhood. *Arch. Surg.* 77:483–491, 1958.
23. Ladd W.E.: Congenital obstruction of the duodenum in children. *N. Engl. J. Med.* 206:277–283, 1932.
24. Ladd W.E.: Surgical diseases of the alimentary tract in infants. *N. Engl. J. Med.* 215:705, 1936.
25. Ladd W.E., Gross R.E.: *Abdominal Surgery of Infancy and Childhood.* Philadelphia, W.B. Saunders Co., 1941.
26. Lewis J.E. Jr.: Partial duodenal obstruction with incomplete duodenal rotation. *J. Pediatr. Surg.* 1:47–53, 1966.
27. Mall F.P.: Development of the human intestine and its position in the adult. *Bull. Johns Hopkins Hosp.* 9:197–208, 1898.
28. McIntosh R., Donovan E.J.: Disturbances of rotation of the intestinal tract. *Am. J. Dis. Child.* 57:116–166, 1939.
29. Porto S.O.: Jaundice in congenital malrotation of the intestine. *Am. J. Dis. Child.* 117:684–688, 1969.
30. Simpson A.J., Leonidas J.C., Krasna I.H., et al.: Roentgen diagnosis of midgut malrotation: Value of upper gastrointestinal radiographic study. *J. Pediatr. Surg.* 7:243–251, 1972.
31. Snyder W.H., Chaffin L.: Embryology and pathology of the intestinal tract: Presentation of 48 cases of malrotation. *Ann. Surg.* 140:368–380, 1954.
32. Stauffer U.G., Herrmann P.: Comparison of late results in patients with corrected intestinal malrotation with and without fixation of the mesentery. *J. Pediatr. Surg.* 15:9–12, 1980.
33. Stewart D.R., Colodny A.L., Daggett W.C.: Malrotation of the bowel in infants and children: A 15-year review. *Surgery* 79:716–720, 1976.
34. Wakefield E.G., Mayo C.W.: Intestinal obstruction produced by mesenteric bands. *Arch. Surg.* 33:47–67, 1936.
35. Wang C.A., Welch C.E.: Anomalies of intestinal rotation in adolescents and adults. *Surgery* 54:839–855, 1963.
36. Waugh G.E.: Congenital malformation of the mesentery: A clinical entity. *Br. J. Surg.* 15:438–449, 1928.
37. Willwerth B.M., Zollinger R.M., Izant R.J.: Congenital mesocolic (paraduodenal) hernia: Embryologic basis of repair. *Am. J. Surg.* 128:358–361, 1974.

90 Howard C. Filston

Other Causes of Intestinal Obstruction

MOST CAUSES of intestinal obstruction in childhood result from complications of congenital anomalies or intestinal inflammation. Intussusception and the other common and significant specific causes of obstruction—congenital, inflammatory, and neoplastic—are covered elsewhere. The most important other intestinal obstruction is the postoperative obstruction, usually due to adhesions and occurring early or, most commonly, late, and occasional acute postoperative intussusception.

Postoperative Obstruction Due to Adhesions

The incidence of obstruction in childhood due to postoperative adhesions is difficult to determine, and the problem has not been extensively addressed in the literature. Festen[10] reported an incidence of 2.2% in 1,476 laparotomies in 1,283 pediatric patients. The problem has been a concern ever since laparotomy became common. Attempts to eliminate intraperitoneal scarring have thus far failed, although there is general agreement on the necessity for gentle handling of the tissues, avoidance of the use of dry pads and sponges, elimination of foreign materials (glove powder, excessive lengths of sutures), and avoidance of gross ligatures of omentum or mesentery, which produce nodules of necrotic fat. Ischemic tissues invite adhesions, and it takes only one adhesion to produce intestinal obstruction in an otherwise adhesion-free abdomen. Festen[10] found that 70% of obstructions in his series were due to a single adhesion.

Janik et al.[13] reported adhesions were the seventh most common cause of intestinal obstruction in the series from the Hospital for Sick Children, Toronto.

Table 90–1 shows the causes of mechanical obstruction in children at the Duke University Medical Center from 1976 to 1983.

TABLE 90–1.—COMPARISON OF SMALL-BOWEL OBSTRUCTION DUE TO ADHESIONS WITH OTHER COMMON INTESTINAL OBSTRUCTIONS, PEDIATRIC SURGICAL SERVICE, DUKE UNIVERSITY MEDICAL CENTER, 1976–1983

Small-bowel obstruction, postoperative	25
Small-bowel obstruction secondary to tumor	3
Small-bowel obstruction secondary to ventriculoperitoneal shunt	2
Imperforate anus	45
Hirschsprung's disease	39
Jejunoileal atresia/stenosis	29
Malrotation with or without volvulus	28
Duodenal atresia	12
Intussusception	9
Meckel's diverticulum	6

Diagnosis

The most important factor in the recognition of small-bowel obstruction due to adhesions is a history, in a patient with abdominal pain, of a previous intraperitoneal surgical procedure and "a scar on the belly." Educational efforts must be directed toward impressing on the primary care physician the importance of this factor in evaluating children with abdominal pain, nausea, and vomiting. Far too often these symptoms are ascribed to the current "flu bug" in the community. Typically, the child with intestinal obstruction due to adhesions complains of a sudden onset of crampy abdominal pain. Anorexia, nausea, and vomiting accompany the pain, or very shortly follow its onset. The bowel below the obstruction may empty once or twice, after which, in the presence of complete obstruction, stools cease. Occasionally, "diarrhea" occurs, a sign of partial intestinal obstruction. Decreased activity and lethargy are common and early.

The findings on physical examination vary with the stage of the condition at the time of presentation. Initially, the abdomen is soft and undistended. Bowel sounds are hyperactive and may be high-pitched. As the child grimaces or cries with each recurrence of cramps, borborygmi may be heard. A little later, one may be able to palpate and perhaps to see individual dilated loops, and the distention becomes apparent. Ultimately, the overdistended bowel is paralyzed and peristaltic pain disappears, to be replaced by the constant pain from distention of the loops and the parietes.

Tenderness of true peritoneal origin is an indication of damaged bowel. Pressure on distended but viable bowel, increasing the tension within it, may cause pain, which may not be differentiable from true tenderness. Since, in either case, the diagnosis is intestinal obstruction and the treatment is immediate operation, the distinction is ordinarily not important. The lower the obstruction, the greater the opportunity for distention, while, with high obstruction, the vomiting may empty the obstructed loops so that distention is not apparent.

While the child is being prepared for operation, proximal decompression by suction tube may relieve the distention significantly, and signs of tenderness and guarding induced by pressure on distended loops now may abate. Janik et al.[13] reported that 100% of patients with gangrene had persistent tenderness after decompression, as, in fact, did 18 children who proved not to have gangrene.

Fever and leukocytosis are suggestive of dead bowel and peritonitis, not of intestinal obstruction.

A chest radiograph, to rule out pneumonia as a cause of paralytic ileus and to show the diaphragm and any free air, and plain supine and upright abdominal views, to show the pattern and position of gas-filled loops, are taken as soon as the child has been examined, a nasogastric tube passed, suction initiated, and intravenous fluids and antibiotics begun. Even early in the course of intestinal obstruction, some dilatation of bowel loops may be evident. The hope is to be able to undertake operation early, before the passage of time produces massive dilatation of loops and multiple air-fluid levels. Air in the colon indicates partial intestinal obstruction, unless the film has been taken so soon after the onset that the air has not yet been evacuated. A prone cross-table lateral film is useful in infants. In infants, it is notoriously difficult to be certain whether a loop distended with gas is colon or small bowel, and only by demonstrating gas in the rectum is it possible to be certain there is gas in the colon.

We have not hesitated to use upper GI barium studies to establish the diagnosis of intestinal obstruction. Barium passes through to the colon within a few hours in cases of partial obstruction, and films taken at frequent intervals may well show the point of obstruction.

CASE REPORT.—A 3½-year-old white girl undergoing chemotherapy after right nephrectomy and radiation therapy for a stage II Wilms' tumor developed nausea, vomiting and watery diarrhea, accompanied by crampy abdominal pain, three days before admission. She was thought to have gastroenteritis, but when her abdomen became tender she was referred to Duke University Medical Center. On arrival, she was passing massive amounts of watery diarrhea with occasional flecks of blood. Her vomitus was bile-stained. Her abdomen was flat and nondistended, but she guarded it. She was approximately 20% dehydrated, irritable, and hallucinating. Her white blood cell count was 22,000 with a shift to the left. Her outside abdominal films showed metal clips from her previous surgical procedure, minimal bowel gas with no evidence of obstruction, and a small amount of gas in her rectum (Fig 90–1,A). The child was rehydrated with balanced salt solution, and, because she was in a phase of bone marrow depression from her latest chemotherapy, she was started on broad-spectrum antibiotic coverage. After several hours of hydration, her BUN level fell from 54 to 20, her creatinine from 2.2 to 1, and her white blood cell count to 8,000. She continued to have watery diarrhea, and a repeat abdominal film showed a nonspecific bowel gas pattern with some gas in the colon and more gas in the rectum (Fig 90–1,B). Because of concern for small-bowel obstruction, a barium upper GI series was performed, which demonstrated dilated proximal loops of bowel and a high-grade small-bowel obstruction approximately in the midjejunum (Fig 90–1,C).

Laparotomy showed a strangulated small-bowel obstruction secondary to postoperative adhesion. She underwent resection and primary anastomosis with lysis of adhesions.

Her postoperative course was uncomplicated.

Comment.—It is often not important whether mechanical obstruction is complete or incomplete. Operative relief is required in any case, and, as in this instance, bowel may be compromised even when obstruction is incomplete.

It is vital to establish the diagnosis of mechanical intestinal obstruction and operate as early as possible. Apart from the deleterious effects on the child of the continued obstruction and the increasing risk of operation with time, a few hours may make the difference between an obstruction easily relieved by snipping a single adhesion and the necessity for resection of large amounts of bowel. The single most dangerous type of mechanical intestinal obstruction, often associated with adhesions, is volvulus. The pain is immediately violent, at a time when there are no physical signs at all. If the volvulus is massive, the proximal bowel is emptied by vomiting, and distention does not appear until the involved loops become gangrenous and suffused with blood. Initial radiographs show no dilated loops. The diagnosis is frequently missed until the bowel has infarcted. Operation may have to be undertaken on informed suspicion.

Treatment

Initial treatment is directed toward rehydrating the patient, correcting electrolyte imbalance, and decompressing the intestine with nasogastric tube suction. Antibiotics should be administered from the time the suspicion of mechanical intestinal obstruction is entertained.[3a] A variety of experimental studies over the last 40 years with each new antibacterial agent in turn have demonstrated that antibiotic therapy prolongs the life of ischemic bowel by limiting the effects of bacterial invasion.

The goal of therapy is to relieve the obstruction before ischemic bowel injury occurs. Nonoperative management is contraindicated unless there is clear evidence of improvement in symptoms, abdominal signs, and radiographic findings. The child referred in good condition can be operated on as soon as all the initial measures have been taken. For a prostrated child, several hours spent in electrolyte correction, antibiotic administration, and decompression are well spent. Extremely severe pain sug-

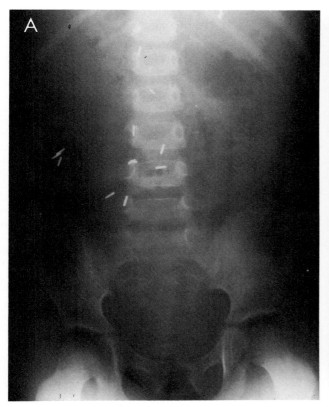

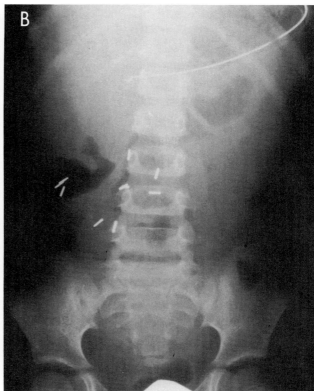

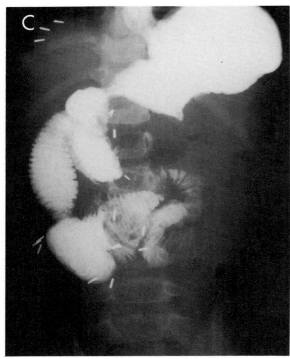

Fig 90–1.—Intestinal gangrene with incomplete intestinal obstruction. **A,** plain abdominal x-ray film showing surgical clips from previous nephrectomy for Wilms tumor and a nonspecific bowel gas pattern with some gas in the rectum. **B,** follow-up plain abdominal film after insertion of a nasogastric tube. There is additional colon gas, more gas in the rectal segment, and no evidence of dilated small bowel. The child had watery diarrhea. **C,** upper gastrointestinal tract contrast study immediately following plain film in **B** shows dilated loops of proximal jejunum with a high-grade mid-small-bowel obstruction. A gangrenous loop of small bowel was found, strangulated by adhesions. In such a high obstruction there is little opportunity for distention. The child recovered.

gests volvulus or another type of closed obstruction, and a few hours may make the difference between live and dead bowel.

A word about long intestinal tubes—we have found them of little help in the typical mechanical intestinal obstruction due to adhesions. They can be useful in the occasional patient with re-

current obstruction, possibly operated on several times before, known to have extensive adhesions, in whom one may hope that there is little possibility of a strangulating obstruction, although even in such cases this should not be relied on. The long tube is difficult to pass in the presence of complete obstruction and should, in any case, be supplemented by a short tube through the other nostril to be sure that the stomach is completely evacuated. Operative relief of the obstruction should not be delayed in an attempt to see whether or not a long tube will be passed and whether or not it will relieve the patient. A long tube, threaded at the end of the operation, either through the nose or directly through a gastrotomy, well into the bowel, will keep it decompressed and possibly lessen the incidence of recurrent obstruction due to adhesions.

When the original operation is remote, an incision, beginning above or below the old one, is often preferable to entering directly through the old scar. The bowel may be adherent to the old incision, making entry into the peritoneal cavity hazardous. The aim of operation is to find a collapsed loop and trace it proximally to the point of obstruction without eviscerating the intestine and unnecessarily handling the dilated and sometimes fragile proximal intestine. With hugely distended bowel, evisceration may indeed by required. To the degree that it is possible, adhesions unrelated to the present obstruction are ignored, lest new injuries result. Great care is required to avoid injury to the intestinal wall. Janik et al.[13] reported that intraoperative injury to otherwise viable bowel required resection in 11% of patients. The surgeon is best advised to assume responsibility for any such injury, rather than to seek refuge in the statement that it was "unpreventable." Particularly shortly after the inciting operation, when the distended bowel is edematous and easily torn by manipulation, such injury is easily inflicted.

It is important to decompress the distended bowel before closure of the wound and sometimes, in the face of massive distention, even immediately upon entering the abdomen. If the bowel can be decompressed by advancing a long tube through nose, mouth, or gastrotomy, so much the better, although it may be difficult to pass the tube beyond the jejunum at operation. Once the tube is in the jejunum, it can be threaded down. This is usually done at the end of the operation. If there is massive distention initially, it is best to evacuate the bowel with a catheter or a large-bore needle inserted through a pursestring, milking the intestinal contents up to the point of suction. Some authors (Festen,[10] Janik et al.[13]) fear such measures. In the series cited, prophylactic antibiotics were not employed. After operation,

nothing is given by mouth until bowel action is restored, and then feeding is carefully begun while the indwelling tube remains in place and clamped off. The survival of a child operated on for severe intestinal obstruction may well depend on the obsessiveness with which the fluid output is monitored and the intake administered.

One of the most difficult diagnoses to make is that of acute mechanical intestinal obstruction occurring in the postoperative period, say, after treatment of a ruptured appendix or laparotomy of any kind (Table 90–2). It may be difficult to differentiate paralytic ileus caused by peritonitis or intestinal handling from mechanical ileus due to adhesions, volvulus, intussusception, trapping in a mesenteric defect, etc. Uniform distribution of air in the small bowel and in the large bowel suggests paralytic ileus. The single best evidence is the evidence of peristaltic pain, cramps, and periodic borborygmi, which are the hallmarks of mechanical intestinal obstruction. Not only is the diagnosis at times difficult to establish but, in the days after operation, there is some place for the hope that the obstruction may be due to "plastic" adhesions, which may yet separate as the bowel regains its tone. Some such patients are well treated by tube decompression and respond. A patient with cramps who does not respond promptly to tube decompression, or whose cramps are extremely severe, should be operated on. Perforation of the bowel in incomplete obstruction is not unknown.

Less Common Causes of Intestinal Obstruction

An intestinal obstruction is generally due to one of the following mechanisms: (1) atresia or stenosis, (2) extrinsic compression, (3) intussusception, (4) anomalies of rotation, (5) inspissation of contents, (6) peristaltic dysfunction, (7) intrinsic mass, or (8) inflammatory lesions. Each will be briefly reviewed. Atresia is purely a neonatal problem. Incomplete duodenal obstruction due to a web, or to annular pancreas may not present until later in infancy or childhood (see Chap. 84).

Extrinsic Compression

Ladd's bands, the peritoneal extensions from the surgical "gutter" to the cecum and ascending colon, found in most cases of

TABLE 90–2.—RELATIVE RISK OF DEVELOPING ADHESIVE SMALL-BOWEL OBSTRUCTION (SBO) AFTER PRIOR IINTRA-ABDOMINAL PROCEDURE, 1968–1979

PROCEDURE	NO. PERFORMED	NO. OF ADHESIVE SBO	RELATIVE RISK (%)
Subtotal colectomy (ulcerative colitis)	48	8	16.6
Resection of symptomatic Meckel's diverticulum	61	7	11.6
Ladd procedure	60	5	8.3
Nephrectomy (Wilms' tumor)	91	7	7.7
Operative reduction/resection of intussusception	96	7	7.3
Hepatectomy (tumor)	30	2	6.6
Fundoplication	97	6	6.2
Oophorectomy (tumor)	18	1	5.5
Gastroschisis repair	60	3	5.0
Bochdalek hernia repair	120	5	4.2
Adrenalectomy (tumor)	48	1	2.1
Appendectomy (with or without drainage)	3,180	16	0.5
With drainage	720	6	0.8
Without drainage	2,460	10	0.4

From Janik J.S. et al.,[13] with permission.

malrotation, are the most common entities producing obstruction by extrinsic compression, in these cases, obstructing the duodenum. Yolk sac remnants, such as Meckel's diverticulum and its extra coelomic extension, the omphalomesenteric duct, obstruct by direct compression of the loop of bowel that herniates beneath them. An inflamed Meckel's diverticulum can become attached to other parts of the mesentery, forming a bridge beneath which a loop of bowel may herniate, or it may cause extensive inflammation and adhesions with subsequent bowel obstruction. The omphalomesenteric duct may compress other loops of bowel or may act as the fixation point for a volvulus of the distal ileum (see Chap. 87).

Vitelline artery and vein remnants, residua of the primitive yolk sac stage, may persist as bands that compress the bowel or act as fixation points for volvulus. The arteries originally extend from the primitive aorta to the yolk sac and persist as branches of the ileal mesenteric arcade system, passing around the ileum to a Meckel's diverticulum or omphalomesenteric remnant, in which case they enter the umbilical cord. The vitelline veins extend from the yolk sac to the sinus venosus and eventually contribute to formation of the portal venous system. The vascular remnants can persist as bands even when the bowel remnants absorb normally; they extend from the umbilicus to the mesentery and obstruct by direct pressure. Kleinhaus et al.[14] reported three cases of obstruction due to vitelline remnants, illustrating compression by the anterior vitelline artery, the posterior vitelline artery, and the vitelline vein (Fig 90–2); the latter usually extends to the inferior mesenteric vein and produces high intestinal obstruction (see Chap. 87).

Preduodenal portal vein results from irregular persistence of an anterior vitelline remnant of the vitelline vein, and whether it causes duodenal obstruction has been frequently questioned. Esscher[8] presented a thorough discussion of the subject and review of the literature questioning whether preduodenal portal vein ever really obstructs the bowel. Our own experience is limited to one case associated with malrotation and Ladd's bands. Because of our concern with the preduodenal vein, we failed to investigate the child for intrinsic obstruction. Her persistent duodenal obstruction proved to be due not to the preduodenal portal vein but to a missed intrinsic duodenal web! The literature suggests that this is a common failing.[8]

Adhesive or congenital bands of origin other than the known anatomical and embryological entities discussed above are rare; usually in utero obstruction or perforation, with meconium peritonitis, is the source. A transomental herniation with strangulation of the bowel has been reported by Luchtman et al.[15]

Intussusception

Spontaneous small-bowel intussusception can occur postoperatively (see Chap. 88) and be very difficult to detect if not included in the differential diagnosis of postoperative ileus. We have seen it in the upper jejunum after a routine infant herniorrhaphy in which the sac was not opened.

Anomalies of Rotation

Anomalies of rotation commonly cause obstruction in infants and are discussed at length in Chapter 89. Volvulus and Ladd's bands are the usual sources of obstruction, but paraduodenal and paracecal herniations[20] and "cocoon" envelopment of the bowel can result from malfixation of the mesentery associated with rotational anomalies (see Fig 89–14). Touloukian,[28] in the third edition of this work, provided a nice discussion of the historical descriptions of various mesenteric hernias. Willwerth et al.[29] presented an excellent review of the embryology, pathogenesis, and treatment of these often confusing obstructive entities, emphasizing the basic rotational anomaly underlying the mesenteric defect.

Inspissation of Contents

Meconium ileus resulting from mucoviscidosis is the common entity in this grouping, but sporadic reports of similar intrinsic obstructions have appeared with documented absence of cystic fibrosis.[6, 25] Cook and Rickham[5] reported eight neonates with neonatal milk curd obstruction, and we have operated on a premature with short-bowel syndrome given cholestyramine who was obstructed by a "Styrofoam" cast of his entire small bowel. Neonatal large bowel obstructions from inspissated meconium present as small left colon syndrome and meconium plug syndrome.

Peristaltic Dysfunction

Hirschsprung's disease is the prototype of dysfunctional obstruction of the distal bowel. Schärli and Meier-Ruge[21] discuss hypoplasia of the myenteric plexus as a possible variant of Hirschsprung's disease that may produce obstruction in short segments, or diarrhea when longer stretches are involved. The entity is characterized by increased acetylcholinesterase activity and represents one of several entities only beginning to be recognized in which ganglion cells are present but dysfunctional. Intestinal pseudo-obstruction is another recently recognized en-

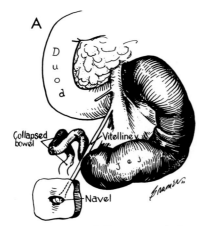
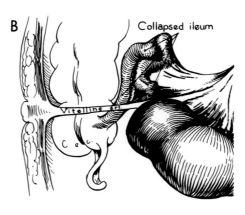

Fig 90–2.—Vitelline artery and vein remnants cause obstruction by extrinsic compression of the jejunum and ileum. (From Kleinhaus et al.[14])

tity in which peristaltic dysfunction is present, despite ganglion cells in the myenteric plexus.[24] Familial forms of pseudo-obstruction or visceral myopathy are recorded.[9, 17] Neonates have presented with megacystis, microcolon, intestinal hypoperistalsis;[1] older children, with chronic idiopathic intestinal pseudo-obstruction, an entity involving chiefly a hypotonic duodenum but frequently progressing to involve other bowel segments as well. Similar problems have been reported in association with gastroschisis and other abdominal wall defects, perhaps representing ischemic injury to the peristaltic control mechanisms.[18] Finally, there have been isolated reports of intestinal obstruction due to segmental absence of one or more layers of the intestinal musculature.[7, 12]

Intrinsic Mass Obstruction

Intrinsic mass obstruction of the intestine usually results from tumors, generally malignant ones. Lymphoma is the most common and should be considered whenever children beyond the usual age group present with unexplained obstruction or intussusception. Remarkably extensive growth of lymphoma in the bowel and mesentery can occur without significant obstructive signs. In four cases of lymphoma that we reported in 1975,[3] only one tumor, which had intussuscepted the bowel, had caused complete obstruction. Other tumors such as leiomyosarcoma[2] occasionally cause intestinal obstruction in children, usually as a result of intussusception. Benign mass lesions such a polyps (including those associated with familial polyposis and Peutz-Jeghers syndrome) hamartomas, hemangiomas, leiomyomas, fibromas, etc., rarely obstruct by mass effect alone. They present with bleeding, anemia, or the crampy recurrent pain of chronic intussusception.

Inflammatory Lesions

Obstruction due to inflammatory lesions of the bowel in infancy usually results from strictures that may form after neonatal necrotizing enterocolitis. Schwartz et al.[22] reported late strictures in seven of 28 medically managed patients with necrotizing enterocolitis, three of whom presented with obstructive symptoms. Two presented with hematochezia and two were asymptomatic, the diagnosis being made by routine radiographic follow-up. In a subsequent prospective study, the same authors[23] identified a 36% incidence of stenosis after necrotizing enterocolitis (ten of 28, seven symptomatic).

Inflammatory etiologies of later childhood include regional enteritis, chronic granulomatous disease,[11] tuberculosis,[19] primary peritonitis, familial Mediterranean fever,[27] and inflammation related to ventriculoperitoneal shunt.[26] The latter can lead to obstruction from infection with subsequent adhesions or from the formation of a pseudocyst at the terminus of the catheter. Obstruction from inflammatory stenosis after radiation for tumors is not a rare phenomenon,[16] and, last, the seat belt has been cited as a cause of bowel injury leading to obstruction stenoses.[4]

REFERENCES

1. Amoury R.A., Fellows R.A., Goodwin C.D., et al.: Megacystis-microcolon-intestinal hypoperistalsis syndrome: A cause of intestinal obstruction in the newborn period. *J. Pediatr. Surg.* 12:1063–1065, 1977.
2. Angerpointner T.A., Weitz H., Haas R.J., et al.: Intestinal leiomyosarcoma in childhood—case report and review of the literature. *J. Pediatr. Surg.* 16:491–495, 1981.
3. Blackburn W.W., Filston H.C.: Common symptoms in children: Routine illness or abdominal lymphoma? *Am. J. Surg.* 130:539–543, 1975.
3a. Blain A. III, Kennedy J.D., Calihan R.J., et al.: Effect of penicillin in experimental intestinal obstruction. *Arch. Surg.* 53:378, 1946.
4. Braun P., Dion Y.: Intestinal stenosis following seat belt injury. *J. Pediatr. Surg.* 8:549–550, 1973.
5. Cook R.C.M., Rickham P.P.: Neonatal intestinal obstruction due to milk curds. *J. Pediatr. Surg.* 4:599–605, 1969.
6. Dolan T.F., Touloukian R.J.: Familial meconium ileus not associated with cystic fibrosis. *J. Pediatr. Surg.* 6:821–824, 1974.
7. Emanuel B., Gault J., Sanson J.: Neonatal intestinal obstruction due to absence of intestinal musculature: A new entity. *J. Pediatr. Surg.* 2:332–335, 1967.
8. Esscher T.: Preduodenal portal vein—a cause of intestinal obstruction? *J. Pediatr. Surg.* 5:609–612, 1980.
9. Faulk D.L., Amuras S., Gardner G.D., et al.: A familial visceral myopathy. *Ann. Intern. Med.* 89:600–606, 1978.
10. Festen C.: Postoperative small bowel obstruction in infants and children. *Ann. Surg.* 196:580–583, 1982.
11. Harris B.H., Boles E.T. Jr.: Intestinal lesions in chronic granulomatous disease of childhood. *J. Pediatr. Surg.* 8:955–956, 1973.
12. Humphry A., Mancer K., Stephens C.A.: Obstructive circular-muscle defect in the small bowel in a one-year-old child. *J. Pediatr. Surg.* 15:197–198, 1980.
13. Janik J.S., Ein S.H., Filler R.M., et al.: An assessment of the surgical treatment of adhesive small bowel obstruction in infants and children. *J. Pediatr. Surg.* 16:225–229, 1981.
14. Kleinhaus S., Cohen M.I., Boley S.J.: Vitelline artery and vein remnants as a cause of intestinal obstruction. *J. Pediatr. Surg.* 9:295–299, 1974.
15. Luchtman M., Berant M., Assa J.: Transomental strangulation. *J. Pediatr. Surg.* 13:439–440, 1978.
16. Marcinski A., Wermenski K., Swiatkowska J., et al.: Intestinal obstruction as a late complication in roentgen therapy of Wilms' tumor. *Z. Kinderchir.* 29:375–377, 1980 (abstr., *J. Pediatr. Surg.* 17:221, 1981).
17. Mjolnerod O.K., Kluge T.: Megaduodenum (familial occurrence of the megaduodenum syndrome with primary degeneration of duodenal muscle layers. *Z. Kinderchir.* 8:53–61, 1970 (abstr., *J. Pediatr. Surg.* 5:487–488, 1970).
18. O'Neill J.A., Grosfeld J.L.: Intestinal malfunction after antenatal exposure of viscera. *Am. J. Surg.* 127:129–132, 1974.
19. Patton J.J., Moore T.C.: Massive megacolon and mega-ileum in childhood due to tuberculous stenosis of the ascending colon. *Surgery* 67:513–518, 1970.
20. Rubin S.Z., Ayalon A., Berlatzky Y.: The simultaneous occurrence of paraduodenal and paracecal herniae presenting with volvulus of the intervening bowel. *J. Pediatr. Surg.* 11:205–208, 1976.
21. Schärli A.F., Meier-Ruge W.: Localized and disseminated forms of neuronal intestinal dysplasia mimicking Hirschsprung's disease. *J. Pediatr. Surg.* 16:164–170, 1981.
22. Schwartz M.Z., Hayden C.K., Richardson C.J., et al.: A prospective evaluation of intestinal stenosis following necrotizing enterocolitis. *J. Pediatr. Surg.* 17:764–770, 1982.
23. Schwartz M.Z., Richardson C.J., Hayden C.K., et al.: Intestinal stenosis following successful medical management of necrotizing enterocolitis. *J. Pediatr. Surg.* 15:890–899, 1980.
24. Shaw A., Shaffer H., Teja K., et al.: A perspective for pediatric surgeons: Chronic idiopathic intestinal pseudoobstruction. *J. Pediatr. Surg.* 14:719–727, 1979.
25. Shigemoto H., Endo S., Isomoto T., et al.: Neonatal meconium obstruction in the ileum without mucoviscidosis. *J. Pediatr. Surg.* 13:475–479, 1978.
26. Sims D.G., Chamberlain J.: Small bowel obstruction following the insertion of a ventriculoperitoneal shunt. *J. R. Coll. Surg. Edinb.* 21:109–111, 1976.
27. Tal Y., Berger A., Abrahamson J., et al.: Intestinal obstruction caused by primary adhesions due to familial Mediterranean fever. *J. Pediatr. Surg.* 15:186–187, 1980.
28. Touloukian R.: Miscellaneous causes of small bowel obstruction, in Ravitch M.M., Welch K.J., Benson C.D. et al. (eds.): *Pediatric Surgery,* ed. 3. Chicago, Year Book Medical Publishers, 1979, pp. 960–964.
29. Willwerth B.M., Zollinger R.M. Jr., Izant R.J. Jr.: Congenital mesocolic (paraduodenal) hernia: Embryologic basis of repair. *Am. J. Surg.* 128:358–361, 1974.

91 STEPHEN L. GANS

Gastrointestinal Endoscopy

IN THE PAST DECADE, trials with prototype instruments demonstrated the value of flexible endoscopy of the gastrointestinal tract in infants and children.[2] Recently, second- and third-generation endoscopes have been developed, and their use has been firmly established. In the upper GI tract, they have been particularly useful in the diagnosis of bleeding conditions and in the differential diagnosis of ulcers. An extended dimension of the new instruments is found in the technique of cannulating the ampulla of Vater for endoscopic retrograde cholangiopancreatography (ERCP). With the development of the flexible colonoscope, the advantages of endoscopy, previously limited to the sigmoid, have been extended all the way to the cecum and terminal ileum, including biopsy of tumors and removal of polyps. The historic background and optical-mechanical principles of these instruments and procedures are described elsewhere.[2]

There are a large number of flexible fiber endoscopes available with varying capabilities and advantages.[1] Selection is particularly important for endoscopy in children, because the restriction in outer diameter of the instrument poses problems. Flexibility and light weight are particularly important in infants and children. The bending tip is provided with two-way or four-way control, and the facility in directing the tip is important. The bending angle and length of the bending segment affect retrograde vision and adaptation to the narrow curves in an infant's stomach and duodenum. Sharpness of vision is directly related to the quality and number of fibers. The ease and capability of aspiration, insufflation, irrigation, biopsy, and the use of other accessories can make the difference between a short, successful procedure and a long, frustrating one.

RADIOLOGY VS. ENDOSCOPY.—Radiology and endoscopy are complementary techniques, the former better demonstrating the topographic relations of the organs under almost physiologic conditions, and the latter providing a more accurate assessment of mucosal lesions and the added possibility of taking tissue samples for biopsy or removing the lesion. The sequence priority, or choice of method, depends on the problem being investigated.

PREPARATION, SEDATION, AND ANESTHESIA.—For diagnosis in small infants, light sedation or no sedation may be adequate. However, as in all endoscopy, complete resuscitation equipment must be on hand to deal with problems such as apnea or laryngospasm. Some procedures, in well-selected children, may be done with sedation only. The surroundings should be pleasant, parents permitted to stand by, and the patient well prepared psychologically. Occasionally, a child may even wish to assist in passing the scope and to look into the eyepiece of a teaching attachment.[1, 5]

In most pediatric centers, general anesthesia is preferred for most diagnostic gastrointestinal endoscopy; the final choice may depend on the availability of adequate instruments, the experience of the endoscopist, and the personal preference of the physician or patient. All agree that painful or delicate procedures in infants and children should be done under general anesthesia.

Gastroduodenoscopy

Indications

Hematemesis and/or melena, unexplained abdominal pain or vomiting, evaluation and biopsy of tumor, and removal of foreign bodies are the principal reasons for endoscopic examination of the stomach and duodenum. Radiologic contrast studies of the gastrointestinal tract are best performed before endoscopy, except in patients with bleeding problems.

The causes of upper GI tract bleeding in children include esophageal varices, esophagitis, Mallory-Weiss syndrome, acute gastritis, peptic ulcer of the stomach (Fig 91–1) or duodenum, angiomata, polyps, and tumors, such as lymphoma. Most of these lesions produce mucosal defects and can be more accurately diagnosed by endoscopy than by contrast radiologic studies. When the cause of abdominal pain and/or bleeding cannot be diagnosed by the usual examinations, endoscopy may demonstrate a missed peptic ulcer or one of the other lesions mentioned above. The importance of evaluation and biopsy of a tumor is evident. Most foreign bodies pass spontaneously, but when abdominal pain or bleeding demands action, the foreign body can sometimes be removed with an endoscope and snare.

Table 91–1 outlines our experience with gastrointestinal endoscopy.

TABLE 91–1.—GASTROINTESTINAL
ENDOSCOPY (109 EXAMINATIONS)

PROCEDURE AND LESIONS DIAGNOSED	NO.
Gastroduodenoscopy	
Esophageal varices	14
Esophagitis	36
Mallory-Weiss syndrome	2
Acute gastritis	6
Duodenitis	2
Peptic ulcer (gastric or duodenal)	4
Angioma	1
Polyp	1
Tumor	
Benign	1
Malignant	2
Foreign body	4
Trauma (esophagus, stomach, or duodenum)	3
ERCP	
Obstructive jaundice	1
Hemobilia	1
Recurrent pancreatitis	2
Colonoscopy	
Inflammatory bowel disease	12
Polyp	14
Hemangioma	2
Foreign body	1

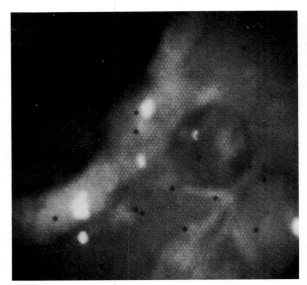

Fig 91–1.—Circular gastric ulcer in a 12-month-old child with repeated hematemesis and a "negative" contrast study.

Technique

For safe and successful gastroduodenoscopy, extended training, experience, patience, gentleness, and good eye-hand coordination are needed. Teaching attachments, auxiliary eyepieces, and capacity for photographic documentation are now available for all endoscopes.

A bite mouthpiece is inserted between the teeth and, under visual control, the tip of the endoscope is introduced smoothly and gently into the esophagus. After examination of the entire length of the esophagus, the tip is cautiously passed into the stomach, using air insufflation. Beginning with retrograde inspection of the cardia and esophageal orifice, the stomach is systematically examined throughout, down to the antrum. With the pylorus in view, the instrument is advanced into the duodenum. Knowledge of anatomy of the duodenum allows appropriate orientation and manipulation around its bends and curves. Biopsy and photography are done for documentation of lesions as needed. Re-examination can be done during withdrawal of the instrument. Polypectomy and foreign body removal are rare procedures. Clinical use of lasers through the instrument channel, for treatment of bleeding lesions, is presently being investigated.[4]

Endoscopic Retrograde Cholangiopancreatography (ERCP)

Technique

This procedure is best performed with a side-viewing endoscope. Because such an instrument is not available in pediatric sizes, experience in this field is limited mostly to older children. Huchzermeyer, however, has reported his experience in 36 patients ranging in age from 6 weeks to 18 years.[3] Whichever endoscope is used, the instrument is advanced into the duodenum as described above, and the papilla identified and cannulated. If the opening is too small to be cannulated, the catheter is placed onto it. Contrast medium is instilled, the examiner watching the screen continuously. Manipulation and probing are helpful in filling preferentially the bile duct or pancreatic duct (Figs 91–2 and 91–3). With improvement of instruments, this procedure should become more feasible in smaller patients.

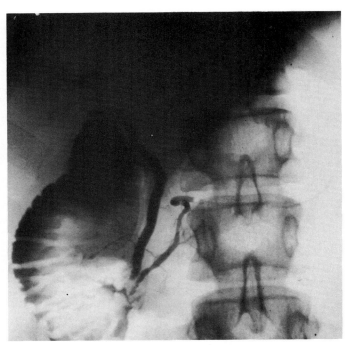

Fig 91–2.—Normal cholangiopancreatogram in a 7-year-old child. Note narrow common duct and hepatic ducts, fine branching of the intrahepatic bile ducts; filling of the gallbladder via the cystic duct; and delicate duct of Santorini. (From Huchzermeyer,[3] with permission.)

Indications

ERCP should be considered only after other diagnostic studies have proved inconclusive. The procedure is most commonly done for difficult biliary tract diagnosis with obstructive jaundice, acute recurrent and chronic pancreatitis, suspected hemobilia, and diagnosis of pancreatic anomalies or rupture (from blunt abdominal trauma). It is contraindicated in patients with acute pancreatitis, pseudocysts of the pancreas, and acute cholangitis (see Table 91–1).

Colonoscopy

Indications

Bleeding from the bowel is a major indication for colonoscopy. Children tolerate rectosigmoid examination better with a flexible scope than with a rigid one. Complete colonoscopy is much more difficult than barium enema but confirms the diagnosis of polyps (Fig 91–4) more effectively than radiologic methods, and the polyps can be expeditiously removed at the same time. Hemangiomas and other tumors may be visualized. Bleeding due to inflammatory bowel disease is appropriately demonstrated, and biopsy can be carried out as required (see Table 91–1).

Diarrhea of abnormally long duration and crampy abdominal pain merit at least limited colonoscopy. If inflammatory bowel disease is found, it can be evaluated by inspection and biopsy and the results of treatment monitored.

Finally, colonoscopy serves as a confirmation of lesions found by x-ray, or may serve to dismiss them.

Technique

Babies and small children are usually examined on their backs, and older children are more comfortable in the left lateral (Sims) position. The instrument is passed gently at all times, coordinating eye and hand manipulation, alternately advancing and retest-

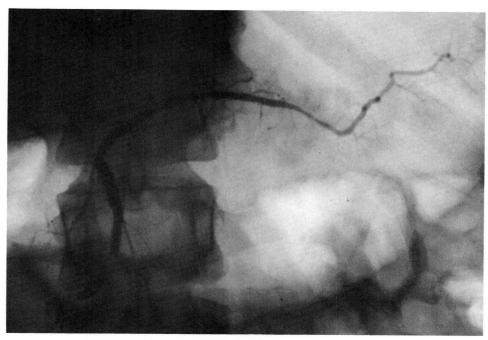

Fig 91–3.—Normal pancreatic duct system in a 9-year-old child (duct of Wirsung, duct of Santorini, and numerous pancreatic branches). (From Huchzermeyer,[3] with permission.)

ing, turning and twisting, steering the instrument with direct vision of the lumen. Air insufflation should be used with judgment to prevent overdistention of the bowel. Fluoroscopy with image intensification is sometimes valuable, particularly in the early stages of one's experience with this procedure. In some instances, the scope can be passed all the way around to the cecum, but this is not always possible and advancement may have to be stopped short of this. The techniques of biopsy, polypectomy, and electrosurgery are comparable to those employed in adult sigmoidoscopy.

Contraindications and Complications

When radiologic or initial-stage direct examination suggest that the bowel might be perforated during the procedure (e.g.,

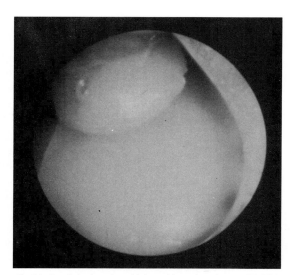

Fig 91–4.—Colonic polyp with broad base in a 4-year-old child.

in cases of deep ulceration, acute fistulation, toxic megacolon, or peritonitis), initiation or continuation of colonoscopy is contraindicated. Perforation is rare in the hands of an experienced endoscopist when these limitations are observed. However, perforation or bleeding from a polypectomy does occur in a small percentage of patients in even the most experienced hands, and must be watched for postoperatively in every infant or child undergoing colonoscopy.

Intraoperative Endoscopy

Under special circumstances, the use of flexible endoscopes, with the abdomen open, can be advantageous. Guided by the surgeon's hands, the end of the scope can be quickly and safely directed at specific targets, or can be passed far down into the upper intestine or far up into the large bowel and ileum. Thus, lesions can be examined and biopsy performed as indicated without opening the bowel, and specific indications for bowel surgery may be demonstrated. Such a combined approach can be planned in advance when there is a known lesion, or may be prompted when operation discloses a lesion. Finally, multiple, scattered polyps or a broad-based polyp may be more safely removed by endoscopy with an open abdomen, for assistance and support.

REFERENCES

1. Cadranel S., Rodesch P.: Fiberendoscopy of the upper gastrointestinal tract, in Gans S.L. (ed.): *Pediatric Endoscopy.* New York, Grune & Stratton, 1983, p. 69.
2. Gans S.L., Ament M., Christie D.L., et al.: Pediatric endoscopy with flexible fiberscopes. *J. Pediatr. Surg.* 10:375, 1975.
3. Huchzermeyer H.: Endoscopic retrograde cholangiopancreatography (ERCP), in Gans S.L. (ed.): *Pediatric Endoscopy.* New York, Grune & Stratton, 1983, p. 87.
4. Peterson W.L.: Laser therapy for bleeding peptic ulcer—a burning issue. *Gastroenterology* 83:485, 1982.
5. Williams C.B., Cadranel S.: Colonoscopy, in Gans S.L. (ed.): *Pediatric Endoscopy.* New York, Grune & Stratton 1983, p. 107.

92 ROBERT M. ARENSMAN

Gastrointestinal Bleeding

IN 1962, Rowena Spencer reported 476 cases of gastrointestinal bleeding in infants and children at Charity Hospital of Louisiana. She concluded that gastrointestinal bleeding was common in children and that the cause was usually diagnosed by careful history and physical examination.[19] Table 92–1 lists causes of gastrointestinal tract hemorrhage in children by age and frequency with which they are encountered. It is apparent that the most common causes of bleeding are benign problems for which good therapeutic modalities are now available. More recent experience in the pediatric surgical services in New Orleans continues to show a similar pattern for this manifestation, and the more widespread use of endoscopic investigations has facilitated rapid diagnosis.

Fortunately, most children with gastrointestinal bleeding do not present with massive hemorrhage. This allows the physician to assess carefully clues from the history and examination and correlate them with patient age and a likely diagnosis. In reviewing the current literature on upper and lower gastrointestinal bleeding in children, it seems appropriate to divide patients into four diagnostic age groups: (1) neonates, (2) infants aged 1 month to 1 year, (3) infants aged 1 year to 2 years, and (4) children older than 2 years.

Neonates

Common Causes of Bleeding

Upper
    Hemorrhagic disease
    Swallowed blood
    Gastritis
Lower
    Fissure
    Necrotizing enterocolitis
    Malrotation and volvulus

We often see children in the nursery or the neonatal intensive care unit for "coffee-ground" gastric aspirate or melena. Usually the amount of aspirate is small, disappears in less than 24 hours, and warrants only careful observation. Even this minor bleeding is sufficient reason to check that the newborn received vitamin K, however we have yet to see a case of gastrointestinal hemorrhage attributable to hemorrhagic disease of the newborn. On occasion, when there is an unusually large neonatal gastric aspirate that is blood-tinged or "coffee-ground" in character,[2, 14] an Apt test is done to confirm swallowed maternal blood as the source.

In premature neonates or those whose delivery histories demonstrate stress, resuscitation, or low Apgar scores, upper gastrointestinal bleeding generally is assumed to represent peptic gastritis. Nasogastric suction, saline lavage, and antacids in small amounts are usually sufficient treatment to clear the aspirates and obviate further evaluation unless bleeding persists or worsens.

Rarely, continued or massive hematemesis heralds peptic ulcer disease. Pediatric endoscopy now allows us to confirm this diagnosis even in children weighing as little as 5 or 6 kg. The same regimen is initially employed when endoscopy confirms an ulcer, but, if treatment is unsuccessful, operation appropriate to the lesion is mandatory, i.e., gastric resection, vagotomy and pyloroplasty, or, rarely, antrectomy and vagotomy.

When evidence of gastrointestinal bleeding occurs rectally, the three most likely diagnoses are fissure, necrotizing enterocolitis, or malrotation with midgut volvulus. Fissures produce a bright-red blood that streaks the stool or occurs in small spots on the diaper, while necrotizing enterocolitis or malrotation produce darker, often maroon or purple stools with varying amounts of mucus.

Simple anal examination, occasionally performed with a nasal speculum, confirms a fissure in ano, which is the most common lesion producing gastrointestinal bleeding in infants under 1 year of age. Further tests are unnecessary, and successful treatment in almost all cases includes stool softeners, rectal dilatation, and topical creams.[3]

Necrotizing enterocolitis in most neonates is suggested by the history. Roentgenograms and, more recently, sonograms[7] confirm the diagnosis and are urgently required so that aggressive medical resuscitation and therapy can be instituted. Seventy percent of these patients recover with antibiotics, bowel rest, and total parenteral nutrition. Recurrent bleeding after apparent recovery can either herald a second occurrence of the disease or can accompany a postnecrotizing enterocolitis stricture. A barium enema may be required for delineation if the child's physical condition permits.

The sudden onset of melena with bilious vomiting in an apparently healthy child, often without abdominal distention, suggests malrotation and midgut volvulus. The early examination is generally negative. Barium enema should be performed immediately to confirm the malrotation and should be followed by mandatory emergency laparotomy so that midgut infarction is avoided, or resected if already present.

Sherman and Clatworthy,[18] as well as Levene,[11] reported that

TABLE 92–1.—CAUSES OF GASTROINTESTINAL
TRACT HEMORRHAGE

DISORDER	PATIENTS <1 YR (N = 158)	PATIENTS >1 YR (N = 119)
Anal fissure	68	15
Intussusception	50	11
Gangrenous bowel	14	0
Duodenal ulcer	10	7
Gastric ulcer	8	9
Meckel's diverticulum	6	2
Ileal hematoma	1	0
Duplication—colon	1	0
Colonic polyp	0	59
Esophageal varices	0	11
Ulcerative colitis	0	3
Regional enteritis	0	1
Hemorrhoids	0	1

Adapted from Spencer R.[19]

at least 50% of neonates with gastrointestinal bleeding have an "unexplained" cause. Sherman and Clatworthy further reported that none of 94 neonates with hematemesis (50%), hematochezia (35%), and melena (17%) required urgent surgical intervention.

Infants 1 Month to 1 Year of Age

Common Causes of Bleeding

Upper
  Esophagitis
  Gastritis
Lower
  Intussusception
  Gangrenous bowel

As children pass beyond the neonatal period, the common sites of gastrointestinal bleeding shift. In children older than 1 month, the two most common causes are esophagitis, usually secondary to reflux, or peptic disease.

The extensive literature on gastroesophageal reflux documents how common this problem is in infants.[13] Johnson and Jolley[9] reported 107 children requiring surgical intervention over a nine-year period, while Tunell et al.[21] encountered 117 children who were operated on for reflux during a 5-year span. In addition to barium esophagogram, a whole array of new tests is available to aid in the diagnosis of esophageal reflux. These include esophagoscopy, intraluminal pH monitoring, esophageal manometrics, and technetium reflux studies.

Bleeding associated with reflux esophagitis can usually be halted by use of antacids in conjunction with thickened feedings and the use of a chalasia board. We have had no patient require an antireflux operation solely to control continued blood loss from uncontrolled esophagitis. In patients usually stressed by failure to thrive and esophagitis, gastroduodenoscopy may reveal concomitant gastric and duodenal erosion. Medical therapy may thus correct more than the esophageal erosions.

In this 1-month-to-1-year age group, hypertrophic pyloric stenosis occasionally causes blood-tinged vomitus.[20] Diagnosis can easily be made on the basis of age, sex, presence of nonbilious vomiting, and the characteristic abdominal mass. Pyloromyotomy corrects the problem and stops the bleeding.

From 6 to 18 months of age, the probable cause of lower gastrointestinal bleeding is intussusception. If the baby has episodic abdominal pain and a sausage-shaped mass, the diagnosis is easily made, but many of these children have minor and irregular pain and no abdominal findings. Venous hypertension in the intussusception results in loss of blood and mucus that produces currant-jelly stools; however, bloody stools from bright red to black are seen almost as frequently. Suspicion based on the infant's age and presentation warrants barium enema diagnosis and treatment. In 60–80% of cases, the intussusception is thus reduced by hydrostatic pressure (see Chap. 88).

The second most common cause of rectal blood loss in this age group is gangrenous bowel. The etiology of the gangrene varies but can usually be attributed to some form of volvulus—either malrotation with volvulus, segmental small-bowel volvulus, Meckel's diverticulum with volvulus, or, rarely, sigmoid volvulus. The rectal bleeding varies from melena to hematochezia. Many of these children when first seen are profoundly ill with dehydration, abdominal distention, masses, and, often, free perforation. If the child is seen early, proctoscopy and barium enema can help diagnose complete malrotation or sigmoid volvulus. More commonly, segmental volvulus and twisting around a Meckel's diverticulum are findings on laparotomy performed for an acute surgical abdomen or persistent small-bowel obstruction.

Infants 1 Year to 2 Years of Age

Common Causes of Bleeding

Upper
  Peptic disease
Lower
  Polyps
  Meckel's diverticulum

After the age of 1 year, peptic ulcer disease is the common cause of hematemesis. Most of these ulcers, gastric or duodenal, occur in children experiencing other problems, such as burns (Curling's ulcer), head trauma (Cushing's ulcer), malignant disease (leukemias), or sepsis. Nevertheless, our surgical service sees two to three children each year with primary duodenal ulcer disease presenting as hematemesis and partial gastric outlet obstruction. Significant hematemesis warrants immediate endoscopy under sedation and topical anesthesia. It has both a higher accuracy of diagnosis and lower incidence of erroneous findings than radiography.

Therapy in children is similar to that in adults and involves suction, antacids, and H_2 antagonists. When there is obstruction or persistent bleeding requiring transfusion, operation is indicated.

Sources of rectal blood in this age group are polyps and bleeding Meckel's diverticulum. The polyps are overwhelmingly of the juvenile type. Most occur in the rectosigmoid and result in painless bowel movements streaked with fresh blood. Proctoscopy can demonstrate many of these polyps, which can be eliminated by simple snare removal and silver nitrate cauterization of the polyp base. This procedure can be done as an outpatient or office procedure, with sedation in some younger patients. Other polyps above the sigmoid area can be demonstrated by colonoscopy or air-contrast barium enema. We prefer colonoscopy, since other polyps can be removed at the same time. Parents seem to reject the thought of allowing polyps to remain and continue bleeding, even when informed that many of these lesions will spontaneously slough. Colonoscopy and biopsy also allow identification of adenomatous polyps (present in about 3% of children with polypoid lesions),[2] which may herald familial polyposis.

Meckel's diverticulum with heterotrophic gastric mucosa results in an ileal ulcer opposite or adjacent to the orifice of the diverticulum. Erosion into a small arteriole leads to painless, brisk, red rectal bleeding.

Technetium scanning for the aberrant gastric mucosa has given results with an overall accuracy of 90% and is generally the first diagnostic test, since the scan must be done before introduction of barium.[6, 15–17] If scanning fails to document the Meckel's diverticulum, other diagnostic tests will probably be tests of exclusion. The diverticulum is seldom seen on small-bowel follow-through or with ileal reflux on barium enema. The patient's age and a large-volume fresh-blood loss suggest the need for exploration even without a definite preoperative diagnosis. Resection of the diverticulum and the ulcer with appropriate closure (wedge or end-to-end) is curative.

Children Older Than 2 Years

Common Causes of Bleeding

Upper
  Varices
Lower
  Polyps
  Inflammatory bowel disease
  Trauma
  All other lesions (Fig 92–1)[2, 5, 6, 12, 18, 19, 22]

Portal vein thrombosis becomes apparent as children approach

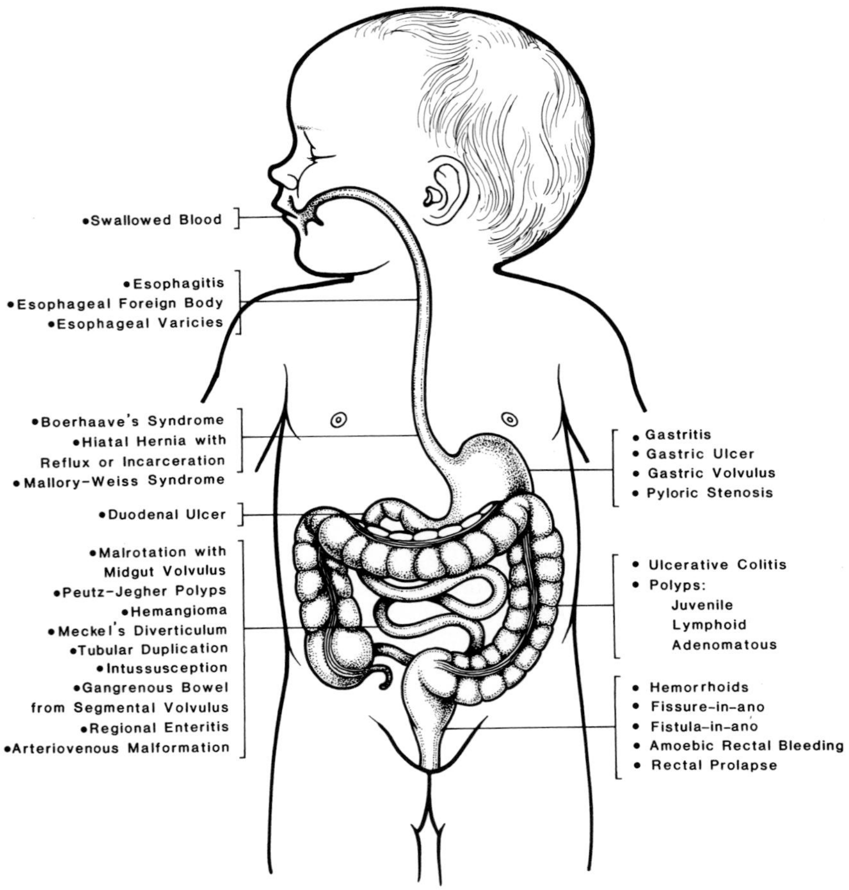

•Swallowed Blood

•Esophagitis
•Esophageal Foreign Body
•Esophageal Varicies

•Boerhaave's Syndrome
•Hiatal Hernia with
Reflux or Incarceration
•Mallory-Weiss Syndrome

•Duodenal Ulcer

•Malrotation with
Midgut Volvulus
•Peutz-Jegher Polyps
•Hemangioma
•Meckel's Diverticulum
•Tubular Duplication
•Intussusception
•Gangrenous Bowel
from Segmental Volvulus
•Regional Enteritis
•Arteriovenous Malformation

• Gastritis
• Gastric Ulcer
• Gastric Volvulus
• Pyloric Stenosis

• Ulcerative Colitis
• Polyps:
Juvenile
Lymphoid
Adenomatous

• Hemorrhoids
• Fissure-in-ano
• Fistula-in-ano
• Amoebic Rectal Bleeding
• Rectal Prolapse

Fig 92–1.—Causes of gastrointestinal bleeding in children. Fortunately, the most common lesions are relatively benign and allow careful evaluation with therapy designed specifically to correct the abnormality encountered.

2–3 years of age. Massive hematemesis is often the first symptom. On more careful examination, these children are found to have splenomegaly, prominent abdominal veins, and, occasionally, hemorrhoids. Presentation of portal hypertension leads to esophagoscopy or esophagogram, which documents varices. Since liver function is preserved and clotting function is normal for most of these children, the bleeding, although heavy, is controllable. With periodic transfusions and sclerotherapy, most of these children can be managed until varices are spontaneously decompressed by portal vein transformation or the child has grown to a size at which portosystemic shunting can be achieved with reasonable expectations of long-term patency.

The most common etiology of rectal bleeding in children over 2 years of age continues to be the juvenile polyp. Not until the teenage years do polyps cease to be a major cause of bleeding. Appropriate diagnostic tests are chosen on the basis of the child's history and physical examination. Because of the frequency and ease of foreign travel today, one must consider such causes of bleeding as amebic and helminthic infestation.[5, 10] In choosing appropriate diagnostic studies, a careful history and examination are crucial, but one should consider gastroduodenoscopy and colonoscopy early[1, 4, 8] because these provide direct observation, are fast, are frequently more accurate than radiography, and allow photographic documentation and biopsy.

When all of these methods—history, examination, diagnostic testing—fail, one faces the dilemma of recommending operation for severe and persistent gastrointestinal bleeding. Unlike patients with chronic abdominal pain, in whom exploratory laparotomy is fraught with great frustration and few findings, at least

half of the children with persistent bleeding have a demonstrable lesion[14] detected at operation. Although gastrointestinal bleeding is only rarely massive and life-threatening in children, patients with persistent, undiagnosed bleeding should be considered for celiotomy and careful intra-abdominal search.

REFERENCES

1. Akasaka Y., Misaki F., Miyaoka T., et al.: Endoscopy in pediatric patients with upper gastrointestinal bleeding. *Gastrointest. Endosc.* 23:199–200, 1977.
2. Andrassy R.J.: Surgical causes of gastrointestinal bleeding in neonates and children. *Pediatr. Emer. Med.* (in press).
3. Berman W.F., Holtzapple P.G.: Gastrointestinal hemorrhage. *Pediatr. Clin. North Am.* 23:885–895, 1975.
4. Chang M., Wang T., Hsu J., et al.: Endoscopic examination of the upper gastrointestinal tract in infancy. *Gastrointest. Endosc.* 29:15–17, 1983.
5. Dalal S.J., Dabhoi-wala N.F.: Rectal bleeding in infancy and childhood: A review of 100 cases. *Indian Pediatr.* 4:37–49, 1967.
6. Duszynski D.O., Jewett T.C., Allen J.A.: ^{99m}Tc Na pertechnetate scanning of the abdomen with particular reference to small bowel pathology. *Am. J. Roentgenol. Radium Ther. Nucl. Med.* 113:258–262, 1971.
7. Goldsmith J.P., Merritt C.R.B., Sharp M.J.: Ultrasound findings in infants with necrotizing enterocolitis. Presented at the 27th Annual Scientific Assembly of the Southern Medical Association, Baltimore, Md., 1983 (submitted for publication).
8. Holgersen L.O., Mossberg S.M., Miller R.E.: Colonoscopy for rectal bleeding in childhood. *J. Pediatr. Surg.* 13:83–85, 1978.
9. Johnson D., Jolley S.G.: Gastroesophageal reflux in infants and children. *Surg. Clin. North Am.* 61:1101–1115, 1981.
10. Kalani B.P., Sogani K.C.: Rectal bleeding in children. *Indian Pediatr.* 14:895–897, 1977.

11. Levene M.I.: Rectal bleeding in the first month of life. *Postgrad. Med. J.* 55:22, 1979.
12. Raffensperger J.G., Luck S.R.: Gastrointestinal bleeding in children. *Surg. Clin. North Am.* 56:413–424, 1976.
13. Randolph J.: Experience with the Nissen fundoplication for gastroesophageal reflux in infants and children. *Ann. Surg.* 198:579–584, 1983.
14. Rittershofer C.R.: Rectal bleeding in children. *Postgrad. Med.* 39:431–437, 1966.
15. Sfakianakis G.N., Conway J.J.: Detection of ectopic gastric mucosa in Meckel's diverticulum and in other aberrations by scintigraphy. I. Pathophysiology and 10-year clinical experience. *J. Nucl. Med.* 22:647–654, 1981.
16. Sfakianakis G.N., Conway J.J.: Detection of ectopic gastric mucosa in Meckel's diverticulum and in other aberrations by scintigraphy. II. Indications and methods—a 10-year experience. *J. Nucl. Med.* 22:732–738, 1981.
17. Sfakianakis G.N., Haase G.M.: Abdominal scintigraphy for ectopic gastric mucosa: A retrospective analysis of 143 studies. *AJR* 138:7–12, 1982.
18. Sherman N.J., Clatworthy H.W. Jr.: Gastrointestinal bleeding in neonates: A study of 94 cases. *Surgery* 62:614–619, 1967.
19. Spencer R.: Gastrointestinal hemorrhage in infancy and childhood: 476 cases. *Pediatr. Surg.* 55:718–734, 1964.
20. Spitz L., Batcup G.: Haematemesis in infantile hypertrophic pyloric stenosis: The source of the bleeding. *Br. J. Surg.* 66:827–828, 1979.
21. Tunell W.P., Smith E.I., Carson J.A.: Gastroesophageal reflux in childhood: The dilemma of surgical success. *Ann. Surg.* 197:560–565, 1983.
22. Yu P.P., White D., Iannuccilli E.A.: The Mallory-Weiss syndrome in the pediatric population. *Rhode Island Med. J.* 65:73–74, 1982.

93 Diller B. Groff, III
Foreign Bodies and Bezoars

THE NATURAL PROCLIVITY for small children to put things in their mouths frequently results in swallowing of the objects. The peak age incidence for such ingestion is between 6 months and 3 years. Adults often contribute to foreign-body ingestion by thoughtlessly giving infants small objects to play with; older children usually swallow foreign bodies accidentally.[1]

Diagnosis

Older children usually report swallowing a foreign body, while adults often witness the ingestion by infants and small children. If the ingestion is unwitnessed, dysphagia, excess drooling, or complaints of substernal discomfort may be the first signs of foreign-body ingestion. Most symptomatic patients have the foreign body lodged at one of three locations in the esophagus: the cricopharyngeus, the middle third where the left main-stem bronchus impinges on the esophagus, or at the esophagogastric junction. After a patient has had an esophageal operation, particularly for correction of esophageal atresia, the site of the anastomosis, where the abnormally functioning lower esophageal segment begins, is usually the point of obstruction. If the foreign body is opaque, it can be followed easily by roentgenograms, remembering to include the pharynx and the rectum in the x-ray field. Finding radiolucent objects in the gastrointestinal system is not as difficult as in the air passages because barium or other contrast materials can be used to outline the object (Fig 93–1). The use of swallowed cotton to outline the object is not recommended because the cotton itself may interfere with subsequent endoscopic removal.

Treatment

Foreign bodies in the esophagus must be removed because of the hazard of esophageal obstruction and subsequent aspiration, and the great danger of eventual erosion through the esophagus. The Foley catheter technique of removal with fluoroscopic control is effective for smooth objects, such as coins.[15] If esophagoscopy is the method of choice, it should be performed by experienced endoscopists under general anesthesia working with a coordinated team of anesthesiologists, nurses, and radiologists.

After a foreign body has passed through the esophagus into the stomach, over 95% will pass through the entire gastrointestinal tract without incident.[8] As long as the patient is asymptomatic, repeat roentgenograms every 7 days should be performed to monitor passage (Fig 93–2). Management of an ingested object that has reached the stomach requires analysis of its configuration. With the exception of alkaline batteries, round or smooth objects, such as coins and stones, can be observed for weeks, since they seldom perforate and eventually pass through the gastrointestinal tract. Long or sharp objects often get stuck in the duodenum, and sharp objects perforate more frequently if lodged in one location for many days. After the foreign body leaves the stomach, it is most likely to impact in the C loop of the duodenum (Fig 93–3) or at the ligament of Treitz. Once past the ligament of Treitz, there is usually clear sailing through the rest of the gastrointestinal tract. In the rectum, some objects assume a transverse position and become impacted at the anus. Rarely, a foreign body enters a Meckel's diverticulum or the appendix and becomes embedded.[19]

If the foreign body is not out of the stomach in 4 weeks, it should be removed with fiberoptic endoscopy.[6, 7] General anesthesia is our choice because the patient remains still while the object is manipulated within the stomach and pulled back out of the esophagus. A contrast upper GI series should be performed before any endoscopy or celiotomy, and this examination itself often causes the object to move out of the stomach or from its lodged position in the small bowel. If any object remains in a fixed position in the duodenum or the small intestine for more than 7 days and cannot be mobilized with cathartics or a GI series, it should be removed operatively. If the object has not moved from the colon after 7 days, enemas should be used to try to evacuate it, and these usually are successful.[10] Foreign bodies impacted in the rectum can be removed by endoscopy through a dilated anal sphincter. Patients who develop fever, vomiting, hematemesis, or bloody stools should be examined immediately;

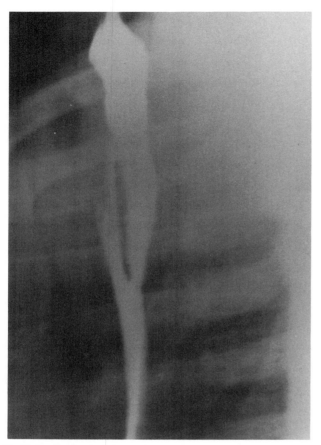

Fig 93–1.—Foreign body in esophagus. Two-year-old with dysphagia had a radiolucent poker chip in the esophagus, as demonstrated by esophagogram in an oblique view. This is readily removed by the balloon catheter technique.

patients with signs of peritonitis or intestinal obstruction should be operated on to remove the foreign body, repair any perforation, and remove sources of entrapment such as antral webs, a Meckel's diverticulum, or the appendix.[12, 19]

Alkaline Disk Batteries

Modern technology has developed the alkaline disk battery, which is easily ingested by children. Reports of perforation within the gastrointestinal system associated with leakage of the alkaline battery contents have made some surgeons recommend aggressive operative removal of all batteries.[18, 19] However, our experience and that of others indicates that a less aggressive approach can be used if there is careful follow-up of the patient.[11, 16]

Recommended Management of Disk Battery Ingestion

1. A child who has ingested an alkaline battery should be given nothing, including emetics, by mouth. Emergency roentgenographic examination from mouth to anus is performed.

2. If the battery is in the oropharynx or the esophagus, it must be removed. If the object has been lodged in the esophagus less than 24 hours and the child is asymptomatic, it can be removed by the Foley catheter technique with roentgenographic guidance. Endoscopic technique for removal is used for all other patients and can always be used instead of the Foley catheter technique.

3. After removal of the disk battery from the esophagus, observation for possible esophageal stenosis is necessary for the first 2–3 weeks. A follow-up esophagogram is not needed in the asymptomatic patient.

4. If the battery is in the stomach or farther along the gastrointestinal tract, and if roentgenograms indicate that the battery case is intact, it is safe to observe the patient as one would for coins and other smooth ingested objects. Cathartics, such as magnesium sulfate or magnesium citrate, may be administered to hasten the transit time. At anytime if the roentgenograms show the battery case to be broken, the battery should be removed operatively.

5. If the intact battery reaches the colon, enemas should be administered to hasten its passage. Stools should be carefully searched to determine that the battery has been passed. If, after 7 days, the battery has not been passed, a follow-up roentgenogram should be made. If the battery is still in the stomach, it is safer to remove it, as ulceration may be associated with abnormalities of the gastric outlet.[12] The battery should be removable by the use of flexible endoscopy, forceps, or snare.[6, 7]

6. If the battery fails to progress beyond a specific location in the small bowel and is in the same position for 5–6 days, cathartics should be administered. If the battery does not move, it should be removed operatively.

7. Any patient with an ingested battery in the gastrointestinal tract who becomes symptomatic, with signs of localized peritonitis or intestinal obstruction, should have the object removed.

Alkaline battery ingestion needs closer follow-up than that of other ingested foreign bodies; however, radical departure from the general principles applied to smooth ingested foreign objects is not necessary.

Bezoars

Most cat owners have found a hair ball, or trichobezoar, which their pet has regurgitated. In the past, these bezoars have been credited with being able to cure gastrointestinal illness. Two papers of Debakey and Ochsner, in which they reported over 303 patients, remain classics.[2, 3] They defined four types of bezoars: trichobezoar of human hair, phytobezoar of vegetable matter, trichophytobezoar, a combination of hair and vegetable matter, and concretions composed of ingested shellac. Contemporary bezoars include congealed formula curds, medication (Kayexalate), and peanuts.[5, 13, 14]

Most bezoars are trichobezoars and are associated with the patient's eating her own hair (90% of patients are female, usually teenaged). Interestingly, most emotionally disturbed patients who eat their hair do not have bezoars.[9] Symptoms are progressive and include a heavy feeling in the stomach, vomiting, inability to eat much, and consequent weight loss and inanition. Jaundice has been an associated finding,[17] and one patient was reported in whom death resulted from perforation and peritonitis while she was undergoing chemical treatment of a gastric trichobezoar.[4]

Physical examination reveals a moveable mass in the epigastrium and left upper quadrant. Upper GI series confirms the diagnosis (Fig 93–4,A). Rarely, a bezoar leaves the stomach and obstructs the small bowel (Fig 93–5).

Treatment of large bezoars is gastrotomy and removal of the mass. Occasionally, the hair ball extends out of the stomach and down through the length of the small intestine (Rapunzel syndrome) (see Fig 93–4,B). Treatment of small bezoars by enzymes such as those found in meat tenderizer (e.g., papain) can be successful, but great care must be used not to give the patient too much salt. Extraction by endoscopy has not been recorded, but this seems a reasonable approach for small gastric bezoars. Treatment of any underlying emotional disorder is important.

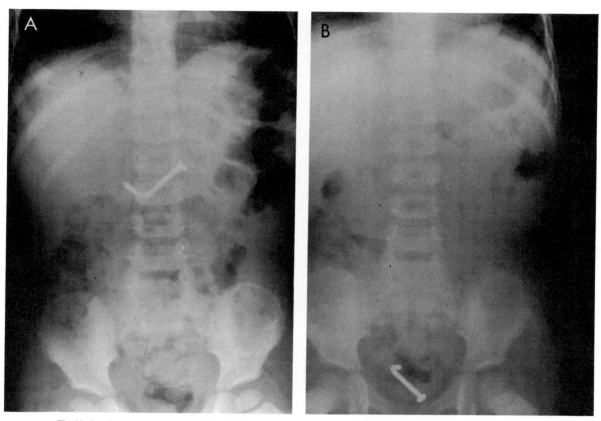

Fig 93–2.—Passage of large ingested foreign body. **A,** large nail ingested by a 4-year-old has reached the stomach. **B,** 7 days later, it is in the rectum and was subsequently passed in the stool.

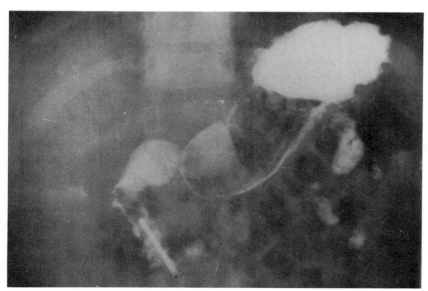

Fig 93–3.—Long rigid foreign body arrested in duodenum. Upper GI series shows a screwdriver impacted in the "C" loop of the duodenum, although it passed through the esophagus and the pylorus. It was removed operatively after 6 days.

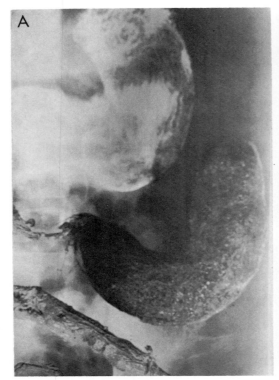

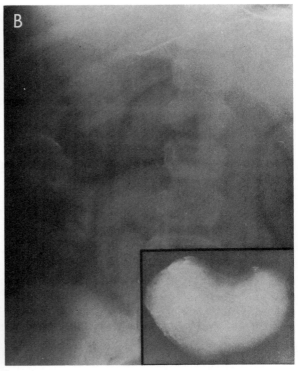

Fig 93–4.—Trichobezoars. **A,** large trichobezoar in the stomach, outlined by barium. The specimen recovered at operation is superimposed on the film. **B,** large trichobezoar with exceptionally long tail (Rapunzel syndrome) removed from the stomach of a 9-year-old girl nearly 4 years after any known or acknowledged trichophagia.

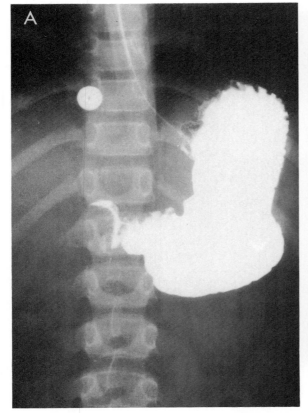

Fig 93–5.—**A,** 8-year-old girl with vomiting and total obstruction in the first portion of the duodenum, thought caused by a duodenal hematoma. **B,** 2 days later, a radiopaque foreign body is impacted in the small bowel. After enterotomy and removal, it was found to be a contrast-coated trichobezoar *(inset).*

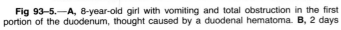

Summary

Removal of foreign bodies impacted in the esophagus is mandatory; however, judicial watchful waiting, cathartics, enemas, and radiographic contrast studies are usually all that is necessary if objects have reached the stomach. Confirmation of final passage, either by finding the object in the stools or by roentgenogram, is essential. Long, sharp, or pointed objects and alkaline disk batteries require special consideration and attention. Early endoscopic removal of ingested objects from the stomach may be justified; however, nonoperative treatment for the majority of ingested foreign bodies is recommended.

REFERENCES

1. Alexander W.J., Kadish J.A., Dunbar J.S.: Ingested foreign bodies in children, in Kaufmann H.J. (ed.): *Progress in Pediatric Radiology*, ed. 2. Chicago, Year Book Medical Publishers, 1969, pp. 256–285.
2. Debakey M., Ochsner A.: Bezoars and concretions. *Surgery* 4:934, 1938.
3. Debakey M., Ochsner A.: Bezoars and concretions. *Surgery* 5:132, 1939.
4. Deslypere J.P., Praet M., Verdonk G.: An unusual case of trichobezoar: The Rapunzel syndrome. *Am. J. Gastroenterol.* 77:467–470, 1982.
5. Duritz G., Oltorf C.: Lactobezoar formation associated with high-density caloric formula. *Pediatrics* 63:674–679, 1979.
6. Euler A.R.: How long should a foreign body stay in the stomach? *Pediatrics* 61:671, 1978.
7. Ghazi A., Tan S., Wolff W.I.: Pediatric fiberoptic instruments—application in removal of foreign body in children's stomachs. *N.Y. State J. Med.* 79:384–386, 1979.
8. Henderson F.F., Gaston E.A.: Ingested foreign body in the gastrointestinal tract. *Arch. Surg.* 36:66, 1938.
9. Hoyt C.S., Burke E.C., Hallenback G.A.: Trichobezoar. *Proc. Staff Meet. Mayo Clin.* 33:298–302, 1958.
10. Kulig K., Rumack C.M., Rumack B.H., et al.: Disk battery ingestion. *JAMA* 249:2502–2504, 1983.
11. Litovitz T.L.: Button battery ingestions. *JAMA* 249:2495–2500, 1983.
12. Mandell G.A., Rosenberg H.J., Schnaufer L.: Prolonged retention of foreign bodies in the stomach. *Pediatrics* 60:460–462, 1978.
13. Menke J.A., Stallworth R.E., Binstadt D.H., et al.: Medication bezoar in a neonate. *Am. J. Dis. Child.* 136:72–73, 1982.
14. Miller S.E., Cox J.A., Majeski J.A.: Acute intestinal obstruction caused by a peanut bezoar in a child. *S. Med. J.* 74:1554, 1981.
15. Nixon G.W.: Foley catheter method of esophageal foreign body removal: Extension of application. *AJR* 132:441–442, 1979.
16. Rumack B.H., Rumack C.M.: Disk battery ingestion. *JAMA* 249:2509–2511, 1983.
17. Schreiber H., Filston H.C.: Obstructive jaundice due to gastric trichobezoar. *J. Pediatr. Surg.* 11:103–104, 1976.
18. Votteler T.P., Nash J.C., Rutledge J.C.: The hazard of ingested alkaline disk batteries in children. *JAMA* 249:2504–2506, 1983.
19. Willis G.A., Ho W.C.: Perforation of a Meckel's diverticulum by an alkaline hearing aid battery. *Can. Med. Assoc. J.* 126:497–498, 1982.

94 Mark M. Ravitch

Duplications of the Gastrointestinal Tract

TERMINOLOGY.—We owe the widespread use of the term "duplications" to the influence of Ladd,[16] who, in 1937, stated, "The term duplications of the alimentary tract is used in the hope of simplifying the nomenclature of these conditions, which has become somewhat confused. The terms in use at the present time to describe these abnormalities are enteric cysts, enterogenous cysts, diverticula, giant diverticula, ileum duplex, jejunum duplex, unusual Meckel's diverticula, and so forth. As all of these names are used to describe the same condition, though occurring in different situations, it would seem desirable to apply one inclusive name." The consideration together of similar developmental anomalies in various parts of the alimentary tract has served a useful purpose. Most duplications might indeed best be called simply "enterogenous cysts," since in only a very special group of these lesions are they, in fact, attempts at doubling of the alimentary tract and therefore properly deserving of the name "duplications." The term is fixed in the literature, however, and not likely to be displaced unless unquestionably acceptable embryologic explanations for the various types lead to designations on the basis of their genesis.

Embryology

The suggestion of an earlier day that these cysts and malformations are developed from the diverticulum of Meckel has been discarded. The diverticulum of Meckel is antimesenteric, whereas these lesions are on the mesenteric border and usually between the leaves of the mesentery. Furthermore, lesions of the kind we are speaking of have been described in patients who had, in addition, typical Meckel's diverticula. Meckel's diverticulum is quite common; duplications are quite rare. It is worth remembering, however, that Meckel's diverticulum, representing the intestinal end of an omphalomesenteric duct and arising from an essentially fixed point in the midgut, often is partially or completely lined by gastric mucosa, which now finds itself at the level of the terminal ileum. The same "migration" of epithelial types occurs in some duplications.

One of the regularly repeated theories of the development of intestinal duplications is that attributed to Lewis and Thyng,[18] although their 1907–1908 paper, like the 1905 paper of Keibel,[13] simply states the embryologic fact without making clinical suggestions with respect to the possible significance of their observations, except in reference to intestinal diverticula. Lewis and Thyng[18] found in the fetal alimentary tract of pigs, rabbits, cats, and sheep, and in human embryos of 4–23 mm, tiny buds of intestinal epithelium protruding into the subepithelial connective tissue. These buds most often appeared as nodes or nodules and occasionally as diverticula.

Bremer,[4] expanding on this observation, stated that exceptionally an individual diverticulum may increase in size, become expanded at the distal end, and either remain connected with the lumen by a narrow pedicle or become separated as a closed cyst. By this time, the muscle layers of the intestinal wall are well established, so that expansion outward is limited by the inner circular muscle layer, and the diverticulum spreads in the lower submucosa, usually in an aboral direction, as noted by Lewis and Thyng. With further expansion the diverticulum may lift the outer layers to form a bulging protuberance of the intestinal wall;

more probably it will bulge inward, lifting the parent mucosa before it to form an intraintestinal cyst, which sometimes nearly fills the intestinal lumen. The expanding cyst or diverticulum is more likely to find a pathway through the inner muscle layer along one of the clefts by which the vessels make their way to supply the mucosa. Once outside the circular muscle, the cyst can spread in the intermuscular tissue and can lift up the outer muscular layer in the form of a dome; finally, the cyst may pierce the longitudinal muscle also and be covered only by the serosa or the adventitia. The presence or the absence of muscle strands in the wall of the cyst indicates which of the methods it has followed.

As described by Lewis and Thyng, these nodes, or diverticula, are found in various positions on the circumference of the bowel and never occur in the colon. Intestinal duplications are invariably on the mesenteric side, usually between the leaves of the mesentery and do occur in the colon as well as in the small bowel. Furthermore, this theory fails to explain the regularity with which duplications have complete muscular coats, although frequently the septum between the duplication and the bowel itself may not have two complete sets of musculature. Also, this theory scarcely explains the long tubular duplications that run to 60–90 cm in length. Nor does it very satisfactorily explain the fact that the mucosa lining a duplication is frequently not that characteristic of the bowel at the level to which the duplication is attached. Bremer himself was inclined to believe that most of the spherical cysts were derived from these embryonic diverticula, but, although the custom of attributing some or all duplications to this mechanism is hallowed by tradition, it seems scarcely supported by the evidence.

The mechanism commonly associated with Bremer's name, and believed by him to account for the majority of the tubular duplications and some of the spherical ones, explains the duplications as originating from an abnormal persistence of the vacuoles normally present among the massed epithelial cells of the "solid stage" of the intestine, normally in the sixth or seventh week. At this time, in the 10-mm embryo, the intestinal tract is increasing in length more rapidly than is the embryo, and it is then that the intestinal tract finds room for itself by extending into the exocoelom of the umbilical cord.

The accelerated growth of the intestine is first indicated by the piling up of the epithelial cells. This occurs to such an extent that in certain regions the lumen of the tube becomes much reduced or even occluded. This is known as the "solid stage." Bremer stated that it never extends throughout the length of the tract at any one time. He suggested that if the increase of the cells fails to occur, the lumen cannot expand properly; a constriction or stenosis of the bowel may then occur, as rapid lengthening of the bowel produces a transverse cleft across the mass of epithelial cells, allowing the ingrowth of submucosa, or even of muscle, to cause atresia. Johnson,[10] in 1910, had shown in wax reconstructions the apparent secretion of fluid by the thickened epithelial mass, creating vacuoles within it. The vacuoles tend to arrange lengthwise in chains or rows and to coalesce with one another, forming the lumen. Bremer suggested that "in rare cases the chains of fused vacuoles may retain their form and cause intestinal duplications." If the vacuoles coalesce only with one another, the resultant cyst does not communicate with the main lumen. If the vacuoles coalesce with one another to form a cyst and then one opens into the main lumen, there will be a communication between the duplication and the lumen of the bowel. Bremer postulated that with growth the two lumina move apart and that the wall of the bowel grows in between them, so that ultimately two complete walls form. Bremer was hard put to explain the fact that, while duplications invariably lie between the layers of the mesentery, the vacuoles seen in the process he

described occur on all sides of the lumen, apparently scattered at random. He did, however, offer a reasonable mechanism for the formation of the extremely long tubular diverticula, which may be as much as 60–90 cm in length. "If one realizes that the length of the small intestine when the vacuoles first appear is from 2.0 to 2.5 mm, whereas at birth the same intestine has attained a length of 2–3 m, and that a duplicate, being an integral portion of the intestine, must share this rapid growth, the lengths reported are not especially remarkable."[4] It is evident that the solid-cord theory explains no better than the diverticulum theory the consistently mesenteric location of the duplications, their muscular wall, and their frequent possession of mucosa unlike that of the adjoining bowel. Furthermore, it is doubtful if the "solid-cord" state occurs anywhere but in the duodenum.

The type of duplication occurring in the mediastinum, and described in Chapter 59, is susceptible of a fairly satisfactory embryologic explanation on the basis of the work of Saunders and others.[19, 24] These malformations occur in the posterior mediastinum, are thick-walled, covered with longitudinal and circular muscle, have characteristic myenteric plexuses and are lined by intestinal epithelium, often gastric. They frequently extend caudally through the diaphragm into the abdomen, there to end blindly or to connect with the lumen of the duodenum or the jejunum (see Figs 59–7 and 59–8). In some instances, the cephalic end is attached to the spine, and Figure 59–8 represents a patient in whom the upper end of the intestinal structure opened into the spinal canal, ultimately resulting in fatal meningitis. It has been repeatedly demonstrated[3, 7, 24] that these mediastinal intestinal duplications are associated with malformations of the cervical and upper thoracic vertebrae. From time to time, there have been clinical descriptions of patients with combined posterior and anterior spina bifida, the anterior cleft being traversed by coils of gut, or with an intestinal fistula penetrating through a dorsal or sacral spinal defect, as the case might be. Saunders, in 1943, clearly stated the embryologic basis for this deformity[24] and restated it during a clinical discussion in 1954.[19]

This split notochord syndrome, described also as "neurenteric canal" or "dorsal intestinal fistula," with its resultant anomaly sometimes mistaken for a spinal cyst or a prevertebral teratoma, dermoid cyst, or sinus, is explained on the basis of partial duplication and separation of the notochord.

The notochord theory of origin for mediastinal enteric cysts is based on events in the third week of embryonic life, when the notochord begins to appear. A proliferation of cells from the primitive streak of the ectoderm produces a narrow rod of cells, which projects ventrally between the ectoderm and the entoderm. This process, the notochordal plate, wedged among the entodermal cells, comes to form part of the wall of the primary entodermal cavity. Normally, the notochordal plate migrates dorsally and is pinched off from the entoderm by ingrowth of mesodermal cells from each side. If the withdrawal of the notochordal elements as a result of ectoentodermal adhesion draws with them some of the adjacent entodermal lining, it becomes impossible for the spinal column to close ventrally; in addition, a tract resembling a diverticulum is established with the primitive gut.

As shown in Figures 59–6 and 59–8, either end or both ends of the intestinal tract so formed may remain open, or both may be closed off from their original communications. At times, the cephalic end may be represented ultimately by no more than a fibrous strand or may disappear altogether, as in most clinical examples. The embryologic and clinical evidence to explain most mediastinal "esophageal duplications" on this basis is very good. Furthermore, unlike the situation in duplications within the abdomen, the mediastinal duplication is often not closely attached to the esophagus. It is possible that some rectal "duplications" are formed in the same way, and both Saunders[24] and Bentley and Smith[3] referred to sacral sinuses and fistulas of this kind. Prop et al.[23] described an infant with a huge cyst dorsal to a bifid lumbosacral spine. The cyst contained a loop of bowel with mesentery, an extreme example of this split notochord mechanism. It is interesting, and probably beyond the bounds of coincidence, that a number of instances have been recorded in which mediastinal cysts of foregut origin have occurred in patients who also had intestinal duplications within the abdomen, quite distant from the mediastinal malformations.

Johnston and associates[11] reported a patient from whom a muscular-walled posterior mediastinal cyst was removed in the presence of failure of fusion of T-4 and T-6. The following year melena developed, and she was found to have a tubular duplication of the jejunum with a communication between the jejunum and the distal end of the duplication and a peptic ulcer in the jejunum at this point. However, a spinal abnormality of the kind under discussion has not been found in association with the usual type of intra-abdominal intestinal duplication, except in the few patients also having a mediastinal cyst.

It seems unlikely that intra-abdominal intestinal duplications owe their existence to a similar mechanism. Fallon and associates,[7] however, believed "that vertebral lesions will eventually be found in association with mesenteric cysts and duplications."

Complete duplication of the colon and rectum is the final type of anomaly generally described under the term "duplications." In this lesion, the entire colon, rectum, and anus, and frequently the terminal ileum as well, are completely double, occasionally triple, up to the point of a Meckel's diverticulum. With this anomaly, doubling of the genitalia and of the bladder and urethra, exstrophy of the bladder, spina bifida, omphalocele, and other lesions are observed with extraordinary frequency. Many of the instances of the complete anomaly are associated with spina bifida, and it seems probable that the condition represents a caudal twinning with duplication of the hindgut and the genital and lower urinary tracts. The same process occurs at the cephalic end of the embryo and results in various double monsters. Double stomatodeum represents such an anomaly.[1]

The report from New Orleans by Paddock and Arensman[22] that, in children with polysplenia, duplications as well as atresias may occur, leads to the thought that duplications may represent a reparative effort gone wrong.

In summary, the origin and formation of the posterior mediastinal enteric cysts is satisfactorily explained on the basis of existing embryologic information and clinical observation. The formation of the traditional enteric cysts is not adequately explained. The extensive doubling of the colon and rectum is adequately explained, but the embryologic bases of the formation of the mediastinal cysts and of the colonic duplications do not satisfactorily explain the intramesenteric intestinal duplications. The entire March 1967 issue of *Annales de chirurgie infantile* was devoted to duplications and carried a most extensive bibliography.

Symptoms and Diagnosis

The manifestations of a duplication of a portion of the gastrointestinal tract depend on its size and location. Posterior mediastinal, "esophageal" duplications may be unexpectedly found only on imaging or may cause dysphagia, respiratory distress, hemoptysis. Many intra-abdominal duplications produce palpable masses. Symptoms are produced by compression of the involved stomach or intestine, torsion and volvulus of the attached bowel,[14, 25] perforation, and bleeding into the intestine. Colonic

and rectal duplications may obstruct the uterus and displace or compress the bladder. Occasionally in an adult, the mucosa of the duplication develops a cancer.[2, 6, 9] For intra-abdominal duplications, sonography has frequently provided more detailed information than conventional contrast radiography.[12, 17] Computed tomography has been employed as well.[27] Technetium scans have shown gastric mucosa in mediastinal duplications and in intestinal duplications.[5, 8, 15, 20, 21, 26]

REFERENCES

1. Abrami G., Dennison W.M.: Duplication of the stomach. *Surgery* 49:794, 1961.
2. Adair H.M., Trowell J.E.: Squamous cell carcinoma arising in a duplication of the small bowel. *J. Pathol.* 133:25, 1981.
3. Bentley J.F.R., Smith J.R.: Developmental posterior enteric remnants and spinal malformations. *Arch. Dis. Child.* 35:76, 1960.
4. Bremer J.L.: Diverticula and duplications of the intestinal tract. *Arch. Pathol.* 38:132, 1944.
5. Curran J.P., Behbahani M., Kim B.H., et al.: Ectopic gastric duplication cyst in an infant. *Clin. Pediatr.* 23:50, 1984.
6. Downing R., Thompson H., Alexander-Williams J.: Adenocarcinoma arising in a duplication of the rectum. *Br. J. Surg.* 65:572, 1978.
7. Fallon M., Gordon A.R.G., Lendrum A.: Mediastinal cysts of foregut origin associated with vertebral abnormalities. *Br. J. Surg.* 41:520, 1954.
8. Ferguson C.C., Young L.N., Sutherland J.B., et al.: Intrathoracic gastrogenic cyst—preoperative diagnosis by technetium pertechnetate scan. *J. Pediatr. Surg.* 8:827, 1973.
9. Hickey W.F., Corson J.M.: Squamous cell carcinoma arising in a duplication of the colon: Case report and literature review of squamous cell carcinoma of the colon and of malignancy complicating colonic duplication. *Cancer* 47:602, 1981.
10. Johnson F T.: The development of the mucous membrane of the esophagus, stomach and small intestine in the human embryo. *Am. J. Anat.* 10:521, 1910.
11. Johnston J.B., Hallenbeck G.A., Ochsner A., et al.: Duplication of two parts of the alimentary tract. *Arch. Surg.* 68:390, 1954.
12. Kangarloo H., Sample W.F., Hansen G., et al.: Ultrasonic evaluation of abdominal gastrointestinal tract duplication in children. *Radiology* 131:191, 1979.
13. Keibel F.: Zur Embryologie des Menschen, der Affen und der Halbaffen. *Anat. Anz.* 27(suppl.):39, 1905.
14. Kleinhaus S., Boley S.J., Winslow P.: Occult bleeding from a perforated gastric duplication in an infant. *Arch. Surg.* 116:122, 1981.
15. Knight J., Garvin P.J., Lewis E. Jr.: Gastric duplication presenting as a double esophagus. *J. Pediatr. Surg.* 18:300, 1983.
16. Ladd W.E.: Duplications of the alimentary tract. *South. Med. J.* 30:363, 1937.
17. Lamont A.C., Starinsky R., Cremin B.J.: Ultrasonic diagnosis of duplication cysts in children. *Br. J. Radiol.* 57:463, 1984.
18. Lewis F.T., Thyng F.W.: The regular occurrence of intestinal diverticula in embryos of the pig, rabbit and man. *Am. J. Anat.* 7:505, 1907–1908.
19. McLetchie N.G.B., Purvis J.K., Saunders R.L.: The genesis of gastric and certain intestinal diverticula and enterogenous cysts. *Surg. Gynecol. Obstet.* 99:135, 1954.
20. Moccia W.A., Astacio J.E., Kaude J.V.: Ultrasonographic demonstration of gastric duplication in infancy. *Pediatr. Radiol.* 11:52, 1981.
21. Newmark H., Ching G., Halls J., et al.: Bleeding peptic ulcer caused by ectopic gastric mucosa in a duplicated segment of jejunum. *Am. J. Gastroenterol.* 75:158, 1981.
22. Paddock R.J., Arensman R.M.: Polysplenia syndrome: Spectrum of gastrointestinal congenital anomalies. *J. Pediatr. Surg.* 17:563, 1982.
23. Prop N., Frensdorf E.L., van de Stadt F.R.: A postvertebral entodermal cyst associated with axial deformities: A case showing the "entodermal-ectodermal adhesion syndrome." *Pediatrics* 39:555, 1967.
24. Saunders R.L.: Combined anterior and posterior spina bifida in a living neonatal human female. *Anat. Rec.* 87:255, 1943.
25. Schwartz D.L., So H.B., Becker J.M., et al.: An ectopic gastric duplication arising from the pancreas and presenting with a pneumoperitoneum. *J. Pediatr. Surg.* 14:187, 1979.
26. Teele R.L., Henschke C.I., Tapper D.: The radiographic and ultrasonic evaluation of enteric duplication cysts. *Pediatr. Radiol.* 10:9, 1980.
27. Thornhill B.A., Cho K.C., Morehouse H.T.: Gastric duplication associated with pulmonary sequestration: CT manifestations. *AJR* 138:1168, 1982.

Duplications of the Stomach

Gastric duplications are infrequent, although not so rare as once thought. Gross[6] had two cases of gastric duplication in a total of 68 intra-abdominal duplications of the gastrointestinal tract. At Children's Hospital of Pittsburgh,[2] of 62 intra-abdominal duplications, five were of the stomach. Izant[10] saw nine cases in 5 years. Abrami and Dennison[1] reported five, one of which is pictured in Figure 94–1. The gastric duplications in most of the reported instances were large cysts that made themselves known in the newborn period or in early infancy by reason of a tense abdomen, vomiting, and a palpable mass. Occasionally, a duplication of the stomach persists into adult life.[8] In one such duplication, a carcinoma developed.[12] Duplications of the stomach are most frequently attached to the greater curvature or to the posterior wall. They apparently do not communicate with the lumen of the stomach except as a result of peptic ulceration, although it is not always clear from the accounts whether there was evidence of peptic ulceration at the site of the communication or not.[10] The duplication reported by Fassbender,[4] of Dortmund, was blind and alongside the length of the stomach and connected with it by three small openings. Endoscopic biopsy of the edge of one showed "peptic necrosis." One of Izant's patients had a gastrocolic fistula, and in one the cyst had ulcerated into the colon. One of Abrami and Dennison's patients had a peptic perforation into the lesser omental bursa; in another, a child with melena and hematemesis, a communication was found between the cyst and the stomach. This might have been congenital but was probably the result of peptic ulceration, since the child had been under observation for some time without prior evidence of the lesion in appropriate studies. Because of the large size or strategic location of the cysts, or the early development of melena and anemia, almost all of the patients reported underwent operation in infancy. Patients have been successfully treated by excision of the cyst in some instances, by wide anastomosis between the cyst and stomach in others, and by resection of the cyst and attached portion of the stomach with reanastomosis of the proximal and distal gastric remnants. The preference should be for an operation that will remove all of the cyst lining.

Occasional cystic duplications lined entirely by gastric mucosa are separate from the stomach and attached to pancreas or mesentery of the bowel.[3, 5, 7] The cyst removed from an adult by Salameh,[13] from Germany, was entirely retroperitoneal, unconnected to the viscera, but in all respects a gastric duplication, both as to mucosa and as to the muscular layer. The cyst of Ocaña,[11] from Cordoba, was bilocular, with a small communication between the two spherical lobes. The 5-week-old patient of Kleinhaus[9] was admitted with distention and ascites. The 10-cm-diameter cyst attached to the greater curvature, and not in communication with the gastric lumen, had "a perforated bleeding ulcer" on the inferior surface. There was bloody fluid in the peritoneal cavity. No histologic description is given.

REFERENCES

1. Abrami G., Dennison W.M.: Duplications of the stomach. *Surgery* 49:794, 1961.
2. Bower R.J., Sieber W.K., Kiesewetter W.B.: Alimentary tract duplications in children. *Ann. Surg.* 188:669, 1978.

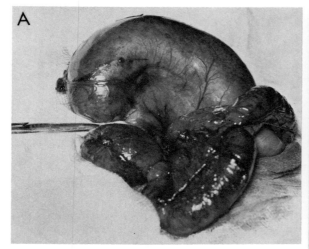

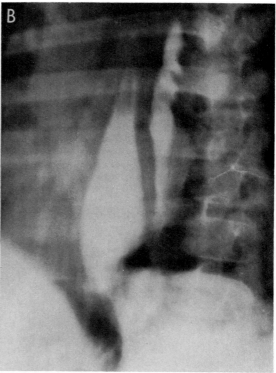

Fig 94–1.—Double esophagus and stomach. An infant, 1 day old, had a tense ovoid mass in the upper abdomen. **A,** photograph showing, *above,* the tense, almost U-shaped gastric duplication four times the size of the stomach, which can be seen bulging from behind the duplication. The spherical mass to the left, below the instrument, is the duodenal duplication, 3 cm in diameter, just distal to the pylorus. It was excised and the stomach and its duplication united by direct gastrogastrostomy. A barium meal 15 days later was said to show a normal esophagus and stomach. **B,** the child was readmitted at age 3 months because of persistent vomiting. After oral administration of barium, pressure on the stomach caused reflux of barium into the two esophaguses, as shown. Esphagoscopy on two occasions revealed only one esophagus connected to the pharynx. This true doubling suggests abortive twinning not related embryogenetically to the common "duplications." (From Abrami and Dennison.[1])

3. Curran J.P., Behbahani M., Kim B.H., et al.: Ectopic gastric duplication cyst in an infant. *Clin. Pediatr.* 23:50, 1984.
4. Fassbender C.W., Gersmann A., Hausamen T.U.: Je ein Fall von vollständiger Duplikatur des Magens und des Duodenums. *Fortschr. Röntgenstr.* 134:304, 1981.
5. Gonzalez B.G.C., Martinez J.G.: A propósito de un caso de reduplicación gástrica y pancreática. *Rev. Esp. Enf. Ap. Digest.* 53:671, 1978.
6. Gross R.E.: *The Surgery of Infancy and Childhood.* Philadelphia, W.B. Saunders Co., 1953.
7. Hélardot P.G., Van Kote G., Barbet P., et al.: Les duplications gastriques séparées de l'éstomac et en relation avec le pancréas. *Chir. Pédiatr.* 23:363, 1982.
8. Kalongi T., Steiner P.: Les duplications gastriques à propos d'un cas observé chez l'adulte. *Ann. Chir.* 28:43, 1974.
9. Kleinhaus S., Boley S.J., Winslow P.: Occult bleeding from a perforated gastric duplication in an infant. *Arch. Surg.* 116:122, 1981.
10. Kremer R.M., Lepoff R.B., Izant R.J. Jr.: Duplication of the stomach. *J. Pediatr. Surg.* 5:360, 1970.
11. Ocaña J.M., Ayala J., Olías J.J., et al.: Duplicatión gástrica con doble formación quística. *An. Esp. Pediat.* 11:888, 1978.
12. Orr M.M., Edwards A.J.: Neoplastic change in duplications of the alimentary tract. *Br. J. Surg.* 62:269, 1975.
13. Salameh S., Terhorst B.: Retroperitonealer Tumor links: Magen-duplex. *Urologe*[A] 22:249, 1983.

Duplications of the Duodenum

Duplications of the duodenum are perhaps a little less common than gastric duplications. Gross[5] listed only four cases, and there had been three at Children's Hospital of Pittsburgh.[7] Sukarochana's[7] paper, in 1970, analyzed 50 cases in the English, French, and German literature. With only an occasional exception, at birth the cysts have caused symptoms of duodenal obstruction, frequently thought to be due to pyloric stenosis unless the palpable mass has been too large, which has often been the case. An occasional patient has been asymptomatic until well into adult life. Dickinson[3] reported a large duodenal diverticulum that perforated freely into the peritoneal cavity and proved to be made up of three separate cysts along the second and third parts of the duodenum, composed of three separate cavities and lined by gastric mucosa, the presumed cause of the perforation. The cyst was successfully peeled from the duodenum. Lesions have been found, for the most part associated with the first and the second portions of the duodenum, in all cases lying behind the duodenum. In four of the 50 collected cases, there was a communication with the duodenum. In 32 of the listed reports, the mucosa type was recorded and five of these had gastric mucosa. As in duplications of the intestinal tract elsewhere, the external appearance is that of bowel; the wall contains both smooth muscle layers.

It was in a large duodenal duplication that Gardner and Hart[4] performed their classic procedure of cystoduodenostomy, subsequently adopted as standard for this lesion. However, there are increasing reports of successful dissection of the cyst from the duodenum, and, in view of the occasional occurrence of gastric mucosa in the cyst wall, this appears to be the preferable technique. External drainage, the so-called marsupialization, is as unsatisfactory for this lesion as for most of the other conditions to which it was once applied. The (adult) patient of Imamoglu and Walt[6] had a large, entirely intrahepatic duplication with an inverted Y connection to the duodenum. The duodenal ends were divided and oversewn, and the hepatic portion drained into a Roux-en-Y jejunal loop.

In the area of the duodenum, but not arising from it, occur occasional cysts that seem so closely related to the biliary and pancreatic ducts that it has been suggested[1] that they have their origin in these ducts. Akers et al.[2] reported three cases. One was in a 9-year-old child with abdominal pain, jaundice, and melena, who had a 2 × 2-cm cyst lined by gastric mucosa, lying immediately inferior to the cystic duct but communicating with the

common duct by a separate stoma. The second was in a 7-year-old boy with abdominal pain, vomiting, and fever, who had a dense 8-cm inflammatory mass on the head of the pancreas. The third was in a 21-month-old girl with abdominal pain and a left abdominal mass, who was found to have a cyst at the juncture of the body and tail of the pancreas that communicated with the duct of Wirsung when she was finally operated on at age 3 years for gross bloody ascites. The opening in the duct of Wirsung was anastomosed to a Roux-en-Y loop, and the patient did well. Wrenn,[9] Williams,[8] Welch,[7a] and others have reported similar cases.

REFERENCES

1. Ackerman N.B.: Duodenal duplication cysts: Diagnosis and operative management. *Surgery* 76:330, 1974.
2. Akers D.R., Favara B.E., Franciosi R.A., et al.: Duplications of the alimentary tract: Report of three unusual cases associated with bile and pancreatic ducts. *Surgery* 71:817, 1972.
3. Dickinson W.E., Weinberg S.M., Vellios F.: Perforating ulcer in a duodenal duplication. *Am. J. Surg.* 122:418, 1971.
4. Gardner C.E. Jr., Hart D.: Enterogenous cysts of the duodenum. *JAMA* 104:1809, 1935.
5. Gross R.E.: *The Surgery of Infancy and Childhood.* Philadelphia, W.B. Saunders Co., 1953.
6. Imamoglu K.H., Walt A.J.: Duplication of the duodenum extending into liver. *Am. J. Surg.* 133:628, 1977.
7. Leenders E.R., Osman M.Z., Sukarochana K.: Treatment of duodenal duplication with international review. *Am. Surg.* 36:6, 1970.
7a. Welch K.J.: The pancreas, in Ravitch M.M., Welch K.J., Benson C.D., et al. (eds.): *Pediatric Surgery,* ed. 3. Chicago, Year Book Medical Publishers, 1979, p. 857.
8. Williams W.H., Hendren W.H.: Intrapancreatic duodenal duplication causing pancreatitis in a child. *Surgery* 69:708, 1971.
9. Wrenn E.L. Jr., Favara B.E.: Duodenal duplication (or pancreatic bladder) presenting as double gallbladder. *Surgery* 69:858, 1971.

Duplications of the Small Intestine

A few duplications, cystic or tubular, are seen in the jejunum, but most all reported enteric cysts are in the ileum. At Children's Hospital of Pittsburgh, there have been 31 small-bowel duplications; only six of those were jejunal. Three were associated with atresia of the intestine, one with jejunal atresia, one with agenesis of the right lung. Only one patient was known to have hemivertebrae. Five of the duplications were tubular, three of these presenting with anemia or bleeding or with a palpable mass, and one with intestinal obstruction.[3]

Single large cysts cause symptoms by virtue of obstruction of the attached bowel, either from distention of the tense cyst or from the visible and palpable mass (Fig 94–2,*A* and *B*). Yanagisawa's[14] patient (Fig 94–2,*C*) was a newborn infant with a volvulus of the intestine apparently caused by a huge cyst. The volvulus had been intrauterine, and the twist had caused necrosis and atresia of the small bowel. Favara, Franciosi, and Akers[1] in a report of 39 duplications, from the tongue to the sigmoid, included four children with atresia of the intestine and what they considered to be associated duplication. On this basis, they proposed that, in rare instances of intrauterine mesenteric vascular insult, an isolated bit of intestine survives to form a cyst with the characteristics of a duplication.

Long tubular cysts give the appearance of attempts at doubling of the intestine. Whereas the spherical cysts do not communicate with the bowel, tubular ones usually have such communications—at the distal end—and are more likely to be lined by gastric mucosa than the spherical cysts, which are usually lined with intestinal mucosa. The tubular cysts, because of their gastric mucosal lining and their communication with the intestine, in many reported instances have caused peptic ulceration of the bowel with melena or perforation, or both. The ulcer may be in the duplication,[7] or in the ileum near the opening of the duplication into the bowel.[2] Occasionally, peptic ulcers are found in globular

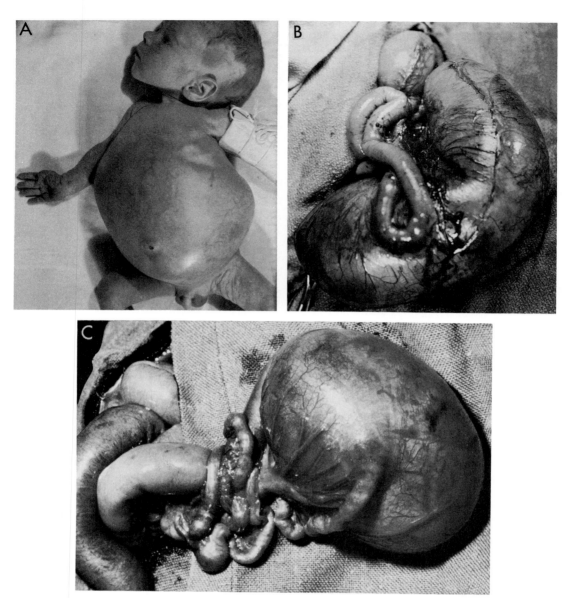

Fig 94–2.—Cystic duplications of the ileum. **A** and **B,** huge duplication causing great abdominal distention in a 12-day-old infant with vomiting, anorexia, and constipation. A huge, tense cyst crossed the abdomen from flank to flank. At either end, the cyst could be dissected from the bowel, but over most of the area of attachment, the muscular walls were common. Cyst and bowel were resected and end-to-end anastomosis performed. **C,** spherical duplication causing fetal volvulus in a baby who vomited from birth and passed no meconium. A tumor "the size of an apple" was palpable in the right lower quadrant. At operation, a spherical cyst was found in the mesentery of the distal ileum. A 720-degree volvulus, when reduced, disclosed atresia at the site of torsion, obviously the result of fetal compression. Cyst with attached bowel was resected and end-to-end anastomosis performed. (Courtesy of Prof. F. Rehbein.[14])

cysts unconnected with the lumen of the bowel.[4] Like the globular cysts, the tubular duplications are usually fused with the attached bowel and have a common muscular wall, so that it is generally necessary to resect the attached bowel together with the malformation. It is sometimes possible to strip the mucosa from the duplication and so avoid a difficult or massive resection; this is done by opening the duplication and peeling off the mucosa, if the duplication is not excessively long.

In 1953, we[8, 9] solved the problem of resecting the blind pelvic end of a complete duplication of the colon by resecting all of it except the portion attached to the functioning rectum, merely stripping the mucosa from that portion. Romualdi,[10] in 1955, applied the same principle in the treatment of imperforate anus,

leaving the distal pouch but stripping it of mucosa; he thus avoided a pelvic dissection, as the proximal bowel was brought down to the perineum inside the denuded distal rectal stump. Wrenn,[13] in 1962, applied the same principle of mucosal stripping to a tubular duplication the entire length of the small intestine to avoid the necessity for a major intestinal resection. After the opening between duplication and small bowel had been closed,

a transverse incision was then made through the seromuscular coat of the duplication. . . . The mucosa was separated from the muscularis and was pulled out as a sleeve. This dissection was carried as far proximally as possible, everting the muscularis as the mucosa was separated from it. After about 15 cm of mucosa had been separated, a second transverse incision was made in the seromuscular coat at the upper end of the separation. The mucosal tube was pulled out through this incision. . . . stripping of the mucosa from the muscularis was then continued upward through multiple transverse incisions in the seromuscular coat.

Gdanietz et al.,[5] from Berlin, successfully applied Wrenn's principle to what was an ileum duplex (Fig 94–3) in an infant with massive bleeding and complete duplication of the ileum, after enlargement of the distal communication between the duplication and the bowel resulted in continued bleeding.

In an occasional tubular duplication of the small bowel with symptoms caused by distention of the long blind sac, relief has been afforded by anastomosis of the distal end of the sac to the main intestinal channel. This has the virtue of avoiding resection of what is, in some patients, a long segment of involved bowel. On the other hand, if the malformation should be lined in whole or in part by gastric mucosa, the risk of peptic ulceration with hemorrhage or perforation, or both, is invited, and Wrenn's mucosal stripping is much to be preferred.

Ileum duplex appears in the literature as a term applied to complete, or all but complete, doubling of the ileum[5, 6, 12] and improperly to ordinary duplication. In rare cases,[11] a separate blood supply to the duplication permits resecting it in toto.

Smaller, essentially intramural, cysts occur usually at or near the ileocecal valve. This is a common variety of small-intestine duplication. A few have caused obstruction by virtue of direct compression of the ileum at its entrance into the cecum. More commonly, these small cysts have precipitated intussusception.

We have had two such (Fig 94–4). Once more, the treatment is resection of the cyst with the attached bowel.

REFERENCES

1. Akers D.R., Favara B.E., Franciosi R.A., et al.: Duplications of the alimentary tract: Report of three unusual cases associated with bile and pancreatic ducts. *Surgery* 71:817, 1972.
2. Aubrey D.A.: An unusual reduplication of the ileum. *Am. J. Surg.* 120:815, 1970.
3. Bower R.J., Sieber W.K., Kiesewetter W.B.: Alimentary tract duplications in children. *Ann. Surg.* 188:669, 1978.
4. Drott C., Jansson R.: Duplication cyst of the jejunum. *Acta Chir. Scand.* 147:731, 1981.
5. Gdanietz K., Wit J., Heller K., et al.: Die komplette Dünndarmduplikatur im Kindesalter. *Z. Kinderchir.* 38:414, 1983.
6. Jewett T.C. Jr., Walker A.B., Cooney D.R.: A long-term follow-up on a duplication of the entire small intestine treated by gastroduplication. *J. Pediatr. Surg.* 18:185, 1983.
7. Niesche J.W.: Duplication of the small bowel with peptic ulcer perforation. *Aust. N.Z. J. Surg.* 42:4, 1973.
8. Ravitch M.M.: Hindgut duplication, doubling of colon and genitourinary tracts. *Ann. Surg.* 137:588, 1953.
9. Ravitch M.M., Scott W.W.: Duplication of the entire colon, bladder, and urethra. *Surgery* 34:843, 1953.
10. Romualdi P.: Una nuova technica operative per la cura di alcune malformazioni del retto. *Soc. Romana Chir.*, May 1955.
11. Schwartz D.L., Becker J.M., Schneider K.M., et al.: Tubular duplication with autonomous blood supply: Resection with preservation of adjacent bowel. *J. Pediatr. Surg.* 15:341, 1980.
12. Schwartz D.L., So H.B., Becker J.M., et al.: An ectopic gastric duplication arising from the pancreas and presenting with a pneumoperitoneum. *J. Pediatr. Surg.* 14:187, 1979.

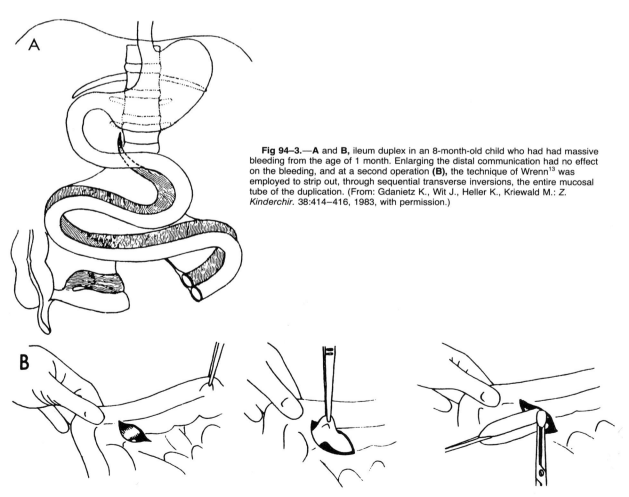

Fig 94–3.—A and **B,** ileum duplex in an 8-month-old child who had had massive bleeding from the age of 1 month. Enlarging the distal communication had no effect on the bleeding, and at a second operation **(B),** the technique of Wrenn[13] was employed to strip out, through sequential transverse inversions, the entire mucosal tube of the duplication. (From: Gdanietz K., Wit J., Heller K., Kriewald M.: *Z. Kinderchir.* 38:414–416, 1983, with permission.)

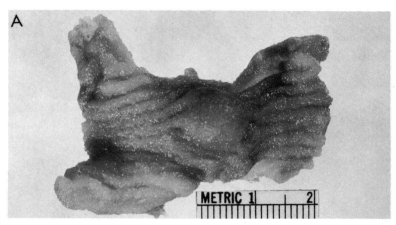

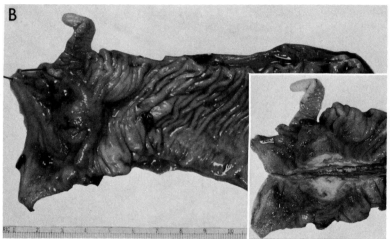

Fig 94–4.—Intramural ileocecal duplication causing intussusception. **A,** 7-year-old boy had repeated attacks of violent colicky pain suggesting intussusception. Barium enema during one attack demonstrated no lesion. Operation was undertaken because the attacks were so convincing. The 1-cm submucosal cystic swelling in the distal ileum was a spherical duplication. The nearby bowel was edematous, suggesting a recent intussusception. **B,** 8-month-old infant gave intermittent evidence of colicky pain and occasionally vomited. A smooth, round, easily movable mass felt in the left upper quadrant was thought to be an intestinal duplication. Operation disclosed a chronic, nonstrangulating intussusception. When reduced, it was found to have been caused by a submucosal enteric cyst, just at the ileocecal valve. The specimen shows the cecum and ascending colon 2 cm of the terminal ileum, the opened appendix, and the cyst just at the ileocecal valve. *Inset* shows the cyst in the fixed and bisected specimen.

13. Wrenn E.L. Jr.: Tubular duplication of the small intestine. *Surgery* 52:494, 1962.
14. Yanagisawa F.: Doppelbildungen des Darmes. *Chirurg.* 30:109, 1959.

Duplications of the Colon

Duplications of the colon occur in a number of forms. The least common, if they occur, are cystic or tubular duplications of the proximal or transverse colon, which have the nonspecific character of the cystic duplications we have been discussing thus far. Sulamaa and Nyberg[11] described an 8-month-old essentially asymptomatic child with an abdominal mass in the transverse mesocolon between stomach and colon, closely attached to the colon, from which it was possible to dissect it. The malformation reported by Higgins[4] was a long "diverticulum" of the transverse colon, running the length of it and producing symptoms from fecal distention. The photograph clearly shows teniae coli and haustrations in the duplication. A similar diverticulum-like tubular duplication of the ascending colon was resected by Kufaas[5] in a 7-month-old infant with chronic vomiting. Torsello[13] resected a "giant duplication" of this kind in the transverse colon. Schwartz's[9] 4-year-old girl presented with a noncommunicating sigmoid duplication which caused volvulus. She also had a tubular duplication of terminal ileum and ascending colon. Yanagisawa[14] described a double sigmoid, the distal end of which connected with the rectum while the proximal end doubled back through the obturator foramen to end in a fistula on the thigh. The supernumerary sigmoid had teniae and appendices epiploicae and was distinct from the normal bowel, suggesting an abor-

tive twinning rather than the ordinary enterogenous cyst. At Children's Hospital of Pittsburgh, there have been seven cystic duplications of the colon and two of the rectum.[1]

The commonest type of cystic duplication of the large bowel actually occurs behind the rectum, usually quite low. It causes symptoms by pressure into the rectum and occasionally by rectal prolapse, so that the cyst, covered by rectal mucosa, is visible through the patulous anus or external to it.[2, 3, 8] These cysts are much less closely attached to the bowel in most cases than cysts situated more proximally along the intestine and have usually been readily excised through para-anal incisions. Obviously they may be mistaken for presacral teratomas; in fact, the name "Middeldorpf's tumor" has been incorrectly given to presacral teratomas, although the lesion that Middeldorpf[6] described is quite obviously an enteric cyst.

Stockman and associates[10] found a 4-year-old girl with rectal bleeding to have a good-sized diverticulum on the anterior wall of the rectum within reach of the finger and containing gastric mucosa. This case is unique.

Carcinoma has been reported arising in duplications of the colon.[7, 12]

REFERENCES

1. Bower R.J., Sieber W.K., Kiesewetter W.B.: Alimentary tract duplications in children. *Ann. Surg.* 188:669, 1978.
2. Cogswell H.D., Thompson H.C.: Duplication of the rectum. *Am. J. Dis. Child.* 73:167, 1947.
3. Custer B.S., Kellner A., Escue H.M.: Enterogenous cysts: Report of case involving the rectum. *Ann. Surg.* 124:508, 1946.

4. Higgins T.T.: A case of reduplication of the transverse colon. *Br. J. Surg.* 38:392, 1951.

5. Kufaas T., Lindman C.R.: Cystic duplication of the colon combined with nonrotation anomaly imitating pyloric stenosis. *Acta Paediatr. Scand.* 72:467, 1983.

6. Middeldorpf K.: Zur Kenntniss der angeborenen Sacralgeschwülste. *Arch. Pathol. Anat.* 101:37, 1885.

7. Orr M.M., Edwards A.J.: Neoplastic change in duplications of the alimentary tract. *Br. J. Surg.* 62:269, 1975.

8. Saugmann-Jensen J.: On enterocystomata of the rectum. *Acta Chir. Scand.* 99:399, 1950.

9. Schwartz D.L., Procaccino M., Becker K.M., et al.: Segmental colonic duplication presenting as a sigmoid volvulus. *Z. Kinderchir.* 38:338, 1983.

10. Stockman J.M., Young V.T., Jenkins A.L.: Duplication of the rectum containing gastric mucosa. *JAMA* 173:1223, 1960.

11. Sulamaa A.M., Nyberg L.O.: On duplications of alimentary tract (two cases). *Acta Chir. Scand.* 98:171, 1949.

12. Tamoney H.J. Jr., Testa R.E.: Carcinoma arising in a duplicated colon: Case report. *Cancer* 20:4, 1967.

13. Torsello G., Pasquale E., Giunta Pasquale S., et al.: Duplicazione gigante del colon trasverso: Presentazione di un case. *Radiol. Med.* 68:668, 1982.

14. Yanagisawa F.: Doppelbildungen des Darmes. *Chirurg.* 30:109, 1959.

Complete Duplication of the Colon, With Duplication of the External Genitalia and Lower Urinary Tract

More than 50 cases have been reported of double colon, anus, bladder, urethra, and external genitalia[1, 2, 10] (Fig 94–5). The colons are usually fused, with a common wall, and the terminal ileum may also be double. In males, there may be two well-developed penises; in females, two vaginas, each with clitoris and labia. In addition, there have been a good many patients with double anus and rectum but not the full constellation of anomalies, probably representing lesser degrees of the same condition. Patients with the full constellation usually present signs of intestinal obstruction because one (or both) of the colons ends blindly or has an inadequate opening in a perineal anus or a rectovaginal or rectourethral fistula. The proximal ends of both colons invariably communicate with the alimentary stream. In some instances, the spina bifida, which is a regular concomitant of this lesion, has gone on to become a myelomeningocele with associated neurologic symptoms. Flye and Izant[4] described a

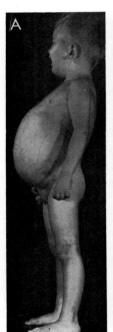

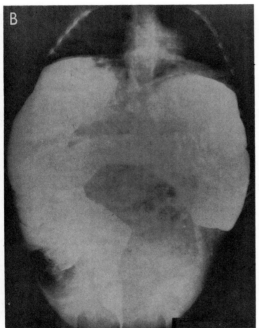

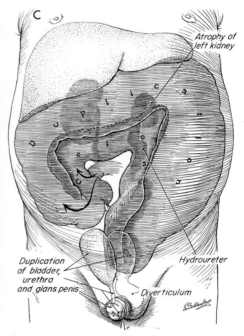

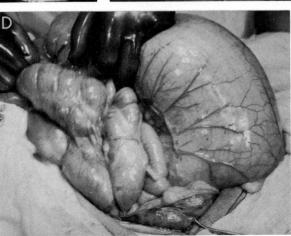

Fig 94–5.—Hindgut duplication: doubling of colon, bladder, and urethra. A 4½-year-old boy had diarrhea in early infancy, followed by persistent, stubborn constipation. Dribbling of urine, plus large voluntary discharges of urine at apparently satisfactory and normal intervals, was a puzzling symptom. **A,** the child, enormously distended with palpable fecal masses, was referred with a diagnosis of Hirschsprung's disease. He had a peculiarly misshapen prepuce and two urethral orifices. Clear urine was voided voluntarily through the right orifice; cloudy urine dripped through the left orifice, the urethra of which contained a visible diverticulum. **B,** barium enema through the single and normal anus outlines one colon; the other, much larger one, displaces the normal colon and is filled with opaque fecal masses. **C,** diagram of the combination of anomalies in this patient. **D,** operative view of the enormously distended supernumerary colon, which began at the cecum and ended blindly, deep in the pelvis. There was only one appendix and one terminal ileum. The great feces-filled sac had obstructed the left ureter at the pelvic brim and destroyed the left kidney. The one ileum can be seen entering the U-shaped cecum and two ascending colons. The tip of the single appendix is visible. The clamp points to the cleft bladder dome. The bladder was septate. In a series of operations, the bulk of the supernumerary colon was excised, mucosa and submucosa stripped from the muscularis of its pelvic portion, and the colon reconstructed. The destroyed left kidney was excised. The left urethra was divided and closed, and the septum between the two bladders was excised. The boy has voided and defecated normally ever since. (From Ravitch M.M., Scott H.W.: *Surgery* 34:843, 1953. Used by permission.)

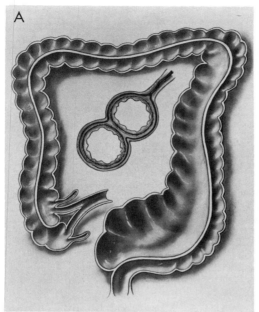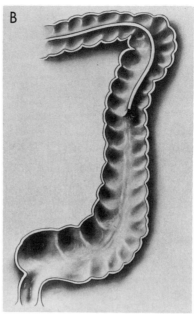

Fig 94–6.—Complete duplication of the colon. A 3-year-old girl with constipation showed poor weight gain and had an intermittent abdominal mass. Sigmoidoscopy revealed no lesion; barium enema and cystography showed displacement of the bladder and rectum. The mass had the characteristics of feces. **A,** findings at operation. The distal ileum bifurcated into two channels and there were two cecums, each with its appendix, and two complete colons. The one along the inner side of the functioning colon ended blindly about 1 inch above the anus and was filled with feces. **B,** through a long colotomy, the distal portion of the septum between the two colons was incised and an anastomosis created between the two. All symptoms were relieved. (Courtesy of Dr. R.T. Soper.) This seems to be the simplest and most satisfactory method of dealing with this problem. The difficulty in reaching the lowest portion of the septum from above required division of the distal portion of the septum from below in a second operation. The automatic instrument for intestinal anastomosis that would divide a septum like this and staple the edges on either side in a single operation would seem ideally suited for this procedure in one stage from above or below.

child who had not only a complete double colon without genitourinary abnormalities but also extralobar pulmonary sequestration communicating with the esophagus. It is obvious that, when the entire length of the colon, and in some instances of the terminal ileum as well, ends blindly, an enormous feces-filled sac results, with production of serious symptoms related to distention of the sac, compression of the other and patent rectum or colon, and compression of the ureter against the pelvic brim. In two cases, all or part of the colon was actually triple.[5]

At Children's Hospital of Pittsburgh, there have been three patients with complete double colons; two had double bladders and one had exstrophy of the bladder. One of the children with double bladder had vertebral anomalies. One of two children with a double appendix had double bladder, urethra, and penis, as well as vertebral anomalies.[3]

Only rarely has it been possible to resect the second colon and reestablish normal continuity.[6] Since the symptoms, quite apart from the various problems imposed by the doubled genitalia, are essentially the result of the doubled intestine, operative efforts have been directed largely to this portion of the deformity.[8] In a number of instances, the rectum of the second colon has been transected, the proximal end being anastomosed to the principal colon. This has left a sac lined by colonic mucosa and emptying into the vagina or through a perineal sinus. The amount of mucus discharged is said not to have been troublesome. In at least two cases, the septum between the two anal openings has been excised, forming the two anal openings into one. Anastomosis of the obstructed colon or rectum to the unobstructed loop has been successful in a number of instances. The best procedure is that suggested by Soper[9] (Fig 94–6).

Treatment of the associated genitourinary anomalies has not been necessary in all cases. Double vagina is not necessarily disadvantageous, and instances of function of both vaginas and subsequent delivery through both are on record.[1] Double male genitalia present a more awkward problem. More instances are on record of this anomaly without associated doubling of the colon than with it. The bladder is usually septate in these patients, each half receiving one ureter and emptying through its own urethra. In the patient of Ravitch and Scott,[8] one urethra was malformed by a huge diverticulum, and the kidney on the same side had been destroyed from compression of the ureter against the pelvic brim by the feces-filled second colon. In this patient, the destroyed kidney was removed, the urethra on this side divided, and the septum between the two bladders excised (see Fig 94–5).

These complicated and extensive anomalies require thorough study before decision as to the proper operative attack.

REFERENCES

1. Beach P.D., Brascho D.J., Hein W.R., et al.: Duplication of the primitive hindgut of the human. *Surgery* 49:779, 1961.
2. Beach P.D., Wright R.H. Jr., Deffer P.A.: Duplication of the primitive hindgut of the human being: An 8-year follow-up of a previous case report. *Surgery* 66:405, 1969.
3. Bower R.J., Sieber W.K., Kiesewetter W.B.: Alimentary tract duplications in children. *Ann. Surg.* 188:669, 1978.
4. Flye W., Izant R.J.: Extralobar pulmonary sequestration with esophageal communication and complete duplication of the colon. *Surgery* 71:744, 1972.
5. Gray A.W.: Duplication of the large intestine. *Arch. Pathol.* 30:1215, 1940.
6. Ravitch M.M.: Hindgut duplication, doubling of colon and genitourinary tracts. *Ann. Surg.* 137:588, 1953.
7. Ravitch M.M., Rivarola A.: Enteroanastomosis with an automatic instrument. *Surgery* 59:270, 1966.
8. Ravitch M.M., Scott W.W.: Duplication of the entire colon, bladder, and urethra. *Surgery* 34:843, 1953.
9. Soper R.T.: Tubular duplication of the colon and distal ileum. *Surgery* 63:998, 1968.
10. Yousefzadeh D.K., Bickers G.H., Jackson J.H. Jr., et al.: Tubular colonic duplication—review of 1876–1981 literature. *Pediatr. Radiol.* 13:65, 1983.

95 Arnold H. Colodny
Mesenteric and Omental Cysts

MESENTERIC AND OMENTAL CYSTS are benign unilocular or multilocular endothelium-lined cysts that contain either chyle or serous fluid.[1, 6, 8] They are uncommon yet interesting intra-abdominal masses that may be difficult to diagnose clinically and often are missed on abdominal palpation.[17] They may present with potential life-threatening complications. Because of their rarity, confusion may occur when they are encountered at operation.

The first recorded description was in 1507 by the Florentine anatomist, Benivieni, who described a mesenteric cyst that he found at autopsy.[3] More than 300 years passed before Rokitansky in 1842 made the first formal description of a mesenteric cyst.[19] The first successful surgical treatment was reported by a French surgeon, Tillaux, in 1880.[21] Several series have indicated 25% of reported cases have been in children.[4, 17, 18, 20, 22, 23]

Etiology

Many varied etiologic theories have been proposed in the past, including those based on parasitic, neoplastic, inflammatory, degenerative and infectious causes, obstruction of the lymphatics, hamartomas of the lymphatics, deviations of the urogenital ridge, pinched-off diverticula of the GI tract, and origin from embryonic totipotential cells.[2, 5, 16, 23]

They probably arise from a congenital, developmental abnormality of the lymphatic system, which results in ectopic lymphatic tissue that proliferates and collects fluid owing to a lack of communication with the central lymphatic system.[9] This developmental theory could account for their occurrence in the newborn. Some believe that these cysts are dynamic in nature, that they grow slowly, representing an imbalance between their afferent and efferent flow. Their endothelial lining is often patchy and incomplete, making it difficult to assess how much the lining membrane contributes to the cyst fluid.[10, 23]

Clinical Features

Experience with 42 patients at Boston Children's Hospital Medical Center since 1930 illustrates the incidence and spectrum of these lesions. Fourteen patients had omental and 28 had mesenteric cysts. The youngest patient was 4 hours old, and the oldest was 11 years of age. Thirty-one of the 42 patients were less than 5 years old. Thirteen presented in the first year of life (Table 95-1). There were 21 females and an equal number of males.

Signs and Symptoms (Table 95-2)

Mesenteric and omental cysts may be asymptomatic or may cause abdominal distention and/or pain or may present with complications such as intestinal obstruction, volvulus, or hemorrhage into the cyst.[24]

Abdominal pain was the most common presenting symptom. Eighteen of the 42 patients had pain as their chief complaint. The pain may be diffuse or localized, dull, aching, or crampy. It may present as an "acute abdomen" with localized peritoneal findings or with a pain pattern characteristic of an acute, mechanical small intestinal obstruction.

Eleven of the 42 patients presented with a chief complaint of a gradually enlarging abdomen. This had frequently been disregarded as normally protuberant. A definite abdominal mass could be palpated in only 18 of the 42 patients (Fig 95-1) (in only two of those with protuberant abdomens).

Five patients in this series presented with an acute mechanical obstruction of the small bowel (see Table 95-2). Three of these five had volvulus, and in all three the mesenteric cyst was in the jejunum. Two of the three had infarcted bowel and had passed gross blood by rectum. The remaining two patients of the five presenting with intestinal obstruction had compression of the bowel stretched out over the cyst in the ileal mesentery. There were no cases of intestinal obstruction caused by omental cysts.

Six of the 42 patients had asymptomatic cysts found on routine physical examination or discovered incidentally during abdominal operation (Fig 95-2).

Two patients with poor appetite and intermittent vomiting presented for failure to thrive. Both had mesenteric cysts and presumably repeated bouts of partial intestinal obstruction or possibly protein loss.[13, 14] The electrolyte and protein content of serous mesenteric cysts is just slightly less than that of plasma. The protein content of chylous cysts is only about one third that of plasma, but fat is present in chyle, of course.[10, 14]

Radiologic Findings

A plain film of the abdomen shows a mass effect that is gasless, homogeneous, and of water density[13] displacing the intestinal tract in a direction dependent on the size and location of the cyst

TABLE 95-1.—AGE DISTRIBUTION

YEARS	NUMBER
0–5	31*
5–10	9
10–15	2

*13 under 1 year of age.

TABLE 95-2.—SIGNS AND SYMPTOMS

	MESENTERIC (N = 28)	OMENTAL (N = 14)
Presenting symptom		
Abdominal pain	12	6
Abdominal distention	6	5
Intestinal obstruction	5	0
Asymptomatic	3	3
Failure to thrive	2	0
Main physical finding		
Abdominal mass	12	6
Abdominal distention	5	4
Intestinal obstruction	5	0
Acute abdomen	3	3
Incidental	3	1

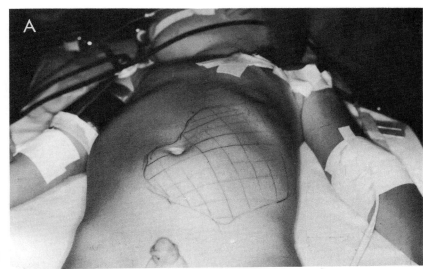

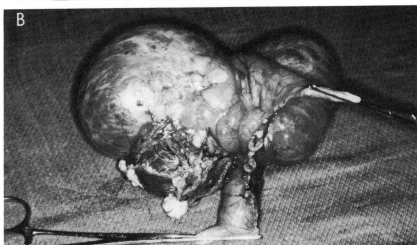

Fig 95–1.—Mesenteric cysts. **A,** 3-year-old boy with a visible, palpable mesenteric cyst. Most cysts are not palpable. **B,** large mesenteric cyst with a mixture of chylous, serous, and hemorrhagic areas, found in the patient pictured in **A.** As is commonly the case, the bowel was so intimately involved that the attached segment was removed en bloc with the cyst.

(Fig 95–3). The cysts are often mobile and may show a small amount of calcification in their wall. Gastrointestinal contrast studies may be helpful in establishing a correct preoperative diagnosis and pinpointing the location of the cysts. Omental cysts displace the stomach posteriorly and/or cephalad (Fig 95–4). The displacement caused by mesenteric cysts depends on their size and location. Occasionally, they may compress the overlying bowel lumen, which appears narrowed and stretched out by an extraluminal mass. In the neonate, total body opacification may be useful.

Ultrasonography reveals a sonolucent transsonic structure with a perimeter well outlined by a smooth wall (Fig 95–5).[11] The cysts may be either unilocular or multilocular and may be located anywhere within the abdomen. Omental cysts are located anteriorly.[15] A large ovarian cyst, a pancreatic cyst, or an enteric duplication may be difficult to differentiate from an omental or mesenteric cyst. Choledochal cysts can usually be differentiated by their location, the associated abnormalities of the biliary tree, and a history of intermittent jaundice. Pancreatic pseudocysts are usually preceded by pancreatitis or abdominal trauma. Ascites is characterized by unencapsulated, shifting transsonic fluid in the flanks with floating intestines, centrally placed. If ascites is loculated in the midabdomen, it may be difficult to differentiate from a cyst.

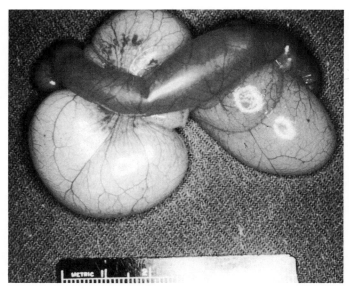

Fig 95–2.—Chylous cyst, found incidentally at laparotomy in an infant with biliary atresia. Note the dumbell shape.

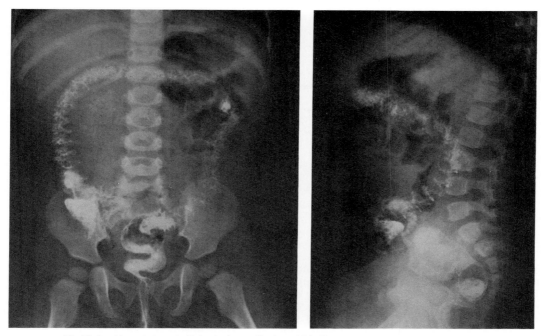

Fig 95–3.—Mesenteric cyst. Abdominal x-ray film in a child with a centrally located mesenteric cyst displacing the colon. On the original films, calcification was visible.

Location of Cysts

Twenty-eight of the 42 patients had mesenteric cysts and 14 had omental cysts. Of the 28 mesenteric cysts, 11 were ileal, 11 were jejunal, and six were in the large bowel mesentery.

Treatment (Table 95–3)

The preferred approach is complete excision of the cyst, and this is possible in the vast majority of patients.[10] Frequently, mesenteric cysts lie in intimate contact with the bowel, which may require resection of the attached bowel with the cyst. In 10

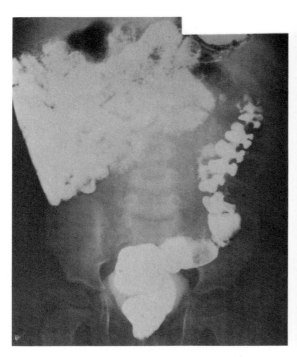

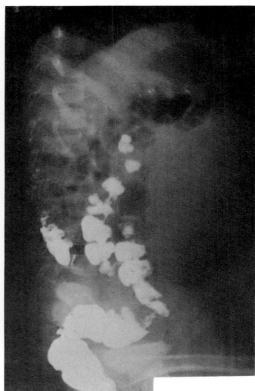

Fig 95–4.—Omental cyst. Typical roentgenographic effects of a large omental cyst, anterior *(left)* and lateral *(right)* views.

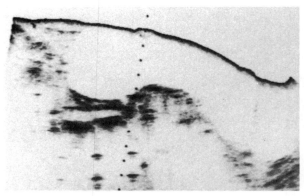 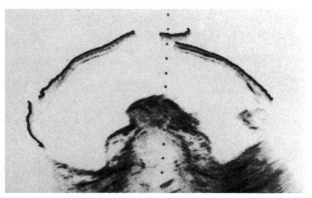

Fig 95–5.—Mesenteric cyst. Ultrasonographic appearance of a large mesenteric cyst just under the abdominal wall. **Left,** sagittal; **Right,** transverse.

of the 28 mesenteric cysts in our series, resection of the cyst alone was performed. In 15 cases, the overlying bowel was resected along with the cyst and primary end-to-end anastomosis performed. It may be impossible at operation to differentiate such a mesenteric cyst from an enteric duplication, although duplications have thick, muscular walls quite different from the thin walls of mesenteric cysts. Pathologic examination showing the smooth muscle wall of a duplication and its epithelial lining will make this differentiation. One patient had multiple cysts that involved the complete small bowel mesentery and could not be completely excised. One infant had volvulus with infarction of the entire midgut. This baby underwent reduction of the volvulus without resection, since the entire midgut would have had to be removed. A second procedure revealed an unsalvageable situation with persistent, progressive gangrene of the midgut. Total excision of the cyst was possible in 39 of the 42 patients.

TABLE 95–3.—OPERATIVE TREATMENT

	MESENTERIC (N = 28)	OMENTAL (N = 14)
Excision	10	13
Partial excision	1	1
Intestinal resection	15	0
Reduction of volvulus	2	0

TABLE 95–4.—POSTOPERATIVE DEATHS AND COMPLICATIONS*

Deaths (none since 1940)	
Intestinal infarction	2
Peritonitis	1
Complications	
Ileoileal intussusception	1
Adhesive obstruction	2 (1 patient)

*N = 42 patients.

TABLE 95–5.—PATHOLOGIC FINDINGS

LOCATION	NO.	SEROUS	CHYLOUS
Omentum	14	13	1
Mesentery			
Jejunal	11	5	6
Ileal	11	6	5
Colonic	6	6	0
Total	42	30	12

Morbidity and Mortality (Table 95–4)

One patient after resection of a cyst developed two episodes of adhesive intestinal obstruction requiring operation, and one patient developed a postoperative small bowel intussusception.

There were three deaths in this series, all before 1940. Two were due to extensive infarction and gangrene, and one was due to perforation and peritonitis. There have been no deaths for the past 44 years.

Pathologic Features

The cysts may be small or large, rounded or ovoid, single or multiple. Single ones may be multiloculated. They are usually thin-walled and flabby, making them difficult to palpate. Some are dumbbell shaped, projecting on either side of the mesentery (see Fig 95–2). The serous cysts are translucent. The inner surface of the cyst wall is usually smooth, but there may be internal strands forming loculi. The contents may be either serous or chylous, with or without various degrees of hemorrhage.[7, 12] Thirteen of the 14 omental cysts were serous, whereas the mesenteric cysts had an almost equal distribution of chylous or serous fluid (Table 95–5). All six cysts in the large-bowel mesentery contained serous fluid.

Microscopically, the cyst wall is composed of a fibrous connective tissue membrane of varying thickness lined by sparse, flat mesothelial cells, which may be smooth, proliferating, irregular, or patchy. It may show dilated lymphatics, and occasionally a few strands of smooth muscle are seen. There may be patchy aggregates of lymphocytes, macrophages, and/or foreign-body giant cells. There may be focal hemorrhages, and, rarely, calcific deposits. Some cysts show evidence of inflammation, with infiltration of polymorphonuclear cells.

REFERENCES

1. Arnheim E.E., et al.: Mesenteric cysts in infancy and childhood. *Pediatrics* 24:469, 1959.
2. Benedict A.L.: Bibliography of chylous cysts of the mesentery. *Surg. Gynecol. Obstet.* 16:666, 1913.
3. Benivieni A.: De abditis nonullis ac mirandis morborum 1 sanationum causis. Quoted by Beahrs O.H., Dockerty M.B.: Primary omental cysts of clinical importance. *Surg. Clin. North Am.* 30:1073, 1950.
4. Burnett W.E., Rosemond G.P., Bucher R.M.: Mesenteric cysts. *Arch. Surg.* 60:699, 1950.
5. Carter R.M.: Cysts of the mesentery. *Surg. Gynecol. Obstet.* 33:544, 1921.
6. Dowd C.N.: Mesenteric cysts. *Ann. Surg.* 32:515, 1900.
7. Engel S., Clagett O.T., Harrison E.G.: Chylous cysts of the abdomen. *Surgery* 50:593, 1961.
8. Estourgie R.J.A., van Beek M.W.: Mesenteric cysts. *Z. Kinderchir.* 32:223, 1981.

9. Friend E.: Mesenteric chylous cysts. *Surg. Gynecol. Obstet.* 15:1, 1912.
10. Gross R.E.: *The Surgery of Infancy and Childhood.* Philadelphia, W.B. Saunders Co., 1953, p. 377.
11. Haller J.O., et al.: Sonographic evaluation of mesenteric and omental masses in children. *AJR* 130:269, 1978.
12. Handelsman J.C., Ravitch M.M.: Chylous cysts of the mesentery in children. *Ann. Surg.* 140:185, 1954.
13. Leonidas J.C., et al.: Mesenteric cyst associated with protein loss in the gastrointestinal tract. *Am. J. Roentgenol.* 112:150, 1971.
14. Messer F.M.: Analysis of fluid from a chylous mesenteric cyst. *J. Lab. Clin. Med.* 23:596, 1938.
15. Mittelstaedt C.: Ultrasonic diagnosis of omental cysts. *Radiology* 117:673, 1975.
16. Mollitt D.L., Ballantine T.V.N., Grosfeld J.L.: Mesenteric cysts in infancy and childhood. *Surg. Gynecol. Obstet.* 147:182, 1978.
17. Moore T.C.: Congenital cysts of the mesentery. *Ann. Surg.* 145:128, 1957.
18. Moynihan B.G.A.: Mesenteric cysts. *Ann. Surg.* 26:1, 1897.
19. Rokitansky C., quoted by Whittlesey R.H., Heidorn C.H., Huntley W.B.: Mesenteric cysts and chylous ascites. *Arch. Pediatr.* 77:357, 1960.
20. Roller C.S.: Mesenteric cysts. *Surg. Gynecol. Obstet.* 60:1128, 1935.
21. Tillaux P.J.: Cyste du mesentére chez un homme. Ablation par la gastrotomie. Quersion. *Rév. Ther. Méd. Chir.*, 47:479, 1880.
22. Vaughn A.M., Lees W.M., Henry J.W.: Mesenteric cysts. *Surgery* 23:306, 1948.
23. Warfield J.O.: A study of mesenteric cysts. *Ann. Surg.* 96:329, 1932.
24. Williams S.A., Ingelfinger J.R., Colodny A.H.: Abdominal enlargement: A parent may be the first to know. *Clin. Pediatr.* 16:1128, 1977.

96 Peter K. Kottmeier

Ascites

HISTORY.—*Askitis*, a derivation from the Greek word *askos*, "bag," refers to the accumulation of excess fluid in the peritoneal cavity, regardless of origin or composition. Hippocrates' assumption that the liver could be the origin of the ascitic fluid was confirmed by Sydenham and Fint over 2,000 years later. The relief of symptoms by paracentesis was common practice for centuries. Paul of Aegina's warning that sudden evacuation of the peritoneal fluid may also lead to the evacuation of the "vital spirit," killing the patient, remains valid.

Diagnosis

Excess fluid accumulation leads to abdominal distention. Free fluid can be detected by ballottement of liver and spleen, shifting dullness, and the presence of a succussion wave. Radiologic signs consist of haziness, bulging of the flank, separation of intestinal loops, and obliteration of the psoas shadow. Medial displacement of the liver or central positioning of the intestine also suggest ascites.[20] Sonography is the most reliable method of differentiation between solid masses, free and loculated fluid. Computed axial tomography can delineate underlying or associated pathology. Paracentesis, with chemical, microscopic, and bacteriologic analysis, history, and clinical findings, should establish the correct diagnosis in most patients (Tables 96–1 and 96–2). Angiography and hepatic wedge pressures may be necessary to differentiate between presinusoidal and postsinusoidal block in children with hepatic ascites.

Causes of ascites are numerous, but a few conditions are responsible in the majority of childhood cases: cardiovascular, hepatorenal, lymphatic, urinary, pancreatic, biliary, and ovarian disease. Both localized and diffuse intraperitoneal cerebrospinal fluid collection have been reported in children following ventriculoperitoneal shunts. The ascites, which may be intermittent, usually resolves spontaneously.[29] Less common causes include postoperative complications (transplantation and dialysis,[30, 42] ventriculoperitoneal shunt[29]), neoplasms,[3] metabolic (fat, amino acids, α-antitrypsin, tyrinosis, vitamin A intoxication,[36] gangliosidosis[1]), serositis, congenital anomalies,[19, 34] and others.

The treatment is directed at the underlying cause or, in cases with refractory ascites, at prevention or control of the accumulation of intraperitoneal fluid. The most common entities of surgical interest leading to ascites are included in this chapter.

Fetal Ascites

The diagnosis can be established by fetal sonography as early as in the second trimester and is usually indicative of a life-threatening fetal condition, although "pseudoascites" or spontaneous disappearance of fetal ascites has been reported.[20, 28] Maternal-fetal Rh incompatibility was the major cause of fetal ascites until the last decade, when the percentage of nonimmune diseases increased.[45] Almost half the cases are associated with congenital anomalies, including cardiovascular, genitourinary, pulmonary, intestinal, achondroplasia, Conradi's disease, and prune belly.[12, 26, 45] Hematological disorders (α-thalassemia, twin transfusion syndrome), α-antitrypsin deficiency,[14] or infection such as toxoplasmosis or cytomegalic virus are other causes.

Chylous Ascites

Morton[27] diagnosed chylous ascites ante mortem in a 2-year-old boy in 1720 and explained his findings as follows:

His belly began to be distended, with shortness of breath, atrophy to the degree of Marasmus—but with a healthy look and countenance—without

TABLE 96–1.—ANALYSIS OF ASCITIC FLUID*

MICROSCOPIC	CHEMICAL	CULTURE
WBC, differential, B-cells	Amylase	Bacterial
RBC	Bile	Fungal
Hematocrit	Triglyceride	Tubercul
Fat globules	Specific gravity	Viral
Sudan III		
Cytology		
Intestinal content		
Bacterial stain		

*Selection of examinations depends on, and should confirm, the clinical diagnosis.

TABLE 96–2.—ANALYSIS OF ASCITIC FLUID*

ASCITES	WBC	B-CELLS	PROTEIN <3 gm/dl	PROTEIN >3 gm/dl	TRIGLYCERIDE	AMYLASE	SPECIFIC GRAVITY <1,015	SPECIFIC GRAVITY >1,015
Chylous	+ +	+ +		+	+ + +			+
Pancreatic	+			+		+		+
Biliary	±			+		(Bile +)		+
Hepatic	±		+				+	

*Correlation of the most important laboratory findings in children with chylous, pancreatic, biliary, and cardiohepatic ascites.

the least tincture of yellowness and a rather greedy appetite to the very day he died. Tapping the child's belly we took out several pints of milky chyle. His dropsy was truly chylous, caused by the chyle flowing into the cavity of the belly by the lacteal vessels which were broke—and the consumption—proceeded merely from an inanition, draining of the nutritious juice.

After 250 years, there is little to add.

Chylous ascites is twice as common in infants as in older children, but the clinical presentation is similar.[49] The mortality in children before total parenteral nutrition was 24%.[39] Chyloperitoneum is rarely present at birth,[48] in contrast to chylous pleural effusion, although we have seen the association of both in the fetus (Fig 96–1).

Vasko and Tapper,[51] in a review of 59 children, listed the following possible causes: congenital malformation 39%, unknown 31%, inflammation 15%, neoplastic 3%. Mechanical obstruction causing chylous ascites has been reported by various authors, mainly due to malrotation, adhesive bands, or incarcerated hernia.[16, 39, 43, 49] Other causes include lymphangiomas, mesenteric

cysts, lymphadenopathy, and blunt trauma. The diagnostic workup should include radiologic examination of abdomen and chest, sonography, and specific examination such as urogram, gastrointestinal series, or CAT scan as indicated. Although pedal lymphangiography will not show mesenteric lymphatic defects, other lymphatic anomalies and intraperitoneal leakage have been reported in older children.[6, 49] The examination of the ascitic fluid yields clear fluid in the neonate and a cloudy, turbid fluid after oral feedings have been started. Ascitic chylous fluid usually shows an increased total fat and triglyceride content, decreased protein, fat globules that often can be stained with Sudan III. Total white blood cell count is usually increased with dominant lymphocytes, particularly B-cells.

Approximately two thirds of infants and children respond to nonoperative therapy. Diets low in fat and high in protein can reduce the lymphatic drainage and therefore the formation of chylous ascites. Although the fat intake has been limited in most series to medium-chain triglycerides (MTC), there is no definite proof for their specific efficacy. The prolonged use of MTC has

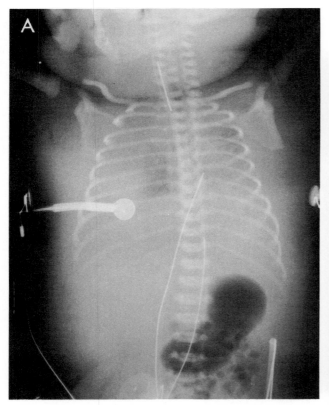

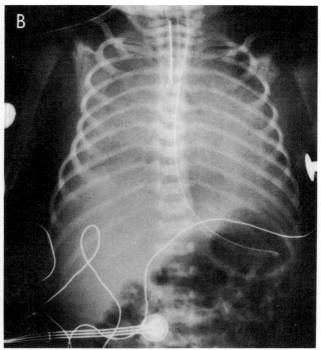

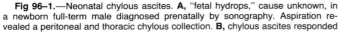

Fig 96–1.—Neonatal chylous ascites. **A,** "fetal hydrops," cause unknown, in a newborn full-term male diagnosed prenatally by sonography. Aspiration revealed a peritoneal and thoracic chylous collection. **B,** chylous ascites responded to nonoperative therapy (MTC diet followed by total parenteral nutrition), but a right chylothorax persisted for 2 months.

reportedly exposed patients to essential fatty acid deficiency.[49] Total parenteral nutrition is therefore preferable. The gastrointestinal tract can be placed completely at rest and nutritional deficiencies avoided. If there is no response after 4–6 weeks, or chylous ascites reaccumulates after a regular diet is resumed, operative intervention should be considered. In patients with identifiable causes, such as mesenteric cysts, malrotation, or trauma, the underlying condition may be repaired without much difficulty. In children without identifiable cause, the identification of a leak can be facilitated through preoperative feedings of heavy cream with a lipophilic dye, such as Sudan black,[43] but our experience and that of others has been disappointing.[49] If no leak can be identified, the area around the root of the mesentery, the most likely site, should be closely inspected after colon, duodenum, and head of the pancreas have been mobilized. In children in whom repeated attempts of nonoperative and operative therapy have failed, a peritoneal-venous shunt, either the LeVeen or Denver type,[7] has been reported to be successful, at least temporarily. The increased viscosity of the chylous ascites[16, 39] has led to more frequent blocking of shunts than is seen with hepatic ascites.[4, 15] Since even the pediatric tubing is too stiff to allow a gentle curve over the clavicle area, we have brought the tubing of the LeVeen shunt past the posterior axillary line over the left shoulder, subcutaneously, and into the jugular vein, thereby completely avoiding a kink in the tubing.

Pancreatic Ascites

Pancreatitis in children is usually caused by trauma and, in decreasing frequency, by infection, drugs, metabolic diseases (hyperlipidemia or aminoacidemia), and pancreatic obstruction. Pancreatic ascites has been reported in infancy.[38] An identifiable cause, obstruction of the ampulla, was found in only one of six infants. The others either had or developed a pancreatic pseudocyst similar to that seen in older children following trauma. Failure to analyze the ascitic fluid for its amylase content appears to be the main cause for delayed or incorrect preoperative diagnosis.[38] External drainage of the associated pseudocyst is effective in most children. Internal drainage is the most commonly used procedure—including cyst gastrostomy, cyst enterostomy, or pancreatectomy with a caudal pancreaticojejunostomy.[5, 11] We use external drainage of traumatic pancreatic pseudocyst as the primary treatment. From 1973 to 1983, eight children with pancreatic pseudocysts were admitted to the pediatric surgical service. Two regressed without treatment. Six were treated with external tube drainage alone, without recurrence. In one of the six, an attempted percutaneous drainage resulted in a colonic injury requiring a secondary tube drainage. Associated ductal obstruction, frequently seen in adults, is rare in children. External drainage, which can occasionally be done percutaneously under radiological control, is therefore more likely to be effective in children.

Biliary Ascites

Fifty cases of biliary ascites in infancy were reviewed by Prevot and associates in 1971.[33] Although symptoms are rarely apparent during the first days of life, the slowly developing signs of biliary ascites may already be present in a considerable number at birth. In contrast to the experience of Hendren,[18] Pinter,[31] and Hansen,[17] distal obstruction was found in only a few cases, although dilatation of the common duct was less rare. The cause of biliary duct perforation is not understood; distal obstruction or congenital weakness of the common duct is assumed to play a role.

In 42 infants with identifiable perforations, the perforation was found in the main biliary tree in 34 infants, and in 16 it was located at the junction of the cystic and common duct. In eight children the perforation was found in an accessory biliary duct.[17, 33]

Two clinical forms of biliary ascites in infants are apparent. Acute biliary peritonitis usually occurs in early infancy with signs of acute peritonitis, abdominal pain, tenderness, vomiting, and occasional icterus. In biliary ascites (chronic biliary peritonitis), the more common form, icterus occurs early, followed by painless abdominal distention, biliary ascites or a "bile sac" formation, and the occasional appearance of an inguinal "hernia" filled with fluid. Although both forms can appear as distinct clinical entities, the perforation of a "bile sac" into the peritoneal cavity can lead to a sudden change from minor clinical symptoms to the more severe and acute symptoms observed with acute biliary peritonitis.[22] Biliary atresia, neonatal hepatitis, or cytomegalic inclusion disease can lead to findings similar to those of early biliary ascites.[13] Intravenous cholangiography has been used to demonstrate intraperitoneal leakage or the presence of a bile sac.[13] Iodine 131 rose bengal studies[17] have been replaced by newer generations of radionuclides, such as PIPIDA ^{99m}Tc or disofenin ^{99m}Tc, diagnostically superior and producing less radiation due to their shorter half-life.[44]

A definitive diagnosis of bile peritonitis can usually be made by peritoneal paracentesis. The biliary ascitic fluid is usually turbid, occasionally green, with a bilirubin content over 400 mg/ml. Laparotomy is necessary in all cases. Operative biliary drainage was employed in 45 patients; 36 survived. The addition of cholecystectomy or attempted repair of the perforation did not appear to influence the operative result. In view of the survival rate of 80% without repair or identification of the distal obstruction, obstruction apparently does not play a significant role in the genesis of spontaneous biliary perforation in the newborn. In older children in whom the most likely cause is trauma, local drainage and repair of the duct are indicated.

Urinary Ascites

Fetal urinary ascites was first described in 1681 by Mauriceau. In 1894, Fordyce reviewed 63 cases, 17 with enlarged bladders. In 1952, Davis and James reported the first surviving infant with fetal urinary ascites and urethral obstruction.[9] Mann et al. reviewed urinary ascites in 36 infants, with a male-to-female ratio of 7:1.[25] Posterior urethral valves were found in 23 children. Other lesions reported include ureteroceles, urethral atresia, bladder neck obstruction, neurogenic bladder, and bladder hamartoma.[49] Perforation of the urinary bladder as the cause of urinary ascites has also been found,[9, 46] including an iatrogenic perforation secondary to an umbilical arterial cutdown.[35] In approximately one fourth of all infants with urinary ascites, abdominal distention was present at birth. Since the site of perforation in Mann's series was found in only 23 of 36 patients (the leak originating in the kidney in 17), he stated, "Failure to find the perforation has led to the assumption that urinary ascites is due to transudation of urine into the peritoneal space," an unlikely explanation for the fact (as in biliary ascites) that some children survive in whom the site of the leak was never found.

Because the vast majority of neonates with obstructive uropathy do not develop ascites, and frank perforation is not found in approximately one fourth of neonates with urinary ascites, additional possible causes have been cited. Retroperitoneal perforation with urinary extravasation can lead to a secondary intraperitoneal transudate. Peritoneal ascites produced in young rats by ureteral ligation does not occur if a simultaneous adrenalectomy is performed, so that humoral factors, such as an altered aldosterone mechanism, have been suspected to be causative or associated factors.[23, 47]

The infant usually presents with abdominal distention and ascites. Peritoneal absorption of the urine usually leads to elevated levels of serum creatinine and urea, but urinary function is usually close to normal. To detect urinary intra-abdominal leakage, both intravenous urography and a voiding cystogram are essential. Dockray,[10] in 1965, described the halo sign, produced by contrast medium in the extravasated urine around the kidney before it ruptures into the peritoneal cavity.

Therapy depends on the identification of the perforation and the level of obstruction. Distal obstruction requires proximal decompression or immediate correction. In most children, except those with posterior urethral valve obstruction, in whom immediate resection of the valve may be adequate, a high proximal decompression should be performed. Nephrostomy or ureterostomy appear to be the procedures of choice.[25]

Ovarian Ascites

Ascites secondary to an ovarian lesion can occur in the fetus, the newborn, and the older child. Large cysts with ascites in 60 neonates led to potentially life-endangering difficulty during delivery. This underlines the importance of a correct prenatal diagnosis to avoid a predictably difficult and dangerous vaginal delivery.[50] The presenting symptoms at birth include abdominal distention and findings suggestive of peritonitis, intraperitoneal hemorrhage, or ovarian torsion. In most instances, the ovarian cysts have been unilateral and either follicular or serous. In the older or adolescent girl, the association of ascites and hydrothorax suggests the possibility of Meigs syndrome, most commonly seen with ovarian tumors such as thecoma.

REFERENCES

1. Abu-Dalu K.I., Tamary H., et al.: GM₁ gangliosidosis presenting as neonatal ascites. *J. Pediatr.* 100:940–943, 1982.
2. Ahmed S.: Neonatal and childhood ovarian cysts. *J. Pediatr. Surg.* 6:702–708, 1971.
3. Aozasa K., Kurokawa K., et al.: Malignant histiocytosis showing ascites and recurrent meningeal infiltration. *Acta Cytol.* 24:228–231, 1980.
4. Bernhoft R.A., Pellegrini A., et al.: Peritoneovenous shunt for refractory ascites. *Arch. Surg.* 117:631–635, 1982.
5. Bloss R.S., Cooley D.A.: Pancreaticojejunostomy for fulminating pancreatitis and pancreatic ascites in a Jehovah's Witness. *J. Pediatr. Surg.* 16:79–81, 1981.
6. Camiel M.R., Benninghoff D.L., et al.: Chylous ascites with lymphographic demonstration of lymph leakage into the peritoneal cavity. *Gastroenterology* 47:188–191, 1964.
7. Chang H.T., Newkirk J., et al.: Generalized lymphangiomatosis with chylous ascites—treatment by peritoneo-venous shunting. *J. Pediatr. Surg.* 15:748–750, 1980.
8. Craven C.E., Goldman A.S., et al.: Congenital chylous ascites: Lymphangiographic demonstration of obstruction of the cisterna chyli and chylous reflux into the peritoneal space and small intestine. *J. Pediatr.* 70:340–345, 1967.
9. Cywes S., Wynne J., et al.: Urinary ascites in the newborn, with a report of two cases. *J. Pediatr. Surg.* 3:350–356, 1968.
10. Dockray K.T.: Perirenal contrast medium: A new roentgenographic sign of neonatal urinary ascites. *JAMA* 193:1121–1123, 1965.
11. Donald J.W., Ozment E.D., et al.: Pancreatic ascites in childhood. *South. Med. J.* 75:1419–1421, 1982.
12. Feeney J.G.: Fetal ascites and congenital heart disease. *Br. Med. J.* 283:934–935, 1981.
13. Frank D.J., DeVaux W.D., et al.: Fetal ascites and cytomegalic inclusion disease. *Am. J. Dis. Child.* 112:604–607, 1966.
14. Ghishan F.K., Gray G.F., et al.: α-antitrypsin deficiency presenting with ascites and cirrhosis in the neonatal period. *Gastroenterology* 85:435–438, 1983.
15. Gullstrand P., Alwmark A., et al.: Peritoneovenous shunting for intractable ascites. *Scand. J. Gastroenterol.* 17:1009–1012, 1982.
16. Guttman F.M., Montupet P., et al.: Experience with peritoneo-venous shunting for congenital chylous ascites in infants and children. *J. Pediatr. Surg.* 17:368–372, 1982.
17. Hansen R.C., Wasnich R.D., et al.: Bile ascites in infancy: Diagnosis with ¹³¹I-rose bengal. *Pediatrics* 84:719–721, 1974.
18. Hendren W.H., Donahoe P.K.: Bile duct perforation in a newborn with stenosis of the ampulla of Vater. *J. Pediatr. Surg.* 11:823–825, 1976.
19. Hertel J., Pedersen P.V.: Congenital ascites due to mesenteric vessel constriction caused by malrotation of the intestines. *Acta Pediatr. Scand.* 68:281–283, 1979.
20. Johnson J.F., Phillips E.L.: Air as a gastrointestinal contrast agent for identifying pseudoascites in the newborn. *AJR* 136:1247–1248, 1981.
21. Kinmonth J.B.: Disorders of the circulation of chyle. *J. Cardiovasc. Surg.* 17:329–339, 1976.
22. Kobayashi A., Obe Y., et al.: Idiopathic acute bile peritonitis in infancy: Report of a case. *Helv. Pediatr. Acta* 25:659–662, 1970.
23. Krane R.J., Retik A.B.: Neonatal perirenal urinary extravasation. *J. Urol.* 111:96–99, 1974.
24. Mackman S., Milburn W.H., et al.: Chylous ascites associated with malrotation of the intestines. *Am. J. Surg.* 113:282–284, 1967.
25. Mann C.M., Leape L.L., et al.: Neonatal urinary ascites: A report of 2 cases of unusual etiology and a review of the literature. *J. Urol.* 111:124–128, 1974.
26. Monie I.W., Monie B.J.: Prune belly syndrome and fetal ascites. *Teratology* 19:111–117, 1979.
27. Morton R.: *Phthissolagus*, ed. 2. London, W & J Innys, 1720.
28. Mueller-Heuback E., Mazer J.: Sonographically documented disappearance of fetal ascites. *Obstet. Gynecol.* 61:253–259, 1983.
29. Ohaegbulam S.C.: Cerebrospinal fluid ascites complicating a ventriculoperitoneal shunt. *Int. Surg.* 65:455–457, 1980.
30. Pascual J.F., Melendez M.T., et al.: Local steroid therapy of refractory ascites associated with dialysis. *J. Pediatr.* 94:319–320, 1979.
31. Pinter A., Pillaszonovich I., et al.: Membranous obstruction of common bile duct. *J. Pediatr. Surg.* 10:839–840, 1975.
32. Press O.W., Press N.O., et al.: Evaluation and management of chylous ascites. *Ann. Intern. Med.* 96:358–364, 1982.
33. Prevot J., Rickham P.P., et al.: Acute biliary peritonitis. *Prog. Pediatr. Surg.* 1:196, 1971.
34. Purohit D.M., Lakin C.A., et al.: Neonatal pseudoascites: An unusual presentation of long tubular duplication of small bowel. *J. Pediatr. Surg.* 14:193–194, 1979.
35. Redman J.F., Seibert J.J., et al.: Urinary ascites in children owing to extravasation of urine from the bladder. *J. Urol.* 122:409–411, 1979.
36. Rosenberg H.K., Berezin S., et al.: Pleural effusion and ascites. Unusual presenting features in a pediatric patient with vitamin A intoxication. *Clin. Pediatr.* 21:435–440, 1982.
37. Rosenthal S.J., Filly R.A., et al.: Fetal pseudoascites. *Radiology* 131:195–198, 1979.
38. Rubin S.Z., Ein S.H.: The unusual presentation of pancreatitis in infancy. *J. Pediatr. Surg.* 14:146–148, 1979.
39. Ryan J.A., Smith M.D., et al.: Treatment of chylous ascites with peritoneo-venous shunt. *Am. Surg.* 47:384–386, 1981.
40. Sanchez R.E., Mahour G.H., et al.: Chylous ascites in children. *Surgery* 69:183–188, 1971.
41. Santoro E., Shaw A.: Chylous ascites secondary to incarcerated inguinal hernia in an infant. *Am. J. Surg.* 119:579–580, 1970.
42. Schnyder P.A., Brasch A.L., et al.: Gastrointestinal complications of renal transplantation in children. *Radiology* 130:361–366, 1979.
43. Schwartz D.L., So H.B., et al.: Recurrent chylous ascites associated with intestinal malrotation and lymphatic rupture. *J. Pediatr. Surg.* 18:177–179, 1983.
44. So S.K., Sharp H.L., et al.: Bile ascites during infancy: Diagnosis using disofenin Tc 99m sequential scintiphotography. *Pediatrics* 71:402–405, 1983.
45. Straub W., Zarabi M., et al.: Fetal ascites associated with Conradi's disease (chondrodysplasia punctata): Report of a case. *J. Clin. Ultrasound* 11:234–236, 1983.
46. Tank E.S., Davis R., et al.: Mechanisms of trauma during breech delivery. *Obstet. Gynecol.* 38:761–767, 1971.
47. Thompson I.M., Burns T.N.C.: Neonatal ascites: A reflection of obstructive disease. *Trans. Am. Assoc. Genitourin. Surg.* 63:154–158, 1971.
48. Ravitch M.M., Rowe M.I.: Surgical emergencies in the neonate. *Am. J. Obstet. Gynecol.* 103:1034–1057, 1969.
49. Unger S.W., Chandler J.G.: Chylous ascites in infants and children. *Surgery* 93:455–461, 1983.
50. Valenti C., Kassner E.G., et al.: Antenatal diagnosis of a fetal ovarian cyst. *Am. J. Obstet. Gynecol.* 123:216–219, 1975.
51. Vasko J.S., Tapper R.I.: Surgical significance of chylous ascites. *Arch. Surg.* 95:355–368, 1967.
52. Wyllie R., Arasu T.S., et al.: Ascites: Pathophysiology and management. *J. Pediatr.* 97:167–176, 1980.

EUGENE S. WIENER

Meconium Peritonitis

HISTORY.—Meconium peritonitis was first described by Morgagni in 1761 in "De Sedibus et Causis Morborum."[11] Agerty et al. described the first successful operation in 1943.[1] In 1968, Boix-Ochoa reviewed a series of 347 cases with a 23% survival.[7]

Meconium peritonitis is a chemical or foreign-body reaction of the peritoneum to *prenatal* perforation of the intestinal tract which may occur as early as the fourth month of gestation. The intestinal perforation may have sealed before birth or may persist. Postnatal intestinal perforation, while resulting in peritonitis that may be associated with leakage of meconium, by definition, is not meconium peritonitis.[11, 21]

Etiology

Intrauterine intestinal perforation may result from various causes, the most common of which is intestinal obstruction. This obstruction may be secondary to meconium ileus, vascular compromise to the fetal intestinal tract resulting in subsequent intestinal atresia or stenosis, intussusception, volvulus, congenital bands, or internal hernias. The perforation may also result from intrauterine appendicitis, Meckel's diverticulitis, or puncture of the intestine during amniocentesis.[11, 15, 21]

We have seen a patient with imperforate anus and vaginal atresia (cloacal deformity) with a dense plastic peritonitis secondary to the combined leak of urine and meconium from the hydrosalpinx. This has also been described by Ceballos and Hicks[10] in infants with neonatal hydrometrocolpos.

Pathology

Meconium is first formed during the third month of intrauterine life and is composed primarily of amniotic fluid, squamous cells, bile salts and pigments, and pancreatic and intestinal enzymes.[11, 15, 21] Hilgier[19] studied the pathophysiology of meconium peritonitis in newborn guinea pigs. During the first 24 hours after meconium exposure, the peritoneum exhibits rapid fibroblastic proliferation. These fibroblastic adhesions envelop the lesion, forming a pseudocyst around the perforated bowel and meconium. Fibrous adhesions occur later, with increased vascularity and formation of mature collagen. Foreign-body granulomas and calcifications develop by the fourth day. In most cases, the perforation seals spontaneously. Calcifications are produced by precipitation of calcium salts by meconium contents, principally pancreatic enzymes.

Microscopically, fibrosis, granulomas with foreign-body giant-cell reaction, and, frequently, calcifications are seen. In some cases, there is no macroscopic evidence of meconium peritonitis, but microscopic evaluation of pathologic specimens demonstrates the classic findings. Tibboel et al.[28] found that, of 69 patients with meconium peritonitis, 14 (20%) had evidence of meconium components in the serosa, mesentery, and peritoneum only on careful microscopic evaluation. Nine of these patients had intestinal atresia, five had no evidence of atresia, and none had meconium ileus.

Calcification has been described in two thirds of patients.[24] While some[2, 12] have described the absence of calcification as a common feature of the meconium peritonitis associated with meconium ileus, calcification has been seen in 30–60% of such infants.[13, 15, 20, 21] Finkel[13] and Xiong[29] found calcifications in 100% of patients with meconium peritonitis not associated with cystic fibrosis. Postoperative sweat tests should be performed in all infants with meconium peritonitis.

The site of perforation, usually in the upper small bowel, is found in two thirds of reported patients with meconium peritonitis.[11, 13, 15, 21] However, there are individual case reports,[4, 17, 27] and certainly many nonreported cases, of asymptomatic calcification in the peritoneum or the scrotum. Most certainly, the incidence of sealed perforations must be higher than reported.

Several classifications of meconium peritonitis have been described.[15, 21, 22, 25, 29] The most practical includes four pathologic types: meconium pseudocyst, generalized adhesive plastic peritonitis, meconium ascites, and infected meconium peritonitis.[22]

TYPE I.—Meconium pseudocyst follows when the perforation is not immediately sealed in utero and meconium continues to enter the peritoneal cavity. A fibrous cyst wall may form entirely from neighboring loops of intestine. More frequently, the gangrenous segment of intestine is a major part of the cyst wall. The remaining free peritoneal cavity is generally devoid of adhesions. The perforation is frequently still present at birth. Calcium may line the wall of the cyst (Fig 97–1).

TYPE II.—Plastic generalized meconium peritonitis results from widespread spillage throughout the peritoneal cavity that may occur at varying times before birth. Scattered peritoneal calcification may be found, and dense fibrous adhesions are present. The site of perforation is frequently sealed off and may not be perceptible. Intestinal obstruction may develop subsequently as the result of the adhesions themselves and may not occur until the child is several weeks of age or even older.

TYPE III.—Meconium ascites results from a perforation that occurs shortly before birth. The perforation may have already sealed, and meconium-stained ascitic fluid fills the abdomen in response to peritonitis. Fine, stippled calcification may be present but may not be detectable if the perforation is very recent.

TYPE IV.—Infected meconium peritonitis results from a perforation that has not sealed before birth. Colonization of the neonatal gut allows secondary bacterial peritonitis. Air, as well as meconium, is present in the free peritoneal cavity. This is the most serious form of meconium peritonitis.

Clinical Presentation

Meconium peritonitis occurs in 1 in 35,000 live births.[21, 22] Of 172 cases of peritonitis in the first 28 days of life, Fonkalsrud[14] found 13 cases of meconium peritonitis. In another series,[5] meconium peritonitis accounted for 50% of cases of neonatal peritonitis seen in the first 5 days.

Hydramnios was present in three of 77 patients.[25] In that series, the birth weight was under 2,000 gm in 13 patients, and associated nonintestinal anomalies were found in only two patients (congenital heart disease and hydronephrosis).[25] Seventy

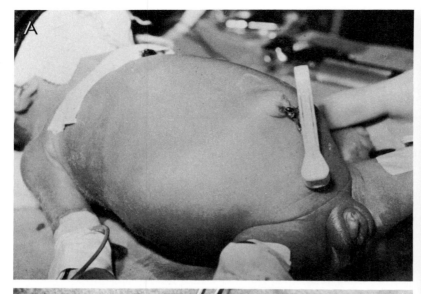

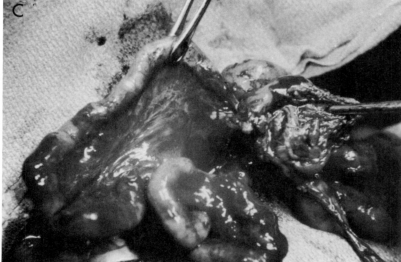

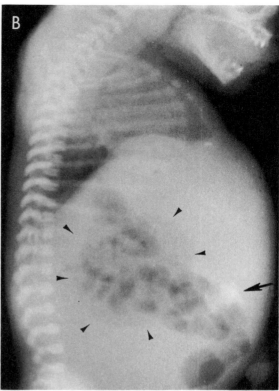

Fig 97–1.—Meconium cyst. **A,** newborn with distended abdomen and tender right abdominal mass. **B,** x-ray demonstration of intra-abdominal calcification *(large arrow)*, air-filled meconium cyst *(small arrows)*. There is no air in the colon. **C,** at operation, there was midileal atresia with a meconium cyst. Resection and end-to-end anastomosis resulted in complete recovery.

of 77 patients presented with signs and symptoms of intestinal obstruction. Vomiting was present on the first day or two of life, although occasionally obstruction, secondary to the meconium peritonitis itself, presented much later.[25]

Meconium peritonitis found incidentally in a hernia sac, presenting as an asymptomatic scrotal mass or as the cause of incidental abdominal or scrotal calcification, has been described with increasing frequency.[4, 17, 21, 27] These patients presumably sustained intrauterine perforations that sealed spontaneously and had no persisting obstruction.

An occasional patient with the ascitic form of meconium peritonitis may present with shock manifested by hypotension, oliguria, and anasarca secondary to capillary leak. Usually, the maternal placenta prevents the fluid and electrolyte imbalance that might be expected from the intense fetal peritoneal inflammation.

Abdominal radiographs usually reveal signs of intestinal obstruction with intra-abdominal calcifications.[24] These calcifications, seen in 67% of cases, must be distinguished from calcifi-

cation in liver, in abdominal tumors, in adrenal hematomas, and from the intraluminal calcifications seen in infants with imperforate anus associated with rectourinary fistulae.[21] Calcification in the scrotum may also be noted on radiographs, with or without intra-abdominal calcification.[28] There are several reports of antenatal diagnosis, made during maternal ultrasound examination.[6, 8, 16, 23, 26]

Indications for Operation

The indications for operation in infants with meconium peritonitis are intestinal obstruction or persistent intestinal leak. Patients who have abdominal or scrotal calcification on x-ray films or calcified meconium found in a hernia sac do not require operation in the absence of intestinal obstruction. Specific indications for operation are radiographic evidence of intestinal obstruction or free intraperitoneal air, the abdominal mass of encysted meconium, localized or general cellulitis of the abdominal wall, sepsis, or generalized deterioration. Infants with meconium ascites or neonatal meconium calcification should be observed closely and not fed until it is certain that they are well and the intestine not obstructed.

Operation

The operations are frequently long and tedious and may involve significant blood loss. The aim of surgical management is to remove all devitalized tissue, preserve adequate intestinal length, and reestablish intestinal continuity. A meconium pseudocyst may be completely or incompletely removed. Every effort should be made to preserve viable bowel. The underlying cause, such as meconium ileus, intestinal atresia, or volvulus, is treated in the manner appropriate to it.

Primary anastomosis, even after extensive dissection and in the presence of generalized meconium peritonitis, is usually well tolerated. If infected meconium peritonitis is present, a temporary enterostomy is frequently required. A Mikulicz enterostomy is preferred by some, but standard enterostomies are usually effective.[11, 21, 22, 25]

Results

Although early reports emphasized a poor outlook,[7] modern anesthetic and postoperative care have significantly altered prognosis. The present survival rate generally depends on the underlying cause. In one series of 77 patients,[25] 44 (57%) survived. Thirteen of the 26 patients (50%) with meconium ileus survived. Results in 51 patients without meconium ileus were somewhat better, 31 (61%) surviving. In another series of 23 infants,[22] meconium pseudocysts were found in five patients, adhesive meconium peritonitis in 12, meconium ascites in two, and infected meconium peritonitis in four. Of these 23, three did not require operation. A fourth infant with scattered calcification, free intraperitoneal air, meconium-stained ascites, and jejunal atresia secondary to volvulus died at 24 hours of age before operation could be performed. Of the remaining 19, 13 (68%) survived. Of the seven who died, three had meconium ileus. Xiong,[29] from China, reported deaths in 49 of 115 cases (42%). None of his patients had meconium ileus.

Careskey et al.[9] reported 100% survival in six infants with giant cystic meconium peritonitis, five of whom had ileal perforations; the other had meconium ileus. They attributed their excellent results to early diagnosis, pseudocyst resection, temporary ileostomy, antibiotics, and careful postoperative care.

REFERENCES

1. Agerty H.A., Ziserman A.J., Shollenberger C.L.: A case of perforation of the ileum in the newborn infant with operation and recovery. *J. Pediatr.* 22:233, 1943.
2. Allouis M., Bracq H., Defawe G., et al.: Les peritonites meconiales antenatales. *Ann. Pédiatr.* 28:635, 1981.
3. Bendel W.L., Michel M.L. Jr.: Meconium peritonitis—review of the literature and report of a case with survival after surgery. *Surgery* 34:321, 1953.
4. Berdon W.E., Baker D.H., Becker J., et al.: Scrotal masses in healed meconium peritonitis. *N. Engl. J. Med.* 277:585, 1967.
5. Birtch A.G., Coran A.G., Gross R.E.: Neonatal peritonitis. *Surgery* 61:305, 1957.
6. Blumenthal D.H., Rushovich A.M., Williams R.K., et al.: Prenatal sonographic findings of meconium peritonitis with pathologic correlation. *J. Clin. Ultrasound* 10:350, 1982.
7. Boix-Ochoa J.: Meconium peritonitis. *J. Pediatr. Surg.* 3:715, 1968.
8. Brugman S.M., Bjelland J.J., Thomasson J.E., et al.: Sonographic findings with radiologic correlation in meconium peritonitis. *J. Clin. Ultrasound* 7:305, 1979.
9. Careskey J.M., Grosfeld J.L., Weber T.R., et al.: Giant cystic meconium peritonitis (GCMP): Improved management based on clinical and laboratory observations. *J. Pediatr. Surg.* 17:482, 1982.
10. Ceballos R., Hicks G.M.: Plastic peritonitis due to neonatal hydrometrocolpos: Radiologic and pathologic observations. *J. Pediatr. Surg.* 5:63, 1970.
11. Cerise E.J., Whitehead W.: Meconium peritonitis. *Am. Surg.* 35:389, 1969.
12. Dodat H., Chappuis J.P., Daudet M., et al.: Les peritonites meconiales. *Chir. Pédiatr.* 20:21, 1979.
13. Finkel L.I., Slovis T.L.: Meconium peritonitis, intraperitoneal calcifications and cystic fibrosis. *Pediatr. Radiol.* 12:92, 1982.
14. Fonkalsrud E.W., Ellis D.G., Clatworthy H.W. Jr.: Neonatal peritonitis. *J. Pediatr. Surg.* 1:227, 1966.
15. Forouhar F.: Meconium peritonitis—pathology, evolution and diagnosis. *Am. J. Clin. Pathol.* 78:208, 1982.
16. Garb M., Rad F.F., Riseborough J.: Meconium peritonitis presenting as fetal ascites on ultrasound. *Br. J. Radiol.* 53:602, 1980.
17. Gunn L.C., Ghionzoli O.G., Gardner H.G.: Healed meconium peritonitis presenting as a reducible scrotal mass. *J. Pediatr.* 92:847, 1978.
18. Heydenruch J.J., Marcus P.B.: Meconium granulomas of the tunica vaginalis. *J. Urol.* 115:596, 1976.
19. Hilgier A.: Observations on the reaction of the peritoneum in newborn guinea pigs to the introduction of meconium and bacterial infection. *Prob. Med. Wieku. Rozwoj.* 4:129, 1975.
20. Leonidas J.C., Berdon W.E., Baker D.H., et al.: Meconium ileus and its complications—a reappraisal of plain film roentgen diagnostic criteria. *Am. J. Roentgenol.* 108:598, 1970.
21. Marchildon M.B.: Meconium peritonitis and spontaneous gastric perforations. *Clin. Perinatol.* 5:79, 1978.
22. Martin L.W.: Meconium peritonitis, in Ravitch M.M., Welch K.J., Benson C.D., et al. (eds.): *Pediatric Surgery*, ed. 3. Chicago, Year Book Medical Publishers, 1979, p. 952.
23. Mayock D.E., Hickok D.E., Guthrie R.D.: Cystic meconium peritonitis associated with hydrops fetalis. *Am. J. Obstet. Gynecol.* 142:704, 1982.
24. Neuhauser E.B.D.: Roentgen diagnosis of fetal meconium peritonitis. *Am. J. Roentgenol.* 51:421, 1944.
25. Santulli T.V.: Meconium ileus, in Holder T.M., Ashcraft K.W. (eds.): *Pediatric Surgery*. Philadelphia, W.B. Saunders Co., 1980, p. 356.
26. Shalev J., Frankel Y., Avigad I., et al.: Spontaneous intestinal perforation in utero: Ultrasonic diagnostic criteria. *Am. J. Obstet. Gynecol.* 144:855, 1982.
27. Thompson R.B., Rosen D.I., Gross D.M.: Healed meconium peritonitis presenting as an inguinal mass. *J. Urol.* 110:364, 1973.
28. Tibboel D., Gaillard J.L.J., Molenaar J.C.: The "microscopic" type of meconium peritonitis. *Z. Kinderchir.* 34:9, 1981.
29. Ya-Xiong S., Lian-Chen S.: Meconium peritonitis—observation in 115 cases and antenatal diagnosis. *Z. Kinderchir.* 37:2, 1982.

Polypoid Diseases of the Gastrointestinal Tract

Polypoid diseases of the gastrointestinal tract include the common lesions of the bowel designated as true polyps (juvenile and adenomatous), a variety of uncommon polyp syndromes, and a number of miscellaneous diseases of the intestinal tract that may present polypoid masses in the lumen of the intestine.

Juvenile Polyps

History.—The important history of juvenile polypoid disease concerns the evolution of the concept established over 25 years ago[54, 65, 84] that this condition represents a distinct pathologic entity easily distinguishable from other polypoid lesions of the colon. Up to that time, these polyps were often identified with adenomas and were even filed in hospital records as adenomatous polyps. Although the juvenile polyp may have been regarded as a benign lesion, so deeply ingrained was (and perhaps still is) the practice of equating intestinal polyp with adenoma[43] that treatment of the juvenile polyp was confused and often unnecessarily radical. The usual juvenile polyp (single or scattered) is currently regarded as a totally benign entity bearing no relation to the adenomatous polyp. In more recent years, this concept has been modified only in two special rare forms of juvenile *polyposis* (not single or multiple scattered polyps): diffuse gastrointestinal juvenile polyposis and familial juvenile adenomatous polyposis, which will be discussed later.[92, 99, 112, 122]

Pathologic Anatomy

Juvenile polyp, also called retention, inflammatory, or cystic polyp, is the most common type of polyp found in the gastrointestinal tract in children, accounting for over 90% of polyps in children under 10 years of age.[54]

Grossly, the lesion is uniformly smooth, glistening, reddish, rounded or oval, ranging from a few millimeters to several centimeters in diameter. The average juvenile polyp is about 1 cm in diameter and ulcerated on the surface. It has a thin stalk or pedicle covered by normal colonic mucosa. The cut surface shows cystic spaces filled with mucus (Fig 98–1).

The histologic picture is distinctive. The surface consists of a single layer of flattened colonic epithelium, often ulcerated. Granulation tissue and inflammatory exudate may replace much of the surface epithelium. The main portion of the mass is made up of an abundant loose and often almost myxomatous vascular and fibrous stroma heavily infiltrated with acute and chronic inflammatory cells consisting of neutrophils, many eosinophils, some lymphocytes, and monocytes. Characteristically, there are many mucus-filled cystic spaces or lakes lined by mature, mucus-secreting tall columnar glandular cells, some of which may appear atrophic. Mitotic figures are extremely rare and there is no evidence of atypism (see Fig 98–1). This is in contrast to the adenomatous polyp, which shows a finely papillary surface with delicate arborization and irregular clefts, little stroma, little inflammation, and no cystic spaces. The glands are neoplastic; many of the cells are atypical and mitoses are present (Fig 98–2).

In our experience, as well as that of others,[52, 65, 71, 96] 70% of the lesions are in the rectum, 15% in the sigmoid colon, and the remainder scattered throughout the more proximal colon to the cecum. Three quarters of the patients have a single polyp, and one quarter have multiple or scattered polyps ranging from 2 to 12 in number, as also reported by others.[31, 45, 67, 72]

Etiology

The pathogenesis of juvenile polyps has been attributed to hereditary,[44] congenital,[62] inflammatory,[28, 54, 118, 120, 121] allergic,[4] and neoplastic[51] causes. Roth and Helwig, in a careful study of their pathologic material,[96] traced the development of these polyps. The first stage is ulceration and inflammation of the mucosa, the duct of a small colonic gland being blocked by the inflammation and ulceration. The blocked gland then proliferates, branches, and dilates, exposing a larger surface of the mucosa, and the ulceration and inflammation progress. Granulation tissue forms, and the cycle continues until the entire lesion is large enough to be held out in the fecal stream by peristalsis and/or the passing of the fecal stream. As a result, a stalk develops. The granulation tissue fibroses, the dilated glands may ulcerate, and the mucus of the cysts mixes with the stroma of the polyp, forming mucous cysts. The final stage may be twisting of the pedicle, infarction, and passage of the polyp in the stool. Horrilleno[54] also explained the formation of the retention mucous cysts by the deposition of fibrin, inflammatory cells, and epithelial debris on the traumatized mucosa, sealing the orifices of many of the mucous glands.

Incidence

The true incidence is probably unknown. Helwig[51] found polyps of the large intestine in 3% of 449 consecutive autopsies in individuals aged less than 21 years. Shapiro[105] found polyps in 3.74% of 2,700 children with proctologic disease. Louw[71] stated that 0.08% of all patients treated at a large children's hospital in Capetown had polyps of the colon.

Juvenile polyps are slightly more common in boys than girls. Although some have been discovered in the first year of life, they are most frequently seen from the ages of 2 to 8 years, with a peak incidence of 4–5 years. There is a spontaneous decline from 12 to 15 years; they are rarely seen thereafter. We have seen juvenile polyps in eight adult patients, and others have reported them in patients up to 61 years of age.[38, 96]

Symptoms and Signs

The most common symptom is bleeding due to inflammation and ulceration of the polyp. This is usually minimal, appearing as streaks of fresh blood on the outside of the stool. The blood from polyps in the proximal colon may be darker and mixed with the stool. Bleeding is intermittent. It is rarely of great magnitude, although this has been reported.[115] Also, rarely, autoamputation may expose a large vessel in the base and bleeding may then be brisk, requiring transfusion, as in one of our patients.

The polyp itself may actually prolapse or protrude at the anus, and may be the cause of prolapse of the anal and rectal mucosa (Fig 98–3). Some patients complain of abdominal cramps due to traction on the polyp during peristaltic activity and, in very rare instances, the lesion may initiate an intussusception. The polyp may undergo autoamputation and be passed by rectum. This has been reported to occur in 10–19% of cases.[49, 63, 67]

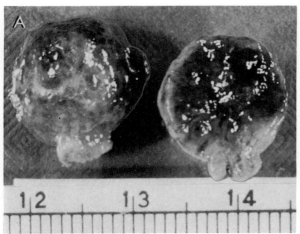

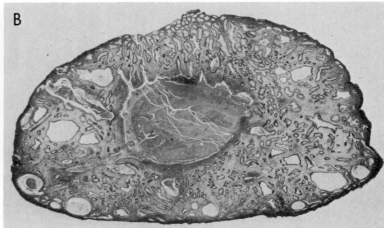

Fig 98–1.—The juvenile polyps. **A,** juvenile polyps with stalk. Note oval, smooth, glistening surface, which is ulcerated. **B,** photomicrograph (×11). Smooth continuous surface of flattened colonic epithelium, much of which is re-placed with granulation tissue and inflammatory exudate. Note large mucous cystic spaces or "lakes" and abundant loose stroma.

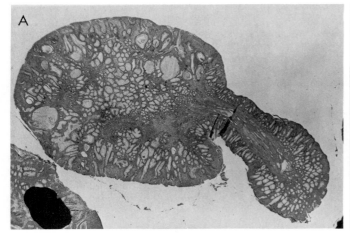

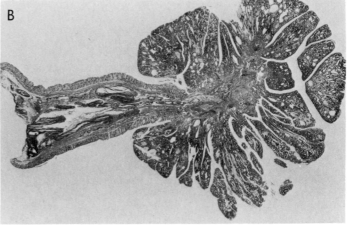

Fig 98–2.—Comparison of juvenile and adenomatous polyps. **A,** juvenile polyp (photomicrograph ×11). **B,** adenomatous polyp and stalk (photomicrograph ×11). Fine papillary surface with arborization and irregular clefts. Little stroma or inflammation. Note absence of cystic spaces. The glands are neoplastic.

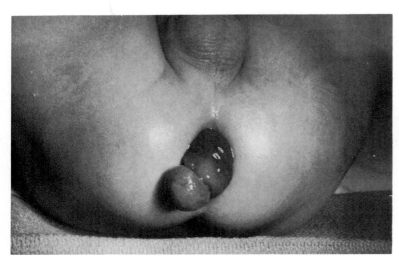

Fig 98–3.—Large juvenile polyp with prolapse protruding from the anus in 7-month-old boy. This is one of the modes of presentation.

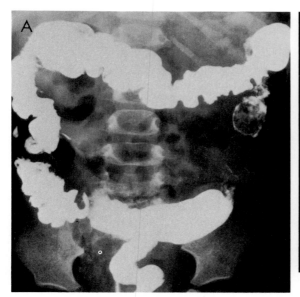
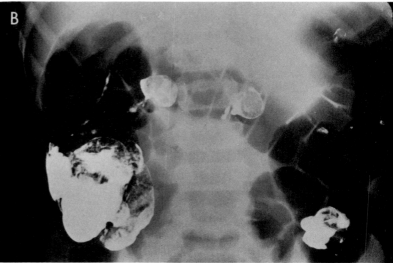

Fig 98–4.—Barium enema demonstration of juvenile polyps. **A,** polyp and stalk in descending colon. Thin coating of barium outlines the lesion. **B,** barium enema with air-contrast technique, showing two large juvenile polyps in the transverse colon.

Diarrhea may occur when many polyps are present.

Digital examination will frequently disclose the lesion. This, together with proctosigmoidoscopy, usually done under general anesthesia except in the older child, has revealed the polyp in over 75% of our cases.[33, 54, 71, 111] In the child, the lithotomy position is used. Most of the polyps are on the posterior rectal wall and best seen in this position. The lateral Sims position may also be used and, in the older child as in the adult, the knee-chest position is advantageous.

A polyp that can be palpated on digital examination should be removed. If it is a juvenile polyp, no further diagnostic evaluation is necessary. If bleeding recurs, or if the polyp proves to be adenomatous or hamartomatous, then careful studies of the colon by barium enema with air-contrast technique or colonoscopy should be performed (Fig 98–4). Postevacuation films are of particular importance in identifying a polyp that may retain a thin coating of barium outlining its surface (Fig 98–4,B). Because of the frequent difficulty of distinguishing a polyp from retained fecal masses in the colon, it is necessary to demonstrate the lesion on at least two separate studies before making a diagnosis of colonic polyp by barium enema.

Diagnosis

The differential diagnosis usually involves the common causes of rectal bleeding, including anal fissures, which can be seen; acute and chronic inflammatory bowel disease, which is usually accompanied by diarrhea; and blood dyscrasias such as Henoch-Schönlein purpura. Bleeding from Meckel's diverticulum or duplication of the bowel is usually of greater magnitude. Bleeding from intussusception is usually darker and accompanied by severe crampy abdominal pain.

The diagnosis is made from the history, the digital rectal examination, proctosigmoidoscopy, and barium air-contrast enema. Laboratory studies should include hemograms for anemia (rare) and, in some instances, blood studies for blood dyscrasias and stool examination for ova and parasites.

Treatment

Polyps in the rectum and lower sigmoid colon can be removed via the proctosigmoidoscope. Many of the lesions can be pulled down into the anus or even out of the anal canal and removed by careful suture ligation of the pedicle at its junction with the normal colon. For lesions that cannot be brought down into the anus, a tonsil snare and cautery are used through the proctoscope for amputation of the entire polyp.

Most, but not all, patients who have one or more polyps above the sigmoid colon will have a polyp in the rectum or lower sigmoid colon, accessible to the proctoscope.[35] In these instances, we remove the lower polyps to establish the diagnosis of juvenile polyp and think it unnecessary to remove the more proximal polyps unless they cause symptoms. Should a polyp not be available by anoscopy or proctosigmoidoscopy, we resort to colonoscopy for removal of the colonic polyp to establish the diagnosis of juvenile polyp (Fig 98–5). Some authors have recommended no treatment in these instances for 3–6 months and then colotomy if the polyp or polyps have not passed spontaneously by the

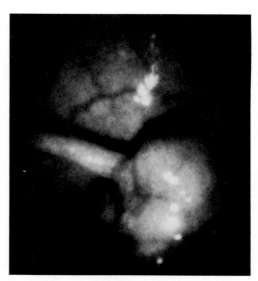

Fig 98–5.—Juvenile polyp with stalk in descending colon as viewed through fiberoptic colonoscope. This was removed with snare and cautery without incident.

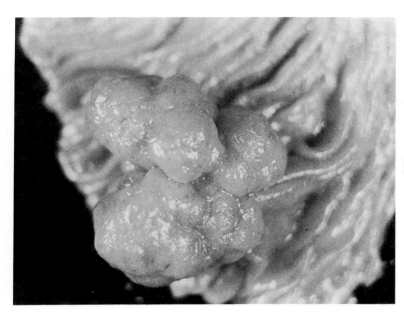

Fig 98–6.—Peutz-Jeghers syndrome. A single large polyp in the jejunum causing intussusception in a 10-year-old boy.

time.[123] We no longer perform colotomy in these cases, relying on the colonoscope. We base our practice on the assumption that adenomatous polyps are not found to coexist with juvenile polyps in the colon in the ordinary case of single or multiple scattered juvenile polyps.[38, 65, 67, 78] However, in the extremely rare syndrome of familial juvenile adenomatous polyposis (discussed later), adenomatous polyps have been found together with juvenile polyps.[61, 71, 122] In these instances, the colon is the seat of *polyposis* and not of several or multiple scattered juvenile polyps.

RESULTS.—There have been no complications following removal of a juvenile polyp via the anoscope or proctosigmoidoscope in our series of patients at Babies Hospital in New York, nor have there been any problems following polypectomy via the colonoscope, which has been employed in recent years. The "recurrence" rate, referring to the appearance of juvenile polyps in new locations, has been 5%; other reports cite figures that vary from 3 to 20%.[54, 65, 120]

The natural history of juvenile polyps is that they are self-limited.[96] Patients who have had polyps left in the colon, after we have established the diagnosis of juvenile polyp by removal of a polyp from the rectum, have usually remained asymptomatic. Most of these polyps will disappear, presumably by autoamputation.[65]

Intestinal Polyposis Associated with Mucocutaneous Pigmentation (Peutz-Jeghers Syndrome)

HISTORY.—The association of intestinal polyps with abnormal mucocutaneous pigmentation was first described by Peutz in 1921.[87] He reported seven cases in a single family and called attention to the hereditary aspects of the condition. Hutchinson[57] had described the distinctive pigmented spots of the lips and mouth in 1896, but he was not aware of intestinal lesions. In 1949, Jeghers and his associates[58] clearly established the syndrome in a classical article that analyzed 22 cases, 10 of their own. In 1957, Dormandy[28] presented an extensive review of the subject. In more recent years information has accumulated on the increased incidence of malignancy in the gastrointestinal tract[2, 27, 29, 39, 53, 86, 93, 94, 127, 131] and elsewhere[16, 30, 56, 104] in these patients.

Pathologic Anatomy

The important pathologic findings are associated with the gastrointestinal polyps. The lesions usually are scattered, but their

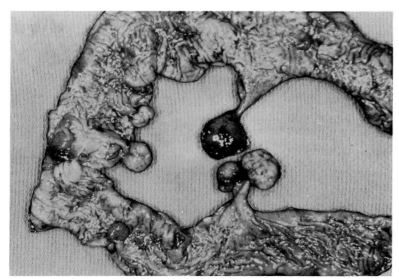

Fig 98–7.—Peutz-Jeghers syndrome. Portion of colon with multiple polyps resected in an 8-year-old boy. Note the variations in size.

location in the small intestine is almost a regular feature of the syndrome, occurring in 93% of cases. They have been found in the rectum and colon in about one third of cases, less frequently in the stomach and duodenum. Although rare cases of a single polyp (Fig 98–6) have been reported, the lesions usually are multiple and located simultaneously in several sites in the gas-

trointestinal tract.[6, 7, 113] They vary in size from a few millimeters to several centimeters (Fig 98–7).

The nature of the polyps is controversial. They were formerly regarded as benign adenomatous lesions, but on the basis of the histologic findings of mitoses, hyperchromatism, and invasion of the muscularis mucosa, some were classified as malignant. Their

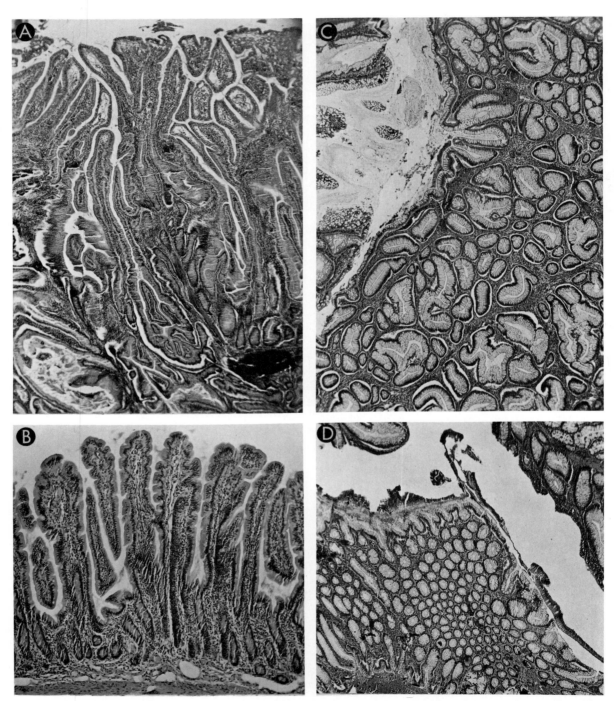

Fig 98–8.—Peutz-Jeghers polyps: microscopic picture. **A,** polyp of the jejunum. Note the villous pattern at the free surface and the small, darkly stained glands in the depths. The topography, as well as the epithelial cells, closely resembles normal small intestinal mucosa. **B,** appearance of nonpolypoid jejunal mucosa adjacent to **A,** for comparison. **C,** polyp of the colon. The glands are neither of the cystic type seen in juvenile polyps nor the true neoplastic glands of the adult adenomatous polyp. Although somewhat enlarged, they are essentially simple mucous glands duplicating the cytology and architecture of the adjacent normal colonic mucosa, shown in **D.**

adenomatous nature was questioned by Bartholomew and his associates,[7] who suggested that they represent tissue excrescences from a developmental abnormality similar to the hamartomas (Fig 98–8).

The mucocutaneous pigmentation due to melanin deposits, and usually distributed on the lip and buccal mucosa, may also occur around the mouth or eyes, across the bridge of the nose, on the tongue, gums, hard palate, and the palmar and plantar surfaces of the fingers and toes (Fig 98–9). The color varies from light brown to black, and the lesions may be linear, oval, or irregular. They are usually small (less than 5 mm in diameter), flat, nonhairy spots that do not coalesce. Microscopically, the pigment is found to be deposited in vertical bands in the basal layer of the epidermis. These pigmented cells are not melanoblasts. The relation of the mucocutaneous pigmentation to the polyposis is unknown. Neither the polyps nor the mucosa of the intestine are pigmented.

Ovarian tumors have been reported in about 5% of females with the syndrome, and it has been suggested that they are related to the same mutant gene.[16, 30, 56, 104]

Incidence

The disease is rare. The sex distribution is about equal, and the syndrome has been described in all racial groups.

A family history has been obtained in half of the patients. The disease is inherited through a Mendelian dominant gene of high penetrance. Probably 50% of descendants of patients with the disease are afflicted.

Symptoms and Signs

Although the syndrome usually is manifest in childhood, the age range in reported cases is from 2 to 82 years, with average age 29. The youngest patients reported to date have been 4 and 11 months.[55, 82]

The cardinal features are the mucocutaneous pigmentation, gastrointestinal polyposis, repeated episodes of abdominal pain due to intussusception, occult blood loss from the intestinal tract, anemia, and a frequent familial incidence.

The pigmented spots are distinctive and should always lead to investigation for intestinal polyps. Pigmentation is often the initial sign, abdominal symptoms generally not becoming apparent before 8–10 years of age.[26]

Recurrent attacks of crampy abdominal pain accompanied by loud borborygmi due to transient intussusception are characteristic. Complete obstruction is rare, the majority of the episodes of intussusception being spontaneously relieved. The pain may be accompanied by an abdominal mass, which may be palpated or seen by the patient. The episodes occur periodically, with intervals of quiescence lasting months to years.

Gastrointestinal bleeding, usually occult, and hypochromic anemia secondary to chronic blood loss, occur in about one third of the cases.

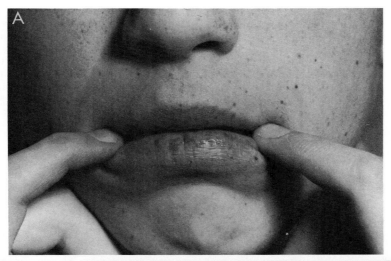

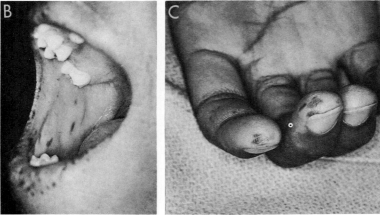

Fig 98–9.—Peutz-Jeghers syndrome. Mucocutaneous spots on, **A,** lips and face; **B,** buccal mucosa; **C,** fingers.

Proctosigmoidoscopy, barium enema studies by the air-contrast technique and gastrointestinal roentgen examinations are necessary (Fig 98–10). Large polyps of the small intestine may be missed in spite of apparently adequate studies. Transient intussusceptions are frequently demonstrated, or there may be segmentation and clumping of the contrast material in the small intestine. Occasionally, gastroscopy is required to confirm the presence of gastric polyps.

The clinical course is characterized by recurrent episodes of crampy abdominal pain due to transient intussusceptions. Melena or the passage of gross blood by rectum, hypochromic anemia, weakness, fainting and stunting of growth may occur. In some patients, the melanin spots of the lips and buccal mucosa begin to fade at puberty.

Differential Diagnosis

Gastric polyposis is occasionally seen in familial colonic polyposis and the Peutz-Jeghers syndrome. In the latter disease, the presence of small intestinal polyps with associated mucocutaneous pigmentation is diagnostic. The melanin spots are distinctive, but they may need to be differentiated from freckles, which show seasonal change, are sparse near the mouth, and rarely involve the palms or buccal mucosa. Histologic examination of one of the polyps will establish the diagnosis.

Treatment

Once the diagnosis has been made, conservative management is preferable. The patient and family should be made acquainted with the disease to avoid needless operations for brief transitory episodes of intussusception.

Operation is necessary for irreducible intussusception or prolonged and serious intestinal bleeding. If resection is not demanded by irreducibility or necrosis, one should be content with reduction of the intussusception and enterotomies to remove any large polypoid masses. In spite of such an approach, multiple operations are often necessary.[89] Radical resections should be avoided when at all possible.

PROGNOSIS.—Patients will live with this disease for many years. The prognosis usually depends on the complications of intussusception, blood loss, and the requisite operations. Most of the deaths are due to these complications.

Although Peutz-Jeghers polyps are considered to be hamartomatous and generally regarded as benign lesions, coincidental hamartomatous and adenomatous polyps have been seen in the small intestine[39] as well as in the colon[94] and stomach.[29] In the long term, Peutz-Jeghers syndrome does carry an increased risk of metastasizing intestinal cancer, albeit small. This has been documented in 2–3% of cases.[29, 39] Such malignancy appears to arise not from the Peutz-Jeghers polyps but from the coincident adenomatous polyps.[69] It occurs most often in the duodenum[93, 94] and has been seen in stomach, jejunum, and colon.

Adenomatous Polyps

These are extremely rare in children. Kottmeier and Clatworthy[67] reported only three in a group of 50 patients with intestinal polyps, and in two of these the polyps were multiple. Knox and his associates[65] did not find any adenomatous polyps in patients under 20 years of age. Louw[71] reported only two solitary adenomas in a large series of polyps in children. We have not seen any adenomatous polyps in a child, except in familial adenomatous polyposis.

The adenomatous polyp, often referred to as the "adult" or "neoplastic" polyp, is made up of a proliferation of glandular elements with much branching and very little stroma and connective tissue. There is usually little evidence of the inflammation frequently seen in the juvenile polyps. The epithelium is often multilayered with atypism, mitotic figures, and hyperchromatic nuclei (see Fig 98–2,*B*). This is a true neoplasm, and the finding of a solitary adenoma in a child requires extensive investigation of the entire colon. This finding may indicate the likely development of familial adenomatous polyposis, and careful follow-up of the patient as well as investigation of members of the family are indicated.[64, 76, 116]

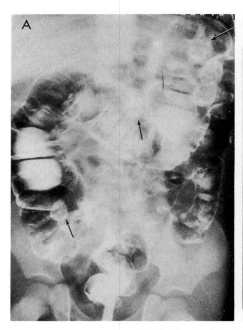
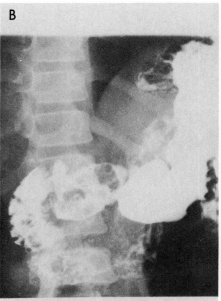
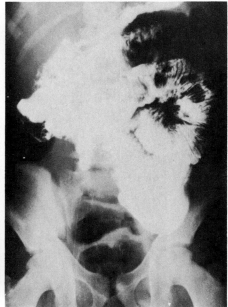

Fig 98–10.—Peutz-Jeghers syndrome in an 8-year-old boy. **A,** barium enema showing multiple polyps. **B,** gastrointestinal barium study demonstrating multiple polyps in duodenum and jejunum in same patient.

Familial Adenomatous Polyposis

HISTORY.—In 1881, Cripps[23] first described the familial history of this disease, and in 1890, Handford[48] first reported the malignant changes. Coffey[19] reported the first total colectomy and ileostomy for familial polyposis in 1926. In 1927, Cockayne[18] reported that the disease was inherited as a Mendelian autosomal non-sex-linked dominant trait. In a study of 68 families and kindred from St. Mark's Hospital, London, in which fairly complete pedigrees were available for three or even four generations, Dukes,[32] in reporting on the genetic pattern of the disease in 1958, made several observations: (1) males and females are equally affected, and either sex can transmit the disease; (2) only those who have the disease themselves are capable of transmitting it to the next generation; (3) in most polyposis families one half of the children are likely to inherit the disease, the remainder being normal;[73] (4) the severity of the disease and the probability of cancer of the rectum or colon developing vary considerably in different families. In families in which polyposis develops early in life, cancer frequently occurs within 10–15 years, whereas in families in which polyposis occurs later the precancerous incubation period is longer, so that the patient may die of natural causes before intestinal cancer has had time to develop. Dukes also reported 11 solitary cases without familial involvement. Bussey[11] has reported the largest series: over 600 patients and 200 affected families.

Pathology

Characteristically, there are innumerable polyps carpeting the bowel from the anus to the cecum, including the appendix.[64] The polyps are of the "adult" adenomatous type, as described in the previous section (see Fig 98–2,B). Lesions under 3 mm in size are usually hyperplastic polyps, do not have malignant potential[68] and need to be differentiated from adenomatous polyps.

Symptoms and Signs

Although the disease has been seen in infancy and early childhood,[1, 45] it is more likely to become symptomatic at puberty or in the late teens.[67] Diarrhea or increased frequency of stools is usually the first symptom, followed by bleeding per rectum, abdominal pain, tenesmus, and anemia. There may be rectal pain and prolapse at the anus.

Early in the disease the patient may be asymptomatic; the polyps are discovered by investigation on the basis of the family history.

Diagnosis

The diagnosis is made by the family history, digital rectal examination, and proctosigmoidoscopy. Excisional biopsy of one of the innumerable polyps will establish the diagnosis. Barium enema with air-contrast examination will demonstrate many filling defects with extensive involvement of the colon (Fig 98–11).

When the diagnosis is made, careful investigation of all members of the family should be carried out. In the long term, members of the family are at high risk of developing carcinoma of the colon, and it will occur at least 20 years earlier than in the general population, as there is an inherited predisposition of the colonic mucosa to undergo malignant change at an early age.[47, 64]

Course

Malignancy is usually not seen until late adolescence or early adult life, though the disease may have been present early in life. In a series of patients less than 13 years of age, carcinoma was found in 6%.[108] In general, all patients with familial adenomatous polyposis will die of carcinoma of the colon or will have advanced malignant disease by the age of 50.[77] Several reports have indicated that 40–66% of patients who came to operation

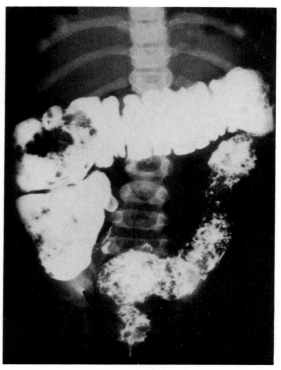

Fig 98–11.—Familial polyposis. Barium enema in an 8-year-old girl. Note the innumerable filling defects, especially in the descending and sigmoid colon and rectum.

as adults had carcinoma.[11, 128] Carcinoma of these colons is frequently multicentric.

Treatment

Colectomy is indicated at any age if the child is symptomatic. Otherwise, colectomy should be done between 10 and 15 years of age once the diagnosis is established.

One of three operations may be done: (1) total colectomy and proctectomy with terminal ileostomy; (2) subtotal colectomy with fulguration of the rectal polyps and ileoproctostomy, preserving the rectum, or (3) total colectomy with an endorectal pull-through procedure in which all of the rectal mucosa is removed and the ileum is brought through the muscular sleeve of the rectum and anastomosed to the anus.[91] Each of the procedures has its advocates. If any rectal mucosa is left behind, the patient must be very carefully followed with frequent examination of the rectum because of the real threat of carcinoma developing in the remaining rectal stump.[9, 42, 50]

Interestingly, when the rectum has been preserved, the polyps of the rectum that have been left behind have sometimes regressed spontaneously and disappeared in these patients, but this may only be temporary.[20, 33, 70, 83, 103]

The safest procedure has been total coloproctectomy (Fig 98–12) with terminal ileostomy. The social advantage of preserving the rectum may be costly, since carcinoma may develop despite frequent and careful follow-up examinations.[98] As many as 60% of patients so treated have had carcinoma develop in the remaining rectum over a period of 2–3 decades.[81] The Ravitch-Soave type of pull-through ileoproctostomy obviates this danger, since all of the rectal mucosa is removed in the procedure.[36, 100, 117, 129, 130]

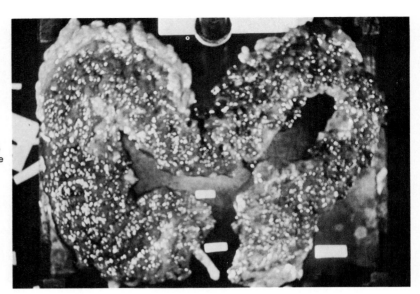

Fig 98–12.—Pancolectomy for familial adenomatous polyposis. Specimen of colon in a 24-year-old man. The entire colon is carpeted with adenomatous polyps. There was no evidence of carcinoma in this colon.

Unusual Polyp Syndromes of the Gastrointestinal Tract

Diffuse Gastrointestinal Juvenile Polyposis

This is a rare but relatively distinct entity seen in infancy. In contrast to children with single or scattered multiple colonic juvenile polyps, there may be involvement of the entire colon (juvenile polyposis coli) or even the entire gastrointestinal tract, with polyposis that carries different clinical or genetic implications.[90, 99, 110, 112, 114] The disease may be familial or nonfamilial, and it appears to be transmitted as a non-sex-linked recessive.

It is characterized by gastrointestinal bleeding, diarrhea, rectal prolapse, intussusception, protein-losing enteropathy producing malnutrition, anasarca, and severe anemia. The prognosis is directly related to the severity and extent of the gastrointestinal involvement with juvenile polyposis. Beyond infancy, accurate histologic interpretation of the polyps is essential to distinguish this syndrome from familial adenomatous polyposis of the colon, familial juvenile adenomatous polyposis and Peutz-Jeghers syndrome.[98]

Although these polyps are benign and histologically of the juvenile type, the rapid downhill course in this life-threatening disease would appear to justify aggressive operative therapy combined with hyperalimentation.[80, 102] Total colectomy with a Ravitch-Soave endorectal pull-through is the recommended procedure.[14, 90, 92, 97, 112]

Familial Juvenile Adenomatous Polyposis

The rare association of juvenile and adenomatous polyps has recently been recognized, but only in *diffuse* colonic or familial juvenile polyposis.[61, 71, 102, 122] In these rare instances the clinical approach differs from that of the usual juvenile polyp, even when histologic identification of the juvenile polyp has been obtained. The retrieval of a single juvenile polyp in *diffuse* juvenile polyposis may not exclude the existence of associated adenomatous polyps. Hence, multiple polyps will have to be sampled. Representative biopsies from several polyps may be obtained by the colonoscope or gastroscope in the upper gastrointestinal tract, eliminating the need for laparotomy.[122]

Since approximately half of all juvenile polyposis is reported to have a familial occurrence, relatives and siblings, in particular, should also be examined.

The coexistence of juvenile and adenomatous polyps has been seen only in *diffuse* colonic polyposis. Hence, the conservative approach in children with single or scattered juvenile polyps (not *polyposis*) should not be changed.

Lymphoid Polyposis (Lymphoid Nodular Hyperplasia)

Sometimes an overgrowth of lymphoid tissue of the intestine may give rise to polypoid masses, which may ulcerate and are thought to cause rectal bleeding. This may be seen in the rectum and colon of children and adults. Called "benign lymphoma" or "pseudoleukemia,"[21, 22] the lesion is not neoplastic.[12]

The gross appearance is that of firm, round, submucosal nodules with smooth or lobulated surfaces. Sometimes the mucosa covering the nodules is ulcerated.[108] The polypoid masses are usually multiple, sessile, and often minute, as seen on proctosigmoidoscopy. Microscopically, they are made up of large hyperplastic lymphoid follicles with large germinal centers covered by colonic mucosa.

Rectal bleeding may be the only symptom, but there may also be crampy pain and diarrhea. The peak incidence is from ages 1 to 3 years.

Barium enema with air-contrast technique reveals multiple small polypoid defects, umbilicated and relatively uniform in size and with smooth margins (Fig 98–13).

The etiology is unknown. The lymphoid hyperplasia may be simply a normal response to a variety of stimuli, including infection and allergy.[15] The lesions usually regress spontaneously or may regress with antibiotics or corticosteroid treatment.[15, 71, 108] Recurrence is rare. The nodular type of lymphoid hyperplasia shows more diffuse involvement of the small and large intestine and selective IgA deficiency.[46]

The lesions may be mistaken for those of familial polyposis, ulcerative colitis, and lymphoma. Total colectomy has been done because of a mistaken diagnosis.[21, 22]

Jona, Belin and Burke[60] have recently reported on two forms of the disease in a series of 12 children. The acute form with involvement of the appendix or terminal ileum presented commonly as acute appendicitis. Appendectomy alone was sufficient in these because of the self-limiting nature of the disease. When

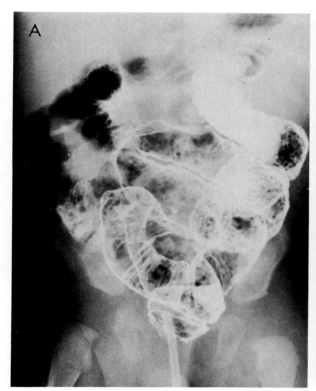
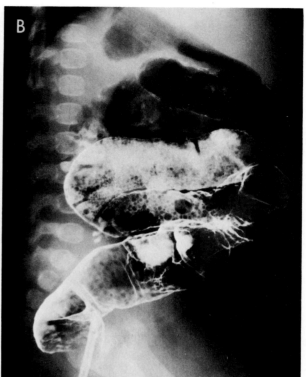

Fig 98–13.—Benign lymphoid nodular hyperplasia of the colon. **A,** anteroposterior and **B,** lateral views of a barium enema in an 8-week-old boy with lymphoid polyposis who presented with frequent stools containing mucus and some blood. He was not treated; the lesions regressed spontaneously, and he remains well 2½ years later.

intussusception was present, resection of the ileum was performed. The chronic form, also common in the terminal ileum, produced disabling symptoms, including recurrent intussusception, chronic anemia, and weight loss. These patients required resection.

Gardner Syndrome

In 1953, Gardner and Richards[41] described a familial form of colonic polyposis that occurs in association with osteomas of the skull and facial bones and, in some instances, with multiple soft tissue tumors such as lipomas, desmoid tumors, leiomyomas, and multiple sebaceous cysts. In 1962, Shiffman[106] reported a case and analyzed 89 others from the literature.

The polyps, which are adenomatous, may also involve the small bowel and duodenum. The syndrome is believed to be inherited as the expression of a single, apparently pleiotropic, dominant gene. The natural history of colonic polyposis in patients with this syndrome is similar to that of familial adenomatous polyposis without soft tissue or bone tumors, and the treatment is the same. Operation is often followed by excessive fibrous reaction, and the resulting intra-abdominal desmoids may be ineradicable and fatal.

Turcot Syndrome

Turcot and his associates[119] reported a brother and sister with diffuse colonic adenomatous polyposis who died of tumors of the central nervous system. The boy died at age 18 years of medulloblastoma involving the spinal cord, and his sister died at age 21 years of glioblastoma multiforme of the frontal lobe. This syndrome may be inherited as an autosomal recessive disorder.[26, 34]

Cronkhite-Canada Syndrome

This rare syndrome, which is mostly seen in patients over 40 years of age, has been reported in children.[66, 97] It is characterized by alopecia, cutaneous hyperpigmentation, atrophic nails, and large bowel polyps resembling juvenile polyps.[24, 97] The syndrome is distinguished from other conditions associated with polyposis because of the late onset, the lack of family history and the unique ectodermal changes.[66]

Other Polyposis Syndromes

Other rare variants of the hereditary pattern of gastrointestinal polyposis with malignant proclivity have been reported in children by Boley[10] and Murphy[85] and their associates.

Miscellaneous Polypoid Diseases

A variety of lesions are found in the gastrointestinal tract of children, some of which may protrude into the lumen of the bowel as polypoid masses but which are not considered to be polyps in the usual sense. These include ectopic pancreatic tissue,[109] polypoid hypertrophy of the gastric rugae on an allergic or hypersensitivity basis,[101] gastric[59, 74, 88, 107] and colonic[3, 5, 13, 17, 79, 126] cancer, gastric heterotopia of the intestine,[39] inflammatory fibroid polyps,[101] fibromas, neurofibromas, ganglioneuromas, lipomas (usually cecal), leiomyomas, and leiomyosarcoma.[84, 95] We have also encountered several hemangiomas of the small bowel and one embryonal rhabdomyosarcoma of the cecum presenting as polypoid masses. Granulation tissue may form polypoid masses in the rectum, which cause bleeding and diarrhea.[116] These granulomas may be traumatic in

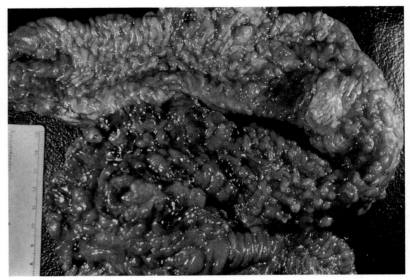

Fig 98–14.—Pseudopolyps in colon resected for ulcerative colitis. The masses represent hypertrophied margins of the numerous ulcers present.

origin. We have had one such patient. The granulomas have recurred after excision and fulguration.

The small intestine is the usual site for primary gastrointestinal lymphomas in children. They may give rise to intussusception. Late in the course of Hodgkin's disease the stomach may be involved.[26]

Pseudopolyps may be seen in inflammatory bowel disease. These masses merely represent hypertrophied and proliferating epithelial margins of the mucosal ulcerations (Fig 98–14).

Colonoscopy

Colonoscopy is a useful procedure in children in certain situations. In skilled hands, the procedure is safe. The complication rate from biopsy or polypectomy with the fiberoptic colonoscope is low. However, these procedures must be carried out with extreme care because of the relative thinness of the bowel wall compared with that of the adult.[8, 37, 40, 115] They should be done under general anesthesia except, perhaps, in some of the more cooperative older children. We have used colonoscopy in place of colotomy to remove more proximal colonic polyps when a polyp was not available by proctoscopy, to establish a diagnosis. We have not used it when a polyp available by proctoscopy proved to be a juvenile polyp. We do not remove the more proximal polyps in these cases unless they cause symptoms. If they do, we remove those polyps by colonoscopy whenever possible and avoid colotomy.

We have also used the technique in investigating young members of familial adenomatous polyposis families.

Colonoscopy has been used to sample various polyps in patients who may have juvenile adenomatous polyposis.[122] However, even in expert hands the diagnosis of carcinoma may be missed in spite of multiple sampling of such polyps.[25]

The colonoscope has been very helpful in locating the source of bleeding in some of our more difficult cases. Probably its most important use for us, so far, has been in the early diagnosis of inflammatory bowel disease and in the assessment of the status and extent (limits) of the disease.

REFERENCES

1. Abramson D.J.: Multiple polyposis in children: A review and a report of a case in a 6-year-old child who had associated nephrosis and asthma. *Surgery* 61:288, 1967.
2. Achord J.L., Proctor H.D.: Malignant degeneration and metastasis in Peutz-Jeghers syndrome. *Arch. Intern. Med.* 111:498, 1963.
3. Alaghemand A.: Carcinoma of the colon and rectum in children. *Am. Surg.* 28:784, 1962.
4. Alexander R.H., Beckwith J.B., Morgan A., et al.: Juvenile polyps of the colon and their relationship to allergy. *Am. J. Surg.* 120:222, 1970.
5. Andersson A., Bergdahl L.: Carcinoma of the colon in children: A report of six new cases and a review of the literature. *J. Pediatr. Surg.* 11:967, 1976.
6. Bailey D.: Polyposis of gastrointestinal tract: The Peutz syndrome. *Br. Med. J.* 2:433, 1957.
7. Bartholomew L.G., Dahlin D.C., Waugh J.M.: Intestinal polyposis associated with mucocutaneous pigmentation. *N.Y. J. Med.* 60:1796, 1960.
8. Behringer G.E.: Polypoid lesions of the colon. *Surg. Clin. North Am.* 54:699, 1974.
9. Bigay D., Plauchu H., Berard P.: Rectocolic familial polyposis: A study of 32 cases. *World J. Surg.* 5:617, 1981.
10. Boley S.J., McKinnon W.M., Marzulli V.F.: The management of familial gastrointestinal polyposis involving stomach and colon. *Surgery* 50:691, 1961.
11. Bussey H.J.R.: *Familial Polyposis Coli: Family Studies, Histopathology, Differential Diagnosis, and Results of Treatment.* Baltimore, Johns Hopkins University Press, 1975.
12. Byrne W.J., Jimenez J.F., Euler A.R., et al.: Lymphoid polyps (focal lymphoid hyperplasia) of the colon in children. *Pediatrics* 69:598, 1982.
13. Cain A.S., Longino L.A.: Carcinoma of the colon in children. *J. Pediatr. Surg.* 5:527, 1970.
14. Cameron G.S., Lau G.Y.P.: Juvenile polyposis coli: A case treated with ileoendorectal pullthrough. *J. Pediatr. Surg.* 14:536, 1979.
15. Capitanio M.A., Kirkpatrick J.A.: Lymphoid hyperplasia of the colon in children. *Radiology* 94:323, 1970.
16. Christian C.D., McLoughlin T.G., Cathcart E.R., et al.: Peutz-Jeghers syndrome associated with functioning ovarian tumor. *JAMA* 190:935, 1964.
17. Clutts G.R., Emmet J.M.: Carcinoma of the colon in children under 16 years of age. *Am. Surg.* 30:671, 1964.
18. Cockayne E.A.: Heredity in relation to cancer. *Cancer Rev.* 2:337, 1927.
19. Coffey R.C.: Colonic polyposis with engrafted malignancy. *Ann. Surg.* 83:364, 1926.
20. Cole J.W., Holden W.D.: Postcolectomy regression of adenomatous polyps of the rectum. *Arch. Surg.* 79:385, 1959.
21. Collins J.E., Falk M., Guibone R.: Benign lymphoid polyposis of the colon: A case report. *Pediatrics* 38:897, 1966.
22. Cosens C.G.: Gastrointestinal pseudoleukemia: A case report. *Ann. Surg.* 148:129, 1958.
23. Cripps W.H.: Two cases of disseminated polyps of the rectum. *Trans. Pathol. Soc. London* 33:165, 1881.
24. Cronkhite L.W. Jr., Canada W.J.: Generalized gastrointestinal pol-

yposis: An unusual syndrome of polyposis, pigmentation, alopecia and onychotrophia. *N. Engl. J. Med.* 252:1011, 1955.

25. Crowson T.D., Ferrante W.F., Gathright J.B. Jr.: Colonoscopy: Inefficacy in early carcinoma detection in patients with ulcerative colitis. *JAMA* 236:2651, 1976.

26. Dehner L.P.: *Pediatric Surgical Pathology.* St. Louis, C.V. Mosby Co., 1975.

27. De Pa Pava S., Cabrira A., Studenski E.R.: Peutz-Jeghers syndrome with jejunal carcinoma. *N.Y. State J. Med.* 62:97, 1962.

28. Dormandy T.L.: Gastrointestinal polyposis with mucocutaneous pigmentation (Peutz-Jeghers syndrome). *N. Engl. J. Med.* 256:1093, 1957.

29. Dozois R.R., Judd E.S., Dahlin D.C.: The Peutz-Jeghers syndrome: Is there a predisposition to the development of intestinal malignancy? *Arch. Surg.* 98:509, 1969.

30. Dozois R.R., Kempers R.D., Dahlin D.C., et al.: Ovarian tumors associated with the Peutz-Jeghers syndrome. *Ann. Surg.* 172:233, 1970.

31. Duhamel J., Bauche P.: Polyps of the colon beyond the reach of the sigmoidoscope. *Arch. Dis. Child.* 40:173, 1965.

32. Dukes C.E.: Cancer control in familial polyposis of the colon. *Dis. Colon Rectum* 1:413, 1958.

33. Eckert C.: Intestinal polyposis, in Ariel I.M., et al. (eds.): *Cancer and Allied Diseases of Infancy and Childhood.* Boston, Little, Brown & Co., 1960, p. 161.

34. Erbe R.W.: Current concepts in genetics: Inherited gastrointestinal polyposis syndromes. *N. Engl. J. Med.* 294:1101, 1976.

35. Euler A.R., Seibert J.J.: The role of sigmoidoscopy, radiographs, and colonoscopy in the diagnostic evaluation of pediatric age patients with suspected juvenile polyps. *J. Pediatr. Surg.* 16:500, 1981.

36. Fonkalsrud E.W.: Endorectal ileal pullthrough with lateral ileal reservoir for benign colorectal disease. *Ann. Surg.* 194:761, 1981.

37. Forde K.A.: Personal communication.

38. Franklin R., McSwain B.: Juvenile polyps of the colon and rectum. *Ann. Surg.* 175:887, 1972.

39. Gannon P.G., Dahlin D.C., Batholomew L.G., et al.: Polypoid glandular tumors of the small intestine. *Surg. Gynecol. Obstet.* 114:666, 1962.

40. Gans S.L., Ament M., Christie D.L., et al.: Pediatric endoscopy with flexible fiberscopes. *J. Pediatr. Surg.* 10:375, 1975.

41. Gardner E.J., Richards R.C.: Multiple cutaneous and subcutaneous lesions occurring simultaneously with hereditary polyposis and osteomatosis. *Am. J. Hum. Genet.* 5:139, 1953.

42. Gingold B.S., Jagelman D.G.: Sparing the rectum in familial polyposis: Causes for failure. *Surgery* 89:314, 1981.

43. Goligher J.C.: *Surgery of the Anus, Rectum and Colon,* ed. 2. London, Bailliere, Tindall & Cassell, 1970.

44. Gowin T.S.: Polyps of colon and rectum in children. *South. Med. J.* 54:526, 1961.

45. Gross R.E.: *The Surgery of Infancy and Childhood.* Philadelphia, W.B. Saunders Co., 1953.

46. Gryboski J.D., Self T.W., Clemett A., et al.: Selective immunoglobulin A deficiency and intestinal lymphoid hyperplasia: Correlating of diarrhea with antibiotics and plasma. *Pediatrics* 42:833, 1968.

47. Haggitt R.C., Pitcock J.A.: Familial juvenile polyposis of the colon. *Cancer* 26:1232, 1970.

48. Handford H.: Disseminated polypi of the large intestine becoming malignant. *Trans. Pathol. Soc. London* 41:133, 1890.

49. Harris J.W.: Polyps of the rectum and colon in children. *Am. J. Surg.* 86:577, 1953.

50. Harvey J.C., Quan S.H.Q., Stearns M.W.: Management of familial polyposis with preservation of the rectum. *Surgery* 84:476, 1978.

51. Helwig E.B.: Adenomas of the large intestine in children. *Am. J. Dis. Child.* 72:289, 1946.

52. Holgersen L.D., Miller R.E., Zintel H.A.: Juvenile polyps of the colon. *Surgery* 69:288, 1971.

53. Horn R.C. Jr., Payne W.A., Fine G.: The Peutz-Jeghers syndrome (gastrointestinal polyposis with mucocutaneous pigmentation): Report of a case terminating with disseminated gastrointestinal cancer. *Arch. Pathol.* 76:29, 1963.

54. Horilleno E.G., Eckert C., Ackerman L.V.: Polyps of the rectum and colon in children. *Cancer* 10:1210, 1957.

55. Howell J., Pringle K., Kirschner B., et al.: Peutz-Jeghers polyps causing colocolic intussusception in infancy. *J. Pediatr. Surg.* 16:82, 1981.

56. Humphries A.L., Shepherd M.H., Peters H.J.: Peutz-Jeghers syndrome with colonic adenocarcinoma and ovarian tumor. *JAMA* 197:296, 1966.

57. Hutchinson J.: Pigmented spots on the lips and mouth in twin sisters. *Arch. Surg.* (London) 7:290, 1896.

58. Jeghers H., McKusick V.A., Katz K.H.: Generalized intestinal polyposis and melanin spots of the oral mucosa, lips, and digits. A syndrome of diagnostic significance. *N. Engl. J. Med.* 241:993, 1949.

59. Johnston D.P., Van Heerden J.A., Lynn H.B., et al.: Carcinoma of the stomach in a 10-year-old boy. *J. Pediatr. Surg.* 10:151, 1975.

60. Jona J.Z., Belin R.P., Burke J.A.: Lymphoid hyperplasia of the bowel and its surgical significance in children. *J. Pediatr. Surg.* 11:997, 1976.

61. Kaschula R.O.C.: Mixed juvenile, adenomatous and intermediate polyposis coli. *Dis. Colon Rectum* 14:368, 1971.

62. Kennedy R.L.J.: Polyps of rectum and colon in infants and in children. *Am. J. Dis. Child.* 62:481, 1941.

63. Kerr J.G.: Polyposis of the colon in children. *Am. J. Surg.* 76:667, 1948.

64. Kissane J.M.: *Pathology of Infancy and Childhood,* ed. 2. St. Louis, C.V. Mosby Co., 1975.

65. Knox W.G., Miller R.E., Begg C.F., et al.: Juvenile polyps of the colon. *Surgery* 48:201, 1960.

66. Koehler P.R., Kyaw M.M., Fenlon J.W.: Diffuse gastrointestinal polyposis with ectodermal changes, Cronkhite-Canada syndrome. *Radiology* 103:589, 1972.

67. Kottmeier P.K., Clatworthy H.W. Jr.: Intestinal polyps and associated carcinoma in childhood. *Am. J. Surg.* 110:709, 1965.

68. Lane N., Kaplan H., Pascal R.R.: Minute adenomatous and hyperplastic polyps of the colon: Divergent patterns of epithelial growth with specific associated mesenchymal changes: Contrasting roles in the pathogenesis of carcinoma. *Gastroenterology* 60:537, 1971.

69. Linos D.A., Dozois R.R., Dahlin D.C., et al.: Does Peutz-Jeghers syndrome predispose to gastrointestinal malignancy? A later look. *Arch. Surg.* 116:1182, 1981.

70. Localio S.A.: Spontaneous disappearance of rectal polyps following subtotal colectomy and ileoproctostomy for polyposis of the colon. *Am. J. Surg.* 103:81, 1962.

71. Louw J.H.: Polypoid lesions of the large bowel in children with particular reference to benign lymphoid polyposis. *J. Pediatr. Surg.* 3:195, 1968.

72. Louw J.H.: Polypoid lesions of the large bowel in children. *S. Afr. Med. J.* 46:1347, 1972.

73. McKusick V.A.: Genetic factors in intestinal polyposis. *JAMA* 182:271, 1962.

74. McNeer G.: Cancer of the stomach in the young. *Am. J. Roentgenol.* 45:537, 1941.

75. Mallam A.S., Thompson S.A.: Polyps of the rectum and colon in children. *Can. J. Surg.* 3:17, 1959.

76. Mauro J., Prior J.T.: Gastrointestinal polypoid lesions in childhood. *Cancer* 10:131, 1957.

77. Mayo C.W., De Weerd J.H., Jackman R.J.: Diffuse familial polyposis of the colon. *Surg. Gynecol. Obstet.* 93:87, 1951.

78. Mazier W.P., Bowman H.E. Sun K.M., et al.: Juvenile polyps of the colon and rectum. *Dis. Colon Rectum* 17:523, 1974.

79. Middelkamp J.N., Haffner H.: Carcinoma of colon in children. *Pediatrics* 32:558, 1963.

80. Middleton P., Ferguson W.: Exsanguinating uncontrollable lower gastrointestinal hemorrhage due to juvenile polyposis. *Dis. Colon Rectum* 20:690, 1977.

81. Moertel C.G., Hill J.R., Adson M.A.: Management of multiple polyposis of the large bowel. *Cancer* 28:160, 1971.

82. Morens D.M., Garvey S.P.: An unusual case of Peutz-Jeghers syndrome in an infant. *Am. J. Dis. Child.* 129:973, 1975.

83. Morganti I., Bellomo R., Franchini A.: Results of total colectomy with ileo-proctostomy in familial polyposis. *Am. J. Proctol.* 22:390, 1971.

84. Morson B.C.: Precancerous lesions of the colon and rectum: Classification and controversial issues. *JAMA* 179:316, 1962.

85. Murphy E.E., Mireles M., Beltran A.: Familial polyposis of the colon and gastric carcinoma. *JAMA* 179:1026, 1962.

86. Payson B.A., Moumgis B.: Metastasizing carcinoma of the stomach in Peutz-Jeghers syndrome. *Ann. Surg.* 165:145, 1967.

87. Peutz J.L.A.: Very remarkable case of familial polyposis of mucous membrane of intestinal tract and nasopharynx accompanied by peculiar pigmentations of skin and mucous membrane. *Ned. Maandschr. Geneeskd.* 10:134, 1921.

88. Phillips R.B.: Gastric malignancy in young people. *Proc. Staff Meetings Mayo Clin.* 14:741, 1939.

89. Pickett L.K., Briggs H.C.: Cancer of the gastrointestinal tract in childhood. *Pediatr. Clin. North Am.* 14:233, 1967.

90. Ravitch M.M.: Polypoid adenomatosis of the entire gastrointestinal tract. *Ann. Surg.* 128:283, 1948.

91. Ravitch M.M.: Anal ileostomy with sphincter preservation in patients requiring total colectomy for benign conditions. *Surgery* 24:170, 1948.

92. Ray J.E., Heald R.J., Chir M.: Growing up with juvenile gastrointestinal polyposis. *Dis. Colon Rectum* 14:375, 1971.
93. Reid J.D.: Duodenal carcinoma in the Peutz-Jeghers syndrome. *Cancer* 18:970, 1965.
94. Reid J.D.: Intestinal carcinoma in the Peutz-Jeghers syndrome. *JAMA* 229:833, 1974.
95. River L., Silverstein J., Tope J.W.: Collective review: Benign neoplasms of the small intestine. *Surg. Gynecol. Obstet.* 102:1, 1956.
96. Roth S.I., Helwig E.B.: Juvenile polyps of the colon and rectum. *Cancer* 16:468, 1963.
97. Ruymann F.B.: Juvenile polyps with cachexia: Report of an infant and comparison with Cronkhite-Canada syndrome in adults. *Gastroenterology* 57:431, 1969.
98. Sachatello C.R., Griffen W.O. Jr.: Hereditary polypoid diseases of the gastrointestinal tract. *Am. J. Surg.* 129:198, 1975.
99. Sachatello C.R., Hahn I.S., Carrington C.B.: Juvenile gastrointestinal polyposis in a female infant: Report of a case and review of the literature of a recently recognized syndrome. *Surgery* 75:107, 1974.
100. Safaie-Shirazi S., Soper R.T.: Endorectal pull-through procedure in the surgical treatment of familial polyposis coli. *J. Pediatr. Surg.* 8:711, 1973.
101. Samter T.G., Alstott D.F., Kurlander C.J.: Inflammatory fibroid polyps of the gastrointestinal tract. *Am. J. Clin. Pathol.* 45:420, 1966.
102. Sandler R.S., Lipper L.: Multiple adenomas in juvenile polyposis. *Am. J. Gastroenterol.* 75:361, 1981.
103. Schutte A.G.: Familial diffuse polyposis of the colon and rectum. *Dis. Colon Rectum* 16:517, 1973.
104. Scully R.E.: Sex cord tumor with annular tubules: A distinctive ovarian tumor of the Peutz-Jeghers syndrome. *Cancer* 25:1107, 1970.
105. Shapiro S.: Occurrence of proctologic disease in infancy and childhood: Statistical review of 2700 cases. *Gastroenterology* 15:653, 1950.
106. Shiffman M.A.: Familial multiple polyposis associated with soft tissue tumors and hard tissue tumors. *JAMA* 179:136, 1962.
107. Siegel S.E., Hays D.M., Romansky S., et al.: Carcinoma of the stomach in childhood. *Cancer* 38:1781, 1976.
108. Silverman A., Roy C.C., Cozzetto F.J.: *Pediatric Clinical Gastroenterology.* St. Louis, C.V. Mosby Co., 1971.
109. Singleton E.B., King B.A.: Localized lesions of the stomach in children. *Semin. Roentgenol.* 6:220, 1971.
110. Smilow P.C., Pryor C.A., Swinton N.W.: Juvenile polyposis coli: A report of three patients in three generations of one family. *Dis. Colon Rectum* 9:248, 1966.
111. Snyder W.H., Jr., Chaffin L., Snyder M.H.: Neoplasms of the colon and rectum in infants and children: A survey of polyps, polyposis and the uncommon malignant lesions of the large bowel. *Pediatr. Clin. North Am.* 3:93, 1956.
112. Soper R.T., Kent T.H.: Fatal juvenile polyposis in infancy. *Surgery* 69:692, 1971.
113. Staley C.V. Schwartz H.: Gastrointestinal polyposis and pigmentation of the oral mucosa (Peutz-Jeghers syndrome). *Int. Abstr. Surg.* 105:1, 1957.
114. Stemper T.J., Kent T.H., Summers R.W.: Juvenile polyposis and gastrointestinal carcinoma. *Ann. Intern. Med.* 83:639, 1975.
115. Stillman A.E., Long P., Komar N.N.: Arteriographic demonstration and colonoscopic removal of a bleeding juvenile polyp. *J. Pediatr.* 88:445, 1976.
116. Swenson O.: *Pediatric Surgery,* ed. 3. New York, Appleton-Century-Crofts, 1969.
117. Telander R.L., Perrault J.: Colectomy with rectal mucosectomy and ileoanal anastomosis in young patients: Its use for ulcerative colitis and familial polyposis. *Arch. Surg.* 116:623, 1981.
118. Todd I.P.: Juvenile polyps. *Arch. Dis. Child.* 39:166, 1964.
119. Turcot J., Despres J.P., St. Pierre F.: Malignant tumors of the central nervous system associated with familial polyposis of the colon: Report of two cases. *Dis. Colon Rectum* 2:465, 1959.
120. Turell R., Maynard A. de L.: Adenomas of rectum and colon in juvenile patients. *JAMA* 161:57, 1956.
121. Veale A.M.O., McColl I., Bussey H.J.R., et al.: Juvenile polyposis coli. *J. Med. Genet.* 3:5, 1966.
122. Velcek F.T., Coopersmith I.S., Chen C.K., et al.: Familial juvenile adenomatous polyposis. *J. Pediatr. Surg.* 11:781, 1976.
123. Ward J.G. Jr., Otherson H.B.: The juvenile polyp of the colon. *Am. J. Surg.* 34:566, 1968.
124. Warren K.W., Kune G.A., Poulantzas J.K.: Peutz-Jeghers syndrome with carcinoma of the duodenum and jejunum. *Lahey Clin. Found. Bull.* 14:97, 1965.
125. Weakley F.L., Hawk W.A., Turnbull R.B. Jr.: What about large-bowel polyps in children? *Cleve. Clin. Q.* 30:199, 1963.
126. Williams C., Jr.: Carcinoma of the colon in childhood. *Ann. Surg.* 139:816, 1954.
127. Williams J.P., Knudsen A.: Peutz-Jeghers syndrome with metastasizing duodenal carcinoma. *Gut* 6:179, 1965.
128. Williams R.D., Fish J.C.: Multiple polyposis, polyp progression and carcinoma of the colon. *Am. J. Surg.* 112:846, 1966.
129. Wolfstein I.H., Dreznik Z.J., Avigad I.S.: Total colectomy and anal ileostomy in multiple polyposis coli. *Arch. Surg.* 113:1101, 1978.
130. Wolfstein I.H., Bat L., Neumann G.: Regeneration of rectal mucosa and recurrent polyposis coli after total colectomy and ileoanal anastomosis. *Arch. Surg.* 117:1241, 1982.
131. Yoshida T., et al.: Case of Peutz-Jeghers syndrome showing malignancy: Bibliographical consideration of polyp malignancy. *Jpn. J. Cancer Clin.* 10:494, 1964.

99   Marc I. Rowe

Necrotizing Enterocolitis

Necrotizing enterocolitis was not a significant cause of infant mortality and morbidity until the mid-1960s, when it rapidly became the preeminent gastrointestinal tract disease encountered in newborn intensive care units. On many surgical services, it is presently the most common newborn surgical emergency and has a mortality that far exceeds that of any other gastrointestinal condition requiring operation. Yet the etiology of this serious illness has eluded extensive clinical and laboratory investigations.

Necrotizing enterocolitis (NEC) is a disease of paradoxes. Classically, it affects the preterm infant 1 week of age. Yet, it can strike the full-term infant and can occur on the first day of life,

or weeks or months after birth. The disease frequently appears sporadically but can present in epidemic-like clusters. The majority of affected infants have been fed, but unfed babies can be attacked. Since 1975, epidemiologic studies comparing risk factors in patients with NEC and matched control infants have identified significant risk factors among the factors common to all critically ill infants. As more information has accumulated from clinical and experimental studies, a better understanding of the disease process and recognition of the various forms of clinical presentation have allowed earlier diagnosis and better selection of operative and nonoperative therapy. With early diagnosis and selective therapy has come a marked reduction in mortality.

HISTORY.—About 160 years ago, cases that resembled NEC began to appear in the literature, but it is impossible to ascertain the first case of true NEC to have been published. Some authors believe that Siebold[126] described the first case in 1825. The patient was a 34-week-gestational-age infant who died at 48 hours of age from peritonitis as a result of perforation of the lesser curvature of the stomach. It is doubtful that a perforation at this site is the result of NEC. Simpson, in 1838,[128] described 24 stillborn and liveborn infants with peritonitis. In each, the process appeared to begin in utero, and these probably were various forms of meconium peritonitis. Zillner, in 1884,[162] reported four newborn infants who died from peritonitis as a result of sigmoid or rectal perforations. Although some have ascribed these lesions to necrotizing enterocolitis, two of the infants were stillborn and the remainder less than 24 hours old at death. The perforations were characterized as "tears" and were thought to be caused by enema tubes. Paltauf,[97] an author seldom cited in historical reviews, may have reported the first true cases of NEC. In 1888, he presented five patients who died of overwhelming peritonitis. Two died at 15 hours of age, early for NEC, but three died at 1 or 2 days of age. The perforations involved the colon and small bowel and, in three of the five patients, there were multiple perforations suggesting NEC. The perforations were described as large, and necrosis affected fairly long segments of bowel.

In spite of this report, many authors credit Genersich[38] with publishing the first case of NEC in 1891, although he himself stated that Plataur had already reported "similar cases" 3 years previously. Genersich's frequently cited patient was cyanotic and had abdominal distention at birth, and died at 45 hours of age. The intestines were matted together into two "egg-sized knots." When the bowel, which was densely adherent, was separated, there was a cavity lined by granulation tissue, and a hole in the ileum 10 cm from the ileocecal valve emptied into the cavity. This almost certainly was a case of meconium peritonitis rather than necrotizing enterocolitis.

By 1939, Thelander[138] had collected 16 cases of perforation of the stomach, 30 of the duodenum, and 39 of the large and small intestine. A number of the patients who had intestinal perforations probably had NEC. The first report of a successfully treated infant with ileal perforation probably due to localized NEC is attributed to Agerty et al. in 1943.[2] The infant was 35 weeks gestational age, was fed on the first day of life, and became distended at 48 hours. A small perforation of the ileum was found at operation. The opening was closed with a pursestring suture, and the patient survived without complications. By 1944, principally due to the work of von Willi,[148] it was recognized that infants suffering from severe infectious enteritis could develop bowel perforation, peritonitis, and death. In 1953,[122] this form of infectious enteritis in the newborn was called necrotizing enterocolitis.

A series of reports from Babies Hospital in New York clearly described the clinical and radiologic picture of NEC and reported a series of experimental studies to clarify the pathogenesis. In 1964, Berdon et al.[12] reported the clinical and x-ray findings of 21 patients with necrotizing enterocolitis. Their introductory paragraph states that 21 cases were seen between 1954 and 1964, and 13 of these were seen in a single 6-month period in 1963. Such a cluster of cases has now been recognized as a common occurrence in NEC. A year later, Mizrahi et al.[92] reported 18 cases of NEC in premature infants. The incidence of NEC in their nursery between 1953 and 1963 was 0.9%, but the disease caused 2.3% of all nursery deaths. During the 1960s, treatment usually consisted of early operation. Most studies were reviews of large uncontrolled series. By 1970, it was recognized that, with early diagnosis, most patients could be managed nonoperatively. The classification of Bell et al.[10] was helpful in establishing a therapeutic pain. From 1964 to 1984, 634 clinical and experimental studies of NEC appeared in the literature. Between 1964 and 1965, only two articles were published, but in 1982 alone, there were 77 reports.

Incidence

The true incidence of NEC still eludes us. It is not a reportable disease, and the incidence varies markedly between institutions and varies over the years within the same institution. Sweet[136] reported an informal nonrandom survey of NEC in 31 newborn intensive care units in the United States and Canada from 1975 to 1977. The average incidence was 24 cases per 1,000 admissions, and he estimated a case rate of 1.2 per 1,000 live births and 40,000 cases annually in the United States. Ryder, Shelton, and Guinan[119] conducted a prospective 12-center investigation of NEC in the United States. The incidence was 2.4 per 1,000 live births and represented 2.1% of all admissions to neonatal intensive care units. Wilson et al.,[155] in an epidemiologic study of infants born in Georgia between 1977 and 1978, identified 148 cases of NEC, an incidence of 1 case per 1,000 live births. Necrotizing enterocolitis accounted for 8% of all deaths occurring in the first day of life and 15% of deaths occurring after 1 week of life in infants below 1,500 gm. They estimated an annual rate in the United States of 2,200 cases per year.

Pathogenesis

The pathogenesis of NEC remains unclear. Until recently, most investigators suggested that it resulted from intestinal mucosal injury from low-flow states, or hypoxia, and bacterial invasion. A large number of conditions that caused hypoxia and low-flow states were identified by retrospective analysis of large series of cases. Recently, a number of workers have re-evaluated the role of these frequently listed risk factors.[69, 119, 132, 159] They utilized studies matching infants with NEC with infants of the same gestational age and weight in the same nursery during the same time period. No significant differences were found between patients with NEC and controls in the rate of prenatal or intrapartum complications, prolonged rupture of membranes, maternal infection, fetal distress, resuscitation at delivery, low Apgar scores, recurrent apnea, hypotension, presence of umbilical vascular catheters, exchange transfusions, patent ductus arteriosus, kind of oral food, age at first feedings, method or type of feeding, or the rate of advancement of feedings. These studies present convincing evidence that most of the factors implicated in the etiology of NEC are simply descriptive of a population of very sick, small, and vulnerable infants.

We believe that the existing evidence supports the concept that NEC is a result of interaction of one or a combination of several factors of different degrees of virulence acting upon hosts of variable vulnerability. The disease may result from a single cause if it is particularly powerful or the host excessively vulnerable. These agents or factors may initiate the disease process by injuring the protective barrier of the intestine—the mucosa. The injury can be direct or indirect. Direct injuries are caused by bacteria or by exposure to hypertonic solutions. Indirect injuries are the result of mucosal cell hypoxia from low-flow states (shock, hyperviscosity, or vascular obstruction) or generalized hypoxia (birth asphyxia, lung or heart disease). Once the mucosa has been injured, bacteria in the lumen, along with their by-products—endotoxins and exotoxins—can enter the bowel wall and cause further damage and eventual intestinal necrosis. Bacteria appear to be an important step in the development of the disease, and certain characteristics of the immature bowel facilitate their growth. Facilitating conditions include the presence of substrate provided by feedings, bowel stasis, and reduction in local mucosal defenses. Initiating factors and factors that affect vulnerability of the host frequently implicated in the pathogenesis of NEC will be discussed below.

Age and Maturity

Necrotizing enterocolitis is predominantly a disease of premature infants of appropriate weight for gestational age. Yu et al.,[161] in a study of 44 patients, found that 82% were below 2,500 gm and 48% under 1,500 gm. In a study of Georgia infants,[155] 58.1% of cases of NEC occurred in infants weighing 1,500 gm or less, and the highest incidence was in infants whose birth weight was 750–1,000 gm. Kliegman and Fanaroff[65] found the mean gestational age of 123 patients with necrotizing enterocolitis was 31 weeks, with an average birth weight of 1,460 gm. Only 7.3% of the patients were full-term, and 10.5% were small for gestational age.

Teasdale and associates[137] reported an inverse relation between age of onset of NEC and gestational age. Infants who developed NEC in the first week of life were more mature, 36.1

weeks gestational age, than those who developed NEC after 1 week of age, 33.4 weeks gestational age. Complications were more common and mortality higher in the early-onset disease. Stoll et al.[132] found a similar inverse relation between gestational age and onset of NEC. All babies of more than 35 weeks gestation were diagnosed within the first 7 days of life. The same age-to-onset relation was found even in very low birth weight babies. Late-onset NEC developed in infants of lower gestational age, 28.3 weeks vs. 30 weeks, and lower body weight, 1,049 vs. 1,177 gm. Sixteen per cent of patients with NEC studied at Denver Children's Hospital[139] presented in the first day of life. These babies were larger (2,624 gm. vs. 1,519 gm.) and more mature (37.9 weeks vs. 32 weeks gestational age).

Wilson et al.[156] calculated the birth weight specific weekly attack rate in NEC. The risk period for NEC decreased as birth weight increased. They also found a consistent pattern of sharply declining risk with attainment of age equivalent to 35–36 weeks gestation. They suggested that the functional maturation of the gastrointestinal tract may play a principal role in determining the risk of NEC. As the infant matures during intrauterine and extrauterine existence, susceptibility to NEC decreases.

The interesting observation of Bauer et al.[6] supports this contention. In a large multicenter collaborative, randomized, and blinded trial to study the effects of prenatal glucocorticoid therapy on fetal lung maturation, they found that infants of mothers receiving corticosteroids had a lower incidence of NEC than infants of mothers given placebo. The incidence of NEC was 2% in the steroid group and 7.1% in the placebo group. Bauer et al. concluded that steroid therapy significantly decreased the incidence of NEC in a very high-risk population and suggested that the protective mechanism might be accelerated intestinal maturation produced by the corticosteroids.

Feedings

Many neonatologists place great emphasis on feedings as a primary factor in the development of NEC. Krouskop et al.[78] even suggested that "feeding is a direct cause of necrotizing enterocolitis or stimulates it to develop." There is a low incidence of necrotizing enterocolitis in unfed infants: 6% in Krouskop's series,[78] 6.8% in Kliegman's study,[65] and 10% in the report of Marchildon et al.[89] These figures supply evidence to link alimentation to NEC but also demonstrate that some infants never fed can develop NEC.

Because of the strong association between feeding and the development of NEC, some have controlled the timing and volume of feedings to prevent the disease. Goldman,[40] in a 13-year review, noted that 25 of 26 cases of NEC developed during the 3 years that infants received large-volume feedings and volume increases were in large increments. The high incidence diminished when feeding volumes were reduced and large volume increases discontinued.

Brown and Sweet[19] also believe that the introduction of feedings is an important etiologic factor in NEC and that the volume and rate of feeding increase is related to the development of the disease. They found that, before they changed to a slowly progressive feeding regimen in July 1974, there were 14 cases of NEC among 1,745 low birth weight infants. From July 1974 to June 1978, when a cautious approach to feeding was practiced, only one case developed among 932 low birth weight infants and 2,557 total patients admitted to the neonatal intensive care unit.

These studies are difficult to interpret because they are longitudinal and use unmatched, historic controls. In a prospective study, Book and colleagues[14] demonstrated no change in incidence of NEC with variations in formula. Yu et al.,[159] in a matched control study, found that the timing and volume of milk

feedings in very low birth weight infants with NEC were the same as in controls. However, in a randomized controlled clinical trial[158] by the same group studying 17 pairs of very low birth weight infants given either total parenteral nutrition or milk feedings, four of the fed babies but none of the unfed babies developed NEC.

The possible role of feedings in the development of NEC has been described by Eidelman and Inwood.[29] They believe that there is a complex relation of a triad of factors: (1) disturbed mucosal integrity, (2) a critical type and number of bacteria, and (3) substrate feedings that promote bacterial growth. They believe that once the bowel mucosa is injured bacterial invasion will be likely if there is rapid growth of bacteria, and that the increased growth is directly related to the availability of substrate formula. Bacteria such as *Escherichia coli*, *Klebsiella*, and *Clostridia* species require carbohydrate for growth. When the bacteria are provided with this substrate, they reproduce rapidly and fermentation produces hydrogen gas, found in pneumatosis intestinalis, the hallmark of NEC. In support of this contention, Marchildon et al., as well as others,[65, 78, 89] have found that unfed infants with NEC seldom had pneumatosis intestinalis.

Reduced Mucosal Blood Flow

Reduced mucosal blood flow leading to cellular injury in the mucosa is one of the most frequently cited etiologic factors. As blood flow decreases, the cells of the intestinal mucosa sustain a hypoxic injury, and damage and death of an increasing number of cells eliminate the barrier to bacterial invasion afforded by protective mucous and intact cell membranes. Bacteria, already present in the bowel lumen, then invade the bowel wall and the combination of the bacterial attack and local ischemia produces clinical NEC. Touloukian et al.[141] as well as others have emphasized the high incidence of perinatal and neonatal factors in infants suffering from NEC that primarily or secondarily lead to intestinal ischemia. Chief among these are hypoxic episodes, exchange transfusions through the umbilical vein, umbilical artery catheters, cardiovascular lesions, and hyperviscosity.

Hypoxia

Lloyd[87] suggested that the response of the neonate to hypoxia was analogous to the diving reflex in birds and mammals. During diving, there is an intense selective vasoconstriction, and blood is preferentially shunted from less vital organs, such as the gut and kidney, to the heart and brain. He found that 80% of newborn infants with gastrointestinal perforation had had a prior asphyxial episode and speculated that these episodes triggered reflex vasospasm in the mesenteric vessels, resulting in ischemia of the bowel. Touloukian et al.,[143] and later Alward et al.,[4] studied changes in mucosal blood flow following asphyxia of the newborn piglet. There was an initial reduction in mucosal blood flow, followed by a "rebound" increased perfusion. Touloukian suggested that these findings and the histologic changes in the bowel were similar to those in early NEC lesions in the human.

Many of the conditions that lead to hypoxia occur in the intrapartum period, or immediately after birth. Kliegman[64] had questioned whether these hypoxic episodes are important in many cases of NEC. He pointed out that the main age of onset of NEC of his patients was 10 days, and 25% of the babies developed the disease after 14 days. This would make most episodes of perinatal hypoxia too remote to be of etiologic importance, since in human neonates the mucosal cell renewal time is 6–9 days.

Several matched control studies have attempted to clarify the relation between hypoxic episodes and NEC. Frantz et al., Kliegman et al., and Stoll et al.[36, 69, 132] comparing infants with NEC and matched controls found no differences in the incidence of hyaline membrane disease, birth asphyxia, or Apgar scores. However, Glider et al. found a higher incidence of Apgar score deterioration in NEC infants than in controls. A conclusion concerning the role of hypoxia episodes and the etiology of NEC is difficult to make because of the lack of a good animal experimental model for NEC and the failure of matched control studies to show a difference in the frequency of hypoxic episodes between NEC babies and controls.

Exchange Transfusions Through Umbilical Vein Catheters

Necrotizing enterocolitis following umbilical venous exchange transfusions has been reported in 1–2% of infants undergoing this procedure.[142] The tip of the umbilical catheter is often located in the umbilical vein, the ductus venosus, or a division of the portal vein rather than the inferior vena cava. It has been theorized that, during the injection phase of exchange transfusion through catheters in these sites, portal venous pressure increases significantly, and the resulting venous congestion impedes arterial flow in the intestines.[140] Five separate matched control studies[36, 69, 132, 139, 159] compared the frequency of exchange transfusion in patients with NEC and controls, and none found any difference between the two groups.

Umbilical Artery Catheterization

Touloukian[141] reported that the frequency of umbilical artery catheterization in babies who develop NEC varied between 25% and 65%. Lehmiller and Kanto[83] proposed an etiologic relation between mesenteric thromboembolism from umbilical artery catheters, feedings, and NEC. They suggested that an indwelling umbilical artery catheter evokes thrombi that intermittently release thromboemboli. If there is great metabolic demand placed on the bowel by feedings, the combination of feedings and multiple thromboemboli leads to intestinal necrosis and NEC. Tyson, De Sa, and Moore[144] and Lehmiller and Kanto[83] found mesenteric thromboemboli at autopsy in patients with necrotizing enterocolitis. However, five matched control studies[36, 69, 132, 139, 159] failed to show a relation between NEC and umbilical artery catheters.

Cardiovascular Abnormalities

Reduced cardiac output as a result of cardiovascular abnormalities may lead to reduced mesenteric blood flow and has been suggested as an etiologic factor in NEC. Bell et al.[11] found increased incidence of NEC in preterm infants who received increased volumes of intravenous fluids and developed patent ductus arteriosus. Congenital heart disease was present in five of 13 term infants with necrotizing enterocolitis studied by Polin et al.[104] There have been two reports[63, 127] of NEC developing after operation for the correction of cardiac lesions. All six of these patients had periods of low flow during operation. Their ages varied from 25 days to 11 months.

Hyperviscosity

Viscosity is a measure of the internal friction resulting when a layer of fluid moves in relation to another layer. Measurements are made at different shear rates and the results recorded as shear force, measured in poise. The major determinant of the viscosity of the blood is the hematocrit. Since blood is a non-Newtonian fluid, as the hematocrit increases above 62% viscosity increases in a nonlinear fashion and is elevated out of proportion to the hematocrit increase. Polycythemia in the newborn has been characterized by a venous hematocrit of 65% or more. Hyperviscosity is whole-blood viscosity of two standard deviations above the mean, defined by Gross and co-workers.[43] In the in-

fant, hyperviscosity is almost always associated with a hematocrit of over 65% but may occur at lower levels depending on the blood pH, body temperature, and protein concentration. Hyperviscosity is relatively frequently encountered in the neonatal period and leads to decreased microcirculatory flow. By reducing intestinal blood flow, it could be an important etiologic factor in NEC.

Hakanson and Oh[47] found that 17.7% of 79 small-for-gestational-age infants had polycythemia and elevated blood viscosity. Thirty-six percent of the infants with hyperviscosity developed NEC, while only 1.5% with normal viscosity developed the disease. In two studies[154, 159] utilizing matched control infants, there was a higher incidence of polycythemia in infants with NEC. Wilson et al.[154] found that polycythemia occurred in 58% of infants with NEC and 16% of controls. Yu et al.[159] reported that 28% of the infants weighing less than 1,500 gm with severe NEC had polycythemia, compared with 10% in control infants.

LeBlanc, D'Cruz, and Pate[82] investigated the relation between polycythemic hyperviscosity and NEC in the newborn dog. In one group, puppies were made polycythemic (hematocrit 70%) by exchange transfusion of packed cells. Those in the control group received an exchange transfusion of whole blood that resulted in a hematocrit of 40%. Gross and microscopic bowel lesions similar to those of NEC in human infants appeared in 58% of the polycythemic animals and 8% of the controls.

Mechanism of Injury Following Mucosal Intestinal Ischemia

Parks and his colleagues[98] in a series of experimental studies found that, after low mesenteric blood flow followed by reperfusion, a reaction between xanthine oxidase, hypoxanthine, and molecular oxygen produces a burst of superoxide radicals. These oxygen-derived free radicals are extremely toxic to cellular structures, damaging the cellular envelope and the membranes of the intracellular organelles such as lysosomes and mitochondria. Their experiments suggest that even brief periods of ischemia followed by reperfusion can alter the mucosal barrier so that the permeability of mucosal cells is markedly increased. Grosfeld and colleagues,[26] in a series of experimental studies in the weanling rat, produced necrosis by sequential intestinal ischemia and reperfusion and prevented the necrosis by intraluminal administration of oxygen-free radical scavengers. Although the super oxide radical mechanism of mucosal damage is attractive, it has yet to be demonstrated that an increased release of oxygen radicals does occur in an experimental model that resembles human necrotizing enterocolitis.

Hyperosmolar Formulas and Medications

In 1974, de Lemos, Rogers, and McLaughlin[28] found that newborn goats fed a hyperosmolar formula developed intestinal lesions resembling those of NEC. Book et al.[13] studied prospectively 16 preterm infants fed either an elemental formula (650 mOsm/kg) or milk formula (350 mOsm/kg). Eighty-eight percent of the infants fed the elemental diet and 25% of the infants fed the milk formula developed NEC. Grantmyre et al.[42] reported a single patient who developed fatal NEC after a Renografin-76 (osmolality 1,900 mOsm/kg) enema for treatment of meconium ileus. In 1977, Willis et al.[153] reported an association between oral administration of hyperosmolar medications and NEC. They noted a significantly higher incidence in infants fed undiluted calcium lactate (osmolality 1,700 mOsm/kg) than in those fed no calcium, or fed calcium lactate diluted with water or formula. White and Harkavy[152] subsequently demonstrated that many oral medications commonly used in the intensive care nursery have very high osmolalities, even when mixed with formula, and that it is usually the vehicle, rather than the medication itself, that is responsible for the high osmolality. Finer et al.[34] reported that the incidence of NEC was 13.4% in preterm infants who received an oral hyperosmolar vitamin E preparation and 5.7% in infants who were given a parenteral vitamin E preparation.

It has been proposed that the introduction of hyperosmolar solutions into the gastrointestinal tract injures the mucosa and contributes to the development of NEC. Neither of the two mechanisms of mucosal injury satisfactorily explains how the mucosal injury develops in the clinical context. Several animal studies[51, 115, 117] have shown that instillation of large volumes of hypertonic solutions intraluminally causes rapid shifts of fluid from the vascular space into the bowel lumen with a resulting decrease in cardiovascular function and an increase in serum osmolality. Presumably, these hemodynamic alterations can reduce intestinal mucosal blood flow and injure the mucosa. However, it is hard to postulate significant changes in blood volume and hemodynamics, given the small doses (1 or 2 ml) of hypertonic medications in the gastrointestinal tract in the circumstances in function.

Application of hypertonic solutions directly to the intestinal mucosa causes mucosal cell damage in the experimental animal.[61, 95] However, most hyperosmolar formulas and medications are given to the patient through the stomach. Considerable dilution occurs in the stomach, duodenum, and small bowel so that it is doubtful that the hypertonic fluid ingested still has an elevated tonicity when it reaches the lower small bowel, the most common site of NEC. In an experimental study in adult humans, Nasrallah et al.[94] found minimal mucosal changes following instillation of large volumes of 15% mannitol into the stomach, in spite of the development of diarrhea in all subjects and symptoms of "dumping" in two.

Infectious Agents

Kliegman has lucidly described the central role of infectious agents in the pathogenesis of NEC. In two recent reviews,[64, 66] he presented evidence that NEC is an infectious disease involving normal or injured bowel in which certain bacteria or viruses are primary agents rather than secondary factors. The evidence supporting an infectious etiology includes: (1) occurrence of clustered epidemics of NEC in which affected patients were related in place and time or had the same infectious agent, (2) association of clostridial species with NEC, (3) occurrence of NEC in infants with no known risk factors, (4) controlled studies that demonstrate no consistent risk factors among infants with NEC paired with unaffected matched infants, and (5) late occurrence of NEC, several weeks or months after perinatal ischemia. Two of the major points, clustered epidemics and clostridial species, will be discussed in detail.

Clustered Epidemics

In most large series, sporadic cases have been followed by the sudden appearance of a cluster of a relatively large number of cases occurring over a short period of time. In many of the epidemics, no specific pathogen has been identified. Virnig and Reynolds, in 1974,[147] reported an outbreak of five cases of NEC in 19 days in the same nursery but found no single pathogen. Book and associates,[16] as part of an ongoing nosocomial-infection surveillance program in the Intermountain Newborn Intensive Care Center, studied prospectively 74 patients who developed NEC between 1972 and 1977. There were six temporally and geographically related clusters of cases of NEC, without isolation of specific organisms. During these episodes, nursery personnel experienced concomitant acute gastrointestinal illnesses. Implementation of infection control measures was associated with a significant decrease in NEC. Similar epidemics without specific

pathogens were noted at Rainbow Babies and Children's Hospital in 1972, 1973, 1974, 1975, and 1978.[64] At Children's Hospital of Philadelphia,[93] there were 11 sporadic cases of NEC in a 12-month period, and in a subsequent 2-month period there were 14 cases. In a case-controlled study[45] of three epidemics in three different nurseries in three different states, investigators found that, in the epidemics, affected infants were of higher birth weight and had higher Apgar scores and fewer perinatal difficulties than the infants with sporadically occurring NEC.

There have been a number of reports of clusters of NEC associated with a single infectious agent. In two such reports[54, 149] *Pseudomonas* was isolated. There have been three outbreaks associated with *Klebsiella* organisms.[52, 56, 109] Powell et al.[105] reported 12 cases of NEC occurring within 3 weeks in a single nursery. *Enterobacter cloacae* was found in the stool or blood of all affected infants. Six weeks after the epidemic, this organism was no longer present in the stools of infants in the nursery.

There have been several reports of epidemic outbreaks of NEC associated with a virus. Rotbart et al.[111] reported a cluster of cases of necrotizing enterocolitis and hemorrhagic gastroenteritis over a 25-day period in their nursery. Rotavirus was detected in the stool of seven of the ten affected patients but in none of the unaffected infants. Eleven staff members had serologic evidence of human rotavirus. Between September 1979 and March 1980, a large outbreak of 91 cases of NEC occurred in two maternity hospitals in Paris.[21, 113] In most patients studied, there was evidence of coronavirus in the stools. Light and electron microscopy done on the intestine of 10 patients revealed coronavirus-like particles in intestinal lesions in all specimens.

Clostridial Species

Clostridial species have been implicated as a cause of NEC. These organisms are obligate anaerobes, invade ischemic tissue, and produce gas and highly destructive toxins. They rapidly colonize the neonatal gut in the first day of life. Epidemics of NEC caused by clostridial organisms have been noted in pigs, lambs, fowl, and cows. Epidemics in newborn piglets caused by *Clostridium perfringens* type C have been stopped by the administration of antitoxin.[22, 33, 129]

Two illnesses directly related to clostridial species and overfeedings, darmbrand[121] and pigbel, resemble NEC. Pathological findings in both cases include pneumatosis intestinalis and intestinal necrosis with minimal inflammatory changes. Darmbrand was seen in postwar Germany and was associated with dietary changes and *Clostridium perfringens* type F endotoxin. Pigbel[80, 81] occurs among children in New Guinea following an infrequent pig feast and is due to type C perfringens endotoxin. It can be prevented by immunization with *Clostridium* toxoid.

Engel, in 1974,[31] reported three cases of NEC associated with Clostridia. Further reports followed.[68, 77, 99] Cases of NEC have also been associated with specific *Clostridium* species. *Clostridium butyricum* was cultured from the bowel, peritoneum, and cerebrospinal fluid of a number of patients with NEC. However, the actual significance of the presence of this bacterium was difficult to determine because the same organism was isolated from stools of unaffected infants.[57, 133] A recent report by Warren, Schreiber, and Epstein[150] describes two infants with severe hemolytic anemia and NEC. *Clostridium perfringens* was isolated from the peritoneal fluid of both babies. This organism is known to elaborate an alpha-toxin that causes massive hemolysis in adults.

A good deal of interest has recently been directed at *Clostridium difficile* as a possible agent in NEC. Han et al.[48] reported an outbreak of NEC involving 13 patients over 2 months. *Clostridium difficile* cytotoxin was detected in the stool of 92.3% of the affected babies, compared with 11.8% of the control infants. The organism was isolated in 61.5% of the infants with NEC and in none of the control babies.

From the reports discussed above, it appears that clostridial species play an important role in some cases of NEC. However, it is not known whether clostridia act as secondary invaders of an existing necrotic focus or by elaborating powerful toxins that initiate intestinal necrosis.

Pathology

The most common site of involvement of NEC is the terminal ileum; the second most common, the colon. The disease can involve a single or multiple segments of intestine. A fulminating form of NEC is characterized by necrosis of the entire gut. Grossly, the affected bowel is markedly distended, often with subserosal collections of gas. The bowel wall is thinned out in areas and varies in color from hemorrhagic to gray. Other areas have a normal appearance. Fibrinous exudate is present on the serosal surface. Peritoneal fluid is bloody if lesions have progressed to necrosis, and brown and turbid after perforation. The mucosa displays ulcerations and wide areas of sloughed mucosa.

The earliest microscopic lesion, bland necrosis of the superficial mucosa, progresses to total necrosis of the mucosa. There is a striking absence of inflammation. The mucosal cells have a ghostlike appearance that resembles postmortem autolysis. Edema and hemorrhage of the submucosa follow complete mucosal necrosis. Pneumatosis is initially seen in the submucosa and later in the muscularis and subserosa. Bacteria in small numbers can be retained in the intestinal wall, and occasionally in gas cysts. Transmural necrosis, characterized by hyaline eosinophilia and loss of nuclear detail in the muscular layers, is present in advanced disease. Mucosal and submucosal fibrosis may be seen adjacent to areas of active mucosal and submucosal necrosis (Fig 99–1). Thrombi in small mesenteric vessels and fibrin thrombi in small arterioles of the submucosa are sometimes seen.[96, 120, 135]

Diagnosis

Clinical Features

The gastrointestinal clinical signs and symptoms of NEC include abdominal distention, gastric retention or vomiting, rectal bleeding, and diarrhea.[55, 110, 130, 146] Abdominal distention, the most common physical finding, occurs in 70–90% of cases. The abdomen is usually soft but, as the disease progresses, may become firm with visible and palpable loops of intestine. Palpation of the abdomen may cause pain. Occasionally, crepitus is felt over a distended loop of intestine. Edema and erythema of the abdominal wall, encountered in approximately 4% of cases, suggest underlying peritonitis. A localized mobile or fixed mass is occasionally felt. Gastric retention or vomiting occurs in over 70% of cases. The aspirate or vomitus may be foul-smelling, and is bile-stained in 32% of cases. Gross and occult rectal bleeding is surprisingly common, 79–86% of cases. Gross blood in the stool is present in 25–63% of cases and occult blood in 22–59%. Bleeding is seldom massive. Diarrhea is the least frequent clinical feature of NEC related to the gastrointestinal tract (15–26%). The nonspecific clinical findings associated with NEC represent physiologic instability. They include lethargy, temperature instability, recurrent apnea, episodes of bradycardia, and shock. Lethargy and temperature instability are the most frequent.

Laboratory Findings

The total white blood cell count is elevated or decreased. It is generally low if there is concomitant gram-negative septicemia. Hutter et al.[58] studied 40 patients with severe NEC. Thirty-seven percent had absolute granulocyte counts below 1,500/m,[3] and the count was significantly lower in the patients who died. Thrombocytopenia commonly accompanies NEC. Eighty-seven percent of the patients of Hutter et al. had platelet counts under 150,000, and 34% of the thrombocytopenic patients bled significantly. Coagulation studies were consistent with disseminated

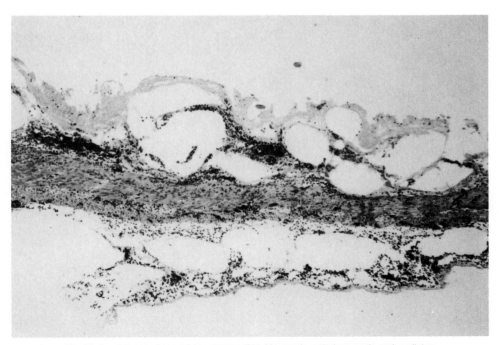

Fig 99–1.—Advanced necrotizing enterocolitis. Mucosa is entirely necrotic and acellular. Extensive pneumatosis is seen in the submucosa and subserosally.

intravascular coagulation in six of 14 thrombocytopenic infants. O'Neill[96] found that, of 40 patients requiring operation for NEC, 95% had platelet counts below 150,000. Rowe and associates[112, 114] found that platelet counts were decreased below 150,000 in patients with blood cultures positive for gram-negative organisms. In piglets, they were able to induce rapid thrombocytopenia by intravenous injection of live *E. coli* and demonstrated that the platelets were destroyed intravascularly. They concluded that thrombocytopenia was a hematologic reaction to gram-negative organisms and their by-products, rather than a specific response to NEC or bowel necrosis.

Although none of the tests to diagnose necrotizing enterocolitis is specific, "positive" results add weight to the diagnosis. Gross examination of stools and tests for occult blood are helpful in confirming the diagnosis because of the high incidence of rectal bleeding. Book, Herbst, and Jung[15] reasoned that, because of mucosal damage in NEC, there should be carbohydrate malabsorption. They tested the stool of formula-fed infants for reducing substances with Clinitest tablets. Seventy-one per cent of formula-fed infants who developed NEC had greater than 2+ reducing substances in their stools.

Garcia and co-workers[37] demonstrated elevated urinary D-lactate excretion in infants with NEC, and not in control infants, suggesting that bacterial fermentation increases production of D-lactate, which is absorbed and excreted by the kidneys. With recovery from NEC or administration of enteral antibiotics, the D-lactate excretion decreased.

Imaging

Because the clinical features of NEC are nonspecific, x-ray findings have served as the cornerstone of the diagnosis. Films that include the abdomen and chest are taken in the anteroposterior projection and left lateral decubitus position. On occasion, upright and cross-table lateral projections are made. The findings most commonly associated with necrotizing enterocolitis are (1) distention of the bowel, (2) intramural gas, (3) portal vein gas, (4) pneumoperitoneum, (5) intraperitoneal fluid, and (6) persistent dilated intestinal loops.[7, 27, 72, 106, 146]

Bowel Distention

Multiple gas-filled loops of intestine with air-fluid levels on lateral decubitus views, an early sign of NEC, are visible in 55–100% of cases. The degree of dilatation and distribution of dilated loops is related to the clinical severity and progression of the disease. In some cases, intestinal dilatation precedes clinical symptoms by several hours.

Pneumatosis Intestinalis

Intramural gas is the most important radiologic feature of NEC, varying in reported frequency from 19% to 98%. Pneumatosis intestinalis, which may appear and disappear rapidly and be present before the clinical manifestations of the disease occur, is commonly an early rather than a late finding. Kliegman et al.[67] noted absence of pneumatosis in 14% of patients when the diagnosis of NEC was strictly documented. Marchildon et al.[89] found that 84% of fed babies developing NEC had intramural gas, but only 14% of unfed babies with NEC had pneumatosis. Pneumatosis coli[86] has been associated with a "benign" form of NEC, responding quickly to medical management (Fig 99–2). Intramural intestinal air has also been found in infants with the enterocolitis of Hirschsprung's disease, inspissated milk syndrome, pyloric stenosis, severe diarrhea, and carbohydrate intolerance.

Two forms of pneumatosis intestinalis are commonly identified—cystic and linear. The cystic form presents as a granular or foamy appearance and is thought to represent an accumulation of gas in the submucosa (Fig 99–2).[100] Linear pneumatosis coexists with the cystic form or develops soon after. Small bubbles form a thin linear or curvilinear pattern outlining a segment of the intestine by the gas within the muscularis and subserosa.

Portal Vein Gas

Portal vein gas, recognized as an arborizing pattern in the right upper quadrant over the liver shadow, represents gas dispersed through the fine radicles of the portal venous system (Fig

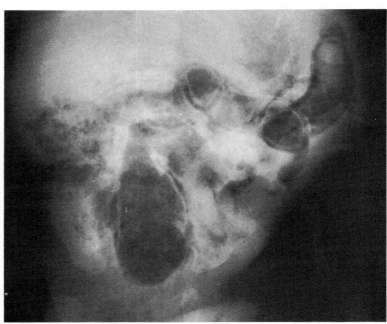

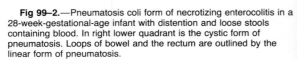
Fig 99–2.—Pneumatosis coli form of necrotizing enterocolitis in a 28-week-gestational-age infant with distention and loose stools containing blood. In right lower quadrant is the cystic form of pneumatosis. Loops of bowel and the rectum are outlined by the linear form of pneumatosis.

99–3).[100] The presence of gas in the portal vein may be fleeting, perhaps accounting for the reported low incidence of this finding (9–20%). Several observers have emphasized that portal vein gas in necrotizing enterocolitis is associated with a poor prognosis, while others have reported survival with or without operative management. The gas may accumulate first in the bowel wall as a result of bacterial invasion, dissect into the venous system, and travel to the fine radicles of the portal vein, or it may represent the action of gas-forming bacteria within the portal venous system.

Pneumoperitoneum

Free air in the peritoneal cavity associated with perforation of the intestine can be demonstrated in from 12% to 32% of all cases of necrotizing enterocolitis. Free air is seen best in the lateral decubitus or upright film of the abdomen. Up to 50% of infants with NEC intestinal perforation proved by operation do not have x-ray evidence of free air.

Intraperitoneal Fluid

X-ray findings suggesting free fluid in the peritoneal cavity are (1) a grossly distended abdomen devoid of gas; (2) gas-filled loops of bowel in the center of the abdomen, surrounded by opacity out to the flanks; (3) increased haziness within the abdomen; (4) separation of bowel loops. These findings have been reported in 11% of cases.

Persistent Dilated Loops

Wexler[151] describes five patients with loops of dilated small bowel that remained unchanged in position and configuration, subsequently developing full-thickness necrosis, and termed this finding the "persistent loop sign." Daneman et al.[27] made similar observations. Others[110] do not believe that this finding indicates bowel necrosis. Leonard et al.[84] found a persistent loop in 33% of 21 patients with proved NEC. Fifty-seven percent of infants with a persistent loop had necrotic intestine at operation or autopsy, but 43% never developed necrosis and recovered with nonoperative treatment.

Contrast Studies

Leonidas et al.[85] suggested that a carefully performed contrast enema may be of value in early or mild forms of NEC presenting diagnostic problems. To avoid the dangers of enema in patients with necrotizing enterocolitis, Cohen and associates[23, 24] used oral metrizamide with subsequent radiographs to delineate the

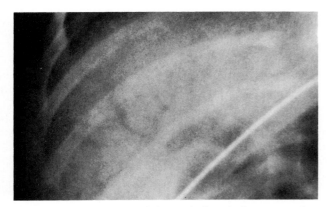

Fig 99–3.—Arborizing pattern of air over the liver shadow, representing gas dispersed through the radicles of the portal venous system.[100]

mucosal pattern of the small and large bowel. They chose this agent because it is isotonic, is nonirritating to tissues, and gives excellent contrast. They studied 28 patients who had clinical and x-ray signs of NEC, including pneumatosis intestinalis. Only four patients showed an altered mucosal pattern consistent with NEC. We believe that presently contrast examinations are not indicated to make the diagnosis of NEC.

Radionuclear Scanning and Ultrasonography

Haase et al.[46] utilized technetium 99 diphosphonate to determine if radionuclide scanning could detect intestinal necrosis in NEC. In 33 scans performed on 23 patients with NEC, there were two false positives and two false negatives, an error rate of 12%. Caride et al.,[20] using the same radionuclide, found positive scans suggesting necrotizing enterocolitis in 10 of 12 patients. At present, nuclide scanning does not increase diagnostic accuracy or aid in selecting operative or nonoperative management.

There have been a few reports of the use of ultrasonography in the diagnosis of NEC or the detection of necrotic bowel. Malin et al.[88] were able to diagnose NEC on the basis of echogenic, intravascular, and hepatic microbubbles detected by ultrasound. Kodroff et al.[71] presented two patients with NEC who had sonographic appearance of abnormal bowel characterized by a hypoechogenic rim with central echogenic focus. They believe these findings were the result of gangrenous bowel with either a walled-off perforation or thickened bowel due to edema and hemorrhage. They also found that sonography is helpful in identifying free fluid in the cul de sac and elsewhere in the peritoneal cavity. Further experience is needed for evaluation of this technique, whose simplicity and avoidance of radiation make it attactive.

Classification

To select appropriate nonoperative and operative treatment and evaluate the effectiveness of various forms of treatment, it is essential that investigators utilize comparable criteria for classifying the stages of NEC. Several classifications have been proposed. German et al.[39] introduced a scoring system based on the duration of symptoms, the x-ray findings, clinical features, and the development of pulmonary insufficiency. Kliegman and Fanaroff[66] utilized a complex clinical classification with seven subgroups.

Bell et al.[10] introduced the most commonly utilized classification. Patients are classified by historical factors, gastrointestinal manifestations, radiologic findings, and systemic signs (Table 99–1).[8] Stage I infants have features suggestive of NEC. Stage II patients are designated as definite cases, and stage III infants are in the advanced stages of NEC with evidence of necrosis of bowel.

Nonoperative Treatment

Unless there is evidence of intestinal necrosis or perforation, the initial treatment of NEC is nonoperative. To prevent further distention and to decompress the gastrointestinal tract, a sump nasogastric tube is maintained on suction. After correction of hypovolemia and electrolyte abnormalities, peripheral or central total parenteral nutrition is started. Intravenous broad-spectrum antibiotics are administered. The group from Babies Hospital in New York[123] utilize ampicillin sodium and gentamicin sulfate. One hundred percent of the predominant organisms recovered in NEC patients in their hospital, *E. coli*, *Klebsiella*, *Proteus*, and 94% of the *Pseudomonas*, are sensitive to gentamicin. Bell, Ternberg, and Bower[9] found that the most common organisms in the blood and peritoneum of infants with peritonitis mainly due

TABLE 99–1.—NEC STAGING SYSTEM*

Stage I (suspected)
Any one or more historical factors producing perinatal stress
Systemic manifestations—temperature instability, lethargy, apnea, bradycardia
Gastrointestinal manifestations—poor feeding, increasing pregavage residuals, emesis (may be bilious or test positive for occult blood), mild abdominal distention, occult blood in stool (no fissure)
Abdominal radiographs showing distention with mild ileus
Stage II (definite)
Any one or more historical factors
Above signs and symptoms plus persistent occult or gross gastrointestinal bleeding, marked abdominal distention
Abdominal radiographs showing significant intestinal distention with ileus, small-bowel separation (edema in bowel wall or peritoneal fluid), unchanging or persistent "rigid" bowel loops, pneumatosis intestinalis, portal vein gas
Stage III (advanced)
Any one or more historical factors
Above signs and symptoms plus deterioration of vital signs, evidence of septic shock, or marked gastrointestinal hemorrhage
Abdominal radiographs showing pneumoperitoneum in addition to findings listed for stage II

*From Bell et al.[8]

to NEC were *E. coli* and *Bacteroides* species. Gentamicin was effective against the *E. coli* and the other gram-negative organisms isolated. Clindamycin was over 90% effective against *Bacteroides* species and other anaerobic organisms cultured. Group D *Streptococcus*, the most common gram-positive organism isolated, was sensitive to ampicillin. They therefore used these three drugs as part of their nonoperative and operative treatment programs. Yu et al.[160] have utilized metronidazole in place of clindamycin to control anaerobic growth.

The use of enteral gentamicin advocated by Bell et al.[8] to prevent perforation during nonoperative treatment has not been universally accepted. They based this treatment on the experimental and clinical observations that ischemic bowel is protected from necrosis if the bacterial flora is suppressed. None of 14 consecutive patients with NEC receiving intragastric kanamycin or gentamicin developed perforation. The study was not controlled. Hansen et al.[49] conducted a randomized, controlled study and found that there was no difference in the course, complications, or mortality between infants receiving gentamicin and those who did not. There was, however, evidence of systemic absorption of gentamicin. Kliegman and Fanaroff[65] similarly found no difference in mortality or incidence of perforation with intragastric kanamycin or gentamicin.

The progress of the disease is monitored by frequent physical examinations, x-ray examination of the abdomen every 6–8 hours, and serial platelet counts, blood cell counts, and blood gas determinations. Antibiotics are usually administered for 10–14 days. Gastric suction is continued while there is evidence of active disease. When the gastric tube is removed, the infant is not immediately fed. The time of resumption of feedings is a point of controversy. We give small volumes of dilute formula several days after the gastric tube has been removed if the baby has not vomited or become distended. Once feedings are resumed, stools are tested for reducing substances and blood. Feedings are discontinued if either test becomes positive.

Indications for Operation

Infants who develop pneumoperitoneum during the course of nonoperative treatment are operated on. Patients with intestinal perforation without pneumoperitoneum, those with full-thick-

ness necrosis of a segment of bowel with impending perforation, and those who have necrotic intestine serving as a source of unrelenting septicemia should be operated on. The major difficulty is identifying these patients. Bell et al.[10] based their therapeutic decisions on clinical staging. All stage III patients were thought to have necrotic bowel and were operated on. They also operated on stage II patients who failed to improve with nonoperative management.

Kosloske, Papile, and Burstein[76] reviewed the indications for operation in 61 patients with NEC. They evaluated ten criteria: (1) clinical deterioration, (2) persistent abdominal tenderness, (3) erythema of the abdominal wall, (4) abdominal mass, (5) profuse GI bleeding, (6) pneumoperitoneum, (7) persistent dilated loop on x-ray films, (8) x-ray evidence of ascites, (9) thrombocytopenia, and (10) positive paracentesis lavage. Clinical deterioration, abdominal tenderness, GI bleeding, x-ray evidence of ascites, and severe thrombocytopenia correlated poorly with the finding of bowel necrosis. A fixed abdominal mass and erythema of the abdominal wall were accurate signs of bowel necrosis. Persistently distended loops of intestine were seen infrequently on serial x-ray films but, when present (three patients), indicated intestinal necrosis. Pneumoperitoneum was always associated with necrosis but occurred with advanced disease. Abdominal paracentesis was positive in 11 of 14 patients who had bowel necrosis. There were no false positive taps. A positive tap was defined as "brown fluid and/or bacteria on smear; volume must be more than 0.5 mm." They recommended abdominal paracentesis for extensive pneumatosis intestinalis seen on radiographs or in patients failing to improve on medical management. Serial paracenteses were done every 4–8 hours. If no peritoneal fluid was encountered, an intestinal lavage was performed by instilling 30 ml/kg of normal saline into the peritoneal cavity, turning the patient from side to side and then withdrawing the fluid.

O'Neill[96] operates on patients who demonstrate continued clinical deterioration despite adequate supportive therapy, or if there is a positive abdominal paracentesis or lavage. The multiple criteria for determining deterioration include redness and edema of the abdominal wall, signs of severe peritonitis on examination, and a marked fall in platelet count. The indication for paracentesis is x-ray evidence of ascites. Ricketts[108] recently reported a survival rate of 72.5% in 51 patients. Sixty-nine percent of the infants weighed less than 1,500 gm, 29% less than 1,000 gm. The indications for operation were pneumoperitoneum, 43%; positive paracentesis or lavage, 47%; stage III disease, 10% (Fig 99–4).[127]

Aside from pneumoperitoneum, it appears that none of the various criteria invariably predicts necrosis of the bowel. Abdominal paracentesis is a safe technique with a high degree of accuracy. Other frequently used criteria are not as accurate. However, when several of these clinical, laboratory, and x-ray findings occur together, the accuracy improves, and this concurrence is an indication for operation.

Operative Management

The patient's general condition must be improved by correcting ventilatory inadequacies and hypoxia, treating shock, and controlling infection. In the operating room, measures should be taken to minimize heat and evaporative water losses. The operating room is kept warm, and a heating mattress is placed on the operating table. The infant's head is covered by an insulated hat, and all preparation solutions and irrigating solutions are kept at 37 to 38 C. A plastic sheet is placed under the infant, and plastic drapes over the infant. During operation, an effort is made to keep as much bowel as possible within the peritoneal cavity. When bowel must be eviscerated, it is placed in a small plastic bag.

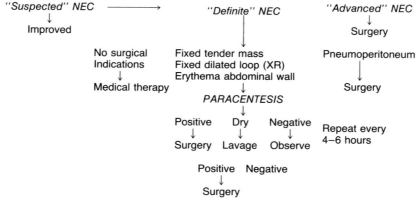

Fig 99–4.—Flow sheet for treatment of necrotizing enterocolitis. (From Ricketts.[108])

The abdomen is opened by a right transverse supraumbilical incision, using the electrocautery to reduce blood loss and operating time. Samples of peritoneal fluid are taken for aerobic and anaerobic culture. The stomach, duodenum, and entire small and large bowel are systematically examined for visible perforations or necrosis. White areas signify ischemic full-thickness necrosis. An area of the intestine that balloons out and is covered by a thinned-out, discolored, semitransparent serosa has undergone necrosis of the mucosa, submucosa, and muscularis and will shortly rupture. There are often long segments of purple or dull greenish-black intestine. It is difficult to determine whether these color changes are due to subserosal hemorrhage and edema or to full-thickness necrosis. Palpation is sometimes helpful. Relatively firm, resilient bowel is usually viable, and lax bowel that dents on compression is often necrotic. A guiding principle is to resect only perforated or unquestionably necrotic tissue and preserve as much bowel as possible. When resecting bowel, it is helpful to observe the cut ends for bleeding.

When a single area of bowel is necrotic, only limited resection is necessary. As Kosloske[73] states, "the cardinal principle of operation for necrotizing enterocolitis is resection of all necrotic bowel and exteriorization of the marginally viable ends." This therapeutic approach is generally agreed on. If there are multiple areas of necrosis separated by viable bowel, multiple stomas are created rather than performing a massive resection. Every effort is made to preserve the ileocecal valve. Once the obviously necrotic bowel has been resected, the residual intestine is measured by sequentially placing a length of thread along the antemesenteric border of the small intestine. The proximal stoma is brought out through a single incision, usually placed in the right lower quadrant, and the distal stoma is placed in the lateral aspect of the wound. To perform the enterostomy, the intestine is attached to the peritoneum and muscle layers with interrupted sutures. About 2 cm of bowel is left protruding from the abdominal wall, and no attempt is made to "mature" the end of the intestine. In the postoperative period, if the viability of the bowel end is questionable, a small portion of the full thickness of the intestine is excised and the cut ends observed for bleeding.

The enterostomy is generally closed in 4 weeks to 4 months. Rothstein et al.[112] described six infants with ileostomies for NEC with recurrent bouts of diarrhea complicated by acidosis and fluid and electrolyte abnormalities. The "salt and water losing states" ceased with reconstitution of bowel continuity, and they recommended early ileostomy closure.

When the area of intestinal necrosis is localized and the remaining intestine appears undamaged, several surgeons have performed resection and primary anastomosis to eliminate the morbidity associated with an enterostomy and to avoid a second operation. Kiesewetter et al.[62] found that 12 of 64 patients with NEC had localized short segments of involved bowel that could be treated by resection and primary anastomosis and performed this procedure on nine patients. Eight survived without complications; one patient had two anastomoses and subsequently developed a leak and peritonitis and died. Twenty-seven patients with necrotizing enterocolitis were treated with resection and primary anastomosis by Harberg et al.[50] The number of patients who had multiple anastomoses, and the extent of the intestinal resections, were not reported. There were three deaths, two early and one late. Two patients required reoperation for anastomotic leaks, and four patients had malabsorption problems postoperatively.

We believe that it is possible to perform resection and primary anastomosis safely in carefully selected patients. The necrotic area of bowel should be sharply localized to a relatively short segment and the surrounding intestine should be healthy. The patient's general condition should be good.

When the majority of the intestine appears to be necrotic, the surgeon is faced with an enormous problem. Massive resection will invariably lead to the short-bowel syndrome, but failure to resect is fatal. Martin and Neblett[90] in one patient performed a high jejunostomy that extensively involved the remaining small bowel and the colon. A major portion of the diseased bowel healed, and the patient survived. Firor[35] treated a single infant with what appeared to be massive necrosis of the small and large bowel by high jejunostomy close to the duodenum. This patient also survived. Diverting the intestinal stream by high proximal enterostomy may facilitate healing of injured bowel by allowing the intestine to decompress, reducing its metabolic demands, and reducing bacterial contamination. With advancements in nutritional and fluid and electrolyte management, the problems previously encountered with high intestinal stomas can now be dealt with satisfactorily. We have utilized high jejunostomies in two patients; both developed multiple distal strictures, had prolonged hospital stays and multiple complications and operations, but survived and now tolerate oral feedings.

In 1977, Ein et al.[30] described the use of peritoneal drainage under local anesthesia to treat extremely ill infants with perforated bowel. By 1980, they had expanded their series to 15 patients.[59] The overall mortality in this high-risk group was 54%. The mortality directly due to necrotizing enterocolitis was 27%. Six of the 15 patients only required the initial drainage and recovered intestinal function. Nine required multiple procedures or died. Two patients required a second drainage procedure and two had a laparotomy because of continued clinical deterioration. Ein et al. stated that laparotomy, resection, and enterostomy is the preferred operative treatment for NEC but recommended peritoneal drainage if the patient weighs less than 1,000 gm and has "marked cardiovascular and homeostatic instability." They further recommended that laparotomy be performed if there is no improvement 24 hours after drainage. More experience with drainage has accumulated over the past 5 years, and most experienced pediatric surgeons have used this procedure occasionally. It is a valuable adjunct to resuscitation of the small high-risk infant with peritonitis, respiratory failure, and shock. Ventilation is improved by the decreased abdominal distention. The drainage of the infected peritoneal fluid under pressure may reduce bacterial invasion and prevent further peritoneal contamination.

Survival

There has been an improvement in survival in the last decade, and survival rates of 60–70% are recorded for both operative and nonoperative treatment (Table 99–2).[100] The improved survival has been attributed to earlier diagnosis, and selective and more effective treatment. The steady progress being made in the physiologic management of the low birth weight and critically ill infant also has contributed to this reduced mortality. It is even possible that the frequency and virulence of the disease is changing.

We do not believe it possible to say that the differences in mortality between series are attributable to differences in the effectiveness of the treatment programs used. In different groups of patients, the disease varies from predominantly localized disease to extensive necrosis. The patient population differs between series. Depending on whether the patient is born locally or referred, and upon birth weight, coexisting disease, and virulence of the disease process, the mortality can vary considerably. The precarious state of patients at risk of developing NEC is emphasized by the fact that, in one series that compared patients with NEC with matched controls, the mortality of the matched control patients was 33%.[131]

Intestinal Strictures

Rabinowitz et al., in 1968,[107] were the first to report the development of intestinal stricture following recovery from acute necrotizing enterocolitis. In 1980, Schwartz et al.[125] collected 73 case reports of strictures after NEC. It is generally believed that the incidence of strictures is increasing with the decrease in the mortality from the disease. Strictures result from healing of an area of intestinal injury. The extent of the stricture is determined by the amount of intestinal wall involved in the necrotic process and the richness of the blood supply to the involved intestinal segment.

The reported overall incidence varies between 11% and 25%,[60, 75, 145] stricture formation being more frequent following

nonoperative treatment. The highest incidence has been reported by Schwartz et al.[124] in a prospective study. They found a 36% incidence of colonic strictures in patients treated nonoperatively. Whether the stricture follows operative or nonoperative therapy, the most common site of involvement has been the colon (70%). The next most common site is the terminal ileum (15%). Sixty percent of the colonic strictures involve the left colon, and the most common colonic site (21%) is the splenic flexure. The majority of patients have single strictures, but multiple strictures are more common after operative management. Multiple strictures were found in 12% of patients without operation and 45% of those operated on.[60, 75, 125, 145]

The resected strictures show varying degrees of inflammation and healing with fibrosis. Lesions examined within 75 days[60] of the onset of necrotizing enterocolitis still showed ulcerations and granulation tissue with moderate fibrosis. Strictures studied after 75 days showed few ulcerations and more mild fibrosis. The degree that the lumen of the intestine is compromised varies from complete obliteration with replacement of the submucosa and muscularis by granulation tissue and fibrosis to moderate narrowing with intact mucosa and muscularis and submucosal granulation and fibrosis. Kosloske et al. and Pokorny et al.[75, 103] both reported patients with evidence of stenosis by barium enema in whom microscopic examination or the resected specimen showed minimal to no fibrosis or granulation tissue, and intact mucosa and no compromise of the lumen. Patients who have required operative treatment of NEC strictures have usually been asymptomatic because the constriction is distal to an intestinal stoma. Of patients treated nonoperatively, slightly over half of those with colonic strictures are symptomatic, presenting with signs and symptoms of intestinal obstruction.

Because of the danger of closing a proximal intestinal stoma in the presence of a distal obstruction, all surgeons perform a contrast study of the distal bowel before closure of a stoma. There is less agreement on the indication for diagnostic studies after nonoperative treatment. Schwartz et al.[124] performed barium enemas on 28 infants following the acute phase of NEC. They found 10 strictures (38%). Four patients were symptomatic and six were asymptomatic. The symptomatic patients were operated on and the asymptomatic patients followed. In one month, three of the six asymptomatic patients required operation. Schwartz et al. and Kosloske advocate routine barium enema in all patients with NEC treated nonoperatively.

If barium enema demonstrates stricture in a symptomatic patient, operation is obviously indicated. Management of an asymptomatic patient with only radiologic evidence of a post-NEC colonic stricture is less clear. Kosloske[75] recommends operation for all patients who have x-ray evidence of a stricture. We agree with the therapeutic approach of Schwartz et al.,[125] operating on symptomatic patients and following asymptomatic ones. A patient who develops gastrointestinal symptoms or fails to thrive is readmitted, radiographs repeated, and operation performed. In most instances, it is possible to prepare the bowel preoperatively and perform resection and primary anastomosis. If the patient presents with acute intestinal obstruction and emergency operation is necessary, we resect the stricture and perform a temporary diverting colostomy.

Prevention

Breast Milk

Infants fed breast milk appear to have less gastroenteritis caused by bacteria and viruses and a lower incidence of neonatal sepsis.[79, 91, 134, 157] Since invasion by infectious agents appears to be a prime factor in the pathogenesis of NEC, breast milk ap-

TABLE 99–2.—SURVIVAL IN NECROTIZING ENTEROCOLITIS*

AUTHORS	INTERVAL	NO. OF CASES	MEDICAL SURVIVAL	SURGICAL SURVIVAL
Touloukian et al.	1955–66	25	2/10 (20%)	4/15 (27%)
Wilson and Woolley	1958–68	16	1/7 (14%)	3/9 (33%)
Stevenson et al.	1962–69	38	13/19 (68%)	12/19 (63%)
Dudgeon et al.	1970–72	63	26/44 (59%)	5/19 (26%)
Bell et al.	1970–72	23	11/14 (78%)	4/9 (44%)
Roback et al.	1970–73	69	13/27 (47%)	14/42 (33%)
O'Neill et al.	1970–74	52	22/32 (69%)	12/20 (60%)
Wayne et al.	1971–74	30	—	21/30 (70%)
Philippart and Rector[100]	1974–76	73	30/41 (73%)	26/32 (81%)
Ricketts[108]	1980–83	51	—	37/51 (72.5%)

*Adapted from Philippart and Rector.[100]

pears to be ideally suited to protect the infant against the disease. The three most important protective actions of breast milk are (1) suppressing growth of *E. coli*, (2) supplying secretory IgA to the gastrointestinal tract, and (3) providing viable leukocytes to the intestine. Breast milk inhibits the growth of *E. coli* by providing an acidic environment and promoting a competitive growth of *Lactobacillus bifidus*.[91] At birth, there are no local mucosal antibodies—secretory IgA. Breast milk contains large quantities of secretory IgA specific for organisms that the mother and her baby are exposed to if the mother remains in contact with her infant.[3, 53] Breast milk also contains a large number of lymphocytes and macrophages capable of antibody formation and phagocytosis.[41, 101] Barlow and associates[5, 102] found that breast-fed, but not formula-fed, newborn rats were protected from experimentally induced NEC, and the protection was related to viable cells in breast milk.

Several clinical trials and retrospective studies have evaluated the use of breast milk to prevent NEC. Several used milk that was frozen or pasteurized, processes that destroy the viable leukocytes. Kliegman, Pittard, and Fanaroff[70] compared infants fed refrigerated breast milk to infants fed formula. There was no difference in the incidence of NEC. This study was retrospective and did not use matched controls. In many instances, the breast milk was obtained from donors or from mothers not exposed to their babies. Eyal et al.[32] found that eight of 129 very low birth weight infants fed expressed breast milk developed NEC. The milk was obtained from the infants' mothers or donated by mothers in the hospital's maternity department. The milk was fed fresh or refrigerated and used within 24 hours. No potentially pathogenic bacteria were grown on culture of the milk.

The concept that breast milk protects against NEC is attractive, but, although there is evidence that it is effective in preventing some infectious diarrheas, there are as yet no studies demonstrating a significant difference in the incidence of NEC in breast-fed and formula-fed infants. A prospective study utilizing matched controls has not been done.[74] Since fresh milk obtained from the infant's own mother who has contact with her infant appears to be important, logistical problems may make such a definitive study difficult.

Feedings

There is little disagreement that NEC is more common in fed infants and that bacterial overgrowth is facilitated by substrate provided by formula. Several groups believe that careful regulation of feeding may prevent NEC. Brown[18] has detailed a feeding regimen for high-risk infants to prevent NEC (Table 99–3). Low birth weight infants and infants with illnesses or prenatal problems are not fed for 7–10 days. Nutrition is provided by peripheral total parenteral nutrition. If no symptoms suggestive of NEC develop, feedings are cautiously begun according to a set routine. Feedings are withheld and the infant evaluated if gastric residuals increase or if any clinical findings associated with NEC develop. Feedings are stopped for 1 week if there is persistent gastric retention.

Enteral Antibiotics

Inhibiting bacterial growth by the administration of nonabsorbable broad-spectrum antibiotics has been used to prevent NEC. Grylack and Scanlon,[44] in a controlled double-blind trial, compared high-risk infants who received oral gentamicin with infants given a placebo. None of the treated babies but four of 22 (19%) of the placebo babies developed NEC. In the study of Rowley and Dahlenburg,[118] 50 patients received gentamicin for 1 week, and 50 matched control infants received placebo. There was no significant difference in the incidence of NEC between

the two groups. Boyle et al.,[17] in a double-blind study using kanamycin found a decrease in gram-negative colonization in the treated infants but an increase in kanamycin-resistant organisms. The incidence of NEC was the same in the treated infants and matched controls. To reduce the colonization of the organism in the nursery, vancomycin[92] has been utilized during an outbreak of NEC related to *Clostridia difficile*. This antibiotic combined with disease control measures led to the disappearance of the organism from the nursery.

The available studies do not support the routine administration of enteral antibiotics to all high-risk premature infants. Effectiveness has not been proved, and resistant organisms may develop. There may be an indication for administering specific antibiotics to infants in nurseries where an outbreak of NEC is associated with a specific organism.

Late Outcome

Stevenson et al.[131] studied 40 necrotizing enterocolitis survivors 1 to 3 years after their illness. The mean birth weight was 1,693 gm, and the average gestational age, 32.4 weeks. Eighteen of the patients had been treated operatively. Height, weight, and head circumference were measured, ophthalmologic examination, audiometry, Stanford-Binet IQ testing, fecal fat determination, and EEG were performed. Forty-eight percent of the children were normal. Fifteen percent had moderate to severe neurologic impairment including spasticity, hydrocephalus, seizures, hearing loss, and retrolental fibroplasia with blindness. Ten percent had gastrointestinal sequelae, strictures, short-gut syndrome, and fat malabsorption, but all tolerated oral feedings. There were no cases of failure to thrive secondary to intestinal dysfunction. When the children were retrospectively matched with control patients without NEC, there was no difference in nongastrointestinal sequelae between the two groups.

Yu et al.[160] evaluated by clinical and neurologic assessment 41 very low birth weight, 2-year survivors of NEC. These patients were compared with 241 2-year-old children who had very low birth weights. Fifteen percent of the children who had NEC and 20% of the control children had developmental or neurologic abnormalities.

Abbasi et al.[1] studied the growth, nutritional status, and gastrointestinal function in 22 1-year survivors of NEC compared

TABLE 99–3.—FEEDING SCHEDULE* FOR NEC PREVENTION

< 1,250 GM		1,250–1,500 GM		> 1,500 GM	
H₂O	2 ml × 2	H₂O	3 ml × 2	H₂O	4 ml × 2
↓	3 ml × 1		4 ml × 1	↓	5 ml × 1
13 cal/oz formula	3 ml × 8	13 cal/oz formula	4 ml × 8	13 cal/oz formula	5 ml × 8
	4 ml × 8		5 ml × 8		6 ml × 8
↓	5 ml × 8	↓	6 ml × 8	↓	7 ml × 8
	6 ml × 8	20 cal/oz formula	6 ml × 8	20 cal/oz formula	7 ml × 8
20 cal/oz formula	6 ml × 8		8 ml × 8		8 ml × 8
	7 ml × 8		10 ml × 8	↓	10 ml × 8
	8 ml × 8		12 ml × 8		12 ml × 8
↓	10 ml × 8	24 cal/oz formula	12 ml × 8	24 cal/oz formula†	12 ml × 8
	12 ml × 8		14 ml × 8		14 ml × 8
24 cal/oz formula	12 ml × 8		16 ml × 8		16 ml × 8
	14 ml × 8		19 ml × 8		19 ml × 8
	16 ml × 8		22 ml × 8		22 ml × 8
	18 ml × 8	↓	25 ml × 8		25 ml × 8
↓	20 ml × 8			↓	29 ml × 8
‡		‡		‡	

*(From Brown.[18] All feedings given via nasogastric tube at 3-hour intervals.

†Infants 2,000 gm or more continue to receive 20 cal/oz formula.

‡Continue to feed according to ordinary nursery routine, based on weight and caloric needs.

with 18 matched control infants. None of the NEC patients had extensive intestinal resections. The studies included anthropometric measurements, serum iron, albumin, prealbumin, retinal binding protein, and liver function measurements. Gastrointestinal function was gauged by vitamin E absorption, bile acid concentrations, and lactose breathing tests. There were no significant differences in any of these studies between the two groups.

Collins et al.[25] postulated that since the terminal ileum, the site of vitamin B_{12} absorption, is frequently resected in NEC, long-term follow-up in patients with ileal resection might detect vitamin B_{12} malabsorption and possibly vitamin B_{12} deficiencies. Of 14 patients studied 1–7 years after resection, six had abnormal vitamin B_{12} absorption, but none had vitamin B_{12} deficiency. Since it takes years to exhaust the hepatic stores of vitamin B_{12}, the deficiency state including megoblastic anemia and hematologic problems is a late finding. They recommend that all infants who had ileal resections for NEC have measurements of vitamin B_{12} absorption, with administration of parenteral vitamin B_{12} considered if malabsorption is present.

REFERENCES

1. Abbasi S., Pereira G.R., Johnson L., et al.: Long-term assignment of growth, nutritional status, and gastrointestinal function in survivors of necrotizing enterocolitis. *J. Pediatr.* 104:550, 1984.
2. Agerty H.A., Ziserman A.J., Shollenberger C.L.: A case of perforation of the ileum in a newborn infant with operation and recovery. *J. Pediatr.* 22:233, 1943.
3. Ahlstedt S., Carlsson B., Fallstrom S.P., et al.: Antibodies in human serum and milk induced by enterobacteria and food proteins, in *Immunology of the Gut.* CIBA Foundation Symposium 46. Amsterdam, Holland Publishing Co., 1977.
4. Alward C.T., Hook J.B., Helmrath T.A., et al.: Effects of asphyxia on cardiac output and organ blood flow in the newborn piglet. *Pediatr. Res.* 12:824, 1978.
5. Barlow B., Santulli T.V., Heird W.C., et al.: An experimental study of acute neonatal enterocolitis—the importance of breast milk. *J. Pediatr. Surg.* 9:587, 1974.
6. Bauer C.R., Morrison J.C., Poole W.K., et al.: A decreased incidence of necrotizing enterocolitis after prenatal glucocorticoid therapy. *Pediatrics* 73:682, 1984.
7. Bell R.S., Graham C.B., Stevenson J.K.: Roentgenologic and clinical manifestations of neonatal necrotizing enterocolitis. *Am. J. Roentgenol. Radium Ther. Nucl. Med.* 112:123, 1971.
8. Bell M.J., Kosloske A., Benton C., et al.: Neonatal necrotizing enterocolitis in infancy: Prevention of perforation. *J. Pediatr. Surg.* 8:601, 1973.
9. Bell M.J., Ternberg J.L., Bower R.J.: The microbial flora and antimicrobial therapy of neonatal peritonitis. *J. Pediatr. Surg.* 15:569, 1980.
10. Bell M.J., Ternberg J.L., Feigin R.D., et al.: Neonatal necrotizing enterocolitis. *Ann. Surg.* 187:1, 1978.
11. Bell E.F., Warburton D., Stonestreet B.S., et al.: High-volume fluid intake predisposes premature infants to necrotising enterocolitis (letter). *Lancet* 2:90, 1979.
12. Berdon W.E., Grossman H., Baker D.H., et al.: Necrotizing enterocolitis in the premature infant. *Radiology* 83:879, 1964.
13. Book L.S., Herbst J.J., Atherton S.O., et al.: Necrotizing enterocolitis in low-birth-weight infants fed an elemental formula. *J. Pediatr.* 87:602, 1975.
14. Book L.S., Herbst J.J., Jung A.L.: Comparison of fast- and slow-feeding rate schedules to the development of necrotizing enterocolitis. *J. Pediatr.* 89:463, 1976.
15. Book L.S., Herbst J.J., Jung A.L.: Carbohydrate malabsorption in necrotizing enterocolitis. *Pediatrics* 57:201, 1976.
16. Book L.S., Overall J.C. Jr., Herbst J.J., et al.: Clustering of necrotizing enterocolitis. *N. Engl. J. Med.* 297:984, 1977.
17. Boyle R., Nelson J.S., Stonestreet B.S., et al.: Alterations in stool flora resulting from oral kanamycin prophylaxis of necrotizing enterocolitis. *J. Pediatr.* 93:857, 1978.
18. Brown E.G.: Prevention, in Brown E.G., Sweet A.Y. (eds.): *Neonatal Necrotizing Enterocolitis.* New York, Grune & Stratton, 1980, p. 179.
19. Brown E.G., Sweet A.Y.: Preventing necrotizing enterocolitis in neonates. *JAMA* 240:2452, 1978.
20. Caride V.J., Touloukian R.J., Ablow R.C., et al.: Abdominal and hepatic uptake of ^{99m}Tc-pyrophosphate in neonatal necrotizing enterocolitis. *Radiology* 139:205, 1981.
21. Chany C., Moscovici O., Lebon P., et al.: Association of coronavirus infection with neonatal necrotizing enterocolitis. *Pediatrics* 69:209, 1982.
22. Clostridia as intestinal pathogens. *Lancet* 2:1113, 1977.
23. Cohen M.D., Schreiner R., Grosfeld J., et al.: A new look at the neonatal bowel-contrast studies with metrizamide (Amipaque). *J. Pediatr. Surg.* 18:442, 1983.
24. Cohen M.D., Smith J.A., Slabaugh R.D., et al.: Neonatal necrotizing enterocolitis shown by oral metrizamide (Amipaque). *AJR* 138:1019, 1982.
25. Collins J.E., Rolles C.J., Sutton H., et al.: Vitamin B_{12} absorption after necrotizing enterocolitis. *Arch. Dis. Child.* 59:731, 1984.
26. Dalsing M.C., Grosfeld J.L., Shiffler M.A., et al.: Superoxide dismutase: A cellular protective enzyme in bowel ischemia. *J. Surg. Res.* 34:589, 1983.
27. Daneman A., Woodward S., de Silva M.: The radiology of neonatal necrotizing enterocolitis. *Pediatr. Radiol.* 7:70, 1978.
28. de Lemos R.A., Rogers J.R. Jr., McLaughlin G.W.: Experimental production of necrotizing enterocolitis in newborn goats (abst.). *Pediatr. Res.* 8:380, 1974.
29. Eidelman A.I., and Inwood R.J.: Necrotizing enterocolitis and enteral feeding. *Am. J. Dis. Child.* 134:545, 1980.
30. Ein S.H., Marshall D.G., Girvan D.: Peritoneal drainage under local anesthesia for perforations from necrotizing enterocolitis. *J. Pediatr. Surg.* 12:963, 1977.
31. Engel R.: Necrotizing enterocolitis in the newborn. Report of 68th Ross Conference on Pediatric Research. Columbus, Ohio: Ross Laboratories 66–71, 1974.
32. Eyal F., Sagi E., Arad I., et al.: Necrotising enterocolitis in the very low birthweight infant: Expressed breast milk feeding compared with parenteral feeding. *Arch. Dis. Child.* 57:274, 1982.
33. Finegold S.M.: *Anaerobic Bacteria in Human Disease.* New York: Academic Press, 1977.
34. Finer N.N., Peters K.L., Hayek Z., et al.: Vitamin E and necrotizing enterocolitis. *Pediatrics* 73:387, 1984.
35. Firor H.V.: Use of high jejunostomy in extensive NEC. *J. Pediatr. Surg.* 17:771, 1982.
36. Frantz I.D., L'Heureux P., Engel R.R., et al.: Necrotizing enterocolitis. *J. Pediatr.* 86:259, 1975.
37. Garcia J., Smith F.R., Cucinell S.A.: Urinary D-lactate excretion in infants with necrotizing enterocolitis. *J. Pediatr.* 104:268, 1984.
38. Genersich A.: Bauchfellentzündung beim Neugeborenen in folge von Perforation des Ileums. *Arch. Path. Anat.* 126:485, 1891.
39. German J.C., Jefferies M.R., Amlie R., et al.: Prospective application of an index of neonatal necrotizing enterocolitis. *J. Pediatr. Surg.* 14:364, 1979.
40. Goldman H.I.: Feeding and necrotizing enterocolitis. *Am. J. Dis. Child.* 134:553, 1980.
41. Goldman A.S.: Human milk, leukocytes, and immunity. *J. Pediatr.* 90:167, 1977.
42. Grantmyre E.B., Butler G.J., Gillis D.A.: Necrotizing enterocolitis after Renografin—76 treatments of meconium ileus. *AJR* 136:990, 1981.
43. Gross G.P., Hathaway W.E., McGaughey H.R.: Hyperviscosity in the neonate. *J. Pediatr.* 82:2004, 1973.
44. Grylack L.J., Scanlon J.W.: Oral gentamicin therapy in the prevention of neonatal necrotizing enterocolitis. *Am. J. Dis. Child.* 132:1192, 1978.
45. Guinan M., Schaberg G., Bruhn F.W., et al.: Epidemic occurrence of neonatal necrotizing enterocolitis. *Am. J. Dis. Child.* 133:594, 1979.
46. Haase G.M., Sfakianakis G.N., Lobe T.E., et al.: Prospective evaluation of radionuclide scanning in detection of intestinal necrosis in neonatal necrotizing enterocolitis. *J. Pediatr. Surg.* 16:241, 1981.
47. Hakanson D.O., Oh W.: Necrotizing enterocolitis and hyperviscosity in the newborn infant. *J. Pediatr.* 90:458, 1977.
48. Han V.K.M., Sayed H., Chance G.W., et al.: An outbreak of *Clostridium difficile* necrotizing enterocolitis: A case of oral vancomycin therapy? *Pediatrics* 71:935, 1983.
49. Hansen T.N., Ritter D.A., Speer M.E., et al.: A randomized, controlled study of oral gentamicin in the treatment of neonatal necrotizing enterocolitis. *J. Pediatr.* 97:836, 1980.
50. Harberg F.J., McGill C.W., Saleem M.M., et al.: Resection with primary anastomosis for necrotizing enterocolitis. *J. Pediatr. Surg.* 18:743, 1983.
51. Harris P.D., Neuhauser E.B.D., Gerth R.: The osmotic effect of water soluble contrast media on circulating plasma volume. *Am. J. Roentgenol. Radium Ther. Nucl. Med.* 91:694, 1964.
52. Hathaway W.: Report of Sixty-eighth Ross Conference on Pediatric Research, 1974.
53. Head J.: Immunobiology of lactation. *Semin. Perinatol.* 1:195, 1977.
54. Henderson A., Maclaurin J., Scott J.M.: Pseudomonas in a Glasgow baby unit. *Lancet* 2:316, 1969.

55. Herbst J.J., Book L.S.: Clinical characteristics, in Brown E.G., Sweet A.Y. (eds.): *Neonatal Necrotizing Enterocolitis.* New York, Grune & Stratton, 1980, p. 25.
56. Hill H.R., Hunt C.E., Matsen J.M.: Nosocomial colonization with Klebsiella, type 26, in a neonatal intensive-care unit associated with an outbreak of sepsis, meningitis, and necrotizing enterocolitis. *J. Pediatr.* 85:415, 1974.
57. Howard F.M., Flynn D.M., Bradley J.M., et al.: Outbreak of necrotizing enterocolitis caused by *Clostridium butyricum. Lancet* 2:1099, 1977.
58. Hutter J.J., Hathaway W.E., Wayne E.R.: Hematologic abnormalities in severe neonatal necrotizing enterocolitis. *J. Pediatr.* 88:1026, 1976.
59. Janik J.S., Ein S.H.: Peritoneal drainage under local anesthesia for necrotizing enterocolitis (NEC) perforation: A second look. *J. Pediatr. Surg.* 15:565, 1980.
60. Janik J.S., Ein S.H., Mancer K.: Intestinal stricture after necrotizing enterocolitis. *J. Pediatr. Surg.* 16:438, 1981.
61. Kameda H., Abei T., Nasrallah S., et al.: Functional and histological injury to intestinal mucosa produced by hypertonicity. *Am. J. Physiol.* 214:1090, 1968.
62. Kiesewetter W.B., Taghizadeh F., Bower R.J.: Necrotizing enterocolitis: Is there a place for resection and primary anastomosis? *J. Pediatr. Surg.* 14:360, 1979.
63. Kleinman P.K., Winchester P., Brill P.W.: Necrotizing enterocolitis after open heart surgery employing hypothermia and cardiopulmonary bypass. *Am. J. Roentgenol.* 127:757, 1976.
64. Kliegman R.M.: Neonatal necrotizing enterocolitis: Implications for an infectious disease. *Pediatr. Clin. North Am.* 26:327, 1979.
65. Kliegman R.M., Fanaroff A.A.: Neonatal necrotizing enterocolitis: A nine-year experience. *Am. J. Dis. Child.* 135:608, 1981.
66. Kliegman R.M., Fanaroff A.A.: Necrotizing enterocolitis. *N. Engl. J. Med.* 310:1093, 1984.
67. Kliegman R.M., Fanaroff A.A.: Neonatal necrotizing enterocolitis in the absence of pneumatosis intestinalis. *Am. J. Dis. Child.* 136:618, 1982.
68. Kliegman R.M., Fanaroff A.A., Izant R., et al.: Clostridia as pathogens in neonatal necrotizing enterocolitis. *J. Pediatr.* 95:287, 1979.
69. Kliegman R.M., Hack M., Jones P., et al.: Epidemiologic study of necrotizing enterocolitis among low-birth-weight infants. *J. Pediatr.* 100:440, 1982.
70. Kliegman R.M., Pittard W.B., Fanaroff A.A.: Necrotizing enterocolitis in neonates fed human milk. *J. Pediatr.* 95:450, 1979.
71. Kodroff M.B., Hartenberg M.A., Goldschmidt R.A.: Ultrasonographic diagnosis of gangrenous bowel in neonatal necrotizing enterocolitis. *Pediatr. Radiol.* 14:168, 1984.
72. Kogutt M.S.: Necrotizing enterocolitis in infancy. *Pediatr. Radiol.* 130:367, 1979.
73. Kosloske A.M.: Operative techniques for the treatment of neonatal necrotizing enterocolitis. *Surg. Gynecol. Obstet.* 149:740, 1979.
74. Kosloske A.M.: Pathogenesis and prevention of necrotizing enterocolitis: A hypothesis based on personal observation and a review of the literature. *Pediatrics* 74:1086, 1984.
75. Kosloske A.M., Burstein J., Bartow S.A.: Intestinal obstruction due to colonic stricture following neonatal necrotizing enterocolitis. *Ann. Surg.* 192:202, 1980.
76. Kosloske A.M., Papile L., Burstein J.: Indications for operation in acute necrotizing enterocolitis of the neonate. *Surgery* 87:502, 1980.
77. Kosloske A.M., Ulrich J.A., Hoffman H.: Fulminant necrotizing enterocolitis associated with Clostridia. *Lancet* 2:1014, 1978.
78. Krouskop R.W., Brown E.G., Sweet A.Y.: The relationship of feeding to necrotizing enterocolitis. *Pediatr. Res.* 8:383, 1974.
79. Larsen S.A. Jr., Homer D.R.: Relation of breast versus bottle feeding to hospitalization for gastroenteritis in a middle-class U.S. population. *J. Pediatr.* 91:417, 1978.
80. Lawrence G., Shann F., Freestone D., et al.: Prevention of necrotising enteritis in Papua, New Guinea by active immunisation. *Lancet* 1:227, 1979.
81. Lawrence G., Walker P.D.: Pathogenesis of enteritis necroticans in Papua, New Guinea. *Lancet* 1:125, 1976.
82. LeBlanc M.H., D'Cruz C., Pate K.: Necrotizing enterocolitis can be caused by polycythemic hyperviscosity in the newborn dog. *J. Pediatr.* 105:804, 1984.
83. Lehmiller D.J., Kanto W.P. Jr.: Relationships of mesenteric thromboembolism, oral feeding, and necrotizing enterocolitis. *J. Pediatr.* 92:96, 1978.
84. Leonard T. Jr., Johnson F., Pettett P.G.: Critical evaluation of the persistent loop sign in necrotizing enterocolitis. *Radiology* 142:385, 1982.
85. Leonidas J.C., Bhan I., Leape L.L.: Barium enema in suspected necrotising enterocolitis: Is it ever indicated? *Clin. Radiol.* 31:587, 1980.

86. Leonidas J.C., Hall R.T.: Neonatal pneumatosis coli: A mild form of neonatal necrotizing enterocolitis. *J. Pediatr.* 89:456, 1976.
87. Lloyd J.R.: The etiology of gastrointestinal perforations in the newborn. *J. Pediatr. Surg.* 4:77, 1969.
88. Malin S.W., Bhutani V.K., Ritchie W.W., et al.: Echogenic intravascular and hepatic microbubbles associated with necrotizing enterocolitis. *J. Pediatr.* 103:637, 1983.
89. Marchildon M.B., Buck B.E., Abdenour G.: Necrotizing enterocolitis in the unfed infant. *J. Pediatr. Surg.* 17:620, 1982.
90. Martin L.W., Neblett W.W.: Early operation with intestinal diversion for necrotizing enterocolitis. *J. Pediatr. Surg.* 16:252, 1981.
91. Mata L.J., Urrutia J.J.: Intestinal colonization of breast-fed children in a rural area of low socioeconomic level. *Ann. N.Y. Acad. Sci.* 176:93, 1971.
92. Mizrahi A., Barlow O., Berdon W., et al.: Necrotizing enterocolitis in premature infants. *J. Pediatr.* 66:697, 1965.
93. Moomjian A.S., Packham G.J., Fox W.W., et al.: Necrotizing enterocolitis—endemic vs. epidemic form. *Pediatr. Res.* 12:530, 1978.
94. Nasrallah S.M., Coburn W.M. Jr., Iber F.L.: The effect of hypertonic mannitol on the intestine of man. *Johns Hopkins Med. J.* 123:134, 1968.
95. Norris H.T.: Response of the small intestine to the application of a hypertonic solution. *Am. J. Pathol.* 73:747, 1973.
96. O'Neill J.A. Jr.: Neonatal necrotizing enterocolitis. *Surg. Clin. North Am.* 61:1013, 1981.
97. Paltauf A.: Die spontane Dickdarm Ruptur der Neugeborenen. *Virchows Arch. Path. Anat.* 111:461, 1888.
98. Parks D.A., Bulkley G.B., Granger D.N.: Role of oxygen-derived free radicals in digestive tract diseases. *Surgery* 94:415, 1983.
99. Pederson P.V., Hansen F.H., Halveg A.B., et al.: Necrotizing enterocolitis of the newborn—is it gas-gangrene of the bowel? *Lancet* 2:715, 1976.
100. Philippart A.I., Rector F.E.: Necrotizing enterocolitis, in Ravitch M.M., Welch K.J., Benson C.D., et al. (eds.): *Pediatric Surgery,* ed. 3. Chicago, Year Book Medical Publishers, 1979, p. 970.
101. Pitt J.: Breast milk leukocytes. *Pediatrics* 58:769, 1976.
102. Pitt J., Barlow B., Heird W.C.: Protection against experimental necrotizing enterocolitis by maternal milk. I. Role of milk leukocytes. *Pediatr. Res.* 11:906, 1977.
103. Pokorny W.J., Harr V.L., McGill C.W., et al.: Intestinal stenosis resulting from necrotizing enterocolitis. *Am. J. Surg.* 142:721, 1981.
104. Polin R.A., Pollack P.F., Barlow B., et al.: Necrotizing enterocolitis in term infants. *J. Pediatr.* 89:460, 1976.
105. Powell J., Bureau M.A., Pare C., et al.: Necrotizing enterocolitis. *Am. J. Dis. Child.* 134:1152, 1980.
106. Rabinowitz J.G., Siegle R.L.: Changing clinical and roentgenographic patterns of necrotizing enterocolitis. *Am. J. Roentgenol.* 126:560, 1976.
107. Rabinowitz J.G., Wolf B.S., Feller M.R., et al.: Colonic changes following necrotizing enterocolitis in the newborn. *Am. J. Roentgenol.* 103:359, 1968.
108. Ricketts R.R.: Surgical therapy for necrotizing enterocolitis. *Ann. Surg.* 200:653, 1984.
109. Roback S.A., Foker J., Frantz I.F., et al.: Necrotizing enterocolitis. *Arch. Surg.* 109:314, 1974.
110. Robertson E.M.: Radiological considerations in the diagnosis of necrotizing enterocolitis in the newborn. *Diagn. Imaging* 50:138, 1981.
111. Rotbart H.A., Levin M.J., Yolken R.H., et al.: An outbreak of rotavirus-associated neonatal necrotizing enterocolitis. *J. Pediatr.* 103:454, 1983.
112. Rothstein F.C., Halpin T.C. Jr., Kliegman R.J., et al.: Importance of early ileostomy closure to prevent chronic salt and water losses after necrotizing enterocolitis. *Pediatrics* 70:249, 1982.
113. Rousset S., Moscovici O., Lebon P., et al.: Intestinal lesions containing coronavirus-like particles in neonatal necrotizing enterocolitis: An ultrastructural analysis. *Pediatrics* 73:218, 1984.
114. Rowe M.I., Buckner D.M., Newmark S.: The early diagnosis of gram negative septicemia in the pediatric surgical patient. *Ann. Surg.* 182:280, 1975.
115. Rowe M.I., Furst A.J., Altman D.H., et al.: The neonatal response to Gastrografin enema. *Pediatrics* 48:29, 1971.
116. Rowe M.I., Marchildon M.B., Arango A., et al.: The mechanisms of thrombocytopenia in experimental gram-negative septicemia. *Surgery* 84:87, 1978.
117. Rowe M.I., Seagram G., Weinberger M.: Gastrografin-induced hypertonicity. *Am. J. Surg.* 125:185, 1973.
118. Rowley M.P., Dahlenburg G.W.: Gentamicin in prophylaxis of neonatal necrotising enterocolitis. *Lancet* 2:532, 1978.
119. Ryder R.W., Shelton J.D., Guinan M.E.: Necrotizing enterocolitis: A prospective multicenter investigation. *Am. J. Epidemiol.* 112:113, 1980.

120. Santulli T.V., Schullinger J.N., Heird W.C., et al.: Acute necrotizing enterocolitis in infancy: A review of 64 cases. *Pediatrics* 55:376, 1975.
121. Sawyer R.B., Sawyer K.C., List J.E.: Infectious emphysema of the gastrointestinal tract in the adult. *Am. J. Surg.* 120:579, 1970.
122. Schmid O., Quaiser K.: Uber eine besondere schwere verlaufende Form von Enteritis beim Saugling. *Oesterr. Z. Kinderh.* 8:114, 1953.
123. Schullinger J.N., Mollitt D.L., Vinocur C.G., et al.: Neonatal necrotizing enterocolitis. *Am. J. Dis. Child.* 135:612, 1981.
124. Schwartz M.Z., Hayden C.K., Richardson C.J., et al.: A prospective evaluation of intestinal stenosis following necrotizing enterocolitis. *J. Pediatr. Surg.* 17:764, 1982.
125. Schwartz M.Z., Richardson C.J., Hayden C.K., et al.: Intestinal stenosis following successful medical management of necrotizing enterocolitis. *J. Pediatr. Surg.* 15:890, 1980.
126. Siebold A.E.: Brand in der kleinen Curvatur des Magens eines atrophischen Kindes. *J. Geburtsh.* 5:3, 1826.
127. Silane M.F., Symchych P.S.: Necrotizing enterocolitis after cardiac surgery. *Am. J. Surg.* 133:373, 1977.
128. Simpson J.Y.: Peritonitis in the fetus in utero. *Edinburgh Med. Surg. J.* 15:390, 1838.
129. Stern M., Batty I.: Pathogenic Clostridia. London, Butterworth, 1975.
130. Stevenson D.K., Graham C.B., Stevenson J.K.: Neonatal necrotizing enterocolitis: 100 new cases. *Arch. Pediatr.* 27:319, 1980.
131. Stevenson D.K., Kerner J.A., Malachowski N., et al.: Late morbidity among survivors of necrotizing enterocolitis. *Pediatrics* 66:925, 1980.
132. Stoll B.J., Kanto W.P. Jr., Glass R.I., et al.: Epidemiology of necrotizing enterocolitis: A case control study. *J. Pediatr.* 96:447, 1980.
133. Sturm R., Staneck J.L., Stauffer L.R., et al.: Neonatal necrotizing enterocolitis associated with penicillin-resistant toxigenic *Clostridium butyricum. Pediatrics* 66:928, 1980.
134. Svirsky-Gross S.: Pathogenic strains of coli (0, 111) among prematures and the use of human milk in controlling the outbreak of diarrhea. *Ann. Pediatr.* 190:109, 1958.
135. Swanson V.L., Landing B.H.: Pathology, in Brown E.G., Sweet A.Y. (eds.): *Neonatal Necrotizing Enterocolitis.* New York, Grune & Stratton, 1980, p. 129.
136. Sweet A.Y.: Epidemiology, in Brown E.G., Sweet A.Y. (eds.): *Neonatal Necrotizing Enterocolitis.* New York, Grune & Stratton, 1980, p. 11.
137. Teasdale F., Le Guennec J.C., Bard H., et al.: Neonatal necrotizing enterocolitis: The relationship of age at the time of onset of prognosis. *CMA J.* 123:387, 1980.
138. Thelander H.E.: Perforation of the gastro-intestinal tract of the newborn infant. *Am. J. Dis. Child.* 58:371, 1939.
139. Thilo E.H., Lazarte R.A., Hernandez J.A.: Necrotizing enterocolitis in the first 24 hours of life. *Pediatrics* 73:476, 1984.
140. Touloukian R.J.: Etiologic role of the circulation, in Brown E.G., Sweet A.Y. (eds.): *Neonatal Necrotizing Enterocolitis.* New York, Grune & Stratton, 1980, p. 41.
141. Touloukian R.J.: Neonatal necrotizing enterocolitis: An update on etiology, diagnosis and treatment. *Surg. Clin. North Am.* 56:281, 1976.
142. Touloukian R.J., Kadar A., Spencer R.P.: The gastrointestinal complications of neonatal umbilical venous exchange transfusions: a clinical and experimental study. *Pediatrics* 51:36, 1973.
143. Touloukian R.J., Posch J.N., Spencer R.P.: The pathogenesis of ischemic gastroenterocolitis of the neonate; selective gut mucosal ischemia in asphyxiated neonatal piglets. *J. Pediatr. Surg.* 7:194, 1972.
144. Tyson J.E., De Sa D.J., Moore S.: Thromboatheromatous complications of umbilical arterial catheterization in the newborn period. *Arch. Dis. Child.* 51:744, 1976.
145. Virjee J.P., Gill G.J., De Sa D.J., et al.: Strictures and other late complications of neonatal necrotising enterocolitis. *Clin. Radiol.* 30:25, 1979.
146. Virjee J.P., Somers S., De Sa D.J., et al.: Changing patterns of neonatal necrotizing enterocolitis. *Gastrointest. Radiol.* 4:169, 1979.
147. Virnig N.L., Reynolds J.W.: Epidemiological aspects of neonatal necrotizing enterocolitis. *Am. J. Dis. Child.* 128:186, 1974.
148. von Willi H.: Ueber eine bösartige Enteritis bei Saüglingen des ersten Trimenons. *Ann. Paediatr.* 162:87, 1944.
149. Waldhausen J.A., Herendeen T., King H.: Necrotizing colitis of the newborn: Common cause of perforation of the colon. *Pediatr. Surg.* 54:365, 1963.
150. Warren S., Schreiber J.R., Epstein M.F.: Necrotizing enterocolitis and hemolysis associated with *Clostridium perfringens. Am. J. Dis. Child.* 138:686, 1984.
151. Wexler H.A.: The persistent loop sign in neonatal necrotizing enterocolitis: A new indication for surgical intervention? *Radiology* 126:201, 1978.
152. White K.C., Harkavy K.L.: Hypertonic formula resulting from added oral medications. *Am. J. Dis. Child.* 136:931, 1982.
153. Willis D.M., Chabot J., Radde I.C., et al.: Unsuspected hyperosmolality of oral solutions contributing to necrotizing enterocolitis in very low-birth-weight infants. *Pediatrics* 60:535, 1977.
154. Wilson R., del Portillo M., Schmidt E., et al.: Risk factors for necrotizing enterocolitis in infants weighing more than 2,000 grams at birth: A case-control study. *Pediatrics* 71:19, 1983.
155. Wilson R., Kanto W.P. Jr., McCarthy B.J., et al.: Epidemiologic characteristics of necrotizing enterocolitis: a population-based study. *Am. J. Epidemiol.* 114:880, 1981.
156. Wilson R., Kanto W.P. Jr., McCarthy B.J., et al.: Short communication: Age at onset of necrotizing enterocolitis: an epidemiologic analysis. *Pediatr. Res.* 16:82, 1982.
157. Winberg J., Wessner G.: Does breast milk protect against septicaemia in the newborn? *Lancet* 1:1091, 1971.
158. Yu V.Y.H., James B., Henry P., et al.: Total parenteral nutrition in very low birthweight infants: a controlled trial. *Arch. Dis. Child.* 54:653, 1979.
159. Yu V.Y.H., Joseph R., Bajuk B., et al.: Perinatal risk factors for necrotizing enterocolitis. *Arch. Dis. Child.* 59:430, 1984.
160. Yu V.Y.H., Joseph R., Bajuk B., et al.: Necrotizing enterocolitis in very low birthweight infants: a four-year experience. *Aust. Paediatr. J.* 20:29, 1983.
161. Yu V.Y.H., Tudehope D.I., Gill G.J.: Neonatal necrotizing enterocolitis: Radiological manifestations. *Aust. Paediatr. J.* 13:200, 1977.
162. Zillner E.: Ruptura flexurae Sigmoidis neonati inter partum. *Virchows Arch. Pathol. Anat.* 96:307, 1884.

100 Robert L. Telander

Crohn's Disease

HISTORY.—In 1932, Crohn and his associates,[9] working at Mt. Sinai Hospital in New York City, described *regional ileitis* and separated it from other inflammatory processes of the small bowel. Because the inflammatory process was soon found to involve all portions of the intestinal tract, it became referred to as *regional enteritis.* Although the initial report described a process localized to the terminal ileum, 4 years later Crohn and Rosenak[10] described several patients in whom both ileum and colon were involved by the granulomatous inflammatory process. However, the common involvement of the colon was not fully accepted until after the report by Lockhart-Mummery and Morson[36] in 1964. As a result, the term "Crohn's disease" often is used to describe the inflammatory process involving all anatomical regions of the gastrointestinal tract.

Crohn's initial report stated that the cause of the disease was unknown, and that statement remains true.

Crohn's disease is a chronic, transmural, inflammatory disease that may involve any portion of the gastrointestinal tract, although most commonly the terminal ileum and colon are involved. The pathologic changes observed in children resemble closely those seen in adults, and the approaches to diagnosis, medical management, and surgical treatment are similar. Freeborn et al.[17] and others[13] observed that approximately 25% of patients with Crohn's disease are diagnosed by age 20 years. Approximately 15% of all cases have their onset before age 15 years.[39, 43] Certain unique characteristics of the child with Crohn's disease demand special consideration—the potential for growth failure, the effect of a severe chronic illness during childhood and adolescence, and the importance of considering the entire family along with the patient in overall management.

For the patient with Crohn's disease, management begins at the patient's first visit. It is important, early on, not to be overly pessimistic when discussing the nature of the disease with the patient and the patient's parents. The discussion must be realistic, of course, but can offer a positive outlook. In a series of children with Crohn's disease, 94% were in fair to excellent health as adults and 71% reported no limitation in activity.[7] We have found that, in patients with involvement of only the small bowel, in a large number the results are good after resection of the affected bowel. The future is not necessarily dismal for these patients.

It is difficult to establish the precise incidence of Crohn's disease in the general population, but it has been reported to be most common in Scandinavia, the United States, and England. It is three to four times more common in Jews than in non-Jews and is rare in black and Hispanic children. Various centers have reported an average incidence of 3.7–4.5 cases diagnosed per year per 100,000 population. Tertiary referral centers have provided most of the reports, and, of course, this immediately introduces a bias in the sampling. Incidence of the disease is more accurately described by the study of stable populations. A recent study by Agrez and his colleagues of a stable population (Olmsted County, Minnesota; population approximately 90,000) identified 103 persons in the county in whom Crohn's disease developed between 1935 and 1975.[1] Forty-two of these 103 patients underwent a surgical procedure.

Etiology

The cause of Crohn's disease remains unknown, but a number of hypotheses have been suggested and studied. The lymphoid tissues of the gut represent approximately 25% of the gut mucosa in spite of the fact that the primary task of the intestine is digestion and absorption of nutrients. This has led to investigations of the role of the cellular and humoral immune systems in Crohn's disease.[14, 27] The colon can participate in the Shwartzman reaction, the Auer phenomenon, and the Arthus reaction. Studies have shown that the colitis associated with these responses clearly differs from Crohn's disease in a number of ways. The lymphocyte subpopulations including T-cells, B-cells, Fc receptor-bearing killer cells, and complement receptor-bearing B-cells also have been studied. The abnormal findings include a diminution of the reactivity to phytohemagglutinin of circulating lymphocytes. Shorter et al. suggested that ulcerative colitis and Crohn's disease represent opposite extremes of a single disease process and that inflammatory bowel disease results from a hypersensitivity to bacterial antigens normally present in the gastrointestinal tract.[47] They postulated that a state of hypersensitivity to enterobacterial antigens and cow's milk develops in infancy, before a normal intestinal mucosal block is established.

Because lymphangiectasia is a prominent pathologic finding in Crohn's disease, obstructing lymphangitis has also been suggested as the basic etiologic process associated with the prominent mesenteric lymphadenopathy.

Specific infectious agents, such as the coliform organisms, and related toxins have always been suspected, but no single organism has been identified as causative. *Clostridium difficile* toxin has been considered.[3] It has been postulated that the bacterial toxin could disrupt the intestinal mucosa, allowing invasion by the resident colonic bacteria. If this were the case, it could lead to a self-perpetuating mechanism: endotoxin-induced Shwartzman reactions, antigen-antibody complexes, or lymphocyte-mediated cytotoxicity. However, there is no evidence that the toxin does initiate the pathologic process.

Psychosocial considerations have been implicated but never demonstrated to cause or to perpetuate the inflammatory process. Familial characteristics, present in at least 10–15%, may predispose a certain portion of the population to the development of inflammatory bowel disease.

Pathology

The earliest visible mucosal changes are small aphthoid ulcers. These small, oval, mucosal ulcerations are made up of a central micro abscess within the lymphoid follicle at the mucosal-submucosal junction.[19, 38] The small ulcers may extend, giving rise to the more characteristic longitudinally directed, penetrating defects. The longitudinal defects vary somewhat in both length and width, and they often penetrate deeply to the serosa (Fig 100–1). They have been referred to as "bear-claw" or "rake" ulcers (Fig 100–2).

The mucosa between the ulcerations may appear normal. Transverse ulcerations may develop as well, resulting in a cobblestone appearance. These findings contrast with those in ulcerative colitis in which, beginning at the rectum and extending continuously cephalad, the mucosa is inflamed and friable, bleeds easily on contact, and has no deep ulcerations until the more serious form has developed.

The most common pattern of involvement in Crohn's disease is thickening and induration of the terminal ileum extending from the cecum proximally, 15–25 cm. There generally is extensive enlargement of the lymph nodes in the adjacent mesentery, and "creeping fat" of the mesentery extends up onto the bowel wall in varying degree. Involvement of the intestine is discontinuous. The ulcers characteristically penetrate the bowel wall and serosa, resulting in a walled-off abscess, an inflammatory mass, or a fistula. Fistulae may extend to any organ; rarely, the penetrating ulcer results in a free perforation. Histologically the associated inflammation contains granulomas in perhaps half to two thirds of patients. These are diagnostic of Crohn's disease, are most commonly in the submucosa, but may be found in all layers of the bowel and, occasionally, in the adjacent lymph nodes.

Clinical Aspects

Diagnosis

The diagnosis of Crohn's disease in a child is made by consideration of the clinical history, physical findings, and, most important, the results of radiologic and endoscopic studies. The similarity between chronic ulcerative colitis and Crohn's disease at times may be remarkable. The demonstration of a granuloma on rectal biopsy is extremely helpful, but this finding is often not present.[25, 32, 38] When the radiologic results are combined with the history and endoscopic findings, the diagnostic accuracy is greater than 90%.

The onset of symptoms in children with Crohn's disease may

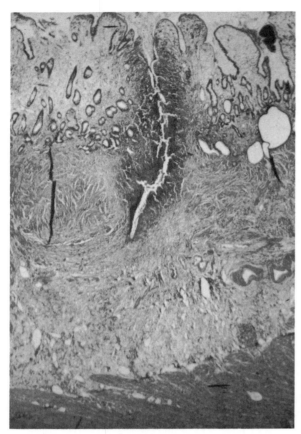

Fig 100–1.—Penetrating ulcer in Crohn's disease. Such sinuses may extend from mucosa to serosa and into adherent viscera or through the abdominal wall, establishing fistulae. Free perforation into the peritoneal cavity is rare.

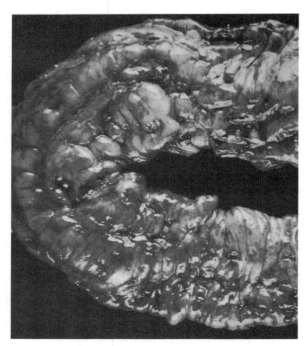

Fig 100–2.—Crohn's disease. Characteristic gross appearance of longitudinal ulceration.

be as early as infancy but is certainly more common in the teens. Although the mean age at onset in adults is approximately 25 years, the mean age at onset of symptoms in several groups of children under 16 was 12–13 years.[7, 41] In a recent study of 177 children 15 years of age or under at the Mayo Clinic, the most common clinical features at the time of diagnosis were abdominal pain (79%), diarrhea (68%), and weight loss (51%)[7] (Table 100–1). The clinical course often was slowly progressive from the time of onset. The patients generally presented with more than one of the common features. Anorexia, fever, fatigability, and growth failure also were common aspects of the clinical presentation. Joint complaints (16%), not uncommon, included arthritis and arthralgias. Twenty percent of these 177 children presented with acute abdominal symptoms and had undergone appendectomy. Perineal discomfort and complaints may be present and include anal fissures or fistulae, which are particularly distressing to the patient who often has a history of unsuccessful attempts at surgical repair of the fistula.

There is often mild to moderate anemia. Patients with the colitis of Crohn's disease often have chronic blood loss and therefore have iron-deficiency anemia. Occasionally, with ileocolitis, vitamin B_{12} absorption may be impaired, leading to megaloblastic anemia. The erythrocyte sedimentation rate was elevated in 85% of children in the Mayo Clinic series (mean, 48.8 mm in 1 hour). The sedimentation rate furnishes a nonspecific reflection of disease activity in the given child and may be used to evaluate response to medical therapy. Serum albumin concentration may be low from loss of protein into the lumen of the bowel and may also be an indicator of disease activity.

There may be a palpable abdominal mass in the right lower quadrant. The patient may have a recent appendectomy scar, and occasionally there may be a fistula to the skin, although this is much less common than it was in the past. There may be evidence of growth retardation and failure of development of the usual secondary sexual characteristics. Although only four of 177 children in the Mayo Clinic study cited growth failure as the chief complaint, it was listed as a problem in 46 patients (26%). Thirty-seven patients (21%) were below the tenth percentile for height at diagnosis.

TABLE 100–1.—CLINICAL FEATURES AT DIAGNOSIS IN 177 PATIENTS 15 YEARS OF AGE OR LESS AT THE MAYO CLINIC*

MANIFESTATION	NO. (%) OF PATIENTS
Abdominal pain	140 (79)
Diarrhea	120 (68)
Asthenic body habitus	109 (62)
Weight loss	90 (51)
Anorexia	75 (42)
Fever	73 (41)
Fatigability	62 (35)
Growth failure (patient's assessment)	46 (26)
Vomiting	43 (24)
Joint symptoms	28 (16)
Perineal inflammation	27 (15)
Hematochezia	24 (14)
Digital clubbing	20 (11)
Right lower quadrant mass	20 (11)
Fistula	18 (10)
Stomatitis	7 (4)

*From Castile R.G., Telander R.L., Cooney D.R., et al.: Crohn's disease in children: Assessment of the progression of disease, growth, and prognosis. *J. Pediatr. Surg.* 15:462–469, 1980. By permission of Grune & Stratton.

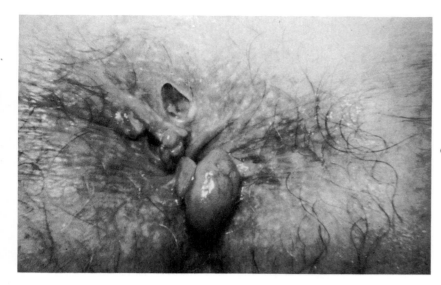

Fig 100–3.—Crohn's disease involving anorectum. Note edematous hyperplastic skin tags.

The anorectal examination, including proctoscopy and colonoscopy, commonly demonstrated abnormalities (50–60%). Perianal disease strongly suggests Crohn's disease rather than ulcerative colitis. The more frequently observed external abnormal findings include perianal disease such as perianal ulcerations, scarring, fistulae, mucosal tags, abrasions, and fissures (Figs 100–3 to 100–5). Endoscopically, a common characteristic of Crohn's disease is discontinuous involvement of the gut. A normal anal canal is common. Rectosigmoid ulcerations are frequently observed. Early observable changes vary from very small aphthoid ulcerations (small, white, oval-shaped ulcers) that bleed easily on

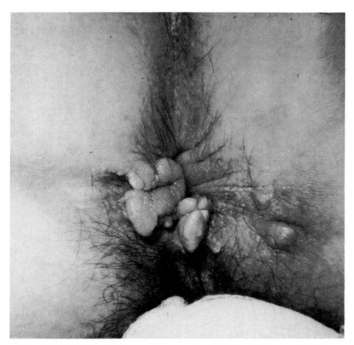

Fig 100–4.—Crohn's disease of anorectum. Note induration and dusky appearance of skin, edematous hyperplastic skin tags, and linear ulcers. Patient had a 5-year history of Crohn's disease. Barium study of colon demonstrated disease limited to rectum, sigmoid, and descending colon, with normal small bowel. After proctocolectomy with Brooke ileostomy, patient's health has remained excellent during 19-year follow-up.

contact to larger, penetrating ulcers. The ulcers tend to have sharp borders and are penetrating. The adjacent mucosa may be edematous but otherwise appears normal.

Biopsy is often not helpful because of the frequent absence of a granuloma or sarcoid type of reaction in the biopsied tissue. A granuloma is a valuable diagnostic histologic feature. Many authors[38] state that the granulomatous reaction to some product of the inflammatory process of Crohn's disease is a part of the reaction to injury and not the initial process. In the acutely ill patient with fever, colonoscopy may result in a worsening of the patient's condition and is often deferred for a time.

Radiologic Features

The findings in children are similar to those in adults. Because any portion of the gastrointestinal tract may be involved, barium studies of the esophagus, stomach, small bowel, and colon are performed at the initial examination. Subsequent examinations are scheduled on the basis of changes in the patient's clinical picture. The patterns of involvement in children are summarized in Figure 100–6. Most reports describe ileocolitis occurring in 40–50%, small-bowel involvement alone in 35–50%, and colon alone in approximately 10%. When the small intestine is involved, the involvement may be limited to the terminal ileum, or there may be discontinuous involvement of the small bowel with or without involvement of the terminal ileum. Duodenal involvement, generally uncommon (3%) in children,[45] occurred in 2% in our series.[7]

The roentgenographic changes observed in the small bowel reflect the presence, in varying degree, of edema and inflammation with ulceration, spasm, fibrosis, and stenosis (Fig 100–7). Minimal changes include thickening and blunting of mucosal folds and some thickening of the bowel wall. Early on, the usual fold architecture and pliability remain relatively normal. With moderate amounts of edema, the folds enlarge somewhat to become mildly distorted. Decreased pliability is evident during fluoroscopy. Some separation of the loops of bowel becomes apparent. With severe degrees of edema and inflammation, the normal mucosal pattern disappears and may be completely effaced. Stenosis of the lumen then commonly develops along with inflexibility and straightening of the loops. The impression of a mass on the cecum may develop as a result of thickening of the terminal ileum and its mesentery, with or without fistulae. The colon is studied most accurately by the double-contrast technique

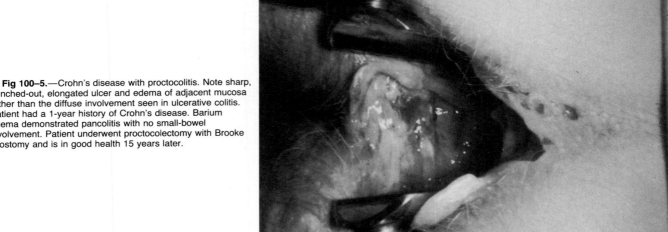

Fig 100–5.—Crohn's disease with proctocolitis. Note sharp, punched-out, elongated ulcer and edema of adjacent mucosa rather than the diffuse involvement seen in ulcerative colitis. Patient had a 1-year history of Crohn's disease. Barium enema demonstrated pancolitis with no small-bowel involvement. Patient underwent proctocolectomy with Brooke ileostomy and is in good health 15 years later.

(Fig 100–8). Barium enema is not carried out if the patient is acutely ill with any evidence of a toxic megacolon.

Ulcerations begin as small aphthoid lesions, often difficult to demonstrate radiologically. They may progress to deeper linear ulcers, which may penetrate the serosa to cause enteric fistulae (Fig 100–9), abscesses, and, in rare instances, free perforation.

Stenosis, which early is minimal, progresses. Multiple fistulae may develop. Edema and inflammation may be replaced by fibrosis that progresses to the point of obstruction.

A "string sign" represents a long stenosis (Fig 100–10). If resolution occurs, it may be assumed that the stenosis was due primarily to edema. Chronicity and proximal dilatation suggest fibrosis and scarring. Extraintestinal masses, represented on the film by areas without bowel loops, generally represented thickened mesentery and bowel wall.

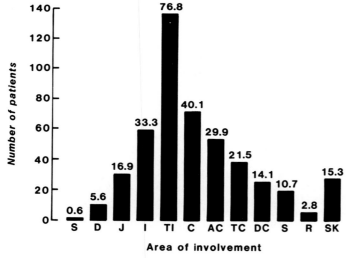

Fig 100–6.—Roentgenographic areas of bowel involvement at time of diagnosis in 177 children. Individual patients may have more than one area of involvement. Numbers above bars are percentages of the 177 patients. *S* indicates stomach; *D*, duodenum; *J*, jejunum; *I*, ileum; *TI*, terminal ileum; *C*, cecum; *AC*, ascending colon; *TC*, transverse colon; *DC*, descending colon; *S*, sigmoid; *R*, rectum; and *SK*, skip areas noted. (From Castile R.G., Telander R.L., Cooney D.R., et al.: Crohn's disease in children: Assessment of the progression of disease, growth, and prognosis. *J. Pediatr. Surg.* 15:462–469, 1980. By permission of Grune & Stratton.)

Medical Therapy

Generally, medical therapy is used initially in all patients and includes attempts to eliminate diarrhea and abdominal cramps and to improve nutrition. Agents that decrease bowel motility, such as diphenoxylate (Lomotil), and occasionally antispasmodics and sedatives, are utilized. Medical therapy for Crohn's disease involving the perianal region has included metronidazole (Flagyl); clinical "improvement" in 15 of 17 patients has been reported.[16] In the more seriously ill patient, sulfasalazine (Azulfidine) may be of benefit. When Azulfidine is not satisfactory, Flagyl can be used with good results, and sometimes administration of both drugs is helpful. For the even more severely ill patient, steroids have been widely utilized but, because of adverse side effects, long-term steroid therapy generally is avoided. Immunosuppressives such as 6-mercaptopurine and azathioprine have been used to control the active disease process but in general have a very small role in the management of children with Crohn's disease.

In addition to standard medical therapy, elemental diets and night-time tube feedings enhance nutrition, correct anemia, and maintain fluid and electrolyte balances. Total parenteral nutrition, in-hospital and at home,[15] has been utilized, with some promise. It may be given at night, leaving the patient free to go to school and participate in daytime activities. Placing the bowel at rest for several weeks with total parenteral nutrition leads to a remission in about 90% of patients.[46] Because most of these patients have some degree of malnutrition, it is of value even for patients who will require operation later. The results of Seashore et al. in children, however, were discouraging, symptoms recurring usually within 3 months[46] and 75% of children followed for more than 1 year requiring operation. Total parenteral nutrition is not a definitive therapeutic modality but does play an important role in medical and surgical therapy.

It is rare (<1%) to find repeated resections leading to a short bowel syndrome in children.[12] When the syndrome does occur, total parenteral nutrition administered at home can be life-saving, minimizes hospitalization, restores health and growth, and permits the patient to return to school.[15] This approach has had good results in our hands and those of others.

The beneficial influence of any of the medical regimens on the long-term progression of the disease has not been clearly established, in part because of the numerous remissions and exacerbations of activity of the disease in patients not receiving medical therapy.

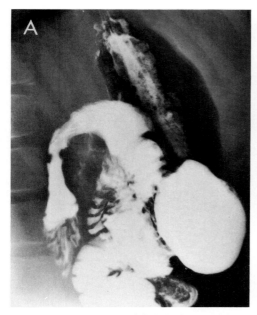 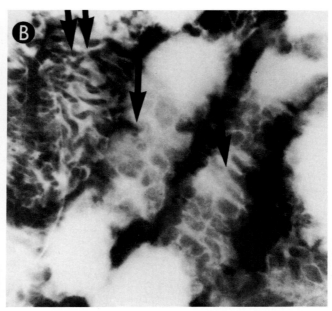

Fig 100–7.—Radiologic appearances of Crohn's disease of the small intestine. **A,** Crohn's disease involving the second portion of the duodenum with localized narrowing and thickening of mucosal folds. **B,** Crohn's disease of the ileum. Note mild thickening of folds *(top arrows),* compared with adjacent normal folds *(lower two arrows).*

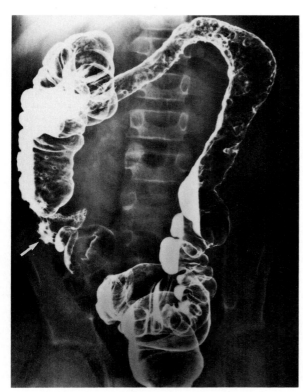

Fig 100–8.—Crohn's disease producing rigidity and decrease in caliber of the transverse and descending colon; the cecum is involved to a lesser degree *(arrow).* (From Hoffman A.D.: The child with diarrhea, in Hilton S.V.W., Edwards D.K., Hilton J.W. (eds.): *Practical Pediatric Radiology.* Philadelphia, W.B. Saunders Co., 1984, pp. 269–325. Used by permission.)

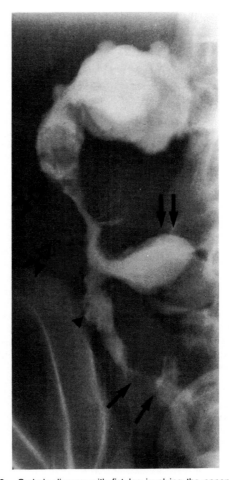

Fig 100–9.—Crohn's disease with fistulae involving the appendiceal stump *(bottom arrows).* Note the marked involvement of proximal ascending colon *(tailed arrows)* and cecum *(arrowhead)* and the patulous terminal ileum *(top arrows).* (From Hoffman A.D.: The child with diarrhea, in Hilton S.V.W., Edwards D.K., Hilton J.W. (eds.): *Practical Pediatric Radiology.* Philadelphia, W.B. Saunders Co., 1984, pp. 269–325. Used by permission.)

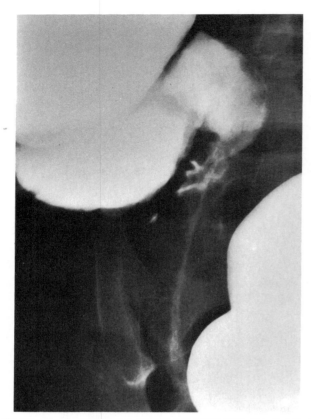

Fig 100–10.—Crohn's disease, terminal ileal involvement. The characteristic "string sign" of involvement of the terminal ileum shown here, with a fixed narrowing for a variable distance, is best demonstrated by barium enema. (From Hoffman A.D.: The child with diarrhea, in Hilton S.V.W., Edwards D.K., Hilton J.W. (eds.): *Practical Pediatric Radiology*. Philadelphia, W.B. Saunders Co., 1984, pp. 269–325. Used by permission.)

Surgical Therapy

Indications

At least 70% of children with Crohn's disease eventually undergo operation.[7, 13] In the recent Mayo Clinic study of children with Crohn's disease (mean follow-up, 8.8 years), 119 (67%) underwent 178 definitive surgical procedures for the disease.[7] An additional 146 nondefinitive procedures, such as drainage of abscesses and treatment of fistulae, were also performed.

Operation is premature in patients with Crohn's disease whose complaints are minor. Resection of involved bowel does not usually cure the disease. Nevertheless, there is benefit to be derived from operation; usually there is a symptom-free period postoperatively, and up to half of the patients will not need another operation for at least 10 years (Fig 100–11), at which time operation offers similar promise. Thus, for these selected patients, good health may be achieved during their adolescence, an important time in their lives.

Operative intervention is indicated for specific complications, or when medical management is ineffective in controlling the disease. In general, there is no controversy regarding surgical intervention in patients who have the dangerous but uncommon complications of toxic megacolon, free perforation, or massive hemorrhage. Occasionally there is more of a question as to the role of operation in the more common problems, as in the child who has intractable disease, internal fistulae, or an inflammatory mass. Decisions concerning operation in such patients require

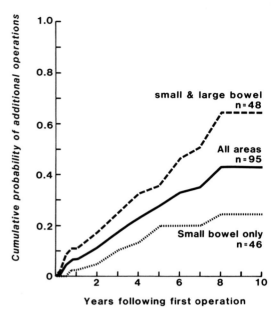

Fig 100–11.—Cumulative probability of additional operation. (From Castile R.G., Telander R.L., Cooney D.R., et al.: Crohn's disease in children: Assessment of the progression of disease, growth, and prognosis. *J. Pediatr. Surg.* 15:462–469, 1980. By permission of Grune & Stratton.)

consideration of a number of factors. The frequency of additional operations becoming necessary is one such factor (Fig 100–11). The removal of minimal amounts of intestine—that is, only those segments with permanent changes—is important. In addition, the patient's state of health is improved after operation, especially important in adolescence, and often remains improved for years. The patient returns to school and to his/her social relationships and activities.

Considerable controversy persists regarding the timing and value of operation in the patient who has growth failure. A number of authors[5, 29, 33, 44] have suggested that the failure is due to chronic malnutrition secondary to inadequate caloric intake. The prevention of growth failure in children with Crohn's disease is of prime importance. In the initial care constant attention must be given to the patient's nutritional status, in addition to episodic medical management. Such medical management includes improved daytime caloric intake orally or by additional night-time tube feedings to reverse growth failure. Total parenteral nutrition may be considered in order to optimize caloric intake and provide complete bowel rest.

If such measures prove inadequate—active disease continues in the intestinal tract and there is no improvement in the rate of growth—elective resection should be strongly considered, particularly for severe growth retardation. These patients, representing only a subgroup of children with Crohn's disease, have a chance of increasing their height percentile if the diseased bowel is resected before the epiphyseal growth plates have closed.[21, 26] In our series, patients who had undergone surgical treatment were found to be in a significantly higher percentile for height, at adult follow-up, compared with the percentile at diagnosis (Fig 100–12). Those who did not undergo operation were at a lower height percentile at follow-up.

The most common specific indications for operation in Crohn's disease include intractability, obstruction, persistence of symptoms in spite of usual medical management, abdominal abscesses or mass, fistulae (internal or external), and perianal disease.

Obstruction, a common indication, is related to the localized

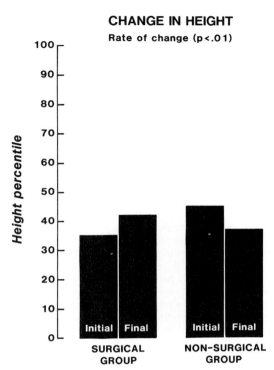

CHANGE IN HEIGHT
Rate of change (p<.01)

Fig 100–12.—Change in mean height percentile from time of diagnosis to adult height in operated and unoperated groups (*P*<.01). (From Castile R.G., Telander R.L., Cooney D.R., et al.: Crohn's disease in children: Assessment of the progression of disease, growth and prognosis. *J. Pediatr. Surg.* 15:462–469, 1980. By permission of Grune & Stratton.)

inflammatory process and its associated edema and encroachment on the lumen of the adjacent bowel. Chronic edema and inflammation progress to fibrosis, irreversible changes, and obstruction. The obstruction for a long time is incomplete, manifested by severe cramps, infrequent stools, occasional vomiting, the episodes tending to occur with increasing frequency. Poor motility of the involved bowel can also contribute to the picture of bowel obstruction. Internal fistulae and an inflammatory mass are commonly associated with the obstructed bowel. The intestinal obstruction is often slowly progressive and chronic. If it is due to early reversible changes, at times it will resolve with nasogastric suction, intravenous fluids, antibiotics, and steroids. If bowel obstruction is not relieved, surgical intervention is essential. Intractability may be viewed in several ways. If the disease is interfering significantly with the patient's quality of life and medical therapy is not providing relief, operation is appropriate. Similarly, if the patient's quality of life is maintained only by the administration of large amounts of medications such as prednisone on a long-term basis, surgical therapy is advisable.

A palpable mass in the right lower abdominal quadrant, encountered in 15–20% of children, represents a localized inflammatory mass associated with severe changes in the terminal ileum. Internal fistulae are a common component of the mass, part of a walled-off perforation into the mesentery and adjacent tissues with associated fever, tenderness, and pain. Such an inflammatory mass or abscess generally requires operation and resection of the involved bowel.

Fistulae secondary to a deep, penetrating ulcer extend between the diseased segment of intestinal tract and an adjacent relatively normal loop of small bowel, cecum, or colon, into the bladder or the perirectal space or may communicate to the skin of abdominal wall or perianal regions. Total parenteral nutrition

has been effective in some patients who had no significant obstruction distal to the fistula. All too often, however, total parenteral nutrition has not eliminated the fistula, although it may enhance the nutritional status of the patient before the necessary operation.

Free perforation is an uncommon, but serious complication in Crohn's disease. The diagnosis may be difficult at times because of high-dose steroid therapy. Operative intervention is essential, with resection of the involved bowel.

Hematochezia, usually episodic and mild, occurs in at least 15% of children with Crohn's disease. Massive hemorrhage is uncommon. In the rare patient with Crohn's colitis and massive hemorrhage, emergency total proctocolectomy and ileostomy is the preferred procedure. Bleeding commonly persists from the rectum if it is allowed to remain in place.

Toxic megacolon, reported in as high as 20% of patients with Crohn's disease, may be associated with severe hemorrhage along with perforation, sepsis, and peritonitis. The complication is an urgent one and frequently requires operation. With medical therapy, the mortality rate tends to be rather high; those patients surviving tend to have recurrent episodes, and the majority will require an operation in the future. Homer and associates recommend early surgical treatment if there is not prompt response to severe colitis, because almost all these patients subsequently require operation within a short time.[26] Gentle handling of the colon is required during operation to avoid rupture, and spillage of stool.

Surgical Considerations

The indications for operation in Crohn's disease are rather straightforward and well established, but the specific choice of surgical procedure can be difficult. We generally resect all bowel grossly involved by disease and perform a primary anastomosis. In our series of 178 definitive procedures in children, the operation was resection with stoma in 33 and bowel bypass in 11. Construction of a Kock pouch is contraindicated because of the potential complications in patients with Crohn's disease. The endorectal pull-through with ileoanal anastomosis is not a good choice because the disease may recur in the rectal muscular sleeve.[49, 50] In general, resection of all gross disease is preferred unless the small bowel is extensively involved by "skip areas." Important considerations in the surgical management of Crohn's disease include removal of only the grossly abnormal bowel with its induration and creeping fat along with approximately 10 cm of proximal normal-appearing bowel without removal of all microscopic residua. It is also important to avoid resection of asymptomatic "skip areas" that may be present at a distance. This approach helps avoid short-bowel syndrome in a patient who may have to undergo additional operations later.

In the recent Mayo Clinic study of children, the probability that a child would undergo an additional operation was related to the time that had passed since the previous operation, the location of the disease in the bowel, and the number of previous surgical procedures.[7] In children who required one operation, the cumulative probability of further operation was 7% within 1 year, 36% within 5 years, and 48% within 10 years (see Fig 100–11). The reoperation rate in children with only small-bowel involvement increased from 3% at 1 year to 23% at 10 years. In contrast, children who had involvement of both the colon and small bowel had a higher rate of recurrence and need for additional operations: approximately 10% at 1 year and 65% at 10 years. Thus, when the small bowel alone was involved, recurrence with reoperation was much less likely than when both ileum and colon were involved. This is in general agreement with several other series.[18, 20, 23, 35, 37]

TABLE 100–2.—Definitive
Surgical Procedures
for Crohn's Disease*

NO. OF OPERATIONS	NO. (%) OF PATIENTS
0	58 (33)
1	70 (40)
2	26 (15)
3	14 (8)
4	6 (3)
5	3 (2)
Total	177

*From Castile R.G., Telander R.L., Cooney D.R., et al.: Crohn's disease in children: Assessment of the progression of disease, growth, and prognosis. *J. Pediatr. Surg.* 15:462–469, 1980. By permission of Grune & Stratton.

More than one operation was performed in 41% of the patients undergoing a definitive surgical procedure (Table 100–2), and the likelihood of an additional operation in a given patient increased as the number of surgical procedures increased. The number of patients having three or more operations was small. In patients undergoing additional procedures, the median interval between procedures was 2.3 years from the first to the second, 2.6 years from the second to the third, and 1.4 years from the third to the fourth.

Recurrent Crohn's disease commonly is seen just proximal to the site of anastomosis, raising interest in the need to have microscopically disease-free margins.[51] Indeed, whether or not microscopic residual at the anastomotic line has any effect upon the incidence of recurrence has been a topic of debate for many years, with evidence suggesting the need to resect all microscopic disease[4, 52] as well as evidence to the contrary.[8, 42] Koch et al.[30] reported that the distribution of recurrent Crohn's disease is related to the initial anatomic location; proximal recurrence is observed most commonly in ileal Crohn's disease, and both proximal and distal recurrence with ileocolitis.

Surgical Procedures

Stomach and Duodenum.—Crohn's disease of the stomach and duodenum may benefit from initial medical therapy consisting of steroids (sulfasalazine may irritate the stomach).[40] Diagnosis may be difficult because of the similarity to peptic ulcer disease. Usually Crohn's disease has been identified distally in the bowel, making the diagnosis clear. The stomach and duodenum themselves are inflamed and indurated, but without creeping fat and lymphadenopathy. Their appearance may suggest peptic ulcer disease or lymphoma. Biopsy may be essential to rule out a malignant process in the third and fourth portions of the duodenum, and peptic ulcer disease must be excluded to ensure that the proper procedure is being performed. Rutgeerts and associates were successful in establishing the diagnosis of Crohn's disease of the duodenum in 73% of patients by endoscopic biopsy (22 of 30 patients).[45] In contrast, Nugent and associates were unsuccessful with endoscopic biopsies in a group of 17 patients with Crohn's disease of the duodenum.[40] The obstructing duodenal Crohn's lesions can best be relieved by gastrojejunostomy or duodenojejunostomy.

Jejunum and Ileum.—The involved terminal ileum or diseased small bowel is resected, along with some of the thickened mesentery, to normal-appearing bowel with normally thin mesentery—approximately 10 cm of grossly normal-appearing bowel

is resected (Fig 100–13). Intestinal continuity usually can be established with an end-to-end anastomosis. All abscesses and inflammatory masses are removed or drained. Fistulous tracts are resected with the diseased bowel. The fistulous tract entering another hollow viscus is separated from it, and the normal viscus is closed primarily. Broe and Cameron reported 13 cases with ileosigmoid fistula in which resection and division of the fistula and simple closure of the colon were performed with excellent results and no anastomotic leaks.[6]

Colon.—When operation is required for severe Crohn's colitis, proctocolectomy and Brooke ileostomy are frequently performed. If there is minimal rectal disease without perianal complications, ileorectostomy or ileosigmoidostomy may be performed. When inflammation is limited to one portion of the colon, that portion may be resected, with colocolostomy. Lindhagen et al.,[34] who attempted to spare the rectum when possible, observed that, when the rectum was primarily involved, the lesions did not disappear after subtotal colectomy. An ileorectal anastomosis was successful only when the rectum was not involved preoperatively. A proximal diverting stoma may be of value in the severely ill patient to shorten the operative procedure, or in the patient recently diagnosed who is not yet mentally ready to consider removal of the rectum. In such patients, subsequent proctectomy can be carried out after the initial colectomy returns the patient to good health.

Patients who are to be operated on for toxic megacolon require aggressive preoperative preparation, with fluid resuscitation and antibiotics. In severely ill children, operation is performed early. A generous incision is required to provide good exposure, but the stoma sites must be considered. Peritoneal fluid is obtained for cultures and Gram stain, the abdomen is irrigated with saline, and all fluid is removed.[31] If the entire colon is involved, it must be handled gently to avoid rupture or perforation. When the rectum has minimal disease, it can be spared and the colon can be removed, with a Brooke ileostomy constructed to allow a subsequent ileoproctostomy. Fulminant colitis, which resembles toxic megacolon without colonic dilatation, also may require proctocolectomy with ileoproctostomy.

Anus and Rectum.—We found perianal disease in approximately 13% and abnormal proctoscopic findings in 63% of children with Crohn's disease.[7] The most common external manifestations included perianal ulcerations and fissures. Less commonly seen were fistulae and mucosal tags (see Figs 100–3 and 100–4). The causal relation of these abnormalities to proximal bowel disease is not clear, and standard surgical methods of treatment of perianal disease lead to failure. Because the perianal region is richly supplied with lymphatics and the abnormal changes include thickening, induration, and duskiness of the tissues, the pathologic process may be similar to the one in the proximal bowel. A linear ulceration in the anal canal (see Fig 100–5) is common, with associated thickened prominent skin tags (see Figs 100–3 and 100–4). The anal canal may be free of ulceration, but the distal rectum often (10–15%) has typical ulcerative changes. When children and young adults have poorly healing anal fistulae and abscesses, the proximal intestinal tract should be investigated for possible Crohn's disease.

A perirectal abscess, with or without fistula, should be widely drained, and any overhanging tissue or skin excised to eliminate premature healing of the superficial portions of the wound. Tub soaks and careful cleansing help to prevent early closure. It has been observed that, when the proximal disease has been controlled or eliminated by medical or surgical means, the anal disease may heal after local treatment. Approximately 60% of patients with ileal or ileocolic Crohn's disease heal perianal lesions after intestinal resection. Perianal disease associated with colonic

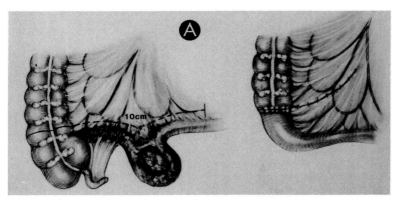

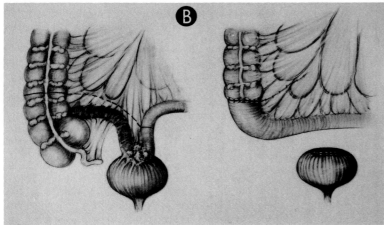

Fig 100–13.—Resection for Crohn's disease. **A,** surgical procedure for treating Crohn's disease of the terminal ileum by resecting terminal ileum with cecum and proximal 10 cm of grossly normal intestine. **B,** a fistula entering the bladder requires, in addition, separation of the fistula from the normal bladder and closure of the bladder. In general, such fistulae lead into viscera not involved by the disease and simple closure suffices for the organ into which the fistula opens.

Crohn's disease, however, tends not to heal. The combination of rectal Crohn's disease and anal fistula invariably led to proctocolectomy in the experience of Hellers et al.[24] If there is no longer inflammation in a shallow or short fistula in ano, there is some chance of slow healing after it is opened. Deeper, more complicated fistulae sometimes are simply observed if the patient is asymptomatic and proximal disease is controlled. If severe perianal disease persists, with fistulae and considerable morbidity, proctocolectomy and ileostomy may be required to relieve the situation. Harper et al.[22] advocated a "split ileostomy" for perianal Crohn's disease. They noted marked relief of perianal disease in 72% (23 of 32 patients) undergoing this procedure. However, only six of the 32 patients eventually had normal bowel continuity restored. A proximal ostomy has not been associated with healing of perianal disease in our experience, or in that of others.[2]

Prognosis

When Crohn's disease is diagnosed in a child, some clinicians wrongly assume an early fatal outcome after a relentless series of operations. This scenario is possible, but we and others have observed restoration of the patient to good health with appropriate surgical therapy. O'Donoghue and Dawson noted that the median relapse time for surgically treated patients is much longer than for patients treated medically, and, to minimize childhood morbidity, operation is often recommended early in children with severe problems.[41] The probability of an additional operation being required is 50% or less in the first 10 years after the initial operation (see Fig 100–11). The removal of hopelessly diseased bowel returns the patient to a good state of health, usually for at least several important teenage years. The psychological

benefits can be great. Growth also may occur during this time if the epiphyses have not closed. The likelihood of repeated operations leading to short-bowel syndrome is less than 1%.

In the recently studied group of children with Crohn's disease treated at the Mayo Clinic, the mean duration of follow-up was almost 9 years, and the mean age of the patient at follow-up was

TABLE 100–3.—PATIENT ASSESSMENT OF STATUS AT FOLLOW-UP (160 PATIENTS)*

PATIENT STATUS	NO. (%) OF PATIENTS
Current state of health	
Excellent	61 (38)
Good	67 (42)
Fair	23 (14)
Poor	7 (4)
Very ill	2 (1)
Patient assessment of disease	
Cured	69 (43)
Present but not an active problem	65 (41)
Currently an active problem	27 (17)
Limitation of daily activities	
Not at all	113 (71)
Moderate	41 (26)
Severe	6 (4)

*From Castile R.G., Telander R.L., Cooney D.R., et al.: Crohn's disease in children: Assessment of the progression of disease, growth, and prognosis. *J. Pediatr. Surg.* 15:462–469, 1980. By permission of Grune & Stratton.

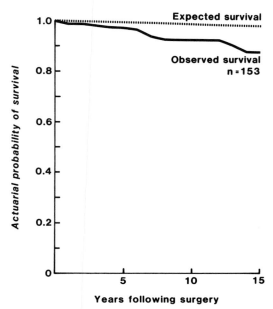

Fig 100–14.—Actuarial probability of survival after onset of disease. (From Castile R.G., Telander R.L., Cooney D.R., et al.: Crohn's disease in children: Assessment of the progression of disease, growth and prognosis. *J. Pediatr. Surg.* 15:462–469, 1980. By permission of Grune & Stratton.)

23 years. The majority of adults (80%) considered their health to be good to excellent (Table 100–3). Others [11, 28, 48] have reported similar findings. An additional 14% reported that their health was fair. There were 43% who regarded themselves cured of the disease and 41% who believed that they had disease but that it was not active. Physical activity was reported as normal by 71% and as somewhat limited by only 26% in their routine daily activities. The limitation was often related to the presence of an ostomy. The remaining 4% reported severe limitation.

Of our 177 children with Crohn's disease, 16 have died. Of these 16, 14 had had previous operations related to their disease. Four died within 1 month after a surgical procedure, but only two of these deaths were considered surgical deaths. The causes of death in these 16 cases were malnutrition in 7, gastrointestinal perforation in 2, bowel obstruction in 2, bleeding in 2, peritonitis in 2, and pulmonary embolus in 1. All deaths were related to complications of regional enteritis. Survival of patients with Crohn's disease compares favorably with that of the normal population (Fig 100–14). After 5 years, the survival rate was 98% (98% of expected), and after 20 years the survival rate was 87% (89% of expected).

REFERENCES

1. Agrez M.V., Valente R.M., Pierce W., et al.: Surgical history of Crohn's disease in a well-defined population. *Mayo Clin. Proc.* 57:747, 1982.
2. Alexander Williams J.: Surgery of the management of Crohn's disease. *Clin. Gastroenterol.* 1:469, 1972.
3. Bartlett J.G.: Clostridium difficile and inflammatory bowel disease (editorial). *Gastroenterology* 80:863, 1981.
4. Bergman L., Krause U.: Crohn's disease: A long-term study of the clinical course in 186 patients. *Scand. J. Gastroenterol.* 12:937, 1977.
5. Block G.E., Moossa A.R., Simonowitz D.: The operative treatment of Crohn's disease in childhood. *Surg. Gynecol. Obstet.* 144:713, 1977.
6. Broe P.J., Cameron J.L.: Surgical management of ileosigmoid fistulas in Crohn's disease. *Am. J. Surg.* 143:611, 1982.
7. Castile R.G., Telander R.L., Cooney D.R., et al.: Crohn's disease in children: Assessment of the progression of disease, growth, and prognosis. *J. Pediatr. Surg.* 15:462, 1980.
8. Crohn B.B., quoted by Hardin C.A., Friesen R.H.: Surgical treatment of regional enteritis. *Am. J. Surg.* 125:596, 1973.
9. Crohn B.B., Ginzburg L., Oppenheimer G.D.: Regional ileitis: A pathologic and clinical entity. *JAMA* 99:1323, 1932.
10. Crohn B.B., Rosenak B.D.: A combined form of ileitis and colitis. *JAMA* 106:1, 1936.
11. De Dombal F.T.: Results of surgery in Crohn's disease. *Proc. R. Soc. Med.* 64:173, 1971.
12. Edwards F.C., Truelove S.C.: The course and prognosis of ulcerative colitis. III. Complications. *Gut* 5:1, 1964.
13. Farmer R.G., Michener W.M.: Prognosis of Crohn's disease with onset in childhood or adolescence. *Dig. Dis. Sci.* 24:752, 1979.
14. Faulk W.P., McCormick J.N., Goodman J.R., et al.: Peyer's patches: Morphologic studies. *Cell. Immunol.* 1:500, 1970.
15. Fleming C.R., McGill D.B., Berkner S.: Home parenteral nutrition as primary therapy in patients with extensive Crohn's disease of the small bowel and malnutrition. *Gastroenterology* 73:1077, 1977.
16. Frank M.S., Bernstein L.H., Brandt L.J., et al.: Healing of perineal Crohn's disease (CD) with metronidazole (abstr.). *Gastroenterology* 76:1135, 1979.
17. Freeborn D.K., Pope C.R., Davis M.A., et al.: Health status, socioeconomic status, and utilization of outpatient services for members of a prepaid group practice. *Med. Care* 15:115, 1977.
18. Goligher J.C., De Dombal F.T., Burton I.: Crohn's disease, with special reference to surgical management. *Prog. Surg.* 10:1, 1972.
19. Gray B.K., Lockhart-Mummery H.E., Morson B.C.: Crohn's disease of the anal region. *Gut* 6:515, 1965.
20. Greenstein A.J., Sachar D.B., Pasternack B.S., et al.: Reoperation and recurrence in Crohn's colitis and ileocolitis: Crude and cumulative rates. *N. Engl. J. Med.* 293:685, 1975.
21. Gryboski J.D., Spiro H.M.: Prognosis in children with Crohn's disease. *Gastroenterology* 74:807, 1978.
22. Harper P.H., Kettlewell M.G.W., Lee E.C.G.: The effect of split ileostomy on perianal Crohn's disease. *Br. J. Surg.* 69:608, 1982.
23. Hellers G.: Crohn's disease in Stockholm County 1955–1974. *Acta Chir. Scand.* (suppl.) 490:1, 1979.
24. Hellers G., Bergstrand O., Ewerth S., et al.: Occurrence and outcome after primary treatment of anal fistulae in Crohn's disease. *Gut* 21:525, 1980.
25. Homan W.P., Tang C., Thorbjarnarson B.: Anal lesions complicating Crohn disease. *Arch. Surg.* 111:1333, 1976.
26. Homer D.R., Grand R.J., Colodny A.H.: Growth, course, and prognosis after surgery for Crohn's disease in children and adolescents. *Pediatrics* 59:717, 1977.
27. Kagnoff M.F.: Effects of antigen-feeding on intestinal and systemic immune responses. I. Priming of precursor cytotoxic T cells by antigen feeding. *J. Immunol.* 120:395, 1978.
28. Kåresen R., Serch-Hanssen A., Thoresen B.O., et al.: Crohn's disease: Long-term results of surgical treatment. *Scand. J. Gastroenterol.* 16:57, 1981.
29. Kelts D.G., Grand R.J., Shen G., et al.: Nutritional basis of growth failure in children and adolescents with Crohn's disease. *Gastroenterology* 76:720, 1979.
30. Koch T.R., Cave D.R., Ford H., et al.: Crohn's ileitis and ileocolitis: A study of the anatomical distribution of recurrence. *Dig. Dis. Sci.* 26:528, 1981.
31. Korelitz B.I., Gribetz D., Kopel F.B.: Granulomatous colitis in children: A study of 25 cases and comparison with ulcerative colitis. *Pediatrics* 42:446, 1968.
32. Korelitz B.I., Sommers S.C.: Rectal biopsy in patients with Crohn's disease: Normal mucosa on sigmoidoscopic examination. *JAMA* 237:2742, 1977.
33. Layden T., Rosenberg J., Nemchausky B., et al.: Reversal of growth arrest in adolescents with Crohn's disease after parenteral alimentation. *Gastroenterology* 70:1017, 1976.
34. Lindhagen T., Ekelund G., Leandoer L., et al.: Crohn's disease in a defined population. Course and results of surgical treatment. I. Small bowel disease. *Acta Chir. Scand.* 149:407, 1983.
35. Lock M.R., Farmer R.G., Fazio V.W., et al.: Recurrence and reoperation for Crohn's disease: The role of disease location in prognosis. *N. Engl. J. Med.* 304:1586, 1981.
36. Lockhart-Mummery H.E., Morson B.C.: Crohn's disease of the large intestine. *Gut* 5:493, 1964.
37. McDermott F.T., Hughes E.S.R., Pihl E.A., et al.: Results of operative management of Crohn's disease: A series of 50 patients managed by one surgeon. *Dis. Colon Rectum* 23:492, 1980.
38. McGovern V.J., Goulston S.J.M.: Crohn's disease of the colon. *Gut* 9:164, 1968.
39. Miller D.S., Keighley A.C., Langman M.J.S.: Changing patterns in epidemiology of Crohn's disease. *Lancet* 2:691, 1974.
40. Nugent E.W., Richmond M., Park S.K.: Crohn's disease of the duodenum. *Gut* 18:115, 1977.

41. O'Donoghue D.P., Dawson A.M.: Crohn's disease in childhood. *Arch. Dis. Child.* 52:627, 1977.
42. Pennington L., Hamilton S.R., Bayless T.M., et al.: Surgical management of Crohn's disease. *Ann. Surg.* 192:311, 1980.
43. Rogers B.H.G., Clark L.M., Kirsner J.B.: The epidemiologic and demographic characteristics of inflammatory bowel disease: An analysis of a computerized file of 1400 patients. *J. Chronic Dis.* 24:743, 1971.
44. Rosenthal S.R., Snyder J.D., Hendricks K.M., et al.: Growth failure and inflammatory bowel disease: Approach to treatment of a complicated adolescent problem. *Pediatrics* 72:481, 1983.
45. Rutgeerts P., Onette E., Vantrappen G., et al.: Crohn's disease of the stomach and duodenum: A clinical study with emphasis on the value of endoscopy and endoscopic biopsies. *Endoscopy* 12:288, 1980.
46. Seashore J.H., Hillemeier A.C., Gryboski J.D.: Total parenteral nutrition in the management of inflammatory bowel disease in children: A limited role. *Am. J. Surg.* 143:504, 1982.

47. Shorter R.G., Huizenga K.A., Spencer R.J.: A working hypothesis for the etiology and pathogenesis of nonspecific inflammatory bowel disease. *Am. J. Dig. Dis.* 17:1024, 1974.
48. Steyn J.P., Kyle J.: Quality of life after surgery for Crohn's disease. *J. R. Coll. Surg. Edinb.* 27:22, 1982.
49. Telander R.L., Dozois R.R.: The endorectal ileoanal anastomosis. *Probl. Gen. Surg.* 1:39, 1984.
50. Telander R.L., Perrault J.: Colectomy with rectal mucosectomy and ileoanal anastomosis in young patients: Its use for ulcerative colitis and familial polyposis. *Arch. Surg.* 116:623, 1981.
51. Wolff B.G.: Surgical management of Crohn's disease. *Probl. Gen. Surg.* 1:51, 1984.
52. Wolff B.G., Beart R.W. Jr., Frydenberg H.B., et al.: The importance of disease-free margins in resections for Crohn's disease. *Dis. Colon Rectum* 26:239, 1983.

101   Lester W. Martin

Ulcerative Colitis

HISTORY.—Ulcerative colitis was probably first described in 1859 by Sir Samuel Wilks,[63] pathologist and physician at Guy's Hospital, London.

The evolution of surgical techniques for the relief of ulcerative colitis began at the end of the 19th century, when fecal diversion became routine in the management. In most cases, improvement was only temporary, but on occasion, spectacular success was achieved. Tube appendicostomy was advocated early in the 20th century,[62] facilitating daily lavage of the colon with warm bicarbonate solution. It is likely that the good results represented spontaneous remissions. Subsequently, ileostomy, suggested by Brown[15] in 1913, became the procedure of choice. It provided total fecal diversion and was vigorously advocated despite significant morbidity and mortality. Prior to World War II, ileostomy appliances were primitive; soiling was inevitable, and patients were unhappy. Physicians as well as patients delayed intervention until many patients were beyond help. Compounding the problem was the limited state of knowledge of fluid, electrolyte, blood, plasma, and antibacterial therapy. Attempts to close the ileostomy in patients in whom initial success had been achieved usually resulted in reactivation of the disease. In many, the diverted bowel did not improve, and in others, extracolonic manifestations persisted. Unsatisfactory results influenced surgeons to proceed to bowel resection rather than diversion.

In 1948, Cattell[16] recommended a three-stage procedure consisting of initial ileostomy followed by a subtotal colectomy with exteriorization of the sigmoid stump and subsequent abdominoperineal resection of the rectum. This remained the procedure of choice until Gavin Miller, of Montreal,[45] suggested a simultaneous ileostomy and partial colectomy in 1949. Two years later, Gardner and Miller[25] reported a mortality rate of only 4.4% in 69 patients thus treated. Improvement in preoperative and postoperative care in the immediate postwar years permitted this more aggressive surgical approach. In 1952, Ripstein[51] and, later, Goligher[27] advocated ileostomy with one-stage proctocolectomy, now considered to be the standard elective operation for the patient with ulcerative colitis.

Two factors have been critical in allowing a satisfactory adjustment to ileostomy life. The first is the eversion technique of ileostomy construction introduced by Brooke[13] in 1952. The second has been the development of a successful adhesive ileostomy appliance.

The search for a sphincter-saving procedure was started early in the 20th century. Devine, of Melbourne,[19] recommended a staged ileosigmoidostomy. During the past two decades, Aylett, of London, has been the leading proponent of colectomy with ileoproctostomy, anastomosing the ileum to the preserved rectum. In 1966,[5] he reviewed his experience with 300 patients operated on for ulcerative colitis. The mortality rate was 5.7%. Five percent of the survivors required conversion to permanent ileostomy. The remainder were evaluated as "successful." Few have been able to duplicate these results, and ileoproctostomy has since been abandoned by most surgeons in the United States. Total coloproctectomy with permanent ileostomy has provided permanent cure of the disease, but delay in patient acceptance of a permanent ileostomy has been responsible for significant operative morbidity and mortality rates. In 1947, Ravitch[49, 50] proposed a technique in which the colon was resected, the rectal mucosa "cored out," and an ileoanal anastomosis performed. The author's 17 years' experience with total colectomy, mucosal proctectomy, and preservation of anorectal continence in 62 patients forms the basis for this chapter.

Etiology

Despite innumerable experimental studies during the past 50 years, the etiology of ulcerative colitis remains a mystery. Research has focused on three major areas: infection, psychological factors, and immune mechanisms.

In 1969, Marcus and Watt[38] produced ulcerative colitis-like lesions in experimental animals with oral administration of a sulfated polysaccharide, carrageenan. It is a common additive found in chocolate products, ice cream, sherbets, custard, dietetic foods, beer, sauces, breads, and toothpaste. Sharratt et al[52] produced mucosal granulomas with this hydrocolloid. In 1970, Mottet[46] confirmed the findings of Marcus and Watt and noted similarities to the pathologic findings of inflammatory bowel disease in man. The finding of ulcerative lesions in one study and granulomas in another is of interest, but the relation to human disease remains uncertain.

Infection

In 1924, Bargen[8] reported the isolation of a *Diplococcus* in 80% of his patients with ulcerative colitis. A variety of microorganisms have subsequently been implicated, but their role has never been substantiated. In 1958, Bacon[7] concluded that bacteria and parasites were more likely secondary invaders than primary agents. Staley[55] introduced *Escherichia coli* into the stomachs of newborn pigs and subsequently demonstrated these organisms in the intestinal wall. There is, however, no evidence to support etiologic roles for the changes in bowel flora of patients with inflammatory bowel disease, nor is there consistent improvement with antibiotic therapy. It is unclear whether sulfasalazine (Azulfidine), introduced 30 years ago, functions as an antimicrobial or as an anti-inflammatory agent. Significant changes in bacterial population do not occur. The efficacy of this drug may not be due to the sulfa radical but to an increase in the concentration of the metabolites of salicylate in intestinal connective tissue.[30]

Psychological Factors

Numerous psychological studies of patients with ulcerative colitis have described a typically infantile, dependent, egocentric, and hesitant personality. Children were described as compulsively neat, restrained in dealing with other children, and excessively demanding when their wants were unmet.[21] MacMahon[37] studied 23 sibling pairs and reported increased neurotic traits in the affected sib, which antedated the onset of the disease, thus supporting the concept of a "premorbid" personality. Physiologic studies by Grace[31] suggested that colonic changes, including frank ulceration, could be produced by emotional stimuli.

Surgeons, however, generally believe that the psychological manifestations of ulcerative colitis are secondary to the stresses of the illness characterized by urgent diarrhea, tenesmus, and inanition. This belief is reinforced by the apparent regression of psychological changes when treatment is successful. Mendeloff[42] studied 227 patients and found no increase in the number of stressful events, compared with a control group. Similarly, a psychoanalytically oriented study by Feldman[22] could not document a significant difference in psychological makeup between 53 patients and their controls. Goligher[29] reported that 86% of more than 400 patients denied any relation between disease onset and emotional stress. They were "normal, well-adjusted individuals whose attitude to life and emotional makeup did not obviously differ from that of the population at large." However, 9% related relapses to emotional trauma, and 5% had had previous psychiatric care.

There is strong evidence to indicate that psychological factors may provoke relapses and contribute to the chronicity of the disease, but controlled studies attempting to relate these same factors to the etiology of disease are inconclusive.

Immune Mechanisms

An immunologic response to an autogenous, bacterial, or chemical antigen is the most attractive etiologic theory at present. It is supported by the clinical and laboratory characteristics of inflammatory bowel disease and by extensive experimental observations. Andresen,[3] in 1942, suggested that milk was related to the pathogenesis; remission occurred when milk was eliminated from the diet of some patients and recurrence observed when it was reintroduced. In 1961 an elevated antibody titer to milk protein was demonstrated in the circulation of patients with ulcerative colitis.[56] Acheson and Truelove[2] reported that breastfeeding had been discontinued in the first month of life in a greater proportion of patients with colitis than in controls. Titers of circulating antibody to cow's milk protein are substantially higher in infants weaned from the breast early in infancy. There is no relation, however, between the height of the titers and the severity of the disease. Beneficial results from milk elimination may be due to the development of lactase deficiency in some patients with chronic diarrheal states.

In 1959, Broberger and Perlmann[12] demonstrated a circulating antibody to fetal human colon in children with ulcerative colitis, but the titer levels did not correspond to the clinical state of the disease. Four years later, they demonstrated in vitro that peripheral lymphocytes from patients with ulcerative colitis were toxic

for colonic epithelial cells.[48] Speculation persists that injury to bowel mucosa by bacterial endotoxin, invasive microorganisms, or certain antibiotics may initiate the immune responses noted.

Pathology

Ulcerative colitis is an inflammatory disease of rectal and colonic mucosa. The macroscopic appearance of the mucosa varies with the clinical state and chronicity of the disease.

Initially, the mucosa has a diffusely erythematous, granular appearance; later, numerous small, shallow ulcers develop and enlarge to result in partial or complete loss of the glandular mucosa, with neutrophilic infiltration, and crypt abscesses and a fibrinopurulent exudate over the surface. As the disease progresses, the wall of the colon becomes thin and diffusely hemorrhagic, which may progress to result in marked dilatation of the colon, further thinning of the wall, and eventual perforation—toxic megacolon. In the more chronic form, the colon becomes stiff, thickened, and foreshortened with atrophic mucosa, pseudopolyp formation, and loss of haustral folds (Fig 101–1). There is no one single microscopic finding that permits the pathologist to state unequivocally that the patient has ulcerative colitis. Crypt abscesses, Paneth cell metaplasia, and disruption of the muscularis mucosa are some of the changes characteristic of ulcerative colitis, but all are nonspecific.

The differential diagnosis includes granulomatous Crohn's colitis, pseudomembranous enterocolitis secondary to antibiotic therapy, irritable colon syndrome, cytomegalic inclusion disease of the colon, amoebic colitis, and benign solitary ulcers of the colon. Only when no evidence for these conditions can be demonstrated, can the microscopic findings be designated as consistent with, and supportive of, the clinical diagnosis of chronic idiopathic ulcerative colitis.

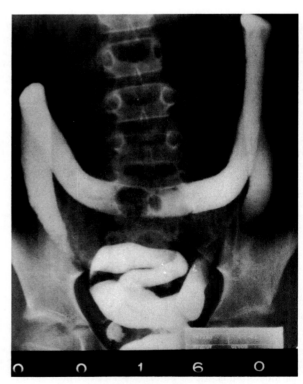

Fig 101–1.—Ulcerative colitis. Radiographic appearance of advanced stage with shortening of the colon and loss of haustral markings—sometimes referred to as a "lead-pipe" appearance.

There is increased incidence of cancer of the colon in patients with ulcerative colitis, particularly in patients who have had the disease longer than 10 years. Goligher reports an increasing rate of malignancy, reaching 41.8% after 25 years.[29] MacDougall[36] found that this high risk of colon cancer was in patients with diffuse disease involving the entire colon (pancolitis), and that, when the colitis was limited to the distal end of the colon, the risk of cancer was little greater than that of the general population. When the onset of the disease is in childhood, the patient has an opportunity to live long enough to enter the high-cancer-risk category.[44] The tumors are often multicentric and invade the bowel wall early, and complicating ulcerative colitis, they are difficult to recognize clinically because the anorexia, bleeding, diarrhea, and weight loss are generally attributed to the colitis until metastasis has occurred. There can be little doubt that the incidence of carcinoma increases in relation to the duration of the colitis.[24] Carcinoma of the colon is less frequent in the child patient but more likely to be fatal, particularly in younger patients. We have been unable to find reported a single long-term survival of colonic carcinoma complicating ulcerative colitis in a patient less than 21 years of age.

Long-standing disease may produce epithelial dysplasia, which eventually gives rise to adenocarcinoma. With increasing experience with colonoscopy and biopsy of suspicious areas, the histologic identification of precancerous changes is becoming a reliable indication for early operation. When carcinomas arise in ulcerative colitis, they are frequently multiple, more common in the proximal colon, flat and difficult to identify radiographically, generally mucin-secreting, and highly anaplastic.

Clinical Manifestations

Ulcerative colitis is characterized by bloody diarrhea, abdominal pain, fever, tenesmus, and vomiting. The course may be acute and fulminant, or more chronic and protracted, characterized by intermittent exacerbations and remissions. The onset of symptoms may be insidious, with only vague abdominal discomfort and slight change in stool frequency, gradually progressing to cramping abdominal pain and bloody diarrhea. In about one third of patients, the onset is abrupt with severe abdominal pain, fever, anorexia, and massive bloody diarrhea. When the disease is limited to the left colon, constipation rather than diarrhea may result, because spasm of the left colon results in retention of stool in the right colon, where the normal capacity to absorb fluid remains unimpaired.

In approximately 10% of patients, the disease begins suddenly, with explosive bloody diarrhea, colonic distention, and rapid clinical deterioration, sometimes with death from toxic megacolon within a matter of hours if not treated. The mucosal inflammation causes distention leading to full-thickness necrosis, thrombosis of submucosal vessels, and often perforation.

In the less fulminant form of the disease, the symptoms may abate spontaneously, with apparent disease-free remission periods of several months or even years. Eventual exacerbation, however, is characteristic.

Indications for Operation

Ulcerative colitis can be cured by removal of the colon. When this implied a permanent ileostomy, operation was often delayed until the operative risk had become prohibitive, and the complication rate was excessive. Since the development of the mucosal proctectomy with restoration of anorectal continence, serious consideration should be given to operation in any patient with chronic ulcerative colitis. Medical treatment of ulcerative colitis is nonspecific and is based on measures designed to give symptomatic relief, correct nutritional deficiencies, restore blood volume, and control the complications of the disease. It is doubtful, however, that the ultimate course of the disease can be altered by nonoperative treatment.

The indications for operation include bleeding, perforation, toxic megacolon, malignancy, failure of nonsurgical management, and a prolonged symptomatic course.[60] Because of the extreme variations of the intensity of the disease, it is not possible to specify a duration of illness as an indication for operation, except to recognize that, after 10 years of the disease, the risk of death from cancer within the next decade is close to 30%. In the chronic form of the disease, if nonoperative management is elected, frequent and regular colonoscopic examination is recommended, with biopsy of any suspicious area to detect a precancerous lesion or an early carcinoma before metastasis. It is probable that ulcerative colitis is never cured without resection. A sweeping recommendation for operation for all patients diagnosed as having ulcerative colitis, however, is not justifiable because of the frequent inability to establish diagnosis conclusively until sufficient clinical data have been accumulated. Most of our patients had had symptoms for several years. One was sick for less than 4 weeks. In fact, the author recalls vividly the details of a case from 33 years ago, of a 17-year-old girl who died of fulminant ulcerative colitis and toxic megacolon with symptoms of less than 12 hours' duration. Bleeding from ulcerative colitis may be mild and intermittent but can also be massive and exsanguinating, to the extent that only emergency operation can prevent death. Other often quoted but less specific indications, including pseudopolyp formation, loss of haustral markings of the colon, and fibrotic shortening of the colon, indicate irreversibility and an advanced stage of the disease process with small likelihood of even a short spontaneous remission.

Every effort should be made to exclude the diagnosis of Crohn's colitis, which is a full-thickness transmural disease and therefore not suitable for mucosal proctectomy, apart from the risk of involvement of the ileum. Table 101–1 lists the clinical features of the two conditions, none of which, however, are conclusive. Indeed, one of our three failures was in a patient with Crohn's colitis which, before operation, we had mistaken for ulcerative colitis.

Surgical Treatment

Total colectomy with a permanent ileostomy has dramatically cured chronic idiopathic ulcerative colitis and obviously prevents subsequent development of colonic carcinoma associated with it. Reluctance to accept a permanent ileostomy has been a major deterrent to colectomy and ileostomy, particularly for the younger patient who is already psychologically labile and is anticipat-

TABLE 101–1.—CHARACTERISTICS OF ULCERATIVE COLITIS AND GRANULOMATOUS COLITIS

CLINICAL FEATURES	ULCERATIVE COLITIS	GRANULOMATOUS COLITIS
Location	Rectum and left colon	Ileum and right colon
Diarrhea	Severe	Moderate
Rectal bleeding	Usual	Intermittent
Rectal involvement	Usual	Rare
Fistula in ano	Absent	Common
Perirectal abscess	Absent	Common
Abdominal wall fistulae	Absent	Common
Toxic megacolon	Common	Absent
Arthritis	Rare	Common
Proctoscopic appearance	Diffuse, granular	Cobblestone
Small-bowel involvement	Absent (except for backwash ileitis)	Common
Microscopic appearance	Limited to mucosa (except abscesses)	Transmural granulomas

ing sports, college, courtship, and marriage, and considers the whole idea of an ileostomy repulsive and totally unacceptable. As a result, the operation is often either rejected or postponed until the operative risk is substantially increased because of the advanced stage of the disease and the poor general condition of the patient.

Initially, considerable enthusiasm was expressed for the Kock continent reservoir which was constructed in conjunction with an ileostomy.[9, 34] It could be emptied by intermittent catheterization, and an ileostomy bag was not required. With further experience and longer follow-up, however, a significant complication rate has become apparent.[57] Of particular significance has been the frequency of spontaneous reduction of the intussuscepting ileal valve that was created surgically to provide continence. The need for reoperation has been reported as approximately 30%, even in experienced hands.

Subtotal colectomy with preservation of the entire rectum and anastomosis of the terminal ileum to the full thickness of the rectum has periodically received enthusiastic support in various centers.[5, 6] Further follow-up, however, demonstrates that at least half of these patients have subsequently developed significant rectal disease requiring further operation. The incidence of problems is so great that preservation of the entire rectum with a direct ileorectal anastomosis has generally been abandoned.

Since ulcerative colitis is a disease that involves primarily the mucosa, surgical ingenuity nearly 50 years ago proposed a total colectomy with preservation of anorectal musculature.[49, 50] Early attempts with this operation, however, were abandoned because of the high incidence of sepsis and the inability to support the patient metabolically. The mucosal stripping procedure was made popular by Soave in 1964, in treatment of Hirschsprung's disease.[54] Our first operation employing these concepts was performed on an 11-year-old boy with ulcerative colitis in February 1967. Ten years later, we reported our generally satisfactory experience with 17 patients with a straight ileoanal anastomosis.[39] The obvious criticism of the operation was excessive perianal excoriation, which persisted for several months following the operation and prevented the patient from attending school or working until accommodation had spontaneously developed as the neorectum gradually dilated. During the past 7 years, we have, in addition, constructed a reservoir from the terminal ileum[23] placed just above the ileoanal anastomosis and below the peritoneal floor. This affords immediate rectal continence, and the pa-

tients can return to work or school within 10–14 days following closure of the temporary ileostomy.[41]

The operation is lengthy and requires meticulous attention to detail as well as strict adherence to basic surgical principles.[40] There is a significant learning curve, and early in the course of a surgeon's experience, many complications are encountered. After the surgeon becomes familiar with various important steps of the operation, however, the results are most gratifying.

Based on our own experience with operation on 62 patients, we are convinced that it is possible to cure the disease and restore anorectal continence in virtually all patients with chronic idiopathic ulcerative colitis. The operation consists of a total colectomy with mucosal proctectomy and construction of a reservoir at the end of the terminal ileum, with anastomosis of the reservoir to the mucosa of the anal canal. A temporary ileostomy for 3–6 months is necessary to divert the fecal stream while the pelvic anastomoses heal.

Before operation, it is necessary that the patient be in positive nitrogen balance and that the rectum be free of gross disease. The success of the operation depends on the surgical removal of the intact sleeve of rectal mucosa, preserving the underlying muscular layer. To do this, the mucosa must be intact, free of ulceration, and free of significant inflammation (Fig 101–2). This can be achieved by 4–6 weeks of intensive medical management. When the disease process is recalcitrant to conventional therapy, the patient is admitted to the hospital, maintained on total parenteral alimentation with nothing by mouth, given systemic steroids and antibiotics, and steroid enemas. A period as long as 6 weeks may be required to heal ulcerated rectal mucosa.

An alternative method is a subtotal colectomy with ileostomy, closing the rectal stump flush with the peritoneal floor. The mucosal proctectomy can then be performed later in a center with expertise in this complicated part of the operation. The indications for this method of management include perforation, severe hemorrhage, toxic megacolon, fulminant disease, obstruction, and the surgeon's inexperience with mucosal dissection. Mucosal proctectomy can then be performed in a separate stage several months later, when the patient is in ideal physical condition.

The initial step of the operation consists of a sigmoidoscopic examination to confirm that the rectal mucosa is free of gross disease. The colon is then irrigated with a large-bore rectal tube, which is left in place for intraoperative irrigation. A generous midline or left paramedian incision is made to mobilize the colon

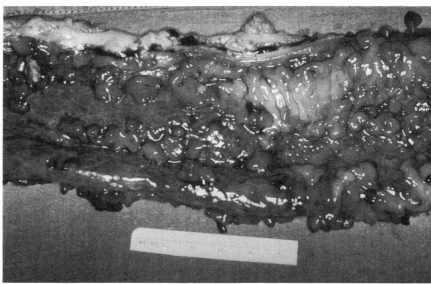

Fig 101–2.—Ulcerative colitis. Photograph of colon demonstrating extensive ulceration. It is important that such ulcerations be healed before attempting to remove intact the mucosal lining of the rectum in the course of the endorectal mucosa-stripping pull-through.

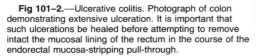

as for a conventional total colectomy. A constricting tape is placed tightly about the upper rectum, and the rectal lumen is thoroughly irrigated with saline to minimize the hazard of contamination if mucosal perforation should occur during dissection. A circumferential incision is made through the muscular wall of the rectum approximately 3 cm below the peritoneal reflection. The rectal mucosa is then dissected free from its muscular wall, operating within the muscular sleeve in order to preserve the nerve supply to the bladder and the ejaculatory mechanism and all muscles necessary for continence. The dissection is carried distal as far as the levator muscles. The proximal portion of the mucosal sleeve is then divided between doubly placed ligatures and the colon removed from the operative field. The mesentery of the terminal ileum is then incised to preserve an adequate blood supply, yet provide sufficient length for the ileum to reach the anus. A sigmoid-shaped reservoir (Fig 101–3), 4 inches long, is then constructed to within 1 cm of the end of the ileum.

From the perineal approach, the anal sphincter is dilated and the dissected mucosal sleeve everted, thoroughly irrigated, and the area prepared as a sterile field. The mucosa is then transected at the top of the anorectal columns. To preserve absolute continence, preservation of the columns is necessary, since they are covered with transitional epithelium, contain involuntary nerve endings, and are not primarily involved in the disease process (Fig 101–4). The end of the ileum is then joined to the mucosa of the anorectal canal with a two-layer anastomosis of absorbable sutures. A Penrose drain is placed inside the rectal cuff between the pulled-through ileum and the denuded rectal wall in order to prevent accumulation of serum in this potential space which, if it became infected, would result in a "cuff abscess." The drain is left in place for 24–48 hours, depending on the amount of drainage. Following completion of the anastomosis, it should be possible for the surgeon to insert a finger through the anal canal into the reservoir. The surgeon then returns to the abdominal field, where a totally diverting ileostomy is performed by dividing the ileum, closing the distal end, and bringing the proximal end out through the right lower quadrant in the area previously selected for the ileostomy. The ileostomy is matured by the Brooke technique immediately following closure of the laparotomy incision. The ileostomy is closed by an

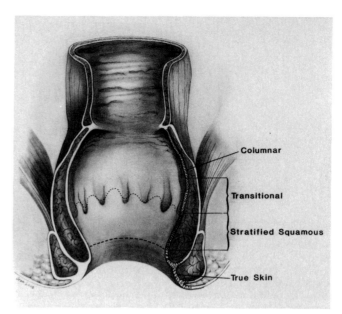

Fig 101–4.—Gross and microscopic anatomy of rectum. Columnar epithelium of rectum ends at the top of the rectal columns, which are covered with transitional epithelium.

end-to-end anastomosis 3–6 months later, after healing and integrity of the distal suture lines have been confirmed by contrast enema and by digital examination.

Results

We have performed this operation on all patients with ulcerative colitis for the past 17 years. Our experience includes 62 patients, with no deaths (Table 101–2). Of 52 patients in whom the operation has been completed (10 currently await ileostomy closure), 49 are continent both day and night, and only one patient requires passage of a catheter to induce evacuation of the reservoir. Early in the course of the development of the procedure, there were three surgical failures resulting in the need for a permanent ileostomy. One was because of misdiagnosed Crohn's colitis, initially thought to be ulcerative colitis. The second failure was because of pelvic sepsis. The third was related to preservation of insufficient anal mucosa, leading to night-time incontinence.

The majority of the complications of the operation occurred early in our series (Table 101–3), only 12 occurring in the last 38 patients.

The reservoir was constructed on 43 patients; 10 are currently awaiting closure of the ileostomy. Initially, we performed a direct end-to-end anastomosis without a reservoir. These patients experienced troublesome diarrhea with perineal excoriation, which generally became tolerable after approximately 1 year. Spontaneous dilatation of the terminal ileum within the pelvis resulted in correction of the problem with a stool frequency of

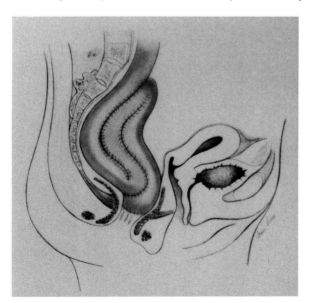

Fig 101–3.—Completed sigmoid reservoir. Shown are the shape and location of completed reservoir, all below the pelvic floor, and the length of ileum connecting reservoir to anal canal only 1 cm.

TABLE 101–2.—TOTAL COLECTOMY
AND MUCOSAL PROCTECTOMY:
RESULTS IN 62 PATIENTS

Deaths	0
Awaiting ileostomy closure	10
Permanent ileostomy	3
Continent—day and night	49

TABLE 101–3.—Total Colectomy and
Mucosal Proctectomy: Operative
Complications in 62 Patients

Rectal stricture requiring operation	3
"Pouchitis"	4
Recurrent anorectal disease	6
Night-time incontinence	1
Reservoir stasis, severe	1
Reservoir stasis, temporary	2
Adhesive bowel obstruction	4
Wound dehiscence	1
Jaundice, temporary	2
Renal calculi	1
Wound infection	3
Cuff abscess	4

two to five daily. In four patients, this spontaneous dilatation did not occur after 2 years, prompting us to perform another operation for construction of a pelvic reservoir, which has given satisfactory results. The reservoir has proved to be a most gratifying addition to the operation and has resulted in a stool frequency of four to six daily, immediately following closure of the ileostomy.

Temporary reservoir stasis with "pouchitis" in three patients responded to dilatation of a distal stricture, irrigation of the pouch, and systemic antibiotics directed at anaerobic organisms. It is our firm belief that "pouchitis" develops secondary to stasis. This may be caused by a distal anastomotic stricture, extension of the reservoir into the abdominal cavity, or placement of the reservoir too far from the end of the ileum that is anastomosed to the anal canal. In all three of our patients, the inflammation of the reservoir was in conjunction with a distal anastomotic stricture and cleared following provision of adequate drainage by dilatation of the stricture.

Permanent reservoir stasis was encountered in one patient early in our series, the reservoir having been made long enough to extend out of the pelvis up into the abdomen. We have, since this experience, paid particular attention to locating the reservoir within the pelvis so that it can be evacuated voluntarily by increasing intra-abdominal pressure. We currently make the reservoir 4 inches long with, preferably, an S-shaped segment of terminal ileum. This utilizes 12 inches of terminal ileum. In two patients, the anatomical arrangement of the blood supply of the terminal ileum precluded the construction of the S-shaped reservoir, and for this reason, we created the J reservoir. Again, we believe it is important, whichever type is used, that it be located below the peritoneal floor so that voluntarily increased intra-abdominal pressure can expel the contents of the reservoir during defecation. We also think it is important that the reservoir extend far enough distally so that an examining finger can be inserted upon rectal examination after completion of the operation. The reservoir should have a capacity of approximately 300 cc immediately following its completion. After a year or two of use, it will hold 500–600 cc.

Night-time Incontinence

Night-time incontinence was encountered in one of our patients in whom the entire mucosa was removed. The mucosa of the area of the rectal columns contains sensory fibers to provide involuntary tightening of the external sphincter and continence during sleep. For this reason, in subsequent patients we have made a point of preserving the mucosa of the area of the rectal columns. If the line of transection is accurately placed, the segment of residual transitional epithelium will measure less than 1 cm in length. Its preservation is necessary for complete conti-

nence. It is important that the surgeon be familiar with both the gross and microscopic anatomy of the anorectal canal before performing this operation. The anal canal is lined with stratified squamous epithelium similar to skin except that it does not contain skin appendages. This slightly discolored area is sometimes referred to as the "vermilion" and is somewhat thinner in texture than normal skin. At the lower extent of the anorectal columns, the epithelium becomes transitional and extends upward to cover the anorectal columns. Above the columns, the epithelium is columnar. Various textbooks refer somewhat casually to the "dentate line," the "pectinate line," and the "anorectal line." It is our distinct impression that preservation of the transitional epithelium covering the anorectal columns is necessary for night-time continence. Our one patient with permanent night-time incontinence as a reason for return to a permanent ileostomy was one in whom the transitional epithelium was removed down to the level of what various textbooks refer to as the "dentate line." We therefore recommend that the transitional epithelium covering the anal columns be carefully preserved.

Recurrent Disease

Ulcerative colitis in the narrow band of retained mucosa has recurred in six of our patients. This condition is suspected on the basis of increasing stool frequency, flecks of blood on the stool, tenesmus, perianal excoriation, or unexplained anemia. Response in five of the six patients was prompt when hydrocortisone suppositories were inserted twice daily. The treatment must be continued, however, for 3 weeks to prevent recurrence of the symptoms. One patient did not return until perianal excoriation and tenderness were so great that she would not cooperate with insertion of the suppositories. For this reason, systemic steroids were administered for 1 week until the symptoms cleared; then suppositories were resumed until the process was completely clear.

It is our distinct impression that recurrent disease of the anorectal canal occurs because of retained columnar epithelium. The columnar epithelium ends at the top of the anorectal columns. Occasionally, the columns appear to be involved with ulcerative colitis before operation. We believe this phenomenon to be one of a "spillover" inflammation secondary to contact similar to what in the ileum has been referred to as "backwash ileitis." If all of the columnar epithelium has been removed above the rectal columns, any minor inflammation of the transitional epithelium appears to be reversible. It is important, therefore, that all of the columnar epithelium be removed and that the transitional epithelium be retained.

Differentiation of Flatus from Stool

Initially, many patients are unable to differentiate flatus from liquid stool. After approximately a year, however, flatus can be passed independently.

Sexual Function

Sexual function in male patients may be adversely affected by the conventional abdominoperineal type of operation performed for cancer. This is probably due to injury to the pelvic nerves during the course of the wide resection necessary for removal of cancer. This complication is encountered less frequently when proctocolectomy is performed for benign disease with the dissection kept closer to the rectal wall. When the mucosa alone is removed, as in the procedure here described for ulcerative colitis, the pelvic nerves are left undisturbed. Sexual function in 14 of our sexually active male patients selected at random has remained undisturbed following operation.

Type of Reservoir

It is now generally recognized that construction of a reservoir is advisable. Different types of reservoirs have been recommended, including simple balloon dilatation of the neorectum, an elliptical-shaped patch of small bowel, the S-shaped reservoir, the J-shaped reservoir, and a double-lumen small-bowel isoperistaltic reservoir.

The exact type of reservoir and its configuration are probably of less importance than certain other requirements of its construction. (1) The reservoir must be located completely in the pelvis below the peritoneal floor so that voluntary increase of abdominal pressure can serve as a means of evacuating the filled reservoir. If the reservoir extends into the abdominal cavity, an increase in abdominal pressure is simply transmitted to the reservoir from all sides and is not effective for evacuation. This will result in stasis and inflammation. (2) The reservoir must be attached directly to the anal canal at the top of the anal columns. If a long segment of small bowel remains between the reservoir and the anastomosis, it will not empty effectively, as demonstrated in the series reported by Parks,[47] in which 50% of patients required intubation of the reservoir for evacuation. (3) The reservoir must be of sufficient diameter to prevent approximation of the valvulae conniventes of the two sides of the small intestine when a peristaltic wave descends. If the two sides of the small intestine can meet, the intestinal stream will be forced to contact the transitional epithelium of the anal canal, which will provide an urge to defecate with each peristaltic wave. (4) The reservoir must be large enough to serve as storage in order to result in an acceptable stool frequency.

Selection of Patients

Initially, we recommended the operation only for children and adolescents, since the original technique required several months for postoperative recovery and accommodation. The addition of the reservoir has eliminated this objectionable feature of the operation and we now recommend the procedure as the operation of choice for adults as well as children. Our youngest patient was 8 years of age and our oldest was 52 years. All patients are seen preoperatively by a gastroenterologist who agrees with the indications for operation. It is particularly important that patients with Crohn's colitis be excluded, since the inflammation in Crohn's disease involves the full thickness of the bowel wall, and mucosal resection cannot, therefore, cure the disease. For this reason, we are suspicious of any patient with a history of perirectal disease, arthritis, iritis, or the systemic manifestations that are so common in Crohn's disease but occur less frequently in patients with ulcerative colitis.

Staging of the Operation

Several of our patients had undergone previous subtotal colectomy for ulcerative colitis and the rectum had been retained, either in the form of a mucous fistula or closure as a Hartmann's pouch. These patients are particularly good candidates for the endorectal stripping procedure. Since they are no longer receiving steroids, they are in good physical condition, and considerable time can be allowed for treatment of the disease in the retained rectal stump, so that the operation can be performed at an elected time. Although we have had only eight patients in this category, they have all tolerated the operation extremely well and have recovered without complications.

Summary

Our experience with operation on 62 patients over 17 years with no deaths indicates that it is possible to remove the diseased colon and restore anorectal continence for virtually all patients with ulcerative colitis and with a minimum of complications. The operation is lengthy and requires meticulous attention to detail and observance of basic surgical principles. It is now being performed in a number of centers,[17, 20, 23, 47, 53, 57] but, even with skilled surgeons and good ancillary facilities, the early complication rate in each center has been significant. The patients are generally highly intelligent, serious, hard-working overachievers. To return them to a productive role in society is a source of great satisfaction to the surgeon.

REFERENCES

1. Acheson E.D.: The distribution of ulcerative colitis and regional enteritis in U.S. veterans with particular reference to the Jewish religion. *Gut* 1:291, 1960.
2. Acheson E.D., Truelove S.C.: Early weaning in the aetiology of ulcerative colitis. *Br. Med. J.* 2:929, 1961.
3. Andresen A.F.R.: Gastrointestinal manifestations of food allergy. *Am. J. Dig. Dis.* 9:91, 1942.
4. Aufses A.H. Jr., Kreel I.: Ileostomy for granulomatous ileocolitis. *Ann. Surg.* 173:91, 1971.
5. Aylett S.O.: Three hundred cases of diffuse ulcerative colitis treated by total colectomy and ileo-rectal anastomosis. *Br. Med. J.* 1:1001, 1966.
6. Aylett S.O.: Symposium on Crohn's disease: Panel discussion. *Proc. R. Soc. Med.* 64:17, 1971.
7. Bacon H.E.: *Ulcerative Colitis.* Philadelphia, J.B. Lippincott Co., 1958.
8. Bargen J.A.: Experimental studies on etiology of chronic ulcerative colitis. *JAMA* 83:332, 1924.
9. Beahrs O.H.: Use of ileal reservoir following protocolectomy. *Surg. Gynecol. Obstet.* 141:363, 1975.
10. Birnbaum D., et al.: Ulcerative colitis among the ethnic groups in Israel. *Arch. Intern. Med.* 105:843, 1960.
11. Broberger O., Lagercrantz R.: Ulcerative colitis in childhood and adolescence, in Levine, S.Z. (ed.): *Advances in Pediatrics.* Chicago, Year Book Medical Publishers, 1966, vol. 14.
12. Broberger O., Perlmann P.: Autoantibodies in human ulcerative colitis. *J. Exp. Med.* 110:657, 1959.
13. Brooke B.N.: The management of an ileostomy including its complications. *Lancet* 2:102, 1952.
14. Brooke B.N., Slaney G.: Portal bacteremia in ulcerative colitis. *Lancet* 1:206, 1958.
15. Brown J.Y.: Value of complete physiological rest of large bowel in ulcerative and obstructive lesions. *Surg. Gynecol. Obstet.* 16:610, 1923.
16. Cattell R.B.: The surgical treatment of ulcerative colitis. *Gastroenterology* 10;63, 1948.
17. Coran A.G., Sarahan T.M., et al.: The endorectal pull-through for the management of ulcerative colitis in children and adults. *Ann. Surg.* 197:99, 1983.
18. Davis L.P., Jelenko C.: Sexual function after abdominoperineal resection. *South Med. J.* 68:422, 1975.
19. Devine H.: Method of colectomy for desperate cases of ulcerative colitis. *Surg. Gynecol. Obstet.* 76:136, 1943.
20. Ekesparre W. von.: Follow-up results of the pull-through operation for ulcerative colitis in children, in: *Progress in Pediatric Surgery,* vol. 7. Baltimore and Munich, Urban & Schwarzenberg, 1978, pp. 1–20.
21. Engel G.L.: Studies of ulcerative colitis. III. The nature of the psychologic processes. *Am. J. Med.* 19:231, 1955.
22. Feldman F. et al.: Psychiatric study of a consecutive series of 34 patients with ulcerative colitis. *Br. Med. J.* 3:14, 1967.
23. Fonkalsrud E.W.: Total colectomy and endorectal ileal pull-through with internal reservoir for ulcerative colitis. *Surg. Gynecol. Obstet.* 150:1, 1980.
24. Gallone L., Olmi L., Marchetti V.: Use of topical rectal therapy to preserve the rectum in surgery of ulcerative colitis. *World J. Surg.* 4:609, 1980.
25. Gardner C. McG., Miller C.G.: Total colectomy for ulcerative colitis. *Arch. Surg.* 63:370, 1951.
26. Glotzer D.J., Silen W.: Indications for surgical treatment in chronic ulcerative colitis and Crohn's disease of the colon, in Kirsner J.B., Shorter R.G. (eds.): *Inflammatory Bowel Disease.* Philadelphia: Lea & Febiger, 1975.
27. Goligher J.C.: Primary excisional surgery in the treatment of ulcerative colitis. *Ann. R. Coll. Surg. Engl.* 15:316, 1954.
28. Goligher J.C., et al.: *Ulcerative Colitis.* Baltimore, Williams & Wilkins, 1968.

29. Goligher J.C., et al.: *Surgery of the Anus, Rectum, and Colon,* ed. 3. London: Bailliere, Tindall & Cox, 1975, p. 843.
30. Gorbach S.L.: in Kirsner J.B., Shorter R.G. (eds.): *Inflammatory Bowel Disease.* Philadelphia, Lea & Febiger, 1975.
31. Grace W.J., et al.: *The Human Colon.* New York, Hoeber, 1951.
32. Helmholz H.F.: Chronic ulcerative colitis in childhood. *Am. J. Dis. Child.* 26:418, 1923.
33. Kelly D.G., Branon M.E., Phillips S.F., et al.: Diarrhea after continent ileostomy. *Gut* 21:711, 1980.
34. Kock N.G.: Intra-abdominal "reservoir" in patients with permanent ileostomy: Preliminary observations on a procedure resulting in fecal "continence" in five ileostomy patients. *Arch. Surg.* 99:223, 1969.
35. Lockhart-Mummery H.E., Morson B.C.: Crohn's disease (regional enteritis) of the large intestine and its distinction from ulcerative colitis. *Gut* 1:87, 1960.
36. MacDougall I.P.M.: The cancer risk in ulcerative colitis. *Lancet* 2:655, 1964.
37. MacMahon A.W., et al.: Personality differences between inflammatory bowel disease patients and their healthy siblings. *Psychosom. Med.* 35:91, 1973.
38. Marcus R., Watt J.: Seaweeds and ulcerative colitis in laboratory animals. *Lancet* 2:489, 1969.
39. Martin L.W., LeCoultre C., Schubert W.K.: Total colectomy and mucosal proctectomy with preservation of continence in ulcerative colitis. *Ann. Surg.* 186:477, 1977.
40. Martin L.W., LeCoultre C.: Technical considerations in performing total colectomy and Soave endorectal anastomosis for ulcerative colitis. *J. Pediatr. Surg.* 13:762, 1978.
41. Martin L.W., Fischer J.E.: Preservation of anorectal continence following total colectomy. *Ann. Surg.* 196:700, 1982.
42. Mendeloff A.I., et al.: Illness experience and life stresses in patients with irritable colon and with ulcerative colitis. *N. Engl. J. Med.* 282:14, 1970.
43. Menguy R.B.: Indications for surgery, in Bercovitz Z.T., Kirsner J.B., Linder A.E., et al. (eds.): *Ulcerative and Granulomatous Colitis.* Springfield, Ill., Charles C Thomas, Publisher, 1973.
44. Michener W.M., Gage R.P., Saver W.G., et al.: The prognosis of chronic ulcerative colitis in children. *N. Engl. J. Med.* 265:1075, 1961.
45. Miller C.G., et al.: Primary resection of the colon in ulcerative colitis. *J. Can. Med. Assoc.* 60:584, 1949.
46. Mottet K.N.: Carrageenan ulceration as a model for human ulcerative colitis. *Lancet* 2:1361, 1970.
47. Parks A.G., Nicholls R.J., Belliveau P.: Proctocolectomy with ileal reservoir and anal anastomosis. *Br. J. Surg.* 67:533, 1980.
48. Perlmann P., Broberger O.: The possible role of immune mechanisms in tissue damage in ulcerative colitis, in Graber P., Miescher P. (eds.): *Mechanism of Cell Tissue Damage Produced by Immune Reactions.* New York, Grune & Stratton, 1962.
49. Ravitch M.M., Sabiston D.C.: Anal ileostomy with preservation of the sphincter. *Surg. Gynecol. Obstet.* 84:1095, 1947.
50. Ravitch M.M.: Anal ileostomy with sphincter preservation in patients requiring total colectomy for benign conditions. *Surgery* 24:170, 1948.
51. Ripstein C.B., et al.: Results of the surgical treatment of ulcerative colitis. *Ann. Surg.* 135:14, 1952.
52. Sharratt M., et al.: Carrageenan ulceration as a model for human ulcerative colitis. *Lancet* 2:932, 1970.
53. Shermeta D.W., Helikson M.A., Haller A.: Continent ileoanal endorectal pull-through. *J. Pediatr. Surg.* 16:171, 1981.
54. Soave F.: A new technique for treatment of Hirschsprung's disease. *Surgery* 46:1007, 1964.
55. Staley T.E., et al.: Early pathogenesis of colitis in neonatal pigs monocontaminated with *Escherichia coli:* Fine structural changes in the colonic epithelium. *Am. J. Dig. Dis.* 15:923, 1970.
56. Taylor K.B., Truelove S.C.: Circulating antibodies to milk proteins in ulcerative colitis. *Br. Med. J.* 2:924, 1961.
57. Taylor B.M., Beart R.W., et al.: Straight ileoanal anastomosis vs. ileal pouch-anal anastomosis after colectomy and mucosal proctectomy. *Arch. Surg.* 118:696, 1983.
58. Telander R.L., Hoffman A., Perrault J.: Early development of the neorectum by balloon dilatations after ileoanal anastomosis. *J. Pediatr. Surg.* 16:911, 1981.
59. Telander R.L., Perrault J.: Colectomy with rectal mucosectomy and ileoanal anastomosis in young patients. *Arch. Surg.* 116:623, 1981.
60. Turnbull R.B. Jr.: Symposium on ulcerative colitis: Management of the ileostomy. *Am. J. Surg.* 86:617, 1953.
61. Zwiren G.T., Andrews H.G., Caplan D.B.: Total colectomy with ileoendomuscular pull-through in the treatment of ulcerative colitis in children. *J. Pediatr. Surg.* 16:174, 1981.
62. Weir R.F.(1902): Quoted by Corbett, R.S.: A review of the surgical treatment of chronic ulcerative colitis. *Proc. R. Soc. Med.* 38:277, 1945.
63. Wilks S., Moxon D.W.: *Lectures on Pathological Anatomy,* ed. 2. London, J. & A. Churchill, Ltd., 1875, pp. 408, 672.

102 Sigmund H. Ein

Primary Peritonitis

PRIMARY PERITONITIS is a diffuse infection of the peritoneal cavity for which there is no obvious focus of infection. It has also come to include those peritoneal infections seen in children with cirrhosis,[4, 6, 11] nephrosis[6, 14] (with and without chronic peritoneal dialysis),[5] and neurosurgical patients with ventriculoperitoneal shunts.[12] The important fact to remember is that most cases arise in previously well individuals.[10]

Primary peritonitis has become less common since the early 1900s, when it made up 10% of all pediatric acute abdominal emergencies. Today, it makes up only 1–2% of all pediatric "acute abdomens" and 13–17% of all infant and childhood peritonitis.[6, 9] It is probably true that the decreased incidence of this peritoneal infection is due to the widespread use of antibiotics for all sorts of extraperitoneal infection.[6, 7, 9, 13] These antibiotics presumably prevent bacterial invasion of the bloodstream and may well abort any beginning primary peritonitis.

It is interesting that in his *Textbook of Pediatric Surgery,*[7] Gross devoted an entire chapter to primary peritonitis, while 30 years later, its successor had no chapter devoted to this disease, and the only mention of it was in the chapter on appendicitis by Cloud,[2] which devoted four lines in the section on differential diagnosis. The three prior editions of this textbook also had no special section devoted to primary peritonitis.

Etiology

The origin of the infecting organism(s) has been the subject of debate.[7, 9] In most cases, no source of the infection can be found outside the peritoneal cavity.[6]

The bloodstream is probably the most common pathway of infection by which the bacteria reach the peritoneum. This conclusion is supported by the frequent occurrence of an upper respiratory tract infection prior to, or along with, the primary peritonitis and the frequent blood culture growth of the same organism(s) found in the peritoneal fluid at laparotomy: Gross[7] found this combination to be present in 50% of his cases.

The female genital tract has been a suspected portal of entry.[7, 9] The Cleveland group[9] had a urinary tract source in almost 60% of their children. In a personal series of 18 infants and children, we found a proved genitourinary tract infection in only one. Nonetheless, the genitourinary tract, so close to the peritoneal cavity, must be considered a potential source of infection.

The transdiaphragmatic lymphatics have been a suggested route of infection, but pneumonia or empyema are seldom associated with primary peritonitis.[7, 9]

Normally, bacteria pass from the lumen of the gut across the mucous membrane and into the tissues.[7, 9] Bacteria that escape the scavenging action of the local neutrophils can gain entrance to the bloodstream, from which they are promptly cleared by an efficient reticuloendothelial filtering system in the liver and spleen, assisted by the body's immune defenses. In infants and children with cirrhosis, the clearance mechanism may be disturbed, and in nephrosis the immune system may be compromised so that the bacteremia can be prolonged.[4] Circulating bacteria are prone to settle out in areas of sluggish blood flow or in collections of protein-rich fluid (ascites) and, once deposited, can establish themselves and initiate an infection.

Clinical Picture

Primary peritonitis tends to be found mostly in females. It is quite rare during the neonatal period but peaks in its incidence between 5 and 10 years of age.

The presenting picture is usually that of short onset with high fever, vomiting, and generalized peritoneal signs. There is sometimes a preceding minor illness like an upper respiratory tract infection. The child looks and acts listless and as if he is suffering toxic effects, and the only difference between this clinical picture of primary peritonitis and that of a ruptured appendix is that the illness develops more rapidly, the child appears sicker, and the white blood cell count may be higher. The urinalysis is usually normal. Abdominal radiographs show a nondiagnostic ileus with some fluid between edematous loops. When no intra-abdominal disease is identified as the source of infection, it is usually too risky to treat the child without operation lest the child have a ruptured appendix or a similar surgical problem. Therefore it is best to resuscitate and treat such a child as if for a ruptured appendix.

If the child has a history of cirrhosis,[4, 6, 11] nephrosis,[6, 14] or has a neurosurgical ventriculoperitoneal shunt,[12] treatment can be with wide-spectrum antibiotics such as cloxacillin and gentamicin, along with the usual intravenous therapy and nasogastric suction. Children with such underlying conditions do not fit into the *true* category of primary peritonitis, since they have intra-abdominal sources of infection. In such cases, a paracentesis[6] smear and culture usually obtains the causative organism of the peritonitis. The organisms should be in pure culture; a mixed flora indicates a perforation peritonitis. By the time the peritoneal organism is recovered from culture, the same organism is often identified from the blood culture taken simultaneously. With the appropriate antibiotic therapy, begun when the presumptive diagnosis is made, the children respond dramatically in 12–24 hours. By the same token, if peritoneal aspiration in a child with nephrosis and peritonitis shows pneumococci in pure culture, antibiotic treatment will suffice.

Operation

After several hours of intravenous rehydration, nasogastric suction, and intravenous administration of antibiotics[3] (e.g., ampicillin, clindamycin, and gentamicin), the child's abdomen should be explored under general anesthesia and through a McBurney incision. The appendix, terminal ileum, and right tube and ovary will all have a diffuse red serositis. The striking thing about this "negative" laparotomy is the peritoneal fluid, which is cloudy and slimy. An immediate Gram stain should be done and both aerobic and anaerobic cultures taken. Primary peritonitis is almost invariably due to a single organism and, if a variety of bacterial forms are seen in the smear from paracentesis or at operation, perforative peritonitis should be suspected. The appendix should be removed. Drainage of the peritoneal cavity is not necessary. Although Gross[7] thought that "appendectomy is a useless, and indeed harmful procedure" in this disease, virtually all present-day pediatric surgeons believe that appendectomy is warranted, indicated, and safe; indeed, it should be done if the abdomen is being explored through a McBurney incision for whatever cause, lest the scar suggest at some future episode that the appendix has been removed.

Postoperative management should be the same as that for a ruptured appendix, with nasogastric suction and intravenous fluids until the postoperative ileus permits oral feedings (usually in 5 days or so). The same antibiotics should be continued until results of the peritoneal fluid and urine cultures are known, and then the antibiotics should be appropriately readjusted, or discontinued if the cultures are negative. These infants and children usually have a smooth recovery, the rare patient having residual intraperitoneal or wound infections.

Bacteriology

The peritoneal exudate at laparotomy is thin and cloudy, with flecks of fibrin if *Streptococcus* is present; the fluid tends to be thicker if *Pneumococcus* is the offending organism. Later on the exudate becomes frankly fibrinopurulent. Specimen collection and culture techniques should be adequate to ensure the isolation of fastidious anaerobes as well as conventional bacteria. In the days of Gross,[7] *Pneumococcus* and *Streptococcus* were the commonest isolated organisms. Nowadays the gram-negative pathogens occur most frequently, *Escherichia coli* the most common.[9] In a personal series of 18 children over the last 14 years, nine peritoneal cultures were negative, five grew *E. coli*, three a streptococcal species, and one *Pneumococcus* and *Meningococcus*.[1] Only one child had two organisms.

The role of anaerobic gram-negative bacteria (*Bacteroides*) is probably underestimated, since few investigators have prospectively sought these organisms with the improved culture techniques; they may well account for the many "negative" cultures obtained in all series.[8, 11] Pneumococci[10] are the commonest causative organisms in nephrotics,[14] and the enteric gram-negative bacteria[9] are the second most frequent; the reverse is true in cirrhotics.[13] Miscellaneous organisms of respiratory or gastrointestinal tract origin account for a small number.[1] Viruses have been identified as causative agents in only a few cases and are probably incriminated far more often than presently recognized. Several alternative antibiotic regimens can provide the desired wide-spectrum coverage.[3]

Results

The mortality rate has fallen dramatically throughout the 20th century, from more than 50% before 1930 to virtually nil in the 1980s. This has almost certainly been due to antibiotics.[6, 7, 9, 13]

REFERENCES

1. Bannatyne R.M., Lakdawalla N., Ein S.H.: Primary meningococcal peritonitis. *Can. Med. Assoc. J.* 117:436, 1977.
2. Cloud D.T.: Appendicitis, in Holder T.M., Ashcraft K.W. (eds.): *Pediatric Surgery.* Philadelphia, W.B. Saunders Co., 1980, p. 498.
3. Condon R.E.: Antibiotics in the management of peritonitis, in Condon R.E., Gorbach S.L. (eds.): *Surgical Infections: Selective Antibiotic Therapy.* Baltimore, Williams & Wilkins Co., 1981, p. 83.
4. Correira J.P., Conn H.O.: Spontaneous bacterial peritonitis in cirrhosis: Endemic or epidemic? *Med. Clin. North Am.* 59:963, 1975.
5. Fine R.N., Salusky I.B., Hall T., et al.: Peritonitis in children undergoing continuous ambulatory peritoneal dialysis. *Pediatrics* 71:806, 1983.
6. Fowler R.: Primary peritonitis, changing aspects 1956–70. *Aust. Paediatr. J.* 7:73, 1971.
7. Gross R.E.: *The Surgery of Infancy and Childhood.* Philadelphia, W.B. Saunders Co., 1953.
8. Matthews P.: Primary anaerobic peritonitis. *Br. Med. J.* 2:903, 1979.
9. McDougal W.S., Izant R.J. Jr., Zollinger R.M. Jr.: Primary peritonitis in infancy and childhood. *Ann. Surg.* 181:310, 1975.
10. Morris I.M., Carter D.J.: Spontaneous pneumococcal peritonitis. *Br. Med. J.* 2:98, 1975.
11. Targan S.R., Chow A.W., Guze L.B.: Role of anaerobic bacteria in spontaneous peritonitis of cirrhosis: Report of two cases and review of the literature. *Am. J. Med.* 62:397, 1977.
12. Tchirkow G., Verhagen A.D.: Bacterial peritonitis in patients with ventriculoperitoneal shunt. *J. Pediatr. Surg.* 14:182, 1979.
13. Weinstein M.P., Iannini P.B., Stratton C.W., et al.: Spontaneous bacterial peritonitis: A review of 28 cases with emphasis on improved survival and factors influencing prognosis. *Am. J. Med.* 64:592, 1978.
14. Wilfert C.M., Katz S.L.: Etiology of bacterial sepsis in nephrotic children, 1963–1967. *Pediatrics* 42:840, 1968.

103 HARRY C. BISHOP
Ileostomy and Colostomy

ENTEROSTOMIES-JEJUNOSTOMIES, ileostomies, and colostomies are commonly used in the management of congenital and acquired surgical diseases in neonates, infants, and older children. Fortunately, most of these enterostomies are needed only temporarily, and it is the rare child who will need to have enterostomy for a lifetime.

Indications for Enterostomies

Atresia

Most uncomplicated atresias of the newborn are repaired by primary anastomosis of the bowel segments. Atresias complicated by in utero perforation with meconium peritonitis and secondary bacterial involvement may require an end enterostomy with the hope of early re-exploration and anastomosis when the peritoneal inflammation has subsided. Colonic atresias are rare, and the massive dilatation of the colon just proximal to the atresia may require an end colostomy to allow the colon to shrink so that a later colocolostomy is possible (see Chap. 104).

Imperforate Anus

Infants with high imperforate anus usually do not undergo definitive reconstruction as neonates and require colostomy. These colostomies should be diverting, to avoid overflow into the distal stoma with subsequent contamination of the urinary tract through the usually present urinary fistula. We prefer to place the colostomy in the upper sigmoid so that the distal colonic segment, with its fistula into the urinary tract, can be irrigated and cleansed, still leaving available a sufficient length of the lower segment of colon for the corrective pull-through procedure at a later date. Others prefer a transverse or splenic flexure colostomy, leaving a longer lower segment of colon for the later pull-through corrective procedure (see Chap. 108).

Hirschsprung's Disease

Hirschsprung's disease usually requires an enterostomy when symptoms are such that the diagnosis is made in the newborn or infant, not only to decompress the megacolon but to avoid or lessen the possibility of enterocolitis. Surgeons preferring the Duhamel or Soave procedures, as we do, perform the colostomy at the transitional zone between the lower aganglionic segment and the upper normally ganglionated bowel. The colostomy is taken down at the definitive operation and the bowel at that level brought down. Advocates of the Swenson procedure prefer a more proximal colostomy, which will be left open as a vent during the healing of the Swenson pull-through procedure. This is subsequently closed, once the pull-through procedure is healed completely.

Meconium Ileus

Infants born with fibrocystic disease of the pancreas complicated by intestinal obstruction from inspissated meconium may be cleared by Gastrografin enemas alone. Many infants with meconium ileus are not relieved by this nonoperative approach, and, when a surgical procedure is necessary, I prefer to resect the massively dilated segment of jejunum with an end-to-side anastomosis of the jejunum to the side of the ileum 4–5 cm distal from its end, which is exteriorized as a single limb ileostomy (Fig 103–1). Postoperatively, catheter irrigation with pancreatic enzymes can be used to liquefy the still impacted meconium in the distal bowel[2] (see Chap. 86).

Necrotizing Enterocolitis

Necrotizing enterocolitis is a devastating complication, usually occurring in distressed premature infants and frequently in infants suffering from respiratory distress syndrome. Although medical management frequently is successful, without full-thickness bowel necrosis, the surgeon is frequently called upon to

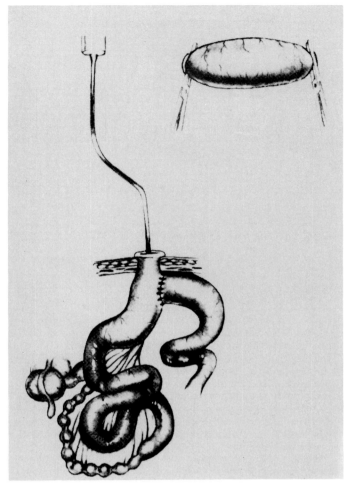

Fig 103–1.—Bishop-Koop procedure for meconium ileus. The maximally dilated segment is resected. End-to-side jejunoileostomy with catheter inserted into still obstructed distal segment for postoperative irrigation. The vent formed by the end of the distal segment may later close spontaneously or may require suture closure.

care for the complications of necrosis and perforation of the small or large bowel, or both. These infants have associated peritonitis, and, if a segment of the bowel is resected, primary anastomosis cannot usually be done safely. Frequently such infants must have a jejunostomy, ileostomy, colostomy, or, on occasion, more than one enterostomy, to conserve as much viable bowel as possible. These enterostomies are usually end ostomies, and the exteriorized bowel may be of borderline viability (see Chap. 99).

Intussusception

Although most ileocolic intussusceptions can be reduced by hydrostatic barium enemas or at laparotomy, on rare occasions an irreducible or perforated intussusception will require resection. The decision must be individualized at the time of resection as to whether primary anastomosis is safe or whether the two ends of the resected bowel should be exteriorized and subsequently closed.

Volvulus of the Midgut

If volvulus of the midgut results in a gangrenous midgut, primary anastomosis of the viable bowel at each end is desirable in order to salvage as much bowel length as possible. Only if perforation with secondary bacterial peritonitis has occurred would a high end jejunostomy be performed (see Chap. 89).

Inflammatory Bowel Disease

The indications for enterostomy must be individualized when caring for patients with Crohn's disease or ulcerative colitis. Every effort should be made to have these enterostomies only temporarily. Even today, however, a permanent ileostomy is occasionally necessary (see Chaps. 100 and 101).

Miscellaneous Indications

TRAUMA AND FOREIGN BODY.—Blunt or penetrating trauma, with disruption of bowel continuity, may require temporary enterostomy in children. Rarely does a gastrointestinal tract foreign body perforate and require exteriorization of the involved bowel segment.

URINARY DIVERSION.—An isolated ileal segment with anastomosis of the ureters to the internal end and exteriorization of the distal end as an ileostomy may be necessary in children, but more and more effort is being made to avoid the need for these ileal diversion procedures (see Chap. 129).

Types and Techniques of Small- and Large-Bowel Enterostomies

Loop Enterostomies

A loop jejunostomy, ileostomy, or loop colostomy[1, 4] is the safest and most popular technique of constructing an abdominal stoma. This is especially true in small infants, for if the bowel and mesentery is divided there is a greater chance for devascularization of the exteriorized ends. An intact loop of bowel can be exteriorized without sacrificing any branch of the mesenteric blood supply, but it is important that it not be brought out through the abdominal wall under tension. Loop enterostomy does have the disadvantages that wound closure may be more difficult, fecal spillover into the distal loop may occur, and prolapse of the distal loop is not uncommon. In most cases, closure requires a formal end-to-end anastomosis.

After a hemostat is passed through the mesentery adjacent to the bowel, a rubber catheter is pulled through to elevate the bowel, avoiding the blood vessels (Fig 103–2,*a*) while the loop is sutured with interrupted nonabsorbable sutures to the peritoneum and then to the deep fascia (Fig 103–2,*b,c*). Since the infant's omentum is flimsy and does not readily adhere to the bowel as it emerges from the abdominal wall, careful suturing of the bowel to the abdominal wall lessens the possibility of dehiscence and escape of another loop of bowel around the ostomy during the postoperative period, especially since the dilated segment of distended bowel will decompress once it is open. These sutures must be carefully placed, using only seromuscular sutures to avoid the possibility of creating an intestinal fistula. No sutures are placed between the bowel and the skin, but the skin should be in contact with the seromuscular coat of the bowel around the full circumference of the stoma. My personal preference is to replace the catheter with a small plastic rod that will lie comfortably on the surface of the skin. A loop of small rubber tubing is attached to either end of the rod, which elevates the back wall of the bowel above the skin surface (Fig 103–2,*d*).

If the bowel is greatly distended, it is opened at operation or decompressed by a catheter sutured into the lumen. If the condition is not acute, opening the bowel only after 12–24 hours allows sealing of the skin to the bowel serosa and avoids contamination of the wound. The bowel should be opened longitudinally

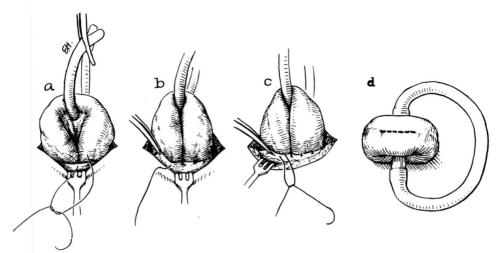

Fig 103–2.—Construction of a loop enterostomy. Loop is held by a catheter *(a)*, and a triangular suture approximates the two limbs and peritoneum. Interrupted silk sutures *(b)* attach the full circumference of bowel to peritoneum and to deep fascia *(c)*. Plastic rod *(d)* beneath loop. The bowel is opened *(dotted line)* longitudinally.

for only a short distance, which will then allow an eversion of the full thickness of the bowel, rolling back to expose each stoma (Fig 103–2,*d*). Leaving the rod beneath the loop for at least a month produces an elevation of this back wall, which will allow the stomas to point away from each other, effectively defunctionalizing the distal bowel. In my experience, this is a most effective means of diverting the bowel content, and it is rare to find evidence of spillover into the distal limb if the loop is properly constructed and opened. Some surgeons prefer a divided loop colostomy in which the bowel is partially opened and allowed to heal for a week or two and then completely divided. This however, leaves the two stomas at roughly the same level, and there is actually a greater chance of overflow and contamination of the distal segment. Other surgeons construct a skin bridge beneath the back wall of the loop. In my experience, the plastic rod more effectively diverts the fecal stream away from the distal stoma. Some surgeons exteriorize the two stomas through separate wounds. This is effective in keeping the distal limb clean but does have the attendant risk of inadequate stomal blood supply and retraction, and certainly requires more operating when the two ends are later reanastomosed.

End Enterostomy

If a segment of bowel has been resected and a primary anastomosis cannot or should not be done, the functioning end of the bowel must be exteriorized. The distal end may be either exteriorized as a mucous fistula or closed and left in the abdominal cavity near the exteriorized limb so it can be easily found for reanastomosis. In small infants, the mesenteric attachment and blood supply are very tenuous and great care must be taken to be sure that the bowel exteriorized through the abdominal wall has an adequate segment of mesentery assuring an adequate blood supply. If a single limb of bowel is exteriorized, it is again important to suture the seromuscular layer to the peritoneum with interrupted sutures, atraumatic 5-0 silk, or 4-0 or 3-0 silk in older children, and then to place a separate row of interrupted sutures from the deep fascia to the seromuscular coat of the bowel. Great care should be taken to assure that the flimsy mesentery is not compressed by the sutures and that there is no tension on the exteriorized limb. When a small-bowel enterostomy is used in infants and children, usually there is no need to mature the end of the bowel by turning its full thickness back

over itself and suturing it to the skin margin. Actually, small patients tolerate the exposed serosa above the skin edge very well, and, although some granulation tissue may form around the stoma, it eventually subsides and stricture is rare. In older children, especially for an ileostomy or colostomy that may be permanent, operative eversion for primary healing between the bowel mucosa and the skin edge is desirable.

If the nonfunctioning segment of the bowel is exteriorized as a mucous fistula, it is generally preferable to bring the limb out through a separate stab incision, away from the functioning stoma, rather than having them exit side by side through the same abdominal wound.

Mikulicz Double-Barreled Enterostomy

Gross,[6] in the early days of pediatric surgery in the United States, popularized the Mikulicz double-barreled enterostomy, but this method is used less frequently now and has been replaced by primary anastomosis or other types of enterostomies.[11] Since the two limbs are sutured together as they emerge through the abdominal wall (Fig 103–3), a spur-crushing clamp can later crush the common wall to create a single lumen that extends below the peritoneum. This allows an extra peritoneal closure, but time has proved that this extra outpouching of the bowel is not desirable, especially in the colon.

Kock Pouches

Reservoir pouches[7] are rarely, if ever, used in small infants but may be considered for the older child who might be faced with a permanent ileostomy following colectomy for ulcerative colitis.

Abdominal Sites for Enterostomies

In newborns and small infants, transverse abdominal incisions are made either a short distance above or below the umbilicus on either side. If a loop colostomy is to be used, the functioning stoma should be as far lateral as will still allow the plastic rod to lie in the body axis without being struck by the flexion of the baby's thigh on the abdomen. Loop colostomies can generally be brought out through the exploratory incision, and ideally the exteriorized loop fills the length of the wound (see Fig 103–2,*d*).

For an end enterostomy, I prefer a separate incision several centimeters above or below the midtransverse exploratory inci-

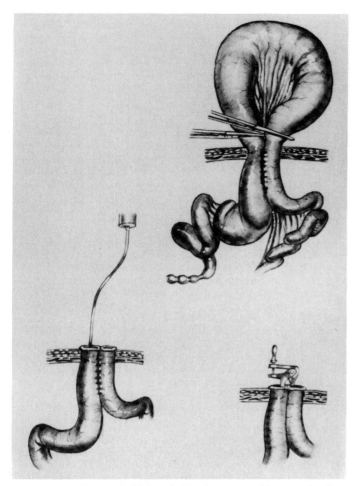

Fig 103–3.—Mikulicz double-barreled ileostomy as used for meconium ileus. Massively dilated loop is resected after the two limbs have been sutured together and exteriorized. Spur crushing clamp creates a common lumen. Extraperitoneal closure is performed when the obstructing spur has been removed. This procedure is no longer commonly used.

sion. In small infants, it is not necessary to remove a "plug" of skin or fascia.

For older children and adolescent patients in elective operations, it is important to find the most desirable spot for an enterostomy by having the youngster wear a colostomy bag and belt preoperatively, marking the area where the stoma should emerge. This assures that the bag will lie on a flat, unscarred area of the abdominal wall and that the belt will be comfortable, above the crest of the ilium and below the costal margins. Usually this site is halfway between the umbilicus and the anterior superior spine. It is important to avoid placing such a stoma close to a depressed or irregular abdominal scar. Colostomy rings and bags fit best on flat surfaces away from scars, bony prominences, and the umbilicus.

Care of Abdominal Enterostomies

The higher in the bowel the enterostomy, the more irritating is the intestinal content to the surrounding skin. Jejunostomies, with a high alkalinity and abundant pancreatic juice, are particularly corrosive. Ileal content is less irritating, but the evacuation is still very liquid and the fluid and electrolyte losses can be quite high until the terminal ileum adapts and is eventually able

to produce a firmer stool. Left-sided colostomies are the easiest to manage, since the stool tends to be more solid and the fluid losses are minimal.[5, 12]

Modern well-fitting enterostomy bags sealed with a karaya gum ring, or Stomadhesive with a ring and bag, are most helpful in keeping the irritating intestinal contents away from the skin. These enterostomy appliances come in many sizes, are sold widely, and are easily applied by the mother or the older patient.

If severe excoriation of the skin occurs, immaculate cleansing, washing with Betadine (povidone-iodine) solution, and exposure to room air are helpful. The heat from an ordinary lamp bulb hastens the healing of the skin surrounding the stoma.

Older youngsters frequently benefit from attending regional "ostomy clubs" and not only learn about the care of their stoma but receive tremendous moral support as well.

Closure of Enterostomies

Ideally, the skin surrounding the enterostomy should be as normal as possible, and closure should not be attempted if the skin is excoriated or ulcerated. Small-bowel enterostomies require little preoperative preparation except for 2 days of clear liquids and 1% neomycin enemas through the functioning enterostomy and the mucous fistula. Ampicillin and gentamicin are started the morning of operation and continued postoperatively. The scarred segment of bowel is resected and a fresh direct anastomosis to the distal segment created. The disparity in size of the two segments is easily managed by anastomosing the end of the larger proximal segment to the "back" oblique end of the distal segment. This is accomplished by resecting part of the antimesenteric wall of the distal bowel, producing an oval opening that will match the size of the lumen of the larger proximal bowel. A smaller oval of the antimesenteric side of the distal bowel can also be used and the antimesenteric wall then incised longitudinally for a distance that will create an opening equal to the proximal lumen. I prefer a two-layer closure with a running, locking, full-thickness suture of chromic catgut (5-0 or 3-0) and then a second interrupted layer of atraumatic 5-0 or 4-0 silk. The mesenteric defect is closed by approximating the edges of the mesentery with a small hemostat on either side and using a free tie to approximate this small amount of tissue. This eliminates the danger of perforating a vessel in the mesentery with the suture needle. After replacing the anastomosed bowel into the peritoneal cavity, the abdominal wall is closed without drainage.

When a colostomy is to be closed, complete preoperative cleansing is important. Clear liquids are given for 2 days before admission and then continued. Saline enemas, three times daily, irrigate the two stomas of the colostomy and the rectum, if indicated. Milk of magnesia (15–30 cc) is given at 9 A.M. and 4 P.M. on the day of admission and repeated the following day, when enemas of 1% neomycin are used three times daily and neomycin (40 mg/kg/24 hr, divided into four doses) is started by mouth. Intravenous fluids are started that day, and antibiotics are given the following morning when the premedications are given. Currently, ampicillin and gentamicin are given intravenously. It is important to resect the scarred segments of the colon and perform a direct two-layer anastomosis. A small width of Penrose drain is usually placed beneath the fascia above the peritoneum and brought out through the subcutaneous tissue and skin at the lateral end of the wound, and the skin is loosely approximated. Antibiotics are continued. The drain is removed 2–3 days later if the wound shows no signs of gross infection. Nasogastric decompression is used until peristalsis returns and gas and/or stool is passed per rectum. If clear oral feedings are tolerated, the diet can be advanced as appropriate for age.

Complications of Abdominal Stomas

Necrosis and Retraction

Necrosis is uncommon when a loop enterostomy has been constructed, since the blood supply to the exteriorized loop has usually not been interfered with. Only if the loop is brought out under tension may necrosis occur. Occasionally, due to tension, the rod underneath the loop colostomy erodes the bowel and allows the limbs to separate, which may permit one or both limbs to retract.[8, 9, 10]

End enterostomies are much more apt to necrose, particularly in infants with necrotizing enterocolitis. If necrosis is superficial to the fascia, revision may not be necessary, particularly if the ostomy is only to be needed temporarily. However, jejunostomies or ileostomies that have necrosed below the skin level are apt to stricture and may need to be revised. If the necrosis is below the fascia, obviously the abdomen needs to be re-explored and a viable segment of bowel exteriorized.

Dehiscence

Dehiscence, and extrusion of another loop of bowel around an enterostomy, usually occurs with inadequate suturing of the peritoneum and deep fascia to the seromuscular coat of the exteriorized bowel. When constructing a loop enterostomy, a triangular suture should be placed, suturing the two limbs and the peritoneum together, for this is a common site for the start of an evisceration (see Fig 103–2,a). The treatment is re-exploration and resuturing of the abdominal wall layers to the exteriorized bowel.

Exuberant Granulation Tissue Around the Enterostomy

Since most enterostomies are not "matured" with suture of the mucosa to the skin, there frequently is excess granulation tissue where the skin abuts the seromuscular coat. This granulation tissue may cause irritation of the surrounding skin and prevent the adequate fitting of an enterostomy bag. The granulations can be cauterized with silver nitrate sticks or by a hyfrecator. It may be necessary to do this repeatedly.

Intestinal Fistula

Occasionally, a fistula occurs between the bowel lumen and the skin surrounding an enterostomy, usually due to placing the seromuscular sutures too deeply and penetrating the mucosa. If such a perforation drains internally into the peritoneal cavity, of course, the enterostomy must be completely revised. An external fistula is often of no consequence.

Incisional Hernia

Weakness of the abdominal wall closure around an enterostomy usually occurs when a segment of dilated bowel has been exteriorized. This is particularly apt to occur in cases of Hirschsprung's disease, when the decompressed bowel shrinks down. Ordinarily, such incisional weakness is of no consequence, although it occasionally produces an irregularity of the skin, making the fitting of a colostomy bag difficult. If an incisional hernia becomes troublesome, revision may occasionally be necessary. I have not seen the incarceration of another loop of bowel in such an incisional hernia.

Stricture

It is rare for an infant or child to develop a stricture around a loop enterostomy unless the bowel has retracted or there have been repeated episodes of infection. Stricture is much more apt to occur with an end enterostomy. For a superficial stricture, excising the skin away from the enterostomy, including the scarred ring, will usually take care of the problem. If it is at the fascial level, radial cuts in the scarred ring will often release the stricture. Rarely, one must redo the enterostomy, pulling out a fresh segment of bowel either through the same wound or elsewhere.

Intestinal Obstruction

Internal hernias between the lateral abdominal wall and the enterostomy rarely occur. More frequently, adhesions around an exteriorized segment of bowel produce intestinal obstruction that requires laparotomy and division of adhesions or reduction of the internal hernia.

Prolapse

End enterostomies rarely prolapse, but prolapses are commonly seen when loop enterostomies are used.[3] Careful suturing of the full circumference of the bowel to the peritoneum and the deep fascia is helpful in preventing prolapse. If prolapse occurs, it usually involves the distal nonfunctioning limb. The degree of prolapse is usually not great, and, although it is unsightly and a nuisance, it is not harmful. Only if it becomes troublesome or impairs the functioning of the proximal stoma is a revision necessary. It is then best to divide the back wall of the loop, reduce the prolapse, and place the distal limb through a separate wound as a mucous fistula or, if possible, close it and replace the closed segment into the abdominal cavity.

Irritation of the Exteriorized Bowel and Surrounding Skin

Occasionally, the exposed bowel mucosa becomes irritated due to the enterostomy apparatus, the gauze, or the patient's clothing. It is very helpful to lay on the exposed mucosa, as a dressing, small squares of an old bed sheet lubricated on one surface with Vaseline, which lessens the irritation and allows healing. Usually any bleeding from the colostomy itself is due to this type of irritation, but the amount of such bleeding is never great. Occasionally a *Monilia (Candida)* infection leads to dermatitis, and Mycostatin powder or ointment is helpful.

Dehydration and Electrolyte Imbalance

Every effort should be made to place an abdominal stoma as far down the intestinal tract as possible, but occasionally high jejunostomies or ileostomies are necessary. Electrolyte imbalance and dehydration are apt to occur in such infants, and adequate replacement and correction with appropriate intravenous solutions are required.[13] Total parenteral nutrition may be necessary and is most helpful to maintain a good nutritional state until the temporary enterostomy can be closed.

REFERENCES

1. Bishop H.C.: Colostomy in the newborn. *Am. J. Surg.* 101:642, 1961.
2. Bishop H.C.: Meconium ileus, in Rob and Smith's *Operative Surgery*, ed. 3. London, Butterworth, 1978.
3. Ein S.H.: Divided loop colostomy that does not prolapse. *Am. J. Surg.* 147:250, 1984.
4. Fazio V.W.: Loop ileostomy and loop-end ileostomy, in Rob and Smith's *Operative Surgery*, ed. 4. London, Butterworth, 1983.
5. Grosfeld J.L., Cooney D.E.: Care of the child with a colostomy. *Pediatrics* 59:469, 1977.
6. Gross R.E.: *The Surgery of Infancy and Childhood*. Philadelphia, W.B. Saunders, 1953.
7. Handelsman J.C., Fishbein R.H.: Permanent ileostomy without external appliance: Kock internal reservoir (pouch) operation. *Johns Hopkins Med. J.* 138:161, 1976.

8. Lister J., et al.: Colostomy complications in children. *Practitioner* 227:229, 1983.
9. Nixon H.H.: Paediatric problems associated with stomas. *Clin. Gastroenterol.* 11:351, 1982.
10. Pearl R.K., et al.: Complications of intestinal stomas. *Contemp. Surg.* 24:17, 1984.
11. Rosenman J.E., Kosloske A.M.: A reappraisal of the Mikulicz enterostomy in infants and children. *Surgery* 91:34, 1982.
12. Rowbotham J.L.: Stomal care. *N. Engl. J. Med.* 279:90, 1968.
13. Schwarz K.B., et al.: Sodium needs of infants and children with ileostomy. *J. Pediatr.* 102:509, 1983.

104 ARVIN I. PHILIPPART

Atresia, Stenosis, and Other Obstructions of the Colon

Colonic Atresia

CONGENITAL COLONIC ATRESIA or stenosis is an infrequent cause of low intestinal obstruction in the neonate. Because these patients present with bilious emesis, marked abdominal distention, and diminished or absent passage of meconium, colonic atresia must be differentiated from other causes of obstruction of the ileum and colon.

History

The first case was recognized in 1673 by Bininger.[14] The first survivor, treated only with colostomy, was reported by Gaub in 1922.[7] Potts, in 1947,[13] reported the first survivor with a primary anastomosis. Few appreciable series have subsequently been reported because isolated colonic atresia or stenosis is an uncommon lesion, and no clearly defined management has emerged.

Incidence

Occurrence rates have been reported as 1 in 1,500 to 1 in 20,000 live births. The former appears inappropriately low and the latter more nearly correct, based on experience in major pediatric surgical centers. In such centers, the occurrence rate approximates one case per year of isolated colonic atresia or stenosis. When associated with other developmental errors, the incidence increases significantly. In the gastrointestinal tract, only gastric atresia is more uncommon. Acquired obstruction of the colon secondary to necrotizing enterocolitis is more common than congenital atresia.

Etiology

Theories of the etiology of atresia and stenosis of the intestine originally were drawn from observation of similar anomalies in the small intestine. Tandler's theory of duodenal stenosis resulting from failure of resorption of the "solid stage" of embryologic events has been questioned.[11, 15] The classic demonstration of Barnard and Louw[1, 9] that jejunoileal atresia results from in utero mesenteric vascular compromise is widely accepted. Congenital colonic atresia and stenosis is similarly considered to be due to vascular compromise.[10] That compromise may occur from a primary in utero vascular event or may be secondary to a mechanical event such as in utero volvulus. Because the types of atresia of the colon differ in frequency, proximal and distal to the splenic flexure, the etiologies may also be different.

Classification

The classification of small-bowel atresias first described by Sutton[16] has been applied to colonic atresia. A type I lesion exhibits external continuity with an intraluminal diaphragm which may be imperforate (atresia) or perforate (stenosis, rare). A type II lesion is characterized by physically separate proximal and distal lumens connected by a fibrous cord with intact mesentery.

The type III lesion is characterized by a gap between the colonic segments, with a mesenteric defect.

The value of such a classification system may exceed pure description. Type III atresias far outnumber type I and II lesions in the right and transverse colon. Conversely, type III lesions are less common than types I and II distal to the splenic flexure.[4, 12, 14]

Associated Anomalies

Isolated colonic atresia is frequently associated with skeletal anomalies such as syndactyly, polydactyly, absent radius, and clubfoot. Ocular and cardiac anomalies have been noted.[14] Associated jejunal atresia was the primary presentation in five of our 36 cases at Children's Hospital of Michigan. Coexistent aganglionosis has been reported[8] and occurred in one of our series. Colonic atresias may be complicated by abdominal wall defects—gastroschisis, omphalocele, or vesicointestinal fissure.[4, 14]

Our series of neonates with congenital colonic atresia, previously reported in part,[2] now numbers 36 from 1945 to 1983. In 22, there were no major associated anomalies. In the remaining 14, there were six with vesicointestinal fissure, three with other abdominal wall defects, and five with jejunal atresia.

Diagnosis

All children with uncomplicated congenital atresia or stenosis present the classic findings of distal intestinal obstruction in the immediate neonatal period. These include marked abdominal distention, bilious vomiting, and absent or unsustained defecation. Variations from this occur in those with a simultaneous jejunal atresia where the clinical presentation is that of jejunal rather than colonic obstruction. Those in whom the colonic atresia is associated with an abdominal wall defect are obvious at the outset.

The plain abdominal film in colonic atresia demonstrates multiple dilated loops with air-fluid levels, consistent with any distal obstruction. However, the terminal dilated loop in colonic atresia is often appreciably larger (Fig 104–1) than that seen in low small-bowel obstruction. Pneumoperitoneum due to colonic perforation is common and was present on admission in four of our 36 patients.

The barium enema reveals a microcolon (Figs 104–1 and 104–2) with incomplete colonic filling. We believe the barium enema is crucial in all presumed small-bowel and colonic atresias because of the frequent association of colonic atresia with clinically apparent more proximal atresias. Failure to recognize the distal lesion may be catastrophic.

Management

The management of colonic atresia is determined by the presence or absence of associated anomalies. Nasogastric decompres-

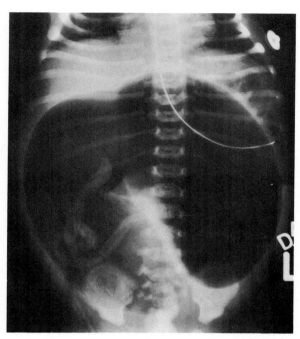

Fig 104–1.—Atresia of the colon at the splenic flexure, Type I. The terminal segment is hugely distended. Residual barium in left microcolon and rectum is from a barium enema.

sion, antibiotics, fluid and electrolyte replacement, and maintenance of normothermia are appropriate in all.

In pure colonic atresia, immediate operation is required to prevent perforation. Alternative management techniques are primary colostomy with later anastomosis, or primary resection and anastomosis as reported in small series.[2, 3, 4, 5, 6, 14] Both have been used successfully. We, and others,[14] prefer to distinguish between colonic atresia proximal and distal to the splenic flexure. Proximal atresias are managed by generous resection of the prox-

imal dilated segment, lesser resection of the distal segment, and primary end-oblique anastomosis. When the atresia occurs in the right colon or hepatic flexure, an ileotransverse colostomy is required. Distal to the splenic flexure, atresia is managed again by resection of the dilated segment and a segment of distal colon. Both ends are exteriorized preparatory to a staged colocolostomy. While much less commonly employed today in newborn intestinal surgery than in previous eras, the Mikulicz spur-crushing technique is well utilized to provide gradual distal colonic dilatation and function. The colostomy is closed later by resection and intraperitoneal anastomosis to obviate the complications that occur with extraperitoneal closure. The Mikulicz technique is preferred to hydrostatic dilatation of the blind-ending distal segment.

Complicated forms of colonic atresia are managed differently. Multiple colonic atresias are resected. The choice of colostomy or anastomosis depends on the site of the most distal atresia and caliber of the bowel. Synchronous jejunal and colonic atresias are managed by jejunojejunostomy and resection of the colonic atresia with a Mikulicz colostomy. Colonic atresia associated with an abdominal wall defect is managed by abdominal wall repair and colostomy, usually in the umbilicus.

Results

Because colonic atresia is so uncommon, the reported series are small and encompass several decades. Experience with this rare lesion as well as marked improvements in supportive care have improved survival, which currently approximates 90%.[4, 14] Deaths now result only from critical associated anomalies or delays in recognition. In our own series of 22 patients with isolated colonic atresia, there were four deaths, all before 1970. Preoperative colonic perforation was present in three of the four nonsurvivors. Delayed function of the distal colonic segment has occurred in several and required intravenous nutritional support. In such cases, rectal biopsy for ganglion cells is appropriate. Late contrast enema may reveal persistent tapering of the distal segment. This is not a concern in asymptomatic patients.

REFERENCES

1. Barnard C.N., Louw J.H.: Continuation studies: The genesis of intestinal atresia. *Minn. Med.* 39:745, 1956.
2. Benson C.D., Lotfi M.W., Brough A.J.: Congenital atresia and stenosis of the colon. *J. Pediatr. Surg.* 3:253, 1968.
3. Berger D., Rehbein F.: Traitement des atresies et stenoses coliques. *Ann. Chir. Inf.* 13:113, 1972.
4. Boles E.T. Jr., Vassy L.E., Ralston M.: Atresia of the colon. *J. Pediatr. Surg.* 11:69, 1976.
5. Coran A.G., Eraklis A.J.: Atresia of the colon. *Surgery* 65:828, 1969.
6. Freeman N.V.: Congenital atresia and stenosis of the colon. *Br. J. Surg.* 53:595, 1966.
7. Gaub O.C.: Congenital stenosis and atresia of the intestinal tract above the rectum: With a report of an operated case of atresia of the sigmoid in an infant. *Trans. Am. S.A.* 40:582, 1922.
8. Johnson J.F., Dean B.L.: Hirschsprung's disease coexisting with colonic atresia. *Pediatr. Radiol.* 11:97, 1981.
9. Louw J.H.: Jejunoileal atresia and stenosis. *J. Pediatr. Surg.* 1:8, 1966.
10. Louw J.H.: Investigations into the etiology of congenital atresia of the colon. *Dis. Colon Rectum* 7:471, 1964.
11. Moutsouris C.: The "solid stage" and congenital intestinal atresia. *J. Pediatr. Surg.* 1:446, 1966.
12. Peck D.A., Lynn H.B., Harris L.E.: Congenital atresia and stenosis of the colon. *Arch. Surg.* 87:428, 1963.
13. Potts W.J.: Congenital atresia of the intestine and colon. *Surg. Gynecol. Obstet.* 85:14, 1947.
14. Powell R.W., Raffensperger J.G.: Congenital colonic atresia. *J. Pediatr. Surg.* 17:166, 1982.
15. Santulli T.V., Blanc W.A.: Congenital atresia of the intestine: Pathogenesis and treatment. *Ann. Surg.* 154:939, 1961.
16. Sutton J.B.: Imperforate ileum. *Am. J. Med. Sci.* 98:457, 1889.

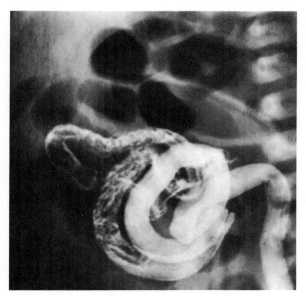

Fig 104–2.—Atresia of the colon, Type III, in a neonate. Barium enema, lateral view, shows microcolon with apple-peel configuration. Dilated loops of small bowel are apparent.

Dysmotility States

Several poorly defined entities have been described over the years that present the clinical appearance of colonic obstruction in the neonate unassociated with a specifically recognized mechanical obstruction. These remain poorly defined because the physiologic alterations that produce these syndromes have not been elucidated.

Meconium Plug Syndrome/Small Left Colon Syndrome

These two entities are discussed together because, while clinically differentiated one from the other, they may represent a continuum of transient neonatal colonic dysfunction. Historically, Clatworthy[1] first described the meconium plug syndrome in 1956, when he reported nine neonates with the clinical presentation of low intestinal obstruction. Seven of the nine patients became normal after anal manipulation or enemas and passage of a large meconium stool (Fig 104–3). Two, for presumed Hirschsprung's disease, had enterostomies, which were later closed. A later report[4] described 30 patients with similar presentation, 17 of whom had narrow left colons on barium enema examination. The original emphasis on abnormalities of the meconium[5] receives less emphasis currently.

In 1974, Davis[2] reported 20 neonates with the clinical features of high-grade partial colonic obstruction. Eight of these patients were infants of diabetic mothers. Contrast enemas revealed a dilated colon proximal to a tapered transition zone at the splenic flexure, much as seen in Hirschsprung's disease, and a narrow left colon, hence the term small left colon syndrome (SLCS). They emphasized that the patient improves after the enema, particularly a Gastrografin enema, but that the narrowed left colon may remain narrowed in follow-up. A later report[3] emphasized the findings in infants of diabetic mothers.

Nixon[6] reported four newborns with intestinal perforations and SLCS. Three of the perforations were in the cecum. We[7] reported nine infants of diabetic mothers, three of whom had had cecal perforation, and emphasized that this syndrome resulted

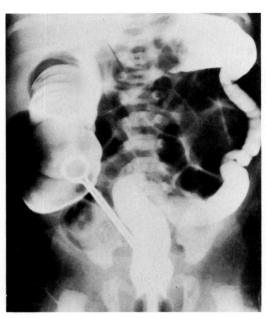

Fig 104–4.—Small left colon syndrome in infant of a diabetic mother. The child had abdominal distention, bilious emesis, and no stools in first 24 hours. Gastrografin enema demonstrates conical transition zone at splenic flexure, narrow left colon without tertiary contractions, and normal rectal caliber. Meconium evacuation was prompt, but symptoms and findings decreased only gradually over ensuing 5 days.

from a transient dysmotility state rather than from mechanical obstruction by meconium. The current series at Children's Hospital of Michigan numbers 28 patients with SLCS. Fifty percent of these neonates were infants of diabetic mothers. The other 50% were septic, and most had been hypoglycemic. None of the recent infants have developed cecal perforation or required colostomy, presumably because of more aggressive management of the hypoglycemia by glucose administration and avoidance of exogenous sympathomimetics.

While the etiology of this syndrome remains uncertain,[2, 7] the management has been standardized. We prefer an initial barium enema to evaluate any distal obstruction. The diagnosis of SLCS is established from maternal history and the radiologic findings of partial colonic obstruction, a conical splenic flexure or proximal left colonic transition zone, absence of tertiary contractions in the narrowed left colon, and a normal-sized rectum (Fig 104–4).

Treatment consists of vigorous management of the hypoglycemia, antibiotics if the infant is septic, nasogastric intubation, and observation. In most infants, the clinical obstruction clears in 24–48 hours, the tube is removed, and feedings initiated over the following 2 days. Dilute Gastrografin enemas are used to promote clearance of meconium in the few patients who have progressive distention or delayed relief of the obstruction. In this group, a rectal suction biopsy is appropriate to exclude the occasional infant with a splenic flexure transition zone of Hirschsprung's disease.

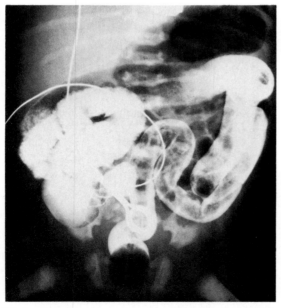

Fig 104–3.—Meconium plug syndrome in neonate with abdominal distention, bilious emesis, and no stools after 24 hours. Barium enema shows meconium in sigmoid and a descending colon of normal caliber. Prompt evacuation of meconium produced relief of all symptoms and findings.

REFERENCES

1. Clatworthy H.W. Jr., Howard W.H., Lloyd J.: The meconium plug syndrome. *Surgery* 39:131, 1956.
2. Davis W.S., Allen R.P., Favara B.E., et al.: The neonatal small left colon syndrome. *Am. J. Roentgenol. Radium Ther. Nucl. Med.* 120:322, 1974.
3. Davis W.S., Campbell J.B.: Neonatal small left colon syndrome. *Am. J. Dis. Child.* 129:1024, 1975.

4. Ellis D.G., Clatworthy H.W. Jr.: The meconium plug syndrome revisited. *J. Pediatr. Surg.* 1:54, 1966.
5. Emery J.L.: Abnormalities in meconium of the foetus and newborn. *Arch. Dis. Child.* 32:17, 1957.
6. Nixon G.W., Condon V.R., Stewart D.R.: Intestinal perforation as a complication of the neonatal small left colon syndrome. *Am. J. Roentgenol.* 125:75, 1975.
7. Philippart A.I., Reed J.O., Georgeson K.E.: Neonatal small left colon syndrome: Intramural not intraluminal obstruction. *J. Pediatr. Surg.* 10:733, 1975.

Neurofibromatosis

Neurofibromatosis is an autosomal dominant neurectodermal dysplasia with frequent mutations. While the disease is common,[5] intrinsic gastrointestinal involvement is uncommon. The stomach and small bowel are affected more often than the colon.[2] Such involvement affects adults more often than children, as evidenced by a review of neurofibromatosis in children by Holt,[3] who did not include gastrointestinal manifestations. Nevertheless, extensive reviews have emphasized that constipation is present and progressive in 10% of patients.[5]

Colonic disease in children may present as polyps with bleeding, obstruction secondary to extrinsic compression by adjacent tumor, or as intrinsic obstruction from autonomic nervous dysfunction analogous to Hirschsprung's disease (Fig 104–5). We have seen children with each of these presentations. The former two presentations rarely present diagnostic or therapeutic difficulties. The latter is a rare presentation with approximately ten cases variably documented.[1, 4, 6, 7] The barium enema picture is similar to that in neglected Hirschsprung's disease but easily distinguished by rectal biopsy, which reveals not only ganglion cells but often increased numbers of ganglion cells, variable in size and associated with an increase in nerve fibers.[6]

While experience with treatment of these lesions is limited, certain standards apply. We have not operated in the absence of symptoms. Polypoid lesions with bleeding or partial obstruction are locally resected. For partially obstructing extrinsic lesions, the bowel is either resected with anastomosis or diverted. The few patients with Hirschsprung's-like presentation have been managed in no consistent way, with variable results. Our approach has been to resect the maximally dilated sigmoid with end colostomy and Hartmann pouch. The pull-through is delayed until colostomy function is clearly normal over a prolonged period of observation. Such an operative approach is delayed until there is demonstrated failure of thorough nonoperative measures and is reserved for those with failure to thrive and episodes of obstructive enterocolitis.

REFERENCES

1. Hassell P.: Gastrointestinal manifestations of neurofibromatosis in children: A report of two cases. *J. Can. Assoc. Radiol.* 33:202, 1982.
2. Hochberg F.H., Dasilva A.B., Galdabini J., et al.: Gastrointestinal involvement in von Recklinghausen's neurofibromatosis. *Neurology* 24:1144, 1974.
3. Holt J.F.: Neurofibromatosis in children. *A.J.R.* 130:615, 1978.
4. Phat V.N., Sezeur A., Danne M., et al.: Primary myenteric plexus alterations as a cause of megacolon in von Recklinghausen's disease. *Pathol. Biol.* 28:585, 1980.
5. Riccardi V.M.: Von Recklinghausen neurofibromatosis. *N. Engl. J. Med.* 305:1617, 1981.
6. Saul R.A., Sturner R.A., Burger P.C.: Hyperplasia of the myenteric plexus. *Am. J. Dis. Child.* 136:852, 1982.
7. Staple T.W., McAlister W.H., Anderson M.S.: Plexiform neurofibromatosis of the colon simulating Hirschsprung's disease. *A.J.R.* 91:840, 1964.

Intestinal Pseudo-obstruction

Uncommon but difficult to deal with is a small group of children with the clinical features of intestinal obstruction, a patent gastrointestinal tract, and ganglion cells present throughout. Attempts to separate subsets of these patients appear arbitrary at present but have resulted in a confused nomenclature, including Sieber syndrome, megacystis-microcolon-intestinal hypoperistalsis syndrome, and chronic idiopathic intestinal pseudo-obstruction syndrome.

Historically, Sieber[6] first reported seven male infants with clinical distal small-bowel obstruction, patent gastrointestinal tracts, and normal ganglion cells. Six of the seven died. Berdon[1] coined the term "megacystis-microcolon-intestinal hypoperistalsis syndrome" in describing five female neonates with these features as well as malrotation. The only survivor required chronic total parenteral nutrition. Puri,[4] in 1983, collected 22 infants with this entity from the literature with the conclusion that they did not survive.

The lack of any recognizable etiology complicates any grouping of afflicted patients. The only feature common to all is the persistence of hypoperistalsis and clinical obstruction, despite currently known diagnostic and therapeutic maneuvers (Fig 104–6). Suggested etiologies include abnormal central and peripheral nerves[5] and degeneration of intestinal smooth muscle.[4, 5]

What is apparent is that there is a spectrum of disease. While certain forms of this entity have a sexual preponderance, there is equal distribution when all forms of pseudo-obstruction are considered. The disease may be familial[1, 2, 5] or sporadic. While most patients present as neonates, others do so in later months or even years. Associated anomalies of the urinary tract include megacystis with or without hydronephrosis. Associated anomalies of the gut include microcolon and malrotation. These are frequent but not uniform and may be persistent or transient. Attempts, as in adults, to categorize patients by level of the gastrointestinal tract involved[5] do not appear useful in infants. However, the recognition in adults does reinforce the observation that there is a spectrum of severity.

Clinical management problems in these children can be formidable. Ideally, the diagnosis should be made without operation. However, that is not currently practical, particularly in the sporadic case presenting neonatally. Evaluation of the urinary

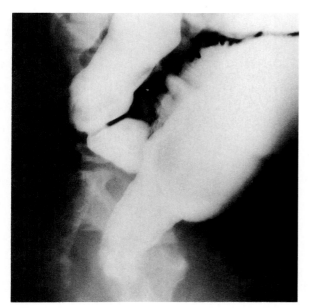

Fig 104–5.—Neurofibromatosis in 8-year-old male with recurrent symptoms of colonic obstruction. Lateral view of barium enema. Note widening of presacral space and transition zone similar to that seen in Hirschsprung's disease. Ganglion cells were found on rectal biopsy.

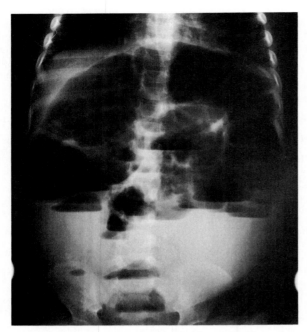

Fig 104–6.—Megacystis microcolon intestinal hypoperistalsis syndrome. Intestinal pseudo-obstruction in 8-month-old female with severe failure to thrive, recurrent bilious vomiting, and constipation. Intravenous pyelography demonstrated megacystis, and contrast studies of the gastrointestinal tract revealed malrotation.

tract and decompression of the bladder relieve the occasionally associated abdominal mass. Children with malrotation require operation because the clinical findings in pseudo-obstruction and uncomplicated malrotation are so similar. The realities are that pseudo-obstruction is recognized only after the first laparotomy for obstruction or malrotation does not relieve the obstruction and intestinal biopsies reveal ganglion cells. In kindreds, rectal biopsy and esophageal manometry are useful and may obviate operation.[2]

Once recognized, management is difficult. Total parenteral nutrition is integral to treatment. Byrne[2] has emphasized home total parenteral nutrition as the only means of survival. However, we have been successful with the use of metoclopramide and senna. Recently, de Lorimier treated two children successfully by intestinal imbrication.[3] These recent successes, while few in number, suggest that not all such patients need have a fatal outcome as suggested[2, 4] without chronic total parenteral nutrition.

REFERENCES

1. Berdon W.E., Baker D.H., Blanc W.A., et al.: Megacystis-microcolon-intestinal hypoperistalsis syndrome: A new cause of intestinal obstruction in the newborn. Report of radiologic findings in five newborn girls. *A.J.R.* 126:957, 1976.
2. Byrne W.J., Cipel L., Euler A.R., et al.: Chronic idiopathic intestinal pseudo-obstruction syndrome in children—clinical characteristics and prognosis. *J. Pediatr.* 90:585, 1977.
3. de Lorimier A.A.: Personal communication.
4. Puri P., Lake B.D., Gorman F., et al.: Megacystis-microcolon-intestinal hypoperistalsis syndrome: A visceral myopathy. *J. Pediatr. Surg.* 18:64, 1983.
5. Schuffler M.D., Deitch E.A.: Chronic idiopathic intestinal pseudo-obstruction. *Ann. Surg.* 192:752, 1980.
6. Sieber W.K., Girdany B.R.: Functional intestinal obstruction in newborn infants with morphologically normal gastrointestinal tracts. *Surgery* 53:357, 1963.

Miscellaneous Lesions

There are additional rare lesions that may produce colonic obstruction in children. Colonic duplications most frequently present as mass lesions rather than obstruction, except in the pelvis where obstruction may be a prominent feature (see also Chap. 94). Another lesion rarely encountered is congenital segmental dilatation of the colon.[3] In this entity, the colon proximal and distal to the dilated segment appears normal fluoroscopically and histologically. The dilated segment is saccular, without taenia, and lacks peristalsis. Constipation from infancy is the dominant feature. Segmental resection is the appropriate therapy.

Volvulus limited to the colon is common in adults but rare in children. In utero volvulus is one of the causes of colonic atresia. Andersen's recent review[1] of postnatal volvulus in children included only 37 cases. The right colon was involved in 12 and the sigmoid in 25. They recommended nonoperative management, as volvulus was an isolated event in their seven cases. Our experience at Children's Hospital of Michigan differs. Symptoms can be chronic with acute exacerbations, and resection has been utilized.

Colonic malignancy is infrequent in pediatric practice.[2] Lymphoma involving the terminal ileum and cecum is well recognized. Adenocarcinomas are rare. Much attention is paid to predisposing lesions such as polyposis, ulcerative colitis, Crohn's colitis, and ureterosigmoidostomies. However, 90% of pediatric colonic adenocarcinomas occur in patients who do not have these predisposing diseases.[2] The reportedly unfavorable prognosis in patients less than 20 years is attributed to delay in diagnosis and to an inordinately high incidence of mucinous and poorly differentiated adenocarcinomas, as compared with adults.[4]

REFERENCES

1. Andersen J.F., Eklof O., Thomasson B.: Large bowel volvulus in children. *Pediatr. Radiol.* 11:129, 1981.
2. Chabalko J.J., Fraumeni J.F. Jr.: Colorectal cancer in children. *Dis. Colon Rectum* 18:1, 1975.
3. Helikson M.A., Schapiro M.B., Garfinkel D.J., et al.: Congenital segmental dilatation of the colon. *J. Pediatr. Surg.* 17:201, 1982.
4. Recalde M., Holyoke E.D., Elias E.G.: Carcinoma of the colon, rectum, and anal canal in young patients. *Surg. Gynecol. Obstet.* 139:909, 1974.

105 Peter K. Kottmeier

Appendicitis

HISTORY.—Howard A. Kelly's monumental work, *The Vermiform Appendix and Its Diseases*, published in 1905, should be read by present-day students, be their interest the etiology of appendicitis, the anatomy and histology of the organ, or its comparative anatomy and embryology. Kelly credited Mestivier's 1759 report of a man operated on for appendiceal abscess, with subsequent death and autopsy, disclosing a pin perforating the appendix, as the first recorded instance of appendicitis. The *Philosophical Transactions of the Royal Society*, in October 1736, carried a report by Claudius Amyand, of St. George's Hospital. He reported a boy 11 years of age with a scrotal hernia from which there was a foul discharging sinus. At operation he found the appendix in the hernial sac, perforated by a pin, allowing the discharge of feces. This was discovered in the course of an operation in which Amyand ligated and amputated the appendix, closed the sac, and packed the wound. " 'Tis easy to conceive that this Operation was as painful to the Patient as laborious to me: It was a continued Dissection attended with Danger on Parts not well distinguished: It lasted near half an Hour, and the Patient bore it with great Courage." The patient recovered well. Heister in 1711 had described the autopsy of a patient with appendicitis, and for several hundred years there had been descriptions of the "passio illiaca." James Parkinson in 1812 reported an early case of appendicitis in English and the first in which perforation was recognized as the cause of death. Thomas Addison in 1839 published a good description of appendicitis. In the remainder of the 18th century and the first half of the 19th century there were numerous autopsy reports of patients dying with right lower quadrant abscesses, peritonitis, and gangrenous appendices. There was much concern with the influence of foreign bodies, stones, concretions, and pins. Louyer-Villermay, in France, in 1824 published the clinical histories and autopsy reports of two patients whom he recognized to have died of rapidly progressing infection in the appendix, with rupture and peritoneal contamination. In 1827, Mélier cited Louyer-Villermay's cases, one of his own, and other reported cases, including Amyand's. He stated: "In my opinion the fecal matter accumulated in the appendix, which then dilated little by little, becoming first inflamed, then gangrenous, and finally perforated. The earliest symptoms, appearing in the form of colic, are probably accounted for by the inflammation and distention of the appendix: its rupture occasioned the effusion, which was responsible in turn, for the peritonitis. The perforation was determined, or at any rate, hastened, by the patient's exertion and taking an enema, since it was at this moment that the intense pain began, and immediately after the peritonitis set in. . . . This disease is considered extremely rare; observe, however, that the five cases which form the basis of this paper have been collected in a short space of time, and that two among them were reported by the same physician; these facts entitle us to believe that if such affections have not been more frequently observed, it is because the appendix has not received sufficient attention, and because lesions situated in it have been overlooked at autopsies. . . . When my friend Monsieur Sévestre was called to the second of the cases, which he reported to me, he was able to state positively that the appendix was affected, so much did the symptoms resemble those of the first case, which had struck him forcibly at the time as characteristic. . . . If it were possible, indeed, to establish the diagnosis of these affections in a certain and positive manner and to show that they are always circumscribed, the possibility of an operation might be conceived: Some day perhaps this result will be reached." Dupuytren, the olympian, tyrannical, and vindictive surgeon-in-chief of the Hotel Dieu, the greatest surgeon in France, in his lectures, through the publications of his students Husson and Dance in 1827 and in his *Leçons Chirurgicales* (1833) attacked Mélier's imputation that right lower quadrant or right iliac abscesses were due to primary disease of the appendix. Ménière in 1820 had similarly attacked Mélier. Dupuytren's opposition plus the misguided concepts of "typhlo-enteritis" and "perityphlitis" substantially delayed, for some 50 years, the proper recognition of the significance of appendicitis. Numerous and significant contributions had been made in the interval when, in 1886, before the Association of American Physicians, Reginald Fitz, pathologist at Harvard, presented his classic paper on the perforating ulcer of the vermiform appendix, with special reference to its early diagnosis and treatment. He insisted upon the primary role of the appendix in perforative peritonitis of the right lower quadrant and coined the term "appendicitis." He stated: "The vital importance of early recognition of perforative peritonitis is unmistakable. Its diagnosis in most cases is comparatively easy. Its eventual treatment by laparotomy generally indispensable. If any good result is to arise from such treatment it must be applied early." Willard Parker in 1867 had demonstrated that iliac abscesses could be drained successfully long before there was evidence of fluctuation. Dupuytren had insisted on incision at the time and point of external fluctuation. Krönlein in 1886 performed the first laparotomy and appendectomy for rupture of the appendix, although the patient died. T. G. Morton, of Philadelphia, in 1887 performed the first successful laparotomy and deliberate appendectomy for ruptured appendix. Within the next 2 or 3 years surgeons everywhere, but particularly in the United States, were operating for appendicitis, and very soon methods were being devised to cover over and suture the stump, in addition to simple ligation. The paper by Charles McBurney in 1889 remains a classic. He strongly re-emphasized the responsibility of the appendix for right lower quadrant abscesses, noted that symptoms were variable, and stated his belief that "in every case the seat of greatest pain, determined by the pressure of one finger, has been very exactly between an inch and a half and two inches from the anterior spinous process of the ilium, on a straight line down from that process to the umbilicus. This may appear to be an affectation of accuracy, but, so far as my experience goes, the observation is correct." He urged early operation, stating that "in the early stage no accurate diagnosis can be made as to whether the appendix is perforated or not. There is no reason to think . . . that diagnosis from symptoms alone will ever reach that perfection . . . if it can be shown by future experience with improved methods of operation, and with more perfect antiseptic precautions, that the exploratory incision for inspection of the diseased appendix is much more free from danger than the expectant treatment, then there could be but one answer to the question: What is the best treatment?"

M. M. RAVITCH

Appendicitis remains the most common condition leading to emergency abdominal operations in children and adolescents.[47] The clinical findings and operative treatment of appendicitis were clearly established over 100 years ago. It is therefore astounding that appendicitis has remained *the* surgical emergency condition with the highest percentage of misdiagnosis leading to operation: "the negative appendix." It surely must also be in the first rank among surgical conditions in which the delay of a proper diagnosis is common, converting a relatively harmless pathologic condition into a potentially lethal one, since perforation of the appendix has occurred before treatment in more than one third of all patients with appendicitis. It is equally alarming that, after the offending appendix has been removed, a postoperative complication rate of up to 40% still occurs and is accepted.

The fact that the mortality of children with appendicitis has drastically declined over the last two decades may have led to a sense of false security. The number of children with appendicitis in the United States is estimated to be 80,000 annually.[4] Since the number of "negative appendices" reported since 1980 has ranged from 11% to 32%,[3, 6, 10, 33, 36, 49] 8,000–30,000 children will undergo an operation at which a normal appendix will be present, and in more than half of these no surgical condition will be found.[6, 36, 49] Thirty percent, or 20,000 children, will not be operated on until the appendix has perforated, leading to a complication in 20–40%, approximately 20,000 children.[33, 40, 58, 59, 62]

Incidence

Appendicitis is rarely seen in third-world countries where diets are high in fiber.[13] While there is no unanimity as to whether the incidence of appendicitis is increasing or decreasing, it appears that factors other than dietary fiber content may be responsible. The incidence of appendicitis in Sweden in 1982 decreased at the same time that the mean dietary fiber content in the Swedish diet was also declining.[3, 48]

Etiology

Wangensteen and Dennis demonstrated in 1939 that the ligation of the appendix was followed by a marked increase in intraluminal pressure, which ultimately surpassed systolic blood pressure.[70] As distention increases, capillaries and venules become clotted, thrombosis and ulceration produce necrosis of the wall, and fluid exudes into the peritoneal cavity. The ulceration of mucosa and muscularis leads to bacterial invasion and finally perforation. Obstruction is the prime cause of appendicitis. The obstruction of the appendix is most often due to inspissated, sometimes calcified, fecal material, which has been documented radiologically in 20% of children with appendicitis. "Inspissated fecal material" was present in 65% of children with perforated appendices, as compared with 25% in nonperforative appendicitis.[60] Obstruction of the appendiceal lumen can also be caused by bacterial infections, including those due to *Yersinia, Salmonella* and *Shigella*.[54, 56, 57] Enteric and systemic viral infections, including measles and chickenpox, can lead to appendiceal edema.[38] Anomalies of mucus-secreting glands, such as seen in cystic fibrosis, are probably responsible for the increased incidence of appendicitis in patients with cystic fibrosis.[46] Local obstruction of the appendix due to the common infestation with pinworms is extremely rare, but *Ascaris* can obstruct, leading to appendicitis.[59] Carcinoid tumors of the appendix rarely cause obstruction, since they are usually located distally. If they are located in the proximal third, they may cause appendicitis.[57] Foreign bodies in the appendix may lead to a perforation, and appendectomy is therefore indicated if such a foreign body is seen in abdominal films (see History section).

Psychological stress has been postulated to lead to an immunologic deficiency, which in turn could lead to a local pathologic reaction with subsequent appendicitis.[16] An increased familial incidence of appendicitis has also been suggested—70% in children with appendicitis as compared with only 13% in a control group.[2]

Diagnosis

The first symptom of the classic triad of pain, vomiting, and fever consists of periumbilical pain. Obstruction of the appendix leads to distention, relaying pain via stretch receptors through visceral nerve fibers to the tenth thoracic ganglion, so that pain is perceived in the umbilical dermatome. The periumbilical pain occurs regardless of the location of the appendix, whether intraperitoneal, retrocolic, or retrocecal. Inflammation follows, with vomiting and fever. The inflammatory exudate causes a localized pain in the immediate area. If the appendix is located in the right lower quadrant, right lower quadrant tenderness develops. Since more than one third of appendices are either retrocolic or retrocecal and/or extend over the pelvic brim, the localization of the inflammation and therefore of the pain may vary.[15] The intensity of the localized pain, however, almost always supersedes the initial periumbilical pain of obstruction. Perforation of the appendix occasionally is accompanied by a short interval of reduced pain, followed by generalized pain and tenderness unless the perforation is sealed off. Intermittent vomiting and/or nausea following the inflammation occur in 80% of children, anorexia in 60%, and diarrhea in 5–10% (usually of a small, mucousy volume, as compared with the more voluminous diarrhea seen in enteritis).[24] In an occasional child, especially in the early phase of appendicitis, intermittent hunger may be present and does not therefore rule out acute appendicitis. While the triad of appendicitis—pain, vomiting, and fever—may be classic, it is not always present. Viral or bacterial infection may precede appendicitis, and therefore the symptoms of the preceding infection may mask the developing appendicitis. In patients with viral or bacterial enteritis, the order of symptoms is usually reversed; nausea, vomiting, and fever precede the abdominal pain.

The review of the patient's history should include preexisting or recurring abdominal symptoms, allergies, systemic disorders, growth and development, and family and social conditions.

Physical Examination

Physical examination of a child with suspected appendicitis follows the cardinal rule: look, listen, feel. The gait of a child with appendicitis, a slight limp, hesitation to climb onto the examining table, inability to stretch the right leg, or scoliosis may suggest acute appendicitis even before the child is examined. Abdominal bruises may indicate unknown, or intentionally withheld, history of trauma. Lower limb infections can cause iliac adenitis, resembling appendicitis. Bowel sounds with early acute appendicitis are usually normal, only occasionally high-pitched, in contrast to the hyperperistalsis usually found in patients with enteritis. Advanced inflammatory changes, such as the perforation of an appendix, usually lead to an ominously quiet abdomen. Examination is required to rule out upper respiratory infections, especially right lower lobe pneumonia. Abdominal palpation, unless gentle, increases abdominal pain and tenderness and therefore increases voluntary guarding, especially in the apprehensive child. Sedation (Nembutal 2 mg/kg) will not mask the underlying process but will allay the anxiety of the child, allowing a more thorough physical examination. Abdominal palpation, sometimes using the stethoscope or the child's own hands, should start in a site opposite the suspected disease, usually the left lower quadrant. The examination gently proceeds to the left upper quadrant, the right upper quadrant, until midabdomen and right lower quadrant are reached. Tenderness at McBurney's point remains the most important finding on physical examination. Voluntary guarding is usually present in the early phase of acute appendicitis, followed by an involuntary spasm with progressive inflammation, and rebound tenderness with the onset of peritonitis. Voluntary guarding is usually overcome by sedation. It is rare that spasm is suppressed by sedation with Nembutal, and persistent spasm is therefore a reliable indicator of peritoneal irritation. Positive obturator or psoas signs suggest a retrocecal or retrocolonic inflammation. Abdominal pain and tenderness extending either into the scrotum, vulva, or past the inguinal ligament may indicate genitourinary causes or radicular nerve pain. Rebound tenderness should not be looked for until the entire physical examination is completed because, if positive, the child will thereafter anticipate pain with any further physical examination and display voluntary guarding at all times.

The diagnostic value of a rectal examination in children with appendicitis has been questioned.[4, 9, 10, 15, 17, 25, 53] Pain and rectal tenderness during rectal examination, indicating appendicitis, are present in only about 50% of patients with appendicitis, but are also present in about half of children without appendicitis.[10, 15] Rectal examination should always be performed in the adolescent female, however, to rule out uterine tubo-ovarian disease. Rectal examination may be helpful, even in early appendicitis, if the appendix extends over the brim of the pelvis.[9] It can also rule out other entities, such as constipation or chronic intestinal inflammatory disease, and allow evaluation of the rectal content. Rectal examination remains an essential part of a complete physical examination.

Appendicitis in Preschool Children

The difficulty in diagnosing acute appendicitis correctly, and early, in preschool children is illustrated by a perforation rate of 50–70%.[8, 24, 63] Delay between the onset of symptoms and admission to the hospital is responsible for perforation in more than one third of these children. The other two thirds, before perforation, however, have been seen at some point during their illness by a physician and treated with antibiotics, antihistamines, or antipyretics.[8, 24] The classic triad of pain, vomiting, and fever is usually not clearly apparent in the young child. Irritability or listlessness may be the first symptom, followed by vomiting. A change in bowel habit is frequently seen, and diarrhea is usually more extensive than in the older child. The physical examination in the small child requires even more patience and gentleness, and sedation plays an even greater role in the apprehensive preschool child.

Neonatal Appendicitis

Fewer than 0.2% of cases of appendicitis occur in children under the age of 1 year and even fewer in neonates.[5] Preterm infants and males are more commonly involved.[31, 61] The cause of neonatal appendicitis is not clear, but an association with other diseases, such as Hirschsprung's disease or necrotizing enterocolitis, has been well established.[5, 12, 25, 42, 61] X-ray and physical findings may be identical to those of necrotizing enterocolitis. In infants without pneumatosis and an abnormal gas pattern, free intraperitoneal fluid, and, occasionally, a fecalith may be apparent. In children beyond the neonatal age but below school age, calcified fecaliths were found in 28%.[25] The most common findings on physical examination consist of abdominal distention followed by local tenderness and occasional abdominal wall erythema.[12, 20, 61] Intra-abdominal neonatal appendiceal perforation led to a mortality rate ranging from 59.5% to 100%.[31, 38] In contrast, survival is much more likely in neonates with scrotal appendicitis.[27, 40]

Laboratory Examination

The total white blood cell count is usually not significantly increased in the early phase of acute appendicitis, and a change in the differential cell count precedes leucocytosis in most children.[11] While a normal white blood cell count is not significant, leukocytosis usually indicates impending or actual perforation.[66] Sedimentation rate, on the other hand, is normal in the first 24 hours during the obstructive phase.[20] Urine microscopic examination is of importance, since urinary tract infection is one of the more common differential diagnoses. It should be kept in mind, however, that the propinquity of appendix and urinary tract can lead to simulation of urinary tract infection in patients with acute appendicitis.[10] Serum amylase levels can also be increased with appendicitis.[68] Since bacterial infections, like *Yersinia*, are frequently associated with appendicitis, a positive serological test result does not rule out acute appendicitis.[6, 45, 56, 58]

X-ray Findings

Radiological examination may be helpful if the clinical diagnosis is in doubt or if perforation is suspected. Suggestive radiological signs of acute appendicitis consist of an abnormal gas pattern in the right lower quadrant, scoliosis, and obliteration of the psoas shadow[25] (Fig 105–1). A fecalith can be visualized in 10–

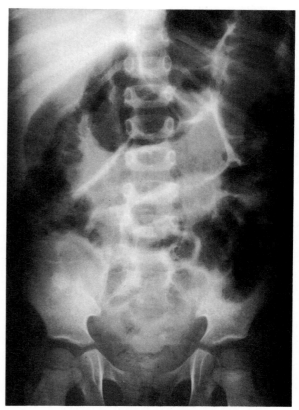

Fig 105–1.—Radiological features of acute appendicitis. A laminated appendiceal fecalith is located in the right lower quadrant. A cecal mass effect is present, with an abnormal gas pattern, localized ileus, and mild right-sided scoliosis.

20% of cases, or more often in younger children. An obstructive pattern develops after an abscess has formed and extraluminal air, usually a small amount, may be present after perforation. In patients with clinical or laboratory findings suggestive of urinary tract infection, an intravenous urogram may be indicated. Barium enema has been recommended as a diagnostic study by various authors.[4, 26, 65] If the entire appendiceal lumen can be visualized, appendicitis is unlikely. False negative interpretations can occur, however, when only part of the lumen is visualized and the distal portion of the appendix is blocked. Since the length of the appendix in an individual patient is not known, additional findings, such as a pressure effect on the ileum or cecum or irritability during fluoroscopy, should be looked for. False-positive findings can occur, since 5–10% of normal appendices cannot be visualized with barium studies. Barium enema, while probably not indicated in most patients, may be helpful in high-risk patients with immune suppression, nephrosis, hemolytic syndrome, or other conditions where operative intervention is dangerous.

In patients with suspected perforation, the radiological localization of a fecalith in an extraluminal position can help the surgeon to retrieve it at operation and avoid a postoperative abscess. Contrast studies showing partial blockage of the appendiceal lumen have been alleged to explain "recurrent crampy abdominal pain." Seventy-two percent of children with recurrent crampy abdominal pain were found to have a fecal cast or distention of the appendix without any evidence of inflammatory changes after the appendix was removed.[60] We believe strongly that diagnoses like "recurrent crampy abdominal pain" or "chronic appendicitis" are not acceptable indications for appendectomy, since their use may create another entity—"chronic remunerative appendicitis."

Laparoscopy and Sonography

Laparoscopy has been advocated in recent years in patients with atypical histories and findings suggestive of appendicitis, especially in females of child-bearing age. While unnecessary open operation may have been avoided, anesthesia is usually used in children.[19, 39, 43] In our experience, the most common finding, uterine tubo-ovarian pathology, can be diagnosed through a noninvasive procedure such as sonography. Sonography can also demonstrate a normal appendix in a child with leukemic typhlitis.[18, 69] It is particularly helpful in children with either preoperative or postoperative appendiceal abscesses.

Differential Diagnosis

The difficulty in arriving at an early, correct diagnosis of acute appendicitis has persisted, and the number of "negative appendices" has remained essentially unchanged over the last 30 years, in spite of the improvement of laboratory and imaging devices. Yet the simple use of an intensive repeat examination in the hospital, as shown by White and Haller in 1975, reduced unnecessary appendectomies from 20% to 6% without increasing the rate of perforation.[71]

The differential diagnoses to be considered include several main groups: intestinal diseases, uterine tubo-ovarian pathology, urinary tract infection, trauma, respiratory and systemic diseases.

Among intestinal diseases, viral and bacterial enteritis are most common. A depressed white blood cell count, part of a preceding viral infection with lymphocytosis rather than leukocytosis, can therefore occur in a patient with acute appendicitis following enteritis. Bacterial enteritis, including *Salmonella, Shigella,* and *Yersinia* may precede, lead to, or exist simultaneously with appendicitis. Chronic inflammatory diseases, including ulcerative colitis, or Crohn's disease, can occur sequentially or simultaneously.[29] If Crohn's disease is suspected at operation, the appendix can be safely removed. The incidence of fecal fistula formation after appendectomy in patients with Crohn's disease is minimal.[29] The histological examination of the removed appendix may ascertain the diagnosis of granulomatous disease. Other intestinal lesions mimicking appendicitis include the occasional Meckel's diverticulum, intussusception, and leukemic typhlitis.[6, 49] Primary peritonitis should be diagnosed or ruled out through paracentesis, especially in patients with nephrotic syndrome.[6, 36] Serositis or primary peritonitis, not associated with the nephrotic syndrome, was found in a surprisingly large number of patients by Bell, who considers it a self-limiting bacterial infection.[6] Vasculitis such as lupus erythematosus or periarteritis nodosa can occasionally present with intestinal symptoms preceding renal symptoms.[37] Infarction of the omentum or fatty appendages has also led to symptoms resembling acute appendicitis.[36] The diagnosis of mesenteric adenitis, a commonly used differential diagnosis, especially after a normal appendix has been removed, should be strictly limited to cases with proved viral cultures. Since most children have large mesenteric nodes, the surgeon's clinical diagnosis of mesenteric adenitis is not acceptable, since other surgical entities leading to the operative diagnosis are then likely to be overlooked. Uterine tubo-ovarian lesions in children include salpingitis, pregnancy, ovarian cysts, torsion, tumors, hematocolpos, and endometriosis.[44] Both upper and lower urinary tract infections, including vesiculitis, can present with findings suggestive of appendicitis. Systemic diseases must be ruled out, largely by an adequate review of the patient's history. They can include hematologic disorders, such as Schön-lein-Henoch purpura, rheumatic fever, juvenile diabetes, abdominal epilepsy, hyperlipemia, porphyria, and sickle cell disease.[6, 36]

Unrecognized trauma, especially in the young abused child, may simulate appendicitis. Foreign bodies, usually an incidental radiological finding, rarely perforate, but since they also tend to remain stagnant in the appendix, an appendectomy is indicated.

Therapy of Nonperforated Appendicitis

Acute nonperforating appendicitis presents a surgical emergency. Once the diagnosis has been established, preparation for the operation can be limited to basic laboratory determinations, such as hematocrit, white blood cell count, BUN, and urinalysis. If the patient has been vomiting, serum electrolytes and urinary specific gravity should be determined. If the patient has not been sedated before the examination, Demerol (1 mg/kg) and Nembutal (1–2 mg/kg) are given intramuscularly to relieve the patient's anxiety. If the patient has vomited or eaten within 6 hours of the operation, a nasogastric tube is inserted and the stomach emptied. A half-isotonic intravenous solution (if the patient has not vomited) or isotonic saline or Ringer's lactate (if the patient has vomited) is administered. If the patient is febrile, the temperature should be controlled after the patient has been sedated, and atropine is withheld until the patient is in the operating room. Depending on the institution's protocol, a limited prophylactic course of antibiotics can be given. The routine use of preoperative antibiotics in children with acute nonperforating appendicitis is still controversial, but the number of wound infections in children with acute appendicitis without perforation has been reported to be relatively high.[22] The use of preoperative antibiotics has lowered the postoperative wound infection in several prospective studies to a rate of 0% to 2%.[14, 72, 73] All prophylactic antibiotics should be limited to a simple preoperative dose or to 24 hours of administration only.[7]

Before the incision is made, the abdomen is re-examined under anesthesia. If no unusual findings are present, the abdomen is opened through a transverse right lower quadrant incision. In girls, we make a skin incision at least 1 inch below McBurney's point and then retract the skin upward to place the muscular incision over McBurney's point. This lowers the unsightly scar to the rather low "belt line" of today's ladies' fashion. After the peritoneum has been opened, the cecum, terminal ileum, and most likely sites of appendiceal location are palpated. If the appendix is found in a normal intraperitoneal position, the cecum is gently mobilized and the appendix brought into the wound. If the appendix cannot be palpated, the incision may have to be enlarged, sometimes transecting the rectus muscle to allow adequate exposure. The technique of appendiceal ligation varies; we have employed Dennis' method of inverting with a single purse-string suture the open appendiceal stump after it has been divided and cauterized. The subserosal branch of the appendiceal artery should be ligated to avoid postoperative bleeding. The open inversion eliminates the potential formation of a mucocele, which may occur if the appendiceal stump is ligated and then inverted. If a normal appendix is found, the abdomen should be thoroughly explored, including uterus and tubo-ovarian structures in girls, large and small bowel in both sexes. In patients with acute appendicitis, where the appendix appears enlarged and firm rather than cystic, the specimen should be opened at the table to rule out neoplasms, such as carcinoid, to assure that the margin of excision is free of tumor. If a gridiron incision is used, peritoneal and fascial layers are closed with running chromic sutures; the wound is not drained. The patient is usually able to eat within 24 hours, and the average hospitalization should be less than 4 days.

Therapy of Perforated Appendicitis

In approximately 30–40% of children, the appendix will have perforated at the time of operation. The previously accepted postoperative complication rate of 20–40% is no longer acceptable. With appropriate surgical technique and parenteral and local antibiotics, the complication rate should be well under 10%.[62] Most postoperative complications are related to infection. Depending on the state of infection, a varying preponderance of bacteria will be found. In the early phase of appendiceal infection, aerobes, with *Escherichia coli,* are dominant. When gangrene or necrosis occurs, anaerobes are 1½ times more common than aerobes.[14, 66, 67] *Bacteroides fragilis* is the most common anaerobic organism and is usually found in early positive blood cultures.[40, 51, 58, 67] Bacteria grown from peritoneal cultures taken at operation are not always indicative of the bacteria causing the postoperative infection.[30] While *E. coli* is usually found as the dominant organism during operation, *Bacteroides* is more common in subsequent wound infections.[30, 66, 67] Stone found that the responsible organism for postoperative anaerobe infections included *Bacteroides* 100%, and, among aerobes, *E. coli* 81%, *Klebsiella* 52%, and *Pseudomonas* 5%.[66] Enterococci, largely a part of a synergistic infection, followed.

The ideal antibiotic should be effective against anaerobes, aerobes, and other most likely encountered bacteria; have a low toxicity; and be cost-effective. Recent studies indicate that various combinations of antibiotics—mainly aminoglycosides, gentamicin, clindamycin, and cephalosporins—have drastically lowered the complication rate from infections.[20, 41, 51, 52, 62] Even a single drug such as metronidazole in patients with perforated appendicitis was effective if given preoperatively and postoperatively for 2 days, reducing wound infections to 7%.[21] Third-generation cephalosporins or supercillins, such as piperacillin, might eventually replace multiple-drug treatment. At present, we have largely adhered to Schwartz's protocol, developed in Boston Children's Hospital.[62] In children with suspected perforated appendicitis, the following antibiotics are given preoperatively: gentamicin (5 mg/kg/24 hr), ampicillin (100 mg/kg/24 hr), clindamycin (40 mg/kg/24 hr). After the appendix has been removed, the peritoneal cavity is then irrigated either with saline or kanamycin (2 gm/L) or cephalothin (4 gm/L). If kanamycin is used, the anesthetist should be informed, to avoid possible respiratory complications. Saline irrigation of the peritoneal cavity has been feared to lead to a wider distribution of the offending bacteria in the presence of peritonitis. It has been clearly shown, however, that intraperitoneal bacteria are found in the diaphragmatic lymphatics within a few minutes after their intraperitoneal instillation. This indicates that, in patients with peritonitis, bacteria have already been diffusely disseminated before operation and that further irrigation is unlikely to increase their distribution. Saline irrigation alone, especially if the saline is left behind in the peritoneal cavity, has been shown to interfere with the peritoneal immune defense by diluting opsonins.[64] Parenteral antibiotics are continued for approximately 1 week. If massive diarrhea occurs following the use of clindamycin, it should be discontinued immediately and vancomycin started.

Operative Therapy of Perforated Appendicitis

The patient is re-examined under anesthesia. If no mass is felt, a standard horizontal muscle-splitting incision is used. In most children, the perforated appendix can be removed. In patients in whom the appendix cannot be safely removed, the appendiceal abscess is drained with Penrose drains exiting through the lateral edge of the wound and an interval appendectomy performed 4–8 weeks later. Drainage of the wound has remained controversial. While delayed wound closure in perforated appendicitis has almost uniformly shown a low infection rate, our results are similar to those with wound drainage and primary closure when covered by multiple antibiotics.[10, 25]

Fowler's position may have reduced the number of multiple intra-abdominal abscesses before the advent of antibiotics by encouraging the formation of pelvic or right lower quadrant abscesses, which at that time were more amenable to operative therapy.[64] Both experimental and clinical evidence indicate that Fowler's position may decrease the absorption of bacteria and lymphatic drainage and therefore increase postoperative complications rather than decrease them. Like others, we therefore no longer encourage the use of Fowler's position.[62]

Appendiceal Abscess

Abscess formation occurs frequently in preschool children with perforation of the appendix.[24] In a few children, an appendiceal abscess may be completely walled off without any signs of peritonitis, toxemia, or obstruction. In these children, primary nonoperative therapy, either with or without antibiotics, has been reported to result in fewer complications than immediate operative intervention.[32, 52] It should be stressed that the primary nonoperative therapy, or "sitting on an appendiceal abscess" is only indicated in an occasional child and must be accompanied by close observation with immediate operative intervention if peritoneal or systemic signs of infection recur.

Postoperative Complications

Even though the postoperative infection rate, using a combination of preoperative and postoperative antibiotics and thorough debridement at the time of operation, has been reduced to as low as 5% in patients with perforated appendicitis, infections still occur.[62] Wound infections are usually due to anaerobic organisms, occasionally *Staphylococcus,* and usually respond to simple drainage. Persistent postoperative fever, pain, and adynamic ileus are common clinical signs of intra-abdominal infection. If the site of the infection cannot be demonstrated by physical examination, radiography, occasionally a gallium scan, sonography, or computed axial tomographic (CAT) scan should help to demonstrate the location. Since in the early stages a differential diagnosis between a phlegmon and abscess may be difficult and operative intervention for a phlegmon not only less effective but potentially more dangerous, an attempt should be made to observe the maturation of an abscess unless the patient's sepsis or toxemia warrants immediate operative intervention.[34] Occasionally, spontaneous drainage of the abscess or a positive response to antibiotics may make an operation unnecessary. Cutaneous fecal fistula, if draining freely and without distal obstruction, rarely requires operative intervention. Early intestinal obstruction, within the first week after operation for a perforated appendicitis, is common and usually responds to nasogastric decompression. If the response is inadequate, the obstruction is usually due to an active inflammation, such as an interloop abscess, rather than to fibrous bands.

Sterility

Although a marked increase of sterility is often said to follow perforative appendicitis in females, we have been unable to find any hard statistical data. Since the hypothesis has been accepted medically, however, the surgeon treating a girl with perforated appendicitis must be aware of the medicolegal aspects.[12]

Pylephlebitis

Pylephlebitis is the result of an appendiceal inflammation spreading into the portal venous system. Multiple liver ab-

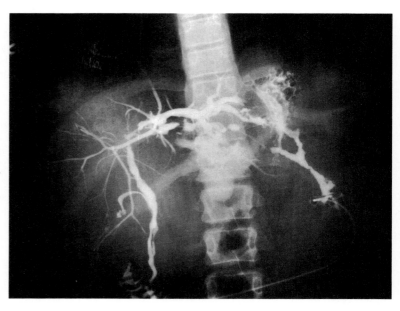

Fig 105–2.—Pylephlebitis due to neglected appendicitis. Cholangiogram in a 10-year-old boy with late sequelae following appendiceal perforation: pylephlebitis and cholangitis. A biliary subdiaphragmatic fistula is located in the right upper quadrant, a hepatogastric fistula in the left upper quadrant, and several biliary cutaneous fistulae in the midabdomen. Intrahepatic and extrahepatic ducts exhibit constrictive changes consistent with chronic cholangitis, which followed perforation of pylephlebitic abscesses into the biliary ductal system. He survived but has poor liver function and portal hypertension.

scesses, sometimes confluent, can occur, leading to liver destruction. Even prompt operative intervention with removal of the perforated appendix may not stop the inflammation in the portal mesenteric veins, which can lead to continuous liver abscesses, septic thrombosis of the portal venous system, and cholangitis. An example of postappendiceal pylephlebitis is shown in Figure 105–2. A 10-year-old boy with symptoms and findings of acute appendicitis was treated as for enteritis, only to return after 3 weeks with jaundice and fever. He survived, after multiple operative interventions and a hepatojejunostomy over the course of a 13-month hospitalization. His liver function is markedly reduced. He has a completely obliterated portal venous system with esophageal-gastric-enteric varices and hypersplenism. His life expectancy is marginal as the result of the missed diagnosis of a simple pathologic entity—acute appendicitis.

REFERENCES

1. Allen D.C., Biggart J.D.: Granulomatous disease in the vermiform appendix. *J. Clin. Pathol.* 36:632–638, 1983.
2. Andersson N., Griffiths H., et al.: Is appendicitis familial? *Br. Med. J.* 2:697–698, 1979.
3. Arnbjornsson E., Asp N.G., et al.: Decreasing incidence of acute appendicitis, with special reference to the consumption of dietary fiber. *Acta Chir. Scand.* 148:461–464, 1982.
4. Ballantine T.V.N.: Appendicitis. *Surg. Clin. North Am.* 6:1117–1124, 1981.
5. Bax N.M.A., Pearse R.G., et al.: Perforation of the appendix in the neonatal period. *J. Pediatr. Surg.* 15:200–202, 1980.
6. Bell M.J., Bower R.J., et al.: Appendectomy in childhood. *Am. J. Surg.* 144:335–337, 1982.
7. Bell M.J., Kosloske A.M., et al.: Antimicrobial prophylaxis in pediatric surgical patients. Communication AAP Committee on Infectious Disease, 1983, pp. 1–7.
8. Boles E.T., Ireton R.J., et al.: Acute appendicitis in children. *Arch. Surg.* 79:447–454, 1959.
9. Bonello J.C., Abrams J.S.: The significance of a "positive" rectal examination in acute appendicitis. *Dis. Colon Rectum* 22:97–101, 1978.
10. Bower R.J., Bell M.J., et al.: Controversial aspects of appendicitis management in children. *Arch. Surg.* 116:885–887, 1981.
11. Bower R.J., Bell M.J., et al.: Diagnostic value of the white blood count and neutrophil percentage in the evaluation of abdominal pain in children. *Surg. Gynecol. Obstet.* 152:424–426, 1981.
12. Buntain W.L.: Neonatal appendicitis mistaken for necrotizing enterocolitis. *South. Med. J.* 75:1155, 1982.
13. Burkitt D.P.: The aetiology of appendicitis. *Br. J. Surg.* 58:695–699, 1971.
14. Busuttil R.W., Davidson R.K., et al.: Effect of prophylactic antibiotics in acute nonperforated appendicitis. *Ann. Surg.* 194:502–509, 1981.
15. Cloud D.T.: Appendicitis. *J. Pediatr. Surg.* 925:498–508, 1980.
16. Creed F.: Life events and appendicectomy. *Lancet* 1:1381–1385, 1981.
17. Daehlin L.: Acute appendicitis during the first three years of life. *Acta Chir. Scand.* 148:291–294, 1982.
18. Deutsch A., Leopold G.R.: Ultrasonic demonstration of the inflamed appendix: Case report. *Radiology* 140:163–164, 1981.
19. Deutsch A.A., Zelikovsky A., et al.: Laparoscopy in the prevention of unnecessary appendicectomies: A prospective study. *Br. J. Surg.* 69:336–337, 1982.
20. Doraiswamy N.V.: Progress of acute appendicitis: A study in children. *Br. J. Surg.* 65:877–879, 1978.
21. Flannigan G.M., Carver R.A., et al.: Antibiotic prophylaxis in acute appendicitis. *Surg. Gynecol. Obstet.* 156:209–211, 1983.
22. Giacomantonio M., Bortolussi R., et al.: Should prophylactic antibiotics be given perioperatively in acute appendicitis without perforation? *Can. J. Surg.* 25:555–556, 1982.
23. Golladay E.S., Roskes S., et al.: Intestinal obstruction from appendiceal abscess in a newborn infant. *J. Pediatr. Surg.* 13:175–176, 1978.
24. Graham J.M., Pokorny W.J., et al.: Acute appendicitis in preschool age children. *Am. J. Surg.* 139:247–250, 1980.
25. Grosfeld J.L., Weinberger M., et al.: Acute appendicitis in the first two years of life. *J. Pediatr. Surg.* 8:285–293, 1973.
26. Hatch E.I., Jr., Naffis D., et al.: Pitfalls in the use of barium enema in early appendicitis in children. *J. Pediatr. Surg.* 16:309, 312, 1981.
27. Heydenrych J.J., Du Toit D.F.: Unusual presentation of acute appendicitis in the neonate. *S. Afr. Med. J.* 62:1003–1005, 1982.
28. Holgersen L.O., Suleman M.: Acute appendicitis in incarcerated inguinal hernia. *N.Y. State J. Med.* 80:1739, 1980.
29. Jacobson S.: Crohn's disease of the appendix, manifested as acute appendicitis with postoperative fistula. *Am. J. Gastroenterol.* 71:592–597, 1979.
30. Jaffers G.J., Pollock T.W.: Intraoperative culturing during surgery for acute appendicitis. *Arch. Surg.* 116:866–868, 1981.
31. Janik J.S., Firor H.V.: Pediatric appendicitis. *Arch. Surg.* 114:717–719, 1979.
32. Janik J.S., Ein S.H., et al.: Nonsurgical management of appendiceal mass in late presenting children. *J. Pediatr. Surg.* 15:574–576, 1980.
33. Jess P., Bjerregaard B., et al.: Acute appendicitis: Prospective trial concerning diagnostic accuracy and complications. *Am. J. Surg.* 141:232–234, 1981.
34. Jordan J.S., Kovalcik P.J., et al.: Appendicitis with a palpable mass. *Ann. Surg.* 193:227–229, 1981.
35. Kassner E.G., Mutchler R.W., et al.: Uncomplicated foreign bodies of the appendix in children: Radiologic observations. *J. Pediatr. Surg.* 9:207–211, 1974.
36. Knight P.J., Vassy L.E.: Specific diseases mimicking appendicitis in childhood. *Arch. Surg.* 116:744–746, 1981.

37. Kumazawa H.: Periarteritis nodosa presenting as acute appendicitis. *Z. Kinderchir.* 32:181–183, 1981.
38. Kwong M.S., Dinner M.: Neonatal appendicitis masquerading as necrotizing enterocolitis. *J. Pediatr.* 96:918, 1980.
39. Leape L.L., Ramenofsky M.L.: Laparoscopy for questionable appendicitis. Can it reduce the negative appendectomy rate? *Ann. Surg.* 191:410–413, 1980.
40. Marchildon M.B., Dudgeon D.L.: Perforated appendicitis: Current experience in a childrens hospital. *Ann. Surg.* 185:84–87, 1977.
41. Marier R.L., Altemeier W.A., et al.: Antibiotic therapy for the surgical patient. Infections in Surgery, roundtable discussion. New York, Surgical Case Publications, Inc., 1983, pp. 1–11.
42. Martin L.W., Perrin E.V.: Neonatal perforation of the appendix in association with Hirschsprung's disease. *Ann. Surg.* 166:799–802, 1967.
43. Meoli F.G., Pinzler D.: Diagnosis of acute appendicitis: A retrospective study of 401 cases. *J. Am. Osteopath. Assoc.* 80:657–661, 1981.
44. Mittal V.K., Choudhury S.P., et al.: Endometriosis of the appendix presenting as acute appendicitis. *Am. J. Surg.* 142:519–521, 1981.
45. Morrison J.D.: Yersinia and viruses in acute non-specific abdominal pain and appendicitis. *Br. J. Surg.* 68:284–286, 1981.
46. Oestreich A.E., Adelstein E.H.: Appendicitis as the presenting complaint in cystic fibrosis. *J. Pediatr. Surg.* 17:191–194, 1982.
47. Peltokallio P., Tykka H.: Evolution of the age distribution and mortality of acute appendicitis. *Arch. Surg.* 116:153–155, 1981.
48. Pieper R., Kager L.: The incidence of acute appendicitis and appendectomy. *Acta Chir. Scand.* 148:45–49, 1982.
49. Pieper R., Kager L., et al.: Acute appendicitis: A clinical study of 1018 cases of emergency appendectomy. *Acta Chir. Scand.* 148:51–62, 1982.
50. Pieper R., Kager L., et al.: Clinical significance of mucosal inflammation of the vermiform appendix. *Ann. Surg.* 197:368–374, 1983.
51. Pieper R., Kager L., et al.: The role of *Bacteroides fragilis* in the pathogenesis of acute appendicitis. *Acta Chir. Scand.* 148:39–44, 1982.
52. Powers R.J., Andrassy R.J., et al.: Alternate approach to the management of acute perforating appendicitis in children. *Surg. Gynecol. Obstet.* 152:473–475, 1981.
53. Puri P., O'Donnell B.: Appendicitis in infancy. *J. Pediatr. Surg.* 13:173–174, 1978.
54. Rabau M.Y., Avigad I., et al.: Rubella and acute appendicitis. *Pediatrics* 66:813, 1980.
55. Raifman M.A., Berant M.: Barium enema re acute appendicitis. *J. Pediatr.* 93:727, 1978.
56. Rodgers B., Karn G.: Yersinia enterocolitis. *J. Pediatr. Surg.* 10:497–499, 1975.
57. Sanders D.Y., Cort C.R., et al.: Shigellosis associated with appendicitis. *J. Pediatr. Surg.* 7:315–317, 1972.
58. Scher K.S., Coil J.A. Jr.: The continuing challenge of perforating appendicitis. *Surg. Gynecol. Obstet.* 150:535–538, 1980.
59. Scher K.S., Coil J.A. Jr.: Appendicitis: Factors that influence the frequency of perforation. *South. Med. J.* 73:1561–1563, 1980.
60. Schisgall R.M.: Appendiceal colic in childhood: The role of inspissated casts of stool within the appendix. *Ann. Surg.* 192:687–693, 1980.
61. Schorlemmer G.R., Herbst C.A. Jr.: Perforated neonatal appendicitis. *South. Med. J.* 76:536–537, 1983.
62. Schwartz M.Z., Tapper D., et al.: Management of perforated appendicitis in children. *Ann. Surg.* 197:407–411, 1983.
63. Siegal B., Hyman E., et al.: Acute appendicitis in early childhood. *Helv. Paediatr. Acta* 37:215–219, 1982.
64. Simmons R.L.: *Peritonitis and Intra-abdominal Abscesses: Principles Governing Treatment.* Kalamazoo, Mich., Upjohn Co., 1982, pp. 1–28.
65. Smith D.E., Kirchmer N.A., et al.: Use of the barium enema in the diagnosis of acute appendicitis and its complications. *Am. J. Surg.* 138:829–834, 1979.
66. Stone H.H.: Bacterial flora of appendicitis in children. *J. Pediatr. Surg.* 11:37–42, 1976.
67. Stone H.H., Kolb L.D., et al.: Incidence and significance of intraperitoneal anaerobic bacteria. *Ann. Surg.* 181:705–715, 1975.
68. Swensson E.E., Maull K.I.: Clinical significance of elevated serum and urine amylase levels in patients with appendicitis. *Am. J. Surg.* 142:667–670, 1981.
69. Ver Steeg K., LaSalle A., et al.: Appendicitis in acute leukemia. *Arch. Surg.* 114:632–633, 1979.
70. Wangensteen O.H., Dennis C.: Experimental proof of the obstructive origin of appendicitis in man. *Ann. Surg.* 110:629–647, 1939.
71. White J.J., Santillana M., Haller J.A. Jr.: Intensive in-hospital observation: A safe way to decrease unnecessary appendectomy. *Am. Surg.* 41:793–798, 1975.
72. Winslow R.E., Dean R.E., et al.: Acute nonperforating appendicitis. Efficacy of brief antibiotic prophylaxis. *Arch. Surg.* 118:651–655, 1983.
73. Wright J.E.: Appendicitis in childhood: Reduction in wound infection with preoperative antibiotics. *Aust. N.Z. J. Surg.* 127–129, 1982.

106 William K. Sieber

Hirschsprung's Disease

HISTORY.—The earliest description of a case of Hirschsprung's disease is an autopsy report on a five-year-old girl by Frederick Ruysch in 1691.[82] Over 20 reports preceded Harald Hirschsprung's[63] classic description of congenital megacolon presented at the 1886 Pediatric Congress in Berlin. Finney's[52] review of 1908 summarized knowledge of this disorder to that time. In 1901, Tittel[144] described the absence of intramural ganglion cells in the rectum of a 15-month-old infant who had been constipated since birth. The term "megacolon" was introduced by Mya in 1894,[95] bringing attention to the then current interpretation of the large colon as the source of the problem. In 1940, Tiffin, Chandler, and Faber,[143] in describing a case of absent ganglion cells in the distal colon, suggested that the megacolon was primarily a disturbance of peristalsis in the ganglion-deficient intestine. Ehrenpreis' 1946[45] doctoral thesis, an exhaustive review of the etiology and pathogenesis of Hirschsprung's disease, pointed out that the diagnosis could be made in the neonate. Zuelzer and Wilson[156] in 1948 and Robertson and Kernohan[111] in 1938 correlated distal aganglionosis with intestinal obstruction in infancy.

Since aganglionic megacolon was not differentiated from other types of megacolon, the literature up to 1950 is confused by the inclusion of inappropriate material. In 1948, Swenson and Bill[134] presented a curative operative technique. Similar studies and conclusions were shortly presented by Hiatt[61] and by Bodian, Stephens, and Ward,[15] who made the definitive and convincingly unequivocal association of aganglionosis with Hirschsprung's disease. Neuhauser's radiologic studies[136] demonstrated the narrow rectum and distal colon, the transition zone, and the proximal dilatation. While many more have contributed to better understanding and management of patients with this anomaly, Duhamel's operative procedure[43] and Soave's[124] application of the endorectal pull-through procedure are outstanding contributions.

Definitions

Megacolon refers to an enlargement of the colon that may be functional, organic, or truly congenital in origin. Organic causes include postoperative strictures in repaired imperforate anus and partial colonic obstruction due to pelvic tumors. Functional causes are chronic constipation and the large colons associated with hypothyroidism and with mental retardation. True congenital megacolon is a congenital anomaly characterized by partial to complete colonic obstruction associated with the absence of intramural ganglion cells in the distal alimentary tract. The aganglionosis may extend proximally to involve the entire colon and, indeed, the entire alimentary tract, with appropriate associated symptoms. This disorder is known as "congenital aganglionosis," "aganglionic megacolon," or "Hirschsprung's disease." While the term "congenital intestinal aganglionosis" is the most accurate designation, "Hirschsprung's disease," the eponymic term of long usage, is here used to designate the disorder.

Pathology

The essential gross pathologic feature of Hirschsprung's disease is a dilated proximal intestine with gradual or abrupt transition to normal-calibered distal intestine. The area of transition is typically funnel-like or cone-shaped (Fig 106–1). The proximal intestinal wall is thickened, due to muscular hypertrophy and, often, edema; the intestine is increased in diameter as well as in length. The degree of proximal hypertrophy and dilatation depends on the duration and degree of obstruction and thus, indirectly, on the age of the patient. Intraluminal fecal concretions and impactions may be present in the dilated portion, and the mucosa may be ulcerated. The distal intestine looks normal. The transition, when it is in the small intestine, is less obvious and easily overlooked unless specifically sought (Fig 106–2). Enterocolitis may obscure the transitional zone.

The fundamental lesion in Hirschsprung's disease is the absence of intramural ganglion cells in the distal intestine. This absence involves both the submucosal and intermuscular nerve plexuses and is associated with an increase in the size and prominence of the nerve fibers. The absence extends for a varying distance proximally and may involve as little as the lower rec-

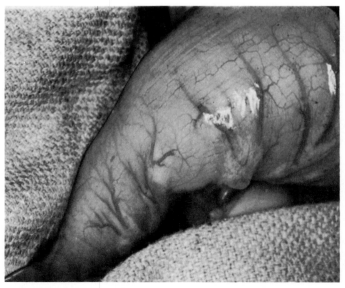

Fig 106–1.—Typical transitional area ("cone") in the rectosigmoid colon of a 2-year-old child with Hirschsprung's disease, as seen at operation.

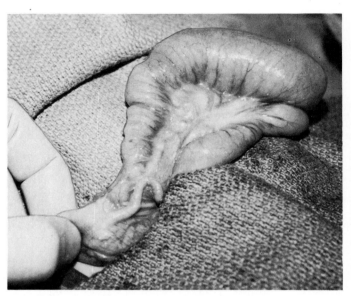

Fig 106–2.—Transitional zone in the ileum of an infant with Hirschsprung's disease, the aganglionosis extending into the terminal ileum (aganglionosis coli).

tum, or as much as the entire colon; in some instances, it extends well into the small intestine, even to include the entire gastrointestinal tract, exclusive of the stomach.[116] Our present concept is that this is an all-or-none phenomenon, that ganglion cells are either present or absent and both plexuses involved or uninvolved, and that the aganglionic section involves the bowel from the anus to the point at which ganglion cells are present more proximally, in normal bowel. This implies that "skip areas" do not occur and that a rectal biopsy containing ganglion cells eliminates the diagnosis of Hirschsprung's disease. Rare instances have been reported of an area of ganglionated bowel within the aganglionic bowel of total colonic aganglionosis.[154]

The histologic appearance of hematoxylin-eosin–stained sections of aganglionic intestine is not dramatically abnormal[151] (Fig 106–3). Ganglion cells, however, are absent from all layers of the bowel wall. The transition to normally innervated intestine may be gradual, with a long segment of intervening hypoganglionic intestine, but more often the transition is short and abrupt.[56] The zone of aganglionosis tends to be at a lower level on the antimesenteric side of the intestine than on the mesenteric side. The proximal extent of aganglionosis does not necessarily correlate with the gross transition to dilated intestine. The aganglionosis may extend well into the cone of dilated intestine. A local increase in the number of ganglion cells at the transition zone has been occasionally reported.[151] Large, predominantly nonmyelinated nerve trunks are commonly found in areas normally occupied by the nerve matrix (Fig 106–3,B). They tend to be most prominent distally. Neuroma-like conglomerations of nerve fibers are sometimes seen near the transition zone. There is no acceptable anatomical explanation for the well-known lack of correlation between the extent of aganglionosis and the severity of symptoms. Garrett et al.[55] noted that infants in whom severe symptoms occurred early tended to have large numbers of nerve fibers in the aganglionic intestine, whereas those with milder symptoms tended to have fewer. Although there are rare reports of aganglionosis of the colon with ganglion cells present distally in the rectum,[143] such a finding is contrary to most recorded experience.

The extent of aganglionosis in 220 patients of the Children's Hospital of Pittsburgh series is presented in Table 106–1. In a

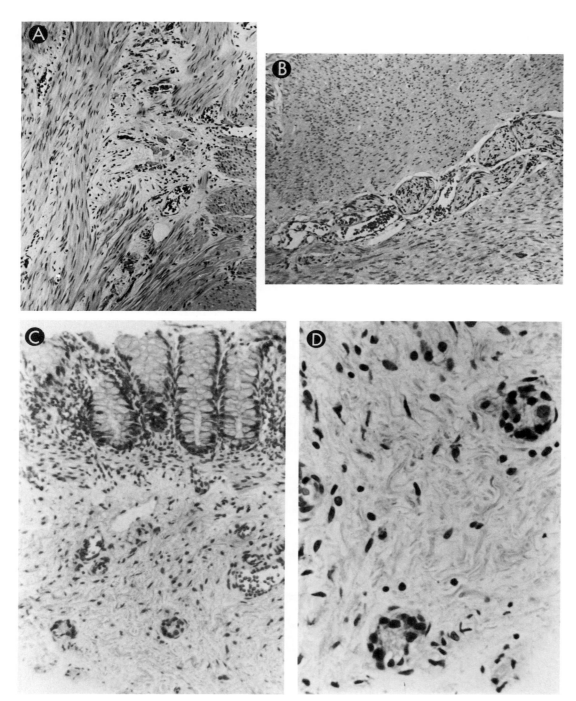

Fig 106–3.—Aganglionosis in Hirschsprung's disease. **A,** normal ganglion cells in a rectal biopsy specimen. **B,** absent ganglion cells in the presence of abnormal nerves in a rectal biopsy specimen from a patient with Hirschsprung's disease. **C,** cluster of ganglion cells in a newly born infant in a rectal biopsy specimen illustrating the similarity to other normal structures in this low-power view. **D,** high-power view of ganglion cells shown in **C.** The importance of experience and persistence in the evaluation of rectal biopsy material in the diagnosis of Hirschsprung's disease is apparent.

comprehensive review of the literature, Ehrenpreis[47] found aganglionosis confined to the rectum and rectosigmoid colon in 77% of patients, and involving the entire colon in 10%. The survey of American experience by Kleinhaus et al.[76] confirms this incidence. Hypoganglionosis, a marked decrease in the number of ganglion cells in the enteric plexuses, is found in the normal internal sphincter and to a variable extent in Hirschsprung's dis-

ease at the site of transition to normal intestine. Bentley[5] and Davidson and Bauer[34] reported cases of distal hypoganglionosis without aganglionosis, with symptoms simulating Hirschsprung's disease.

Histopathologic studies[49, 67, 68] have demonstrated an increase in the enzyme acetylcholinesterase in the aganglionic colon. This increase is greatest distally and appears to be less as the normally

TABLE 106–1.—Extent of Aganglionosis in 220 Patients, Children's Hospital of Pittsburgh Series

	TOTAL NO. (%) OF CASES	MALE	FEMALE
Short segment			
Rectosigmoid	117		
Sigmoid	54		
Total	171 (77.73)	143 (83.5)	28 (16.5)
Long segment			
Descending colon	11 (5.0)	6	5
Splenic flexure	9 (4.10)	7	2
Transverse colon	5 (2.27)	3	2
Hepatic flexure	1 (0.45)	1	0
Total colon and above	23 (10.45)	13 (56.5)	10 (43.5)
Total	49 (22.27)	30 (62.0)	19 (38.0)
Grand total	220	173 (78.7)	47 (21.3)

innervated area is approached. In the normal colon, acetylcholinesterase staining delineates the ganglia, and the nerves in both muscle layers. In aganglionic intestine, such staining demonstrates increased numbers of oversized nerve fibers in the muscularis mucosa, in the lamina propria of the mucosa, and in the submucosa, as well as in the musculature (Fig 106–4).

Hirschsprung's disease, as a maldevelopment of tissue derived from the neural crest, can be considered one of the neurocrestopathies. These hamartomatous, dysgenetic, and neoplastic conditions include pheochromocytoma, neuroblastoma, neurofibromatosis, medullary carcinoma of the thyroid gland, carcinoid tumors, and perigangliomas.[16] The common neuroectodermal origin of these seemingly diverse entities is reflected in their association as syndromes or clinical entities. Thus, neurofibromatosis (von Recklinghausen's disease) may be associated with megacolon[140] and neuroblastoma with Hirschsprung's disease.[31]

Hirschsprung's disease is usually a solitary anomaly in a full-term, otherwise healthy infant. Associated anomalies do occur with significant frequency (Table 106–2). Down syndrome occurs in approximately 5% of cases.[58] Congenital deafness[121] and an increased incidence of diabetes[23] have been observed. Congenital genitourinary anomalies are present in less than 5% of patients with Hirschsprung's disease.[48] Other alimentary tract anomalies are unusual. It is tempting to ascribe the acquired megacolon of repaired anorectal anomalies to associated Hirschsprung's disease. The combination of Hirschsprung's disease and anorectal anomalies is actually unusual enough to be the subject of single case reports.[75, 149] When a life-threatening associated anomaly is present, the infant rarely survives, and in these instances the diagnosis of Hirschsprung's disease is often made only at necropsy. The reported incidence of associated anomalies varies from less than 5% to 21%,[65] the great variation being due to the diligence with which they are sought and the manner in which they are reported.

Embryology

Nerve cells of the alimentary tract can be detected, as early as 5 weeks of gestation, as immature neuroblasts in the well-formed cervical vagal trunks that supply nerve fibers to the esophagus.[100] The neurenteric ganglion cells migrate from the neural crest to the upper end of the alimentary tract and then follow the vagal fibers caudally. Neuroblasts are recognized intramurally in the esophagus by the sixth week of gestation. By the seventh week, they are found as far distally as the midgut, and they have arrived at the mid-transverse colon by the eighth week. Migration to the most distal portion of the alimentary tract is completed by the 12th week of gestation. Intramural migration from the circular muscle layer to the submucosal area completes the distribution of neuroblasts. Smith[122] pointed out that maturation of neuroblasts into ganglion cells continues well into the second

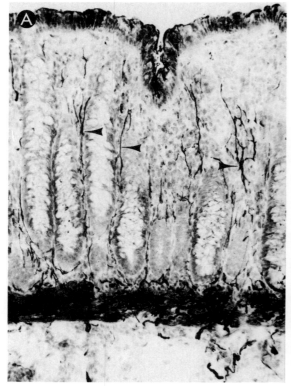

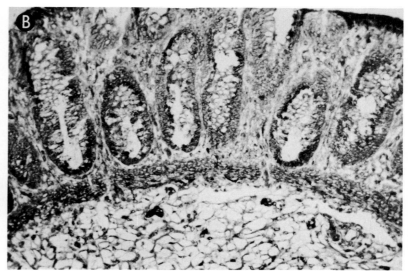

Fig 106–4.—Acetylcholinesterase staining in Hirschsprung's disease. **A,** section stained for acetylcholinesterase in a patient with Hirschsprung's disease. *Arrows* point to the stained nerve fibers in the lamina propria. There is dense staining in the muscularis mucosa. **B,** rectal suction mucosal biopsy specimen of normal rectum, stained for acetylcholinesterase. No nerve fibers are seen and there is little staining in the normal intestine of this patient.

TABLE 106–2.—CONGENITAL ANOMALIES NOTED IN 42
OF 220 PATIENTS WITH HIRSCHSPRUNG'S DISEASE,
CHILDREN'S HOSPITAL OF PITTSBURGH SERIES

Alimentary tract		9
Esophageal atresia with tracheoesophageal fistula	1	
Imperforate anus	1	
Malrotation	1	
Pyloric stenosis	1	
Stenosis (duodenal)	1	
Meckel's diverticulum	4	
Nervous system		21
Down syndrome	11	
Microcephaly	5	
Retarded (hydrocephalus, 2)	5	
Genitourinary system		7
Hydronephrosis with ureteropelvic obstruction	2	
Dysplastic kidney	1	
Double collecting system	2	
Undescended testis	2	
Cardiovascular system		7
(Down syndrome)	2	
Skeletal system		6
Chest wall deformity	1	
Polydactyly	1	
Talipes equinovarus	4	
Endocrine system		2
Congenital goiter with hypothyroidism	1	
Diabetes mellitus	1	
Respiratory system		1
Agenesis of right lung	1	
Special senses		2
Congenital deafness	1	
Agenesis of left eye	1	
Total		55

year of life. Three distinct intramural nerve plexuses are recognized.[3] Auerbach's or the myenteric plexus lies between the circular and longitudinal muscle layers. Henle's plexus (deep submucosal plexus) is found in the submucosa at the inner margin of the circular muscle. Meissner's submucosal plexus (superficial submucosal plexus) is located just beneath the muscularis mucosa.

Physiology

Propulsive colonic motility involves a contraction preceded by a wave of relaxation. This muscular activity is regulated by the intrinsic innervation of the intestine, which includes the classic cholinergic excitatory fibers and adrenergic inhibitory fibers. The intrinsic intestinal innervation has been shown to include noncholinergic excitatory and nonadrenergic inhibitory fibers. The neurons of the nonadrenergic inhibitory system are in the myenteric plexus of Auerbach. They are associated with some extrinsic innervation in the upper and lower intestine, but in the greater part of the intestine these neurons have only short intramural connections. This system is thought to be responsible for the relaxation phase of peristalsis and for the relaxation of the internal anal sphincter.[26, 54] Burnstock[25] suggests that the transmitter released from such nerves is adenosine triphosphate and that the system should therefore be called the "purinergic system" and the nerves, "purinergic nerves."

RESEARCH MODELS.—Study and evaluation of methods of treatment of Hirschsprung's disease have been hampered by the lack of research models. The natural occurrence of aganglionosis in several strains of mice has been reported and extensively studied.[17, 110, 150] However, an animal model with aganglionosis and increased intramural nerve fibers is not presently available.

Etiology

Hirschsprung's disease results from arrested caudal migration of neuroblasts in the alimentary tract. In 3–5% of cases, a genetic or familial factor can be implicated.[101]

Acquired forms of megacolon with aganglionosis are recognized. In Chagas' disease (American trypanosomiasis), seen in South America,[78] destruction of intramural ganglion cells can result in both cardiospasm and megacolon. Ehrenpreis[46] documented a case of recurrent congenital aganglionosis in which selective aganglionosis of the distal pulled-through colon was believed to have been caused by anoxia due to vascular insufficiency. Instances of newborn infants with clinical Hirschsprung's disease and ganglion cells in a suction rectal biopsy, who later proved to have an aganglionic rectum, probably represent technical errors in the suction biopsy procedure rather than cases of acquired Hirschsprung's disease as reported.[38]

Pathophysiology

Balloon studies show normal motor activity in the proximal, ganglion-containing colon. Spasm, lack of propulsive peristalsis, or both, could account for the functional obstruction caused by the aganglionic bowel. Hiatt[62] identified by balloon motility studies a mass contraction of the aganglionic segment of intestine. He concluded that the lack of an adrenergic inhibitory mechanism resulted in constant spasm of this segment, making propulsive peristalsis unlikely. Others[33] have been unable to confirm spasm in the aganglionic area but have shown lack of relaxation. Normal progressive peristalsis through the aganglionic area cannot be demonstrated by motility studies and the tonus, as determined by the baseline pressure, does not appear to be elevated. The aganglionic area shows no evidence of muscular hypertrophy, as one might expect if there were constant spasm. It is likely that both mechanisms are operative, but that lack of peristalsis is the most consistent cause of the obstruction. Pressure studies of the anal sphincteric mechanism in patients with Hirschsprung's disease have disclosed that, rather than distention of the rectum causing reflex internal sphincteric relaxation, contraction and increased internal sphincter pressure result.[145] This finding correlates with the clinical observation of a sphincteric as well as a colonic abnormality. While the absence of intramural ganglion cells is the fundamental congenital anatomical defect in Hirschsprung's disease, how this alters smooth muscle activity is not known. Cannon's law of denervation could explain the abnormal smooth muscle function in aganglionic megacolon.[47] However, the demonstration of adrenergic innervation,[147] the lack of verification of a truly spastic aganglionic segment, the response of the aganglionic intestine to various drugs, and the variable course of the disease challenge the validity of this simple explanation. In vitro studies of fresh specimens of colon from patients with aganglionic megacolon[26, 54] show that both adrenergic and cholinergic nerve fibers are markedly increased in the aganglionic segment, and that nonadrenergic inhibitory nerves are absent. Our present concept of the pathophysiology of Hirschsprung's disease is that there is disruption of the normal mechanism of colonic motility and defecation.[20] Absence of the intramural ganglia and of the nonadrenergic inhibitory fibers interferes with the normal relaxation mechanism of peristalsis and with internal sphincter relaxation. The extrinsic innervation may also be involved. Disruption of these control mechanisms may be complete, as in total aganglionosis, or may be of lesser degree, as in ultrashort-segment Hirschsprung's disease wherein only the internal sphincter mechanism is interfered with. Increased cholinergic excitatory activity, increased adrenergic excitatory activity, and loss of adrenergic inhibitory activity may be additional factors in promoting the lack of propulsive peristalsis and obstruction. Such mechanism of action could explain the presence of a Hirschsprung-like clinical course in patients who have intramural ganglion cells.

Incidence

The incidence of Hirschsprung's disease is around 1 in every 5,000 live births.[47] Thus, each year approximately 700 infants with Hirschsprung's disease are born in the United States. In the Children's Hospital of Pittsburgh series, there were 201 white children, (91.55%), 18 black children (8%), and one Oriental child (0.45%). One survey[76] showed equal incidence in blacks and whites. Eighty percent of patients with Hirschsprung's disease are boys. This preponderance of males is not seen in long-segment Hirschsprung's disease, in which there is also a familial occurrence. The genetics of Hirschsprung's disease has been studied by Passarge,[101] who favors the hypothesis of a multifactorial genetic system. The risk of the disease developing in siblings of a patient varies from 0.6% for sisters of males with a short aganglionic segment to 18% for brothers of females with long aganglionic segments. Carter[30] found two affected of 103 offspring of parents who had been surgically treated for short-segment Hirschsprung's disease, and two of four offspring of parents with long-segment Hirschsprung's disease, giving an estimated risk of 2% for offspring of short-segment patients and a much higher risk for offspring of long-segment patients.

Clinical Course

The history begins at birth with delayed passage of meconium and subsequent constipation. Evacuation may occur after a rectal examination. When the passage of the first meconium is delayed beyond 48 hours in a full-term, otherwise healthy infant, aganglionic megacolon should be suspected.[137] In our series, birth weights were available in 190 infants. Of these, the birth weight was less than 5 pounds (2,500 gm) in only five (2.6%) infants. Abdominal distention may be present early. It may occur gradually or suddenly, accompanied or preceded by vomiting. These episodes may disappear abruptly and spontaneously, or may be terminated by an enema or a suppository. The baby strains ineffectively, but defecation is painless. During early life the abdomen is distended and constantly tympanitic; it becomes tense, shiny, and round during attacks of acute obstruction (Fig 106–5). Diarrhea with foul, liquid stools may be the first and only symptom. Edema, periorbital and later generalized,[24] is uncommon but occurs as part of a protein-losing enteropathy associated with chronic diarrhea. Cecal perforation[127] with pneumoperitoneum may be the initial finding. Acute appendicitis in the newly born is often associated with Hirschsprung's disease.[93] Infants with Hirschsprung's disease may follow one of five more or less distinct clinical courses:[120]

1. There is complete obstruction at birth, with vomiting, abdominal distention, failure to pass meconium, and roentgenographic evidence of low intestinal obstruction.

2. There is delayed passage of meconium followed by repeated periods of obstruction relieved either spontaneously or by enema. The infants are chronically ill with episodes of fecal impaction, vomiting, and dehydration. They often have multiple hospitalizations.

3. Infants in this group have initially mild symptoms for several weeks or months, constipation being succeeded by complete, acute intestinal obstruction.

4. In this group with initially mild symptoms of constipation, there is an abrupt onset of enterocolitis with diarrhea, distention, fever, and prostration. Diarrhea may be the only sign.

5. In the final group, mild constipation may be the only sign.

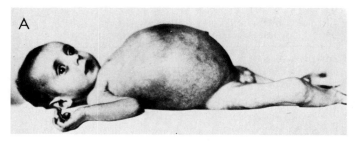

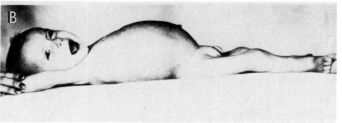

Fig 106–5.—**A,** appearance of a 9-month-old infant with Hirschsprung's disease. **B,** after 1 month of daily enemas.

Deflation by digital rectal examination may be dramatic and diagnostic. Variations in the severity of constipation have no correlation with the length of the aganglionic segment or with the development of enterocolitis.

The most serious complication in the neonatal period is ischemic enterocolitis. The abdomen distends tensely within a few hours, and the child vomits profusely while passing large amounts of foul-smelling gas and putrid, loose stools, which may be bloody. The lesion is ischemic necrosis of the mucosa of the bowel above the aganglionic segment, often extending into the small intestine. Intestinal pneumatosis, pericolic abscess, perforation, and septicemia commonly lead to death. If such an infant with Hirschsprung's disease survives, the obstructive crises become less frequent, stubborn constipation continues, and a huge potbelly develops, with visible peristaltic waves and palpable fecalomas. A flared lower costal cage, raised diaphragm, poor nutrition, and chronically ill appearance were once common in the older child with classic Hirschsprung's disease (Fig 106–6). Such patients are now rarely seen. The classic appearance may not be present if the aganglionic segment is very short or if the constipation is well managed by the parents. These children are not incontinent, and they do not soil. They do pass much flatus and may have tremendous gaseous distention of the abdomen. Current reports of a 25–30% mortality emphasize the lethal nature of unrecognized Hirschsprung's disease in infancy.[65]

Differential Diagnosis

Hirschsprung's disease must be differentiated from other causes of intestinal obstruction with distention and either delayed or absent passage of meconium. Of 97 infants admitted to Children's Hospital of Pittsburgh with such symptoms, absent ganglion cells in rectal suction biopsy confirmed the diagnosis of Hirschsprung's disease in 77 infants—ganglion cells being present in the remaining 20, of which 14 had meconium plug syndrome and six had small left colon syndrome. Delayed passage of meconium, associated with distention, suggests the possibility of obturation obstruction due to meconium ileus or to meconium plug syndrome. Meconium ileus is distinguished by a familial history of cystic fibrosis, the tendency of babies with meconium ileus to be small, and by the characteristic roentgenographic findings of an unused, so-called microcolon. In meconium plug

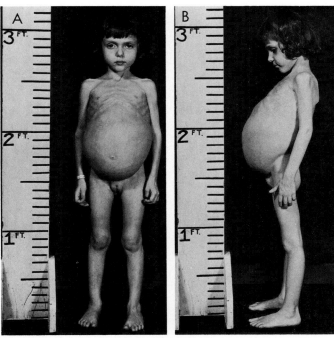

Fig 106–6.—Hirschsprung's disease. Classic appearance in an 8-year-old girl. The potbelly, flared lower rib cage, thin limbs, and general malnutrition are typical. Neglected cases of this kind, once common, and thought "typical," are now rare.

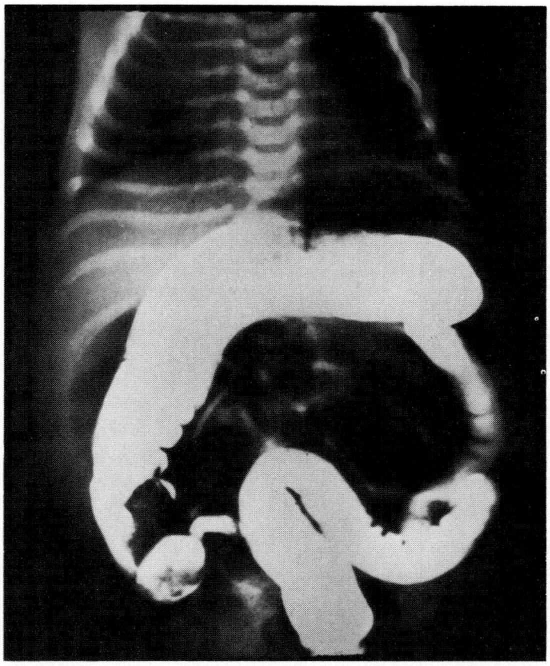

Fig 106–7.—Small left colon syndrome. Barium enema in a 48-hour-old infant with abdominal distention, vomiting, and no passage of meconium. Note pseudotransitional zone at the splenic flexure area.

syndrome,[50] a contrast enema is diagnostic and curative. Passage of the meconium plug is followed by prompt relief of distention and by normal defecation. A rectal biopsy is mandatory in all patients with meconium plug syndrome, since occasional infants with Hirschsprung's disease may have an associated meconium plug and appear well for a period of time following its passage.

In the neonatal small left colon syndrome,[37] clinical low intestinal obstruction is associated with a small-caliber, smooth, rounded left colon and a sudden increase in the size of the colon proximal to the splenic flexure (Fig 106–7). In contrast to the meconium plug syndrome, barium flows easily past the splenic flexure into the dilated proximal colon with very little hold-up at the splenic flexure. Many of these infants have diabetic mothers. The barium enema appears to be curative. The condition was originally described as benign, but more recent reports[97] urge prompt relief of the obstruction by enemas, since delay has resulted in perforation of the cecum. The left colon does not immediately become normal, but gradually increases to normal caliber over a period of weeks to months. LeQuesne and Reilly[84] suggest that the meconium plug syndrome, the small left colon syndrome, and the transient obstructions seen in premature infants may represent different manifestations of functional immaturity of the colon rather than distinct entities.

Sepsis in the newborn, adrenal insufficiency, hypothyroidism, and cerebral injury have all been associated with low intestinal obstruction in infancy[37, 50] and may simulate neonatal Hirschsprung's disease. An increasing number of functional obstructions have been noted because, with better obstetric and neonatal care, more prematurely born and medically ill babies survive.[84, 105] Kapila, Haberkorn, and Nixon[73] have described a form of chronic adynamic bowel that simulates Hirschsprung's disease. In older children, the classic picture of Hirschsprung's disease is that of the potbellied chronically ill child with palpable abdominal fecalomas, an empty rectum, and no evidence of fecal soiling,

with the history of bowel trouble going back to early life. In functional megacolon, or the enlarged colon due to chronic constipation, the onset is rarely before 6 months of age. Vomiting almost never occurs, and the child is not ill. Abdominal distention is rare. There is usually fecal soiling or frank overflow incontinence, and, upon rectal examination, a huge fecaloma fills the rectum down to the anal canal.[146] The perianal region is often smeared with feces. There is often a history of early and difficult toilet training. Personality disorders in parent and child are readily apparent on questioning. Roentgenographic examination shows the pear-shaped, hugely dilated rectum. Huge bowel movements occur at infrequent intervals. Rectal biopsy may be necessary to rule out short-segment Hirschsprung's disease.

Huge megacolon in mentally defective children may require roentgenographic study and rectal biopsy for diagnosis. Schärli has described patients with colonic neuronal dysplasia whose course resembles that of patients with Hirschsprung's disease.[118]

Diagnostic Procedures

The history and physical findings may suggest the disease and indicate appropriate roentgenographic studies. The barium enema is usually confirmative and assesses the length of the aganglionic segment. Anorectal pressure studies may be helpful, but the definitive diagnosis of Hirschsprung's disease rests on the demonstration of the absence of intramural ganglion cells.

Roentgen Examination

In the first few days of life, colonic distention with absence of air in the rectum on a plain abdominal roentgenogram is suggestive of Hirschsprung's disease, especially when confirmed in the lateral view (Fig 106–8). Contrast studies employing a thin barium-water mixture and the technique originally described by Neuhauser[136] may, even in the newborn, identify an area of tran-

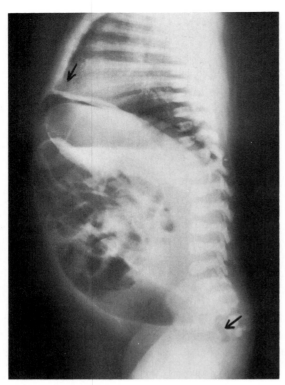

Fig 106–8.—Plain lateral roentgenogram of the abdomen in a 12-hour-old male infant with Hirschsprung's disease. Note the small rectum *(lower arrow)* and the subdiaphragmatic intraperitoneal air *(upper arrow)*. This infant had a rectal perforation, presumably from a rectal tube. Pneumoperitoneum in the neonate with Hirschsprung's disease is more generally due to appendiceal or cecal perforation.

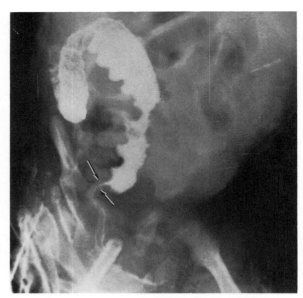

Fig 106–9.—Barium enema in a 3-day-old male infant with Hirschsprung's disease. Note the saw-toothed appearance of the colon proximal to the inert rectum, due to spasm, not ulceration.

sition to dilated, proximally obstructed bowel. Repeated rectal examinations and enemas will obscure such findings in an infant as well as in the older child. Pediatric radiologists emphasize the importance of using a plain catheter inserted just beyond the anal sphincter, introducing the contrast material by means of a hand syringe and under fluoroscopic control, with the restrained infant or child initially in the lateral position. The examination should be terminated when the transitional zone is identified. Rectal perforation is a real danger. For this reason, and to avoid obscuring the contour of the distal rectum, inflatable catheters are not used. In infancy, a saw-toothed appearance of the sigmoid may be noted in the absence of a well-defined transitional zone[7] (Fig 106–9). Barium retention in the colon for 2 or 3 days may be the only suggestive sign of disease in infants. In older children, an easily identifiable transition zone is usually apparent (Fig 106–10). Roentgenographic studies may not be diagnostic when aganglionosis is low or when it extends to include the entire colon.[113] Total colonic aganglionosis manifests itself as incomplete low small-bowel obstruction. The colon may be short and the hepatic and splenic flexures rounded. An elongated, dilated, right-sided sigmoid colon on the plain film or on contrast studies strongly suggests aganglionic megacolon. A short sigmoid colon in the presence of incomplete low small-bowel obstruction, with retention of barium for 2 or 3 days, may be the most specific radiologic finding in total colonic aganglionosis. Hirschsprung's disease may be associated with enterocolitis, and pneumatosis may be apparent in the plain film. The colonic mucosa of such infants is thickened, edematous, and may contain multiple pseudopolyps. As enterocolitis develops, the aganglionic portion dilates, the mucosa becomes ulcerated, and the outline of the co-

lon more irregular (Fig 106–11). The transition zone may be obscured. Perforation is recognized by pneumoperitoneum. The colon distal to a colostomy presents a striking roentgenographic appearance[83] of nondistensibility, thickness, and nodularity of the mucosal relief. These changes appear to be most marked in patients with enterocolitis. The Gastrografin enema, an effective treatment for simple obturation obstruction in meconium ileus, has been used extensively for diagnostic contrast enemas in the newborn. This medium, by virtue of its high osmolarity, may cause dangerous, abrupt, extracellular fluid volume loss and has, in our experience, obscured the radiologic diagnosis of Hirschsprung's disease. A thin barium-water mixture is preferable. When the ratio of the widest diameter of the rectum to the widest diameter of the sigmoid is greater than or equal to one, the rectosigmoid index is said to be normal.[106] In Hirschsprung's disease, the ratio is less than one. Such measurements may be helpful in the newborn, or when the transition is not easily seen.

Rectal Biopsy

The histologic demonstration of the absence of ganglia and of the presence of excess nonmyelinated nerves in the distal intestine in an adequate rectal biopsy establishes the diagnosis of Hirschsprung's disease. Swenson et al.[135] introduced rectal biopsy for definitive diagnosis in patients with a colostomy performed for the relief of colonic obstruction in early life, and in newborn infants in whom Hirschsprung's disease was suspected but not radiographically evident, for short-segment disease, and for unusual cases. Nixon[98] and Swenson and co-workers[137] did not consider rectal biopsy a routine requirement for diagnosis, and Ehrenpreis[47] rarely used the procedure. Others[40, 119] have felt that a tissue diagnosis is mandatory before definitive operation. In the past, when older patients with well-established transitional zones were commonly seen, barium enemas were usually diagnostic and few rectal biopsies were done in our series. In recent years, most patients are seen in the neonatal period when diagnosis is difficult, and rectal biopsy is always necessary.

To be valid, the biopsy specimen must be obtained at least 1.5 cm above the pectinate line. The anus is dilated and a full-thickness specimen of the posterior rectal wall is taken 2–3 cm above

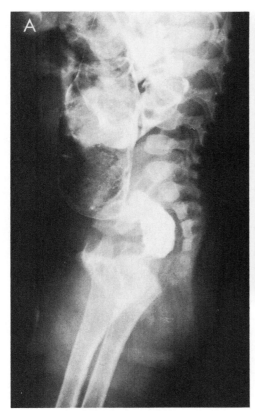

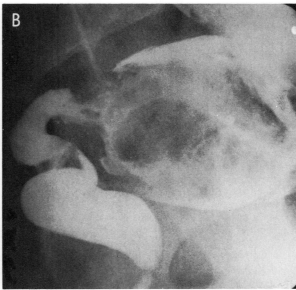

Fig 106–10.—Roentgen picture in Hirschsprung's disease. **A,** barium enema findings in an 8-month-old boy. The transition from small-caliber aganglionic rectum to dilated, normally innervated colon is clearly illustrated. **B,** barium enema in a 16-year-old boy illustrates the characteristic transitional area from normal-caliber rectum to fecaloma-containing, dilated, normally innervated colon.

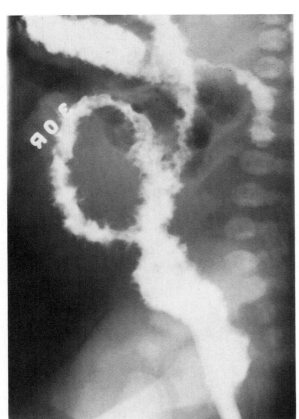

Fig 106–11.—Barium enema in an infant with enterocolitis. There is no transitional zone.

the pectinate line. Hemostasis is accomplished by ligature or electrocautery, and the mucosal defect is sutured. The procedure may be difficult in infants and in older patients with a small anus that cannot be easily dilated. In reporting 100 consecutive biopsies done over a 5-year period, Swenson emphasized the low morbidity and the accuracy of the procedure. An incision along the pectinate line, either posteriorly or laterally, permits submucosal dissection of the distal rectal wall for adequate biopsy, in a variation of the technique described by Bill et al.[9]

The procedure devised by Thomas and associates[141] has been used in older children with megarectum. It is a major operation, requiring endotracheal anesthesia in an awkward position for the patient. The posterior rectal wall is exposed through a vertical incision at the tip of the coccyx in the posterior midline, the pubococcygeus separated from the coccyx, and the retrorectal space entered. By submucosal dissection a generous strip of muscularis of the rectum can be removed. The procedure results in a myectomy—which may be therapeutic. The extension of rectal biopsy into a therapeutic procedure for so-called short-segment aganglionosis by the transrectal excision of a narrow longitudinal strip of the posterior rectal wall musculature has been practiced by Bentley,[5] Lynn,[87] and Nissan and Bar-Maor.[96] Open rectal biopsy requires a general anesthetic and a 24-hour delay for permanent histologic section examination. Serial sections are cut and thoroughly examined before the absence of ganglion cells can be accepted. An important part of the procedure is proper orientation of the removed specimen by the surgeon for the pathologist.

Simplification of the method has been sought. As early as 1950, Bodian[14] recommended a biopsy taken as a 1 × 2-cm sheet of mucosa and submucosa properly oriented and serially sectioned. Shandling and Auldist[119] use a punch biopsy of the lowest valve of Houston to secure a specimen. The technique involves the use of a biopsy forceps, such as a Hartmann forceps, and subsequent intraluminal pressure to control bleeding.

Shandling[119] and Burrington and Wayne[27] consider this technique diagnostically reliable and free of significant complications.

Suction biopsy techniques using special apparatus such as the all-purpose Rubin[40] tube or the Noblett[99] instrument are now common. The specimen obtained is a 3 × 1-mm piece of mucosa and submucosa. The reliability of the method depends on the quality of the specimen received. An adequate biopsy produces approximately 20 serial sections, each containing submucosa and muscularis mucosa, where the submucosal (Meissner) plexus should be located. The histologic identification of nerve cells is more difficult there than in the myenteric plexus. The interpretation of ganglion cells rests on the identification of nerve units rather than large triangular ganglion cells.[153] Because nerve cells mature as the infant grows, the appearance as well as the number of ganglion cells is altered as the infant becomes older.[122]

Since the histologic diagnosis is one of exclusion rather than of finding a positive feature, some believe the suction biopsy should be used as a screening test only, insisting on a conventional rectal biopsy for the definitive diagnosis. The procedure is simple and relatively safe;[2] however, perforation of the rectosigmoid colon, and excessive bleeding can occur.[108] In our series of over 200 procedures, suction biopsy was followed by septicemia and meningitis in three infants and by bleeding that required transfusion and suturing in one, older, patient.

The uncertainty and dissatisfaction with a diagnosis arrived at by exclusion generated a search for positive diagnostic methods. With the development of practical histochemical staining techniques that identify acetylcholinesterase in biopsy material, an accurate positive diagnostic procedure was introduced. Meier-Ruge[94] recommends the identification of large amounts of acetylcholinesterase in the mucosa and muscularis mucosa of the distal rectum by the method of Karnofsky and Raitz as the diagnostic method of choice. He considers the method simple and reliable. Pease et al.[102] have found the method unreliable, the 2-hour processing time of no particular advantage, and they no longer use it. It has not been widely adopted for general use in this country. Lake et al.[79, 80] found acetylcholinesterase staining the most reliable means of diagnosing Hirschsprung's disease, especially when used in conjunction with conventionally stained paraffin sections. Only recently has this staining method been routine in this country.[69] Our current preference for the definitive diagnosis of Hirschsprung's disease is an adequate suction rectal mucosal biopsy stained for acetylcholinesterase, as well as hematoxylin-eosin–stained paraffin sections. Histological verification of the diagnosis is required before surgical therapy. Full-thickness rectal biopsy is rarely necessary unless the specimen is inadequate or the level of origin of the specimen is in doubt.

Anorectal Manometry

Drawing on an extensive experience with anorectal and colonic manometry, Schuster et al.[145] devised a nonoperative manometric diagnostic test for Hirschsprung's disease. In normal individuals, transient rectal distention causes relaxation of the internal anal sphincter. In Hirschsprung's disease, contraction rather than relaxation occurs. El Shafie et al.[51] simplified the apparatus to make the method more available. Aaronson and Nixon[1] consider anorectal manometry a simple and safe diagnostic test of special value as an outpatient screening procedure. They believe it should be available for the routine investigation and management of Hirschsprung's disease, just as are barium enemas and rectal biopsies. Holzschneider et al.[66] have shown that manometry excludes Hirschsprung's disease from the first day of life on, but that it can be diagnostic of Hirschsprung's disease only after the 12th day of life.

Comparison of Methods of Definitive Diagnosis

Aaronson and Nixon[1] compared the available diagnostic procedures on 100 consecutive patients. The overall diagnostic reliability of anorectal manometry was 85%. They concluded that anorectal manometry was more reliable for the diagnosis of ultrashort-segment disease than the barium enema examination and that its chief usefulness was in excluding Hirschsprung's disease (90%) rather than in confirming its presence (74%). Radiologic diagnosis was 83% correct, inaccurate in total aganglionosis, short-segment disease, and patients with a colostomy. In those three groups of patients, manometry was superior. Tobon and Schuster,[146] in 100 patients with megacolon, noted 95% diagnostic accuracy with rectal biopsy, 80% with barium enema, but 100% with manometry. Holzschneider,[64] comparing the accuracy of diagnostic methods, concluded that an acetylcholinesterase-stained suction biopsy was the most accurate, manometric examination more accurate than roentgen or conventional histological studies, but unreliable in those under 1 month of age. Anorectal manometry, although not available in many institutions, is valuable in diagnosis.

Enterocolitis

Ulcerative enterocolitis is the usual cause of death in infants with unrelieved intestinal obstruction due to Hirschsprung's disease.[10] The syndrome varies in onset and course, from persistent troublesome diarrhea over many weeks or months without systemic manifestations, to the sudden onset of gross abdominal distention with explosive, liquid, foul diarrhea, progression to listlessness, high fever, prostration, hypovolemic shock, and death within 24 hours. Crises of enterocolitis may occur, with in-between periods of relatively good health. The diarrhea seen in Hirschsprung's disease may be a mild form of enterocolitis, but progression to fatal enterocolitis is, in our experience, unusual. More commonly, the infant with periodic acute obstruction suddenly develops the rapidly progressive symptoms described. No specific pathogen can be cultured from stool or blood. Thomas et al.,[142] noting the similarity to pseudomembranous enterocolitis, suggested an association with *Clostridium difficile* and were able to detect high titers of cytotoxin in four and positive cultures of *C. difficile* in the feces of five of six children with Hirschsprung's enterocolitis. At necropsy, the colitis was in the obstructed intestine, proximal to the aganglionic segment. There is no consistent correlation between the length of the aganglionic segment and the incidence of enterocolitis.

Enterocolitis can occur before and after definitive operation for aganglionosis. It may appear before and after colostomy. When present in the neonates, it almost always recurs during the postoperative period. Pneumatosis intestinalis and mucosal ulcerations with hypermotility suggest enterocolitis. Barium enema studies of the by-passed intestine following colostomy[83] and examination of resected intestine following recovery from enterocolitis[8] demonstrate residual, often extensive, mucosal changes such as polypoid mucosa, persistent granulation tissue, and extensive lymphoid hyperplasia. These persistent changes probably explain the tendency to recurrence and may well constitute an indication for lifelong surveillance for possible neoplasia.

Until recently, enterocolitis accounted for most of the deaths in infants with Hirschsprung's disease. The severity of this serious complication has decreased in recent years. The treatment is the release of the obstruction by rectocolonic irrigation every 6–8 hours as described and advised by Swenson et al.[138] or by prompt emergency transverse colostomy after fluid replacement and correction of hypovolemic shock. Ehrenpreis[47] cautioned against emergency colostomy unless conservative measures fail, pointing out that the mortality for colostomy under these circumstances is excessive. It is our firm conviction that, when Hirschsprung's disease is diagnosed in infancy, lethal enterocolitis can be prevented by prompt colostomy.[120] Table 106–3 presents statistical data concerning enterocolitis at Children's Hospital of Pittsburgh in infants under 6 months of age.

Branski[22] recognized small-bowel mucosal damage with disaccharide deficiency, accompanying enterocolitis, and suggests the routine addition of parenteral alimentation in treatment. Arhan et al.[4] noted increased elasticity and prolongation of the time for accommodation to distention in the rectal wall of patients with Hirschsprung's disease. They used such measurements of the elastic properties of the rectal wall to assess the severity of the illness and indirectly to predict those at risk for the development of enterocolitis and best treated by prompt colostomy.

Medical (Nonoperative) Treatment

The treatment of aganglionic megacolon is operative relief of the intestinal obstruction. Medical treatment is ineffectual and dangerous. Procrastination is dangerous. The only effective nonoperative treatment is decompression by enemas, which can result in perforation of the thin-walled aganglionic segment. Soapsuds enemas and tap-water enemas have caused water intoxication from massive circulatory overloading due to absorption from the huge mucosal surface of the dilated colon.[129] For this reason, isotonic solutions should be used in cleansing enemas for these infants and children. Retention enemas of liquid Colace solution followed by cleansing saline irrigation in 12–24 hours are effective in removing fecal concretions. In 19 patients in the Children's Hospital of Pittsburgh series, treatment was not directed to the relief of intestinal obstruction. Ten of these patients died, three following exploratory laparotomy. The remaining nine children with biopsy-proved short-segment aganglionosis are mildly constipated and require only occasional enemas.

Surgical Treatment

Definitive surgical treatment of aganglionotic megacolon involves bringing normal bowel as low in the rectum as is technically possible by resecting or bypassing the aganglionic bowel. Preliminary decompression by an appropriately placed enterostomy is mandatory in long-segment aganglionosis, in those with poor nutrition from prolonged obstruction, in the newborn, and in enterocolitis. The definitive surgical procedure is deferred until the infant is approximately 1 year of age or until the older patient is returned to good nutritional status. The definitive procedure is followed in 3–4 weeks by colostomy closure, unless the initial procedure was a terminal colostomy and a two-stage rather than a three-stage procedure was performed. A primary definitive operation without colostomy is indicated in the older infant or child who remains nutritionally well with minimal colonic enlargement and who is having adequate daily evacuations with the use of suppositories, rectal dilatations, and enemas.

TABLE 106–3.—ENTEROCOLITIS IN INFANTS UNDER AGE 6
MONTHS, CHILDREN'S HOSPITAL OF PITTSBURGH SERIES

	1950–57	1958–68	1969–73	1974–83
No. of patients	25	56	47	66
With enterocolitis	5 (20%)	14 (25%)	3 (6%)	10 (15%)
Died of enterocolitis	2 (10%)	5 (9%)	1 (2%)	0 (0%)

Preliminary Decompression

The colostomy is ideally located in the normally innervated intestine just proximal to the aganglionic gut. This requires frozen-section control of the placement of the colostomy, and a pathologist experienced in the detection of intramural ganglion cells in frozen-section material. The obstructed gut, just above the transition, may be so large that colostomy at that level would be impractical and dangerous. In such instances, a right transverse colostomy can be more easily and safely done. Preoperative diagnosis should be sufficiently accurate to obviate exploratory laparotomy through large incisions and extensive handling and biopsy of the intestine at colostomy, except for biopsy at the level of colostomy. Many surgeons regularly perform a right transverse colostomy as a first stage procedure in all cases. Routine transverse colostomy may set the stage for later problems if the aganglionic area is long. The distal portion of normal intestine and its mesentery tend to remain short, a handicap in reconstruction at the time of definitive repair. The transverse colostomy is usually done as a loop colostomy, taking care to keep the opening in the mesentery close to the bowel wall and preserving the marginal artery. This is of great importance to prevent necrosis of the distal colon should pull-through complications occur. The peritoneum and posterior rectus sheath are sutured circumferentially to the serosa of the exteriorized colon and brought together beneath the colon through the mesenteric defect. The anterior rectus sheath is also brought together beneath the exteriorized colon, which is now opened longitudinally. Delaying the opening of the colostomy for 24 hours is inconsistent with the concept of emergency decompression to prevent the development of enterocolitis. In infants with a low area of aganglionosis for whom a two-stage procedure is anticipated, or when the aganglionic segment is long and grossly difficult to distinguish, biopsy can be carried out by excision of a small segment and distal closure, bringing the proximal end out as a terminal single-barreled colostomy. Ileostomy should be done without hesitation in infants with aganglionosis coli. A right upper abdominal transverse incision permits adequate exploration; a small segment of the terminal ileum is removed to verify the location of ganglion cells; and the two ends of intestine are exteriorized, in either end of the incision, suturing the mesentery to the peritoneal closure between.

Many believe that colostomy or ileostomy should be performed on all infants with congenital aganglionosis, postponing the definitive procedure until the infant is 1–1½ years of age. The decrease in the incidence and severity of enterocolitis, with earlier diagnosis and prompt decompression, has encouraged earlier definitive operation, often without preliminary enterostomy. Carcassonne et al.[29] used Swenson's procedure successfully in infants 5 to 61 days of age. So et al.[123] employed the endorectal pull-through procedure in newborns. Table 106–4 summarizes the Children's Hospital of Pittsburgh experience with preliminary decompression procedures for congenital aganglionosis.

Indications for Definitive Surgical Treatment

Do all patients with Hirschsprung's disease need a major operation? There are instances of patients who have lived to adulthood with minimal impairment of health or inconvenience. More commonly, at some time these patients have an acute abdominal emergency such as volvulus or enterocolitis. Rarely, patients are encountered in whom, without operation, the general health is good and regular bowel movements were reestablished after the diagnosis was made in early life.[98]

TABLE 106–4.—COLOSTOMY, ENTEROSTOMY FOR CONGENITAL
AGANGLIONIC MEGACOLON, CHILDREN'S HOSPITAL OF
PITTSBURGH SERIES

TIME PERIOD	NO.	DIED	CAUSE OF DEATH	
1950–64	70	15 (21%)	Enterocolitis	11
			Postoperative wound dehiscence	2
			Enterostomy in aganglionic bowel	2
1965–73	69	6 (8.7%)	Aspiration	1
			Enterostomy in aganglionic bowel (adult)	1
			Total aganglionosis	3
			Enterocolitis (sepsis)	1
1974–83	64	4 (6.25%)	Total aganglionosis (sepsis)	2
			Neuroblastoma	1
			Down-CV	1

The verified diagnosis of Hirschsprung's disease is an indication for corrective operation. Patients with a short segment are probably best treated by myectomy.[87] If adequate improvement does not result, a resection and pull-through procedure is indicated. Some mentally retarded patients respond poorly to resection and pull-through procedures. Permanent colostomy may be the most practical solution for them.

Preoperative Care

After verification of the diagnosis, the bowel is emptied and cleansed with enemas or colonic irrigations. A clear liquid diet, the administration of a saline cathartic, and irrigations will accomplish this in colostomy patients, but copious and prolonged colonic irrigations may be necessary to remove fecalomas from the distal colon in those without a colostomy or in older patients with a colostomy. A 24-hour antibiotic bowel preparation (neomycin and erythromycin base) and a parenteral broad-spectrum antibiotic before operation are standard. The preoperative intravenous pyelogram has been replaced by a renal sonogram. Preoperative preparation should include daily anal dilatations. Common to all operations for Hirschsprung's disease are the insertion of a nasogastric tube into the stomach, a urethral catheter into the bladder, and a large-bore needle into an arm vein for the administration of fluids during the procedure. The patient is placed in the lithotomy position with the knees bent and the feet on holders projecting from the end of the table, so that the abdomen and perineum may be simultaneously exposed. In older patients, or by preference of the surgeon, the legs may be elevated only later, for the perineal part of the procedure.

Surgical Techniques

The following surgical procedures are available for the definitive surgical treatment of aganglionosis. Excellent descriptions by the major proponents are given later in this chapter.

Swenson's Procedure

This is the procedure originally devised for the definitive treatment of Hirschsprung's disease[132] (Fig 106–12,A). The technique is illustrated in Figure 106–13. The essential features of the operation include freeing of the rectum by precise dissection close to the rectal wall down to the sphincteric mechanism, resection of the aganglionic intestine, temporary closure of both the distal aganglionic rectum and the proximal normally innervated colon, eversion of the closed rectal stump through the anus, and a precise two-layer anastomosis of the pulled-through normal colon to the everted rectum, performed perineally. At the conclusion of the procedure, the levators pull the anastomosis up above the anus. The resection should leave 1.5 cm of rectal wall anteriorly, and almost none posteriorly, so as actually to perform a posterior sphincterotomy. The procedure is lengthy, requiring precise technique, patience, and a meticulous and methodical surgeon. In the past, as surgeons unacquainted with these requirements performed this operation, the overall complication rate was excessive. At present, in the hands of competent surgeons, this operation carries no special hazards. Because of the high incidence of postoperative enterocolitis, Swenson[133] altered the original procedure to the more extensive resection described above, which actually involves a posterior sphincterotomy. Hiatt[61] modified the procedure by intussuscepting the devascularized bowel through the anus and then resecting the extruded bowel, thus avoiding possible intra-abdominal contamination. This procedure proved cumbersome and unnecessary and is not now commonly employed. Lavery[81] used the circular end-to-end stapling instrument for the anastomosis. The 21-mm diameter of the presently available instrument limits its use to older infants.

Duhamel's Procedure

Duhamel[43] devised an operation (see Fig 106–12,B) that eliminates much pelvic dissection and preserves the aganglionic rectum. This technique, as modified by Martin, is illustrated in Figure 106–14. The aganglionic intestine is resected down to the peritoneal reflection and the rectum is sutured closed. The proximal normal intestine is then brought through a retrorectal tunnel and through an incision in the posterior half of the circumference of the distal rectal wall. The posterior wall of the rectum above this level and the anterior wall of the pulled-through colon are then apposed by a crushing clamp, which results in a wide anastomosis of the end of the colon to the posterior wall of the rectum. This ingenious procedure is remarkably free of complications, requires little pelvic dissection, and can be safely done in adults as well as in infants.

The original procedure was modified by placing the anastomosis above rather than through the internal sphincter to avoid incontinence (Grob et al.[59]). While Duhamel has not been concerned about the length of the retained rectal pouch, and, in-

---

Fig 106–12.—A, Swenson's procedure removes the aganglionic intestine, leaving only 1–2 cm anteriorly; a sphincterotomy is done posteriorly. This results in normally innervated intestine down to the sphincter mechanism. **B,** Duhamel's procedure removes the aganglionic intestine down to the peritoneal reflection, preserving the aganglionic rectum. Bringing the normally innervated intestine down behind the rectum and anastomosing this in the fashion illustrated provides normally innervated intestine for half the circumference of the rectum. The sphincter mechanism is not disturbed. **C,** Roviralta's procedure is a modification of the Duhamel without intestinal resection. A long, defunctionalized distal intestinal segment remains in place. To eliminate the rectal "pouch," Martin originally anastomosed the tip of the rectum to the front of the pulled-through colon. **D,** Grob and Bowring, in a modification of the Duhamel, place clamps to eliminate the rectal pouch and simulate the Swenson procedure in end result, but with a longer anterior aganglionic wall. **E,** Martin, in patients with total aganglionosis of the colon, in addition to eliminating the spur, anastomoses side by side the pulled-through ileum to a long length of colon. **F,** Soper and Ikeda modify the Duhamel procedure by eliminating the common wall completely and anastomosing half the circumference of the anterior aganglionic rectal wall to the anterior half of the circumference of the pulled-through colon. **G,** the Soave procedure resects the aganglionic intestine submucosally, leaving the aganglionic muscular wall of the rectum through which the normally innervated intestine is pulled. This results in normally innervated intestine anastomosed to the sphincter mechanism but surrounded above this level by an aganglionic muscular cuff. The sphincter mechanism is dilated by the procedure but is otherwise left undisturbed. **H,** State removes the left colon, including the splenic flexure, and anastomoses the mid-transverse colon to the rectum just above the peritoneal reflection. This extended anterior resection preserves much of the aganglionic rectum in continuity and does not disturb the sphincter mechanism.

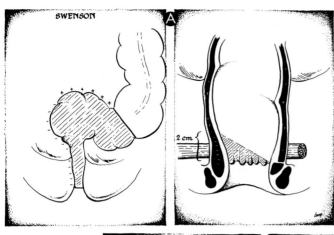

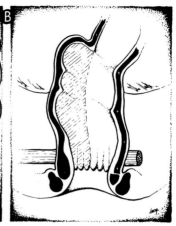

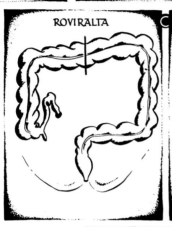
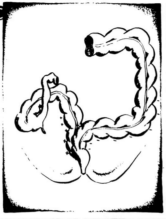
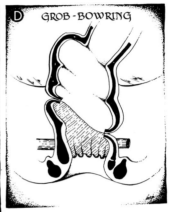

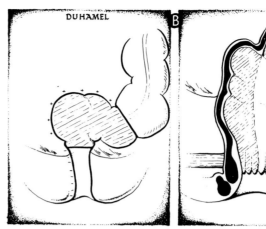

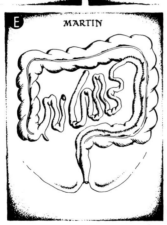
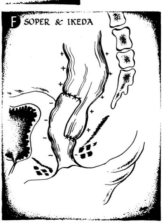

Fig 106–12.—See legend on facing page.

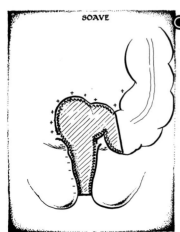
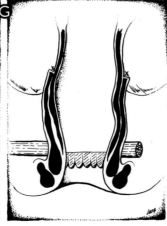
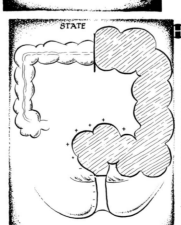
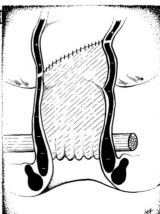

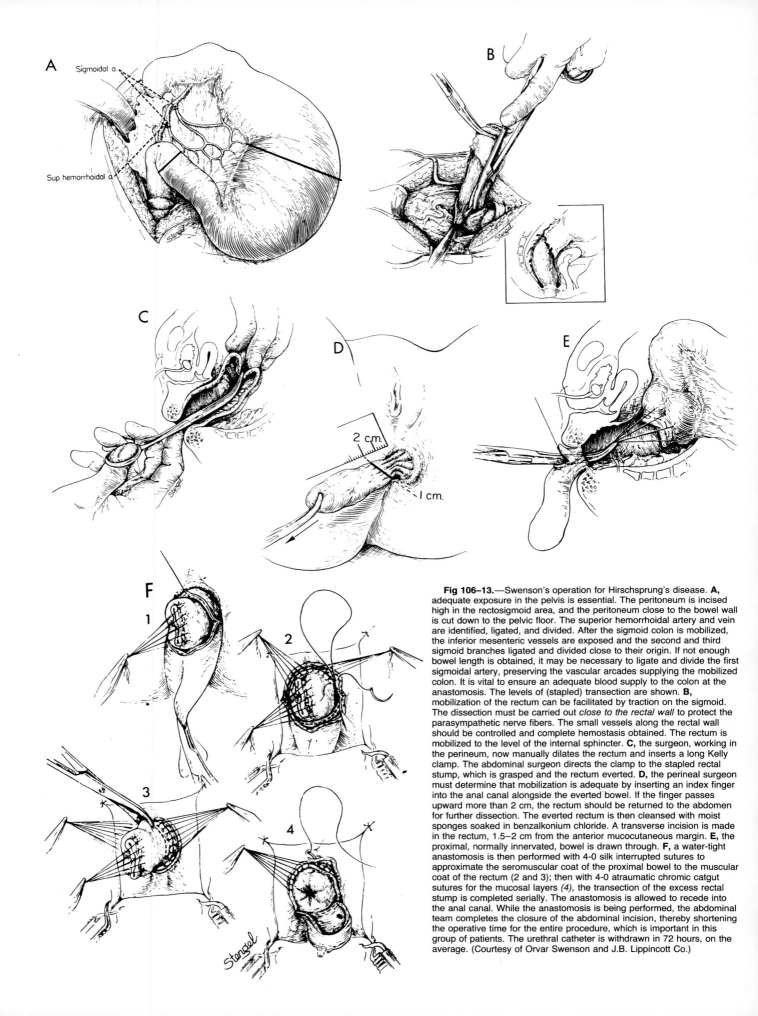

Fig 106–13.—Swenson's operation for Hirschsprung's disease. **A,** adequate exposure in the pelvis is essential. The peritoneum is incised high in the rectosigmoid area, and the peritoneum close to the bowel wall is cut down to the pelvic floor. The superior hemorrhoidal artery and vein are identified, ligated, and divided. After the sigmoid colon is mobilized, the inferior mesenteric vessels are exposed and the second and third sigmoid branches ligated and divided close to their origin. If not enough bowel length is obtained, it may be necessary to ligate and divide the first sigmoidal artery, preserving the vascular arcades supplying the mobilized colon. It is vital to ensure an adequate blood supply to the colon at the anastomosis. The levels of (stapled) transection are shown. **B,** mobilization of the rectum can be facilitated by traction on the sigmoid. The dissection must be carried out *close to the rectal wall* to protect the parasympathetic nerve fibers. The small vessels along the rectal wall should be controlled and complete hemostasis obtained. The rectum is mobilized to the level of the internal sphincter. **C,** the surgeon, working in the perineum, now manually dilates the rectum and inserts a long Kelly clamp. The abdominal surgeon directs the clamp to the stapled rectal stump, which is grasped and the rectum everted. **D,** the perineal surgeon must determine that mobilization is adequate by inserting an index finger into the anal canal alongside the everted bowel. If the finger passes upward more than 2 cm, the rectum should be returned to the abdomen for further dissection. The everted rectum is then cleansed with moist sponges soaked in benzalkonium chloride. A transverse incision is made in the rectum, 1.5–2 cm from the anterior mucocutaneous margin. **E,** the proximal, normally innervated, bowel is drawn through. **F,** a water-tight anastomosis is then performed with 4-0 silk interrupted sutures to approximate the seromuscular coat of the proximal bowel to the muscular coat of the rectum (2 and 3); then with 4-0 atraumatic chromic catgut sutures for the mucosal layers *(4),* the transection of the excess rectal stump is completed serially. The anastomosis is allowed to recede into the anal canal. While the anastomosis is being performed, the abdominal team completes the closure of the abdominal incision, thereby shortening the operative time for the entire procedure, which is important in this group of patients. The urethral catheter is withdrawn in 72 hours, on the average. (Courtesy of Orvar Swenson and J.B. Lippincott Co.)

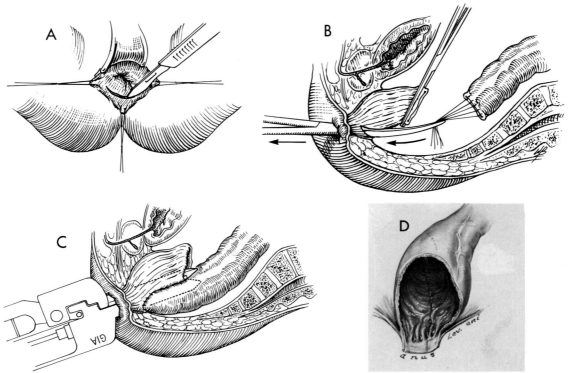

Fig 106–14.—Duhamel's procedure–Martin's method. **A,** the rectum having been divided just above the peritoneal floor and the proximal, aganglionic, colon resected, a transverse incision is made around the posterior half of the rectal wall 1 cm from the mucocutaneous junction. **B,** the posterior rectal wall is separated from the puborectalis muscle, and the presacral space (previously opened from above) is entered. A clamp passed through from below draws the proximal colon through the rectal incision. **C,** the colon has been sutured to the incision in the posterior rectal wall with fine catgut and a circular anastomosis performed. The GIA stapler is inserted so that the prong in the rectum extends out through the open proximal end. Operation of the instrument staples rectum and colon together and divides the resulting septum for its entire length. **D,** the open upper end of the rectum has been sutured to the end of the incision in the colon so that there is no superior pouch. The cutaway shows the completed result.

deed, Roviralta[112] has recommended no resection, merely transecting the colon well above the site of transition (see Fig 106–12,*C*), leaving a long aganglionic standpipe closed, or as a mucous fistula, most experienced surgeons believe the pouch should be as small as possible and have modified the procedure to accomplish this (see Fig 106–12,*D*). Martin and Altemeier[91] emphasize delayed opening of the pulled-through colon (48–72 hours) in patients without a protecting colostomy and careful placement of the clamps to include the very tip of the common wall, leaving no rectal pouch whatsoever. Ochsner forceps, the Gross spur-crushing clamp modified by Bill,[11] and special clamps by Zachary and Lister,[155] Sulamaa,[131] and Ikeda[70] have been used to crush the common wall. The GIA stapling machine has been used to divide and suture the common wall.[139] Soper[126] and Ikeda[70] (see Fig 106–12,*E*) have eliminated the rectal pouch completely by anastomosing the intra-abdominal anterior half of the circumference of the pulled-through colon to the anterior rectal wall, after completely removing the spur of common wall.

Martin[89, 90] applied the procedure to long-segment aganglionosis (see Figs 106–12,*E,* and 106–16), adding an extended side-to-side anastomosis between normal pulled-through intestine and aganglionic colon to provide additional absorptive surface and a further reservoir. Recent reports[35, 104] suggest late complications and few virtues of this complicated procedure. The final evolution of this procedure is a modification[21] wherein anterior and lateral dissection is avoided, only the posterior wall being freed to the internal sphincter. The resulting anastomosis is long and oblique and resembles the original Swenson procedure in concept.

Soave's Operation

The endorectal pull-through procedure, described by Soave[124] and illustrated in Figures 106–12,*G,* and 106–15, involves removal of the mucosa of the distal bowel by submucosal dissection to the anus and the passage of the normally innervated colon through the remaining rectosigmoid muscular tube. The procedure is done preferably without a colostomy, allowing a segment of the pulled-through colon to protrude well beyond the anal skin margin for removal at a second stage 2 weeks later. This procedure has been modified by Boley[18] to a one-stage procedure by primary anastomosis of the pulled-through colon to the muscular cuff at the anal verge. Soave's operation is easy to perform and avoids all pelvic dissection by passing through rather than removing the abnormal bowel. The circular end of the muscle tube is palpable for some time postoperatively; in the original procedure, vigorous, repeated dilatation was essential. Marks[88] advocates splitting the muscular cuff posteriorly to avoid this. Mucosal dissection is simple in infants, more difficult in older patients because of bleeding, and may be quite difficult in patients with previous enterocolitis. Coran and Weintraub[32] have modified the procedure, everting the mucosal tube and employing the Swenson technique, for ease of anastomosis. Blanchard et al.[13] use an intraluminal Foley catheter blown up beyond the anus and pulled up from below to aid in the distal endorectal dissection.

State's Operation

Extended anterior resection of the colon, as advised by State[128] (see Fig 106–12,*H*), includes resection of the left colon well

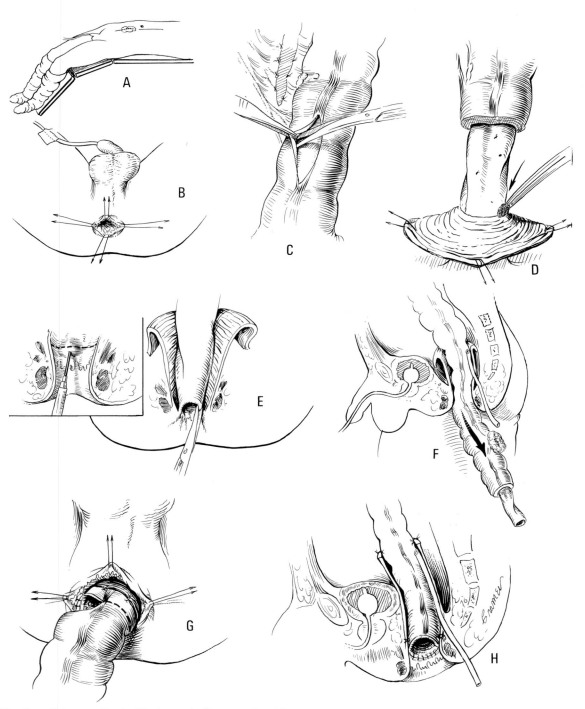

Fig 106–15.—Soave-Boley operation for Hirschsprung's disease; endorectal pull-through with primary anastomosis. **A,** pelvis is dorsiflexed 30 degrees over the table break for the abdominal stage. **B,** position for perineal stage. Traction sutures are placed parallel to the anal circumference at the anocutaneous junction. **C,** dissection of the mucosal tube is begun through a longitudinal incision 4–8 cm above the peritoneal reflection. **D,** the muscular sleeve is transected and the blunt dissection carried down to within 1–2 cm of the dentate line. **E,** the mucosal dissection is completed from below, transanally, through a circumferential incision in the mucosa 1 cm above the dentate line. This is facilitated by a submucosal injection of 0.5% procaine solution *(inset).* **F,** after irrigation of the muscular cuff with kanamycin solution and placement of a Penrose drain, the normal colon is pulled down through the cuff. **G,** four to six 3–0 chromic catgut sutures are placed between the muscular cuff and the seromuscular layer of the colon 1 cm above the transected rectal mucosa. The pulled-through colon is then divided 1 cm below these sutures and an anastomosis performed with 3–0 chromic catgut between the rectal mucosa 1 cm above the dentate line and all layers of the colon. **H,** completed anastomosis. The upper end of the muscular cuff is loosely approximated to the enclosed colon with interrupted 4–0 silk sutures.

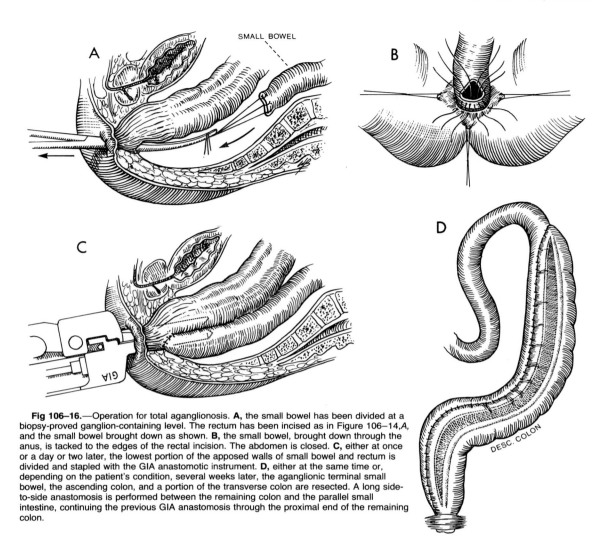

Fig 106–16.—Operation for total aganglionosis. **A,** the small bowel has been divided at a biopsy-proved ganglion-containing level. The rectum has been incised as in Figure 106–14,*A,* and the small bowel brought down as shown. **B,** the small bowel, brought down through the anus, is tacked to the edges of the rectal incision. The abdomen is closed. **C,** either at once or a day or two later, the lowest portion of the apposed walls of small bowel and rectum is divided and stapled with the GIA anastomotic instrument. **D,** either at the same time or, depending on the patient's condition, several weeks later, the aganglionic terminal small bowel, the ascending colon, and a portion of the transverse colon are resected. A long side-to-side anastomosis is performed between the remaining colon and the parallel small intestine, continuing the previous GIA anastomosis through the proximal end of the remaining colon.

proximal to the mid-transverse colon and primary anastomosis of the transverse colon to the upper rectum. The rectum is retained and remains in continuity without alteration. In the modification by Rehbein,[109] the resection includes a greater portion of the rectum.

Two-Stage Pull-Through Techniques

Black,[12] Turnbull,[148] and Pellerin[103] have each independently devised a two-stage operation in which the rectum is divided at the level of the internal sphincter mechanism and the normally innervated intestine pulled through the everted rectal stump with fixation by serosal sutures or clips. In 1–2 weeks, a secondary suture anastomosis or cautery removal of the redundant colon is done. Retraction of the pulled-through colon and doughnut-like strictures requiring prolonged dilatation have made these procedures unpopular, although a place remains for their use in the patient with primary pull-through failure.

Other Procedures

Kasai et al.[74] combined colectomy and posterior transanal myectomy abdominally and perineally. Satomura[117] describes a unique endorectal pull-through procedure with a nonsuture anastomosis. Lernan and Nissan[85] performed a low anterior resection joining the colon to a long posterior anorectal myectomy

and sphincterectomy. This was followed by good results in six of nine patients, without complications. Such procedures have not been widely used in this country.

Postoperative Complications

Conditions essential for successful surgical treatment of Hirschsprung's disease are those common to any successful colon operation and include adequate blood supply to the two anastomosed ends of intestine, lack of tension on the suture line, good hemostasis, and adequate resection of the aganglionic intestine. A complication common to all of the operations has been postoperative intestinal obstruction from adhesions, volvulus, or intussusception. Leakage from the anastomosis may be especially hazardous in the Swenson procedure, since the anastomosis is above the levator mechanism but below the peritoneal floor. A resulting abscess may not be apparent before sudden rupture into the peritoneal cavity. Suture line leakage in the endorectal pull-through procedure results in a sleeve abscess between the pulled-through colon and the muscular cuff of the rectum. This may be difficult to diagnose until chronic sepsis or fistula indicates the source of the trouble. Patients undergoing the Swenson procedure appear to be prone to enterocolitis, the disorder often appearing for the first time postoperatively. Enterocolitis occurs in a significant number of patients following the Duhamel procedure. In our experience, such patients have always had enterocolitis before the definitive procedure. Endorectal procedures have, according to Boley,[19] the lowest incidence of postoperative enterocolitis. Late postoperative enterocolitis in treated Hirschsprung's disease may mimic the symptoms of untreated Hirschsprung's disease. Prolonged decompression by rectal tubes, anal dilatation, and anal sphincterotomy provide relief. The temptation to do a second, different type of pull-through procedure should be resisted unless there is clear evidence of a previously inadequate resection. Anastomotic leaks represent a real hazard. When suspected, prompt emergency colostomy is mandatory. Procrastination and lesser procedures allow continuing infection to result in granulomas and scarring, with permanent destructive changes, and incontinence. Emergency transverse colostomy was done in 18 of our patients. Late complications include stenosis and soiling. Enlargement and inadequate emptying of the rectal pouch with subsequent stenosis, fecalomas, and soiling were peculiar to the original Duhamel procedure. Modification of the Duhamel operation have practically eliminated this problem. Simple further division of the common wall provides dramatic, lasting improvement. Re-formation of the common wall when divided by the stapler has been reported[42] but must be rare. Anastomotic stenosis is a hazard peculiar to the Swenson operation.

Operative Results

What results can be achieved by these operative procedures? Functional constipation, with spontaneous improvement and later complete recovery, is common, so that early functional evaluation may be erroneous. A follow-up period of less than 5 years is probably meaningless for the final evaluation of the various operative procedures.

Swenson's Procedure

Swenson et al.,[138] in a comprehensive review of 483 patients undergoing the Swenson procedure, recorded an overall mortality rate of 3.3% (16 of 483). The mortality varied with age, being greatest (28.5% or eight of 28) in those under 4 months of age at operation. Immediate postoperative complications included wound infection (4.6%), wound dehiscence (1.2%), anastomotic leaks (5%), pelvic abscesses (2.9%), and intestinal obstruction (2.7%). Late postoperative complications were rectal strictures (6.2%) and temporary soiling (13.3%). Ten (2.1%) of the patients died of other causes. The mortality and complication record must be viewed with appreciation of the fact that this is the report of a total experience going back to 1947. The follow-up period for 435 of these patients extended from less than 1 year to as long as 25 years. Of 282 patients interviewed 5 or more years after operation, 90% had normal bowel habits. Nine patients (3.2%) had permanent soiling, and two patients had permanent colostomies because of rectal strictures due to delayed colostomy for anastomotic leaks and other extenuating circumstances. None had urinary incontinence or impotence. Eighty of the patients are married and have children. Enterocolitis occurred immediately postoperatively in 79 (16.4%) of the patients and late in 100 (27%). Six patients (1.2%) died from enterocolitis 3–36 months postresection. This comprehensive report sets a standard for future reporting of results of other operative procedures. No comparable reports have appeared.

Duhamel's Operation

Duhamel[43] reported a personal series of 28 patients undergoing the Duhamel procedure, with a 2.6% mortality, a 10% complication rate, and a satisfactory result in 96% of the survivors. Ehrenpreis[47] and others[21, 27, 28, 60, 86, 126, 139] achieved similar results with low mortality and minimal postoperative complications. The Duhamel operation is a relatively simple, complication-free procedure, providing an uneventful early postoperative course. Late fecalomas, once a problem, are now avoided by eliminating or reducing the size of the residual rectal pouch.

Soave's Procedure (Endorectal Pull-Through)

Franco Soave[124] kindly provided information concerning his overall experience with 147 patients. He reported three immediate postoperative deaths; 87.9% of 71 patients followed more than 10 years postoperatively had a good result, judged by function, physical examination, and, in most instances, roentgen studies. The remaining 12.1% have mild residual strictures, persistent constipation, or intermittent staining. The experience of others has been variable.[39] Davies, Cywes, and Louw[36] reported four deaths in 24 patients undergoing the two-stage Soave procedure. There were early complications in more than half the patients. The endorectal pull-through with primary anastomosis (Boley) or unsutured (Soave) technique was free of initial complications and resulted in excellent function in 12 of 13 patients reported by Klotz.[77] Davies et al.[36] used the Boley technique in 45 consecutive cases, finding it superior to the two-stage technique. Small series of patients treated by primary suture and the endorectal technique have been reported by many,[32, 57, 107, 114, 115, 117] emphasizing simplicity of the technique and trouble-free immediate postoperative course. Long-term follow-up reports are lacking.

State's Operation

Eighteen patients treated by one-stage extended left colon resection by State[128] were reported as having spontaneous bowel movements and being in good health over 10 years later. Sterioff et al.[130] found only one of three patients well 24 years later following a similar resection. Rehbein's procedure,[109] differing from State's in that the resection includes more of the rectum distally and usually only the rectosigmoid proximally, has resulted in 72% very good, 22% good, and 6% poor results in 267 patients followed more than 5 years.[65] All were continent. This procedure leaves 3–7 cm of aganglionic rectum. An essential part of the postoperative care is forcible dilatation of the anus.

Comparison of Different Procedures

In comparing results of various operative procedures, it is pertinent to point out that many surgeons performing these procedures began their experience with the Swenson operation. The many details necessary for success in the definitive operation were worked out by these surgeons with the Swenson operation before the new procedures were introduced. Personal bias and experience are difficult to assess, and the total number of patients in any personal experience is small.

Louw and Cywes,[86] in as closely controlled a study as possible, compared 40 patients with Swenson operations to 40 Duhamel-treated patients. Mortality and complications were similar. They concluded that Swenson's operation is more suitable for older children and Duhamel's better for those under 1 year of age. Dorman et al.[41] reported on 61 children, 31 having Swenson's operations and 30 Duhamel's, and concluded that completely normal bowel function was preserved more often in patients treated by the Duhamel technique. Soper and Figueroa[125] compared a series of patients who had a modified Duhamel procedure with a similar series having the Boley technique and concluded that both procedures are technically easy to perform, associated with little morbidity or mortality, and are acceptable treatment for Hirschsprung's disease. San Filippo et al.,[114] discussing results of definitive procedures in the treatment of 56 patients with Hirschsprung's disease, concluded that the highest complication rate was in the Duhamel-treated group. The endorectal pull-through procedure was deemed superior because it had the fewest complications and the best long-term results.

Holzschneider's[65] comprehensive evaluation of 439 patients from 16 pediatric surgical departments in the United States and Europe, examined 1–18 years following definitive surgical treatment, confirms reports of others. According to his studies, the best results were achieved with the Duhamel-Grob procedure, using the stapler. Khan and Nixon,[72] reviewing a group of 62 patients followed more than 5 years postoperatively, favored the Duhamel procedure but indicated that the differences in results following the Swenson, Duhamel, and sutured Soave procedures were not great. Progressive improvement in function and bowel control with time is noted in all.

The survey of American surgeons' experience[76] with Hirschsprung's disease indicated a preference for Swenson's procedure by 23% of the surgeons, Duhamel's procedure by 30%, and an endorectal pull-through by 47% (39% primary anastomosis, 8% two-stage procedure). The survey concluded that all procedures were being used successfully for the treatment of Hirschsprung's disease, that Swenson's procedure was followed by a 15% incidence of enterocolitis, and that the incidence of this complication was lower with the other operative procedures.

Postoperative Roentgen Studies

The barium enema[71] following Swenson's operation shows reduced colon length with straightening of the left colon and often downward displacement of the splenic flexure. The suture line cannot usually be identified, and the colon returns in most instances to near-normal caliber by 4 months postoperatively. In the lateral view, increased prerectal space seen preoperatively persists for several months, but there is no evidence of a small rectum. Many patients have no roentgen abnormalities other than shortening of the colon. In the Duhamel patients, a distinctive roentgen appearance after operation is apparent in the anteroposterior projection—a double barium density as the rectal pouch is superimposed on the proximal colon. The lateral projection clearly outlines the anterior rectum. In the modifications of the Duhamel procedure, the postoperative films show no rectal pouch and often appear remarkably normal. Following the Soave operation, the appearance on barium enema examination depends on the length of time since operation. The lateral view initially demonstrates a wide presacral space, and the canal in the anteroposterior projection may appear stiff, straight, and narrow. After some time, the appearance may be quite normal.

Experience—Children's Hospital of Pittsburgh

Table 106–5 contrasts our recent with our previous experience. Enterocolitis appeared commonly (25%) 2–6 months postoperatively after Swenson's procedure in the early series and continues to be a postoperative problem in the current series (three of 12 patients, 25%). The single death in the recent series was due to a bizarre anaerobic abdominal wall infection that caused death 24 hours following an uneventful Swenson procedure. Our early experience[39] (1973) with the endorectal pull-through procedure was disappointing, with three deaths from enterocolitis and many serious complications in our first 20 patients. Current experience with an additional 25 patients, using Boley's primary suture technique, has proved this to be a safe, effective procedure. Duhamel's operation has been followed by a low initial mortality and morbidity and by generally good functional results. This procedure has been used in all patients with aganglionosis coli—a particularly difficult group of patients. Enterocolitis was encountered after all procedures but was less frequent and less severe after the Duhamel procedure. The functional result of the operation improved with time, regardless of the type of operation done,[72] so that in our series 122 (81%) of 151 patients followed beyond 5 years have normal evacuation and continence. Extensive aganglionosis involving the entire colon was present in 31 patients. Fifteen of these are now alive; two of them with almost total aganglionosis have jejunostomies and require intravenous alimentation. Seven of these patients appear to have a good result, are continent, but have occasional increase in stool frequency.

Personal Approach to Hirschsprung's Disease

Hirschsprung's disease, when diagnosed in the newborn and in infants under 3 months of age, is treated by prompt right transverse colostomy. If the infant's abdomen is not grossly distended, and if the colon is promptly and persistently decompressed by anal dilatations, a regimen of dilatation and rectal irrigation is begun and continued until a primary pull-through procedure is done after 1 year of age. If aganglionosis extends beyond the low or middle sigmoid area, an enterostomy is placed just proximal to the transition zone, as determined by frozen section at the time of operation. For long-segment aganglionosis, including aganglionosis coli, the Duhamel operation is used. Myectomy is used for low aganglionosis when clear radiologic evidence of a transition zone is lacking. In adults, the Duhamel operation is preferred, preceded by colostomy.

With Duhamel's operation, since the rectum is not removed, the morbidity is minimal. The initial and long-term results com-

TABLE 106–5.—HIRSCHSPRUNG'S DISEASE: TOTAL EXPERIENCE, 1950–1973, CONTRASTED WITH 1974–1982, CHILDREN'S HOSPITAL OF PITTSBURGH

	NO. 1950–73	NO. 1974–82	DEAD 1950–73	DEAD 1974–82	LIVING 1950–73	LIVING 1974–82
Dead on arrival	2	0	2	—	0	—
No. of operations	8	0	0	—	8	—
Nondefinitive operation only	34	4	33	4	1	0
Definitive operation elsewhere	7	2	—	—	7	2
Definitive operation						
Unorthodox procedure	2	0	2	—	0	—
State	1	0	0	—	1	—
Swenson	80	12	9	1	71	11
Duhamel	68	34	1	—	67	34
Endorectal	23	25	4	—	19	25
Total	174	71	16	1	158	70
Grand total	225	77	51	5	174	72

pare favorably with those of the Swenson procedure. For these reasons, our preference is for the Duhamel operation for treatment of Hirschsprung's disease.

REFERENCES

1. Aaronson I., Nixon H.H.: A clinical evaluation of anorectal pressure studies in the diagnosis of Hirschsprung's disease. *Gut* 13:138, 1972.
2. Andrassy R.J., Isaacs H., Weitzman J.J.: Rectal suction biopsy for the diagnosis of Hirschsprung's disease. *Ann. Surg.* 193:419, 1981.
3. Aldridge R.K., Campbell P.E.: Ganglion cell distribution in the normal rectum and anal canal: A basis for the diagnosis of Hirschsprung's disease by anorectal biopsy. *J. Pediatr. Surg.* 3:475, 1968.
4. Arhan P., DeVroede G., Davis K., et al.: Viscoelastic properties of the rectal wall in Hirschsprung's disease. *J. Clin. Invest.* 62:82, 1978.
5. Bentley J.F.R.: Posterior excisional anorectal myotomy in management of chronic fecal accumulation. *Arch. Dis. Child.* 41:144, 1966.
6. Bentley J.F.R., Nixon H.H., Ehrenpreis T., et al.: Seminar on pseudo-Hirschsprung's disease and related disorders. *Arch. Dis. Child.* 41:143, 1966.
7. Berdon W.E., Baker D.H.: The roentgenographic diagnosis of Hirschsprung's disease in infancy. *Am. J. Roentgenol.* 93:432, 1965.
8. Berry C.L.: Persistent changes in the large bowel following the enterocolitis associated with Hirschsprung's disease. *J. Pathol.* 97:131, 1969.
9. Bill A.H., Creighton S.A., Stevenson J.K.: The selection of infants and children for the surgical treatment of Hirschsprung's disease. *Surg. Gynecol. Obstet.* 104:151, 1957.
10. Bill A.H., Chapman N.D.: The enterocolitis of Hirschsprung's disease: Its natural history and treatment. *Am. J. Surg.* 103:70, 1962.
11. Bill A.H., Donald J.C.: Modified procedure for Hirschsprung's disease to eliminate rectal pouch. *Surg. Gynecol. Obstet.* 128:831, 1969.
12. Black M.B., Botham R.J.: Combined abdominorectal resection for lesions of the mid and upper parts of the rectum. *Arch. Surg.* 76:688, 1958.
13. Blanchard H., Collin P.P., Braun P.: Maneuver for easy dissection during the endorectal pull-through procedure in children. *Surg. Gynecol. Obstet.* 138:607, 1974.
14. Bodian M.: Pathological aids in the diagnosis and management of Hirschsprung's disease, in Dyke S.C. (ed.): *Recent Advances in Clinical Pathology.* London, J. & A. Churchill, Ltd., 1960, 3d series.
15. Bodian M., Stephens F.D., Ward B.L.H.: Hirschsprung's disease and idiopathic megacolon. *Lancet* 1:6, 1949.
16. Bolande R.P.: Neurocrestopathies. *Hum. Pathol.* 5:409, 1974.
17. Bolande R.P.: Animal model of human disease: Hirschsprung's disease, aganglionic or hypoganglionic megacolon. *Am. J. Pathol.* 79:189, 1975.
18. Boley S.J.: New modification of the surgical treatment of Hirschsprung's disease. *Surgery* 56:1015, 1964.
19. Boley S.J.: Hirschsprung's Disease: Choice of operation, in Mangot R.: *Abdominal Operations,* ed. 6. New York, Appleton-Century-Crofts, 1974, p. 1732.
20. Boley S.J.: Editorial: The pathophysiology of Hirschsprung's disease—a continuing search. *J. Pediatr. Surg.* 10:861, 1975.
21. Bowring A., Kern I.B.: The management of Hirschsprung's disease in the neonate. *Aust. Paediatr. J.* 8:121, 1972.
22. Branski D., Lebenthal E.: Small intestinal changes in enterocolitis complicating Hirschsprung's disease. *J. Clin. Gastroenterol.* 1:237, 1979.
23. Bugaighis A.G., Lister J.: Incidence of diabetes in families of patients with Hirschsprung's disease. *J. Pediatr. Surg.* 6:620, 1970.
24. Burke J.A., Belin R.P.: Hirschsprung's disease associated with anasarca and hypoproteinemia. *South. Med. J.* 68:1011, 1975.
25. Burnstock G.: Purinergic nerves. *Pharmacol. Rev.* 24:509, 1972.
26. Burnstock G.: Costa M.: Inhibitory innervation of the gut. *Gastroenterology* 64:141, 1973.
27. Burrington J.D., Wayne E.R.: Modified Duhamel procedure for treatment of total aganglionic colon in children. *J. Pediatr. Surg.* 11:391, 1976.
28. Canty T.G.: Modified Duhamel procedure for treatment of Hirschsprung's disease in infancy and childhood: Review of 41 consecutive cases. *J. Pediatr. Surg.* 17:773, 1982.
29. Carcassonne M., Morisson G., LaCombe, et al.: Primary corrective operation without decompression in infants less than three months of age with Hirschsprung's disease. *J. Pediatr. Surg.* 17:241, 1982.
30. Carter C.O., Evans K., Hickman V.: Children of those treated surgically for Hirschsprung's disease. *J. Med. Genetics* 18:87, 1981.
31. Chatten J., Voorhees M.L.: Familial neuroblastoma. *N. Engl. J. Med.* 277:1230, 1967.
32. Coran A.G., Weintraub W.H.: Modification of the endorectal procedure for Hirschsprung's disease. *Surg. Gynecol. Obstet.* 143:277, 1976.
33. Davidson M.: Alimentary canal, in Code C.F., Werner H. (eds.): *Handbook of Physiology,* ed. 5. Baltimore, Williams & Wilkins, 1970, p. 2783.
34. Davidson M., Bauer C.H.: Studies of distal colonic motility. IV. Achalasia of the distal rectal segment despite presence of ganglia in the myenteric plexus in this area. *Pediatrics* 21:746, 1958.
35. Davies M.R.Q., Cywes S.: Inadequate pouch emptying following Martin's pull-through procedure for intestinal aganglionosis. *J. Pediatr. Surg.* 18:14, 1983.
36. Davies M.R.Q., Cywes S., Louw J.H.: Franco Soave's operation. *S. Afr. J. Surg.* 13:223, 1975.
37. Davis W.S., Allen R.P., Favara B.E., et al.: Neonatal small left colon syndrome. *Am. J. Roentgenol.* 120:322, 1974.
38. Dimler M.: "Acquired" Hirschsprung's disease. *J. Pediatr. Surg.* 16:844, 1981.
39. Doedhar M., Sieber W.K., Kiesewetter W.B.: A critical look at the Soave procedure for Hirschsprung's disease. *J. Pediatr. Surg.* 8:249, 1973.
40. Dobbins W.O., Bill A.H.: Diagnosis of Hirschsprung's disease excluded by rectal suction biopsy. *N. Engl. J. Med.* 272:990, 1965.
41. Dorman G.W., Votteler T.P., Graivier L.: A preliminary evaluation of the results of treatment of Hirschsprung's disease by the Duhamel-Grob modification of the Swenson pull-through operation. *Ann. Surg.* 166:783, 1967.
42. Dudgeon D.L., Coran A.G., Rosenkrantz J.G.: Septum reformation: A complication of the Duhamel procedure. *Surgery* 73:274, 1973.
43. Duhamel B.: Retrorectal and transanal pull-through procedure for the treatment of Hirschsprung's disease. *Dis. Colon Rectum* 7:455, 1964.
44. Dunn P.M.: Intestinal obstruction in the newborn with special reference to transient functional ileus associated with respiratory distress syndrome. *Arch. Dis. Child.* 38:459, 1963.
45. Ehrenpreis T.: Megacolon in the newborn: A clinical and roentgenological study with special regard to the pathogenesis. *Acta Chir. Scand.* 94:(suppl. 112), 1946.
46. Ehrenpreis T.: Acquired megacolon as a complication of rectosigmoidectomy for Hirschsprung's disease. *Arch. Dis. Child.* 40:180, 1965.
47. Ehrenpreis T.: *Hirschsprung's Disease.* Chicago: Year Book Medical Publishers, 1970.
48. Ehrenpreis T., Ericsson N.O., Livaditis A.: Anomalies of the urinary tract in patients with Hirschsprung's disease. *Z. Kinderchir.* 8:89, 1970.
49. Elema J.J., deVries J.A., Vos L.J.J.: Intensity and proximal extension of acetylcholinesterase activity in the mucosa of the rectosigmoid in Hirschsprung's disease. *J. Pediatr. Surg.* 8:361, 1973.
50. Ellis D.G., Clatworthy H.W. Jr.: The meconium plug syndrome revisited. *J. Pediatr. Surg.* 1:54, 1966.
51. El Shafie M., Suzuki H., Schnaufer L., et al.: A simplified method of anorectal manometry for wider clinical application. *J. Pediatr. Surg.* 7:230, 1972.
52. Finney J.: Congenital idiopathic dilatation of colon. *Surg. Gynecol. Obstet.* 6:624, 1908.
53. Fraser G.C., Berry C.: Mortality in neonatal Hirschsprung's disease: With particular reference to enterocolitis. *J. Pediatr. Surg.* 2:205, 1967.
54. Frigo G.M., DelTacco J., Lecchini S., et al.: Some observations on the intrinsic nervous mechanism in Hirschsprung's disease. *Gut* 14:35, 1973.
55. Garrett J.R., Howard E.R., Nixon H.H.: Autonomic nerves in rectum and colon in Hirschsprung's disease. *Arch. Dis. Child.* 44:406, 1969.
56. Gherardi G.J.: Pathology of the ganglionic-aganglionic junction in congenital megacolon. *Arch. Pathol.* 69:650, 1960.
57. Gordan F.T., Coran A.G., Wesley J.R.: Modified endorectal procedure for management of long-segment aganglionosis. *Ann. Surg.* 194:70, 1981.
58. Gravier L., Sieber W.K.: Hirschsprung's disease and mongolism. *Surgery* 60:458, 1966.
59. Grob M., Genton N., Vontobel V.: Erfahrungen in der Megacolon congenitum and Vorschlag einer neuen Operationstechnik. *Zentralbl. Chir.* 84:1781, 1959.
60. Grosfeld J.L., Ballantine V.N., Csiko J.F.: A critical evaluation of the Duhamel operation for Hirschsprung's disease. *Arch. Surg.* 113:454, 1978.

61. Hiatt R.B.: The surgical treatment of congenital megacolon. *Ann. Surg.* 133:321, 1951.
62. Hiatt R.B.: A further description of the pathologic physiology of congenital megacolon and the results of surgical treatment. *Pediatrics* 21:825, 1958.
63. Hirschsprung H.: Stuhlträgheit Neugeborener in Folge von Dilatation und Hypertrophie des Colons. *Jahrb. Kinderh.* 27:1, 1887.
64. Holzschneider A.M., Kraeft H.: The value and reliability of anorectal electro-manometry. *Z. Kinderchir.* 33:25, 1981.
65. Holzschneider M.: *Hirschsprung's Disease.* Stuttgart: Hippokrates-Verlag; New York, Thieme-Stratton, 1982.
66. Holzschneider A.M., Kellner E., Streibl P., et al.: The development of anorectal continence and its significance in the diagnosis of Hirschsprung's disease. *J. Pediatr. Surg.* 11:151, 1976.
67. Howard E.R.: Hirschsprung's disease: A review of the morphology and physiology. *Postgrad. Med. J.* 48:471, 1972.
68. Howard E.R.: Histochemistry in the diagnosis and investigation of congenital aganglionosis (Hirschsprung's disease). *Ann. Surg.* 39:602, 1973.
69. Huntley C.C., Shaffner L. deS., Challa V.R., et al.: Histochemical diagnosis of Hirschsprung's disease. *Pediatrics* 69:755, 1982.
70. Ikeda K.: New techniques in the surgical treatment of Hirschsprung's disease. *Surgery* 61:503, 1967.
71. James E.A. Jr., Greenfield J.B., Pfister R.C., et al.: The roentgenologic appearance of postoperative congenital megacolon (Hirschsprung's disease). *Am. J. Roentgenol.* 109:351, 1970.
72. Khan O., Nixon H.H.: Results following surgery for Hirschsprung's disease: A review of three operations with reference to neorectal capacity. *Br. J. Surg.* 67:436, 1980.
73. Kapila L., Haberkorn S., Nixon H.H.: Chronic adynamic bowel simulating Hirschsprung's disease. *J. Pediatr. Surg.* 10:885, 1975.
74. Kasai M., Suzuki H., O'Hi R., et al.: Rectoplasty with posterior triangular colonic flap—a radical new operation for Hirschsprung's disease. *J. Pediatr. Surg.* 12:207, 1977.
75. Kiesewetter W.B., Sukarochana K., Sieber W.K.: The frequency of aganglionosis associated with imperforate anus. *Surgery* 58:855, 1965.
76. Kleinhaus S., Boley S.J., Sheraw M., et al.: Hirschsprung's disease: A survey of the members of the Surgical Section of the American Academy of Pediatrics. *J. Pediatr. Surg.* 14:588, 1979.
77. Klotz D.H. Jr., Volcek T.T., Kottmeier P.H.: Reappraisal of the endorectal pull-through operation for Hirschsprung's disease. *J. Pediatr. Surg.* 8:595, 1973.
78. Koberle F.: Enteromegaly and cardiomegaly in Chagas' disease. *Gut* 4:399, 1963.
79. Lake B.D., Puri P., Nixon H.H., et al.: Hirschsprung's disease: An appraisal of histochemically demonstrated acetylcholinesterase activity in suction rectal biopsy specimens as an aid to diagnosis. *Arch. Pathol. Lab. Med.* 102:244, 1978.
80. Lake B.D., Claireaux A.E.: Acetylcholinesterase and Hirschsprung's disease (letter). *Arch. Path. Lab. Med.* 107:661, 1983.
81. Lavery I.C.: The surgery of Hirschsprung's disease. *Surg. Clin. North Am.* 63:161, 1983.
82. Leenders E., Sieber W.K.: Congenital megacolon observation by Frederick Ruysch—1691. *J. Pediatr. Surg.* 5:1, 1970.
83. Leonidas J.C., Krasna I.H., Strauss L., et al.: Roentgen appearance of the excluded colon after colostomy for infantile Hirschsprung's disease. *Am. J. Roentgenol.* 112:116, 1971.
84. LeQuesne G.W., Reilly B.J.: Functional immaturity of the large bowel in the newborn. *Radiol. Clin. North Am.* 13:331, 1975.
85. Lernan O.Z., Nissan S.: Low anterior resection with a long posterior anorectal myectomy and sphincterectomy for Hirschsprung's disease. *J. Pediatr. Surg.* 15:613, 1980.
86. Louw J.H., Cywes S.: Treatment of Hirschsprung's disease. *S. Afr. J. Surg.* 5:69, 1967.
87. Lynn H.B.: Rectal myectomy in Hirschsprung's disease, a decade of experience. *Arch. Surg.* 110:991, 1975.
88. Marks R.M.: Endorectal split sleeve pull-through procedure for Hirschsprung's disease. *Surg. Gynecol. Obstet.* 136:627, 1973.
89. Martin L.W.: Surgical management of total colonic aganglionosis. *Ann. Surg.* 176:343, 1972.
90. Martin L.W.: Total colonic aganglionosis preservation and utilization of entire colon. *J. Pediatr. Surg.* 17:635, 1982.
91. Martin L.W., Altemeier W.A.: Clinical experience with a new operation (modified Duhamel procedure) for Hirschsprung's disease. *Ann. Surg.* 156:678, 1962.
92. Martin L.W., Caudill D.R.: A method for elimination of the blind rectal pouch in the Duhamel operation for Hirschsprung's disease. *Surgery* 62:951, 1967.
93. Martin L.W., Perrin E.V.: Neonatal perforation of the appendix in association with Hirschsprung's disease. *Ann. Surg.* 166:799, 1967.
94. Meier-Ruge W.: Hirschsprung's disease: Its aetiology, pathogenesis and differential diagnosis. *Curr. Top. Pathol.* 59:131, 1974.
95. Mya G.: Due osservazioni di dilatazione ed ipertrofia congenita del colon. *Sperimentale* 48:215, 1894.
96. Nissan S., Bar-Maor J.A.: Further experience in the diagnosis and surgical treatment of short-segment Hirschsprung's disease and idiopathic megacolon. *J. Pediatr. Surg.* 6:738, 1971.
97. Nixon G.W., Condon V.R.: Intestinal perforation as a complication of the neonatal small left colon syndrome. *Am. J. Roentgenol.* 125:75, 1975.
98. Nixon H.H.: Megacolon and other congenital anomalies of the colon, in Goligher J.C. (ed.): *Surgery of the Anus, Rectum and Colon,* ed. 3. Springfield, Ill.: Charles C Thomas, Publisher, 1975.
99. Noblett H.R.: A rectal suction biopsy tube for use in the diagnosis of Hirschsprung's disease. *J. Pediatr. Surg.* 4:406, 1969.
100. Okamoto E., Ueda T.: Embryogenesis of intramural ganglia of the gut and its relation to Hirschsprung's disease. *J. Pediatr. Surg.* 2:437, 1967.
101. Passarge E.: Genetics of Hirschsprung's disease. *Clin. Gastroenterol.* 2:507, 1973.
102. Pease P.W.B., Corkery J.J., Camero N.A.H.: Diagnosis of Hirschsprung's disease by punch biopsy of rectum. *Arch. Dis. Child.* 51:541, 1976.
103. Pellerin D.: Le traitement chirurgicale de la maladie de Hirschsprung par la resection-anastomose exteriorisée sans suture. *J. Int. Coll. Surg.* 37:691, 1962.
104. Perrault J., Stockwell M., Stephens C., et al.: Malabsorption and pouch ulceration following the Martin repair for total colonic aganglionosis. *J. Pediatr. Surg.* 14:458, 1979.
105. Philippart A.I., Reed J.O., Georgeson K.E.: Neonatal small left colon syndrome: Intramural not intraluminal obstruction. *J. Pediatr. Surg.* 10:733, 1975.
106. Pochaczevsky R., Leonidas J.C.: Recto-sigmoid index. *Am. J. Roentgenol.* 123:770, 1975.
107. Pomerantz M., Sabiston D.C.: Modified operation for the treatment of Hirschsprung's disease. *Am. J. Surg.* 115:198, 1968.
108. Rees B.I., Azma A., Nigam M., et al.: Complications of rectal suction biopsy. *J. Pediatr. Surg.* 18:273, 1983.
109. Rehbein F., Morger R., Kundert J.G., et al.: Surgical problems in congenital megacolon (Hirschsprung's disease). *J. Pediatr. Surg.* 1:526, 1966.
110. Richardson J.: Pharmacological studies of Hirschsprung's disease on murine model. *J. Pediatr. Surg.* 10:875, 1975.
111. Robertson H.E., Kernohan J.W.: The myenteric plexus in congenital megacolon. *Proc. Staff Meet. Mayo Clin.* 13:123, 1938.
112. Roviralta E.: Congenital megacolon: Colon exclusion: Procedure of choice in the infant. *Rev. Esp. Pediatr.* 22:297, 1966.
113. Sane S.M., Girdany B.R.: Total aganglionosis coli. *Radiology* 107:397, 1973.
114. San Filippo J.A., Allen J.E., Jewett T.C.: Definitive surgical management of Hirschsprung's disease. *Arch.* 105:245, 1972.
115. SanLuis J.L., Nemoto T., Beardmore H.E.: Surgical treatment of Hirschsprung's disease. *Surgery* 63:331, 1968.
116. Saperstein L., Pollack J., Beck A.R.: Total intestinal aganglionosis. *Mt. Sinai J. Med.* 47:72, 1980.
117. Satomura K.: Follow-up study of the endorectal pull-through operation for the treatment of Hirschsprung's disease with special reference to intestinal anastomosis. *Surgery* 76:581, 1974.
118. Schärli A.F., Meier-Ruge W.: Localized and disseminated forms of neuronal dysplasia mimicking Hirschsprung's disease. *J. Pediatr. Surg.* 16:164, 1981.
119. Shandling B., Auldist A.W.: Punch biopsy of the rectum for the diagnosis of Hirschsprung's disease. *J. Pediatr. Surg.* 7:546, 1972.
120. Sieber W.K.: Hirschsprung's disease. *Curr. Prob. Surg.* June 1978.
121. Skinner R., Irvine D.: Hirschsprung's disease and congenital deafness. *J. Med. Genet.* 10:337, 1973.
122. Smith B.: Pre- and postnatal development of the ganglion cells of the rectum and its surgical implications. *J. Pediatr. Surg.* 3:386, 1968.
123. So H.B., Schwartz D.L., Becker J.M., et al.: Endorectal "pull-through" without preliminary colostomy in neonates with Hirschsprung's disease. *J. Pediatr. Surg.* 15:470, 1980.
124. Soave F.: Hirschsprung's disease: A new surgical technique. *Arch. Dis. Child.* 39:116, 1964.
125. Soper R.T., Figueroa P.R.: Surgical treatment of Hirschsprung's disease: Comparison of modification of the Duhamel and Soave operations. *J. Pediatr. Surg.* 6:761, 1971.
126. Soper R.T., Miller F.E.: Modification of Duhamel procedure: Elimination of rectal pouch and colorectal septum. *J. Pediatr. Surg.* 3:376, 1968.

127. Soper R.T., Opitz J.M.: Neonatal pneumoperitoneum and Hirschsprung's disease. *Surgery* 51:527, 1961.
128. State D.: Segmental colon resection in the treatment of congenital megacolon (Hirschsprung's disease). *Am. J. Surg.* 105:93, 1963.
129. Steinbach H.L., Rosenberg R.H., Grossman M., et al.: The potential hazard of enemas in patients with Hirschsprung's disease. *Radiology* 64:45, 1955.
130. Sterioff S. Jr., White J.J., Ravitch M.M.: Hirschsprung's disease: Long-term results of resection of the proximal dilated segment. *J. Pediatr. Surg.* 8:309, 1973.
131. Sulamaa M.: Anastomotic clamp for retro-rectal transanal pull-through procedure in Hirschsprung's disease—a new modification of Duhamel's operation. *Ann. Chir. Inf.* 9:63, 1968.
132. Swenson O.: *Pediatric Surgery,* ed. 2. New York, Appleton-Century-Crofts, 1962.
133. Swenson O.: Sphincterotomy in the treatment of Hirschsprung's disease. *Ann. Surg.* 160:540, 1964.
134. Swenson O., Bill A.H.: Resection of rectum and rectosigmoid with preservation of the sphincter for benign spastic lesions producing megacolon: An experimental study. *Surgery* 24:212, 1948.
135. Swenson O., Fisher J.H., Gherardi G.J.: Rectal biopsy in the diagnosis of Hirschsprung's disease. *Surgery* 45:690, 1959.
136. Swenson O., Neuhauser E.B.D., Pickett L.K.: New concepts of etiology, diagnosis and treatment of congenital megacolon (Hirschsprung's disease). *Pediatrics* 4:201, 1949.
137. Swenson O., Sherman J.O., Fisher J.H.: Diagnosis of congenital megacolon: An analysis of 501 patients. *J. Pediatr. Surg.* 8:587, 1973.
138. Swenson O., Sherman J.O., Fisher J.H., et al.: The treatment and postoperative complications of congenital megacolon: A 25 year follow-up. *Ann. Surg.* 182:266, 1975.
139. Talbert J.L., Seashore J.H., Ravitch M.M.: Evaluation of modified Duhamel operation for correction of Hirschsprung's disease. *Ann. Surg.* 179:671, 1974.
140. Ternberg J., Winters K.: Plexiform neurofibromatosis of the colon as a cause of congenital megacolon. *Am. J. Surg.* 109:663, 1965.
141. Thomas C.G., Bream C.A., DeConnick P.: Posterior sphincterotomy and rectal myotomy in the management of Hirschsprung's disease. *Ann. Surg.* 171:796, 1970.
142. Thomas D.F.M., Fernie D.S., Malone M., et al.: Association between *Clostridium difficile* and enterocolitis in Hirschsprung's disease. *Lancet* 1:78, 1982.
143. Tiffin M.E., Chandler L.R., Faber H.K.: Localized absence of ganglion cells of the myenteric plexus in congenital megacolon. *Am. J. Dis. Child.* 59:1071, 1940.
144. Tittel K.: Uber eine angeborene Missbildung des Dickdrmes. *Wien Klin. Wochenschr.* 14:903, 1901.
145. Tobon F., Nigel C.R., Reid W., et al.: Non-surgical test for the diagnosis of Hirschsprung's disease. *N. Engl. J. Med.* 278:188, 1968.
146. Tobon F., Schuster M.: Megacolon: Special diagnostic and therapeutic features. *Johns Hopkins Med. J.* 135:91, 1974.
147. Touloukian R.J., Morgenroth V.H. III, Roth R.H.: Sympathetic neurotransmitter metabolism in Hirschsprung's disease. *J. Pediatr. Surg.* 10:593, 1975.
148. Turnbull R.B.: Pull-through resection of the rectum with delayed anastomosis, for cancer or Hirschsprung's disease. *Surgery* 59:498, 1966.
149. Vanhouette J.J.: Primary aganglionosis associated with imperforate anus: Review of the literature pertinent to one observation. *J. Pediatr. Surg.* 4:468, 1969.
150. Webster W.: Aganglionic megacolon in piebald-lethal mice. *Arch. Pathol.* 97:111, 1974.
151. Weinberg A.G.: Hirschsprung's disease—a pathologist's view. *Perspect. Pediatr. Pathol.* 2:207, 1975.
152. Young L.W., Yunis E.J., Girdany B.R., et al.: Megacystis-microcolon-intestinal hypoperistalsis syndrome: Additional clinical, radiological, surgical and histopathological aspects. *AJR* 137:749, 1981.
153. Yunis E.J., Dibbins A.W., Sherman F.E.: Rectal suction biopsy in the diagnosis of Hirschsprung's disease in infants. *Arch. Pathol. Lab. Med.* 100:329, 1976.
154. Yunis E.J., Sieber W.K., Akers D.R.: Does zonal aganglionosis really exist? Report of a rare variety of Hirschsprung's disease and review of the literature. *Pediatr. Pathol.* 1:33, 1983.
155. Zachary R.B., Lister J.: Crushing instrument for Duhamel's procedure in Hirschsprung's disease. *Lancet* 1:476, 1964.
156. Zuelzer W.W., Wilson J.L.: Functional intestinal obstruction on congenital neurogenic basis in infancy. *Am. J. Dis. Child.* 75:40, 1948.

Swenson's Procedure
Jordan J. Weitzman

In 1948, a landmark article was published describing the first curative operation for Hirschsprung's disease.[3] This operation, known as the Swenson procedure, with only one modification[4] is still employed by surgeons throughout the world.

Most patients with Hirschsprung's disease are diagnosed during infancy and should initially be treated with colostomy. Although the colostomy may be performed months before the pull-through, it should be regarded as the first stage of the pull-through and should be placed in the terminal portion of the normal ganglionic colon. The final step of the Swenson procedure is a two-layered anastomosis, which will be more difficult if the muscular wall of the pulled-through bowel has atrophied because it was distal to the colostomy. The reader is directed to more detailed discussions of colostomy placement.[6, 8] If a child older than 6 months is diagnosed as having Hirschsprung's disease, is in good general health, and has minimal proximal colonic distention, the preliminary colostomy can be eliminated.

Preoperative preparation in children with a colostomy is mechanical, with a clear liquid diet for 2–3 days and saline enemas of the colostomy stomas. The operation is deferred until the child is 1 year old, weighs at least 20 lb, and has been free of symptoms of enterocolitis for at least 6 months.

The technique is illustrated in Figure 106–13. Some points not illustrated need emphasis. The operation is carried out with the patient in the lithotomy position with drapes arranged so that the perineum can be exposed without contaminating the abdominal field. In the older child, especially one who has not had a preliminary colostomy, it can be very difficult to remove all fecal material from the colon preoperatively. This retained fecal material will cause no problems if the Swenson procedure is performed with the abdominal and perineal fields draped separately. The step shown in Figure 106–13,*C* can be performed without contaminating the abdomen and the proximal colon, which may contain retained feces, if the rectum is not opened until the final step shown in Figure 106–13,*F* (steps 3 and 4). Separate operative teams and instruments must be employed for the abdomen and perineum. Of all the pull-through procedures, the Swenson technique is the only one that can be used without soiling the operative field in the patient with rock-hard fecal impaction in the colon and/or retained fecal material in the aganglionic rectum. Because the consequences of an anastomotic leak can be so serious, a diverting colostomy or ileostomy is performed in all patients, no matter how perfect the anastomosis appears. It must be kept in mind that a diverting colostomy will not prevent the catastrophic complication of a severe rectal stricture, resulting from a poorly performed anastomosis. The colostomy and closure of the abdomen are performed by the second team while the rectal anastomosis is being performed. Digital examination of the rectum is not done until the tenth postoperative day. The protective colostomy is closed 4–6 weeks after the rectal anastomosis has completely healed.

Our results have been excellent. A frequent early postoperative problem is perineal excoriation, which always clears up after a few months. Bladder and ejaculatory dysfunction have not occurred in any of our 65 patients nor in other large series.[1, 5] We have had no rectal strictures and no immediate postoperative deaths, but two late deaths—one very early in our series due to fulminating enterocolitis and one due to a closed-loop bowel obstruction managed at another institution. It is essential that toilet training not be forced on the patient. Toilet training is for the convenience of the parents. Children who are otherwise normal physically, emotionally, and mentally will 90% of the time train themselves by the age of 5 years. Bowel habits improve with age, and problems are virtually absent in the teenager. The most common serious postoperative complication, enterocolitis,[8] occurred in 15% of our patients. The radical rectal resection resulting in a partial internal sphincterectomy (see Fig 106–13,*D*) has not reduced the incidence of postoperative enterocolitis, as Swenson hoped it would, but we believe it should still be done because it has resulted in a higher percentage of normal anorectal reflexes.[2] It is important that the operating surgeon and the parents understand the possibility of enterocolitis so that it can be detected early. With anal dilatation, colon irrigation, and, occasionally, posterior anal sphincterotomy, the problem can be controlled. Fortunately, recurrent enterocolitis almost always disappears by the age of 5 years.[7]

The Swenson procedure is a difficult operation. A well-trained surgeon who masters its technical details[6, 9] can expect good results. Optimal rectal function is best achieved if the operating surgeon personally sees the patient over a period of years, so that the parents as well as the patient have support when any problem regarding bowel function arises. Performing an operation that should provide a child with a lifetime of normal rectal function is an enormous responsibility.

REFERENCES

1. Clausen E.G., Davies O.G. Jr.: Early and late complications of the Swenson pull-through operation for Hirschsprung's disease. *Am. J. Surg.* 106:372, 1963.
2. Holzschneider A., Kellner E., Streibl P., et al.: The development of anorectal continence and its significance in the diagnosis of Hirschsprung's disease. *J. Pediatr. Surg.* 11:151, 1976.
3. Swenson O., Bill A.H.: Resection of rectum and rectosigmoid with preservation of the sphincter for benign spastic lesions producing megacolon. An experimental study. *Surgery* 24:212, 1948.
4. Swenson O.: Partial internal sphincterectomy in the treatment of Hirschsprung's disease. *Ann. Surg.* 160:540, 1964.
5. Swenson O., Sherman J.O., Fisher J.H., et al.: The treatment and postoperative complications of congenital megacolon. *Ann. Surg.* 182:166, 1975
6. Swenson, O.: Hirschsprung's disease, in Raffensperger J.G. (ed.): *Swenson's Pediatric Surgery*, ed. 4. New York, Appleton-Century-Crofts, 1980, p. 519.
7. Weitzman J.J., Hanson B.A., Brennan L.P.: Management of Hirschsprung's disease with the Swenson procedure. *J. Pediatr. Surg.* 7:157, 1972.
8. Weitzman J.J.: Complications of Hirschsprung's disease and its management, in de Vries P.A., Shapiro S.R. (eds.): *Complications of Pediatric Surgery*. New York, John Wiley & Sons, 1982, p. 269.
9. Weitzman J.J.: Hirschsprung's disease: Definitive surgical management with the Swenson procedure. Motion Picture, ACS-843. American College of Surgeons, Surgical Film Library, 1 Casper Street, Danbury, CT 06810.

Duhamel's Procedure—Martin's Method
Lester Martin

The first step of our operative management consists in establishing a diverting colostomy, sufficiently proximal to permit its preservation following the definitive operation, in order to protect the anastomosis. In the event of preoperative enterocolitis, it is our impression that diversion of the fecal stream for at least 6 months will minimize the likelihood of recurrence of enterocolitis following closure of the colostomy. For the usual patient, a right transverse colostomy, with the colon completely divided, is the method of choice.

Definitive Operation

The three currently popular operations originally described by Swenson, Soave, and Duhamel have each undergone modifications so that they now differ considerably less than in their original descriptions. Probably of greater importance than the method employed are the skill and the experience of the individual surgeon.

The operation we use is our modification of the Duhamel procedure. We have eliminated the blind proximal rectal stump by creating an anastomosis from the end of the rectal stump to the side of the pulled-through colon, and we have emphasized a meticulous anastomosis to the anal canal. The aganglionic rectum is left in place but constitutes only half the circumference of the new rectal wall. The sensory function of the rectum is therefore preserved. Dissection within the pelvis is minimal, in order to minimize the risk of injury to the delicate nerve fibers of the bladder and the ejaculatory mechanism.

TECHNIQUE.—Operation (see Fig 106–14) is carried out with the patient in the lithotomy position. A generous left paramedian rectus-retracting incision is used to open the abdomen. The rectum is divided just above the peritoneal floor, with the anastomosis clamps placed obliquely to preserve a longer segment of rectum anteriorly. The proximal aganglionic colon is resected and the proximal end examined microscopically to confirm the presence of ganglion cells. The end of the proximal colon is then closed and inverted with interrupted sutures, the ends of which are left long for subsequent use in drawing the colon down into the pelvis. The presacral space is opened and, by blunt finger dissection, a space created between the rectum and the sacrum as far distally as the levator muscles.

The surgeon then proceeds to the perineal portion of the operation. The anal sphincter is gently dilated, the rectum thoroughly irrigated with sterile saline solution followed by a mild antiseptic, and the area draped. A transverse incision is made with an electrocautery around the posterior half of the rectal wall 1 cm from the mucocutaneous junction. The posterior rectal wall is separated from the puborectal muscle and the presacral space, previously opened from above, is entered. A long curved hemostat is inserted and the end of the proximal colon withdrawn into the pelvis posterior to the rectum through the incision in the posterior rectal wall, to which it is sutured with interrupted fine catgut sutures about the circumference. The sutures closing the end of the colon are then removed and an open anastomosis accomplished from the end of the colon to the opening in the posterior wall of the rectum. The common wall between the native rectum and the pulled-through colon is then resected by applying the GIA stapling instrument twice to remove a triangular-shaped segment of the common wall (Fig 106–17). The cut edges are oversewn in order to prevent any adherence of these edges.

The surgeon then returns to the abdominal part of the operation for the proximal portion of the anastomosis between the proximal end of the rectal stump and the side of the adjacent colon. Both the colon and the end of the rectal stump are opened and the side-to-side anastomosis between the two within the pelvis is completed by inserting the GIA anastomotic stapler from above. The anterior half of the anastomosis between the rectum and the side of the colon is then completed by manual suture, and the peritoneal floor is repaired.

The previously established proximal colostomy is closed 4–6 weeks later after the pelvic anastomosis is completely healed.

ADVANTAGES OF PROCEDURE.—There appear to be several advantages of this operative technique: (1) The entire rectum is preserved and incorporated in the new rectum, preserving the

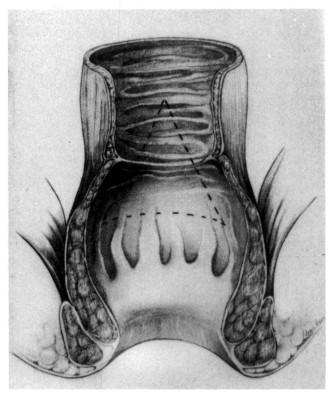

Fig 106–17.—Illustration of triangular-shaped segment, on common wall between rectum and pulled-through ileum, that is removed during Martin's operation. The base of the triangle is the line of incision of the posterior rectal wall through which the proximal, normally ganglionated bowel, is drawn and to the edges of which the end of the proximal bowel is carefully sutured. The sides of the triangle indicate the two lines of application of the GIA™ stapler to produce a wide open anastomosis.

sensory portion of the reflex arc (perception of fullness) for the urge to defecate. (2) The minimal pelvic dissection permits preservation of the nerves supplying the ejaculatory apparatus in the male. (3) Blood loss during the operation is minimal and rarely is there a need for blood transfusion. (4) Half the circumference of the new rectum, which is normally ganglionated, serves to propel the fecal stream. (5) The operation does not leave a residual aganglionic cuff encircling the rectum. (6) An indwelling urethral catheter is rarely necessary following operation unless considerable retraction on the bladder has occurred during the operation.

No deaths have followed this operation, and transfusion during operation has not been necessary. The incidence of postoperative complications has been minimal. All 37 patients experienced relief of constipation and have remained remarkably free of postoperative symptoms.

Soave's Operation—Boley's Technique
Scott J. Boley

The technique of endorectal pull-through for Hirschsprung's disease was adapted from procedures by Ravitch[7] for familial polyposis and ulcerative colitis and by Rehbein[8] and Romualdi[9] for

imperforate anus. The basic principle is bringing proximal normal colon through the aganglionic rectum, stripped of its mucosa. Soave[11] originally described, and continued to employ, a staged technique of endorectal pull-through and delayed anastomosis (see previous section). As suggested in 1964, we have advocated a primary anastomosis.[1]

The advantages of the endorectal pull-through are absence of pelvic dissection (as all dissection below the peritoneal reflection is done within the rectal muscular sleeve), presence of normal propulsive colon down to the anus, intact sensory receptors in the rectal muscular cuff and puborectalis muscle, preservation of all sphincters, few anastomotic problems, and simple postoperative care. Primary anastomosis obviates the prolonged hospitalization, postoperative dilatations, and complications of the protruding colonic stump associated with Soave's procedure. Endorectal pull-through with primary anastomosis does not require the degrees of skill and experience necessary to perform a Swenson procedure properly while providing results that are equal or better. The modified Duhamel procedure is as easy, or easier, to perform as the endorectal pull-through but has been associated with more postoperative incontinence and enterocolitis. Endorectal pull-through with primary anastomosis is our operation of choice for all children with Hirschsprung's disease except those with "ultrashort-segment" disease, in whom anorectal myectomy is preferred.[2, 3] For total colonic aganglionosis, the ileal pull-through is combined with a reservoir fashioned from an antiperistaltic segment of right colon.[4] While we have performed our operation in infants as young as 8 weeks of age, it can be more satisfactorily done at 4–6 months of age. The mucosal dissection is rapid and bloodless when the diagnosis has been made in the neonatal period and a colostomy performed at that time. In older children in whom the diagnosis has been delayed, the hypertrophied bowel makes the dissection more difficult but it still can be performed with only moderate blood loss.

When Hirschsprung's disease is diagnosed in infants under 4 months of age, it is our practice to perform a colostomy immediately and the definitive operation at 4–6 months. In older children, a colostomy is not performed unless the colon cannot be adequately emptied and decompressed. Initially, we placed the colostomy in the most distal ganglionic colon, but a right transverse colostomy is now used except when long-segment aganglionosis is present. While this change adds a third stage to the procedure, it provides protection against infection when the definitive operation is done.

Preoperative preparation consists of a clear liquid diet for 2–3 days and mechanical and antibiotic cleansing of the colon. If a colostomy is present, warm saline enemas are administered into the proximal stoma the morning and evening before operation and the defunctionalized bowel is irrigated with kanamycin solution through the rectum and distal stoma. Kanamycin is given orally for 36 hours before operation.

Technical points to be emphasized are : (1) preservation of the blood supply to the rectal muscular cuff, (2) carrying the transabdominal mucosal dissection low enough (1–2 cm above the dentate line), (3) preservation of 1 cm of rectal mucosa above the dentate line, (4) avoidance of tension on the anastomosis, (5) placement of the sutures between the muscular cuff and colon 1 cm above the colo-anal anastomosis, and (6) avoidance of excess colon between the two layers of sutures to prevent mucosal prolapse. The drain in the cuff must be removed within 48 hours, and digital examination is avoided for 7–10 days (see Fig 106–15).

Our results have been very satisfactory. Defecation usually begins within 48 hours, and most children have been discharged in 7–10 days. In more than 50 patients operated on by this technique, there have been no deaths or major anastomotic complications. Early minor complications have included cuff abscess, minor mucosal prolapse, transient perianal excoriation, and anal stenosis, relieved by dilatation. One patient had mild enterocolitis 1 year postoperatively, and one child developed intestinal obstruction. Delayed bowel training occurred in three children—one with mental retardation, one with α_1-antitrypsin deficiency, and one with a severe emotional problem. The ease and safety of the endorectal pull-through with primary anastomosis and the good immediate and late results have led to its wide acceptance and popularity.[6] According to the Survey on Hirschsprung's disease (1976) of the Section of Surgery of the American Academy of Pediatrics, this procedure is employed by more responding pediatric surgeons than are the Swenson, Duhamel, or Soave procedures.[5, 10, 12]

REFERENCES

1. Boley S.J.: New modification of the surgical treatment of Hirschsprung's disease. *Surgery* 56:1015, 1964.
2. Boley S.J.: Technique of endorectal pull-through with primary anastomosis for Hirschsprung's disease. *Surg. Gynecol. Obstet.* 127:353, 1968.
3. Boley S.J., Kleinhaus S.: Hirschsprung's disease: Choice of operation, in Maingot R.: *Abdominal Operations.* New York, Appleton-Century-Crofts, 1974, p. 1706.
4. Boley S.J.: A new operative approach to total colonic aganglionosis. *Surg. Gynecol. Obstet.* 159:481, 1984.
5. Davies M.R.Q., Cywes S., Louw J.H.: Franco Soave's operation. *Suid-Afrikaanse Tydskrif vir Chirurgie* 13:223, 1975.
6. Klotz D.H., Velcek F.T., Kottmeier P.H.: Reappraisal of the endorectal pull-through operation for Hirschsprung's disease. *J. Pediatr. Surg.* 8:595, 1973.
7. Ravitch M.M., Sabiston D.C.: Anal ileostomy with preservation of the sphincter. *Surg. Gynecol. Obstet.* 93:87, 1951.
8. Rehbein F.: Operation der anal und Rectumatresie mit Rectourethral-fistel. *Chirurg.* 30:417, 1959.
9. Romualdi P.: Eine neue Operationstechnik Für die Behandlung einigen Rectummissbildungen. *Langenbecks Arch. Klin. Chir.* 296:371, 1960.
10. San Filippo J.A., Allen J.E., Jewett T.C.: Definitive surgical management of Hirschsprung's disease. *Arch. Surg.* 105:245, 1972.
11. Soave F.: A new surgical technique for the treatment of Hirschsprung's disease. *Surgery* 56:1007, 1964.
12. Soper R.T., Figueroa P.R.: Surgical treatment of Hirschsprung's disease: Comparison of modifications of the Duhamel and Soave operations. *J. Pediatr. Surg.* 6:761, 1971.

Total Colonic Aganglionosis—Martin's Operation
Lester Martin

In approximately 5% of infants with Hirschsprung's disease, the aganglionosis involves the entire colon. In a smaller percentage of patients, the distal small intestine is likewise devoid of ganglion cells.[9, 13, 15] Preservation and utilization of the aganglionic descending colon has proved feasible and appears to be a satisfactory means of recapturing some of the reabsorptive capacity of the colon.[1, 2, 9, 10] The operation (see Fig 106–15) that we developed for this purpose has been successfully completed for 17 infants during the past 22 years.

Operative Technique

Diagnosis is suspected by radiologic examination and confirmed by rectal biopsy.[14] The extent of the aganglionosis is determined at the time of laparotomy by microscopic examination of multiple extramucosal biopsy specimens of the seromuscular layer of bowel wall. At the level where ganglion cells are identi-

fied, the small bowel is transected and an ileostomy established through a separate incision appropriately placed to accommodate an appliance. The distal end is brought out as a mucous fistula either through a separate stab wound or through the end of the working incision.

The definitive operation may then be performed at an elected time, preferably at approximately 1 year of age. Before operation, both proximal and distal stomas should be thoroughly irrigated to remove gross bowel contents. A large-caliber catheter placed in the rectum before opening the abdomen can be used for intraoperative irrigation of the colon, with direct manual manipulation to dislodge and remove any residual stool. The ileostomy is taken down and the proximal small bowel mobilized sufficiently to provide adequate length to reach the perineum without tension. The pelvic peritoneum is opened and the space behind the rectum entered. A passageway is created between the rectum and sacrum to the level of the levator muscles.

The surgeon then proceeds to the perineum with the patient's legs in the modified lithotomy position. After appropriate skin preparation and draping, a transverse incision is made in the posterior half of the anal canal, approximately 0.5 cm from the mucocutaneous junction. The posterior wall of the rectum is mobilized and a passageway created between the wall of the rectum and the puborectal muscle posteriorly and continued superiorly into the previously opened presacral space. The closed proximal end of small bowel is then drawn through the presacral space and into the incised opening in the posterior rectal wall, where it is attached with several fine catgut sutures (Fig 106–16,A and B). The end of the pulled-through ileum is then opened and sutured to the edges of the opening in the posterior rectal wall with mucosa-to-mucosa approximation. The common wall between the rectum and pulled-through ileum is then resected with two applications of the GIA stapler, removing a triangular-shaped segment of the common wall, as illustrated in Figure 106–17. The staple line is then oversewn with a running lock stitch of absorbable suture. The surgeon then returns to the abdominal portion of the operation where the side-to-side anastomosis is continued proximally to the level of the splenic flexure (see Fig 106–16,D). The proximal aganglionic colon and small bowel are excised. In four instances, we continued the anastomosis proximally to incorporate and preserve the transverse and ascending colon,[16] but the long-term functional results were not improved over those when only the left colon was utilized.

Results

In 10 of the 17 infants, the aganglionic segment involved a portion of the small intestine. The only death was in one infant early in the series who died of sepsis 3 months following ileostomy and before the definitive operation. The operation was completed on 17 infants. All survived, and the time since operation now ranges from a few months up to 22 years. Initially, following operation, the stools were liquid and nonformed and occurred as often as every 2 hours. Gradually over a period of several months, the number decreased and the consistency thickened. A bowel movement at night during sleep was not uncommon during the first postoperative year. Certain vegetables such as corn, beans, or peas occasionally cause crampy abdominal pain and diarrhea. Their elimination from the diet is advised for the first 3 or 4 years. Viral enteritis has caused dehydration more rapidly than for the usual child and has necessitated hospitalization on one or more occasions for intravenous fluid administration. If the anastomosis is created too high on the posterior wall of the rectum, recurrent bouts of abdominal distention and diarrhea will be experienced. We have encountered this in two children in whom the initial operation was performed elsewhere. We have also encountered one child in whom the anastomosis was accomplished too low on the posterior wall of the rectum. This resulted in incontinence that was subsequently corrected by means of a posterior approach to plicate the most distal portion of the terminal ileum. In one of our patients, the anastomosis was completed, but the right and transverse colon were left in continuity, the anastomosis extending only to the splenic flexure. Inspissated stool accumulated in the defunctionalized proximal colon with subsequent erosion through the wall and the development of a jejunocolic fistula. Resection of the involved segment of jejunum and defunctionalized portion of the colon corrected the diarrhea, which initially had been erroneously attributed to enterocolitis. In one infant, protracted diarrhea was found to be related to regrowth of the septum between the small bowel and the rectum. The septum had initially been divided with the stapling device but not oversewn. Division of the recurrent septum corrected the problem.

Previous operations for total colonic aganglionosis have been successful,[14] but the reported mortality rate has averaged 40–50%.[4–7, 13] With our operation, the risk has been minimal and the results generally satisfactory.[1, 2, 9–11] Growth and development are normal for all of the children. It appears that the colon reintroduced into the intestinal tract in this manner recaptures its function of reabsorption. In two infants, the distal half of the small intestine was aganglionic; yet, in both there was satisfactory salvage by the operation. The procedure is recommended for infants with total colonic aganglionosis as well as for those in whom the aganglionic segment involves up to as much as half of the small intestine.

REFERENCES

1. Belloli G., Frigiola A., DaGiau F., et al.: L'operasione di Lester Martin nell'aganglionosi ileo-colica. *Minerva Pediatr.* 27:1535, 1975.
2. Burrington J.D., Wayne E.R.: Modified Duhamel procedure for treatment of total aganglionic colon in children. *J. Pediatr. Surg.* 11:391, 1976.
3. Coran A.G., Bjordal R., Eck S., et al.: Surgical management of total colonic and partial small intestine aganglionosis. *J. Pediatr. Surg.* 4:531, 1969.
4. Desjardings J., Simpson J.: Neonatal Hirschsprung's disease (treatment of complete aganglionosis of the colon by the Duhamel operation). *Arch. Surg.* 87:1019, 1963.
5. Dorman G.: Universal aganglionosis of the colon. *Arch. Surg.* 75:906, 1957.
6. Edelman S., Strauss L., Becker J., et al.: Universal aganglionosis of the colon. *Surgery* 47:667, 1960.
7 Freeman N.V.: Long-segment Hirschsprung's disease. *Proc. R. Soc. Med.* 64:378, 1971.
8. Gerald B.: Aganglionosis of the colon and terminal ileum: Long-term survival. *Am. J. Roentgenol.* 95:230, 1965.
9. Martin L.W.: Surgical management of Hirschsprung's disease involving the small intestine. *Arch. Surg.* 97:183, 1968.
10. Martin L.W.: Surgical management of total colonic aganglionosis. *Ann. Surg.* 176:343, 1972.
11. Pellerin D., Nihoul-Fekete C., Bertin P., et al.: An extensive form of Hirschsprung's disease treated by Lester Martin's ileocoloplasty. *Ann. Chir. Infant.* 12:71, 1971 (abstr. *J. Pediatr. Surg.* 6:788, 1971).
12. Sandegard E.: Hirschsprung's disease with ganglion cell aplasia of the colon and terminal ileum. *Acta Chir. Scand.* 106:369, 1953.
13. Soltero-Harrington L.R., Garcia-Rinaldi R., Able L.W.: Total aganglionosis of the colon: Recognition and management. *J. Pediatr. Surg.* 4:330, 1969.
14. Swenson O., Fisher J.H.: Treatment of Hirschsprung's disease with the entire colon involved in the aganglionic defect. *Arch. Surg.* 70:535, 1955.
15. Walker A.W., Kempson R.L., Ternberg J.: Aganglionosis of the small intestine. *Surgery,* 60:449, 1966.
16. Martin L.W.: Total colonic aganglionosis: Preservation and utilization of the entire colon. *J. Pediatr. Surg.* 17:635, 1982.

107   James A. O'Neill, Jr.
Colorectal Tumors

Although Kern and White reported adenocarcinoma of the colon in a 9-month-old infant and others have reported cases in patients less than 10 years of age, the vast majority of cases have been in children over 10 years of age. For all intents and purposes, carcinoma of the colon in childhood is a disease of adolescents.[7, 9] There appear to be three different forms of the disease—that which is sporadic, that which is associated with genetic disorders, and that which is associated with chronic colitis. Colorectal carcinoma is common in individuals over 50 years of age and extremely uncommon in individuals under 20 years of age.[1, 11, 14] Only about 1% of colorectal malignancies are found in individuals under 30 years of age. Nonetheless, colorectal carcinoma is the most common gastrointestinal cancer of childhood.[3]

Signs and Symptoms

The signs and symptoms of cancer of the colon and rectum in childhood are really no different from those in adults, but the expectation and recognition of these findings leads clinicians in directions other than toward diagnosis of malignancy. The most common symptoms are abdominal pain, vomiting, constipation, weight loss, and anorexia. The most common signs are bloody stools, anemia, and abdominal distention. Physical findings include an abdominal mass, abdominal distention, weight loss, and abdominal tenderness, in that order.[3, 7] Overall, the signs, symptoms, and physical findings when taken together usually indicate long-standing disease and, frequently, intestinal obstruction. Because of the age of the subject, the findings and symptoms usually lead to preoperative diagnoses such as peritonitis of uncertain origin, intestinal obstruction, appendicitis, intussusception, and possible retroperitoneal malignancy. The differences in children and in adults with colonic carcinoma will be detailed below, but with regard to recognition based on signs, symptoms, and physical findings, a delay in diagnosis of as long as 2 years has been common up to this point in children, perhaps partly explaining the poor prognosis in them.[3]

Pathology

In virtually every review of colocarcinoma in childhood, all varieties of cancer have been seen, ranging from well-differentiated adenocarcinoma to highly malignant mucin-secreting carcinoma with signet-ring formation.[7] One essential difference in children, as compared with adults, is that up to 50% of children have mucin-secreting carcinoma, while in adults the incidence of this form of colonic malignancy is only about 5%.[2] This pathologic factor, associated with poor prognosis, may further explain the lower survival rate in children. There is no information for children regarding the production of carcinoembryonic antigen (CEA). The factors having to do with staging of disease related to treatment and prognosis appear to be no different in children than in adults.

Entities Associated With Colorectal Carcinoma in Childhood

Chabalko and Fraumeni, in an epidemiologic study, reported that the frequency of precancerous lesions in young people with colorectal cancer is about 10%, far higher than in older patients.[4] This, nevertheless, means that 90% of children reported with cancer of the colon have "spontaneous" malignancy. However, since some of those children with spontaneous colon cancer have had second malignancies, and in others the cancer is found in unusually occurring adenomatous polyps or villous adenomas, it is reasonable to speculate that the incidence of premalignant conditions in childhood is higher than the 10% figure.[2]

Genetic Disorders

Gardner syndrome (adenomatous polyps with various tumors of soft tissue and bone),[10] Turcot syndrome (familial adenomatous polyps associated with central nervous system tumors),[16] Peutz-Jeghers syndrome (multiple hamartomatous polyps),[8] and the familial polyposis coli[12] have all been reported to be associated with the later development of colorectal carcinoma, usually in adolescence or later. The association between these familial genetic disorders and later development of colonic malignancy has led to the recommendation that such individuals except for the Peutz-Jeghers patients should have elective prophylactic proctocolectomy. The development of sphincter-saving operations, discussed in Chapter 101, has made it easier to recommend such procedures in children.

Inflammatory Bowel Disease

The best recognized relation of inflammatory bowel disease and the later development of colonic malignancy is in ulcerative colitis. The relation of chronic inflammation of any type to subsequent development of cellular metaplasia, and later outright malignancy, has been well known for decades. Devroede and colleagues, in a long-term study of a large number of patients from the Mayo Clinic, found that the incidence of carcinoma of the large bowel in a group of patients with chronic ulcerative colitis starting in childhood was 20% per decade in those at risk, beginning after the first 10 years of the disease.[6] In a long-term study from the same institution, Weedon and co-workers followed over 400 patients with various forms of Crohn's disease and demonstrated that the incidence of colorectal cancer was 20 times greater in those patients than in a control population.[17] Until that time, the relation of cancer to Crohn's disease and its chronic inflammation was unclear. The more extensive the disease, the more likely is malignancy. The same is true of ulcerative colitis, although carcinoma is rare if the disease is localized

exclusively to the rectum and left colon,[6] presumably because in such cases the disease is of shorter duration.

While barium enema examination is useful in patients with ulcerative colitis or Crohn's colitis, probably the best method of intensive follow-up is flexible colonoscopy performed yearly, with random biopsies performed at 10-cm intervals from the rectum. Certainly any atypia indicates that resection is in order, but duration of disease over 10 years, even if it is mild, is another indication for colectomy.

Another form of chronic inflammation, which has recently been noted to be associated with the later development of malignancy, is colitis due to parasitic diseases such as amebiasis or schistosomiasis.[7] Untreated parasitic disease, as seen in children in poor socioeconomic conditions, appears to have the same potential for production of malignancy as ulcerative colitis and with the same relation to duration of disease.

Ureterosigmoidostomy

Urinary diversion is required for the treatment of a number of genitourinary disorders in childhood, but particularly for exstrophy of the bladder and for neurogenic bladder. The oldest form of internal urinary diversion is ureterosigmoidostomy, and a good number of patients who have undergone this procedure have now been followed for many years. Ureterosigmoidostomy is still preferred by a number of experienced urologists, particularly for exstrophy of the bladder. However, a number of patients who have had ureterosigmoidostomy performed for bladder exstrophy have developed adenocarcinoma at the junction of the ureteral stoma and the sigmoid colon.[15] It has been shown experimentally that the combination of urine and feces over a long period of time, perhaps associated with chronic inflammation, may lead to the development of carcinoma.[5] Patients with ureterosigmoidostomy should, after puberty, have twice-yearly stool guaiac determinations and yearly sigmoidoscopy with biopsy. Visualization of the anastomoses is facilitated by the use of indigo carmine. If the incidence of colonic carcinoma in patients who have had ureterosigmoidostomy continues to rise, use of this procedure will have to be reevaluated. As yet, the statistical likelihood of malignant transformation with this procedure is not known.

Treatment and Results

The surgical treatment of colorectal carcinoma, once it has been recognized, is really no different in children than in adults. Emphasis is appropriately placed on prophylactic surgical procedures for premalignant conditions. On the other hand, the prognosis in children is far worse than in adults, probably because of several factors—generally delayed recognition, a much higher incidence of highly malignant mucin-secreting tumors, and the potential for more rapid tumor growth in a subject who is actively growing.[2] Recalde and his group found a 17.5% five-year survival rate in patients with all pathologic types of colorectal carcinoma, and other reviews have shown similar findings.[13] Fluorouracil and a variety of other chemotherapeutic agents have been tried, as well as radiotherapy, but none of these measures has had any curative or palliative value.

REFERENCES

1. Alaghemand A.: Carcinoma of the colon and rectum in children. *Am. Surg.* 28:784, 1962.
2. Anderson A., Bergdahl L.: Carcinoma of the colon in children: A report of six new cases and a review of the literature. *J. Pediatr. Surg.* 11:967, 1976.
3. Cain W.S., Longino L.A.: Carcinoma of the colon in children. *J. Pediatr. Surg.* 5:527, 1970.
4. Chabalko J.J., Fraumeni J.F.: Colorectal cancer in children: Epidemiologic aspects. *Dis. Colon Rectum* 18:1, 1975.

5. Crissey M., Steele G., Gittes R.: Rat model for carcinogenesis in ureterosigmoidostomy. *Science* 207:1079, 1980.
6. Devroede G.J., Taylor W.F., Sauer W.G., et al.: Cancer risk and life expectancy of children with ulcerative colitis. *N. Engl. J. Med.* 285:17, 1971.
7. Goldthorn J.F., Powars D., Hays D.M.: Adenocarcinoma of the colon and rectum in the adolescent. *Surgery* 93:409, 1983.
8. Horn R.C., Payne W.A., Fine G.: The Peutz-Jeghers syndrome. *Arch. Pathol.* 76:41, 1963.
9. Kern W.H., White W.C.: Adenocarcinoma of the colon in a 9-month-old infant. *Cancer* 11:855, 1958.
10. Kottmeier P.K., Clatworthy H.W.: Intestinal polyps and associated carcinoma in childhood. *Am. J. Surg.* 110:709, 1963.
11. Middlecamp J.N., Haffner H.: Carcinoma of the colon in children. *Pediatrics* 32:558, 1963.
12. Peck D.A., Watanabe K.S., Trueblood H.W.: Familial polyposis in children. *Dis. Colon Rectum* 15:23, 1972.
13. Recalde M., Holyoke E.D., Elias E.G.: Carcinoma of the colon, rectum, and anal canal in young patients. *Surg. Gynecol. Obstet.* 139:909, 1974.
14. Sessions R.T., Riddell D.H., Kaplan H.J.: Carcinoma of the colon in the first two decades of life. *Ann. Surg.* 162:279, 1965.
15. Spence H.M., Hoffman W.W., Fosmire G.P.: Tumor of the colon as a late complication of ureterosigmoidostomy for exstrophy of the bladder. *Br. J. Urol.* 51:466, 1979.
16. Turcot J., Despres J.P., St. Pierre F.: Malignant tumors of the central nervous system associated with familial polyposis of the colon. *Dis. Colon Rectum* 2:465, 1959.
17. Weedon D.D., Shorter R.G., Ilstrup D.M., et al.: Crohn's disease and cancer. *N. Engl. J. Med.* 289:1099, 1973.

108   John M. Templeton / James A. O'Neill, Jr.

Anorectal Malformations

HISTORY.—In the 7th century A.D., Paulus Aegineta recommended incising anal obstructions with a scalpel, followed by systematic dilatation.[8] This operative approach remained in vogue as late as the mid-1800s. The first more precise surgical dissection was performed in 1787 by Benjamin Bell in England. He described a formal perineal dissection designed to establish continuity of the rectum with the perineum but without formal repair.[45]

In 1835, Amussat[2] described a procedure for repair of high imperforate anus in a female. Through a T-shaped incision in the perineum he exposed the rectal ampulla. After detaching it from the surrounding tissues and evacuating its contents, he drew it down to the perineum, where he sutured the rectal mucosa to the skin in order to avoid contraction and stricture. He was the first to emphasize a formal repair with sutures for this purpose. Later, he switched to a midsagittal incision, which he extended up to the sacrum by excising the coccyx.[22] In 1854, Pughe,[7] following the earlier guidelines of Amussat, operated on a boy with imperforate anus who had passed meconium in the urine. On follow-up 6 years later, the child was found to be thriving. Matas,[23] in 1897, noted improved exposure by extending a midline incision from the center of the anus up to the sacrum and, where necessary, by excising the coccyx and the fourth and fifth sacral vertebrae.

In 1710, Littre[22] proposed an iliac colostomy for obstruction of the rectum. This approach was first utilized for infants with imperforate anus by French surgeons in the late 1700s. In most cases, the children died. However, in 1856, Chassaignac[6] succeeded in utilizing a previously made iliac colostomy to pass a probe down the distal colon until it lay against the perineum, which was then incised and an anal opening created. The colostomy was subsequently closed. Nevertheless, colostomies in infancy continued to be a problem. Therefore, McLeod, in 1880, suggested combining abdominal exploration with a perineal dissection when the rectum could not be found on perineal dissection. With the finger deep in the pelvis as a guide, the perineal wound could be deepened, allowing the rectum to be grasped and brought down to the perineum.[22] Hadra, in Germany, first performed this operation in 1884, but the patient died.[8]

In the early 1900s, a perineal operation for both high and low anomalies was generally favored because of continued high mortality rates with staging colostomies and primary abdominoperineal repairs.[8, 22] In 1930, Wangensteen and Rice[52] originated the "invertogram" whereby an infant with imperforate anus was held upside down and a lateral radiograph of the pelvis was taken to demonstrate the end of the rectum. This technique was designed "to determine whether the atresic bowel may be reached from below or not." When lesions above the pubococcygeal line were encountered, they suggested a colostomy. This technique, however, stimulated renewed interest in primary abdominoperineal repair of high imperforate anus in the newborn. In 1948 and 1949, Rhoads[31] and Norris[26] independently reported success with a one-stage abdominoperineal operation in the newborn. In 1953, Stephens published his experience with an operative approach based on blunt dissection of a plane

anterior to the levator ani in order to pass the neorectum anterior to the puborectalis muscle.[43] In 1967, Rehbein[30] reported a procedure whereby the blind rectal pouch denuded of mucosa was used as a channel for the pull-through of the neorectum. While agreeing with Stephens' emphasis on the importance of the levator musculature and puborectalis sling, Rehbein thought that use of the muscular sleeve of the blind rectal pouch safely indicated the way through the levator mechanism while avoiding possible nerve damage due to sacral dissection. He emphasized nonmobilization of the blind rectal pouch and no specific ligature of the rectourethral fistula. In 1967, Kiesewetter[18] combined Stephens' direct exposure of the levator mechanism with Rehbein's endorectal procedure. He believed that this approach best preserved the sensation and reflex mechanisms essential to fecal continence. In 1981, de Vries and Pena[9] reported their posterior, sagittal anorectoplasty technique for repair of high and intermediate imperforate anus.

Embryology

By the 4-mm (4-week) embryonic stage, the cloaca and cloacal membrane are present. The membrane lies transversely and separates the internal from the external cloaca. The internal cloaca at this stage receives the allantois, wolffian ducts, and rectum. Between the 4-mm and 16-mm (6-week) stages, the internal cloaca is divided in a coronal plane by the urorectal septum, which starts cranially and ends caudally. This downgrowth of the urorectal septum (Tourneux's fold) is paralleled by lateral ingrowths (Rathke's plicae) and results in two chambers, one receiving the allantois and wolffian ducts and the other receiving the rectum.[47] Failure of the urorectal septum to develop probably results in a rectourinary fistula in the male and rectocloacal or rectovaginal fistula in the female.[4] Also, between the 4-mm and 16-mm stages, mesoderm builds up on the surface of the perineum, resulting in the formation of the genital tubercle on the ventral aspect, genital folds on either side, and anal tubercles posteriorly. The depression produced thereby is the external cloaca. When the urorectal septum reaches the cloacal membrane at the 16-mm stage, the membrane begins to atrophy. When this atrophy is complete, the future urogenital tract and future rectum both issue into the external cloaca.[45]

During growth of the embryo from 16 mm to 50 mm, the uroanal septum grows caudally into the external cloaca. It does so by growth of the perineal mound, which is an extension of the urorectal septum, and by inward migration of the inner genital folds on either side. These folds grow medially until they fuse with the perineal mound to form the perineum separating the urinary and anal canals.[47] The anal orifice itself arises as a separate entity by the ringlike fusion of the right and left anal tubercles. By the 19-mm stage, patency of the anal canal is usually established.[4] From then until the 50-mm stage, further elongation of the urethra and anal canal occurs, but external differentiation of male and female genital structures is not yet apparent. This differentiation becomes clear, however, by the 56-mm stage. In the male, the outer portions of the genital folds also migrate medially until they meet in the midline, forming the perineal raphe from the midpoint of the anus to the frenulum of the glans. Defects in the development of these anal wrappings and perineal components may result in anocutaneous, anourethral, or rectobulbar fistulae. In the female, the perineal mound is covered only by the inner genital folds. The urogenital part of the external cloaca remains open and is flanked by the labia minora (inner folds) and the labia majora (outer folds). Since the outer genital folds do not fuse, they play no part in the development of the anus and the perineum, and there is no perineal raphe.[47] Defects in the fusion of the inner genital folds may result in anocutaneous or anovestibular fistulae.

Anatomy and Physiology of Fecal Continence

Development of the neuromuscular structures essential to fecal continence parallels the embryologic development of the rectum and anus. Neurologic control is provided from nerves arising in the second, third, and fourth sacral segments. Varying degrees of continence are possible even if there is some damage to the third or fourth sacral segments, but bilateral loss of innervation from the second through the fifth sacral segments usually results in uncorrectable fecal incontinence.[45] Traditionally, the muscular components of fecal continence include the levator ani muscles and the external sphincter muscles. Stephens thought that, by themselves, the levators were sufficient to provide complete fecal control. He described the levators as a funnel, the lowest point of which was a muscular sling, the puborectalis muscle. This sling was thought to be the most significant portion of the levators in providing fecal continence.[44] In contrast to the levators, Stephens and Smith[45] discounted the importance of the external sphincter muscles.

Other investigators,[1, 10, 17, 36] however, continued to suggest that the external sphincters play an important part in fecal control. Beginning in 1980, the work of de Vries and Pena[8, 9] has provided evidence of the importance of these muscles and their relation to the levator ani muscles. By completely dividing these muscles posteriorly, and with frequent electrostimulation, they have identified four recognizable muscle groups: the subcutaneous and superficial external sphincter muscle layers, the proximal levator ani, and the striated muscle complex (Fig 108–1). This muscle complex is composed of a fusion of the puborectal portion of the levator ani and the external sphincter muscles, including a deep external sphincter component, which cannot be identified clinically. Dorsal to the muscle complex, the subcuta-

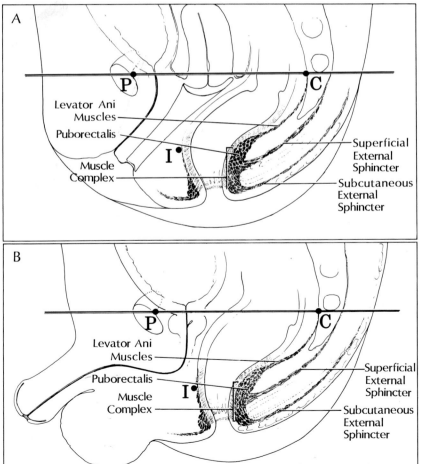

Fig 108–1.—Normal female and male rectal anatomy. In normal females **(A)** and males **(B)**, the distal rectum is invested by a muscle complex that represents a fusion of the levator muscles and the longitudinal fibers of the external sphincter muscles. The distal portion of the muscle complex is composed of circular fibers of the external sphincter. These longitudinal and circular fibers insert into the distal rectal wall. Shown are the pubococcygeal *(PC)* line and the *"I"* (ischium) point and their relation to normal pelvic structures.

neous and superficial external sphincter muscles extend upward toward the coccyx as separate layers of longitudinal muscle fibers. Deep to the superficial external sphincter layer is the upper portion of the levator ani muscles. Stimulation of the levators results in a strong ventral contraction in contrast to the weaker contraction of the longitudinal fibers of the two external sphincter layers, which pull in a cephalocaudal direction. Where the external sphincter muscles fuse with the levators marks the beginning of the striated muscle complex. The muscle complex and the anorectal canal within it course posteriorly to exit through the anal opening.

The action of the levator ani, in general, is to elevate the rectum, whereas the action of puborectalis and the deep external sphincter muscle is to pull the anal canal ventrally. The result is compression of the rectum against the triangular ligament, thereby increasing the angulation of the proximal anorectal canal. Circular fibers of the external sphincter muscle squeeze the anal canal from the pectinate line outward. Pull-through procedures in which the rectum is misplaced outside the muscle complex discard the benefit of both this squeezing action and the ventral pull in the anal canal.

The third component essential to successful fecal control is sensation and proprioception.[35] In the anal canal, numerous sensory fibers denote pain, touch, cold, pressure, and friction. These sensory receptors occur both in the mucosal layer and in the deeper muscular layers. Distally in the anal canal, sensation regarding the presence of fecal contents is fairly precise.[45] Patients with fecal incontinence following pull-through operations in which little attention was given to the external sphincter often complain that they are not aware of stool exiting the anal canal until it touches the skin, by which time soilage has occurred.

In contrast to sensation, proprioception in the rectum and anus is mainly perceived within the muscle and connective tissue of the levator ani and the muscle complex.[17] The puborectalis and the external sphincter muscles both respond briskly to even slight distention in the distal rectum. This reflex contraction is essential to successful fecal continence. The puborectalis can also respond with short conscious peaks of contraction.[35] The external sphincter provides fine control, especially with regard to the passage of flatus and liquid stool, but it does so only by means of short bursts of activity. The muscle complex produces an anorectal resistance zone 3.5–5.0 cm long in normal older children or in adults. If the reflex contraction of the puborectalis muscle is impaired and/or the anorectal resistance zone is shortened, incontinence usually occurs.[35]

Incidence and Frequency

The usual reported incidence of anorectal malformations is 1 per 5,000 live births. There is a slight preponderance of males. In a collective series of 3,645 cases, 57% were male and 43% were female.[45] In our own series of 313 patients with anorectal malformations seen over 22 years at Children's Hospital of Philadelphia,[51] there was a male-to-female preponderance of 58% to 42%. Of the 120 patients with intermediate or high lesions, 72% were male and 28% were female. In general, the male-to-female ratio of patients with intermediate or high lesions is 2:1. In patients with low lesions, the ratio is 1:1.[34] In males with an intermediate or high anomaly, 80% have a fistula between the rectum and urethra and 6.6% have a fistula between the rectum and the bladder. In males with a low anomaly, 35% have a thin membrane covering the anus or stenosis of the distal anorectal canal. Another 58% have a discernible fistula at birth, in most cases an anocutaneous fistula along the perineal or scrotal raphe. Of females with a high or an intermediate anomaly, 78.6% have a fistula to the genitourinary tract. Of females with a low anomaly,

93% have an external fistula.[45] The incidence of these anomalies is not affected by the parity of the mother, the mother's age, or the race or nationality of the child's family. Although there is no strong genetic predisposition for these disorders, there are reports of imperforate anus occurring in more than one sibling or in members of a family over three different generations.[54]

Classification

Anorectal malformations are best defined in anatomical terms. An anatomical approach simplifies decision-making for the surgeon when confronted with a patient with imperforate anus. In 1984, at the Wingspread Workshop on Anorectal Malformations organized by Stephens and Smith,[46] a classification was established to define these malformations according to the patient's sex and the level at which arrest of rectal descent occurred (Table 108–1). While many rare malformations are not included, the system is easy to understand and to teach. In addition, workshop participants endorsed the use of standardized registration forms for each patient with diagnosed imperforate anus so that in the future the results of different surgical procedures can be compared.[14]

From the work of Stephens and Smith, it is clear that anorectal malformations exist as a spectrum. From a functional viewpoint, however, these lesions can be grouped according to whether the end of the rectum is supralevator (high), partially translevator (intermediate), or fully translevator (low). As shown in Figure 108–2, there are two important landmarks to identify when reviewing the invertogram proposed by Wangensteen and Rice:[52] the classic pubococcygeal line and the "I" (ischium) point,[45] represented by the lowest quarter of the ossified ischium. A rectum that ends above the pubococcygeal line is clearly supralevator, or "high." If the rectum ends below the pubococcygeal line, but not below the "I" point, it is "intermediate." The rectum in the intermediate zone has entered the upper funnel portion of the levator mechanism but has not passed completely beyond and distal to the puborectalis muscle. By contrast, a rectal pouch that is clearly below the "I" point has penetrated the entire levator

TABLE 108–1.—ANATOMICAL CLASSIFICATION
OF ANORECTAL MALFORMATIONS

FEMALE	MALE
High	High
Anorectal agenesis	Anorectal agenesis
With rectovaginal fistula	With rectoprostatic urethral fistula*
Without fistula	Without fistula
Rectal atresia	Rectal atresia
Intermediate	Intermediate
Rectovestibular fistula	Rectobulbar urethral fistula
Rectovaginal fistula	Anal agenesis without fistula
Anal agenesis without fistula	
Low	Low
Anovestibular fistula*	Anocutaneous fistula*
Anocutaneous fistula*†	Anal stenosis*‡
Anal stenosis‡	
Cloacal malformations§	
Rare malformations	Rare malformations

*Relatively common lesion.
†Includes fistulae occurring at the posterior junction of the labia minora often called "fourchette fistulae" or "vulvar fistulae."
‡Previously called "covered anus."
§Previously called "rectocloacal fistulae." Entry of the rectal fistula into the cloaca may be high or intermediate, depending on the length of the cloacal canal.

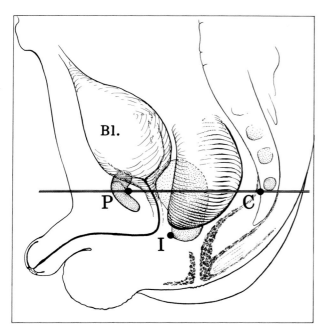

Fig 108–2.—Imperforate anus. The rectal pouch is shown in relation to the pubococcygeal *(PC)* line and the *"I"* point. The *PC* line represents the upper limits of the levator musculature. It is not until the rectum has passed well below the *"I"* point that it can be considered to be translevator, i.e., a low anomaly. In this drawing, the rectal pouch lies between the *PC* line and the *"I"* point and this should, therefore, be considered an intermediate anomaly. *Bl* indicates bladder.

mechanism and may, therefore, be properly referred to as "low" (Fig 108–3,*A* and *B*).

Clinical Investigation

Physical Examination

The appearance of the perineum does not necessarily predict whether the lesion is low, intermediate, or high. Some children, for example, have a clearly delineated anal area and yet have a high anomaly. In the rare child with rectal atresia, the distal 1– 2 cm of the anal canal may be completely formed, and yet the distal rectal pouch is in an intermediate or high position. One group of children, however, have characteristic physical features that confirm suspected high imperforate anus: (1) complete absence of any anal features in the presence of a flat bottom (i.e., little or no buttocks crease), (2) no external sphincter contraction on scratching the perineum. Such children usually have major sacral anomalies with absence of the sacrum below S-1 or S-2. Sacral innervation is, therefore, likely to be severely deficient, and the poor prognosis for eventual fecal continence is poor.

As shown in Figure 108–3,*A* and *B*, there is an obvious fistulous tract in the region of the perineal body. A fistula in this region in both males and females usually, but not always, indicates a low imperforate anus. In males, the fistula may be denoted by a whitish or dark-stained subcuticular tract along the perineal raphe and occasionally along the scrotal raphe as well. In the absence of a perineal fistula in a male, the presence of a well-developed bucket-handle deformity in the anal area often indicates anal stenosis (covered anus). Re-evaluation of such a patient 12–24 hours after birth may reveal a dark spot of meconium in the center of the anal structures, indicating a stenotic or covered anus. In contrast, if a male newborn has a cleft scrotum or an atypical hypospadias, or if he passes meconium or flatus via the penis, one should suspect intermediate or high rectal agen-

esis. Passage of meconium in the urine is usually associated with a fistula in the bulbar urethra. This fistula is usually larger than the more common proximal urethral fistula. A urethral catheter inserted in such a patient generally goes into the rectum rather than into the proximal urethra or the bladder. In spite of this, patients with a bulbar fistula are less likely to get urinary tract infections than are patients with a prostatic urethral fistula.[40]

In females, the external appearance of the perineum and vaginal introitus usually indicates whether the lesion is low or high. A fistula in the perineum of a female is usually open and easy to see, although its opening may be quite small. If the fistula is close to the center of the external sphincter, an imperforate anus may not be recognized until weeks later when the child is evaluated for chronic constipation. In the absence of an obvious fistula in the perineum, careful inspection of the posterior edge of the vulva or of the vestibule just distal to the hymen often reveals a fistula. These fistulae are usually longer (Fig 108–3,*A*), but most are still associated with a low lesion. A fistula at the level of the vulva or the vestibule may be assessed by gentle probing with a no. 5F or no. 8F catheter. If the catheter appears to enter a fistulous tract, it will usually have meconium on its tip when it is withdrawn. In such a patient, pressure at the usual site of the anus often extrudes meconium through the small fistulous opening. As a further test for a low lesion, one can insert a curved hemostat into the fistulous tract and determine how close the rectal pouch is to the skin by palpating the hemostat through the skin at the level of the external sphincter. These simple diagnostic maneuvers usually confirm the presence of a low-lying lesion, allowing one to plan for early correction and to reassure the family. One should be alert, however, for the occasional male with a perineal fistula or the female with a vestibular fistula in whom the rectal pouch is not low but intermediate (Fig 108–3,*C*). Probing these long fistulae with a small hemostat usually demonstrates that the fistulous tract remains narrow and ascends deep into the pelvis. Whenever there is any doubt regarding the level of the rectal pouch, a contrast study of the fistula should be performed. It would be a mistake to perform a perineal dissection for what in reality is an intermediate lesion.

In the female, complete absence of any externally visible fistula almost always indicates an intermediate or high lesion. Just as in the male who passes meconium or gas in the urine, passage of either meconium or gas from above the hymen in a female accurately indicates that the lesion is intermediate or high. If one can identify a normal urethra and hymen in a female with no visible fistula, the rectum most commonly enters the lower third of the posterior vaginal wall.[3] Occasionally, however, the rectal fistula may enter the vagina as high as the posterior fornix.[45] On the other hand, if the vulvae are abnormal and there is no hymen, it is likely that the patient has a cloacal anomaly.[3] In this anomaly, a urethra is usually not visible and the patient often passes both urine and stool via a single orifice. In such patients, entry of the rectal fistula into the posterior wall of the cloaca may be high or intermediate, depending on the length of the cloacal canal. Also, many of these patients may have no sign of an anal dimple but instead have just a fine raphe extending posteriorly along the perineal body.[45] Although patients with cloacal anomalies have a high incidence of associated genitourinary anomalies, cloacal anomalies in general represent a spectrum of severity in which rectal problems predominate in one patient and genitourinary problems predominate in another.[11] Carefully planned diagnostic studies are especially important in these instances.

Diagnostic Studies

The purposes of specific diagnostic studies are: (1) to determine the level of the blind rectal pouch, (2) to identify any as-

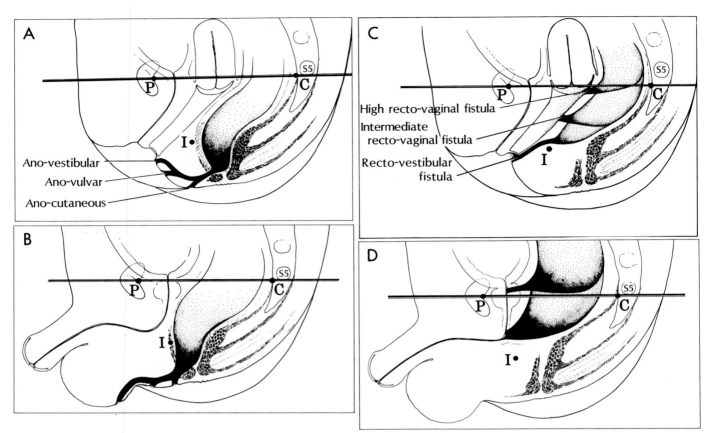

Fig 108–3.—Imperforate anus. Kinds of fistulae. **A,** low imperforate anus anomalies in the female almost always have an external fistulous tract. The tract is named for the point at which it exits: cutaneous (perineal), vulvar (labia majora), or vestibular (just distal to the hymen). A hemostat placed inside all these fistulous tracts will pass posteriorly before turning cephalad to enter the rectum. **B,** low imperforate anus anomalies in the male usually have an external fistulous tract. The tracts are all anocutaneous, but they vary in how far removed the exit site is from the true anus. When the fistula extends up to and along the scrotal raphe, meconium can often be seen through the thin overlying skin. **C,** interme- diate and high imperforate anus lesions in the female are usually associated with a fistula to the posterior vagina. The passage of stool from above the hymen confirms the presence of an intermediate or high lesion. Patients with a vestibular fistula should be carefully evaluated because the underlying rectal pouch may be intermediate and not low. **D,** intermediate and high imperforate anus in the male is usually associated with a fistula to the urinary tract. Most of these fistulae involve the prostatic urethra; the rectal pouch is therefore high. A few involve the bulbous urethra. Fistulae at this level are usually larger and enter the urethra more obliquely.

sociated fistulous communications, and (3) to determine the presence or absence of any other congenital anomalies. Much of this information can be obtained by simple, relatively noninvasive studies and maneuvers. The urine should be examined for meconium or squamous epithelial cells. A voided urine specimen is more informative because it is more likely to reflect contents in the urethra than would a specimen obtained by placing a catheter in the bladder. Passage of a nasogastric tube helps rule out associated esophageal atresia. Chest films in conjunction with a cardiac examination suggest any underlying cardiac, upper vertebral, or rib anomalies. Any suspicion of cardiac anomalies may be verified by electrocardiograms and echocardiograms. A supine film of the abdomen and pelvis may reveal anomalies of the lumbosacral spine and any abnormal bowel pattern. Anomalies of the limbs, particularly the forearm, may be assessed clinically and radiographically. Finally, an ultrasound scan of the neonate's abdomen is very helpful in assessing renal anomalies and/or agenesis.

The presence of two or more of these anomalies in a patient with imperforate anus is not uncommon and has led to the use of the term VATER association. The acronym VATER does not refer to a syndrome but rather reflects the tendency of certain anomalies to occur more frequently in the same patient, specifically vertebral defects (*V*), anal atresia (*A*), tracheoesophageal fis-

tula (*TE*), and radial and renal anomalies (*R*). This association has been expanded to VACTERL, in which *C* stands for cardiac lesions, particularly ventricular septal defects, and *L* stands for limb deformities.[16] Recognition of a potential VACTERL association in a patient with imperforate anus is important, since it mandates a careful search for anomalies in other organ systems. Recognition and timely treatment of many of these anomalies are the key to lowered mortality and better outcome.

Accurate interpretation of Wangensteen-Rice invertograms of the pelvis requires some thought and planning:

1. It is important to allow enough time for adequate bowel gas to pass to the end of the blind rectum. Frequently, x-ray films taken at 12 hours of life show a rectal pouch that is lower than it appeared to be at 6 hours of life. If the bowel is not overly distended with air, one may wait 4–6 hours before placing a nasogastric tube for gastric decompression that will permit enough air to pass down the gastrointestinal tract. One should guard against overdistention of the bowel, however. Newborns with imperforate anus and unrelieved massive bowel distention have developed spontaneous bowel perforation or sigmoid volvulus by 24 hours of life.[13]

2. The child should be held vertically upside down for 3 minutes before the film is taken. Moreover, it is very important to obtain a true lateral view of the pelvis, where both the right and

the left ischium overlie each other exactly. The hips should be kept relatively straight so that the femora do not obscure the pubic bone. Placing a thin smear of barium paste in the buttocks cleft at the level of the external sphincter helps to denote the cutaneous level of the anus.

3. Interpretation of the invertogram requires proper placement of the pubococcygeal line and the "I" point (see Fig 108–2). The coccyx in an infant is usually not calcified. If all five sacral segments appear to be present on the anteroposterior projection, one can place a mark for the coccyx about 0.5 cm. below the ossified portion of S-5. A line drawn between the latter point and the center of the pubic bone will define the pubococcygeal line. If S-5 and S-4 are missing, the pubococcygeal line should be drawn so as to approximate the level at which the coccyx would usually be. Structures lying approximately at the level of the pubococcygeal line include the bladder neck, the verumontanum, the anterior peritoneal reflection of the rectum in the male, and the external os of the cervix in the female.

If the air in the blind rectal pouch ends at or above the pubococcygeal line, the lesion is considered to be high (Fig 108–3,*C* and *D*). If the air in the rectum ends between the pubococcygeal line and the "I" point, the lesion is considered intermediate. If the gas shadow lies much higher than expected, one should obtain another film because there may have been some contraction of the puborectalis muscle when the picture was obtained. Likewise, if the gas shadow is not smooth and rounded, it may be due to active contraction of the puborectalis muscle when the film was taken or to meconium in the distal rectum.

4. Miscellaneous problems in the interpretation of the invertogram include the following: (*a*) in a female, the invertogram may not accurately reveal the level of the blind rectal pouch because of the escape of gas and stool through a vaginal fistula; (*b*) if the child is straining excessively, or if there is excessive pressure on the abdomen, some intermediate lesions will appear to have a gas shadow below the "I" point. Occasionally, this may be seen in a male child with an intermediate-level lesion in association with a rectobulbar fistula.

5. The invertogram may show air in the bladder, which, in a female, indicates a rectovesical fistula and, in a male, may be seen with either a rectovesical fistula or, more commonly, a proximal urethral fistula.[45] Other procedures for evaluation of the level of the rectal pouch include percutaneous injection of soluble contrast material through the perineum, and ultrasound scanning.[37] A properly performed and interpreted invertogram usually makes such studies unnecessary.

Because urinary anomalies occur frequently in patients with imperforate anus, renal ultrasound should be performed on admission. Also, before discharge one should obtain a pyelogram to assess structure and function of the upper urinary tract and a voiding cystourethrogram to detect possible vesicoureteral reflux, which is surprisingly common in children with imperforate anus.[32] In children with an intermediate or high lesion who have undergone a colostomy, injection of the distal colostomy with soluble contrast often helps to define any associated rectourinary or rectovaginal fistulae.

Surgical Management

Neonates face similar medical and surgical risks whether they are undergoing a perineal anoplasty or a colostomy. Preoperative studies should include routine blood tests, chest x-ray films, and an assessment of urinary function. A nasogastric tube is important to minimize abdominal distention and prevent possible vomiting and aspiration. Although meconium in the distal colon is relatively sterile, the patient should be given broad-spectrum antibiotics directed especially against gram-negative organisms. The patient should also receive vitamin K.

Low-Lying Lesions

Although most forms of low imperforate anus require a surgical procedure, many of the less severe varieties can be handled in the newborn nursery. Some children with anal stenosis (covered anus) can be managed by progressive dilatation of the anus up to a size that allows satisfactory evacuation of stool. If the anal opening still appears to be stenotic, however, a limited cutback procedure or anoplasty to divide the external sphincter muscle in one area is often required. In children with a perineal body fistula 1–2 cm anterior to the external sphincter muscle, a cutback procedure (Fig 108–4,*A*) or posterior perineal anoplasty (Fig 108–4,*B*) should be performed. Occasionally, a child may have a fistulous opening near the true anus, and not be recognized as having an imperforate anus. As the child gets older and begins to eat solid foods, the stools may become more firm, resulting in chronic constipation. Close inspection reveals that posterior to the fistulous orifice the perineum bulges outward when the infant strains downward. Dilatation and enemas may often help temporarily, but, once the rectum is clean, a perineal anoplasty should be performed.

In males with a low imperforate anus and a long subcutaneous fistulous tract along the raphe, the tract should be thoroughly opened and a more formal anoplasty performed in the center of the external sphincter mechanism. In females with a low imperforate anus and an anocutaneous fistula, surgical management becomes more difficult as the fistulous orifice reaches the vulva or passes inside the vaginal introitus (see Fig 108–3,*A*). Most fistulae in the vestibule of the vagina just external to the hymen still qualify as a low imperforate anus.[45] With a curved hemostat, one can usually demonstrate that the rectum has descended quite distally and often lies fairly close to the true external sphincter mechanism. A cutback procedure in children with anovulvar or anovestibular fistula usually results in adequate stool passage. Stephens and others have maintained that long-term fecal continence in such children is good.[45] However, because the anal margin remains so anterior, the child may face several long-term complications, including soilage of the vagina, urinary tract infections, and posterior vaginal lacerations if vaginal delivery is attempted in adulthood. Anal transposition is therefore recommended to avoid such problems (Fig 108–5). If the newborn is too small or is otherwise ill, this procedure can be delayed several weeks or months. A 5–10-mm limited cutback procedure followed by daily dilations with a no. 24F catheter usually assures adequate stool discharge until the child is older.

Following repair of a low imperforate anus, daily dilatations for several months to a year will help to prevent stricture formation, thereby avoiding long-term complications of constipation and fecal impaction. Stretching the posterior anal margin with a finger is particularly helpful in maintaining an adequate channel. In addition, lubricants, such as mineral oil given by mouth, can be helpful in children who continue to strain at stools. An occasional child will require a repeated cutback procedure if symptoms do not resolve. Rectal biopsy should be performed at the same time in such instances to rule out the rare occurrence of Hirschsprung's disease in a child with imperforate anus.[21, 45] As shown in Figure 108–6, failure to prevent a pattern of recurring bouts of fecal impaction can lead to massive megacolon, necessitating a pull-through procedure.[29]

Intermediate and High-Lying Lesions

Most cases of intermediate or high imperforate anus are recognized on the first day of life. In the past, anatomical variations in these patients have led to different clinical approaches in the newborn period. For example, a female infant often has an intermediate-level rectovaginal fistula large enough to permit defeca-

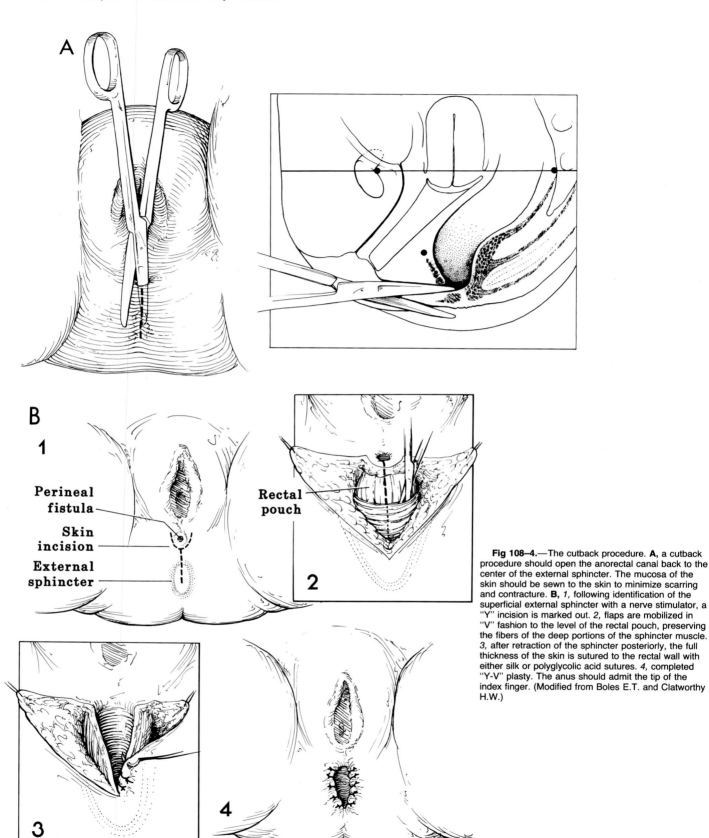

Fig 108—4.—The cutback procedure. **A,** a cutback procedure should open the anorectal canal back to the center of the external sphincter. The mucosa of the skin should be sewn to the skin to minimize scarring and contracture. **B,** *1,* following identification of the superficial external sphincter with a nerve stimulator, a "Y" incision is marked out. *2,* flaps are mobilized in "V" fashion to the level of the rectal pouch, preserving the fibers of the deep portions of the sphincter muscle. *3,* after retraction of the sphincter posteriorly, the full thickness of the skin is sutured to the rectal wall with either silk or polyglycolic acid sutures. *4,* completed "Y-V" plasty. The anus should admit the tip of the index finger. (Modified from Boles E.T. and Clatworthy H.W.)

Perineal fistula

Skin incision

External sphincter

Rectal pouch

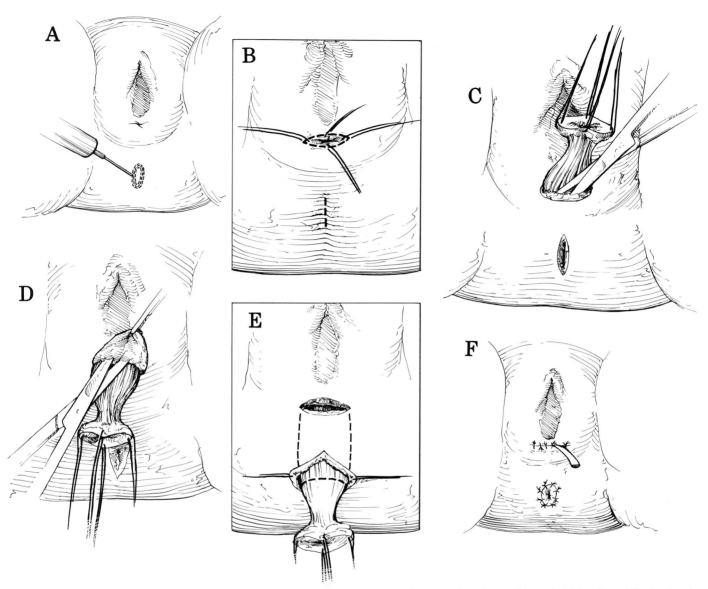

Fig 108–5.—Anal transposition is most suited for anovulvar and anovestibular fistulae. **A,** stimulation to define center of true anus. **B,** traction sutures on margin of fistula; mobilization begun with a small transverse oval incision. **C** and **D,** rectum carefully mobilized on all sides with care to avoid injury to vagina. **E,** following midline opening of anorectal canal, fistula with mobilized rectum is brought down from above. **F,** after amputation of the distal end of fistula, primary suture of rectal wall to skin; upper wound drained and closed.

tion through the vagina with little difficulty. Eventually, however, problems develop—including vaginitis, skin excoriation, urinary tract infection, and stool impaction above the level of the fistula. One 7-year-old girl we saw had been allowed to defecate through her vagina from birth. She was admitted with severe megacolon and malnutrition. Attempts to dilate such fistulae usually tear the thin vaginal wall surrounding the fistula.

If there is any doubt about the presence of an intermediate or high lesion, a vaginogram in a female and a retrograde urethrogram in a male, with or without a voiding cystourethrogram, will usually delineate the underlying anatomy. In a female, if there is a rectal fistula to the vagina above the hymen, or, in a male, if there is a fistula into the bladder or urethra, the rectal pouch is *not* translevator. Such patients are best managed by a formal pull-through procedure. Some surgeons have favored primary pull-through procedures without a colostomy in the newborn pe-

riod, but the operative mortality with these early pull-throughs has proved to be four to five times as high as that in older children undergoing the same operation.[45] Hence, the first procedure in any child with an intermediate or high anomaly should be a diverting colostomy.

Colostomy as a Staging Procedure

Although a colostomy in a neonate with imperforate anus is considered protective, it may be associated with a number of serious complications: (1) stenosis of the colostomy with enterocolitis,[42] (2) a high incidence of urinary tract infections in the presence of a fistula from the rectum to the urinary tract,[39, 53] (3) hyperchloremic acidosis in patients with proximal colostomies and rectourinary fistulae,[12, 38, 49] and (4) persistent diarrhea.

The high incidence of urinary tract infections in patients with

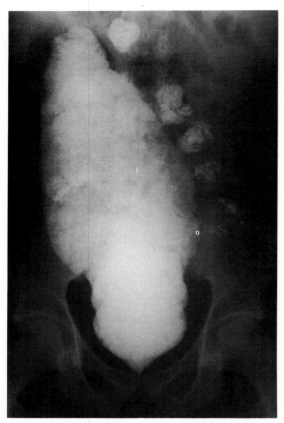

Fig 108–6.—Megarectum consequent upon strictured anoplasty. Barium enema in an 18-year-old with persistent constipation since undergoing a cutback procedure as a newborn. He had not received anorectal dilatations postoperatively, and the area of the cutback procedure had become stenotic.

a fistula from the distal colon to the genitourinary tract has led some investigators[39, 40] to emphasize the use of repeated distal colon washouts and suppressive antibiotics. Such efforts have not been uniformly successful for two reasons. First, patients who had urinary fistulae plus vesicoureteral reflux or other urinary anomalies had an incidence of urinary tract infections almost twice that of patients with urinary fistulae but no urinary anomalies.[40] Second, transverse colostomy resulted in a long defunctionalized distal colonic segment in which stasis of urine and colonic secretions could occur in spite of repeated washouts. Other investigators[5, 24] have therefore favored placing the colostomy in the sigmoid colon and dividing the colostomy to assure complete diversion of the fecal stream. They emphasize that a shorter defunctionalized distal colon segment provides less opportunity for stasis and bacterial overgrowth. In addition, such a colostomy appears to protect the patient from hyperchloremic acidosis, which has only been seen in patients with transverse colostomy.[12, 38, 49]

Because of these multiple concerns, the following guidelines are suggested in planning a colostomy in a newborn with an imperforate anus: (1) perform a completely divided colostomy in the proximal sigmoid colon; (2) make sure that there is adequate laxity in the distal colon segment in order to permit the option of a definitive pull-through procedure via the sacral route alone; (3) before discharge in the newborn period, thoroughly lavage the distal colon until it is clear; (4) if the child has a known or suspected fistula to the urinary tract, give 100,000 units of penicillin G suspension by mouth twice a day. This prophylaxis is espe-

cially important in children with other urinary tract disorders such as vesicoureteral reflux or structural anomalies.

Assessment and Preparation for a Pull-through Procedure

Previously, children with Down syndrome or moderately severe sacral anomalies were often not considered for a definitive pull-through procedure. However, with recent emphasis on precise anatomical reconstruction of both the levator and the external sphincter mechanisms,[8, 9] such patients should now be considered as possible candidates for operation. One group of patients, though, should be carefully assessed before undergoing a pull-through procedure: those with neurogenic bladder. This condition is almost always present in patients with an absent sacrum below S-1 or S-2 or in patients with a lumbosacral myelomeningocele.[40] Children with either of these severe spinal anomalies may show one or more of the following features: (1) no evidence of episodic voiding; the diapers are constantly wet due to continual dribbling of urine from an overly distended bladder or a bladder without sphincteric control; under these circumstances, the bladder can be easily emptied by compression; (2) a chronically distended bladder requiring frequent Credé maneuvers to achieve voiding; (3) marked weakness or absence of external sphincter muscle function in response to electrical stimulation. These features suggest a severe deficiency of sacral innervation. In such children, the prospects for fecal continence are poor, and a pull-through procedure should probably not be attempted.

Nevertheless, for the vast majority of patients with a high imperforate anus, a pull-through procedure is indicated. The choice of when to do the procedure varies according to individual surgeons and the approach they use. Stephens and Kiesewetter advised waiting until the patient was at least 6–12 months of age. De Vries and Pena performed a posterior sagittal anorectoplasty with good results in an otherwise healthy infant of 3 months. In their experience, the blind rectal pouch, even at 3 months of age, has an excellent intramural blood supply, permitting the rectum to be safely mobilized, tapered, and sewn to the anal skin.

Regardless of the patient's age, several studies should be performed shortly before the planned pull-through even if they were previously done in the neonatal period. These studies help to define the relation of the rectum to the pelvic anatomy and to identify any unexpected problems. (1) A distal colostogram done with soluble contrast in a lateral view often reveals the anatomy of an associated fistula more clearly than was possible in the newborn period. (2) A voiding cystourethrogram may also contribute information regarding a fistula, but, more important, it delineates any underlying bladder dysfunction. For example, if significant vesicoureteral reflux is identified, it may be wiser to repair this disorder before proceeding with a pull-through procedure. (3) In the female, endoscopy may demonstrate a septate vagina or other genital anomalies that may not have been well delineated by contrast studies. In the male, endoscopy is usually not indicated because most of the information obtained by this study can be obtained by a voiding cystourethrogram and a colostogram.

Surgical Techniques

Classic approaches to high- or intermediate-level lesions include those reported by Stephens,[43, 44] Swenson and Donnellan,[48] Rehbein,[30] Kiesewetter,[18] and Mollard.[25] Until recently, the preferred approach in most centers was that described by Stephens. At present, we prefer the posterior sagittal anorectoplasty, which is described in detail by de Vries and Pena later in this chapter (pp. 1035–1037).

Many early repairs suffered because they did not define a precise route to the perineum anterior to the so-called puborectal sling. This was true of both two-stage and single-stage repairs such as the original Rhoads repair[31] and later variations described by Gross and by Santulli.[33] For these reasons, most workers in the field preferred the Stephens procedure.[45] The essential principles of this technique involve the identification of the proximal portions of the levator ani via a posterior approach through the sacrococcygeal junction. Identification of the space anterior to the levator ani was thought to be the key element in passing the pulled-through rectum anterior to the puborectal muscle. In rectal anomalies in which the pouch lies at or distal to the pubococcygeal line, it may be possible to divide the fistula and mobilize the rectum via the sacrococcygeal route alone, thus making abdominal exploration unnecessary. On the other hand, when the rectal pouch is above this line, following definition of the puborectal sling, the rectosigmoid is dissected via the abdominal route and a rectourethral, rectovaginal, or rectovesical fistula divided from above bringing the colon through the already defined puborectal sling. Thus, with high-lying lesions, a sacroabdominoperineal rectoplasty is performed. The main difference between the Stephens operation and the operation recently described by de Vries and Pena[9] is that the original principles of the Stephens operation are extended to include precise definition of rectal sphincter components at and below the puborectalis sling, including the entire striated muscle complex.

Swenson and Donnellan[48] stressed the important role of the puborectalis sling in the repair, but with their technique the space anterior to the puborectalis was defined principally from below, and then the dissection was joined with the abdominal portion. Rehbein[30] devised an endorectal dissection within the rectal pouch to avoid damage to the urinary tract and pelvic nerves. With his approach, an attempt is made to palpate the levator with a finger above and below, but the space anterior to the puborectalis is bluntly dissected without direct visualization. For this reason, Kiesewetter tried an approach that combined Stephens' sacral dissection and definition of the puborectalis sling with Rehbein's endorectal dissection of the rectum done through the abdomen.[18] Regardless of the form of dissection and pull-through of the rectal pouch, however, most surgeons preferred to define the puborectalis portion of the levator mechanism via a posterior approach in order to preserve the muscle in its entirety and to allow for accurate pull-through anterior to the puborectalis.

In 1978, Mollard[25] described a surgical treatment of high imperforate anus with definition of the puborectal sling by an anterior perineal approach. Once again, attention was paid to the puborectalis sling, but Mollard and co-workers believed that, with an anterior perineal approach, the sling could be clearly visualized while damage to the urethra, puborectal muscle, and nervi erigentes could be minimized. In his description, Mollard referred to the approaches described by a number of previous workers, including Swenson and Donnellan, Rehbein, and Santulli. The essentials of the Mollard operation involve an abdominoperineal procedure with the patient in the lithotomy position. A bougie is passed into the urethra for identification purposes. Following this, a curved anterior perineal incision is made approximately 1 cm lateral and anterior to the site of the new anus. This flap can then be dissected and reflected posteriorly, and it is then possible to dissect upward along the bulbous and membranous urethra so that all muscle fibers encountered along the way can be gently retracted laterally and posteriorly, thus creating a small tunnel anterior to the puborectal sling. Mollard believes that the puborectalis sling can be easily perceived via this approach. Next, an abdominal dissection is performed, using Rehbein's technique described above. Following completion of

the endorectal dissection, the colon to be pulled through is brought downward, anterior to the previously identified levators and out through a separate posterior stellate incision made exactly in the spot where the new anus is to be. The anterior perineal flap incision is then closed. Mollard and co-workers have been using this procedure for all cases of high imperforate anus and some cases of intermediate anomalies. They prefer to do the pull-through at 9–18 months of age following a neonatal colostomy, as is the case with most of the other operative approaches. They have also used this approach for remedial operations in cases of a prior pull-through where the puborectalis sling had been missed.

Complications

Mortality

The cause of death in most children with imperforate anus is related to associated congenital anomalies. Some anomalies, such as renal aplasia, are intrinsically fatal. In reports published since 1960, combined mortality rates for patients with high and low imperforate anus lesions vary from 11.1% to 34.7%.[45] In Stephens' series, the mortality in patients with high lesions was 45.6%, whereas the mortality in patients with low lesions was 22%. In general, males had a mortality rate twice that of females for both high lesions and low lesions. Most of these deaths were directly attributable to anomalies of the cardiovascular, genitourinary, and central nervous systems.

Genitourinary Complications

Genitourinary anomalies can produce morbidity both before and after a definitive pull-through procedure that can hinder a child's growth and development. The importance of minimizing urinary tract infections in patients with a fistula from the colon to the urinary tract has already been emphasized. Another important cause of urinary tract infections in patients with imperforate anus is vesicoureteral reflux. Investigators noted reflux in patients with imperforate anus, and these infants were routinely studied with voiding cystourethrograms in the neonatal period.[32, 40] Females had a higher incidence of reflux than males. Also, patients with high imperforate anus had a high incidence of reflux. In one series,[27] routine voiding cystourethrograms showed that 39% of patients with high-lying lesions had reflux, vs. only 4% of patients with low lesions. Routine pyelography, however, is not an adequate technique for evaluation of the neonate with imperforate anus. Rickwood[32] noted that vesicoureteral reflux was missed in 75% of patients with imperforate anus in whom a pyelogram was the only surveillance study performed. When both procedures were performed routinely, the incidence of abnormalities of the upper tracts was 2.5 times greater in children with high lesions than in children with low lesions. Current experience now suggests that high-quality ultrasonography may replace routine pyelography in the neonatal period. Assessment of the upper tracts can be performed shortly after birth, and thereby contribute to preoperative planning.

Following a definitive pull-through procedure, recurrent genitourinary problems—many of them iatrogenic in nature—may arise. Frequently, one becomes aware of these problems because of recurring urinary tract infections. A neurogenic bladder may be found on cystourethrogram even though such findings were not present preoperatively. Excessive dissection in the pelvis is thought to be the cause of this problem.[53] Urethral stricture may occur if the urethra is damaged when the fistula is divided, and this may require repeated dilatation or secondary repair. On the other hand, inadequate resection of the fistula may lead to the development of a urethral diverticulum. These diverticula have occurred with equal frequency in patients undergoing abdominoperineal and after sacroperineal pull-through procedures of the types described by Stephens[45] and Kiesewetter.[53] Patients with these diverticula usually present a number of years after the pull-through procedure with recurring urinary tract infections and episodes of pain and/or apparent infection in the pelvic area. Occasionally, large calculi may develop within these diverticula. If a diverticulum does become infected, a secondary fistula to the new rectum may develop. Currently, we believe that the optimal treatment for all these complications is a midline sagittal sacral approach, allowing identification and preservation of the muscles of continence.

Gastrointestinal Complications

Stenosis of the anus or anorectal canal may result from a compromised blood supply to the pulled-through segment of colon or from pelvic infection, leading to fibrosis of the pericolic soft tissue. In most cases, however, stenosis of the anus or anorectal canal is the result of simple wound contracture. A number of surgeons therefore favor anorectal dilatation for several months until complete healing has taken place. In an infant a size 12 or 13 Hegar dilator is usually sufficient, and in an older child a size 14 or 15. Following the procedure developed by de Vries and Pena, prolonged dilatation is essential because of the tapering of the bowel that is employed. With appropriate dilatations, impactions or constipation are usually not a problem.

Prolapse of the anal mucosa usually results when the anus is made too large, particularly when cruciate incisions have been made at right angles to the perineal raphe. Extensive prolapse of the mucosa leads to perineal rash, excoriation, and bleeding. Mucous soiling can also be a problem. Such patients require a revision of the anoplasty in order to recess the mucosa below the level of the skin. Following this revision, dilatation should be performed daily until the scar is soft, in order to prevent anal stricture.

In spite of anorectal dilatation and laxatives, persistent constipation may still be a problem. Several recent series[29, 41] have drawn attention to a megarectum condition called "terminal reservoir syndrome" or "primary rectal ectasia," which is thought to exist at birth in some children with either high or low imperforate anus. Months or years after repair, these patients present with persistent constipation and eventual massive accumulation of stool. Barium enema shows massive dilatation of the bowel, usually limited to the terminal rectosigmoid colon. Even with a proximal diverting colostomy, the megarectum does not resolve. These patients usually require tapering or resection of the abnormal bowel and a Swenson or Duhamel pull-through procedure.[29]

In assessing a child with unexplained constipation following appropriate treatment of imperforate anus, one should also consider the possibility of coincidental Hirschsprung's disease. Most authors[21, 45] report only rare instances of this phenomenon. When a higher incidence of associated Hirschsprung's disease has been reported, most of those patients were erroneously said to have low-segment Hirschsprung's disease. Rectal biopsies in these patients revealed no ganglion cells, but specimens were usually taken from the distal 1–2 cm of the rectum and often were composed largely of tissue from the distal fistula. However, there are patients with imperforate anus who have proved to have long-segment Hirschsprung's disease. The length of aganglionic colon has ranged from 7 to 10 cm in most patients to total aganglionosis coli in one patient. These patients are identified in two ways. First, if a pull-through procedure utilizing aganglionic colon was done in a newborn, constipation will ensue. Second, if

a temporizing colostomy was done distal to an unrecognized transition zone, as occurred in one of our own cases,[21] the patient will have recurring bouts of abdominal distention and constipation. A biopsy of the colostomy and a barium enema will confirm the diagnosis. For this reason, when imperforate anus is definitively corrected, specimens should be sent for routine pathologic assessment of ganglion cells.

Follow-up Results and Patient Care

Fecal Continence

CRITERIA.—The criteria of normal fecal continence are clear: no accidents or soiling with either solid or diarrheal stool; controlled passage of flatus; rare constipation; and no medications, cathartics, or enemas needed to control or regulate defecation. Although fecal continence following repair of low imperforate anus is generally good, the results following repair of high imperforate anus are not uniformly good. When comparing one author's results with another's, the criteria for distinguishing "good" from "fair" and "fair" from "poor" results are not always the same. Moreover, some authors stress only the mechanics of fecal control (e.g., accidents with diarrheal stool),[19] while others stress the social impact on the patient (e.g., number of days absent from school).[41] Others have graded imperforate anus patients according to a numerical system based on the presence or absence of fecal leakage, rectal sensation, and normal levator indentation on contrast studies.[15] Finally, other authors have stressed the importance of meticulous physiologic assessment of patients following imperforate anus operation including manometrics, electromyography, and perineal electrostimulation.[35, 36, 50] There is no general agreement regarding which tests are most clinically useful.

At the recent Wingspread Workshop on Anorectal Malformations,[46] the participants agreed that a common standard for evaluating postoperative results was essential in order to compare one procedure with another. A descriptive nonscoring system was proposed, with emphasis on whether the patient is clean, whether stool can be retained, and whether therapy is needed.

RESULTS.—The literature reveals a wide disparity of results in patients who have undergone repair of high imperforate anus. As shown in Table 108–2, the best results have been in Mollard's limited series of 15 patients with high imperforate anus.[25] In our experience[51] and that of others,[24, 41, 45] the next best results were seen in patients in whom the rectal pouch was low enough to permit a sacral approach alone. In contrast, Kiesewetter's own results, reported in 1977, were better following abdominoperineal than sacroperineal or sacroabdominal perineal procedures.[19] In our experience, females have better fecal continence results than do males. This may be due to a higher percentage of females with intermediate lesions.

Of historical interest, Partridge's experience was with a mixture of newborn patients and patients staged with an initial colostomy, all of whom had their definitive pull-through procedure done by an abdominoperineal approach.[45] His poor results contrasted with the good results of Swenson and Donnellan,[48] who strongly advocated abdominoperineal procedures done in the newborn period. Their technique stressed division of any fistula via an abdominal approach and the use of the entire intact colon and rectum as the pull-through segment. This approach may well preserve autonomic reflex function in the distal bowel. They also stressed an anterior perineal dissection to mobilize the space between the urethra and puborectalis muscle under direct visualization, the approach now used by Mollard with such good results.

TABLE 108–2.—FUNCTIONAL RESULTS IN HIGH IMPERFORATE
ANUS REPAIR

STUDY AND DATE	NO. OF CASES	NO. (%) GOOD	NO. (%) FAIR	NO. (%) POOR
Partridge and Gough (1961)[45]	63	21 (33)	27 (43)	15 (24)
Kiesewetter and Turner (1963)[45]	39	15 (38)	6 (15)	18 (46)
Swenson and Donnellan (1967)[48]	22	14 (64)	5 (23)	3 (13)
Rehbein (1967)[30]	45	18 (40)	13 (29)	14 (31)
Stephens and Smith (1971)[45]				
Total	25	14 (56)	8 (32)	3 (12)
Sacroperineal	11	7 (64)	3 (27)	1 (9)
Sacroabdominoperineal	10	6 (60)	4 (40)	
Kiesewetter and Chang (1977)[19]				
Total	78	40 (51)	20 (26)	18 (23)
Sacroperineal or sacroabdominoperineal	43	18 (42)	16 (37)	9 (21)
Abdominoperineal	35	22 (63)	4 (11)	9 (26)
Mollard et al. (1978)[25]	15	12 (80)	1 (7)	2 (13)
Children's Hospital of Philadelphia[51]				
Total	61	31 (51)	24 (39)	6 (10)
Sacroperineal	10	7 (70)	3 (30)	0 (0)
Sacroabdominoperineal	13	5 (38.5)	5 (38.5)	3 (23)
Abdominoperineal	38	19 (50)	16 (42)	3 (8)

Conservative Management of Soiling Problems

Very few patients have perfect fecal continence following operation for high imperforate anus. Many patients with a "good" continence score have problems with diarrheal stools and flatus. For the child with only "fair" fecal continence, considerable resources and perseverance are required of both the child and the family in order to achieve a good quality of life. A number of experienced investigators have developed guidelines and maneuvers[19] to help their patients cope.

1. Parents need to understand that successful fecal control may not be achieved until the child is aged 10 years or older. Parents often report that girls seem to have more interest in being clean than boys, but that both boys and girls often have better fecal continence when they are away from home. Motivation is a major factor and generally improves with time.[19]

2. In general, a child who is clean between occasional episodes of soiling has a better long-term outlook than does a patient who soils continually. It is very helpful with such a child to establish a pattern by encouraging defecation after meals, especially breakfast, to provide an opportunity for the child consciously to evacuate the rectum, and therefore be clean until after lunch or supper. Success with such controlled bowel movements should be reinforced with praise.

3. Certain foods with a laxative effect—plums, prunes, peaches, chocolate, tomato products, nut products, or corn—should be avoided. Some foods with a binding effect—cheese, peanut butter, bran products, or hot cereals—may make the consistency of the stool easier to manage.

4. Persistent perianal rashes inhibit fecal control because of accompanying pain and swelling. Liberal use of substances like Desitin, Fasteeth, Balmex, cornstarch, or even Maalox, may provide a barrier between the skin and the irritating stool.

5. Of all the specific antidiarrheal medications, Immodium provides the most sustained effect in slowing gastrointestinal tract transit time with the fewest side effects.

6. Some children have poor fecal control, not on the basis of frequent accidents, but because of rectal inertia with or without stenosis of the anorectal canal. These patients tend to develop fecal impaction in the rectosigmoid colon and then may soil due to liquid overflow. Some of these patients may benefit from bis-acodyl suppositories once or twice a day. Others with this problem find that they can manage with a cleansing enema once every 2–4 days and then be completely clean in between.

Secondary Procedures for Fecal Incontinence

Before deciding to reoperate on a patient with continued fecal incontinence, one should determine the likely cause of the poor fecal control. If the patient has major anatomic or physiologic problems, such as severe agenesis of the sacrum or meningomyelocele or a neurogenic bladder, the pelvic musculature may not be capable of fecal control. Such a patient should have a thorough assessment with manometry, electromyography, and electrical stimulation of the perineum. Fortunately, patients with severe intrinsic deficiency of the pelvic musculature are not common.

Much more common are patients in whom the rectum was not properly pulled through anterior to the levator musculature, or in whom the striated muscle complex was completely missed during the anoplasty portion of the previous operation. In these patients, careful assessment of the perineum by electrical stimulation often shows that the anus is anterior to the true center of the external sphincter mechanism and even lateral to the true midline. Digital rectal examination may demonstrate definite "voluntary" contraction of the puborectalis sling behind the rectum, and yet there is a patulous anal canal distal to the sling. In these patients, the anorectal zone of resistance is shorter than the required 3.5 cm.[35]

The indications for attempting a secondary procedure for incontinence should be clinical and social. In general, a patient of any age with constant fecal soiling or a patient older than 8 years with intermittent soiling in spite of therapy should be considered for a possible secondary procedure. If the patient is functioning at the best possible level and if the anorectum is clearly misplaced, this patient should be offered reoperation. Fecal continence should be graded preoperatively so that one can assess the result of the secondary procedure.

A number of secondary procedures are available for such patients. Most emphasize adherence to the basic principles stressed in doing a primary procedure. Repeated procedures of Stephens[45] and Mollard[25] emphasize mobilizing a misplaced rectum and placing it anterior to an intact puborectalis sling. If the puborectalis is partially severed during Stephens' approach, he urges that the severed portions be drawn together and sutured behind the rectum. Pena,[28] when reexploring the rectum by the posterior midline sagittal approach, endeavors to identify and preserve the striated muscle complex and the proximal levators. The rectum is often tapered so that it will fit comfortably within the muscle complex. Pena recommends that secondary procedures of this type be protected by a completely diverting colostomy.

Another operative approach is to rearrange the anatomy of the muscular pelvis in order to bring more effective muscle contraction to bear against the rectum. A variety of muscle slings have been designed to wrap pedicles of striated muscle with intact neurovascular bundles around the distal rectum to provide voluntary muscular control. The most commonly used has been the gracilis sling. Results have not been uniformly successful, owing perhaps to the fact that, while muscle tone and control may be increased, sensation is often not improved. Another mode of rearranging pelvic anatomy has been advocated by Kottmeier.[20] In his procedure, the levator sling is released from its posterior attachments by excising the coccyx and splitting the ileococcygeus muscle laterally on both sides. The upper portion of the ileococcygeus is then sewn tightly behind the rectum, producing a more acute anterior angulation of the rectum. Kottmeier's results with this approach have been quite successful in patients with fecal incontinence secondary to trauma. For patients who are incontinent following a repair of imperforate anus, sacral levatorplasties are less successful. One third become continent, one third are improved, and one third are unchanged.[28]

REFERENCES

1. Arhan P., Faverdin C., Devroede G., et al.: Manometric assessment of continence after surgery for imperforate anus. *J. Pediatr. Surg.* 11:157, 1976.
2. Amussat J.J.: Anus artificiel créé par un nouveau procédé. *Gaz. Méd.* (Paris) 654, 1835.
3. Bill A.H., Hall D.G., Johnson R.J.: Position of rectal fistula in relation to the hymen in 46 girls with imperforate anus. *J. Pediatr. Surg.* 10:361, 1975.
4. Bill A.H. Jr., Johnson R.J.: Failure of migration of the rectal opening as the cause for most cases of imperforate anus. *Surg. Gynecol. Obstet.* 106:643, 1958.
5. Boles E.T.: Imperforate anus. *Clin. Perinatol.* 5:149, 1978.
6. Chassaignac M.: Presentation de malades, Bulletin de la Société de Chirurgie de Paris, 410, Feb. 20, 1856.
7. Cule J.H.: John Pughe 1814–1874: A scholar surgeon's operation on imperforate anus in 1854. *Ann. R. Coll. Surg. Engl.* 37:247, 1965.
8. de Vries P.A.: The surgery of anorectal anomalies: Its evolution, with evaluations of procedures. *Curr. Prob. Surg.* May 1984.
9. de Vries P.A., Pena A.: Posterior sagittal anorectoplasty. *J. Pediatr. Surg.* 17:638, 1982.
10. Eisner M.: Functional examination of rectum and anus in normals, in disturbances of continence and defecation, and in congenital malformation. *Scand. J. Gastroenterol.* 7:305, 1972.
11. Hendren W.H.: Urogenital sinus and anorectal malformation: Experience with 22 cases. *J. Pediatr. Surg.* 15:628, 1980.
12. Iwai N., Ogita S., Shirasaka S., et al.: Hyperchloremic acidosis in an infant with imperforate anus and rectourethral fistula. *J. Pediatr. Surg.* 13:437, 1978.
13. Janik J.S., Humphrey R., Nagaraj H.S.: Sigmoid volvulus in a neonate with imperforate anus. *J. Pediatr. Surg.* 18:636, 1983.
14. Japan Study Group of Anorectal Anomalies: A group study for the classification of anorectal anomalies in Japan with comments to the international classification (1970). *J. Pediatr. Surg.* 17:302, 1982.
15. Kelly J.H.: The clinical and radiological assessment of anal continence in childhood. *Aust. N.Z. J. Surg.* 42:62, 1972.
16. Khoury M.J., Cordero J.F., Greenberg F., et al.: A population study of the VACTERL association. *Pediatrics* 71:815, 1983.
17. Kiesewetter W.B., Nixon H.H.: Imperforate anus. I. Its surgical anatomy. *J. Pediatr. Surg.* 2:60, 1967.
18. Kiesewetter W.B.: Imperforate anus. II. The rationale and technic of the sacro-abdomino-perineal operation. *J. Pediatr. Surg.* 2:106, 1967.
19. Kiesewetter W.B., Chang J.H.T.: Imperforate anus: a five to thirty year follow-up perspective, *Prog. Pediatr. Surg.* 10:111, 1977.
20. Kottmeier P.K., Dizadiw R.: Complete release of the levator ani sling in fecal incontinence. *J. Pediatr. Surg.* 2:111, 1967.
21. Mahboubi S., Templeton J.M. Jr.: Association of Hirschsprung's disease and imperforate anus in a patient with "cat-eye" syndrome: A report of one case and review of the literature. *Pediatr. Radiol.* 14:441, 1984.
22. Mastin W.M.: A résumé of the surgical treatment of anorectal imperforation in the newborn. *Surg. Gynecol. Obstet.* 7:316, 1908.
23. Matas R.: The surgical treatment of congenital ano-rectal imperforation considered in the light of modern operative procedures. *Trans. Am. Surg. Assoc.* 15:453, 1897.
24. Miller R.C., Izant R.J. Jr.: Sacrococcygeal perineal approach to imperforate anus. *Am. J. Surg.* 121:62, 1971.
25. Mollard P., Marechal J.M., de Beaujeu M.J.: Surgical treatment of high imperforate anus with definition of the pubo-rectalis sling by an anterior perineal approach. *J. Pediatr. Surg.* 13:499, 1978.
26. Norris W.J., Brophy T.W. III, Brayton D.: Imperforate anus: A case series and preliminary report of the one-stage abdomino-perineal operation. *Surg. Gynecol. Obstet.* 88:623, 1949.
27. Parrot T.S., Woodard J.R.: Importance of cystourethrography in neonates with imperforate anus. *Urology* 13:607, 1979.
28. Pena A.: Posterior sagittal anorectoplasty as a secondary operation for the treatment of fecal incontinence. *J. Pediatr. Surg.* 18:762, 1983.
29. Powell R.W., Sherman J.O., Raffensperger J.G.: Megarectum: A rare complication of imperforate anus repair and its surgical correction by endorectal pull-through. *J. Pediatr. Surg.* 17:786, 1982.
30. Rehbein F.: Imperforate anus: Experiences with abdomino-perineal and abdomino-sacro-perineal pull-through procedures. *J. Pediatr. Surg.* 2:99, 1967.
31. Rhoads J.E., Pipes R.L., Randall S.P.: A simultaneous abdominal and perineal approach in operation for imperforate anus with atresia of the rectum and rectosigmoid. *Ann. Surg.* 127:552, 1948.
32. Rickwood A.M.K., Spitz L.: Primary vesicoureteric reflux in neonates with imperforate anus. *Arch. Dis. Child.* 55:149, 1980.
33. Santulli T.V.: The treatment of imperforate anus and associated fistulas. *Surg. Gynecol. Obstet.* 95:601, 1952.
34. Santulli T.V., Schullinger J.N., Kiesewetter W.B., et al.: Imperforate anus: A survey from the members of the Surgical Section of the American Academy of Pediatrics. *J. Pediatr. Surg.* 6:484, 1971.
35. Scharli A.F., Kiesewetter W.B.: Defecation and continence: Some new concepts. *Dis. Colon Rectum* 13:81, 1970.
36. Schnaufer L., Talbert J.L., Haller J.A., et al.: Differential sphincter studies in the diagnosis of anorectal disorders of childhood. *J. Pediatr. Surg.* 2:538, 1967.
37. Schuster S.R., Teele R.L.: An analysis of ultrasound scanning as a guide in determination of "high" and "low" imperforate anus. *J. Pediatr. Surg.* 14:798, 1979.
38. Shepard R., Kiesewetter W.B.: Hyperchloremic acidosis as a complication of imperforate anus with recto-urinary fistula. *J. Pediatr. Surg.* 1:62, 1966.
39. Singh M.P., Haddadin A., Zachary R.B., et al.: Renal tract disease in imperforate anus. *J. Pediatr. Surg.* 9:197, 1974.
40. Smith E.D.: Urinary anomalies and complications in imperforate anus and rectum. *J. Pediatr. Surg.* 3:337, 1968.
41. Smith E.I., Tunell W.P., Williams G.R.: A clinical evaluation of the surgical treatment of anorectal malformations. *Ann. Surg.* 187:583, 1978.
42. Smith E.I., Gill C.C.: Prestenotic enteritis and enterocolitis in children. *South. Med. J.* 68:427, 1975.
43. Stephens F.D.: Congenital imperforate rectum, recto-urethral and recto-vaginal fistulae. *Aust. N.Z. J. Surg.* 22:161, 1953.
44. Stephens F.D.: Malformation of the anus. *Aust. N.Z. J. Surg.* 23:9, 1953.
45. Stephens F.D., Smith E.D.: *Anorectal Malformations in Children.* Chicago, Year Book Medical Publishers, 1971.
46. Stephens F.D.: Wingspread Conference on Anorectal Malformations, Racine, Wis., May 1984 (to be published).
47. Stephens F.D.: *Congenital Malformations of the Urinary Tract.* New York, Praeger Publishers, 1983.
48. Swenson O., Donnellan W.L.: Preservation of the puborectalis sling in imperforate anus repair. *Surg. Clin. North Am.* 47:173, 1967.
49. Tank E.S., Watts H.: Hyperchloremic acidosis from urethrorectal fistula and imperforate anus. *Surgery* 63:837, 1968.
50. Taylor I., Duthie H.L., Zachary R.B.: Anal continence following surgery for imperforate anus. *J. Pediatr. Surg.* 8:497, 1973.
51. Templeton J.M. Jr., Ditesheim J.A.: High imperforate anus: Quantitative results of long-term fecal continence. *J. Pediatr. Surg.* 1985, in press.

52. Wangensteen O.H., Rice C.O.: Imperforate anus. *Ann. Surg.* 92:77, 1930.
53. Wiener E.S., Kiesewetter W.B.: Urologic abnormalities associated with imperforate anus. *J. Pediatr. Surg.* 8:151, 1973.
54. Winkler J.N., Weinstein E.D.: Imperforate anus and heredity. *J. Pediatr. Surg.* 5:555, 1970.

Posterior Sagittal Anorectoplasty for Intermediate and High Imperforate Anus Anomalies

Pieter A. De Vries / Alberto Pena

The vast majority of intermediate and high imperforate anus anomalies can be repaired via a posterior sacral approach. This includes the majority of patients with cloacal anomalies. In patients who require an abdominal approach, a posterior sagittal dissection can still be done first. Therefore, in virtually every case, the following sequence can be employed.

The distal colon should be thoroughly cleansed. This is facilitated when a patient has previously undergone a divided sigmoid colostomy. In a male patient, a Foley catheter should be placed in the bladder. In a female patient, one may elect to place a Foley into the bladder after the operation has begun for ready access to the urethra in the operative field. If endoscopy has not been previously performed, it may be done at the start of the

procedure to identify the anatomy of the vagina and urethra. Then the patient should be placed prone with 60–80 degrees of flexion at the hips. It is very important to provide a generous amount of padding between the patient and the table, particularly under the hips in order to avoid compression injury to the femoral nerves.

Electrical stimulation will be used extensively throughout the procedure, so it is important to be certain that no paralyzing agents are used as a part of the anesthetic management. Before the incision is made, the center of the site for the anus is mapped out carefully with transcutaneous electrostimulation. This is facilitated by wetting the skin with saline for better conduction. The center of the anus may be marked with a small scratch in the skin.

A midsagittal skin incision is then made from the mid-sacrum down to, and through, the anterior margin of the anus (Fig 108–7,A). With a needle tip Bovie on cutting current, the dissection is carried down mid-sagitally through the subcutaneous and superficial external sphincter muscle layers. Frequent electrical stimulation serves as a guide to divide the muscles exactly in the midline. Prolapse of portions of fat through muscle on the surface of the wound may indicate that one has wandered off the midline.

The fibers of the external sphincter layers and levators join together to contribute to the striated muscle complex. The subcutaneous external sphincter layer extends most of the way from the anus to the coccyx, whereas the superficial external sphincter layer inserts on the tip and posterior surface of the coccyx (Fig 108–7,B).

The coccyx is split midsagittally for exposure and to preserve

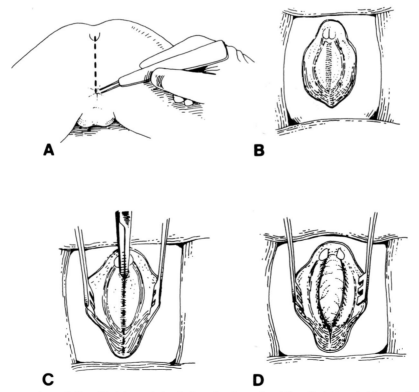

A **B** **C** **D**

Fig 108–7.—Posterior sagittal anorectoplasty. **A,** line of incision and electrical stimulation to determine appropriate anal site. **B,** midsagittal incision through the coccyx and the external sphincter fibers of the anus, showing the striated muscle complex deep to the anal site; subcutaneous external sphincter extending about halfway to the coccyx; superficial external sphincter inserting on the coccyx; levator deeper in midline. **C,** right-angled forceps beneath levator ani. **D,** all layers of striated muscle partially retracted laterally exposing visceral endopelvic fascia. (From de Vries P.A., Posterior sagittal anorectoplasty, in Hofmann v. Kap-herr S. (ed.): *Anorektale Fehlbildungen.* Stuttgart, Gustav Fischer Verlag, 1984. Reprinted with permission.) Continued.

the insertions of the superficial external sphincter. The dissection is then continued down through a layer of fatty tissue beneath this muscle to the level of the levator ani, which arises from the ventral surface of the coccyx. By means of a midsagittal split of the coccyx, one can place a right-angle clamp into the pelvis deep to the levator ani (Fig 108–7,*C*). The levator ani layer is split from the undersurface of the coccyx down to, and through, its contribution to the striated muscle complex (Fig 108–7,*D*). Next, overlying the bowel is the visceral endopelvic fascia, which must be incised to reach the longitudinal smooth muscle layer of the bowel.

Depending on how high or low the rectal pouch is, one may be able to dissect around the proximal rectum near the level of the peritoneal reflection. On the other hand, it is often easier to open the rectum first directly in the midline (Fig 108–8,*A*). This approach allows one to visualize any associated fistulae and to avoid injury to autonomic nerves and ganglia in the perirectal area. The bowel should subsequently be mobilized from the genitourinary tract in a plane between the muscularis and submu-

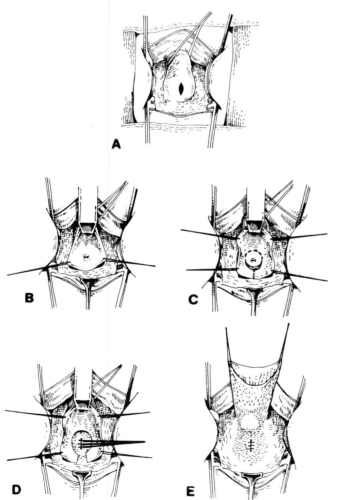

Fig 108–8.—Posterior sagittal anorectoplasty (cont.). **A,** sagittal incision in terminal bowel after proximal dissection around rectum and placement of a tape around the rectum proximally. **B,** retracted rectotomy showing fistula site. **C,** hemicircumferential incision through mucosa-submucosa for placement of first sutures to close fistula. **D,** completed closure of the fistula orifice. **E,** stippled area where muscular bowel wall is left in place and clear area above where peritoneum may be encountered. (From de Vries P.A., Posterior sagittal anorectoplasty, in Hofmann v. Kap-herr S. (ed.): *Anorektale Fehlbildungen.* Stuttgart, Gustav Fischer Verlag, 1984. Reprinted with permission.) Continued.

cosa of the rectum in order to protect these autonomic structures.

The fistula to the urethra can now be seen and probed from within the bowel lumen (Fig 108–8,*B*). The rectal orifice of the fistula is circumferentially incised through only the mucosa-submucosa, half the circumference at a time (Fig 108–8,*C*). Mobilization of the ventral wall of the rectum is aided by placing a number of fine silk traction sutures on the mucosal edges of the bowel and around the cut edges of the fistula. Also, these sutures through the cut edges of the fistula prevent retraction of the fistula ventrally. The mucosa of the fistula is closed by interrupted absorbable sutures. The surrounding edges of the muscular coat are then approximated over the fistula area with interrupted 5-0 proline sutures (Fig 108–8,*D*). This approach allows virtually complete excision of the fistula, thereby preventing the complication of developing a posterior urethral diverticulum.

In mobilizing the anterior surface of the rectum, the plane of dissection is kept between the smooth muscle coat and the submucosa until one reaches the level of the seminal vesicles. By leaving the muscular coat of the rectum on the urethra and prostatic capsule, one can avoid damage to the ganglia supplying the genitourinary tract that are located in that area. This dissection is facilitated by traction sutures on the cut edge of the terminal bowel (Fig 108–8,*E*). Above the level of the seminal vesicles one can dissect through the muscularis of the anterior rectal wall until one achieves complete mobilization of the full-thickness rectal wall. Mobilization of the remainder of the anterior rectal wall and the posterior and lateral portions of the rectum is then performed along a plane directly on the surface of the bowel so as to avoid damage to the pelvic visceral nerves, which lie close to the posterior and lateral surfaces of the rectum. This mobilization involves division of numerous small branches of the middle hemorrhoidal vessels, which must be carefully electrocoagulated on both ends to avoid retraction of a bleeding vessel into the deep pelvic tissues.

Following adequate mobilization of the ectatic rectum, the bowel must usually be tapered to permit its placement both anterior to the levators and in the center of the striated muscle complex. As shown in Figure 108–9,*A* and *B,* de Vries believes that an elongated wedge of the ventral surface, which is largely devoid of muscularis, should be excised. He also thinks that tapering the ventral surface minimizes mobilization of the terminal bowel. Pena prefers to taper the dorsal surface of the bowel in order to avoid placing the suture line adjacent to the suture line closure of the urinary fistula.

The amount of rectal tapering depends on the size of the rectum itself and the size of the muscle complex that will be used to envelop the rectum during closure of the muscle layers. The mucosa of the tapered edges is approximated with 5-0 absorbable sutures. The muscularis is then approximated with 5-0 interrupted proline (Fig 108–9,*B*). The narrowed rectum now constitutes the future anorectal canal. Before the tapered rectum is secured within the striated muscle complex, de Vries thinks that the bowel should accommodate a no. 12 Hegar dilator. Pena prefers a more narrowed tapering, which will accommodate a no. 9 or 10 Hegar dilator.

Reconstruction of the striated pelvic musculature around the rectum begins with 5-0 and 4-0 proline sutures reuniting the divided edges of the levator muscle (Fig 108–9,*C*) at a point where the distal portion of the levator ani muscles join with the external sphincter layers. Sutures are placed both through the two edges of the muscle and through the smooth muscle coat of the rectum to provide a tethering mechanism. In the male, this secures the new rectum in a position close to the urethra. The proximal margins of the divided levator muscle are then also closed with 5-0 or 4-0 proline sutures, but these do not include seromuscular suturing of the bowel.

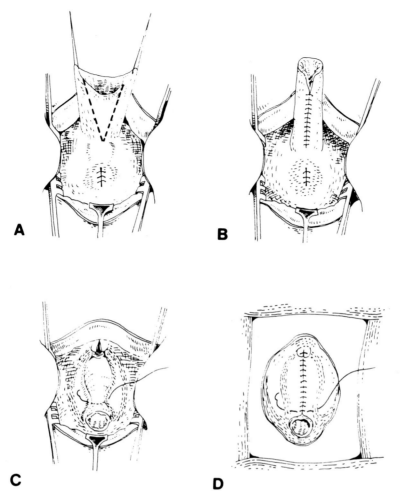

Fig 108–9.—Posterior sagittal anorectoplasty (cont.). **A,** *dotted line,* the extent of anterior wedge resection for tapered repair of rectum. **B,** approximation of the tapered edges of rectum. **C,** first and deepest suture for approximation of the levators to establish the beginning of the canal. **D,** after reapproximation of the levator ani to the coccyx, interrupted sutures are placed in the edges of the superficial external sphincter muscle. (From de Vries P.A., Posterior sagittal anorectoplasty, in Hofmann v. Kap-herr S. (ed.): *Anorektale Fehlbildungen.* Stuttgart, Gustav Fischer Verlag, 1984. Reprinted with permission.)

Reconstruction of the tapered rectum within the center of the distal portion of the striated muscle complex is facilitated by the use of frequent electrical stimulation. As the front and back edges of the muscle complex are reconstructed with the new rectum lying in between, 5-0 proline sutures are used to incorporate seromuscular portions of the bowel wall in order to keep the bowel well secured inside the muscle complex. These sutures are used all the way to the level of the anus. In this repair, the course of the distal tapered rectum (the new anorectal canal) changes direction from a point close to the urethra or vagina to pass posteriorly to the level of the anus. Next, the lateral halves of the coccyx and the muscle edges of the superficial external sphincter muscle are similarly reapproximated (Fig 108–9,*D*). Before suturing the skin edges of the anus to the terminal bowel, any excess length of bowel is trimmed back to a point level with the skin. Sutures of 5-0 proline are used to secure the edges of full-thickness bowel to the skin. The subcutaneous external sphincter is closed with additional sutures of interrupted 5-0 proline, and the skin is closed with running absorbable subcuticular sutures.

In patients with a very high rectal pouch (e.g., those with a rectovesical fistula), an abdominal component to the repair may be needed after an initial posterior sagittal dissection. In such patients, a rubber tube of appropriate size for the patient's muscle complex is placed through the pelvis; one end lies just inside the peritoneal cavity, the other end exits through the center of the anus. The muscle layers are approximated dorsal to the tube, leaving enough space to allow subsequent approximation of the bowel to the muscles of the muscle complex. The tube is sutured temporarily to the skin where it exits from the anus. Then the patient is turned supine. After the abdomen is opened, the rectum is separated from the bladder and appropriately tapered. The tapered bowel is sewn to the rectal tube, which is then drawn out through the anal orifice, bringing the bowel with it. The rectoplasty is then completed by suturing the bowel to the surrounding muscle complex in several tiers for tethering. Then final approximation of the sagittally divided muscle layers, primarily dorsally, is carried out and the anoplasty completed.

The monofilament sutures at the anal orifice are left in place for at least 2 weeks. They are usually well tolerated. After 2–3 weeks, under general anesthesia, the sutures are removed, the anal orifice is calibrated with Hegar dilators, and the integrity of the muscle function of the anus is assessed by electrical stimulation. Dilatations with increasingly larger Hegar dilators are carried out over 3 months so that at the end of this period the anus will admit a no. 12 or no. 13 Hegar dilator in a small infant and a no. 14 or no. 15 dilator in an older child. At this time, the colostomy can be closed.

Other Disorders of the Rectum and Anus

Fecal Continence

Fecal continence results from the coordinated interaction of several complex mechanisms.[28] Four components are of major significance: the rectum, the puborectalis muscle sling, the internal and external sphincters, and the anal mucosa (Fig 109–1).

The *rectum* is basically not a reservoir but is normally empty or contains only a small amount of stool. In the normal resting state of the rectum, contraction waves are higher and motor activity greater than in the sigmoid, producing a reversed gradient that serves as a pressure barrier to the progress of stool. The sensory function of the rectum may be even more critical: pressure sensors respond to dilatation when there is rectal filling, resulting in the conscious perception of the need to defecate and triggering reflexive relaxation of the internal sphincter.

The *puborectalis* muscle has long been recognized to be of critical importance in continence, hence the need to ensure that the rectum is brought down within the puborectalis sling during operations for high imperforate anus (see Chap. 108). The puborectalis muscle is part of the external sphincter apparatus, not of the levator ani complex as was previously supposed. It forms a sling, open anteriorly, that produces a sharp anterior angulation of the rectum. Both voluntary (white) and involuntary (red) fibers are found in its striated muscle. It is normally in a state of tonic contraction that maintains the anorectal angle. With sudden increases of intra-abdominal pressure, as with coughing or straining, this tonic contraction increases automatically, probably the major mechanism of prevention of stress incontinence. The muscle contracts reflexly when the anal mucosa is stimulated and voluntarily when the urge to defecate is consciously suppressed. During defecation, it is consciously relaxed. The puborectalis muscle also contains pressure sensors that function much like those in the rectal wall to provide both conscious perception of rectal fullness and relaxation of the internal sphincter.[15] This function is particularly important in patients who have had the rectum removed (e.g., in the pull-through procedures for Hirschsprung's disease or polyposis).

The *internal anal sphincter*, part of the muscle wall of the anorectum, is smooth muscle, not under voluntary control. It is normally in a state of near maximum tonic contraction but relaxes reflexly in response to rectal distention. This reflex is independent of external innervation and is thought to be mediated via the myenteric plexus. It is absent in patients with Hirschsprung's disease (and persistent increased sphincter tone may be a cause of postoperative enterocolitis or stool retention in these patients).

The *external sphincter* has three components: subcutaneous, superficial, and deep. The subcutaneous fibers account for the anal "pucker," while the superficial fibers provide concentric sphincteric contraction external to the internal sphincter. The deep external sphincter fibers are arranged in a sling open posteriorly, thus oriented opposite the puborectalis.[29] Like the puborectalis, it is composed of striated muscle with both red and white fibers. All three parts of the external sphincter contract reflexly in response to stimulation of the anal mucosa, as well as to a number of other stimuli, such as increased intra-abdominal pressure, rectal distention, postural change, perianal scratch, and anal dilatation. The external sphincters may be voluntarily contracted or relaxed, together with the puborectalis, to suppress or assist defecation.

The *anal mucosa*, densely innervated, is exquisitely sensitive to a variety of stimuli (unlike the rectal mucosa, which is essentially inert). This sensory apparatus permits discrimination of solid, liquid, or gas.

Mechanism of Continence

In a normal person, the gastrocolic reflex and normal colonic propulsion gradually deliver stool to the sigmoid. As pressure increases, it overcomes the resistance in the rectum, which then fills. Receptors in the rectal wall and puborectalis generate signals that lead to the conscious perception of the urge to defecate and to reflex relaxation of the internal sphincter. This permits temporary passage of stool into the anal canal where it contacts the highly sensitive anal mucosa. At the same time, reflex contraction of the external sphincters and the puborectalis empty the rectum retrograde. The colon then accommodates to a larger volume, stretch receptors are no longer activated, and the sensation of the need to defecate disappears.

Normal Defecation

In normal defecation, voluntary response to the sensation of rectal filling results in contraction of the abdominal muscles, closure of the glottis, and descent of the diaphragm, together with voluntary relaxation of the pelvic muscles, puborectalis, and external sphincter. The internal sphincter relaxes reflexly in response to rectal distention. After expulsion of stool, sphincteric contraction empties the anorectum, and the contraction of the puborectalis and the levator ani muscles obliterates the rectal lumen and reestablishes the acute angle.

Constipation

The term "constipation" is best used to describe the situation in which stools are passed infrequently. This is related to difficulty in defecation and to particularly hard stools—often spoken of as "constipation." The three conditions are interrelated, for infrequent defecation results in large, hard stools that are difficult to pass. There is considerable variation among normal individuals in frequency of evacuations, but 99% of adults and children have three or more bowel movements a week, the majority, one or two a day.

Etiology

Constipation may result from anatomic or physiologic abnormalities of the anorectum or colon, or be due to systemic causes such as metabolic derangements, drugs, or feeding problems.

Anatomic Abnormalities

These are neurogenic or mechanical. Neurogenic abnormalities that cause constipation may be extrinsic (such as *myelomen-*

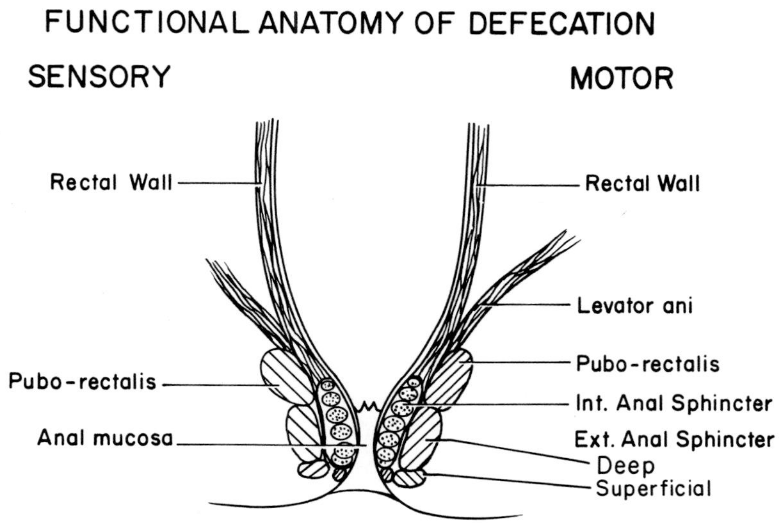

FUNCTIONAL ANATOMY OF DEFECATION

SENSORY   MOTOR

Fig 109–1.—Main anatomical mechanisms responsible for fecal continence.

ingocele, in which there is deficient innervation of the sphincters and other pelvic muscles), or intrinsic (such as *Hirschsprung's disease,* in which the ganglion cells of the myenteric plexuses are absent).

Mechanical causes of obstruction are more common than neurogenic abnormalities. *Anal stenosis* and forms of *imperforate anus* with a perineal or vulvar fistula are usually apparent on physical examination. *Anterior ectopic anus* is obvious on inspection if the anal opening is close to the vulva or scrotum, but some patients appear externally normal.[18]

The majority of constipated children have no recognizable anatomic abnormality. Far more common are constitutional or psychogenic causes of constipation.

Constitutional Constipation

Many children appear to have a congenital predisposition to infrequent bowel movements: "functional" or "constitutional" constipation or "sluggish bowels." Recent studies have shown that many of these patients have physiologic abnormalities. Anorectal manometric studies have demonstrated increased resting pressures in the anorectum and increased anal sphincter tone in some.[2, 8, 20] Others have significantly delayed colon transit ("colon inertia").[2, 18] As infants, some have great difficulty moving their bowels, while others have only one bowel movement a day but are otherwise free of symptoms. They do not come to medical attention until later when stool frequency decreases further, and hard stools develop. Frequently, a parent is similarly afflicted.

Psychogenic Constipation

The largest group of children with significant constipation have fecal retention as a result of emotional factors. Stool patterns may be normal until the beginning of toilet training, the arrival of a new sibling, or another stressful event. These patients may also have physiologic abnormalities.

Metabolic Abnormalities

Metabolic abnormalities include hypothyroidism, hyperparathyroidism, hypercalcemia, cystic fibrosis, and lead poisoning. Drugs such as opiates, anticholinergics, and phenothiazines sometimes cause constipation. Prolonged breast feeding may be associated with infrequent and small stools. Infants may have infrequent stools if they are underfed, have insufficient fluid or sugar in the diet, or have inadequate intake because of vomiting. Constipation was part of the clinical picture of pyloric stenosis 100 years ago.

Pathophysiology

Regardless of the cause, chronic fecal retention results in decompensation of the defecatory apparatus. Failure to eliminate stool regularly results in its accumulation in the rectum, while the dehydrating action of the colon progressively hardens the retained stool with each passing day. As large amounts accumulate, the puborectalis and the external and internal sphincters stretch and become less effective. The continuing activation of stretch receptors produces sensory decompensation, and the child loses the perception of the urge to defecate. The combination of sensory loss and sphincter decompensation, as well as the increased proximal peristalsis due to the obstructing stool, may result in encopresis. When a bowel movement is finally achieved, the great effort required may cause stretching and tearing of the anus, bleeding, and the formation of an anal fissure. This in turn causes additional pain with defecation, and the child understandably avoids bowel movements, which he knows will be painful. Efforts in suppressing the urge to defecate, such as stiffening or crossing the legs, or dancing about on the toes, are sometimes misinterpreted as efforts to have a bowel movement. The involuntary escape of a small amount of stool and the resultant soiling are frequently the major complaint, but such encopresis is in part merely overflow incontinence.

Diagnosis

The patient's age is a critical factor in determining the cause of constipation. Neonates are more likely to have an anatomical abnormality, whereas older children who develop constipation rarely have it for mechanical reasons.

The Neonate

Several readily identifiable patterns of abnormal defecation may be recognized in the neonate: intestinal obstruction, straining, "sluggish" bowels, and hard stools.

Intestinal obstruction is the characteristic mode of presentation of Hirschsprung's disease, which approximately 50% of the time is symptomatic in the neonatal period. The diagnosis can be established or eliminated by rectal biopsy.

Straining, sometimes with complete inability to move the bowels even when the stools are soft, usually results from an obstructive lesion—anal stenosis or anterior ectopic anus—or from increased anal tone. These babies may be in great discomfort and seem to be constantly trying to move their bowels. Anal stenosis is obvious on digital examination if the anus will not accept the examiner's little finger. Anterior ectopic anus may be obvious on inspection or on digital examination that reveals a posterior cul-de-sac. Increased sphincter tone may be difficult to detect on digital examination.

A *sluggish bowel*, or "constitutional" constipation, frequently appears early in life. Bowel movements are normal or firm, but the infant defecates only once a day or less. The cause is probably colonic inertia, with prolonged transit time. There is often a family history of similar complaints.

Hard stools result from decreased frequency of defecation from any cause, iron supplements, or inadequate water in the formula.

The Older Child

If symptoms began in early infancy, an anatomical or functional abnormality must be suspected. Physical examination usually identifies an anorectal malformation or neurologic abnormality. *Hirschsprung's disease* should be considered (and punch rectal biopsy obtained) if there is no evidence of anal obstruction, the rectal ampulla is empty, and there is no straining or fecal soiling. Barium enema and sigmoidoscopy are usually of little help in evaluating constipation and should not be routinely performed. Short-segment Hirschsprung's disease may suggest "constitutional" constipation, and rectal biopsy should be performed if there is inadequate response to therapy.[8]

Children who develop difficulty moving their bowels after having previously established a normal pattern almost always have *psychogenic constipation*. The diagnosis is suggested by establishing a temporal connection between a significant psychic event and the onset of constipation. Classically, this type of constipation begins with toilet training, the birth of a sibling, or other significant disruption in the family. Excessive parental concern over defecation, or punitive or artificial attempts to enforce a regular bowel pattern, results in willful or subconscious suppression of defecation by the child and progressive fecal retention.

Treatment

Correction of an underlying anatomic or metabolic abnormality usually eliminates the constipation. Anal stenosis responds to dilation, which can be done by the parent, twice daily for the first month, then daily until the anus is of adequate size. These patients rarely need operative treatment. Anterior ectopic anus requires posterior sphincterotomy and anoplasty[18] (Fig 109–2). Operation is not indicated if symptoms are relieved by stool softeners. Newborns and infants who have no anatomic abnormality usually respond to stool softening. Dark Karo syrup, ¼ to ½ tsp, two to three times daily in the formula is frequently sufficient. Maltsupex or milk of magnesia may also be used. Patients with neurogenic disorders may require a regular schedule of rectal emptying with suppositories or enemas. Adjustment of stool consistency by dietary manipulation or small doses of milk of magnesia may be necessary to prevent the extremes of incontinence or retention.

Patients with mild "constitutional" constipation respond to stool softening with twice-daily milk of magnesia, Metamucil, or bran. If there is colon inertia or persistent increased anal sphinc-

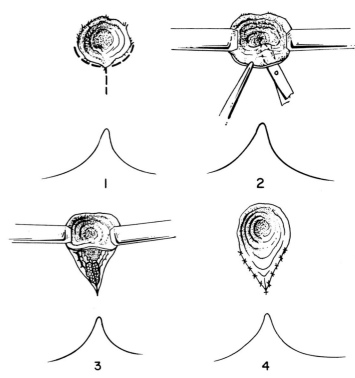

Fig 109–2.—Posterior sphincterotomy for anterior ectopic anus or anal hypertonia. *1*, incision. *2*, elevation of mucosal flap. *3*, incision through skin and all sphincter fibers in midline posteriorly. *4*, advancement of mucosal flap with two-layer closure. (From Leape.[18])

ter tone and the patient cannot be weaned from laxatives, sphincterotomy or myectomy should be considered.[19, 29]

Chronic Fecal Retention

The treatment of chronic fecal retention is more complicated. Whether psychogenic or "constitutional," it results in physical decompensation that is not easily reversed. By the time the child is seen by the surgeon, any potential benefit that withholding of stool may have had in the psychological struggle with the parent has been lost, and the child and parent are usually both anxious to get things under control. If the child is motivated, successful treatment is relatively easy. If not, it is difficult to establish a normal defecatory pattern.

Successful treatment of chronic fecal retention must address the problems of decompensation and discomfort. The program must enable the bowel to recover its sensory and motor function. It must also enable the child to have a painless bowel movement, so that he can relax and actively participate in the development of a normal bowel pattern. The physician's role is to help the parent and child understand the problem, provide a program for its successful correction, and give emotional support. This cannot be accomplished in a 15-minute office visit, which may partly account for the high failure rate of the usual treatment of constipation.

An essential ingredient in enlisting the cooperation of parent and child is that they understand what is wrong. This requires a description of normal colon physiology and an explanation of the abnormality in constipation. The child is unable to move his bowels because the rectal muscles are stretched; he is unable to tell when he has to go because his nerves are fatigued; and he loses control because his sphincters are decompensated.

The treatment is explained in this context: that it will permit the rectal nerves and muscles to recover, after which the child will be able to have normal bowel movements voluntarily. Although some have recommended psychotherapy, it is far more time-consuming and expensive than simple physical measures and should be reserved for the occasional child with a serious behavioral disorder that precludes cooperation in the treatment program.

There are three essential features in treatment: evacuation of retained feces, effective stool softening, and the development of a normal defecatory pattern.

EVACUATION.—The colon must be emptied of retained fecal material. If there is an impaction, manual extraction may be needed (rarely requiring a general anesthetic). Several large-volume (1–2 qt) soapsuds enemas are usually necessary. In the younger child, saline should be used. In refractory cases, a milk and molasses enema (4 oz molasses in 1 qt milk) is almost always effective.

EFFECTIVE STOOL SOFTENING.—Prevention of dehydration and stool hardening is essential for obtaining painless movements. Although many agents are available for this purpose, none is as effective, as safe, or as inexpensive as milk of magnesia. Its primary action is to increase water in the stool, and it has only a very mild stimulatory effect. The dose must be titrated to produce stool that is the consistency of cooked oatmeal. Milk of magnesia must be given *twice* daily for uniform effect. A starting dose for a 4-year-old child is 1 tablespoon, twice daily. This dosage may be doubled or halved every 2 or 3 days until proper stool consistency is obtained, after which it does not usually need to be changed. The only purpose of the milk of magnesia is to keep the stools soft, and the parent must understand that the dose should *not* be decreased or increased according to the *frequency* of bowel movements.

PATTERNING.—Developing the habit of normal daily defecation may take several months. This is best accomplished by choosing a consistent time of day when defecation will be voluntarily attempted. After the evening meal is most convenient, since usually parent and child are both at home, and the timing also takes advantage of the gastrocolic reflex. If the child is unable to have a bowel movement within 5 or 10 minutes, a large-volume soapsuds enema is given to empty the rectum. Both parent and child must understand that the only purpose of the enema is to ensure regular daily emptying of the rectum so that the muscles and nerves can regain control. Enemas must be viewed as an aid in defecation, not punishment. It is necessary that the rectum be emptied either by an adequate bowel movement or an enema *every day* without fail until the problem is resolved. Although in most cases enemas are seldom needed after the first week or two, the program must be continued for at least 6 months to establish a normal pattern. The dose of milk of magnesia is then gradually reduced until it is eliminated.

Successful treatment of fecal retention requires that the physician be an active partner in helping the child solve his problem. Although it is emphasized that only the child can move his bowels, it is equally important that he feel the doctor and his parents are allies in helping him work out his problem. Monthly follow-up visits are necessary to reinforce these messages and to ensure that the program is being properly followed. In the vast majority of cases, response is rapid and dramatic, but the program must be followed for months if the new pattern is to be established.[24a]

In an occasional patient, particularly one with constitutional constipation, long-term use of small doses of milk of magnesia or other softening agents may be necessary to assure regular bowel movements. In patients who cannot be weaned from laxatives, there has been some success with anorectal myectomy or sphincterotomy.[18, 29]

Fecal Incontinence

Probably no aberration of bodily function is as socially unacceptable as the inability to control one's stools. The term *encopresis* is traditionally used for fecal incontinence that results from either chronic fecal retention or from a behavioral disorder, although, strictly defined, the term implies incontinence of psychic origin only.

Etiology

Myelomeningocele is the most common congenital abnormality resulting in fecal incontinence. Other disorders of the spinal cord such as *diastematomyelia* and *lipomeningocele* may also be responsible. Patients with high (supralevator) *imperforate anus* frequently have associated imperfect development of the pelvic nerves and hypoplasia of the sphincters, which result in incontinence even when a technically perfect repair has been carried out.

The most frequent form of *acquired* fecal incontinence is that associated with *chronic fecal retention* due to psychogenic or constitutional constipation. Encopresis in the absence of constipation or an anatomic abnormality of the anorectum is a sign of a severe *behavioral disorder*.

Fecal incontinence may occur as a postoperative complication following repair of high *imperforate anus* if the rectum is not properly placed through the puborectalis sling and the external sphincters. Damage to the muscles or nerves during the repair of high or low imperforate anus may also result in incontinence. Rarely, fecal incontinence is seen in *pull-through operations* for Hirschsprung's disease, ulcerative colitis, or polyposis, especially if the postoperative course has been complicated by perirectal sepsis.

In adults, fecal incontinence has been reported after virtually every type of anorectal procedure, including hemorrhoidectomy, fistulectomy, repair of prolapse, and excision of tumors. Trauma to the spinal cord or to the anorectum may cause incontinence. Various diseases, but rarely in pediatric practice, may also cause fecal incontinence: multiple sclerosis, scleroderma, radiation proctitis, Crohn's disease, and diabetes.

Diagnosis and Assessment

A complete history and physical examination usually reveal the nature of the abnormality causing fecal incontinence. In a child who has not been operated on, a history of normal bowel movements eliminates congenital abnormalities as a cause. Incontinence that is sporadic or associated with bizarre behavior, such as hiding of soiled underpants, is usually psychogenic in origin. A neurologic abnormality is readily identified by the presence of a lax anus, decreased perianal sensation, absent pucker to pinprick, prolapse of the rectum, urinary incontinence, or associated paraparesis. Especially in postoperative pull-through patients, digital rectal evaluation of the sphincters and of the position and tone of the puborectalis muscle is essential.

X-ray films of the lumbosacral spine reveal bony abnormalities (such as absence or incomplete development of the sacrum or occult spina bifida) that may be associated with neurologic impairment. Anorectal manometry[21] is the most helpful study, permitting assessment of sphincteric function, rectal sensation, and anorectal sphincteric reflexes. Electromyographic studies[31] are sometimes indicated to evaluate the sphincters. Defecography[15] provides specific information as to puborectalis function and rectal emptying.

Treatment

There are three primary methods of treatment of fecal incontinence: dietary and medicinal control of stool consistency, operant conditioning ("biofeedback"),[7, 23, 32] and sphincter reinforcing ("sling") operations.[5, 13, 17, 24, 25,]

Neurogenic incontinence associated with myelomeningocele or other major spinal abnormality or with high imperforate anus is usually controllable by dietary alteration of stool consistency and a pattern of regular rectal emptying, either by abdominal pressure or the use of suppositories or enemas. Anorectal manometry should always be carried out in these patients to determine if there is rectal filling sensation and reflex relaxation of the internal sphincter. If these are present, biofeedback conditioning may enable the patient to develop voluntary control.[32] Rare successes have been reported with muscle transplant procedures in those fortunate patients whose lower limbs are spared neurologic impairment.[24]

Incontinence secondary to *chronic fecal retention* disappears with its treatment (see Constipation, pp. 1038–1039). In children with *behavioral incontinence*, the use of biofeedback is quicker and has a higher success rate than psychotherapy, although the latter may also be indicated. Olness reported success with biofeedback in 38 of 40 patients with "functional" incontinence.[23]

Some degree of incontinence is found in almost all patients following repair of *high imperforate anus*. If the sacrum is intact and the sphincters and puborectalis muscles appear to be functioning properly, control will usually be spontaneously achieved by the time the patient is 5 or 6 years of age. Biofeedback may accelerate this process. Improper positioning of the pulled-through rectum outside the puborectalis or external sphincters must be corrected surgically. If incontinence persists after such correction, or muscle tone is weak, but sensory perception is intact, a trial of biofeedback is worthwhile. If that fails, muscle transplant might be considered. The modified gracilis sling, in which one or both gracilis muscles are wrapped around the external anal sphincters, has been successful in most reported cases.[5, 24, 25] An alternative is the free muscle transplant of Hakelius.[13]

Artificial sphincters and electrical stimulation have been effective experimentally in the control of fecal incontinence. At present, it is unclear what role either will have in the treatment of fecal incontinence.

Rectal Prolapse

Prolapse of the rectum is herniation of the rectum through the anus. This herniation may be merely mucosal, or involve all layers of the rectum, so-called complete prolapse, or procidentia. Mucosal prolapse is common after operations for imperforate anus, while spontaneous prolapse of the rectum in a child is almost invariably full-thickness or complete. The studies of Fowler[11] have confirmed this observation by demonstrating that radiopaque markers injected through the apex of the prolapse will appear in the peritoneal cavity. Characteristically, mucosal prolapse produces radial folds at the junction with the anal skin, whereas full-thickness prolapse is characterized by circular folds in the prolapsed mucosa. Prolapse of an inch or more is almost invariably of the full thickness of the rectal wall (Fig 109–3).

Etiology and Pathophysiology

In the vast majority of children with rectal prolapse, the etiology is unknown. Debilitating disease and malnutrition, the usual predisposing factors in adults, are not found in most children who present with protrusion of the rectum. Conditions in which there is an abnormality of the innervation of the support muscles

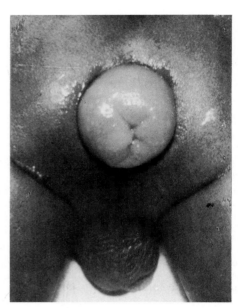

Fig 109–3.—Rectal prolapse in a 2-year-old boy. The smooth, glistening, edematous appearance is common in children.

of the perineum, particularly the levator ani muscle complex, the puborectalis, and the anal sphincters, do predispose to prolapse. *Myelomeningocele* or any condition leading to sacral nerve impairment may be responsible. *Exstrophy* of the bladder may be associated with defects in the pelvic support mechanism and lead to prolapse. A number of patients with cystic fibrosis develop rectal prolapse for reasons that are unclear; it is not necessarily associated with bulky stools or difficult defecation and can occur in patients who are otherwise well-controlled with pancreatic enzyme supplements.

Most children with "idiopathic" rectal prolapse are preschoolers, with a peak incidence in the second year of life. This age predilection has led to speculation that prolapse results from a combination of developmental events that take place at this time: assumption of erect posture, decrease in body fat, and institution of voluntary control over defecation. If the child is required to spend long periods of time on the toilet while learning to move his bowels, the straining may stretch the support mechanisms and result in prolapse.

Any condition that results in straining at stool is probably of etiologic significance. Rectal polyps or worms may be causes of straining that result in prolapse.

Clinical Features

The appearance of part of a child's "insides" protruding through the anus is a frightening experience for a mother. Prolapse usually occurs during or after defecation, and in most cases reduces spontaneously. The physician may have to rely on the mother's description to make the diagnosis. In simple prolapse, normal healthy pink mucosa protrudes a centimeter or more through the anus. If spontaneous reduction does not occur, the bowel becomes edematous and engorged, and begins to bleed.

In patients in whom initial prolapse is extensive or recurs immediately after reduction, the (rare) possibility of intussusception must be considered. In prolapse, it is not possible to insert the finger in the sulcus between the prolapsed bowel and the anus, whereas, with intussusception, the finger can be inserted into the rectum between the intussusceptum and the anal opening.

In some patients, prolapse may occur at relatively infrequent intervals (weeks or months). In others, it occurs with every bowel movement. Particularly in babies, prolapse may occur between bowel movements and in association with crying or straining. If the underlying cause of straining is eliminated, episodes of prolapse tend to diminish in frequency and disappear spontaneously.

Management

An acute prolapse is usually reduced easily if reduction is undertaken promptly before there is edema formation. The herniated bowel is grasped with the tips of the fingers of the gloved hand applied circumferentially and pushed in. If there is edema, firm, steady pressure of the fingertips for several minutes may be necessary to reduce the swelling and permit reduction of the prolapse. Digital rectal examination should follow to ensure that reduction has been complete. If prolapse recurs immediately, the buttocks may be strapped together with a single band of adhesive tape for several hours.

The parent should be taught how to reduce the prolapse and encouraged to do it promptly whenever it recurs. Plastic sandwich bags are an inexpensive, familiar, readily available substitute for surgical gloves. A lubricant is not necessary.

Conditions predisposing to straining, most commonly constipation or diarrhea, should be corrected, and their correction usually leads to disappearance of the problem. All patients with prolapse should have a sweat test to rule out cystic fibrosis, which may be otherwise totally unsuspected and asymptomatic. Neurologic abnormalities causing prolapse are usually obvious on physical examination. Patients with recurring prolapse without apparent cause should undergo barium enema examination and sigmoidoscopy to rule out polyps or other rectal lesions. These are rare.

Management of Recurrent Prolapse

Injection Treatments

Simple, inexpensive, and highly effective, this is the treatment of choice. We use a modification of the technique described by Wyllie[33] (Fig 109–4). The operation can be performed on an outpatient basis, although general anesthesia is required. Immediately preoperatively, the rectum is emptied with a suppository (not an enema). With the patient in the lithotomy position, linear injections of 5% phenol in glycerine or peanut oil are made in the rectal submucosa at four different sites. A no. 19 spinal (8-cm) needle attached to an injection syringe is inserted through the skin just outside the mucocutaneous junction and guided to the proper position by a finger in the rectum. Two to three milliliters of solution are injected in a linear track as the needle is slowly withdrawn. The injection is repeated in four quadrants. The patient may be discharged on recovery from anesthesia. The procedure is painless and immediately effective. Complications such as bleeding or infection are rare. None have been seen by the author, nor in Wyllie's series of 100 patients.[33]

Prolapse is cured in approximately 90% of patients by a single treatment, and in almost all of the others by a second injection. Wyllie reported no failures, although there were no patients with myelomeningocele or other neurologic disorders in his series. Since this form of treatment is the simplest, safest, cheapest, and has the highest success rate, it is difficult to understand why other forms of therapy have been recommended. Use of other sclerosing solutions, such as 30% saline,[16] deposition of the sclerosing solution outside the rectum, and transmucosal injection have been associated with a higher failure rate and increased incidence of complications.

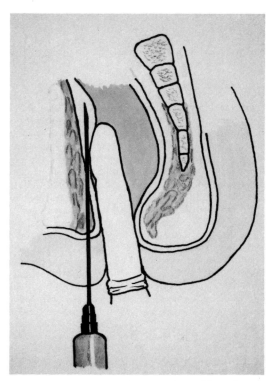

Fig 109–4.—Injection treatment of rectal prolapse. Finger in rectum guides needle. (From Wyllie.[33])

Linear Electrocauterization

This technique produces a perirectal inflammatory response with electrocautery rather than injection of sclerosing solutions. The reported success rate is similar to that achieved by injections (7% recurrence), but the procedure required a 4–5-day hospital stay for preparation and postoperative care, and was associated with a 10% incidence of complications, including rectal bleeding and narrowing of the anorectal canal, requiring subsequent dilatation.[14]

Operations for Rectal Prolapse

In 1965, Altemeier noted that more than 50 different operative procedures had been described for rectal prolapse in adults.[1] Since that time, still other techniques have been described. If two or three injection treatments are unsuccessful and operative treatment is required, probably the Ripstein procedure is most likely to be successful.[26] Through a transabdominal approach, the rectum is fixed to the hollow of the sacrum by a prosthetic or fascia lata graft sutured to the bowel and the presacral fascia, creating a new pelvic "floor" and securing the rectum to the hollow of the sacrum. Other operations that have been recommended include rectal suspension and levator repair through a posterior sagittal approach,[3] the Lockhart-Mummery procedure,[22] and radical perineal excision.[1] The diversity of approach reflects the lack of satisfaction with any single surgical technique in the treatment of prolapse of the rectum. Fortunately, operation is rarely required.

Anorectal Trauma

Unlike adults—in whom gunshot wounds, motor vehicle accidents, and foreign bodies account for the majority of injuries to the anorectum—in children, sexual abuse is the most common cause of anorectal trauma.[4] Iatrogenic causes are second, including broken thermometers, enemas, barium enema examination, and anorectal dilatations. Rectal trauma from motor vehicle accidents and gunshot wounds is much less frequent. Impalement or straddle injuries are occasionally seen, as are foreign bodies.

Pathophysiology

Often, anorectal trauma is superficial. If the injury is not full-thickness, it is not more serious than a biopsy and will heal without further treatment. Penetrating injuries are most usefully classified according to location above or below the levator ani muscle complex. Distal injuries are unlikely to result in perianal sepsis. Penetrating injuries above the levator ani muscle may result in an ischiorectal abscess with extension into the retroperitoneal space. Penetrating injuries above the peritoneal reflection result in peritonitis. Impalement injuries in infants (as from enema, anal dilator, or sigmoidoscope) are more likely to be intraperitoneal because of the short length of the rectum. Vehicular accident victims and those with gunshot wounds of the rectum should always be suspected of having an intraperitoneal injury. Bacteriologically, a broad mixture of both aerobic and anaerobic organisms has been found in rectal injuries, including *Escherichia coli, Enterococcus, Bacteroides, Klebsiella,* and *Pseudomonas,* as well as *Proteus, Staphylococcus,* and *Streptococcus.*[27]

Because the rectum is relatively insensitive, in the absence of external anal injury, serious rectal trauma may be asymptomatic until peritonitis or an ischiorectal abscess develops.

Diagnosis

The child who is brought for medical care because of a rectal complaint or bleeding with a vague history and the presence of perineal or other body bruises should be suspected of being a victim of sexual assault. The presence of condylomata acuminata in the perianal area is strong evidence of sexual abuse.[20] If the child has multiple injuries, as from a motor vehicle accident, attention must be given to the basic principles of trauma management first: establishment of an airway, control of hemorrhage, assessment of head injury and spinal fractures, etc. In the absence of penetrating injuries of the pelvis or the perineum, rectal trauma is unusual. The presence of fresh blood on rectal examination demands a full evaluation. Similarly, a gunshot wound in the pelvis, perineum, or upper thigh also requires careful evaluation to exclude rectal injury.

After establishing the time and cause of injury, a thorough examination of the perineum, buttocks, anus, and rectum should be performed, as well as assessment of anal sensation and sphincter tone. Any patient in whom rectal injuries are suspected should have a sigmoidoscopic examination. Stools should be removed with suction and gentle saline irrigation, but the usual distention with air should be avoided, if at all possible, to avoid potential peritoneal contamination. Upright abdominal x-ray examination may reveal free air. If sigmoidoscopy is negative and rectal injury is still suspected, water-soluble contrast examination of the rectum may be helpful. Contrast study of the urinary tract may also be indicated.

Treatment

Treatment depends on location of the injury, its depth, and its age and follows the principles established for adults.

Foreign Bodies

In children, foreign bodies in the rectum are usually swallowed ones that have passed uneventfully through the intestinal tract. Fishbones and straight pins are particularly likely to become lodged in the rectal wall. Considerable ingenuity may be required for their removal, but in most cases the trauma is superficial and no further treatment is necessary.

Miscellaneous Anal Disorders

Anal Fissure

Superficial, acute tears in the anal mucosa and skin are common in infancy and are a common cause of anorectal bleeding at any age. In most children, anal fissures result from constipation, the large, hard stool causing superficial tearing during bowel movements. Because of the sensitivity of the anal epithelium, subsequent acts of defecation are exquisitely painful, leading to holding of stools, making them harder still, and increasing the pain even more when defecation does occur. In occasional patients, there is no history of hard stools, and the etiology of the fissures is obscure.

Chronic anal fissure may result from nonhealing of an acute fissure, or from a superinfection that converts it to a chronic ulceration. Chronic fissure may also be the first symptom of Crohn's disease, appearing long before the intestinal manifestation. Anal fissures are common in patients undergoing chemotherapy for leukemia. Chronic fissures are usually painful, but bleeding is less common than with acute fissures.

The diagnosis of a fissure is easily made by inspecting the anus. The skin must be drawn away from the anus, facilitated by the patient's bearing down during the examination, so that the pectinate line is exposed. Fissures are not readily seen with the proctoscope or the sigmoidoscope. The acute fissure appears as a longitudinal "split," typically posteriorly. Chronic fissures are typically associated with hypertrophy of the proximal anal papilla and may include a "sentinel" skin tag distally as well. Granulation tissue may be present, or, if there is indolent infection, there will be a shaggy base to the ulcer.

Treatment

Stool softening is the most important treatment for an acute fissure. In the infant, the simple addition of Karo syrup to the formula may be all that is necessary. In the older child, milk of magnesia is most effective. Warm sitz baths help relax the sphincter and may provide some relief. In severe cases, application of an analgesic ointment is appropriate. Acute fissures usually heal within a week or two and do not recur if stool consistency is controlled. The treatment of a chronic fissure is excision to eliminate the granulation tissue and scar. Sphincterotomy or dilatation is performed at the same time. Excision is not recommended for chronic fissures or ulcerations in patients with leukemia, whose wounds do not heal well.

Anorectal Infection

Perianal abscess is most common in infants. A superficial abscess or furuncle in the perianal skin results from an infected diaper rash. The causative organism may be *Staphylococcus* or enteric bacterium.[10] Infection in the anal canal or perirectal region is more likely to result from a crypt abscess that burrows into the intersphincteric plane, to present subcutaneously at the anus or in the ischiorectal fossa. These abscesses are due to enteric organisms, especially anaerobes, and may result from minor anomalies at the mucocutaneous junction.[6] There is no clear association with abnormalities of defecation or stool consistency. In the older child, the development of a perianal abscess may be an indication of inflammatory bowel disease, chronic granulomatous disease, immunodeficiency state, or leukemia.

The diagnosis of perianal abscess is usually apparent on examination (Fig 109–5). Intersphincteric or perirectal extension may be detected by rectal examination. An ischiorectal abscess may initially be detectable only by rectal palpation. External swelling, edema, and erythema are inconspicuous at first, but induration can be palpated early.

Perianal or ischiorectal abscesses should be incised and drained on diagnosis. Fluctuation is not to be waited for. General anesthesia may be required in some individuals with large abscesses. Antibiotics are seldom necessary.[10] In most cases, adequate drainage is followed by prompt healing, but recurrence is not unusual. Approximately 25% of patients will subsequently develop a fistula in ano.

Fistula In Ano

Fistula in ano results from extension of a perianal abscess to the skin and to the inside of the anal canal (Fig 109–6). It almost invariably follows a perianal abscess and should be suspected as the cause of a recurrent perianal infection. The fistulous communication may extend between the inner and external sphincters or be trans-sphincteric, exiting lateral to the external sphincter. They are most common in infancy and, for reasons that are unknown, are more likely to occur in males. In children, unlike adults, the fistulous tract is usually fairly straight, exiting on the skin on the same bearing as the crypt opening. There may be chronic drainage of mucus, with very little pus, but with recurring flare-ups.

Treatment of fistula in ano is fistulotomy: opening the sinus tract throughout its length. This requires general anesthesia and careful, gentle passage of a probe through the fistulous tract, taking care not to make a false passage. Simple opening is all that is required unless there is a great deal of granulation tissue and chronic inflammatory reaction, in which case excision of the tract results in quicker healing. Sitz baths, good anal hygiene, and maintenance of soft stools are all that are required for healing in most cases.

Condyloma Acuminatum

Condyloma acuminatum has been reported in children in increasing numbers in the past decade. It is caused by the papil-

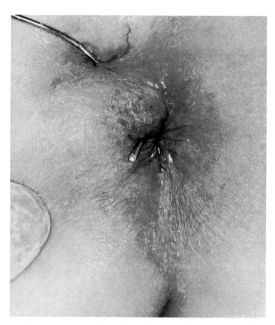

Fig 109–6.—Fistula in ano in 18-month-old boy that developed after incision and drainage of a perianal abscess. A probe connects the external and internal openings of the fistula. Operation consists in cutting down on the probe, opening the entire tract.

lomavirus, closely related to laryngeal papilloma and to the common skin wart viruses. The condylomata have a predilection for moist skin areas, particularly the perianal region (Fig 109–7). In most cases, condyloma acuminatum in a child results from sexual abuse,[20] although transmission from infected mothers during delivery has been reported.[9] The local child protection agency should be contacted to evaluate the possibility of sexual abuse.

Treatment of condyloma acuminatum with podophyllum resin is effective. For children, it should be diluted to 10–15% to avoid excessive skin reaction. Surgical excision or cauterization is also effective and preferable if there are a large number of lesions. Autoimmunization with autogenous vaccine made from ground-up papillomas has been recommended.

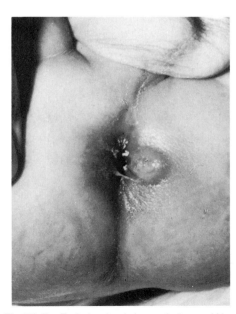

Fig 109–5.—Typical perianal abscess in 1-year-old boy.

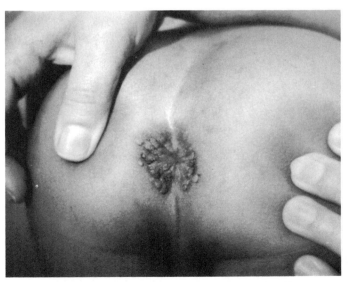

Fig 109–7.—Condylomata acuminata. (From De Jong.[9])

Hemorrhoids

Internal hemorrhoids are seldom seen in children, except in patients with severe portal hypertension. Thrombosis of external hemorrhoids may occur, particularly in teenagers, and require incision and evacuation of the painful clot. In most cases, the diagnosis is inaccurate and the patient actually has mucosal prolapse, a polyp, or a local anal infection.

REFERENCES

1. Altemeier W.A., Culbertson W.R.: Technique for perineal repair of rectal prolapse. *Surgery* 58:758, 1965.
2. Arhan P., Devroede G., Jehannin B., et al.: Idiopathic disorders of fecal continence in children. *Pediatrics* 71:774, 1983.
3. Ashcraft K.W., Amoury R.A., Holder T.M.: Levator repair and posterior suspension for rectal prolapse. *J. Pediatr. Surg.* 12:241, 1977.
4. Black C.T., Pokorny W.J., McGill C.W., et al.: Anorectal trauma in children. *J. Pediatr. Surg.* 17:501, 1982.
5. Brandesky G., Holschneider A.M.: Operations for the improvement of fecal incontinence. *Prog. Pediatr. Surg.* 9:105, 1976.
6. Brook I., Martin W.J.: Aerobic and anaerobic bacteriology of perirectal abscess in children. *Pediatrics* 66:282, 1980.
7. Cerulli M.A., Nikoomanesh P., Schuster M.M.: Progress in biofeedback conditioning for fecal incontinence. *Gastroenterology* 76:742, 1979.
8. Clayden G.S., Lawson J.O.N.: Investigation and management of long-standing chronic constipation in childhood. *Arch. Dis. Child.* 51:918, 1976.
9. De Jong A.R., Weiss J.C., Brent R.L.: Condyloma acuminata in children. *Am. J. Dis. Child.* 136:704, 1982.
10. Enberg R.N., Cox R.H., Burry V.F.: Perirectal abscess in children. *Am. J. Dis. Child.* 128:360, 1974.
11. Fowler R.: The anatomy and treatment of rectal prolapse in childhood. *Aust. Paediatr. J.* 3:90, 1967.
12. Grasberger R.C., Hirsch E.F.: Rectal trauma. *Am. J. Surg.* 145:795, 1983.
13. Hakelius L., Gierup J., Grotte G., et al.: A new treatment of anal incontinence in children: Free autogenous muscle transplantation. *J. Pediatr. Surg.* 13:77, 1978.
14. Hight D.W., Hertzler J.H., Philippart A.I., et al.: Linear cauterization for the treatment of rectal prolapse in infants and children. *Surg. Gynecol. Obstet.* 154:400, 1982.
15. Holschneider A.M.: The problem of anorectal continence. *Prog. Pediatr. Surg.* 9:85, 1976

16. Kay N.R.M., Zachary R.B.: The treatment of rectal prolapse in children with injections of 30 percent saline solution. *J. Pediatr. Surg.* 5:334, 1970.
17. Kottmeier P.K.: A physiological approach to the problem of anal incontinence through use of the levator ani as a sling. *J. Pediatr. Surg.* 60:1262, 1966.
18. Leape L.L., Ramenofsky M.L.: Anterior ectopic anus: A common cause of constipation in children. *J. Pediatr. Surg.* 13:627, 1978.
19. Martelli H., Devroede G., Arhan P., et al.: Mechanisms of idiopathic constipation: Outlet obstruction. *Gastroenterology* 75:623, 1978.
20. McCoy C.R., Applebaum H., Besser A.S.: Condyloma acuminata: An unusual presentation of child abuse. *J. Pediatr. Surg.* 17:505, 1982.
21. Meunier P., Marechal J.M., DeBeaujeu M.J.: Rectoanal pressures and rectal sensitivity studies in chronic childhood constipation. *Gastroenterology* 77:330, 1979.
22. Nwako F.: Rectal prolapse in Nigerian children. *Int. Surg.* 60:284, 1975.
23. Olness K., McParland F.A., Piper J.: Biofeedback: A new modality in the management of children with fecal soiling. *J. Pediatr.* 96:505, 1980.
24. Pickrell K., Georgiade N., Richard E.R., et al.: Gracilis muscle transplant for correction of neurogenic incontinence. *Surg. Clin. North Am.* 39:1405, 1959.
24a. Ravitch M.M.: Pseudo Hirschsprung's disease. *Ann. Surg.* 147:781, 1958.
25. Raffensperger J.: The Gracilis sling for fecal incontinence. *J. Pediatr. Surg.* 14:794, 1979.
26. Ripstein C.B., Lanter B.: Etiology and surgical therapy of massive prolapse of the rectum. *Ann. Surg.* 157:259, 1963.
27. Robertson H.D., Ray J.E., Ferrari B.T., et al.: Management of rectal trauma. *Surg. Gynecol. Obstet.* 154:161, 1982.
28. Schuster M.M.: Progress in gastroenterology, the riddle of the sphincters. *Gastroenterology* 69:249, 1975.
29. Shafik A.: A new concept of the anatomy of the anal sphincter mechanism and the physiology of defecation. *Inves. Urol.* 12:412, 1975.
30. Shandling B., Desjardins J.G.: Anal myomectomy for constipation. *J. Pediatr. Surg.* 4:115, 1969.
31. Ustach T., Hambrecht T., Bass D., et al.: Patterns of anal sphincter response to electrical stimulation in humans. *Gastroenterology* 56:1202, 1969.
32. Wald A.: Use of biofeedback in treatment of fecal incontinence in patients with meningomyelocele. *Pediatrics* 68:45, 1981.
33. Wyllie G.G.: The injection treatment of rectal prolapse. *J. Pediatr. Surg.* 14:62, 1979.

110

JOHN R. LILLY

Biliary Atresia: The Jaundiced Infant

HISTORY.—The first to describe accurately the different forms of biliary atresia and formally designate it as a specific disease entity was Thomson[90] in 1891. In 1916, Holmes[32] published a comprehensive review of all reported cases and found that 16% were theoretically susceptible to operative correction. It was not until 1928, however, that the first successful reconstruction of the correctable form of biliary atresia was reported by Ladd.[45] One of his early patients was reported doing well 37 years later.[61] In 1953, Gross[27] documented that biliary atresia was by far the most common condition responsible for obstructive jaundice in infancy. Only a handful of Gross's patients had patent ducts permitting operative reconstruction. In the majority of the bile ducts at the liver were occluded, and the patients' conditions were considered noncorrectable.

A number of ingenious, if, in retrospect, hopeless or absurd, operations for noncorrectable biliary atresia were attempted in the 1950s and early 1960s. The liver was impaled with metal tubes,[84] incised with valvulotomes,[72] and partially amputated[60] in heroic attempts to achieve drainage of bile. Except occasionally in the inventors' hands, these procedures failed, as did indirect operations that attempted drainage of the liver by lymphatics.[24, 94] The inability to help the great majority of patients operatively gradually led to procrastination in the decision to operate on jaundiced infants. Consequently, even infants with remediable lesions were operated on so late that irreversible liver damage had already occurred. This kind of tragedy led Swenson and Fisher[88] to advocate brief diagnostic laparotomy and operative cholangiography in infants with unexplained jaundice. A contradictory recommendation was made in 1968 by Thaler and Gellis.[89] At that time, most cases of biliary atresia could not be differentiated from neonatal hepatitis. They contended that infants with neonatal hepatitis would be harmed by operation, and, therefore, surgical procedures should be postponed until the patient was 4 months old. The surgeons' case for early operation also was weakened by their own reports describing "spontaneous" cure of biliary atresia.[22, 35, 44, 88] In many of these examples, the surgeon was uncertain of the diagnosis, often because operative cholangiography had not been performed, thus casting considerable doubt on the accuracy of the laparotomy findings. Nonetheless, the rather mystical belief that a totally fibrotic extrahepatic ductal system may subsequently become patent is still held by some.

During the same year that Thaler and Gellis publicly recommended operative delay, Kasai et al.[38] reported operative relief of biliary obstruction in infants traditionally considered to have noncorrectable biliary atresia. An analysis of their results indicated that biliary drainage might be anticipated in many infants having operations before 3 months of age, whereas surgical failure was almost universal in those satisfying the Thaler and Gellis conditions, i.e., operation undertaken after 4 months.

The early American experience with Kasai's operation was mixed, controversial, and, on occasion, emotional. Campbell and colleagues[17] reported outright failure in 12 consecutive patients; death was thought to be hastened by the procedure. Arcari[10] wondered aloud if Kasai's operation should continue to be performed. Gellis,[26] who at first recanted his original position of procrastination, subsequently reversed field and would not recommend the operation. On the other hand, confirmation of Kasai's results, albeit in small numbers, was reported by Bill[14] and by Lilly and Altman.[52] At the height of the controversy, Adelman,[1] in a painstaking follow-up of 89 surgically uncorrected patients with biliary atresia, reported a single survivor, in this an atypical case. The "spontaneous cure" concept was undone; most surgeons began performing hepatic portoenterostomies. Fully 90% of infants born with biliary atresia in the 1980s had Kasai's operation.[53]

Biliary atresia is a condition in which the extrahepatic bile ducts are grossly nonpatent. Its incidence is about 1 in 15,000 live births.[78] There is a slight predominance of the disease in females.[53] Formerly, it was believed the Japanese were more often afflicted, but evidence for this is inconclusive.[78] Traditionally, the disease has been arbitrarily divided into a "correctable" type, in which the proximal extrahepatic bile ducts are patent (and the distal ducts occluded), and a "noncorrectable" type, in which the proximal extrahepatic ducts are occluded.

Pathology

Biliary atresia was long thought to be a congenital malformation—a fault in ductal embryogenesis due to failure of the extrahepatic biliary system to develop patency.[95] The fundamental concept of Kasai's operation directly challenged this hypothesis. If the procedure was successful during the first months of life and failed thereafter, a dynamic disease rather than a static phenomenon was implicated. Support for an ongoing disease is found in histologic analyses of the surgically excised extrahepatic bile ducts. Microscopic biliary structures (which communicate with the intrahepatic biliary tree[19]) are present in the otherwise grossly occluded hepatic duct in most infants under 2 months old. These structures gradually disappear over the next several months, and at 4 months only fibrous tissue remains.[36]

The loss of gross patency of the biliary system appears to be a gradual process, not completed until sometime around birth. Few patients with biliary atresia are born notably jaundiced. Furthermore, we have treated several patients who had minimal jaundice in the newborn period but had the gross findings of biliary atresia recorded during neonatal operations for intestinal atresia. Subsequently, progressive jaundice led to reoperation and confirmation of the diagnosis.[82] Also, gradual biliary occlusion is the most rational explanation for the occasional patient with a bile cyst of the extrahepatic ducts with atresia at both ends.[43]

The sclerotic process in biliary atresia is panductal, afflicting the intrahepatic biliary tree as well as the extrahepatic system. The intrahepatic bile ducts are narrow, distorted in configuration, and irregular in shape.[52, 67] The damage to the intrahepatic biliary system is responsible for much of the morbidity after Kasai's operation. In most patients this component of the disease appears self-limited, but in some it may continue, accounting for late surgical failure.

Etiology

The biliary duct system originates from the hepatic diverticulum of the foregut at 4 weeks of embryonic life and differentiates into a caudal and cranial component. The gallbladder, cystic duct, and common bile duct derive from the caudal component, and the proximal extrahepatic ducts (as well as most of the intrahepatic biliary system) derive from the cranial component. Although considerable variation occurs, the three most common anatomical manifestations of biliary atresia (Fig. 110–1) roughly follow this embryologic pattern. That is, in correctable biliary atresia, the proximal extrahepatic bile ducts (cranial diverticulum) are patent and the distal ducts (caudal diverticulum) oblit-

Supported in part by Grant RR-69 from the General Clinical Research Centers Program, Division of Research Resources, National Institutes of Health.

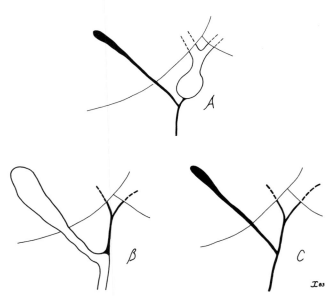

Fig 110–1.—Drawing of the three most common anatomical expressions of biliary atresia. **A,** "correctable" biliary atresia. The proximal bile ducts are patent although hypoplastic. **B,** variant (15%) of "noncorrectable" biliary atresia, in which the gallbladder, cystic duct, and common bile duct are patent but the proximal bile ducts are occluded. **C,** most common type of noncorrectable biliary atresia, in which the entire extrahepatic bile ducts are nonpatent. (Courtesy of Dr. Jack Chang.)

erated. The reverse is seen in about 15% of patients with noncorrectable biliary atresia, i.e., the gallbladder, cystic duct, and common bile duct (caudal diverticulum) are patent and the proximal hepatic duct occluded.[53] In the third and largest category, the entire duct system is diseased (both cranial and caudal hepatic diverticula).

While the hepatic diverticulum is undergoing differentiation, a number of other important events in organogenesis take place. The inferior vena cava and portal vein form, intestinal rotation begins, and the spleen begins to form. That 10–15% of patients with biliary atresia have associated anomalies in these organs (absent inferior vena cava, preduodenal portal vein, intestinal malrotation, and polysplenia)[54] suggests that the developmental insult causing biliary atresia may occur at this time, quite early in embryonic life.

The trigger mechanism, however, is still unknown. Malunion of the pancreatic and biliary systems has been implicated,[63] as has a fetal vascular accident.[25] Recently, a reovirus type 3 infection has been incriminated by Morecki as the pathologic event.[65]

Although a cause-effect relation has not been documented, the circumstantial evidence is impressive.

Diagnostic Evaluation

Jaundice in the first months of life may be on a mechanical, obstructive basis or on a hepatic parenchymal basis from infectious, hematologic, or metabolic disease. Formerly, careful investigations of all hepatocellular causes of jaundice were prerequisite to operative exploration. These included tests for syphilis, toxoplasmosis, listeriosis, hepatitis B, galactosemia, fructosemia, and α_1-antitrypsin deficiency, to list but a few. Percutaneous needle biopsy was also considered necessary.

Aside from the expense, the completion of the aforementioned studies consumed at least a week, and often 2 weeks of potentially invaluable time. For the past 3 years, we have employed the newer technetium 99m iminodiacetic acid (IDA) radiopharmaceuticals as an early diagnostic study in all cases of unexplained jaundice in infants.[69] These agents greatly improve visualization of the hepatobiliary system and allow independent evaluation of hepatocyte clearance, hepatobiliary transit, and excretion. In the patient with biliary atresia, the primary disease process is in the bile ducts. Hepatocyte clearance of the isotope is relatively well maintained (Fig 110–2,A) early in the course of the disease, i.e., the first 3 months. In contrast, in hepatocellular jaundice, the primary target is the hepatocyte and imaging demonstrates a decrease in hepatocyte clearance and a parallel decrease in excretion (Fig 110–2,B).

Thus, radioisotope imaging with IDA agents often permits a rapid and clear distinction between obstructive and nonobstructive jaundice. For nonobstructive jaundice, the full complement of diagnostic studies outlined earlier is initiated. For obstructive jaundice, ultrasonography is undertaken, often confirming the diagnosis by demonstrating enhanced hepatic parenchymal echoes and the tiny or empty gallbladder of biliary atresia. One final diagnostic study must be done before operative cholangiography, α_1-antitrypsin determination. The radioisotope and ultrasonographic findings in the phenotype Pi ZZ may be indistinguishable from those of biliary atresia.[47]

Operative Cholangiography

Diagnostic work-up should be completed by the sixth week of life, and no later than the eighth week, so that operative cholangiography may be done promptly thereafter. A small right subcostal incision is used. In most cases of biliary atresia, the gallbladder is fibrotic, the lumen at least partially occluded, and cholangiography is impossible. If the gallbladder is patent, dilute contrast material is injected under just enough pressure to demonstrate continuity of the biliary tree between liver and duo-

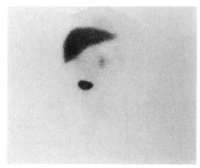

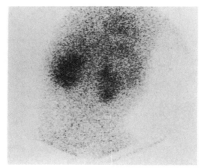

Fig 110–2.—Iminodiacetic acid (IDA) isotope study in a 2-month-old patient with biliary atresia *(left)* and a 3½-month-old infant with neonatal hepatitis *(right)*. Contrast the excellent hepatocyte clearance of the patient with biliary atresia to that of the poor hepatic isotope uptake in the patient with hepatocellular disease. Clinical and serologic studies in the two patients were remarkably similar. (Courtesy of Dr. William Klingensmith.)

denum. Although it has been advocated, it is probably dangerous to clamp the distal common duct and inject the gallbladder again if reflux of contrast material into the intrahepatic radicles is not demonstrated. Instead, if the gallbladder contains bile, it is wiser to desist and close the wound, since biliary hypoplasia (see below) is probably the diagnosis. If the gallbladder contains "white bile" (and biliary continuity cannot be demonstrated), full exploration of the extrahepatic biliary tree should be undertaken.

Correctable Biliary Atresia

The form of biliary atresia correctable by conventional reconstruction has been reported to occur in 12%[34] to 16%[32] of patients. The true incidence is a good deal lower, since many cases of hilar bile cysts (without gross communication to the intrahepatic bile ducts) and choledochal cyst in infants were formerly included in these compilations. In our consecutive series, of almost 100 infants with biliary atresia followed, there were only two examples of a correctable lesion.[82]

Roux-en-Y intestinal anastomosis to the proximal bile duct is the recommended treatment. The limb of the Roux-en-Y should be anastomosed, not to the bulbous end of the hepatic duct, but to normal ductal tissue above it. Excision of the patent duct, often to the liver hilus, may be required.[49] Failure to remove all the diseased portion of the duct results in anastomotic stricture, cholangitis, and eventual cirrhosis.[42]

In the large survey conducted by the Surgical Section of the American Academy of Pediatrics, only half the patients with correctable lesions were alive at the time of the report.[34] The reason for the guarded long-term prognosis is coexisting intrahepatic disease. Although intestinal drainage of the patent duct segment is occasionally curative,[15, 20] most infants with correctable biliary atresia have some degree of residual liver disease.[53]

Noncorrectable Biliary Atresia

The great majority of patients with biliary atresia have grossly nonpatent bile ducts at the liver hilus and were previously considered noncorrectable. About 15% have residual patency of the distal biliary tree, i.e., gallbladder, cystic duct and common bile duct.[53] In either case, bile flow from the liver is impossible.

Hepatic Portoenterostomy

In Kasai's operation, the extrahepatic bile ducts are totally removed and bile drainage established by anastomosis of an intestinal conduit to the transected duct at the liver hilus. Operative success depends on the presence of microscopic biliary structures at the liver hilus and is inversely proportional to the age of the patient.[38] The microscopic biliary structures drain bile into the approximated intestinal conduit, and in time, we believe,[82] an autoanastomosis between the intestinal and ductal epithelial elements occurs (Fig 110–3).

The essential technical maneuvers for constructing a functional bilioenteric anastomosis are depicted in Figure 110–4. Briefly, they are: (1) Precise identification of the extrahepatic duct remnant at the porta hepatis. A semblance of the common hepatic duct almost always can be found at the hilar bifurcation of the portal vein (Fig. 110–5). (2) High (proximal) transection of this biliary structure. The proper level is confirmed by frozen-section examination of the hilar end of the surgical specimen. True "bile ducts" must be seen histologically[70] (Fig 110–6). (3) Meticulous anastomosis of the intestinal conduit to the transected duct at the porta hepatis. We have found a double-layered anastomosis[38] to be of no advantage over a single running layer of absorbable suture.

A number of options are available for reestablishing gastrointestinal tract continuity. Most involve temporary exteriorization of the conduit. Exteriorization of the biliary conduit decreases its intraluminal pressure and, consequently, lessens the pressure gradient the hepatic secretory pressure has to overcome. The likelihood of biliary stasis is decreased, thus lessening the susceptibility to postoperative cholangitis. The exteriorization procedures used most commonly are (1) "double-Y" anastomosis of Kasai,[36] (2) Sawaguchi's[76] total exteriorization of the conduit, and (3) double-barreled exteriorization of the midportion of a Roux-en-Y biliary conduit[52, 86] (Fig 110–7).

The presence of a still patent gallbladder, cystic duct, and distal common duct (see Fig 110–1,B) eliminates the necessity for an intestinal conduit. If the gallbladder, instead of a jejunal Roux loop, is brought up for anastomosis, the risk of postoperative cholangitis is almost eliminated.[36, 42, 57, 67] On the other hand, persistent anastomotic bile leak[67] and biliary obstruction[36] have been reported with the gallbladder conduit. Consequently, we[57]

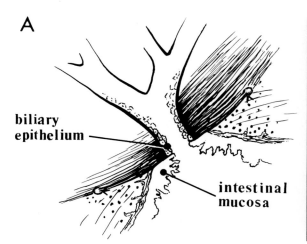

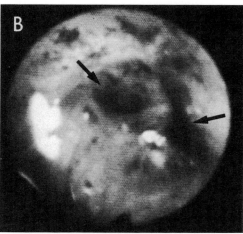

Fig 110–3.—Nature of bilio-intestinal anastomosis. **A,** author's conception of the eventual hilar anastomosis following Kasai's hepatic portoenterostomy operation. We believe an autoanastomosis occurs between the intestinal mucosa and the intrahepatic biliary epithelium, accounting for a permanent biliary fistula. (Courtesy of Dr. Jack Chang.) **B,** hilar anastomosis in a 10-month-old infant with biliary atresia treated by Kasai's hepatic portoenterostomy. The photograph was taken through a flexible endoscope in the bilioenteric conduit. The main right and left intrahepatic ducts *(arrows)* are visible, and bile was seen exiting from both. Note the uninterrupted epithelial lining of intestine and bile duct. (Courtesy of Dr. Arnold Silverman.)

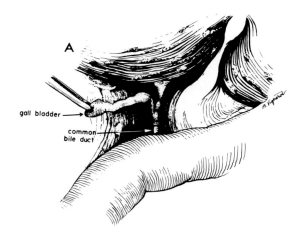

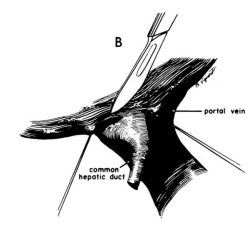

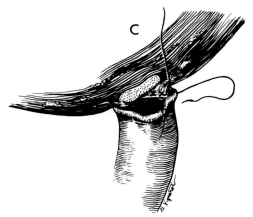

Fig 110–4.—Author's technique of hepatic portoenterostomy. **A,** the gallbladder is dissected free from the liver and traced to the obliterated common bile duct. The common duct is transected immediately distal to its junction with the cystic duct. Using the gallbladder as a handle, the proximal hepatic duct is dissected from the other portal structures to the liver hilus. **B,** two guy sutures of fine absorbable material are placed in the liver capsule just at the medial and lateral sides of the common hepatic duct remnant. This structure is located at the bifurcation of the portal vein and somewhat posterior to it. **C,** previously placed guy sutures are sutured, full thickness, to the mesenteric and antimesenteric borders of the open end of a Roux-en-Y jejunal conduit. A running anastomosis is done between the full thickness of the intestine and the available adventitial structures surrounding the transected duct.

have employed temporary catheter decompression of the gallbladder (Fig 110–8) until the anastomosis has healed and the diminutive distal biliary structures have dilated and become capable of carrying the full bile load.

With Kasai's operation, most surgeons report successful bile drainage in about half the infants operated on under 4 months of age,[5, 55, 57, 64, 86] and success may approach 80% in infants less than 10 weeks old.[36] Biliary drainage is generally sluggish for

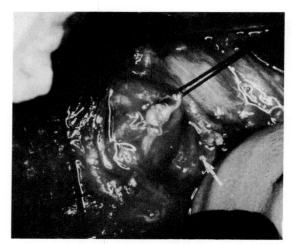

Fig 110–5.—Remnant of the common hepatic duct in a patient with biliary atresia. A 6-0 silk suture has been placed in the stump of the duct, which was found and dissected from the portal vein bifurcation *(arrow)*. The surgeon's finger *(bottom)* provides size comparison.

several weeks after operation, and jaundice does not resolve significantly in most infants for 6–12 weeks. In patients with an exteriorized biliary conduit, bile volume and its quantity of bilirubin and biliary lipids can be monitored, permitting an almost day-to-day evaluation of the status of the biliary anastomosis.[55]

Postoperative Management

If a conduit has been exteriorized, bile drainage must be replaced when volumes reach more than 100 ml daily. Failure to do so has resulted in acute dehydration and electrolyte aberrations, which may be lethal.[8] In the double-barreled conduit, bile drainage from the proximal conduit stoma is refed into the distal stoma periodically throughout the day. The bile salts in the conserved bile may aid absorption of fats and fat-soluble vitamins.

About 3–6 months after operation, when bile flow has reached a steady state, the exteriorized conduit is closed operatively, reestablishing direct flow of bile to the gastrointestinal circuit. To avoid postoperative cholangitis, we have employed temporary catheter decompression of the bilioenteric conduit,[83] thus permitting a more gradual adaptation of the conduit to the abrupt increase in bile flow and consequent heightened intraluminal pressure after stomal closure.

Complications

Cholangitis

Cholangitis is an almost universal complication after hepatic portoenterostomy. Predisposing to the infection are (1) intrahepatic duct stasis, an inherent part of biliary atresia for at least

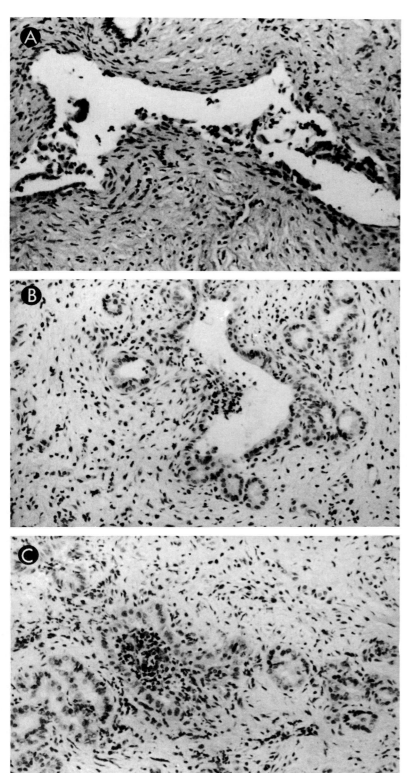

Fig 110–6.—Three specific types of biliary structures seen microscopically at the hilar end of the excised common hepatic duct. Only "bile ducts" communicate with the intrahepatic biliary system and drain bile after operation. Proper identification of biliary structures is essential at operation. (Courtesy of Dr. Ryoji Ohi and Dr. Robert H. Shikes.) **A,** bile duct. The lumen is irregular. The epithelium is partly denuded; elsewhere it varies from low cuboidal to atypical. Not seen here was a clearly demarcated wall with concentrically arranged ductules and glands (hematoxylin and eosin stain; × 100). **B,** collecting ductule and biliary glands. The epithelium is cuboidal and generally intact. The wall is not discrete and merges with the surrounding stroma (hematoxylin and eosin stain; × 100). **C,** biliary glands. The glands are scattered in nests within the stroma (hematoxylin and eosin stain; × 100).

several months after operation, and (2) bacterial contamination of the intestinal conduit. Complete colonization of the conduit with enteric bacteria occurs within 1 month of operation.[31] The two required ingredients for cholangitis, i.e., bacterial organisms and biliary stasis, are present in almost all patients.

Cholangitis is manifested by fever, leukocytosis, and decreased quantity and quality of bile. Aminoglycoside and cephalosporin antibiotics are effective. Fever usually resolves in 24–48 hours, but resumption of high-quality bile flow may take 5–7 days. Antibiotics are continued until then.

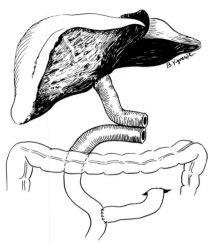

Fig 110–7.—Bilioenteric conduit constructed by the author. The proximal (hepatic) aspect of the defunctionalized limb of the Roux-en-Y jejunostomy is exteriorized as a double-barreled jejunostomy.

During the first weeks after operation cholangitis may, on infrequent occasions, be intractable. Fever persists despite adequate antibiotic treatment, or the infant develops a pattern of recurrent attacks of cholangitis, separated by only a few days of good health. During this early postoperative period, cholangitis may be followed by cessation of bile flow. In such circumstances we have employed short, 3–5-day, bursts of systemic steroid treatment[56] (prednisolone 10 mg/kg/day, reduced by half each day) primarily for its anti-inflammatory and secondarily for its choleretic effect. This kind of steroid treatment is successful in about 25% of patients.[82]

If antibiotic and steroid therapy are ineffective, reoperation is undertaken. The anterior wall of the hilar-intestinal anastomosis is taken down and the hilar area scored many times with a no. 12 blade. Any detritus is removed and the anterior anastomotic wall is reconstituted. Our belief is that, by so doing, microabscesses at the hilus are drained, or patent intrahepatic bile ducts are opened just proximal to the anastomotic site.[82] Bile flow re-

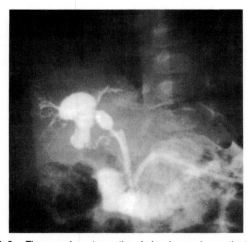

Fig 110–8.—Three-week postoperative cholangiogram in a patient with biliary atresia treated by hepatic portocholecystostomy ("gallbladder Kasai"). The distal ductal system has tripled in caliber since the definitive operation, thereby permitting safe removal of the anastomotic decompression catheter. There is some extravasation of contrast material. Note the characteristically distorted, irregular, narrow intrahepatic ductal system. (Courtesy of Dr. Carol H. Rumack.)

sumes in over half of infants reoperated on during this early postoperative period.[6, 68, 87] In our hands, reoperation for recalcitrant cholangitis has not been as rewarding as that for cessation of bile flow.[51] Finally, we have not been successful in preventing recurrences of cholangitis by the long-term "prophylactic" use of antibiotics.

Six to nine months after operation, as biliary stasis resolves and bile flow reaches normal, the liability to cholangitis wanes. In fact, cholangitis is unusual after the first postoperative year and then is a consequence of mechanical factors, e.g., partial obstruction of the conduit, stomal cicatrix, and not intrahepatic biliary stasis.[82]

To lessen the risk of cholangitis, the Roux-en-Y biliary construction has been modified by a variety of maneuvers, most commonly by temporarily exteriorizing the conduit. Creation of intestinal conduit "valves" to prevent intestinal reflux, as reported by Strauss[85] as early as 1951 ("ascending" infection theory), and omentopexy to the porta hepatis (lymphatic theory) also have advocates.[21, 62, 74] To date, no large series has been free of cholangitis.

Portal Hypertension

A variable degree of hepatic fibrosis is already present in patients with biliary atresia at the time of initial operation; the extent of liver damage may be quite different in individual patients of the same age.[46] Portal hypertension has been documented in most of those in whom pressures were taken.[92] Moreover, either as a consequence of ongoing intrahepatic disease or the only gradual resolution of biliary obstruction, hepatic damage is often progressive during the first several postoperative years.[7] Most authors have incriminated postoperative cholangitis as the key factor responsible for progressive liver damage and portal hypertension.[40, 41, 64, 91] However, the liability to cholangitis is due to intrahepatic biliary stasis and is thus more likely a reflection of the severity of the underlying disease.

The three principal clinical expressions of portal hypertension are splenomegaly (sometimes proceeding to frank hypersplenism), esophageal variceal hemorrhage, and variceal hemorrhage from the exteriorized conduit. Ascites is unusual. Manifestations are usually delayed until the patient is about 3 years old. Eleven of 47 patients (23%) with sustained bile drainage developed major variceal hemorrhage in our Denver series.[58]

Investigators in Sendai[39] and Bicetre[66] have documented spontaneous alleviation of portal hypertension in many patients. Kasai and colleagues[40] correlated reduction in portal pressure with improvement in liver histology. Another factor may be the spontaneous development of new portosystemic shunts. A large splenorenal shunt appeared spontaneously in one of our patients,[58] and a similar example was noted by Odievre.[66] Whatever the reasons, the improvement of portal hypertension in many patients with ongoing bile drainage suggests that drastic interventional procedures such as portal shunts,[4, 40, 66] gastric devascularization,[41, 91] or splenectomy[41] may be unnecessary. We have treated our patients with esophageal variceal hemorrhage by endosclerosis, those with hypersplenism by splenic embolization, and those with conduit variceal hemorrhage by disconnection of portosystemic shunts at the stomal site.[58] Subsequent hemorrhage has been minor and infrequent.

Other Complications

Absorption of fat-soluble vitamins requires a critical level of bile salts for micelle formation. Because of impaired normal bile flow to the gut for many months (both before and after operation), most children with biliary atresia have fat-soluble vitamin deficiencies for several years.[9] Rickets (vitamin D), ataxic neuromyopathy (vitamin E), and hemorrhage (vitamin K) have been reported.[9, 28, 79] Thus far, vitamin A deficiency has not been associated with a specific clinical problem. Specific guidelines for replacement of the fat-soluble vitamins have not yet been established.

Although not reported after Kasai's operation, the specter of hepatic malignancy exists in long-term survivors of biliary atresia.[30, 93] Among the first 40 patients with uncorrected biliary atresia undergoing liver transplantation in Denver, three had hepatomas.[80] Follow-up at this time is insufficient to determine if surgical relief of biliary obstruction by hepatic portoenterostomy removes the risk.

Prognosis

Survival

Survival in the combined New York City–Denver–Washington, D.C., series is shown in Figure 110–9. Of the 185 patients treated by Kasai's hepatic portoenterostomy since 1973, 90 are alive for at least 1 and as long as 10 years after operation. Twenty-three of these 90 survivors are alive 5 or more years from operation, 18 (78.3%) of whom are without jaundice and have normal or nearly normal growth and development.

The survival rate during the first 5-year period was 19.4%, and during the second, 62.4%. Although many factors contributed to the tripling of survival, including improved surgical technique and more aggressive reoperation, the primary reason for the difference between these two time frames is the younger age of the patients at operation. Because of the spreading recognition of the direct relation of patient age to operative success, infants with biliary atresia are undergoing operation at an earlier age.

Quality of Life

The first several years after portoenterostomy operations in many patients with biliary atresia are marred by repeated attacks of cholangitis, manifestations of portal hypertension, and recurrent and prolonged hospitalizations. Thereafter, complications decrease to a considerable extent. Despite the early tribulations, most children develop surprisingly normally, in both cognitive and motor skills.[5, 40, 66] A slower rate of growth and development characteristically occurs for 8 to 24 months, followed by a "catch-up" period.[11, 16]

Liver Transplantation

Liver transplantation, discussed in Chapter 40, is briefly referred to here as another form of treatment for biliary atresia. The dramatic improvement in short-term survival after liver transplantation with cyclosporin A immunosuppression[33, 81] raises the legitimate question of the feasibility of the procedure for biliary atresia. For reasons to be discussed, liver transplantation is rarely an alternative to hepatic portoenterostomy but is, instead, a complementary operation.

A rather prosaic categorization of "post-Kasai" patients would be: (1) Patients who are straight-out operative failures. With our present state of knowledge, a 10% failure rate is probably an irreducible figure. (2) Patients who achieve bile drainage but because of the severity of the underlying liver damage and intrahepatic ductal disease remain moderately jaundiced, fail to thrive, and develop multiple clinical manifestations of portal hypertension. (3) Patients who have normal bile drainage, grow and develop according to normal standards and have only mild hepatic sequelae of biliary atresia. The relative percentage of patients in each category depends on many factors, e.g., age at operation, disease severity, postoperative management.

Patients in the first category are generally not appropriate candidates for transplantation because of the relative rapidity of their death, about 18 months in untreated biliary atresia,[53] and the absolute scarcity of suitable infant donors. Children in the third category, obviously, are not transplant candidates. Thus, liver transplantation has its greatest applicability in patients who have only partially successful operations, i.e., biliary obstruction is relieved but not cured, and survival is prolonged but limited.

The patient in this intermediate category demands the most surgical effort, attention, and care. For instance, because of persistent biliary stasis and recurrent cholangitis, hilar debridement or conduit revision, including reexteriorization of the bowel, may be required. For progressive portal hypertension and life-threatening variceal hemorrhage, some form of operative intervention may be required. Other surgical procedures may be necessary to prevent the further degradation of life or for actual survival (sometimes with surprisingly gratifying results).[19, 41, 86] In so doing, the surgeon runs counter to the recommendations of the National Institutes of Health[77] (NIH) that secondary Kasai procedures should be avoided because they complicate and thereby endanger the success of the transplant operation. However, until

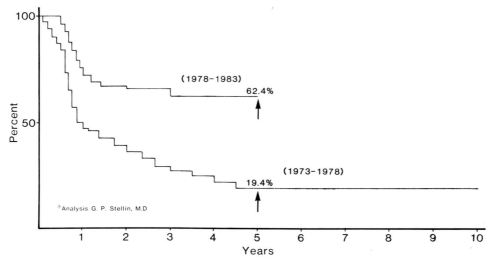

Fig 110–9.—Life survival curves of 185 New York City–Denver–Washington, D.C. patients with biliary atresia treated by Kasai's hepatic portoenterostomy operation. Survival in 80 patients in the first 5-year period (1973–1978) was 19.4% at five years. Survival rates in 105 patients more than tripled (62.4%) during the second 5-year period (1978–1983) primarily due to the much lower mortality rates after the first 2 postoperative years. Follow-up is a minimum of 1 year.

infant hepatic donors become readily available, the NIH rules are self-defeating. The very operations warned against are those responsible for sufficient prolongation of life to permit organ procurement. Consequently, we believe the best interests of the patient are served by providing expeditious surgical solution of complications. Obviously, if alternative forms of treatment (e.g., esophageal endosclerosis rather than portocaval shunt operations for variceal hemorrhage) are feasible, they should be utilized.

Other Surgical Lesions Responsible for Jaundice in Infants

Other than biliary atresia, the major surgical lesions that may be encountered at surgical exploration are: (1) biliary hypoplasia, (2) inspissated bile syndrome, (3) choledochal cyst, and (4) neonatal perforation of the extrahepatic bile ducts.

Biliary Hypoplasia

Biliary hypoplasia is a lesion characterized by an exceptionally small but grossly visible and radiographically patent extrahepatic biliary duct system. The diagnosis is almost invariably made at exploration for jaundice in infancy. Biliary hypoplasia is not a specific disease entity but a manifestation of a variety of hepatobiliary disorders, e.g., neonatal hepatitis, α_1-antitrypsin deficiency, intrahepatic biliary atresia, Alagille syndrome, paucity of intrahepatic bile ducts, arteriohepatic dysplasia.

The hypoplastic biliary tree has been attributed to disuse atrophy because of diminished bile flow,[29, 71] but an element of actual structural damage may coexist.[29] The miniscule ducts may also subsequently completely disappear.[82] In this context, we formerly believed that on occasion, biliary hypoplasia could represent an early stage of biliary atresia. That is, hypoplasia was an intermediary between normal patency and full occlusion. Two patients who apparently followed this progressive course[47] were later found to have a primary intrahepatic duct disorder at subsequent review of hepatic pathology.

Biliary hypoplasia cannot be improved by surgical maneuvers. In patients with paucity of the intrahepatic bile ducts, however, Alagille[2] has recommended that the cholecystostomy catheter be left in place postoperatively to decompress the biliary system. The prognosis is highly variable, depending on the primary disease. Some infants recover, some die in infancy, and others live to adolescence, often with jaundice, pruritus, and stunted growth.[3]

Inspissated Bile Syndrome

In neonates, massive hemolysis secondary to Rh and ABO blood group incompatibility or thick, tenacious bile in patients with cystic fibrosis may lead to mechanical obstruction as a consequence of sludge in the bile ducts. On occasion, inspissation may proceed to the point of production of biliary calculi.[12] Usually operative therapy consists of simple irrigation of the biliary tree.[75] In exceptional cases with bile pigment stones, manual removal of the calculi is required.[13, 50] Because of early diagnosis and exchange transfusion for the precipitating disease, the inspissated bile syndrome is now rarely seen.

Choledochal Cyst

In infants with choledochal cyst, the distal common bile duct is often totally obstructed. The hepatic histologic resemblance is to biliary atresia.[46] Total excision of the cyst and mucosa-to-mucosa anastomosis by Roux-en-Y choledochojejunostomy is the treatment of choice.[23] Anastomotic drainage of the cyst into the duodenum or jejunum results in a high incidence of late anastomotic stricture, recurrent cholangitis, and the risk of cyst malig-

nancy.[23] Technically, excision may be made a good deal easier and safer by approaching the cyst from its inside and leaving a strip of the posterior wall, denuded of mucosa (overlying the hepatic artery and portal vein).[48] If the diagnosis is made early and biliary obstruction corrected, reversal of minor degrees of hepatic damage is anticipated.[96] Liver damage and cirrhosis may be progressive in infants, however, despite adequate biliary drainage.[37]

Idiopathic Perforation of the Extrahepatic Bile Ducts

In neonates with biliary ascites, the almost invariable location of the duct perforation at the union of the common bile and cystic ducts suggests this junctional site may be particularly vulnerable to developmental error. At operation, sterile bilious ascites[18] and a bile-filled pseudocyst are usually found. The operative cholangiogram is sometimes misleading in that phantoms (e.g., stenosis, calculi) may be seen in the distal common duct.[59] In most cases these merely represent biliary sludge that resolves spontaneously. The lesion is self-limited and seals several weeks after operation, and most patients are best treated by simple drainage of the area of perforation. We leave a cholecystostomy catheter in place after operation to assess healing of the duct perforation, and drains are not removed until that has been demonstrated.[59] Intestinal anastomosis to the pseudocyst, mistaking the lesion for a ruptured choledochal cyst, is associated with significant mortality.[73] Spontaneous perforation of the common bile duct is an isolated error in duct development, and residual hepatobiliary disease has not been reported (see Chap. 96).

REFERENCES

1. Adelman S.: Prognosis of uncorrected biliary atresia: An update. *J. Pediatr. Surg.* 4:389, 1978.
2. Alagille D.: Personal communication, 1983.
3. Alagille D., Odievre M., Gauntier M., et al.: Hepatic ductular hypoplasia associated with characteristic facies, vertebral malformations, retarded physical, mental, and sexual development, and cardiac murmur. *J. Pediatr.* 86:63, 1975.
4. Altman R.P.: Portal decompression by interposition mesocaval shunt in patients with biliary atresia. *J. Pediatr. Surg.* 11:809, 1976.
5. Altman R.P.: The portoenterostomy procedure for biliary atresia. *Ann. Surg.* 188:3, 1978.
6. Altman R.P.: Results of re-operation for correction of extrahepatic biliary atresia. *J. Pediatr. Surg.* 14:305, 1979.
7. Altman R.P., Chandra R., Lilly J.R.: Ongoing cirrhosis after successful porticoenterostomy in infants with biliary atresia. *J. Pediatr. Surg.* 10:685, 1975.
8. Anderson K.A.: Oral communication, 1982.
9. Andrews W.S., Pau C.M.L., Chase H.P., et al.: Fat soluble vitamin deficiency in biliary atresia. *J. Pediatr. Surg.* 16:284, 1981.
10. Arcari F.: Discussion of Altman R.P., Chandra R., Lilly J.R.: Ongoing cirrhosis after successful porticoenterostomy in infants with biliary atresia. *J. Pediatr. Surg.* 10:690, 1975.
11. Barkin R.M., Lilly J.R.: Biliary atresia and the Kasai operation: Continuing care. *J. Pediatr.* 88:1015, 1980.
12. Benson C.D., Lofti M.W., Hertzler J.H.: Surgical aspects of biliary tract disease in the infant and child. *Trans. West. Surg. Assoc.* 1966.
13. Bernstein J., Braylan R., Brough A.J.: Bile-plug syndrome: A correctable cause of obstructive jaundice in infants. *Pediatrics* 43:273, 1969.
14. Bill A.H., Brennom W.S., Huseby T.L.: New concepts of pathology, diagnosis, and management of biliary atresia. *Arch. Surg.* 109:367, 1974.
15. Bunton G.L., Cameron R.: Regeneration of liver after biliary cirrhosis. *Ann. N.Y. Acad. Sci.* 111:412, 1963.
16. Burgess D.B., Martin H.P., Lilly J.R.: The developmental status of children undergoing the Kasai procedure for biliary atresia. *Pediatrics* 70:624, 1982.
17. Campbell D.P., Poley J.R., Alaupovic P., et al.: The differential diagnosis of neonatal hepatitis and biliary atresia. *J. Pediatr. Surg.* 9:699, 1974.
18. Caulfield E.: Bile peritonitis in infancy. *Am. J. Dis. Child.* 52:1348, 1936.
19. Chiba T., Kasai M., Sasano N.: Histopathological studies on intrahepatic bile ducts in the vicinity of porta hepatis in biliary atresia. *Tohuku J. Exp. Med.* 118:199, 1976.

20. Danks D.M., Campbell P.E., Clarke A.M., et al.: Extrahepatic biliary atresia. *Am. J. Dis. Child.* 128:684, 1974.
21. Donahoe P.K., Hendren W.H.: Roux-en-Y on-line intussusception to avoid ascending cholangitis in biliary atresia. *Arch. Surg.* 118:1091, 1983.
22. Finlayson C.: Congenital obliteration of the bile ducts in a child who lived for three years and three months. *Arch. Dis. Child.* 12:153, 1937.
23. Flanigan D.P.: Biliary cysts. *Ann. Surg.* 182:635, 1975.
24. Fonkalsrud E.W., Kitagawa S., Longmire W.P.: Hepatic lymphatic drainage to the jejunum for congenital biliary atresia. *Am. J. Surg.* 112:188, 1966.
25. Gautier M.: L'Atrésie des voies biliaires extrahepatiques: Hypothèse étiologique basée sur l'étude histologique de 130 réliquats fibreux. *Arch. Franc. Pédiat.* 36(suppl. 3), 1979.
26. Gellis S.S.: Biliary atresia commentary. *Pediatrics* 55:8, 1975.
27. Gross R.E.: *The Surgery of Infancy and Childhood.* Philadelphia, W.B. Saunders Co., 1953.
28. Guggenheim M.A., Jackson V., Lilly J., et al.: Vitamin E deficiency and neurologic disease in children with cholestasis: A prospective study. *J. Pediatr.* 102:577, 1983.
29. Hays D.M., Woolley M.M., Snyder W.H.: Diagnosis of biliary atresia: Relative accuracy of percutaneous liver biopsy, open liver biopsy, and operative cholangiography. *J. Pediatr.* 71:598, 1967.
30. Henriksen N.T., Drabos P., Aagenaes Q.: Cholestatic jaundice in infancy: The importance of familial and genetic factors in etiology and prognosis. *Arch. Dis. Child.* 56:622, 1981.
31. Hitch D.C., Lilly J.R.: Identification, quantification, and significance of bacterial growth within the biliary tract after Kasai's operation. *J. Pediatr. Surg.* 13:563, 1978.
32. Holmes J.B.: Congenital obliteration of the bile ducts—diagnosis and suggestions for treatment. *Am. J. Dis. Child.* 11:405, 1916.
33. Iwatsuki S., Shaw B.W. Jr., Starzl T.E.: Liver transplantation for biliary atresia. *World J. Surg.* 8:51, 1984.
34. Izant R.J. Jr., Akers D.R., Hays D.M., et al.: Biliary atresia survey, Surgical Section, Proceedings of the American Academy of Pediatrics, 1965.
35. Kanof A., Donovan E.J., Berner H.: Congenital atresia of the biliary system: Delayed development of correctability. *Am. J. Dis. Child.* 86:780, 1953.
36. Kasai M.: Treatment of biliary atresia with special reference to hepatic portoenterostomy and its modifications. *Prog. Pediatr. Surg.* 6:5, 1974.
37. Kasai M., Asakura Y., Taira Y.: Surgical treatment of choledochal cyst. *Ann. Surg.* 182:844, 1970.
38. Kasai M., Kimura S., Asakura Y., et al.: Surgical treatment of biliary atresia. *J. Pediatr. Surg.* 3:665, 1968.
39. Kasai M., Okamoto A., Ohi R., et al.: Changes of portal vein pressure and intrahepatic blood vessels after surgery for biliary atresia. *J. Pediatr. Surg.* 16:152, 1981.
40. Kasai M., Watanabe I., Ohi R.: Follow-up studies of long-term survivors after hepatic portoenterostomy for "noncorrectable" biliary atresia. *J. Pediatr. Surg.* 10:173, 1975.
41. Kimura S., Nakamura S., Araki S., et al.: Long-term results of hepatic portoenterostomy for biliary atresia. *Z. Kinderchir.* 26:42, 1979.
42. Kimura K., Tsugawa C., Matsumoto Y., et al.: The surgical management of the unusual forms of biliary atresia. *J. Pediatr. Surg.* 14:653, 1979.
43. Klotz D., Cohn B.D., Kottmeier P.K.: Choledochal cysts: Diagnostic and therapeutic problems. *J. Pediatr. Surg.* 8:271, 1973.
44. Kravetz L.J.: Congenital biliary atresia. *Surgery* 47:453, 1960.
45. Ladd W.E.: Congenital atresia and stenosis of the bile ducts. *JAMA* 91:1082, 1928.
46. Landing B.H.: *Considerations of the Pathogenesis of Neonatal Hepatitis, Biliary Atresia and Choledochal Cyst: The Concept of Infantile Obstructive Cholangiography.* Baltimore, University Park Press, 1972.
47. Lilly J.R.: The surgery of biliary hypoplasia. *J. Pediatr. Surg.* 11:815, 1976.
48. Lilly J.R.: Total excision of choledochal cyst. *Surg. Gynecol. Obstet.* 146:254, 1978.
49. Lilly J.R.: Discussion of Kimura K., Tsugawa C., Matsumoto Y., et al.: The surgical management of the unusual forms of biliary atresia. *J. Pediatr. Surg.* 14:653, 1979.
50. Lilly J.R.: Common bile duct calculi in infants and children. *J. Pediatr. Surg.* 15:577, 1980.
51. Lilly J.R.: Discusson of: Altman R.P., Anderson K.D.: Surgical management of intractable cholangitis following successful Kasai procedure. *J. Pediatr. Surg.* 17:894, 1982.
52. Lilly J.R., Altman R.P.: Hepatic portoenterostomy (the Kasai operation) for biliary atresia. *Surgery* 78:76, 1975.
53. Lilly J.R., Altman R.P., Hays D.M., et al.: Biliary Atresia Registry, American Academy of Pediatrics. Unpublished data, 1984.
54. Lilly J.R., Chandra R.S.: Surgical hazards of co-existing anomalies in biliary atresia. *Surg. Gynecol. Obstet.* 139:49, 1974.
55. Lilly J.R., Javitt N.B.: Biliary lipid excretion after hepatic portoenterostomy. *Ann. Surg.* 184:369, 1976.
56. Lilly J.R.: Liver, gallbladder, and extrahepatic bile ducts, in Welch K.J. (ed.): *Complications of Pediatric Surgery.* Philadelphia, W.B. Saunders Co., 1982.
57. Lilly J.R., Stellin G.P.: Catheter decompression of hepatic portocholecystostomy. *J. Pediatr. Surg.* 17:904, 1982.
58. Lilly J.R., Stellin G.: Variceal hemorrhage in biliary atresia. *J. Pediatr. Surg.* 19:476, 1984.
59. Lilly J.R., Weintraub W.H., Altman R.P.: Spontaneous perforation of the extrahepatic bile ducts and bile peritonitis in infancy. *Surgery* 75:664, 1974.
60. Longmire W.P., Sanford M.C.: Intrahepatic cholangiojejunostomy with partial hepatectomy for biliary obstruction. *Surgery* 24:264, 1948.
61. Lou M.A., Schmutzer K.J., Regan J.F.: Congenital extrahepatic biliary atresia. *Arch. Surg.* 105:771, 1972.
62. Luck S., Raffensperger J.: Oral communication, 1983.
63. Miyano T., Suruga K., Suda K.: Abnormal choledocho-pancreatico ductal junction related to the etiology of infantile obstructive jaundice disease. *J. Pediatr. Surg.* 14:16, 1979.
64. Miyata M., Satani M., Ueda T., et al.: Long-term results of hepatic portoenterostomy for biliary atresia: Special reference to postoperative portal hypertension. *Surgery* 76:234, 1974.
65. Morecki R., Slaser J., Cho S., et al.: Biliary atresia and reovirus type 3 infection. *N. Engl. J. Med.* 307:481, 1982.
66. Odievre M.: Long-term results of surgical treatment of biliary atresia. *World J. Surg.* 2:589, 1978.
67. Odievre M., Valayer J., Razemon-Pinta M., et al.: Hepatic portoenterostomy or cholecystostomy in the treatment of extrahepatic biliary atresia. *J. Pediatr.* 88:774, 1976.
68. Ohi R., Hanamatsu M., Mochizuki I., et al.: Reoperation in patients with biliary atresia. *J. Pediatr. Surg.* 20:256, 1985.
69. Ohi R., Klingensmith W.C., Lilly J.R.: Diagnosis of hepato-biliary disease in infants and children with Tc-99m-diethyl-IDA imaging. *Clin. Nucl. Med.* 6:297, 1981.
70. Ohi R., Shikes R.H., Stellin G.P., et al.: In biliary atresia duct histology correlates with bile flow. *J. Pediatr. Surg.* (in press).
71. Porter C.A., Mowat A.P., Cook P.J.L., et al.: Alpha₁-antitrypsin deficiency and neonatal hepatitis. *Br. Med. J.* 3:435, 1972.
72. Potts W.J.: *The Surgeon and the Child.* Philadelphia, W.B. Saunders Co., 1959.
73. Prevot J., Babut J.M.: Spontaneous perforations of the biliary tract in infancy. *Prog. Pediatr. Surg.* 3:187, 1971.
74. Rickham P.P., Hirsig J.: Biliary atresia: Recent advances in aetiology, diagnosis and treatment. *Z. Kinderchir.* 26:114, 1979.
75. Rickham P.P., Lee E.Y.C.: Neonatal jaundice: Surgical aspects. *Clin. Pediatr.* 3:197, 1964.
76. Sawaguchi S.: The treatment of congenital biliary atresia, with special reference to hepatic portoenteroanastomosis. Presented at annual meeting of the Pacific Association of Pediatric Surgeons, Tokyo, Japan, 1972 (personal communication).
77. Schmidt R., Berwick D.M., Combes B., et al.: Liver transplantation. *Nat. Inst. Health Consensus Dev. Conf. Summary* 4:7, 1983.
78. Shim W.K.T., Kasai M., Spence M.A.: Racial influence on the incidence of biliary atresia. *Prog. Pediatr. Surg.* 6:53, 1974.
79. Sokol R.J., Bove K.E., Heubi J.E., et al.: Vitamin E deficiency during chronic childhood cholestasis: Presence of sural nerve lesion prior to 2-1/2 years of age. *J. Pediatr.* 103:197, 1983.
80. Starzl T.E.: Personal communication, 1977.
81. Starzl T.E., Iwatsuki S., Van Thiel D.H., et al.: Evolution of liver transplantation. *Hepatology* 2:614, 1982.
82. Stellin G.P., Lilly J.R.: Unpublished data.
83. Stellin G.P., Ueda J.E., Lilly J.R.: Conduit decompression in biliary atresia. *J. Pediatr. Surg.* 18:782, 1983.
84. Sterling J.A.: Artificial bile ducts in the management of congenital biliary atresia. *J. Int. Coll. Surg.* 36:293, 1961.
85. Strauss A.A.: Congenital atresia of the bile ducts. *J. Mt. Sinai Hosp.* 17:552, 1951.
86. Suruga K., Nagashima K., Kohno S., et al.: A clinical and pathological study of congenital biliary atresia. *J. Pediatr. Surg.* 7:655, 1972.
87. Suruga K., Miyano T., Kimura K., et al.: Reoperation in the treatment of biliary atresia. *J. Pediatr. Surg.* 17:1, 1982.
88. Swenson O., Fisher J.H.: Utilization of cholangiogram during exploration for biliary atresia. *N. Engl. J. Med.* 249:247, 1952.
89. Thaler M.M., Gellis S.S.: Studies in neonatal hepatitis and biliary atresia. *Am. J. Dis. Child.* 116:257, 1968.
90. Thomson J.: On congenital obliteration of bile ducts. *Edin. Med. J.* 37:523, 1891.

91. Toyosaka A., Okamoto E.: Portal hypertension after successful hepatic porto-enterostomy for biliary atresia. *Jpn. J. Pediatr. Surg.* 11:537, 1979.
92. Valayer J.: Hepatic porto-enterostomy: Surgical problems and results, in Berenberg S.R. (ed.): *Liver Diseases in Infancy and Childhood.* The Hague, Martinus Nijhoff Medical Division, 1976.
93. Van Wyk J., Halgrimson C.G., Giles G., et al.: Liver transplantation in biliary atresia with concomitant hepatoma. *S. Afr. Med. J.* 46:885, 1972.
94. Williams L.F., Dooling J.A.: Thoracic duct-esophagus anastomosis for relief of congenital biliary atresia. *Surg. Forum* 14:189, 1963.
95. Ylppo A.: Zwei Fälle von kongenitalem Gallengangsverschluss. Z. *Kinderh.* 9:319, 1913.
96. Yeong M.L., Nicholson G.I., Lee S.P.: Regression of biliary cirrhosis following choledochal cyst drainage. *Gastroenterology* 82:332, 1982.

111 JAMES A. O'NEILL, JR.
Choledochal Cyst

CHOLEDOCHAL CYST, or congenital cystic dilatation of the common bile duct, is a relatively rare abnormality first reported clinically by Douglas in 1852.[4] Alonzo-Lej and his group described a classification of choledochal cysts into three types, based on anatomy.[1] Since that time, other forms and subgroups have been described, based on cholangiographic findings.[24] The common varieties are as follows:

Type I—segmental or diffuse fusiform dilatation of the extrahepatic bile duct
Type II—diverticulum of the extrahepatic bile duct
Type III—choledochocele
Type IV—multiple cysts of the intra- or extrahepatic duct, or both
Type V—single or multiple intrahepatic cysts.

Such intrahepatic cysts associated with hepatic fibrosis have been referred to as Caroli's disease.[3] Over 90% of choledochal cysts are of the type I variety, being either fusiform or saccular dilatations of the extrahepatic ductal system[1] (Fig 111–1).

In almost all reported series, Orientals, particularly Japanese, outnumber Caucasian patients. Almost two thirds of all reported cases are in the Japanese literature. Females, for no known reason, outnumber males three or four to one.

Choledochal cysts of all types, except type III, are similar from a histologic point of view.[28] The wall is generally quite thick, consisting of dense connective tissue with some smooth muscle. Varying degrees of inflammation are present and ordinarily there is no mucosal lining, although at times patchy areas of columnar epithelium may be found. The choledochocele form of cyst is usually lined by duodenal mucosa, although in some the lining resembles that of the bile duct. At times, type I choledochal cysts are associated with intrahepatic cysts or biliary atresia. Cirrhosis is common in infants who present with complete biliary obstruction, and the outlook is guarded under these circumstances.

Etiology

A number of theories have been offered to explain the occurrence of choledochal cysts, and most of them attribute the formation to obstructive factors. Other theories suggest some sort of primary weakness or abnormality of the bile duct itself, and still others indicate that both obstruction and intrinsic bile duct defects were contributory. Alonzo-Lej discussed these various etiologic possibilities in detail.[1] Yotsuyanagi postulated that there may be an inequality of proliferation of epithelial cells when primitive bile ducts are still solid, such that, if cellular proliferation of the proximal end is more active than that of the distal portion of the duct, canalization will leave an abnormally dilated proximal end.[28] With the advent of accurate cholangiographic techniques, particularly endoscopic retrograde cholangiopancreatography, Todani and others suggested that an anomalous arrangement of the pancreatobiliary ductal system, which allows reflux of pancreatic enzymes and dissolution of the ductal wall, is responsible.[25] In this type of arrangement, the union of the pancreatic duct and distal common bile duct is located a distance from the duodenum, with a long common channel and abnormal angle resulting in reflux of pancreatic juice into the bile duct, due to the absence of the sphincter of Oddi around the union. Babbitt was the first to suggest this factor as a possible cause.[2] Ito and his group, as well as others, emphasized the significance of a narrow distal segment of the dilated common duct as a form of stenosis, with resultant proximal dilatation.[12] In the infant, if reflux of pancreatic enzymes is responsible for degeneration of the wall of the bile duct, trypsin is most likely to be responsible, since the newborn produces little, if any, amylase.[16] However, few convincing experimental preparations have been devised, so the exact etiology is still obscure. As the abundant Japanese literature on choledochal cyst suggests, the condition is much more common in the Orient than in the West. It is impossible to ignore the fact that this great difference in frequency and in distribution is true also of biliary atresia. It is tempting to ascribe both diseases to the same, possibly viral, cause.

Clinical Findings

Choledochal cysts are generally classified as infant or adult. In the infant group, babies ranging from one to three months of age present with obstructive jaundice, acholic stools, and hepatomegaly, in a clinical picture indistinguishable from that of biliary atresia.[20] At times, even in the young patients, characteristic signs of cirrhosis are present. Such patients do not have abdominal pain, and a mass is not palpable. Low-grade fever may be present however, just as it is in patients with biliary atresia, although not in a pattern suggestive of cholangitis.

In the so-called adult type of choledochal cyst, clinical mani-

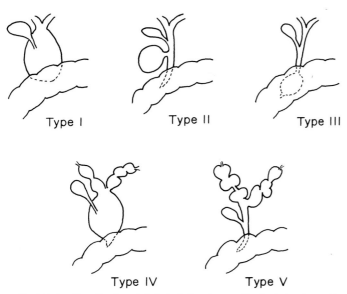

Fig 111–1.—Classification of choledochal cysts according to cholangiographic appearance.

festations generally do not become evident until after 2 years of age. It is in this group of patients that the classic triad of pain, mass, and jaundice may be present. Intermittent jaundice is the rule, usually associated with vague right upper quadrant and occasional back pain. While hepatomegaly may be present, it is less prominent than that associated with the infant form of choledochal cyst, in which biliary obstruction is usually complete. The pain pattern has been described as similar to that of recurrent pancreatitis, and evidence has been adduced that the acute attacks represent bouts of pancreatitis.[21] If the diagnosis is not made early, older patients will present with cirrhosis and manifestations of portal hypertension. Fever and vomiting, suggestive of recurrent cholangitis, are frequently present in older patients with this problem. It is important to note that symptoms in older patients are subtle and intermittent enough so that the diagnosis frequently goes unrecognized.

Diagnosis

Regardless of the form of anatomic abnormality, some form of imaging technique is the preferred approach to diagnosis.[22] In the past, upper gastrointestinal tract contrast x-ray studies were used in an attempt to show indentation of the superior and posterior aspects of the duodenum by a choledochal cyst, but the technique was useless in the infant and not reliable in older subjects. Ultrasonography is probably the best screening study, followed by ^{99}Tc DISIDA scintigraphy, if a choledochal cyst is suspected.[13] Of all the iminodiacetic acid (IDA)-derivative scans available, the DISIDA scan is probably best, because the agent is lipophilic and less bound to bilirubin than other forms of the isotope. This sequence is noninvasive and thus particularly valuable in the newborn. Two of our patients had a diagnosis of choledochal cyst made prenatally, during the third trimester of pregnancy.[10] An alternative to ultrasound demonstration of choledochal cyst is computerized tomography (CT). In one of our patients, CT scanning was combined with intravenous cholangiography, but this particular technique was selected because intrapancreatic disease was suspected, and we thought that CT scanning might be more accurate than ultrasound. In most cases, abdominal ultrasonography is probably the best screening study,

since it can demonstrate changes in the caliber of bile ducts and also provide information about the status of the liver. Percutaneous transhepatic cholangiography is probably best reserved for older individuals with a suspected choledochal cyst, especially patients with a suspected intrahepatic biliary cyst.[8] Another technique that may be useful in older subjects with a suspected ductal anomaly is endoscopic retrograde cholangiopancreatography.[19] It is this technique that has given evidence to suggest that a common channel syndrome is responsible for dilatation of the bile ducts. Whatever combination of techniques is used for preoperative diagnosis, an intraoperative cholangiogram should always be performed, since it is likely to provide the most accurate anatomical information as the operative repair is being undertaken. The injection may be performed either through the gallbladder or directly into the dilated duct itself, but it is important to reflux dye into the intrahepatic ductal system to determine whether or not intrahepatic anomalies coexist (Figs 111–2 and 111–3).

Postoperatively, abdominal ultrasound and the DISIDA scan are helpful follow-up tools, capable of showing duct size compared with preoperative status, rate of bile excretion, the degree of stasis, and whether stones or sludge are present.

Liver biopsy generally is not very helpful as a preoperative study, except to indicate the status of cirrhosis. Liver function tests are only helpful when they are deranged.

Other entities that come into the diagnostic picture, and are differentiable by various combinations of the abovementioned diagnostic imaging studies, include congenital hepatic fibrosis, Caroli's disease with hepatic fibrosis, primary sclerosing cholangitis, congenital cirrhosis, and congenital stricture of the common hepatic or common bile duct.

Treatment

In the first period following recognition of this condition, aspiration, marsupialization, and external drainage were attempted as the simplest techniques. After this, the era of internal drainage began, and the most popular approach for many years was cyst-duodenostomy, as originally proposed by Ladd and Gross.[7] While patients who had this operation rarely had any significant problem in the immediate postoperative period, long-term follow-up series reported by Alonzo-Lej, by Hays, and by O'Neill indicated that the longer the follow-up, the higher the incidence of symptomatic complications.[1, 9, 20] Generally, symptoms were characteristically mild and usually considered insignificant, particularly because the incidence of complications did not become significant until several years had passed. Generally, the pattern was one of reflux from the duodenum into the cyst and biliary tree, followed by stricture and repeated bouts of cholangitis. In fact, it appeared as if duodenobiliary reflux without stricture and delayed emptying was also associated with cholangitis. For these reasons, the procedure of choice then became cyst jejunostomy, using a Roux-en-Y limb of sufficient length to obviate reflux into the biliary tree. Some, such as Spitz, still prefer the latter procedure, since over two thirds of patients undergoing Roux-en-Y cyst jejunostomy have excellent results on long-term follow-up.[23] This has been our experience as well.

McWhorter first reported excision of a choledochal cyst with internal drainage in 1924.[18] The procedure carried too high a mortality rate in the early years to be acceptable, so that internal drainage of the cyst was preferred. Alonzo-Lej, in 1959, performed and used primary resection.[1] In 1970, Kasai and his group reported a series of 21 patients, 14 of whom had resection with Roux-en-Y hepaticojejunostomy. The results were sufficiently favorable to stimulate others around the world to use this procedure.[5, 11, 14, 26] In the last 5 years, cyst excision with Roux-

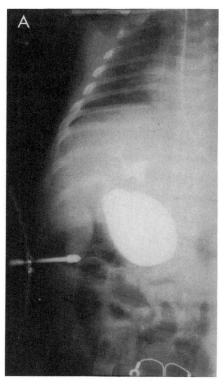

Fig 111–2.—A, operative cholangiogram done by injection into the choledochal cyst demonstrates cystic dilatation of the cystic and common hepatic bile ducts in a 3-month-old girl. **B,** at operation, the extrahepatic ducts were found uniformly dilated, and no opening could be found into the duodenum. **C,** the choledochal cyst was completely excised and the distal end closed by suture ligation. One can see just enough of a proximal cuff left to allow an adequate anastomosis to a Roux-en-Y limb of jejunum, which was performed. The child has been well for 2 years.

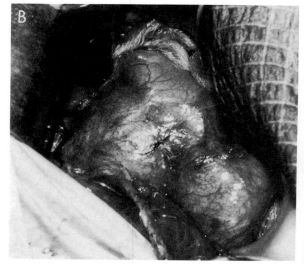

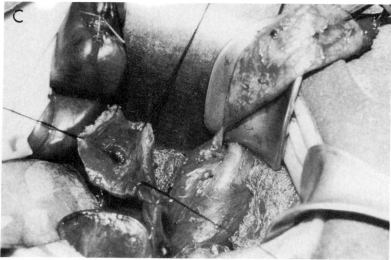

en-Y hepaticojejunostomy has been the only procedure used in our institution.

Lilly and Todani had each reported cyst excision using a plane of dissection between the inner and outer layers of the cyst, beginning at the confluence of the cystic and common ducts.[17, 27] The cystic duct is used as a guide to the correct layer for dissection, or the cyst may be opened in its midportion, anterolaterally, and the plane determined under direct vision. Blunt dissection is carried out around the entire wall of the midsegment of the cyst. The outer layer of the cyst, as well as the portal vein and hepatic artery, are left undisturbed. A Penrose drain may then be placed completely around the freed cyst wall, and the dissection is continued superiorly and inferiorly. The small terminal duct, which is usually connected with the pancreatic duct,

is then suture-ligated and transected. Excision of the cyst is completed by transection of the common hepatic duct at the level of its bifurcation. If an incision is then made along the lateral wall of both the right and left hepatic ducts for approximately 5 mm, one may then obtain a wider anastomotic stoma. We have used this technique of excision in older patients with thick-walled cysts and extensive inflammation, but have preferred total cyst excision in younger patients, as shown in Figure 111–2,*B* and *C.* We have had no problems with total cyst excision in young patients.

Todani et al. prefer hepaticoduodenostomy following cyst excision, but we and most others prefer Roux-en-Y hepaticojejunostomy, because of concern for the possible late deleterious effects of duodenobiliary reflux.[26] We prefer anastomosis of the

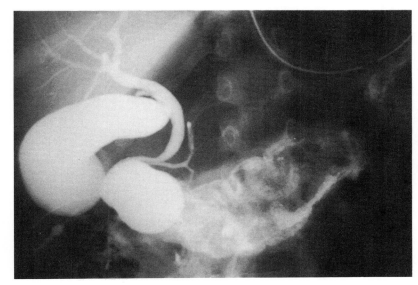

Fig 111–3.—Operative cholangiogram via the gallbladder in a 4-year-old boy demonstrates a choledochocele (type III choledochal cyst) within the duodenum, which was opened so that the choledochocele could be unroofed and the edges oversewn. Sphincteroplasty of the pancreatic and common bile ducts was performed as well. The patient, who had recurrent preoperative bouts of abdominal pain, mild jaundice, and pancreatitis, has had no problem for 3 years.

jejunum to the hepatic remnant of the dilated duct, with an inverting interrupted suture line of 4-0 or 5-0 silk.

The abovementioned techniques are applicable to the vast majority of patients with type I cysts. The remaining types of choledochal cysts must be treated as indicated by their anatomy. Type II cysts or diverticula may either be excised or drained into the duodenum, depending on their presentation. Choledochocele is most easily treated by unroofing the cyst, oversewing the edges to prevent bleeding, and performing sphincteroplasty of the pancreatic and bile ducts, if indicated. In those instances where intrahepatic cysts are not accessible and easily drained, hepatic resection, by lobectomy or segmentectomy, is the most successful approach, as shown by Todani and others.[24]

Cholecystectomy is indicated in all patients with type I choledochal cysts, whether or not the cyst is excised, since stasis and late stone formation are otherwise the rule.

Results and Complications

The most extensive long-term analysis of patients operated on for choledochal cyst was reported by Flanigan in 1975.[6] In a review of 235 cases, he found that the incidence of recurrent pain, jaundice, and stricture formation associated with cholangitis was 58% following cyst duodenostomy, 34% after Roux-en-Y cyst jejunostomy, and only 8% following complete cyst excision. In recent years, mortality with cyst excision in all reported series has been virtually nil, except when the cyst was associated with biliary atresia. Another reason for excising the cyst, in addition to the fact that it appears to be followed by a much lower incidence of cholangitis, is the potential late occurrence of carcinoma in the cyst wall. Over 50 such cases of cyst carcinoma have been reported in the literature.[27] In the survey of the Surgical Section of the American Academy of Pediatrics on choledochal cysts reported by Kim in 1981, 14 of 198 patients were dead because of biliary atresia, cholangitis with sepsis, hepatic failure, or carcinoma.[15] Thirty-six patients were lost to follow-up, and 138 were followed up to 22 years. Of these, 115 were alive without liver disease. The common late complications were cholangitis, in a third of the patients, and various complications of cholangitis, such as obstructive jaundice, pancreatitis, GI tract bleeding, and stone formation in an additional one fourth of the patients. Portal hypertension developed in 12% of patients.

Our own series over the last 8 years consists of 14 patients,

ten female and four male. Seven of the patients presented as infants, ranging from newborn to 6 months of age, with obstructive jaundice characteristic of biliary atresia. The other seven presented from 3 years to 16 years of age. Three had pain and an apparent mass; one had pain with jaundice but no mass; and two in the older age group had the classic triad of pain, mass, and jaundice. Two patients initially had cyst duodenostomies, both requiring revision, one to Roux-en-Y cyst jejunostomy and the other to excision of the cyst with hepaticojejunostomy. Six patients had primary Roux-en-Y cyst jejunostomies; one of these was revised to excision with hepaticojejunostomy because of stenosis of the original anastomosis, associated with jaundice. Four patients had primary excision of the cyst with hepaticojejunostomy, two by intramural resection, and two by total resection. One patient with cystic dilatation of the left intrahepatic ducts was treated by left hepatic lobectomy, and another with a choledochocele was treated by unroofing of the choledochocele and sphincteroplasty of the pancreatic and common bile ducts, both of which were stenotic. In this 8-year period there have been no deaths, and no long-term complications have yet been encountered. Our results support the preference for excision of a choledochal cyst with Roux-en-Y hepaticojejunostomy reconstruction, but we are also impressed with how well the patients who have had Roux-en-Y cyst jejunostomies have done. Of course, the long-term possibility of carcinoma in the cyst wall has not been eliminated. Cholecystectomy has been performed in all patients. Despite these initial favorable results, it must be kept in mind that many patients do not begin to have trouble for as long as 10 years, and some patients have not had difficulty for up to 30 years before presenting with recurrent cholangitis, biliary stones, and similar related problems.

REFERENCES

1. Alonzo-Lej F., Revor W.B., Pessagno D.J.: Congenital choledochal cyst, with a report of 2, and an analysis of 94 cases. *Surg. Gynecol. Obstet. Internat. Abst. Surg.* 108:1, 1959.
2. Babbitt D.P.: Congenital choledochal cyst: New etiological concept based on anomalous relationships of common bile duct and pancreatic bulb. *Ann. Radiol.* 12:231, 1969.
3. Caroli J., Soupalt R., Kossakowski J., et al.: La dilatation polykystique congénitale des voies biliaires intrahepatiques. Essai de classification. *Sem. Hôp. Paris* 34:488, 1958.
4. Douglas A.H.: Case of dilatation of the common bile duct. *Monthly J. Med. Sci.* (London) 14:97, 1852.

5. Filler R.M., Stringel G.: Treatment of choledochal cyst by excision. *J. Pediatr. Surg.* 15:437, 1980.
6. Flanigan D.P.: Biliary cysts. *Ann. Surg.* 182:635, 1975.
7. Gross R.E.: *The Surgery of Infancy and Childhood.* Philadelphia, W.B. Saunders Co., 1953, p. 524.
8. Hashimoto T., Yura J.: Percutaneous transhepatic cholangiography (PTC) in biliary atresia with special reference to the structure of the intrahepatic bile ducts. *J. Pediatr. Surg.* 16:22, 1981.
9. Hays D.M., Goodman G.N., Snyder W.H., et al.: Congenital cystic dilatation of the common bile duct. *Arch. Surg.* 98:457, 1969.
10. Howell C.G., Templeton J.M., Weiner S., et al.: Antenatal diagnosis and early surgery for choledochal cyst. *J. Pediatr. Surg.* 18:387, 1983.
11. Ishida M., Tsuchida Y., Saito S., et al.: Primary excision of choledochal cysts. *Surgery* 68:884, 1970.
12. Ito T., Ando H., Nagaya M., et al.: Congenital dilatation of the common bile duct in children—the etiologic significance of the narrow segment distal to the dilated common bile duct. *Z. Kinderchir.* 39:40, 1984.
13. Kangarloo H., Sarti D.A., Sample W.F., et al.: Ultrasonographic spectrum of choledochal cysts in children. *Pediatr. Radiol.* 9:15, 1980.
14. Kasai M., Asakura Y., Taira Y.: Surgical treatment of choledochal cyst. *Ann. Surg.* 172:844, 1970.
15. Kim S.H.: Choledochal cyst: Survey by the Surgical Section of the American Academy of Pediatrics. *J. Pediatr. Surg.* 16:402, 1981.
16. Lebenthal E., Lee P.C.: Development of functional response in human exocrine pancreas. *Pediatrics* 66:556, 1980.
17. Lilly J.R.: The surgical treatment of choledochal cyst. *Surg. Gynecol. Obstet.* 149:36, 1979.
18. McWhorter G.L.: Congenital cystic dilatation of the common bile duct. *Arch. Surg.* 8:604, 1924.
19. Okada A., Oguchi Y., Kamata S., et al.: Common channel syndrome—diagnosis with endoscopic retrograde cholangiopancreatography and surgical management. *Surgery* 93:634, 1983.
20. O'Neill J.A., Clatworthy H.W.: Management of choledochal cysts: A fourteen-year follow-up. *Am. Surg.* 37:230, 1971.
21. Ravitch M.M., Snyder G.B.: Congenital cystic dilatation of the common bile duct. *Surgery* 44:752, 1958.
22. Scharschmidt B.F., Goldberg H.I., Schmid R.: Approach to the patient with cholestatic jaundice. *N. Engl. J. Med.* 308:1515, 1983.
23. Spitz L.: Choledochal cyst. *Surg. Gynecol. Obstet.* 147:444, 1978.
24. Todani T., Narusue M., Watanabe Y., et al.: Management of congenital choledochal cyst with intrahepatic involvement. *Ann. Surg.* 187:272, 1978.
25. Todani T., Watanabe Y., Fujii T., et al.: Anomalous arrangement of the pancreaticobiliary ductal system in patients with a choledochal cyst. *Am. J. Surg.* 147:672, 1984.
26. Todani T., Watanabe Y., Mizuguchi T., et al.: Hepaticoduodenostomy at the hepatic hilum after excision of choledochal cyst. *Am. J. Surg.* 142:584, 1981.
27. Todani T., Watanabe Y., Narusue M., et al.: Congenital bile duct cysts—classification, operative procedures, and review of thirty-seven cases including cancer arising from choledochal cyst. *Am. J. Surg.* 134:263, 1977.
28. Yotsuyanagi S.: Contribution to aetiology and pathology of idiopathic cystic dilatation of the common bile duct with report of three cases. *Gann* 30:601, 1936.

112   GEORGE W. HOLCOMB, JR.

Gallbladder Disease

GALLBLADDER DISEASE in infants, children, and adolescents consists primarily of acute distention with hydrops, acalculous cholecystitis, and cholelithiasis of hemolytic and nonhemolytic origin. In some respects gallbladder disease in children parallels that of adults, but in other areas the differences are substantial.

Hydrops of the Gallbladder

Acute hydrops with marked distention of the gallbladder is no longer considered unusual in infancy or childhood and is being recognized with increasing frequency. Noncalculous, enlargement of the gallbladder has been associated with a number of diseases such as scarlet fever, mucocutaneous lymph node syndrome (Kawasaki's disease), diarrhea, mesenteric adenitis, leptospirosis, and familial Mediterranean fever.[45, 68, 72, 77, 83] Hydrops has been described in neonates secondary to cystic duct agenesis and to temporary obstruction of the cystic duct by lymph node enlargement.[6, 63, 72] It also has been found in a newborn with septicemia.[59] Initially, dark green bile accumulates; if obstruction is prolonged, bile is resorbed and a clear serous transudate collects.

The availability of ultrasound studies and the awareness of this condition have contributed to an increasing frequency of diagnosis. With ultrasonography, one can usually distinguish acute gallbladder distention from other disorders such as intussusception and subhepatic appendicitis.[39]

Observation, in the absence of complications, has proved successful in dealing with milder cases of hydrops without sepsis. During the observation period, gallbladder size can be monitored by serial sonography. Early resumption of oral feedings will stimulate evacuation of the gallbladder. If distention persists and tenderness increases, abdominal exploration may be necessary. At laparotomy, edema around the gallbladder, ducts, bile ducts and enlarged lymph nodes are often observed. Histologic examination of the gallbladder wall shows little or no inflammation.[16] Cholecystectomy is advised for obstruction of the cystic duct or when gangrene has developed in the gallbladder wall. In the absence of cystic duct obstruction or evidence of infarction, cholecystostomy may be employed for temporary decompression of the biliary tract. Subsequent tube cholecystography will indicate patency of the extrahepatic biliary duct system.

Acalculous Cholecystitis

Inflammation of the gallbladder without stones, rarely diagnosed in the past, is being recognized with increasing frequency today. Noncalculous cholecystitis may occur independently[2, 46, 48] but is often found in patients with other diseases such as septicemia, typhoid fever, *Salmonella* infection, giardiasis, pneumonia, and otitis media.[25, 55, 72, 76] Kawasaki's disease is associated with serious complications in children, including cystic duct obstruction from edema and gallbladder infarction. The essential lesion producing this necrosis in a patient reported by Mercer and Carpenter was arteritis.[47] Partial obstruction of the cystic duct, by enlarged lymph nodes in mesenteric adenitis or by congenital stenosis, has been thought to be an etiological factor.[6, 20, 38]

In addition, cholecystitis without calculi has been found in postoperative patients, in severe trauma cases, and following extensive burns, massive blood transfusions, or hyperalimentation.[17, 53, 55, 58, 76, 81] The condition has been observed in all ages, from the neonatal to the elderly patient.[2, 43, 49, 51] One 16-year-old girl in our series recently developed bile peritonitis from a perforated gallbladder without previous symptoms. This occurred 3 weeks following an extensive two-stage operation for removal of a recurrent acoustic neuroma, which required transfusion of 12 units of packed cells. Infants with gangrenous gallbladders, some with perforation and others with primary purulent cholecystitis, have also been reported.[2, 48, 49, 59, 76]

Multiple factors involved in development of acalculous cholecystitis include sepsis, dehydration, gallbladder stasis, prolonged parenteral alimentation, gastrointestinal ileus, and blood transfusions. Perhaps the most frequent combination of contributory factors is dehydration, absent gallbladder contractions, and gastrointestinal ileus.

Diagnosis

Usually with acalculous cholecystitis there is tenderness and muscle guarding localized in the right upper quadrant or extending to the right lower abdomen. Pain is the most common symptom, although nausea and vomiting, diarrhea, and fever may be noted. There may be leukocytosis, and patients may show jaundice with acholic stools. Pancreatitis may be associated.[46, 55] It is said that acute cholecystitis without stones is most common in young children. The sex distribution is about equal.

Plain roentgenograms of the abdomen seldom provide evidence of the diagnosis. Oral or intravenous cholangiograms may not show the gallbladder. Ultrasonography accurately depicts gallbladder distention and possible echogenic debris, which calls attention to acalculous cholecystitis. The examination can be performed quickly on seriously ill children. Diagnosis is often delayed because clinical findings suggest hepatitis, acute appendicitis, or intussusception.

Treatment

Although milder forms of noncalculous cholecystitis may be managed with nasogastric suction, intravenous fluids, and antibiotics, these patients should be monitored by a surgeon so that evidence of peritoneal irritation and impending necrosis will not go unnoticed. With progressive deterioration, persistence of a tender mass in the right subcostal region, and ultrasonic evidence of increasing gallbladder distention, the need for surgical intervention becomes evident. Cultures of bile obtained during laparotomy may be negative in spite of the frequent association of the condition with other septic diseases. Cholecystostomy has proved successful when the gallbladder is distended but not markedly inflamed. Cholecystectomy is preferred for advanced stages or when there is patchy gangrene. Pieretti and associates reported cholecystectomy performed in 11 children, 14 days to 14 years of age, without important technical difficulties or postoperative complications.[55] Cholecystostomy was deemed advisable in two patients initially, but one of these required removal of the gallbladder 3 months later. Any jaundice is related not to biliary calculi but to periductal inflammatory edema. Operative cholecystography or exploration of the common duct is seldom indicated. Postoperatively, the serum amylase and bilirubin values gradually return to normal as edema subsides.

Clinical presentation, history, and even the operative findings, bacteriologic studies, and histopathologic changes may be remarkably similar in what is called hydrops and what is called acalculous cholecystitis. Insistence on a nonoperative course solely because "hydrops" has been diagnosed is clearly not justifiable.

Cholelithiasis and Hemolytic Disease

In the past, it was widely held that the most frequent cause of gallstone development in children was hemolytic disease.[3, 25, 27, 41, 44, 54, 65, 74] However, during the last two decades the proportion of children and adolescents reported with "idiopathic" cholelithiasis has increased to over 80%, and the recognized frequency of stones resulting from hemolysis has diminished to 20% or less.[10, 18, 24, 29, 30, 31, 64, 71] Hereditary spherocytosis, sickle cell anemia, and thalassemia remain the most common hemolytic disorders associated with development of gallstones.

The male-female incidence in *hereditary spherocytosis* is either about equal or slightly higher for females. The incidence of pigment stones in children with this disorder has been estimated to range as high as 60%, but in most series is approximately 30%.[42] Several years are usually required for pigment stones to develop, although they have been noted in infants under 1 year of age. Since jaundice occurs intermittently, because of the basic hemolytic process, its development does not necessarily suggest the presence of common duct calculi.

Pigment stones may be symptomatically silent and detected only by appropriate diagnostic studies. An ultrasound evaluation is recommended for children over 2 years of age who have spherocytosis and are candidates for splenectomy. It is advisable for the surgeon to palpate the gallbladder when splenectomy is performed for hemolytic disease. Confirmation of stones or gravel indicates the need for simultaneous cholecystectomy. An upper midline or left subcostal incision with extension to the right of the midline is satisfactory in both procedures.

Sickle cell disease is one of the most serious hereditary disorders. There are about 50,000 children with this condition in the United States.[12] The public is aware of the prevalence of this disease in the American black community. About 10% carry genes for sickle cell disease. Recent studies have confirmed the increased frequency of gallstones in sickle cell disease. Calculi may be discovered in children as young as 4 years of age. The occurrence of stones rises from 10% in patients under age 10 to as high as 55% in those between 10 and 18.[40] The high incidence of cholelithiasis associated with this disease indicates the need to screen all children for gallstones who complain of upper abdominal pain before labeling them as suffering from recurrent sickle cell crisis.[1]

Cholecystectomy is advised in children with sickle cell disease and symptoms from stones, but not routinely for those without symptoms.[12, 14, 36] Preferably, cholecystectomy should be performed as an elective procedure and not during a hemolytic crisis. Before the operation, precautions should be taken to reduce the hemoglobin-S level to less than 40% by partial exchange transfusion. This will help minimize the complications that may occur during the operative and postoperative periods. In addition, children with sickle cell anemia require close attention to maintenance of hydration and normothermic conditions, adequate oxygenation, and prevention of acidosis during and after the procedure.

Gallstones now occur in only 2.3% of children with *thalassemia major* because of the current use of a hypertransfusion regimen.[8] However, ultrasonographic studies should be obtained in those who develop abdominal symptoms.

Cholelithiasis in the Absence of Hemolytic Disease

Idiopathic cholelithiasis occurs in infancy, in childhood, and during the adolescent years with sufficient frequency to warrant its consideration in the differential diagnosis of upper abdominal discomfort. Traditionally, it has been emphasized that hemolytic anemia was the primary cause of gallstones in most young patients.[3, 25, 27, 41, 44, 65, 74] In recent years, however, increasing numbers of investigators have reported that cholelithiasis occurs more frequently in children unrelated to hemolytic diseases.[10, 18, 24, 29, 30, 31, 64, 71, 73]

History

Although cholelithiasis is seen most commonly in adults, it has been known for over 250 years to occur in children. One of the early descriptions of gallstones in a child was recorded by Gibson of Leith in 1721[21] (Fig 112–1). From a 12-year-old boy, Gibson removed "three Scotch pints of water of a greenish hue" by paracentesis from the child's abdomen about 18 months after an injury. The boy died 2 days later, and autopsy revealed a distended gallbladder and common duct filled with many spongy yellow stones. Little interest in childhood cholelithiasis was evident until Blalock's report in 1924[5] and Potter's in 1938.[56] Ulin et al. completed a comprehensive study of cholecystitis in children in 1952 and accepted 326 cases reported in the literature as having a valid diagnosis.[79]

Until 1960, about 500 cases had been described, but most authors reviewed other reports and added only a few from their own personal experience. Since 1960, increasing numbers of children and adolescents with cholelithiasis have been reported in individual reviews, the largest single study being of 83 patients.[31] Interest in this subject has risen rapidly in the past decade, and two misconceptions that formerly prevailed, namely that the condition is uncommon and that most gallstones in children result from hemolytic disease, have been corrected.

Etiology

DEMOGRAPHIC FEATURES.—The occurrence of gallstones varies from country to country, as well as in different races and with varying genetic influences. Nonhemolytic cholelithiasis is relatively uncommon in American black children.[7] In Chile, 5–8% of adolescent girls and 25–30% of young women develop gallstones from cholesterol hypersecretion.[80] The female Pima Indians of Arizona, who secrete supersaturated bile, reach an 80% incidence of cholesterol stones as they get older.[61, 62] In contrast, the Masai in Africa, whose bile is only half-saturated, rarely develop biliary calculi.[4, 62] The hereditary influence is reinforced by the discovery that sisters of young women with cholesterol stones have more highly saturated bile than sisters of controls.[19] Caucasians are second only to the American Indian in developing biliary concretions. The prevalence of gallstones among adult whites in Europe and the United States varies between 10% and 20% and increases to as high as 40% with advanced age. In the western world, high-cholesterol and low-fiber diets predominate, very likely contributing to the high occurrence of this disease. Glenn stated that the development of gallstones has reached epidemic proportions in the adult population in this country.[23]

AGE.—Cholelithiasis is found in increasing numbers in each decade of life from before birth to old age. Although rare, gallstones in infants have recently been reported, often in association with some anatomic deformity of the biliary system, extensive small-bowel resection, or long-term parenteral nutrition. A 6-week-old infant and a 6-day-old neonate without these associated conditions have been described with stones, perforation of the gallbladder, and bile peritonitis.[33, 70] Cholecystostomy and choledochotomy with removal of small nonpigmented stones was performed in another 4-month-old infant. Four years later, cholecystectomy was required for cystic duct obstruction from another stone.[15]

SEX.—The female-male ratio of adults who develop stones is generally accepted as 4:1. The ratio is considerably higher in adolescents. Soderlund and Zetterstrom[71] reported a 19:1 ratio; Odom et al., 22:1;[50] Holcomb et al., 14:1;[31] and Strauss, 11:0.[73]

PREGNANCY.—As early as 1966, attention was called to the frequent association of biliary calculi and teenage pregnancy.[38] In a more recent study of 14–18-year-old girls with gallstones, 65% were or had been pregnant, and none had hemolytic anemia.[31] Thirteen developed symptoms during pregnancy, 23 within 6 months of delivery and nine more than 6 months postpartum.

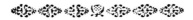

XXX. *An extraordinary large Gall-Bladder and hydropick Cystis; by Mr.* JOSEPH GIBSON *Surgeon in* Leith, *Member of the Society of Surgeon Apothecaries of* Edinburgh, *and City Professor of Midwifery.*

WILLIAM GORDON, of a healthy Habit, when about twelve Years of Age, in *October* 1721, fell from a Wall of three Yards perpendicular Height a-cross an old Tree, on which his right Side struck; and he immediately complained of an acute Pain all over the Bastard Ribs

His Legs, which only pitted towards the Evening, during eight Months after his Fall, were in *November* 1721, constantly swelled, as were his Thighs and Belly. About the Middle of *January* following, Water was felt fluctuating in his *Abdomen*, and, till the Beginning of *April* thereafter, all his Symptoms increased daily, especially the Difficulty of breathing, which did not allow him to sit, far less to ly down;

but some Days before his Death he was obliged to stand erect, supported by Chairs, Tables, or the People about him, while he slumbered.

and of Mr. *Adam Lindsay* Chirurgeon-Apothecary in *Edinburgh*, I drew off by the Trocar near three *Scots* Pints or twelve Pounds of Water, of a greenish Hue, having a gross Sediment of the same Colour.

Wound was dressed as usual. He died the second Day after the Operation, being the 3d of *April*, and I was allowed to inspect his Body on the 5th.

The *Ductus communis cholidochus* was larger than usual, and was filled with many small spongy Stones of a yellowish Hue that swam in Water.

Fig 112–1.—Excerpt from the article by Mr. Joseph Gibson, surgeon in Leith (Scotland), describing events following an injury to a 12-year-old boy in 1721.

Similar observations have been made by others.[18, 24, 50, 64] Honore found a history of recent pregnancy in 18 of 31 (58.1%) teenagers with gallstones, but in only five of 112 (4.5%) control patients of the same ages who underwent other operative procedures.[32]

Indeed, pregnancy has been determined to be cholestatic.[67] In addition, twice as many women of childbearing age who use oral contraceptives have developed gallbladder disease as have nonusers.[7] Gallstones have been produced experimentally in rabbits by the prolonged injection of progesterone and estradiol, simulating the hormones manufactured by the placenta during pregnancy.[34]

Although the exact physiologic mechanism of stone formation is not known, pregnancy, gallbladder stasis, and obesity seem to accentuate the hereditary predisposition of females.

OBESITY.—Body weight in excess of 10% of normal for height and age has been reported in association with gallstones in 33–54% of patients.[31, 32] Honore concluded that obesity in adolescents predisposes to the formation of cholesterol calculi.[32]

TOTAL PARENTERAL NUTRITION (TPN).—Bile stasis, resulting in elevation of total and direct bilirubin, has been observed in infants receiving long-term parenteral hyperalimentation.[78] Several reports have described stones in premature infants treated for respiratory distress syndrome who received total parenteral nutrition (TPN) and furosemide.[9, 13, 82] Some authors, however, claim that cholestasis and hepatobiliary dysfunction in premature infants are related more to fasting within the first few weeks of life than to parenteral nutrition.[57]

In a prospective evaluation of 21 children receiving long-term intravenous nutrition, nine (43%) developed cholelithiasis and five have since undergone cholecystectomy.[60] Two thirds of these children had pre-existing ileal disease or had undergone extensive small-bowel resection. The mean age of this group was 52.3 months, the youngest only 8 months of age. There appears to be a direct correlation between duration of hyperalimentation and development of calculi. Children in this study who developed gallstones had received TPN more than twice as long as their counterparts who did not develop stones. Concretions have been detected as soon as 8 months after institution of TPN, but the average time in Roslyn's report was 36 months.[60] Analysis by infrared spectroscopy in four of the children indicated the stone consisted mainly of calcium bilirubinate. The cholesterol content was less than 20% by weight. Although TPN diminishes gallbladder evacuation, the absence of oral feedings also contributes to gallbladder stasis and, in turn, the development of noncholesterol stones.

The diagnosis of gallbladder disease in infants and children receiving TPN may be very difficult. Symptoms often are confusing or absent. Liver function tests are frequently abnormal with hyperalimentation and are therefore unreliable for diagnostic determinations. Ultrasonography or radionuclide scans combined with constant clinical suspicion assist greatly in the diagnosis. Periodic surveillance with ultrasonography should be obtained in patients receiving hyperalimentation longer than 6 weeks. Cholecystectomy should be considered for children who develop gallstones while receiving TPN, particularly those with symptoms.

POSTOPERATIVE.—Of the patients receiving prolonged parenteral nutrition, those who appear to be at greatest risk have had ileal disorders or resection of the terminal ileum. Pellerin and associates reported two 1-year-old infants and a 7-year-old child who developed gallstones following ileal resection.[52] The stones were detected 8 months, 18 months, and 27 months following the initial operation. The role of the distal small intestine in the enterohepatic transport of bile salts is essential for normal balance of bile circulation. Resection or disease involving the terminal ileum alters this cycle and disrupts the equilibrium among cholesterol, bile salts, and lecithin. The implication that ileal resection might contribute to gallstone formation has special meaning for pediatric surgeons who find it necessary to do ileocolectomies for necrotizing enterocolitis, midgut volvulus, irreducible intussusception, and other conditions. Cholelithiasis also has developed following cardiac valve replacement, duodenal operations, and gastrectomy, particularly in association with vagotomy.[7, 41, 75]

Children at risk for developing calculi following these operative procedures should be evaluated annually and appropriate sonographic studies obtained to detect gallstones.

BILIARY PANCREATITIS.—Pancreatitis secondary to intermittent passage of calculi down the common duct, producing temporary or prolonged obstruction at the sphincter of Oddi, is uncommon in teenagers. A recent review of pancreatitis in 30 children indicated no instances of biliary pancreatitis.[11] In the Vanderbilt Children's Hospital study, however, six teenagers were diagnosed as having biliary pancreatitis.[31] All six were girls whose ages ranged between 13 and 18 years. Each complained of epigastric or right upper quadrant pain with midback radiation, and the diagnosis was confirmed with the finding of hyperamylasemia. None were clinically jaundiced, although some had slightly elevated bilirubin levels.

The acute pancreatitis was allowed to subside with nasogastric suction and intravenous fluids. At cholecystectomy, small stones were found in the gallbladder in each patient. Pancreatitis promptly subsided, did not recur, and the convalescence of each was uneventful.

CONGENITAL DEFORMITIES.—Major developmental anomalies of the gallbladder described by Gross include agenesis, duplication, bilobation, floating gallbladder, diverticulum, and ectopia.[26] Formation of calculi has been recorded in association with several of these conditions, also in fusiform choledochal cysts and diverticula of the gallbladder or of the cystic duct.[20, 28] Forshall and Rickham described two children with gallstones and congenital stenosis of the cystic duct.[20]

INFECTION.—As early as 1892, Naunyn thought superimposed infection played a part in the development of cholelithiasis.[7] Rather than causing the stones, it seems more probable that infection and secondary inflammatory changes result from the presence of these stones.

Pathology

COMPOSITION OF STONES.—Most idiopathic gallstones in children and teenagers are composed of varying proportions of pigment (calcium bilirubinate), cholesterol, and calcium. Calculi removed from adult Americans consist predominantly of cholesterol, while in Orientals pigment stones are more commonly found. Why stones form is not known. One popular belief is that bile supersaturated with cholesterol is responsible for calculus formation.[69] Pure cholesterol stones are soft, pale yellow, usually smaller in size, and occur infrequently. Most nonpigment stones are of the mixed cholesterol variety and vary in size from sandy concretions to aggregates up to 2.5 cm in diameter. Pigment calculi, from hemolysis, are composed largely of calcium bilirubinate, usually shaped like a mulberry, and black in color. Such stones develop in infants and children receiving prolonged parenteral hyperalimentation and following extensive distal small-bowel resection (Fig 112–2).

Histologic evaluation of the gallbladder in chronic cholelithiasis shows scarring and thickening, but occasionally acute in-

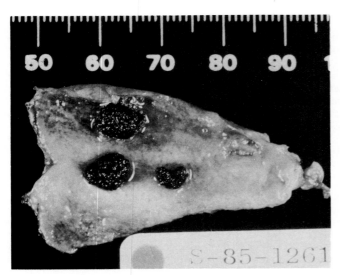

Fig 112–2.—This gallbladder, from a 3-year-old boy, contains varying-sized stones. The largest stone measured 7.2 mm and was composed of 100% calcium carbonate. As a neonate with necrotizing enterocolitis, he had an ileal resection and received hyperalimentation.

flammation, or even normal mucosa, is associated with stones in young people.

Clinical Features

SYMPTOMS.—While some children in the Vanderbilt study complained of food intolerance, especially greasy foods, many did not experience these symptoms.[31] Although nausea, vomiting, and anorexia were noted, the most common complaint was abdominal pain. Sometimes this pain was intermittent or colicky with maximal discomfort in the right upper quadrant, right lower, or left upper abdomen. Radiation to the back and right shoulder was sometimes noted, particularly by the older teenagers. Many of the younger children could not localize pain well but often described a general midabdominal or periumbilical dis-

comfort. Gallstones may exist without recognized symptoms, particularly if they are too large to pass into the cystic duct.

DIAGNOSIS.—An indication of the difficulty in diagnosing gallbladder disease in children is the fact that 15–20% have had an appendectomy for the original symptoms.[37] Soderlund and Zetterstrom reported that disease of the gallbladder was suspected initially in only half of their cases (30/60).[71] In the other half, up to 10 years elapsed before the correct diagnosis was made. Reports of a 4-year-old girl and of a teenager being referred for psychiatric guidance because of unexplained abdominal pain, later diagnosed as gallstone colic, give additional support to the difficulty of this diagnosis.[31, 66] Both patients experienced complete relief following cholecystectomy.

Physical examination usually shows some tenderness in the right subcostal area with or without muscle guarding. On occasion, a tender, distended gallbladder can be palpated. Temperature may be slightly elevated as may the leukocyte count or sedimentation rate. Jaundice is not often encountered unless associated with common duct obstruction or hemolytic disease. Serum cholesterol level is seldom elevated, and serum lipid values have been reported below normal.[29] The differential diagnosis should include hepatitis, appendicitis, intussusception, pancreatitis, chronic constipation, and abdominal epilepsy.

GALLBLADDER ASSESSMENT.—Plain abdominal roentgenograms may accurately identify opaque gallstones, but lucent calculi must be diagnosed by other studies. Oral cholecystography in the past has proved to be the most accurate diagnostic test (Fig 112–3), but ultrasonography is rapidly supplanting this modality as the first choice of most clinicians, in spite of occasional false-negative observations. Oral cholecystography is not the most appropriate diagnostic study in infants and young children unable to swallow tablets, nor is it useful in the presence of jaundice or following extensive bowel resection. In these situations, ultrasonic imaging is definitely preferred. Gray-scale and, in particular, real-time ultrasonography provide an early, accurate, and noninvasive method of diagnosing cholelithiasis in children. When the gallbladder can be identified by ultrasound studies, a stone discovery rate as high as 98% is expected[22] (Fig 112–4).

Although ultrasound imaging is successful in delineating ana-

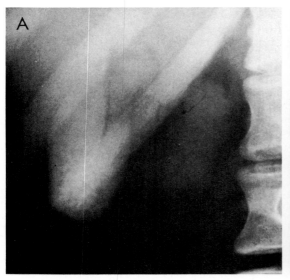
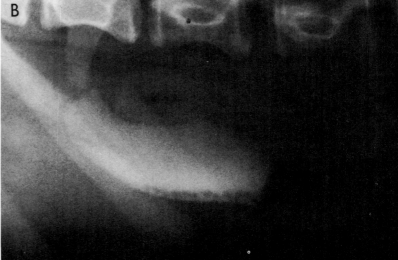

Fig 112–3.—The oral cholecystogram in cholelithiasis. **A,** oral cholecystogram in a 16-year-old girl with multiple small nonpigment stones, who developed acute cholecystitis 2 months postpartum. Symptoms started during the last month of pregnancy. **B,** lateral decubitus view of the cholecystogram illustrating layering effect that confirms presence of multiple calculi.

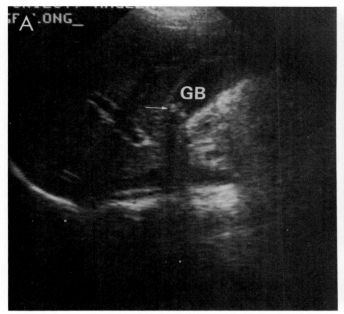

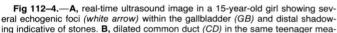

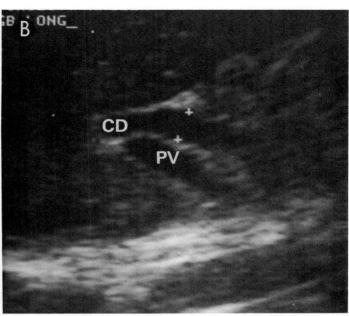

Fig 112–4.—**A,** real-time ultrasound image in a 15-year-old girl showing several echogenic foci *(white arrow)* within the gallbladder *(GB)* and distal shadowing indicative of stones. **B,** dilated common duct *(CD)* in the same teenager measures 0.93 cm in its greatest diameter. The portal vein *(PV)* is just below the common duct.

tomical structures such as the gallbladder and the extrahepatic ducts and for detecting calculi and their size, it is not a test of function and cannot be used to diagnose acute cholecystitis. Cholescintigraphy, with one of the technetium 99m-labeled acetanilide iminodiacetic acid (^{99m}Tc IDA) derivatives, is currently the most accurate method of evaluating the patient with acute cholecystitis, notably one with obstruction of the cystic duct.[35] Cholescintigraphy is also useful in determining patency of the common duct in the presence of jaundice, assessing traumatic and postoperative biliary extravasation, and detecting congenital choledochal cysts.

Cholecystography and ultrasonography are recommended for evaluation of children and adolescent girls who complain of vague, otherwise unexplained epigastric and right abdominal pain.

Treatment

STONE DISSOLUTION.—Nonoperative dissolution of gallstones is undergoing intense research, but the success rate has been a disappointing 13.5% in the high-dose chenodeoxycholic acid (CDCA) group. There are no reports of its use in children.

OPERATIVE TREATMENT.—In the absence of inflammation in the gallbladder wall, some surgeons have advised cholecystostomy and simple removal of stones. The experience with adults has indicated that gallbladder disease recurs and may require subsequent operative procedures. This disappointing recurrence has also been reported for children who have undergone cholecystostomy.[15, 71] Elective removal of the gallbladder by a well-trained pediatric surgeon who is careful to identify the anatomical structures carries a very low risk. Most children tolerate cholecystectomy very well, and this is the procedure of choice.

Operative cholangiograms should be obtained if the gallbladder contains stones small enough to pass through the cystic duct, if there is a history of jaundice, or when the common duct is dilated (Fig 112–5). In many institutions, cholangiography is always performed during cholecystectomy for stone.

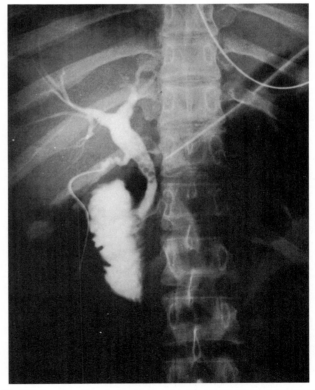

Fig 112–5.—Operative cholangiogram in a 15-year-old girl convalescing from biliary pancreatitis with an initial serum amylase level of 9,600 Somogyi units. Symptoms had recurred several times during the previous 12 months. Multiple lucent defects suggest either stones or air bubbles in the common duct. The proximal segment of the common duct and the common hepatic duct are dilated. Choledochotomy revealed no calculi, but the gallbladder contained several stones.

Complications such as biliary dyskinesia are seldom noted in young postcholecystectomy patients. In one study, only three of 59 children developed moderate biliary dyskinesia following gallbladder removal.[71] In the Vanderbilt group of 73 patients 18 years of age and under who underwent cholecystectomy for idiopathic stones, morbidity was minimal and mortality was zero.[31] Two wound infections developed, and one girl required enterolysis for relief of intestinal obstruction.

REFERENCES

1. Ariyan S., Shessel F.S., Pickett L.K.: Cholecystitis and cholelithiasis masking as abdominal crises in sickle cell disease. *Pediatrics* 58:252, 1976.
2. Arnspiger L.A., Martin J.G., Krempin H.O.: Acute non-calculous cholecystitis in children. *Am. J. Surg.* 100:103, 1960.
3. Barnett H.L. (ed.): *Pediatrics*, ed. 15. New York, Appleton-Century-Crofts, 1972, p. 709.
4. Biss K., Ho K.J., Mikkelson B., et al.: Some unique biologic characteristics of the Masai of East Africa. *N. Engl. J. Med.* 184:694, 1971.
5. Blalock A.: A statistical study of 888 cases of biliary tract disease. *Bull. Johns Hopkins Hosp.* 35:391, 1924.
6. Bloom R.A., Swain V.A.J.: Non-calculous distention of the gall-bladder in childhood. *Arch. Dis. Child.* 41:503, 1966.
7. Bockus H.L.: *Gastroenterology*, vol. 3. Philadelphia, W.B. Saunders Co., 1976, p. 752.
8. Borgna-Pignatti C., de Stefano P., Pajno D., et al.: Cholelithiasis in children with thalassemia major: An ultrasonic study. *J. Pediatr.* 99:243, 1981.
9. Boyle R.J., Sumner T.E., Volberg F.M.: Cholelithiasis in a three-week small premature infant. *Pediatrics* 71:967, 1983.
10. Brenner R.W., Stewart C.F.: Cholecystitis in children. *Rev. Surg.* 21:327, 1964.
11. Buntain W.L., Wood J.B., Woolley M.M.: Pancreatitis in childhood. *J. Pediatr. Surg.* 13:143, 1978.
12. Burrington J.D., Smith M.D.: Elective and emergency surgery in children with sickle cell disease. *Surg. Clin. North Am.* 56:55, 1976.
13. Callahan J., Haller J.O., Cacciarelli A.A., et al.: Cholelithiasis in infants. *Radiology* 143:437, 1982.
14. Cameron J.L., Maddrey W.C., Zuidema G.D.: Biliary tract disease in sickle cell anemia: Surgical considerations. *Ann. Surg.* 174:702, 1971.
15. Carswell W.R., Willis J.D.: Cholecystitis with gall-stones in infancy and childhood. *Br. J. Surg.* 56:547, 1969.
16. Chamberlain J.W., Hight D.W.: Acute hydrops of the gallbladder in childhood. *Surgery* 68:899, 1970.
17. Chen P.S., Aliapoulios M.A.: Acute acalculous cholecystitis—ultrasonic appearance. *Arch. Surg.* 113:1461, 1978.
18. Crichlow R.W., Seltzer M.H., Jannetta P.J.: Cholecystitis in adolescents. *Dig. Dis.* 17:68, 1972.
19. Danzinger R.G., Gordon H., Shoenfield L.J., et al.: Lithogenic bile in siblings of young women with cholelithiasis. *Mayo Clin. Proc.* 47:762, 1972.
20. Forshall I., Rickham P.P.: Gallbladder disease in childhood. *Br. J. Surg.* 42:161, 1955.
21. Gibson J.: An extraordinary large Gall-Bladder and hydropick Cystis: Medical Essays and Observations. *Philosoph. Soc. Edin.* 2:352, 1737.
22. Gibson J.Y., Pomeroy C.: Evaluation of the gallbladder by gray scale ultrasonography. *South. Med. J.* 72:1285, 1979.
23. Glenn F.: An update on our epidemic of gallstones. *Med. Times* 106:38, 1978.
24. Goodman, D.P.: Cholelithiasis in persons under twenty-five years old. *JAMA* 236:1731, 1976.
25. Gravier L., Dorman G.W., Votteler T.P.: Gallbladder disease in infants and children. *Surgery* 63:690, 1968.
26. Gross R.E.: Congenital anomalies of the gallbladder. *Arch. Surg.* 32:131, 1936.
27. Gross R.E.: *The Surgery of Infancy and Childhood.* Philadelphia, W.B. Saunders Co., 1953, p. 531.
28. Haff R.C., Andrassy R.J., Legrand D.R., et al.: Gallbladder disease in the young male. *Am. J. Surg.* 131:232, 1976.
29. Hagberg B., Svennerholm L., Thoren L.: Cholelithiasis in childhood. *Acta Chir. Scand.* 123:307, 1962.
30. Harned R.K., Babbitt D.P.: Cholelithiasis in children. *Radiology* 117:391, 1975.
31. Holcomb G.W. Jr., O'Neill J.A. Jr., Holcomb G.W. III: Cholecystitis, cholelithiasis and common duct stenosis in children and adolescents. *Ann. Surg.* 191:626, 1980.
32. Honore L.H.: Cholesterol cholelithiasis in adolescent females. *Arch. Surg.* 115:62, 1980.
33. Hughes R.G., Mayell M.J.: Cholelithiasis in a neonate. *Arch. Dis. Child.* 50:815, 1975.
34. Imamoglu K., Wangensteen S.L., Root H.D., et al.: Production of gallstones by prolonged administration of progesterone and estradiol in rabbits. *Surg. Forum* 10:246, 1960.
35. Johnson D.G., Coleman R.E.: New techniques in radionuclide imaging of the alimentary system. *Radiol. Clin. North Am.* 20:635, 1982.
36. Karayalcin G., Hassani N., Abrams M., et al.: Cholelithiasis in children with sickle cell disease. *Am. J. Dis. Child.* 133:306, 1979.
37. Kiesewetter W.B.: Cholecystitis and cholelithiasis, in Benson C.D., Mustard W.T., Ravitch M.M., et al. (eds.): *Pediatric Surgery*, ed. 2. Chicago, Year Book Medical Publishers, 1969, p. 745.
38. Kirtley J.A. Jr., Holcomb G.W. Jr.: Surgical management of diseases of the gallbladder and common duct in children and adolescents. *Am. J. Surg.* 111:39, 1966.
39. Kumari S., Lee W.J., Baron M.G.: Hydrops of the gallbladder in a child: Diagnosis by ultrasonography. *Pediatrics* 63:295, 1979.
40. Lackman B.S., Lazerson J., Starshak R.J., et al.: The prevalence of cholelithiasis in sickle cell disease as diagnosed by ultrasound and cholecystography. *Pediatrics* 64:601, 1979.
41. Lau G.E., Andrassy R.J., Mahour G.H.: A thirty year review of the management of gallbladder disease at a children's hospital. *Am. Surg.* 49:411, 1983.
42. Lawre G.M., Ham J.M.: The surgical treatment of hereditary spherocytosis. *Surg. Gynecol. Obstet.* 139:208, 1974.
43. Lucas C.E., Walt A.J.: Acute gangrenous acalculous cholecystitis in infancy. *Surgery* 64:847, 1968.
44. MacMillan R.W., Schullinger J.N., Santulli T.V.: Cholelithiasis in childhood. *Am. J. Surg.* 127:689, 1974.
45. Magilavy D.B., Speert P., Silver T.M., et al.: Mucocutaneous lymph node syndrome: Report of two cases complicated by gallbladder hydrops and diagnosed by ultrasound. *Pediatrics* 61:699, 1978.
46. Marks C., Espinosa J., Hyman L.J.: Acute acalculous cholecystitis in childhood. *J. Pediatr. Surg.* 3:608, 1968.
47. Mercer S., Carpenter B.: Surgical complications of Kawasaki's disease. *J. Pediatr. Surg.* 16:444, 1981.
48. Mukamel E., Zer M., Avidor I., et al.: Acute acalculous cholecystitis in an infant: A case report. *J. Pediatr. Surg.* 16:521, 1981.
49. Oates G.D.: Perforated empyema of the gallbladder in an infant. *Br. J. Surg.* 48:686, 1961.
50. Odom F.C., Oliver B.B., Kline M., et al.: Gallbladder disease in patients 20 years of age and under. *South. Med. J.* 69:1299, 1976.
51. Orlando R., Gleason E., Drezner A.D.: Acute acalculous cholecystitis in the critically ill patient. *Am. J. Surg.* 145:472, 1983.
52. Pellerin D., Bertin P., Nihoul-Féketé C., et al.: Cholecystitis and ileal pathology in childhood. *J. Pediatr. Surg.* 10:35, 1975.
53. Peterson S.R., Sheldon G.F.: Acute acalculous cholecystitis: A complication of hyperalimentation. *Am. J. Surg.* 138:814, 1979.
54. Pickett L.K.: Liver and biliary tract, in Benson C.D., Mustard W.T., Ravitch M.M., et al. (eds.): *Pediatric Surgery*, ed. 1. Chicago, Year Book Medical Publishers, 1962, p. 628.
55. Pieretti R., Auldist A.W., Stephens C.A.: Acute cholecystitis in children. *Surg. Gynecol. Obstet.* 140:16; 1975.
56. Potter A.H.: Biliary disease in young subjects. *Surg. Gynecol. Obstet.* 66:604, 1938.
57. Rager R., Finegold M.J.: Cholestasis in immature newborn infants: Is parenteral alimentation responsible? *J. Pediatr.* 86:264, 1975.
58. Rice J., Williams H.C., Flint L.M., et al.: Posttraumatic acalculous cholecystitis. *South. Med. J.* 73:14, 1980.
59. Robinson A.E., Erwin J.H., Wiseman H.J., et al.: Cholecystitis and hydrops of the gallbladder in the newborn. *Radiology* 122:749, 1977.
60. Roslyn J.J., Berquist W.E., Pitt H.A., et al.: Increased risk of gallstones in children receiving total parenteral nutrition. *Pediatrics* 71:784, 1983.
61. Sampliner R.E., Bennett P.H., Comess L.J., et al.: Gallbladder disease in Pima Indians. *N. Engl. J. Med.* 283:1358, 1970.
62. Schiff L., Schiff E.R.: *Diseases of the Liver*, ed. 5. Philadelphia, J.B. Lippincott Co., 1982, pp. 1513–1521.
63. Scobie W.G., Bentley J.F.R.: Hydrops of the gallbladder in a newborn infant. *J. Pediatr. Surg.* 4:457, 1969.
64. Sears H.F., Golden G.T., Horsley J.S.: Cholecystitis in childhood and adolescence. *Arch. Surg.* 106:651, 1973.
65. Seiler I.: Gallbladder disease in children. *Am. J. Dis. Child.* 99:662, 1960.
66. Shrand H., Ackroyd F.W.: Gallstones in children. *Clin. Pediatr.* 12:191, 1973.
67. Simcock M.J., Forster F.M.C.: Pregnancy is cholestatic. *Med. J. Aust.* 2:971, 1967.
68. Slovis T.L., Hight D.W., Philippart A.I., et al.: Sonography in the

diagnosis and management of hydrops of the gallbladder in children with mucocutaneous lymph-node syndrome. *Pediatrics* 65:789, 1980.

69. Small D.M., Rapo S.: Source of abnormal bile in patients with cholesterol gallstones. *N. Engl. J. Med.* 283:53, 1970.
70. Snyder W.H. Jr., Chaffin L., Oettinger L.: Cholelithiasis and perforation of the gallbladder in an infant, with recovery. *JAMA* 149:1645, 1952.
71. Soderlund S., Zetterstrom B.: Cholecystitis and cholelithiasis in children. *Arch. Dis. Child.* 37:174, 1962.
72. Strauss R.G.: Scarlet fever with hydrops of the gallbladder. *Pediatrics* 44:741, 1969.
73. Strauss R.G.: Cholelithiasis in childhood. *Am. J. Dis. Child.* 117:689, 1969.
74. Swenson O.: *Pediatric Surgery.* New York, Appleton-Century Crofts, 1958, p. 280.
75. Tchirkow G., Highman L.M., Shafer A.D.: Cholelithiasis and cholecystitis in children after repair of congenital duodenal anomalies. *Arch. Surg.* 115:85, 1980.

76. Ternberg J.L., Keating J.P.: Acute acalculous cholecystitis. *Arch. Surg.* 110:543, 1975.
77. Todd D.W., Rosen W.C., Miller R.H.: Hydrops of the gallbladder in children—diagnosis and management. *Minn. Med.* 66:81, 1983.
78. Touloukian R.J., Downing S.E.: Cholestasis associated with long-term parenteral hyperalimentation. *Arch. Surg.* 106:58, 1973.
79. Ulin A.W., Nosal J.L., Martin W.L.: Cholecystitis in childhood. *Surgery* 31:312, 1952.
80. Valdivieso V., Palma R., Nervi F., et al.: Secretion of biliary lipids in young Chilean women with cholesterol gallstones. *Gut* 20:997, 1979.
81. Wald M.: Gangrenous cholecystitis with bile peritonitis as a complication of burns in a 14-year-old boy. *Med. J. Aust.* 48:553, 1961.
82. Whitington P.F., Black D.D.: Cholecystitis in premature infants treated with parenteral nutrition and furosemide. *J. Pediatr.* 97:647, 1980.
83. Wong M.L., Kaplan S., Dunkle L.M., et al.: Leptospirosis: A childhood disease. *J. Pediatr.* 90:532, 1977.

113 ROBERT J. TOULOUKIAN

Nonmalignant Liver Tumors and Hepatic Infections

PEDIATRIC HEPATIC TUMORS are the third most common abdominal solid tumors in children, following Wilms tumor and neuroblastoma.[7] Benign hepatic cysts and tumors account for approximately one third of all cases. Young and Miller[51] and Dehner[5] report the incidence of these lesions to be about 0.7 per million population per year.

The largest collected series of liver tumors in children, reported by members of the Surgical Section of the American Academy of Pediatrics, represents the combined 20-year experience of some 200 pediatric surgeons[12] (Table 113–1). This and recent reports from single institutions[10, 11] indicate that the three main categories of benign liver tumors are: (1) congenital cysts; (2) solid tumors, including those of epithelial origin, such as liver cell or bile duct adenomas, hamartomas composed of both epithelial and mesenchymal elements, and "pseudo" tumors, such as focal nodular hyperplasia; (3) vascular lesions, including cavernous hemangiomas and hemangioendothelioma of infancy.

In almost every case, the diagnosis of a benign liver tumor can be made by detecting clinical enlargement of the abdomen and an upper abdominal mass that may be ill-defined if the tumor is large enough to involve an entire lobe, particularly the right. Extension of the mass into the right posterior abdomen may make the tumor appear to be of flank origin. Associated symptoms, including a sense of fullness, satiety, or abdominal pain, depend on the degree and rapidity of enlargement. An acute abdominal crisis with severe pain and hypotension signals rupture of the tumor with intraperitoneal hemorrhage. The combination of hepatic enlargement and congestive heart failure with a bruit over the liver is clearly diagnostic of a vascular lesion arising from the liver. Rapid assessment of liver tumors and prompt diagnosis are essential, since the differential always must include the possibility of malignancy. Initial work-up includes plain abdominal films and ultrasonography. Ultrasound is the simplest way to determine the consistency of the lesion. Solid tumors should be further studied by computerized tomography for better differentiation of their internal structure. Angiography before resection is required by some to assess the arterial supply of the liver.

Cysts

Simple *congenital* cysts of the liver are often large enough to be detected on physical examination and are easily distinguished from solid tumors by ultrasonography. Symptoms are uncommon and related to compression of adjacent viscera.[17] Hemorrhage, perforation, or torsion are very rare complications.[13] The cyst is lined by cuboidal epithelium, probably of biliary origin, contains clear serous fluid, may be loculated, and only rarely communicates with the biliary tree. Epidermoid cysts of the liver—ex-

TABLE 113–1.—BENIGN LIVER TUMORS IN CHILDREN*

TUMOR	NO. OF PATIENTS	
Hemangioma	54	
Cavernous		38
Hemangioendothelioma		16
Hamartoma	37	
Cysts	16	
Simple		10
Hydatid		6
Adenoma	7	
Focal nodular hyperplasia	5	
Lymphangioma	2	
Eosinophilic granuloma	1	

*From Exelby P.R. et al.[12]

tremely rare—are believed to be derived from accessory foregut buds.[46] Treatment of a solitary cyst varies according to its size and location within the liver. Operative cholangiography is useful in determining the exact relation of the bile ducts to the cyst and whether or not a biliary communication exists. Operative excision of the cyst alone may be difficult because of adjacent major bile ducts and vessels. Under such circumstances, wedge resection or lobectomy is appropriate. For large cysts involving both lobes of the liver, internal drainage to a Roux-en-Y limb of jejunum is preferable. Alternatively, the cyst may be completely unroofed and the edges secured with a running absorbable suture. In the absence of a biliary communication, this maneuver merely results in a little serous drainage into the peritoneal cavity, from which the cyst fluid is resorbed (Fig 113–1).

Polycystic disease of the liver is an inherited defect of unknown etiology,[47] associated with polycystic kidney in over 50% of affected patients. Liver function is generally well preserved despite extensive hepatic replacement by cysts. When extensive cystic replacement results in hepatic failure, there is, at present, no treatment except hepatic transplantation.

Solid Tumors

Hepatoadenoma

Hepatoadenoma is a rare, benign, encapsulated tumor, usually accompanied by glycogen storage disease, type I (von Gierke's disease).[15] The tumor is generally a solitary mass located in the right lobe, and presents more commonly in females during the second decade of life. Nuclear scanning shows an area of decreased uptake. These tumors are vascular, and angiography is likely to demonstrate large feeding vessels. Nearly one quarter of reported patients have had an acute abdominal crisis due to an intraperitoneal hemorrhage from infarction and rupture.

Wedge resection or lobectomy is indicated and is usually technically feasible. The cut surface of this tumor reveals a homogeneous brownish parenchyma. Microscopy shows well-differentiated large hepatocytes with no discernible portal structures or portal veins.[5] The risk of recurrence following resection is low. Mitoses are rarely seen, and there is no evidence that the lesion is premalignant.

Mesenchymal Hamartoma

Mesenchymal hamartoma has also been referred to as cystic mesenchymal hamartoma, hamartoma, lymphangioma, cavernous lymphangiomatoid tumor, and solitary bile cell fibroadenoma. The term "mesenchymal hamartoma" was initially used by Edmondson[9] to describe a large mass composed of multiple cysts of various sizes filled with clear fluid or mucoid material. On occasion, the tissue is discolored due to old hemorrhage. A connective tissue stroma combined with bile ducts, liver cells, and angiomatous components characterizes the hamartoma, which is defined as a benign malformation composed of disordered tissue cells normally present in the involved organ. The tumor is detected during the first year of life in about 80% of patients. Plain abdominal films show a soft tissue mass, the cystic nature of which may be confirmed by ultrasonography. The degree of vascularity varies, depending on the prominence of the angiomatous components (Fig 113–2). Significant numbers of vascular channels may precipitate congestive heart failure from arteriovenous shunting,[43] and the histopathologic distinction from hemangiomas of the liver is difficult. Resection is the treatment of choice. For predominantly cystic lesions of large size, internal drainage may be feasible and desirable. This can be accomplished by Roux-en-Y technique. Alternatively, the cyst may be opened into the free peritoneal cavity for drainage and reabsorption.[26]

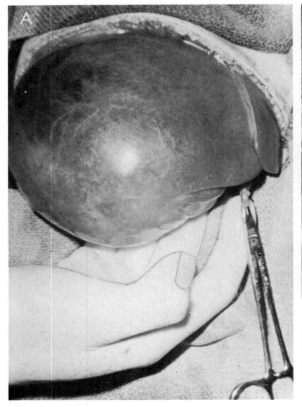
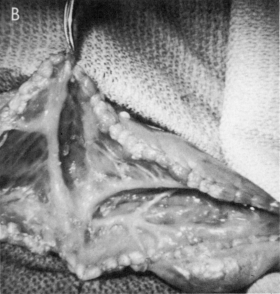

Fig 113–1.—Simple cyst of liver. **A,** simple congenital cyst occupying most of the right lobe of the liver. **B,** cyst of liver surgically prepared for permanent intraperitoneal drainage. Note internal anatomical architecture of liver viewed through the posterior cyst wall. The edge of the liver has been whipped with a running locked absorbable suture. The secretion is serous, and there is no communication with the biliary tree. (Courtesy of Dr. J. Randolph and Dr. R.P. Altman.)

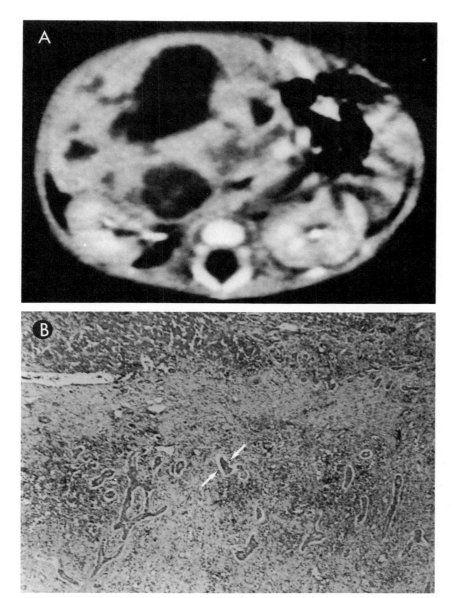

Fig 113–2.—One-month-old infant with an immense cystic mesenchymal hamartoma, occupying most of the right lobe. **A,** some areas opacify on CT scan following injection of Renografin-60, while others remain clear, suggesting necrosis. The tumor is multilobulated and vascular. Parenchymal staining as well as lucencies are consistent with tumor necrosis. A lobectomy was performed. The patient has survived and has done well. **B,** microscopy shows proliferating bile ducts entrapped *(arrows)* within a vascularized fibrous stroma.

Focal Nodular Hyperplasia

The etiology of focal nodular hyperplasia remains obscure. This tumor is believed to arise in response to a focal hepatic injury[9] or to arterialization by an anomalous artery.[49] It also has been reported in a child with sickle cell disease.[28] The lesion occurs in all age groups, but in a recent review of liver tumors,[10] the three children with focal nodular hyperplasia were between 2 and 5 years of age. The tumor is usually large enough to be palpable. Abdominal pain is an infrequent presenting finding caused variably by torsion of a pedunculated mass or from rupture with intraperitoneal bleeding. Ultrasonography shows a solid hepatic mass, but filling defects may be detected on nuclear scans. The lesions are quite vascular, large veins coursing across the surface of the visible portion of the tumor (Fig 113–3). The appearance resembles that of a hepatoblastoma, but the tumor is always benign. For this reason, a preliminary biopsy and frozen section should be obtained to avoid extended lobectomy or other major resection when a wedge or localized resection might be curative. The cut surface of the tumor shows nodules with central areas of fibrosis, and the histologic picture is one of micronodular cirrhosis with hyperplastic regenerative nodules.

Vascular Tumors

Solitary cavernous hemangioma and multiple infantile hemangioendotheliomas represent the ends of a broad spectrum of composite benign vascular tumors of the liver. The lesions tend to be detected early during infancy and generally no later than the second or third year of life, although asymptomatic hemangiomas of the liver have been found in older patients.[6]

Children with cavernous hemangiomas usually have a large

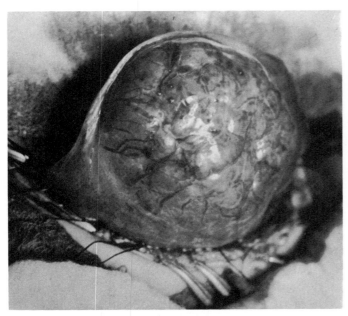

Fig 113–3.—Focal nodular hyperplasia in right lobe of liver in a 1-year-old child. Note the large veins coursing over the surface, characteristic of focal nodular hyperplasia. Only the discrete peripheral 6 × 6-cm mass was resected.

hepatic tumor, which may be symptomatic. Instances of rupture, hemoperitoneum, and shock have been recorded.[6, 21] These hemangiomas tend to be localized to one lobe, usually the right, but both lobes are affected in approximately 20% of children.[6] Many appear "hypovascular" on nuclear scan, but angiography reveals a large feeding artery to a solitary tumor (Fig 113–4). Arteriovenous shunting is often seen. Treatment of a solitary vascular tumor depends principally on the presence or absence of associated symptoms and on its resectability. Spontaneous resolution does occur, and a period of supportive medical treatment, as described for infantile hemangioendothelioma is indicated, but such cavernous hemangiomas may not regress as rapidly as cutaneous hemangiomas.[27] If the lesion is well localized, resection can be performed[29, 44] to avoid the risk of late rupture. Approximately one third of patients coming to operation have additional smaller hemangiomas. The tumors are well demarcated with a tan, smooth, outer surface and a spongy consistency. The vascular channels are lined by one or several layers of endothelium and separated by pale myxoid-appearing connective tissue containing fibroblasts and a few smooth muscle cells. Focal areas of inflammation, thrombosis, hemorrhage, fibrosis, necrosis, and interstitial calcification are common.[6, 20]

Capillary hemangioendotheliomas of the liver are known as infantile hemangioendotheliomas because of their pronounced cellularity. These lesions may be solitary but characteristically are multiple and produce a nodular deformity of the entire liver. The nodules have a red-purple central color, a whitish gray outer surface, and usually pulsate because of arteriovenous connections. Stout[45] described these tumors as having a "formation of vascular tubes lined by immature endothelial cells with a delicate framework of reticular fibers and pronounced tendency for the lumens to anastomose." The cellularity and multiplicity of the hepatic hemangiomas in the presence of cutaneous lesions could be taken as evidence of malignancy with multiple metastases.[41] However, the presence of the cutaneous lesions at birth, the pattern of organ involvement, and the occasional but unpredictable

spontaneous involution of cutaneous and hepatic lesions suggest a multicentric origin.

The diagnosis of hepatic hemangioendothelioma must be suspected when an infant has high-output congestive heart failure and hepatomegaly with a systolic bruit over the epigastrium, in the absence of myopathic congestive heart failure. Cutaneous hemangiomas, when present, become part of a diagnostic clinical triad. The association with thrombocytopenia[25, 42] is less common in hepatic hemangiomas than is congestive heart failure. Obstructive jaundice is rare.

Physical findings are characteristic of high-output congestive heart failure with left-to-right shunting through the angioma. Those presenting within the first month or two, often have intractable failure with severe tachypnea, tachycardia, and evidence of cyanosis. The onset in older infants tends to be more subtle, and symptoms improve with cardiotonic drugs and diuretics, while such routine medical measures fail to help the younger patients.

Further diagnostic work-up for patients suspected of having a hepatic hemangioendothelioma should include selective angiography of the celiac axis and hepatic artery. These vessels are particularly large, and a tapering of the proximal aorta at the celiac axis is consistent with preferential flow to the liver (Fig 113–5,A and B). Multiple abnormal branches from the hepatic artery give rise to the characteristic opacifying "blush" of an arteriovenous shunt (Fig 113–5,C). Small ectatic vessels with localized pooling are seen during the venous phase. These findings confirm the presence of a hepatic hemangioma, and further diagnostic work-up, including needle or open wedge biopsies, is both unnecessary and dangerous because of the risk of uncontrolled hemorrhage.

Steroids and irradiation have been advocated, but the initial enthusiasm for their use has diminished, particularly in patients who show little or no improvement with digitalis and diuretic therapy. Results with irradiation alone have not been impressive. Park[35] recently reported high fever as a dangerous complication following irradiation up to 1,500 rad. Success with steroids, given as prednisone in doses up to 5 mg/kg/day, has been reported[2, 16, 48] and such a trial is advocated in patients with mild failure who begin to improve on cardiotonic drugs. The mechanism of action of systemic corticosteroids on hemangiomas is unknown, but it is believed the drug increases the reactivity of the vascular bed, reduces the shunting, and hastens obliteration of the vascular channels.[52]

If congestive heart failure is not rapidly controlled by supportive medical measures, including steroids, then either ligation or embolization of the hepatic artery should be undertaken, since a mortality of up to 50% has been reported in the 2 weeks following the onset of sustained heart failure.[23, 32] Successful outcome following ligation of the common hepatic artery was first reported by de Lorimier[8] in a 20-day-old infant with mild congestive heart failure. Similar reports have followed.[22, 30, 33, 37] The procedure, as described, avoids dissection of the porta hepatis. More distal ligation of the right and left hepatic artery may prevent a "steal" of blood flow through either the gastroduodenal or right gastric artery entering beyond the ligature in the hepatic artery. Restitution of flow through the hepatic artery was reported by Mattioli et al.[30] 8 months after hepatic artery ligation. Intrahepatic shunting by similarly directed blood flow from these or other collaterals may recur within days of the ligation procedure. Our personal experience includes one such neonate having recurrent shunts from various sources, including the right phrenic artery, which was eliminated by balloon embolization (Fig 113–6). Increasing experience with selective angiography makes either balloon or microsphere embolization of the hepatic artery an alter-

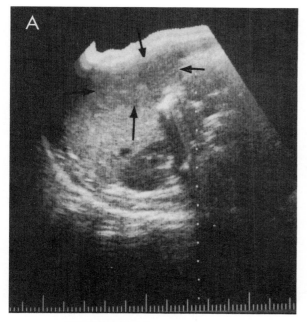

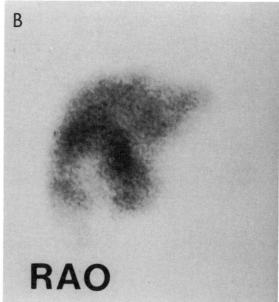

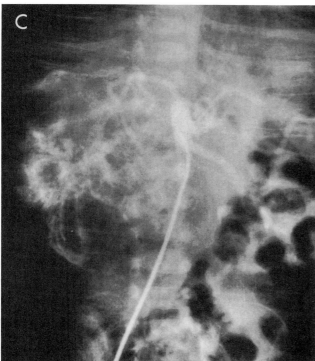

Fig 113–4.—Cavernous hemangioma in the right lobe of a 4-month-old with a bruit over the liver. **A,** tumor appears echolucent by ultrasound and **B,** "hypovascular" on nuclear scan. **C,** right hepatic artery, arising from the superior mesenteric artery in this case, supplies a large sharply circumscribed mass. Diffuse vascular blushes indicate presence of extensive arteriovenous communications. Gradual involution of tumor was monitored by ultrasound over 2 years.

native to hepatic artery ligation in selected cases of congestive heart failure from intrahepatic arteriovenous shunts.

Hepatic Infections and Abscess

Chronic Granulomatous Disease

In the preantibiotic era, pyogenic hepatic abscess occurred most often following perforated appendicitis,[19] a sequence rarely encountered in modern practice. Currently, chronic granulomatous disease (CGD) of childhood is the principal predisposing condition leading to formation of a hepatic abscess. This condition, caused by genetically transmitted deficient killing of phagocytized catalase-producing bacteria by circulating polymorphonuclear leukocytes (PMN),[36] presents during the first few months of life with episodic lymphadenitis, eczema, pneumonia, and hepatosplenomegaly. Failure of normal bactericidal function leads to a granulomatous as well as a suppurative response in the

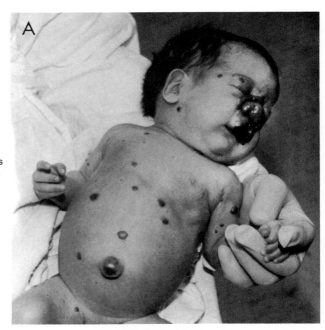

Fig 113–5.—Hemangioendothelioma in a neonate with a large liver, bruit, and severe congestive heart failure. **A,** cutaneous hemangiomas have enlarged, and the lesions on lip and palate are ulcerated. **B,** aorta tapers at the celiac axis, and blood is diverted through the liver. **C,** arteriovenous shunting opacifies the entire parenchyma. The patient underwent hepatic artery ligation but died shortly after, from congestive heart failure. (From Touloukian R.J.: *Pediatrics* 45:71, 1970. Reprinted with permission.)

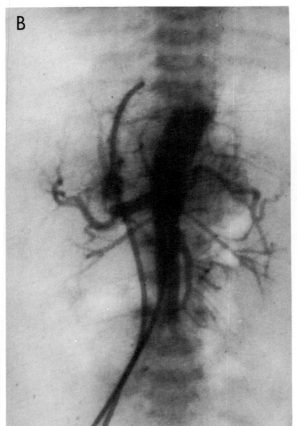

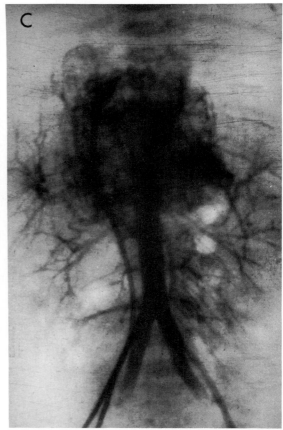

host tissue, which is infiltrated with large numbers of PMN, mononuclear cells, and histiocytes.[18] Abscess formation commonly occurs in regional nodes, usually the cervical and axillary group, soft tissues, lung, and liver.

Forty percent of all pyogenic liver abscesses are formed in children with CGD, while 30% of the remainder have a defect of host-systemic defense, most commonly acute leukemia.[3] Other causes are umbilical vein catheterization,[50] omphalitis, sickle cell disease, and biliary tract operations.[24] Cryptogenic hepatic abscesses in uncompromised children have also been reported.[13]

Presenting clinical findings include evidence of systemic infection, particularly high fever accompanied by hepatosplenomeg-

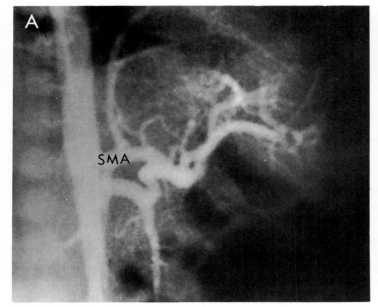

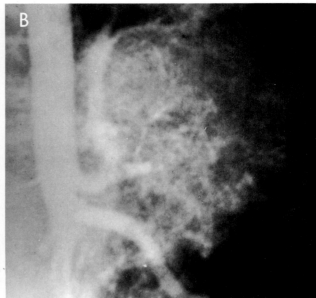

Fig 113–6.—Hemangioendothelioma in a 7-week-old with a large liver, bruit, and intractable congestive heart failure. **A,** arterial blood to liver comes through the large hepatic artery with collateral from superior mesenteric artery (SMA). Shunting and heart failure recurred following hepatic artery ligation and division of collateral flow from SMA. **B,** subsequent angiogram reveals demonstrable large phrenic artery as the principal source of hepatic artery blood. Infant recovered after selective catheterization and embolism of the phrenic artery.

aly, local tenderness, and jaundice. Localization of the infection to the liver is not always obvious, particularly in a patient without a known immune deficiency or CGD. The diagnosis of a solitary liver abscess has been facilitated by the various imaging techniques. Gray-scale ultrasonography or CT should be the initial examination in search for an abscess, followed by gallium scan and hepatic scintigram.[46] Lesions as small as 2 cm in diameter have been detected by radionuclide scan.[34] Failure to identify a defect on any one of the available studies should not rule out the possibility of very small or microscopic abscesses, which account for about half of liver abscesses in children without CGD.

Staphylococcus aureus, Streptococcus pyogenes, and *Escherichia coli* are organisms cultured in both CGD and non-CGD cases.[3, 24] In cryptogenic infection, anaerobic bacteria are likely to be responsible.[13] Antibiotic coverage should take this consideration into account.

Open surgical drainage combined with long-term antibiotic therapy is essential in controlling infection. A transverse incision should be placed directly over the cavity to minimize the risk of intraperitoneal spillage. Overlying liver tissue is unroofed with the electrocautery and the cavity debrided and drained or packed. Excision of peripheral abscesses is preferred in patients with CGD,[38] since the wall of the cavity is formed by granulomatous tissue containing many viable intracellular organisms. Selection of antibiotic combinations, based on the sensitivity of the cultured organisms and given intravenously for 4–6 weeks, precludes the need for excising deep-seated cavities and the risk incurred by this extensive procedure. Early diagnosis and adherence to the principles of adequate open surgical drainage with effective antibiotics should reduce the most recently quoted mortality rates of 27% in children with CGD and 42% in other children with pyogenic hepatic abscesses.[3]

Amebic Infection

Amebic infections of the liver are caused by the protozoan *Entamoeba histolytica,* which enters the liver through the portal circulation of patients with amebic dysentery. Most pediatric cases occur during early infancy. The infection may cause thrombosis and liver cell injury, leading to an abscess in a small minority of cases, usually immunosuppressed or steroid-treated children. Uncommon in the United States, this condition is endemic in Latin America, much of Asia, and South Africa. The clinical course is characterized by low-grade fever, malaise, and local tenderness over the liver. The abscess is usually within the right lobe and can be identified by a nuclear scan. Some urgency in detection is indicated because of the 10% risk of spontaneous rupture.

The diagnosis of invasive amebic infection can be made by either a serologic soluble antigen fluorescence antibody test or immunoelectrophoresis study.[31] Preoperative suspicion of the diagnosis is essential since antiamebic and antibiotic drugs result in a dramatic response in a few days. The most effective currently employed therapeutic agent is metronidazole (Flagyl).[4] Closed multiple aspiration of cyst contents under fluoroscopic direction is the preferred method for evacuating the pus. Collapse of the cavity with healing makes open surgical drainage unnecessary. Prevention of secondary infection by pyogenic organisms is essential.

Hydatid Disease

Hydatid disease rarely occurs in the United States, but has been cited in a recent Canadian series[11] and is endemic throughout much of South America and the Near East. Patients are febrile and possibly toxic on presentation.[1] Detection of multicompartmented cysts with calcification noted on plain film or ultrasound scan is highly suggestive of this parasitic cyst, and the diagnosis is confirmed by the Casoni skin test. The cyst fluid is generally under tension. The risk of intra-abdominal recurrence from seeding of "daughter" cysts is great, and complete resection or exteriorization with prekilling of the embryos by injecting hypertonic saline or aqueous iodine into the cyst is indicated to minimize this possibility.[39]

REFERENCES

1. Amis-Jahed A.K.: Clinical echinococcosis. *Ann. Surg.* 182:541, 1975.
2. Brown S.H., Neerhout R.C., Fonkalsrud E.W.: Prednisone therapy in the management of large hemangiomas of infants and children. *Surgery* 71:168, 1972.
3. Chusid M.: Pyogenic hepatic abscess in infancy and childhood. *Pediatrics* 62:554, 1978.
4. DeBakey M.E., Jordan G.L. Jr.: Hepatic abscesses, both intra- and extra-hepatic. *Surg. Clin. North Am.* 57:325, 1977.
5. Dehner L.P.: Hepatic tumors in the pediatric age group: A distinctive clinicopathologic spectrum. *Perspect. Pediatr. Pathol.* 4:217, 1978.
6. Dehner L.P., Ishak K.G.: Vascular tumors of the liver in infants and children: A study of 30 cases and review of the literature. *Arch. Pathol.* 92:101, 1971.
7. de Lorimier A.A.: Hepatic tumors of infancy and childhood. *Surg. Clin. North Am.* 57:443, 1977.
8. de Lorimier A.A., Simpson E.B., Baum R.S.: Hepatic artery ligation for hepatic hemangiomatosis. *N. Engl. J. Med.* 277:33, 1967.
9. Edmondson H.A.: Differential diagnosis of tumors and tumor-like lesions of liver in infancy and childhood. *J. Dis. Child.* 19:168, 1956.
10. Ehren H., Mahour G.H., Isaacs H. Jr.: Benign liver tumors in infancy and childhood: Report of 48 cases. *Am. J. Surg.* 145:325, 1983.
11. Ein S.H., Stephens C.A.: Benign liver tumors and cysts in childhood. *J. Pediatr. Surg.* 9:847, 1974.
12. Exelby P.R., Filler R.M., Grosfeld J.L.: Liver tumors in children in the particular reference to hepatoblastoma and hepatocellular carcinoma: American Academy of Pediatrics Surgical Section Survey, 1974. *J. Pediatr. Surg.* 10:329, 1975.
13. Harrington E., Bleicher M.: Cryptogenic hepatic abscess in two uncompromised children. *J. Pediatr. Surg.* 15:660, 1980.
14. Henson S.W. Jr., Gray H.K., Docherty M.B.: Benign tumors of the liver. III. Solitary cysts. *Surg. Gynecol. Obstet.* 103:607, 1956.
15. Howell R.R., Stevenson R.F., Ben-Menachem Y., et al.: Hepatic adenomata with type I glycogen storage disease. *JAMA* 236:1481, 1976.
16. Jackson C., Green H.L., O'Neill J.A., et al.: Hepatic hemangioendothelioma. *Am. J. Dis. Child.* 131:74, 1977.
17. Johnston P.W.: Congenital cysts of the liver in infancy and childhood. *Am. J. Surg.* 116:184, 1968.
18. Johnston R.B., Baehner R.L.: Chronic granulomatous disease: Correlation between pathogenesis and clinical findings. *Pediatrics* 48:730, 1971.
19. Keefer C.S.: Liver abscess: A review of 85 cases. *N. Engl. J. Med.* 211:21, 1934.
20. Kissane J.M.: *Pathology of Infancy and Childhood*, ed. 2. St. Louis, C.V. Mosby Co., 1975, p. 296.
21. Kissinger C.C., Sternfeld E., Zuker S.D.: Rupture of cavernous hemangioma of the liver as a cause of death in newborn infants. *Ohio Med. J.* 36:383, 1940.
22. Laird W.P., Friedman S., Koop C.E., et al.: Hepatic hemangiomatosis: Successful management by hepatic artery ligation. *Am. J. Dis. Child.* 130:657, 1976.
23. Larcher V.F., Howard E.R., Mowat A.P.: Hepatic hemangiomata: Diagnosis and management. *Arch. Dis. Child.* 56:7, 1981.
24. Larsen L.R., Raffensperger J.: Liver abscess. *J. Pediatr. Surg.* 14:329, 1979.
25. Leonidas J.C., Strauss L., Beck A.R.: Vascular tumors of the liver in newborns: A pediatric emergency. *Am. J. Dis. Child.* 124:507, 1973.
26. Lin T., Chen C., Wang S.: Treatment of non-parasitic cystic disease of the liver. *Ann. Surg.* 168:921, 1968.
27. Margileth A.M., Museles M.: Cutaneous hemangiomas in children: Diagnosis and conservative management. *JAMA* 194:523, 1965.
28. Markowitz R.I., Harcke H.T., Ritchie W.G.M., et al.: Focal nodular hyperplasia of the liver in a child with sickle cell disease. *AJR* 134:594, 1980.
29. Matolo N.M., Johnson D.G.: Surgical treatment of hepatic hemangioma in the newborn. *Arch. Surg.* 106:725, 1973.
30. Mattioli L., Lee K.R., Holder T.M.: Hepatic artery ligation for cardiac failure due to hepatic hemangioma in the newborn. *J. Pediatr. Surg.* 9:859, 1974.
31. McCarty E., Pathmanand C., Sunakorn P., et al.: Amebic liver abscess in childhood. *Am. J. Dis. Child.* 126:67, 1973.
32. McLean R.H., Moller J.H., Warwick W.J., et al.: Multi-nodular hemangiomatosis of the liver in infancy. *Pediatrics* 49:563, 1972.
33. Moazam F., Rodgers B.M., Talbert J.L.: Hepatic artery ligation for hepatic hemangiomatosis of infancy. *J. Pediatr. Surg.* 18:120, 1983.
34. O'Mara R.E., McAfee J.G.: Scintillation scanning in the diagnosis of hepatic abscess in children. *J. Pediatr.* 77:211, 1970.
35. Park W.C., Phillips R.: The role of radiation therapy in the management of hemangiomas of the liver. *JAMA* 212:496, 1970.
36. Quie P.G., White J.G., Holmes B., et al.: In vitro bactericidal capability of human polymorphonuclear leukocytes—diminished activity in chronic granulomatous disease of childhood. *J. Clin. Invest.* 46:668, 1967.
37. Rake M.O., Liberman M.M., Dawson J.L., et al.: Ligation of the hepatic artery in the treatment of heart failure due to hepatic hemangiomatosis. *Gut* 11:512, 1969.
38. Roback S., Weintraub W.H., Good R.A., et al.: Chronic granulomatous disease of childhood: Surgical considerations. *J. Pediatr. Surg.* 6:601, 1971.
39. Saidi F.: *Surgery of Hydatid Disease*. Philadelphia, W.B. Saunders Co., 1976.
40. Schullinger J.N., Wigger H.J., Price J.B., et al.: Epidermoid cyst of the liver. *J. Pediatr. Surg.* 18:240, 1983.
41. Schwartz A.R.: Multiple malignant hemangioendothelioma in infant: Report of case. *Arch. Pediatr.* 62:1, 1945.
42. Shim W.C.T.: Hemangiomas of infancy complicated by thrombocytopenia. *Am. J. Surg.* 116:896, 1968.
43. Smith W.L., Ballantine T.V.N., Gonzalez-Cruissi F.: Hepatic mesenchymal hamartoma causing heart failure in the neonate. *J. Pediatr. Surg.* 13:183, 1978.
44. Sompii E., Niemi K., Ruuskanen O.: Cavernous hepatic hemangioma in the newborn infant: Case report of a successful resection. *J. Pediatr. Surg.* 9:239, 1974.
45. Stout A.P.: A tumor of blood vessels featuring vascular endothelial cells. *Ann. Surg.* 118:445, 1943.
46. Sty J.R., Starshak R.J.: Comparative imaging in the evaluation of hepatic abscesses in immunocompromised children. *J. Clin. Ultrasound* 11:11, 1983.
47. Thaler M.M., Ogata E.S., Goodman J.R., et al.: Congenital fibrosis and polycystic disease of liver and kidneys. *Am. J. Dis. Child.* 126:374, 1971.
48. Touloukian R.J.: Hepatic hemangioendothelioma during infancy: Pathology, diagnosis, and treatment. *Pediatrics* 45:71, 1970.
49. Whelan T.J. Jr., Baugh J.H., Chandor S.: Focal nodular hyperplasia of the liver. *Ann. Surg.* 177:150, 1973.
50. Williams J.W., Rittenberry A., Dillard R., et al.: Liver abscess in newborn: Complications of umbilical vein catheterization. *Am. J. Dis. Child.* 125:111, 1973.
51. Young J.L. Jr., Miller R.W.: Incidence of malignant tumors in U.S. children. *J. Pediatr.* 86:254, 1975.
52. Zweifach B.W., Shorr E., Black M.M.: The influence of the adrenal cortex on behavior of terminal vascular bed. *Ann. N.Y. Acad. Sci.* 56:626, 1953.

Portal Hypertension

HISTORY.—In 1888, Eck[40] successfully created a portosystemic shunt in a laboratory animal. Pavlov[50a] recognized a neurologic syndrome of "meat intoxication" in 1895. Banti (1898) described the syndrome of splenomegaly and gastrointestinal bleeding that became known as "the portal hypertensive state." There followed almost a half-century of inactivity until the 1940s, when protein intolerance in cirrhotic patients was studied by Sherlock.[92] The first clinical application of portosystemic shunt, splenorenal shunt, was performed by Alan Whipple[108] in 1945. Portal decompression for the management of bleeding esophageal varices was accomplished soon after by portacaval and splenorenal shunts by Blakemore,[78] Rousselot,[86] Linton,[66] and Child.[27a] The neurologic and metabolic consequences of these shunts have been the subject of intense investigation. Hemodynamic studies suggested that encephalopathy might be the result of depriving the lumen of portal blood. This prompted Warren and others to emphasize the importance of maintaining antegrade hepatic portal inflow, leading eventually to the development of the selective splenorenal shunt. Technical obstacles imposed by the size of vessels available for shunting in children have been largely overcome, and both selective and nonselective portosystemic shunting have been successful in small subjects. The past decade has seen a resurgence of interest in surgical options other than portosystemic shunt. Esophageal devascularization procedures as well as direct obliteration of varices by endoscopic sclerosis have recently gained favor.

Causes of Portal Hypertension

The consequences of obstruction to portal flow may be subtle and readily compensated, or alarming and life-threatening. The management of the child with portal hypertension is, to a large extent, determined by the etiology of obstruction to portal venous flow.

Extrahepatic Obstruction

Formerly, most cases of portal hypertension seen in children resulted from extrahepatic obstruction to portal flow.[90] Thrombosis of the portal vein secondary to perinatal omphalitis, or as a complication of exchange transfusions through the umbilical vein, was usually implicated. Intra-abdominal sepsis and dehydration has also resulted in portal vein thrombosis. The occluded portal vein is ultimately replaced with a lacework of recanalized and collateral venous channels, referred to as cavernomatous transformation of the portal vein (Fig 114–1). Isolated defects involving the portal vein, such as congenital atresia, are rare causes of extrahepatic portal obstruction.[21]

Intrahepatic Obstruction

Liver disease, the most common cause of portal hypertension in adults, is now seen with increasing frequency in children. A 1982 survey of pediatric surgeons revealed that the incidence of portal hypertension resulting from liver disease (cirrhosis) was approximately equal to that seen consequent to portal vein obstruction[2] (Table 114–1). This change is accounted for by the population of patients born with biliary atresia and in whom jaundice is relieved by portoenterostomy; but liver disease progresses, eventually resulting in clinically significant portal hypertension.[4] Additional causes of cirrhosis in children are seen in Table 114–2. Congenital hepatic fibrosis, a disease of obscure etiology, occurs in two forms: (1) familial, with an associated renal tubular anomaly; and (2) sporadic, in which kidney involvement is unusual.[56, 57] Significant portal hypertension with consequent gastrointestinal hemorrhage develops in nearly all these patients. The liver parenchyma is generally spared, and, thus, liver function remains relatively unimpaired.[19] Approximately 10–15% of patients with cystic fibrosis will develop focal biliary cirrhosis and portal hypertension.[38] Cirrhosis consequent to the metabolic abnormality, α_1-antitrypsin deficiency, or as an endstage of chronic active viral hepatitis, is a further etiologic consideration in children.[88, 92]

Suprahepatic Obstruction (Budd-Chiari Syndrome)

Hepatic vein obstruction, not uncommon in Central and South America, is a rare cause of portal hypertension in North America and Europe.[1] The association between hepatic vein thrombosis and oral contraceptives is now recognized. In the Orient, suprahepatic vena caval obstruction frequently results from intraluminal webs or diaphragms.[77]

In most cases, a specific etiologic factor is not identified.[44] The onset of the condition is insidious and the course indolent. Often months or years elapse between the first symptoms and the recognition of the syndrome. The disease is refractory to treatment. An acute form of Budd-Chiari syndrome has been recognized, but most patients follow a progressively downhill course characterized by abdominal pain, ascites, hepatosplenomegaly, and,

TABLE 114–1.—PORTAL HYPERTENSION

ETIOLOGY	NO. OF PATIENTS
Extrahepatic	36
Hepatic (cirrhosis)	38
Suprahepatic (Budd-Chiari)	1
Other (etiology?)	1
Total	76

From Altman and Krug.[2]

TABLE 114–2.—CAUSES OF CIRRHOSIS

FACTOR	NO. OF PATIENTS
Biliary atresia	10
Congenital hepatic fibrosis	8
Cystic fibrosis, focal biliary cirrhosis	6
α_1-antitrypsin deficiency	3
Radiation, chemotherapy	3
Chronic active hepatitis	3
Sclerosing cholangitis	1
Histiocytosis X	1
Galactosemia	1
Congenital biliary cirrhosis	1
Etiology unknown	1
Total	38

From Altman and Krug.[2]

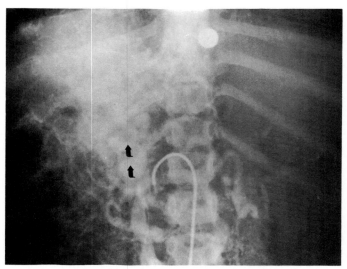

Fig 114–1.—Extrahepatic portal vein thrombosis (superior mesenteric artery injection, venous phase). The recanalized portal vein is demonstrated (cavernomatous transformation). Despite portal vein thrombosis, portal flow is hepatopetal *(arrows)*.

finally, death from hepatic failure or gastrointestinal hemorrhage.[81] The hepatic parenchyma is subject to extensive destruction because of the high-grade outflow block.[20] Attempts to relieve thrombosis in the hepatic veins by systemic anticoagulation or the administration of fibrinolytic agents such as streptokinase have had only limited success.

In some cases, ascites is refractory to pharmacologic management. In this circumstance the peritoneovenous (LeVeen) shunt has proved effective and is recommended as an alternative.[64]

Additionally, partially diverting portosystemic shunts—side-to-side portacaval, splenorenal, mesocaval—have been applied with amelioration of symptoms and extended survival in up to 60% of affected patients.[73] Cameron described a mesoatrial shunt for portal decompression in patients with significant narrowing of the inferior vena cava.[24] By this technique, the portal flow is directed to the systemic circulation by a prosthetic graft running from the superior mesenteric vein to the right atrium. Survival after mesocaval and mesoatrial bypass has been reported by Huguet et al.[53] Orthotopic liver transplantation has also been used in a patient with end-stage liver disease from Budd-Chiari syndrome secondary to hepatic vein occlusion.[82] Thus, surgical intervention by peritoneovenous shunt, portal decompression, or, in special circumstances, liver replacement is appropriate for selected patients with Budd-Chiari syndrome in whom inexorable deterioration leading to death is predictable. Side-to-side portacaval shunt to relieve portal pressure has resulted in resolution of symptoms and extended survival in selected patients.[63]

Gastrointestinal Hemorrhage From Esophageal Varices

Whether portal venous flow is obstructed consequent to portal vein thrombosis or to intrahepatic disease, collateral venous channels inevitably develop. The life-threatening complication of portal hypertension is hemorrhage from the variceal collaterals in the esophagus and stomach.

When gastrointestinal hemorrhage is the presenting symptom in a previously well child, a history of abdominal infection or umbilical vein cannulation in the perinatal period suggests the diagnosis of portal vein thrombosis. Stigmata of cirrhosis (jaundice, ascites, spider angiomata, hepatosplenomegaly) indicate the

likelihood that the portal hypertension is a consequence of intrinsic liver disease (cirrhosis).

The essentials of management of the patient with gastrointestinal hemorrhage are the same regardless of the etiology. Central venous access is obtained and a nasogastric tube is positioned in the stomach for gastric lavage with iced half-normal saline. To avoid water intoxication, particularly in small children, it is important that the volume of solutions used for irrigation be monitored and the stomach aspirated completely after each flush with irrigant.

Congestive splenomegaly is a common accompaniment of portal hypertension, but in children clinically significant thrombocytopenia is unusual. Vitamin K is given parenterally if clotting factors are abnormal. Transfusions of fresh frozen plasma and washed packed red cells are alternated with whole blood to replace volume and provide clotting factors.

Balloon tamponade in infants or small children is hazardous. There is an appreciable risk of aspiration of secretions blocked by the balloon. The accidental dislodgment of the tube in an agitated child can result in disastrous airway obstruction. When balloon tamponade is employed, the margin of safety is increased by securing the airway by endotracheal intubation. Formal diagnostic studies are begun when the patient's condition is stable.

ENDOSCOPY.—Direct visualization of the esophagus, stomach, and duodenum through the flexible endoscope is now the most accurate and reliable technique for assessing the patient with upper gastrointestinal hemorrhage.

SPLENOPORTOGRAPHY.—Percutaneous splenoportography is applicable in children.[45, 72] A manometric determination of portal pressure is possible through a needle or catheter inserted into the splenic pulp. The splenic pulp pressure is generally somewhat higher than that recorded by direct cannulation of a portal or mesenteric vein tributary. A splenic pressure greater than 250 mm water indicates portal hypertension. Injection of contrast material directly into the spleen provides brilliant studies of the patency and caliber of the splenic and portal veins (Fig 114–2) as well as the size and location of collaterals.

ANGIOGRAPHY.—The risks inherent in percutaneous splenic puncture in patients with elevated portal pressure and clotting disorders are obviated by the use of more direct angiographic techniques. Mesenteric artery cannulation is feasible in most infants and children, and sequential films obtained after injection usually demonstrate the venous anatomy (Fig 114–3), including collateral channels and esophageal varices, although not usually the source of bleeding. The instillation of vasoactive agents into the superior mesenteric artery is effective in controlling variceal bleeding.[12, 13, 79, 89] Vasopressin (Pitressin) infused into the mesenteric circulation reduces visceral blood flow, as seen in Figure 114–4. The vasoconstrictive effect of vasopressin is independent of the autonomic nervous system, and sustained infusion is well tolerated. Vasopressin infusion via a peripheral vein is equally effective in reducing splanchnic blood flow, and this is now the preferred route for administration.[28] The infusion of vasopressin is initiated at 0.2 unit/ml/min, but, to control refractory bleeding or to restrict volume, the concentration can be increased. Vasopressin infusion is an important adjunct in the management of children with persistent bleeding from esophageal varices. Coronary artery spasm from vasopressin injection, often a limiting factor in adults, is not usually a consideration in children. However, the strong antidiuretic action of vasopressin can result in iatrogenic fluid overload, hyponatremia, and water intoxication, so that careful monitoring is required. Bleeding can almost always be controlled in children, providing an interval during which resuscitative measures can be completed.

The prognosis for the patient with portal hypertension de-

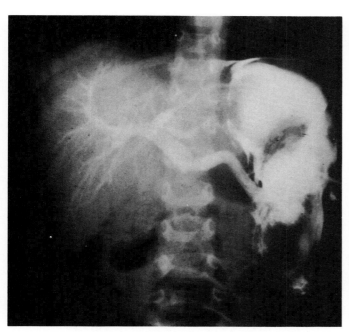

Fig 114–2.—Percutaneous splenoportogram. The spleen is large, the liver small (cirrhotic). Both the splenic and portal veins are visualized. The splenic pulp pressure was slightly higher than actual portal pressure determined at operation.

pends, among other factors, on the presence or absence of underlying liver disease. Decisions regarding the advisability of portosystemic shunts or nonshunt therapeutic options are often difficult and are based on the clinical status of the patient, the underlying mechanism of the portal hypertension, and the experience and resources of the institution.

Shunt Therapy

Effective and reliable portal decompression in small subjects has taxed the surgeon's ingenuity. The concept of shunting blood from the high-pressure portal to the low-pressure systemic system was conceived by Eck[40] and pioneered by Whipple,[108, 109] Linton,[66] Blakemore,[18] Child,[26, 27] and Rousselot.[86] Through their efforts, the end-to-side and side-to-side portacaval and splenorenal shunts were developed, and proved to be effective in decompressing the portal system and controlling hemorrhage from esophageal varices. Refinements in shunt techniques for application in children were made by Clatworthy and Boles,[31] who developed the central splenorenal shunt. Clatworthy[32] and Marion[70, 71] independently described the mesocaval shunt, which is particularly useful in patients in whom neither the portal nor the splenic veins are available for shunting. The interposition mesocaval shunt, popularized in adults by Drapanas,[39] has been utilized successfully in infants and children.

In the past, the premise was accepted that, until a child reached the age of 6 or 7 years, the vessels available for shunting were too small for successful anastomosis and that the technical obstacles precluded this option.[42, 43] Recently, several centers

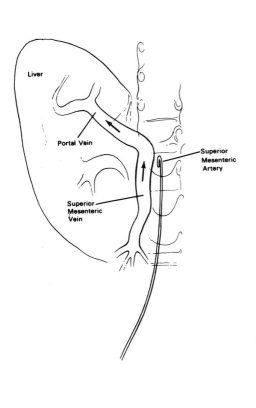

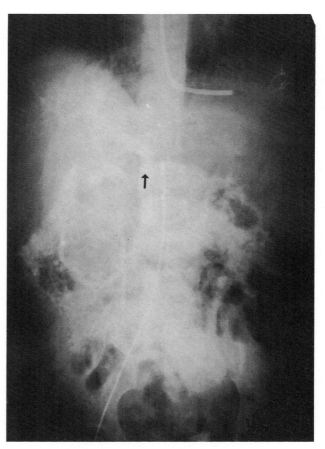

Fig 114–3.—Transfemoral mesenteric angiogram (right), venous phase. Normal superior mesenteric vein *(arrow)*. In this patient with cirrhosis, portal flow is hepatopetal.

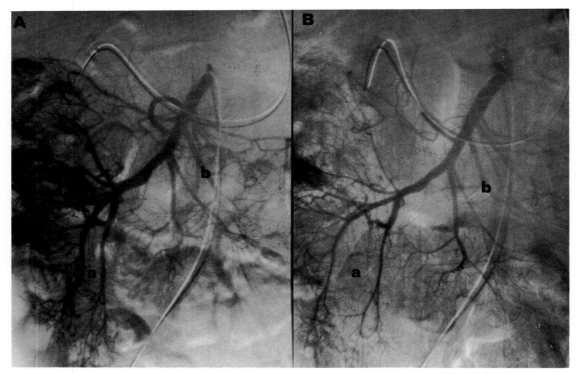

Fig 114–4.—Effect of vasopressin infusion in superior mesenteric artery. Selective superior mesenteric arteriogram before **(A)** and after **(B)** a 20-minute infusion of vasopressin, 0.1 μg/ml/min. Angiograms were made at the same flow rate of contrast and exposed 4 seconds after the start of injection. Note marked decrease in caliber of ileal *(a)* and jejunal *(b)* arteries and decreased capillary stain, reflecting markedly reduced visceral blood flow following vasopressin infusion. This effect can be obtained as well by peripheral intravenous infusion of vasopressin.

have reported favorable experience with shunts in small subjects and have achieved a remarkably high patency rate. Alvarez[6, 7] reports an experience with shunt procedures in 76 children with portal hypertension, of whom 64 had shunts after gastrointestinal hemorrhage. In 12, the shunt was prophylactic. Shunt patency was confirmed in 70 of the 76 patients (92%), a remarkable outcome, particularly since the mean age of the patients was under 7 years. Similar excellent results were achieved by Bismuth,[15, 16] who treated 90 children by portal diversion. Fifty-two had extrahepatic portal vein obstruction, and 38 had cirrhosis. The type of shunt performed varied, but a central splenorenal shunt was favored (59 patients). The shunt patency rate was 94%, and there were no complications in the group of children with extrahepatic portal block, despite the fact that the diameter of the veins used for portosystemic anastomosis was less than 10 mm in two thirds of patients.[15, 16] Thus, it seems that neither age nor size is a limiting factor.

The surgical decisions are compounded by the inability to foretell which patients will rebleed in spite of medical treatment and which will develop aggravated liver failure or en-

cephalopathy[91] with or without a portosystemic shunt. Child's criteria for assessing hepatic reserve have been useful in predicting the patient's tolerance to portal diversion and the results to be expected from shunting portal flow[26] (Table 114–3). In Figure 114–5, the clinical status of patients with extrahepatic portal hypertension is compared to a group of children with elevated portal pressure and gastrointestinal hemorrhage secondary to cirrhosis.[2] It is apparent that most of those with portal vein obstruction have essentially normal liver function and are in the Child's A category, whereas those with cirrhosis have impaired liver function and are more often grouped in the Child's B or C category.[27] Clatworthy[30] has aptly contrasted extrahepatic and intrahepatic portal hypertension, referring to the former as "good livers, bad veins" and the latter as "bad livers, good veins."

Predictive criteria based on hemodynamic and clinical factors have also been utilized.[23, 75, 94] However, surgical judgments must also take into account the overall status of the child, including growth, achievement of developmental milestones, and prognosis of the underlying disease.

TABLE 114–3.—Child's Criteria for Assessment
of Hepatic Reserve

CRITERION	A Good Risk	B Moderate Risk	C Poor Risk
Serum bilirubin (mg/100 ml)	<2.0	2.0–3.0	>3.0
Serum albumin (gm/100 ml)	>3.5	3.0–3.5	<3.0
Ascites	None	Easily controlled	Poorly controlled
Encephalopathy	None	Minimal	Advanced
Nutrition	Excellent	Good	Poor

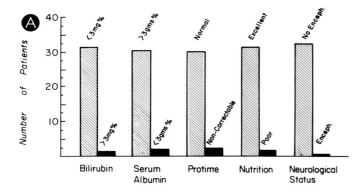

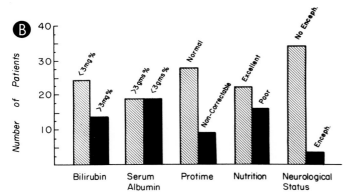

Fig 114–5.—Comparison of the clinical status of patients with extrahepatic portal hypertension **(A)** and patients with elevated portal pressure and gastrointestinal hemorrhage secondary to cirrhosis **(B)**.

Extrahepatic Portal Obstruction

These patients usually present between the ages of 2 and 4 years, and hemorrhage is often the first indication of the underlying disorder. Because the obstruction to portal flow is extrahepatic, liver function is unimpaired and bleeding is relatively well tolerated. Bleeding episodes are frequently self-limited and, as collateral venous channels develop spontaneously, the need for surgical decompression is rarely pressing.[9, 80] Alvarez et al.[7] and Bismuth et al.[15, 16] have demonstrated the feasibility of early shunting, with extended long-term patency in this group of patients, and advocate portosystemic shunts as the treatment of choice even for the first episode of bleeding. This is in contrast to the traditional recommendation that collaterals will eventually decompress the portal system, obviating the need for an operation in all but a few patients.[31, 33, 41, 43, 49, 97]

Intrahepatic Obstruction—Cirrhosis

As cirrhosis progresses, the likelihood of bleeding increases. In patients with compromised liver function, recurrent bleeding is ominous. Here, too, the status of the child influences the therapy. Thus, in children with cystic fibrosis the pulmonary status is often the determining factor. Those with severe pulmonary disease are obviously not good candidates, whereas those with adequate lung reserve can be expected to benefit from portosystemic shunt. In patients with biliary atresia, relieved of jaundice, with stable hepatic histology, when hemorrhage represents the principal threat to life, portosystemic shunting may be appropriate. The mesocaval H graft has proved particularly applicable in patients in whom portacaval or splenorenal shunts have failed or

in those who have had previous operations in the porta hepatis[3, 11] (i.e., Kasai portoenterostomy) (Fig 114–6). The H graft can also be applied in a patient who has had a previous splenectomy. Autogenous internal jugular vein is preferred for creation of the shunt, since this obviates the need for a slender vascular prosthesis that may tend to clot as neointima develops within the graft.[3, 78]

Stomal bleeding secondary to local trauma compounded by elevated portal pressure has been troublesome in some patients whose portoenterostomy procedure involved external cutaneous venting of the conduit. Usually the bleeding can be controlled by local measures—pressure or suture. In a few patients, bleeding from the conduit has followed stomal closure, especially when this is accomplished by a simple turn-in procedure after crushing the Mikulicz spur.[106] Resection of the stomas with the terminal few centimeters of bowel and formal end-to-end jejunojejunostomy accomplishes resection of the potentially hazardous jejunal varices and probably eliminates the risk of hemorrhage from within the conduit after stomal closure.

The ideal portosystemic connection preserves liver function while shunting the high pressure portal flow to the systemic circulation. All of the techniques mentioned above, when properly applied, shunt portal blood effectively and decompress esopha-

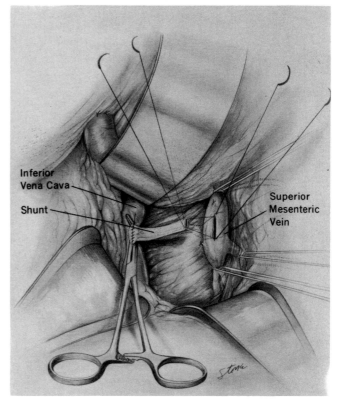

Fig 114–6.—Interposition mesocaval shunt operation in a 14-month-old child. After portoenterostomy (Kasai) performed at age 8 weeks, the serum bilirubin was normal and the child's growth was in the 50th percentile. Three episodes of life-threatening hemorrhage from esophageal varices led to interposition mesocaval shunt, employing autogenous internal jugular vein. The relation between the superior mesenteric vein and inferior vena cava is seen. The duodenum is retracted superiorly and the biliary conduit retracted toward the left. The caval anastomosis is completed first. The caval and mesenteric venotomies are twice the diameter of the vein graft, which will distend after flow is restored. The patient is now 11 years old (born March 1974), 10 years postshunt, and 11 years post-Kasai for biliary atresia. Current status is excellent. No jaundice (bilirubin normal). No further bleeding since shunt. Shunt patency has been confirmed by transfemoral venography. (From *J. Pediatr. Surg.* 11:809, 1976. Used by permission.)

geal varices. Boles reports a favorable long-term experience after portosystemic shunting in children.[17] In his series of 41 patients followed up for 30 years, the presenting event was upper gastrointestinal bleeding in 19 patients. All patients were symptomatic by their thirteenth year and most by age 6 years. Twenty-nine portosystemic shunt procedures were carried out in 26 patients with a success rate of 54%. Direct operations included resections (11) and devascularization procedures (7) with moderate success (5/11) in the former group, but no long-term favorable results with the latter. However, many others have voiced serious concerns about the high incidence of undesirable side effects following conventional shunt therapy. The hemodynamic patterns and physiologic consequences to the patient vary with the type of shunt constructed (Fig 114–7). Thus, the end-to-side por-

tacaval shunt directs all portal flow around the liver. The side-to-side portacaval shunt and all splenorenal and mesocaval shunts theoretically direct only a portion of the splanchnic flow to the systemic circulation. Reversal of blood flow in the portal vein, allowing the portal to act as an outflow tract, is a potential but infrequent consequence of any of these hemodynamically similar shunts (Fig 114–7).[61, 62, 87, 112] This phenomenon has been implicated as a factor in the development of postshunt hepatic encephalopathy, which can result in disabling cerebral deterioration.[74, 76] Voorhees et al.[103] described serious late neuropsychiatric complications in adolescents and adults previously subjected to portosystemic shunt. These complications and the frequency of hospitalization for neuropsychiatric sequelae years after creation of the shunt, although without evidence of hyper-

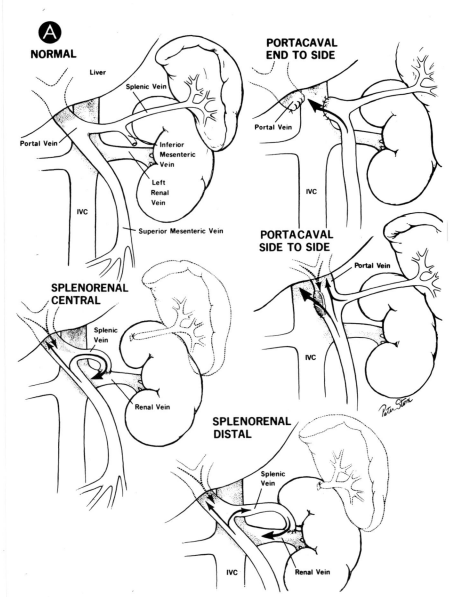

Fig 114–7.—Types of portosystemic shunts. **A,** in the end-to-side portacaval shunt, all portal flow is diverted to systemic circulation. In the side-to-side portacaval shunt, the major direction of portal flow is to the systemic circulation, but the capacity for hepatic portal perfusion is retained, depending on the resistance within the liver. Flow dynamics are such that there is a potential for reversal of flow in the portal vein (hepatofugal), shown by *broken arrow*. In central splenorenal shunt, the principal direction of portal flow is to the systemic circulation. Placing the shunt centrally minimizes angulation of the splenic vein (spleen removed). In distal splenorenal shunt, major direction of portal flow is to systemic circulation. Perfusion of the liver with portal blood and potential hepatofugal flow is shown (spleen removed). *(Continued.)*

ammonemia, raise serious questions about the advisability of shunting portal blood flow in children. It has recently been suggested that alterations in intestinal absorption following portosystemic shunt also contribute to the pathogenesis of encephalopathy.[83] Maintenance of high pressure in the portal system may be a further advantage of the distal splenorenal shunt, and the beneficial effects on intestinal absorption with respect to late psychoneurologic function may be important in preventing post-shunt encephalopathy.

These concerns have led to intensive investigations into alternative techniques of shunting designed to eliminate these undesirable physiologic consequences. Warren,[104, 105] followed by Zeppa[111] and others,[22, 47] proposes "selective shunting" (Fig 114–

7). By this technique the portal circulation is partitioned into two components: (1) antegrade portal flow to the liver, and (2) selective transsplenic flow from the esophageal varices via the short gastric veins, through the splenic vein into the renal vein and systemic circulation. Thus, the portal inflow to the liver is maintained while the collateral esophageal varices are selectively decompressed.[54] This operation has been applied successfully in children.[84] Extended patency, up to 10 years after selective distal splenorenal shunt, was confirmed in 17 of 27 patients (63%) operated by Maksoud and Mies.[69] The patients were between 4 and 12 years of age, and seven were less than 8 years old. The etiology of portal hypertension was extrahepatic obstruction in four and intrahepatic in the remainder. The largest component of

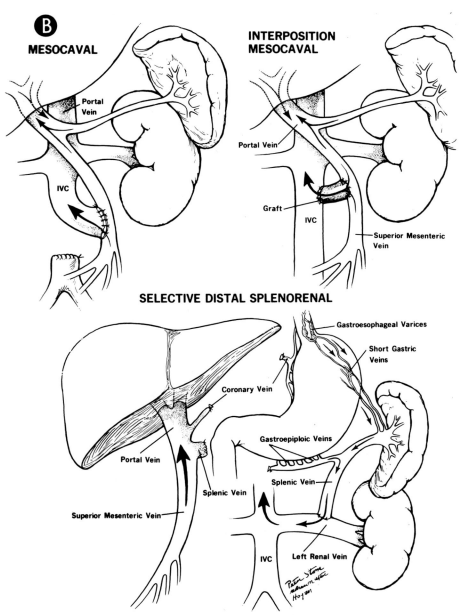

Fig 114–7 Cont.—B, mesocaval shunt. Vena cava is transected and proximal cava is anastomosed to side of superior mesenteric vein. Major direction of visceral flow is toward vena cava. Hepatopetal, as well as potential for hepatofugal, flow is depicted. Interposition mesocaval shunt is hemodynamically similar to mesocaval shunt. Autogenous vein graft is preferred for creation of this shunt in infants and children. In selective distal splenorenal shunt, the portal flow is partitioned. Portal inflow to the liver is preserved, while gastroesophageal varices are simultaneously decompressed through short gastric veins and then to systemic circulation by a distal splenorenal shunt.

those with hepatic disease was schistosomiasis (10 patients). This experience seems to confirm the feasibility of such shunt procedures, even in small subjects.

Nonshunt Alternatives

Alternatives to rerouting portal blood flow, developed in adults, have had trials in children. Transthoracic ligation of esophageal varices[67] or direct ligation by an abdominal approach[85, 107] provides only short-term palliation.[36] Esophageal transection,[48, 52, 60] esophagogastrectomy, short-segment colon[59] or small-bowel interposition,[50] transplantation, and translocation of the spleen[102] and omentum have all been utilized as temporizing or definitive procedures in young patients. Many of these operations have been abandoned, and are now of only historic interest. However, technical factors and the concerns over adverse sequelae late after portosystemic shunt have renewed interest in nonshunt procedures for the management of gastrointestinal hemorrhage from esophageal varices.

Sugiura and Futagawa[98, 99] advocate extensive esophagogastric devascularization combined with esophageal transection and reanastomosis. Johnston[55] and others use a stapling device for dividing and reanastomosing the esophagus. Ligation procedures, or interruption of varices utilizing direct suture or staplers, combined with devascularization have been recommended by others.[34, 37] A modification involving dissection and Vosschulte ligature of the esophagus has been successfully applied in children by Berger et al.[14, 113] The operations tend to be long and tedious. Some can be expedited by the use of staplers. Devascularization procedures are effective in controlling and preventing future bleeding from varices.

There has been renewed enthusiasm for direct obliteration of esophageal varices by endoscopic sclerotherapy, first described by Crafoord in 1939.[35] Since the underlying portal hypertension was unmodified, new collaterals developed and bleeding usually recurred. Thus, for many years injection procedures were out of favor. The recent resurgence of interest in endoscopic sclerotherapy was stimulated by the work of Terblanche.[100, 101]

Direct injection of sclerosant (sodium morrhuate) has been utilized effectively for the emergency management of acute hemorrhage from esophageal varices.[51] It is, however, preferable to employ this procedure after bleeding has been controlled and the patient resuscitated. Injection procedures can be made utilizing rigid endoscopic equipment[65] or through a flexible endoscope, depending on the experience and skill of the operator.[96] Using a modified slotted rigid esophagoscope, the varix to be injected is trapped and 0.5–2.5 ml of sclerosant is injected directly. The esophagoscope is rotated so that the solid side can effect tamponade of the injection site. Several clusters of varices are treated similarly. Visualization is somewhat easier and perhaps safer through the flexible endoscope, but postinjection tamponade is not possible. Both techniques are effective. Serial injections are well tolerated and are usually required to obliterate the varices[10] (Fig 114–8). Relatively infrequent but serious complications of this procedure include hemorrhage, mucosal ulceration, esophageal stricture, and perforation with mediastinitis. In experienced hands, the procedure is relatively safe and has been used successfully both in children with portal hypertension secondary to portal vein thrombosis and in those with cirrhosis whose long-term prognosis is poor.[29] In the former group, sclerotherapy may serve as a temporizing procedure, allowing the patient to grow, increasing the likelihood that a successful portosystemic shunt can be performed should that option be elected.

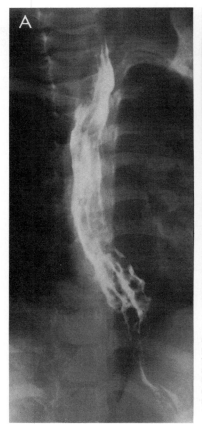

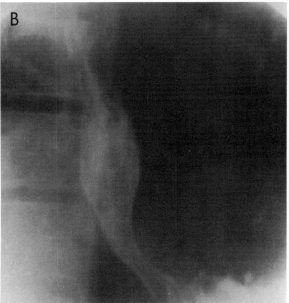

Fig 114–8.—Sclerotherapy for esophageal varices. **A,** barium swallow shows linear irregularities, varices in distal esophagus. The patient, an 11-year-old female, has portal hypertension from portal vein thrombosis (see Fig 114–1). She was treated by endoscopic sclerotherapy after numerous episodes of upper gastrointestinal tract hemorrhage. **B,** barium esophagram 6 months after a series of endoscopic sclerotherapy. The esophageal varices have been successfully obliterated.

Endoscopic sclerotherapy has also been utilized in conjunction with splenic embolization when gastrointestinal hemorrhage is associated with significant hypersplenism secondary to splenomegaly. The disadvantage of total removal of the spleen, particularly in children, was first recognized by King and Schumacker[58] and later emphasized by Singer.[93] This led to the evolution of methods to reduce hypersplenism while conserving some splenic function. Maddison[68] first performed embolization of the spleen for hypersplenism in 1973.

The spleen has been embolized by numerous techniques.[8, 95, 110] The one currently favored utilizes minute Gelfoam particles embolized directly into the peripheral branches of the splenic artery. This results in near total splenic infarction with reduction of most, but not all, of the splenic mass (Fig 114–9). To minimize potential infectious complications the patient is given antibiotics prophylactically. Fever and tenderness over the infarcting spleen are common, but if proper precautions are observed abscess formation is rare.

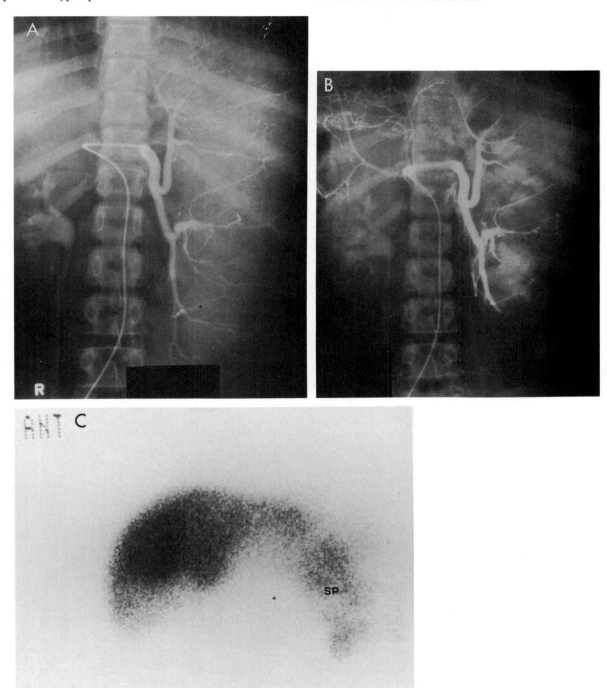

Fig 114–9.—A, selective splenic arteriogram of patient in Figures 114–1 and 114–8. Massive enlargement of spleen is demonstrated before embolization. The patient had hypersplenism with a platelet count of 25,000–35,000/mm³. **B,** selective splenic arteriogram after splenic artery embolization. Distal branches are occluded by minute Gelfoam fragments, resulting in near total splenic infarction. **C,** nuclear scan (⁹⁹ᵐTc sulfur colloid) 6 months after embolization. Most of the spleen *(SP)* is infarcted, but there is some residual splenic tissue. The platelet count is consistently greater than 250,000/mm³.

Ascites

An additional, and often particularly troublesome, consequence of obstructed portal blood flow is the development of ascites.[25] In some patients ascites is refractory to pharmacologic management, including administration of albumin, furosemide, and the aldosterone antagonist spironolactone.[46] For some of these children the peritoneovenous shunt technique of LeVeen[64] has been successful.[5] In small subjects, the shunt is seated in the iliac fossa, which is approached extraperitoneally. From this position, the peritoneum is easily reached for placement of the collecting tubing while the venous cannula is tunneled laterally to the neck for placement in the superior vena cava via the internal jugular vein (Fig 114–10).

Elevation of portal venous pressure per se is not life-threatening. It is the secondary consequences of portal hypertension, especially hemorrhage from esophageal varices, that are potentially lethal. Today the surgeon has several options, pharmacologic and operative, that can be effective alone or in combination

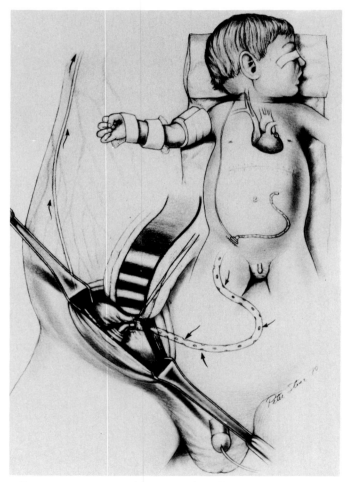

Fig 114–10.—Illustration of 1-year-old infant with cirrhosis, portal hypertension, and intractable ascites. A portoenterostomy was carried out at 4 months, but liver disease progressed despite good flow of bile. The LeVeen valve was accommodated easily in the right iliac fossa, which was approached extraperitoneally (age 10 months). The venous tubing is tunneled laterally to enter the superior vena cava via a jugular cutdown. Paracentesis was performed just before the procedure to minimize leakage of ascitic fluid and to avoid sudden circulatory overload. The LeVeen shunt functioned for approximately 4 months, then clotted. The baby died of cirrhosis and liver failure shortly thereafter. (From *J. Pediatr. Surg.* 16:965, 1981. Used by permission.)

to control or minimize this hazard and thereby improve the quality of life for these children.

REFERENCES

1. Alagille D., et al.: Syndrome de Budd-Chiari et maladie veno-occlusive chez l'enfant. *Arch. Fr. Pédiatr.* 25:1039, 1968.
2. Altman R.P., Krug J.: Portal hypertension: American Academy of Pediatrics, Surgical Section Survey. *J. Pediatr. Surg.* 17:567, 1982.
3. Altman R.P.: Portal decompression by interposition mesocaval shunt in patients with biliary atresia. *J. Pediatr. Surg.* 11:809, 1976.
4. Altman R.P., Chandra R., Lilly J.R.: Ongoing cirrhosis after successful porticoenterostomy in infants with biliary atresia. *J. Pediatr. Surg.* 10:685, 1975.
5. Altman R.P., Cavett C.M.: The retroperitoneal approach for peritoneal venous shunting in infants and small children. *J. Pediatr. Surg.* 16:965, 1981.
6. Alvarez F., Bernhard O., Brunelle F., et al.: Portal obstruction in children. I. Clinical investigation and hemorrhage risk. *J. Pediatr.* 103:696, 1983.
7. Alvarez F., Bernhard O., Brunelle F., et al.: Portal obstruction in children. II. Results of surgical portosystemic shunts. *J. Pediatr.* 103:703, 1983.
8. Almwark A., Bengmark S., Gullstrand P., et al.: Evaluation of splenic embolization in patients with portal hypertension and hypersplenism. *Ann. Surg.* 196:518, 1982.
9. Aoyama K., Myers N.A.: Extrahepatic portal hypertension: The significance of variceal haemorrhage. *Aust. Paediatr. J.* 18:17, 1982.
10. Atkinson J.B., Woolley M.M.: Treatment of esophageal varices by sclerotherapy in children. *Am. J. Surg.* 146:103, 1983.
11. Auvert J., Weisgerber G.: Immediate and long-term results of superior mesenteric vein–inferior vena cava shunt for portal hypertension in children. *J. Pediatr. Surg.* 10:901, 1975.
12. Baum S., et al.: Gastrointestinal hemorrhage. II. Angiographic diagnosis and control. *Adv. Surg.* 7:149, 1973.
13. Baum S.I., Nusbaum M.: The control of gastrointestinal hemorrhage by selective mesenteric arterial infusion of vasopressin. *Radiology* 98:497, 1971.
14. Berger D., Produit S., Genton N.: Alternative therapeutique pour le traitement de l'hypertension portale infantile. *Chirurg. Pédiatr.* 24, 1983.
15. Bismuth H., Franco D.: Portal diversion for portal hypertension in early childhood. *Ann. Surg.* 180:439, 1976.
16. Bismuth H., Franco D., Alagille D.: Portal diversion for portal hypertension in children, the first ninety patients. *Ann. Surg.* 192:18, 1980.
17. Boles E.T. Jr., Birken G.: Extrahepatic portal hypertension in children: Long-term evaluation. *Chir. Pédiatr.* 24:23, 1983.
18. Blakemore A.H.: Portacaval anastomosis: A report of 14 cases. *Bull. N.Y. Acad. Med.* 22:254, 1946.
19. Boley S.J., Arlan M., Magilner L.J.: Congenital hepatic fibrosis causing portal hypertension in children. *Surgery* 54:356, 1963.
20. Bonnette J., et al.: Cirrhosis in a 15-month-old child suggesting Budd-Chiari syndrome. *Ann. Pédiatr.* 12:548, 1965.
21. Britton R.C., Mahoney E.B., Hogg L. Jr.: Congenital stricture of the portal vein. *Arch. Surg.* 61:713, 1950.
22. Britton R.C., Voorhees A.B. Jr., Price J.B. Jr.: Selective portal decompression. *Surgery* 67:104, 1970.
23. Burchell A.R., et al.: Hemodynamic variables and prognosis following portacaval shunt. *Surg. Gynecol. Obstet.* 138:359, 1974.
24. Cameron J.L., Maddrey W.C.: Mesoatrial shunt: A new treatment for the Budd-Chiari syndrome. *Ann. Surg.* 187:401, 1978.
25. Castell D.O.: Ascites in cirrhosis: Relative importance of portal hypertension and hypoalbuminemia. *Am. J. Dig. Dis.* 12:916, 1967.
26. Child C.G.: Portal hypertension as seen by 17 authorities, in Child C.G. (ed.): *Major Problems in Clinical Surgery*, vol. 14. Philadelphia, W.B. Saunders Co., 1974.
27. Child C.G.: *The Liver and Portal Hypertension*. Philadelphia, W.B. Saunders Co., 1964.
27a. Child C.G., Zuidema G.C.: Experimental surgery of the portal vein, hepatic artery and hepatic veins, in Child C.G. (ed.): *The Liver and Portal Hypertension*. Philadelphia, W.B. Saunders Co., 1964, pp. 189–224.
28. Chojkier M., Groszmann R.J., Atterbury C.E., et al.: A controlled comparison of continuous intra-arterial and intravenous infusions of vasopressin in hemorrhage from esophageal varices. *Gastroenterology* 77:540, 1979.
29. Clark A.W., MacDougall B.R.D., Westaby D., et al.: Prospective controlled trial of injection sclerotherapy in patients with cirrhosis and recent variceal hemorrhage. *Lancet* 2:552, 1980.
30. Clatworthy H.W. Jr.: Extrahepatic portal hypertension, in Child C.G. (ed.): *Major Problems in Clinical Surgery*, vol. 14. Philadelphia, W.B. Saunders Co., 1974.

31. Clatworthy H.W. Jr., Boles E.T. Jr.: Extrahepatic portal bed block in children: Pathogenesis and treatment. *Ann. Surg.* 150:371, 1959.

32. Clatworthy H.W. Jr., Wall T., Watman R.N.: A new type of portal-to-systemic shunt for portal hypertension. *Arch. Surg.* 71:588, 1955.

33. Cohen D., Mansour A.: Extrahepatic portal hypertension. Long-term results. *Prog. Pediatr. Surg.* 10:129, 1977.

34. Cooperman A.M., Hermann R.E.: Ligation procedures in the management of portal hypertension. *Surgery* 81:382, 1977.

35. Crafoord C., Frenckner P.: New surgical treatment of varicose veins of the oesophagus. *Acta Oto-laryng.* (Scand.) 27:422, 1939.

36. Crile G. Jr.: Transesophageal ligation of bleeding esophageal varices. *Arch. Surg.* 61:654, 1950.

37. Delaney J.P.: A method for esophagogastric devascularization. *Surg. Gynecol. Obstet.* 150:899, 1980.

38. di Sant'Agnese P.A., Blanc W.A.: A distinctive type of biliary cirrhosis of the liver associated with cystic fibrosis of the pancreas: Recognition through signs of portal hypertension. *Pediatrics* 18:387, 1956.

39. Drapanas J.T.: Interposition mesocaval shunt for the treatment of portal hypertension. *Ann. Surg.* 176:435, 1972.

40. Eck N.V.: On the question of ligature of the portal vein. *Voyenno Med.* 130:1, 1877, translated in Child C.G. *Surg. Gynecol. Obstet.* 137:210, 1973.

41. Fonkalsrud E.W.: Shunt operations for portal hypertension in children (editorial). *J. Pediatr.* 103:742, 1983.

42. Fonkalsrud E.W.: Surgical management of portal hypertension in childhood. *Arch. Surg.* 115:1042, 1980.

43. Fonkalsrud E.W., Myers N.A., Robinson M.J.: Management of extra-hepatic portal hypertension in children. *Ann. Surg.* 180:487, 1974.

44. Fonkalsrud E.W., Linde L.M., Longmire W.P.: Portal hypertension from idiopathic superior vena caval obstruction. *JAMA* 196:129, 1966.

45. Foster J.H., et al.: Splenoportography: An assessment of its value and risk. *Ann. Surg.* 179:773, 1974.

46. Fuller R.K., Khambatta P.B., Gobezie G.C.: An optimal diuretic regimen for cirrhotic ascites. *JAMA* 237:972, 1977.

47. Galambos J.T., Warren W.D., et al.: Selective and total shunts in the treatment of bleeding varices: A randomized controlled trial. *N. Engl. J. Med.* 295:1089, 1976.

48. George P., et al.: Emergency oesophageal transection in uncontrolled variceal haemorrhage. *Br. J. Surg.* 60:635, 1973.

49. Grauer S.E., Schwartz S.I.: Extrahepatic portal hypertension: A retrospective analysis. *Ann. Surg.* 189:566, 1979.

50. Habif D.: Treatment of esophageal varices by partial esophagogastrectomy and interposed jejunal segment. *Surgery* 46:212, 1959.

50a. Hahn M., Massen O., Nencki M., et al.: Das Eck der Fistel zwischen der unteren Hohlvene und der Pfortader und ihre Folgen fur den organismus. *Arch. Exper. Path. Parmakol.* 32:161, 1983.

51. Hennessy T.P.J., Stephens R.B., Keane F.B.: Acute and chronic management of esophageal varices by injection sclerotherapy. *Surg. Gynecol. Obstet.* 154:375, 1982.

52. Hirashima T., Hara T., Takeuchih H., et al.: Transabdominal esophageal mucosal transection for the control of esophageal varices. *Surg. Gynecol. Obstet.* 151:36, 1980.

53. Huguet C., Thierry D., Olivier J.M.: Budd-Chiari syndrome with thrombosis of inferior vena cava: Long-term patency of mesocaval and cavoatrial prosthetic bypass. *Surgery* 94:108, 1983.

54. Hutson D.G., Pereiras R., Zeppa R., et al.: The fate of esophageal varices following selective distal splenorenal shunt. *Ann. Surg.* 183:496, 1976.

55. Johnston G.W.: Treatment of bleeding varices by oesophageal transection with the SPTV gun. *Ann. R. Coll. Surg. Engl.* 59:404, 1977.

56. Kerr D.N.S.: Congenital hepatic fibrosis. *Q. J. Med.* 30:91, 1961.

57. Kerr D.N., Warrick C.K., Hart-Mercer J.: A lesion resembling medullary sponge kidney in patients with congenital hepatic fibrosis. *Clin. Radiol.* 13:85, 1962.

58. King H., Shumacker H.B.: Splenic studies: Susceptibility to infection after splenectomy performed in infancy. *Ann. Surg.* 136:239, 1952.

59. Koop C.E., Roddy R.: Colonic replacement of distal esophagus and proximal stomach in the management of bleeding varices in children. *Ann. Surg.* 147:17, 1958.

60. Koyama K., Takagi Y., Ouchih K., et al.: Results of esophageal transection for esophageal varices: Experience in 100 cases. *Am. J. Surg.* 139:204, 1980.

61. Kraft R.O., Fry W.J.: The demonstration of hepatofugal flow following side-to-side portacaval anastomosis. *Surg. Gynecol. Obstet.* 118:124, 1964.

62. Lambert M.J., Tank E.S., Turcotte J.G.: Late sequelae of mesocaval shunts in children. *Am. J. Surg.* 127:19, 1974.

63. Langer B., et al.: Clinical spectrum of the Budd-Chiari syndrome and its surgical management. *Am. J. Surg.* 129:197, 1975.

64. LeVeen H.H., Wapnick S., Grosberg S., et al.: Further experience with peritoneovenous shunt for ascites. *Ann. Surg.* 184:574, 1976.

65. Lilly J.R., Van Stiegmann G., Stellin G.: Esophageal endosclerosis in children with portal vein thrombosis. *J. Pediatr. Surg.* 17:571, 1982.

66. Linton R.R., Jones C.M., Volwyler W.: Portal hypertension: Treatment by splenectomy and splenorenal anastomosis with preservation of the kidney. *Surg. Clin. North Am.* 27:1162, 1947.

67. Linton R.R., Warren R.: The emergency treatment of massive bleeding from esophageal varices by transesophageal suture of those vessels at the time of acute hemorrhage. *Surgery* 33:243, 1953.

68. Maddison F.: Embolic therapy of hypersplenism. *Invest. Radiol.* 8:280, 1973.

69. Maksoud J.G., Mies S.: Distal splenorenal shunt (DSS) in children. *Ann. Surg.* 195:401, 1982.

70. Marion P.: Traitement chirurgical de l'hypertension portal. *Helv. Med. Acta* 21:375, 1954.

71. Marion P.: Mesoenterico-caval anastomosis. *J. Cardiovasc. Surg.* (suppl.) 70:70, 1966.

72. Melhem R.E., Rizk G.K.: Splenoportographic evaluation of portal hypertension in children. *J. Pediatr. Surg.* 5:522, 1970.

73. Mitchell M.C., Boitnott J.K., Kaufman S., et al.: Budd-Chiari syndrome: Etiology, diagnosis and management. *Medicine* 61:199, 1982.

74. McDermott W.V. Jr., et al.: Postshunt encephalopathy. *Surg. Gynecol. Obstet.* 126:585, 1968.

75. McDermott W.V., Jr.: Evaluation of the hemodynamics of portal hypertension in the selection of patients for shunt surgery. *Ann. Surg.* 176:449, 1972.

76. McDermott W.V. Jr., Adams R.D.: Episodic stupor associated with ECK fistula in human with particular reference to the metabolism of ammonia. *J. Clin. Invest.* 1:1, 1954.

77. Nakamura T., et al.: Inferior vena cava and hepatic vein thrombosis (Budd-Chiari syndrome): Characteristics of Japanese cases, including 18 authors' cases and 165 literature cases. *Jpn. J. Clin. Med.* 25:705, 1967.

78. Nay H.R., Fitzpatrick H.F.: Mesocaval "H" graft using autogenous vein graft. *Ann. Surg.* 183:114, 1976.

79. Nusbaum M., et al.: Pharmacologic control of portal hypertension. *Surgery* 62:299, 1967.

80. O'Donnell B., Maloney M.A.: Development and course of extrahepatic portal obstruction in children. *Lancet* 1:789, 1968.

81. Parker R.G.F.: Occlusion of the hepatic veins in man. *Medicine* 38:369, 1959.

82. Putnam C.W., Porter K.A., Weill R., et al.: Liver transplantation for Budd-Chiari syndrome. *JAMA* 236:1142, 1976.

83. Rikkers L.F.: Portal hemodynamics, intestinal absorption, and postshunt encephalopathy. *Surgery* 94:126, 1983.

84. Rodgers B.M., Talbert J.L.: Distal splenorenal shunt for portal decompression in children. *J. Pediatr. Surg.* 14:33, 1979.

85. Romero-Torres R.: Hemostatic suture of the stomach for the treatment of massive hemorrhage due to esophageal varices. *Surg. Gynecol. Obstet.* 153:710, 1981.

86. Rousselot L.M., et al.: Experience with portacaval anastomoses: Analysis of 104 elective end-to-side shunts for prevention of recurrent hemorrhage from esophago-gastric varices (1952–1961). *Am. J. Med.* 34:297, 1963.

87. Sarfeh I.J., Rypins E.P., Conroy R.M., et al.: Portacaval H-grafts: Relationships of shunt diameter, portal flow patterns, and encephalopathy. *Ann. Surg.* 197:422, 1983.

88. Schaefer J.W., et al.: Progression of acute hepatitis to postnecrotic cirrhosis. *Am. J. Med.* 42:348, 1967.

89. Shaldon S., Sherlock S.: The use of vasopressin (Pitressin) in the control of bleeding from oesophageal varices. *Lancet* 2:222, 1960.

90. Shaldon S., Sherlock S.: Obstruction to the extrahepatic portal system in children. *Lancet* 1:63, 1962.

91. Sherlock S., et al.: Portal systemic encephalopathy: Neurological complications of liver disease. *Lancet* 2:453, 1954.

92. Sherlock S.: Post-hepatitis cirrhosis. *Lancet* 1:817, 1948.

93. Singer D.B.: Postsplenectomy sepsis, in Rosenberg H.S., Bolande R.P. (eds.): *Perspectives in Pediatric Pathology*, vol. 1. Chicago, Year Book Medical Publishers, 1973.

94. Smith G.W.: Use of hemodynamic selection criteria in the management of cirrhotic patients with portal hypertension. *Ann. Surg.* 179:782, 1974.

95. Spigos D.G., Tan W.S., Mozes M.F., et al.: Splenic embolization. *Cardiovasc. Intervent. Radiol.* 3:282, 1980.

96. Stamatkis J.D., Howard E.R., Psacharopoulos H.T., et al.: Injection sclerotherapy for oesophageal varices in children. *Br. J. Surg.* 69:74, 1982.

97. Starzl T.: Portal vein thrombosis and portal thrombosis (editorial). *J. Pediatr.* 103:741, 1983.

98. Sugiura M., Futagawa S.: Further evaluation of the Sugiura procedure in the treatment of esophageal varices. *Arch. Surg.* 112:1317, 1977.

99. Sugiura M., Futagawa S.: A new technique for treating esophageal varices. *J. Thorac. Cardiovasc. Surg.* 66:677, 1973.

100. Terblanche J., Yakoob H.I., Bornman P.C., et al.: Acute bleeding varices: A 5-year prospective evaluation of tamponade and sclerotherapy. *Ann. Surg.* 194:521, 1981.

101. Terblanche J., Northover J.M.A., Bornman P., et al.: A prospective controlled trial of sclerotherapy in the long-term management of patients after oesophageal variceal bleeding. *Surg. Gynecol. Obstet.* 148:323, 1979.

102. Turunen M., Pasila M., Sulamaa M.: Supradiaphragmatic transposition of the spleen for portal hypertension. *Ann. Surg.* 157:127, 1963.

103. Voorhees A.B., Chaitman E., Schneider S., et al.: Portasystemic encephalopathy in the non-cirrhotic patient. *Arch. Surg.* 107:659, 1973.

104. Warren W.D.: Control of variceal bleeding: Reassessment of rationale. *Am. J. Surg.* 145:8, 1982.

105. Warren W.D., Zeppa R., Foman J.J.: Selective transplenic decompression of gastroesophageal varices by distal splenorenal shunt. *Ann. Surg.* 166:437, 1967.

106. Weiner E.: Personal communication, 1984.

107. Welch C.S.: Ligation of esophageal varices by the transabdominal route. *N. Engl. J. Med.* 255:677, 1956.

108. Whipple A.O., Blakemore A.H., Lord J.E.: The problem of portal hypertension in relation to the hepatosplenopathies. *Ann. Surg.* 122:449, 1945.

109. Whipple A.O.: The rationale of portacaval anastomosis. *Bull. N.Y. Acad. Med.* 22:251, 1946.

110. Witte C.L., Ovitt T.W., Van Vyck D.B., et al.: Ischemic therapy in thrombocytopenia from hypersplenism. *Arch. Surg.* 111:1115, 1976.

111. Zeppa R., Warren W.D.: The distal splenorenal shunt. *Am. J. Surg.* 122:300, 1971.

112. Zuidema G.D., Kirsch M.M.: Hepatic encephalopathy following portal decompression: Evaluation of end-to-side and side-to-side anastomoses. *Am. Surg.* 31:567, 1965.

113. Vosschulte K.: Place de la section par ligature de l'oesophage dans le traitement de l'hypertension portale. *Lyon Chir.* 53:519, 1957.

115 Kenneth J. Welch

The Pancreas

Embryology

The pancreas forms from paired primordia between the fourth and the seventh weeks of fetal life. The dorsal pancreas arises from the dorsal wall of the duodenum. The ventral pancreas develops to the right of the midline and grows caudally. As gut rotation proceeds, the common bile duct is displaced to the right; the ventral pancreas grows around the right side of the duodenum and comes into juxtaposition with the dorsal pancreas, which contributes the body and tail. The independent duct systems fuse. The dorsal duct (Santorini) opens directly into the duodenum, and the ventral duct (Wirsung) opens into the duodenum by way of the common bile duct. The dorsal duct persists, draining the body and tail, fusing with the ventral duct just to the right of the mesenteric vessels. Occasionally, the ventral duct disappears and the entire gland is drained by the duct of Santorini.

The islets of Langerhans arise from the epithelial cords that give rise to the secretory acini. They separate at an early stage and differentiate independently.

Annular pancreas is the commonest developmental error encountered by the surgeon, followed in frequency by anomalies of the duct system, duplication, fusion with spleen, duodenum, and stomach, and encapsulated structures contributed by adjacent intestinal primordia. Heterotopic pancreatic primordia may account for the Zollinger-Ellison syndrome. One may encounter atresia, severe hypoplasia, or suppression of either pancreatic bud, resulting in absence of the body and tail or absence of the head, with corresponding changes in duct anatomy (Table 115–1).

Pancreatitis

Acute Pancreatitis

Acute pancreatitis was first described by Fitz[20] in 1889, and the essential pathologic features recognized by Rich and Duff[41] in 1936. The literature contains reports of fulminant or even fatal disease, the diagnosis being made at laparotomy or autopsy.[7, 14, 21] The diagnosis can be made in most instances early in the disease by determining serum and urinary amylase levels, which are three to five times normal. After 2 or 3 days, amylase levels can be normal or only mildly elevated.

Etiology and Pathogenesis

Frey and Redo[21] reported 14 cases of diffuse, hemorrhagic pancreatitis discovered at autopsy. The children had a history of poor oral intake, nausea, vomiting, diarrhea, abdominal pain, and some form of intercurrent infection. Several children were first seen with tachycardia, jaundice, and coma. The idiopathic form of pancreatitis accounts for 50% of reported cases, although recent reports provide a greater range of etiology. In the usual case, pancreatitis comes on rapidly after, or in association with, a febrile illness and a period of poor intake, often associated with vomiting and dehydration. Blumenstock et al.[7] first called attention to the idiopathic variety, included in all recent reports. Hendren et al.[26] encountered six idiopathic cases in 15 children with pancreatitis, and Frey and Redo[21] found six in 18. Fifty-six cases of pancreatitis seen at the Boston Children's Hospital are considered to be idiopathic (Table 115–1).

TABLE 115–1.—DISORDERS OF THE PANCREAS IN 300
CHILDREN (CHILDREN'S HOSPITAL, BOSTON, 1938–1984)

Pancreatitis		135 (45%)
Acute idiopathic	56	
Acute traumatic	38	
Pseudocyst	17	
Chronic fibrosing	10	
Chronic familial	6	
Calcifying	5	
Hyperlipidemia	3	
Idiopathic spontaneous hypoglycemia (ISH)		77 (26%)
Medically treated	49	
Nesidioblastosis, surgically treated	28	
Congenital abnormalities		58 (19%)
Annular pancreas	36	
Atresia of ducts	5	
Intrapancreatic gastric duplication	4	
Hypoplasia	3	
Dextroposition, pancreas and stomach only	2	
Duplication, complete	2	
Pancreaticoduodenal duplication	2	
Fusion with spleen	2	
Intrapancreatic accessory spleen	1	
Absence of body and tail	1	
Tumors		30 (10%)
Insulinoma, benign	8	
Cyst, developmental	6	
Choristoma, hamartoma	6	
Adenocarcinoma (duct cell)	4	
Adenocarcinoma (acinar cell)	3	
Islet cell carcinoma (nonfunctioning)	1	
Adenoma (acinar cell)	1	
Cyst, papillary	1	

The association of steroid administration and pancreatitis was documented by Baar and Wolff[3] and subsequently confirmed by Oppenheimer and Boitnott,[36] among others. Fifteen percent of children with end-stage renal disease have evidence of pancreatitis. Secondary hyperparathyroidism and hypercalcemia undoubtedly play a role. The incidence increased to 40% in a group of children with renal disease who received steroids. A similar situation exists in children with primary liver disease who are treated with steroids. Extrahepatic biliary tract disease is, however, uncommon in children with pancreatitis. Cholelithiasis was encountered twice in our series and once in 48 cases collected from the literature.[32] Pancreatitis may be associated with familial aminoaciduria and hyperlipidemia.[15] The hereditary and familial varieties tend to be recurrent, ultimately producing pancreatic cirrhosis or calcinosis, or both. Postoperative pancreatitis, from injury to the pancreas at the time of operation, is less common in children than in adults because of the relative infrequency of operations on the biliary tract, stomach, and duodenum. Injury to the tail of the pancreas during splenectomy causes a milder, usually self-limited, form. Diffuse pancreatic calcinosis in a 1-year-old child was reported by Martin and Canseco.[31] We encountered it in three children with cystic fibrosis and one each with familial chronic pancreatitis and hyperparathyroidism (Table 115–1). Acute hemorrhagic pancreatitis has been reported following the administration of chlorothiazide, tetracyclines, oral contraceptives, azothioprine, L-asparaginase, and the new anticonvulsant drug, valproic acid.[33, 45] Mumps pancreatitis is rare, or certainly mild, in children; amylase elevation is not diagnostic because of simultaneous bilateral sialadenitis.[8] In 12 of 17 reported cases in adults, there was a predisposing biliary or pancreatic factor.[37] One case of pancreatitis has been described associated with polyarteritis nodosa.[21] Invasion of the pancreatic

ducts by *Ascaris lumbricoides* with resultant pancreatitis has been reported in children in this country and abroad.[22] Pancreatitis in the burn patient treated with steroids was described by Baar and Wolff.[3] Marczynska-Robowska reported pancreatic necrosis in patients with adrenocorticotropin (ACTH)-treated Still's disease.[30] Pancreatitis after renal transplantation was reported in five of 68 patients.[40] The patients were receiving prednisone, azothioprine, and antilymphocyte globulin (ALG). Pancreatitis has not been reported in children after liver transplantation, perhaps because the use of cyclosporin A has sharply reduced the dosage of steroids employed.[44]

Recent additions to causes of pancreatitis are infectious mononucleosis, hyperlipidemia types 1 and 5, scorpion bite, and acute intermittent porphyria. Pancreatitis occurred in two patients undergoing hyperalimentation; however, both cases occurred postoperatively, and both patients were receiving steroids.

About half the patients with pancreatitis do not have elevated serum amylase levels. If the suspicion is high, the amylase-creatinine clearance ratio is useful:

$$\frac{\text{urine amylase}}{\text{serum amylase}} \times \frac{\text{serum creatinine}}{\text{urine creatinine}} \times 100.$$

Normally, it is less than 5; above this, pancreatitis is likely. Combining lipase and amylase determinations gives a higher accuracy of diagnosis of pancreatitis. Up to 60% of adults and children with an increased amylase level do not have pancreatitis and have a normal amylase-creatinine clearance value. Amylase-creatinine clearance is abnormally high in patients with burns, diabetes, renal failure, and following cardiac surgery. Deoxynuclease, ribodeoxynuclease, and the pancreozymin secretin tests are still experimental. Improved diagnosis is credited to the use of the body computed tomographic (CT) scan with selenium or tellurium 123/methionine enhancement.[2] Ultrasonography confirms the CT findings. With both techniques, the gland appears enlarged. Gross ductal enlargement may be demonstrated on ultrasound scans, but ductal anatomy is not well demonstrated by either technique. Diagnostic peritoneal lavage has been recommended,[29] if only to rule out a major intra-abdominal catastrophe other than pancreatitis, although perforated or dead bowel will leak amylase. Finally, exploratory laparotomy during the acute phase may become necessary to rule out other surgical conditions. Thirty-two such laparotomies among 231 lavaged adult patients with pancreatitis were performed within the first 36 hours of onset.[29] Mortality in this group was 12%, compared with 10% for medical treatment only without laparotomy. Therefore, laparotomy should not be withheld if the diagnosis is in doubt about another equally or more serious surgical condition.

In childhood, pancreatitis of known etiology is most frequently due to trauma.[49] In approximately one of five patients, a pseudocyst develops. In 38 cases of traumatic pancreatitis, we have found seven pseudocysts.

Medical Management

Traditional therapy has been supportive—including pain relief, administration of parenteral fluids, maintenance of caloric intake, and inhibition of pancreatic secretion. Meperidine rather than morphine is used to control pain (0.5 mg/kg every 4 hours). Nasogastric decompression is of uncertain value. If laparotomy became necessary for diagnosis or drainage, most would perform a gastrostomy. Anticholinergic drugs have fallen into disuse. Calcium supplementation is reserved for patients with tetany. The cause of the low blood levels of calcium has been variously attributed to saponification of necrotic fat, glucagon-related thyrocalcitonin release, and hypomagnesemia. Glucagon, aprotinin, (Trasylol), and cimetidine have not altered the course of the disease in any way and are no longer used. Krauste et al.[29] report experience with peritoneal lavage as a primary treatment method in acute fulminating pancreatitis. The acute fulminant necrotic or hemorrhagic form of pancreatitis is seldom seen in children and usually involves patients who are immunocompromised in one form or another. The clinical course, as in adults, is rapid and catastrophic. They treated 21 adult patients with acute fulminant pancreatitis out of a total of 269 adult patients, most of whom had the mild form of disease. During the same period, 28 laparotomies were performed during the acute phase of fulminant hemorrhagic pancreatitis for clinical deterioration and for certainty of diagnosis. There were 10 deaths, a mortality rate of 35%. Predicted mortality in this group was 80%. All had three or more Ranson criteria for potentially fatal issue.[39] When operation was performed, it consisted of near-total pancreatectomy.

A reduction of circulating blood volume due to loss of large amounts of blood and plasma from the intravascular compartment is the major physiologic disturbance in acute pancreatitis. Errors of undertreatment and overtreatment are common. Urine output must be monitored, and central venous pressure should be maintained in the range of 8–12 cm H_2O by infusion of electrolyte solutions, plasma, or albumin.

As the disease wears on, there is an increasing respiratory demand, with reduction of pulmonary reserve. Retroperitoneal edema, elevation of the diaphragm, pleural effusion, and abdominal splinting combine to produce basal atelectasis, leading to intrapulmonary shunting of blood. Liberated enzymes cause direct pulmonary parenchymal injury. A vicious cycle of increasing metabolic demand and decreasing pulmonary reserve leads to respiratory failure and cessation of cardiac activity when arterial pH falls below 6.8. Arterial blood gas determinations are essential for adjustment of FIO_2 to PaO_2 levels. Assisted respiration diminishes the work of breathing and minimizes the effects of pulmonary edema. Some degree of pancreatic necrosis is inevitable and with it, secondary infection. The antibiotic of choice is cefazolin (Ancef), 25–50 mg/kg/day. Repeated cultures may detect the emergence of *Pseudomonas,* for which the drugs of choice are clindamycin and gentamicin (Garamycin).

Hyperalimentation during the period of intravenous therapy has made feeding jejunostomy obsolete. An elemental diet after return to oral feedings has been found helpful.

Surgical Treatment

Surgical intervention is rarely indicated in the acute phase of pancreatitis if the diagnosis is certain. Although surgical complications are common, they seldom appear before the end of the second week. Because pancreatitis is seldom suspected in childhood, the usual preoperative diagnosis is acute appendicitis. When the abdomen is opened, fat necrosis and a large volume of intraperitoneal fluid of high colloid content and high pancreatic enzyme activity are encountered. The surgeon should not attack the ampulla, common duct, or pancreatic duct. Even if anomalies of the duct are present, they are best diagnosed and corrected later. Coincident biliary tract disease with cholelithiasis is rare. The lesser sac should be thoroughly drained through the divided gastrocolic ligament. Large Penrose sump drains are brought out through a separate stab wound in the flank. Operation for late complications, usually signaled by high fever and toxicity, includes near-total pancreatic resection or debridement and drainage of pancreatic abscess.

The cause of death in reported series, mostly involving adults, has been a combination of factors: infection, hemorrhage, shock, and cardiopulmonary, renal, and hepatic failure. Howard and Ravdin[27] were among the first to define the pathophysiology of

pancreatitis and in 1948 reported a mortality of 76% in 80 consecutive patients. Nugent and Atendido[34] in 1967, reporting a mortality of 17.4%, recommended limited surgical intervention. Romer and Carey[43] noted a 23% mortality in 100 consecutive patients with acute hemorrhagic pancreatitis. In recent series, the mortality has varied from 5% to 15%.[11, 12] Krauste et al. in 1983 reported a 10% mortality in 269 patients.[29]

Similar success can be achieved in children by calling attention to this uncommon disorder, especially in immunocompromised patients, and placing it higher on the list of acute surgical conditions of the abdomen.

Chronic Relapsing Pancreatitis

Relatively few reports of chronic relapsing pancreatitis in childhood are available, although it is being more frequently suspected in children with recurring abdominal pain. Ghishan et al.[23] encountered 10 such children. All had endoscopic retrograde cholangiopancreatography (ERCP); they were placed in three groups. Group 1, four patients, had hereditary pancreatitis. Group 2, two patients, had similar courses and findings but no family history. Group 3, four children, all of them jaundiced, had fibrosing pancreatitis. One had hyperlipidemia type 1. ERCP was helpful in four patients, groups 1 and 2. In group 3, duct anatomy was normal and serum amylase levels were normal in three of four patients. All patients with chronic relapsing pancreatitis of the familial or hereditary type required internal drainage of the distal pancreatic duct with Roux-en-Y, either as an end-to-end pancreaticojejunostomy (Duval) or a longitudinal pancreaticojejunostomy (Puestow).[38] Children with chronic fibrosing pancreatitis had relative stenosis of the distal common duct and were treated by sphincteroplasty. One produced obstruction and required a choledochoduodenostomy. Seven of 10 patients were asymptomatic 8 months to 4 years following operation. The report stresses the importance of determining duct anatomy by ERCP or intraoperative pancreatography. In all cases, the distal common duct should be studied, recording the opening pressures. For complete common duct obstruction, a Roux-en-Y choledochojejunostomy is required.

Comfort and Steinberg[15] reported 29 cases without associated biliary or gastrointestinal disease, and others[18, 28, 48, 51] have reported additional cases of chronic pancreatitis in children. Such children must be suspected of having heredofamilial disease with aminoaciduria or hyperlipidemia type 1 or 5, or both. Hyperparathyroidism, more common in adults than in children, must be ruled out. The symptoms, other than recurring abdominal pain, are variable, and laboratory findings are inconclusive. Changes in the pancreas discovered at laparotomy consist of diffuse hardening and nodularity involving the entire gland. Biopsy, although seldom performed because of its hazard, shows fibrosis and loss of acini, initially sparing the islets of Langerhans. Symptoms increase in frequency and severity. Eventually, there is evidence of pancreatic exocrine insufficiency, with steatorrhea and weight loss. The gland may become calcified. Diabetes appears late in some cases.

Appropriate studies include measurements of serum lipase, amylase and calcium, fasting blood sugar, serum cholesterol, phospholipids, free fatty acids, stool fat, and trypsin activity in the duodenum and/or stools. Plain x-ray films may reveal calcification (Fig 115–1). A barium meal should be given to outline the duodenum. There is usually some enlargement of the C loop. Ultrasonography and CT show diffuse enlargement of the gland, cysts, or dilated ducts. Direct injection of the pancreatic ducts, utilizing the flexible fiberoptic gastroscope ERCP (under general anesthesia to age 5 years, diazepam sedation in older children), may show bizarre ductal architecture with areas of stricture and dilatation—the beading or chain-of-lakes appearance (Fig 115–

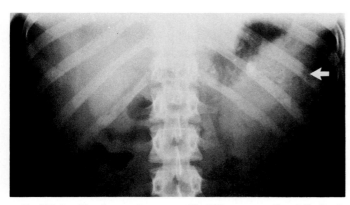

Fig 115–1.—Chronic recurring pancreatitis. Diffuse pancreatic calcification is seen in the left upper quadrant *(arrow)* in this roentgenogram of an 11-year-old girl with familial pancreatitis. The ^{99}Tc radionuclide scan showed minimal uptake in the body and tail of the pancreas. The transduodenal pancreatogram showed an essentially normal pancreatic duct. Treatment consisted of a 75% distal resection and Puestow's procedure.

2). Pancreatography should not be performed during the active phase of pancreatitis. Percutaneous pancreatography under ultrasonic guidance is reported.[23] Septic complications, including perforation, cholangitis, and pancreatitis, have followed retrograde pancreatic duct injection in a small percentage of cases, especially with overfilling or proximal obstruction. However, this is not a high price to pay for essential anatomical information.

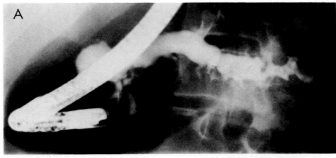

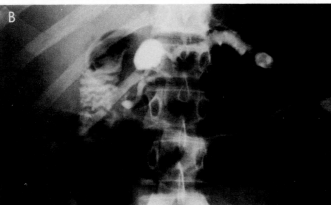

Fig 115–2.—Chronic recurring hereditary pancreatitis in a 14-year-old girl. **A,** endoscopic retrograde pancreatography demonstrates proximal stenosis of the pancreatic duct with distal ectasia and calcification. **B,** further details of pancreatic duct anatomy in the same patient after removal of the flexible fiberoptic gastroscope. This study has replaced open operation for pancreatic duct evaluation except in those instances in which the pancreatic duct cannot be catheterized or identified. The patient was treated by distal pancreatectomy and Roux-en-Y Puestow pancreaticojejunostomy.

Cotton[17] and Becker[4] also recommend the use of ERCP in children with pancreatitis. Bluestone et al.[6] reported on five children, 5–15 years of age, with relapsing pancreatitis, all of the hereditary type, studied by ERCP. The Olympus JFB sideviewing duodenoscope and 50% Hypaque contrast medium were used. Intravenous glucagon was used to diminish duodenal peristalsis during the study. All but one were performed under intravenous diazepam (Valium) sedation. In four of five patients, there was a dilated ventral duct with beading and calculi. Treatment consisted of either end-to-end or longitudinal pancreaticojejunostomy. At times, especially in small children, it is not possible to catheterize the pancreatic ducts, and laparotomy is necessary to demonstrate the type and degree of involvement. Intraoperative evaluation should include a cholangiogram, with opening biliary infusion pressure, and direct pancreatography. Because of the possibility of stone or stricture at the ampulla, a buried duplication, or an anomalous duct system such as pancreas divisum, it is important to mobilize the duodenum, incise its wall vertically, directly evaluate the ampulla, and select the proper surgical drainage procedure.

Pancreas Divisum

Pancreas divisum results when the dorsal and ventral components of the pancreas fail to fuse.[5, 16] The dorsal component is drained by the duct of Santorini and the ventral component by the duct of Wirsung, which ordinarily joins the distal common duct and enters the duodenum as a common channel. The usual residual of the dorsal component is probably the uncinate process. The Santorini branch usually drains this area exclusively. The finding of separate duodenal entry of the two pancreatic ducts is not unusual, about 20% in children according to Vawter. On routine ERCP studies of asymptomatic patients, the incidence is 5%. Yet 25% or more of such patients ultimately develop recurring pancreatitis. Britt et al.[10] described six patients with recurring pancreatitis and pancreas divisum. Five were treated with sphincteroplasty of the ampulla. None of his patients were children, but, as with other reports of chronic relapsing pancreatitis, the disease often dated from early childhood or adolescence. Of 44 patients from the literature, none were children at the time of surgical treatment.[10, 25, 42] ERCP studies uniformly showed a short or absent ventral duct of Wirsung. Attempts to catheterize the dorsal duct of Santorini were usually unsuccessful. The cause of pancreatitis in this group is thought to be a relative stenosis and obstruction of a dorsal duct small in comparison to the volume of pancreas drained, although no pressure flow studies have been recorded to date. We encountered one child with pancreas divisum who required surgical treatment—a 14-year-old girl with pancreatitis recurring over a 6-month period. Amylase levels ranged from 200 to 6,000 units/l. Ninety percent of the gland was drained by the duct of Santorini (Fig 115–3). Both ducts were treated by sphincteroplasty; neither was dilated. The patient is asymptomatic, and amylase levels remain in a normal range 1 year later. Yedlin and Philippart[52] described a case of pancreas divisum in a 10-year-old boy with recurring pancreatitis, pleural effusion, and a central pseudocyst. Neither duct was dilated on ERCP study. Treatment consisted of sphincteroplasty of the minor duct and internal drainage of the pseudocyst. The patient did well. Silen doubts the significance of pancreas divisum because of the absence of flow measurements in this system and the absence of dilatation of the duct in all reported cases.[46] Whether the entity is fact or myth has not been determined, and the experience in childhood is small. Long-term follow-up of these patients operated on in childhood will be of interest. Bernstein et al.[5] reviewed the evidence for the association of pancreas divisum with recurrent pancreatitis

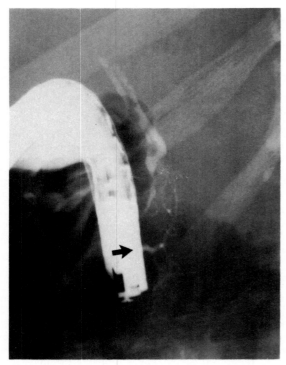

Fig 115–3.—Pancreas divisum in a 14-year-old girl with recurrent pancreatitis. ERCP study shows a short branching ventral duct of Wirsung *(arrow)*. Ninety percent of the gland, including the body, tail, and uncinate process, is drained by the duct of Santorini. The high-volume flow and relatively small proximal dorsal duct are said to account for pancreatic enzyme extravasation and recurring pancreatitis.

and found it supportable in six patients operated on for pancreas divisum, the youngest aged 17 years. Treatment of choice was sphincteroplasty of one or both ducts. The gallbladder was removed in all patients. Cholecystectomy is wise following sphincteroplasty, since, because of bile stasis in the gallbladder, all adult patients ultimately develop stones.[6, 46] Follow-up ranged from 13 to 34 months. Good results were obtained in five patients; one continues to have recurring pancreatitis. As in most other reports, ERCP and operative pancreatography failed to show dilatation of either system. If there is a dilated duct, sphincteroplasty should probably be combined with the Puestow procedure[38] or a modification of Duval's pancreaticojejunostomy for direct ductal decompression. Bluestone et al.[6] stressed that the duct system be studied by ERCP immediately before operation. Some dilatations of the pancreatic duct have proved to be temporary, the duct returning to normal following medical treatment of the pancreatitis. Pancreatography is, of course, required in all cases of pancreatic duct obstruction to determine the surgical procedure of choice regardless of etiology.

Our experience with chronic relapsing pancreatitis has increased to eight patients. Three have been previously reported. Three patients had a positive family history. For pancreatic duct ectasia and calculi, all required distal duct drainage by the Puestow method of longitudinal pancreaticojejunostomy. Four patients had chronic fibrosing pancreatitis, as designated by O'Neill et al.[35] All required sphincteroplasty and all did well. Follow-up ranged from 3 months to 7 years. All have been relieved of pain and recurring pancreatitis. Ghishan et al.[23] estimated that there are 195 proved cases of familial or hereditary pancreatitis with 40 affected kindred. The youngest patient operated on to date was aged 4 years. Chronic relapsing pancreati-

tis due to one form or another of hyperlipidemia type 1, 2B, 3A, or 5 is rare and reportable. Parenchymal destruction is progressive. More information is needed, but thus far sphincteroplasty has been effective in selected cases. Although rare in children, causative biliary tract pathology must always be ruled out. Junction of the common bile duct and main pancreatic duct, a common finding, led to distal ampullary obstruction by a stone and reflux pancreatitis in Hendren's[26] patient with congenital spherocytosis. It is estimated that less than 4% of pancreatitis in children is caused by a biliary tract disorder. Arima and Akita[1] described anomalous junction of the pancreaticobiliary duct system in 25% of patients with congenital biliary tract dilatation. One patient, a 13-year-old boy, had recurring pancreatitis. Williams, Caldwell, and Wilson[50] report a family with seven members having idiopathic hereditary pancreatitis. Three required duct drainage and were relieved of symptoms. In one patient, pancreatitis began at age 11, in another at 15, and in another at 17. In a review of the literature, they found total pancreatectomy required in three, unspecified drainage in nine, and pancreaticojejunostomy in 14 with 13 good results. Sphincterotomy was employed in six, three with good results and three with no improvement. The review includes childhood and adult experience.

Pancreatic remnants in ectopic foci have caused pancreatitis within the esophagus (reported by Briceno et al.[9]), multiple omental sites (Fam[19]), and gastric bleeding from accessory pancreas (Carcassonne[13]). Ectopic pancreas within the spleen and stomach, with bleeding, is reported by Goldfarb.[24]

REFERENCES

1. Arima E., Akita H.: Congenital biliary tract dilatation and anomalous junction of the pancreaticobiliary duct system. *J. Pediatr. Surg.* 14:9, 1979.
2. Arndt R.D.: Iodopamide enhanced CT (computed tomography) of the pancreas. *Radiology* 139:491, 1981.
3. Baar H.S., Wolff O.H.: Pancreatic necrosis in cortisone-treated children. *Lancet* 1:812, 1957.
4. Becker M., et al.: ERCP in children. *Dtsch. Med. Wochenschr.* 25:1055, 1980.
5. Bernstein D., Ferrera J., Caren L.: The medical and surgical management of pancreas divisum. *Surgical Rounds* 7:64, 1983.
6. Bluestone P.K., Gaskin K., Filler R., et al.: Endoscopic retrograde cholangiopancreatography in pancreatitis in children and adolescents. *Pediatrics* 68:387, 1981.
7. Blumenstock D.A., Mithoefer J., Santulli T.V.: Acute pancreatitis in children. *Pediatrics* 19:1002, 1957.
8. Bole G.G. Jr., Thompson O.W.: Acute mumps pancreatitis. *Univ. Mich. Med. Bull.* 24:442, 1958.
9. Briceno L.T., Grases P.J., Gallegos J.: Pancreatic remnants causing esophageal stenosis. *J. Pediatr. Surg.* 16:731, 1981.
10. Britt J.L., Samuels A.D., Johnson J.W.: Pancreas divisum. *Ann. Surg.* 197:654, 1983.
11. Camer S.J., Eric G.C., Warren K.W., et al.: Pancreatic abscess: A critical analysis of 113 cases. *Am. J. Surg.* 129:427, 1975.
12. Cameron J.L.: Acute pancreatitis, in Shackelford R.T., Zuidema G.D. (eds.): *Surgery of the Alimentary Tract.* Philadelphia, W.B. Saunders Co., 1983, pp. 31–61.
13. Carcassonne M., Daou N.: Gastric bleeding and accessory pancreas in children. *Chir. Pediatr.* 21:357, 1980.
14. Collins J.: Pancreatitis in young children. *Arch. Dis. Child.* 33:432, 1958.
15. Comfort M.W., Steinberg A.G.: Pedigree of a family with hereditary chronic relapsing pancreatitis. *Gastroenterology* 21:54, 1952.
16. Cooperman M., Ferrera J.J., Fromkes J.J., et al.: The surgical management of pancreas divisum. *Am. J. Surg.* 143:107, 1982.
17. Cotton P.B., Laage N.J.: ERCP in children. *Arch. Dis. Child.* 57:131, 1982.
18. Dean J., Scott H.W. Jr., Law H.: Chronic relapsing pancreatitis in childhood: Case report and review of the literature. *Ann. Surg.* 173:443, 1971.
19. Fam S., O'Brien D.S., Borger J.A.: Ectopic pancreas with acute inflammation. *J. Pediatr. Surg.* 17:86, 1982.
20. Fitz R.H.: Acute pancreatitis. *Med. Rec.* (New York), 1889, p. 35.
21. Frey C., Redo S.F.: Inflammatory lesions of the pancreas in infancy and childhood. *Pediatrics* 32:93, 1963.

22. Gallie W.E., Brown A.: Acute hemorrhagic pancreatitis resulting from roundworms: Report of a case. *Am. J. Dis. Child.* 27:192, 1924.
23. Ghishan F.K., Greene H.L., Avant G., et al.: Chronic relapsing pancreatitis in childhood. *J. Pediatr. Surg.* 102:514, 1983.
24. Goldfarb W.B.: Carcinoma in heterotopic gastric pancreas. *Ann. Surg.* 37:77, 1971.
25. Gregg J.A.: Pancreas divisum: Its association with pancreatitis. *Am. J. Surg.* 134:539, 1977.
26. Hendren W.H. Jr., Greep J.M., Patton A.S.: Pancreatitis in childhood: Experience with 15 cases. *Arch. Dis. Child.* 40:132, 1965.
27. Howard J.M., Ravdin I.S.: Acute pancreatitis: Study of 80 patients. *Am. Pract.* 2:385, 1948.
28. Ingomar C.J., Terslev E.: A case of chronic pancreatitis in early childhood. *Danish Med. Bull.* 12:91, 1965.
29. Krauste A., Hockestedt K., Ahonen J., et al.: Peritoneal lavage as a primary treatment in acute form of pancreatitis. *Surg. Gynecol. Obstet.* 156:458, 1983.
30. Marczynska-Robowska M.: Pancreatic necrosis in a case of Still's disease. *Lancet* 1:815, 1957.
31. Martin L., Canseco J.D.: Pancreatic calculosis. *JAMA* 135:1055, 1947.
32. Molander D.W., Bell E.T.: Relation of cholelithiasis to acute hemorrhagic pancreatitis. *Arch. Pathol.* 11:17, 1946.
33. Nogueira J., Freedman M.A.: Acute pancreatitis as a complication of Imuran therapy in regional enteritis. *Gastroenterology* 62:1040, 1972.
34. Nugent F.W., Atendido W.A.: Aggressive treatment of hemorrhagic pancreatitis. Scientific exhibit, Lahey Clinic Foundation, Boston, 1967.
35. O'Neill J.A., Green H., Ghishan F.K.: Surgical implications of chronic pancreatitis. *J. Pediatr. Surg.* 17:920, 1982.
36. Oppenheimer E.G., Boitnott J.K.: Pancreatitis in children following adrenal corticosteroid therapy. *Bull. Johns Hopkins Hosp.* 107:297, 1961.
37. Paxton J.R., Payne J.H.: Acute pancreatitis: A statistical review of 307 established cases of acute pancreatitis. *Surg. Gynecol. Obstet.* 86:69, 1948.
38. Puestow C.B., Gillespie W.J.: Retrograde drainage of pancreas for chronic relapsing pancreatitis. *Am. Surg.* 76:898, 1958.
39. Ranson J.H.C., Spencer F.C.: The role of peritoneal lavage in severe acute pancreatitis. *Ann. Surg.* 187:565, 1978.
40. Renning J.A., Warden G.D., Stevens L.E., et al.: Pancreatitis after renal transplantation. *Am. J. Surg.* 123:293, 1972.
41. Rich A.R., Duff G.L.: Pathogenesis of acute hemorrhagic pancreatitis. *Bull. Johns Hopkins Hosp.* 58:212, 1936.
42. Richter J.M., Schapiro R.H., Mulley A.G., et al.: Association of pancreas divisum and pancreatitis, and its treatment by sphincteroplasty of the accessory ampulla. *Gastroenterology* 81:1104, 1981.
43. Romer J.F., Carey L.C.: Pancreatitis, a clinical review. *Am. J. Surg.* 111:795, 1966.
44. Rowe M.I.: Personal communication.
45. Shanklin D.R.: Pancreatic atrophy apparently secondary to hydrochlorothiazide. *N. Engl. J. Med.* 266:1097, 1962.
46. Silen W.: Gastrointestinal and biliary conditions. *Bull. Am. Coll. Surg.* 69:15, 1984.
47. Stickler G.B., Yonemoto R.H.: Acute pancreatitis in children. *Am. J. Dis. Child.* 95:206, 1958.
48. Warwick W.J., Leavitt S.R.: Chronic relapsing pancreatitis in childhood. *Am. J. Dis. Child.* 99:648, 1960.
49. Welch K.J.: The pancreas, in Ravitch M.M., et al. (eds.): *Pediatric Surgery*, ed. 3. Chicago, Year Book Medical Publishers, 1979, pp. 857–876.
50. Williams R.A., Caldwell B.F., Wilson S.E.: Idiopathic hereditary pancreatitis, experience with surgical treatment. *Arch. Surg.* 117:408, 1982.
51. Williams T.E., Sherman N.J., Clatworthy H.W. Jr.: Chronic fibrosing pancreatitis in childhood: A cause of recurrent abdominal pain. *Pediatrics* 40:1019, 1967.
52. Yedlin S.T., Philippart A.I.: Pancreas divisum: A cause of pancreatitis in childhood. Presented at the 15th annual meeting, American Pediatric Surgical Association, Marcos Island, Florida, May 11, 1984.

Pancreatic Cysts and Pseudocysts

Cyst formation in and around the pancreas, unless posttraumatic, is infrequently encountered in childhood. Priestley and ReMine[26] classified pancreatic cysts as (1) congenital and developmental, (2) retention, (3) pseudocysts, (4) neoplastic, and (5) parasitic. To this, we would add heterotopic enteric duplications. There is unavoidable inaccuracy in such a classification because, with time or infection, the epithelial lining that makes the diagnosis possible may be lost or destroyed.

Congenital and Developmental Cysts

In a 1959 review of the literature, Miles[20] found eight examples of true congenital cyst in children under age 2 and three in infants under age 6 months, including one newborn. Pilot et al.[24] reported obstruction of the common bile duct by a pancreatic cyst in a newborn. Six children with simple cysts have been encountered at Children's Hospital, Boston, among 25 patients with cysts and tumors, second in frequency only to choristoma or hamartoma. Multiple heterotopic cysts were scattered over the length of the pancreas in one recent patient. Sweat test results were negative. The multiple cysts that occur with cystic fibrosis are excluded. Decourcy[7] reported a dermoid cyst of the pancreas.

Congenital or developmental cysts may be unilocular or multilocular. Four examples of multiloculated cysts appear in the literature. Ours were unilocular. Cysts have been reported to simultaneously occur in other organs. Hippel-Lindau disease is characterized by hereditary cerebellar cysts, hemangiomas of the retina, and cysts of the pancreas and other organs.

Developmental cysts are lined by epithelium backed up with acinar tissue. They are most common in the body and tail of the pancreas and may achieve considerable size. They contain cloudy yellow fluid, usually sterile and without high enzyme activity. A developmental cyst, unless critically located, seldom gives rise to symptoms until it is quite large. As it enlarges, it presses through the gastrohepatic or gastrocolic omentum, more often the latter. The stomach is displaced upward and anteriorly while the transverse colon is pushed downward and anteriorly, readily demonstrated in barium x-ray studies and by sonography. Symptoms are due to extrinsic pressure on neighboring organs.

These cysts are rarely associated with infection or adhesions. Surgical treatment consists of total excision of the cyst with a rim of normal pancreatic tissue, or internal drainage of those in the pancreatic head. Drainage of the pancreatic stump through a separate stab wound in the left flank is always advisable.

Retention Cysts

Retention cysts of the pancreas are found occasionally in children and are said to result from chronic obstruction of the duct system. Outwardly, they resemble congenital cysts but contain cloudy fluid with a high concentration of pancreatic enzymes. There is a lining epithelium unless it has been destroyed by long-standing pressure or inflammation. At operation, and depending on the location of the cyst, the decision must be made between excision with a margin of adjacent pancreas or some form of internal drainage, most conveniently Roux-en-Y.

Enteric Duplication Cysts

Intrapancreatic or juxtapancreatic gastric duplications with ductal communication, and separate from the stomach, have been encountered in four patients at Children's Hospital, Boston. Hélardot et al.[14] added two cases and surveyed the literature to 1982, identifying 13 cases in all.[1, 14, 16, 26] This does not include the cases of Hendren,[15] or of Peters and Filston,[23] unique in that the lesion was identified by ERCP. The history in our children was that of failure to thrive, lack of interest in food, abdominal pain, and documented attacks of pancreatitis with elevated serum amylase levels. One patient presented with bleeding into the duplication followed by rupture beneath the diaphragm. The lesion and the intraoperative pancreatogram are seen in Figure 115–4. Surgical treatment consisted of resection

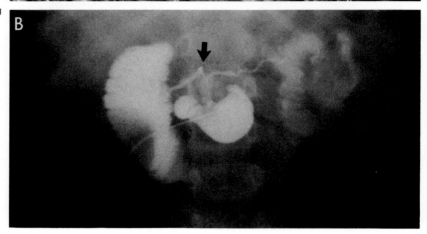

Fig 115—4.—Intrapancreatic gastric duplication in a 7-year-old boy with recurring pancreatitis. **A,** intraoperative photograph. *Arrow* indicates location of fluid-filled noncompressible structure within the head of the pancreas. **B,** direct injection with Hypaque 50 shows the extent of the duplication and an anomalous pancreatic duct *(arrow)* that joins the duplication and the main pancreatic duct of Wirsung. The gastric duplication was enucleated and the interconnecting duct ligated.

of the duplication alone in 10 patients, distal pancreatectomy (tail or body and tail) in five, and pancreaticoduodenal resection in two. Identification of such lesions is possible with ERCP, real-time sonography, or CT. The lesion is usually small and not palpable before operation. Exploration is required to identify the mass and because of the repeated attacks of pancreatitis. The duplication should be excised as close to the duplication wall as possible. Any communicating duct must be identified and ligated. Failure to do so in one of our cases and in the case of Peters[23] resulted in prolonged pancreatic drainage and necessitated reoperation for closure of the fistula. Patients ranging in age from 2 months to 17 years have been reported by Akers,[1] Katz,[18] and Huguier.[16] Pancreatitis with rupture and hemorrhage has also been reported by Akers.[1] In four patients, a "pseudocyst" had been diagnosed. The true nature of the process is identified, at operation and by light microscopy, by its intestinal-structured wall. All patients are free of symptoms following distal pancreatic resection or resection of the duplication and closure of the communicating duct. Hendren reported a large duodenal duplication buried in the head of the pancreas, successfully treated by pancreaticoduodenectomy.[15]

Neoplastic Cysts

Papillary neoplastic cysts, rarely encountered in childhood, must be presumed to be premalignant.[1] Their true nature can only be established by microscopic examination after excision. They are easily ruptured, and the contents are extremely irritating to the peritoneal cavity. In one patient, an inadequately excised cystadenoma degenerated to rhabdomyosarcoma was reported by Grosfeld et al.[10] Gunderson and Javis[11] reported cystadenoma in a 16-month-old infant. Lewis and Dormandy[19] reported cystadenoma in a 13-year-old girl. The subject has been classically reviewed by Becker et al.[2]

Pseudocysts

A pseudocyst of the pancreas is a cystic structure located primarily in the lesser sac, the wall composed of granulation tissue in varying stages of maturity and the lining devoid of epithelium. The boundaries of the pseudocyst are determined by the organs that outline the omental bursa. The pseudocyst may or may not communicate with the pancreatic duct system. When it does, amylase levels in excess of 3,000 units/l are common. It is usually unilocular, and volumes in excess of 1,000 ml are found. We have previously called attention to the prevalence of traumatic pancreatitis in childhood, which in approximately 20% of cases results in pancreatic pseudocyst. Cooney and Grosfeld[5] reviewed the literature to 1975 and found 60 well-documented pediatric cases, adding 15 of their own. Reports of pseudocysts due to trauma in children, and, to a lesser degree, following idiopathic pancreatitis, are increasing. Drennen[8] in 1922 recognized the role of trauma in pancreatitis.

Carswell[4] reported four cases from Africa, in children. Single case reports in addition to our own bring the total of childhood cases[6, 9, 17, 25] to 93. Seventeen children with pseudocysts have been seen at Children's Hospital, Boston, two of which were previously reported by Hendren et al.[15] and two by Tank et al.[28]

ETIOLOGY.—The etiology of pancreatic pseudocysts in children is shown in Table 115–2. Age as a factor in the etiology of pancreatic pseudocysts is seen in Table 115–3. Biliary tract disease existed in only one patient, a 13-year-old girl with congenital spherocytosis whose family had refused splenectomy; a stone became impacted in the common duct, simultaneously obstructing the pancreatic duct. A pseudocyst formed in the body and tail of the pancreas. One patient had a critically placed duplication. Three patients had antecedent mumps. The patients of Udekwu[29] had ethionine- and kwashiorkor-induced pancreatitis. Pancreatitis in African children has been reported by Owor.[22] Carswell[4] reported four African children with pseudocysts; all had antecedent pancreatitis. In the idiopathic group, many patients had a history of febrile illness with deprivation of food, nausea, vomiting, and abdominal pain. Of patients in all groups, 88% had serum amylase levels elevated to three times normal or higher.

DIAGNOSIS.—The diagnosis of pancreatic pseudocyst is suggested by a history of blunt abdominal trauma or an illness resembling pancreatitis followed by a free interval of weeks to months. The child then complains of epigastric abdominal pain and anorexia progressing to nausea, vomiting, and weight loss. Eventually or suddenly, one is able to palpate a spherical epigastric mass. The enlarging pseudocyst displaces the stomach upward and anteriorly and the colon downward and anteriorly (Fig 115–5). Examination after a barium meal shows this displacement and also a posterior gastric depression defect (Figs 115–6 and 115–7). The C loop of the duodenum may or may not be widened, and the duodenum in its retroperitoneal portion may be compressed or obstructed. Ascitic fluid may be present, with pancreatic enzyme levels higher than those in the serum. In one patient who developed chylous ascites, cystogastrostomy resulted in disappearance of the ascites and spectacular nutritional improvement. Selective arteriography has not helped in showing even large pseudocysts. Ultrasound and/or CT are generally diagnostic.[13]

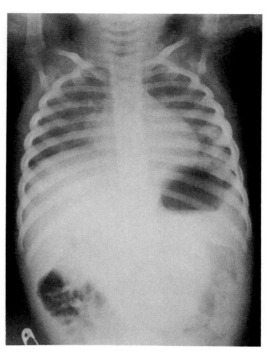

Fig 115–5.—Pancreatic pseudocyst. Roentgenogram of a 3-year-old girl with this complication of idiopathic pancreatitis. Note downward displacement and broad U-shape of the transverse colon due to fixation at the splenic and hepatic flexures. The opaque spherical mass indents the stomach and obscures the antrum and proximal duodenum. Posterior cystogastrostomy was performed.

TREATMENT.—Small cysts not interfering with gastrointestinal tract function can be followed with serial sonography, body CT, or pancreatic scans until they ultimately disappear. Complications from untreated large pseudocysts include hemorrhage, secondary infection, perforation with peritonitis, and mechanical in-

TABLE 115–2.—ETIOLOGY OF PANCREATIC PSEUDOCYSTS IN CHILDREN

	BOYS	GIRLS	NO. PATIENTS	%
Trauma	32	18	50	54
Idiopathic pancreatitis	14	22	36	38
Hereditary pancreatitis	1	1	2	3
Miscellaneous			5	5
Mumps	3			
Duplication	1			
Cholelithiasis	1			
Totals	52	41	93	

TABLE 115–3.—ETIOLOGY OF PANCREATIC PSEUDOCYSTS IN CHILDREN BY AGE

AGE (YR.)	NO. PATIENTS	TRAUMA	PANCRE-ATITIS	MISC.
0–5	38	15	20	3
5–10	30	19	10	1
10–15	25	17	7	1
Totals	93	51	37	5

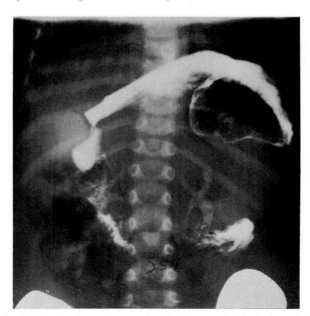

Fig 115–6.—Posttraumatic pseudocyst. Upper gastrointestinal roentgenogram of a 7-year-old boy, showing indentation of stomach, distorted duodenum, and central filling defect corresponding to the pseudocyst occupying most of the body and tail of the pancreas. Point of injury occurs where the pancreas crosses the vertebral column. The intravenous pyelogram was normal. The patient was treated by posterior cystogastrostomy.

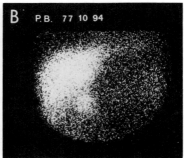

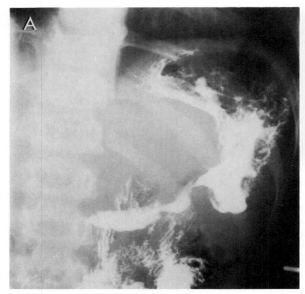

Fig 115–7.—Pancreatic pseudocyst due to chronic recurring pancreatitis. The cyst is indistinguishable from those resulting from blunt trauma. Surgical management is identical in the two conditions. The outlook, however, is much less favorable with pseudocyst due to pancreatitis because of greater involvement of the gland to the right of the superior mesenteric vessels. **A,** barium meal showing gastric displacement by the huge cyst. **B,** ^{99}Tc radionuclide scan of the same patient shows concentration of the material in the head and uncinate process of the pancreas with no uptake to the left of L-2.

terference with gastrointestinal, pancreatic, or biliary function. The operative procedures utilized in children are indicated in Table 115–4. Most recent patients have been treated with internal drainage by cystogastrostomy or Roux-en-Y cystojejunostomy, excision, or merely observation to ultimate disappearance (Figs 115–8 and 115–9).

Spontaneous resolution of pancreatic pseudocysts has been reported in five patients by Bradley[3] among 38 patients with pancreatitis studied with ultrasound. This has particular application in children with pseudocyst due to blunt trauma in whom laparotomy may not otherwise be indicated. We have confirmed this observation in six children whose pseudocysts ultimately disappeared. van Heerden et al.[30] reported on 71 patients, the number of children not stated. In their series, posterior cystogastrostomy was the treatment of choice in 32 patients with one death, Roux-en-Y cystojejunostomy in 16, resection in 10, external drainage in nine with one death and cystoduodenostomy or Puestow's procedure in four. Excellent results were obtained in

TABLE 115–4.—Operative Treatment of Pancreatic Pseudocysts in Children

PROCEDURE	NO. OF PATIENTS
Posterior cystogastrostomy	31
Roux-en-Y cystojejunostomy	17
Excision	13
Marsupialization	9
Drainage only	9
No operation*	7
Tube drainage	6
Puestow I or II with excision	3
Cystoduodenostomy	2
Laparotomy only†	1
Total	98

*One discovered at autopsy; six followed to disappearance (recent).
†Cyst ruptured; cardiac arrest.

93% of patients. In two children not operated on, the pseudocyst was discovered at autopsy. One, reported by Oeconomopoulos and Lee,[21] received irradiation of a suspected solid retroperitoneal malignancy without substantial effect. The child died of nutritional failure and sepsis. The other, a 14-month-old boy, was discovered to have a pseudocyst of the pancreatic body and tail without a history of antecedent illness.

Recent experience with 116 pseudocysts in children was reported by Kagan et al.[17] They estimated that simple drainage was performed in 23%, excision and distal pancreatectomy in 13%, cystogastrostomy in 46% and cystojejunostomy in 18%. Dahmen and Stephens report 11 children treated from 1960 to 1976.[6] Six were posttraumatic, and five had a history of pancreatitis. Pokorny et al.[25] reported six patients treated with external drainage only. Success must be explained by diminishing drainage from the disruption at the site of injury. At our institution, five patients since 1978 required surgical treatment. One required cystogastrostomy in combination with sphincteroplasty of the ampulla of Vater. Six others were observed ultrasonically to resolution, the treatment of choice if at all possible. Windell[31] reported a 13-year-old boy with a posttraumatic pseudocyst drained with an ultrasonically guided 20-cm 16-gauge Teflon needle; 1,000 cc of high-amylase fluid was recovered. A second tap was required, leaving the Teflon sheath on drainage 24 hours. The lesion resolved. Hancke and Jacobsen (Copenhagen) also recommend ultrasonically guided puncture of pseudocysts.[12] Of 40 lesions so treated, 31 resolved after first aspiration, nine after two to four aspirations. There were no recurrences. Harkányi reports similar success.[13]

With the universal availability of hyperalimentation, a more conservative management of this condition is probably justified. Observation to involution is possible in many cases, traumatic or idiopathic in origin. Teflon sheath drainage with ultrasonic guidance seems to be effective in the treatment of even mature pseudocysts. Long-term follow-up is necessary before discarding the eminently satisfactory techniques of internal drainage.

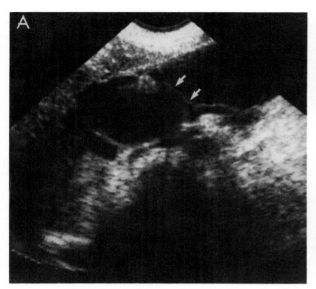

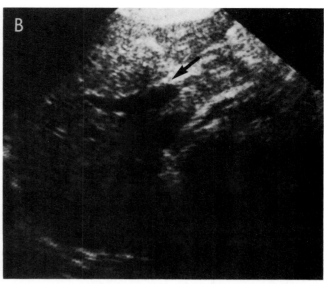

Fig 115–8.—Posttraumatic pseudocyst in a 16-year-old boy. **A,** transverse ultrasonogram of the upper abdomen showing a large posttraumatic pseudocyst surrounding the hepatic artery *(arrows).*

B, repeat ultrasonogram following surgical drainage shows complete evacuation of the cyst. *Arrow* points to portal vein with normal pancreatic head below and to the right.

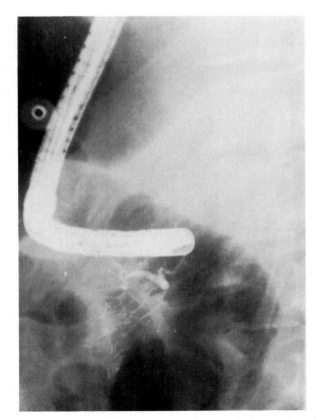

Fig 115–9.—Pancreatitis with pseudocyst. Postoperatively, normal proximal pancreatic duct is demonstrated on transduodenal pancreatogram. This 17-year-old girl previously had posterior cystogastrostomy for pseudocyst, multiple episodes of idiopathic pancreatitis, and ultimate distal pancreatectomy. Drug addiction was suspected.

REFERENCES

1. Akers D.R., Favara B.E., Franciosi R.A., et al.: Duplication of the alimentary tract: Report of three unusual cases associated with bile and pancreatic ducts. *Surgery* 71:817, 1972.
2. Becker W.F., Welsh R.A., Pratt H.: Cystadenoma and cystadenocarcinoma of the pancreas. *Ann. Surg.* 161:845, 1965.
3. Bradley E.L.: Spontaneous resolution of pancreatic pseudocysts. *Am. J. Surg.* 129:23, 1975.
4. Carswell J.: Pancreatic pseudocysts in children: 4 cases from Uganda. *Gr. J. Surg.* 62:360, 1975.
5. Cooney D.R., Grosfeld J.L.: Operative management of pancreatic pseudocysts in infants and children: A review of 75 cases. *Ann. Surg.* 182:590, 1975.
6. Dahmen B., Stephens C.A.: Pseudocyst of the pancreas after blunt trauma in children. *J. Pediatr. Surg.* 16:17, 1981.
7. Decourcy J.L.: Dermoid cyst of the pancreas. *Ann. Surg.* 118:394, 1943.
8. Drennen E.: Traumatic pancreatitis. *Ann. Surg.* 76:488, 1922.
9. Garel L., Brunelle F., Lallemand D., et al.: Pseudocyst of the pancreas in children which require surgery. *Pediatr. Radiol.* 13:120, 1983.
10. Grosfeld J.L., Clatworthy H.W., Hamoudi A.B.: Pancreatic malignancy in childhood. *Arch. Surg.* 101:370, 1970.
11. Gunderson A.E., Javis J.F.: Pancreatic cystadenoma in childhood: Report of a case. *J. Pediatr. Surg.* 4:478, 1969.
12. Hancke S., Jacobsen C.K.: Puncture of pancreatic mass lesions, in Holm H.H., Cristenson J.K. (eds.): *Ultrasonically Guided Puncture Technique.* Copenhagen, Munksgaard, 1980, pp. 61–65.
13. Harkányi Z., Végh M., Hittner I., et al.: Grey-scale echography of traumatic pancreatic cysts in children. *Pediatr. Radiol.* 11:81, 1981.
14. Hélardot P.G., Van Kote G., Barbet P.: Les duplications gastriques séparées de l'estomac et en relation avec le pancréas. *Chir. Pédiatr.* 23:363, 1982.
15. Hendren W.H. Jr., Greep J.M., Patton A.S.: Pancreatitis in childhood: Experience with 15 cases. *Arch. Dis. Child.* 40:132, 1965.
16. Huguier M., Luboinski J.: Duplication gastrique communiquant avec les canaux pancréatiques. *Arch. Fr. Mal. App. Dig.* 64:153, 1975.
17. Kagan R.J., Reyes H.M., Sangarappillai A.: Pseudocyst of the pancreas in childhood. *Arch. Surg.* 116:1200, 1981.
18. Katz W., Annessa G., Read R.C.: Gastric duplication with pancreatic communication. *Minn. Med.* 1175–1179, 1967.
19. Lewis A., Dormandy J.: Cystadenoma of the pancreas: A report of two cases. *Br. J. Surg.* 58:420, 1971.
20. Miles R.M.: Pancreatic cyst in the newborn. *Ann. Surg.* 149:576, 1959.
21. Oeconomopoulos C.T., Lee C.M. Jr.: Pseudocysts of the pancreas in infants and young children. *Surgery* 47:836, 1960.

22. Owor B.: Chronic pancreatic disease in African children. *Uganda Med. J.* 1:7, 1972.
23. Peters G.: Personal communication.
24. Pilot L.M., Gooselaw J.G., Isaacson P.G.: Obstruction of the common bile duct in the newborn by a pancreatic cyst. *Lancet* 84:204, 1964.
25. Pokorny W.J., Raffensperger J.G., Harberg F.J., et al.: Pancreatic pseudocysts in children. *Surg. Gynecol. Obstet.* 151:182, 1980.
26. Priestley J.J., ReMine W.H.: Problems in the surgical treatment of pancreatic cysts. *Surg. Clin. North Am.* 47:1313, 1958.
27. Schwartz D.L., So H.B., Becker J.M., et al.: An ectopic gastric duplication arising from the pancreas and presenting with a pneumoperitoneum. *J. Pediatr. Surg.* 14:187, 1979.
28. Tank E.S., Eraklis A.J., Gross R.E.: Blunt abdominal trauma in infancy and childhood. *J. Trauma* 8:439, 1968.
29. Udekwu F.A.O.: Pancreatic pseudocysts in children. *J. Int. Coll. Surg.* 44:123, 1965.
30. van Heerden J.A., ReMine W.H.: Pseudocysts of the pancreas: Review of 71 cases. *Arch. Surg.* 110:500, 1975.
31. Windell R.L.: Needle aspiration and the treatment of pancreatic pseudocyst in childhood. *Ann. R. Coll. Surg. Engl.* 65:331, 1983.

Pancreatic Neoplasms

Malignant tumors of the pancreas in infants and children are rare. All but two of the reported cases are carcinomas.[12, 32] English-language reports total 38 cases (Table 115–5). Early reports are ambiguous because of the random histologic classification.[17] The disease was uniformly fatal before Whipple[37] introduced pancreatoduodenectomy, subsequently modified by Cattell and Warren[6] and by Child.[7]

SYMPTOMS AND SIGNS.—The symptoms and signs in 62 reported cases of carcinoma of the pancreas in children, including Japanese cases, are listed in Table 115–6. Forty-four percent were males and 56% were females. Age at the time of diagnosis ranged from 3 months to 18 years, with an average of 9.2 years.

Islet Cell Carcinoma

There were 10 children with islet cell carcinoma, six girls and four boys. Percutaneous biopsy was performed in one patient.

Two children had bypass procedures; one was followed by interval pancreatoduodenectomy. Six had initial pancreatoduodenectomy. One patient had a recurrence 3 years after pancreatoduodenectomy. Five patients are living and well 3–16 years after pancreatoduodenectomy. Some early cases of acinar cell adenocarcinoma have been reclassified as islet cell carcinoma. One should not compromise with partial resection or a bypass procedure unless there is evidence of regional spread or distant metastasis.

Adenocarcinoma

Twelve children had adenocarcinoma involving acinar tissue only. In two patients, no operation was performed because of terminal disease; three had biopsy only, one had a bypass procedure, and one, partial resection. Two had pancreatoduodenectomy. All died within 10 months of the onset of symptoms. Duct cell carcinoma was encountered in six patients; three patients had biopsy only and died in 1 week to 16 months; two had pancreatoduodenectomy and were alive and well at 7 and 29 years. One had local resection, three times, and is alive with disease at age 12 years.

Miscellaneous Carcinomas

Undifferentiated carcinoma was found in three patients. Two had no operation because of advanced disease; one had biopsy only. All died within 6 months of onset of symptoms. Two cancers were cylindrical cell tumors. One patient had no operation, and the other had biopsy only; both died within 6 weeks. Carcinoma simplex and medullary carcinoma were encountered in one child each; one had biopsy only and one had no operation. Both died within 3 months. Results in this mixed carcinoma group are difficult to evaluate because they represent early reported cases. Three children would probably have benefited from pancreatoduodenectomy. Grosfeld[12] reported sarcomatous (rhabdomyosarcoma) degeneration of a pancreatic cystadenoma. The case ap-

TABLE 115–5.—PANCREATIC MALIGNANCY IN INFANTS AND CHILDREN*

MALIGNANCY	NO. OF PATIENTS	AGES	SEX M	SEX F	OPERATION PERFORMED None	Biopsy Only	Bypass	Pancreato-duodenectomy	RESULT
Nonfunctioning islet cell carcinoma	9	1, 3, 4, 6, 6, 9, 11, 12, 14	3	6	1	1	2	5 (total) 1 (partial)	Alive and well: 3, 4, 6, 11, 16 yr Recurred: 3 yr Dead: 2 wk, 6 mo, 20 mo, 2 yr, 3 yr
Adenocarcinoma	9	$^3/_{12}$, $^5/_{12}$, 3, 4, 6, 9, 12, 14, 15	5	4	2	3	1	2 (total) 1 (partial)	Dead: 1 wk, 1 mo, 4 mo, 5 mo, 5 mo, 5 mo, 6 mo, 10 mo, 10 mo
Undifferentiated carcinoma	3	8, 13, 14	2	1	2	1			Dead: 10 wk, 4 mo, 6 mo
Cylindric cell carcinoma	2	$^7/_{12}$, 2		2	1	1			Dead: 2 wk, 6 wk
Duct cell carcinoma	2	4, 10	1	1		1		1 (total)	Alive and well: 1 yr Dead: 1 wk
Carcinoma simplex	1	$^7/_{12}$		1	1				Dead: 6 wk
Medullary carcinoma	1	9	1			1			Dead: 3 mo
Cystadenosarcoma	1	2		1				1 (partial)	Dead: 2 mo
Total	28		12	16	7	8	3	8 (total) 3 (partial)	Alive: 6 patients Dead: 22 patients

*See references 1, 9, 11, 12, 15, 16, 18, 20, 22, 23, 25, 26, 27, 28, 30, 33, 35, 36.

TABLE 115–6.—ADENOCARCINOMA OF THE PANCREAS IN CHILDHOOD (CHILDREN'S HOSPITAL, BOSTON, 1955–1984)

CASE NO.	AGE	SEX	SYMPTOMS	LOCATION	SIZE (cm)	CELL TYPE	TREATMENT	RESULT*
1	18	M	Jaundice, obstruction	Head	4	Duct cell	Biopsy only	DOD 18 mo
2	10	F	Abdominal pain, duodenal ulcer	Entire gland	20	Duct cell	Biopsy only	DOD 6 mo
3	9	F	Abdominal pain	Head	8	Duct cell	Pancreatoduodenectomy	NED 29 yr
4	12	F	Abdominal pain	Body and tail	20	Duct cell (papillary type)	Local resection × 3	AWD
5	3	F	Palpable tumor	Head	8	Acinar cell	Pancreatoduodenectomy	DOD 30 mo
6	7	F	Palpable tumor	Tail	20	Acinar cell	Local resection	DOD 19 mo
7	15 mo	M	Melena, hematemesis	Head	8	Islet cell	Pancreatoduodenectomy	DOD 35 mo

*Abbreviations: DOD indicates dead of disease; NED, no evidence of disease; and AWD, alive with disease.

pears to be unique. Neurofibrosarcoma of the duodenum treated by pancreatoduodenectomy has been reported.

The Children's Hospital (Boston) experience with malignant tumors of the pancreas in children consists of seven patients—five girls and two boys ranging in age from 15 months to 18 years, with an average age of 8.7 years[19] (Table 115–6). Tumors were resected in five of seven cases. Three had some modification of the Whipple procedure, and two had local resections. Three tumors were adenocarcinomas of the duct cell type, two were adenocarcinomas of the acinar cell type, one a papillary cystadenocarcinoma, and one an islet cell carcinoma without endocrine function. One undifferentiated acinar cell carcinoma developed in a field of orthovoltage radiation approximately 15 years after treatment for left Wilms tumor. As with adult experience, results were poor. Five patients died with regional or distant metastasis documented at autopsy. The original tumors were large—on average, 13.6 cm. Patients most commonly presented with abdominal pain and an epigastric mass (Table 115–7). The usual preoperative diagnoses were pancreatic pseudocyst, abdominal lymphoma, neuroblastoma and Wilms tumor. Primary pancreatic malignancy was not suspected in any case. None were ampullary or preampullary in location.

In adult experience, 85% of malignant tumors of the exocrine pancreas are adenocarcinomas, predominantly of duct cell origin. Acinar cell adenocarcinomas account for less than 10%. Acinar cell tumors are proportionately more common in children. Diagnosis can be established by demonstrating PAS-positive cytoplasmic granules and by ultrastructural identification of electron-dense zymogen granules (Fig 115–10). It appears that children with an acinar cell tumor have a somewhat better prognosis than

TABLE 115–7.—PANCREATIC
CARCINOMA IN INFANTS AND
CHILDREN: SYMPTOMS AND
SIGNS IN 62 PATIENTS

SYMPTOM	NO. OF PATIENTS
Epigastric mass	31
Abdominal pain	26
Anorexia	14
Icterus	11
Vomiting	10
Weight loss	10
Anemia	9
Steatorrhea	8
Fever	7
Melena	3
Diarrhea	3
Hematemesis	2

those with an adenocarcinoma of the duct cell type. Six of 13 children with acinar cell tumors are alive with no evidence of disease 2 months to 16 years following operation. Prognosis for children with adenocarcinoma of the duct cell type is similar to that for adults, with the 5-year survival rate approximately 1%.[34] Patients with papillary cystic tumors and islet cell carcinoma, like our long-term survivors (one of each), seem to have a better prognosis, as reported by Boor[4] and by Compagno.[8]

Review of the world literature on cancer of the pancreas in children is difficult because of the varied terminology. Horie et al.[13] coined the term "pancreatoblastoma" for certain carcinomas of the pancreas in childhood. Classification according to cell or origin (e.g., islet cell, duct cell, or acinar cell carcinoma) seems preferable and is adhered to in the English-language reports.[3, 10, 20, 21, 24, 31, 38]

An extraordinary report on pancreatic carcinoma in Japanese children is that by Tsukimoto and Tsuchida.[32] Their 24 children, ranging in age from 2 to 14 years, bring world experience to 62 cases. Average age at diagnosis was 7 years; 12 were males and 12 were females. The mode of clinical presentation was identical to that of cases reported elsewhere and is included in Table 115–6. Only one patient had jaundice, stressing the location of these tumors in the main parenchymal organ, no cases involving the periampullary area. Of the 24 Japanese patients, 14 had resection of the tumor (two by pancreatoduodenectomy); few patients received radiotherapy. Treatment with cyclophosphamide, vincristine, and mitomycin was of no apparent value. Of 13 patients encountered since 1974, seven were alive with no evidence of disease 8 months to 16 years after operation. The histopathologic diagnosis was adenocarcinoma in 13 cases; five were classified as pancreatoblastoma because of primitive features. There was one cystadenocarcinoma; three tumors were highly undifferentiated and unclassifiable. Three patients had nonfunctioning islet cell carcinoma, and two had functioning islet cell carcinoma; one had sarcoma of the pancreas similar to that described by Grosfeld.[12] Difference in survival between the Japanese and English language series is unexplainable on the basis of the histopathologic classification. Many tumors were located in the tail of the gland, permitting adequate resection. Horie et al.[13] believed that tumors in this location indicated embryonal endocrine origin from ventral primordia and had a better prognosis. The reason for the theory is not fully explained. Patients having the primitive features of pancreatoblastoma did well, four of five surviving. These tumors show organoid acinar differentiation and discrete squamoid nests. Zymogen-like granules on electron micrography (Fig 115–10) appear to be adenocarcinomas of the acinar cell type.

Hurez,[14] Stokes,[29] and Tsukimoto[32] encountered four children with hypoglycemia and islet cell carcinoma. All had resection with long-term survival.

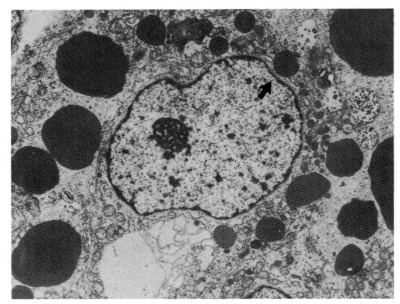

Fig 115–10.—Identification of electron membrane-bound dense zymogen granules permits classification of the tumor as acinar cell adenocarcinoma. (From Kissane J.M.[17])

Chemotherapeutic regimens used for adults might be appropriate for children with pancreatic carcinoma: SMF (streptozotocin, mitomycin C, fluouracil), FAM (fluouracil, Adriamycin [doxorubicin], mitomycin C) and FAM-S (FAM plus streptozotocin). All three regimens are equivalent, with a wide range of response. Children tolerate streptozotocin better than adults.[5] Megavoltage irradiation for pancreatic adenocarcinoma should follow resection or debulking of the tumor. High doses with accurate localization are required.

REFERENCES

1. Becker W.F.: Pancreatoduodenectomy for carcinoma of the pancreas in an infant: Report of a case. *Ann. Surg.* 145:864, 1957.
2. Becker W.F., Welsh R.A., Pratt H.: Cystadenoma and cystadenocarcinoma of the pancreas. *Ann. Surg.* 161:845, 1965.
3. Benjamin E., Wright D.H.: Adenocarcinoma of the pancreas of childhood: A report of two cases. *Histopathology* 4:87, 1980.
4. Boor P.J., Swanson M.R.: Papillary-cystic neoplasm of the pancreas. *Am. J. Surg. Pathol.* 3:69, 1979.
5. Broder L.E., Carter S.K.: Pancreatic islet cell carcinoma. II. Results of therapy with streptozotocin in 52 patients. *Ann. Intern. Med.* 79:108, 1973.
6. Cattell R.B., Warren K.W.: *Surgery of the Pancreas.* Philadelphia, W.B. Saunders Co., 1953.
7. Child C.G.: Radical one-stage pancreaticoduodenectomy. *Surgery* 23:492, 1948.
8. Compagno J., Oertel J.E.: Mucinous cystic neoplasms of the pancreas with overt and latent malignancy (cystadenocarcinoma and cystadenoma): A clinicopathologic study of 41 cases. *Am. J. Clin. Pathol.* 69:573, 1978.
9. Corner B.D.: Primary carcinoma of the pancreas in an infant aged 7 months. *Arch. Dis. Child.* 18:106, 1943.
10. Dynan R.W., Neerhout R.C., Johnson T.S.: Pancreatic carcinoma in childhood: Case report and review. *J. Med.* 65:711, 1964.
11. Fonkalsrud E.W., Wilderson J.A., Longmire W.P.: Pancreatoduodenectomy for nonfunctioning islet cell tumor of the pancreas in infancy and childhood. *JAMA* 197:158, 1966.
12. Grosfeld J.L., Clatworthy H.W., Hamoudi A.B.: Pancreatic malignancy in childhood. *Arch. Surg.* 101:370, 1970.
13. Horie A., Yano Y., Kotoo Y., et al.: Morphogenesis of pancreatoblastoma, infantile carcinoma of the pancreas: Report of two cases. *Cancer* 39:247, 1977.
14. Hurez A., Bedouelle A., Debray A., et al.: Carcinoma of the islet of Langerhans with severe hypoglycemic manifestations in a 9-year-old child—subtotal pancreatectomy. *Arch. Fr. Pédiatr.* 18:625, 1961.
15. Jaubert de Beaujeu M., Chabal B., Metairs R., et al.: Duodeno-pancreatectomie céphalique pour tumeur pancréatique chez un enfant de 4 ans et demi. *Pédiatrie* 19:369, 1964.
16. Kaletcheff A.: Carcinoma of the pancreas in a girl 14 years old. *Gac. Méd. Caracas* 46:393, 1939.
17. Kissane J.M.: Tumors of the exocrine pancreas in childhood, in McGuire W.L. (ed.): *Cancer Treatment and Research,* vol. 8. The Hague, Martinus Nijhoff, 1982, pp. 99–127.
18. Kuhn, A.: Primary pancreatic carcinoma in infancy. *Klin. Wochenschr.* 24:494, 1887.
19. Lack E.E., Cassady J.R., Levey R., et al.: Tumors of the exocrine pancreas in children and adolescents. A clinical and pathological study of 7 cases. *Am. J. Surg. Pathol.* (In Press).
20. May P.T., Loo D.C., Tock E.P.: Pancreatic acinar cell carcinoma in childhood. *Am. J. Dis. Child.* 128:101, 1974.
21. Miecarek P.A.: Primary adenocarcinoma of the pancreas in a 15-year-old boy. *Am. J. Pathol.* 11:527, 1935.
22. Morlock C.G., Dockerty M.C.: Carcinoma of the pancreas during the first 2 decades of life: Report of 2 cases. *Postgrad. Med.* 26:239, 1959.
23. Moynan R.W., Neerhout R.C., Johnson T.C.: Pancreatic carcinoma in childhood. *J. Pediatr.* 65:711, 1964.
24. Osborne B.M., Culbert S.J., Cangir A., et al.: Acinar cell carcinoma of the pancreas in a 9-year-old child; case report with electron microscope observations. *South. Med. J.* 70:370, 1977.
25. Simon R.: Pancreatic Carcinoma in a 13-Year-Old Child (inaugural dissertation) (Griefswald: J. Abel, 1889).
26. Smith W.R.: Primary carcinoma of the pancreas in children: Report of a case in a boy 14 1/2 years of age with generalized metastasis. *Am. J. Dis. Child.* 50:1482, 1935.
27. Stein M.L., Rossi V.C., de Almeida A.M.C.: Carcinoma of the pancreas in the infant: Presentation of a case. *Pediatr. Prat.* 33:75, 1962.
28. Stewart S.C., Stewart L.F.: A case of cancer of the pancreas in a 9-year-old boy. *Int. Clin.* 2:118, 1915.
29. Stokes J.M., Wohltmann H.J., Hartmann A.F.: Pancreatectomy in children. *Arch. Surg.* 93:40, 1966.
30. Stout B.F., Todd D.A.: Report of a case of primary adenocarcinoma of the pancreas in a 4-year-old child. *Tex. J. Med.* 28:464, 1932.
31. Taxy J.B.: Adenocarcinoma of the pancreas in childhood. Report of a case and a review of the English language literature. *Cancer* 37:1508, 1976.
32. Tsukimoto I., Tsuchida M.: in Humphrey G.B., Grindey G.B., Dehner L.P., et al. (eds.): *Pancreatic Tumors in Children.* Amsterdam, Martinus Nijhoff, 1982, pp. 150–157.
33. Warren K.W.: Nonfunctioning islet cell carcinoma in an 11-year-old child treated by pancreato-duodenectomy. *Lahey Clin. Bull.* 9:155, 1955.
34. Warren K.W., Christophi C., Armendariz R., et al.: Current trends in the diagnosis and treatment of carcinoma of the pancreas. *Am. J. Surg.* 145:813, 1983.

35. Warthen R.O., Sanford M.D., Rice E.C.: Primary malignant tumor of the pancreas in a 15-month-old boy. *Am. J. Dis. Child.* 83:663, 1952.
36. Wastell C.: Malignant nonfunctioning islet cell tumor of the pancreas in a 14-year-old girl. *Proc. R. Soc. Med.* 58:432, 1965.
37. Whipple A.O., Parsons W.B., Mullins C.R.: Treatment of carcinoma of the ampulla of Vater. *Ann. Surg.* 102:763, 1935.
38. Wright S.: Pancreaticoduodenectomy in infancy: A case report. *Surgery* 69:389, 1971.
39. Zollinger R.M., Ellison E.H.: Primary peptic ulcerations of the jejunum associated with islet cell tumors of the pancreas. *Ann. Surg.* 142:709, 1955.

Multiple Endocrine Adenomatosis

Zollinger-Ellison Syndrome

In 1955, Zollinger and Ellison[18] proposed that a humoral ulcerogenic factor of pancreatic islet cell origin might be responsible for the severe ulcer diathesis seen in patients with primary jejunal ulceration. Gregory[8] was the first to demonstrate the presence of a potent gastric secretagogue in pancreatic islet cell tissue, identified as gastrin. Thirty-five percent of patients have diarrhea, usually associated with gastric hypersecretion.

Operative procedures other than total gastrectomy have been unsuccessful. More than 400 cases of pancreatic islet cell tumors and gastric hypersecretion with peptic jejunal ulceration and diarrhea have been collected, of which some 24 have been in children. Two hundred and fifty patients were operated on. Only 27% were living without gastrectomy. Fox et al.[4] reported 137 patients with Zollinger-Ellison syndrome treated by total gastrectomy. Of these, 75% were alive and well at 1 year and 42% at 10 years; 73 patients had liver metastases, yet 68% were alive and well at 1 year and 30% at 10 years. Protection by total gastrectomy, then, is neither complete nor permanent.[5] Successful treatment of malignant Zollinger-Ellison tumors with streptozotocin and fluouracil has been reported.[10]

Ellison and Wilson,[3] investigating the question of benign versus malignant tumors in the Zollinger-Ellison syndrome, found 152 of 249 tumors (61%) to be malignant, 44% with metastasis; 72 patients (29%) had adenomas and 25 (10%) hyperplasia alone. The head-body-tail ratio was 4:1:4. Lesions were multiple and involved two anatomical areas in 29%. The entire gland was involved in 19%. Eighty patients had involvement of lymph nodes, 67% had local spread, 48% had lesions in the liver, and two patients had lung involvement.

Wilson and Schulte[16] reported 15 children with Zollinger-Ellison syndrome and ulcerogenic islet cell tumors. All had undergone gastric resection before their 15th birthdays. Seven underwent total gastrectomy. All were living and well for periods of up to 9 years, but presumably had residual tumor since the primary lesion was not removed. Eight children had less than total gastrectomy; six of these died. Patients' ages ranged from 7 to 15 years; 13 were boys. Several had already developed hyperparathyroidism. Buchta[1] reports one case and found three additional children treated by total gastrectomy, all alive and well. Four of eight children whose fathers had Zollinger-Ellison syndrome have inherited the syndrome in a budding or full form.

Ulcerogenic pancreatic islet cell tumors may grow slowly, and clinically are slow to evolve. The first manifestation, in children with multiple endocrine neoplasias, may be hyperparathyroidism. Shafer[13] first saw a child with non-beta islet cell carcinoma at age 14; the presenting complaint was diarrhea. A year later, a peptic ulcer developed. Total gastrectomy was performed, and the patient was well 2 years later. Unrecognized Zollinger-Ellison syndrome may contribute to excessive mortality in children unless appropriately treated by total gastrectomy and resection of the neoplasm if it occupies the body or tail of the pancreas and has not spread. All children with Zollinger-Ellison syndrome have been 7 years of age or older and can tolerate total gastrectomy.

The international Zollinger-Ellison syndrome registry continues to access childhood cases. Five cases since Wilson's report emphasize the high incidence of multiple tumors within the pancreas and of metastatic disease at the time of diagnosis. Elevated gastrin levels reported up to 11 years after operation presumably indicate residual metastatic disease.[12]

Other Endocrine Lesions of the Pancreas

Other pancreatic endocrine lesions include gastropancreatic and enteropancreatic (GEP) tumors, insulinomas (discussed below), gastrinomas (discussed under the Zollinger-Ellison syndrome), and familial gastrinoma (multiple endocrine neoplasia [MEN-1]). Schmidt's[11] case appears to be unique in that it is pancreatic in origin—a mixed islet cell tumor with ectopic ACTH production and Cushing syndrome as the predominant clinical feature.

Glucagonoma has been reported by Palmer et al.,[9a] an apudoma by Johnson[9] and a child with VIP syndrome by Ghishan.[7] Percutaneous transhepatic venous sampling (THVS) has been reported in several adult series. The hormone content in the venous effluent establishes the site of the tumor and its specific product.[15] Similar studies have been reported in children by Gauderer[6] and by Carcassonne[2] in the management of children with nesidioblastosis. C-terminal peptide assay has been added to preoperative testing for insulin-producing states. It is always below 0.2 pmol/L in the normal individual. MEN-1 patients have a higher incidence of microadenomatosis and, like nesidioblastosis patients, require extensive pancreatic resection. They present at a very young age with hypergastrinemia and peptic ulceration. Substances measured by THVS sampling include gastrin, glucagon, vasoactive intestinal polypeptide (VIP), motilin, somatostatin, insulin, and pancreatic polypeptide (PEP), the substance thought to cause diarrhea. Excess PEP secretion has been designated *apudoma*. Multiple endocrine adenomatosis (MEA type 1), Werner syndrome, is a familial disorder characterized by hyperplastic or neoplastic, synchronous or asynchronous (MEN-1)[14] involvement of the pituitary, pancreas, and parathyroid glands. One or more polypeptide hormones are involved.

Synchronous involvement of the pituitary, parathyroid, and pancreas is infrequent in children. A parathyroid disorder is usually the first abnormality, followed by pancreatic islet cell disease. The pituitary is least, and last, involved presenting as Cushing's disease. Some have Zollinger-Ellison syndrome due to islet cell hyperplasia and peptic ulcer disease due to gastrin hypersecretion. Thompson believes children will develop all of the above, providing they live long enough, but generally multihormone production is not seen before age 20 years.[14] Others may have glucagonomas, VIP-omas, somatostatinomas, and pancreatic polypeptide (PEP)-secreting tumors. PEP is a screening marker for islet cell hyperplasia.

Children with nesidioblastosis have not, to date, developed the MEN-1 syndrome. Periodic PEP assays may be the way to follow MEN-1 patients in looking for altered regulation of other hormones.

REFERENCES

1. Buchta R.M., Kaplan J.M.: Zollinger-Ellison syndrome in a 9-year-old child: A case report and review of the entity in childhood. *Pediatrics* 47:594, 1971.
2. Carcassonne M., DeLarue A., LeTourneau J.N.: Surgical treatment of organic pancreatic hypoglycemia in the pediatric age. *J. Pediatr. Surg.* 18:75, 1983.
3. Ellison E.H., Wilson S.D.: The Zollinger-Ellison syndrome: Reappraisal and evaluation of 260 registered cases. *Ann. Surg.* 160:512, 1964.

4. Fox P.S., Hoffman J.W., Decosse J.J., et al.: The influence of total gastrectomy on survival in malignant Zollinger-Ellison tumors. *Ann. Surg.* 180:559, 1974.

5. Friesen S.: In discussion of Wilson D., Schulte W.J., Meade R.C.: *Arch. Surg.* 103:108, 1971.

6. Gauderer M., Stanley C.A., Baker L., et al.: Pancreatic adenomas in infants and children: Current surgical management. *J. Pediatr. Surg.* 13:591, 1978.

7. Ghishan F.K.: Infant diarrhea due to pancreatic vasoactive intestinal polypeptide (VIP) secretion. *Pediatrics* 64:46, 1979.

8. Gregory R.A., Tracy H.J.: The preparation and properties of gastrin. *J. Physiol.* 149:70, 1959.

9. Johnson T.L.: Apudoma of pancreas. *Br. J. Surg.* 29:123, 1982.

9a. Palmer J.P., Werner P.L., Benson J.W., et al.: Dominant inheritance of large molecular weight immunoreactive glucagon. *J. Clin. Invest.* 61:763, 1978.

10. Ruffner B.W. Jr.: Chemotherapy for malignant Zollinger-Ellison tumors: Successful treatment with streptozotocin and fluouracil. *Arch. Intern. Med.* 136:1032, 1976.

11. Schmidt J.H., Pysher T.J.: Ectopic Cushing's syndrome in an adolescent, in Humphrey G.B., Grindey G.B., Dehner L.P., et al. (eds.): *Pancreatic Tumors in Children.* Amsterdam, Martinus Nijhoff, 1982, p. 173.

12. Schwartz D.L., White J.J., Saulsbury F., et al.: Gastrin response to calcium infusion: An aid to the improved diagnosis of Zollinger-Ellison syndrome in children. *Pediatrics* 54:599, 1974.

13. Shafer W.H.: Non-beta islet cell carcinoma of the pancreas presenting as diarrhea. *Ann. Intern. Med.* 61:539, 1964.

14. Thompson N.W.: Surgical considerations in the MEA I syndrome, in Johnston I.D., Thompson N.W. (eds.): *Endocrine Surgery (Surgery,* vol. 2). London, Butterworth's International Medical Reviews, 1983, pp. 144–164.

15. Vinik A.I., Glowniak B., Glazer B., et al.: Localization of gasteroentero pancreatic (GEP) tumors, in Johnston I.D., Thompson N.W. (eds.): *Endocrine Surgery (Surgery,* vol. 2). London, Butterworth's International Medical Reviews, 1983, pp. 164–182.

16. Wilson D., Schulte W.J., and Meade R.C.: Longevity studies following total gastrectomy in children with the Zollinger-Ellison syndrome. *Arch. Surg.* 103:108, 1971.

17. Zollinger R.M.: Islet cell tumors of the pancreas and the alimentary tract. *Am. J. Surg.* 129:102, 1975.

18. Zollinger R.M., Ellison E.H.: Primary peptic ulcerations of the jejunum associated with islet cell tumors of the pancreas. *Ann. Surg.* 142:709, 1955.

Hypoglycemia

History

In 1869, Langerhans,[19] while still a medical student, identified the pancreatic islets. In 1902, Nicholls,[22] a pathologist, described the first islet cell adenoma. In 1908, Lane,[18] employing better histologic techniques, differentiated the alpha and beta cells of the islets. Banting and Best[2] discovered insulin in 1921 and postulated its role in hypoglycemia. The term "hyperinsulinism" has proved to be an oversimplification. W.J. Mayo, in 1927, first excised a functioning islet cell tumor. The tumor was malignant, and there was metastasis at the time of operation. Graham and Hartmann recommended subtotal pancreatectomy for hypoglycemia in 1934.[12]

Diagnosis

The approach to the evaluation of hypoglycemia is seen in Table 115–8. The necessity for early diagnosis and treatment, once hypoglycemia is suspected, is underscored by the high incidence of neurologic sequelae in infants affected before 1 year of age.

The suggested baseline studies obtained on a fasting morning specimen and during a symptomatic period should facilitate the exclusion of primary extrapancreatic endocrine disorders such as panhypopituitarism, isolated growth hormone deficiency, adrenal insufficiency, hypothyroidism, and congenital adrenal hyperplasia (adrenogenital syndrome). Growth hormone, cortisol, thyroxine, triiodothyronine, and thyroid-stimulating hormone can all be measured by radioimmunoassay. Physical findings usually identify endocrinopathies involving the hypothalamus, pituitary, adrenals, and thyroid.

The Beckwith-Wiedemann syndrome (exomphalos-macroglossia-gigantism), has a high association with hypoglycemia. Glycogen storage disease is suggested by hepatomegaly, lactic acidemia, and absent glycemic response to exogenous glucagon. Inborn errors of gluconeogenesis (e.g., fructose 1,6-diphosphatase deficiency) are differentiated by their positive response to exogenous glucagon but absent glycemic response to alanine, glycerol, and fructose. The enzyme deficiency results in lactic acidemia rather than glucose production. Ketotic hypoglycemia is suggested by a history of low birth weight, onset of symptoms after 18 months of age, thinness, small stature, early-morning symptoms following an overnight fast, and concomitant ketonemia and ketonuria. These children have been reported to have abnormally low alanine levels and may possibly have a gluconeogenic substrate-limited disorder.[25, 29] Patients show a positive glycemic response to alanine infusion, 250 mg/kg over 30 minutes, and a positive response to exogenous glucagon after being fed. Their hypoglycemia tends to resolve spontaneously with age.

Leucine sensitivity describes a particular response associated with insulinoma, nesidioblastosis, and beta-cell hyperplasia. It should be regarded as an indicator of organic hyperinsulinism rather than a diagnosis in itself. Sensitivity is demonstrated by a fall in blood glucose of ≥40% from the fasting level when L-leucine is administered orally at 150 mg/kg. Maximal lowering of blood glucose occurs within 20–45 minutes, secondary to insulin stimulation; and simultaneous glucose insulin and glucagon levels should be obtained. As with any test provocative of hypoglycemia, 50% dextrose (2 ml/kg/dose, given intravenously) should be available to treat hypoglycemic symptoms.

Organic hyperinsulinism can be suspected when circulating insulin levels are absolutely elevated or are inappropriately elevated for the simultaneous glucose level, an insulin level ≥10 μU/ml associated with a simultaneous glucose level of ≤50 mg/dl. It should be suspected in any infant presenting with hypoglycemia in the first year of life. Thyroid profile, growth hormone and cortisol levels, 24-hour excretion of catecholamines, and the glycemic response to exogenous glucagon are normal. Serial preprandial glucose and glucoregulatory hormone levels should be obtained for at least 2 days, with the child on a normal diet and a regular feeding schedule. If glucose is required to maintain normoglycemic levels or a symptom-free state, the rate is frequently more than 0.5 gm/kg/hr, and reliable infusion via a central venous catheter is required. Whenever glucose infusion is required to control hypoglycemic symptoms, serial monitoring is necessary (1) to provide a baseline for comparison once intervention is initiated, (2) to document inappropriate insulin and blood glucose levels, and (3) to correlate blood glucose variation with insulin, glucagon, growth hormone, and intake. A 4–6-hour fast is sufficient in young infants; careful monitoring is necessary to prevent glucose levels from reaching the dangerous level of 30 mg/dl. There is growing evidence that organic hyperinsulinism accounts for most cases of "idiopathic" hypoglycemia. Presently available diagnostic studies do not permit differentiation of one endocrine cell abnormality from another. Histopathology does not explain the true pathophysiology of hyperinsulinism.

Nesidioblastosis (Greek *nesidion* [islet], *blastos* [germ] implies neoformation of islet tissue from pancreatic ductules or epithelium. Yakovac et al.[37] in 1971, first reported the specific histopathologic findings in infants with hypoglycemia (Fig 115–11). Numerous reports followed.[1, 11, 16, 17] The true incidence has probably been underestimated. A clear distinction among nesidioblastosis, islet hyperplasia, and microadenomatosis is not always possible.[20] Identification of all four known islet cells—al-

TABLE 115–8.—Outline of Medical Work-up for Hypoglycemia
of Infants and Children

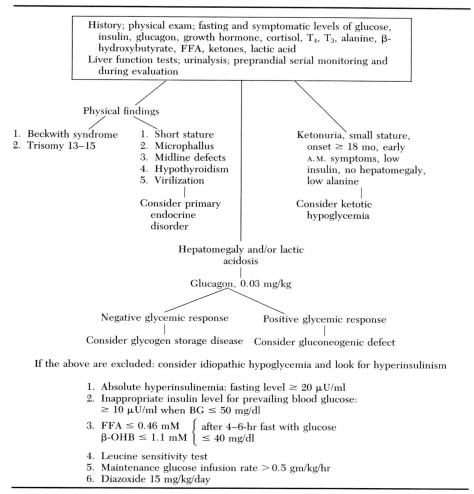

History; physical exam; fasting and symptomatic levels of glucose, insulin, glucagon, growth hormone, cortisol, T_4, T_3, alanine, β-hydroxybutyrate, FFA, ketones, lactic acid
Liver function tests; urinalysis; preprandial serial monitoring and during evaluation

Physical findings

1. Beckwith syndrome
2. Trisomy 13–15

1. Short stature
2. Microphallus
3. Midline defects
4. Hypothyroidism
5. Virilization

Consider primary endocrine disorder

Ketonuria, small stature, onset ≥ 18 mo, early A.M. symptoms, low insulin, no hepatomegaly, low alanine

Consider ketotic hypoglycemia

Hepatomegaly and/or lactic acidosis

Glucagon, 0.03 mg/kg

Negative glycemic response

Consider glycogen storage disease

Positive glycemic response

Consider gluconeogenic defect

If the above are excluded: consider idiopathic hypoglycemia and look for hyperinsulinism

1. Absolute hyperinsulinemia: fasting level ≥ 20 μU/ml
2. Inappropriate insulin level for prevailing blood glucose: ≥ 10 μU/ml when BG ≤ 50 mg/dl
3. FFA ≤ 0.46 mM after 4–6-hr fast with glucose
   β-OHB ≤ 1.1 mM ≤ 40 mg/dl
4. Leucine sensitivity test
5. Maintenance glucose infusion rate > 0.5 gm/kg/hr
6. Diazoxide 15 mg/kg/day

pha, beta, delta, and pancreatic polypeptide cells—requires immunofluorescent methods with specific antisera or ultrastructural characterization of the various secretory granules through electron microscopy (Fig 115–12). The pathogenesis of hypoglycemia may reside in the disorganized islet structure in nesidioblastosis. Recent studies indicate that intraislet relationships and islet architecture (Table 115–9) may be just as important in glucose homeostasis as the quantitative dispersal of islet components.

The clinical spectrum of hypoglycemia due to nesidioblastosis is quite broad and does not differ from that of hypoglycemia in general. Infants may present with frank seizures or subtle behavioral and minor motor signs, such as quivering of the lip or episodic disconjugate gaze. Occasionally, patients may be asymptomatic until stressed by a minor infection that interferes with oral intake. Preprandial blood glucose levels are invariably less than 40 mg/dl, even in asymptomatic infants. In more severely affected infants, blood glucose levels may be lower than 30 mg/dl. There is no sex predominance. Birth weight tends toward the high side, and frequently a history of maternal illness in the third month of pregnancy can be elicited. Vance et al.[35] reported multiple endocrine adenomatosis in eight family members with nesidioblastosis.

Medical Management

In infants and children unable to maintain blood glucose levels above 40 mg/dl on a frequent feeding schedule, or in whom symptoms persist even at higher glucose levels, glucose should be administered intravenously. Infusion should be continuous and regulated at the minimal rate, providing continuous relief of symptoms and/or maintenance of normoglycemia. The rate of infusion may range from 0.2 gm to as much as 1 gm/kg/hr. Regardless of whether glucose or diazoxide (15 mg/kg/day), preferred by some, is being infused, pretreatment and posttreatment blood sugar, insulin, glucagon, and growth hormone levels should be obtained. If intravenous administration of glucose or diazoxide does not maintain normoglycemia, intramuscular or subcutaneous injection of glucagon (0.03 mg/kg, 1 mg maximal dose) results in euglycemia, provided liver glycogen stores are normal.

Assuming hyperinsulinism is present, and that extrapancreatic endocrine function is normal, we believe management should consist of supportive therapy to assure normoglycemia or at least asymptomatic hypoglycemia. A properly functioning central venous line is mandatory. Fluid overload, common in these infants, must be avoided. Feedings should be given at least every 4 hours but may be adjusted, depending on serial monitoring of the blood glucose level.

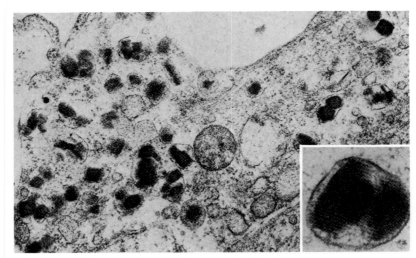

Fig 115–11.—Nesidioblastosis. Electron micrograph showing beta cell membrane-bound insulin inclusions (×50,000); inset (×80,000) shows crystalline array of insulin. (From Yakovac et al.[37])

Surgical Management

Numerous reports of neurologic impairment in hypoglycemia of infancy unresponsive to medical management and the rapidly growing evidence of specific histopathology in hyperinsulin states in infancy, especially nesidioblastosis, suggest that pancreatectomy should be performed early rather than as a last resort. Follow-up of our earlier cases has shown that pancreatectomy is curative in a significant proportion of patients and that the risk of pancreatic insufficiency or diabetes mellitus is low. Nearly complete pancreatectomy is mandatory when medical treatment fails to control symptoms or succeeds only at the expense of serious and significant side effects, i.e., in an unstable patient despite high glucose load.

An upper abdominal transverse incision dividing both rectus muscles provides good exposure. The lesser sac is entered and the duodenum mobilized by the Kocher maneuver. The pancreas is then inspected for its entire length. Occasionally, a solitary functioning islet cell adenoma may be found, especially in children older than 4 years. If such a lesion is found, it is removed by distal pancreatectomy with preservation of the spleen. Liver biopsy and biopsies from the head, body, and tail of the pancreas should be obtained for electron and immunofluorescent microscopic studies. Insulinoma in the infant may not be a discrete surgical lesion, as previously thought. Coexistent beta-cell hyperplasia or multifocal microadenomatosis may occur and be indistinguishable from nesidioblastosis. If a discrete adenoma is identified and removed, and insulin levels remain high and glucose levels low, a 95% pancreatectomy is required. If no localized lesion is found, the pancreas is mobilized from left to right. The short gastric vessels should be preserved, to protect the spleen. Multiple vessels between the splenic vein, splenic artery, and the superior border of the pancreas are divided and

disposed of with suture ligatures or bipolar coagulation. Mobilization is continued until the superior mesenteric vessels come into view and the junction of the splenic vein and the portal or interior mesenteric vein is established. Resection should be carried out well to the right of these vessels, removing the uncinate process and continuing to the point of origin of the superior and the inferior pancreaticoduodenal arteries. These vessels mark the superior and inferior limits of the dissection and transection. Carcassonne,[5] who checks portal venous insulin levels before pancreatectomy, recommends a second portal venous insulin level at this point in the operation. He also recommends insertion of a tube through the common duct into the duodenum to be sure the duct is protected during the final phase of the dissection and to provide postoperative biliary tract decompression. The duct of Wirsung and any accessory pancreatic duct that has been transected are closed with nonabsorbable sutures. A postresection cholangiogram is worthwhile to demonstrate the patency of the common bile duct. Drainage of the bed of the pancreatic resection is optional. Ninety-five percent pancreatic resection as the initial procedure has been recommended by Thomas,[34] Hamilton,[14] Harken et al.,[15] Gauderer,[10] Carcassonne,[5] and Shermeta;[32] and we agree.

Hypoglycemia is to be expected postoperatively and may require diazoxide (15 mg/kg/day). Usually it can be managed with close monitoring of input and output and of blood sugars, and by appropriate fluid therapy. Once oral intake is established, gradual weaning from the glucose infusion can be attempted, again with serial monitoring of glucose, insulin, and glucagon levels. Normoglycemia without intravenous supplementation and after 8- or 12-hour fasts indicates surgical success.

EXPERIENCE AND RESULTS.—Subtotal resection of the pancreas for hypoglycemia was first reported in 1934 by Graham and Hartmann.[12] The patient, a 1-year-old girl, underwent exploration for islet cell tumor. When none was found, 80% subtotal pancreatectomy was carried out. The pancreas was normal histologically. The patient survived but was mentally retarded.

Of 78 cases collected from the literature, plus 28 from Boston Children's Hospital, 1939–1984, 64 achieved normoglycemic levels postoperatively. Twenty-three remained normoglycemic following pancreatectomy and medical therapy. Fourteen children were considered not to be improved by 80–85% pancreatic resection. Six of our patients required reoperation and near-total

TABLE 115–9.—ENDOCRINE CELLS OF THE PANCREAS

TYPE	%	PRODUCT	SECONDARY
Alpha (α)	30	Glucagon	
Beta (β)	40	Insulin	Raises Δ
Delta (Δ)	10	Growth hormone	Blocks α and β
MG	10–18	Mixed granular cells	Unknown
X	3	Pancreatic polypeptide	Insulinoma

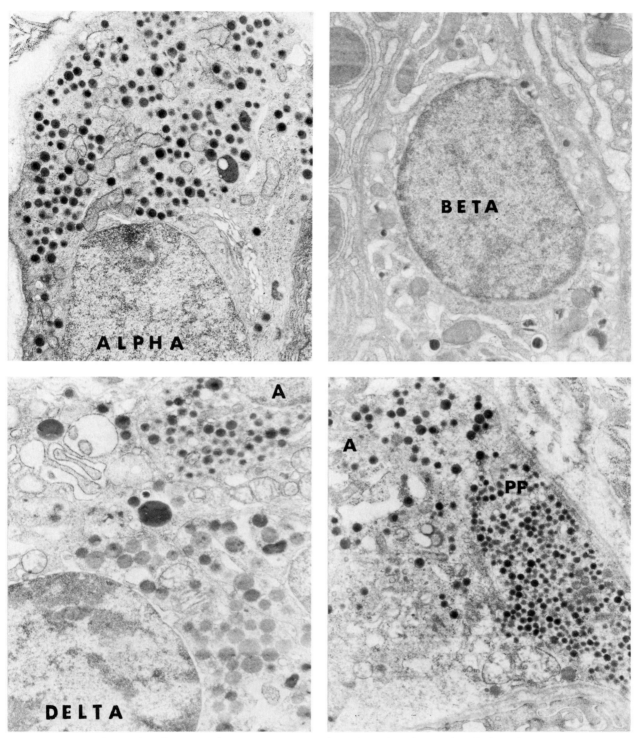

Fig 115–12.—The islets of Langerhans form a complex endocrine system containing at least four other hormone-producing cells in addition to the insulin-producing beta cells *(top right)*. The alpha cell *(top left)* produces glucagon, a hormone that causes stored liver glycogen to break down and provide glucose and controls the manufacture of glucose in the liver from precursors such as amino acids. The newly recognized delta cell *(bottom left)* produces somatosta-tin, which regulates the secretion of both insulin and glucagon. Recently Gabbay et al. described two additional cells in the human islets, one containing a newly recognized pancreatic polypeptide *(bottom right),* whose function is still unknown. The fifth cell is as yet unidentified as to content or function. (From *Children's World* 4 [no. 2], 1977.)

pancreatectomy; four required pancreatin; and three required insulin. It is evident that 95% of the pancreas must be resected to obtain the maximal surgical benefit, as first suggested by Thomas et al.[34] in 1977. Unfortunately, in the collected experience 24 children were already neurologically impaired before operation and remained so postoperatively, indicating that the surgical procedure came too late. Seven patients died of infection, months to years after operation. The role of splenectomy in these cases is not clear but is highly suspect.

All truly resistant hypoglycemia develops before the age of 1 year, and usually before the age of 6 months. The patients show little response to medical therapy, including glucagon and somatostatin (pituitary growth hormone). The defect seems to be one of insulin regulation. In time, some become frankly diabetic. A second operation removing all but a rim of pancreas in the duodenal curve is recommended for patients not improved by less extensive initial resection.

Of our 28 patients undergoing pancreatic resection for idiopathic hypoglycemia, 16 had nesidioblastosis, nine had islet cell hyperplasia, two had a normal pancreas, and one had diffuse adenomatosis. Sixteen of the patients have been the subjects of previous reports. We have not employed formal pancreatoduodenectomy, as recommended by McFarland et al.[21]

Recent experience at Boston Children's Hospital (1977–1983) consists of five additional patients: all were infants, the youngest 6 weeks old; all had nesidioblastosis; none had a localized lesion. Four of five underwent 95% resection as the first and definitive procedure. One patient underwent an 85% resection and subsequently came to 95% resection because of continued symptoms and unrelieved hypoglycemia. All 12 patients operated on between 1970 and 1983 are normoglycemic and neurologically intact. We did not encounter hypoglycemia due to focal islet cell adenoma (uncommon until the end of the first decade of life) in this period.

Carcassonne[5] reported six patients: two, aged 12 and 14, had islet cell adenoma; three, aged 1–14 months, had diffuse nesidioblastosis; one had normal pancreatic tissue. In a survey of the literature from 1975 to 1981, he identified 218 children with hypoglycemia and placed them in two groups: (1) infant type (123 patients with diffuse pancreatic lesions, 37 lesions localized); (2) childhood type (17 had diffuse lesions; 47 had localized tumors). No diffuse lesions were encountered in patients after age 8. Among 72 infants undergoing subtotal pancreatectomy for organic hyperinsulinism, 28 had mental retardation. Eighty-five percent resection resulted in 54 recurrences of hypoglycemia and necessitated 36 reoperations to the 95% level. Eight recurrences were observed in 22 patients who underwent 95% pancreatectomy. Thirteen patients requiring reresection did not develop exocrine gland insufficiency, but four developed diabetes requiring insulin. Carcassonne concludes that, after age 4, 95% of patients have a localized lesion permitting less radical pancreatic resection.

Carcassonne suggests that focal distal pancreatic lesions can be treated by distal pancreatectomy with preservation of the spleen. If this reduces insulin in the portal vein to normal, no further resection is required. If there is no change in the insulin level, dissection is continued to the right of the superior mesenteric vein. A second portal vein insulin sample is obtained and, if normal, the operation stops here. If frozen sections still show nesidioblastosis, islet cell hyperplasia, or diffuse microadenomatosis, operation continues, as outlined above, to the 95% level. Insulinemia ceases in all cases at this level of transection, but hyperglycemia may ensue. Intravenous insulin infusion may be necessary at 0.1 mg/kg/hr.

Ortiz et al.[24] described reimplantation of the ampulla of Vater after total pancreatectomy for nesidioblastosis, thus ensuring survival of the distal common duct and permitting one to extend the resection. Langer et al.[20] reported on recent (1977–1982) experience from Toronto. The patients with organic hyperinsulinemia were operated on; five underwent 95% pancreatectomy. One required choledochojejunostomy following injury to the distal common duct. All patients were rendered normoglycemic; none showed evidence of diabetes, exocrine deficiency, or developmental delay. Average follow-up was 16 months. Five patients underwent 85% pancreatectomy leaving the uncinate process: two did well; two went on to 95% pancreatic resection. One did well early but became hypoglycemic 3 years later, apparently due to regrowth of residual pancreas, and required total pancreatectomy. Mean follow-up was 36 months. Nine of 10 patients had nesidioblastosis; one had a normal pancreas. A functioning spleen was preserved in all cases.

Campbell et al.[4] reported 11 patients ranging in age from 4 to 10 years. Light or electron microscopy showed normal pancreas in three, nesibioblastosis in two, islet cell hyperplasia in two, and diffuse microadenomas in four. Symptoms persisted in six patients: two still require diazoxide; one required total pancreatectomy. All patients had 80–85% resection initially. In this 15-year study, the spleen was sacrificed in the early patients and preserved in four recent patients.

Woolley et al.[36] stated that, of 16 patients undergoing pancreatectomy for hypoglycemia, none had a localized lesion. Five patients with islet cell hyperplasia were cured after 85% pancreatectomy. One showed improvement and one no change. Two patients with nesidioblastosis were cured, and three were improved but were not euglycemic. Two ultimately required total pancreatectomy. Neurologic status was not reported.

Schiller et al.[30] reported seven infants with 85% resection. One was extended to 95% and another to total pancreatectomy. None are neurologically impaired. Analysis of the problem may be too simplistic. Shermeta and Mendelsohn[32] reported three infants who had persistent hypoglycemia following 90% pancreatectomy and yet showed no elevation of serum insulin levels. They suggested that the problem might not be entirely due to excess secretion of insulin but rather to a hyperglucagon state. Total pancreatectomy might be inappropriate therapy. Davidson et al.[6] also issued a word of caution about total pancreatectomy in these failed patients. They reported two infants with recurrent hypoglycemia after extensive resection who were treated successfully with mesoxalyl urea (Alloxan), a cytotoxic drug specific to beta cells that has long been known to cause diabetes in animals. It has no demonstrable effect on other cells of the pancreas. The patients' exocrine function remains intact. In the short term, neither has become diabetic. This option in medical management is a hopeful development.[33] Aynsley-Green et al.[1] reported three infants who were glucose-drip–dependent at infusion rates of 10 mg/kg/minute despite diazoxide, 20–25/kg/day, and chlorothiazide. All three underwent 95% pancreatectomy. All required insulin within 24 hours of operation initiated as insulin infusion 0.1 units/kg/hr. One must be concerned about the ultimate price of euglycemia achieved by extended resection. The spleen should be spared to avoid the risk of postsplenectomy sepsis.

Islet Cell Adenoma

Hypoglycemia that appears initially in the older child is uncommon, and organic hyperinsulinism must be strongly considered. It is difficult, if not impossible, to rule out islet cell adenoma if the lesion occurs in a newborn (Fig 115–13), or is less than 0.5 cm. in diameter. The diagnosis of islet cell adenoma, as of idiopathic hypoglycemia, is one of exclusion when a specific etiology cannot be established. Celiac arteriography followed by

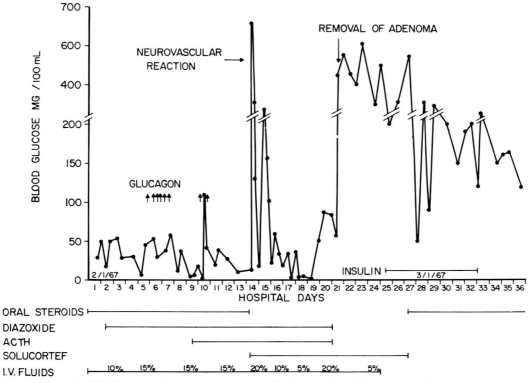

Fig 115–13.—Islet cell adenoma in a newborn. Chart summarizing failure of medical therapy, and cure following surgical removal of the neoplasm. (From Salinas et al.[29])

selective injection of the dorsal pancreatic artery, first described by Olsson[23] and later by Boijsen,[3] has been useful in identifying these small tumors with their enormously rich blood supply (Fig 115–14). The lesion is most difficult to demonstrate when it overlies L-2 or when it is obscured by the spleen. Gastric insufflation, magnification, and subtraction techniques permit identification in 70% of patients. These tumors usually occur in children over 4 years of age, although 14 cases have been reported in the neonatal period. We have encountered six children with islet cell adenoma at Boston Children's Hospital. In four, surgical removal resulted in dramatic cure. In two, the adenoma was discovered at autopsy; like Robinson's patient, who died at age 4 days,[28] these were early cases.

Islet cell adenoma of the pancreas is being reported with increasing frequency in children; 68 cases have been reported to date.[8, 10, 13, 26, 27] The islet cell tumor has a firmer consistency than the surrounding normal pancreas. Because of the rich capillary network, it has a pinkish color as compared with the more ivory tint of normal pancreatic tissue. The tumor is round, firm, discrete, and usually encapsulated. The cells of the adenoma are primarily beta cells. There is no clear histologic difference between functioning and nonfunctioning tumors. The tumor is multicentric in 14% of cases; 25% are located in the head of the pancreas; 73% are found in the body or tail; 2% are ectopic.

The age distribution, to age 15 years, of patients with functioning islet cell tumors is listed in Table 115–10. Seven children had benign islet cell tumors diagnosed at autopsy. Two patients had exploration only, two had biopsy only, and 23 had excision of the tumor with little if any margin of adjacent pancreas. Subtotal pancreatic resection, with amounts ranging from 25% to 90% of the gland, was performed in 35 patients, some with intraoperative insulin monitoring. Ten had multiple adenomas. Ec-

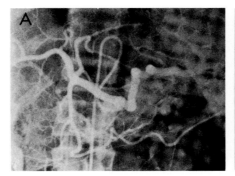
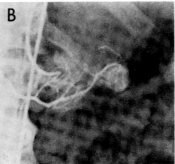

Fig 115–14.—Insulinoma: arteriographic demonstration. Celiac arteriography (A) followed by selective injection of dorsal pancreatic artery (B) showing insulinoma in tail of pancreas. (From Edis et al.[7])

TABLE 115–10.—AGE AND SEX
DISTRIBUTION OF 68 CHILDREN WITH
FUNCTIONING ISLET CELL TUMORS

AGE (YR)	NO. OF PATIENTS	SEX M	F
0–2	31 (15 newborn)	30	38
2–4	7		
4–6	6		
6–8	4		
8–10	7		
10–12	8		
12–15	5		
	68		

topic tumor in the liver occurred once. Forty-eight children with islet cell adenoma were cured, but 23 had some degree of mental retardation. Six were improved but required supplemental steroids, 11 died, and follow-up was not available for two.

In 12% of cases, tumors are multiple. Most are located in the body and tail. If an adenoma is found in the body or tail of the pancreas, it is advisable to carry out a subtotal resection of the gland, preserving the spleen, rather than enucleating the tumor itself.

REFERENCES

1. Aynsley-Green A., Polak J.M., Bloom S.R., et al.: Nesidioblastosis of the pancreas. Definition of the syndrome and the management of severe neonatal hyperinsulinemic hypoglycemia. *Arch. Dis. Child.* 56:496, 1981.
2. Banting F.G., Best C.H.: The internal secretion of the pancreas. *J. Lab. Clin. Med.* 7:251, 1922.
3. Boijsen E., Samuelson L.: Angiographic diagnosis of tumors arising from pancreatic islets. *Acta Radiol. (Diagn.)* 10:161, 1970.
4. Campbell J.R., Rivers S.P., Harrison N.W., et al.: Treatment of hypoglycemia in infants and children. *Am. J. Surg.* 146:21, 1983.
5. Carcassonne M., DeLarue A., LeTourneau J.N.: Surgical treatment of organic pancreatic hypoglycemia in the pediatric age. *J. Pediatr. Surg.* 18:75, 1983.
6. Davidson P.M., Young D.G., Logan R.W., et al.: Alloxan therapy for nesidioblastosis. *J. Pediatr. Surg.* 19:87, 1984.
7. Edis A.J., McIlrath D.C., van Heerden J.A., et al.: Insulinoma—current diagnosis and management. *Curr. Probl. Surg.* October 1976.
8. Fischer G.W., Vasquez A.M., Buist N.R., et al.: Neonatal islet cell adenoma: Case report and literature review. *Pediatrics* 53:753, 1974.
9. Fonkalsrud E.W., Trout H.H., Lippe B., et al.: Idiopathic hypoglycemia in infancy. *Arch. Surg.* 108:801, 1974.
10. Gauderer M., Stanley C.A., Baker L., et al.: Pancreatic adenomas in infants and children: Current surgical management. *J. Pediatr. Surg.* 13:591, 1978.
11. Gould B.E., Memoli V.A., Dardi L.E., et al.: Nesidiodysplasia and nesidioblastosis of infancy. *Scand. J. Gastroenterol.* 16:129, 1981.
12. Graham E.A., Hartmann A.F.: Subtotal resection of the pancreas for hypoglycemia. *Surg. Gynecol. Obstet.* 59:474, 1934.
13. Grosfeld J.: Surgical management of islet cell adenoma in infancy. *Surgery* 84:519, 1978.
14. Hamilton J.P., Baker L., Kaye R., et al.: Subtotal pancreatectomy in the management of severe persistent idiopathic hypoglycemia in children. *Pediatrics* 39:49, 1967.
15. Harken A.H., Filler R.M., AvRuskin T.W., et al.: The role of "total" pancreatectomy in the treatment of unremitting hypoglycemia in infancy. *J. Pediatr. Surg.* 6:284, 1971.
16. Heitz P.U., Kloppel G., Hacki W.H., et al.: Nesidioblastosis: The pathologic basis of persistent hyperinsulinemic hypoglycemia in infants. *Diabetes* 26:632, 1977.
17. Hirsch H.J., Loo S., Evans N., et al.: Hypoglycemia of infancy and nesidioblastosis: Studies with somatostatin. *N. Engl. J. Med.* 296:1323, 1977.
18. Lane M.A.: The cytologic characters of the islands of Langerhans. *Am. J. Anat.* 7:409, 1908.
19. Langerhans P.: Dissertation. Berlin, G. Lange, 1869.
20. Langer J.C., Filler R.M., Wesson D.E., et al.: Surgical management of persistent neonatal hypoglycemia due to islet cell dysplasia (nesidioblastosis). Presented at the 15th Annual Meeting, American Pediatric Surgical Association, Marcos Island, Florida, May 11, 1984.
21. McFarland J.O., Gillette F.S., Zwemer R.J.: Total pancreatectomy for hyperinsulinism in infants. *Surgery* 57:313, 1965.
22. Nicholls A.G.: Simple adenoma of the pancreas arising from an island of Langerhans. *J. Med. Res.* 8:385, 1902.
23. Olsson O.: Angiographic diagnosis of an islet cell tumor of the pancreas. *Acta Chir. Scand.* 126:346, 1963.
24. Ortiz V.N., Haase F.M., Jotes J.F., et al.: Reimplantation of the ampulla of Vater after total pancreatectomy for nesidioblastosis. *J. Pediatr. Surg.* 13(82):722, 1978.
25. Pagliara A.S., Karl I.E., Haywood M., et al.: Hypoglycemia in infancy and childhood. Part II. *J. Pediatr.* 82:558, 1973.
26. Rich R.H., Dehner L.P., Okinaga K.: Surgical management of islet cell adenoma in infancy. *Surgery* 84:519, 1978.
27. Rickham P.O.: Islet cell tumors in childhood. *J. Pediatr. Surg.* 1:83, 1975.
28. Robinson M.J., Clarke A.M., Gold H., et al.: Islet cell adenoma in the newborn: Report of two patients. *Pediatrics* 48:232, 1971.
29. Salinas E.D., Mangurten H.H., Roberts S.S., et al.: Functioning islet cell adenoma in the newborn. *Pediatrics* 41:646, 1968.
30. Schiller M., Krausz M., Meyer S., et al.: Neonatal hyperinsulinism—surgical and pathologic considerations. *J. Pediatr. Surg.* 15:16, 1980.
31. Shermeta D.W., Mendelsohn G.: Hyperinsulinism and hypoglycemia in the neonate: Therapeutic choices. *J. Pediatr. Surg.* 15:398, 1980.
32. Shermeta D.W., Mendelsohn G., Haller J.A.: Hyperinsulinemic hypoglycemia of the neonate associated with persistent fetal histology and function of the pancreas. *Ann. Surg.* 191:182, 1980.
33. Talbot N.B., Crawford J.D., Bailey C.C.: Use of mesoxalyl urea (Alloxan) in treatment of an infant with convulsions due to idiopathic hypoglycemia. *Pediatrics* 1:337, 1948.
34. Thomas C.G., Underwood L.E., Carney C., et al.: Neonatal and infantile hypoglycemia due to insulin excess. *Ann. Surg.* 185:505, 1977.
35. Vance J.E., Stoll R.W., Kitabachi A.E., et al.: Familial nesidioblastosis as the predominant manifestation of multiple endocrine adenomatosis. *Am. J. Med.* 52:211, 1972.
36. Woolley M.: In discussion of Campbell J.R., et al. *Am. J. Surg.* 146:21, 1983.
37. Yakovac W.C., Baker L., Hummeler K.: Beta cell nesidioblastosis in idiopathic hypoglycemia of infancy. *J. Pediatr.* 79:226, 1971.

116 E. Thomas Boles, Jr.

The Spleen

THE SPLEEN was long held to be an organ unessential to life and to good health, and one whose loss was of little consequence. This view has changed as important functions of the spleen have become better defined and as the evidence that its loss may be life-threatening, particularly during infancy and early childhood, has become widely accepted.[57] Three functions of the spleen have been clearly identified: (1) clearance and phagocytosis of particulate matter from the blood, (2) antibody formation, and (3) hematopoiesis. The microcirculation of the spleen is ideally constituted to provide a relatively prolonged exposure of blood cells and other particulate matter to splenic macrophages and other phagocytic cells. About 90% of the arterial blood circulating through the spleen passes first into the open circulation of the red pulp, after which the cells and other particulate matter can enter the venous sinuses only by passing through pores between endothelial cells.[7] During this passage through the red pulp, the splenic phagocytes remove microorganisms. These include both those bacteria to which the individual has antibody and, more importantly, those to which it has no pre-existing antibody. Although the liver has more reticuloendothelial tissue than the spleen and is highly efficient in removing bacteria coated with specific antibody, clearance of bacteria without specific antibody occurs largely in the spleen.[3] This seems to be particularly true of encapsulated bacteria such as the *Pneumococci*. Humoral immunity (antibody) against such organisms is transmitted to the newborn through the placenta, but this passive maternal antibody protection largely disappears within a few months. Active immunity, from the development of immunoglobulins against these bacteria, develops later in childhood; and during the interim, protection against blood-borne bacteria depends largely on the phagocytic ability of the splenic macrophages.

Also during passage through the red pulp, reticulocytes are converted to normal biconcave red blood cells, pits and Howell-Jolly bodies are removed from erythrocytes, and acanthotic red cells are removed from the circulation. Old erythrocytes are destroyed and phagocytosed. In addition, abnormal red cells (spherocytes and fixed sickle cells) are trapped and removed in the red pulp.[11, 17]

The germinal centers of the white pulp are important sites of antibody production.[50, 51] They have a particularly vital and unique role in the production of antibodies against blood-borne bacteria. Those bacteria to which the individual has little or no immunity are transported from the red pulp to the germinal centers of the white pulp, and specific immunoglobulin M (IgM) antibody is produced. With absence of the spleen or in hyposplenic states, this normal antibody response to blood-borne bacteria is diminished or absent.[17]

Two important opsonizing proteins, tuftsin and properdin, also are manufactured in the spleen. The first of these acts on neutrophils to enhance phagocytosis; the second is an important element in the alternate pathway of complement elaboration.[6, 42, 43] The importance of these factors to the defense mechanism has not been definitely determined.

Finally, in intrauterine life the spleen is a blood-forming organ, and this activity persists up to about 5 months of age, after which the bone marrow exclusively takes over the function of hematopoiesis. Rarely, this function resumes again with extramedullary hematopoiesis in children or adults.

Abnormal Splenic Function

Hypersplenism

Sequestration and phagocytosis of particulate matter in the red pulp increase to abnormal degrees when the red pulp is expanded, as in many types of splenomegaly, or when the reticuloendothelial cellular function increases. The term "hypersplenism" denotes a concept to explain a number of hematologic states benefited by splenectomy. The overactive spleen traps and destroys one or more of the formed elements in the blood. This results in a deficiency of that element in the peripheral blood and in its increased production in the bone marrow. Hypersplenism may be primary or secondary to some other disease that results in splenomegaly.

In secondary hypersplenism, splenomegaly secondary to another disease results in an expanded red pulp with increased sequestration and phagocytosis of the formed elements of the blood as a consequence of increased pooling of blood.[17] In childhood, the most common example of this phenomenon is congestive splenomegaly secondary to portal hypertension, in which neutropenia is common and pancytopenia not unusual. Other diseases that may produce secondary hypersplenism in children include thalassemia major, reticuloendotheliosis, histoplasmosis, Boeck's sarcoid, and Gaucher's disease. If the hypersplenic state can be well documented and is severe, splenectomy may be helpful, by correcting a specific cytopenia or pancytopenia, without affecting the basic underlying disease. Motulsky et al. lucidly described the "big spleen" syndrome insofar as erythrocyte destruction is concerned.[41] They pointed out the difficulties in hemolytic states of distinguishing between increased splenic destruction of red cells and conditions in which red cells coated by antibodies are more vulnerable to hemolysis.

Hyposplenism

Diminished to absent splenic function results from surgical or congenital absence of the organ, and from diseases that impair the microcirculation of the spleen (sickle cell anemia) or that infiltrate the parenchyma (sarcoidosis).[9] Hematologic abnormalities occurring promptly after splenectomy include a marked increase in the platelet count and granulocytosis. Long-term effects include red blood cell morphological abnormalities such as Howell-Jolly bodies. A number of diseases can result in functional asplenia or hyposplenism, although the spleen is intact. These include sickle cell anemia and sarcoidosis, diseases which do occur in childhood and in which the spleen is often enlarged. Chronic ulcerative colitis and celiac disease are other conditions in which hyposplenism may be seen and in which the spleen may become atrophic.[17] Radiation therapy, as in the treatment of lymphomas, may seriously impair or even destroy normal splenic function.[13]

The normal splenic functions of trapping and destroying bacteria and of antibody production are obviously impaired whether the spleen is anatomically missing or is functionally damaged or destroyed. The major clinical hazard in all such patients is impairment of defense mechanisms against infection.

Postsplenectomy Sepsis

Following splenectomy, or with marked hyposplenism, children have an increased risk of episodes of overwhelming infection. Morris and Bullock, in 1919, postulated, on the basis of experimental studies, that splenectomy increases the risk of infection.[40] King and Shumacker, in 1952, first documented this clinical relation in their report of five infants who developed episodes of severe sepsis following splenectomy for hereditary spherocytosis.[34] Two of these infants died of sepsis. Subsequent reports have amply confirmed and expanded these findings.[8, 19, 20, 28, 30, 58]

Clinically typical postsplenectomy infections are rapid in onset, fulminating in course, and fatal in about 50% of cases.[15] Most occur within two years of splenectomy, but the complication has been reported as long as 25 years later.[23] The risk is greatest in infancy, continues to be substantial throughout the preschool years, and remains a lesser but definite hazard during the remainder of childhood and adult life.

In addition to age, the disease for which splenectomy is performed is another factor affecting the risk of infection. Eraklis and Filler reviewed the courses of 467 children who had had splenectomy and divided these children into three groups according to the risk of postsplenectomy sepsis.[19] When splenectomy was done for traumatic laceration, idiopathic thrombocytopenic purpura, and other such benign diseases, no patients in the series developed sepsis. The risk was low in hereditary spherocytosis and aplastic or hypoplastic anemias. However, in serious diseases affecting the reticuloendothelial system, such as Cooley's anemia, Wiskott-Aldrich syndrome, and histiocytosis, the risk became high. Chilcote et al. reviewed the collected experience of the Children's Cancer Study Group with children who had had splenectomies as part of staging laparotomies for Hodgkin's disease.[8] Twenty episodes of sepsis in 18 children occurred among the total group of 200 children, and ten died.[8] The fulminant nature of the disease, as well as the predominance (50%) of *Pneumococcus* as the infecting organism, was documented. Not only was the postsplenectomy rate very high, but also the risk of such infection was as high in the 10–19-year-old group as in the younger children, half of the infections occurring in each group.

The excellent, comprehensive review of the subject by Singer documented an overall postsplenectomy sepsis rate of 4.25% and a mortality rate of 2.52% in a collected series of 2,796 patients.[57] The calculated rate of fatal sepsis in asplenic children was 200 times that of the population of children at large. He also found marked variability in the risk of postsplenectomy sepsis depending on the primary disease. The risk was lowest in trauma (1.45%) and highest in thalassemia (24.8%), other conditions (idiopathic thrombocytopenic purpura, hereditary spherocytosis, portal hypertension, reticuloendothelial disease) falling between these extremes. However, in every category of primary disease, the risk of subsequent sepsis following splenectomy increased many times. *Pneumococcus* was the organism responsible for approximately 50% of the postsplenectomy septic episodes. Other responsible organisms included *Meningococcus, Escherichia coli, Hemophilus influenzae, Staphylococcus,* and *Streptococcus.*[57]

In response to bacterial infections, the spleen enlarges by vascular engorgement, and phagocytosis of bacteria in the red pulp increases. Many experimental studies have shown that antibody production in response to intravenously administered antigen is impaired following splenectomy, although antibody response to antigen given by other routes is not affected. Rowley showed this by administering sheep red cells to rats, both normal and asplenic.[50] He gave the same antigen intravenously to human volunteers and demonstrated normal antibody response in controls but no response in those whose spleens had been removed.[51] Another impairment of the immune state is the consistently reduced level of immunoglobulin M (IgM) documented in a number of studies of patients following splenectomy.[29, 54, 60] Following splenectomy, these phagocytic and antibody-producing defense mechanisms are obviously lost or deficient. Although reliable data are not available for humans, approximately 25% of normal splenic tissue has been shown experimentally to be adequate for preservation of these antibacterial defense functions.[47]

Prevention or reduction of the risk of postsplenectomy sepsis obviously is a vital consideration, particularly in the young child. Three approaches have been advocated: (1) active immunization against *Pneumococcus*, (2) prophylactic penicillin therapy, and (3) prompt, aggressive therapy of infections. An effective, safe, and commercially available polysaccharide antipneumococcal vaccine affords protection against 14 of the serotypes of pneumococci and is estimated to afford protection against about 85% of all pneumococcal infections.[45] This should be used in all asplenic children. The vaccine is less antigenic for children under 2 years of age.[49] Drawbacks include lack of protection against some pneumococcal strains. Reports of fatal pneumococcal sepsis in patients who have received the vaccine document this problem.[1, 2] Obviously no protection is afforded against the other types of bacteria responsible for such sepsis. Antibody levels persist for at least $3\frac{1}{2}$ years at satisfactory levels.[61] Because of this, plus a marked increase in the number of reactions to second vaccine injections, booster doses are not currently recommended.[49, 52]

Prophylactic penicillin, either daily by the oral route or monthly by intramuscular depot, is a second reasonable approach. Essentially all pneumococcal strains, and many but not all of the other bacteria responsible for such infections, are penicillin-sensitive. Effectiveness of such a program has not thus far been demonstrated. In addition to insensitive bacteria, patient compliance is a significant problem.

Education of the parents, and later the child, following splenectomy as to the significance of infection and of the importance of early and aggressive treatment is clearly an essential part in the management of this problem. In such a program, advocated by Pearson, parents are instructed to bring the child to a hospital emergency department whenever a fever of 102 F or more develops. The child is evaluated, blood cultures drawn, and an intravenous loading dose of penicillin given. The child is observed for 3–6 hours. If deterioration occurs or other evidence of a typical postsplenectomy septic episode develops, the child is admitted to an intensive care unit. This program has some limitations because of its attempt to balance safety against false alarms, but emphasizes parental education and the necessity of alertness to any signs of infection.[45]

Perhaps the most fruitful approach is a critical re-evaluation of indications for, and timing of, splenectomy. These will be considered in the sections on diseases for which splenectomy has traditionally been recommended.

Hematologic Diseases and Splenectomy

The spleen plays a central role in two relatively common hematologic diseases of childhood, hereditary spherocytosis and idiopathic (immune) thrombocytopenic purpura.

Hereditary Spherocytosis

In this hemolytic anemia, inherited as an autosomal dominant trait, the basic defect is in the erythrocyte whose shape is spherical, apparently because of a defect in the cellular membrane. Because of their shape, the red cells are unable to pass freely through the red pulp, and sequestration and phagocytosis take place there at a more rapid rate than normal.[63]

The disease is characterized by chronic anemia, which is usually mild but with occasional "crises" of rapidly developing severe anemia. These crises, usually secondary to intercurrent infection, are caused by temporary failure of bone marrow production to keep pace with the high demand for erythrocytes.[12] Jaundice is usually mild or absent, tending to parallel the degree of anemia. The spleen is characteristically large, easily palpable, and firm. Pigment gallstone formation, which eventually occurs in most adults, is rare in the prepubertal child.

Diagnostic laboratory results include: (1) spherocytes and a high reticulocyte count on blood smear examination, (2) increased erythropoiesis on bone marrow study, (3) increased osmotic fragility of the red cells in hypotonic saline, (4) increased mechanical fragility of freshly drawn red cells, and (5) a negative Coombs test.[64]

Splenectomy invariably results in permanent relief of anemia and jaundice by removing the site of the increased erythrocyte destruction and restoring the red cell life span to normal.[55] Splenectomy does not affect the basic structural abnormality of the erythrocytes. The appropriate age for operation should be individualized. In neonates with severe hemolysis and high indirect bilirubin levels, exchange transfusions are the treatment of choice. Children up to school age usually can be managed by transfusions during crises. Generally speaking, splenectomy can and should be avoided before the age of 5 or 6 years, and in some children who are in good health and without severe anemia the operation can be further postponed.[45]

Idiopathic (Immune) Thrombocytopenic Purpura (ITP)

This disease is characterized by bleeding into the skin, a low platelet count, a spleen of normal size, and bone marrow with megakaryocytes in normal or increased numbers. Usually the disease manifests abruptly with purpura. Epistaxis is less frequent, and renal and gastrointestinal bleeding occur in less than 10% of cases.[59] By far the most dangerous complication is intracranial bleeding, which develops in 1–2% of these children. The majority of affected children have had a viral infection of some sort preceding the purpuric state by one to six weeks.

The platelet count is below 40,000/mm³ in about three fourths of the children and less than 20,000/mm³ in those with more severe manifestations.[62] Bleeding time, clot retraction, and capillary fragility are abnormal in proportion to the thrombocytopenia. Platelet survival time is markedly reduced from a normal of 8–10 days to a few hours or even minutes. Normal or increased numbers of megakaryocytes in the bone marrow is an important finding that excludes diseases with secondary thrombocytopenia, due to decreased megakaryocytes, in conditions such as leukemia.

The exact pathogenesis of the disease is still uncertain, but clearly there is an important immunologic factor. Harrington and his colleagues first demonstrated a thrombocytopenic factor in the blood of affected patients, and this observation has been confirmed.[24, 25, 53] This antiplatelet factor appears to be an immunoglobulin.[3] The exact mechanism of platelet destruction is not known. The antigen may well be virus related, and a number of hypotheses have been advanced in an effort to explain the relation in this disease between platelets, virus, and antibodies.[62] The spleen is the major site of destruction of the sensitized platelets.[53] Furthermore, the spleen probably is important as an organ of production of the antiplatelet antibody.[32, 36]

The disease is self-limiting and relatively brief in at least 70%

of patients, complete clinical and laboratory recovery occurring within 3–6 months.[35, 59, 62] In the remaining 20–30%, the disease persists for longer than 6 months and occasionally for several years with platelet counts below 100,000/mm³. Exacerbations of purpura with low platelet counts (below 25,000/mm³) are seen in children with the chronic form in association with intercurrent viral diseases.

The mortality of ITP of less than 1% is caused almost entirely by intracranial, rarely from gastrointestinal, bleeding. Intracranial bleeding typically occurs within the first 2 or 3 weeks of the disease, and the risk of this complication is much less later in the acute as well as in the chronic form.[35]

In the child with acute ITP with only mild purpura and ecchymoses, no treatment other than restriction of activity is necessary. In the presence of severe bruising, spontaneous bleeding from mucosal surfaces, and hematuria, steroid therapy is usually recommended during the first 2–4 weeks. This treatment probably does not influence the ultimate course of the disease but often produces a more rapid rise in the platelet count to reasonably safe levels than would occur spontaneously. Steroids also reduce the bleeding tendency by improving capillary integrity.[59] Steroid therapy may also be wise in the active preschool child. If evidence of intracranial bleeding develops, the child should be managed on an emergency basis with platelet transfusions and splenectomy. Such therapy is also appropriate in the rare instance of severe gastrointestinal bleeding.[35] Splenectomy under these circumstances is effective in restoring a normal platelet count and preventing further bleeding. The immediate risk of the procedure is very low.

In the child with chronic thrombocytopenia, a low risk of serious bleeding remains, and the necessity for restricted physical activity is a burden to both child and parents. If the platelet count remains in the 20,000–40,000/mm³ range, splenectomy is indicated at about 6 months after diagnosis.[59] If the platelet count is above 50,000/mm³, the decision in regard to splenectomy can be deferred for a year or longer.[45] The results of splenectomy in the chronic form of this disease are generally excellent, with reported cure rates between 65% and 90%.[10, 59, 62]

Hypersplenism

A number of conditions, noted previously, result in splenomegaly and secondary hypersplenism. In childhood, portal hypertension with congestive splenomegaly is the most common. Splenectomy may be a part of a shunting or devascularization procedure in the management of esophageal varices but rarely, if ever, is indicated solely because of hypersplenism. Thalassemia major is the next most common condition in this group, and severe hypersplenism is very common in this disease. The indication for splenectomy primarily concerns the effect of the spleen on blood requirements and hence the progressive iron loading.[38] The procedure is effective in markedly reducing blood requirements when these become excessive, and furthermore corrects the associated and often severe thrombocytopenia. Other conditions in which secondary hypersplenism may develop include histiocytosis, acquired hemolytic anemia, and lymphomas.

In all instances of these uncommon conditions in which splenectomy is a consideration, the hematologic evaluation is of primary concern. A careful assessment to balance the benefits to be gained against the risks of the operation itself and the subsequent asplenic state obviously is essential.

Hodgkin's Disease

Most treatment protocols for Hodgkin's disease are based on the stage of the disease. It is therefore essential to stage the extent of the disease as accurately as possible in order to select the most appropriate radiotherapy, chemotherapy, or combination of both. Thus far, clinical, laboratory, and imaging studies have not permitted precise staging; and a staging laparotomy with multiple node biopsies, liver biopsies, and splenectomy remains essential for the most accurate staging.[21, 26, 27, 31] The procedure primarily is for the purpose of determining the presence or absence of intra-abdominal disease, although subgroups that may influence therapy also are determined.

The question of splenic involvement is important and is best based on microscopic examination. Intra-abdominal disease is found in 30–40% of patients with clinical stage I to stage III disease. The problem with total splenectomy has been the high resultant incidence of postsplenectomy sepsis, and clearly these children have depressed immune defense mechanisms on the basis both of their disease and of its treatment.[8, 48] Active immunization with polyvalent pneumococcal vaccine has apparently decreased this risk substantially. An alternative to total splenectomy in the presence of a grossly uninvolved spleen is partial splenectomy, removing about one third and leaving sufficient spleen to minimize functional loss and hence, in all likelihood, prevent subsequent sepsis.[5] The loss in diagnostic accuracy by a procedure short of total splenectomy is uncertain, but this accuracy probably remains greater than 95%.[5, 14, 45]

If the spleen is grossly involved with nodules, total removal for diagnosis alone is clearly unnecessary; and splenectomy is not therapeutic. However, removal does decrease the area receiving radiation therapy under these circumstances—a significant advantage, since the left kidney and lower left lung can then be avoided. Furthermore, radiation therapy to the spleen may depress its function to a degree comparable to that of splenectomy.[13] Whether or not a reasonable degree of splenic function returns following radiotherapy remains undetermined.

Trauma

Until the last decade, laceration of the spleen probably constituted the single most common indication for splenectomy in childhood. Widespread acceptance of the important role of the spleen in prevention of infection plus the realization that hemorrhage from splenic injury is usually self-limited and that the spleen heals remarkably well have altered this situation. Splenic injuries caused by blunt trauma are now managed in many pediatric surgical centers by a spleen-conserving approach.

The cause of the injury is blunt trauma in more than 95% of cases, and injuries secondary to automobile accidents are the most frequent. Bicycle accidents and falls are also relatively common. Penetrating wounds were responsible in only 3% of splenic injuries in our series.[33] Half or more of all the children had associated injuries, of which central nervous system injuries were both the most common and the most serious, occurring in 31%

in our experience.[33, 44, 56] This is a particularly dangerous situation, since the child's obtunded state masks the clinical picture of the splenic injury. Renal, musculoskeletal, and chest injuries were less common; and other abdominal injuries were noted in only 10% of the children.

The diagnosis is made on clinical grounds, supplemented by nuclear scans. Abdominal pain occurs in nearly all responsive patients but may be generalized rather than confined to the left upper quadrant. Abdominal tenderness and muscle guarding in the left upper quadrant are the most helpful physical findings. Evidence of significant hypovolemia with hypotension, tachycardia, and pallor is evident at initial evaluation in about half the cases. One fifth of the patients in our experience were initially unresponsive because of head injuries. A number of imaging diagnostic tests, including computerized tomography and angiography, may be used to establish the diagnosis. However, the radionuclide liver-spleen scan using technetium 99m is both highly accurate and convenient and has become the standard confirmatory study on our service (Fig 116–1).

Management of these children has evolved over the past decade from routine splenectomy to a policy of splenic preservation whenever possible. Laparotomy and splenic repair are feasible, safe, and effective.[37, 39] These procedures can be done safely after 12–24 hours of resuscitation and observation rather than as true emergency procedures. Patients handled in this fashion rarely show evidence of continued bleeding after initial correction of hypovolemia, and at operation a high proportion are found to have single splenic lacerations that are no longer bleeding. Such experiences have led to a policy of nonoperative management for most patients in many pediatric surgical services.[16, 18, 33] Laparotomy is performed when there is evidence of continued significant bleeding, when possible peritonitis from associated gastrointestinal injuries is suspected, and when the nuclear scan shows loss of vascularization of a major portion of the spleen, or severe fragmentation.

Children managed in this fashion clearly must be observed frequently and monitored closely in an intensive care unit. Intravenous fluids, including blood if necessary, are given to correct hypovolemia and to maintain normal cardiovascular stability. The liver-spleen radionuclide scan is performed on the unit as resuscitation progresses, using a portable gamma camera. Moving the patient to a radiology department is thereby avoided. If facilities for such close monitoring are not available, the patient should either be transferred to an institution with such facilities, or laparotomy and splenic repair performed.

Results of treatment based on a philosophy of splenic conservation have been excellent. In a recent 4-year experience with 49 patients with splenic injuries, splenectomy was required in only six, two of whom had penetrating wounds.[33] Splenic repair

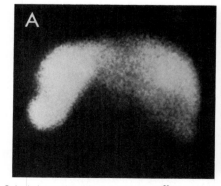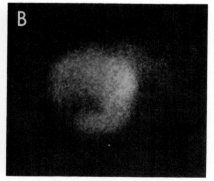

Fig 116–1.—Splenic laceration. Liver-spleen scan (^{99m}Tc-sulfur colloid). **A,** posterior view shows defect in lateral aspect of spleen. **B,** left lateral view shows defect in spleen corresponding to laceration.

was performed in 15, and the remaining 28 were managed by observation alone. The complication rate was low (10%), and there were no deaths. Deaths that do occur in children with splenic trauma are usually caused by associated head injuries.

Although the risk of sepsis is low following removal of an injured spleen, some risk remains and it is long-lasting.[4, 22, 44, 57] Perhaps one reason for the low rate of subsequent sepsis is the demonstration by Pearson et al., of return of splenic function together with demonstrable splenic nodules on nuclear scanning.[46] The exact incidence of such residual splenic nodules and their function in prevention of subsequent infection are unanswered questions. The results with techniques of splenic preservation are excellent in terms of mortality and early morbidity, so that adoption of such a philosophy of management appears clearly justified.

Operative Techniques

The preoperative care of a child scheduled for splenectomy depends largely on the diagnosis and, to a lesser extent, on the urgency of the procedure. Two measures are applicable in all instances. First, the tragedy of vomiting and aspiration can be eliminated by passing a nasogastric tube, emptying the stomach, and connecting the tube to an appropriate source of suction. Such a measure adds to the technical ease of the procedure by keeping the stomach decompressed. Second, an intravenous cannula of adequate size ensures prompt replacement of lost blood.

Elective splenectomy is performed with the patient supine, the left side elevated 20–30 degrees. A transverse incision in the left upper quadrant just above the level of the umbilicus is used. The technique is illustrated in Figure 116–2. A careful search for accessory spleens should be made before closure, particularly when the indication is a hematologic disease.

For splenic operations either for trauma or as a part of a staging laparotomy for Hodgkin's disease, the patient is best placed supine and the laparotomy performed through a vertical upper midline abdominal incision. In a staging laparotomy, the incision may be extended below the umbilicus to facilitate removal of iliac lymph nodes.

In a laparotomy for splenic trauma, the spleen should be mo-

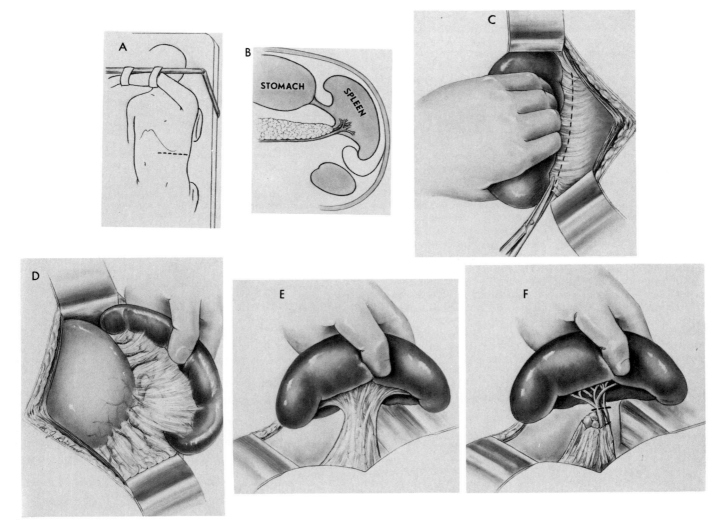

Fig 116–2.—Elective splenectomy. **A,** patient supine with elevated left side and moderate reverse Trendelenburg position. **B,** cross-sectional view illustrates attachments of spleen and relationships to stomach, pancreas, and left kidney. Note the posterior peritoneal reflection. **C,** spleen held downward and medially, exposing the posterior peritoneal reflection, which is divided posteriorly and superiorly. **D,** spleen lifted out of incision and held laterally, demonstrating the short gastric vessels between spleen and stomach. These are individually divided and ligated. **E,** spleen attached only by hilus. Posterior aspect of hilus is exposed by reflecting spleen and tail of pancreas medially. **F,** posterior dissection of hilus completed, showing the splenic vessels skeletonized and the close relation of the tail of the pancreas.

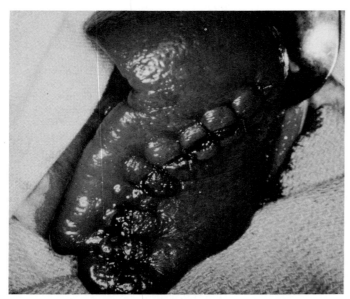

Fig 116–3.—Operative photograph showing long laceration of spleen without devascularization. Repair by simple interrupted sutures.

bilized by division of the lateral peritoneal reflection, as with an elective procedure, and delivered into the surgical wound. In most instances splenic lacerations are simply repaired with interrupted sutures (2-0 polyglycolic acid sutures work well) (Fig 116–3). Any devascularized segment is removed. Only very rarely, as when the spleen is completely avulsed from its blood supply or when fragmentation is extreme, is total splenectomy necessary.

In a laparotomy for the staging of Hodgkin's disease, the spleen again is mobilized as previously described. The spleen is measured and the presence of gross tumor nodules noted. For total splenectomy, the technique shown in Figure 116–2 is followed. For partial splenectomy, the artery extending down from the hilus and supplying the lower splenic segment is ligated in continuity. The lower third of the spleen is then resected, using a fish-mouth incision. The edges of this incision are then approximated with interrupted 2-0 absorbable sutures. Bleeding during the procedure is not troublesome with this technique, nor has postoperative bleeding been a complication.[5] The remaining splenic remnant is then returned to its normal bed and omentum draped over the suture line.

REFERENCES

1. Ahonkhai V.I., Landesman S.H., Fikrig S.M., et al.: Failure of pneumococcal vaccine in children with sickle-cell disease. *N. Engl. J. Med.* 301:26–27, 1979.
2. Appelbaum P.C., Shaikh B.S., Widome M.D., et al.: Fatal pneumococcal bacteremia in a vaccinated, splenectomized child. *N. Engl. J. Med.* 300:203–204, 1979.
3. Baldini M.G.: Idiopathic thrombocytopenic purpura and the ITP syndrome. *Med. Clin. North Am.* 56:47–64, 1972.
4. Balfanz J.R., Nesbit, M.E. Jr., Jarvis C., et al.: Overwhelming sepsis following splenectomy for trauma. *J. Pediatr.* 88:458–460, 1976.
5. Boles E.T. Jr., Haase G.M., Hamoudi A.B.: Partial splenectomy in staging laparotomy for Hodgkin's disease: An alternative approach. *J. Pediatr. Surg.* 13:581–586, 1978.
6. Carlisle H.N., Saslaw S.: Comparison of properdin levels in medical and hematologic patients. *Am. J. Med. Sci.* 242:271–278, 1961.
7. Chen L.: Microcirculation of the spleen: An open or closed circulation? *Science* 201:157–159, 1978.
8. Chilcote R.R., Baehner R.L., Hammond D., et al.: Septicemia and meningitis in children splenectomized for Hodgkin's disease. *N. Engl. J. Med.* 295:798–800, 1976.
9. Crosby W.H.: Hyposplenism: An inquiry into normal functions of the spleen. *Annu. Rev. Med.* 14:349–370, 1963.
10. Crosby W.H.: Splenectomy in hematologic disorders. *N. Engl. J. Med.* 286:1252–1254, 1972.
11. Crosby W.H.: Splenic remodeling of red cell surfaces. *Blood* 50:643–645, 1977.
12. Dacie J.V.: *The Haemolytic Anemias*, ed. 2. New York, Grune & Stratton, 1960.
13. Dailey M.O., Coleman C.N., Kaplan H.S.: Radiation-induced splenic atrophy in patients with Hodgkin's disease and non-Hodgkin's lymphomas. *N. Engl. J. Med.* 302:215–217, 1980.
14. Dearth J.C., Gilchrist G.S., Telander R.L., et al.: Partial splenectomy for staging Hodgkin's disease: Risk of false-negative results. *N. Engl. J. Med.* 299:345–346, 1978.
15. Diamond L.K.: Splenectomy in childhood and the hazard of overwhelming infection. *Pediatrics* 43:886–889, 1969.
16. Douglas G.J., Simpson J.S.: The conservative management of splenic trauma. *J. Pediatr. Surg.* 6:565–570, 1971.
17. Eichner E.R.: Splenic function: Normal, too much and too little. *Am. J. Med.* 66:311–320, 1979.
18. Ein S.H., Shandling B., Simpson J.S., et al.: Nonoperative management of traumatized spleen in children: How and why. *J. Pediatr. Surg.* 13:117–119, 1978.
19. Eraklis A.J., Filler R.M.: Splenectomy in childhood: A review of 1413 cases. *J. Pediatr. Surg.* 7:382–388, 1972.
20. Eraklis A.J., Kevy S.V., Diamond L.K., et al.: Hazard of overwhelming infection after splenectomy in childhood. *N. Engl. J. Med.* 276:1225–1229, 1967.
21. Filler R.M., Jaffe N., Cassady J.R., et al.: Experience with clinical and operative staging of Hodgkin's disease in children. *J. Pediatr. Surg.* 10:321–328, 1975.
22. Gopal V., Bisno A.L.: Fulminant pneumococcal infections in "normal" asplenic hosts. *Arch. Intern. Med.* 137:1526–1530, 1977.
23. Grinblat J., Gilboa Y.: Overwhelming pneumococcal sepsis 25 years after splenectomy. *Am. J. Med. Sci.* 270:523–524, 1975.
24. Harrington W.J., Minnich V., Hollingsworth J., et al.: Demonstration of thrombocytopenic factor in blood of patients with thrombocytopenic purpura. *J. Lab. Clin. Med.* 38:1–10, 1951.
25. Harrington W.J., Sprague C.C., Minnich V., et al.: Immunologic mechanisms in idiopathic and neonatal thrombocytopenic purpura. *Ann. Intern. Med.* 38:433, 1963.
26. Hays D.M., Hittle R.E., Isaacs H. Jr., et al.: Laparotomy for the staging of Hodgkin's disease in children. *J. Pediatr. Surg.* 7:517–527, 1972.
27. Hellman S.: Current studies in Hodgkin's disease: What laparotomy has wrought. *N. Engl. J. Med.* 290:894–898, 1974.
28. Horan M., Colebatch J.H.: Relation between splenectomy and subsequent infection: A clinical study. *Arch. Dis. Child.* 37:398–411, 1962.
29. Hosea S.W., Burch C.G., Brown E.J., et al.: Impaired immune response of splenectomized patients to polyvalent pneumococcal vaccine. *Lancet* 1:804–807, 1981.
30. Huntley C.C.: Infection following splenectomy in infants and children. *Am. J. Dis. Child.* 95:477–480, 1958.
31. Kaplan H.S., Dorfman R.F., Nelsen T.S., et al.: Staging laparotomy for Hodgkin's disease: Analysis of indications and patterns of involvement in 285 consecutive, unselected patients. *Natl. Cancer Inst. Monogr.* 36:291–301, 1973.
32. Karpatkin S., Strick N., Siskind G.W.: Detection of splenic antiplatelet antibody synthesis in idiopathic autoimmune thrombocytopenic purpura (ATP). *Br. J. Haematol.* 23:167–176, 1972.
33. King, D.R., Lobe T.E., Haase G.M., et al.: Selective management of the injured spleen. *Surgery* 90:677–682, 1981.
34. King H., Shumacker H.B. Jr.: Splenic studies. I. Susceptibility to infection after splenectomy performed in infancy. *Ann. Surg.* 136:239–242, 1952.
35. McClure P.D.: Idiopathic thrombocytopenia purpura in children: Diagnosis and management. *Pediatrics* 55:69–74, 1975.
36. McMillan R., Longmire R.L., Yelenosky R., et al.: Quantitation of platelet binding IgG produced in vitro by spleens from patients with idiopathic thrombocytopenic purpura. *N. Engl. J. Med.* 291:812, 1974.
37. Mishalany H.: Repair of the ruptured spleen. *J. Pediatr. Surg.* 9:175–178, 1974.
38. Modell B.: Total management of thalassemia major. *Arch. Dis. Child.* 52:489–500, 1977.
39. Morgenstern L., Shapiro S.J.: Techniques of splenic conservation. *Arch. Surg.* 114:449–454, 1979.
40. Morris D.H., Bullock F.D.: The importance of the spleen in resistance to infection. *Ann. Surg.* 70:513–521, 1919.
41. Motulsky A.G., Casserd F., Giblett E.R., et al.: Anemia and the spleen. *N. Engl. J. Med.* 259:1164–1169, 1215–1219, 1958.
42. Najjar V.A., Nishioka K.: "Tuftsin": A natural phagocytosis stimulating peptide. *Nature* 228:672–673, 1970.

43. Najjar V.A., Schmidt J.J.: The chemistry and biology of tuftsin. *Lymphokine Reports* 1:157–179, 1980.
44. Oakes D.D.: Splenic trauma. *Curr. Probl. Surg.* 18:342–401, 1981.
45. Pearson H.A.: Splenectomy: Its risks and its roles. *Hosp. Prac.* August 1980, pp. 85–94.
46. Pearson H.A., Johnston M.T., Smith K.A., et al.: The born-again spleen. *N. Engl. J. Med.* 298:1389–1392, 1978.
47. Perla D., Marmorston J.: *The Spleen Resistance.* Baltimore, Williams & Wilkins Co., 1935.
48. Ravry M., Maldonado N., Velez-Garcia E., et al.: Serious infection after splenectomy for the staging of Hodgkin's disease. *Ann. Intern. Med.* 77:11–14, 1972.
49. Recommendation of the Immunization Practices Advisory Committee. Center for Disease Control, Department of Health and Human Services; Atlanta, Georgia: Pneumococcal polysaccharide vaccine. *Ann. Intern. Med.* 96:203–205, 1982.
50. Rowley D.A.: The effect of splenectomy on the formation of circulating antibody in the adult male albino rat. *J. Immunol.* 64:289–295, 1950.
51. Rowley D.A.: The formation of circulating antibody in the splenectomized human being following intravenous injection of heterologous erythrocytes. *J. Immunol.* 65:515–521, 1950.
52. Rytel M.W.: Pneumococcal infections and pneumococcal vaccine: An update. *Infect. Control* 3:295–298, 1982.
53. Schulman N.R., Weinrach R.S., Libre E.P., et al.: The role of the reticuloendothelial system in pathogenesis of idiopathic thrombocytopenic purpura. *Trans. Assoc. Am. Phys.* 78:374, 1965.
54. Schumaker M.J.: Serum immunoglobulin and transferrin levels after childhood splenectomy. *Arch. Dis. Child.* 45:114, 1970.
55. Schwartz S.I., Adams J.T., Bauman A.W.: Splenectomy for hematologic disorders. *Curr. Probl. Surg.* May 1971.
56. Sherman R.: Management of trauma to the spleen, in Shires G.T. (ed.): *Advances in Surgery.* Chicago, Year Book Medical Publishers, 1984, pp. 37–71.
57. Singer D.B.: Postsplenectomy sepsis. *Perspect. Pediatr. Pathol.* 1:285–311, 1965.
58. Smith C.H., Erlandson M., Schulman I., et al.: Hazard of severe infections in splenectomized infants and children. *Am. J. Med.* 22:390–404, 1957.
59. Stuart M.J., McKenna R.: Diseases of coagulation: The platelet and vasculature, in Nathan D.G., Oski F.K. (eds.): *Hematology of Infancy and Childhood.* Philadelphia, W.B. Saunders Co., 1981.
60. Sullivan J.L., Ochs H.D., Schiffman G., et al.: Immune response after splenectomy. *Lancet* 1:178–181, 1978.
61. Vella P.P., McLean A.A., Woodhour A.F., et al.: Persistence of pneumococcal antibodies in human subjects following vaccination. *Proc. Soc. Exp. Biol. Med.* 164:435–438, 1980.
62. Willoughby M.L.N.: Thrombocytopenia, in *Paediatric Haematology.* New York, Churchill Livingstone, 1977.
63. Young L.E., Izzo M.J., Platzer R.F.: Hereditary spherocytosis I. Clinical, hematologic, and genetic features in 28 cases. *Blood* 6:1073–1098, 1951.
64. Young L.E., Izzo M.J., Platzer R.F.: Hereditary spherocytosis. II. Observations on the role of the spleen. *Blood* 6:1099–1113, 1951.

117 Eric W. Fonkalsrud

The Adrenal Glands

Anatomy

THE ADRENAL GLANDS are situated posteriorly along the anteromedial border of the superior poles of the kidneys, embedded in the perirenal adipose tissue. The right adrenal is partially covered by the vena cava and the liver, and lies on the lower extensions of the diaphragm. The left adrenal is covered by the peritoneum of the lesser omental bursa, the splenic vessels, and the tail of the pancreas. The glands are located in the upper extension of a compartment enclosed by Gerota's fascia and are held in position by numerous fibrous bands and vascular attachments. They are darker yellow and firmer than the perirenal fat in which they lie. Average weight is 3–5 gm, varying with age. Although close to the kidneys, the adrenals are supported independently and remain in a relatively fixed position when the kidney is depressed.

The abundant arterial supply to the glands may be variable, although its source is generally the phrenic artery superiorly, the aorta medially, and the renal artery inferiorly (Fig 117–1). Branches from the ovarian or internal spermatic artery on the left, and from the intercostal arteries bilaterally, are occasionally present. On entering the gland, the arterioles enter sinusoids devoid of endothelial lining, which extend as small twigs into the medulla. A subcapsular arterial plexus sends small capillary loops to the cortex. Venous blood drains into large lacunae in the medulla, from which it is collected by a central vein that empties into the renal vein on the left and directly into the vena cava on the right. Accessory adrenal veins may communicate with the azygos and portal venous systems. Arteriography of the adrenal

glands has defined many variations from the classic blood supply. Despite the ample vascularity of the adrenal, the blood flow to the normal adult gland measures only about 10 ml/minute.

The adrenal lymphatics form two plexuses, one directly beneath the capsule and the other within the medulla. On the right, the adrenal lymphatics extend into the periaortic lymph nodes near the crus of the diaphragm. The left adrenal lymphatics drain to nodes near the origin of the left renal artery.

The adrenal nerve supply, derived from the celiac and renal splanchnic plexuses, enters the lower midportion of the capsule to traverse the cortex and terminate in the medulla, where there are many small ganglia. Stimulation of the adrenal nerves produces a prompt release of medullary hormones without influencing cortical activity.[16] Few, if any, nerve fibers are present in the adrenal cortex.

The adrenal cortex is divided into three sections: (1) the zona glomerulosa or outer zone, (2) the zona fasciculata, a wide intermediate zone, and (3) the zona reticularis, a narrow inner zone adjacent to the medulla. The zona glomerulosa is the site of aldosterone production, while the zona fasciculata and zona reticularis produce other glucocorticoids. It is likely that androgen precursors, as well as small amounts of testosterone and estrogens, are produced by cells within the zona fasciculata and zona reticularis.

Embryology

The development of the adrenal gland represents the union of ectodermal chromaffin cells from the neural crest, which form

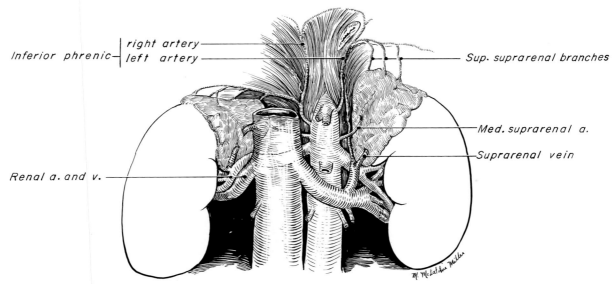

Inferior phrenic ⎰ right artery ——————— Sup. suprarenal branches
⎱ left artery ———————

Med. suprarenal a.

Suprarenal vein

Renal a. and v. ——————

Fig 117–1.—Anatomical relation of the adrenal glands, showing major vascular supply.

the adrenal medulla, and cells from the splanchnic mesoderm, which form the cortex. The sympathetic ganglion cells separate from the adrenal precursor cells very early and migrate ventrally where they form the aortic paraganglia. The cortical cells develop by proliferation of the coelomic mesothelium on either side of the root of the foregut mesentery medial to the upper ends of the wolffian bodies. These cells, arising in numerous places in the suprarenal ridge, lose their connection with the mesothelium and constitute a complete layer of mesoderm around the pheochromocytes of the medulla. The pheochromocytes become the mature chromaffin gland cells that produce the neurohormones, epinephrine and norepinephrine.

The fetal adrenal at 3 months is larger than the kidney. The inner fetal zone, also known as the provisional cortex and the androgenic zone, is the major portion of each developing gland. It involutes after birth and undergoes changes similar to those occurring in the uterus and the breast.

During the course of development, medullary or cortical tissue may remain in various locations to form accessory collections of cells. The most common sites for accessory adrenal tissue are shown in Figure 117–2. In fetal life, extra-adrenal paraganglionic chromaffin masses are numerous and bulky and usually lie along the aorta and its branches. Large chromaffin masses near the origin of the inferior mesenteric artery are known as the organs of Zuckerkandl. They may be paired or fused masses, and produce norepinephrine only. Following birth, the chromaffin cells within the medulla differentiate, while the extra-adrenal chromaffin bodies usually involute.

Adrenocortical rests are common in children and are most often found as bright yellow nodules within the kidney or the liver, along the route of descent of the gonads, in hernial sacs, or within the gonads themselves. Adrenocortical rests are believed to be present in 50% of newborn infants and to atrophy and disappear within a few weeks. Their persistence in patients with adrenogenital syndrome is due to continued ACTH stimulation. In the male with adrenogenital syndrome, there is often a well-developed adrenal rest within the testis; this may be mistaken for a normal-sized gonad, since the testis is likely to be atrophic and the adrenal cortical tissue hyperplastic. The anomalous locations of the adrenal cortical rests are important, since hyperplasia in the accessory tissue may produce tumorous swellings in the presence of sustained ACTH secretion, as in congenital adrenal hyperplasia. Adrenal insufficiency occasionally develops when misplaced normal adrenal glands are inadvertently removed, as during nephrectomy.

Physiology

Although more than 50 different steroids have been isolated from the adrenal cortex, most are precursors, and only a few are actually secreted into the circulation.[19] The general structure of the steroids secreted by the adrenal cortex is shown in Figure 117–3. The corticosteroids are C-21 compounds and include both the glucocorticoids and mineralocorticoids. The androgens are C-19 steroids, and the estrogens are C-18 steroids. The entire cortex normally contains all enzyme systems necessary for the conversion of cholesterol to cortisol. The zona glomerulosa contains 18-hydroxylase and dehydrogenase, which are responsible for conversion of corticosterone to aldosterone. The secretion rates of the adrenal steroids have been determined in man. The two most important corticosteroids are cortisol, the major glucocorticoid, and aldosterone, the major mineralocorticoid.[17]

Under normal conditions, the hypothalamus secretes corticotropin-releasing factor (CRF), which serves to release ACTH from the anterior pituitary. As the blood levels of cortisol rise, a feedback regulatory mechanism inhibits further release of CRF from the hypothalamus except in periods of stress. Androgens are also dependent on ACTH secretion for their release; however, they are not capable of inhibiting ACTH secretion in a regulatory manner. There is a normal diurnal variation in the secretion rate of CRF, and consequently of ACTH and cortisol. This regulatory mechanism may be altered by metyrapone (Metopirone), which interferes with 11-beta-hydroxylation in the cortex. Cortisol synthesis then decreases, and there is thus no feedback to limit continued pituitary secretion of ACTH. The metyrapone test is used to determine whether the pituitary is capable of secreting increased amounts of ACTH. Cortisol and androgens are metabolized in the liver and excreted in the urine.

Secretion of aldosterone depends primarily on stimulation by renin and angiotensin. When renal artery pressure decreases, the renal juxtaglomerular cells release renin. Renin acts on angiotensinogen from the liver to form angiotensin I, which in turn

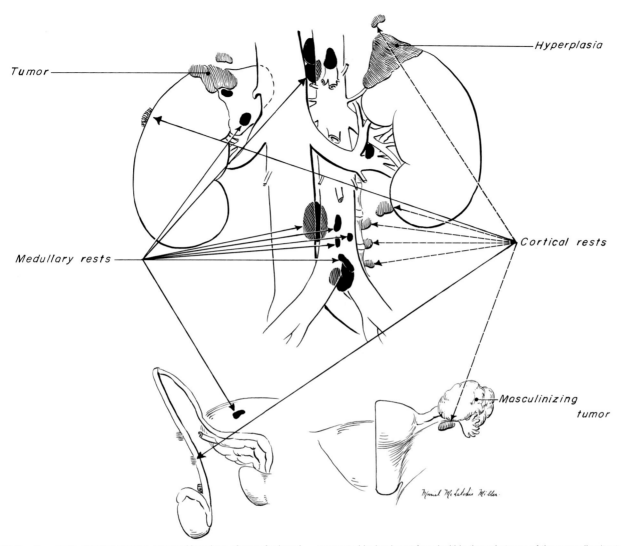

Fig 117–2.—Composite drawing showing reported locations of rest of adrenal cortical and medullary tissues. These sites have surgical significance when the suspected lesion is not found within the substance of the normally situated adrenal glands.

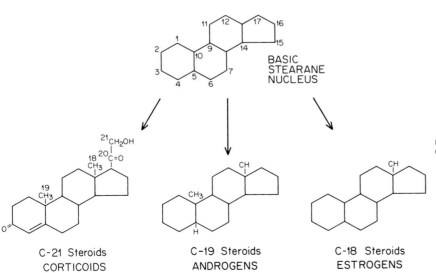

Fig 117–3.—Structure of adrenal steroids showing modification of basic stearane nucleus to form the C-21, C-19, and C-18 steroids.

is converted by a circulating enzyme into angiotensin II. Angiotensin II stimulates the adrenal cortex to release aldosterone, which in turn is regulated by aldosterone-induced renal retention of sodium that increases the blood volume and reduces the production of renin. Secondary aldosteronism may result from renal artery obstruction that causes hypersecretion of renin by the juxtaglomerular cells, and consequently excess aldosterone with sodium retention, and hypertension.

There is considerable overlap in terms of sodium and potassium metabolism between the glucocorticoids and mineralocorticoids. Cortisol enhances gluconeogenesis which, when excessive, produces protein depletion and diabetes. Cortisol also induces a centripetal distribution of fat, hyperlipemia, enhances water diuresis, and assists in maintaining the homeostasis of extracellular fluid volume by preventing the shift of water into the cell. Cortisol also sensitizes arterioles to the pressor effects of norepinephrine and related compounds. Glucocorticoids reduce the inflammatory process and the cellular response to injury and inhibit hypersensitivity responses to antigen-antibody complexes.

In contrast to cortical steroid secretion, there is no known direct hormonal control over medullary secretion. Epinephrine, norepinephrine, and dopamine are secreted by at least two types of chromaffin cells in the medulla. These catecholamines are synthesized from tyrosine. The extra-adrenal chromaffin tissues (including sympathetic ganglia and nerve endings) chiefly produce norepinephrine and dopamine. Although there is considerable pharmacologic overlap between the catecholamines, epinephrine has greater excitatory, hyperglycemic, and metabolic effects than does norepinephrine. The catecholamines are normally metabolized rapidly, and about 40% is excreted in the urine as conjugated 3-methoxy,4-hydroxymandelic acid (vanillylmandelic acid [VMA]). The principal pathway for the production of epinephrine from phenylalanine and tyrosine is shown in Figure 117–4. When epinephrine and norepinephrine are injected intravenously, only small amounts appear in the urine, most of the urinary excretion consisting of the metabolites metanephrine, normetanephrine, and vanillylmandelic acid.

Pheochromocytoma

Although Frankel,[18] in 1886, reported the first case of a hypertensive syndrome with retinitis and bilateral adrenal tumors in an 18-year-old girl, it was not until 1922 that a clear relation between paroxysmal hypertension and adrenal medullary tumors was established by Labbe and associates.[25] In 1912, Pick[35] named the tumor for its predominant cell, the pheochromocyte.

Pheochromocytomas produce symptoms by secreting large amounts of epinephrine and norepinephrine in widely varying proportions. The proportion of norepinephrine is greater in childhood than in adult cases.[8] The overall incidence of pheochromocytoma is estimated to be 1 in 6,000 hypertensive patients,[24] and responsible for approximately 1% of the cases of childhood hypertension, typically occurring between the ages of 8 and 9 years.[4] Stackpole and associates, in 1963,[40] reported 100 cases of pheochromocytoma in children under the age of 14 years. The right adrenal is involved about twice as often as the left. Whereas 7% of pheochromocytomas are bilateral in adults, Hume[21] observed that 24% are bilateral in children. Others have seen an incidence of bilateral pheochromocytomas as high as 70% in children followed over the course of many years.[4] Extra-adrenal pheochromocytomas are present in approximately 30% of the cases in children, about twice as common as in adults. They are chiefly found in the paraganglia, the organs of Zuckerkandl, and the bladder. Extra-abdominal tumors may develop in the brain, thorax, or neck. Unlike adults, in whom there is a female pre-

dominance, in preadolescent children pheochromocytoma is usually encountered in males. After the onset of puberty, the tumor tends to occur in females, suggesting a possible hormonal influence associated with growth and menarche.[40]

Malignancy develops in fewer than 6% of children with pheochromocytoma, less than half the incidence in adults. In patients who experience a recurrence, symptoms are usually noted within a year of resection.

In 1947, a familial relation in pheochromocytoma was described, and now its association with various endocrine conditions is commonly recognized.[3] (Indeed, 10% of childhood tumors are familial, four times the frequency in adults.) This familial occurrence has been noted in a variety of syndromes that are attributed to genetic derangements of neural crest derivatives. The common cell of origin of a number of endocrine tumors was regarded by Pearse as a part of the neuroendocrine group. On the basis of the function of the cells, he termed these APUD tumors (for *a*mine *p*recursor *u*ptake and *d*ecarboxylation).[39] These cells are believed to be totipotential, migratory, and capable of secreting a variety of polypeptide hormones.[42]

Sipple syndrome, multiple endocrine adenomatosis II (MEA II) or multiple endocrine neoplasia (MEN II), is a genetic disorder involving multifocal tumor formation in the system of polypeptide-secreting cells. Its expressions can include pheochromocytoma, medullary carcinoma of the thyroid, parathyroid hyperplasia or tumors, and multiple mucosal neuromas.[42] The neuroma associated with Sipple syndrome develops primarily in the lip and is a true neuroma, rather than the nerve sheath tumor that characterizes von Recklinghausen's disease. Patients whose disease complex is characterized by medullary carcinoma of the thyroid; pheochromocytoma; multiple mucosal neuroma of lips, tongue, and upper eyelids; and pathognomonic facies are subclassified as MEA IIb.[45] The only true clinical overlap with von Recklinghausen's neurofibromatosis is the association of pheochromocytoma, usually bilateral.

Adrenal medullary hyperplasia has been documented as a probable precursor of pheochromocytoma in the MEA II syndrome.[7] Serum calcitonin determinations have been utilized for screening potential MEA II patients for the medullar thyroid cancers. In occult cases, the pentagastrin stimulation test of calcitonin secretion may prove more reliable.[12] The association of pheochromocytoma with parathyroid hyperplasia or adenomas in the MEA II syndrome may be secondary or compensatory in nature, representing reactive stimulation of the parathyroid to maintain normal calcium concentrations in response to the calcium-lowering effects of calcitonin.

It is estimated that approximately 4% of patients with pheochromocytomas have accompanying neurocutaneous syndromes, including von Recklinghausen's disease, tuberous sclerosis, Sturge-Weber syndrome, and von Hippel-Lindau disease.[45] The 12% incidence of other anomalies in such children's families (hydrocephalus, neurofibromas, ganglioneuromas, megacolon, megaureter, cryptorchidism) suggests a genetic trait having characteristics of a malformation syndrome. Pheochromocytomas have an increased incidence in patients suffering from congenital heart disease. Moon and associates[32] have produced medullary hyperplasia and pheochromocytomas in rats by continued intraperitoneal injection of growth hormone; however, this relation has not been demonstrated in human subjects.

Symptoms

Age at onset of signs and symptoms averages 9½ years. The preponderance of females as well as the common occurrence in adolescents suggest that the hormonal influences of puberty and growth may be important etiologic factors.

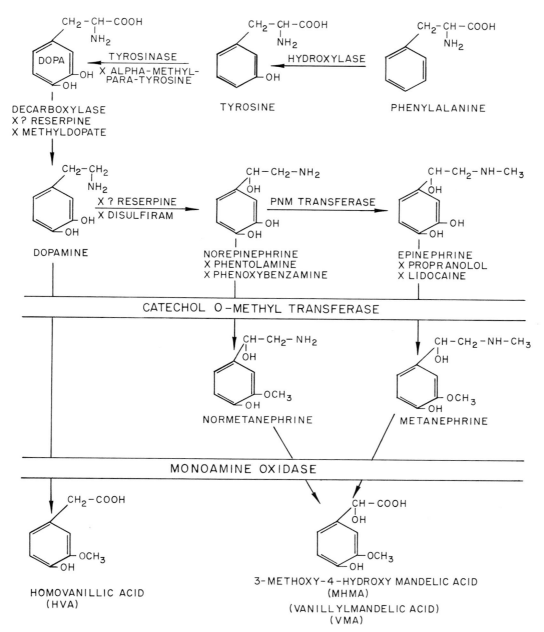

Fig 117–4.—Biosynthetic pathway showing metabolism, excretion, and sites of blockage *(X)* of the catecholamines by various drugs.

Tumors arising in the adrenal medulla produce both epinephrine and norepinephrine, whereas most extra-adrenal pheochromocytomas yield only norepinephrine. The catecholamines manufactured by pheochromocytomas may directly or indirectly activate the alpha- and/or beta-adrenergic receptors, resulting in the adrenergic syndrome (apprehension, hypertension, tachycardia, diaphoresis, manifestations of increased metabolism, constipation, and gastrointestinal tract bleeding). A functioning tumor in a child usually causes sustained hypertension.

By contrast, adults generally experience paroxysmal hypertension. Nevertheless, periods of high pressures may occur in children during paroxysmal crises. Episodes of tachycardia, systolic hypertension, and arrhythmia reflect the muscular beta-receptor effects of epinephrine secretion, whereas bradycardia and diastolic hypertension are evidence of the increased peripheral vasoconstriction by the alpha-adrenergic receptors stemming from circulating norepinephrine. The contracted vascular system leads to decreased plasma volume, reduced red cell mass, and, occasionally, orthostatic hypotension.[6] Norepinephrine is predominantly alpha in effect, whereas epinephrine elicits a mixture of alpha and beta actions. Most pheochromocytomas contain (but do not secrete) substantial quantities of dopamine. The relative proportions of norepinephrine and epinephrine may influence the signs and symptoms produced by pheochromocytomas.[12] Characteristically, epinephrine and norepinephrine are produced by adrenal medullary tumors, whereas norepinephrine alone is secreted by extra-adrenal tumors. In general, higher levels of norepinephrine are encountered in most childhood tumors, possibly reflecting a higher incidence of extra-adrenal pheochromocytomas, which do not possess the capacity for methylation of norepinephrine.

The onset of symptoms in children is often rapid, with diaphoresis unrelated to environmental temperature, usually preceded by pallor. Throbbing headaches with flushing may occur, and the hands may show a puffy redness, cyanosis, and mottling. Elevated body temperature, dilated pupils, and heat intolerance may become evident. Weight loss is common, despite a ravenous appetite. Substernal, precordial, abdominal, lumbar, or femoral pain may be constant or colicky. Epistaxis, hematemesis, melena, nausea, and vomiting may be associated with abdominal pain, which may simulate or actually be caused by colitis or appendicitis.[15] Partial intestinal obstruction may stem from fecal impaction. Polyuria, polydipsia, microscopic hematuria, and glycosuria with elevated fasting blood sugar levels are typical of pheochromocytoma. Convulsions and coma may result from hypertensive encephalopathy, and vision may be blurred by hypertensive retinitis. Despite these alarming symptoms, sudden death due to pheochromocytoma is uncommon in childhood. Peripheral vasoconstriction, bradycardia, and sweating characterize the alpha effects, while the beta effects include tachycardia, increased cardiac contractile force, bronchodilatation, and peripheral vasodilatation with lowered diastolic blood pressure.

Hypertension from pheochromocytomas may be differentiated from that due to coarctation of the aorta by the presence of bounding femoral pulses in pheochromocytoma. Many renal lesions, including intrinsic and extrinsic tumors, unilateral and bilateral pyelonephritis, glomerulonephritis, and renal artery stenosis may be associated with hypertension in childhood. Urinalysis, renal function studies, and arteriography can, in most cases, distinguish these conditions from pheochromocytoma. Other causes of hypertension in childhood that should be differentiated from pheochromocytoma are hyperthyroidism, adrenogenital syndrome, Cushing's syndrome, acrodynia, brain tumor, lead poisoning, and essential hypertension. In children with paroxysmal hypertension, the diagnosis of familial autonomic dysfunction (Riley-Day syndrome) should be ruled out.

Diagnostic Studies

Intravenous pyelography, abdominal ultrasonography, and computerized axial tomographic (CAT) scans can contribute to localizing a pheochromocytoma. Aortography, with selective arterial catheterization, may be particularly helpful in children whose tumor is not readily discoverable through less invasive studies, although this procedure could also serve as a provocative test, and precautions therefore must be taken to manage reactions (Fig 117–5). Any child suspected of having a pheochromocytoma should be evaluated in hospital, where accurate urine collection can be obtained and the hazards of special procedures can be minimized. Overzealous and prolonged diagnostic efforts to localize a tumor may seriously delay treatment.

The histamine provocative test introduced by Roth and Kvale[37] in 1945, as well as other such tests to increase catecholamine secretion, have largely been eliminated from the diagnostic armamentarium because of risks associated with increasing catecholamine secretion in an already hypertensive patient. The phentolamine (Regitine) test originally introduced in 1949 by Longino and co-authors[29] is useful only in patients with sustained hypertension, but should rarely be employed. A positive result produces a 35/25 mm/Hg fall of pressure within 5–10 minutes after the intravenous injection of 5 mg of Regitine.

More recently, in diagnosing pheochromocytoma, direct chemical methods of measuring the level of catecholamines and metabolites in plasma have largely replaced the indirect pharmacologic tests. Secretion of the catecholamines is initiated by acetylcholine released from neurons that embrace the secretory cell. After a brief period of activity in the circulation, these catecholamines are reduced by oxidation to 3-methoxy, 4-hydroxymandelic acid (VMA). Only 2–4% of norepinephrine and epinephrine are excreted directly into the urine, whereas more than one third of the total secreted catecholamines appears as VMA and one half is excreted as free or conjugated metanephrines.[22] A significant linear relation between the rate of urinary excretion of VMA and the size of a pheochromocytoma has been demonstrated.[14] Because of their higher concentrations, urinary assay for the metabolites of epinephrine or norepinephrine has proved easier and more reliable. A pheochromocytoma may often be lo-

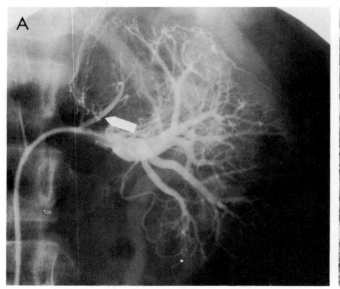
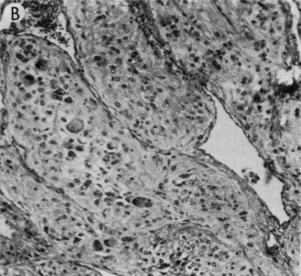

Fig 117–5.—Pheochromocytoma of left adrenal gland in a 15-year-old boy. **A,** aortogram shows tumor above left kidney. **B,** microscopic appearance of pheochromocytoma from same patient; hematoxylin-eosin stain; ×240.

calized by determining catecholamine levels in blood samples obtained at various levels of the inferior vena cava.[30]

The prevailing diagnostic tests in children are 24-hour collections of urine for free catecholamines, VMA, and metanephrines. For screening purposes, an overnight urine collection can be used. The catecholamine quantities are related to the amount of creatinine in the sample (usually as micrograms of metabolite per milligram of creatinine). Although VMA assays are widely available, they are subject to interference by various medications and dietary components. Assays of urinary catecholamines and VMA have been associated with an approximate 25% incidence of false-negative findings, whereas such results occur in only 4% of metanephrine determinations. Measurement of urinary homovanillic acid (HVA), the major end-product of dopamine metabolism, may help to diagnose malignant dopamine-secreting pheochromocytomas. Patients with neuroblastoma characteristically secrete high levels of dopamine metabolites.

Measurement of plasma catecholamines by radioenzyme assay may be more effective than either 24-hour urinary VMA or metanephrine determinations.[5] Patients must remain supine while blood samples are obtained; nonetheless, the catecholamine assay offers the major advantage of obviating 24-hour urine collection, which can be difficult in young children.

Plasma renin activity may increase in some 70% of patients with pheochromocytomas, possibly leading to an erroneous diagnosis of renal artery stenosis in children.[1]

Treatment

Medical therapy for patients with functioning pheochromocytomas is limited almost exclusively to preoperative preparation. Phentolamine and phenoxybenzamine (Dibenzyline) act to block the alpha-adrenergic receptors of epinephrine and norepinephrine. Because of the potential danger of hypertensive paroxysms, the patient should be started on alpha-blocking agents as soon as the diagnosis of pheochromocytoma has been confirmed. Phenoxybenzamine is the most effective alpha-adrenergic blocker because its 12–24-hour duration of action allows oral administration twice daily. The recommended starting dose of phenoxybenzamine is 1–2 mg/kg/24 hr in four divided doses; the dose should be increased until the blood pressure returns to normal. Phentolamine can be used for rapid alpha-adrenergic blockade, whereas phenoxybenzamine therapy for 1–2 weeks can be employed when operation is not urgent.[33] Congestion of nasal mucosa is a minor side effect, indicating blockage of the vasoconstrictors.

The beta-adrenergic blocker propranolol (Inderal) has been used to prepare patients for operation or intraoperatively to control tachycardia and prevent arrhythmias resulting from alpha-adrenergic blockade. The routine preoperative use of beta blockade has been somewhat controversial because occasional severe cardiovascular crises have occurred after this procedure. Nitroprusside has occasionally been used preoperatively and intraoperatively in patients who have become refractory to oral and intravenous alpha blockers. Patients with pheochromocytomas tend to be hypovolemic, experiencing an average 15% reduction of normal plasma volume. Carefully monitored preoperative reexpansion of the vascular system helps to minimize intraoperative fluctuations in blood pressure and intractable cardiac arrhythmias. Use of drugs that decrease catecholamine synthesis, such as alpha methylparatyrosine (AMPT), an inhibitor of tyrosine hydroxylase, has been recommended as an alternate preoperative treatment regimen.[22] Prolonged medical therapy for pheochromocytoma has no current place.

It is generally recognized that children with pheochromocytoma who have a high basal metabolic rate, and high plasma levels of catecholamines, are the poorest anesthesia risks. General anesthesia for excision of a pheochromocytoma may be divided into two stages. The first is characterized by efforts to keep the systemic blood pressure down, while the tumor is isolated and its blood supply and drainage ligated. The second involves efforts to keep the systemic blood pressure up thereafter. For safe anesthetic management, it is considered essential to use arterial and central venous pressure catheters as well as a urinary catheter, and to monitor the electrocardiogram continuously. The following drugs must be available to reduce systemic hypertension: phentolamine, nitroprusside and diazoxide. To control tachycardia and cardiac arrhythmias, xylocaine and propranolol are necessary. It is recommended that the anesthesiologist accompany the patient from the ward and administer Innovar, 0.04 ml/kg, intravenously at this time, repeating the dose after 5 minutes if the patient remains anxious. The induction of general anesthesia is particularly critical, because inadequate sedation may produce severe hypertension while excessive alpha blockade with inadequate blood volume re-expansion may result in severe hypotension. Enflurane has become the anesthetic drug of choice in recent years, although the plane of anesthesia is probably more important than the agent employed. Enflurane does not sensitize the myocardium to exogenous catecholamines, nor does it stimulate the release of catecholamines. Pancuronium, a nondepolarizing, long-acting muscle relaxant administered intravenously, is preferred over succinylcholine or curare. After intubation, anesthesia can also be maintained by a combination of nitrous oxide and oxygen with methoxyflurane. Innovar may also be administered if additional analgesia is required during operation. Halothane is not employed because of its propensity to sensitize the myocardium to the arrhythmic activity of catecholamines. Blood and, if necessary, norepinephrine or angiotensin II should be used to control hypotension that may occur precipitously after removal of the tumor.[41, 44]

More than 95% of childhood pheochromocytomas are located in the abdomen, even though the tumor site may occasionally be inaccurately determined. A bilateral subcostal incision that can be extended into the flank or across the lower costal margin into the chest for large tumors has provided satisfactory exposure for children. An abdominal exploration encompassing both adrenal glands, the periaortic sympathetic ganglia, the small-bowel mesentery, and the pelvis reveals more than 95% of all pheochromocytomas. Gentle dissection with early control of venous drainage and minimal manipulation of the tumor or involved gland should be employed to avoid flooding the circulation with an excess of catecholamines. The tumor is usually encapsulated and may have small remnants of normal adrenal tissue contiguous with it. The entire adrenal gland should be removed. Pheochromocytomas rarely adhere to the kidney, so that a concomitant nephrectomy is seldom required.

The right adrenal (where tumors are likely to occur) is exposed by reflecting the transverse colon inferiorly and mobilizing the duodenum medially to expose the upper kidney and adrenal gland (Fig 117–6,*A*). The liver is elevated superiorly and/or medially, and the lateral border of the vena cava is rolled medially to facilitate exposure of the gland, which is partially tucked under the vena cava. The risk of hemorrhage is greater on this side, where the adrenal vein is short and easily torn.

The left adrenal is exposed by reflecting the transverse colon inferiorly, dividing the gastrocolic ligament and elevating the stomach (Fig 117–6,*B*). The posterior peritoneum along the lower edge of the pancreas is incised, and the tail of the pancreas is then elevated to expose the renal and adrenal veins. An alternative technique for exposing the left adrenal is to divide the peritoneum lateral to the splenic flexure of the colon and mobilize the colon medially. The adrenal is then exposed by incising

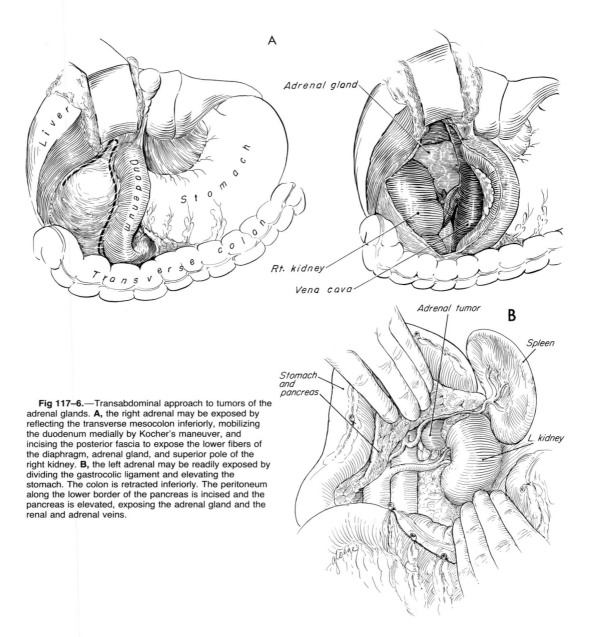

Fig 117–6.—Transabdominal approach to tumors of the adrenal glands. **A,** the right adrenal may be exposed by reflecting the transverse mesocolon inferiorly, mobilizing the duodenum medially by Kocher's maneuver, and incising the posterior fascia to expose the lower fibers of the diaphragm, adrenal gland, and superior pole of the right kidney. **B,** the left adrenal may be readily exposed by dividing the gastrocolic ligament and elevating the stomach. The colon is retracted inferiorly. The peritoneum along the lower border of the pancreas is incised and the pancreas is elevated, exposing the adrenal gland and the renal and adrenal veins.

the perirenal fascia. In most instances, when the adrenal veins are interrupted and the pheochromocytoma is removed, hypotension ensues, requiring a norepinephrine infusion for varying periods of time, ranging up to several days. The reduced blood volume resulting from long-term catecholamine secretion should be corrected by appropriate transfusions of plasma, albumin, blood, or electrolyte solutions, as indicated. Exploration of the contralateral adrenal gland is mandatory in all children; clear visualization of the entire gland is essential, and some authors have recommended biopsy because of the high incidence of bilateral tumors.[4] Adrenal cortical insufficiency is unlikely if the major portion of one adrenal gland is left in place. If both adrenals are removed or if the remaining gland is atrophic, intravenous hydrocortisone should be given promptly.

In occasional patients, the blood pressure may not return to normal levels for several days after removing the tumor. In our experience, if blood pressure fails to normalize within 2 to 3 weeks, or if hypertension returns, a second tumor is likely. Hypertension due to a second pheochromocytoma is apt to occur within 5 years subsequent to removal of the initial tumor. Children who undergo resection of the pheochromocytoma should undergo follow-up examinations at least twice annually, including measurement of blood pressure, and urine catecholamine determinations. The progeny and siblings of patients with pheochromocytoma should also be periodically evaluated for hypertension because of the high familial incidence.

Although malignancy in pheochromocytomas is approximately 10%, it is uncommon in children and usually diagnosed by the finding of distant nonfunctioning metastases. On the basis of its histology, it is difficult to predict whether a pheochromocytoma in a child will behave as a malignant tumor, since pleomorphism and lymphatic, vascular, and capsular invasion are frequently evident.[11] A combination of local excision, radiation, chemotherapy, and anti-adrenergic agents has provided symptomatic palliation for many years in these rare patients. The most common sites for metastatic lesions are the skeleton, liver, lymph nodes, lung, and central nervous system.

Cortical Lesions of the Adrenal Glands

Cushing Syndrome

In 1932, Cushing[10] described a syndrome in which patients manifested adiposity, amenorrhea, purplish striae, hypertension, polydipsia, and polyphagia, believed to stem from basophil adenomas of the pituitary. Anderson and associates,[2] in 1938, showed that hyperactivity of the adrenal cortex was the common etiology in all cases of Cushing syndrome. It has subsequently been established that the condition results primarily from excessive production of adrenal cortical hormones owing to bilateral adrenal cortical hyperplasia induced by increased adrenocorticotrophic hormone (ACTH) secretion in the pituitary (possibly containing an adenoma), or to an ectopic ACTH-producing neoplasm. Adrenal adenoma, adrenal carcinoma, and nodular dysplasia of the adrenals are less likely causes of Cushing syndrome. The incidence of spontaneous Cushing syndrome is estimated to be approximately 6 per million population, occurring mainly in young adult females, and it is rare in childhood. Cushing's disease is potentially fatal, usually within 5 years of the time the disease first becomes apparent.

In a review of 110 patients with Cushing syndrome in 1971, Orth and Liddle[34] noted that 59% had pituitary-dependent hypercortisolism (Cushing's disease), 26% had hypercortisolism due to adrenocortical tumors, and 15% had hypercortisolism stemming from nonendocrine tumors that produced ACTH. It is difficult to distinguish the hyperplastic gland grossly at operation, or even microscopically from the normal gland. Patients with adrenal hyperplasia have normal plasma and ACTH values, but cortisol secretion is suppressed after administering dexamethasone. Unlike adults, in children manifesting Cushing syndrome the source is often iatrogenic administration of pharmacologic doses of glucocorticoids or, rarely, ACTH.

Among patients whose adrenocortical tumors caused Cushing syndrome, one third of the tumors proved to be carcinomas, often producing a florid manifestation of the disease. More than half of the children with Cushing syndrome had carcinoma. Widespread metastases may occur and frequently show hyperfunction. Malignancy may be difficult to demonstrate histologically, the best criteria being invasion into veins, extension through the capsule, and distant metastases.

Although preoperative diagnosis of the rare ectopic ACTH-secreting tumors in children can be difficult, such patients usually have Cushing's symptoms without the characteristic fat distribution. They also have higher plasma ACTH levels and cortisol excretion, not suppressed with dexamethasone. Such ectopic tumors are usually found in the lung, parotid, liver, thymus, thyroid, pancreas, and adrenal medulla. In patients with adrenocortical adenoma or carcinoma, dexamethasone fails to suppress cortisol secretion, and low plasma ACTH levels are typical.

Clinical Manifestations

The symptoms of Cushing syndrome in adolescents include truncal obesity with characteristic fat pads in the upper back (buffalo hump), adipose accumulation in the face (moon facies), plethora, hypertension with headaches, peripheral edema, muscular weakness and growth retardation, capillary fragility, ecchymoses, osteoporosis and pathologic fractures, as well as skin fragility with abdominal striae due to protein depletion (Fig 117–7). Indeed, the skin is often so fragile that removal of adhesive tape may de-epithelialize areas. Since cortisol promotes reten-

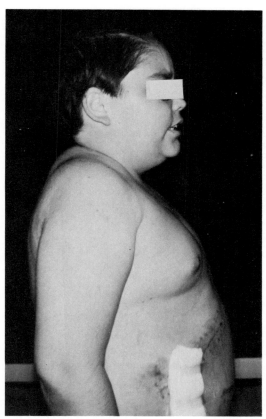

Fig 117–7.—Cushing syndrome secondary to adrenal adenoma in 14-year-old boy. The characteristic fat distribution, with "buffalo hump" and "moon facies," is seen.

tion of salt and water, electrolyte imbalance usually occurs, with metabolic alkalosis and hypokalemia, even though aldosterone secretion is normal.[31] Androgen secretion may be increased, accounting for the amenorrhea, hirsutism, and acne that frequently occur in adolescent girls, and the virilization often appearing in boys. These patients tend to manifest a diabetic glucose tolerance curve with glycosuria and diabetes due to accelerated protein breakdown and increased gluconeogenesis. The white blood cell count can be elevated, with mild leukocytosis, lymphopenia, and eosinopenia. Emotional instability is characteristic. The serum gamma-globulin level is reduced, which, when combined with abnormal protein and carbohydrate metabolism, makes these patients particularly subject to infections. Bone and height age are retarded in cases of Cushing syndrome, whereas in children who are simply obese they are usually advanced.

Diagnostic Studies

An outline of studies designed to diagnose Cushing syndrome has been presented by Scott and associates[38] (Fig 117–8). In many patients with Cushing syndrome, the normal diurnal variation of blood ACTH and cortisol levels may be absent, and secretion of the two hormones is constant throughout the day. Patients with adrenocortical hyperplasia usually experience a greater rise in plasma cortisol levels after intravenous administration of ACTH over a 4–6-hour period than found in the normal patient.[36] Measurement of urinary 17-hydroxycorticosteroids has been a useful method of determining cortisol secretion. While normal adults excrete between 3 and 12 mg of 17-hydroxycorti-

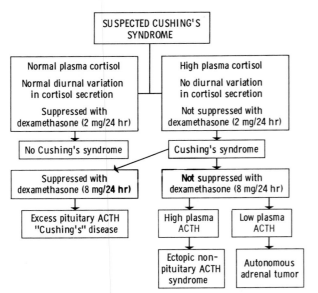

SUSPECTED CUSHING'S SYNDROME

Normal plasma cortisol	High plasma cortisol
Normal diurnal variation in cortisol secretion	No diurnal variation in cortisol secretion
Suppressed with dexamethasone (2 mg/24 hr)	Not suppressed with dexamethasone (2 mg/24 hr)

No Cushing's syndrome → Cushing's syndrome

| Suppressed with dexamethasone (8 mg/24 hr) | Not suppressed with dexamethasone (8 mg/24 hr) |

Excess pituitary ACTH "Cushing's" disease

High plasma ACTH → Ectopic non-pituitary ACTH syndrome

Low plasma ACTH → Autonomous adrenal tumor

Fig 117–8.—Protocol for evaluation of patients with suspected Cushing syndrome. (From Scott et al.[38])

costeroids in the urine in 24 hours, patients with Cushing syndrome usually excrete more than 12 mg.

The dexamethasone suppression test developed by Liddle[26] to determine the etiology of adrenocortical hyperfunction is based on the fact that small doses of this synthetic steroid can block ACTH release in the normal patient. During the 6-day test period, the patient undergoes continuous 24-hour urine collection for corticosteroids. The first 2 days are used as a control; during the second 2 days the patient receives 0.5 mg of dexamethasone orally every 6 hours for a total of 2 mg/day, and on the final 2 days, the patient is given 2 mg of dexamethasone orally every 6 hours for a total of 8 mg/day. The normal individual experiences a suppression of 17-hydroxycorticosteroid excretion of more than 50% on the 2-mg/day dose of dexamethasone. Patients with Cushing syndrome who have bilateral adrenal hyperplasia do not evidence a suppression until 8 mg/day of dexamethasone is given; those with adrenocortical adenoma or carcinoma show no suppression with dexamethasone. Nonetheless, the dexamethasone suppression test is not completely reliable.

The rapid dexamethasone suppression test may be more reliable than the standard test. It consists of administering 1 mg dexamethasone orally at 11 P.M. and, after adequate sedation, measuring plasma cortisol values the following morning at 8 A.M. A level of 17-hydroxycorticosteroids in the plasma above 5 μg/100 ml suggests nonsuppressibility of ACTH secretion and is diagnostic of Cushing syndrome. (The level falls to nearly zero in the normal patient.) The ratio of urinary corticosteroids to creatinine can be used instead of plasma cortisol levels to indicate suppression by dexamethasone.

The standard ACTH stimulation test may provide additional diagnostic information. After an 8-hour infusion of 50 units of ACTH (adult dose), the normal response is the excretion of 20–40 mg of 17-hydroxycorticosteroids in the urine during the next 24 hours; patients with Cushing syndrome secondary to adrenocortical hyperplasia excrete over 50 mg of urinary 17-hydroxysteroids over the next 24 hours.[36]

The metyrapone (Metopirone) test was also developed by Liddle[26] to evaluate pituitary and adrenal function. Metyrapone blocks 11-beta-hydroxylation in the adrenal cortex, effecting a fall in cortisol production that increases ACTH secretion in the nor-

mal person. In children with Cushing's disease caused by adrenal hyperplasia, steroids increase markedly in the urine over amounts seen in normal individuals. Adrenal cortical adenomas that produce Cushing syndrome show no increase unless they also respond to ACTH stimulation.

Roentgenograms of the sella turcica should be made in all patients with Cushing syndrome, particularly those with hyperpigmentation, to investigate the possibility of a pituitary tumor. Bone roentgenograms may disclose osteoporosis and pathologic fractures, both common in children with this syndrome. The CAT scan and ultrasound study have been particularly helpful in identifying adrenal tumors, even those that are very small. Additional assistance in localizing adrenal tumors or in showing occasional adrenal hyperplasia may be obtained from selective renal arteriograms or venograms. Retroperitoneal pneumograms with tomography are rarely used.

Treatment

In patients with Cushing syndrome secondary to excess pituitary secretion of ACTH and resultant adrenal hyperplasia, bilateral adrenalectomy has been performed effectively for many years, although the treatment is directed at the target organ, not the inciting organ. The transabdominal approach for bilateral adrenalectomy has had favorable results in children, although some surgeons prefer the bilateral posterior retroperitoneal approach while others employ the bilateral flank approach, particularly in obese patients. The resultant adrenal insufficiency is effectively managed with replacement therapy. Less than bilateral total adrenalectomy is usually followed by recurrent symptoms of Cushing syndrome.[13]

Pituitary irradiation with cobalt-60 can control Cushing's disease, although it may take as long as 6 months before the response is observed. In some centers, adrenalectomy is now used only for patients whose conditions are refractory to pituitary irradiation, possibly 50%.[28]

Transnasal resection of pituitary adenomas under control of the microscope, so commonly used in adults, has, until recently, been considered inapplicable to the problem in children with their small hypophyses and still smaller tumors. The report of Styne and collaborators from the University of California, San Francisco, puts a new light on this.[42] In 15 children, ages 7 to 13 years, a transsphenoidal microadenectomy was performed. There were no deaths. Ten patients had mild diabetes insipidus for less than 3 days, and two children had diabetes insipidus for 1 and 4 months. All were discharged by 6 days after operation. An adenoma was found in 14 of the 15 patients. One patient required a second operation and was well after removal of a second adenoma.

When a benign adenoma is suspected on the basis of preoperative studies, the involved gland should be resected and the contralateral gland submitted for biopsy. Adrenocortical carcinomas should be widely excised and the abdomen thoroughly searched for metastases. Prolonged drug treatment is used primarily for Cushing syndrome resulting from inoperable carcinoma of the adrenal cortex with metastases. Ectopic ACTH-producing tumors should be resected, but if this is not feasible, bilateral adrenalectomy should be performed, depending on the patient's prognosis for life in relation to the primary tumor. Most adrenal tumors are relatively radioresistant. Preliminary experience suggests responsiveness to multidrug regimens as adjunctive treatment.[20] The adrenocorticolytic drug o,p-DDD has proved helpful in managing the inoperable or recurrent hormonally active tumor by producing involution of the secretory function and ameliorating the associated endocrine symptoms.

Feminizing Tumors

Feminizing adrenal tumors are rare in children, almost invariably occur in males, and usually are malignant. Gynecomastia is the most common symptom. A palpable tumor is present in many of the patients. The testes show marked alterations of the spermatogonia and absence of spermatogenesis.

Hyperaldosteronism

Rare in children, primary aldosteronism as described by Conn[9] may be caused by a benign adrenal cortical adenoma or by bilateral adrenal hyperfunction, with or without hyperplasia. Adenomas, which account for almost 90% of cases of primary aldosteronism, are usually small, well encapsulated, and solitary. Hyperaldosteronism resulting from adrenal cortical carcinoma is rare. Primary aldosteronism is characterized by excessive amounts of aldosterone in the urine (over 175 μg/24 hr) with normal amounts of 17-hydroxycorticoids and 17-ketosteroids. The most prominent features of the syndrome include hypertension without retinopathy, antidiuretic hormone-resistant polyuria, muscle weakness, severe headaches, tingling and paresthesias of the limbs and extremities. These patients usually manifest hypokalemia and alkalosis. The urine output is large and dilute, often containing protein. The plasma renin is usually normal, in contrast to patients with secondary aldosteronism who have elevated renin secretion. A comprehensive review of the many causes of secondary aldosteronism has been presented by Kaplan.[23]

Bilateral adrenal exploration is indicated for patients with primary aldosteronism, in the hope of removing an adenoma. If an adrenal adenoma cannot be found, the course is not clear, since primary aldosteronism may be managed medically with good success. Bilateral hemiadrenalectomy (with careful sectioning of the gland in a search for adenoma or hyperplasia to be followed by complete adrenalectomy if a tumor is found on the involved side) is recommended by many. Total adrenalectomy is the procedure of choice for definite hyperplasia; however, unilateral adrenalectomy and 50–75% resection of the contralateral gland may be optimal for patients with clear primary aldosteronism in whom neither adenoma nor hyperplasia can be found. Liddle[27] has shown that aminoglutethimide inhibition of steroid synthesis is effective in treating patients with primary aldosteronism.

Cysts and Stromal Tumors

Small hemorrhagic cysts of the fetal adrenal cortex are not uncommon, are frequently bilateral, and are occasionally noted incidentally at laparotomy for other conditions, or at post mortem.[46] Most small cysts are absorbed spontaneously. Adrenal hemorrhage in the newborn due to fetal anoxia or difficult labor may produce adrenal insufficiency with shock and sepsis that, if not treated by adrenal cortical hormone replacement, may be fatal. A large cyst, although rare, may be sufficiently big to be first noted as an abdominal mass (Fig 117–9). These cysts may be seen to displace the kidneys inferiorly on intravenous pyelogram and should be removed because of the difficulty in distinguishing them from solid tumors.[17] Occasionally, large adrenal cysts in the newborn may contain malignant tumor.[43]

Stromal tumors of the adrenal are exceedingly rare and usually asymptomatic. These tumors include fibroma, lipoma, hamartoma, neurofibroma, osteoma, hemangioma, lymphangioma, melanoma, and sarcoma. Excision is required because of the difficulty in distinguishing this type of lesion from neuroblastoma and other neoplasms.

Adrenal Insufficiency

Acute adrenal cortical insufficiency may result from adrenal hemorrhage due to trauma, infection, tumor, or adrenal vascular occlusion. The Waterhouse-Friderichsen syndrome may occur with meningococcus septicemia or be caused by *Pneumococcus, Staphylococcus,* or hemolytic *Streptococcus* and occasionally other bacterial and viral infections. These patients may experience fever, hypotension, emesis, headache, diarrhea, hypoglycemia, dehydration, weakness, lethargy, and abdominal pain. Investigation usually shows hyponatremia, hyperkalemia, hypoglycemia, and azotemia.

Treatment should include cortical hormone replacement, including prompt intravenous infusion of 50 mg of hydrocortisone followed by daily maintenance infusions of 100–200 mg. Appropriate antibiotics should be given, and refractory hypotension may require administration of vasopressor drugs.

Children with chronic adrenal insufficiency following bilateral adrenalectomy or other causes usually require maintenance steroid replacement with approximately 10–40 mg of hydrocorti-

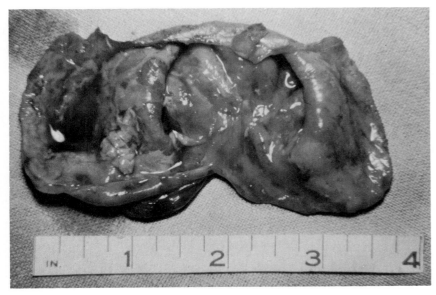

Fig 117–9.—Large hemorrhagic right adrenal cyst from 3-week-old female that was recognized as a large abdominal mass. Neuroblastoma cells were present in the cyst wall.

sone daily. Nausea, emesis, and other gastrointestinal symptoms can be accurate indicators of need for increased steroid replacement. A guideline for other corticosteroid replacement for addisonian patients has been reviewed by Frawley.[19]

REFERENCES

1. Altman A.J., Schwartz A.D.: Tumors of the sympathetic nervous system, in Altman A.J., Schwartz A.D. (eds.): *Malignant Diseases of Infancy, Childhood and Adolescence*. Philadelphia, W.B. Saunders Co., 1978, p. 326.
2. Anderson E., Parson W., Bloomberg E.: Therapy in Cushing's syndrome. *J. Clin. Endocrinol.* 13:375, 1941.
3. Atuck N.O., McDonald T., Wood T., et al.: Familial pheochromocytoma, hypercalcemia, and von Hippel-Lindau disease. *Medicine* 58:209, 1979.
4. Bloom D.A., Fonkalsrud E.W.: Surgical management of pheochromocytoma in children. *J. Pediatr. Surg.* 9:179, 1974.
5. Bravo E.L., Tarazi R.C., Gifford R.W., et al.: Circulating and urinary catecholamines in pheochromocytoma. *N. Engl. J. Med.* 301:682, 1979.
6. Brunjes J., Johns V.J. Jr., Crane M.D.: Pheochromocytoma: Postoperative shock and blood volume. *N. Engl. J. Med.* 262:393, 1960.
7. Carney J.A., Sizemore G.W., Tyce G.M.: Bilateral adrenal medullary hyperplasia in multiple endocrine neoplasia, Type II: The precursor of bilateral pheochromocytoma. *Mayo Clin. Proc.* 50:3, 1975.
8. Cone T.E. Jr., Allen M.S., Pearson H.A.: Pheochromocytoma in children: Report of three familial cases in two unrelated families. *Pediatrics* 19:44, 1957.
9. Conn J.W.: Primary aldosteronism: A new clinical syndrome. *J. Lab. Clin. Med.* 45:6, 1955.
10. Cushing H.: The basophil adenomas of the pituitary body and their clinical manifestations. *Bull. Johns Hopkins Hosp.* 50:137, 1932.
11. Dahner L.P.: Endocrine system with exocrine pancreas—adrenal, in Dahner L.P.: *Pediatric Surgical Pathology*. St. Louis, C.V. Mosby Co., 1975, p. 432.
12. Dibbins A.W., Wiener E.S.: Retroperitoneal tumors in children. *Curr. Probl. Surg.*, October, 1973.
13. Egdahl R.H., Melby J.D.: Recurrent Cushing's disease and intermittent functional adrenal cortical insufficiency following subtotal adrenalectomy. *Ann. Surg.* 166:586, 1967.
14. Farndon J.R., Davidson H.A., Johnston I.D.A., et al.: VMA excretion in patients with pheochromocytoma. *Ann. Surg.* 191:259, 1980.
15. Fee H.J., et al.: Fatal outcome in a child with pseudomembranous colitis. *J. Pediatr. Surg.* 10:959, 1975.
16. Forsham P.H.: The adrenals, in Williams R.H. (ed.): *Textbook of Endocrinology*, ed. 3. Philadelphia, W.B. Saunders Co., 1962, p. 383.
17. Forsham P.H., Melmon K.L.: The adrenals, in Williams R.H. (ed.): *Textbook of Endocrinology*, ed. 4. Philadelphia, W.B. Saunders Co., 1968, p. 287.
18. Frankel F.: Ein Fall von doppelsseitigen, völlig laten verlaufenen Nebennierentumor und gleichzeitiger Nephritis mit Veränderungen am Circulationsapparat und Retinitis. *Arch. Pathol. Anat.* 103:244, 1886.
19. Frawley T.F.: Adrenal cortical insufficiency, in Eisenstein A.B. (ed.): *The Adrenal Cortex*. Boston, Little, Brown & Co., 1967, p. 439.
20. Gold E.M.: The Cushing's syndrome: Changing views of diagnosis and treatment. *Ann. Intern. Med.* 90:829, 1979.
21. Hume D.M.: Pheochromocytoma in the adult and in the child. *Am. J. Surg.* 99:458, 1960.
22. Javadpour N., Woltering E.A., Brennan M.F.: Adrenal neoplasm. *Curr. Probl. Surg.* 17:No. 1, 1980.
23. Kaplan N.M.: Secondary aldosteronism: With observations on the definition of hypokalemia. *Am. J. Clin. Pathol.* 54:315, 1970.
24. Kvale W.F., et al.: Present-day diagnosis and treatment of pheochromocytoma. *JAMA* 164:854, 1957.
25. Labbe M., Tinel J., Doumer A.: Crises solaires et hypertension paroxysmique en rapport avec une tumeur surrenale. *Bull. Soc. Med. Hop. Paris* 46:982, 1922.
26. Liddle G.W.: Tests of pituitary-adrenal suppressibility in the diagnosis of Cushing's syndrome. *J. Endocrinol.* 33:515, 1965.
27. Liddle G.W.: Management of aldosteronism. *Am. J. Clin. Pathol.* 54:331, 1970.
28. Lipsett M.B.: Rationale for chemotherapy of Cushing's syndrome, in Astwood E.B., Cassidy C.E. (eds.): *Clinical Endocrinology II*. New York, Grune & Stratton, 1968, p. 489.
29. Longino F.H., et al.: Effects of a new quarternary amine and a new imidazoline derivative on the autonomic nervous system. *Surgery* 26:421, 1949.
30. Mahoney E.M.: Localization of (adrenal and extra-adrenal) pheochromocytomas by vena cava blood samplings. *Surg. Forum* 14:405, 1963.
31. Migeon C.J., Green O.C., Eckert J.P.: Study of adrenocortical function in obesity. *Metabolism* 12:718, 1963.
32. Moon H.D., et al.: Pheochromocytomas of adrenals in male rats chronically injected with pituitary growth hormone. *Proc. Soc. Exp. Biol. Med.* 93:74, 1956.
33. Moore T.J., Williams G.H.: Adrenal causes of hypertension. *Compr. Ther.* 4:46, 1978.
34. Orth D.N., Liddle G.W.: Results of treatment in 108 patients with Cushing's syndrome. *N. Engl. J. Med.* 285:243, 1971.
35. Pick L.: Das Ganglioma Embryonale Sympathicum. *Klin. Wochenschr.* 19:16, 1912.
36. Ronald A.E., et al.: The use of intravenous ACTH: A study of quantitative adrenocortical stimulation. *J. Clin. Endocrinol.* 12:763, 1952.
37. Roth G.M., Kvale W.F.: Tentative test for pheochromocytoma. *Am. J. Med. Sci.* 210:653, 1945.
38. Scott H.W. Jr., et al.: Surgical management of adrenocortical tumors with Cushing's syndrome. *Ann. Surg.* 173:892, 1971.
39. Scott H.W., Jr., Oates J.A., Nies A.S., et al.: Pheochromocytoma: Present diagnosis and management. *Ann. Surg.* 183:587, 1976.
40. Stackpole R.H., Melicow M.M., Uson A.C.: Pheochromocytoma in children: Report of 9 cases with followup studies. *J. Pediatr. Surg.* 63:314, 1963.
41. Stringel G., Ein S.H., Creighton R., et al.: Pheochromocytoma in children: An update. *J. Pediatr. Surg.* 15:496, 1980.
42. Styne D.M., Grumbach M.M., Kaplan S.L., et al.: Treatment of Cushing's disease in childhood and adolescence by transsphenoidal microadenomectomy. *N. Engl. J. Med.* 310:889, 1984.
43. Sundaram M., Srivisal F., DeMello D., et al.: Angiography of multiple asynchronously manifest pheochromocytomas: The APUD concept. *AJR* 130:1168, 1978.
44. Van de Water J.M., Fonkalsrud E.W.: Adrenal cysts in infancy. *Surgery* 60:1267, 1966.
45. Van Heerden J.A., Shops S.G., Hamberger B., et al.: Pheochromocytoma: Current status and changing trends. *Surgery* 91:367, 1982.
46. Wander J.V., Das Gupta T.K.: Neurofibromatosis. *Curr. Probl. Surg.* 14:No. 2, 1977.
47. Zintel H.A., Schuh F.D.: Surgical diseases of the adrenal glands. *Am. J. Gastroenterol.* 44:515, 1965.

PART VIII

Genitourinary System

PLATE V

A. Newborn boy with abdominal muscular deficiency syndrome, "prune belly." Such infants have a spectrum of associated disorders mostly involving the genitourinary tract. The visible megacystis with grade 3 to 4 bilateral ureteral reflux was treated with bilateral ureteral tapering and reimplantation and by reduction cystoplasty. Bilateral orchiopexies are required usually at age 3 years. A pectus excavatum deformity is evident.

B. Splenogonadal fusion, the rarest of inguinal anomalies, presents as a mass that is often misinterpreted, as was true in this case, as a form of testicular malignancy and treated by orchiectomy with initial ligation of the vas and vessels high in the inguinal canal. No bilateral cases have been reported.

C. Hydronephrosis (ureteropelvic obstruction). The nonfunctioning right kidney shown here was removed from a 2½-year-old girl. There is advanced hydronephrosis, and several cortical cysts are present. The ureter below the level of the obstruction is of normal caliber. When the kidney functions and infection has not supervened, a suitable form of pelviplasty should be attempted before resorting to nephrectomy.

D. Unilateral multicystic dysplastic kidney with proximal ureteral atresia. This condition results from an overproduction of convoluted tubules in relation to collecting tubules, with cyst formation and pressure atrophy of adjacent nephrons. Function is rare. Renal scintigraphy and abdominal ultrasonography provide the diagnosis. Treatment, usually in early infancy, is ipsilateral nephrectomy. Function of the opposite kidney is normal, with compensatory hypertrophy.

E. Exstrophy of the urinary bladder. This newborn male shows the irregularity of bladder mucosa that is typical of exstrophy—the mucosa bulging forward on straining. The penis is epispadiac. No suitable reservoir could be devised, and the patient was treated by bilateral nonrefluxing isolated-segment ureterosigmoidostomies. Bladder augmentation will be attempted if volume and pressure flow studies permit the interval repair of the epispadias.

F. Hydrocolpos in newborn. This condition, apparent on inspection of the introitus, is treated by simple excision of the diaphragm and external drainage. The vaginal and uterine cavities are greatly dilated, and often there is a considerable, but reversible, bilateral hydronephrosis.

PLATE V

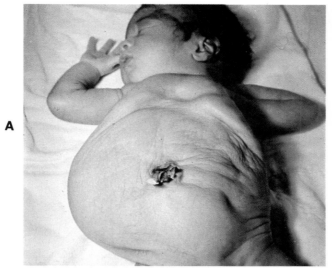

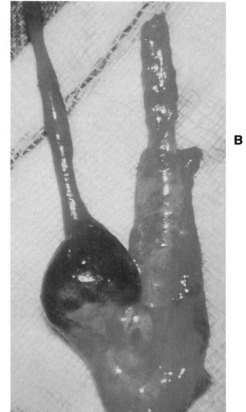

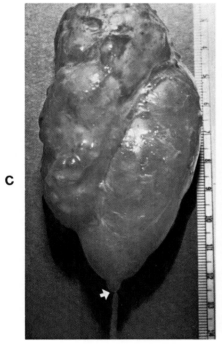

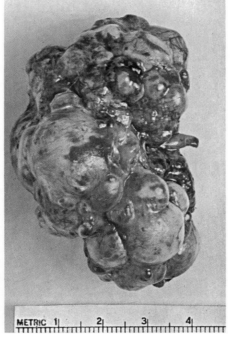

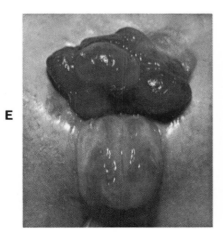

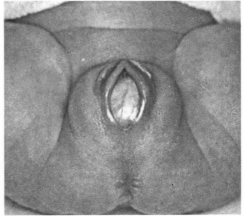

A

B

C

D

E

F

118   Howard McC. Snyder III

Cystic Disease of the Kidney, Dysplasia, and Agenesis

THE KIDNEY is one of the organs most commonly involved in cystic disease. The etiologic mechanisms of many of the types of renal cystic disease, the majority of which are congenital, are unknown.

Microdissection studies by Osathanondh and Potter[73] revealed that renal cysts are in continuity with the nephron and demonstrated which part of the uriniferous tubule was involved in the cystic process. This discovery discounts a previously held theory that renal cysts were the result of nonunion between the nephron and the collecting duct.[48]

Research has contributed to understanding of the development of renal cystic disease in a variety of experimental animals.[10, 32, 50] Although none of the models bears any direct resemblance to human cystic disease, this research has been valuable in providing theories as to the possible causes of renal cystic disease.[85]

Classification of Cystic Disease

Renal cystic disease classifications vary greatly. The classifications of Bernstein,[13, 16] Osathanondh and Potter,[73] and Spence and Singleton[92] have been the most valuable. Other classifications continue to be reported.[56] The number of different classifications indicates that no system is perfect or uniformly applicable. We believe that the Spence and Singleton classification[92] has the greatest clinical application:

Renal dysplasia
  Congenital unilateral multicystic kidney
  Segmental and focal renal dysplasia
  Renal dysplasia associated with congenital lower tract obstruction
Congenital polycystic kidney disease
  Infantile type
  Adult type
Cystic disorders of renal medulla
  Sponge kidney
  Medullary cystic disease
  Renal cystic disease with congenital hepatic fibrosis
Caliceal cyst
Simple cyst
Peripelvic cyst
Perinephric cyst
Cysts associated with neoplasm
  Cystic degeneration of parenchymal tumors
  Malignant change occurring in wall of simple cyst
  Cystadenoma and multilocular cysts
Cysts secondary to nonmalignant renal disease
Miscellaneous

Although medullary cystic disease (juvenile nephronophthisis) has been suggested to be one of the leading causes of idiopathic renal failure among adolescents, it is best considered a form of interstitial nephritis with associated cysts[38] and will not be discussed here, nor will renal cysts in hereditary syndromes. The reader is referred to other texts and articles for information on these conditions.[14, 15, 47, 87] Unilateral multicystic kidney is discussed under Renal Dysplasia (pp. 1130–1132).

Infantile Polycystic Kidney Disease (Autosomal Recessive)

Infantile polycystic disease is the single most common genetically determined cystic disease of the kidneys in childhood but is nonetheless rare. The disease is inherited as an autosomal recessive trait and occurs in about 1 in 10,000 live births.[18]

The newborn with infantile polycystic disease typically presents with bilateral, massive (12 to 16 times normal), hard, kidney-shaped, nonbosselated flank masses.

Other diseases that cause bilateral flank masses and need to be excluded are hydronephrosis (with or without hydroureter), renal malignancies (Wilms tumor, mesoblastic nephroma), and renal vein thrombosis. The initial intravenous urogram in the infantile polycystic kidney has a characteristic appearance, showing a very prolonged nephrogram phase with a diagnostic "sunburst" or streaked appearance of the contrast material (Fig 118–1,D). Kidneys that cannot be visualized urographically warrant other investigations, such as voiding cystography ultrasonography, isotope study, prograde pyelography, blood coagulation study, vanillylmandelic acid (VMA) determination, or arteriography.

Formerly, the newborn with infantile polycystic kidneys died within the first 2 months of life. Death was secondary either to renal failure[18] or respiratory insufficiency.[63] Lieberman et al.[63] believe that, with improved respiratory care, longer survival is possible.

Autopsy confirms the massive enlargement of the kidneys. The renal subcapsular surface shows multiple small cysts (Fig 118–1, A). Sectioning of the kidney reveals a radial arrangement of the dilated tubules, extending from the medulla to the subcapsular zone (Fig 118–1,B and C). Microdissection[73] has shown that the cysts are fusiform dilatations of the collecting ducts and tubules. Every patient with infantile polycystic kidney disease also has an abnormal liver. Microscopy demonstrates a proliferation and dilatation of the bile ducts and a variable degree of periportal fibrosis. Macroscopic cysts of the liver are uncommon. Lieberman et al.[63] state that cystic disease of other viscera is neither predictable nor common. Only about 30% of patients with adult onset of adult polycystic kidney disease have a cystic liver.

Blyth and Ockenden[18] believe that infantile polycystic disease involves spectra of both degree of severity and role of inheritance. They subdivide the disease into four groups, including congenital hepatic fibrosis. Such an inclusion is a contentious issue[16, 63] and raises the point of the tendency of some authors to "lump" diseases together or to split them by subdivisions. Blyth and Ockenden state also that the less severe forms of infantile

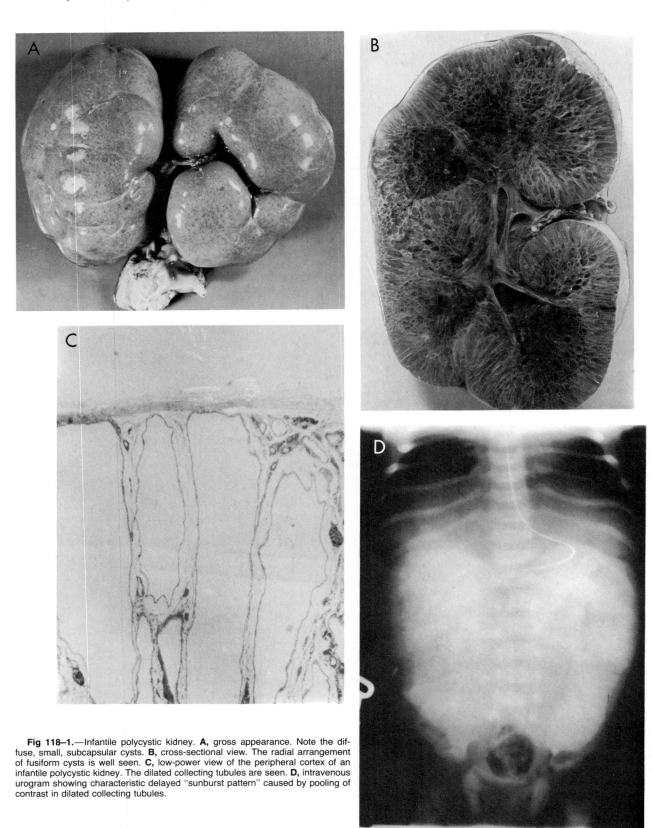

Fig 118–1.—Infantile polycystic kidney. **A,** gross appearance. Note the diffuse, small, subcapsular cysts. **B,** cross-sectional view. The radial arrangement of fusiform cysts is well seen. **C,** low-power view of the peripheral cortex of an infantile polycystic kidney. The dilated collecting tubules are seen. **D,** intravenous urogram showing characteristic delayed "sunburst pattern" caused by pooling of contrast in dilated collecting tubules.

polycystic disease can pass undiagnosed until childhood. There is an inverse correlation of the degree of renal and hepatic involvement. The older the age at diagnosis, the more likely that the presenting symptom will be one of the complications of liver disease (cirrhosis) rather than renal problems (renal mass, hypertension, renal failure). Lieberman et al.[63] do not believe there is a spectrum of infantile polycystic disease. Instead, they imply that all children are equally affected. Those who survive infancy undergo radiologic and histologic changes of the kidney to the point where it is difficult to differentiate the kidneys histologically from adult polycystic kidneys. They noted that the fusiform cysts were rounded and irregular.

Initially, the newborn with infantile polycystic kidneys requires respiratory care and management of renal insufficiency. In the future, dialysis and renal transplantation will have to be considered. However, the clinician must remember that the longer the survival, the greater the chance that the patient will suffer the complications of cirrhosis.

Adult Polycystic Kidney Disease (Autosomal Dominant)

This condition is the most common form of cystic disease in humans, occurring once in every 1,250 live births, and accounting for about 10% of all end-stage renal disease.[37] The disease typically presents after the age of 40 with flank pain, hematuria, hypertension, pyelonephritis, nephrocalcinosis, or progressive renal failure. Although Landing et al.[62] did not see presymptomatic adult polycystic disease in any of the more than 5,000 consecutive autopsies done on infants and children, computerized tomography (CT) and sonography can reveal cysts as small as 0.3 cm in size,[45, 89] and this condition is now being diagnosed more often and managed early in life.[72] There are reports of autosomal dominant polycystic disease in children[18, 54, 70, 94] that clearly justify the use of the term "adult polycystic disease." The intravenous urogram characteristically shows renal enlargement with distortion of the caliceal pattern by spherical cysts of varying sizes. Section of the kidneys confirms the presence of rounded or irregular cysts in all parts of the nephron.

The pattern of this disease in childhood has raised the question of whether adult polycystic kidney disease presents with a spectrum of functional severity as well. Patients have reportedly died in childhood from uremia[18] and myocardial infarction;[70] cerebrovascular accidents have occurred.[82]

Adult polycystic disease differs from infantile polycystic disease in its mode of inheritance, which is autosomal dominant, its radiologic and histologic appearance, and the less common involvement of the liver (a third have cysts, but cirrhosis is not seen). Although not seen in infantile polycystic renal disease, about a third of patients with adult polycystic renal disease have intracranial berry aneurysms that are an important cause of death before end-stage renal disease has developed.

Treatment of the childhood presentation of adult polycystic disease includes genetic counseling and management of hypertension, congestive cardiac failure, and renal failure. Dialysis and renal transplantation are rarely necessary before adulthood.

Multilocular Cysts of the Kidney

A problem in reviewing this disease is the confusing terminology that has been used in the past, i.e., polycystic nephroblastoma, benign multilocular cystic nephroma, focal or partial polycystic kidney, lymphangioma, and cystadenoma. As with adult polycystic disease, patients with multilocular cysts of the kidney are being reported more frequently. There are two peak ages of incidence: boys in childhood and women in adulthood.[68] There is no familial tendency. Although the lesion is usually unilateral, bilateral cases have been reported.[23] Potter[73] considers this disease to be a segmental dysplasia, but other authors[19, 24, 97, 98] believe that it is tumorous and possibly neoplastic.

Patients with this disease usually present with an abdominal or flank mass, which may be asymptomatic. More than half of the reported patients are less than 4 years of age,[6] and the disease has been reported in infants.[97, 98] The intravenous urogram generally reveals a unilateral renal mass, which may be polar and which distorts the collecting system.[7] Isotope and ultrasound studies do not yield specific diagnostic features. Renal angiography demonstrates a relatively avascular, well-delineated mass. However, Austin and Castellino[4] found neovascularity in four of nine patients studied by angiography.

The tumors are round, well encapsulated and noninfiltrating, distorting and displacing normal renal tissue (Fig 118–2). The cut surface of the kidney may have a cyst-within-cyst configuration.[58] Microscopically, the cysts are lined by uniform, flattened-to-cuboidal epithelial cells. The components of the septal stroma vary from small, round, primitive cells to elongated, mature fibroblasts and occasional smooth muscle cells.[19, 81] Some authors, confronted with such atypia of the stroma, have diagnosed malignancy, i.e., Wilms tumor.[24, 97, 98] Renal cell carcinoma has been reported also.[25, 77, 78] Despite these interpretations, no multilocular cyst has been demonstrated to exhibit malignant behavior.

The inability to make an accurate preoperative diagnosis of multilocular cystic disease necessitates exploration of the affected kidney. Although a nephrectomy is usually performed if the diagnosis is suspected, enucleation of the multilocular mass constitutes adequate treatment. Chemotherapy and irradiation are inappropriate.

Simple Cysts

Simple cysts can be single or multiple and are usually situated in the cortex of the kidney. In childhood, this disease is rare,[29, 49, 84] but Kissane and Smith[57] state that 50% of adults over age 50 years have simple cysts, suggesting that simple renal cysts are an acquired disease. They may be retention cysts developing in persistent early rudimentary glomeruli or may result from tubular obstruction from inflammation or local ischemia.[90] Males are affected more frequently than females. There is a higher in-

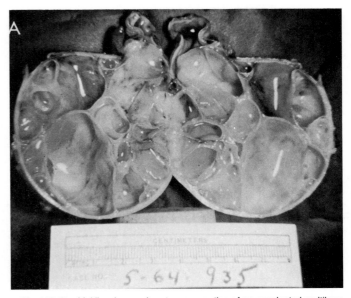

Fig 118–2.—Multilocular renal cyst: cross-section of an enucleated multilocular cyst. Note thick capsule and characteristic overall round configuration.

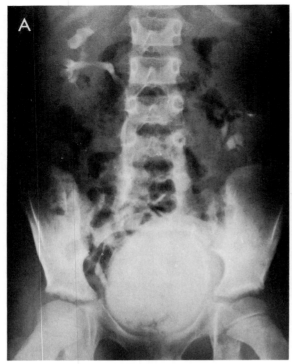

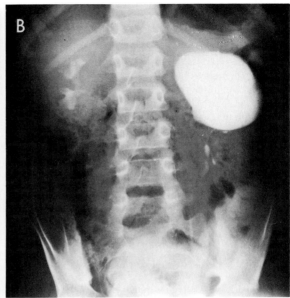

Fig 118–3.—Simple renal cyst. **A,** intravenous pyelogram shows lucent, spherical shadow and caliceal displacement. **B,** puncture of the cyst and instillation of contrast material demonstrate the large, smooth-walled cyst. A simple cyst, diagnosed by ultrasonography, pyelography, or contrast injection (rarely needed), may be ignored, or at most merely unroofed.

cidence of the disease in the left kidney. The disease is not familial.

Simple cysts are often diagnosed during the evaluation of an abdominal mass or flank pain or may be found incidentally during an intravenous urogram.[59] Hypertension has been reported.[5] Included in the differential diagnosis of a space-occupying lesion are Wilms tumor, duplication anomalies of the upper tract, and multilocular cysts. In addition to an intravenous urogram, tomogram, isotope and ultrasound studies, cyst puncture, and injection of contrast material (Fig 118–3), selective renal angiography may be necessary (rarely) for complete evaluation.[9, 41] If the diagnosis of a simple cyst can be made on the basis of these investigations, the cyst can be followed or treated by simple aspiration. If treatment is operative, unroofing of the cyst is adequate. Nephrectomy is not indicated unless the adjacent renal parenchyma has insufficient function.[29]

Caliceal Diverticula (Pyelogenic Cysts)

Caliceal diverticula usually are small and situated at one pole of the kidney. They are lined by transitional epithelium and communicate by a narrow connection with the fornix of a calix (the upper calix most commonly).[100] They are sporadic, usually unilateral, and uncommon in childhood.[39, 99] They may be associated with vesicoureteral reflux.[1]

Most caliceal diverticula are diagnosed incidentally on intravenous urography. Occasionally, a narrowed connection to the calix may lead to stasis, stone formation, or infection, which in turn may cause symptoms. Operation is rarely necessary and is indicated only for symptomatic patients. The caliceal diverticulum is resected either by wedge excision or partial nephrectomy. Intraoperative ultrasound may assist in locating the diverticulum if the overlying parenchyma is normal.

Medullary Sponge Kidney (Medullary Tubular Ectasia)

It is uncommon for this disease to be diagnosed in childhood. Although some authors believe this is a genetically transmitted

disease,[26, 83] in most cases, there is no family history and the mode of inheritance (if inheritance indeed exists) remains to be determined.

Medullary sponge kidney is often diagnosed incidentally on intravenous urography carried out in a patient with ureteral colic, hematuria, or urinary tract infection. The radiologic appearance is one of marked enlargement of the collecting tubules, giving the impression of a bunch of flowers. Tiny cysts, 1–5 mm in diameter, are seen occasionally within the renal pyramids. The disease is bilateral in more than 75% of patients.[60] In some patients, the disease is demonstrated only within one papilla of the kidney.[43] Nephrocalcinosis can be seen in the medullary pyramids of about half the patients[60] and may lead to the symptomatic passage of calculi.

Microdissection[73] has shown a diffuse and uniform enlargement of the collecting ducts. The renal cortex and glomerular filtration are normal in the absence of stones or infection.

Treatment is directed toward management of the complications of the disease, i.e., calculi and urinary tract infection.

Renal Dysplasia (Dysgenesis)

Renal dysplasia is a histologic diagnosis that describes the presence of primitive metanephric structures within the kidney.[12, 31, 33, 86] Tubules lined by primitive epithelium and surrounded by swirls of mesenchyme constitute the most specific histologic feature of renal dysplasia (Fig 118–4). Other structures such as primitive glomeruli, tubules, and foci of hyaline cartilage may be seen, but they are not unique to the dysplastic kidney.[12, 95]

In the past, the term "renal dysplasia" has been used too broadly, especially when describing the appearance of bizarre pelvicaliceal systems. The result was the erroneous impression that histologic renal dysplasia can be diagnosed from an x-ray film. To the present, no publication supports this belief. To resolve this false assumption, Williams[99] recommended the term "renal dysmorphism" to describe the radiologic appearance of bizarre pelvicaliceal systems.

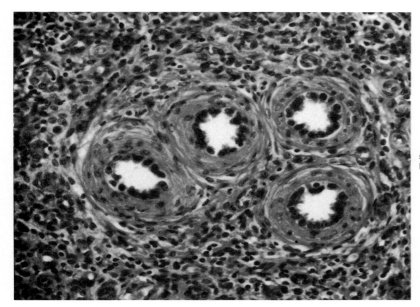

Fig 118–4.—Renal dysplasia. Primitive tubules surrounded by swirls of mesenchyme are the pathologic hallmark of this diagnosis.

Renal dysplasia may involve the kidney totally, segmentally, or focally. Further, the dysplasia can be subdivided into solid and cystic varieties. Usually, renal dysplasia is associated with an obstructive anomaly of the urinary tract, i.e., urethral valves, ureteroceles, ectopic ureters, or ureteropelvic junction obstructions.[33, 86] Uncommonly, renal dysplasia can be seen in kidneys associated with ureteral reflux.[34, 66, 67] Potter[80] has seen undeniable renal dysplasia in the complete absence of any distal obstruction of the urinary tract. Except for the rare patient with familial renal dysplasia,[12, 15] there appears to be no pattern of inheritance of the disease.

Theories of the development of renal dysplasia include the possibilities of teratogenic causes[80] and congenital distal obstruction.[34, 40] Maizels and Simpson[69] produced histologic dysplasia by denuding the ureteral bud of metanephric mesenchyme, suggesting that a nonobstructive phenomenon may be important. Another interesting theory was proposed by Mackie and Stephens,[66, 67] which maintains that dysplasia is the result of either a high or low origin of the ureteric bud from the wolffian duct. The ureter then grows into metanephric tissue which lacks the potential for normal renal development, leading to the formation of a dysplastic kidney.

Pyelonephritis is said to be more common in patients with dysplastic kidneys,[31, 76] but the association has been questioned by others.[33, 86]

Multicystic Kidney

Multicystic kidney is the classic example of renal dysplasia. It is the most common renal cystic disease of the newborn[58] and is considered to be either the most common or the second most common abdominal mass in the newborn.[64, 71]

Schwartz[88] was the first to propose the term "multicystic kidney." In 1955, Spence[91] described the specific features of the multicystic kidney and emphasized the need to distinguish it from the other cystic diseases of the kidney. Previously, misnomers such as "congenital polycystic kidney disease" and "unilateral polycystic kidney disease" were commonly applied to this condition.

Although the etiology of the multicystic kidney remains to be proved, Stephens[93] suggests that, in the migration of the developing kidney from the sacral to the lumbar level, the normal shift

of vasculature may not occur, leading to an ischemic insult producing both the multicystic kidney and the usually associated ureteral atresia. In the past, the disease usually presented as a unilateral flank mass. At present, an increasing number of cases are being detected by antenatal fetal ultrasound performed for obstetric indications. Careful palpation can reveal an irregular, bosselated surface caused by the cysts, which typically feel like a bunch of grapes. Transillumination indicates the mass to be lucent. However, a cystic hydronephrotic kidney also transmits light. Not all multicystic kidneys are found in the lumbar area; there are reports of the kidney in a pelvic location as well.[74, 75] Multicystic kidney disease carries no sex or racial predilection and is not familial. The left kidney is more commonly involved than the right.[33] Even though Spence[91] stressed the unilaterality of the multicystic kidney, there are reports of the disease being bilateral.[42, 52, 80] Obviously, children with bilateral multicystic kidneys are either stillborn or die early in the neonatal period.

Today, investigation of a patient with suspected multicystic kidney often begins with a renal ultrasound examination, which is often diagnostic[11] (Fig 118–5,*C*). An intravenous pyelogram or renal scan fails to demonstrate the affected kidney. There are exceptions, though; Kaplan and Miller[53] have seen a multicystic kidney become visible 24–48 hours after injection of contrast material. A urogram is done as well to assess the status of the contralateral upper tract, which has a 20% or greater chance of being abnormal.[33, 42, 74, 75] Interestingly, if the ureteral atresia is low,[28] or if the multicystic kidney is small,[22] there is an increased likelihood of contralateral abnormality. The lower urinary tract should also be evaluated with a voiding cystogram because it is subject to a greater than normal incidence of anomalies.[33]

Contrary to one report,[61] we and most others do not believe that cystoscopy and retrograde pyelography and/or angiography are necessary. Computerized axial tomography requires an anesthetic in an infant and usually adds little useful diagnostic information.

Multicystic kidneys differ in size and external appearance. Grossly, the kidney shows a number of cysts, ranging in size from a few millimeters to several centimeters (Fig 118–5,*A*). The renal artery is usually atretic. Sectioning the kidney most often shows a random arrangement of noncommunicating cysts. Occasionally, there is a more solid central core (Fig 118–5,*B*). Histologically, primitive structures suggesting abortive nephrogenesis

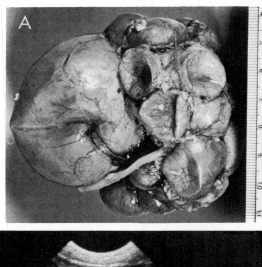

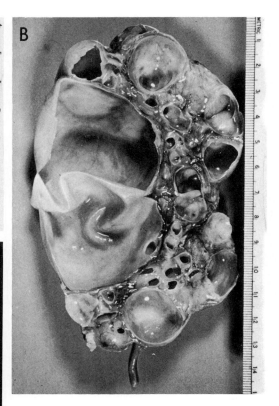

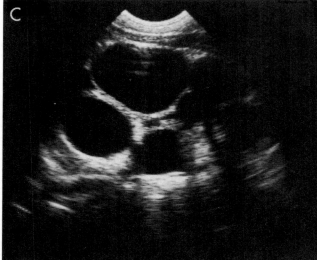

Fig 118–5.—Unilateral multicystic kidney. **A**, external appearance of a multicystic kidney and its atretic ureter. Notice the variations in cyst size. **B**, cross-sectional appearance. **C**, ultrasound of multicystic kidney. Note random arrangement of noncommunicating cysts. The commonest retroperitoneal mass in the newborn, it is usually resected electively—our preference.

are seen within a stroma that is cellular and loosely arranged. Cartilage may be present. The kidney is totally abnormal, unlike the multilocular cystic kidney.

Virtually every multicystic kidney has ureteral atresia, which can be found anywhere along the course of the ureter. Cystoscopy usually reveals a ureteric orifice in a normal location and retrograde pyelography (if performed) confirms a blind-ending ureter. Less commonly, the cystoscopy may only show a ureteral dimple or no orifice at all.[35]

In the past, most children with a multicystic kidney underwent exploration to rule out a nonfunctioning renal tumor or a severe ureteropelvic junction obstruction with little renal function. Today, the diagnosis of a multicystic kidney is usually established without operation. As the child grows, most multicystic kidneys become relatively smaller and many actually shrink in size. This then raises the issue of whether these kidneys need to be removed. Although rare, hypertension in childhood has been associated with a multicystic kidney.[51] Malignant renal neoplasms have arisen later in life in multicystic kidneys.[8, 46] Other adults with multicystic kidneys have presented with a mass, local pain, hematuria, urinary tract infection, and hypertension.[2] It is not clear how many asymptomatic adults may harbor a missed multicystic kidney. Our view, which is in accord with that of most surgeons performing urologic operations in children,[17] is that removal of multicystic kidneys is prudent. We usually do this electively at 6–12 months of age.

Renal Agenesis

Renal agenesis must be differentiated from renal aplasia; the latter refers to an extremely rudimentary kidney with severe corticomedullary dysplasia. The aplastic kidney is devoid of normal gross architectural arrangement, but histologic study may demonstrate a few well-differentiated nephrons. Renal agenesis is the complete absence of any identifiable renal tissue. Agenesis can be unilateral or bilateral. Usually, the ureter on the affected side is absent or atretic. It is difficult to be precise about the incidence of unilateral renal agenesis because there are differences between autopsy[20] and urography series. Nevertheless, a reasonable incidence seems to be between 1 in 500 and 1 in 1,000 at autopsy.[65]

Unilateral agenesis occurs with greater frequency than bilateral renal agenesis. The diagnosis is usually made incidentally during intravenous urography. Contralateral anomalies have a greater than normal incidence.[27, 30]

The question arises as to how completely a patient with a solitary, hypertrophied, but otherwise normal kidney should be evaluated. Tomography, ultrasonography, and isotope studies may be necessary. If these tests confirm renal agenesis, cystoscopy and retrograde pyelography are difficult to justify.

In girls, unilateral renal agenesis is well known to be associated with anomalies of the genital tract.[44] The most common anomaly is a unicornuate or bicornuate uterus.[96] Absence or aplasia of the vagina and absence or hypoplasia of the Fallopian tubes and ovaries are known to occur. Kelalis[55] reports that a significant number of genital anomalies are found in boys who have been diagnosed as having unilateral renal agenesis. These anomalies affect the penis, testes, and seminal vesicles.

Bilateral renal agenesis is incompatible with survival. The infant is either stillborn or dies in the early neonatal period from pulmonary insufficiency or uremia. Typical Potter facies is seen.[79] The bladder is either atretic or dysplastic. Anomalies of other organ systems are reported.[3, 21]

REFERENCES

1. Amar A.D.: The clinical significance of renal caliceal diverticulum in children: Relation to vesicoureteral reflux. *J. Urol.* 113:255, 1975.
2. Ambrose S.S., Gould R.A., Trulock T.S., et al.: Unilateral multicystic renal disease in adults. *J. Urol.* 128:366, 1982.
3. Ashley D.J.B., Mostofi F.K.: Renal agenesis and dysgenesis. *J. Urol.* 83:211, 1960.
4. Austin S.R., Castellino R.A.: Multilocular cysts of the kidney. *Urology* 1:546, 1973.
5. Babka J.C., Cohen M.S., Sode J.: Solitary intrarenal cyst causing hypertension. *N. Engl. J. Med.* 291:343, 1974.
6. Baldauf M.C., Schultz D.M.: Multilocular cyst of the kidney: Report of three cases with review of the literature. *Am. J. Clin. Pathol.* 65:93, 1976.
7. Banner M.P., Pollack H.M., Chatten J., et al.: Multilocular renal cysts: Radiologic-pathologic correlation. *A.J.R.* 136:239, 1981.
8. Barrett D.M., Wineland R.E.: Renal cell carcinoma in multicystic dysplastic kidney. *Urology* 15:152, 1980.
9. Bartone F.F., Mazer M.J., Anderson J.C. et al.: Diagnosis and treatment of fluid-filled renal structures in children with ultrasonography and percutaneous puncture. *Urology* 16:432, 1980.
10. Baskin G.B., Roberts J.A., McAfee R.D.: Infantile polycystic renal disease in a rhesus monkey (Macaca mulatta). *Lab. Anim. Sci.* 31:181, 1981.
11. Bearman S.B., Hine P.L., Sanders R.C.: Multicystic kidney: A sonographic pattern. *Radiology* 118:685, 1976.
12. Bernstein J.: Developmental abnormalities of the renal parenchyma—renal hypoplasia and dysplasia. *Pathobiol. Annu.* 3:213, 1968.
13. Bernstein J.: The classification of renal cysts. *Nephron* 11:91, 1973.
14. Bernstein J., Kissane J.M.: Hereditary disorders of the kidney. *Perspect. Pediatr. Pathol.* 1:117, 1973.
15. Bernstein J., et al.: The renal lesion in syndromes of multiple congenital malformations. *Birth Defects* 10:35, 1974.
16. Bernstein J.: A classification of renal cysts. *Perspect. Nephrol. Hypertens.* 4:7, 1976.
17. Bloom D.A., Brosman S.: The multicystic kidney. *J. Urol.* 120:211, 1978.
18. Blyth H., Ockenden B.G.: Polycystic disease of kidneys and liver presenting in childhood. *J. Med. Genet.* 8:257, 1971.
19. Boggs L.K., Kimmelstiel P.: Benign multilocular cystic nephroma: Report of two cases of so-called multilocular cyst of the kidney. *J. Urol.* 76:530, 1956.
20. Campbell M.F.: Congenital absence of one kidney: Unilateral renal agenesis. *Ann. Surg.* 88:1039, 1928.
21. Campbell M.F., Harrison J.H.: *Urology*, ed. 2. Philadelphia, W.B. Saunders Co., 1970.
22. Cendron J., Gubler J.P., Valayer J., et al.: Dysplasie multikystique du rein chez l'enfant. *J. Urol. Nephrol.* 79:773, 1973.
23. Chatten J., Bishop H.C.: Bilateral multilocular cysts of the kidneys. *J. Pediatr. Surg.* 12:749, 1977.
24. Christ M.L.: Polycystic nephroblastoma. *J. Urol.* 98:570, 1968.
25. Cole A.T., Gill W.B.: Dual renal cell carcinoma in a unilateral polycystic kidney. *J. Urol.* 109:182, 1973.
26. Copping G.A.: Medullary sponge kidney: Its occurrence in a father and daughter. *Can. Med. Assoc. J.* 96:608, 1967.
27. Dees J.E.: Prognosis of the solitary kidney. *J. Urol.* 83:550, 1960.
28. DeKlerk D.P., Marshall F.F., Jeffs R.D.: Multicystic dysplastic kidney. *J. Urol.* 118:306, 1977.
29. DeWeerd J.H., Simon H.B.: Simple renal cysts in children: Review of the literature and report of five cases. *J. Urol.* 75:912, 1956.
30. Emmanuel B., Nachman R., Aronson N., et al.: Congenital solitary kidney: A review of 74 cases. *Am. J. Dis. Child.* 127:17, 1974.
31. Ericsson N.O., Ivemark B.I.: Renal dysplasia and pyelonephritis in infants and children I and II. *Arch. Pathol.* 66:255, 1958.
32. Filmer R.B., Caron F.A., Rowland R.G., et al.: Adrenal corticosteroid-induced renal cystic disease in the newborn hamster. *Am. J. Pathol.* 72:461, 1973.
33. Filmer R.B., Taxy J.B., King L.R.: Renal dysplasia: Clinicopathological study. *Trans. Am. Assoc. Genitourin. Surg.* 66:18, 1974.
34. Filmer R.B., Taxy J.B.: Cysts of the kidney, renal dysplasia and renal hypoplasia, in Kelalis P.P., King L.R. (eds.): *Clinical Pediatric Urology*. Philadelphia, W.B. Saunders Co., 1976.
35. Fine M.G., Burns E.: Unilateral multicystic kidney: Report of six cases and discussion of the literature. *J. Urol.* 81:42, 1959.
36. Gardner K.D. Jr.: Juvenile nephronophthisis and renal medullary cystic disease, in Gardner K.D. Jr.: *Cystic Diseases of the Kidney.* New York, John Wiley & Sons, 1976, pp. 173–185.
37. Gardner K.D., Evan A.P.: Cystic kidneys: An enigma evolves. *Am. J. Kid. Dis.* 3:403, 1984.
38. Gardner K.D. Jr.: Juvenile nephronophthisis and renal medullary cystic disease. *Perspect. Nephrol. Hypertens.* 4:173, 1976.
39. Gleason D.C., McAlister W.H., Kissane J.: Cystic disease of the kidney in children. *Am. J. Roentgenol.* 100:135, 1967.
40. Glick P.L., Harrison M.R., Noall R.A., et al.: Correction of congenital hydronephrosis in utero. III. Early mid-trimester ureteral obstruction produces renal dysplasia. *J. Pediatr. Surg.* 18:681, 1983.
41. Gordon R.L., Pollack H.M., Popky G.L., et al.: Simple serous cysts of the kidney in children. *Radiology* 131:357, 1979.
42. Greene L.F., Feinzaig W., Dahlin D.C. Multicystic dysplasia of the kidney: With special reference to the contralateral kidney. *J. Urol.* 105:482, 1971.
43. Greene L.F., Barrett D.M.: Renal cystic disease: Radiological appearance. *Perspect. Nephrol. Hypertens.* 4:91, 1976.
44. Griffin J.E., Edwards C., Madden J.D., et al.: Congenital absence of the vagina. *Ann. Intern. Med.* 85:224, 1976.
45. Grossman H., Rosenberg E.R., Bowie J.D., et al.: Sonographic diagnosis of renal cystic disease. *AJR* 140:81, 1983.
46. Gutter W., Hermanek P.: Maligner Tumor der Nierengegend unter dem Bilde der Knollenniere. *Urol. Int.* 4:164, 1957.
47. Habib R.: Nephronophthisis and medullary cystic disease, in Strauss J. (ed.): *Pediatric Nephrology: Current Concepts in Diagnosis and Management.* New York, Intercontinental Medical Book Corp., 1974.
48. Hildegrand O.: Weiterer Beitrag zur Pathologischen Anatomie der Nierengeschwulste. (Additional contribution concerning the pathological anatomy of cystic disease of the kidney.) *Arch. Klin. Chir.* 48:343, 1894.
49. Holl W.H., Delporto G.B., Keegan G.T., et al.: Case report: Simple renal cyst in child. *J. Urol.* 115:465, 1976.
50. Iverson W.O., Fetterman G.H., Jacobson E.R., et al.: Polycystic kidney and liver disease in the springbok. I. Morphology of the lesions. *Kidney Int.* 22:146, 1982.
51. Javadpour N., Chelouhy E., Moncada L., et al.: Hypertension in a child caused by a multicystic kidney. *J. Urol.* 104:918, 1970.
52. Johannessen J.V., et al.: Bilateral multicystic dysplasia of the kidneys. *Beitr. Pathol.* 148:290, 1973.
53. Kaplan G.W., Miller K.E.: Unpublished data.
54. Kaye C., Lewy P.R.: Congenital appearance of adult-type (autosomal dominant) polycystic kidney disease: Report of a case. *J. Pediatr.* 85:807, 1974.
55. Kelalis P.P.: Anomalies of the urinary tract, in Kelalis P.P., King L.R. (eds.): *Clinical Pediatric Urology.* Philadelphia, W.B. Saunders Co., 1976.
56. Kendall A.R., Pollack H.M., Karafin L.: Congenital cystic disease of the kidney: Classification and manifestations. *Urology* 4:635, 1974.
57. Kissane J.M., Smith M.G.: *Pathology of Infancy and Childhood.* St. Louis, C.V. Mosby Company, 1967.
58. Kissane J.M.: Congenital malformations, in Heptinstall J. (ed.): *Pathology of the Kidney*, ed. 2. Boston, Little, Brown & Co., 1974.
59. Kramer S.A., Hoffman A.D., Aydin G., et al.: Simple renal cysts in children. *J. Urol.* 128:1259, 1982.
60. Kuiper J.J.: Medullary sponge kidney. *Perspect. Nephrol. Hypertens.* 4:151, 1976.
61. Kyaw M.M., Koehler P.R.: Congenital multicystic kidney. *Perspect. Nephrol. Hypertens.* 4:115, 1976.
62. Landing B.H., Gwinn J.L., Lieberman E.: Cystic diseases of the kidney in children. *Perspect. Nephrol. Hypertens.* 4:187, 1976.
63. Lieberman E., Salinas-Madrigal L., Gwinn J.L., et al.: Infantile polycystic disease of the kidneys and liver: Clinical, pathological and radiological correlations and comparison with congenital hepatic fibrosis. *Medicine* 50:277, 1971.
64. Longino L.A., Martin L.W.: Abdominal masses in the newborn infant. *Pediatrics* 21:596, 1958.
65. Longo V.J., Thompson G.J.: Congenital solitary kidney. *J. Urol.* 68:63, 1952.
66. Mackie G.G., Awang H., Stephens F.D.: The ureteric orifice: The embryological key to radiologic status of duplex kidneys. *J. Pediatr. Surg.* 10:473, 1975.

67. Mackie G.G., Stephens F.D.: Duplex kidneys: A correlation of renal dysplasia with position of the ureteral orifice. *J. Urol.* 114:274, 1975.
68. Madewell J.E., Goldman S.M., Davis C.J., et al.: Multilocular cystic nephroma. *Radiology* 146:309, 1983.
69. Maizels M., Simpson S.B.: Primitive ducts of renal dysplasia induced by culturing ureteral buds denuded of condensed renal mesenchyme. *Science* 21:509, 1983.
70. Mehrizi A., Rosenstein B.J., Pusch A., et al.: Myocardial infarction and endocardial fibroelastosis in children with polycystic kidneys. *Bull. Johns Hopkins Hosp.* 115:92, 1964.
71. Melicow M.M., Uson A.C.: Palpable abdominal masses in infants and children: A report based on a review of 653 cases. *J. Urol.* 81:705, 1959.
72. Milutinovic J., Phillips I.A., Bryant J.L., et al.: Autosomal dominant polycystic kidney disease: Early diagnosis and data for genetic counselling. *Lancet* 1:1203, 1980.
73. Osathanondh V., Potter E.L.: Pathogenesis of polycystic kidneys: Historical survey. *Arch. Pathol.* 77:459, 1964.
74. Parkkulainen K.V., Hjelt L., Sirola K.: Congenital multicystic dysplasia of kidney: Report of nineteen cases with discussion of the etiology, nomenclature and classification of the cystic dysplasias of the kidney. *Acta Chir. Scand.* (suppl.) 244:5, 1959.
75. Pathak I.G., Williams D.I.: Multicystic and cystic dysplastic kidneys. *Br. J. Urol.* 36:318, 1964.
76. Perrin E.V., Persky L., Tucker A., et al.: Renal duplication and dysplasia. *Urology* 4:660, 1974.
77. Pfister R.C., Galli S.J.: Multicystic renal mass in a 43-year-old woman (Case records of the Massachusetts General Hospital). *N. Engl. J. Med.* 292:415, 1975.
78. Posso M., Safadi D., Van Dyk O.J.: Unilateral polycystic or multicystic kidney associated with focal mural renal cell carcinoma: Presentation of a case. *J. Urol.* 109:559, 1973.
79. Potter E.L.: Facial characteristics of infants with bilateral renal agenesis. *Am. J. Obstet. Gynecol.* 51:885, 1946.
80. Potter E.L.: *Normal and Abnormal Development of the Kidney.* Chicago, Year Book Medical Publishers, 1972.
81. Powell T.: Multilocular cysts of the kidney. *Br. J. Urol.* 23:142, 1951.
82. Proesmans W., Van Damme B., Casaer P., et al.: Autosomal dominant polycystic kidney disease in neonatal period: Association with a cerebral arteriovenous malformation. *Pediatrics* 70:971, 1982.
83. Pyrah L.N.: Medullary sponge kidney. *J. Urol.* 95:274, 1966.
84. Redman J.F., Scriber L.J., Bissada N.K.: Simple renal cyst in a child. *J. Pediatr. Surg.* 11:117, 1976.
85. Resnick J.S., Brown D.M., Vernier R.L.: Normal development and experimental models of cystic renal disease. *Perspect. Nephrol. Hypertens.* 4:221, 1976.
86. Risdon R.A.: Renal dysplasia. I. A clinicopathological study of 76 cases. *J. Clin. Pathol.* 24:57, 1971.
87. Royer P.: Malformations of the kidney. *Major Probl. Clin. Pediatr.* 11:9, 1974.
88. Schwartz J.: An unusual unilateral multicystic kidney in an infant. *J. Urol.* 35:259, 1936.
89. Segal A.J., Spataro R.F.: Computed tomography of adult polycystic disease. *J. Comput. Assist. Tomogr.* 6:777, 1982.
90. Siegel M.J., McAlister W.H.: Simple cysts of the kidney in children. *J. Urol.* 123:75, 1980.
91. Spence H.M.: Congenital unilateral multicystic kidney: An entity to be distinguished from polycystic kidney disease and other cystic disorders. *J. Urol.* 74:693, 1955.
92. Spence H.M., Singleton R.: Cysts and cystic disorders of the kidney: Types, diagnosis, treatment. *Urol. Survey* 22:131, 1972.
93. Stephens F.D.: *Congenital Malformations of the Urinary Tract.* New York, Praeger, 1983, p. 195.
94. Stickler G.B., Kelalis P.P.: Polycystic kidney disease: A recognition of the "adult form" (autosomal dominant) in infancy. *Mayo Clin. Proc.* 50:547, 1975.
95. Taxy J.B., Filmer R.B.: Metaplastic cartilage in nondysplastic kidneys. *Arch. Pathol.* 99:101, 1975.
96. Thompson D.P., Lynn H.B.: Genital anomalies associated with solitary kidney. *Mayo Clin. Proc.* 41:538, 1966.
97. Uson A.C., Del Rosario C., Melicow M.M.: Wilms' tumor in association with cystic renal disease: Report of two cases. *J. Urol.* 83:262, 1960.
98. Uson A.C., Melicow M.M.: Multilocular cysts of kidney with intrapelvic herniation of a "daughter" cyst: Report of 4 cases. *J. Urol.* 89:341, 1963.
99. Williams D.I.: *Urology in Childhood.* New York, Springer-Verlag, 1974.
100. Wulfsohn M.A.: Pyelocaliceal diverticula. *J. Urol.* 123:1, 1980.

119   W. Hardy Hendren / Patricia K. Donahoe

Renal Fusions and Ectopia

Several malformations of clinical importance result from failure of normal renal embryogenesis. These include horseshoe kidney, crossed renal ectopia, pelvic kidney and lump or discoid kidney.

Embryology

The ureters arise as buds from the wolffian duct at the 5–8-mm stage of the embryo (end of the fourth week of gestation). The ureteric buds join the developing metanephrogenic masses in the pelvis and ascend as the retroperitoneum elongates. During ascent, each kidney rotates from its original position with the renal pelvis pointing anteriorly to its final position with the pelvis located medially. If ascent of the kidney is arrested by failure of absorption of the primitive vessels or arrest in development of the metanephric mass, the kidney remains in the pelvis and fails to rotate.[9]

The two renal masses may fuse across the midline. If one metanephric mass is larger than the other, it can ascend more rapidly, pulling up with it a smaller renal mass from the opposite side; this results in crossed fused ectopia. In crossed ectopia the better renal moiety tends to occupy the upper pole. The crossed fused moiety is smaller and positioned at the lower pole. Fusion with crossover occurs after the sensory nerves develop, so that pain from a stone in the upper ureter of a crossed renal unit in later life will be referred to the normal sensory distribution on the opposite side.[19]

During ascent of the kidney, the wolffian duct from which the ureter arose migrates caudally along the urogenital sinus, carrying the ureter with it to the bladder. Often, when there is an abnormality of upward migration and rotation of the kidney, there is simultaneously an abnormality of downward migration of the ureter into the urogenital sinus.

Horseshoe Kidney

Horseshoe kidney is the most common fusion defect encountered in clinical practice. In 95% of cases, the lower poles of the two kidneys are joined by a bridge of normal kidney tissue. Occasionally the bridge is fibrous tissue. In about 40% of cases the isthmus lies at the level of L-4, just beneath the origin of the inferior mesenteric artery. In 20% the isthmus is in the pelvis; in the rest it lies at the level of the lower poles of normally placed kidneys. The blood supply to a horseshoe kidney is usually anomalous, which must be borne in mind during operation. A small number of horseshoe kidneys have fusion at the upper poles. In horseshoe kidney there is failure of rotation of the kidney as well as fusion, so that the renal pelves are located anteriorly and are often extrarenal. Ureteral duplication is not uncommon. Campbell[3] placed the incidence of horseshoe kidney at 1 in 425 autopsies and noted that men are affected about 2½ times as often as women, although our clinical experience has been very different.

Horseshoe kidney can usually be diagnosed by intravenous pyelography (IVP); the kidneys are rotated and tilted so that the upper poles point outward and the lower poles point toward the spine. The classic operation described in the literature for horseshoe kidney has been division of the isthmus and outward fixation of the lower pole of each kidney. We have not encountered a case in childhood where this appeared necessary and have never performed such an operation. There have been several reviews of the problem of horseshoe kidney.[4, 8, 10, 14, 18, 20] Gutierrez[10] stressed that no permanent cure or relief of symptoms could be obtained without division of the isthmus, which was described in 1911. Culp and Winterringer[4] reported 106 patients aged 5–65 who underwent operation at the Mayo Clinic for horseshoe kidney from 1912 through 1963. More than half of the patients were in the third and fourth decades. Males predominated 4:1. Removal of half the horseshoe kidney was the commonest procedure. More than 60% of the patients had stones. Hydronephrosis was the next most common problem, due to ureteropelvic junction (UPJ) obstruction. The combination of symphysiotomy, pyeloplasty and nephropexy was recommended. Glenn[8] reported on 51 patients seen at Duke Hospital over a 25-year period from 1933 to 1958, with approximately equal sex distribution. Twelve of the 51 patients were operated on, usually for hydronephrosis and calculus formation. Correction involved division or section of the isthmus, nephropexy and pyeloplasty. Kölln et al[14] reported on 105 patients with horseshoe kidney, of whom 18% required operation. Segura, Kelalis, and Burke,[20] in a review of 34 children in whom horseshoe kidney was diagnosed at the Mayo Clinic from 1935 to 1970, emphasized that vesicoureteral reflux was found in eight of 10 children investigated by cystography. Two thirds of the children required some surgical procedure. These authors stressed that diagnosis of horseshoe kidney should initiate a thorough urologic evaluation, including cystography and cystoscopy. Pitts and Muecke[18] described their experience with 170 patients with horseshoe kidney seen at the New York Hospital during a 40-year period. Hydronephrosis secondary to stones and/or UPJ obstruction was responsible for most of the operations. Foley Y-V pyeloplasty was successful in most cases of UPJ obstruction. The authors believed that advocacy of division of the isthmus was probably due to a slight improvement in drainage from the renal pelvis after an extensive dissection of connective tissue from around the UPJ, rather than any benefit from division of the isthmus per se.

Case Material

In the past 20 years our personal clinical case material has included 31 children with horseshoe kidney, ranging in age from newborn (eight were less than 1 year of age) to 18 years; 21 were females and only 10 were males. Horseshoe kidney was discovered during urinary evaluation for the following reasons: 17, infection; 2, hematuria; 3, abdominal pain; 4, abdominal mass (1 had Wilms tumor); 3, imperforate anus (1 of these had multiple anomalies, including esophageal atresia); 1, hypertension, and 1 case of urethral valves in an infant presenting with urinary ascites. All these children had a complete urologic investigation, including cystography. Ten had vesicoureteral reflux. In two, the reflux was minimal, not requiring ureteral reimplantation; the other eight underwent ureteral reimplantation. Of these, one had previous severe upper tract changes, eventually necessitating renal transplantation.

Primary UPJ obstruction was the most common anatomical malformation most often on the left side. Nine children had left pyeloplasty but no procedure on the right side, which drained normally. Two patients had bilateral pyeloplasty for bilateral ureteropelvic junction obstruction. One infant had UPJ atresia on the right side, presenting as an abdominal mass; right nephrectomy was performed; 6 years later left pyeloplasty was performed. One infant with hypertension had UPJ atresia on the left side, with a dysplastic renal moiety. Left nephrectomy cured the hypertension. Five children had urethral meatotomy for distal urethral narrowing. One boy with urethral valves, who as an infant had urinary ascites and had received an ileal loop, underwent urinary tract undiversion. In five patients, no operation was performed. One of these was an infant with multiple anomalies who died of enterocolitis with perforation of the bowel after colostomy for imperforate anus and division of tracheoesophageal fistula. The child with Wilms tumor underwent partial nephrectomy.

Examples of horseshoe kidney are shown in Figures 119–1 to 119–4. In cases with UPJ obstruction, there was high insertion of the ureter on the renal pelvis. In each case this was managed by either a long side-to-side anastomosis between the ureter and the adjacent renal pelvis (Fig 119–3) so that the functional UPJ was placed in a dependent position (Fig 119–4), or a standard dismembering pyeloplasty. Satisfactory drainage resulted in each case. Although in most cases of UPJ obstruction we favor dismembering pyeloplasty, this side-to-side nondismembering tech-

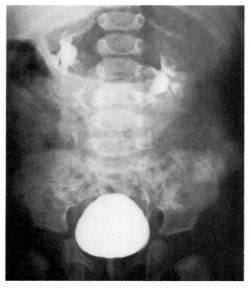

Fig 119–1.—Horseshoe kidney. Female infant with imperforate anus. Note duplex collecting system on the right; on the left there is rotation of the collecting system, and the upper pole is tipped outward. This patient had vesicoureteral reflux. Anoplasty was performed at 8 months of age, followed by colostomy closure. Ureteral reimplantation was performed at age 3 years because of persisting reflux and recurrent urinary infection. There was no ureteropelvic junction abnormality in this case.

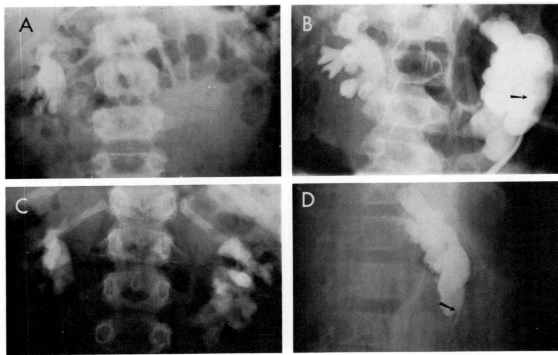

Fig 119–2.—Horseshoe kidney in a boy, 7 years old, with left ureteropelvic junction obstruction. The patient had sudden onset of left flank pain as presenting symptom. **A,** on preoperative IVP there is nonvisualization of left side. **B,** preoperative bilateral retrograde pyelogram shows high insertion of left ureter *(arrow)* and severe hydronephrosis. **C,** IVP 8 months after pyeloplasty shows satisfactory function and less left hydronephrosis. **D,** retrograde examination 8 months postoperatively showing dependent position of ureteropelvic junction *(arrow).*

nique can be used in some patients with horseshoe kidneys. Some authors have employed the Foley Y-V pyeloplasty with satisfactory results. We prefer a large direct anastomosis of the ureter to the renal pelvis in dependent position.

We have not encountered a case in which the ureter appeared in any way obstructed by the renal isthmus and, therefore, have not performed division of the isthmus. Long-term follow-up will be necessary to observe whether stone formation, so common in adult patients, will be a problem in later life despite apparently adequate pyeloplasty during childhood. No stones have been seen to date in these patients, half of whom have been operated on more than 10 years ago.

Our experience in horseshoe kidney leads us to agree completely with Segura, Kelalis and Burke[20] from the Mayo Clinic that all children with horseshoe kidney deserve complete urologic investigation. Like Pitts and Muecke,[18] we question whether division of the isthmus is of any benefit, at least in children.

Crossed Renal Ectopia

Crossed fused renal ectopia is a rare anomaly, estimated to occur in about 1 in 7,500 autopsies. An extensive review of the literature in 1947 disclosed only 384 cases.[1] Several authors have pointed out the presence of hydronephrosis, stones and infection in their series.[2, 15-17] In our experience, however, there is impor-

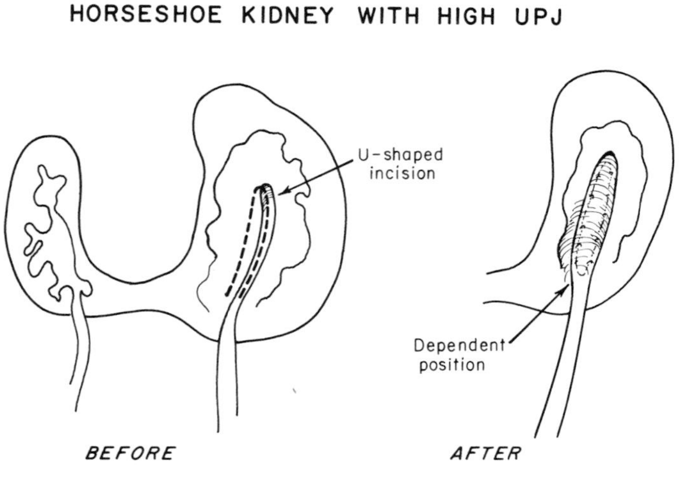

Fig 119–3.—Horseshoe kidney. Preoperative anatomy and technique for pyeloplasty in patient shown in Figure 119–2. It is just as satisfactory to dismember the actual ureteropelvic junction and to perform a larger, dependent anastomosis.

HORSESHOE KIDNEY WITH HIGH UPJ

U-shaped incision

Dependent position

BEFORE   *AFTER*

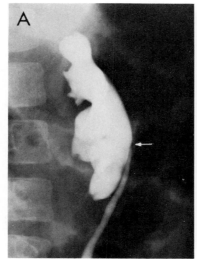

Fig 119–4.—Horseshoe kidney, left side, with high insertion of ureteropelvic junction. Right nephrectomy had been performed in neonatal period for ureteropelvic atresia. Left side was followed until age 6 years; there was increasing dilatation. **A,** preoperative retrograde pyelogram, oblique view to show high in- sertion of ureter on renal pelvis *(arrow).* **B,** antegrade pyelogram performed via temporary postoperative nephrostomy catheter 10 days after pyeloplasty. Note open ureteropelvic junction and its dependent position *(arrow).*

tant correctable lower tract pathology in the majority of cases in children.[13]

Case Material

Our clinical experience with crossed fused renal ectopia in children includes 21 cases in the past 20 years, nine of which have been described in detail;[13] 11 were boys and 10 were girls. Radial clubbed hand was seen in two patients, an association with crossed renal ectopia that has been reported previously. Nine of the patients did not require a major urologic reconstructive procedure. One of these, a male infant, had vesicoureteral reflux, which disappeared on prolonged follow-up. Two males had urethral valves, one with hypospadias. In 2 boys, the con-

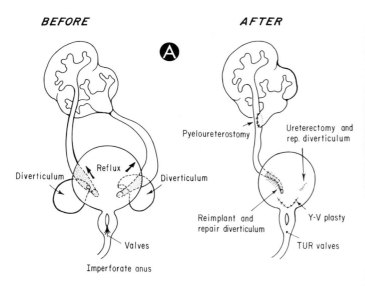

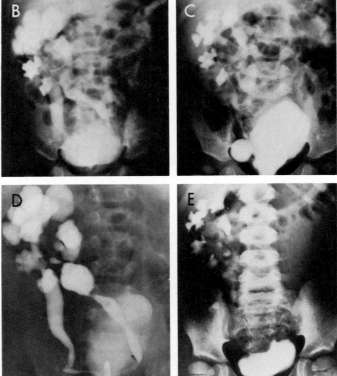

Fig 119–5.—Crossed renal ectopia, case 1: urethral valves and diverticula. **A,** preoperative and postoperative anatomy. **B,** preoperative IVP at age 6 months. **C,** 6 months after resection of valves, showing improvement in the upper tracts; reflux persisted. **D,** retrograde study showing upper tract anatomy and ureteropelvic junction stenosis of lower pole moiety. **E,** an IVP 3 years after reconstruction was completed.

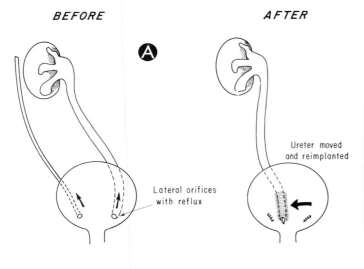

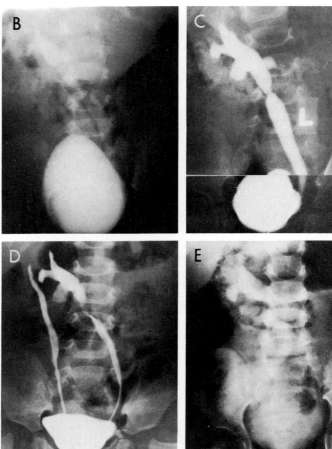

Fig 119–6.—Crossed renal ectopia, case 2: reflux and hydronephrosis. **A,** preoperative and postoperative anatomy. **B,** preoperative IVP. **C,** preoperative cystogram showing reflux up crossed ureter. There was minimal reflux into the other ureter on other films not shown here. **D,** preoperative retrograde examination. **E,** an IVP 18 months postoperatively.

dition was discovered incidentally during a screening IVP for cryptorchidism. The fifth, a female with esophageal atresia and multiple hemivertebrae, had distal urethral stenosis treated by meatotomy. The other three cases with noncomplicated crossed ectopia included two in whom the kidney was felt on abdominal examination and one girl who had a urogenital sinus defect that prompted study of the urinary tract.

The remaining 12 patients had other serious anomalies of the urinary tract requiring major reconstruction, some shown in Figures 119–5 to 119–11. Ectopic ureter was seen in seven patients; in two cases the ectopic ureter emptied into a seminal vesicle. Ureteropelvic junction obstruction was seen in five patients; five males had urethral valves. In one case the original pathology leading to the construction of an ileal loop was not known. Vesicoureteral reflux was seen in 13 of the 21 cases.

CASE 1.—A 5-month-old boy was referred for correction of an anal malformation. Urinary tract evaluation showed urethral valves, reflux, paraureteral diverticula, and crossed fused ectopia with UPJ stenosis (Fig 119–5). The urethral valves were destroyed endoscopically. At age 10 months, the bladder neck was incised endoscopically because the bladder was not emptying completely. At age 17 months, the lower renal pelvis was anastomosed to the right ureter to correct moderate ureteropelvic junction obstruction. At age 21 months, the refluxing right ureter was reimplanted; the crossed ectopic left ureter was removed and the bilateral bladder diverticula repaired; Y-V plasty was performed on the anterior bladder neck (which would no longer be done today).

CASE 2.—A 10-month-old girl had urinary tract screening because of marked failure to thrive and urinary infection. There was crossed renal ectopia with hydronephrosis and reflux (Fig 119–6). Reflux was corrected

in one ureter, and the other, which drained no renal parenchyma, was removed. This patient also had Fanconi's anemia and marked hypoplasia of the left thumb.

CASE 3.—A 5-year-old boy admitted to the hospital for surgical correction of radial clubbed hand was found to have elevation of the BUN (50 mg/100 ml) and serum creatinine (1.5 mg/100 ml). Evaluation disclosed type III urethral valves, reflux into a dilated seminal vesicle into which emptied an ectopic ureter, reflux up a dilated crossed ectopic ureter, and severe dysplasia of the lower pole of a crossed fused kidney. A single-stage operative correction was performed (Fig 119–7).

CASE 4.—A 3-year-old boy underwent a screening IVP because he had minimal subcoronal hypospadias (Fig 119–8). No right kidney was seen. Cystogram showed reflux. There was an episode of epididymitis. With the child under anesthesia, the examiner's finger in the rectum revealed a palpable seminal vesicle; massaging it drained pus into the urethra, visible endoscopically. A one-stage reconstruction was performed.

CASE 5.—A 2-year-old girl had urologic investigation after repair of imperforate anus. An IVP showed a solitary right kidney with crossed ectopia (Fig 119–9); cystogram showed reflux. A single-stage reconstruction was performed, reimplanting the crossed ectopic ureter and removing an ectopic megaureter filled with pus and connected to a dysplastic nubbin of tissue in the hilus of the functional kidney.

CASE 6.—A 14-year-old girl (Fig 119–10) was referred for possible restoration of urinary tract continuity.[11, 12] At age 16 months, an ileal conduit had been performed, but details regarding the indications were not available. The bladder was tiny, holding only 10 ml. The lower renal moiety was nonfunctional and filled with stones. A longer ileal loop was fashioned, the destroyed renal moiety was removed, and a tube was inserted into the bladder to begin stretching it. The conduit was later tapered and implanted into the bladder, but reflux resulted because the

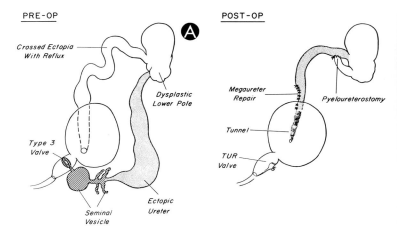

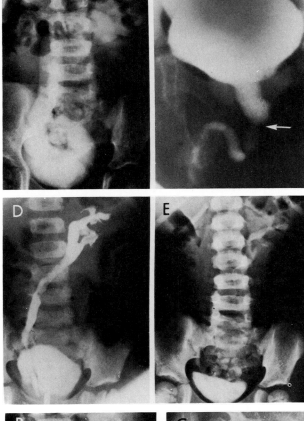

Fig 119–7.—Crossed renal ectopia, case 3: urethral valves, reflux and dysplasia of lower pole. **A,** preoperative and postoperative anatomy. **B,** preoperative IVP. **C,** preoperative cystogram. *Arrow* points to type III valves. Note faint opacification of the large, round structure (seminal vesicle) behind the prostatic urethra and bladder neck. **D,** postoperative retrograde study showing tapered and reimplanted ureter and pyeloureterostomy. **E,** IVP 2 years postoperatively.

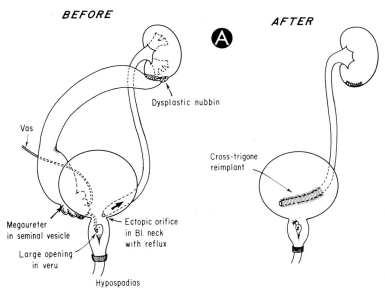

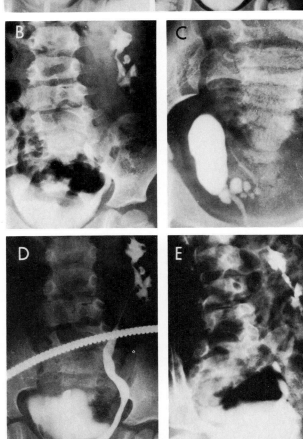

Fig 119–8.—Crossed renal ectopia, case 4: reflux, megaureter and dysplastic lower pole. **A,** preoperative and postoperative anatomy. **B,** preoperative IVP. **C,** retrograde injection of right seminal vesicle; there is opacification of lower 3 in. of megaureter. **D,** retrograde injection of refluxing left ureter, which entered bladder neck. **E,** an IVP 1 year postoperatively.

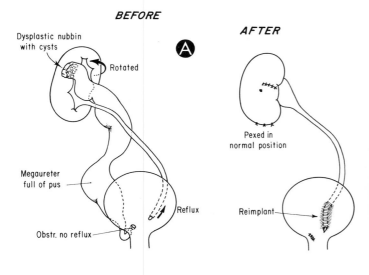

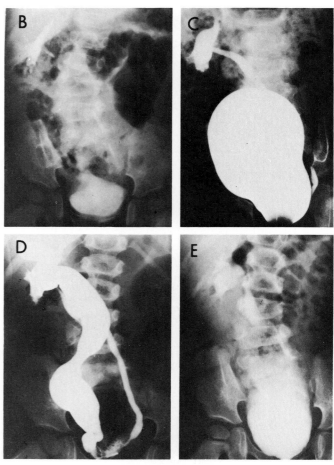

Fig 119–9.—Crossed renal ectopia, case 5: imperforate anus, dysplastic crossed element, reflux and megaureter. **A,** preoperative and postoperative anatomy. **B,** preoperative IVP. **C,** cystogram preoperatively. **D,** retrograde injection of both ureters during operation. **E,** IVP 6 months postoperatively.

bladder remained too small and contracted to accomplish a satisfactory nonrefluxing tunnel. Ultimately ileocecal cystoplasty was performed.

Case 7.—An 8-year-old boy underwent investigation (Fig 119–11) after an episode of urinary infection. An IVP showed a solitary right hydronephrotic kidney. Cystogram showed massive reflux up an ectopic, dilated ureter draining into a prostatic urethra. Cystoscopy showed a unilateral type I valve. An extensive single-stage reconstruction was performed. It included transurethral resection of the valve, removal of the ectopic ureter and its dysplastic nubbin of tissue, and pyeloplasty by the technique used in cases of horseshoe kidney.

These case histories show the coexistence of serious lower tract malformations in patients with anomalies resulting from migration and fusion defects of the renal masses. They serve to underscore the principle that, whenever screening IVP shows a fusion defect, complete urologic investigation is mandatory to rule out the presence of a surgically correctable malformation, such as those seen in the majority of these patients.

Pelvic Kidney

A pelvic kidney is one located ectopically in the pelvis; it has a congenitally short ureter and aberrant blood supply. In addition to its abnormal location, a pelvic kidney is frequently small, with irregular shape, variable rotation and extrarenal caliceal drainage.[5-7, 21, 22] Solitary pelvic kidney is a common finding in girls with congenital absence of the vagina (Fig 119–12). Pelvic kidney is commonly associated with multiple congenital anomalies (Fig 119–13). It may be an incidental finding that requires no operation, or it may be associated with a problem of impaired

drainage or reflux requiring surgical correction (Fig 119–14). In the past 20 years, we have encountered 16 patients with a pelvic kidney. Nine were girls; seven were boys. Nephrectomy was performed in one patient and pyeloplasty in five patients. Six patients had pyeloplasty for UPJ obstruction. One patient had megaureter repair of his solitary pelvic kidney. Two patients had operation for reflux as well as pyeloplasty of the pelvic kidney. Two patients had operations for urinary incontinence, not related to the pelvic kidney. Five patients had no need of operation.

Discoid Kidney

The discoid, lump, or pancake kidney, as these terms suggest, is abnormal in shape as well as in location. This rare anomaly occurs in about 3 of 50,000 autopsies, according to Campbell.[3] The blood supply is variable and anomalous; the collecting system is largely extrarenal, and as in horseshoe kidney it lies anteriorly. These kidneys are discovered by palpation of an abdominal mass in an infant or during investigation for urinary infection.

Case Material

In the past 20 years, we have encountered 10 children with discoid kidney. Seven were male and three were female. Seven of these children had pyeloplasty for UPJ obstruction. Two males had urethral valves; one had an operation for reflux. One patient had no problem with the discoid kidney, discovered as a palpable mass. One of these lump or discoid kidneys is shown in Figure

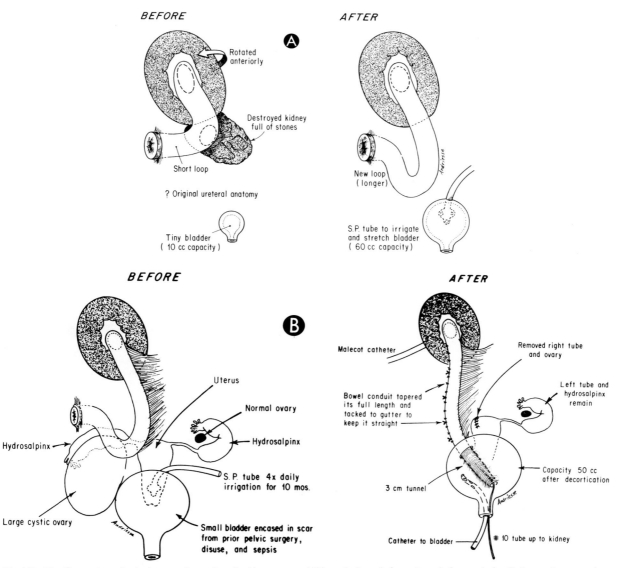

Fig 119–10.—Crossed renal ectopia, case 6: previous ileal loop, crossed kidney destroyed. **A,** anatomy before and after first operative procedure. **B,** anatomy before and after second operation. *(Continued)*

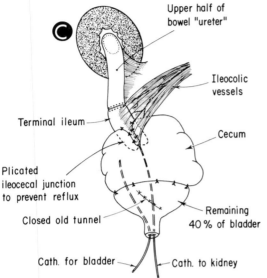

Upper half of bowel "ureter"

Ileocolic vessels

Terminal ileum

Cecum

Plicated ileocecal junction to prevent reflux

Closed old tunnel

Remaining 40 % of bladder

Cath. for bladder — Cath. to kidney

Fig 119–10 (cont).—**C,** final reconstruction, using cecal augmentation of contracted bladder. **D,** preoperative loopogram and cystogram to assess anatomy. **E,** IVP after undiversion. Note tapered bowel segment joined to bladder. Bladder remained small; there was reflux. Therefore, cecal cystoplasty was performed. **F,** IVP 3 weeks after cecal cystoplasty. Increased experience with undiversion has proved that bowel implantation can be done successfully only with a good bladder in which a very long tunnel can be made. Today, this patient would be managed by performing a cecal cystoplasty (see Chap. 130). She is now age 24 years, and is in excellent health. Cystogram shows no reflux; IVP is stable with excellent function.

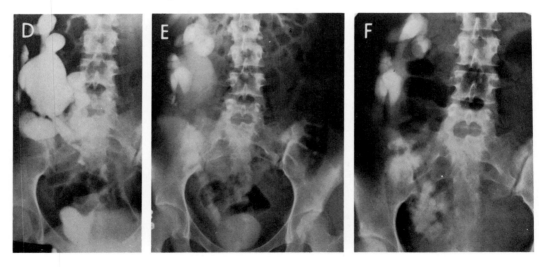

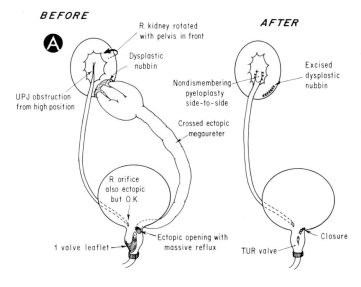

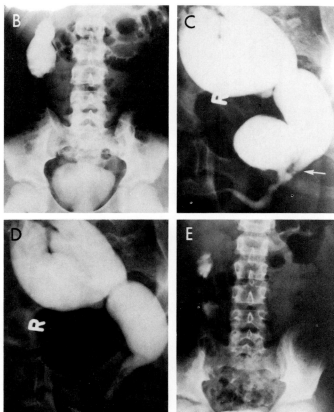

Fig 119–11.—Crossed renal ectopia, case 7: urethral valve, reflux, ureteropelvic junction obstruction, ectopic megaureter and dysplastic crossed element. **A,** preoperative and postoperative anatomy. **B,** preoperative IVP. **C,** voiding cystourethrogram; *arrow* points to ectopic megaureter entering prostatic urethra. Note peculiar trident-like collecting system at upper end of this ectopic ureter; there was no renal parenchyma associated with it. **D,** postvoiding cystogram films showing massive trapping of dye in ectopic ureter and its collecting system. **E,** an IVP 2 months after reconstructive procedure.

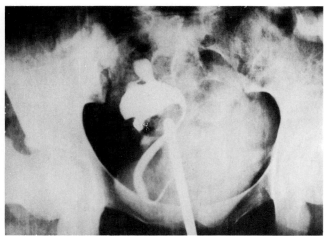

Fig 119–12.—Solitary pelvic kidney seen on IVP in 18-year-old girl with congenital absence of vagina, a common association. This pelvic kidney required no operation, i.e., there was no obstruction to its drainage and no vesicoureteral reflux.

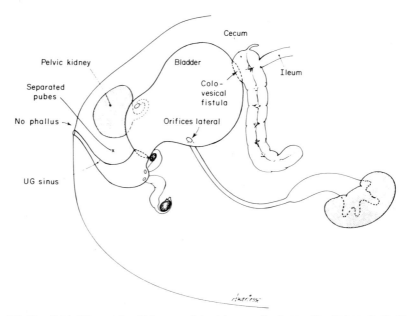

Fig 119–13.—Pelvic kidney and multiple congenital pelvic anomalies in neonate with imperforate anus.

PELVIC KIDNEY, BILATERAL REFLUX, BILATERAL UPJ OBSTRUCTION, VALVES

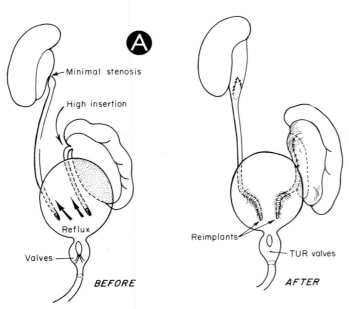

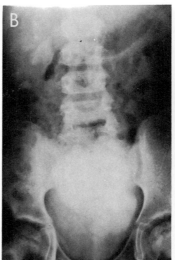

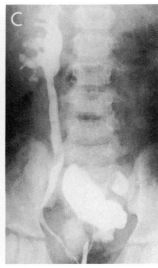

Fig 119–14.—Pelvic kidney with both massive reflux and ureteropelvic junction obstruction from high insertion of ureter on renal pelvis. **A,** anatomy before and after reconstruction. **B,** preoperative IVP. **C,** postoperative retrograde pyelogram. Pelvic kidney was not removed despite severe hydronephrosis because this patient has limited total renal function, i.e., the right kidney is severely damaged from chronic pyelonephritis.

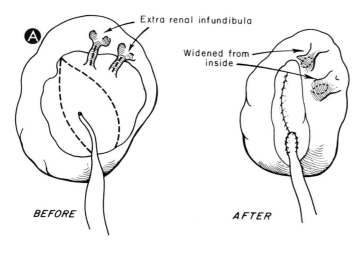

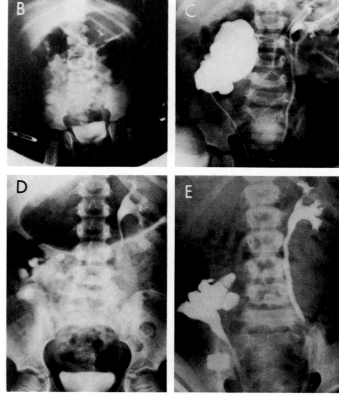

Fig 119–15.—Discoid "lump" kidney in right lower quadrant. **A,** preoperative and postoperative anatomy. **B,** preoperative IVP. **C,** preoperative retrograde pyelogram. Left side normal; severe right hydronephrosis. **D,** postoperative IVP. **E,** postoperative retrograde pyelogram.

119–15 with UPJ obstruction from high insertion of the ureter on the renal pelvis. This is the most common problem in horseshoe kidneys and ectopic kidneys. It is reparable by pyeloplasty.

Summary

When investigation of the urinary tract discloses an abnormality in the position or shape of a kidney or a fusion anomaly, a complete evaluation should be undertaken. This should include an IVP, a cystogram, and often cystoscopy and retrograde pyelography. (Aortography can be useful to define abnormal vasculature.) The evaluation will often disclose a correctable problem such as UPJ obstruction, ectopic ureters, vesicoureteral reflux, or bladder outflow obstruction. Concomitant malformations at both ends of the urinary tract, i.e., upper and lower, were seen in the majority of cases. This is not surprising in view of the complex embryology of the kidney and ureter.

REFERENCES

1. Abeshouse B.S.: Crossed ectopia with fusion. *Am. J. Surg.* 73:658, 1947.
2. Boatman D.L., Culp D.A. Jr., Culp D.A., et al.: Crossed renal ectopia. *J. Urol.* 108:30, 1972.
3. Campbell M.F.: Anomalies of the kidney, in Campbell M.F., Harrison G.H. (eds.): *Urology,* vol. 2. Philadelphia, W.B. Saunders Co., 1970, chap. 36.
4. Culp O.S., Winterringer J.R.: Surgical treatment of horseshoe kidney: Comparison of results after various types of operations. *J. Urol.* 73:747, 1955.
5. Downs R.A., Lane J.W., Burns E.: Solitary pelvic kidney: Its clinical implications. *Urology* 1:51, 1973.
6. Dretler S.P., Olsson C., Pfister R.C.: The anatomic, radiologic and clinical characteristics of the pelvic kidney: An analysis of 86 cases. *J. Urol.* 105:623, 1971.
7. Dretler S.P., Pfister R.C., Hendren W.H.: Extrarenal calyces in the ectopic kidney. *J. Urol.* 103:406, 1970.
8. Glenn J.F.: Analysis of 51 patients with horseshoe kidney. *N. Engl. J. Med.* 261:684, 1959.
9. Gray S.W., Skandalakis J.E.: The kidney and ureter, in *Embryology for Surgeons.* Philadelphia, W.B. Saunders Co., 1972, p. 443.
10. Gutierrez, R.: *The Clinical Management of the Horseshoe Kidney.* New York, Paul B. Hoeber, Inc., 1934.
11. Hendren W.H.: Urinary tract refunctionalization after prior diversion in children. *Ann. Surg.* 180:494, 1974.
12. Hendren W.H.: Reconstructive surgery of the urinary tract in children. *Curr. Probl. Surg.,* May 1977.
13. Hendren W.H., Donahoe P.K., Pfister R.C.: Crossed renal ectopia in children. *Urology* 7:135, 1976.
14. Kölln C.P., Boatman D.L., Schmidt J.D., et al.: Horseshoe kidney: A review of 105 patients. *J. Urol.* 107:203, 1972.
15. Kretschmer H.L.: Unilateral fused kidney. *Surg. Obstet. Gynecol.* 40:360, 1925.
16. McDonald J.H., McClellan D.S.: Crossed renal ectopia. *Am. J. Surg.* 93:995, 1957.
17. Mayers M.M.: Crossed renal ectopia. *J. Urol.* 36:111, 1936.
18. Pitts W.R. Jr., Muecke E.C.: Horseshoe kidneys: A 40-year experience. *J. Urol.* 113:743, 1975.
19. Romans D.G., Jewett M.A.S., Robson C.J.: Crossed renal ectopia with colic: A clinical clue to embryogenesis. *Br. J. Urol.* 48:171, 1976.
20. Segura J.W., Kelalis P.P., Burke E.C.: Horseshoe kidney in children. *J. Urol.* 108:333, 1972.
21. Vincent E.: A propos des malformations urinaires et génitales féminines associées: La réposition sanglante du rein ectopique pelvien. *J. Urol. Nephrol.* 81:237, 1975.
22. Ward J.N., Nathanson B., Draper J.W.: The pelvic kidney. *J. Urol.* 94:36, 1965.

120 David A. Lloyd
Renal Vein Thrombosis

Thrombosis of the renal venous system results in varying degrees of renal infarction, characterized by hematuria, thrombocytopenia, and a palpable kidney. Newborn infants are particularly vulnerable. The designation *renal vein thrombosis* includes thrombosis of the primary renal vein, in addition to the more common involvement of the intrarenal vein.

History.—Rayer[42] is credited with the first description of renal vein thrombosis in 1839. The first report of renal venous thrombosis in a child was probably that of Bednar in 1850.[30] In Europe during the latter half of the nineteenth century, the condition was a common finding at autopsy of children dying of gastroenteritis,[96] but it was not until 90 years after Rayer's description that the first report appeared in English. In 1926, Aschner[2] presented five patients, including an infant, to the American Urological Association, and other reports followed.[24, 35] The mortality was high, and most patients were diagnosed at autopsy or at operation. Campbell and Matthews, in 1941, claimed to be the first to make the preoperative diagnosis of renal vein thrombosis.[12] They strongly advocated urgent nephrectomy for unilateral disease and predicted a 75% survival rate following nephrectomy, compared to the prevailing 95% mortality without operation. This aggressive surgical approach was generally supported until 1964, when Stark[48] reported full recovery of three infants treated without operation and drew attention to earlier reports of recovery with supportive treatment alone. With the realization that renal venous thrombosis is often a manifestation of a pre-existing illness and is not necessarily lethal, the emphasis has swung away from operative management to focus on correcting the underlying disorder. The roles of anticoagulation, thrombolysis, and thrombectomy have yet to be clarified. Recent developments are the use of noninvasive diagnostic techniques, notably ultrasonography and computerized tomography.

Pathogenesis

Typically, renal vein thrombosis is preceded by hemoconcentration and decreased renal perfusion, leading to renal venous stasis. The newborn kidney is particularly vulnerable, because the low renal perfusion pressure in the neonate and the combined resistance of two consecutive intrarenal capillary beds predispose to venous stasis. Venous congestion of the tissues drained by the occluded vein leads to local tissue hypoxia, cellular disruption, and hemorrhage into the renal parenchyma, manifested as hematuria. With severe renal congestion, arterial perfusion is impaired, if not halted. If both kidneys are affected, there may be oliguria.

Renal vein thrombosis may involve the small intrarenal veins, the larger renal veins, or both.[24] The origin of the thrombotic process is determined histologically by the degree of maturation of the thrombus in the different veins.[7] Intrarenal thrombosis usually commences in the arcuate and interlobar veins at the corticomedullary junction. The thrombotic process propagates peripherally to the smaller tributaries of the renal cortex, and centrally along the interlobar veins to the main renal vein and the inferior vena cava.[1, 7] Less commonly, thrombosis commences in the renal vein, with or without peripheral extension into the smaller tributaries; if the collateral venous circulation is adequate, there will be minimal renal infarction.[23, 27, 51, 56]

The entire kidney or a localized renal segment may be infarcted, depending on the level of venous obstruction, the collateral venous circulation, and the rate of propagation of the thrombus through the renal venous system. In animals, acute renal vein occlusion causes a rapid rise in renal venous pressure and a fall in renal arterial pressure.[23] With the development of collateral venous circulation, the renal swelling decreases and blood flow increases. The left kidney is theoretically more likely to recover than the right, because of the rich collateral venous drainage of the left renal vein via the gonadal, suprarenal, phrenic, and lumbar veins.[5] On the right, these veins drain directly into the inferior vena cava.

Histologically, the thrombus initially consists almost entirely of platelets, later there is organization and fibrosis, and recanalization may occur.[1, 11] Infarction of the kidneys with death of cells results in scarring, distortion, and contraction. When the process begins before birth, calcification frequently occurs.

Bilateral venous thrombosis probably occurs more commonly than is generally recognized. In the apparently normal contralateral kidney, minor thrombosis of the intrarenal veins, undetected clinically, has been identified at autopsy. Cases are on record in which one kidney has been removed because of renal vein thrombosis, only to be followed by similar involvement of the contralateral kidney.[52]

The renal vein thrombus may extend into the inferior vena cava[33, 51] and cause pulmonary embolism.[17] The incidence of inferior vena cava thrombosis is higher with bilateral renal vein thrombosis[21] and in patients with the nephrotic syndrome.[14] Renal vein thrombosis secondary to primary inferior vena cava thrombosis is uncommon.[1, 17, 53]

Etiology

The causes of thrombosis of the renal venous system are different in the newborn infant and the older child (Table 120–1). In the newborn, renal vein thrombosis occurs usually in the absence of primary renal disease; rare exceptions include infants with congenital nephrotic syndrome.[21, 29] Factors leading to impaired renal blood flow in the newborn include perinatal stress, severe infection, diarrhea, and congenital cardiac disease. Acute hypoxia and hypovolemia cause hypotension, reflex vasoconstriction diverting blood away from the kidney, and hemoconcentration. As a result, renal perfusion is decreased. Perinatal asphyxia, neonatal septic shock, gastroenteritis, neonatal necrotizing enterocolitis, concentrated hyperosmolar feedings,[21, 25] and cytomegalic viral infection[55] have been implicated in renal vein thrombosis. Gastroenteritis has become a less common etiologic factor as the treatment of dehydrated infants has improved but remains an associated finding in approximately 11% of newborns with renal vein thrombosis.[1]

With cyanotic congenital heart disease, there is a high risk of renal venous stasis because of hypoxia, polycythemia, and poor renal perfusion due to cardiac failure.[1, 27] This may be aggravated by cardiac catheterization,[34] since the contrast medium increases blood viscosity, both directly and by provoking an osmotic diuresis; further, the contrast medium itself may be nephrotoxic in susceptible patients.[4]

In newborns with no apparent predisposing illness, the cause of renal vein thrombosis remains unknown. Avery[3] drew atten-

TABLE 120–1.—CLINICAL DATA ON 40 INFANTS WITH RENAL VEIN THROMBOSIS, CHILDREN'S HOSPITAL OF PITTSBURGH, 1956–1983

	AGE			
	Under 1 mo	1–12 mo	Over 1 yr	TOTAL
No. patients	25	3	12	40
Obstetric data				
Maternal diabetes	4	—	—	4
Maternal diuretics	4	—	—	4
Preeclampsia	1	—	—	1
Hydramnios	4	—	—	4
Fetal distress	5	—	—	5
Traumatic birth	2	—	—	2
Associated disorders				
None	3	—	—	3
Nephrotic syndrome	—	1	3	4
Cyanotic cardiac disease	5	1	—	6
Other cardiac disease	4	—	1	5
Respiratory distress	9	—	4	13
Diarrhea	3	1	3	7
Dehydration	4	1	4	9
Hypotension	6	1	3	10
Wilms tumor	—	—	2	2
CNS defects	4	—	2	6
Miscellaneous	3	—	3	6

tion to the association between neonatal renal venous thrombosis and maternal diabetes. In a review by Oppenheimer[40] of 4,000 infants who died within 2 weeks of birth, the incidence of venous thrombosis in those born of diabetic mothers was 15.8%, and in those with nondiabetic mothers was 0.8%; the most frequent sites of thrombosis were the renal and adrenal veins. Maternal prediabetes may also be a significant factor.[51] Nonetheless, renal vein thrombosis is an uncommon occurrence, even in infants of diabetic mothers, and some reviews have failed to confirm the association.[1]

Maternal use of drugs during pregnancy, notably steroids and thiazide diuretics, has been linked with renal venous thrombosis. Steroids may induce a prediabetic state with pancreatic hyperplasia,[7, 9] which is also found in infants born of mothers with maternal diabetes and prediabetes. Other factors associated with renal vein thrombosis include maternal toxemia, hydramnios, and birth trauma.[40]

Renal vein thrombosis may occur before birth. Evidence for this includes the finding of organized renal vein thrombi and calcification in newborns, including stillborn infants.[9, 54] The cause of such intrauterine thrombosis is unknown; associated predisposing factors are maternal diabetes[3, 40, 51] and maternal trauma.[46]

In infants more than 1 month of age, renal vein thrombosis is usually associated with hypovolemia, in particular with acute fluid loss from gastrointestinal disorders or thermal burns.[1, 17, 21] In older children, as in adults, there is an increasing association with underlying renal disease, notably the nephrotic syndrome. The causal relationship between renal vein thrombosis and the nephrotic syndrome remains uncertain: renal vein thrombosis may precede signs of the nephrotic syndrome[11, 29] but occurs in most patients as a complication of pre-existing nephrotic syndrome.[26, 31] Coagulation abnormalities, causing a hypercoagulable state and decreased fibrinolytic activity,[29] are common in patients with the nephrotic syndrome, who are liable to renal and extrarenal thrombotic complications, including pulmonary embolism.[14, 26]

Renal tumors may invade the renal veins, initiating thrombosis that propagates into the inferior vena cava. Other causes of renal vein thrombosis include accidental or operative blunt trauma and extrinsic pressure on the renal vein. Primary inferior vena caval thrombosis has occurred following prolonged use of a central venous catheter;[21] in some patients the etiology is not apparent.[17, 53]

Incidence

The incidence of renal vein thrombosis in life is not known; based on autopsy data, the condition is uncommon but not rare. Among 1,569 autopsies on children in Glasgow,[1] the incidence of renal vein thrombosis was 0.4%; this included 585 neonates, in whom the incidence of renal vein thrombosis was 2.7%. Cruikshanks[16] reported a 1.9% incidence of renal vein thrombosis in 800 autopsies on newborns, and in another autopsy study on children the incidence was 0.4%–0.6%.[48] From these data, the incidence of renal vein thrombosis in autopsied children of all ages is approximately 0.5%, and in newborns is approximately 2%–2.5%. The male-to-female ratio is 1.6 to 1, and in newborns the predominance of males is even greater.[1, 33] Renal vein thrombosis occurs at all ages. Fifty-six to 74% of affected children are less than 4 weeks of age, and 31%–38% are less than 1 week old.[1, 17, 28, 33, 34]

Clinical Features

Clinically, there are three groups of patients.[37, 44] (1) Apparently healthy, full-term newborn infants, with no obvious predisposing illness. The renal vein thrombosis may be present at birth[56] or may manifest acutely, often with a febrile illness. (2) Infants or young children with a preceding illness or disease that predisposes to formation of thrombus in the renal veins. This is the most common type. The underlying illness may obscure the evidence of renal vein thrombosis, which may remain undetected clinically, either to resolve spontaneously or to be identified at autopsy. (3) Children with pre-existing renal disease, notably the nephrotic syndrome. Generally occurring in older children, the presentation is usually acute, with flank pain, a palpable kidney, and proteinuria or hematuria (unlike the asymptomatic chronic presentation in adults).[31] There may be extrarenal thromboembolic lesions, particularly pulmonary embolism. In all groups the clinical course varies, some children manifesting a progressive illness with shock, consumptive coagulopathy, and deteriorating renal function.

The typical clinical features of renal vein thrombosis are a palpable renal mass and hematuria. These are not consistent findings and are more common in newborn infants. The incidence of a palpable renal mass was 56% in Arneil's review (unilateral, 38%; bilateral, 18%)[1] and 43% in the Children's Hospital of Pittsburgh series (unilateral, 25%; bilateral, 18%).[32] Among affected newborn infants, 56%–60% had a palpable mass, compared with 20%–45% of the older children.[1, 32] The importance of identifying a mass in order to make the diagnosis is suggested by the fact that a mass was palpated in 13 (87%) of 15 children in whom renal vein thrombosis was diagnosed during life, and in only four (16%) of 25 children in whom the diagnosis was made at autopsy.[32] Even with bilateral disease, the kidneys may not be palpable; of 14 patients known to have bilateral disease, eight (57%) had bilateral masses, and in one a unilateral mass could be palpated.[21] The presence of a mass, with or without hematuria, is not pathognomonic of renal vein thrombosis and should lead to evaluation of the kidneys. In the newborn, the differential diagnosis of a flank mass includes congenital renal abnormalities (hydronephrosis, multicystic disease, renal dysplasia), renal tumor, renal trauma with hemorrhage, acute adrenal hemorrhage, and neuroblastoma.

Hematuria was recorded in 63% of patients with renal venous thrombosis at Children's Hospital of Pittsburgh, where 72% of affected newborn infants and 43% of older children had gross or microscopic hematuria.[32] In Arneil's review, 61% of the children had hematuria; 64% in newborn infants and 47% in children over 1 month of age.[1] Emanuel[18] identified renal vein thrombosis in seven (20%) of 35 newborns with hematuria. In three patients, the hematuria preceded detection of a renal mass.

Inferior vena cava thrombosis is suspected when there is edema of the lower limbs and dilated superficial abdominal wall veins, but these are uncommon findings, since collaterals are usually adequate.[21, 33] Varicocele may follow occlusion of the left renal vein.[32] The blood pressure is usually normal or low, depending on the nature of the predisposing disease. Hypertension is a late complication, seldom seen in the acute phase.[19]

Diagnosis

Laboratory Investigations

Thrombocytopenia is a frequent finding in renal vein thrombosis. Arneil[1] found that 18 of 20 patients (90%) had a platelet count less than 75,000/mm.[3] At Children's Hospital of Pittsburgh,[32] 50% of affected patients had fewer than 100,000 platelets/mm;[3] 50% of these were below 50,000/mm.[3] The thrombocytopenia is chiefly the result of platelet entrapment in the renal thrombus.[1, 43] Coagulation studies usually characterize consumptive coagulopathy, namely prolonged thromboplastin and prothrombin times, decreased platelet count and serum fibrinogen and factor V levels, elevated serum fibrin degradation products, and an abnormal peripheral smear with fragmented red blood cells, burr cells, and target cells.[43] The white blood cell count is commonly elevated. Anemia is not a constant finding and was present in 32% of newborns and 62% of older patients.[1] These hematologic abnormalities are not specific, and blood cultures are recommended to exclude septicemia.

Serum sodium, potassium, and urea levels vary widely, depending on associated disorders and the degree of renal dysfunction. There may be hypernatremia or hyponatremia.[1, 32] The blood urea level is usually elevated, particularly with bilateral renal vein thrombosis.[21, 22] The number of patients with blood urea in excess of 100 mg/dl varies from 8%[32] to 55%.[1]

Urinalysis shows hematuria and proteinuria when the onset of renal vein thrombosis is acute, as in most neonates. In older children with nephrotic syndrome, the urine more commonly contains protein, and not blood.

Imaging and Radiographic Studies

Plain abdominal radiographs may show renal enlargement but are usually normal. Calcification in organized intrarenal thrombi has a characteristic lace-like pattern, corresponding with the renal venous tree.[9] In newborns, this is evidence of intrauterine thrombosis. Calcification in the vena cava is typically bullet-shaped.[33]

Ultrasonography is the procedure of choice for the diagnosis of renal vein thrombosis[36] and in the newborn is superior to computerized tomography. The diagnostic features are thrombus in the renal vein (Fig 120–1,A) and renal enlargement. A variety of renal echo patterns have been described, nonspecific and varying with the distribution of the renal lesion.[8] The inferior vena cava should be evaluated for evidence of extension of the renal vein thrombus (Fig 120–1,B). Other causes of renal or adrenal enlargement, including multicystic renal disease, congenital hydronephrosis, and tumor, may be identified or excluded. The safety of ultrasonography favors its use for subsequent follow-up.

Computerized tomography demonstrates renal enlargement and thrombus in the renal vein and inferior vena cava, and a

coexisting renal or pararenal abnormality may be identified. Injection of contrast allows simultaneous evaluation of renal function.[15, 22]

Radionuclide renal scanning permits quantitative evaluation of renal function, and in the acute phase shows renal enlargement with decreased function.[13, 38] This is a valuable method of monitoring the function of the recovering kidney.

Contrast radiography, notably intravenous pyelography, inferior vena cavography, retrograde pyelography, and renal angiography, has been superseded by ultrasonography, computerized tomography, and radionuclide scanning. The intravenous pyelogram is abnormal in over 90% of patients with renal vein thrombosis,[1] showing delayed opacification and renal enlargement. With extensive renal infarction, the kidney is not visualized by pyelography and its presence should be confirmed by ultrasound. To avoid further hemoconcentration, there should be no fluid restriction before the pyelogram. Inferior vena cavography demonstrates vena caval thrombus and collateral venous circulation; renal vein thrombus may be seen extending into the inferior vena cava.

Management

Following the report in 1942 by Campbell and Matthews[12] of two patients with renal vein thrombosis successfully treated by nephrectomy, this procedure was recommended as the treatment of choice for acute unilateral renal vein thrombosis.[27] Reasons for removing the infarcted kidney were that the kidney was a nidus for infection, that there was a risk of transcaval spread of the thrombus to the contralateral renal vein, and that hypertension was prevented.

The subsequent documentation of survival without nephrectomy raised doubts about the need for early operation and placed the emphasis on early, vigorous correction of fluid and electrolyte derangements. In a strong plea for nonoperative management, Stark[48] reviewed the literature and pointed out that, of the patients whose recovery had been attributed to nephrectomy, many had been operated on after the acute phase, while well on their way to recovery. Further, nephrectomy, with or without thrombectomy, did not prevent subsequent infarction of the opposite kidney, since the disease process usually commenced in the intrarenal veins. Although there are some who continue to advocate early operation, in general, nephrectomy has been abandoned in favor of nonoperative therapy. Nephrectomy may be required for delayed complications, notably hypertension and infection, but the rarity of these argues against prophylactic nephrectomy.[47]

Currently, the acute management of renal vein thrombosis in children consists of correcting fluid and electrolyte abnormalities, preventing propagation of the thrombus, and, in selected patients, disobliteration of thrombosed major veins. These recommendations are based on a wide spectrum of retrospective reviews, since the very nature of renal vein thrombosis, in particular its infrequent occurrence and sometimes subtle presentation, has thus far precluded prospective evaluation.

General Measures

Initial management is directed at correcting abnormalities of fluid, electrolyte and acid-base balance by appropriate intravenous therapy. In severely ill infants, this should be done before embarking on contrast studies, which may aggravate pre-existing hypovolemia and hemoconcentration. Underlying conditions such as infection or cardiac failure require specific treatment. Careful monitoring of critically ill newborn infants is essential, particularly with regard to renal function. Hypertonic infusions and nephrotoxic antibiotics and drugs should be avoided. Di-

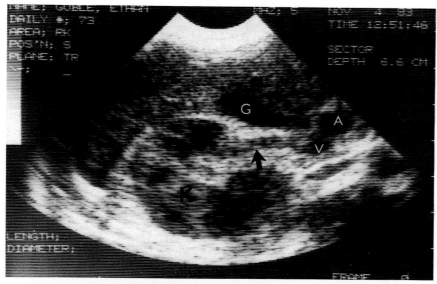

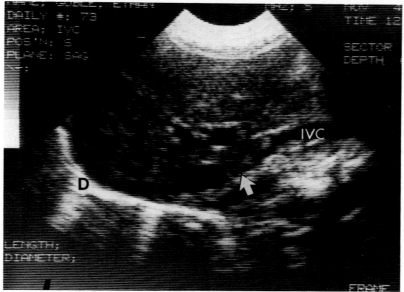

Fig 120–1.—Renal vein thrombosis. **Top,** transverse renal sonogram. Thrombus in the renal vein *(arrow)* extends into the inferior vena cava *(V).* Aorta *(A),* gallbladder *(G),* kidney *(K).* **Bottom,** longitudinal sonogram. Thrombus *(arrow)* is seen in the inferior vena cava *(IVC).* Diaphragm *(D).* This infant with transposition of the great vessels presented 2 days after cardiac catheterization with fever, frank hematuria, and a right flank mass. Sonography confirmed right renal venous thrombosis, and renal scan showed decreased function in the enlarged right kidney. Right renal function returned to normal under nonoperative management.

uretics are of limited, if any, value. Bilateral renal infarction may result in progressive renal failure necessitating modification of fluid and electrolyte infusions. Rarely, peritoneal dialysis is indicated.[1] Antimicrobial therapy is required when there is evidence of infection, and infective foci are eradicated.

Prevention of Thrombus Propagation

In many patients, correction of hemoconcentration prevents further propagation of the thrombus and is followed by full recovery.[45] In high-risk patients (e.g., with the nephrotic syndrome), and those with evidence of disseminated intravascular coagulation, intravenous heparin may be of value,[43, 45] but the role of anticoagulant therapy has not been clearly defined. Heparinization has been recommended when the diagnosis is made early,[1] or when there is evidence of bilateral involvement;[1, 17] this would include almost all newborn patients. At Children's

Hospital of Pittsburgh, heparin therapy is not employed for acute renal vein thrombosis. Long-term anticoagulation may be appropriate for patients with the nephrotic syndrome who exhibit multifocal thromboembolism.

Thrombectomy and Thrombolysis

Since the intrarenal veins are frequently occluded by thrombus, clearing the main renal vein often does not alleviate the renal infarction. In some patients, thrombectomy of the renal vein has been followed by maintained improvement of renal blood flow, probably when the thrombus was limited to the main renal vein and its larger tributaries. At present, there is no simple method of identifying these patients before operation. For unilateral renal venous thrombosis, the outcome without operation is usually good, and there is general agreement that operation offers no advantage if the patient is stable.

With bilateral renal vein thrombosis, particularly when associated with inferior vena caval thrombosis, the dramatic clinical picture prompted some to adopt an aggressive surgical approach.[17] Satisfactory, prolonged restoration of renal flow after bilateral renal vein and inferior vena caval thrombectomy has been reported by Thompson.[52] He recommends routine inferior vena cavography and advises thrombectomy when this demonstrates renal vein and inferior vena cava thrombus. On the other hand, many patients with bilateral renal vein thrombosis and inferior vena cava thrombosis have recovered without operation, and the benefit of thrombectomy remains to be proved. Without thrombectomy, the inferior vena cava may remain permanently occluded, but collateral veins develop, providing adequate alternative venous drainage.[33]

Thrombolysis offers a more logical approach to clearance of thrombi, since patency of the smaller intrarenal veins may also be achieved. In a few isolated cases, systemic urokinase[21, 45] or streptokinase[10, 20] has been used in combination with heparin, apparently with good results. Thrombolysis may be applicable to patients with bilateral renal vein thrombosis, particularly when there is associated vena caval thrombosis.[21]

Outcome

Survival

In Arneil's large review,[1] the overall survival rate was 34%, but it is not clear how many patients were diagnosed during life. In reported series of children of all ages diagnosed during life,[17, 32, 33, 34] the overall survival rates ranged between 45% and 86%. In general, there are two groups of patients: those in whom the renal vein thrombosis is a minor incident in the course of some other major disease and characteristically is identified at autopsy, and those in whom renal venous thrombosis occurs as a major complication of an otherwise mild or moderate illness. The second group includes most cases in neonates, and the prognosis is usually good. In the Pittsburgh series, 15 patients were diagnosed during life, and 12 (80%) survived. There were 12 newborn infants, of whom 10 (83%) recovered, and three older children with one survivor (33%). Others have reported survival rates of 86% and 75% for newborn infants with renal vein thrombosis.[7, 25] It has become apparent that most deaths are due to the underlying disease and not the renal infarction, and the improved survival rate is mainly a reflection of improved management of the predisposing disorder.

Sequelae

The extent to which the kidney recovers after infarction varies widely, from full recovery with normal function through a spectrum of abnormal function. The prognosis can be inferred from radioisotope renography during the acute phase, which appears to correlate well with the ultimate outcome.[33, 41] Marked renal edema and severely impaired renal blood flow are associated with significant permanent renal damage. Isotope renography permits longitudinal evaluation of renal function.

The possible long-term sequelae have been defined[49] as: (1) a nonfunctioning, completely fibrosed, shrunken kidney; (2) a partially fibrosed kidney with impaired function; (3) renovascular hypertension; (4) nephrotic syndrome; (5) chronic renal infection; (6) chronic renal tubular dysfunction. Many patients in whom the injured kidney is not removed do not develop these complications.[1] Occasional older patients presenting with chronic renal dysfunction have radiologic changes suggesting previously undetected neonatal renal venous thrombosis.[27, 50] Of surgical significance are hypertension and chronic renal infection, which may necessitate nephrectomy.[20]

Hypertension, an uncommon but serious complication, may be associated with elevated plasma-renin levels. The kidney is usually atrophic, and nephrectomy is curative.[17, 47] In one instance, renin-mediated hypertension diagnosed at birth, following intrauterine renal venous thrombosis, was cured by nephrectomy.[19] There is no correlation between the morphologic abnormalities demonstrated radiographically and the degree of functional impairment.[25] Not all patients with small scarred kidneys develop hypertension. Further, hypertension may develop without an associated increase in plasma-renin levels; in such patients, the hypertension is probably not related to activation of the renin-angiotensin system, and nephrectomy may not be appropriate,[25] particularly as spontaneous resolution of the hypertension has been reported.[41]

REFERENCES

1. Arneil G.C., MacDonald A.M., Murphy A.V., et al.: Renal venous thrombosis. *Clin. Nephrol.* 1:119, 1975.
2. Aschner P.W.: Thrombosis and thrombophlebitis of the renal vein. *J. Urol.* 17:309, 1927.
3. Avery M.E., Oppenheimer E.H., Gordon H.H.: Renal-vein thrombosis in newborn infants of diabetic mothers. *N. Engl. J. Med.* 256:1134, 1957.
4. Avner E.D., Ellis D., Jaffe R., et al.: Neonatal radiocontrast nephropathy simulating infantile polycystic kidney disease. *J. Pediatr.* 100:85, 1982.
5. Baum N.H., Moriel E., Carlton C.E. Jr.: Renal vein thrombosis. *J. Urol.* 119:443, 1978.
6. Beckmann V.O.: Ueber Thrombose der Nierenvene bei Kindern. *Verhandlungen der Physikalisch Medizenische Gessellschaft in Wurzburg* 9:201, 1858.
7. Belman A.B.: Renal vein thrombosis in infancy and childhood. *Clin. Pediatr.* Nov., 1976:1033.
8. Bowen A.D., Smazal S.F.: Ultrasound of coexisting right renal vein thrombosis and adrenal hemorrhage in a newborn. *J. Clin. Ultrasound* 9:511, 1981.
9. Brill P.W., Mitty H.A., Strauss L.: Renal vein thrombosis: A cause of intrarenal calcification in the newborn. *Pediatr. Radiol.* 6:172, 1977.
10. Burrow C.R., Walker W.G., Bell W.R., et al.: Streptokinase salvage of renal function after renal vein thrombosis. *Ann. Intern. Med.* 100:237, 1984.
11. Cade R., Spooner G., Juncos L., et al.: Chronic renal vein thrombosis. *Am. J. Med.* 63:387, 1977.
12. Campbell M.F., Matthews W.F.: Renal thrombosis in infancy. *J. Pediatr.* 20:604, 1942.
13. Chapman C.N., Szilklas J.J., Spencer R.P., et al.: Radionuclide study of functional resolution of unilateral renal vein thrombosis. *Clin. Nucl. Med.* 8:56, 1983.
14. Chugh K.S., Malik N., Uberoi H.S., et al.: Renal vein thrombosis in nephrotic syndrome—a prospective study and review. *Postgrad. Med. J.* 57:566, 1981.
15. Coleman C.C., Saxena K.M., Johnson K.W.: Renal vein thrombosis in a child with the nephrotic syndrome: CT diagnosis. *AJR* 135:1285, 1980.
16. Cruikshanks J.N.: Causes of 800 neonatal deaths. *Special Report Series, Medical Research Council*, 145, 1930.
17. Duncan R.E., Evans A.T., Martin L.W.: Natural history and treatment of renal vein thrombosis in children. *J. Pediatr. Surg.* 12:639, 1977.
18. Emanuel B., Aronson N.: Neonatal hematuria. *Am. J. Dis. Child.* 128:204, 1974.
19. Evans D.J., Silverman M., Bowley N.B.: Congenital hypertension due to unilateral renal vein thrombosis. *Arch. Dis. Child.* 56:306, 1981.
20. Friolet V.B., Gugler E., Bettex M., et al.: Uber 6 Fälle von Nierenvenenthrombosen im Kindesalter. *Helv. Paediat. Acta* 19:243, 1964.
21. Gonzalez R., Schwartz S., Sheldon C.A., et al.: Bilateral renal vein thrombosis in infancy and childhood. *Urol. Clin. North Am.* 9:279, 1982.
22. Greene A., Cromie W.J., Goldman M.: Computerized body tomography in neonatal renal vein thrombosis. *Urology* 20:213, 1982.
23. Harris J.D., Ehrenfeld W.K., Lee J.C., et al.: Experimental renal vein occlusion. *Surg. Gynecol. Obstet.* 126:555, 1968.
24. Hepler A.B.: Thrombosis of the renal veins. *J. Urol.* 31:527, 1934.
25. Jobin J., O'Regan S., Demay G., et al.: Neonatal renal vein thrombosis—long-term follow-up after conservative management. *Clin. Nephrol.* 17:36, 1982.

26. Kaplan B.S., Chesney R.W., Drummond K.N.: The nephrotic syndrome and renal vein thrombosis. *Am. J. Dis. Child.* 132:367, 1978.
27. Karafin L., Stearns T.M.: Renal vein thrombosis in children. *J. Urol.* 92:91, 1964.
28. Kaufmann H.J.: Renal vein thrombosis. *Am. J. Dis. Child.* 95:377, 1958.
29. Lewy P.R., Jao W.: Nephrotic syndrome in association with renal vein thrombosis in infancy. *J. Pediatr.* 85:359, 1974.
30. Llach F.: *Renal Vein Thrombosis.* New York, Futura Publishing Co., 1983.
31. Llach F., Papper S., Massry S.G.: The clinical spectrum of renal vein thrombosis: Acute and chronic. *Am. J. Med.* 69:819, 1980.
32. Lloyd D.A., Ricci M.: Renal venous thrombosis in newborns and children. Submitted for publication, 1985.
33. McDonald P., Tarar R., Gilday D., et al.: Some radiologic observations in renal vein thrombosis. *Am. J. Roentgenol.* 120:368, 1974.
34. McFarland J.B.: Renal venous thrombosis in children. *Q.J. Med.* 34:269, 1965.
35. Marshall S., Whapham E.: Case of bilateral renal infarction in a newly born infant. *Lancet* 2:428, 1936.
36. Metreweli C., Pearson R.: Echographic diagnosis of neonatal renal venous thrombosis. *Pediatr. Radiol.* 14:105, 1984.
37. Moeller E.R.: Unilateral renal vein thrombosis. *U.S. Armed Forces Med. J.* 9:992, 1958.
38. Nielander A.J.M., Bode W.A., Heidendal G.A.K.: Renography in diagnosis and follow-up of renal vein thrombosis. *Clin. Nucl. Med.* 8:56, 1983.
39. Olson D.: Renal vein thrombosis in infants, in Lieberman E. (ed.): *Clinical Pediatric Nephrology.* Philadelphia, J.B. Lippincott Company, 1976.
40. Oppenheimer E.H., Esterly J.R.: Thrombosis in the newborn: Comparison between infants of diabetic and nondiabetic mothers. *J. Pediatr.* 67:549, 1965.
41. Rasoulpour M., McLean R.H.: Renal venous thrombosis in neonates. *Am. J. Dis. Child.* 134:276, 1980.
42. Rayer P.R.O.: *Traité des maladies des reins.* Paris, J.B. Bailliere, 1839–1841.
43. Renfield M.L., Kraybill E.N.: Consumptive coagulopathy with renal vein thrombosis. *J. Pediatr.* 82:1054, 1973.
44. Sandblom P.H.: Renal thrombosis with infarction in the newborn: Two different forms. *Acta Pediatr.* 35:161, 1948.
45. Seeler R.A., Kapadia P., Moncado R.: Nonsurgical management of thrombosis of bilateral renal veins and inferior vena cava in a newborn infant. *Clin. Pediatr.* 9:543, 1970.
46. Siegal A., Hertz M., Lindner A.: Renal vein thrombosis in a newborn: A case report with emphasis on pathological and radiological features. *J. Urol.* 118:464, 1977.
47. Smith J.A. Jr., Lee R.E., Middleton R.G.: Hypertension in childhood from renal vein thrombosis. *J. Urol.* 122:389, 1979.
48. Stark H.: Renal vein thrombosis in infancy. *Am. J. Dis. Child.* 108:430, 1964.
49. Stark H., Geiger R.: Renal tubular dysfunction following vascular accidents of the kidneys in the newborn period. *J. Pediatr.* 83:933, 1973.
50. Sutton T.J., Leblanc A., Gauthier N., et al.: Radiological manifestations of neonatal renal vein thrombosis on follow-up examinations. *Radiology* 122:435, 1977.
51. Takeuchi A., Benirschke K.: Renal venous thrombosis of the newborn and its relation to maternal diabetes. *Biol. Neonate* 3:237, 1961.
52. Thompson I.M., Schneider R., Lababidi Z.: Thrombectomy for neonatal renal vein thrombosis. *J. Urol.* 113:396, 1975.
53. Touloukian R.J.: Idiopathic vena caval thrombosis with renal infarction in the newborn infant: Survival following nephrectomy. *Surgery* 65:978, 1969.
54. Tseng C.H., Chang G.K.J., Lora F.: Congenital calcified thrombosis of inferior vena cava, bilateral renal veins and left spermatic vein. *Pediatr. Radiol.* 6:176, 1977.
55. Vorlicky L.N., Balfour H.H. Jr.: Cytomegalovirus and renal vein thrombosis in a newborn infant. *Am. J. Dis. Child.* 127:742, 1974.
56. Zuelzer W.W., Kurnetz R., Fallon R.: Thrombosis of renal veins. *Am. J. Dis. Child.* 1:81, 1951.

121 R. H. WHITAKER
Pyeloureteral Obstruction

Hydronephrosis

ONE OF THE MAJOR recent changes in our attitude toward hydronephrosis has been a much more careful analysis of the degree of obstruction and its likely effects on renal function. All too commonly, a pyeloplasty was performed for almost any significant degree of dilatation, regardless of the symptoms; more often, an operation was performed for symptoms alone, with inadequate dynamic assessment of the system.

We have come to accept the term "hydronephrosis" as simply a description of the radiologic findings of a larger than normal renal pelvis, with or without a degree of caliceal distention. "Hydronephrosis" should then be modified as either obstructed or nonobstructed. If it is accepted that it is either infection or raised pressure (or both) that damages a kidney with a dilated system, then the only reasons for operating on the hydronephrosis are to reduce the overall volume, and hence reduce the likelihood of urinary tract infection, or to relieve obstruction and lower the pressure. This fundamental concept implies that, if infection is not a problem and there is no obstruction, there is nothing to be gained by performing a pyeloplasty. Conversely, the combina-

tion of abnormally high pressure and infection left untreated leads to disaster.

Clinical Types of Hydronephrosis

To list the various clinical presentations of this disease is more than an academic exercise. The classification into which a patient falls determines the investigation, management, and expected results. Each group can be categorized by its clinical and radiologic findings.[25]

Chronic Hydronephrosis

The child often presents with vague, nonspecific symptoms of dull ache in the loin or with urinary tract infection. Indeed, the condition may be a chance finding during investigation of the urinary tract for other problems or may even be found on a prenatal ultrasound study. Neonates may present with an asymptomatic abdominal mass. Unless infected, the kidney is not usually tender but may be palpable in a thin older child. Ultrasonography shows a dilated renal pelvis, and this is confirmed with an intravenous urogram (IVU). The pelvis is larger than normal and has a rounded outline as the diuretic effect of the contrast material expands it; the calices are usually, but not always, clubbed. If there *is* a marked degree of caliectasis, the changes are permanent, and after operation there is usually no improvement in the urographic appearance of the calices.

Acute or Intermittent Hydronephrosis

This is probably the more common type in children. One is confronted with an infant or young child who is clearly in pain and is tender in the loin. In an older child, the pain may be localized, and vomiting, hematuria, and urinary tract infection are common accompaniments. The situation often resolves within 24 hours so that by the time radiologic studies are performed the appearance may be back to near normal. Occasionally, the IVU shows an entirely normal kidney between attacks,[25] but more often there is a slight fullness of the renal pelvis, with normal calices and rapid transit of the contrast medium, at least on the early films (Fig 121–1). However, the diuretic effect of the contrast medium, or of an administered diuretic, may rapidly change the situation. The renal pelvis may double in size and become rounded; contrast is no longer seen in the ureter, and the calices become distended (see Fig 121–1). Erect, prone, or oblique roentgenograms may help to clarify the situation. The kidney may even become palpable and painful during these x-ray studies.

These measures do not always precipitate such an acute hydronephrotic state, and to see the true situation it is necessary to perform an IVU during an attack of pain. The findings during acute urography are often even more dramatic. The early films may show a negative pyelogram, while later on there is delay in the appearance of contrast in the collecting system, followed by delay in its clearance. A prone film is particularly useful here, as it shows contrast pooling in the pelvis.

In any child with a history of recurrent attacks of abdominal pain, the question of an intermittent hydronephrosis should be considered; once considered, the diagnosis is not difficult to prove. It cannot be overemphasized that it may only be during the attack that an IVU gives the correct diagnosis.

Equivocal Hydronephrosis

Many children do not fit into either of the above categories—the symptoms, signs, and radiologic findings are indefinite. Many such children present with infection, but with no symptoms directly related to the kidneys, and it may be difficult to correlate the clinical picture with the equivocal x-ray findings. The IVU may show some fullness of the pelvis, and possibly some caliectasis, but there is no delay in the appearance of contrast and minimal delay in emptying; the ureter is seen on many of the films, but the thickness of the renal parenchyma may be a little less than in the uninvolved kidney. Clearly, the kidney is not entirely normal, but at the same time there is no clear indication for a pyeloplasty.

The equivocal hydronephrosis has been the subject of intensive investigation over the past 10 years, and the lines of investigation are now clarified. In a few children, a further IVU with the administration of a diuretic during the study may show the "acute" changes in the appearance of the kidney described above, thus suggesting obstruction. Diuresis renography,[10, 17] using ^{99m}Tc-labeled DTPA (diethylenetriaminepentaacetic acid) or ^{123}I hippuran, may give a clear demonstration of the absence or presence of obstruction, but even these sophisticated studies may be misleading in 15% of children. The methods are influenced by the size of the system and the ability of the kidney to respond to a diuretic load. I have turned increasingly to a direct urodynamic analysis using percutaneous pressure flow studies and have found this to be a useful and accurate method of quantative assessment of the degree of obstruction.[22, 26]

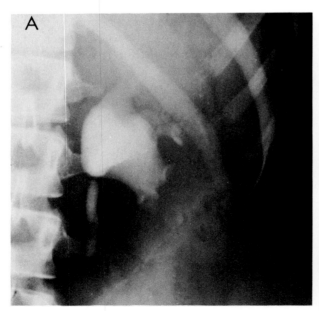
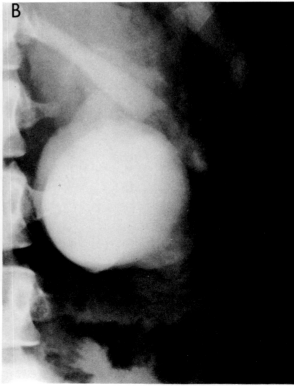

Fig 121–1.—Intermittent hydronephrosis. **A,** intravenous urogram of patient with intermittent hydronephrosis, taken between attacks of pain. **B,** intravenous urogram in same patient, after administration of a diuretic, showing acute hydronephrosis.

Reflux-Induced Hydronephrosis

Although distention of the renal pelvis caused by sudden massive reflux of urine or contrast medium from the bladder is common enough, it is most unusual to see a true obstruction develop at the pelviureteral junction as a result of such reflux.[11, 24] To make a definite diagnosis of reflux-induced obstruction, the renal pelvis at micturating cystourethrography must remain overfilled long after the ureter beneath it has emptied; in the child old enough to stand, the renal pelvis should remain full, even with the child upright. It is only during voiding that a sufficient volume of urine ascends the ureter to cause such distention. Reimplantation of the ureter may cure this problem, and a pyeloplasty is necessary only if the urographic appearances suggest continuing obstruction thereafter.

Etiology of Pelviureteric Junction Obstruction

Given the volume of past research, it is surprising that no definite theory has arisen to explain the "idiopathic" type of obstruction. At operation, a variety of kinks, angulations, and adhesions are seen,[25] as are blood vessels adjacent to the ureter. Undoubtedly, these may on occasion be the primary obstructive factors, but far more commonly the obstruction is still apparent after these have been dealt with.

Angulations and Adhesions

Johnston[6] performed intraoperative pressure flow studies before and after freeing adhesions from the pelviureteral region and found that in 24 of 32 children this completely relieved the obstruction. He admitted, however, that such angulations and adhesions might be secondary to some other underlying pathology.

Aberrant Vessels

Johnston et al.[7] and Uson et al.[21] found a lower branch of the renal artery apparently compressing the ureter in children with hydronephrosis in approximately 20% of cases. It is my experience that displacement of this vessel allows free drainage in only a small number of affected children. More commonly, the aberrant vessel is simply an exacerbating factor in an already obstructed renal pelvis, which tends to prolapse over such a vessel.

Ureteral Stenosis or Hypoplasia

A true stricture or severe narrowing is most unusual, although relative thinning of the ureteric wall for a centimeter or so is common enough. Extensive histologic investigation of these segments has been performed by many workers, and a variety of opinions expressed as to the findings—the quantity and arrangement of muscle fibers or the preponderance of fibrous tissue being most commonly implicated.[4, 5, 14, 16]

Polyp, Papilloma, or Valve

Benign connective tissue polyps are occasionally encountered at the pelviureteral junction. With the increasing resolution of x-ray techniques, polyps are now sometimes diagnosed preoperatively; simple excision and pyeloplasty solves this problem. Very rarely, a true papillary tumor is encountered in this region.[13] Occasionally, a valvular mucosal fold in the upper ureter seems to be the primary obstructive factor, but as this is often found only during a pyeloplasty, it is difficult to be sure that the fold is not secondary to an "idiopathic" obstruction.

Persistent Fetal Ureteral Folds

Johnston[6] has described the natural history of these folds, which occur during fetal life as invaginations of the musculature and mucosa[18] (Fig 121–2). They usually disappear with growth and only rarely cause a true obstruction. They appear more convincing on x-rays than by direct inspection of the ureter at operation. They are associated with a dependent renal pelvis, and it is important to avoid excising more ureter than is absolutely necessary.

Idiopathic Obstruction

In the vast majority of patients with ureteropelvic obstruction, there is no obvious cause for the obstruction, but the findings at operation are consistent. Instead of a normal funnel-shaped ureteropelvic junction, there is an abrupt change in the size of the system between the pelvis and upper ureter. With an increased fluid load (for example, from injection of saline into the pelvis), this discrepancy in size is exaggerated. If the upper ureter is cut across 0.5 cm below the ureteropelvic junction in preparation for a dismembered pyeloplasty, the pelvis does not empty; but a probe inserted up the ureter into the pelvis passes easily, excluding a true stenosis. On withdrawing the probe, there is a squirt of urine which, seconds later, becomes a drip and then stops completely. This phenomenon suggests abnormal muscular activity and supports the theory that I have propounded elsewhere.[23]

The theory suggests that it is the shape and distensibility of

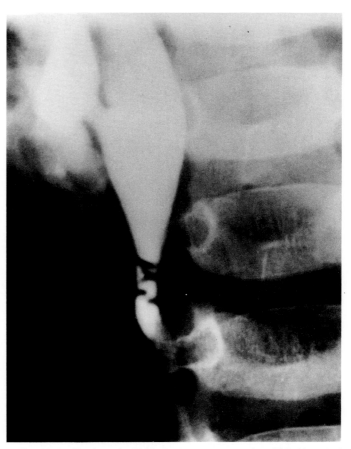

Fig 121–2.—Persistent fetal folds. Intravenous urogram in a child with marked fetal folds. These were excised and a pyeloplasty performed.

the renal pelvis itself that prevents normal bolus formation and that the circular component of the contraction wave, having missed the opportunity to form a bolus, finally occludes the lumen at the ureteropelvic junction. A vicious circle then ensues; the more the obstruction, the greater the pressure in the pelvis, the stronger the contraction wave, and the greater the resulting degree of obstruction. This theory, difficult as it is to prove, fits most of the known dynamic facts of this condition.[9, 15]

Diagnostic Methods

The methods involved can be summarized as follows.

Ultrasound

Routine prenatal ultrasound has become increasingly popular, and many hydronephroses are now being detected before they might otherwise have presented. Similarly, children with a first urinary tract infection are now screened conveniently with ultrasound, which may detect even small degrees of pelvicaliceal dilatation.

Intravenous Urography

This is usually the only investigation needed, although the standard IVU may need to be supplemented by the use of diuretics, prone films, and "acute" urography (see Fig 121–1). The radiologic indices of obstruction constitute a subject in themselves, but suffice it to say that in some patients it is difficult to be sure if the system is truly obstructed; other methods of investigation are needed in such patients.

Scintigraphy

Frequently it is important to know the contribution of each kidney to overall renal function. Dimercaptosuccinate (DMSA) or ^{123}I hippuran scintigraphy is ideal for this purpose. A nephrectomy might be considered the proper management in the older child if the kidney in question contributes less than 15% of an overall normal function. The finding in the obstructed kidney of 15% of a compromised overall function might suggest that the kidney should be preserved if at all possible. DMSA or ^{123}I hippuran scintigraphy is ideal for this purpose.

Radionuclide studies (^{123}I hippuran or ^{99m}Tc DTPA) can assess transit through the kidney, and in 85% of patients this correlates well with the presence or absence of obstruction. Interpretation of these studies is more difficult in solitary, grossly dilated, or poorly functioning kidneys.

Retrograde Ureterography and Micturating Cystourethrography

In children, it is particularly important to be sure that the ureter below a hydronephrotic kidney is normal, and this may not be obvious from the IVU. An associated obstructed megaureter or a refluxing ureter can complicate the postoperative course of a pyeloplasty. If the ureter is seen to be normal on the IVU, neither of these studies is essential; if the ureter is not seen or seems to be wide, one undertakes one of them, or both. Clearly, in a small boy it is best to avoid urethral instrumentation, and a percutaneous antegrade approach may be more suitable.

Percutaneous Nephrostomy

This technique can be used both therapeutically and diagnostically. In the acutely or chronically obstructed kidney, when the urogram gives insufficient information, the dilatation is confirmed with ultrasound, and the system is then cannulated for drainage and further radiologic evaluation. In the child with a doubtful degree of obstruction, the system can be perfused via a thin cannula at a known flow rate and pressures measured.[4, 5] This allows an accurate and quantitative assessment of the degree of obstruction which, together with scintigraphic evaluation of renal function, allows a logical clinical approach.

The Opposite Kidney and Associated Anomalies

Hydronephrosis is frequently bilateral, especially in infants. In a large series of children,[7, 8] bilaterality was found in 10%–20%. In infants under 6 months, the incidence may be as high as 25%–40%.[19, 27] The kidney contralateral to the one with hydronephrosis has a much-increased risk of being absent or multicystic. Similarly, children with other developmental anomalies such as imperforate anus, spina bifida, and congenital heart diseases are more prone to hydronephrosis. Noninvasive investigation with ultrasound is justified in all such children. Hydronephrosis is commonly encountered in horseshoe and ectopic kidneys, where the pelvis is often sufficiently deformed to make operation more difficult.

Complications

Stones and infection are common, secondary to obstruction and stasis. Stones are reported in 2%–5% of children with hydronephrosis.[7, 8, 21] A well-executed pyeloplasty usually absolves the kidney from further stone formation, but this is not always the case. Pyonephrosis with severe obstruction of the hydronephrotic kidney is much less often seen in children than adults. Rupture of a hydronephrosis may occur with even minor trauma in a child[7] and makes an IVU essential in any child with a renal injury or an abdominal injury associated with hematuria. Hypertension is a recognized but uncommon complication of hydronephrosis, especially in a solitary functioning kidney.[3, 7] Unfortunately, relief of the obstruction rarely cures the hypertension.

Treatment

Principles

Initially, it must be decided if the kidney is worth keeping. As a general rule, the younger the child the more likely is a return of useful function, so that in an infant one considers a pyeloplasty, unless the kidney is no more than a thin sac. Unfortunately, the function of the obstructed kidney as estimated by radionuclide studies cannot predict the extent of recovery. The final decision is often made at operation, when not only the thickness but the overall mass of the kidney can be assessed; if there is any doubt, it is wise to err on the side of preserving the kidney. The ultimate aim of all pyeloplasties is to achieve a funnel-shaped ureteropelvic junction that allows normal peristaltic activity with coaption and propulsion of a bolus.

Preliminary Nephrostomy

In adults with acute symptoms, it is often advantageous to drain the kidney temporarily by percutaneous nephrostomy. This is only occasionally applicable in children, in whom exploration of the kidney is usually indicated as a first procedure following cystoscopy and ureterography.

Pyeloplasty

The renal pelvis and upper ureter are most easily approached via an anterior subcostal incision from the tip of the twelfth rib to the edge of the rectus sheath or just beyond, displacing the peritoneum. This incision allows the pyeloplasty to be performed without extensive mobilization of the kidney. Others prefer the wider access of a loin incision.

The site of obstruction is usually obvious, but if there is doubt, the renal pelvis can be distended by injecting saline. The loose fat and fascia are dissected off the upper ureter and pelvis so that factors determining the choice of operative procedure can be assessed. These include: (1) the presence or absence of an aberrant lower pole vessel, (2) the angle between the pelvis and the ureter (Fig 121–3), (3) the height of ureteral insertion into the pelvis, (4) the extent of narrowing (apparent or real) of the upper ureter.

A vessel crossing the ureter indicates the need for a "dismembered" pyeloplasty, usually of the Anderson-Hynes type[1] (Fig 121–4), but occasionally all that is needed is an oblique anastomosis (Fig 121–5); the vessels themselves should be displaced behind the ureter and not divided. In a pyeloplasty in continuity, the angle between the pelvis and ureter is of importance (see Fig 121–3). The last two factors have a bearing on the design of the reconstruction of the renal pelvis and the extent to which the ureter is excised, or incised in the case of a flap pyeloplasty.

Dismembered Pyeloplasty

The redundant renal pelvis is excised, with careful preservation of the flap that is to be anastomosed to the ureter (see Fig 121–4). It is not essential to remove all the extrarenal pelvis, and, indeed, great care should be taken to avoid cutting close to the caliceal necks. The ureter is mobilized just enough to allow it to lie alongside the pelvic flap and is then spatulated for approximately 1.5 cm. The anastomosis is performed with chromic catgut or polyglycolic acid sutures, the size depending on the age of the child. In infants, 5-0 or 6-0 is best. In older children, 4-0 may be more appropriate. I use a continuous fine suture and lock it every 4–5 bites. Although others favor an interrupted suture line, I believe a continuous closure is more watertight. A drain should always be left close to, but not in contact with, the anastomosis and removed only when nothing has drained for 2–3 days. Splinting is not essential but has several advantages. A fine polyethylene tube through the anastomosis for 8 days prevents the two edges of the suture line from sticking together and prevents the ureteropelvic junction from kinking in the immediate postoperative period. A nephrostomy, or pyelostomy if preferred, should always accompany the splint to allow proximal drainage. That tube can be removed a day or so after the splint. In an older child, a Cummings tube is ideal, as it serves both purposes (Fig 121–6). If no splint is used, proximal diversion

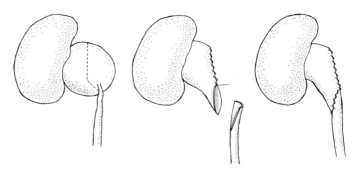

Fig 121–4.—Anderson-Hynes pyeloplasty.

should not be used either, as that prevents urine from draining through the anastomosis; such a "dry" anastomosis may narrow during the healing process.

Pyeloplasty in Continuity

If the ureteropelvic junction is dependent, or if there is a narrowing of the upper ureter, a dismembered pyeloplasty is not often practical. Instead, a flap of renal pelvis is used to put a "gusset" into the upper ureter. This achieves the basic aim of any pyeloplasty—producing a funneled ureteropelvic junction (see Fig 121–3). The direction of the flap to be cut from the pelvis depends on the angle of the upper ureter and the lower border of the pelvis. If this approximates a right angle, the flap is vertical;[20] if the angle is obtuse, a curved flap is needed.[2] The principles of splintage and drainage are the same as for dismembered pyeloplasty.

Bilateral Hydronephrosis

Bilateral pyeloplasties performed at the same time via an intraperitoneal approach are perfectly feasible, but a more conservative approach uses two separate extraperitoneal loin or subcostal incisions, allowing an interval of perhaps 2–3 weeks between operations.

Duplex Kidneys

It is not unusual to see a hydronephrosis in the lower moiety of a duplex system. This poses no special surgical problems unless the ureters join very close to the ureteropelvic junction of the lower moiety. The techniques already described must be modified to obtain the most efficient drainage. This may involve

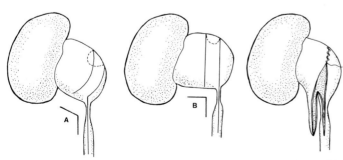

Fig 121–3.—Pyeloplasty in continuity. **A,** if the angle is greater than a right angle, a curved pelvic flap is needed. **B,** if it is a right angle, a vertical flap is best.

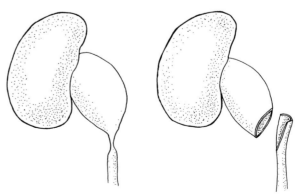

Fig 121–5.—Pyeloplasty using oblique anastomosis.

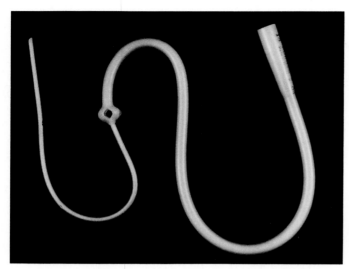

Fig 121–6.—Cummings tube for combined splintage and nephrostomy drainage.

an anastomosis between the lower pelvis and the upper ureter, which in infants can be of minute caliber, and calls for great care and fine suturing.

Horseshoe and Ectopic Kidneys

Because of the direction in which the pelvis points in these abnormal kidneys, it is often technically difficult to obtain dependent drainage of the anastomosis. In a dismembered pyeloplasty, the pelvic flap may lie awkwardly or the anastomosis may abut the parenchyma of the lower pole or isthmus. A nephropexy with rotation of the lower pole of the kidney backward, upward, and laterally often allows the ureteropelvic junction to lie more nearly correctly (Fig 121–7). This is not always an easy procedure, due to the multiplicity and complexity of the renal vessels, and may require division of the isthmus in a horseshoe kidney.

Pyeloplasty in the Presence of Reflux

Vesicoureteral reflux may complicate the postoperative course after a pyeloplasty. It may be necessary to place a urethral catheter in the bladder, or even to perform a temporary suprapubic cystostomy to prevent this reflux from harming the anastomosis.

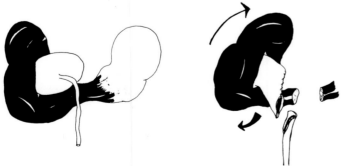

Fig 121–7.—Horseshoe kidney with hydronephrosis. It is often necessary to divide the isthmus and rotate the lower pole of the kidney outward, backward, and upward to allow the pelvis to become dependent.

Follow-Up

If a splint through the anastomosis is used, there is no place for clamping the nephrostomy tube or performing a nephrostogram (which invites leakage and provides little information). When the splint and nephrostomy tube are removed, there may be a little urinary leakage for 24 hours, occasionally somewhat longer. Provided this stops and the child remains well, no further investigations are necessary at this stage. A diuresis renogram at 1 month is reassuring, but an equivocal one is unhelpful. An IVU at 6 months is most important; if this is satisfactory, there is little need for further investigations without specific indications.

Results

Pyeloplasty is a remarkably effective operation in terms of relief of symptoms and resolution of the radiologic signs of obstruction; based on those criteria a 93% success rate is reported.[8] This is not to say that the caliceal appearances always return to normal; such structural alterations are permanent.

Diuresis radionuclide renography is a satisfactory way of assessing the result of operation, but if there is doubt as to the presence or absence of continuing obstruction, a percutaneous pressure flow study may become necessary.[26] In children under 1 year, some improvement in renal function can be expected. Over that age, stabilization of function is the best that can be achieved.[12]

REFERENCES

1. Anderson J.C.: *Hydronephrosis.* London, William Heinemann, Ltd., 1963.
2. Culp O.S., De Weerd J.H.: A pelvic flap operation for certain types of ureteropelvic obstruction: Preliminary report. *Proc. Mayo Clin.* 26:483, 1951.
3. Davis R.S., Manning J.A., Branch G.L., et al.: Renovascular hypertension secondary to hydronephrosis in a solitary kidney. *J. Urol.* 110:724, 1973.
4. Foote J.W., Blennerhasset J.B., Wiglesworth F.W., et al.: Observations on the ureteropelvic junction. *J. Urol.* 104:252, 1970.
5. Gosling J.A., Dixon J.S.: The structure of the normal and hydronephrotic upper urinary tract, in O'Reilly P.H., Gosling J.A. (eds.): *Idiopathic Hydronephrosis.* Heidelberg, Springer-Verlag, 1982, p. 1.
6. Johnston J.H.: The pathogenesis of hydronephrosis in childhood. *Br. J. Urol.* 41:724, 1969.
7. Johnston J.H., Evans J.P., Glassberg K.I., et al.: Pelvic hydronephrosis in children: A review of 219 personal cases. *J. Urol.* 117:97, 1977.
8. Kelalis P.P., Culp O.S., Stickler G.B., et al.: Ureteropelvic obstruction in children: Experiences with 109 cases. *J. Urol.* 106:418, 1971.
9. Kiil F.: *The Function of the Ureter and Renal Pelvis.* Oslo, Oslo University Press., 1957.
10. Koff S.A., Thrall J.H., Keyes J.W. Jr.: Assessment of hydroureteronephrosis in children utilising diuretic radionuclide urography. *J. Urol.* 123:531, 1980.
11. Lebowitz R.L., Blickman J.G.: The coexistence of ureteropelvic junction obstruction and reflux. *AJR* 140:231, 1983.
12. Mayor G., Genton N., Torrado A., et al.: Renal function in obstructive nephropathy: Long-term effect of reconstructive surgery. *Pediatrics* 56:740, 1975.
13. Mirandi D., De Assis A.S.: Transitional cell papilloma of ureter in young boy. *Urology* 5:559, 1975.
14. Murnaghan G.F.: The dynamics of the renal pelvis and ureter with reference to congenital hydronephrosis. *Br. J. Urol.* 30:321, 1958.
15. Murnaghan G.F.: The mechanism of congenital hydronephrosis with reference to the factors influencing surgical treatment. *Ann. R. Coll. Surg. Engl.* 23:25, 1958.
16. Notley R.G.: The structural basis for normal and abnormal ureteric motility. *Ann. R. Coll. Surg. Engl.* 49:248, 1971.
17. O'Reilly P.H., Lawson R.S., Shields R.A., et al.: Idiopathic hydronephrosis—the diuresis renogram: A new non-invasive method of assessing equivocal pelviureteral junction obstruction. *J. Urol.* 121:153, 1979.

18. Ostling K.: Genesis of hydronephrosis. *Acta Chir. Scand.* (suppl. 86) 72:5, 1942.
19. Roth D.R., Gonzales E.T. Jr.: Management of ureteropelvic junction obstruction in infants. *J. Urol.* 129:108, 1983.
20. Scardino P.L., Prince C.L.: Vertical flap ureteropelvioplasty: Preliminary report. *South. Med. J.* 46:325, 1953.
21. Uson A.C., Cox, L.A., Lattimer J.K.: Hydronephrosis in infants and children. *JAMA* 205:323, 1968.
22. Whitaker R.H.: Methods of assessing obstruction in dilated ureters. *Br. J. Urol.* 45:15, 1973.
23. Whitaker R.H.: Some observations and theories on the wide ureter and hydronephrosis. *Br. J. Urol.* 47:377, 1975
24. Whitaker R.H.: Reflux induced pelviureteric obstruction. *Br. J. Urol* 48:555, 1976.
25. Whitaker R.H.: Hydronephrosis. *Ann. R. Coll. Surg. Engl.* 59:388, 1977.
26. Whitaker R.H.: The Whitaker test. *Urol. Clin. North Am.* 6:529, 1979.
27. Williams D.I., Karlaftis C.M.: Hydronephrosis due to pelvi-ureteric obstruction in the newborn. *Br. J. Urol.* 38:138, 1966.

122 F. Douglas Stephens

Bifid and Double Ureters, Ureteroceles, and Fused Kidneys

When two ureters issue from a double kidney, they may form a Y junction with long or short common stems or a V junction with negligible stem, in both cases being referred to as bifid ureters, or they may open separately into the urinary or genital tracts as double ureters. These are common developmental and often inherited abnormalities and, as such, may be entirely symptom-free.[2, 34] Atwell and Allen[3] demonstrated a high incidence of duplex and reflux ureters in first-degree relatives of patients who were found to have a paraureteral diverticulum. They considered these three conditions interrelated and the mechanisms of inheritance similar. Some ureters have defective insertions into the bladder or urethra, resulting in vesicoureteral reflux; others exhibit obstructive lesions that promote stasis and infection, back pressure or wetting problems.

It seems likely that there is a close embryologic correlation between the morphology of the renal segments and the position of orifices in the lower tract. On the basis of this correlation, accurate identification of orifice position will help the clinician and radiologist to explain the nature of the abnormal shapes and sizes of the kidneys of the duplex systems and will guide them in the management of children with these troublesome abnormalities.[20]

Embryology

These curious developmental misadventures may be explained on the basis of normal and abnormal development of both single and double ureters.

Five key steps in the normal embryology of the ureter require individual consideration. These are: (1) budding of the ureter from the wolffian duct, (2) caudal migration of the ureteral orifices, (3) expansion of the vesicourethral canal from a tubular to a globular shape, (4) nephrogenic cord and blastema from which the permanent kidney is derived, and (5) atrophy of the wolffian or müllerian ducts.

In step 1, the ureter begins at the 4-mm stage of development as a bud arising from the wolffian (mesonephric) duct, a short distance from the entry of the duct into the urethra; this bud further divides into upper and lower calices and collecting ducts

and penetrates the adjacent metanephric tissue that forms the renal parenchyma.

In step 2, between 4-mm and 10-mm stages, the terminal part of the wolffian duct, at and including that part from which the ureteral bud arises, expands in trumpet fashion and is taken up or absorbed into the vesicourethral canal. The orifice of the ureter in this way separates from that of the wolffian duct, and comes to lie craniolateral to the wolffian orifice in the urethra. Further migration of the ureteral orifice is normally to the lateral cornu of the trigone in which the ureterovesical valve subsequently develops (Fig 122–1).

In step 3, at the time that the ureters are separating and migrating from the wolffian ducts, the tubular vesicourethral canal undergoes an accelerated expansion to form the bladder and prostatic urethra. This takes place in embryos of 6–16 mm crown-rump length.

In step 4, the nephrogenic cord, the terminal section of the wolffian ridge, gives rise first to the pronephros at the cranial end of the embryo, then to the mesonephros in the midpart of the embryo, and, finally, to the metanephros in the sacral area. The wolffian duct begins cranially in the lateral aspect of the pronephros, continues caudally alongside the mesonephros and the nephrogenic cord, and then angulates medially and anterior to the cord to enter the internal cloaca and subsequently its anterior urinary compartment. The pronephros and mesonephros are temporary structures; the metanephros, or permanent kidney, develops in a specific section of the nephrogenic cord alongside the angulated section of the wolffian duct from which the ureteral bud arises and enters the metanephric blastema. Presumably, the unwanted sections of the cord to either end of the metanephric section also atrophy. The renal blastema differentiates around the bud and moves cranially, elongating the ureter, while the ureteral bud orifice migrates caudally as described (Fig 122–2).

In step 5, the wolffian ducts act as the guides to the müllerian ducts, which arise near the gonads on the wolffian ridge and come to issue into the urethra, between the orifices of the wolffian ducts near the bladder neck, at or about the 30-mm stage. In the male, the wolffian duct develops into the vas deferens and

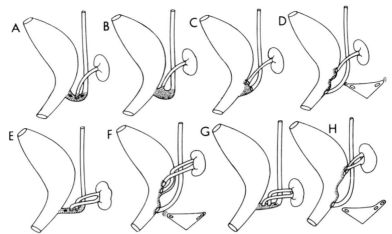

Fig 122–1.—Embryologic rearrangement of ureteral orifices in single and double systems from wolffian duct to urinary tract. **A–D,** single ureter arising from normal site on wolffian duct *(middle black dot)* and migrating to the lateral cornu of trigone. **E** and **F,** double ureters arising from two sites on the duct *(black dots)* and migrating to two sites in urinary tract, rearranging themselves so that the upper pole ureteral orifice lies caudal to that of the lower pole ureter. **G** and **H,** another combination with upper pole ureteral orifice migrating to the normal position on the trigone and the lower pole ureter issuing laterally. Ureteral buds arising from points high on wolffian duct may not be absorbed into the urinary tract and remain attached to the wolffian (seminal) duct.

the müllerian ducts atrophy, except for the utriculus prostaticus. In the female, the wolffian ducts wither and become incorporated, as Gartner's ducts, in the lateral walls of the rapidly growing müllerian ducts. They may eventually disappear altogether.

The müllerian ducts in the female fuse and migrate distally, carrying in their lateral walls the wolffian ducts, and shifting the vaginal orifice from its hidden pelvic location to the exposed position in the vestibule (Fig 122–3).

Ureteral Bud Deformities

The ureteral bud, with its inherent powers of molding to shapes and sizes of the ureter, pelvis, calices and ducts of Bellini, may develop abnormally. It may arise as a mega- or microureter, the orifice or all or any part being larger or smaller than normal.

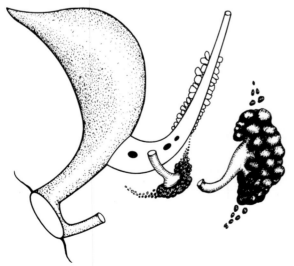

Fig 122–2.—Wolffian duct at 4-mm stage entering vesicourethral canal. Note expansion of terminal end and the ureteral bud emerging from the "knee" bend to enter the main mass of renal blastema. *Black dots* represent alternate sites of budding and corresponding dwindling nephrogenic blastema. Mesonephric structures abut the cranial end of the metanephros and the buds that arise high on the duct.

The bud may divide to form a bifid system, or two buds may arise to form two separate ureters. When the ureters are duplicated, both may be normal in all other respects, or either or both may be abnormal.

With double ureters, the ureteral bud nearest to the terminal end of the wolffian duct is taken up, first into the bladder, and preforms the trigone on which the second ureter issues on the ectopic pathway.[25]

Upper pole ureters that open on the trigone, urethra, or vestibule lie together with the lower pole ureter as they traverse together the common tunnel through the bladder wall.[24] Only the rare bud that retains its very high attachment to the wolffian duct takes a totally extravesical course to the vas or vesicle in the male, and to Gärtner's duct embedded in the lateral wall of the vagina (Fig 122–3). If Gärtner's duct remains patent, the urine is led distally to emerge at the orifice of the duct near the hymen; if Gärtner's duct is atrophic, the urine will be trapped in the ureter and that part of the adjoining duct that has remained patent, forming a bulging, soft, cyst-like structure in the side wall of the vagina.

BIFID URETERS.—At the 4-mm stage, a single bud issues from the wolffian duct and (1) splits immediately to form two ureters, the V junction coming to lie in the intramural tunnel of the bladder, or (2) splits after the formation of a single stem of variable length, the Y junction being extravesical (Fig 122–4). If splitting occurs at the region of the hilus of the kidney, the pelvis may be replaced by two or three calices.

If the orifice of the bifid ureters lies within the confines of the normal trigone, the stem and urethra are normal in caliber, and the renal substance is structurally normal also. The two ureters, however, may be larger than the common stem with hydronephrosis.[26] If the ureteral orifice is misplaced laterally on the bladder base, the intravesical portion of the ureter is shortened and vesicoureteral reflux is likely to ensue. The parenchyma of the two parts of the bifid kidney is structurally similar because the site of origin of the common stem bud is the same for each part.[20]

Other uncommon abnormalities that may affect bifid ureters with a common stem include stenosis of either limb of the bifid system, a ureteral valve, renal hypoplasia, obstruction to either ureter by hilar vessels, and simple ureterocele formation (Fig 122–5).[16, 19]

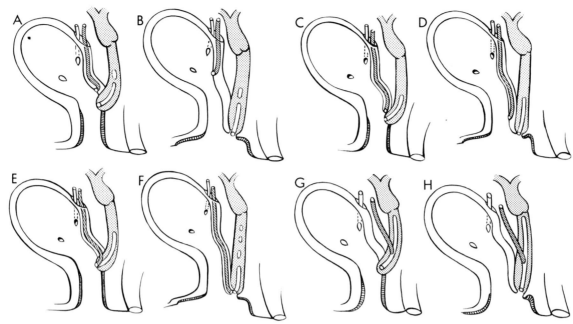

Fig 122–3.—Embryologic rearrangement of ectopic ureters of duplex systems caused by involvement with müllerian ducts at 30-mm stage. The ectopic orifice, being well clear of the wolffian duct orifice **(A)** at the time of arrival of the müllerian ducts, migrates cranially **(B)** uninfluenced by the müllerian ducts. **C** and **D,** when the ectopic orifice is adjacent to the wolffian orifice at the time of arrival of the müllerian ducts, it becomes involved in the caudal müllerian migration and is transposed part way along the urethra. **E** and **F,** if the ectopic orifice is contiguous with the wolffian orifice **(E)** it will "hitchhike" on Gärtner's and müllerian ducts, issuing on the hymen **(F)**. **G** and **H,** the ectopic ureter that retains its connection at a high level with the wolffian duct takes a course posterior to the bladder to enter Gärtner's duct in the lateral wall of the vagina.

DOUBLE URETERS.—Two buds representing, respectively, the major calices to the cranial and caudal renal segments arise separately from the wolffian duct. Both buds grow out into the adjacent nephrogenic blastema to induce the development of two separate, but contiguous, kidney segments. The origins of the two buds migrate caudally into the urethra and somersault into the bladder, while the renal ends of the buds migrate cranially.

The positions of the ureteral orifices of double ureters in the urinary tract are dictated by the sites of origin of the respective ureteral buds on the terminal part of the wolffian duct. These, in turn, are very closely related to the nephrogenic cord that lies alongside the duct, and hence the position of the orifice and budding may have direct bearing on the point of contact of the bud with the nephrogenic cord and the quality of the developing kidney (Fig 122–6).

ORIFICE POSITION AND RENAL MORPHOLOGY.—To explain the correlation of orifice position and renal morphology, the terminal part of the wolffian duct and nephrogenic cord may be divided into three short sections. The middle section of the duct, when absorbed into the vesicourethral canal, is transposed, together with the ureteral buds that arise from it, to the normal trigone

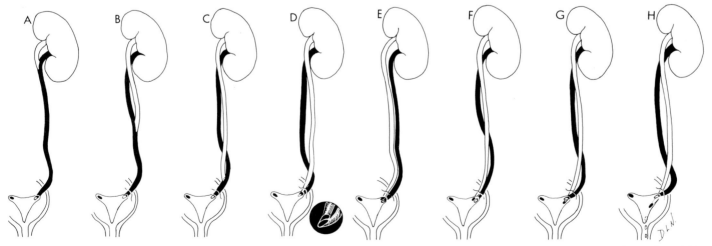

Fig 122–4.—Course of bifid and double ureters. **A,** bifid pelvis. **B** and **C,** bifid ureters with midureter and distal Y junctions; note anterior relationship of upper pole ureter (UPU) to lower pole ureter (LPU). **D,** intravesical V junction. **E,** uncrossed double ureters with UPU orifice cranial to orifice of LPU. **F** and **G,** junctional bud ureters on medial arc of ectopic pathway; note that in **G** the UPU crosses behind the LPU in the intramural tunnel to achieve an opening caudal to the orifice of the LPU. **H,** locations of UPU orifices on lateral border of trigone and in urethra.

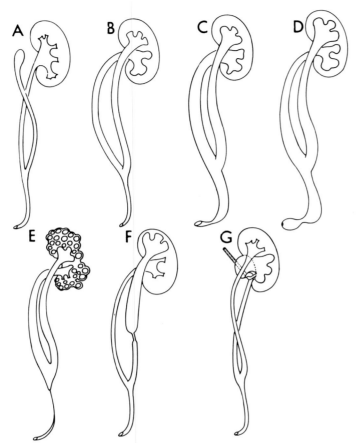

Fig 122–5.—Bifid ureters complicated by additional anomalies: **A,** blind-ending ureter; **B,** megaureters and normal-caliber stem; **C,** megaureter with vesicoureteral reflux; **D,** ureterocele; **E,** atresia; **F,** ureteral stenosis; **G,** lower hilar vessel obstructing lower pole ureter.

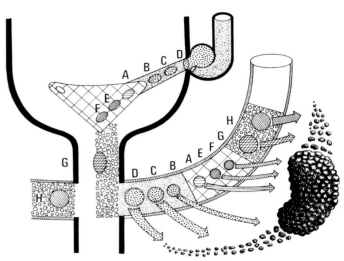

Fig 122–6.—Composite diagram depicting three sections of the distal end of the wolffian duct from which the ureteral buds may arise, the corresponding sections of the nephrogenic cords that the buds penetrate to induce the permanent kidney, and the sites on the bladder base, trigone, urethra, and genital ducts to which the orifices of the ureteral buds migrate. The **A, E,** and **F** buds penetrate the main mass of renal blastema, predestined for the development of the normal permanent kidney; **B, C,** and **D** buds enter progressively smaller amounts of blastema, and the **G** and **H** buds strike the nephrogenic cord that adjoins the mesonephros and that undergoes atrophy, involution, and dysplasia.

area in the bladder. The buds penetrate the adjoining nephrogenic cord in that section earmarked for the normal development of the kidney. The most distal section of the duct is transposed onto the bladder base, craniolateral to the trigone, and the third section arranges itself in the urethra and bladder neck regions. The orifices of buds arising from these two sections are transposed with them, accounting for the lateral ectopic and urethral ectopic locations, respectively. These stray buds penetrate the corresponding extraneous nephrogenic cord sections, the distal being the depleted tail end of the cord and the other adjoining the mesonephros, which is destined to undergo atrophy or involution (Fig 122–6).

Mackie, Awang, and Stephens[21] found a close correlation between the orifice position in the bladder, urethra, or genital ducts and the renal radiographic appearance and morphology in patients with bifid and double ureters. The orifices of ureters lying on the normal trigone were associated with normal kidneys and ureters, whereas those lying lateral to the normal trigone, were accompanied by larger than normal ureters and thinner kidneys; and those sited in the urethra or genital ducts had large and tortuous ureters and small dysplastic kidneys (Fig 122–7).

The greater the distance of origin of the buds either way from the middle section, and hence the greater the distance of the ureteral orifices from the normal trigonal area, the more abnormal were the renal segments and the clearer the distinguishing

line or groove between the two parts of the double kidney. With borderland orifices, the accompanying kidney segments show less obvious changes.

Symptoms and Treatment of Bifid and Double Ureters

Urinary infections with dysuria, suprapubic or loin pains, or failure to thrive bring the patient to notice. Pain alone, without infection, is rare.

The junction site of bifid ureters, the presence of vesicoureteral reflux, and the anatomy of both components of the double system should be determined by intravenous pyelography, voiding cystoureterography, or retrograde pyelography. Sometimes percutaneous antegrade urography may help to define the presence and course of the upper pole ureter. Differential function of the two renal segments can be assessed by nuclear imaging techniques.

Bifid ureters may exhibit stasis due to ureter-to-ureter reflux, and are then more prone to episodes of infection if the limbs of the Y are long or wider than normal in caliber, or if the common stem also is abnormally wide and permits vesicoureteral reflux. Infections are uncommon when the Y junction of normal caliber ureters is above the pelvic brim and also in the V-type bifid ureters.[18]

For those with repeated infections in the upper tract, whether the bifid ureters are normal or larger than normal in caliber, the upper pole ureter should be anastomosed to the pelvis or ureter of the lower renal segment with excision of the upper pole ureter down to the Y junction.[22] Reimplantation of the common stem may be indicated when infection is associated with vesicoureteral reflux.

Patients with double ureters issuing into the bladder present with infection, chiefly because of reflux into the lower pole ureter and less often into the upper pole ureter or the opposite ureter or ureters. Long-term, low-dose antibiotic therapy is indicated if infections can be prevented while reflux persists. Ne-

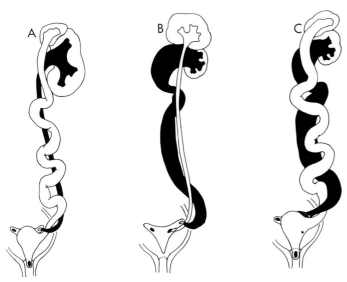

Fig 122–7.—Ureteral orifice position and predictable renal morphology. **A,** LPU in *A* position of Figure 122–6, kidney is structurally normal; UPU orifice in *G* position with or without ureterocele; kidney segment is small and dysplastic. **B,** LPU in *C* position, kidney is thin and hypoplastic; calices are clubbed, and ureteromegaly is present: UPU in *A* position, kidney is structurally normal. **C,** LPU in *C* position and lifted onto ureterocele results in ureterocaliectasis and thin hypoplastic kidney; UPU orifice in *G* (or *H*) position results in ureterocaliectasis with or without ureterocele and small dysplastic kidney. Note that UPU is anterior to LPU in extravesical course and behind in the intramural tunnel.

phroureterectomy or heminephrectomy may be indicated for hypofunction of renal segments. Reimplantation of reflux ureters should be undertaken when the function of the kidney segment is sound, breakthrough infections occur, and reflux seems long-term or permanent in either ureter. Both ureters can usually be reimplanted together in their common sheath.[4, 9] A ureteroureteral anastomosis may be indicated instead of reimplantation if only one of the two ureters is incompetent and both are near normal in caliber.[22]

Infection also results from stasis caused by obstruction of the upper pole ureter due to stenosis or to the squeeze of the urethral sphincters on the ectopic ureter or ureterocele.

Reimplantation of Double Ureters

In the transplantation procedure to be described, anatomical concepts of the fasciae of the ureter described by Elbadawi[7] facilitate the technical steps in the dissection of single ureters; and, with minor modifications, the descriptions of the fasciae apply to operations on double ureters. An intravesical approach gives adequate access to most double ureters and their fasciae inside and outside the hiatus for mobilization and implantation of the ureters, ensuring sufficient elongation of the reset submucosal segment. A racquet incision is made, encircling the two orifices with the cranial handle extension over the hiatus onto the posterior wall. The mucosal lining of the bladder is lifted off the ureters and undercut widely. Waldeyer's sheath within the bladder and hiatus, which is formed by fibers attached to the hiatal muscle and the ureter, is incised and split apart to expose the ureters, which are lifted from the common bed. The distal attachments to the trigone around the floor and orifices are picked up and divided (Fig 122–8).

The hiatus is then incised in a cranial direction, cutting through the muscle of the bladder for a distance of 2 cm. The extravesical space is cleared so that Waldeyer's fascia can be lifted off the ureters laterally. The two ureters lie in a delicate

"see-through" sheath, which is common to and free from both until it blends at the hiatus with the ureters, binding them firmly together in the submucosal segment. Laterally, where the ureters glide freely inside the "see-through" sheath, an incision in the line of the ureters is made and a plane of separation is developed all around the two ureters without separating them individually. This sheath is then divided circumferentially, and the ureters will then slide out of the cranial part of the sheath for about 2–3 cm, with only very light traction. Enough ureter length is gained for reimplantation by this maneuver. The caudal aspect of the hiatus is repaired and forms the new muscular bed for the ureters; the orifices are advanced onto or across the trigone, and the bladder mucosa is sewn back over the ureters.

When the upper pole ureter takes a long submucosal course to issue into the urethra or urethrovaginal bridge, both the ureter and calix are dilated and the renal segment is hypoplastic or dysplastic, though some functioning nephrons may be present. Male and female patients in whom the orifice of the ectopic ureter lies in the upper third of the urethra, cranial to the point of highest threshold of the urethral pressure profile, are continent because the urine secreted by the upper pole overflows back into the bladder; such ureters are usually dilated, and 20% exhibit reflux.[25]

When, as in some females, the orifice lies in the distal two thirds of the urethra or beyond, urine dribbles incontinently, although the patient will void normally at regular intervals. Urinary infections, pus discharge on the diaper, or pus appearing in the vulva, especially after fluid loading of the patient, are all typical features.

If the renal segment is sound and the orifice of the ureter is in the region of the bladder neck and does not permit reflux, minimal deroofing by transurethral resection to shift the orifice back into the bladder is indicated. In most children, the renal segment is defective and should be removed, together with its dilated and tortuous ureter. Excision of the intravesical extension of the ureter may be undertaken through a separate incision at the same operation. Some surgeons prefer to excise the distal ureter later, and only if symptoms recur.

Ureteroceles in Double Ureters

A ureterocele is a globular expansion of the submucosal section of the ureter. On the basis of location of orifice, ureteroceles may be divided into simple and ectopic types.[8, 16] A third miscellaneous group comprises the blind ureterocele and the cecoureterocele[24] (Fig 122–9).

Stenosis and ureterocele may well be regarded as cause and effect. However, the combination is not always present, and then the cause is not clear. For example, in many instances, the ectopic ureter runs submucosally along the trigone and urethra and is partly obstructed by the urethral sphincters, yet does not exhibit ureterocele formation. Furthermore, the ureter on which a large ureterocele is present may exhibit a large orifice in the urethra or bladder. It appears that the factors operating to form the ureterocele in such examples exist in the early developmental phase when the ureteral orifice is migrating from the wolffian duct to the urethra or bladder, and before urine is excreted from the kidney. The orifice and the adjoining ureter may become involved in the process, which expands the vesicourethral tube into the globular shape of the bladder, imparting this expansion stimulus to the ectopic ureter that lies within its walls.[25] Tanagho[29] postulates that the ureteral bud undergoes a focal dilatation to produce the giant ureterocele before it begins its migration from the wolffian duct.

The simple type of ureterocele has a stenotic orifice situated on the trigone within the bladder. The orifice may occur on the

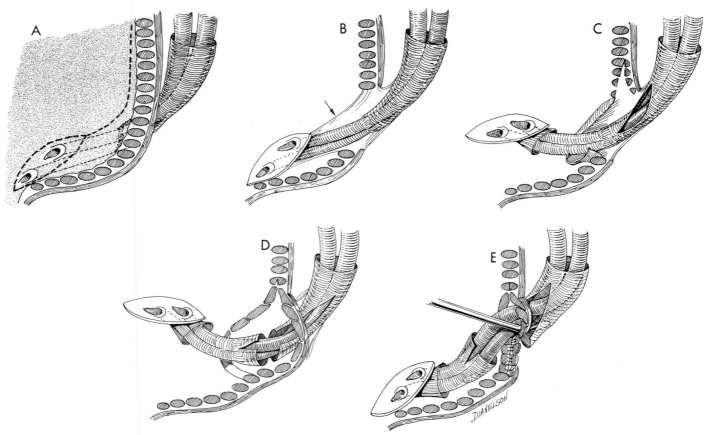

Fig 122–8.—Reimplantation of double ureters. **A,** the heavy broken line indicates the line of incision of the mucosa of the bladder. **B,** Waldeyer's fascia attaches circumferentially to the bladder muscle of the hiatus, clothes the ureters inside the bladder to their orifices, and runs on into the deep trigone and outside the bladder to the fascial sheath of the ureters. Waldeyer's fascia is incised longitudinally in the direction of the ureters *(arrow)* and then divided circumferentially around the ureters in their common sheath. **C,** the hiatus is then identified and enlarged by division of bladder muscle in a craniolateral direction. Through this widened hiatus, the lateral extension of Waldeyer's fascia can be gently separated from the juxtavesical ureters, bringing them in their "see-through" common sheath into view. This sheath blends with the muscle coats of the ureters at the hiatus and binds the ureters individually and together inside the bladder. **D,** this delicate "see-through" fascia is picked up lateral to the hiatus, incised, and elevated from the ureters and divided circumferentially without separating the ureters. **E,** the ureters glide freely for several centimeters out of the sheath into the bladder, with gentle traction. The hiatus is repaired on the caudal aspect of the ureters, snugging up the bladder muscle and using an 8 F calibrator to avoid undue tightness. The orifices are then advanced along the trigone and sutured into place. The bladder mucosa is finally approximated over both ureters in their new intravesical bed.

common stem of the bifid ureter, but more frequently it issues at some point on the trigone, caudal to the orifice of the lower pole ureter. The ectopic ureterocele is of giant size and issues at the bladder neck or beyond in the urethra, and its orifice may be stenotic, normal or very wide in caliber. The cecoureterocele is characterized by a wide, reflux orifice in the bladder and a tubular submucosal tongue extending along the urethra. In the cecoureterocele the orifice is situated on the dome of the ureterocele, and permits in and out flow of bladder urine into the ureterocele. The dilated submucosal ureter in the trigonal area forms the ureterocele, which is moderately large, and the lumen of the ureterocele extends distally beyond the level of the internal urethral meatus in the submucosal plane (Fig 122–9). Sometimes, this submucosal extension of the lumen may reach to the level of the external urinary meatus. The ureterocele fills with urine chiefly by reverse flow from the bladder during voiding, and the tongue obstructs the urethra.[21] The blind ureterocele is self-explanatory, but it usually has a submucosal extension into the urethra.

Diagnosis and Treatment of Simple Ureterocele

The simple ureterocele is sessile or pedunculated, and the orifice may be situated at the caudal end of the ureterocele or surmounted on its convexity (Fig 122–9). The muscle of the ureterocele may be thick and hypertrophic, and extend to the rim of the orifice. It may, however, be thin or absent around the orifice and roof of the ureterocele.

Simple ureteroceles may be symptomless until complicated by infection, stone formation or prolapse into the urethra. Then the symptoms lead to urologic investigation. The diagnosis is usually made on the IVP series. The kidney being of good function, the terminal ureter fills with radiopaque material and may exhibit a "cobra-head" appearance in the base of the bladder.

Micturition cystourethrography may demonstrate other features, such as reflux into the ureterocele or into the lower pole ureter, or the prolapsed ureterocele, if pedunculated, may be apparent as a nonopaque, rounded, filling defect in the bladder neck or urethra[28] (Fig 122–9).

In most instances of simple ureterocele, the orifice lies on the trigone and the renal morphology is structurally and functionally sound, though somewhat depleted by the effects of back pressure. Treatment, therefore, focuses on the ureterocele: (1) if the orifice is end on and visible endoscopically, it may be enlarged by ureteral dilatation if catheters can be inserted, or by minimal diathermy of the margin and roof around the orifice. If the orifice is slightly tilted onto the dome, it may be enlarged by diathermy of its 6 o'clock margin, as described by Hutch and Chisholm.[15]

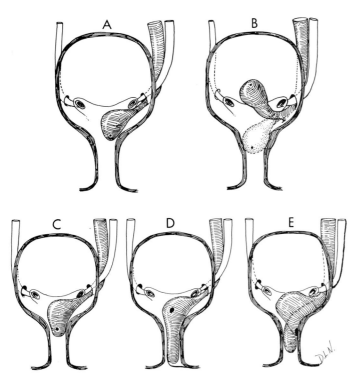

Fig 122–9.—Ureterocele types, and the effects of ureterocele on ipsilateral and contralateral ureters (assuming both open on the trigone in the *A* position of Fig 122–6). **A** and **B,** show a simple ureterocele with stenotic orifice in **E** and **F** positions in the bladder; **A** is sessile and **B** is pedunculated and liable to prolapse along the urethra. Ipsi- and contralateral ureters are usually normal in caliber, but the LPU may be mildly compressed and dilated. **C,** ectopic stenotic ureterocele remains dilated at all times and obstructs the bladder neck with moderate dilatation of the LPU and contralateral ureter. **D,** cecoureterocele, which fills during voiding by reflux, and "cecum" partially blocks the urethra; the LPU and the contralateral ureters are mildly dilated. **E,** ectopic ureterocele with wide orifice empties during voiding; minimal urethral obstruction and minimal dilatation of other ureters (diagram also shows the ureterocele prolapsed into the urethra).

(2) If the orifice is not visible endoscopically, the bladder should be opened, the ureterocele excised, and both ureters mobilized and advanced onto midtrigone to prevent reflux.

Diagnosis and Treatment of Ectopic Ureterocele

Urinary infection, uremia with failure to thrive, urethral obstruction with voiding difficulties or sudden prolapse of the ureterocele at the external meatus bring the child with ureterocele deformity for evaluation.

The cystogram may show a large, rounded filling defect of the ureterocele distended by its nonopaque urine content at the bladder base. During voiding, the filling defect may remain unchanged if its orifice is stenotic, disappear if its orifice is not obstructed, prolapse into the urethra, or fill with radiopaque medium. Reflux may occur into the lower pole ureter or opposite ureter, which may be larger than normal in diameter.

The IVP depicts the renal segments of the kidneys. Characteristically, the upper segment is hydronephrotic with poor function and may displace the lower renal segment laterally and caudally. The dilated upper pole calix and ureter may opacify, and the lower pole segment and ureter may show normal or abnormal features. The upper tracts on both sides, in young children, are governed in their appearance and renal morphology chiefly by the positions of the orifice, but obstruction and infection may also complicate the radiologic interpretations. Combinations are shown in Figure 122–7.

Cystoscopy is important in determining the type and management of the ectopic ureterocele; the location and size of the orifices and the dynamics of the ureterocele serve as guides in management. If the ureterocele can be seen to contract actively and change its shape to that of a ureter lying invisible beneath the trigonal mucosa, surgical transposition of the orifice from urethra to trigone by minimal deroofing, using the resectoscope for the purpose, is appropriate. This maneuver corrects the ureteral obstruction, cures the ureterocele, and permits the ureteral musculature to maintain competence.

When the ureterocele on prolonged cystoscopic observation fails to show contractility but merely collapses, resection of the roof would induce reflux, so incision alone is not adequate treatment in this situation. For an acute crisis of infection in the upper pole system, incision of the roof of the ureterocele and catheter drainage of the bladder is a suitable temporizing maneuver.

The renal segments of most ectopic ureteroceles are defective and should usually be removed, together with the attached ureter, unless total renal function is so depleted that preservation of even this poorly functioning segment is important. Heminephrectomy combined with ureterectomy is adequate if the accompanying and contralateral ureters and kidneys are normal in size and function. To ensure that the blood supply to the remaining segment of the double kidney is not inadvertently impaired during the heminephrectomy procedure, the renal pedicle or the branches supplying the segment to be resected should be temporarily compressed with a gentle bulldog clamp. Then, after peeling back the capsule, the segment is separated by sharp and blunt dissection from lateral to medial sides, isolating, ligating, and dividing the hilar vessels of supply as they come free with the detached segment of the kidney. By this lateral-to-medial separation, the vessels to both parts of the double kidney are clearly identified before division, and the risks of ischemia to the remaining segment averted.

A second operation, however, to remove the ureterocele, reimplant ureters, and correct any other intravesical anomalies should be undertaken if infections persist or recur, if the bladder outlet or ipsilateral ureter are obstructed by the ureterocele, or if other ureters are incompetent and exhibit potential hazard to the remaining kidneys.[12, 17, 31, 33]

Blind Ureters

With either bifid or double ureters, one ureter may be blind at its cranial end. The upper pole ureter is most commonly affected. The lower pole ureter appears to subserve a whole kidney with full complement of calices. The blind ureter may be short, long, slim or bulbous, and opens distally at a Y junction or onto the ectopic pathway in the bladder or urethra. It may have a normal orifice in the bladder or may exhibit reflux or ureterocele formation (Fig 122–10).

The blind ureter in the bifid system may give rise to stasis and infection or recurrent pain.[1] The blind unit of a double system may be found incidently when investigations are carried out for infections resulting from stasis and reflux in the other ureters. Rarely, a dilated aborted ureter may have a wide orifice at the bladder neck, causing a flap valve obstruction of the urethra. Treatment is indicated for repeated infection or pain or in conjunction with surgery for reflux in the ureters or obstruction.

Excision of a blind limb of a bifid system down to the Y junction or excision of the blind double ureter for its own intrinsic pathologic state or in combination with reimplantation of other ureters is sometimes necessary.

Single Ectopic Ureters

Ureters are generally regarded as ectopic when the orifice issues elsewhere but in the cornu of the normal trigone. Lateral ectopia is the most common form and is associated with vesi-

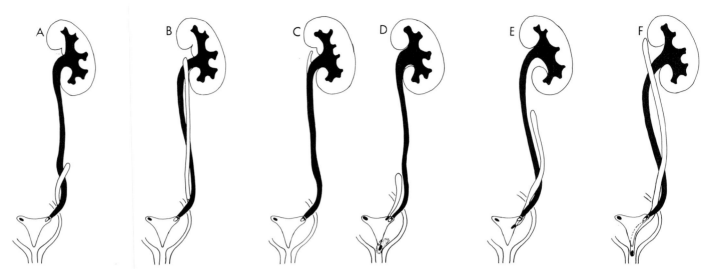

Fig 122–10.—Blind ureters. **A–C,** examples found in bifid systems. **D–F,** blind UPUs of double system. **D** shows an isolated ureterocele in the UPU system of another patient.

coureteral reflux. However, the term "ectopic" is generally applied to ureters that open in the bladder neck, urethra, or genital tracts. Most examples are associated with duplex kidneys and have already been described. Ectopic ureters, when single, issue in similar sites, have similar symptomatology, and require similar surgical corrective procedures.

Single ectopic ureters are dissimilar in the following ways: The ureter subserves the whole kidney, which may itself be ectopic or abnormal; the vesicoureteral hiatus through which the ureter enters into the submucosal plane of the bladder is nearer to or at the bladder neck, and the trigone on that side is small or absent; when the hiatus is at the bladder neck, the internal sphincter mechanism may be impaired in its function, inducing leakage, which remains apparent after nephrectomy or reimplantation of the ureter; when both right and left ureteral orifices enter in the distal part of the urethra, all the urine dribbles to the exterior; the bladder does not fill with urine, and it remains small in capacity and its sphincter is impaired in function. Reimplantation of the ureters into the bladder may be followed by urinary incontinence because of the sphincteric deficiency. If after reimplantation the bladder increases in size to more normal capacity and incontinence persists, attention can be directed to surgical repair of the bladder neck.[14, 23, 32]

Horseshoe Kidneys

The kidneys may be symmetrically placed and fused by a bridge of renal parenchyma connecting their lower poles, or asymmetrically situated when the lower pole of one kidney leans across the midline to impact onto the lower pole or hilus of the opposite kidney. The bridge of connecting parenchyma may be thin or wide, with or without a demarcating line or notch at the junction of the two components.[27]

The renal pelvis may be fully rotated to face medially, especially when the connecting isthmus is narrow. The wider the isthmus and the more asymmetric the kidney, the more anterior or lateral the orientation of the pelvis.

In this deformity, it is postulated that one or both nephrogenic cords are medially displaced, jamming together to one side or in the midline. They retain this fusion as they migrate to the lumbar region, carrying with them their ipsilateral ureters. Kidneys with asymmetric and wide fusions are more prone to added anomalies, such as ureteropelvic obstruction by high insertion of

the ureter on the pelvis or stenosis, blood vessel tangles with the ureter, duplications, reflux megaureters, or complex deformities of the cloaca, spinal cord, or vertebrae.[6]

Many children with horseshoe kidneys are symptom-free, and their kidneys and ureters function normally. Obstruction or reflux in others lead to stasis, infection, or stone formation with the corresponding symptomatology. Occasionally, the patient will present with hematuria or a dull pain caused by the bridge alone. Alleviation of pain may follow division of the isthmus and separation of the kidneys.

The diagnosis of horseshoe kidneys is made on routine urologic investigations, including palpation of the bridge; IVP, which characteristically demonstrates the medially directed calices in the lower poles and bridge; and micturition cystourethrography for defects of the ureterovesical junction and lower tract.

Surgical access to the bridge, ureteropelvic junction, and pelvis of the kidney is anterior and extraperitoneal. Conventional surgical techniques are suitable for ureteropelvic obstructions, especially the Foley Y and the side-to-side anastomosis for high insertion of the ureter to an anterior pelvis. Fortunately, division of the isthmus is rarely necessary in children and is contraindicated when the bridge is wide and when one kidney impinges widely onto the other. Nephrectomy is only indicated if one kidney is functionless and hypoplastic or is hydronephrotic or involved in serious trauma or tumor formation. Because of the multiplicity of arteries and veins that supply the back, front, and isthmus of horseshoe kidneys, hemorrhage at operation is likely to be a serious hazard.

Crossed Renal Ectopia

A crossed, fused ectopic kidney is one that crosses the midline to fuse with the opposite kidney and lies almost entirely on the opposite side of the body from that on which its ureteral orifice opens in the bladder.

Although crossed, fused kidneys are commonly arranged so that the contralateral kidney is caudal, they sometimes appear in tandem, and occasionally the contralateral kidney is cranial. The orientation of the pelvis of the fused kidneys varies; both may face medially, anteriorly, or laterally, or the pelves may face each other.

Other abnormalities of the urinary and other tracts occur commonly, namely hydronephrosis associated with vesicoureteral reflux or obstruction, duplication, cystic disease of the kidney, and genital, cloacal and spinal anomalies.[30]

The embryologic explanation is probably unlike that of horseshoe kidneys. Here, it is postulated that the terminal ends of the wolffian ducts and the vesicourethral canal are deviated to one side of the midline by excessive flexion and rotation of the hind end when the ureteric buds are developing. The ducts and both buds are displaced to one side and overlie and penetrate the nephrogenic cord on that side. Thus, the two ureters induce two kidneys from the same nephrogenic cord and ascend to the lumbar region from the same side. The ureters, however, issue into the urinary tract from opposite sides.[6]

The total renal function and the drainage may be adequate and the deformity symptomless and harmless, but superimposed troublesome anomalies may require chemotherapy for infection, or surgery for obstruction, vesicoureteral reflux, or renal hypoplasia.[12, 13]

Retrocaval Ureter

Partial obstruction of the ureter in the upper third on the right side, together with medial angulation and dilatation, are "cardinal" features of retrocaval ureter, which was described by Harrill in 1940.[11] This is a very rare anatomical twist of the ureter behind and around an inferior vena cava developed predominantly from the right subcardinal vein, which lies ventral to the ureter, instead of from the supracardinal vein, which is dorsal and harmless to the ureter. It is a wonder that variations are not more common because of the complex makeup of the inferior vena cava in segments from three temporary veins, namely the right sub-, and supra- and posterior cardinals.[16]

Right-sided loin or abdominal pain of renal or ureteral colic or the effects of infection are the presenting features. Uroradiographic demonstration of the hydronephrosis and dilated ureter above the twist by IVP and of the undilated, retrocaval, compressed and medially deviated ureter below it by retrograde ureterography are the chief diagnostic features of the condition.

Renal function is generally sound at the time of diagnosis, and surgery is directed to relief of obstruction. The ureter around the vena cava is mobilized, divided, unwound, and reanastomosed anterior to the vena cava.[5, 11]

REFERENCES

1. Albers D.D., Geyers J.R., Barnes S.D.: Clinical significance of blind ending branch of bifid ureter: Report of 3 additional cases. *J. Urol.* 105:634, 1971.
2. Atwell J.D., Cook P.L., Howell C.J., et al.: Familial incidence of bifid and double ureters. *Arch. Dis. Child.* 49:390, 1974.
3. Atwell J.D., Allen N.H.: The interrelationship between paraureteric diverticula, vesicoureteric reflux and duplication of the pelvicaliceal collecting system: A family study. *Br. J. Urol.* 52:269, 1980.
4. Barrett D.M., Malek R.S., Kelalis P.P.: Problems and solutions in surgical treatment of 100 consecutive ureteral duplications in children. *J. Urol.* 114:126, 1975.
5. Considine J.: Retrocaval ureter: A review of the literature with a report on two new cases followed for fifteen years and two years respectively. *Br. J. Urol.* 38:412, 1966.
6. Cook W.A., Stephens F.D.: Urinary system malformations in children, in Bergsma D., Duckett J.W. (eds.): *International Pediatric Urology.* New York, Alan R. Liss, Inc., 1977.
7. Elbadawi A.: Anatomy and function of the ureteral sheath. *J. Urol.* 102:224, 1972.
8. Ericsson N.O.: Ectopic ureterocele in infants and children: A clinical study. *Acta Chir. Scand.* (suppl.) 197:1, 1954.
9. Fehrenbaker L.G., Kelalis P.R., Stickler G.B.: Vesicoureteral reflux and ureteral duplication in children. *J. Urol.* 107:862, 1972.
10. Gosalbez R., Garat J.M., Piro C., et al.: Congenital ureteral valves in children. *Urology* 21:237, 1983.
11. Harrill H.C.: Retrocaval ureter: Report of a case with operative correction of the defect. *J. Urol.* 44:450, 1940.
12. Hendren W.H.: Recent advances in the management of low urinary obstruction in the newborn, in Rickham P.P., Hecker W.C., Prevot J. (eds.): *Progress in Pediatric Surgery*, vol. 2. Baltimore, University Park Press, 1971, p. 115.
13. Hendren W.H., Donahoe P.K., Pfister R.C.: Crossed renal ectopia in children. *Urology* 7:135, 1976.
14. Hutch J.A., Amar A.A.: in *Vesicoureteral Reflux and Pyelonephritis.* New York, Appleton-Century-Crofts, 1972, p. 165.
15. Hutch J.A., Chisholm E.R.: Surgical repair of ureterocele. *J. Urol.* 96:445, 1966.
16. Kelalis P.P., King L.R., Belman A.B.: *Clinical Pediatric Urology*, ed. 2. Philadelphia, W.B. Saunders Co., 1985, p. 486.
17. King L.R., Kozlowski M., Schacht M.J.: Ureteroceles in children: A simplified and successful approach to management. *JAMA* 294:1461, 1983.
18. Lenaghan D.: Bifid ureters: An anatomical, physiological and clinical study. *J. Urol.* 87:808, 1962.
19. Libert M., Wespes E., Schulman C.C.: Pelviureteric junction obstruction of the lower collecting system in incomplete ureteric duplication. *Eur. Urol.* 8:329, 1982.
20. Mackie G.G., Stephens F.D.: Duplex kidneys: A correlation of renal dysplasia with position of ureteral orifice. *J. Urol.* 114:274, 1975.
21. Mackie G.G., Awang H., Stephens F.D.: The ureteric orifice: The embryologic key to radiologic status of duplex kidneys. *J. Pediatr. Surg.* 10:473, 1975.
22. Ratner I.A., Fisher J.H., Swenson O.: Double ureters in infancy and childhood. *Pediatrics* 28:810, 1961.
23. Stephens F.D.: A form of stress incontinence in children: Another method of bladder neck repair. *Aust. NZ J. Surg.* 40:124, 1970.
24. Stephens F.D.: Caecoureterocele and concepts on the embryology and aetiology of ureteroceles. *Aust. NZ J. Surg.* 40:239, 1971.
25. Stephens F.D.: *Congenital Malformations of the Rectum, Anus, and Genito-Urinary Tracts.* Edinburgh: E. & S. Livingstone, Ltd., 1963, p. 191.
26. Stephens F.D.: Idiopathic dilatations of the urinary tract. *J. Urol.* 112:819, 1974.
27. Stephens F.D.: *Congenital Malformations of the Urinary Tract.* New York, Praeger Publishers, 1983, pp. 391, 404.
28. Subbiah N., Stephens F.D.: Stenotic ureterocele. *Aust. NZ J. Surg.* 41:257, 1972.
29. Tanagho E.A.: Embryologic basis for lower ureteral anomalies: A hypothesis. *Urology* 5:451, 1976.
30. Vitko R.J., Cass A.S., Winter R.S.: Anomalies of the genito-urinary tract associated with congenital scoliosis and congenital kyphosis. *J. Urol.* 108:655, 1972.
31. Williams D.I., Fay R., Lille J.G.: Functional radiology of ectopic ureterocele. *Br. J. Urol.* 44:417, 1972.
32. Williams D.I., Lightwood R.G.: Bilateral single ectopic ureters. *Br. J. Urol.* 44:267, 1972.
33. Williams D.I., Woodard J.R.: Problems in management of ectopic ureteroceles. *J. Urol.* 92:635, 1964.
34. Whitaker J., Danks D.M.: A study of the inheritance of duplication of the kidneys and ureters. *J. Urol.* 95:176, 1966.

123 W. Hardy Hendren
Megaureter

"MEGAURETER" IS A descriptive term for a ureter that is abnormally wide or dilated; synonyms include megaloureter and hydroureter. Until relatively recently megaureters were not treated surgically.[2, 4, 29, 31, 35] In the past 20 years, however, ample evidence has accumulated that most such ureters should be surgically corrected and that excellent results can be accomplished most of the time.[1, 3, 8, 10–12, 21–24, 28, 39]

Causes

Megaureter is not a pathologic entity, but an abnormal enlargement of the ureter that can have several causes. There may be outlet obstruction, as in patients with urethral valves, which can cause abnormally high pressures in the bladder, as well as tremendous secondary hypertrophy of the bladder wall. This in turn can cause back pressure on the upper tracts. Much or all of this dilatation can subside if the urethral valves are removed. In some patients with valves there is also an abnormality at the lower end of the ureter, with intrinsic obstruction of the lower ureter or massive reflux.

Neurogenic bladder is another condition in which there can be abnormal dilatation of the ureters. Neuromotor dysfunction of the bladder causes secondary back-pressure changes in the ureters and upper tracts.

In some cases of megaureter there is an elongated, fibrous terminal segment, similar in some respects to ureteropelvic junction obstruction at the other end of the ureter. Some authors have referred to this as an adynamic segment of ureter, or achalasia of the ureter. Microscopic cross-section of the ureter usually shows fibrosis and absence of normal muscle. The terminal ureter can also be obstructed by a ureterocele, causing severe dilatation and tortuosity of the ureter above; there is usually an associated dysplastic renal segment. An ectopic ureter entering the bladder neck, urethra, or elsewhere can be abnormally wide.

Excessive flow through an otherwise normal ureter, seen in diabetes insipidus, can cause widening of the ureter as a secondary manifestation of the high flow burden.

In the abdominal muscle deficiency, prune belly syndrome, there is usually abnormal development of the entire urinary tract, including the ureters, which are very tortuous. A microscopic section of the ureteral wall may show decreased musculature and excessive connective tissue.

Obstructive vs. Refluxing Megaureter

In general, wide ureters can be divided into those with obstruction and those with massive reflux (Fig 123–1). However, a few ureters have, paradoxically, both reflux and obstruction. For example, in an ectopic ureter located in the bladder neck or proximal urethra, obstructed most of the time when the bladder neck is closed, there may be massive reflux when the bladder neck opens during micturition. In obstructive megaureter with an adynamic distal segment, or if there is a paraureteral diverticulum just above the ureteral orifice (there is no muscle behind the ureter), reflux is occasionally observed during voiding, although the ureteral orifice looks normal. These exceptions are uncommon.

In obstructive megaureter, or so-called primary megaureter, the ureteral orifice is usually normal in appearance. The terminal ureter is small for a length of 1–2 cm; however, a ureteral catheter can be passed through it with ease. It can be hazardous to pass a ureteral catheter, however, for this can produce enough edema to cause complete obstruction several hours later, precipitating a crisis that requires immediate nephrostomy. If a catheter is passed, it should be only when planning immediate operation under the same anesthesia; this safeguard applies also to passing a catheter from below through a ureteropelvic junction obstruction.

In recent years we have preferred to define the anatomy preoperatively in most cases, using prograde study from above. A needle is inserted into the kidney, under local anesthesia, with the patient in the prone position. Contrast medium is infused under fluoroscopic control, while spot films are taken to show the obstructed segment. Simultaneously ureteral peristalsis can be observed. Pressure determinations can be obtained by a second needle placed into the renal pelvis, connected to a transducer and recording device, as described by Whitaker.[38]

In refluxing megaureter, the orifice is generally dilated, with the appearance of a golf hole. It is often laterally located in the side wall of the bladder, instead of the trigone. There is usually no muscle backing behind the ureter, so that it lacks a valve-like action, and this results in massive reflux. In some cases a panendoscope can be passed through the dilated orifice and several centimeters up the ureter. Indeed, a panendoscope can readily be passed all the way to the kidney in some instances if the ureter is not tortuous.

There is frequently a paraureteral diverticulum just above the orifice in both obstructive and refluxing megaureter. It is easy to mistake the ostium of the diverticulum for the ureteral orifice. Ureteral peristalsis can be active in both types of megaureter, but in some cases of refluxing megaureter it can be sluggish or absent, particularly if urinary infection has caused secondary fibrosis of the ureteral wall. The kidney parenchyma may be less well preserved in refluxing megaureter than in obstructive megaureter.

Megaureter in some patients is an isolated, unilateral problem, and there is a normal bladder and normal contralateral ureter. Often, however, the problem is bilateral. Frequently, too, the bladder is very abnormal, especially in boys with urethral valves. When operation on the dilated ureter is needed, the surgeon's task is similar in dealing with both obstructed and refluxing megaureter. It involves resecting the terminal ureter, tapering it appropriately, and reimplanting it into the bladder so that it is not obstructed and does not allow vesicoureteral reflux. This is difficult surgery! Ureteral tapering and reimplantation offers great possible benefit; however, great harm can result if the procedure is performed unskillfully. In urologic surgery, a bad technical performance often results in renal failure many years later, less

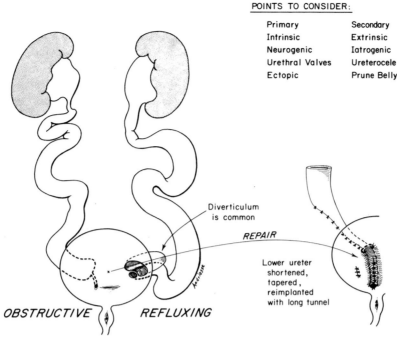

POINTS TO CONSIDER:

Primary	Secondary
Intrinsic	Extrinsic
Neurogenic	Iatrogenic
Urethral Valves	Ureterocele
Ectopic	Prune Belly

Diverticulum is common

REPAIR

Lower ureter shortened, tapered, reimplanted with long tunnel

OBSTRUCTIVE   REFLUXING

Fig 123–1.—Main types of megaureter and some etiologic factors to consider.

readily identified as the aftermath of a poorly performed operation. The end result can be preceded by several years of life of poor quality.

Correction of Megaureter

Indications

Today there is general agreement that primary lower ureteral malfunction should be corrected; i.e., if there is primary obstruction or massive reflux with great dilatation of the ureter, operation on the ureter itself is warranted.

In some cases, the ureter and its renal segment are best removed, such as those cases of ureterocele with duplex collecting system, usually in females. Generally the lower pole of the kidney is well preserved, although there is often reflux up that ureter. Most commonly, the megaureter drains a dysplastic upper pole, which is best removed. Occasionally, the large ureter is removed but pyelopyelostomy is performed if the upper pole has a reasonable amount of function. In our experience it is seldom best to taper the enlarged upper pole ureter and reimplant it along with the adjacent lower pole ureter.

Most controversial are those cases of megaureter seen in boys with urethral valves. Many have been treated by temporary ureterostomy of various types (loop ureterostomy, circle ureterostomy, Roux-en-Y ureterostomy, end ureterostomy).[5, 6, 7, 9, 22, 25–27, 30, 31, 33, 34, 36, 37, 40] It is our opinion that ureterostomy has been greatly overdone in the past.[18] Currently it seems to be on the decline. There is a spectrum of pathology in boys with urethral valves. In some cases only endoscopic resection of the valves is needed; impressive ureteral dilatation can subside in time after relief of valve obstruction. In other cases there will be some improvement, but massive reflux or lower ureteral obstruction may remain. This can be dealt with electively later, as the child is followed closely. In some extreme cases with massive decompensation of the upper tracts we have preferred to pursue an immediate total lower urinary tract reconstruction, dealing with the

valve and the lower ureters in the same operative session.[13–15] It should be underscored that total reconstruction is never done in an acutely ill infant. First, a small plastic feeding catheter is passed into the bladder, and the child is treated for dehydration, acidosis, and infection. Only after restoration of metabolic equilibrium would it be reasonable to proceed with a major reconstructive procedure. In boys with urethral valves, it is now possible to destroy the valves endoscopically with the new pediatric fiberoptic panendoscopes. Open resection of valves by the former method of splitting the symphysis pubis is entirely outmoded and is apt to result in stress incontinence in later life. Indeed, we have not encountered a case in the past 10 years in which perineal urethrostomy was needed, owing to the efficiency of the modern pediatric endoscopes.

Figure 123–2 shows data concerning megaureter repair from 1960 to November 1984. There were 338 ureters repaired in 249 patients. Almost one third of the patients were under 2 years of age; the remainder were distributed throughout childhood. There were a small number of adults; they usually presented with infection or stones and less severe upper tract problems that had allowed them to pass through childhood before clinical detection. Of the 338 ureters repaired, 173 were obstructed and 165 had reflux. In 156 cases, there was a unilateral megaureter, and in 91 the problem was bilateral. Some had normal bladders, but in more than half the bladder was abnormal, such as in boys with urethral valves or girls with ureteroceles.

Technique of Operation

In most cases, only the lower ureter needs to be repaired. Although the upper ureter may be initially tortuous, it will often straighten out in time if the lower ureter is repaired, thereby relieving obstruction or reflux. Early in our experience, we tended to repair tortuous upper ureters somewhat more often than today. We believe that there are a few cases in which both ends require operation. In any event, the lower end should always be done first. In four instances in which there was ischemia

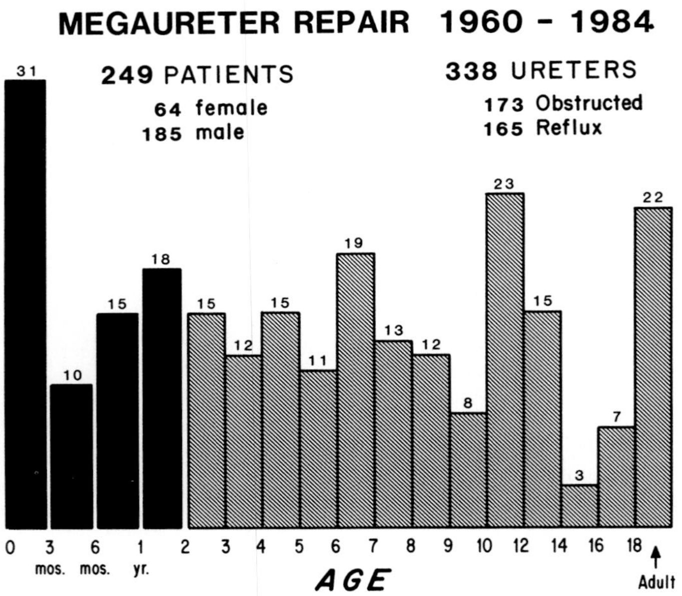

MEGAURETER REPAIR 1960 – 1984

249 PATIENTS
64 female
185 male

338 URETERS
173 Obstructed
165 Reflux

Fig 123–2.—Data on author's series of patients with megaureter, repaired from 1960 to November 1984.

of the lower ureter, an upper ureteral repair had been done first, so that the collateral blood supply of the ureter was not ideal. When a lower ureter is mobilized and tapered, one must rely heavily on its collateral blood supply from above. In cases with severe hydronephrosis and urosepsis, it may occasionally be necessary to provide temporary nephrostomy drainage to stabilize the child's condition before proceeding with reconstruction. I believe the surgeon should resist the temptation to shorten and straighten a tortuous upper ureter at that time, for this may jeopardize the all-important lower tract repair to be done later.

There are technical points to which attention must be paid in reimplanting ureters, whether they are of normal size, moderately dilated, or megaureters. There should be minimal handling of the ureter with forceps, which can injure its delicate wall. The ureter should be mobilized enough to reimplant it into the bladder without angulation or tension. Its blood supply must be preserved. The entry into the bladder must be at a point where it will not be obstructed or angulated as the bladder fills. The ratio of tunnel length to diameter of the ureter must be high enough to prevent reflux, usually four or five to one.

Operative steps in megaureter repair are shown in Figure 123–3. Usually a transverse suprapubic skin incision is made (Fig 123–3,A), opening the fascia vertically to expose the bladder. In a reoperative case, however, wider exposure is necessary, and so a vertical transperitoneal approach is preferred. The same is true if the lower ureter is very tortuous.

The bladder is opened through a vertical midline cystostomy, stopping its lower end just short of the bladder neck. Formerly we used a Y-V plasty almost routinely, but this resulted in stress incontinence in some males. It should be emphasized that the bladder neck can be extremely hypertrophied in some males with urethral valves. It is better to leave it intact, because experience has shown that operation, either open or endoscopic, to open the bladder neck can result in stress incontinence, especially in these thick-walled, muscular, sometimes noncompliant bladders. Indeed, in some cases in which the bladder neck was altered during infancy, it has been necessary to narrow it later to correct stress incontinence. Some of these cases may require augmentation of the bladder with bowel to increase bladder volume and lower voiding pressures.

The Denis Browne Universal retractor is of great help in performing these lower tract reconstructions. Four traction sutures on the edges of the cystostomy aid in the exposure (Fig 123–3,B). A surgical gauze is placed in the trigone and retracted upward by one hand-held retractor. A no. 5 infant feeding catheter is sewn into the ureteral orifice. The orifice is circumscribed and the ureter mobilized intravesically for several centimeters (Fig 123–3,C). In some very tortuous ureters 6–8 inches of ureter can be delivered through this intravesical mobilization. Some surgeons prefer to mobilize the dilated ureter extravesically. This may require a good deal of dissection paravesically, which can injure some of the nerve supply to the bladder. We have seen this result in a partially neurogenic bladder that emptied poorly. After the initial intravesical mobilization for as great a length as proceeds easily, the ureter is pulled out of the bladder and the dissection carried upward outside of the bladder. First, the obliterated hypogastric ligament is ligated and divided so that the peritoneum can be retracted upward and medially to afford access to the posterior gutter. To pull the ureter up to this point, scissors are passed along its anterior aspect, breaking through the adventitia above the level of the paravesical web and pulling the ureter through to that point. This technique gives minimal disturbance of bladder innervation.

In mobilizing the ureter (Fig 123–3,D), it is important to preserve its periureteral adventitia, which carries collateral blood supply and lymphatics. A skeletonized ureter may be ischemic. Obviously, some of the small blood vessels to the lower ureter must be divided, but this should be as far from the ureter as possible, so that despite considerable mobilization there is ample adventitia surrounding the ureter. The amount of mobilization will vary with the degree of tortuosity of the ureter. Some megaureters are quite dilated but not very tortuous. Others are moderately dilated but very tortuous. The lower mobilization is seldom carried much higher than the external iliac vessels. If the ureter is particularly tortuous, dissecting it free at that level may deliver several inches of ureter coiled up in the pelvis.

The length of ureter that is to be tapered does not generally need to be extensive (Fig 123–3,E). Usually, it includes that segment of the ureter that will be reimplanted in the trigone of the bladder, plus a few centimeters of that part of the ureter that will lie outside the bladder. If a tortuous lower ureter is being straightened out, particularly important is its blood supply, which runs longitudinally along its medial aspect, close to its attachment with the peritoneum, which can restrict straightening of the ureter. The peritoneum can be dissected away from the ureter without injuring the ureter and its adventitia.

In reducing the caliber of the ureter (Fig 123–3,F), there are several important points to be made. First, the trimming is done laterally, opposite the main, longitudinal blood supply. Second, the strip removed should not be too wide. If the remaining ureter is too narrow, it can become ischemic. The ureter will be like a pedicle flap of any tissue, i.e., its width must not be made too narrow compared to the length. Furthermore, an additional 3–4 mm of ureteral wall will be taken up in the suture line closure. Although the ureter may appear still a bit too large after trimming and closure, it will become smaller in time if it is reimplanted in a satisfactory manner so that there is no reflux or obstruction. It is helpful to place a catheter in the lumen of the ureter during its trimming, no. 10, 12 or 14 F, depending on the size of the patient. Allis clamps can be applied to facilitate trimming, but it is far easier to use the special ureteral clamps made for us by V. Mueller Company, 6600 Touhy Ave., Chicago, IL 60648. They fit comfortably down into the pelvis, and by rotating them 90 degrees the cut edge of ureter can be brought up into view to facilitate suturing the ureter.

Closure (Fig 123–3,G) is accomplished with a 4-0 or 5-0 chromic, running lock suture, locked to prevent reefing or short-

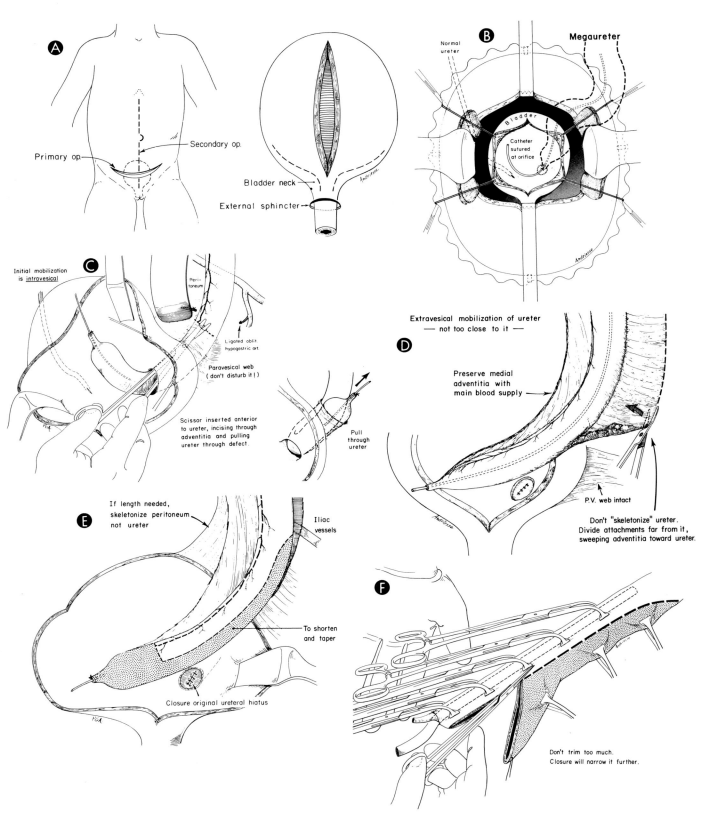

Fig 123–3.—Technique for repair of lower megaureter. See text. *(Continued)*

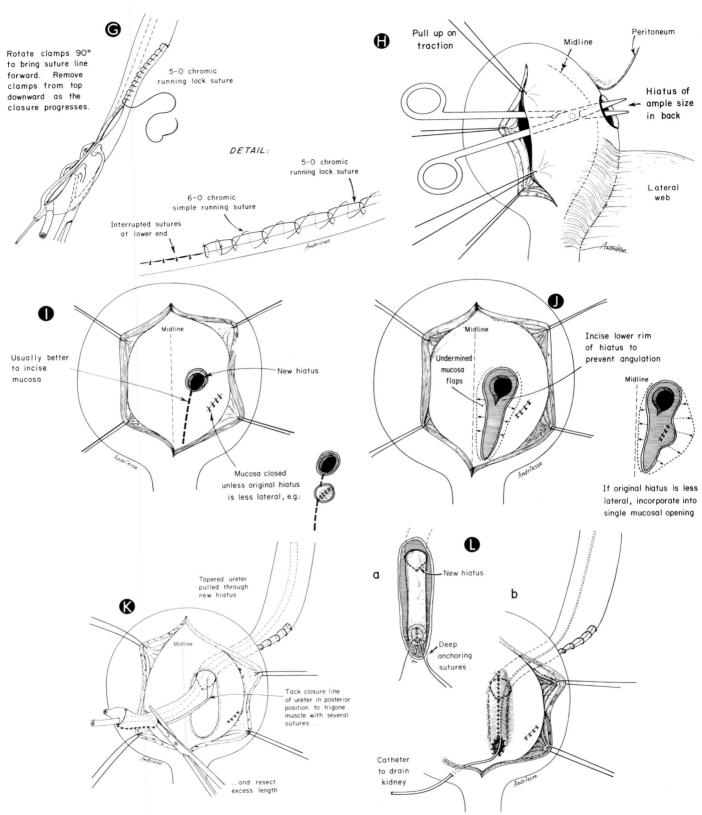

G

Rotate clamps 90° to bring suture line forward. Remove clamps from top downward as the closure progresses.

5-0 chromic running lock suture

DETAIL:

5-0 chromic running lock suture

6-0 chromic simple running suture

Interrupted sutures at lower end

H

Pull up on traction

Midline

Peritoneum

Hiatus of ample size in back

Lateral web

I

Midline

Usually better to incise mucosa

New hiatus

Mucosa closed unless original hiatus is less lateral, e.g.:

J

Midline

Undermined mucosa flaps

Incise lower rim of hiatus to prevent angulation

Midline

If original hiatus is less lateral, incorporate into single mucosal opening

K

Tapered ureter pulled through new hiatus

Midline

Tack closure line of ureter in posterior position to trigone muscle with several sutures...

...and resect excess length

L

a

New hiatus

Deep anchoring sutures

b

Catheter to drain kidney

Fig 123–3.—(cont.).—Technique for repair of lower megaureter. See text.

ening of the closure. The lower several centimeters are closed with interrupted sutures to permit trimming away any excess length of ureter without cutting the running suture closure. The running lock suture is usually not watertight. Therefore, a fine 6-0 chromic simple suture is run along the edge of the closure, quite superficially, to make it watertight.

Of prime importance in the operation is the location of the new muscle hiatus through which the ureter will enter the bladder (Fig 123–3,*H*). A common mistake is to make it too lateral, which can result in angulation and obstruction when the bladder fills. To select this hiatus we choose a point near the vertical midline of the trigone, an appropriate distance upward from the bladder neck. A hole is made through the mucosa, through the back wall of the bladder and to the cul-de-sac peritoneum, but not through it. Pulling upward on the traction sutures in the bladder wall, the operator can see the scissor points emerging through the back wall of the bladder, between it and the cul-de-sac peritoneum. In the male, this is near the vas deferens, which should be spared. In the female, this is just anterior to the upper vagina. This opening should be large enough to avoid constricting the ureter. Incising the inferior rim will prevent angulation of the ureter where it enters the bladder. This is especially true in hypertrophied bladders, as in boys with urethral valves, where heavy strands of muscle across the ureter can act as obstructing bands.

A bed should be prepared for implanting the ureter (Fig 123–3,*I* and *J*). Sometimes this can be done by making a submucosal tunnel, as in other types of ordinary ureteral reimplantation. In most cases in recent years, we have found it better to incise the mucosa downward, laying back mucosal flaps, to prepare a bed for the ureter next to the trigone. The original ureteral hiatus should be closed. If a diverticulum is present, it is nearly always through this hiatus. To repair it, the mucosa protruding through the hiatus must be mobilized before closure of the hiatus. Sometimes the new bed for the ureter is medial to the previous hiatus if the original hiatus was far lateral. In other cases the original hiatus closure will lie on the back wall of the bed for reimplanting the trimmed ureter.

The trimmed ureter is then brought through the new hiatus in the back wall of the bladder (Fig 123–3,*K*), placed in its bed, and adjusted to lie without tension. At this point retractors in the bladder and on the peritoneum should be released temporarily, to make certain there is no tension between the bladder in its collapsed state and the ureter as it is to be implanted. The suture line closure of the ureter should be in back next to the bladder muscle, so that a fistula will not occur between it and the bladder. The ureter is tacked with fine chromic sutures to its bed in the trigone. Excess length is then resected.

In anchoring the ureter at its new hiatus (Fig 123–3,*L*) we place the most distal sutures deep in the trigone, taking both mucosa and muscle to anchor the tip of the ureter. The remaining sutures around the circumference of the orifice fasten the bladder mucosa to the full-thickness edge of the ureter. If the diameter of the orifice is still too large, its upper rim can be deliberately narrowed a little during the closure. The mucosa flaps of trigone are then closed over the ureter, incorporating a superficial bit of adventitia of the ureter to help obliterate some of the dead space in the tunnel. The reimplanted megaureter usually has a tunnel 3–4 cm long. The kidney is drained for about 12 days by a plastic no. 5 or 8 F feeding catheter with extra holes cut in it. This catheter is placed through a stab wound in the lower abdomen, through the opposite side of the bladder wall, and up the ureter to the kidney. We seldom use nephrostomy today in megaureter repair except in the occasional child with massive hydronephrosis who presents with infection. In those circumstances, immediate percutaneous nephrostomy may

be indicated, and this decompression tube should be left in place until the lower ureter repair is completed.

Figure 123–4 shows an alternative method we have used in the past several years for trimming the caliber of the dilated ureter by freehand technique instead of using special clamps. This method is currently my preference because (1) the ureter is not clamped at all, which is possibly better than applying even a relatively gentle clamp and (2) it preserves all of the periureteral tissue, which is so important for blood supply of the ureter.

In patients with bilateral megaureters we routinely repair both lower ureters at once. This is a prolonged, tedious procedure. The plastic feeding catheters are removed 10–12 days later, always one side at a time. Another small plastic catheter drains the bladder. A Foley catheter is not used for this, as we do not like to have a Foley balloon pressing on a repaired ureter and the mucosa closure over it. Rarely are suprapubic tubes used, unless we have narrowed the urethra and the bladder neck extensively, as in a patient undergoing epispadias repair or other operation for incontinence.

REPAIR OF THE UPPER URETER.—Occasionally, repair of the upper ureter should be considered if it remains tortuous and elongated, especially if there is apparent functional obstruction at the ureteropelvic junction. Several points should be stressed regarding the upper ureter. Considerable spontaneous improvement in a very tortuous upper ureter can occur after successful repair of a lower end that was once obstructed or refluxing. Kinks can straighten out, and dilatation can recede. If the patient is doing well clinically, it is best to wait for several months or longer to make this decision. The upper ureter may be alarmingly dilated immediately after repair of the lower ureter; this is caused by edema surrounding the reimplantation. Repeat pyelography should be performed to follow this. The edema should improve in several weeks.

Prograde perfusion with fluoroscopic observation of emptying, together with pressure measurements, can be helpful. It is interesting to watch some of these dilated ureters fluoroscopically. Active peristalsis may be present but ineffective if the walls of the ureter cannot coapt. The urine may churn back and forth with passage of each peristaltic wave, instead of being milked effectively down into the bladder.

If on follow-up the upper ureter remains dilated and tortuous and exhibits inadequate peristaltic emptying as well as delayed emptying, upper ureteral repair may be indicated. It is much easier to perform and is much less standard in technique than a lower repair (Fig 123–5). In some, it is merely resection of a tortuous ureteropelvic junction. In others, modest tapering of the lower ureter is included. The part of the ureter that will remain should never be mobilized generously away from its bed, for this will jeopardize its blood supply. If a tortuous ureteropelvic junction is resected, only the segment to be resected is mobilized, and an oblique anastomosis is then performed between the upper end of the remaining ureter and the lower renal pelvis. A dilated renal pelvis may be partially resected, just as in any pyeloplasty, if it is too large.

Clamps are not used during upper ureter repair. The ureter is incised longitudinally in situ, the operator trimming away an appropriate width of its edge; ordinary or angled scissors with straight blades are used. Like the lower ureter, the upper one should not be made too narrow. A Malecot catheter is placed in the lower pole of the kidney to drain the kidney and its ureter temporarily. Contrast medium is injected through this catheter 10–12 days later to make certain there is good drainage and there are no leaks. Before withdrawing the catheter, 0.5% neomycin solution is instilled into the kidney as added protection against bacteremia when the tube is withdrawn.

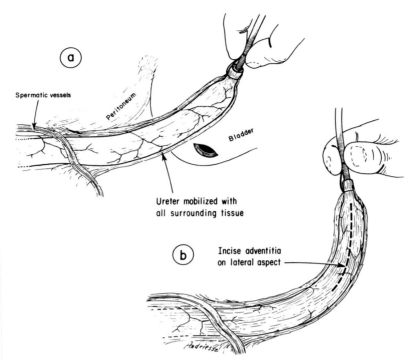

Fig 123–4.—Alternate method of trimming the caliber of the dilated ureter freehand without using clamps. **A**, the ureter is mobilized intra- and extravesically as usual, preserving as much of the surrounding tissue as possible. During this mobilization the hypogastric vessels on the lateral pelvic wall are swept clean. The ureter is free from the peritoneum anteromedial to it, laying clean the peritoneum, not the ureter. At the start of this extravesical dissection of ureter, the obliterated umbilical artery ligament crossing the ureter is divided, which allows forward retraction of the peritoneum. **B**, the periureteral tissue is opened to expose that segment of the wall to be excised. Generally, the strip to be excised is about one half the circumference of the ureter. *(Continued.)*

Complications

Megaureter repair for an isolated anomaly, in a patient with a normal bladder, should be possible with a very low complication rate, probably no greater than 2%–3%. When dealing with very abnormal bladders, seen in boys with urethral valves when endoscopic resection of valves is not sufficient, even meticulous technique will give some failures, in the range of about 5%. This is acceptable when compared to the alternative of urinary diversion. Most failures can be repaired by reoperation.[16, 17] Major reconstruction carries the risk of major potential complications. It should be emphasized that most complications do not occur spontaneously. They are created in the operating room from failure to pay sufficient attention to technical details. Intravesical mobilization of the lower ureter reduces the likelihood of causing neurogenic bladder. Preserving the adventitia of the ureter and its intramural blood supply reduces the chance of ischemic necrosis. The ureter should not be trimmed too narrow. The hiatus should be properly located. The reimplanted tunnel must be long enough to prevent reflux. A soft catheter stent for drainage must be used; we have seen several cases of ureterovesical fistula from the anterior wall of the ureter to the bladder at the top of the tunnel, where a stiff catheter eroded the ureter. The upper ureter should never be operated on first, for the reasons given earlier.

Case Material

The following cases are presented as examples of megaureter and the spectrum of its clinical presentation.

Case 1.—A 7-year-old boy was referred with an obstructed left megaureter (Fig 123–6) but a well-preserved kidney on that side; the opposite side was normal. The problem had been discovered during a laparotomy for abdominal pain. An intubated ureterotomy of the narrow terminal ureter had failed to relieve the obstruction.

The narrow distal ureter was resected, with tapering and implantation of the terminal ureter. The result was satisfactory during a 24-year follow-up. The patient is now 31 years of age and completely well.

Comment.—With a unilateral obstructive megaureter like this, particularly when the bladder is normal, an excellent result should be possible in most cases. The upper tract is often relatively well preserved, so that an almost normal kidney can be salvaged. Apparent partial ureteropelvic junction obstruction secondary to tortuosity disappeared after obstruction of the lower ureter was eliminated.

Case 2.—A 4-month-old girl was referred with a left flank mass, thought to be a tumor. An IVP showed a hydronephrotic, solitary left kidney (Fig 123–7). Cystogram showed a normal bladder; there was no reflux. The lower ureter was resected, shortened, tapered and reimplanted. The upper ureter remained tortuous. It drained poorly on retrograde filling, so 1 year later it was repaired also. The tortuous ureteropelvic junction was resected, and the upper ureter was tapered. Creatinine clearance preoperatively was 15 L/sq m of body surface area. It rose to 104 L following operation and has remained in that range during a 20-year follow-up.

Comment.—This case shows the remarkable capacity of a hydronephrotic kidney to improve in childhood, especially if repair is done early. Although the child was only 4 months of age, direct repair was undertaken without resorting to a preliminary diversion such as ureterostomy, pyelostomy, or nephrostomy. Renal function in normal infants is relatively low compared to that of older individuals, on the basis of creatinine clearance related to body surface area. Values comparable to those in the adult are reached generally by about 1 year of age. It is our impression that when severe obstructive uropathy can be relieved early, the eventual return in renal function may be greater than in similar cases where repair is not accomplished until a later age. This patient is now a completely well young woman.

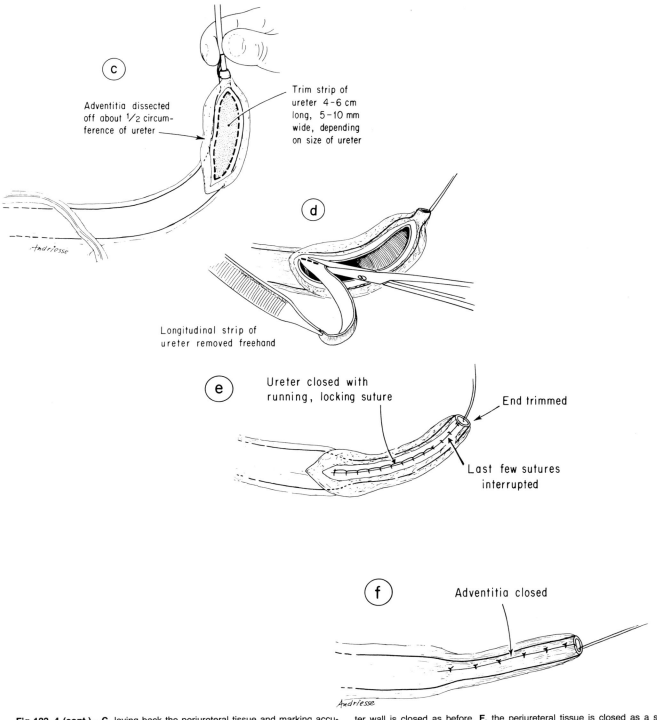

Fig 123–4 (cont.)—**C,** laying back the periureteral tissue and marking accurately with a skin pencil the strip to be removed is facilitated by having the ureter distended with saline. **D,** excision is performed with straight scissors. **E,** the ure-

ter wall is closed as before. **F,** the periureteral tissue is closed as a separate layer over the ureter.

CASE 3.—A 2½-year-old boy had one episode of urinary infection. A cystogram (Fig 123–8) showed massive bilateral reflux and very dilated, tortuous ureters. Intravenous pyelogram showed bilateral severe hydronephrosis, megaureters, and a large bladder that emptied poorly. Bilateral lower ureteral tapering and reimplantation was performed. An IVP taken immediately postoperatively showed severe dilatation of both upper tracts, especially the left side, but the patient was clinically well. Retrograde pyelogram 2 months later showed satisfactory lower ureters, continued dilatation of the upper tracts, and persisting tortuosity of the

left upper ureter, which emptied poorly on radiographic evaluation. Nothing further was done with the right side. The left upper ureter required resection for tortuosity, with tapering of the midureter.

Comment.—The patient has been well and free of urinary infection during a 20-year follow-up. At age 15 years he was at the 75th percentile for height and 60th percentile for weight. Laboratory values showed blood urea nitrogen (BUN) of 15 mg/100

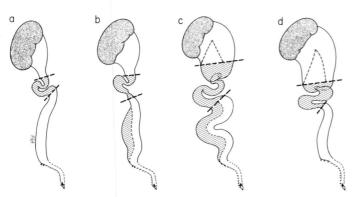

Fig 123–5.—Techniques of upper ureteral repair used in some cases of megaureter.

ml, creatinine 1.1 mg/100 ml, and creatinine clearance 100 L absolute, although the original IVP showed bilateral poor upper tract visualization and severe hydronephrosis.

The right upper ureter, which was less involved, became normal in appearance without further operation. It is possible that the left upper ureteral tortuosity and dilatation might have improved spontaneously if we had permitted a longer period of observation in this case, which was relatively early in our experience with operative correction of megaureter.

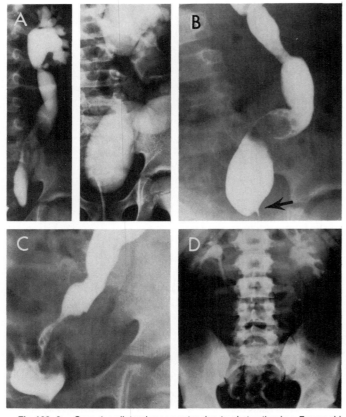

Fig 123–6.—Case 1: unilateral megaureter due to obstruction in a 7-year-old boy. **A,** retrograde study preoperatively. **B,** prograde study before repair (*arrow* points to obstructed segment). **C,** prograde study outlining lower ureter tapered and reimplanted 2 weeks previously. Note modest length of tapering, which included intravesical ureter and 3–4-cm segment outside the bladder. **D,** an IVP 14 years later is close to normal. The patient is well 24 years after this repair.

CASE 4.—A 1-week-old boy was referred with gram-negative septicemia and palpable bladder and kidneys. Catheter drainage with a 5 F plastic feeding catheter, antibiotics, and intravenous therapy improved the clinical status immediately. An IVP showed severe bilateral hydronephrosis and poor visualization of the upper tract (Fig 123–9). A voiding cystourethrogram showed severe type I urethral valves and multiple cellules of the bladder, but no reflux. One week after admission, the valves were resected endoscopically. Retrograde pyelograms at that time outlined dilated upper tracts and ureters, particularly on the right side.

The patient thrived under close observation. Follow-up films showed partial obstruction on the right at both the ureterovesical junction and the ureteropelvic junction, and continuing reflux on the left side. At age 1 year, an elective procedure was done to correct these problems, with satisfactory outcome. The patient, now aged 15 years, is well.

Comment.—This child is typical of many infant boys with severe urethral valves. He responded well to catheter drainage followed by endoscopic resection of valves and required no other immediate treatment. There was persisting reflux on the left side, however, and partial obstruction on the right. Therefore, a delayed reconstructive procedure was indicated. The left ureter required only simple reimplantation, no longer being so dilated as to require tapering. The right ureter remained dilated, and so a lower megaureter repair was performed. After the lower tract was repaired at age 1 year, the upper tracts were followed. Hydronephrosis remained on the right, and 7 months later the right ureteropelvic junction was resected. Prograde pyelography and pressure measurements were not performed in those days (15 years ago); however, in light of current practice, if pressure determination showed normal pressures, perhaps in retrospect it might have been reasonable to follow the right upper tract for a longer time before proceeding with repair. As experience has been gained with greater numbers of megaureter repairs, we have tended to operate less often on the upper ureter than we did 25 years ago, when we began this type of reconstructive surgery.

CASE 5.—A 3-month-old boy was referred with acute urinary infection. Laboratory values showed BUN 70 mg/100 ml and creatinine 3.6 mg/100 ml. An IVP (Fig 123–10) showed poor visualization bilaterally and an enlarged bladder. A cystogram showed urethral valves; there was massive reflux up dilated and tortuous ureters. His condition improved dramatically during 4 days of drainage and vigorous medical management. At cystoscopy, the ureteral orifices were widely dilated, confirming that massive reflux would likely persist despite endoscopic resection of valves. Therefore, in addition to resection of the valves transurethrally, the lower ureters were shortened, tapered and reimplanted. Follow-up films showed persisting severe hydronephrosis of the upper tracts with dilated, tortuous ureters, and so the upper tracts were repaired 6 weeks later. There were two complications on the left side: (1) partial obstruction of the lower ureter after its implantation, requiring temporary nephrostomy drainage, and (2) a suture line leak after tapering of the upper ureter, requiring an additional week of nephrostomy drainage before it closed. The patient has remained well during 16-year follow-up. Values for BUN and creatinine are normal. Renal function measures 70% of predicted normal for his age.

Comment.—A direct reconstructive procedure of the lower ureters was performed in this case because conditions observed at cystoscopy were expected to result in continuing massive reflux, which this patient could ill afford. Repeated urosepsis could have quickly destroyed the already badly damaged and hydronephrotic upper tracts. The patient did very well despite the complications of partial obstruction of one lower ureter immediately after its tapering and reimplantation and temporary leakage from the upper ureter on the same side after its revision.

Lesser degrees of reflux can be expected to disappear after valves have been resected. In the overall spectrum of boys with reflux and urethral valves, in our experience the reflux will disappear in about 50% of cases during prolonged follow-up. The decision regarding which cases require ureteral reimplantation should be made individually and should be based on the state of the upper tracts, the amount of reflux, presence or absence of

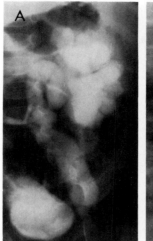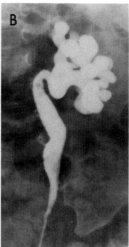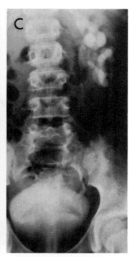

Fig 123–7.—Case 2: megaureter due to obstruction in a 4-month-old girl with a single kidney. **A,** IVP before repair of lower megaureter at age 4 months. **B,** retrograde pyelogram 6 months after lower ureteral repair. Upper ureteral repair was deferred to see if this tortuosity would recede. Because it did not, the upper ureter was shortened and tapered. **C,** IVP at age 10 years. Note ureter of normal appearance at both lower and upper ends. Recent IVP (20 years after repair) was stable.

urinary infection and the question of whether the patient has sufficient renal function to withstand further episodes of infection that may occur if reflux remains.

CASE 6.—A 9-year-old boy was referred with severe bilateral hydronephrosis and presumed urethral stricture. Antegrade voiding cystourethrogram (Fig 123–11) showed intermittent dilatation of the prostatic urethra, which on some frames of the study was not very impressive and on other frames was typical of severe type I urethral valves. There was no reflux. There was also a small filling defect in the bulbous urethra, which proved at cystoscopy to be a cyst of Cowper's duct. An IVP showed severe bilateral hydronephrosis. Laboratory studies showed BUN value of 36 mg/100 ml and creatinine 2 mg/100 ml. The patient had been previously unaware that his stream was abnormal.

Cystoscopy showed severe type I urethral valves; they were opened up endoscopically with a cutting electrode. The cyst on the floor of the bulbous urethra was unroofed. The ureteral orifices looked normal, but the bladder was trabeculated and the bladder neck quite hypertrophied, consistent with secondary changes from urethral valves. Serial antegrade perfusion studies of the upper tracts were performed when the patient first presented, 3 months later and 8 months later (Fig 123–12). Although there was slight improvement in the degree of dilatation of the upper tracts and upper ureters, both lower ureters remained quite dilated. There was a narrow terminal segment of ureter visible on both sides. Perfusion pressures remained slightly dilated, although the patient was clinically well.

Eight months after removal of the valves, a modest resection and tapering of each lower ureter was performed. Perfusion of the upper tracts 3 months later showed normal lower ureters and normal perfusion pressures. An IVP 7 years later looks excellent.

Comment.—Megaureters in boys with urethral valves but no reflux may improve remarkably on prolonged follow-up after resection of valves. However, we are convinced that in some there is also pathology at the lower end of the ureter, as in this case, and that it should be corrected. Prograde pyeloureterography with simultaneous pressure recording with doubtless help define better which of these patients without reflux will require a lower ureteral reconstructive procedure and which can be safely followed with the expectation that there will be spontaneous resolution of upper tract dilatation. Normal and abnormal pressure flow relations in these ureters are not yet well established. In some cases there has been unquestionable partial obstruction, judging by the degree of upper tract dilatation, even though pressures were not very elevated. We believe that some of these points will be clarified with greater experience in this type of case.

It is interesting that this boy was unaware of his bladder outlet obstructive problem. His initial intravesical voiding pressures were 50 mm Hg, with a voiding rate of only 3 ml/second! Two days after valve resection, voiding pressures had dropped to 35 mm Hg, and the rate increased to 9 ml/second. Three months later voiding pressures measured only 9 mm Hg, and the flow rate was 12 ml/second. Histologic examination of the lower ureters showed fibrosis and lack of muscle in the wall of the terminal ureter. Now an 18-year-old student in college, the patient is well.

CASE 7.—A 2-month-old boy was referred with pseudomonas septicemia; there were peripheral septic skin lesions. He had the typical lax, wrinkled abdomen of prune belly syndrome, with palpable bladder, ureters, and kidneys. Immediate treatment included catheter drainage of the bladder, intravenous fluids, and antibiotics. An IVP 4 days later showed massively dilated upper tracts and poor visualization (Fig 123–13). Cystogram showed massive reflux. In 5 days his status had improved markedly, and reconstruction was undertaken. Somewhat unusually for the prune belly syndrome, typical type I urethral valves were seen, causing marked obstruction of the prostatic urethra. They were destroyed endoscopically. The ureteral orifices were gaping holes on the side wall of the bladder, often seen in the prune belly syndrome. Immediate reconstruction was elected.

When mobilized, the ureters reached to below the baby's knees! About 8–10 inches of excess ureteral length was removed; the remaining lower ureters were tapered and reimplanted into the bladder. The infant's postoperative course was unremarkable. Cystogram showed no reflux. Postoperative evaluation included antegrade pyelography, because an IVP did not outline the upper tracts well. The upper ureters remained tortuous, with sluggish emptying (Fig 123–13,C). Therefore, bilateral upper ureteral shortening and tapering was performed 2 years after the lower ureteral procedure. Each kidney was noted to be dysplastic, with many small cortical cysts, not uncommon in these babies. The dome of the bladder was quite dilated and emptied poorly, like a large diverticulum. Subsequently this was resected. Bilateral intra-abdominal undescended testes were brought into the scrotum.

The patient is now 12 years old and has amazingly good renal function despite his original status: BUN 27 mg/100 ml, creatinine 1.1 mg/100 ml, creatinine clearance 63 liters/sq m body surface area. His height is at 25th percentile and weight at 15th percentile. The IVP is stable.

Comment.—This child has severely dysplastic kidneys and will probably require renal transplantation eventually. Major operative reconstruction afforded him an infection-free infancy, preserving what little renal function there was when he first presented. With no operative intervention, he would likely have died of recurrent infection. We prefer direct reconstruction in a

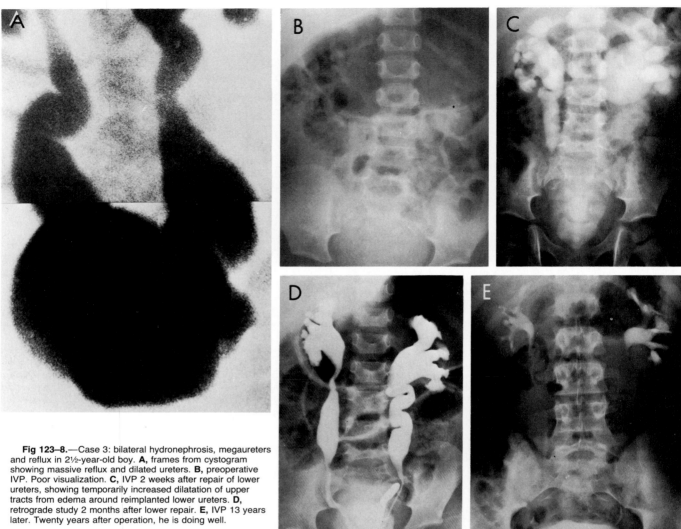

Fig 123–8.—Case 3: bilateral hydronephrosis, megaureters and reflux in 2½-year-old boy. **A,** frames from cystogram showing massive reflux and dilated ureters. **B,** preoperative IVP. Poor visualization. **C,** IVP 2 weeks after repair of lower ureters, showing temporarily increased dilatation of upper tracts from edema around reimplanted lower ureters. **D,** retrograde study 2 months after lower repair. **E,** IVP 13 years later. Twenty years after operation, he is doing well.

severely decompensated case like this rather than resorting to prolonged ureterostomy, vesicostomy, etc. If orchidopexy is contemplated in boys with the prune belly syndrome, it should be done during infancy, when the testes can in some cases be brought down into the scrotum. If orchidopexy is deferred for a number of years, the spermatic vessels are relatively shorter and the testicles cannot be brought down into the scrotum except by dividing the spermatic vessels, relying on the collateral blood supply accompanying the vas deferens.

We have performed reconstructive procedures in 27 patients with the prune belly syndrome, including 16 who had undergone previous urinary diversion. These are among the most difficult reconstructive procedures, but operation can be of considerable benefit to most of these boys despite the poor condition of the urinary tracts when first seen. The prune belly syndrome represents, like all conditions, a spectrum in severity. Some of the most severely affected patients have such severe renal dysplasia that they will die of renal insufficiency despite surgical efforts. In other cases, the relatively good renal function warrants every possible salvage maneuver.

I do not agree, for several reasons, with the watch-and-wait philosophy advocated by some for patients with the prune belly syndrome because (1) stasis and a large volume of urine in the upper tracts predisposes to infection in "prunes" just as in other cases; (2) massive reflux, which many have, predisposes to infection and should be corrected; (3) most of these patients ultimately become infected if the above problems remain uncorrected; (4) we don't see many "old prunes"; there must be a reason for that!

CASE 8.—This 9-year-old boy was referred for secondary reconstruction of megaureter (Figs 123–14 and 123–15). During infancy he was uremic; right nephrostomy and then bilateral ureterostomies were performed. He remained in that state for 8 years, draining through both flanks, although mainly from the left kidney.

Six months previously closure of the ureterostomies and left ureteral reimplantation had been performed. The left ureter became obstructed; T-tube ureterostomy was done. Injection of the T tube showed that the left ureter was dilated, but it had good peristalsis. A cystogram showed type I urethral valves with elongation and dilatation of the prostatic urethra. There was a periureteral diverticulum on each side.

The valves were destroyed by means of a cutting electrode. Reoperation was performed through a long midline incision. The lower ureter was mobilized with difficulty because there was a great deal of surrounding inflammatory reaction associated with the inlying tube. The ureter

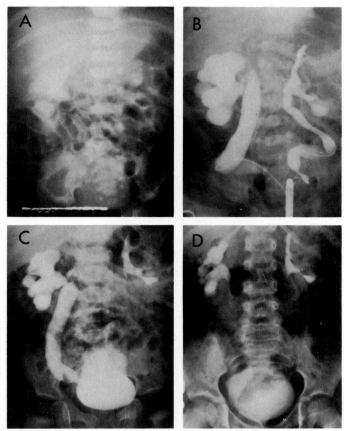

Fig 123–9.—Case 4: urethral valves and obstructive uropathy in a 1-week-old boy. **A,** IVP on admission with bilaterally poor function and severe hydrone-phrosis. **B,** retrograde pyelogram at time of endoscopic resection of valves shows bilaterally dilated, tortuous ureters, worse on the right than the left. **C,** IVP at age 5 months. There was considerable left-sided reflux as well as partial obstruction at both ends of the right ureter. A reconstructive operation was therefore per-formed at age 1 year. **D,** IVP at age 6 years.

from that level downward was not usable. Adequate length of ureter for reimplantation could be obtained only by extensive mobilization, because it was tethered upward at the site of the previous ureterostomy. To mo-bilize this ureter widely, all tissues along the pelvic wall, the great ves-sels and the gutter were swept toward the ureter as one would do during a radical retroperitoneal dissection for cancer, to leave the ureter all of its surrounding blood supply as well as the spermatic vessels. The kidney was similarly mobilized outside of Gerota's fascia, as one would do during radical nephrectomy. This allowed it to be pulled downward about 2 in.; its lower pole was fixed to the psoas muscle. These maneuvers gave enough length to achieve satisfactory ureteral reimplantation. The ureter was 15 mm in diameter, too wide to obtain a satisfactory tunnel length ureter diameter ratio. Therefore, it was tapered to half its original size for a length of about 3 in. It was brought through a new hiatus in the back wall of the bladder and laid into a long muscle bed made by incising open the mucosa. Psoas hitch was performed as an aid to this difficult lower ureteral reconstruction; this immobilized the bladder at the site of the new ureteral hiatus, and gave added length to the reimplant tunnel. The rudimentary right kidney was removed; however, its normal ureter was saved in case the left repeat reimplantation did not succeed.

Nine years following this reconstruction, the patient, now aged 18 years, is well, free from infection, attends college, and has normal blood chemical values.

Comment.—Ureterostomy, which has been advocated so widely in children with urethral valves and megaureter, did tide this child through early infancy, but it greatly complicated the eventual reconstruction. The continuing presence of unrecog-nized type I urethral valves undoubtedly precluded success of the previous operation. We have seen many similar cases where

valves were not originally recognized. Initial failure of the left ureteral tapering and reimplantation was doubtless because the ureter was too short, since it was tethered upward at the site of the original ureterostomy.

Many cases of secondary megaureter repair like this have shown that it is possible to perform reconstruction by one means or another and avoid urinary diversion. Maneuvers to be em-ployed include: (1) wide mobilization of the ureter, with metic-ulous preservation of all surrounding tissues for its blood supply; (2) downward displacement of a kidney in some cases; and (3) the psoas hitch procedure, which can make up for a certain loss in length of terminal ureter. We avoid using the Boari bladder flap technique in these cases because the results we have seen have been inconsistent. (4) As a last resort a segment of bowel can be used to replace a deficient ureter, tapering and tunneling the bowel as if it were a megaureter.

CASE 9.—A 5-year-old boy was referred for secondary megaureter re-construction (Fig 123–16). At age 9 months he had had a urinary infec-tion. He was found to have bilateral hydronephrosis, which was treated by nephrostomies. At age 4 years bilateral lower megaureter repair was performed, but bilateral obstruction occurred, requiring continued bilat-eral nephrostomy drainage.

Reoperation was performed through a vertical midline incision to gain extensive transabdominal exposure of both ureters. They had been im-planted too far laterally through the bladder wall, causing obstruction, and the ureter ends were fibrotic. At operation they were mobilized ex-tensively, taking care to preserve their blood supply from above. The previously tapered segments were excised, and the ureter just above that point on each side was shortened, tapered, and reimplanted, each through a new hiatus that was more medial and closer to the midline of the trigone. The upper tracts improved greatly. Cystogram showed no reflux.

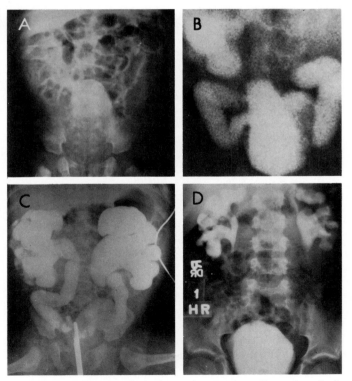

Fig 123–10.—Case 5: urethral valves and megaureters with massive reflux in a boy aged 3 months. **A,** preoperative IVP showing large bladder and poor vi-sualization of the upper tracts. **B,** preoperative cystogram (taken from cinecys-togram study performed in that era). Note massive reflux up dilated, tortuous ureters. **C,** retrograde pyelogram 1 week after admission, during cystoscopy to resect severe type I urethral valves. Note massive hydronephrosis. It was judged best to proceed with immediate reimplantation of the ureters in this case. **D,** IVP at age 9 years. A recent IVP (16 years after operation) was stable.

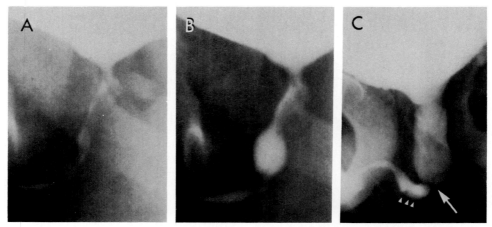

Fig 123–11.—Case 6: urethral valves and megaureters in a 9-year-old boy. Frames from preoperative voiding study, accomplished by suprapubic filling of the bladder through a transcutaneous needle. **A,** relatively normal-appearing urethra with a poor stream. **B,** moderate dilatation of prostatic urethra as stream is beginning to flow with greater force. **C,** typical appearance of severe type I ure-thral valves *(large arrow)* as patient is straining with abdominal effort, disclosing dilated, elongated prostatic urethra. *Small arrows* point to a slight filling defect in the floor of the bulbous urethra, which proved to be a cyst of Cowper's duct origin, probably not significant in this case.

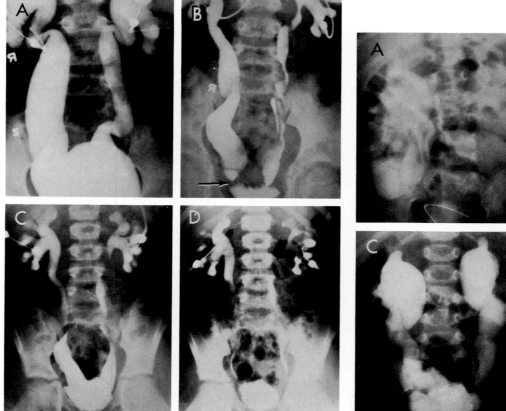

Fig 123–12.—Case 6: serial prograde perfusion studies in same patient as in Figure 123–11. **A,** study done when patient was first seen, showing bilaterally dilated upper tracts and ureters, greater on the right than on the left. **B,** repeat study 3 months after resection of valves. Perfusion pressures were unchanged from original study. Note narrow terminal ureter *(arrow)* visible on the right side. **C,** repeat study 8 months after valve resection. Upper tracts slightly improved in degree of dilatation, but little change in lower ureters. Perfusion pressures were the same. **D,** study 3 months after lower ureteral resection, tapering, and reimplantation. Note normal appearance of lower ureters and further improvement in the upper tracts. Perfusion pressures were normal. Now, 9 years later, IVP shows excellent upper tracts.

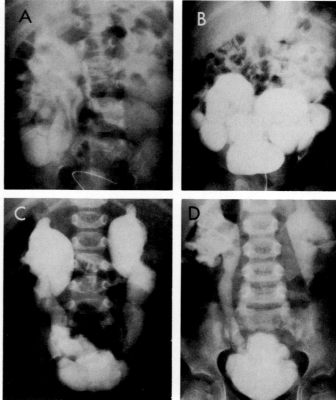

Fig 123–13.—Case 7: prune belly syndrome and urethral valves in a 2-month-old boy. **A,** IVP and **B,** cystogram 4 days after admission with pseudomonas septicemia. Endoscopic destruction of valves and reconstruction of lower ureters were performed. **C,** prograde study of upper tracts at age 2 years, showing still ballooning renal pelves and tortuous, dilated upper ureters that emptied poorly. Peristalsis was very sluggish. The upper ureters were now shortened and the volume of each renal pelvis reduced. **D,** IVP at age 5 years. The patient is free of urinary infection but has polydipsia and polyuria secondary to a renal concentrating defect. Current IVP is stable.

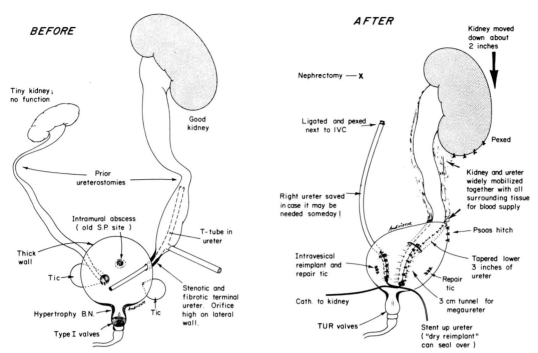

BEFORE

Tiny kidney; no function

Good kidney

Prior ureterostomies

Intramural abscess (old S.P. site)

T-tube in ureter

Thick wall

Tic

Stenotic and fibrotic terminal ureter. Orifice high on lateral wall.

Hypertrophy B.N.

Tic

Type I valves

AFTER

Kidney moved down about 2 inches

Nephrectomy — **X**

Pexed

Ligated and pexed next to IVC

Kidney and ureter widely mobilized together with all surrounding tissue for blood supply

Right ureter saved in case it may be needed someday !

Psoas hitch

Intravesical reimplant and repair tic

Tapered lower 3 inches of ureter

Repair tic

Cath. to kidney

3 cm tunnel for megaureter

TUR valves

Stent up ureter ("dry reimplant" can seal over)

Fig 123–14.—Case 8: anatomy before and after reconstructive procedure for left megaureter in 9-year-old boy with unrecognized urethral valves, previous nephrostomy, and bilateral ureterostomies.

It has now been 10½ years since this secondary salvage procedure. Current IVP is much improved. Blood chemical values include BUN 13 mg/100 ml, creatinine 1.1 mg/100 ml, and creatinine clearance 86 liters/sq m of body surface area. A college senior, he is completely well.

Comment.—This case illustrates two important complications that can occur during megaureter correction: (1) The ureters were obstructed because they had been brought through the bladder wall at a point that was too far lateral; and (2) the lower ureters had been tapered excessively, leading to ischemic fibrosis. A permanent urinary diversion had been considered for this child, but reoperation made that unnecessary. The difficulty of a secondary reconstruction should not be underestimated; this procedure lasted for 8 hours. However, the boy is much better off with his kidneys draining into the bladder instead of into a urinary diversion appliance. There is increasing evidence that with permanent urinary diversion, especially ileal conduits, there is continuing damage to the upper urinary tract from bacilluria and reflux. Furthermore, there is no question that the quality of life with a bag does not measure up to that without a bag.

There are some cases in which two satisfactory ureteral reimplantations are difficult or impossible to accomplish, especially if the ureter requires tapering and long tunnel reimplantation, i.e., megaureter repair. Most often, in my experience, these have been reoperative cases where the ureters were shortened and scarred. In a series of such cases[19] a good solution to this problem has been to rereimplant the better ureter into the bladder, hitching the bladder on that side to the psoas muscle, which allows creating a longer tunnel; fixation of the bladder adjacent to the new ureteral hiatus prevents angulation of the ureters as the bladder fills and empties. The less good ureter is drained via transureteroureterostomy (TUU) into the opposite side.[20] This approach of one reimplant and TUU of the other ureter has proven so helpful than in recent years I have extended it to a smaller number of new cases in which two megaureter repairs might prove difficult, such as prune belly syndrome cases with huge, tortuous ureters and an abnormal bladder, and urethral valve cases with an especially abnormal bladder.

The following two cases, one reoperative and one new, illustrate this approach.

CASE 10.—A 15-year-old boy was referred for secondary reconstructive ureteral surgery. At age 2 months, hydronephrosis and megaureter had been discovered; right ureteral reimplantation was performed. At age 2 years, bilateral reimplantation and bladder neck revision were performed. At age 4 years, lysis of the right ureteropelvic junction and bilateral ureteral reimplantation were performed. At 6 years, bladder neck revision was carried out; and at age 7 years, the patient underwent reduction cystoplasty and left ureteral reimplantation.

Preoperative evaluation at the time of referral showed massive reflux on the left side and obstruction on the right during prograde perfusion (Figs 123–17 and 123–18). At operation, cystoscopy disclosed type I urethral valves. The bladder was trabeculated. Through a transabdominal incision from the pubis to the xyphoid process, the full length of the urinary tract was exposed. The right colon was reflected medially and the right ureter was mobilized all the way to the kidney, leaving attached to it the spermatic vessels for collateral blood supply. The left ureter was similarly dissected completely, sweeping all of the retroperitoneal tissue toward the ureter, including the spermatic vessels. The kidney was mobilized completely, together with its perirenal fat, so that its only remaining attachment was at the hilus. This made it possible to slide the kidney down about 3 inches to gain additional length for a fourth reimplantation of the left ureter. Right-to-left transureteroureterostomy was performed to drain the right side. A psoas hitch was performed as an adjunct to reimplantation, obtaining a 6-cm cross-trigone tunneled reimplantation. The operation lasted 12 hours.

The patient convalesced uneventfully. During 6 years of follow-up, the urine has been sterile. Cystograms show no reflux; prograde perfusion of the upper tracts showed emptying at normal pressures. The patient leads a normal life. His only restriction is to avoid contact sports and other activities in which there is a high likelihood of flank trauma, since he could ill afford to lose a kidney.

Comment.—Total exposure and revision of the entire urinary tract, as in this case, is a lengthy, difficult undertaking that should be attempted only in medical centers where procedures of this magnitude are commonplace. Anesthesia management, intraoperative fluid administration, and maintenance of both normal blood gases and pH are vital to success. Fluid volume re-

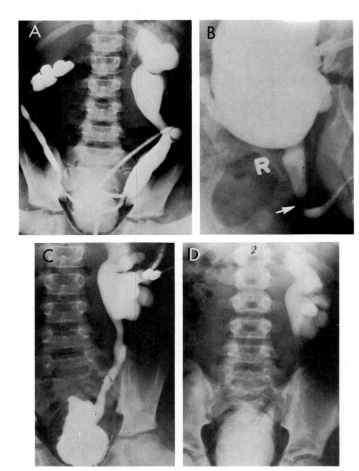

Fig 123–15.—Case 8: same patient as in Figure 123–14. **A,** preoperative filling of entire urinary tract by injection of T tube in left ureter. Note sites of previous ureterostomies in mid-left megaureter and upper right ureter, where both ureters had been temporarily exteriorized and later closed. **B,** preoperative voiding study, showing typical urethral valve obstruction *(arrow)*. **C,** prograde pyelogram during pressure perfusion study 6 months postoperatively. Pressures were normal. There was no reflux on cystogram. **D,** IVP 6 months after secondary reconstructive procedure. Patient is clinically well 9 years later.

placement in these cases is usually in the range of 20–25 ml per kilogram of body weight per hour, much more than is required in most operations.

CASE 11.—An 8-month-old male infant with prune belly syndrome was referred for reconstructive surgery, (Fig 123–19). There had been recurrent urinary infections with febrile seizure and probable brain damage secondary to the febrile seizures. At operation, the two ureters were shortened, tapering and reimplanting the better one and draining the other into it. This procedure lasted 9 hours but was well tolerated. In 20 months since operation, the patient has been well. Postoperative cystogram showed no reflux. An IVP showed great improvement in the upper urinary tract (Fig 123–20).

Comment.—This unusual approach should be considered when one ureter is much more favorable for ureteral tapering and reimplantation than the other, and the bladder is so abnormal that two excellent reimplants may be difficult to accomplish. Transureteroureterostomy can be done with a negligible complication rate if the ureter to be drained is brought across into the recipient ureter without tension and is anastomosed to it with care.

CASE 12.—A 24-year-old medical student was referred for reconstruction because of severe recurrent infection, which had caused him to drop out of school. At age 8 years, he had had hydronephrosis and bilateral

obstructive megaureter. Urethral valves were fulgurated, and suprapubic drainage of the bladder was maintained for a time. At age 11 years, an ileal loop was constructed to drain the midportion of each ureter, leaving the ureters connected to the bladder. He continued in this way for 13 years in good health. At age 23 years, the ileal loop was resected, together with the lower ureters, implanting the midureters into a bladder pedicle flap (Fig 123–21).

Although the original problem was relatively straightforward, i.e., bilateral obstructive megaureters, this patient's eventual reconstruction was extremely complex because both of the lower ureters had been removed, leaving insufficient length for a standard reconstructive procedure. The distance was too great to be bridged by sliding a kidney downward and utilizing a psoas hitch procedure. Autotransplantation was not felt justifiable, for two reasons: (1) it would be dangerous to perform vascular anastomoses in a contaminated field; and (2) it would represent an unjustifiable risk to transplant a kidney with already greatly diminished function. We chose, therefore, to use a small bowel conduit to join the right kidney to the bladder, and left-to-right transureteropyelostomy to drain the left kidney into the right side. The right ureter was fashioned into a nipple to give a second line of defense against reflux should there be reflux into the tapered and reimplanted small bowel conduit. This difficult reconstruction lasted for 13 hours. The patient's convalescence was uneventful except for serum hepatitis 6 weeks later. Ten years postoperatively, he voids normally, there is no reflux, and antegrade perfusion of the drainage system via the left kidney shows normal emptying pressures from the upper tract into the bladder.

The patient is now a practicing anesthesiologist working full time in good health. The IVP is stable (Fig 123–22).

Comment.—Most failures in operations for megaureter can be solved by procedures of lesser magnitude, as illustrated in Cases 8 and 9. However, in some instances a segment of bowel will be

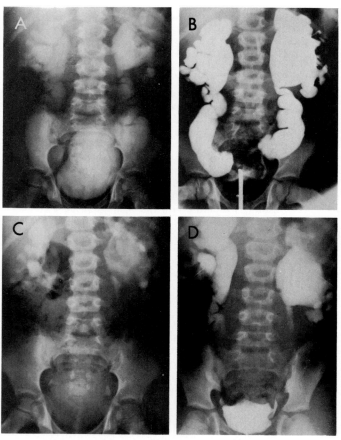

Fig 123–16.—Case 9: secondary operation for failed reimplantation. **A,** preoperative IVP before reoperation on lower ureters. **B,** preoperative retrograde examination, showing both ureters obstructed at the ureterovesical junction. **C,** an IVP and **D,** prograde pyelogram 9 months following reoperation, with now satisfactory lower ureters and less upper tract dilatation. Note spontaneous straightening of the upper ureters. The patient is well now, 10½ years later.

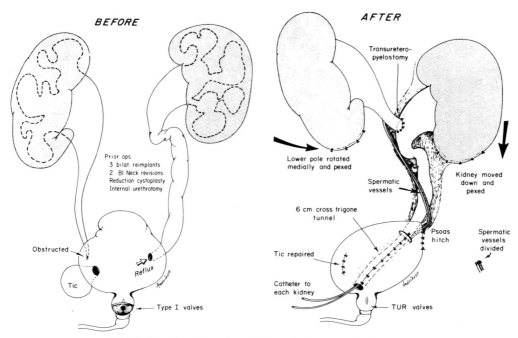

BEFORE

AFTER

Prior ops
3 bilat. reimplants
2 Bl Neck revisions
Reduction cystoplasty
Internal urethrotomy

Obstructed

Reflux

Tic

Type I valves

Transuretero-
pyelostomy

Lower pole rotated
medially and pexed

Spermatic
vessels

Kidney moved
down and
pexed

Spermatic
vessels
divided

6 cm cross trigone
tunnel

Psoas
hitch

Tic repaired

Catheter to
each kidney

TUR valves

Fig 123–17.—Case 10: anatomy before and after reoperation to correct
right ureteral obstruction and left ureteral reflux.

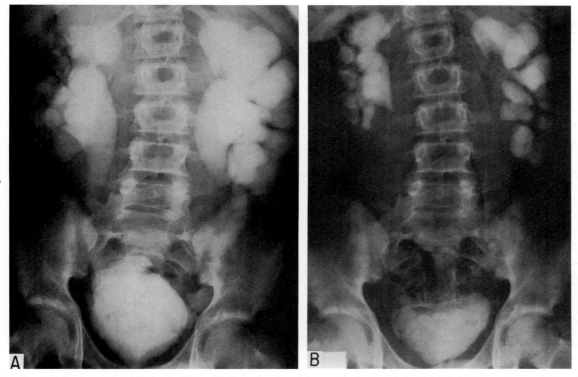

Fig 123–18.—Case 10. **A,** preoperative IVP showing bilateral hydronephrosis
from obstruction on the right and reflux on the left. **B,** IVP 4 months after repeat
left ureteral reimplantation and right-to-left transureteropyelostomy. The patient is
now completely well 6 years later.

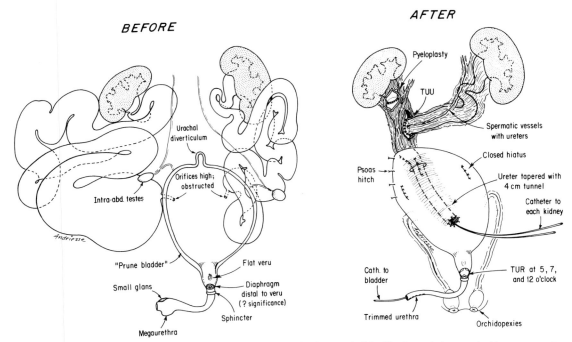

Fig 123–19.—Case 11: prune belly syndrome—preoperative and postoperative anatomy. Note extreme ureteral tortuosity, typical of prune belly syndrome. Note that it is possible to operate on both ends plus the middle of the ureter

required. It is important that a nonrefluxing mechanism be incorporated when bowel is used, or reflux and pyelonephritis can result. Transureteroureterostomy or transureteropyelostomy has proved to be of great value in managing one side of the urinary tract when the other is draining into the bladder. In performing transureteroureterostomy, there must be no tension on the anastomosis, and the blood supply must be carefully maintained for the ureter that is being brought across the retroperitoneum to be joined to the opposite side. We have used this maneuver in more than 100 complex reconstructive cases with satisfactory results.

The nipple technique shown in this case for the upper "ureter"

simultaneously if its blood supply is spared with great care, i.e., all periureteral tissue and the gonadal vessels are kept with the ureters to avert their devascularization.

has proved unreliable, for some of them disappear in time. Experience with bowel ureter has underscored that to prevent reflux the bowel must be tapered to reduce its caliber; a long tunnel (8–10 cm) must be constructed; and the bladder must be ideal, not one which is small, scarred, and noncompliant. Other options must be used in such cases, as described in Chapter 130.

Conclusion

Megaureter occurs with two main clinical manifestations, obstruction and massive reflux. When the bladder is normal, repair of megaureter is a relatively straightforward undertaking; results

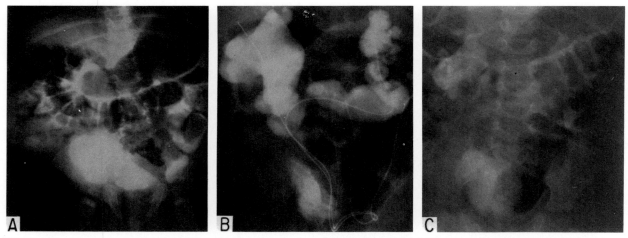

Fig 123–20.—Case 11: massive ureteral tortuosity and hydronephrosis. **A,** preoperative IVP. There was no reflux in this case, which is unusual. **B,** outlining repaired urinary tract anatomy 10 days postoperatively by injecting contrast medium into the ureteral drainage stent catheters, showing shortened ureters and transureteroureterostomy. **C,** IVP 3 months after repair, showing great improvement. No reflux on cystography. This is a well patient, urologically, 3 years later.

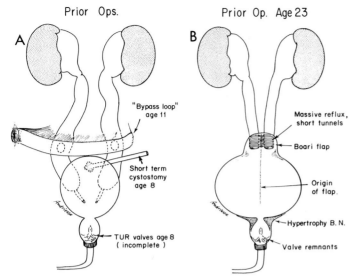

Prior Ops.

Prior Op. Age 23

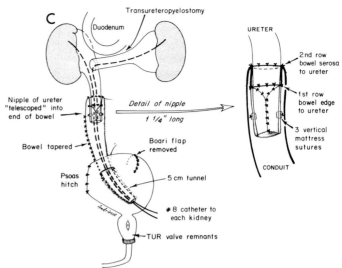

Fig 123–21.—Case 12: secondary operation in 24-year-old man with multiple previous procedures. **A,** original condition of bilateral obstructive megaureters, treated by short-term cystostomy at age 8 years and bypass ileal loop at age 11.

B, anatomy when patient was referred at age 24 years with massive reflux after operation 1 year before. **C,** technique for reconstruction. Right ureter was connected to bladder by ileal conduit; left ureter was connected to right renal pelvis.

should be successful in most cases. Even the severely decompensated ureter, with tortuosity and elongation, can be repaired. However, this can be an extraordinarily difficult task, especially when the bladder is abnormal, as in boys with urethral valves.

There are major pitfalls to avoid. The most common of these are: (1) devascularizing the ureter; (2) trimming it excessively; (3) implanting it in the lateral wall of the bladder, where it may be obstructed or have persisting reflux; and (4) temporarily exteriorizing the ureter as a ureterostomy, which introduces other potential complications. In the majority of these cases there is a better surgical alternative than performing a urinary diversion procedure. This is demanding surgery that should not be attempted on an occasional basis. Results can be satisfactory in more than 95% of cases if the surgeon adheres to certain technical guidelines, which have been described.

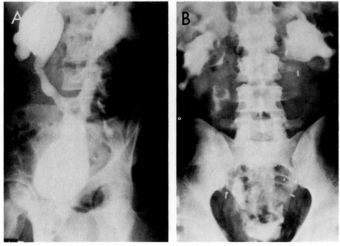

Fig 123–22.—Case 12. **A,** preoperative cystogram showing bladder, Boari flap, and reflux. **B,** IVP 6 months postoperatively, showing satisfactory drainage of the upper tracts into the bladder via tapered bowel conduit. There was no reflux on voiding cystogram examination.

REFERENCES

1. Belman A.B.: Megaureter classification, etiology and management. *Urol. Clin. North Am.* 1:497, 1974.
2. Bergman H.: *The Ureter.* New York, Harper & Row, 1967.
3. Bischoff P.: Operative treatment of megaureter. *J. Urol.* 85:268, 1961.
4. Derrick F.C., Jr.: Management of the large, tortuous, adynamic ureter with reflux. *J. Urol.* 108:153, 1972.
5. Dwoskin J.Y.: Management of the massively dilated urinary tract in infants by temporary diversion and single-stage reconstruction. *Urol. Clin. North Am.* 1:515, 1974.
6. Eckstein H.B., and Kapila, L.: Cutaneous ureterostomy. *Br. J. Urol.* 42:306, 1970.
7. Feminella J.G. Jr., Lattimer J.K.: A retrospective analysis of 70 cases of cutaneous ureterostomy. *J. Urol.* 106:538, 1971.
8. Flatmark A.U., Maruseth K., Knutrud O.: Lower ureteric obstruction in children. *Br. J. Urol.* 42:434, 1970.
9. Ghazali S.: Experience with the Sober ureterostomy. *J. Urol.* 112:142, 1974.
10. Hendren W.H.: Ureteral reimplantation in children. *J. Pediatr. Surg.* 3:649, 1968.
11. Hendren W.H.: Operative repair of megaureter in children. *J. Urol.* 101:491, 1969.
12. Hendren W.H.: Restoration of function in the severely decompensated ureter, in Johnston J.H., Scholtmeijer R.J. (eds.): *Problems in Paediatric Urology.* Amsterdam, Excerpta Medica, 1972, chap. 1.
13. Hendren W.H.: A new approach to infants with severe obstructive uropathy: Early complete reconstruction. *J. Pediatr. Surg.* 5:184, 1970.
14. Hendren W.H.: Posterior urethral valves in boys: A broad clinical spectrum. *J. Urol.* 106:298, 1971.
15. Hendren W.H.: Complications of urethral valve surgery, in Smith R.B., Skinner D.G. (eds.): *Complications of Urologic Surgery.* Philadelphia, W.B. Saunders Co., 1976.
16. Hendren W.H.: Reoperation for the failed ureteral reimplantation. *J. Urol.* 111:403, 1974.
17. Hendren W.H.: Complications of megaureter repair in children. *J. Urol.* 113:238, 1975.
18. Hendren W.H.: Complications of ureterostomy. *J. Urol.* 120:269, 1978.
19. Hendren W.H.: Reoperative ureteral reimplantation: Management of the difficult case. *J. Pediatr. Surg.* 15:770, 1980.
20. Hendren W.H., Hensle, T.W.: Transureteroureterostomy: Experience with 75 cases. *J. Urol.* 123:826, 1980.
21. Hendren W.H.: Megaureter, in Bergman H., (ed.): *The Ureter,* ed. 2. New York, Springer-Verlag, 1981.
22. Johnston J.H.: Temporary cutaneous ureterostomy in the manage-

ment of advanced congenital urinary obstruction. *Arch. Dis. Child.* 38:161, 1963.

23. Johnston J.H.: Reconstructive surgery of megaureter in childhood. *Br. J. Urol.* 39:17, 1967.

24. Kalicinski Z., Kansy J., Kotarbinska B., et al.: Surgery of megaureters—modification of Hendren's operation. *J. Pediatr. Surg.* 12:183, 1977.

25. Leape L.L., Holder T.M.: Temporary tubeless urinary diversion in children. *J. Pediatr. Surg.* 5:288, 1970.

26. Lome L.G., Howat J.M., Williams D.I.: The temporary defunctionalized bladder in children. *J. Urol.* 107:469, 1972.

27. Lome L.G., Williams D.I.: Urinary reconstruction following temporary cutaneous diversion in children. *J. Urol.* 108:162, 1962.

28. McLaughlin A.P., Leadbetter W.F., Pfister R.C.: Reconstructive surgery of primary megaloureter. *J. Urol.* 106:186, 1971.

29. Nesbit R.M., Withycombe J.F.: The problem of primary megaloureter. *J. Urol.* 72:162, 1954.

30. Perlmutter A.D., Tank E.S.: Loop cutaneous ureterostomy in infancy. *J. Urol.* 99:559, 1968.

31. Perlmutter A.D., Patil J.: Loop cutaneous ureterostomy in infants and young children: Late results in 32 cases. *J. Urol.* 107:655, 1972.

32. Pfister R.C., Newhouse J.H., Hendren W.H.: Percutaneous pyeloureteral urodynamics. *Urol. Clin. North Am.* 9:41, 1982.

33. Schmidt J.D., Hawtrey C.E., Culp D.A., et al.: Experience with cutaneous pyelostomy diversion. *J. Urol.* 109:990, 1973.

34. Sober I.: Pelviureterostomy-en-Y. *J. Urol.* 107:473, 1972.

35. Stephens F.D.: Treatment of megaureters by multiple micturition. *Aust. N.Z. J. Surg.* 27:130, 1957.

36. Straffon R.A., Kyle K., Corvalen J.: Technique of cutaneous ureterostomy and results in 51 patients. *J. Urol.* 103:138, 1970.

37. Wasserman D.H., Garrett R.A.: Cutaneous ureterostomy: Indications in children. *J. Urol.* 94:380, 1965.

38. Whitaker R.H.: Methods of assessing obstruction in dilated ureters. *Br. J. Urol.* 45:15, 1973.

39. Williams D.I., Hulme-Moor I.: Primary obstructive megaureter. *Br. J. Urol.* 42:140, 1970.

40. Williams D.I., Cromie W.J.: Ring ureterostomy. *Br. J. Urol.* 47:789, 1975.

124 CASIMIR F. FIRLIT

Vesicoureteral Reflux

VESICOURETERAL REFLUX (VUR) is the retrograde flow of urine from the bladder into the upper urinary tract, associated with abnormalities of the ureterovesical junction. These abnormalities may be congenital—primary reflux, or acquired—secondary reflux. VUR is not a normal phenomenon of the urinary tract and is significant because of its association with renal dysfunction and parenchymal scarring, particularly in the presence of infection. Almost all patients with radiographic evidence of renal scarring have or have had VUR, while 30%–60% of children with VUR will have parenchymal scars.[12, 30, 45, 46] Whether sterile reflux has the same effect is presently unresolved. It should also be noted that normal individuals may reflux transiently, but that persistence is pathologic.[5, 27, 38] The precise incidence of vesicoureteral reflux in the general population is not well established. Accepted figures for the general pediatric population are 1%–2%.[39] Among patients with urinary tract infections, 29%–50% have VUR. In asymptomatic patients, approximately 0.5% have VUR. The frequency with which VUR is detected is inversely proportional to the age of the population.[27, 28, 30] The highest incidence, up to 70%, is thought to be during the first 2 years of life,[39] eight times more common in females than males, more commonly unilateral than bilateral, and rare in blacks. There is a familial distribution, affecting 8%–26% of siblings of children with VUR. The severity of this familial reflux is variable.[34]

Etiology

Primary or congenital reflux results from an inadequate intravesical submucosal tunnel for the ureter, resulting in a lack of posterior buttress support. The "flap" mechanism is mainly passive, and it is the ratio of submucosal tunnel length to ureteral diameter which is the main determinant of its effectiveness.[30, 32] This ratio should be 4–5:1 for an effective mechanism. There is often a large, poorly developed trigone with lateral placement of the ureteral orifice.[4] When a complete ureteral duplication is present, the same mechanism may result in reflux in the lower pole ureter in up to 50% of cases.[39] The role of congenital vesical outlet obstruction in primary reflux has been the source of some debate.[2] Initial reports showed a 50%–95% incidence; later work stated that it was a rare to nonexistent occurrence.[44] Presently, it is thought that posterior urethral valves or urethral stricture may be associated with VUR.[39] Secondary reflux occurs when the valvular mechanism has been iatrogenically rendered incompetent, usually due to transurethral surgery. Such procedures as transurethral resection of bladder tumors or the prostate, failed ureteral reimplantation, ureteral meatotomy, or unroofing of a ureterocele may result in reflux.

Classifications of VUR

Present-day preference for the classification of VUR is based on one of two systems; the Dwoskin-Perlmutter[10] and International Reflux Study Committees.[30] Currently, the latter is being used more, although the relation between the two can be seen in Figure 124–1. Grade I involves the ureter only; grade II the ureter, pelvis, and calices with no dilatation, and normal caliceal fornices; grade III represents mild or moderate dilatation and/or tortuosity of the ureter and mild or moderate dilatation of the renal pelvis but none or slight blunting of the fornices. Grade IV reflux demonstrates moderate dilatation and/or tortuosity of ureter and moderate dilatation of the renal pelvis and calices, with complete obliteration of the sharp angle of fornices but maintenance of papillary impressions in the majority of the calices. Grade V reflux shows gross dilatation and tortuosity of the ureter, with gross dilatation of the renal pelvis and calices, and loss of papillary impressions in the majority of calices. These classifications are made on the basis of a contrast cystogram. One cystogram alone may be insufficient to diagnose a lesser grade of reflux. The hydronephrosis seen in association with VUR may give a picture easily confused with that of a ureteropelvic junction obstruction (pseudoureteropelvic junction obstruction).[22, 26]

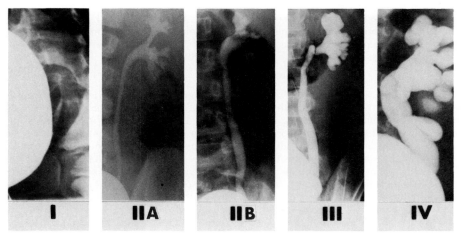

Fig 124–1.—Classification of ureteral reflux. *Grade I,* lower ureteral filling; *grade IIA,* ureteral and pelvicaliceal filling, without other changes; *grade IIB,* ureteral and pelvicaliceal filling with mild caliceal blunting but without clubbing and without dilatation of the pelvis or tortuosity of the ureter; *grade III,* ureteral and pelvicaliceal filling, caliceal clubbing, and minor to moderate pelvic dilatation with slight tortuosity of the ureter; *grade IV,* massive hydronephrosis and hydroureter. (From Dwoskin and Perlmutter.[10])

Natural History

The natural history of untreated vesicoureteral reflux is not known in its entirety because urinary infections signal the presence of VUR in most cases and medical or surgical therapy is usually instituted. From older studies, we know that some cases of reflux resolve spontaneously without treatment and without renal damage.[5, 27, 28] On the other hand, other cases progress to end-stage renal disease with or without treatment.[12, 21, 41] Most patients with vesicoureteral reflux fall between these extremes and are managed successfully by current modes of therapy.

Lenaghan's series of 102 children treated before the recognition that continuous antibiotic prophylaxis can prevent renal damage represents the closest approximation available to the natural history of untreated vesicoureteral reflux.[45, 46] Children with reflux associated with ureteral duplication, vesical diverticulum, urethral valves, or neurogenic bladder were excluded. In addition, patients with the severest forms of reflux were excluded by virtue of early intervention to correct their reflux. This select group, with uncomplicated reflux followed for 5–18 years, was managed on a regimen of multiple micturition and intermittent antibiotic therapy when surveillance cultures were positive. Reflux stopped spontaneously in 83 (45%) of 167 ureters. Age at diagnosis and the caliber of the refluxing ureter correlated best with the cessation of reflux. In this series, the younger the age at the time of diagnosis, the more likely the patient was to outgrow the reflux. For example, of 22 children presenting with reflux during the first year of life, 68% ceased to reflux by age 14. This is in contrast to 44% of 18 ureters and 37% of 19 ureters diagnosed in patients between ages 1 and 2 and 2 and 3, respectively. Ureteral caliber was measured on the voiding cystourethrogram. Normal caliber was defined as under 1 cm maximum width. Moderate and gross dilatation were defined as 1–2 cm and greater than 2 cm width, respectively. Reflux ceased in 66% of 98 normal caliber ureters, compared with 33% of 48 moderately dilated ureters and 14% of 21 grossly dilated ureters. Cumulatively, reflux ceased spontaneously in 42% of the 102 patients. Reflux ceased in 65% of 37 patients with unilateral reflux and 50% of 31 patients with bilateral reflux, both into normal-caliber ureters. Bilateral reflux into dilated ureters was distinctly unfavorable, with cessation of reflux in only 9% of 34 patients. Comparative radiographs of sufficient quality to evaluate progressive renal damage were available for 120 of the 167 renal units drained by ureters with reflux. Renal damage occurred in 37.5% of the 120 renal units. Progressive renal damage was more likely in kidneys in which scars were already present than in kidneys that were initially normal (66% vs. 21%). Renal deterioration was more likely in the presence of dilated ureters. In 12 of 13 cases with initially normal kidneys, deterioration was associated with infection.

The place of operation in the treatment of vesicoureteral reflux has been controversial.[39] Most of the controversy has focused on the difficulty in identifying patients who would benefit most from operation. Furthermore, the impact of surgical intervention on the natural history of vesicoureteral reflux has not been clearly documented.[21, 39, 46] With surgical correction of reflux, accelerated renal growth was noted in previously unscarred kidneys. In kidneys with extensive pyelonephritic scars, no change was observed unless the opposite kidney also had scars.[37] Improvement in renal function after successful antireflux procedures as defined by concentrating ability has been documented.[43] On the other hand, Babcock et al. could not demonstrate any significant change in renal growth patterns after successful operation.[6] These conflicting results can be explained by patient selection, as some of the patients in Babcock's series improved with operation. The explanation for the lack of improvement after operation was that a defect in the embryologic development of these kidneys resulted in fixed abnormalities of the renal parenchyma, known as renal dysplasia.[6] Stephens proposed the "ureteral bud theory" to explain the association of vesicoureteral reflux with renal dysplasia.[42] An abnormal origin of the ureteral bud from the wölffian duct leads to lateral ectopia of the ureteral orifice on the trigone and vesicoureteral reflux. Because of its abnormal origin, the ureteral bud also encountered derelict renal blastema during its ascent, and a dysplastic kidney was formed. If the association of vesicoureteral reflux with dysplasia is strong, the role of operation in the severest cases of reflux must be questioned. In these patients, chronic renal failure may be inevitable, and an operation would not prevent the development of uremia as the child outgrew his limited renal reserve.[40]

Hypertension and chronic renal failure are infrequent, although well-recognized, long-term sequelae of vesicoureteral reflux. Persistent urinary tract infection after cessation or correction of reflux is not well recognized. Long-term reflux with failure to empty the upper tracts is thought to lead to increased bladder capacity and diminished bladder tone. These floppy bladders empty poorly and are therefore more prone to recurrent infections. The incidence of this sequel of vesicoureteral reflux is not known. In an attempt to prevent this complication, however, some surgeons have liberalized their indications for reflux surgery to include abnormally large bladder capacity.

Diagnosis

An intravenous pyelogram (IVP) and voiding cystourethrogram (VCUG) should be performed in all children with febrile urinary tract infections. Febrile urinary tract infections and those associated with loin pain and gastrointestinal complaints are more likely to be a consequence of VUR. Urinary tract infections in children are manifest by a wide spectrum of symptoms, which vary considerably with age. In neonates, most urinary tract infections are asymptomatic and may be suspect if weight loss and/or failure to thrive are evident. In toddlers and in older children, symptoms specific to the urinary tract such as urgency, frequency, and incontinence are more likely.

Vesicoureteral reflux is a radiologic diagnosis confirmed by the voiding cystourethrogram.[25] The extent of reflux and the amount of upper tract dilatation on the VCUG are used to grade the reflux and numerous grading systems have been proposed. The most commonly used classification to this day remains that described by Dwoskin and Perlmutter.[10] Recent attempts to substitute an international grading (1–5) system appear to be gaining momentum. Adequate studies require complete bladder filling, patient cooperation, and personnel attuned to the pediatric patient.

The role of the IVP in the evaluation of VUR is to document renal parenchymal scarring. The amount of ureteral dilatation is usually greater in the VCUG than on the IVP, and it is the amount of dilatation on the former test on which the grading of reflux is based. An occasional patient with hydronephrosis presents with the radiologic appearance of ureteropelvic junction (UPJ) obstruction on IVP when VUR has caused ureteral dilatation, elongation, and tortuosity which mimicked UPJ obstruction.[22, 26] Such cases illustrate the need for visualization of the complete ureter either by VCUG retrograde pyelography or renal scan to rule out vesicoureteral reflux before proceeding with pyeloplasty.

In most major pediatric centers, the use of cystoscopy in the evaluation of vesicoureteral reflux has declined sharply. Endoscopic evaluation of the ureterovesical junction was used in the past to assess orifice configuration and location. These data were then used to predict the eventual spontaneous resolution or its failure. Vesicoureteral junction morphology assessed endoscopically has been shown to be an unreliable predictor for a number of reasons: (1) It is highly subjective, with interobserver variability; and (2) even in the best of hands it has no better than a 50% chance of indicating cessation. Further, ureteral orifice configuration, location, and tunnel length can be reliably ascertained from the contrast cystogram alone (Fig 124–2). At Children's Memorial Hospital, Chicago, cystoscopy is reserved for patients in whom reflux has failed to cease following 2–3 years of surveillance. The nuclear voiding cystourethrogram (NVCUG) is replacing the contrast cystogram as the best method for following patients with vesicoureteral reflux. Besides the advantage of low-dose radiation exposure (up to 200 times less than with contrast studies), NVCUG is a more sensitive test because of its longer exposure and study time.[9] Further, the NVCUG supplies the clinician with quantitative information such as bladder volumes at which reflux occurs and bladder capacity. These measurements, serially compared with those of previous studies, demonstrate the status of the reflux. If improvement is occurring, the reflux occurs at progressively larger volumes before it disappears. Increasing bladder capacities alone, in the presence of persistent or slowly improving reflux, indicate early operation to

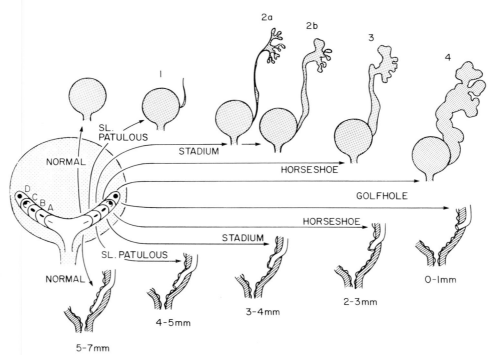

Fig 124–2.—Comparison of the radiographic cystogram *(upper register)*, ureteral orifice configuration, and trigonal location *(central figure)* with their respective submucosal tunnel lengths *(lower register)*. The illustration clarifies descriptive and prognostic criteria used for the assessment of reflux ureters. Consequently, a radiographic cystogram, with the bladder filled to capacity for age, will of itself allow for staging orifice appearance, location, and submucosal tunnel length. This staging will establish the initial assessment and aid in proper management. These relations are correct in children from neonates to age 15 years. The only variable is tunnel length, which increases with age. This illustration is correct for children to age 7 years.

prevent recurrent cystitis problems associated with the poorly emptying large-capacity bladders in some long-term reflux patients. Children who demonstrate cessation of VUR but persist with large bladders appear to be candidates for recurrent cystitis.[7]

A role for urodynamic studies has been proposed in the evaluation of VUR.[29] Koff demonstrated dramatic improvement by pharmacologic therapy in VUR with diagnosis of vesicosphincter dyssynergia and hypertonic neurogenic bladder in patients with reflux who are otherwise neurologically normal. Currently, the incidence of dyssynergia and nonneurogenic bladder associated with VUR is not known. However, in patients with strangury, incontinence, or frequency, the diagnosis may be suspected, and micturition flow studies and cystometry should be performed.

The current management of vesicoureteral reflux is based largely on the initial voiding cystourethrogram. Cystoscopy has not been necessary in most cases because of our confidence in the relation between the degree of ureteral dilatation and the degree of abnormality of the ureterovesical junction (Fig 124–2). For long-term assessment, we rely on the NVCUG performed at yearly intervals. We operate for reflux if it consistently occurs at decreasing or low bladder volumes, or if vesical decompensation (megacystis) occurs. Further, since the incidence of spontaneous resolution of VUR beyond 10–11 years of age is extremely low, we recommend operation for children in this age group to eliminate the need for prolonged close surveillance and/or antibiotic prophylaxis into adolescence and adulthood. Issues of compliance, cost, frequent irradiation, and antibiotics all must enter into the surgical equation.

Operative Management of Vesicoureteral Reflux

The indications for the surgical management of reflux are listed below.

    Principal indications
        Absent intravesical submucosal tunnel
        Persistent or recurrent urinary infection, despite antibacterial prophylaxis.
        Renal growth arrest
        Progression of renal scarring
        Poor patient or parental compliance with nonoperative therapy
        Persistent ipsilateral reflux following corrective operation
        Failure of submucosal tunnel growth for 2–4 years
    Other indications
        Intrarenal reflux (grade IV reflux, international system; see Fig 124–1)
        Reflux into the lower segment of a duplicated kidney
        Reflux associated with a paraureteral diverticulum
        Reflux in children over age 10 years
        Persistent reflux after relief of outlet obstruction

The "principal" category includes indications that are generally agreed upon. Indications in the second category are equally valid but less commonly cited. The operative management of vesicoureteral reflux is never a surgical emergency. Antibiotic prophylaxis allows for elective planning without undue parental emotional stress. As long as the child remains uninfected, risk to the kidney is negligible. Above all, active urinary infection is an absolute contraindication to immediate operation. The urine should be sterilized first and the bladder inflammatory response allowed to subside. Operating in the face of active or unrecognized cystitis places the child's life at risk and adversely influences the result of surgical correction.

In the past, neurovesical dysfunction was also believed to be an absolute contraindication to the performance of antireflux procedures. Presently, with the accepted practice of clean intermittent catheterization, operative correction of reflux is indicated when spontaneous correction fails to result in cessation of reflux. Proper antimicrobial prophylaxis, specific autonomic pharmacotherapy, and close surveillance appear to optimize spontaneous resolution.[24] When nonoperative mangement fails, surgical involvement is appropriate. The nonneurogenic neurogenic bladder syndrome with its associated hydronephrosis or vesicoureteral reflux requires extreme caution in considering operation for reflux.[1] This disorder, characterized by incontinence, elevated intravesical resting and voiding pressure, trabeculation, and dilatation of the upper urinary tract, appears at first to be appropriate for correction, but pronounced hydroureteronephrosis will result and renal function may become seriously jeopardized. This disorder should be suspected when vesical enlargement, deformity, trabeculation, and/or detrusor hypertrophy are demonstrated radiographically or cystoscopically, in the absence of neurologic defects on detailed examination. The correction of vesicoureteral reflux in patients with moderate or moderately severe renal insufficiency (serum creatinine 3–4 mg/dl) is more controversial. The controversy revolves around the expected outcome. Certainly, in renal dysplasia with reflux, or in reflux nephropathy, improvement in renal function, demonstrated by a reduction in serum creatinine, will not occur. However, I have favored operating for reflux in these situations when the potential for urinary infection appears great—particularly in young girls who void infrequently and/or have large bladder capacities.[29] The concept is that severe episodes of pyelonephritis may add sufficient insult to an already compromised kidney to accelerate its rate of renal impairment. Here, we hope to buy time, but not prevent the inevitable.

Many operative procedures have been described[12, 16, 18, 37, 38] to correct reflux. They may be categorized as intravesical or extravesical. Further, each category may be subcategorized to include either a hiatal recession, ureteral meatal advancement, or both. The surgical indication for these procedures varies and is influenced by ureteral meatal, and/or ureteral hiatal positions, trigonal configuration, neuropathic bladder, (i.e., spina bifida), and the surgeon's preference. The purpose of any surgical approach must be to alter the intravesical ureteral length to stop reflux without producing obstruction. When creating the submucosal tunnel in preparation for ureteral reimplantation, this length must be a minimum four to five times the ureteral diameter. This relation is a "urophysiologic law" and must be respected. Less than this will result in reflux, while more may result in obstruction. Further, a thick or slightly dilated ureter requires a longer than usual submucosal tunnel. Distal ureteral fixation on the trigone is necessary to properly immobilize the ureter to achieve lengthening and support against a solid muscle buttress during bladder filling and emptying.

Probably the most commonly performed antireflux procedure is the intravesical ureteroneocystostomy as described by Politano and Leadbetter.[2, 36, 37] This procedure is predominantly an intravesical approach to the ureter and its hiatus. The bladder is approached through a transverse suprapubic skin-crease incision, which allows excellent extraperitoneal exposure of the bladder. The bladder is opened with cutting cautery and held open with stay sutures suspended over a Denis Browne ring retractor. The dome of the bladder is packed with one or several gauze sponges in order to keep the posterior bladder wall comfortably taut. This maneuver is critical, because it determines ultimately the position of the "new" ureteral hiatus. If too lax, the "new" hiatus may have too much mobility, which may result in a J-hook obstruction during filling. The bladder is inspected and the ureteral meatus identified. Reflux is typically associated with a laterally situated meatus (ectopia lateralis) on a splayed or asymmetric trigone.

I then insert an 8 F red rubber catheter into the reflux ureter and suture the meatus to the catheter. This allows for fixation and manipulation without extensive trauma. The perimeatal area is then infiltrated with 0.5% lidocaine with 1/200,000 epinephrine to facilitate dissection and reduce oozing. A circumscribing incision frees the ureter from the mucosa. Interval fibrous or vascular strands may be carefully electrocoagulated. Extreme care is necessary to avoid ureteral injury.[11] The dissection is carried proximally to the detrusor hiatus and then through to the perivesical adventitia. At this point, I prefer to continue the dissection extravesically. The ureter is transferred to the extravesical space and freed proximally to the area of the obliterated umbilical artery. It is critical to keep in mind that the blood supply to the distal, transected ureter must come via segmental ureteral sleeve and intramural vessels. The ureter must be handled minimally and the ureteral vascular areolar sleeve left intact. Violation of these principles causes ureteral ischemia, which results in stricture, hydronephrosis, ureteral slough, persistent reflux, or urinary extravasation.[11] Once mobilization has been accomplished, the hiatus is approximated with two or three chromic sutures. The mucosa superiorly and medially is elevated with a pair of tenotomy scissors for 3.5–4 cm. At the uppermost recess of the "new" submucosal tunnel, a counterincision is carried through the mucosa and detrusor to the extravesical space. This maneuver forms the "new" hiatus. The transected end of the ureter is manipulated through the new hiatus and submucosal tunnel, and terminates at the original meatal site or more distally on the trigone toward the bladder neck. Before the ureter is fixed, its extravesical and transmural course is carefully inspected for twisting, kinking, or obstruction. The ureteral hiatus should accept the tip of a right-angled clamp. Intravesically, the terminal ureter is trimmed, spatulated, and sutured to the trigone with one to two 4-0 chromic sutures. The remainder of the anastomosis is accomplished with interrupted 5-0 chromic sutures. Generally, ureteral stenting is not used but may be necessary when ureteral edema occurs or if tapering[19] or folding[23] of megaureters is undertaken. The bladder is closed in three layers and drained via Foley (Silicone) urethral catheter for 3 days postoperatively.

The procedure combines ureteral meatal advancement with hiatal recession. This ability to vary the intravesical ureteral length in two directions proves most versatile. However, it is tempting to increase this length by placing the hiatus "too lateral" or "too superior," particularly if the ureter is dilated. The technique has stood the test of time and is the most widely used procedure in this country.

Ureteral Advancement

Ureteral advancement alone is suitable if the trigone is extremely broad and the refluxing ureter laterally positioned.[12-15] Since acquisition of intravesical length is the object of this procedure, a broadly based trigone is critical. This procedure utilizes a temporary ureteral stent, 6–8 F, sutured to the ureteral meatus for mobilization and identification. The area circumscribing the ureteral meatus is infiltrated with 1 or 2 ml of 0.5% lidocaine with 1/200,000 epinephrine. The ureter is circumscribed sharply and dissected submucosally to the hiatus (Fig 124–3). The ureter must be freed circumferentially at the hiatus and extravesically for 2–3 cm. This allows for sufficient ureteral freedom for the eventual advancement. The mucosa distally and medially is infiltrated and a submucosal tunnel developed. A point for fixation is determined and the mucosa over this point fenestrated. The ureter is then manipulated distally and submucosally

to the fenestrated area. Two 4-0 chromic sutures anchor the ureteral meatus to the trigonal musculature. Finer chromic sutures approximate the ureteral mucosa to bladder mucosa. The stent is removed and the mucosa at the original site is reapproximated over the advanced ureter. Ureteral stents are rarely used.

Intravesical ureteral advancement is useful in selected situations (Fig 124–4). A broadly based trigone, lateral ureteral ectopia, and a ureter of reasonably normal caliber are criteria for this technique. As in all situations of ureteral surgery, fine sutures and extremely delicate manipulation of tissue are vital to a successful outcome.

The two foregoing techniques are the most frequently used operations for vesicoureteral reflux. Less frequently employed but equally as reliable, are the extravesical techniques.[17, 31] These techniques totally avoid the bladder lumen and achieve hiatal recession, which results in an increased tunnel length. Further, a modification adds a ureteral advancement maneuver with hiatal recession as a refinement of this technique. The Lich technique of extravesical ureteroplasty utilizes a standard suprapubic extravesical approach.[21] The perivesical space is developed gently and a Balfour retractor inserted. The ureter is identified as it emerges beneath the obliterated umbilical artery and courses toward the bladder. A sling such as used in vascular surgery is passed beneath it for gentle traction. Careful and deliberate periureteral and perihiatal dissection is performed to free the ureter and express the bladder mucosa (Fig 124–5). The detrusor is incised 3–4 cm superiorly and the incision carried through to the mucosa, avoiding mucosal punctures. The medial and lateral detrusor edges are then stabilized with forceps and the mucosa separated with a "pusher" from its detrusor backing. The mobilized ureter is then positioned into this detrusor-submucosal trough and the detrusor reapproximated over the ureter with interrupted 4-0 chromic sutures. This procedure recedes the ureteral hiatus while adding additional detrusor buttress. On the average, a 3- or 4-cm tunnel is achievable. Bilateral procedures are easily performed at the same time. Postoperatively, because it avoids the vesical lumen, the extravesical approach is extremely easy on the patient. Bladder signs and symptoms, which include hematuria, urgency, spasm, incontinence, and pain, are remarkably reduced in comparison with intravesical procedures. The overall subjective morbidity of this procedure is very low.

Recently, I have used extravesical ureteral advancement to manage reflux in normal or slightly dilated ureters[20] (Fig 124–6). This technique has several advantages. First, it is purely an extravesical procedure, so postoperative morbidity is greatly reduced. Children walk freely by the next day. Since catheter drainage is minimal, urethral symptoms are absent. Generally, affect and appetite are normal within 24 hours of operation. Hospital stay is 36–48 hours for unilateral and 48–96 hours for bilateral procedures. The only significant complaints are referable to the abdominal incision, easily managed with mild analgesics. Second, this procedure combines all the principles necessary for a precise anatomical correction of the ureterovesical junction. The surgical procedure involves a suprapubic, extravesical approach to the ureter and hiatus. After gentle perivesical manipulation, a self-retaining retractor with blades of dissimilar length is positioned to allow the longer blade to rest against and rotate the bladder as it is extended. This maneuver is critical because it rotates the bladder and allows for anteromedial migration of the ureteral hiatus. If the retractor is positioned properly, the surgeon looks directly at the hiatus throughout the entire procedure. The ureter is manipulated with the aid of a sling for the sharp and blunt perihiatal dissection, which is continued until all detrusor fibers are transected and the ureter remains attached only to bladder mucosa (Fig 124–6,*B*). Four stay-sutures are now

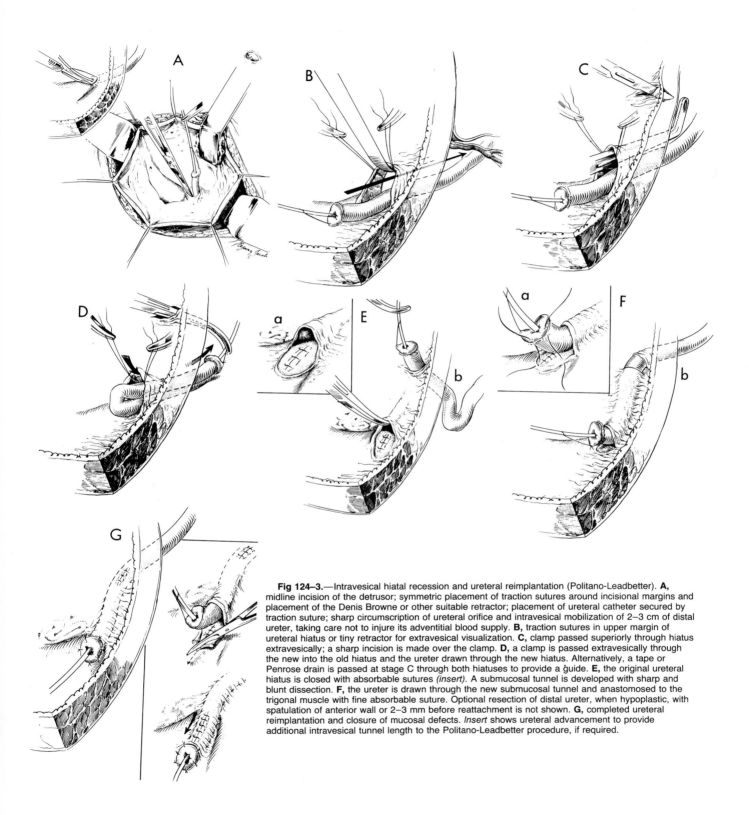

Fig 124–3.—Intravesical hiatal recession and ureteral reimplantation (Politano-Leadbetter). **A,** midline incision of the detrusor; symmetric placement of traction sutures around incisional margins and placement of the Denis Browne or other suitable retractor; placement of ureteral catheter secured by traction suture; sharp circumscription of ureteral orifice and intravesical mobilization of 2–3 cm of distal ureter, taking care not to injure its adventitial blood supply. **B,** traction sutures in upper margin of ureteral hiatus or tiny retractor for extravesical visualization. **C,** clamp passed superiorly through hiatus extravesically; a sharp incision is made over the clamp. **D,** a clamp is passed extravesically through the new into the old hiatus and the ureter drawn through the new hiatus. Alternatively, a tape or Penrose drain is passed at stage C through both hiatuses to provide a guide. **E,** the original ureteral hiatus is closed with absorbable sutures *(insert).* A submucosal tunnel is developed with sharp and blunt dissection. **F,** the ureter is drawn through the new submucosal tunnel and anastomosed to the trigonal muscle with fine absorbable suture. Optional resection of distal ureter, when hypoplastic, with spatulation of anterior wall or 2–3 mm before reattachment is not shown. **G,** completed ureteral reimplantation and closure of mucosal defects. *Insert* shows ureteral advancement to provide additional intravesical tunnel length to the Politano-Leadbetter procedure, if required.

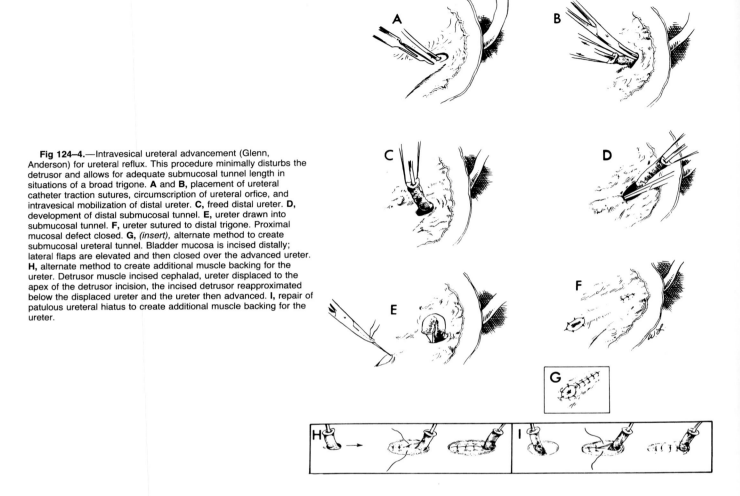

Fig 124–4.—Intravesical ureteral advancement (Glenn, Anderson) for ureteral reflux. This procedure minimally disturbs the detrusor and allows for adequate submucosal tunnel length in situations of a broad trigone. **A** and **B,** placement of ureteral catheter traction sutures, circumscription of ureteral orfice, and intravesical mobilization of distal ureter. **C,** freed distal ureter. **D,** development of distal submucosal tunnel. **E,** ureter drawn into submucosal tunnel. **F,** ureter sutured to distal trigone. Proximal mucosal defect closed. **G,** *(insert),* alternate method to create submucosal ureteral tunnel. Bladder mucosa is incised distally; lateral flaps are elevated and then closed over the advanced ureter. **H,** alternate method to create additional muscle backing for the ureter. Detrusor muscle incised cephalad, ureter displaced to the apex of the detrusor incision, the incised detrusor reapproximated below the displaced ureter and the ureter then advanced. **I,** repair of patulous ureteral hiatus to create additional muscle backing for the ureter.

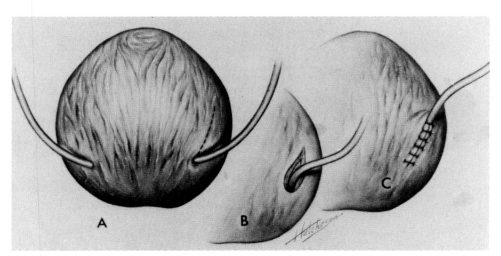

Fig 124–5.—Lich-Grégoir technique of ureteroneocystostomy. **A,** extravesical ureteroplasty—hiatal recession. *Dashes* indicate the suprahiatal area for detrusor incision. **B,** superior lateralmost extent of this incision and dissection will be the new hiatus. **C,** submucosally insinuated ureter, covered by the reapproximated detrusor. (From Kelalis P.P., King L.R. (eds.): *Clinical Pediatric Urology.* Philadelphia, W.B. Saunders Co., 1976. Reprinted with permission.)

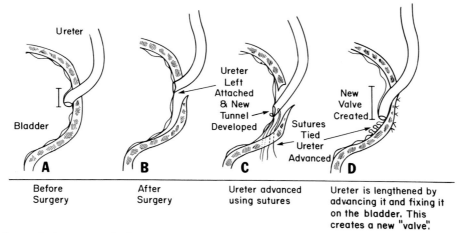

Ureter

Bladder

A
Before
Surgery

B
After
Surgery

Ureter
Left
Attached
& New
Tunnel
Developed

Sutures
Tied
Ureter
Advanced

C
Ureter advanced
using sutures

New
Valve
Created

D
Ureter is lengthened by
advancing it and fixing it
on the bladder. This
creates a new "valve".

Fig 124–6.—Extravesical ureteral advancement. **A,** abnormal relation of the ureter and the bladder, with short submucosal tunnel and minimal buttress. **B,** initial perihiatal dissection liberating the ureter and bladder mucosa from the detrusor. **C,** once circumferential mobility is achieved, two traction sutures are placed as indicated, tied, and the ureter advanced. **D,** completed extravesical advancement and detrusor reconstruction, resulting in normal relation between submucosal ureter and detrusor.

placed, two caudad and two laterally. The caudad stays are stabilized with traction and the mucosa is carefully "peeled" off the detrusor with a dorsal and horizontal stroke. This action develops the submucosal space caudad to the orthotopic ureteral insertion (Fig 124–6,*C*). This submucosal space is developed for 1½–2 cm. Two horizontal 4-0 chromic mattress sutures, placed at the 5 and 7 o'clock position, penetrate the detrusor extravesically, traverse the "new" submucosal space, bite the ureter extravesically at its orthotopic extravesical juncture, and return along the same course to exit through the detrusor near their point of entry. Traction on the two sutures results in a caudad advancement of the ureteral orifice onto the trigone, where they are tied. The free edges of the detrusor are then reapproximated with interrupted 4-0 chromic sutures, completing the detrusor backing. These maneuvers result in an anatomical relocation—advancement—of the ureter onto the trigone, and precisely reconstruct the ureterovesical junction. Bilateral procedures can be easily performed. The reduced postoperative morbidity with this extravesical approach makes it extremely appealing.

All patients are continued on antibacterial suppression for 3 months postoperatively. I usually perform an excretory urogram (IVP) (one 20-minute film) and a nuclear voiding cystogram at that time.[9] If the studies are normal, the antibiotic is discontinued 1 week later. Follow-up assessment is with an excretory urogram annually for 2 years. Following 2 years of health and evidence of renal stability or growth, these children are discharged from my surveillance, to remain under the observation of their primary physician.

Duplex Ureters

Vesicoureteral reflux into duplex collecting systems is found in approximately 4%–5% of children undergoing antireflux operations.[4] General experience has indicated that spontaneous cessation of reflux in duplex ureters is considerably less frequent than in single systems. The duplex ureters resolve reflux in only 25% of instances when observed for 4 years. Single-system reflux controls, in comparison, resolve reflux in 70%–75% of instances in a comparable period.

Duplicated ureters lie in a common fibromuscular sheath. Because of their common blood supply, the surgical correction of reflux in one requires the reimplantation of both ureters in a common-tunnel technique (Fig 124–7). The approach is a combination of intra- and extravesical mobilization. The new hiatus is created by incision superior and medial to the original site. Both ureters are manipulated intravesically and through a developed 3–4-cm submucosal tunnel terminating distally and medially on the trigone. The common sheath is transected, exposing the two ureters, which in turn are sutured to the trigone.

Duplex ureteral surgery involves operation on the involved ureter and on the noninvolved ureter as well. It is an intravesical procedure and, although reliably successful in correcting reflux,

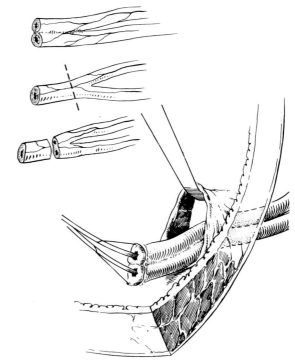

Fig 124–7.—Completely duplicated ureters, lying within a single muscular sleeve in the most distal portion. They are reimplanted as a common sheath. *Insert* shows appearance of complete duplication; low incomplete duplication, with juxtavesical union of the ureters, treatment of low incomplete duplication by resection of common stem to level of double lumina, to be followed by common-sheath reimplantation.

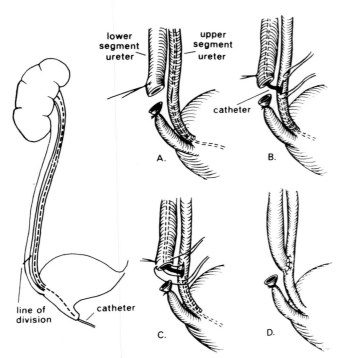

Fig 124–8.—Ipsilateral lower ureteroureterostomy. **A,** transected extravesical reflux ureter. Proximal ureteral stump is tied. **B,** ureterostomy and corner 5–0 chromic sutures to be tied before completing a running watertight anastomosis, **D,** completed anastomosis of reflux ureter to orthotopic (nonreflux) ureter. Note ureteral stump of reflux ureter is suture-ligated. (From Amar A.D.[3] Reprinted with permission.)

is disconcerting because of the extent of the surgical procedure. I have, over the last several years, favored an extravesical approach to the terminal ureters to perform a lower ipsilateral ureteroureterostomy (Fig 124–8). Here, the previously catheterized involved ureter is easily identified, separated from its mate, and transected. The recipient, normal, ureter is incised and the ureterotomy held open with four 5-0 chromic sutures. The transected end of the "reflux ureter" is then anastomosed to the recipient ureter with 5-0 chromic catgut. Ureteral stents are not used. A small Penrose drain is left. An indwelling urethral catheter is used for 24 hours. Hospital stay is 2–3 days. This technique is as reliable as the more extensive intravesical approach, and morbidity is greatly reduced. There have been no problems reported secondary to the retained ureteral stump. These procedures represent the most successfully applied operative techniques to correct vesicoureteral reflux in children.[3, 8] Our reference to extravesical procedures, as reliable as the traditional intravesical procedures, constitutes a balanced presentation. It is ultimately the judgment, knowledge, experience, and skill of the surgeon that dictates the choice of procedure.

Results

Any one of the procedures described will reliably correct vesicoureteral reflux in over 95% of patients. Urinary infections and/or asymptomatic bacteriuria will decrease to less than 18%. However, since reflux has been corrected, the risk of upper urinary tract or kidney infection is negligible. A group of these patients were studied from our experience and variable factors found to explain their infections. Seventy-three percent had bladders larger than normal. Compared with an age-matched control group, 24% had neurovesical voiding disturbances and the remainder had either normal evaluations or were suspected

of being immunologically deficient. The children with large bladder volumes were the ones plagued with recurrent lower urinary tract infections. Since then, we have been keenly aware of bladder volume. Particularly in the child with mild (grade II) reflux, reflux and increasing bladder volume are related and reflect, in our opinion, a decompensating urinary transport system. In these cases, we now intervene surgically much earlier than in the past.

If the surgical attempt to correct vesicoureteral reflux fails, endoscopic reassessment is necessary to evaluate the ureteral orifice and tunnel.[33] However, if acute obstruction at the ureterovesical junction occurs, ipsilateral "high" ureteral diversion would be preferable to intravesical manipulation.[35] This type of emergency drainage procedure is reserved for patients with acute infections, severe pain, or extensive hydronephrosis, despite intravenous antibiotic therapy. Surgical manipulation of the "healing" ureteroneocystostomy results in severe ischemic injury and eventual fibrosis. The potential for renal compromise under such circumstances is quite significant. Fortunately, in the hands of an experienced surgeon, ureteroneocystostomy is a highly effective and safe form of therapy for vesicoureteral reflux.

REFERENCES

1. Allen T.D.: The non-neurogenic neurogenic bladder. *J. Urol.* 117:232, 1977.
2. Allison R.C., Leadbetter G.W. Jr.: The effect of urethrotomy on vesicoureteral reflux. *J. Urol.* 108:480, 1972.
3. Amar A.D.: Ipsilateral ureteroureterostomy for single ureteral disease in patients with ureteral duplication: A review of eight years of experience with 16 patients. *J. Urol.* 119:472, 1978.
4. Ambrose S.S., Nicolson W.P.: The causes of vesicoureteral reflux in children. *J. Urol.* 87:688, 1962.
5. Ambrose S.S., Nicolson W.P.: Ureteral reflux in duplicated ureters. *J. Urol.* 92:439, 1964.
6. Babcock J.R., Keats G.K., King L.R.: Renal changes after an uncomplicated antireflux operation. *J. Urol.* 115:720, 1976.
7. Berger R.M., Maizels M., Moran G.C., et al.: Bladder capacity (ounces) equals age (years) plus 2 predicts normal bladder capacity and aids in diagnosis of abnormal voiding patterns. *J. Urol.* 129:347, 1983.
8. Bockrath J.M., Maizels M., Firlit C.F.: The use of lower ipsilateral ureteroureterostomy to treat vesicoureteral reflux or obstruction in children with duplex ureters. *J. Urol.* 129:543, 1983.
9. Conway J.J., Belman A.B., King L.R.: Direct and indirect radionuclide cystography. *Semin. Nucl. Med.* 4:197, 1974.
10. Dwoskin J.Y., Perlmutter A.D.: Vesicoureteral reflux in children: A computerized review. *J. Urol.* 109:888, 1973.
11. Filly R.A., Friedland G.W., Fair W.R., et al.: Late ureteric obstruction following ureteral reimplantation for reflux: A warning. *Urology* 4:540, 1974.
12. Filly R., Friedland G.W., Govan D.E., et al.: Development and progression of clubbing and scarring in children with recurrent urinary tract infections. *Radiology* 113:145, 1974.
13. Glenn J.F., Anderson E.E.: Distal tunnel ureteral reimplantation. *J. Urol.* 97:623, 1967.
14. Glenn J.F., Anderson E.E.: Complications of ureteral reimplantation. *Urol. Surv.* 23:243, 1973.
15. Glenn J.F., Anderson E.E.: Distal tunnel ureteral reimplantation. *Trans. Am. Assoc. Genitourin. Surg.* 58:37, 1976.
16. Gonzales E.T., Glenn J.F., Anderson E.E.: Results of distal tunnel ureteral reimplantation. *J. Urol.* 107:572, 1972.
17. Gregoir W., Van Regemorter G.: Le reflux vesico-ureteral congenital. *Urol. Int.* 18:122, 1964.
18. Hendren W.H.: Ureteral reimplantation in children. *J. Pediatr. Surg.* 3:649, 1968.
19. Hendren W.H.: Operative repair of megaureter in children. *J. Urol.* 101:491, 1969.
20. Daines S.L., Hodgson N.B.: Management of reflux in total duplication anomalies. *J. Urol.* 105:720, 1971.
21. Hodson C.J., Maling T.M.J., McManamon P.J., et al.: The pathogenesis of reflux nephropathy (chronic atrophic pyelonephritis). *Br. J. Radiol.* (suppl. 13), 1975.
22. Jimenez-Mariscal J.L., Moussali Flah L.: Ureteropelvic junction obstruction secondary to vesicoureteral reflux: Later complications after successful vesicoureteral reimplant. *Urology* 18:203, 1981.
23. Kalicinski H., Kansy J., Kotarbinska B.: Surgery of megaureters—modification of Hendren's operation. *J. Pediatr. Surg.* 12:183, 1977.

24. Kaplan W.E., Firlit C.F.: Management of reflux in the myelodysplastic child. *J. Urol.* 129:1195, 1983.
25. Kelalis P.P.: The present status of surgery for vesicoureteral reflux. *Urol. Clin. North Am.* 1:457, 1974.
26. King L.R.: Apparent ureteropelvic junction obstruction caused by vesicoureteral reflux. III. *Med. J.* 133:711, 1968.
27. King L.R., Kazmi S.O., Belman A.B.: Natural history of vesicoureteral reflux—outcome of a trial of nonoperative therapy. *Urol. Clin. North Am.* 1:441, 1974.
28. King L.R., Surian M.A., Wendel R.M., et al.: Vesicoureteral reflux: Classification based on cause and the results of treatment. *JAMA* 203:169, 1968.
29. Koff S.A.: Effect of uninhibited bladder contractions on UTI and reflux, *Dialogues in Pediatric Urology.* Pearl River, N.Y., W.J. Miller Assoc., Inc., 1983.
30. Lenaghan D., Whitaker J.G., Jensen F., et al.: The natural history of reflux and long-term effects of reflux on the kidney. *J. Urol.* 115:728, 1976.
31. Lich R. Jr., Howerton L.W., Davis L.A.: Recurrent urosepsis in children. *J. Urol.* 86:554, 1961.
32. McGovan J.H., Marshall V.F.: Reimplantation of ureters into the bladders of children. *J. Urol.* 99:572, 1968.
33. Martin D.C., Kaufman J.J.: Pitfalls in ureterovesicoplasty for the prevention of reflux. *J. Urol.* 97:846, 1967.
34. Miller H.C., Caspari E.W.: Ureteral reflux as genetic trait. *JAMA* 220:842, 1972.
35. Pokorny M., Pontes J.E., Pierce J.M. Jr.: Ureterostomy in situ: Technique for temporary urinary diversion. *Urology* 8:447, 1976.
36. Politano V.A.: One hundred reimplantations and five years. *J. Urol* 90:696, 1963.
37. Politano V.A., Leadbetter W.F.: An operative technique for the correction of vesicoureteral reflux. *J. Urol.* 79:932, 1958.
38. Ransley P.G., Risdon R.A.: Renal papillae and intrarenal reflux in the pig. *Lancet* 2:1114, 1974.
39. Ravitch M.M., Welch K.J., et al.: *Pediatric Surgery.* Chicago, Year Book Medical Publishers, ed. 3. 1979, p. 1212.
40. Salvatierra O. Jr., Kountz S.L., Belzer F.O.: Primary vesicoureteral reflux and end-stage renal disease. *JAMA* 226:1454, 1973.
41. Segura J.W., Kelalis P.O., Stickler G.B., et al.: Urinary tract infection in children: Retrospective study. *J. Urol.* 105:591, 1971.
42. Stephens F.D., Lenaghan D.: The anatomical basis and dynamics of vesicoureteral reflux. *J. Urol.* 87:669, 1962.
43. Uehling D.T.: Effect of vesicoureteral reflux on concentrating ability. *J. Urol.* 106:947, 1971.
44. Waterhouse R.K., Hackett R.E.: Congenital anomalies of the kidney, urethra, bladder, in Kendall A.R., Karafin L. (eds.): *Urology.* Hagerstown, Md., Harper & Row, 1979, p. 66.
45. Williams D.I.: The natural history of reflux—a review. *Urol. Int.* 26:350, 1971.
46. Williams D.I., Scott J., Turner-Warwick R.R.: Reflux and recurrent infection. *Br. J. Urol.* 33:435, 1961.

125 John W. Duckett
Prune Belly Syndrome

PRUNE BELLY SYNDROME is the term given by William Osler[45] in 1901 to the wrinkled, wizened, prunelike appearance of the abdomen in patients with congenital deficiency of the abdominal wall musculature. Parker,[47] in 1895, correlated the congenital triad of (1) abdominal wall musculature deficiency, (2) urinary tract abnormalities, and (3) cryptorchidism. Prune belly syndrome is currently the most widely accepted designation;[3, 7, 25, 33, 49, 58, 64, 71, 72, 80, 87] synonymous terms are the Eagle-Barrett syndrome,[16] absence of abdominal musculature,[8, 10, 36, 40] abdominal muscular deficiency syndrome,[74] triad syndrome,[66, 68] and mesenchymal dysplasia syndrome.[30, 44] Stephens[68] has asserted that, although the triad of this anomaly is graphically etched in the medical literature as the prune belly syndrome, the term is rather harsh when used in conversation with patients or parents and more so when the person with this syndrome is called "a prune." He, therefore, for years has advocated that the term "triad" be used in conversation with patients and families.

Since cryptorchidism is part of the triad, the fully developed syndrome must occur exclusively in males. In rare instances, a girl may be affected by deficient abdominal musculature;[54] however, it is unusual to find the characteristic urinary tract anomalies at the same time. It is also possible in males to have a urinary tract quite typical of those associated with prune belly syndrome and yet not have dramatic abdominal wall musculature deficiency or bilaterally undescended testes. For this reason, the term "pseudoprune"[15] has been applied to the patient with the incomplete triad. Perhaps females should also be included in this subgroup.

Spectrum

The prune belly syndrome is a disease with a wide spectrum, ranging from very severe manifestations leading to stillbirth, or death in early infancy, to the mild appearances in children whose prognosis is excellent even with little or no definitive therapy. In the past, mortality has been reported as high as 20% in early infancy and 50% within 2 years. This previously grave prognosis has led, we think, to excessive use of early operative intervention, which may in itself contribute to the poor survival. We believe that the dilated urinary tract seen with prune belly syndrome does not require the aggressive therapy indicated for a baby with obstructive uropathy, such as posterior urethral valves. Welch and Kearney[75] attributed their early 70% mortality figure to the disastrous use of upper and lower urinary tract catheter drainage and subsequent development of urosepsis and uremia. Although there continue to be a few advocates of aggressive surgical intervention, the available data do not suggest that operative procedures have altered the course of events.[6] On the basis of our experience with 53 patients, we have concluded that selective surgical intervention, with appropriate antibiotic management, will continue to improve the prognosis for this perplexing group of patients.

Etiology

Explanations of the embryopathy of prune belly syndrome remain speculative. Many have considered the laxity of the abdominal wall to be caused by pressure atrophy or deformity of the abdominal muscles by obstructed, enlarged urinary organs.[42] Since not all patients have severe degrees of dilatation of the urinary tract, it is claimed that the obstruction or dysfunction may have been a transient event in utero.

Another explanation suggests a defect in the lateral plate mesenchyme, so that these thoracic somite buds fail to differentiate into myoblasts, and the myoblasts fail to continue their ventral and caudal migration to form the abdominal wall. The presence of fibrous tissue enclosed by fascia that should surround muscle suggests faulty differentiation. The dystrophic and sporadic appearance of muscle in the wall speaks for a haphazard differentiation, incomplete migration, or partial degeneration of already formed muscles.[5, 77]

A third and novel theory based on an error of embryogenesis of the yolk sac and allantois could account for the spectra of redundancy and vesicourachal enlargement.[68] This theory incriminates the yolk sac and its relation to the lateral folds of the discoid embryo. As the embryo enlarges and folds into the chorionic cavity, the yolk sac normally shrinks and constricts the umbilicus. One can envision that a much greater part of the yolk sac may be retained inside the embryo, leaving the abdominal walls redundant and allowing the intra-abdominal contents to expand. The spectrum of redundancy may depend on the volume of yolk sac retained temporarily inside the abdomen. This theory does not per se account for the dilatation and errors of the development of the ureters and genital tract. However, it does explain the unusual anomalies of the bladder, and urachus and prostatic urethra.

Heredity

Ives[30] delved into the genetics, chromosomes, and twinning in patients with the prune belly syndrome. He found no evidence of single gene or autosomal recessive genetic inheritance. Harley et al.,[27] however, reported two siblings with prune belly syndrome and chromosomal mosaicism.

The incidence of twinning in pregnancies resulting in prune belly syndrome is 1 in 23, as opposed to the spontaneous occurrence rate in all pregnancies of 1 in 80. Six pairs of monozygotic twins have been discordant for the prune belly syndrome. An explanation for this may be an unequal division of the mesodermal cells during the critical primitive streak formation during the third week. Riccardi and Grum[57] proposed that a heritable component may be the primary insult involving a two-step autosomal dominant mutation with sex-limited expression. In certain circumstances, an X-linkage inheritance may be possible also. Chromosomal anomalies are the exception.[20, 24]

Clinical Manifestations

Prune belly syndrome is a disorder of variable severity. Efforts have been made to classify the clinical manifestations in order to correlate their management, morbidity, and mortality.[50, 74, 83] It has been difficult to accept these classifications when the spectrum of the disease is so varied. If the clinician is aware of the wide spectrum of the disease, management can be individualized for each patient.

The prognosis of the patient with prune belly syndrome is not related to the degree of urinary tract dilatation, but to the relative preponderance of renal dysplasia. It is possible to have significant somatic disarrangements and still have a physiologically functional urinary tract. The dilatation of the urinary tract in prune belly syndrome is quite characteristic and does not behave like urinary tract dilatation in other circumstances. It is this difference that has confounded clinicians in the past.

Oligohydramnios and Compression Anomalies

Oligohydramnios is more frequently seen with prune belly syndrome than would be expected from chance occurrence and is an explanation for many of the orthopedic deformities and for the pulmonary hypoplasia. Many patients exhibit signs of intrauterine compression, particularly in the limbs and thorax, resulting from the oligohydramnios.[77] The degree of compression varies. In those with good renal excretion and no leakage of urine from the amniotic cavity, the compression signs are absent. Others exhibit only faint dimples at the knee and elbow joints and minimal molding of feet and thoracic cage. Some, however, have Potter's syndrome[53] with low-set ears, bowed limbs, dislocated hips, deformed digits, talipes, and indented thorax. Complete urethral atresia may be seen in severe manifestations of prune belly syndrome. In the past, it was thought this would not permit a viable fetus.[62] However, we now have seen several children with urethral atresia in whom a patent urachus has allowed the urine to flow into the amniotic space. In these children, the volume of amniotic fluid was normal and the kidneys well-developed.

Abdominal Musculature

The abdominal wall epaxial and hypaxial trunk muscles develop normally. However, the muscles of the lateral and ventral walls are diffusely deficient (Fig 125–1) in a variable patchy and asymmetric fashion. The three layers are poorly defined, the lower medial aspects of the abdominal wall consisting of skin, fat, and the condensation of fibrous tissue onto the peritoneum.[1, 41] The upper rectus muscles are better developed than the lower rectus muscles, and the outer oblique muscles in the upper abdomen are usually better developed than those in the lower abdomen.[56] The umbilicus is pulled upward by the intact upper recti. The abdominal wall is quite pliable, and the viscera can easily be palpated. In babies, intestinal peristalsis is readily visible. If one side of the abdomen is more lax than the other, this is generally the side with the more severe urinary tract involvement.

In most cases, the abdominal skin in the newborn infant is typically wrinkled, resembling a prune. The wrinkling smooths out as the subcutaneous tissues develop so that the prune belly appearance disappears after the first year. As time passes, more abdominal tone develops, and when the child is standing, a pear-shaped, "potbellied" appearance is seen. These children are usually unable to sit up directly from the supine position, due to their lack of abdominal musculature, and must turn prone in order to use their limbs to get up. This muscular weakness may cause delays in learning to walk.

Kidneys

Prognosis for these patients depends in large part on the relative degree of renal dysplasia.[53] At least four theories have been proposed to explain the abnormal hypoplastic and dysplastic development of the kidneys;[68] (1) the intermediate cell mass and metanephros may lack its full share of mesoderm from the primitive streak; (2) the ureteric bud may arise from an ectopic location on the wolffian duct and lack the capability for induction; (3) the stepwise substitution of ladder-like mesonephric vessels by the ascending kidney and elongation of the ureter may fail, leading to ischemia of the ureter and kidney, ureteric atresia or stenosis, and renal hypoplasia or dysplasia; (4) a less likely consideration is that early fetal obstruction to urine flow causes the developmental changes.

Dysmorphism of the renal structures includes characteristic

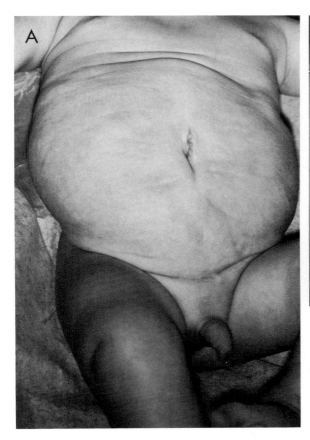

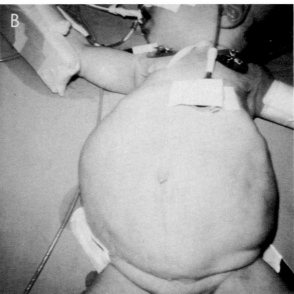

Fig 125–1.—A, and **B,** abdominal wall laxity in two patients with prune belly syndrome.

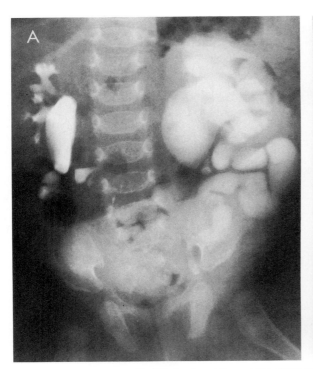

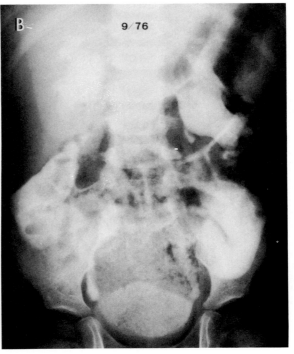

Fig 125–2.—A and **B,** examples of kidneys in patients with prune belly syndrome. Note the dilatation with blunted calices without evidence of obstruction.

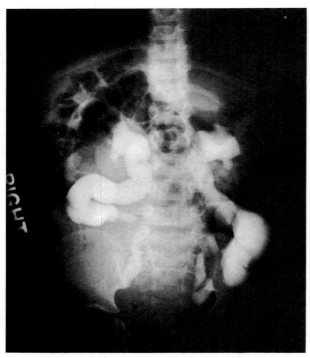

Fig 125–3.—Tortuous, dilated ureters are the hallmark of prune belly syndrome. Note the greater involvement of the distal portion of the ureter. (From Duckett J.W.: Prune belly syndrome, in Holder T.M., Ashcraft K.W. [eds.]: *Pediatric Surgery.* Philadelphia, W.B. Saunders Co., 1980, p. 812. Reprinted with permission.)

cystic calices, narrowing of the infundibula, blunted calices without evidence of obstruction, irregular renal contour, and incomplete rotation of the kidney (Fig 125–2). There is a tendency to equate the degree of dysplasia with the bizarre caliceal appearance. Dysplasia is a histologic diagnosis and should not be read into radiographs. Care must also be taken in interpretation of renal biopsies, since segmental dysplasia may be present.

All grades of dysplasia may be found within renal tissue.

Congenital hydronephrosis, with the usually grossly dilated pelvis and calices and thinning of the parenchyma, is not the usual picture with prune belly syndrome. Even with a large redundant pelvis, there is seldom evidence of ureteropelvic obstruction, although many reports include hydronephrosis as a finding. We have seen three patients with ureteropelvic dysfunction who have benefited from pyeloplasty. The dilated pelvis is a result of the basic mesenchymal defect of deficient smooth muscle and not of obstruction.

The solid dysplastic kidneys studied by Stephens[68] in postmortem specimens exhibited hypoplasia of renal units and dysplastic structures such as embryonic tubules, cartilage, cysts, and mesenchymal connective tissue. In some, the structure was composed of near-normal cortex and medulla with minimal dysplasia, while in others, the cortex and medulla were in part or wholly dysplastic and hypoplastic. Kidneys associated with urethral atresia were small, solid, and dysplastic. These autopsy specimens were, of course, from patients most severely affected by prune belly syndrome.

Ureters

The ureters are characteristically elongated, tortuous, and dilated, the distal portion more coiled and affected[4, 23] (Fig 125–3). The diagnosis may frequently be made by the radiologic appearance of the ureter. In some ureters, there is saccular dilatation of the midportion. Fluoroscopic monitoring shows ineffective peristalsis. As the patient grows, the ureters seem to straighten and their propulsive function improves.

Most of the histologic studies have been of postmortem specimens, which obviously are from more severely affected patients. Stephens[68] found the walls of the ureter composed of fibrocytes, collagen, and smooth muscle in mixed proportions. The total thickness of the ureters in some parts was accounted for by thick hyaline ground substance, which was acellular collagen.[17, 26, 46] Segments of the ureter with either large or small diameters were similarly affected.

The ureters display a remarkable variation in size and tortuosity. Some have multiple pleat valves in the distal parts.[39] Due to the redundancy of the ureters, those who perform reconstructive

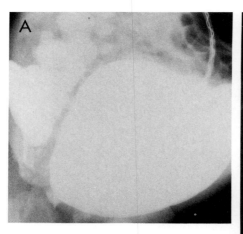
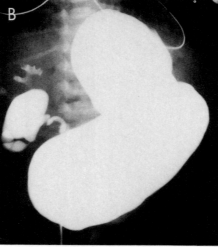
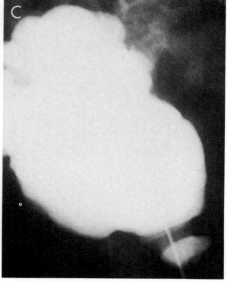

Fig 125–4.—Examples of prune belly syndrome bladders. Note the smooth-walled dilated bladder with an occasional urachal diverticulum. Reflux is frequently seen. Trabeculation is usually absent. Note the multiple diverticula in **C.**

surgery for prune belly syndrome can provide photographs of straightened ureters reaching to the patient's knees, or even to the feet.

Because the distal portion of the ureter is commonly the most dilated and tortuous, it is recommended, if operation is to be performed, that the lower portions be removed and the upper ureters be brought down to the bladder for reimplantation. High-loop cutaneous ureterostomies are not recommended in these children. If a high diversion is indicated, a pyelostomy is the better method. If the distal ureters are brought to the skin as end ureterostomies, poor peristalsis is likely not to overcome the resistance at the stoma, and stasis persists. We have not recommended ureteral or upper tract cutaneous diversion in children with prune belly syndrome.

Bladder

The bladder is of exceptionally large capacity, irregular in outline with thickened walls, but without hypertrophy of the muscles. There are no trabeculations, even in the more severe forms with obstruction by an associated urethral stenosis. The apex of the bladder is often capped with a urachal diverticulum (Fig 125–4) attached to the umbilicus. Occasionally, the urachus is patent. Histologically, the smooth muscles are intermixed with fibrocytes and collagen, which contribute largely to the thickness of the bladder. In some portions, the walls are devoid of muscle and are composed of large or small plaques of collagen, which, under pressure, form a bulge or diverticulum. Cussen[11] and Stephens[67] measured the muscle cells in ureters and bladders of prune belly syndrome patients and found them normal in dimension, indicating the absence of hypertrophy.

The trigone is usually large, often asymmetric, with narrow and elongated cornua. The ureteral orifices are lateral and sometimes asymmetric. The ureterovesical hiatus may be up to 5 cm from the internal urethral meatus, and the ureteral orifice may be found in a large paraureteral diverticulum. In most cases, the orifices are large and gaping, admitting free reflux in at least 75% of cases.[15] This positioning of the ureteral orifice in prune belly syndrome supports the bud theory[38] for poor renal development with lateral ectopia of the ureterovesical unit.

The bladder neck is quite wide at the junction of the dilated prostatic urethra. Measured intravesical pressures are low, with normal voiding and urine flows.[44, 81] Many of these children are capable of emptying their bladders completely. In some, significant urine residual is the only indication of faulty bladder urodynamics.[65] The urine can usually be kept sterile with suppressive antibacterials, even when residual urine is present. The tonicity of the bladder seems to improve with age.[37]

We have treated two children with bladders that, despite absence of demonstrable outlet obstruction, would not spontaneously expel urine per urethram, although the urine could quite easily be expressed manually. These children were treated with cutaneous vesicostomy.

Prostate

The maldeveloped prostate gland contains very few normal epithelial elements.[12] Stephens[66] found prostatic tubules in only one of seven specimens, and in this instance the number present was much smaller than normal. These were, of course, in postmortem specimens.

Sexual Function

As the children grow into adulthood, a common complaint in sexual function is absence of ejaculation.[2, 84] They do, however, have normal erections and orgasms. A fertile patient with prune belly syndrome has never been reported.

Prostatic Urethra

Prune belly syndrome can be diagnosed from the typical appearance of the prostatic urethra. The bladder neck is quite wide, with a tapering dilatation of the prostate down to the membranous urethra. Even though the internal meatus of the bladder neck is widely open, there is usually a demarcated shallow collar at the bladder neck. There is frequently more posterior bulging and occasionally a small utricular diverticulum. The prostatic urethra is expanded to three to four times the size of the membranous urethra, which is of normal caliber. The anterior wall of the posterior urethra is shorter than the posterior wall, and, in some, infolding occurs. The posterior wall pouches posteriorly, particularly at the point of ejaculatory ducts. The verumontanum is usually small, absent, or replaced by local umbilication of the pouched posterior wall (Fig 125–5).

The lack of prostatic tissue has been one explanation for the marked dilatation of the posterior urethra. Another is a deficiency of smooth muscle and the similar dilatation of the rest of the urinary tract.

Prostatic urethral funneling down to the junction of the membranous urethra causes the voiding cystourethrogram to appear as though a posterior urethral valve were present. In the majority of cases, this is not the case, although there are instances in which obstruction occurs at the membranous urethra due to atresia or stenosis. This membranous urethral obstruction has a different embryologic origin than that of classic posterior urethral valves.

Wigger and Blanc[77] concluded from autopsy material and previously published cases that urethral obstruction occurred in one third of patients with prune belly syndrome. The lesions were stenosis, atresia, diaphragm, diverticulum, and valves. With careful endoscopic evaluation of the prostatic apex and the membranous urethra in several patients with high residual urines, Stephens[68] found an obstructing fold at the junction of the membranous urethra and dilated prostatic urethra in four instances. The fold is best seen on the dorsum of the urethra, and it seems to represent redundancy of the dilated proximal urethra, which overrides and partially closes the membranous urethra as the posterior urethra distends. When this fold or curtain is resected at the 12 o'clock position, voiding is improved. To these lesions, Stephens assigned a "type IV valve" classification.

Anterior Urethra

In the very severe forms of prune belly syndrome, there may be a severe stenosis or atresia of the membranous and bulbous urethra. If the patient with atretic urethra survives, a patent urachus is generally found. We have seen a number of patients with this condition who were stillborn or died shortly after birth, and only two that have survived with vesicostomy.

Kroovand et al.[35] reported that seven out of 19 boys with prune belly syndrome had fusiform dilatations of the bulbous urethra and that two had fusiform dilatation of the pendulous urethra. We do not think this was a significant finding and would not consider this dilatation a malformation.

Megalourethra

Two types of megalourethra are associated with prune belly syndrome: fusiform and scaphoid.[60] We reviewed 31 well-documented cases, including five of our own.[62] Approximately half of the 26 patients with scaphoid megalourethra were clearly recognized as having prune belly syndrome, and the five with fusiform megalourethra most likely had the syndrome. Megalourethra is truly a saccular dilatation of the anterior urethra and not an anterior urethral diverticulum, as some have indicated (Fig

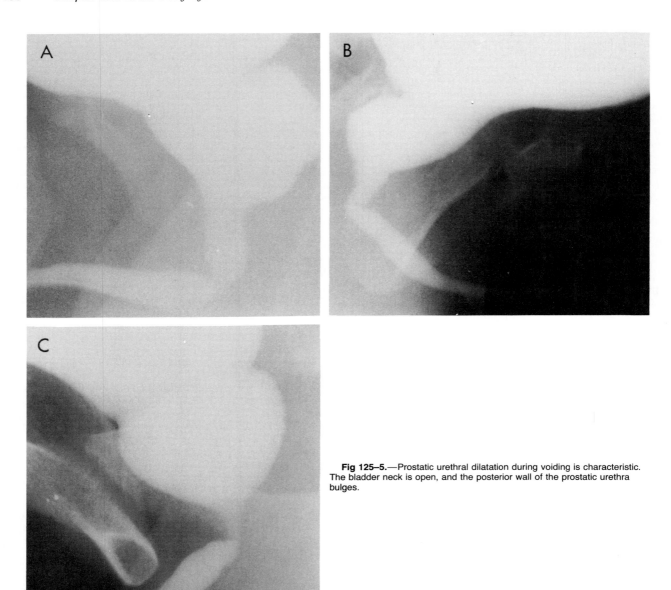

Fig 125–5.—Prostatic urethral dilatation during voiding is characteristic. The bladder neck is open, and the posterior wall of the prostatic urethra bulges.

125–6). The corpus spongiosum is deficient, whereas the distal glans and fossa navicularis are normal. Surgical correction, using the principles of hypospadias repair, is successful. Marsupialization was needed early in two of our four patients, owing to infection and stasis. Instrumentation of a megalourethra for radiographic studies should be avoided. Two of our four patients became septic from this inappropriate action.

Cryptorchidism

Except in the "pseudoprune" forms of prune belly syndrome, both testes lie in the abdomen, at about the level of the iliac vessels on the posterior abdominal wall, overlying the ureters.

Histologically, the germinal epithelium consists of solid cords of cells indistinguishable from the features of a normal testis of the same age. The gubernacula are elongated, attached proxi-

mally to the body of testis or to the tail of the epididymis and distally to the pubic tubercle. The tails of the gubernacula in all instances pass along the inguinal canal to reach the tubercle. The structure of the gubernacula revealed no unusual features.[70]

The epididymis is frequently detached from the testis, with the typical epididymal deformities of cryptorchidism. The ductus deferens in some specimens has thick walls, composed of collagen with sparce or rudimentary muscle. In several specimens, the vas was irregularly tortuous and thin-walled with segments of atresia.

There have been two reported cases of teratocarcinoma developing in patients with prune belly syndrome, one at age 24[86] and the other at age 30.[61] Whether orchiopexy is indicated in these children stirs considerable controversy. If orchiopexy is performed, normal spermatogenesis may occur, although there is very little evidence that there will be prostatic and seminal fluid

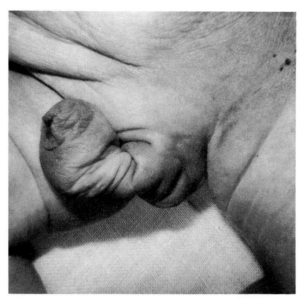

Fig 125–6.—Megalourethra in a patient with prune belly syndrome.

to support sperm activity. It is our practice to bring the testes to the scrotum in early childhood.[88]

Orthopedic Problems

Talipes equinovarus, absence of a limb, dysplastic hips, congenital hip dislocation, polydactyly, and arthrogryposis have been reported. It is important to note dislocation of the hips early and institute treatment.

Gastrointestinal Anomalies

Malrotation has been reported, with duodenal bands and midgut volvulus.[63] Rectal atresia or imperforate anus, as seen in the very severe forms, requires colostomy early on.[43] At the same time, it is wise to see and perform biopsy on both kidneys. Gastroschisis[78] and omphalocele[52] have been reported. There have also been reports of splenic torsion.[29]

Lung Malformation

Congenital cystic adenomatoid malformation of the lung has been reported.[73] Pneumothorax and pneumomediastinum with hypoplastic lungs are common with the severe forms. Because of the splayed-out ribs, deformities of the chest, and weak abdominal musculature, these children are quite prone to pulmonary infections. Pulmonary toilet is difficult.

Cardiovascular Defects

Ventricular and atrial septal defects occur and require appropriate correction. With the exception of nonurologic complications such as pneumothorax, pneumomediastinum, pulmonary and cardiac abnormalities, or imperforate anus, investigation of a child with prune belly syndrome is not a neonatal emergency.

Antenatal Diagnosis

A great deal of attention has recently been given in the literature to antenatal diagnosis and antenatal treatment of the urologic "obstructive" lesions in the prune belly syndrome. In utero intervention[19, 22] and even termination of pregnancy[51] have been undertaken on the basis of antenatal ultrasound evidence of

prune belly syndrome. A computer search of publications in the last 5 years has not demonstrated a single case in which antenatal treatment of prune belly syndrome yielded any benefit. Kramer[34] reviewed this topic extensively and noted the difficulties of ultrasound diagnosis in utero. False negative and false positive findings are complicated by the unobstructed nature of the prune belly syndrome urinary tract. With the high error rate associated with in utero ultrasound and the extremely small chance of benefit to the fetus, we believe that antenatal intervention holds no place in the prune belly syndrome. There may be a case where dystocia occurs because of a distended urinary tract at the time of labor and delivery, which might be relieved by percutaneous decompression,[19] but antenatal urinary drainage procedures should be discouraged.

Management

Radiographic Investigations

Excretory urography and voiding cystourethrography should be delayed for at least a few days and then performed with the utmost care to avoid infection. Antibiotic coverage is important during this period.

A voiding cystogram generally reveals most of the anatomical picture because reflux is so common. It also gives an idea of bladder function.

Ultrasound may give an impression of the density of renal tissue and suggest the parenchyma is normal, dysplastic, or cystic.

Finally, functional imaging of the upper urinary tract by intravenous pyelogram or renal scan has its place after the first several days of life.

Observation

We prefer to have the baby feed normally and to observe the clinical course over the first several weeks, monitoring levels of blood urea, creatinine, and electrolytes, all of which indicate the degree of renal dysplasia. Despite enormous dilatation of the urinary tract and apparent poor emptying of the bladder, the temptation for early surgical intervention should be suppressed. Injudicious creation of nephrostomy drainage, cutaneous ureterostomies, or cystostomy tube drainage may convert a balanced, although dilated, urinary tract into one completely dependent on future extensive surgical reconstruction. A good measure of renal function is the serum creatinine level. During the first week to 10 days, a rising serum creatinine value is ominous.

Therapeutic Considerations

Various approaches have been espoused; (1) doing as little as possible,[15] (2) early high urinary diversion, (3) high-loop ureterostomy with subsequent urinary tract reconstruction, (4) nephrostomies with later reconstruction, and (5) immediate reconstruction without prior diversion.[28, 31, 48, 55, 75,84, 85] All of these alternatives, save the first, are based on what we think are erroneous concepts for the prune belly syndrome: (1) these approaches presuppose that obstruction is present and (2) that massive reflux and residual urine in the urinary tract lead to renal damage and should be eliminated.

Those who encourage extensive surgical reconstruction, particularly in the neonatal period, do so in babies they classify as mildly to moderately affected. The operation includes excision of the distal half of the ureters, with tapering reimplantation into the bladder of the less involved upper portion of the ureters. In addition, the bladder is reduced in size and the testes are brought into the scrotum. The results in some of these reports are quite satisfactory in terms of improvement in the radio-

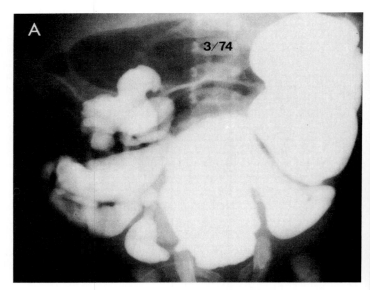
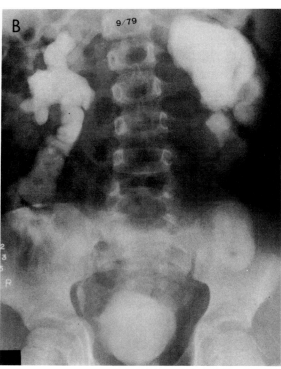

Fig 125–7.—Prune belly—obstruction at uretero-pelvic junction. **A** and **B,** this patient initially had a vesicostomy. A left ureteropelvic junction obstruction was identified and a left pyeloplasty performed. The vesicostomy was taken down and the abdominal wall revised. Due to recurrent obstruction at the left ureteropelvic junction, a left ureterocalicostomy was performed. Renal function has remained normal.

graphic appearance of the urinary tract. However, the necessity for such reconstruction is still debatable.

We prefer a policy of "watchful waiting" in most cases, based on the observation that the dilatation of the urinary tract in prune belly syndrome is not due to obstruction (Figs 125–7 and 125–8), as is the case with posterior urethral valves. Rather, it is a congenital deficiency of smooth muscles of the pelvis, ureters, and bladder. This lack of tone allows the collecting system to distend to alarming proportions without the significant increase

in pressure associated with obstruction. With the urinary tract full of urine and easily palpable through a lax abdominal wall, it is indeed difficult to avoid the temptation to operate to achieve better drainage. Certainly, there are bona fide indications for surgical intervention. Before embarking on such a course, however, one should remember that there are quite a few reported, and unreported, technical failures leading to permanent diversion or rapid renal failure.[13]

If a baby does not do well over the course of several weeks,

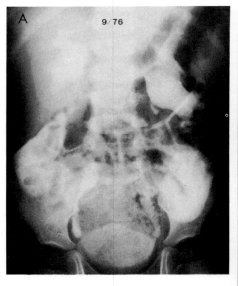
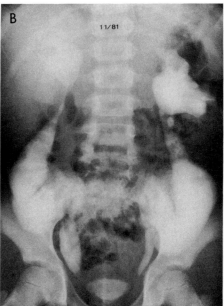
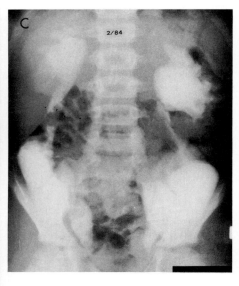

Fig 125–8.—Prune belly—normal renal function in spite of megaloureter and megacystis. This patient has had an 8-year follow-up of "watchful waiting" and has maintained normal renal function.

and the serum creatinine level rises, we recommend flank explorations to assess the kidneys visually and to perform biopsy. Pyelostomy[59] is considered only if the systems are redundant and stagnant. Cutaneous ureterostomies are offered only if the ureters are enormously dilated up near the kidney and the pelves are quite small. The degree of renal dysplasia is the limiting factor in these cases, not the amount of dilatation in the collecting system. Since the dysplasia may be segmental, the entire kidney should be assessed. Severely affected children are the ones likely to go into chronic renal failure early and to die in the next several years unless a renal transplant is performed.

Infection

Infection is, of course, the "spoiler" in this stagnant but balanced system. Antibiotics in the neonatal period and long-term prophylactic antibacterial therapy with a sulfonamide or nitrofurantoin should be given as prevention. When urosepsis is present, the already poor peristalsis of the ureter and poor contractility of the bladder are suppressed even more, and surgical drainage may become necessary.

Cutaneous Vesicostomy

When diversion is needed, we prefer to use a tubeless and temporary bladder drainage by way of a cutaneous vesicostomy.[14] This creates a vent for the entire system, and in nine patients has provided quite satisfactory decompression. This procedure is performed through a small transverse incision across the midline, midway between the symphysis and umbilicus. A button of skin and rectus fascia is excised and the dome of the bladder delivered into the incision and fixed to the rectus fascia and skin. A rather generous stoma is made (as opposed to the smaller one we make for myelomeningocele), since stenosis is more of a problem with a vesicostomy in prune belly syndrome. In some cases, the urachal diverticulum may be excised in forming the stoma. Urine then drains into diapers, and no collection bag is used. Closure of this temporary vent at a later date is simple. Prolapse of the stoma has not been a problem, but stenosis may lead to revisions.

Of our nine patients who have had vesicostomies, the vesicostomy has been closed satisfactorily in seven.

Vesicoureteral Reflux

Although vesicoureteral reflux is present in about three fourths of these children, we do not recommend reimplantation of the ureters for the indications accepted in primary vesicoureteral reflux.[76] Ureteral capacity is such that voiding pressures are not transmitted directly to the kidney. It is technically difficult to prevent reflux and yet not cause some obstruction at the ureterovesical junction, because of the poor peristaltic function of these ureters. It is very easy to overtaper these ureters and produce stenosis. Imbrication of the ureter may be a preferred method for reimplantation of these floppy, atonic ureters.

If reimplantation is required, it is best to use the highest portion of the ureter that will reach the bladder comfortably, excising the redundant distal portion. It may be appropriate to use a good portion from one side to get a proper reimplantation, crossing over the other proximal ureter for a transureteroureterostomy.

Abdominal Wall Plication

In our earlier experience,[15] we undertook six vertical abdominal wall plications and questioned their benefit. No improvement in urinary drainage can be expected with a plication procedure. Cosmetic improvement may be achieved, but in general, the results were not gratifying.[69] The patients in whom this plication was done in the past were quite seriously affected and many returned to a lax state after an initially successful result.

Since the report by Randolph et al.,[56] we have developed renewed interest in the procedure. Previously, plication was done with a vertical incision from the xiphoid process to the symphysis, with excision of redundant tissue and imbrication for support. Randolph reported a U-shaped abdominal incision excising a wedge of the weaker lower abdominal musculature, skin, and peritoneum. In ten cases now, we have done this and the patients and parents have been very pleased with the cosmetic result. The fact that a waist has been created that was never there before allows pants to be worn with a belt, and other clothing appears more normal. The boys tire of wearing overalls or suspenders.

Urethrotomy (Sphincterotomy)

Cukier[9] noted that, in some older children, bladder emptying became more of a problem and residual urine was quite significant. He resected with a hot knife the area of the narrowed portion of the membranous urethra and achieved improvement in voiding, with reduction in residual urine. Williams[79] concurred that improvement in the urodynamics could be achieved with this procedure; however, he used the Otis urethrotome through a perineal urethrotomy.

We have used the hot knife to cut at 12 o'clock in eight patients with success in seven. We have made no child incontinent.

The procedure of urethrotomy or sphincterotomy theoretically must reduce the outlet resistance through a relatively normal membranous urethra. The bladder detrusor contraction is too weak to overcome the membranous and bulbous elasticity. A relaxing incision is required to diminish this resistance without creating incontinence. Stephen's[68] concept of a "type IV" valve may be relevant in this regard. Our previous skepticism of this has now developed into optimism, and we use this technique in selected older children.

Reduction Cystoplasty

Some[49, 82] have recommended a reduction of the volume of these enormous bladders, particularly in patients with large urachal diverticula. Perlmutter[49] reported marked improvement in three patients with excision cystoplasty. Williams and Parker[82] suggested that plication of the detrusor may be successful. Hanna et al.[26] excised the mucosa and used a detrusor flap to augment the bladder thickness to facilitate better emptying. We have not been impressed that cystoplasty offers much improvement.

Respiratory Care

There are special anesthetic considerations in children with impaired pulmonary development.[32] Due to the inefficient cough mechanism, special postoperative surveillance is in order to obviate pneumonia.

Clinical Experience

Over the past 12 years, we have managed 53 children with the prune belly syndrome. Seven have died: four in the newborn period with severe dysplasia, three of whom had urethral atresia. Two others succumbed to renal failure, one at age 6 years and the other at age 19 after unsuccessful transplantation. One patient with good renal function died of pulmonary complications, a tracheostomy having been in place for 5 years. Twelve patients have incomplete prune belly syndrome. The classic urinary tract characteristics of prune belly syndrome were found in ten of these patients; yet some have one or both testes descended and thus are classified as "pseudoprunes." Three females are included in the group of those with the incomplete syndrome, two with moderately severely affected upper tracts. The third is severely affected, with an elevated creatinine level.

Our policy of nonintervention in the urinary tract unless specific indications present is generally reflected in this review of our clinical experience. Since 35% of our patients have had more aggressive management elsewhere, it is difficult to compare results of management schemes.

Of 21 patients managed totally at Children's Hospital of Philadelphia, nine have had cutaneous vesicostomies as an effective temporary diversion in the early years of life. Seven of the vesicostomies have already been closed, with success in maintaining a stable clinical course.

Eight have had sphincterotomies in order to reduce the relative outlet resistance for more effective detrusor emptying. This procedure was successful in seven. Two patients required a second sphincterotomy.

Ureteral reconstructions were done in five patients in this group of 21, four for apparent ureterovesical obstruction, the other because a large paraureteral diverticulum of the bladder was removed.

Pyeloplasty for ureteropelvic dysfunction was done in three. One of these required a ureterocalicostomy later. All were successful. Three had nephroureterectomy for nonfunction and dysplasia.

Twelve children presented with some form of urinary diversion: four with end cutaneous ureterostomies, four with loop ureterostomies, one with pyeloileal cutaneous diversion. Three had tubed diversions. Of this group, all but one have been successfully undiverted.

Two patients had major primary ureteral reconstructions, with tapering and reimplantation. One died of renal failure at age 6 years, while the other underwent a successful renal transplant from his sister at age 15 years. Neither patient benefited from the reconstruction.

Abdominal wall reconstructions were done in 16 patients. Six had vertical midline resections with imbrication. The results were not worth the effort. Recently, since Randolph[56] suggested a resection of the lower abdominal wall with a transverse incision below the umbilicus extending into each flank, we have attempted ten more cases with much more satisfactory results.

Orchidopexies were done by the Fowler-Stephens[18] technique of dividing the spermatic vessels and fixing the testis in the scrotum, based on a wide peritoneal flap surrounding the undisturbed vasal vessels in 27 testes.[21] Five became atrophic (20%). Sixteen testes were brought down by conventional orchidopexy.[85]

Two patients with urethral atresia of the membranous urethra have had a reconstruction using an island flap urethroplasty of skin from the penis or foreskin. Their course is early; however, we are optimistic that both will void per urethram.

Conclusions

The prune belly syndrome is a disorder of wide spectrum. The characteristic urinary tract dilatations are secondary to smooth muscle deficiency and developmental arrest. Thus, the dilatation is entirely different from the normally developed system that becomes obstructed. The surgical experience derived from treating children with obstruction does not necessarily apply to this entity.

Certainly, stasis of urine because of the increased capacity may lead to infection. With today's effective antibacterial agents, we should easily be able to manage this.

We have found that temporary cutaneous vesicostomy is best in the first line of treatment for venting the system. This easily drains the ureters and kidneys and can be readily reversed later. In most cases, reconstructive ureteral surgery to improve the radiographic appearance or to eliminate reflux does not seem warranted. There is significant risk of worsening the urodynamics of a tenuously balanced system in the face of smooth muscle deficiency.

The degree of renal differentiation appears to be the yardstick for prognosis. We believe that a more optimistic outlook for these children can be expected if a more conservative approach to their management is followed, employing carefully selected surgical intervention only when necessary.

REFERENCES

1. Afifi A.K., Rebeiz J.M., Andonia S.J., et al.: The myopathy of the prune belly syndrome. *J. Neurol. Sci.* 15:153–165, 1972.
2. Asplund J., Laska J.: Prune belly syndrome at the age of 37. *Scand. J. Urol. Nephrol.* 9:297–300, 1975.
3. Barnhouse D.H.: Prune belly syndrome. *Br. J. Urol.* 44:356, 1972.
4. Berdon W.E., Baker D.H., Wigger H.J., et al.: The radiologic and pathologic spectrum of the prune belly syndrome. *Radiol. Clin. North Am.* 15:83–92, 1977.
5. Bruton O.C.: Agenesis of abdominal musculature with genitourinary and gastrointestinal tract anomalies. *J. Urol.* 66:607, 1951.
6. Burke E.C., Shin M.H., Kelalis P.P.: Prunebelly syndrome. *Am. J. Dis. Child.* 117:668, 1969.
7. Carter T.C., Tomskey G.C., Ozog L.S.: Prunebelly syndrome. *Urology* 3:279–282, 1974.
8. Cremin B.J.: The urinary tract anomalies associated with agenesis of the abdominal walls. *Br. J. Radiol.* 44:767, 1971.
9. Cukier J.: Resection of the urethra in the prune belly syndrome. *Birth Defects* 13:95–96, 1977.
10. Culp D.A., Flocks R.H.: Congenital absence of abdominal musculature. *J. Iowa State Med. Soc.* 44:155, 1954.
11. Cussen L.J.: The morphology of congenital dilatation of the ureter: Intrinsic ureteral lesions. *Aust. N.Z. J. Surg.* 41:185, 1971.
12. Deklerk D.P., Scott W.W.: Prostatic maldevelopment in the prune belly syndrome: A defect in prostatic stromal epithelial interaction. *J. Urol.* 120:341, 1978.
13. Dreikorn K., Palmtag H., Robal L.: The prune belly syndrome: Treatment of terminal renal failure by hemodialysis and renal transplantation. *Eur. Urol.* 3:245–247, 1977.
14. Duckett J.W. Jr.: Cutaneous vesicostomy in childhood. *Urol. Clin. North Am.* 1:485–495, 1974.
15. Duckett J.W.: The prune-belly syndrome, in Kelalis P.P., King L.R., Belman A.B. (eds.): *Clinical Pediatric Urology.* Philadelphia, W.B. Saunders Co., 1976, pp. 615–635.
16. Eagle J.F., Barrett G.S.: Congenital deficiency of abdominal musculature with associated genitourinary abnormalities: A syndrome. Reports of 9 cases. *Pediatrics* 6:721–736, 1950.
17. Ehrlich R.M., Brown W.J.: Ultrastructural anatomic observations of the ureter in the prune belly syndrome. *Birth Defects* 13:101–103, 1977.
18. Fowler R., Stephens F.D.: The role of testicular vascular anatomy in the salvage of the high undescended testis. *Aust. N.Z. J. Surg.* 29:92–106, 1959.
19. Gadziala N.A., Kavada C.Y., Doherty F.J., et al.: Intrauterine decompression of megalocystis during the second trimester of pregnancy. *Am. J. Obstet. Gynecol.* 144:355, 1982.
20. Garlinger P., Ott J.: Prune belly syndrome: Possible genetic implications. *Birth Defects* 10:173–180, 1974.
21. Gibbons M.D., Cromie W.J., Duckett J.W. Jr.: Management of the abdominal undescended testicle. *J. Urol.* 122:76, 1979.
22. Glazer G.M., Filly R.A., Callen P.W.: The varied sonographic appearance of the urinary tract in the fetus and newborn with urethral obstruction. *Radiology* 144:563, 1982.
23. Grossman H., Winchester P.H., Waldbaum R.S.: Syndrome of congenital deficiency of abdominal wall musculature and associated genitourinary anomalies. *Prog. Pediatr. Radiol.* 3:327, 1970.
24. Halbrecht I., Komlos L., Shabtai F.: Prunebelly syndrome with chromosomal fragment. *Am. J. Dis. Child.* 123:518, 1972.
25. Hammonds J.A., Van Den Ende E.W., Boardman R.G., et al.: Prune belly syndrome. *S. Afr. Med. J.* 48:839–840, 1974.
26. Hanna M.K., Jeffs R.D., Sturgess J.M., et al.: Ureteral structure and ultrastructure. III. The congenitally dilated ureter (megaureter). *J. Urol.* 117:24, 1977.
27. Harley L.M., Chen Y., Rattner W.H.: Prune belly syndrome. *J. Urol.* 108:174, 1972.

28. Hendren W.H.: Restoration of function in the severely decompensated ureter, in Johnson J.H., Scholtmeijer R.J. (eds.): *Problems in Paediatric Urology.* Amsterdam, Excerpta Medica, 1972, pp. 1–56.
29. Heydenrych J.J., DuToit D.E.: Torsion of the spleen and associated prune belly syndrome—a case report and review of the literature. *S. Afr. Med. J.* 53:637–639, 1978.
30. Ives E.J.: The abdominal muscle deficiency triad syndrome—experience with ten cases, in Bergsma D. (ed.): *Birth Defects* 10(4):127–137, 1974.
31. Jeffs R.D., Comisarow R.H., Hanna M.K.: The early assessment for individualized treatment in the prune belly syndrome. *Birth Defects* 13:97–99, 1977.
32. Karamanian A., Kravath R., Nagashima H., et al.: Anaesthetic management of "prune belly" syndrome: Case report. *Br. J. Anaesth.* 46:897, 1974.
33. King C.R., Prescott G.: Pathogenesis of the prune-belly anomalad. *J. Pediatr.* 93:273–274, 1978.
34. Kramer S.A.: Current status of fetal intervention for hydronephrosis. *J. Urol.* 130:641, 1983.
35. Kroovand R.L., Al-Ansari R.M., Perlmutter A.D.: Urethral and genital malformations in prune belly syndrome. *J. Urol.* 127:94, 1982.
36. Lattimer J.K.: Congenital deficiency of the abdominal musculature and associated genitourinary anomalies: A report of 22 cases. *J. Urol.* 79:343, 1958.
37. Lee S.M.: Prunebelly syndrome in a 54-year-old man. *JAMA* 237:2216–2217, 1977.
38. Mackie G.G., Stephens F.D.: A correlation of renal dysplasia with position of the ureteral orifice. *J. Urol.* 114:274, 1975.
39. Maizels M., Stephens F.D.: Valves of the ureter as a cause of primary obstruction of the ureter: Anatomic, embryologic and clinical aspects. *J. Urol.* 123:742, 1980.
40. McGovern J.H., Marshall V.F.: Congenital deficiency of the abdominal musculature and obstructive uropathy. *Surg. Gynecol. Obstet.* 108:289, 1959.
41. Mininberg D.T., Montoya F., Okada K., et al.: Subcellular muscle studies in the prune belly syndrome. *J. Urol.* 109:524–526, 1973.
42. Moerman P., Fryns J.P., Goddeeris P., et al.: Pathogenesis of the prune belly syndrome: A functional urethral obstruction caused by prostatic hypoplasia. *Pediatrics* 73:470, 1984.
43. Morgan C.L. Jr., Grossman H., Novak R.: Imperforate anus and colon calcification in association with the prune belly syndrome. *Pediatr. Radiol.* 7:19–21, 1978.
44. Nunn I.N., Stephens F.D.: The triad syndrome: A composite anomaly of the abdominal wall, urinary system and testes. *J. Urol.* 86:782, 1961.
45. Osler W.: Congenital absence of the abdominal musculature with distended and hypertrophied urinary bladder. *Bull. Johns Hopkins Hosp.* 12:331, 1901.
46. Palmer J.M., Tesluk H.: Ureteral pathology in the prune belly syndrome. *J. Urol.* 111:701, 1974.
47. Parker R.W.: Case of an infant in whom some of the abdominal muscles were absent. *Trans. Clin. Soc. Lond.* 28:201, 1895.
48. Parrott T.S., Woodard J.R.: Obstructive uropathy in the neonate. *J. Urol.* 116:508, 1976.
49. Perlmutter A.D.: Reduction cystoplasty in prune belly syndrome. *J. Urol.* 116:356, 1976.
50. Perlmutter A.D., Kroovand R.L.: Prune belly syndrome. *Weekly Urology Update Series,* lesson 45, vol. 2. Princeton, N.J., Biomedia, 1979.
51. Pescia G., Cruz J.M., Werhs D.: Prenatal diagnosis of prune belly syndrome by means of raised maternal AFP levels. *J. Genet. Hum.* 30:271, 1982.
52. Peterson D.S., Fish L., Cass A.S.: Twins with congenital deficiency of abdominal musculature. *J. Urol.* 107:670–672, 1972.
53. Potter E.L.: Abnormal development of the kidney, in Potter, E.L. (ed.): *Normal and Abnormal Development of the Kidney.* Chicago, Year Book Medical Publishers, 1972, pp. 154–220.
54. Rabinowitz R., Schillinger J.F.: Prune belly syndrome in the female subject. *J. Urol.* 118:454–456, 1977.
55. Randolph J.G.: Total surgical reconstruction for patients with abdominal muscular deficiency (prune belly) syndrome. *J. Pediatr. Surg.* 12:1033–1043, 1977.
56. Randolph J.G., Cavett C., Eng G.: Abdominal wall reconstruction in the prune belly syndrome. *J. Pediatr. Surg.* 16:960, 1981.
57. Riccardi V.M., Grum C.M.: The prune belly anomaly: Heterogeneity and superficial X-linkage mimicry. *J. Med. Genet.* 14:266–270, 1977.
58. Rogers L.W., Ostrow P.T.: The prune belly syndrome. *J. Pediatr.* 83:786, 1973.
59. Schmidt J.D., Hawtrey C.E., Culp D.A., et al.: Experience with cutaneous pyelostomy diversion. *J. Urol.* 109:990–992, 1973.
60. Sellers B.B. Jr., McNeal R., Smith R.V., et al.: Congenital megalourethra associated with prune belly syndrome. *J. Urol.* 16:814, 1976.
61. Shockley K.F.: Personal communication, 1983.
62. Shrom S.H., Cromie W.J., Duckett J.W.: Megalourethra. *Urology* 17:152, 1981.
63. Silverman F.M., Huang N.: Congenital absence of the abdominal muscle associated with malformation of the genitourinary and alimentary tracts: Report of cases and review of literature. *Am. J. Dis. Child.* 80:9, 1950.
64. Smith D.W.: Recognizable patterns of human malformation, in Smith D.W. (ed.): *Major Problems in Clinical Pediatrics,* vol. 70. Philadelphia, W.B. Saunders Co., 1976, p. 5.
65. Snyder H.M., Harrison N.W., Whitfield H.M., et al.: Urodynamics in the prune belly syndrome. *Br. J. Urol.* 48:663, 1976.
66. Stephens F.D.: *Congenital Malformations of the Rectum, Anus and Genitourinary Tracts.* Edinburgh, E. & S. Livingstone, Ltd., 1963.
67. Stephens F.D.: Idiopathic dilatations of the urinary tract. *J. Urol.* 112:819, 1974.
68. Stephens F.D.: *Congenital Malformations of the Urinary Tract.* New York, Praeger, 1983.
69. Stephenson K.L.: A new approach to the treatment of abdominal musculature agenesis and plastic reconstruction. *Surgery* 2:413, 1953.
70. Tayakkanonta K.: The gubernaculum testis and its nerve supply. *Aust. N.Z. J. Surg.* 33:61, 1963.
71. Tuch B.A., Smith T.K.: Prune belly syndrome: A report of 12 cases and review of the literature. *J. Bone Joint Surg.* 60:109–111, 1978.
72. Waldbaum R.S., Marshall V.F.: The prune belly syndrome: A diagnostic therapeutic plan. *J. Urol.* 103:668, 1970.
73. Weber M.L., Rivard G., Perreault G.: Prune belly syndrome associated with congenital cystic adenomatoid malformation of the lung. *Am. J. Dis. Child.* 132:316–317, 1978.
74. Welch K.J.: Abdominal muscular deficiency syndrome (prune belly), in Ravitch, M.M. et al. (eds.): *Pediatric Surgery,* ed. 3. Chicago, Year Book Medical Publishers, 1979, pp. 1220–1232.
75. Welch K.J., Kearney G.P.: Abdominal musculature deficiency syndrome: Prune belly. *J. Urol.* 111:693, 1974.
76. Welch K.J., Stewart W., Lebowitz R.L.: Nonobstructive megacystitis and refluxing megaureter in pre-teen enuretic boys with minimal symptoms. *J. Urol.* 114:449, 1975.
77. Wigger H.J., Blanc W.A.: The prune belly syndrome. *Pathol. Annu.* 12:17–39, 1977.
78. Wilbert C., Cohen H., Yu Y.T., et al.: Association of prune belly syndrome and gastroschisis. *Am. J. Dis. Child.* 132:526–527, 1978.
79. Williams D.I.: Prune-belly syndrome, in Harrison J.H., Gittes R.F., Perlmutter A.D., et al. (eds.): *Campbell's Urology,* ed. 4. Philadelphia, W.B. Saunders Co., 1979, pp. 1743–1755.
80. Williams D.I.: The prune belly syndrome, in Williams D.I., Johnston J.H. (eds.): *Paediatric Urology.* London, Butterworth & Co., 1982.
81. Williams D.I., Burkholder G.V.: The prune belly syndrome. *J. Urol.* 98:1244, 1967.
82. Williams D.I., Parker R.M.: The role of surgery in the prune belly syndrome, in Johnson J.H., Goodwin W.F. (eds.): *Reviews of Paediatric Urology.* Amsterdam, Excerpta Medica,1974, pp. 315–331.
83. Woodard J.R.: The prune belly syndrome. *Urol. Clin. North Am.* 5:75, 1978.
84. Woodard J.R., Parrott T.S.: Orchiopexy in the prune belly syndrome. *Br. J. Urol.* 50:348–351, 1978.
85. Woodard J.R., Parrott T.S.: Reconstruction of the urinary tract in prune belly uropathy. *J. Urol.* 119:824–830, 1978.
86. Woodhouse C.R., Ransley P.G.: Teratoma of the testes in the prune belly syndrome. *Br. J. Urol.* 55:580, 1983.
87. Woodhouse C.R., Ransley P.G., Williams D.I.: Prune belly syndrome—report of 47 cases. *Arch. Dis. Child.* 57:856, 1982.
88. Woodhouse C.R., Snyder H.M., Duckett J.W.: Testicular function in adults with PBS. *J. Urol.* 133:607–609, 1985.

126 Evan J. Kass
Congenital Neuropathic Bladder

Neuropathic bladder dysfunction as a consequence of myelodysplasia (myelomeningocele, lipomeningocele, sacral agenesis, spinal dysraphism, or neuroenteric cysts) is one of the most common significant congenital disabilities. The most frequent manifestation of these neural tube defects is myelomeningocele, which has a prevalence of 1–2 in 1,000 live births in the United States. The potential for a second child in a family being born with this condition is 50-fold greater. Although the etiology is unknown, both environmental and genetic factors are thought to be operational.[37]

Until 1960, most children with congenital neurospinal dysraphism (myelodysplasia) died of complications of central nervous system disease within the first few years of life. Since then, early repair of the myelomeningocele, combined with successful shunting procedures for management of hydrocephalus, has significantly altered the previously bleak prognosis.[36] However, along with improved longevity has come the necessity for long-term urologic, orthopedic, psychologic, and social care.

Normal Micturition

Micturition in the normal infant involves a simple spinal reflex arc. At bladder capacity, the urethral sphincter mechanism is completely inhibited, coincident with contraction of the detrusor smooth muscle, facilitating evacuation of the bladder at a low intravesical pressure. At the completion of micturition, the tone of the urethral sphincter returns and detrusor contractions cease. Intravesical pressure remains low throughout bladder filling while urethral resistance progressively increases, until at capacity voiding is once more initiated.[31] The sensory and motor innervation to both the bladder and urethral sphincter originate from parasympathetic ganglia located in the second, third, and fourth segments of the sacral spinal cord. Ascending and descending spinal pathways integrate this sacral reflex center with the basal ganglia and cerebral cortex, which provide both facilitating and inhibitory impulses to the reflex micturition center.[10] There is also sympathetic innervation originating from T10-L2 supplying the detrusor and urethral sphincter. Any lesion that directly injures the sacral spinal cord or interferes with the spinal pathways to the higher centers can result in a neuropathic bladder.

Identification of the Group at Risk

Virtually all children with congenital neuropathic bladder dysfunction have a normal excretory urogram at birth,[35] and it is only with the passage of time that hydronephrosis, vesicoureteral reflux, renal parenchymal damage, and bladder diverticula develop[11, 14, 33] as a consequence of a functional neurologic obstruction of the bladder outlet.[6, 53] The severity of the obstructive uropathy and the rate at which it develops are related to the degree of urethrovesical obstruction, much as in the child with posterior urethral valves.

The potential for the development of obstructive uropathy should be recognized in every child born with a soft tissue swelling (Fig 126–1), hairy patch, nevoid mass, or dermal sinus overlying the lumbosacral region, as well as in any child discovered to have spinal dysraphism.[49] In children with congenital neuropathic bladder dysfunction, neither the anatomical level of the neurologic lesion nor the apparent level of the motor or sensory impairment correlates with the severity of bladder involvement.[15] In addition, some children with imperforate anus or sacrococcygeal teratoma may have neuropathic bladder involvement, either as a consequence of the primary disease or secondary to surgical intervention. When evaluating a child with any of the aforementioned conditions, the potential for neurologic bladder involvement must be considered, and when there is any question of a neuropathy, appropriate neurologic and urologic investigations should be undertaken.

Urologic Evaluation

The purpose of the urologic evaluation is to identify neuropathic voiding dysfunction and to classify the neuropathy so that appropriate therapy can be instituted. The specific elements included in such an evaluation are the neurourologic history and physical examination, radiographic investigations, and specific urodynamic studies to assess both vesical and urethral sphincter function.

The neurourologic history should include a careful delineation of the pattern of bladder function, including frequency of micturition, caliber and force of the urinary stream. Is the child able to initiate and interrupt a urinary stream? Does the child strain to void? Is there a history of urinary tract infection? What are the characteristics of the urinary incontinence (when it occurs, severity, influence of activity, frequency, length of the dry interval, etc.)? One should ascertain whether there are associated disturbances of gait or problems with bowel control.[9]

The neurourologic examination should be directed specifically to any abnormalities that may suggest the possibility of neurovesical dysfunction, including cutaneous manifestations of congenital spinal dysraphism, poor anal tone, ankle deformity, leg-length discrepancy, diminished ankle jerk reflexes, weakness of the lower extremities or diminished perineal or scrotal sensation.[1, 48] The absence of a bulbocavernosus reflex (elicited by squeezing the glans penis or clitoris, normally resulting in a reflex contraction of the anal sphincter) is very suggestive of neuropathy.

Urologic radiographic studies, such as an excretory urogram or a voiding cystourethrogram, may first suggest the presence of occult spinal dysraphism. In such children, the interpedicular distances of vertebrae may be widened, or there may be absence of or deformity of several sacral segments[1, 16, 52] (Fig 126–2). A thick-walled bladder with severe trabeculation, cellules, or diverticula in the absence of any anatomical urethral obstruction also suggests the presence of neuropathy (Fig 126–3).

A variety of urodynamic testing techniques to assess bladder and urethral sphincter function have been described. Most investigators employ a combination of cystometry and electromyography of the periurethral striated muscle to classify the specific type of urethrovesical dysfunction present.[5, 8, 23] The cystometrogram is a clinical test of bladder function designed to

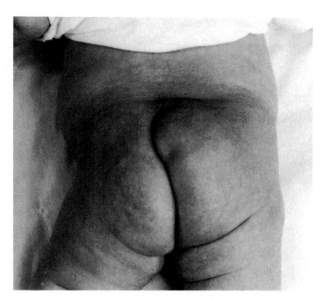

Fig 126–1.—Lipomeningocele with neuropathic bladder. Infant with a soft tissue swelling, a lipomeningocele, in the buttock. The only obvious neurologic abnormality was perineal anesthesia, but there was neuropathic bladder dysfunction.

measure the postvoiding residual, the effective bladder storage capacity, the presence or absence of involuntary contractions, and the ability to perceive bladder fullness. If involuntary contractions occur, the bladder volume at which they become manifest is recorded, and anticholinergic medications (oxybutynin hydrochloride or propantheline bromide) may be administered to assess their efficacy in abolishing these contractions, thereby increasing the effective bladder storage capacity. Electromyography is employed to determine the level of activity present

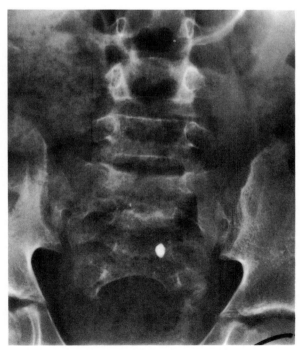

Fig 126–2.—Unsuspected sacral agenesis. This 6-year-old girl presented with urinary incontinence and fecal soiling. Because she walked normally, a neuropathic bladder was not suspected until the sacral abnormalities were detected.

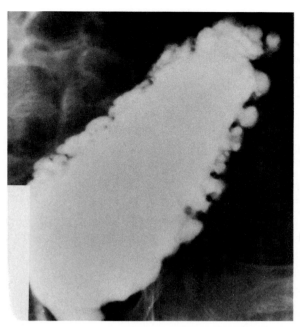

Fig 126–3.—Neuropathic bladder. Voiding cystourethrogram demonstrating typical appearance of a neuropathic bladder with diverticulum-like cellules between the trabeculations. The cystogram in the newborn period was normal.

in the striated external urethral sphincter and is routinely performed in conjunction with the cystometrogram to record the sphincter activity during progressive bladder filling, as well as during micturition. In a neurologically intact individual, sphincteric activity is minimal with an empty bladder; there should be a progressive increase in the level of sphincter activity as the bladder fills, until bladder capacity is reached. When the detrusor contracts, sphincteric activity is completely inhibited until evacuation is complete[30] (Fig 126–4,*A*). Failure to demonstrate this progressive change in sphincteric activity, the presence of abnormal electrical activity (positive waves or fibrillations) and overall decrease in the expected amount of electrical activity, or the failure to inhibit electrical activity completely during voiding are all characteristics of neuropathic voiding dysfunction.[22] The failure of the urethral sphincter mechanism to relax during micturition (Fig 126–4,*B*) is responsible for the development of increased intravesical pressures and incomplete bladder emptying, which in turn results in the development of vesicoureteral reflux, hydronephrosis, renal parenchymal damage, and urinary tract infection.[41] Similarly, severe sphincteric denervation (Fig 126–4,*C*) as manifested by electromyographic activity typically results in a continual dribbling incontinence[43] and because intravesical pressure remains low, urinary tract damage is uncommon. Electromyography of the striated muscle urethral sphincter permits identification of two separate and distinct prognostic groups: (1) children with a nonrelaxing urethral sphincter mechanism (dyssynergia) who are at high risk of urinary infection and upper tract damage; and (2) those with an incompetent urethral closing mechanism or one that appropriately relaxes in concert with the detrusor contraction (synergy) who do not share this increased risk.[15]

Management Options

The primary treatment objectives in children with neuropathic urethrovesical dysfunction are to preserve the integrity of the upper urinary tracts, prevent urinary infection, and control uri-

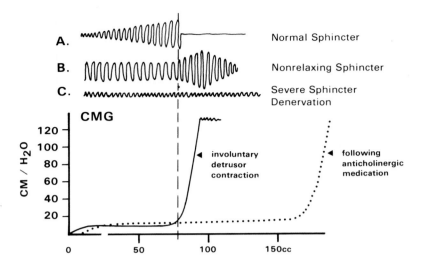

A. Normal Sphincteric activity completely ceases coincident with detrusor contraction.

B. Nonrelaxing Sphincter mechanism either fails to relax or actually contracts in response to the detrusor contraction.

C. Severe Sphincter Denervation results in decreased urethral resistance.

Fig 126–4.—Electromyogram of periurethral striated musculature.

nary incontinence. Early attempts at management were focused upon improving bladder emptying with a variety of techniques, including manual expression (Credé's maneuver), urethral dilatation, or internal urethrotomy to lower urethral resistance and the use of indwelling bladder catheters (urethral or suprapubic). While short-term success might have been achieved by these methods, progressive renal damage was frequent and control of urinary incontinence was often impossible, so that these measures have fallen into disfavor. Suprapubic compression is contraindicated in children with neuropathic bladder dysfunction, particularly in the presence of vesicoureteral reflux, because, while it may produce adequate bladder emptying, it does so by increasing the intravesical pressure without a concomitant decrease in urethral resistance.[8] In children with reflux, this elevated intravesical pressure is transmitted directly to the kidney and may cause renal parenchymal damage.

In the late 1950s and 1960s, permanent cutaneous urinary diversions (ileal or colon conduits) were thought to be an excellent method of protecting the kidney from the effects of the abnormal bladder function, while simultaneously eliminating urinary incontinence.[42] Large numbers of children underwent urinary diversion for control of urinary incontinence, or management of urinary infection and hydronephrosis, before it became obvious that the initial optimism for such surgical diversions was unfounded.[51] Not only did pyelonephritis and renal damage (Fig 126–5) occur in up to 50% of children with previously normal urinary tracts,[39] but urinary leakage from ill-fitting abdominal wall collecting devices was an all too frequent occurrence, imposing on many children the social stigma of a strong uriniferous odor. Permanent cutaneous urinary diversion is presently required only when no other form of management is possible. When such diversion is necessary, antireflux colon conduits[2] are preferred because of their reduced potential for renal damage compared with ileal conduits, which do not have an antireflux mechanism.[46] For children with dilated ureter(s), a cutaneous ure-

terostomy combined with a transureteroureterostomy is a simple and safe alternative to permanent urinary diversion.[38] Recently, continent forms of urinary diversion employing the ileocecal valve to provide a sphincter mechanism have been described.[40, 54]

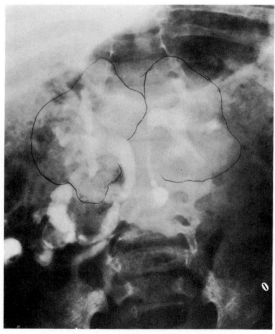

Fig 126–5.—Renal deterioration after urinary diversion. Eight-year-old child with an ileal conduit. The extretory urogram demonstrates bilateral renal parenchymal damage that had not been present prior to the urinary diversion.

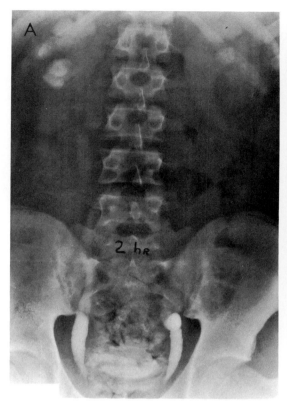
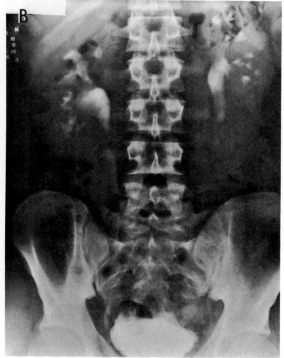

Fig 126–6.—Neuropathic bladder, response of hydronephrosis to clean intermittent catheterization. **A,** 13-year-old child with bilateral hydroureteronephrosis secondary to neuropathic bladder dysfunction. **B,** same child 1 year later, after management with clean intermittent catheterization.

Today, most children with congenital neuropathic bladder dysfunction are managed by clean intermittent catheterization, a technique first promulgated by Lapides in 1972.[32] Since its introduction, intermittent catheterization has radically altered both the management and the long-term prognosis for these children, because for the first time it became possible simultaneously to eliminate urinary incontinence and preserve renal function without a major operation. Initially, because of the fear that repeated unsterile catheterizations of the bladder would inevitably lead to urinary infection, there was a general reluctance to employ this technique. However, the experience to date demonstrates that, while asymptomatic bacilluria may occur in up to 60% of children, fresh renal damage has been documented in fewer than 3% of the kidneys at risk, and febrile urinary tract infections have occurred in less than 10% of the children.[12, 25] In addition, many children with pre-existing hydronephrosis (Fig 126–6) or vesicoureteral reflux have demonstrated radiographic improvement, or resolution of the reflux, when managed by clean intermittent catheterization. In order to achieve this success, a high level of patient compliance is requisite because the keystone of the entire intermittent catheterization program is frequent, complete emptying of the bladder while avoiding elevated intravesical pressures. Unless these goals are met, the periodic introduction of an unsterile catheter into the bladder may not be innocuous and can be responsible for serious urinary infection and renal damage. It is important to emphasize that when febrile urinary infections and renal damage have occurred, it has been almost exclusively in children who are either unable to comply with the catheterization program, or in those with high-grade vesicoureteral reflux.[25]

Management of Vesicoureteral Reflux

Clean Intermittent Catheterization

Renal damage in children with neurologic urethrovesical dysfunction is the direct result of urinary infection and obstruction combined with vesicoureteral reflux.[28] In the absence of reflux and obstruction, urinary tract infection does not produce renal damage, and, similarly, reflux alone without obstruction and infection is not responsible for parenchymal injury.[25] Clean intermittent catheterization permits the effective control of urinary obstruction by completely emptying the bladder at regular intervals before there is an unphysiologic increase in the intravesical pressure. In children subject to involuntary detrusor contractions, it is imperative that the catheterizations occur before the involuntary contraction, otherwise, the elevated intravesical pressures will continue unabated, perpetuating the conditions responsible for the development of vesicoureteral reflux and obstruction. To facilitate control of this process, anticholinergic medications are required to decrease the frequency of the involuntary, high pressure, contractions, thus increasing the effective low-pressure urinary storage capacity of the bladder (see Fig 126–4). Once this abnormal bladder function is successfully managed by intermittent catheterization, the protocol for management of the vesicoureteral reflux proceeds as in children with normal bladder function. Spontaneous resolution of the reflux can be expected in up to 50% of children with moderate degrees of reflux (grade I, II, III)[21] managed by clean intermittent catheterization. Nonoperative management consisting of clean intermittent catheterization (Fig 126–7), appropriate pharmacologic

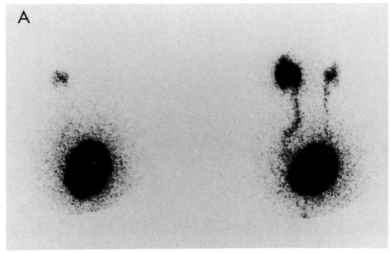

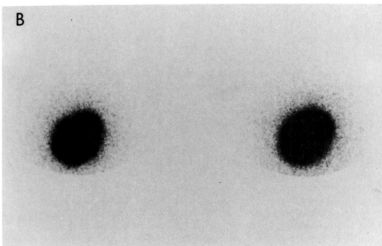

Fig 126–7.—Neuropathic bladder. Response of vesicoureteral reflux to clean intermittent catheterization. **A,** isotope cystogram demonstrating bilateral vesicoureteral reflux. **B,** repeated cystogram 2 years later demonstrating resolution of the reflux. The condition was managed with clean intermittent catheterization, anticholinergic medication, and antimicrobials.

agents, prophylactic antimicrobials, and periodic urine cultures to exclude the possibility of occult infection is preferred for moderate degrees of reflux.[26] This protocol is continued unless there is evidence of breakthrough infection or progressive renal damage, at which point surgical alternatives should be considered. Children with higher grades of reflux (grade IV and V)[21] usually require surgical correction of the reflux. Antireflux operations employing standard techniques can be highly successful in children with neurovesical dysfunction, provided an effective program of bladder management is instituted.[26] If one attempts to manage vesicoureteral reflux as a problem independent of the bladder dysfunction and does not provide simultaneous effective bladder management, the results of medical or surgical treatment will be unsatisfactory.

Cutaneous Vesicostomy

Cutaneous vesicostomy is a safe and effective method of providing low-pressure bladder drainage.[7] The indications overlap with those for clean intermittent catheterization, namely: (1) ineffective bladder emptying. (2) hydronephrosis, and (3) vesicoureteral reflux. Several factors must be considered when deciding between those two management alternatives, including the age of the child, severity of the reflux, renal function, and psychosocial circumstances. In a young child, or whenever intermittent

catheterization is not a reasonable alternative, vesicostomy is preferred, particularly when renal function is compromised. The operation is simple, easily tolerated by even small infants, and requires little additional parental care. Clean intermittent catheterization, with or without an antireflux procedure, is a better alternative in the older, cooperative child, who is able to perform intermittent catheterization.

The decision to close the vesicostomy should be made jointly by the patient, family, and physician. Closure should be undertaken only when it is possible to institute an adequate program of intermittent catheterization. If the vesicoureteral reflux has not resolved, an antireflux procedure should be performed at the time of closure.

Management of Urinary Incontinence

Clean intermittent catheterization is employed to manage incomplete bladder emptying, hydronephrosis, urinary tract infection, vesicoureteral reflux, and urinary incontinence. When incontinence alone is the primary target of management, a catheterization program is usually started when the child is mature enough to accept responsibility and expresses a genuine interest (usually between 4 and 8 years of age). Incontinence is a result of a failure to store urine effectively as a consequence of involuntary detrusor contractions, inadequate urethral resistance, or, more commonly, both.[15] Anticholinergic medications will, in most individuals, effectively control the involuntary detrusor contractions and increase the effective low-pressure reservoir capacity of the bladder.[47] When urethral resistance is low, α-adrenergic medication (ephedrine sulfate or phenylpropanolamine) is administered to stimulate alpha receptors in the bladder neck and urethra, increase the intraurethral pressure, and reduce urinary incontinence. Achieving satisfactory urinary continence has been possible in up to 90% of children, with intermittent catheterization in combination with the appropriate uropharmacologic agents.[27]

The management of children who have failed to achieve satisfactory continence must be individualized. Some children remain incontinent despite a good bladder capacity and adequate sphincter activity because they are unable or unwilling to comply with the catheterization program. As long as these children are not at risk of urinary tract injury, no surgical intervention is required and they can be managed with diapers or an external collecting device until compliance improves. Unfortunately, some children, despite adequate compliance and appropriate dosages of pharmacologic agents, are not completely dry. When the family or the child is satisfied, no additional therapeutic intervention is required. However, if incontinence is a significant problem additional surgical alternatives may be considered. When incontinence results from a small-capacity bladder with involuntary de-

trusor contractions unresponsive to anticholinergic medications, or a small-capacity noncompliant bladder, augmentation enterocystoplasty can improve urinary continence, particularly when the urethral sphincter mechanism is adequate.[24] When incontinence results from an inadequate sphincter mechanism unresponsive to pharmacologic manipulation, two surgical alternatives are available. The first is to create an adequate sphincter mechanism as described by Dees[13] and Leadbetter.[34] Experience with these procedures for children with neuropathic incontinence has been mixed.[28] The most commonly employed surgical alternative for management of urinary incontinence is the artificial urinary sphincter described by Scott and associates.[50] This prosthetic device consists of an inflatable Silastic cuff placed around the bladder neck and periodically deflated by a pump control mechanism placed in the labial folds or scrotum. When the cuff is full, it compresses the bladder neck, preventing leakage of urine. When deflated, it permits the bladder to empty in a relatively normal fashion. Intermittent catheterization may be employed in conjunction with this device if the child is unable to empty the bladder completely. The criteria for patient selection include adequate bladder capacity, absence of vesicoureteral reflux, intellectual and mechanical competence to reliably manipulate the pump mechanism, and the absence of urinary infection. Complications include mechanical device problems, which necessitate reoperation for repair, as well as infection or cuff ero-

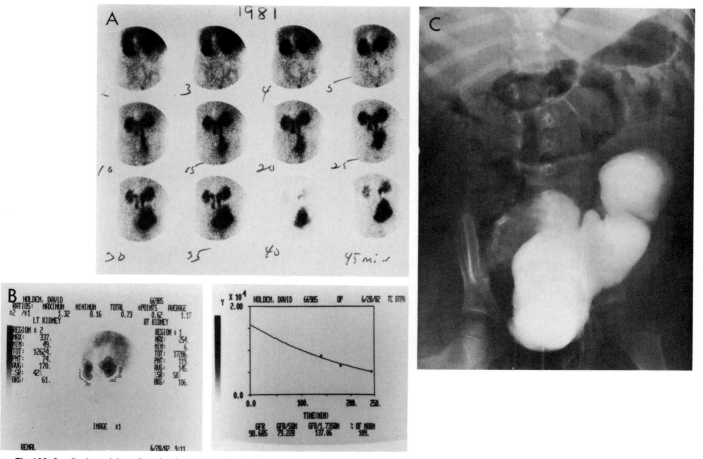

Fig 126–8.—Ileal conduit undiversion in neuropathic bladder. This 8-year-old boy with ileal conduit underwent urinary undiversion by combining a right ureteral reimplantation into the bladder with a left-to-right transureteroureterostomy, a colonic bladder augmentation, and a Young-Dees-Leadbetter bladder neck reconstruction. **A,** follow-up renal scan 1 year after operation demonstrates good renal function bilaterally. **B,** differential renal function and GFR remain excellent 2 years following operation. **C,** voiding cystourethrogram demonstrates the bladder deformity resulting from the colon enterocystoplasty.

sion, which may require removal of the device.[18] The success rate for the artificial sphincter in children with myelodysplasia has been reported to be as high as 90%.[3]

Bowel Control

By utilizing a combination of dietary manipulation, bulk stool softeners, and suppositories, bowel control should be possible in virtually all children with neuropathic bladder dysfunction. There is no indication for the routine use of colostomy in these children.

Reconstruction of the Urinary Tract

During the past 10 years, the techniques and principles of urinary tract reconstruction in individuals with normal bladder function, who had previously been diverted, have become well established.[19, 20] More recently, the same techniques, when coupled with clean intermittent catheterization and pharmacologic manipulation of the urinary tract, have been extended to children with neuropathic bladder dysfunction (Fig 126–8) with excellent success.[24, 40, 45] Before such operations are contemplated, all children should undergo an extensive evaluation, including tests of renal function, radiographic studies of the urinary tract, and urodynamic testing.[4] The only absolute contraindication to reconstruction or undiversion is an unwillingness on the part of the family or the child to perform clean intermittent catheterization according to the prescribed schedule.

Protocol for Evaluation and Management

All children with neuropathic bladder disease require periodic uroradiographic investigation for early detection of hydronephrosis and vesicoureteral reflux.[29] The particular imaging techniques employed will vary with the capabilities of the individual institution. A protocol for evaluation of children with neuropathic bladder dysfunction must have as its goal the early identification of the three major risk factors implicated in the development of renal parenchymal damage: (1) a nonrelaxing sphincter mechanism, (2) vesicoureteral reflux, and (3) urinary tract infection. In order to achieve this goal, all children with neuropathic bladder dysfunction should undergo periodic radiographic studies, urine culture, and, in addition, have urodynamic bladder studies as soon as possible after the diagnosis of neuropathic bladder dysfunction is first considered.[15]

In a newborn with myelodysplasia, a renal scan,[44] nuclear cystogram (IVP, VCUG are acceptable alternatives), renal function studies, urine culture, and urodynamic studies are performed before the child is discharged from the hospital. Children whose urodynamic studies demonstrate a nonrelaxing urethral sphincter mechanism are at increased risk of developing renal damage and should have a follow-up renal scan or renal ultrasound[17] and a nuclear cystogram at 6 months of age and yearly thereafter. A urine culture is obtained every 3 months and with any febrile episode. Should hydronephrosis, vesicoureteral reflux, incomplete bladder emptying, or recurrent urinary tract infections be documented, clean intermittent catheterization is begun or a cutaneous vesicostomy is performed. The choice of therapy depends on the severity of the problem, age of the child, and psychosocial factors. Children with a relaxed or denervated sphincter mechanism are at lower risk of developing renal damage, and in them a lower intensity of surveillance is warranted. After the initial newborn studies, follow-up renal scan or ultrasound is performed annually. Nuclear cystograms are not routinely performed unless hydronephrosis or urinary tract infection is documented. Urine cultures are routinely obtained every 3 months for the first 2 years of life and every 6 months thereafter. As long as the urinary system remains normal and free from in-

fection, clean intermittent catheterization is not instituted until the family or child expresses a sincere desire to start and is willing to accept the responsibilities involved. Should hydronephrosis, incomplete bladder emptying, or vesicoureteral reflux develop, management proceeds as previously described for children with a nonrelaxing sphincter mechanism.

REFERENCES

1. Aghasi M., Eidelman A., Yuval E.: Sacrococcygeal dysgenesis. *Eur. Urol.* 5:48, 1979.
2. Althausen A.F., Hagen-Cook K., Hendren W.H.: Non-refluxing colon conduit: Experience with 70 cases. *J. Urol.* 120:35, 1978.
3. Barrett D.M., Furlow W.L.: The management of severe urinary incontinence in patients with myelodysplasia by implantation of the 791/792 urinary sphincter device. *J. Urol.* 128:484, 1982.
4. Bauer S.B., Colodny A.H., Hallet M., et al.: Urinary undiversion in myelodysplasia: Criteria for selection and predictive value of urodynamic evaluation. *J. Urol.* 124:89, 1980.
5. Blaivas J.G., Labib K.B., Bauer S.B., et al.: Changing concepts in the urodynamic evaluation of children. *Birth Defects* 13:153, 1977.
6. Blaivas J.G., Sinha H.P., Zayed A.H., et al.: Detrusor external sphincter dyssynergia: A detailed electromyographic study. *J. Urol.* 125:545, 1981.
7. Blocksom B.: Bladder pouch for prolonged tubeless cystostomy. *J. Urol.* 78:398, 1957.
8. Borzyskowski M., Mundy A.R., Neville B.G.R., et al.: Neuropathic vesicoureteral dysfunction in children. *Br. J. Urol.* 54:641, 1982.
9. Borzyskowski M., Neville B.G.R.: Neuropathic bladder and spinal dysraphism. *Arch. Dis. Child.* 56:176, 1981.
10. Bradley W.E.: Innervation of the detrusor muscle and urethra. *Urol. Clin. North Am.* 1:3, 1974.
11. Cass A.S.: Urinary complications in myelomeningocele patients. *J. Urol.* 115:102, 1976.
12. Crooks K.K., Enrile B.G.: Comparison of the ileal conduit and clean intermittent catheterization for myelomeningocele. *Pediatrics* 72:203, 1983.
13. Dees J.E.: Congenital epispadias with incontinence. *J. Urol.* 62:513, 1949.
14. Devens K., Pompino H.J., Kubler F.: The upper urinary tract in neurogenic bladders without diversion—a ten year follow-up. *Prog. Pediatr. Surg.* 10:177, 1977.
15. Diokno A.C., Kass E.J., and Lapides J.: New approach to myelodysplasia. *J. Urol.* 116:771, 1976.
16. Duhamel B.: From mermaid to anal imperforation: The syndrome of caudal regression. *Arch. Dis. Child.* 36:152, 1961.
17. Gates G.F.: Ultrasonography of the urinary tract in children. *Urol. Clin. North Am.* 7:215, 1980.
18. Gonzalez R., Sheldon C.A.: Artificial sphincters in children with neurogenic bladders: Long-term results. *J. Urol.* 128:1270, 1982.
19. Hendren W.H.: Reconstruction of previously diverted urinary tracts in children. *J. Pediatr. Surg.* 8:135, 1973.
20. Hendren W.H.: Reoperative ureteral reimplantation: Management of the difficult case. *J. Pediatr. Surg.* 15:770, 1980.
21. International Reflux Study Committee: Medical versus surgical treatment of primary vesicoureteral reflux: A prospective international study in children. *J. Urol.* 125:277, 1981.
22. Kass E.J.: Pediatric urodynamics: Evaluation for neuropathy. *Dial. Pediatr. Urol.* 6:4, 1983.
23. Kass E.J., Koff S.A.: Bethanechol denervation supersensitivity testing in children. *J. Urol.* 127:75, 1982.
24. Kass E.J., Koff S.A.: Bladder augmentation in the pediatric neuropathic bladder. *J. Urol.* 129:552, 1983.
25. Kass E.J., Koff S.A., Diokno A.C., et al.: The significance of bacilluria in children on long-term intermittent catheterization. *J. Urol.* 126:223, 1981.
26. Kass E.J., Koff S.A., Diokno A.C.: Fate of vesicoureteral reflux in children with neuropathic bladders managed by intermittent catheterization. *J. Urol.* 125:63, 1981.
27. Kass E.J., McHugh, T., Diokno A.C.: Intermittent catheterization in children less than 6 years old. *J. Urol.* 121:792, 1979.
28. Klauber G.T.: Combined surgery and intermittent catheterization for neurogenic bladder dysfunction in children. *Birth Defects* 13:107, 1977.
29. Klauber G.T., and Action Committee on Myelodysplasia: Current approaches to the evaluation and management of children with myelomeningocele. *Pediatrics* 63:663, 1979.
30. Koff S.A., Kass E.J.: Abdominal wall electromyography: A new noninvasive technique to improve pediatric urodynamic accuracy. *J. Urol.* 127:736, 1982.
31. Lapides J.: Symposium on neurologic bladder. *Urol. Clin. North Am.* 1:1, 1974.

32. Lapides J., Diokno A.C., Silber S.J., et al.: Clean intermittent self-catheterization in the treatment of urinary tract disease. *J. Urol.* 107:458, 1972.
33. Lawrence K.M.: The natural history of spina bifida cystica: A detailed analysis of 407 cases. *Arch. Dis. Child.* 39:41, 1964.
34. Leadbetter G.W. Jr.: Surgical correction of total urinary incontinence. *J. Urol.* 91:261, 1964.
35. Levitt S.B., Sandler H.J.: The absence of vesicoureteral reflux in the neonate with myelodysplasia. *J. Urol.* 114:118, 1975.
36. Lorber J.: Results of treatment of myelomeningocele: An analysis of 524 unselected cases, with special reference to possible selection for treatment. *Dev. Med. Child. Neurol.* 13:279, 1971.
37. McLaughlin J.F., Shurtleff D.B.: Management of the newborn with myelodysplasia. *Clin. Pediatr.* 18:463, 1979.
38. Mahoney E.M., Kearney G.P., Prather G.C.: An improved non-intubated cutaneous ureterostomy technique for the normal and dilated ureter. *J. Urol.* 117:279, 1977.
39. Middleton A.W., Hendren W.H.: Ileal conduits in children at the Massachusetts General Hospital from 1955–1970. *J. Urol.* 115:591, 1976.
40. Mitchell M.E.: The role of bladder augmentation in undiversion. *J. Pediatr. Surg.* 16:790, 1981.
41. Mollard P., Meunier P.: Urodynamics of neurogenic bladder in children—a comparative study with clinical and radiological conclusions. *Br. J. Urol.* 54:239, 1982.
42. Nash D.F.E.: Ileal loop bladder in congenital spinal palsy. *Br. J. Urol.* 28:387, 1956.
43. Nordling J., Meyhoff H.H., Hald T.: Neuromuscular dysfunction of the lower urinary tract with special reference to the influence of the sympathetic nervous system. *Scand. J. Urol. Nephrol.* 15:7, 1981.
44. Palomar J.M., Duck G.B., Evans B.B., et al.: Renal quantitative scintillation camera studies in the management of myelodysplasia. *J. Urol.* 123:211, 1980.
45. Perlmutter A.D.: Experiences with urinary undiversion in children with neurogenic bladder. *J. Urol.* 123:402, 1980.
46. Richie J.P., Skinner D.G., Waisman J.: The effect of reflux on the development of pyelonephritis in urinary diversion: An experimental study. *J. Surg. Res.* 16:256, 1974.
47. Rickwood A.M.K., Thomas D.G., Philip N.H., et al.: A system of management of the congenital neuropathic bladder based upon combined urodynamic and radiologic assessment. *Br. J. Urol.* 54:507, 1982.
48. Rubenstein M.A., Bucy J.G.: Caudal regression syndrome: The urologic implications. *J. Urol.* 114:934, 1975.
49. Scott J.E.: Bladder function in congenital non-cystic spinal abnormalities. *Chir. Pediatr.* 23:348, 1982.
50. Scott F.B., Bradley W.E., Timm G.W.: Treatment of urinary incontinence by an implantable prosthetic urinary sphincter. *J. Urol.* 112:75, 1974.
51. Shapiro S.R., Lebowitz R., Colodny A.H.: Fate of 90 children with ileal conduit urinary diversion a decade later: Analysis of complications, pyelography, renal function and bacteriology. *J. Urol.* 114:289, 1975.
52. Smith E.D.: Congenital sacral anomalies in children. *Aust. N.Z. J. Surg.* 29:165, 1959.
53. Sunder G.S., Parsons K.F., Gibbon N.O.K.: Outflow obstruction in neuropathic bladder dysfunction: the neuropathic urethra. *Br. J. Urol.* 50:190, 1978.
54. Zinman L., Libertino J.A.: Antirefluxing ileocecal conduit. *Urol. Clin. North Am.* 7:503, 1980.

127

Brian E. Hardy / Kenneth J. Welch

Enuresis

Enuresis is that form of urinary incontinence that is normal in very young children but becomes abnormal if it continues. The problem, really only a symptom, is frequently referred to as a disease. If it has persisted, uninterrupted, since birth, it is called primary enuresis. If there has been a dry period, it is secondary enuresis. If it occurs by day, it is diurnal enuresis.

Much of the uncertainty about the nature and treatment of enuresis stems from confusion in terminology. It is also obvious that there are gaps in our knowledge. Despite all the attention directed to this subject, the prevalence of nocturnal enuresis does not seem to have altered much in the past 40 years.[34]

Etiology and Natural History

Enuresis is normal for the young, neurologically intact, immature child. With increasing age, myelinization advances and the potential for neurologic control of micturition is acquired. Thus it becomes increasingly rare for the older child to be wet. Other indices of myelinization, e.g., motor progress and the age of walking, suggest that maturation probably varies from child to child. The degree of maturation required for complete day and night bladder control occurs in some children before age 1 year, in many children by age 3 and in most by age 5.[38, 63] Children who are not *consistently* dry at night but who have sometimes been dry at night have demonstrated the presence of the neurologic potential to control micturition; secondary nocturnal enuretics do not suffer from delayed maturation.

Although there is wide variation in reported figures, nocturnal enuresis can be expected in approximately 15% of 5-year-olds, 5% of 10-year-olds and in 1% of children 15 years or older[44, 49] (Fig 127–1).

Nocturnal enuresis is rarely a symptom of delayed neurologic maturity in children at or beyond 5 years of age. It can be associated with emotional problems or organic disease, but neither is common; however, a greater percentage of enuretics have a detectable emotional problem than the 10–15% found in the general population.[67] Results of treatment make it unlikely that many or most enuretics have an emotional cause for their wetting. The incidence of organic disease in enuretic children is again close to the incidence in the nonenuretic population. Hallgren[26] could not detect any statistically significant difference in the incidence of genitourinary pathology between enuretics and nonenuretic controls. Perlmutter[49] also found organic pathology to be an uncommon cause of enuresis. In the vast majority of school-age children with nocturnal enuresis, the problem is due to an unusual irritability of the detrusor mechanism that occurs during sleep, quite possibly a sleep disorder.[2, 6, 21, 30, 37] The problem is almost certainly multifactorial. Sleep arousal is difficult in enuretics, and they show detrusor contractions during non-REM sleep, when such autonomic activity should be basal.[6, 20] In addition to abnormal bladder activity during sleep, many enuretics have a functionally small-capacity, irritable bladder while awake.[5, 36, 50, 56] Of particular significance is the observation that while undergoing urodynamic testing, a high per-

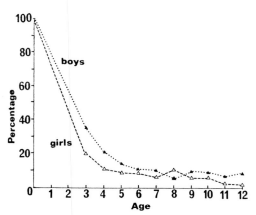

Fig 127–1.—Ages at which 3,013 Oxford schoolchildren achieved urinary continence. (From Salmon.[51])

centage of enuretics have a poor cerebral appreciation of the degree of bladder filling.[42] The observed differences in cultural, familial, and sex incidence have not been adequately explained.

Appropriate Investigation

Any evaluation that satisfies the anxieties of the enuretic child and the chagrined parents has therapeutic value.[36] Beyond that, it is obligatory that the physician dealing with an enuretic child be satisfied that the patient is or is not suffering from an emotional disorder or an organic lesion. With adequate history-taking and thorough physical evaluation, these disorders can be ruled out in the vast majority of cases.[22, 67] There is no characteristic association of enuresis with any specific psychiatric syndrome, and there is no evidence of an association with thumb-sucking or other such behavior. Previous studies showing such associations were conducted before the era of modern statistical analysis.[52] The current feeling is that nocturnal enuresis is generally a monosymptomatic disorder.[49] It has been suggested that enuretic patients with behavior problems seek medical consultation, whereas enuretics without behavior problems do not.[54] Assessment must be made of the patient's psychological state, largely independent of the coexisting enuresis. Emotional disturbances are more common in children who wet both day and night.[52]

Enuresis can be the sole symptom of organic disease,[64] but, as with other forms of urinary incontinence, this is unlikely. Usually there will be other symptoms, such as a poor urinary stream, frequency, or dysuria. Nocturnal enuresis alone is even more unlikely to be secondary to organic disease, as this implies that the child has instinctively learned timed voiding or some other maneuver to compensate for the defect while awake.

In the child with nocturnal enuresis alone, without other symptoms or signs and without a history of urinary tract infections, elaborate investigation is usually unrewarding. Urinalysis and urine culture are, however, essential for all enuretics. Dodge[16] has clearly shown that enuretic girls are more likely to have infections than nonenuretic controls, by a factor of almost 4:1. There was no difference between the two corresponding groups of boys; in fact, infection was rare in boys. Meadow[43] reported that approximately one out of two schoolgirls with symptomless urinary tract infections had a significant genitourinary abnormality. The incidence of upper urinary tract pathology among children with both enuresis and urinary tract infection has been found to be in 1 in 4;[32] thus, urinary tract infection presenting as enuresis may in a high percentage of cases be part of a more serious problem. If a urinary infection has occurred or is detected, further work-up is required. In any instance in which an organic lesion is suspected, uroradiologic imaging is mandatory. Urodynamic studies are indicated if a neurologic lesion is suspected. Cystoscopy is performed if an outflow tract obstruction is suggested by these studies.

If an emotional disturbance is suspected, help from a trained psychotherapist may be required. Before instituting such a referral, however, one must perform radiologic studies to document the absence of correctable lesions.

Increasing age in itself is an indication for complete and aggressive investigation. The older the enuretic, the more isolated he or she becomes in the peer group, and the greater are parental anxiety and patient suffering. Increased demand for reassurance that nothing correctable has been overlooked, plus a concomitant need for explanation, can force further studies. Unnecessary investigation is certainly to be avoided in young enuretics of either sex. The vast majority of enuretics can be safely and adequately managed without formal and extensive studies. Uroradiologic studies will rule out or confirm the presence of any anatomical abnormality (Fig 127–2). With the marked recent improvement in technology, ultrasonography has supplanted intra-

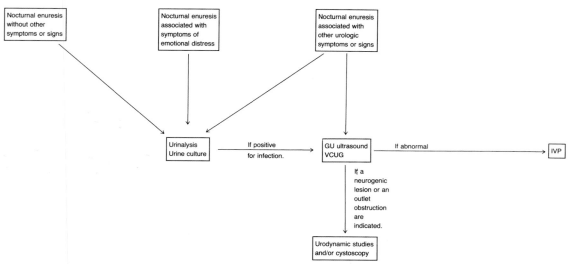

Fig 127–2.—Steps in the management of nocturnal enuresis.
Increasing age of the patient moves the level of investigation to the right.

venous pyelography in screening the upper urinary tract for abnormalities. An intravenous pyelogram is still indicated if an exact anatomical definition is required, once an abnormality has been detected.

Treatment

Idiopathic Pernicious Nocturnal Enuresis

Patients with this problem constitute the great majority of enuretics. Many modes of therapy have been advocated. It is essential to realize that all methods of treatment have time as their ally. This is most true in the young child and becomes less true with increasing years; 98% of enuretics will have spontaneous cures by their mid-teens.[29] (see Fig 127–1). In many instances, no treatment at all is indicated. If the child is still young and the major reason for seeking consultation is reassurance "that nothing serious is wrong," many parents demand no more, and many parents will refuse treatment once they have this reassurance, understand the natural history of the problem, and are confronted with any proposed therapy. If treatment is indicated, proposed, and accepted, there are four most commonly advocated modes.

Drug Therapy

Because it causes the least disruption of the family routine, drug therapy continues to be our primary approach in an enuretic requiring treatment.

IMIPRAMINE (TOFRANIL).—Although there are those who dispute its efficacy,[46] imipramine has been shown in several controlled series to be helpful in nocturnal enuretics.[1, 13, 41] Approximately 50% of enuretics will be initially controlled with this medication; however, because there is a considerable relapse rate once therapy is stopped, only 30% appear to be cured by imipramine. The basis for the beneficial pharmacologic action of imipramine is not clear; when it is effective, an increase in functional bladder capacity can be measured.[17] The drug also alters sleep patterns. By increasing the duration of stage 2 non-REM sleep, it decreases those shifts in sleep levels that are associated with enuretic episodes.[41] Clinicians using imipramine should be aware of certain side effects.[3] They are rare but are potentially hazardous: namely electrocardiographic changes—cardiac arrhythmias, congestive failure, and seizure disorders. Dosage should not exceed 2.5 mg/kg/day. Concurrent use of monoamine oxidase inhibitors is contraindicated. Weekly communication with patients and parents is recommended. Imipramine is currently widely used in patients of all ages; it is not recommended for children under 6 years of age. It can affect enuresis in the presence of organic disease, and in so doing can mask underlying pathology[11] (Fig 127–3). Other tricyclic antidepressants (e.g., amitriptyline) produce comparable results and have similar side effects and hazards.

OXYBUTYNIN (DITROPAN).—This drug exerts a direct antispasmodic effect on smooth muscle and inhibits the muscarinic action of acetylcholine.[14] Reports suggest that it is at least as effective as imipramine.[59] Its side effects and contraindications are mainly related to its paralytic effect on smooth muscle other than the bladder detrusor. The drug is not recommended for children under 5 years, as no data are yet available for this age group. We currently use Ditropan when imipramine has failed to control enuresis or has been stopped because of unpleasant side effects.

MISCELLANEOUS DRUGS.—Theoretically, a wide range of drugs should be useful in nocturnal enuresis, particularly the belladonna alkaloids and ephedrine. Although many of these drugs are of help in isolated cases, they are only rarely used.[44, 45]

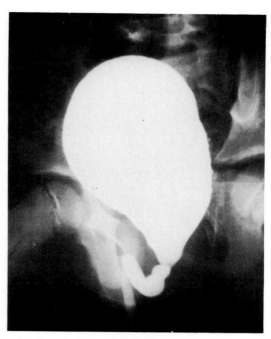

Fig 127–3.—Enuresis in association with an organic lesion—urethral valve. This 7-year-old boy was referred because of pernicious nocturnal enuresis that had responded transiently to imipramine. He was observed to have difficulty in initiating voiding with an otherwise good stream. A VCUG showed classic and unsuspected type III posterior urethral valves. Following transurethral resection of the valves, he gained total continence. However, most enuretics have no such organic lesion.

Vasopressin and its analogues appear to control enuresis very effectively, but relapse seems to be almost universal once the drug is stopped.[1, 58]

Responsibility-Reinforcement

In principle, children are taught to assume responsibility for their own bodies and are instructed about bodily functions. Enuresis charts are kept, and patients are encouraged to become aware of the feelings associated with bladder fullness and the factors that lead to it. Reinforcement is by reward for progress: both the parents and the physician must be involved. It is, in essence, behavior modification therapy and requires reward for every level of progress. Improvement is generally slow. Marshall[39] found that 70% of patients showed marked improvement (defined as a greater than 80% reduction in enuretic episodes); the relapse rate was 5%.

Bladder Training

Enuresis can be eliminated by increasing functional bladder capacity. One way of attaining this is by a combination of forcing fluids and making a concurrent attempt to extend the time between daytime voidings. With this method, 30% of enuresis patients have been cured.[57] Obviously responsibility-reinforcement is incorporated in this form of bladder training.

Conditioned Response Therapy

This form of treatment is gaining popularity. The act of voiding completes an electric circuit and sets off an awakening device, either an alarm or a light. Eventually, conditioning occurs with awakening before voiding. Results are again variable, but, even allowing for relapse and variation in the definition of success, it is probably the most effective treatment available, with cure

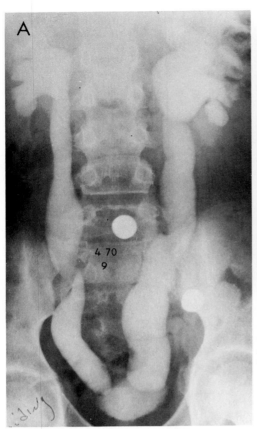

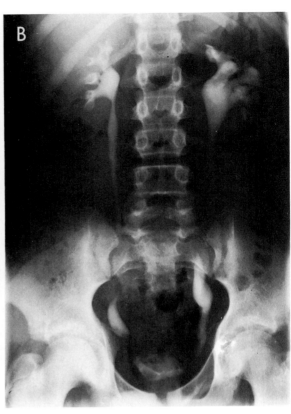

Fig 127–4.—Enuresis in association with organic lesion—Megalocystis and ureteral reflux. **A,** postvoiding IVP showing bilateral grade III reflux in a 9-year-old male nocturnal enuretic. Pyuria was discovered in a pretonsillectomy urinalysis. The VCUG showed megalocystis with reflux but no evidence of intravesical obstruction; he voided to completion. (From Welch et al.[64]) **B,** result in same patient at age 12 following reduction cystoplasty, bilateral reimplantation and right lower and left upper and lower ureteral tapering. The patient is now totally continent and free of infection.

rates in the 40% range.[4, 10, 15, 62, 65, 66] With conditioned response therapy, treatment must be expected to be prolonged, with an average period of 3–4 months.[65, 68]

Enuresis Due to Organic Disease

Enuresis is generally monosymptomatic and unexplained. It can, however, coexist with major genitourinary tract disease, which may itself require treatment. Such treatment should be undertaken without high expectation that a cessation of enuresis will result.

In evaluating any group of nocturnal enuretics, an incidence of organic pathology is to be expected. Although such patients are rare, the danger of encountering a major treatable and potentially destructive lesion of the genitourinary tract increases with patient age (Figs 127–3 and 127–4). Many patients referred with "nocturnal enuresis" can, on initial evaluation, be determined to have a more complex problem because of additional symptoms. Nevertheless, a high index of suspicion is mandatory, and full investigation is required in the child approaching 7 years of age who is still wet at night. Structural abnormalities of the urinary tract that threaten renal function (e.g., vesicoureteral reflux) (Fig 127–5) may demand operation. If obstructive lesions (e.g., posterior urethral valves) are found, they should be surgically removed. Neurogenic lesions will more frequently require either drug therapy or intermittent catheterization than urologic surgery.

Miscellaneous Forms of Therapy

PSYCHOTHERAPY.—Psychotherapy is enormously expensive and time-consuming and at best is only minimally successful in enuresis. It has been shown to have little advantage over no active treatment.[65] Psychotherapy would not seem to be indicated for enuresis unless other symptoms indicate a significant emotional disorder that needs treatment.[54] Psychiatrists should, however, treat patients who have identifiable psychopathology.[19]

HYPNOTHERAPY.—Hypnotherapy produces excellent results in selected patients with secondary enuresis. If the onset of wetting was temporally related to family tension or other acute precipitating stress,[12] the relief of nervous tension afforded by the hypnotherapy cures the enuresis in greater than 90% of cases. Although claims are made for a less selective utilization of hypnotherapy, no results are offered to justify this approach.[61]

ALLERGY.—Serum IgE levels have not yet been found to be elevated in enuretics, as compared with controls. However, there seems no doubt that an "allergic cystitis" can be the cause of enuresis in a small number of patients.[17] An increased incidence of allergic manifestations in enuretics has been reported by some[69] but disputed by others.[53] Trial restriction of the sensitizing food product seems to be indicated if an enuretic has a positive allergy history.

ELIMINATION OF INFECTION.—In children with both enuresis

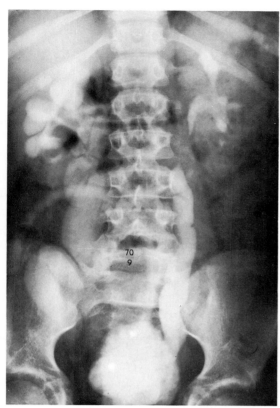

Fig 127–5.—Megaureter in 9-year-old boy presenting with nocturnal enuresis. There were no other urinary symptoms or signs. Postvoiding IVP showed right grade III reflux and left grade II B reflux. Treatment consisted of reduction cystoplasty for megacystis, bilateral ureteral reimplantation, and right upper and lower and left lower ureteral tapering. The patient is now continent and free of infection.

and a urinary tract infection, successful treatment of the infection will cure the enuresis in about 30% of cases.[55] This suggests that in the remaining 70% the infection did not play a role. The poor response of enuretics to the treatment of infection in no way minimizes the need to detect and treat infection in such patients.

REFERENCES

1. Aladjem M., Wohl R., Boischis H., et al.: Desmopressin in nocturnal enuresis. *Arch. Dis. Child.* 57:137, 1982.
2. Anders T.F., Weinstein P.: Sleep and its disorders in infants: A review. *Pediatrics* 50:312, 1972.
3. Bennett H.J.: Imipramine and enuresis: Never forget its dangers (letter). *Pediatrics* 69:831, 1982.
4. Berg I., Forsythe I., McGuire R.: Response of bedwetting to the enuresis alarm: Influence of psychiatric disturbance and maximum functional bladder capacity. *Arch. Dis. Child.* 57:394, 1982.
5. Booth C.M., Gosling J.A.: Histological and urodynamic study of the bladder in enuretic children. *Br. J. Urol.* 55:367, 1983.
6. Broughton R.J.: Sleep disorders: Disorders of arousal? *Science* 159:1070, 1968.
7. Bieger P.P.: Enuresis nocturna in het lager. *Ned. Tijdschr. Geneeskd.* 98:1839, 1954.
8. Bloomfield J.M., Douglas J.W.B.: Bedwetting; prevalence among children aged 4–7 years. *Lancet* 1:850, 1956.
9. Bransby E.R., Blomfield J.M., Douglas J.W.B.: The prevalence of bedwetting. *Med. Officer* 94:5, 1955.
10. Cohen M.W.: Enuresis. *Pediatr. Clin. North Am.* 22:545, 1975.
11. Cole A.T., Fried F.A.: Favourable experiences with imipramine in the treatment of neurogenic bladder. *J. Urol.* 107:44, 1972.
12. Collison D.R.: Hypnotherapy in the management of nocturnal enuresis. *Med. J. Aust.* 1:52, 1970.
13. Dinello F.A., Champelli J.: The use of imipramine in the treatment of enuresis: A review of the literature. *Can. Psychiatr. Assoc. J.* 13:237, 1968.
14. Diokno A.C., Lapides J.: Oxybutynin, a new drug. *J. Urol.* 108:307, 1972.
15. Dische S., Yule W., Corbett J., et al.: Childhood noctural enuresis: Factors associated with outcome of treatment with an enuresis alarm. *Dev. Med. Child Neurol.* 25:67, 1983.
16. Dodge W.F., et al.: Nocturnal enuresis in 6- to 10-year-old children: Correlation with bacteriuria, proteinuria and dysuria. *Am. J. Dis. Child.* 120:32, 1970.
17. Esperanca M., Gerrard J.W.: Nocturnal enuresis: Comparison of the effect of imipramine and dietary restriction on bladder capacity. *Can. Med. Assoc. J.* 101:721, 1969.
18. Forrester R.M., Stein Z., Susser M.W.: A trial of conditioning therapy in nocturnal enuresis. *Dev. Med. Child Neurol.* 6:158, 1964.
19. Fritz G.K., Armbrust J.: Enuresis and encopresis. *Psychiatr. Clin. North Am.* 5:283, 1982.
20. Gastaut H., Broughton E.: A clinical and polygraphic study of episodic phenomena during sleep, in Wortis, J. (ed.): *Recent Advances in Biological Psychiatry.* New York, Plenum Publishing Corp., 1965, p. 197.
21. Gillin J.C., Rapoport J.L., Mikkelsen E.J., et al.: EEG sleep patterns in enuresis: A further analysis and comparison with normal controls. *Biol. Psychiatry* 17:947, 1982.
22. Graham P.: Enuresis: A child psychiatrist's approach, in Kolvin I., MacKeith R.C., Meadow S.R. (eds.): *Bladder Control and Enuresis.* London, William Heinemann, Ltd., 1973, p. 276.
23. Groenhart P.: Enuresis nocturna. Thesis, Utrecht, 1943.
24. Hallgren B.: Enuresis, I. A study with reference to the morbidity risk and symptomatology. *Acta Psychiatr. Neurol. Scand.* 31:379, 1956.
25. Hallgren B.: Enuresis, II. A study with reference to certain physical, mental, and social factors possibly associated with enuresis. *Acta Psychiatr. Neurol. Scand.* 31:405, 1956.
26. Hallgren B.: Enuresis: A clinical and genetic study. *Acta Psychiatr. Neurol. Scand.* (suppl. 117), 1957.
27. Hawkins D.N.: Enuresis: A survey. *Med. J. Aust.* 49:979, 1962.
28. Jonge G.A. de: *Kinderen met Enuresis; Een Epidemiologisch en Klinisch Onderzoek.* Assen, van Goreum, 1969.
29. Jonge G.A. de: Epidemiology of enuresis: A survey of the literature, in Kolvin I., MacKeith R.C., Meadow S.R. (eds.): *Bladder Control and Enuresis.* London, William Heinemann, Ltd., 1973, p. 39.
30. Kales A., Kales J.D.: Sleep disorders: Recent findings in the diagnosis and treatment of disturbed sleep. *N. Engl. J. Med.* 290:487, 1974.
31. Kardash S., Hillman E.S., Werry J.: Efficacy of imipramine in childhood enuresis: A double-blind study with placebo. *Can. Med. Assoc. J.* 99:263, 1968.
32. Kuzemko J.A.: Enuresis and urinary tract infection. *Practitioner* 198:688, 1967.
33. Klackenberg G.: Primary enuresis—when is the child dry at night? *Acta Paediatr.* 44:513, 1955.
34. Leading article: Bed wetting. *Br. Med. J.* 1:4, 1977.
35. Levine A.: Enuresis in the Navy. *Am. J. Psychiatry* 100:320, 1943.
36. Linderholm B.E.: The cystometric findings in enuresis. *J. Urol.* 96:718, 1966.
37. Lowy F.H.: Recent sleep and dream research: Clinical implications. *Can. Med. Assoc. J.* 102:1069, 1970.
38. MacKeith R., Meadow R., Turner R.K.: How children become dry, in Kolvin I., MacKeith R.C., Meadow S.R. (eds.): *Bladder Control and Enuresis.* London, William Heinemann, Ltd., 1973, p. 3.
39. Marshall S., Marshall H.H., Lyon R.P.: Enuresis: An analysis of various therapeutic approaches. *Pediatrics* 52:813, 1973.
40. Martin C.R.A.: *A New Approach to Nocturnal Enuresis.* London, H.K. Lewis & Co., Ltd., 1966.
41. Martin G.I.: Imipramine pamoate in the treatment of childhood enuresis: A double-blind study. *Am. J. Dis. Child.* 122:42, 1971.
42. McGuire E.J., Savastano J.A.: Urodynamic studies in enuresis and the nonneurogenic neurogenic bladder. *J. Urol.* 132:299, 1984.
43. Meadow R., White R.H.R., Johnston N.M.: Prevalence of symptomless urinary tract disease in Birmingham schoolchildren. I. Pyuria and bacteriuria. *Br. Med. J.* 4:81, 1969.
44. Meadow R.: Childhood enuresis. *Br. Med. J.* 4:787, 1970.
45. Meadow R.: Practical aspects of the management of nocturnal enuresis, in Kolvin I., MacKeith R.C., Meadow S.R. (eds.): *Bladder Control and Enuresis.* London, William Heinemann, Ltd., 1973, p. 181.
46. Meadow R., Berg I.: Controlled trial of imipramine in diurnal enuresis. *Arch. Dis. Child.* 57:714, 1982.
47. Notschaele L.A.: Bedwateren bij kinderen van de kleuter- en lagere school. *Tijdschr. Sociale Geneeskd.* 42:226, 1964.

48. Oppel W.C., Harper P.A., and Rider R.V.: The age of attaining bladder control. *Pediatrics* 42:614, 1968.
49. Perlmutter A.D.: Enuresis, in Kelalis P.P., King L.R., Belman A.B. (eds.): *Clinical Pediatric Urology.* Philadelphia, W.B. Saunders Co., 1976, p. 166.
50. Ringertz H.: Bladder capacity, urethral sensation and lumbosacral anomalies in children with enuresis. *Acta Radiol. (Diagn.)* 25:45, 1984.
51. Salmon M.A.: The concept of day-time treatment for primary nocturnal enuresis, in Kolvin I., MacKeith R.C., Meadow S.R. (eds.): *Bladder Control and Enuresis.* London, William Heinemann, Ltd., 1973, p. 189.
52. Shaffer D.: The association between enuresis and emotional disorders: A review of the literature, in Kolvin I., MacKeith R.C., Meadow S.R. (eds.): *Bladder Control and Enuresis.* London, William Heinemann, Ltd., 1973, p. 118.
53. Siegel S., et al.: Relationship of allergy, enuresis, and urinary tract infection in children 4 to 7 years of age. *Pediatrics* 57:526, 1976.
54. Simonds J.F.: Enuresis. *Clin. Pediatr.* 16:79, 1977.
55. Stansfeld J.M.: Enuresis and urinary tract infection, in Kolvin I., MacKeith R.C., Meadow S.R. (eds.): *Bladder Control and Enuresis.* London, William Heinemann, Ltd., 1973, p. 102.
56. Starfield B.: Functional bladder capacity in enuretic and nonenuretic children. *J. Pediatr.* 70:777, 1967.
57. Starfield B.: Enuresis: Its pathogenesis and management. *Clin. Pediatr.* 2:343, 1972.
58. Terho P., Kekomäki M.: Management of nocturnal enuresis with a vasopressin analogue. *J. Urol.* 131:925, 1984.
59. Thompson I.M., Lauvetz R.: Oxybutynin in bladder spasm, neurogenic bladder, and enuresis. *Urology* 8:452, 1976.
60. Thorne F.C.: The incidence of nocturnal enuresis after age 5 years. *Am. J. Psychiatry* 100:686, 1944.
61. Tilton P.: Childhood enuresis: Hypnosis suggested [letter]. *Postgrad. Med.* 74:44, 1983.
62. Wagner W., Johnson S.B., Walker D., et al.: A controlled comparison of two treatments for nocturnal enuresis. *J. Pediatr.* 10:302, 1982.
63. Weir K.: Night and day wetting among a population of three-year-olds. *Dev. Med. Child Neurol.* 24:479, 1982.
64. Welch K.J., Stewart W., Lebowitz R.L.: Non-obstructive megacystis and refluxing megaureter in pre-teen enuretic boys with minimal symptoms. *J. Urol.* 114:449, 1975.
65. Werry J., Cohrssen J.: Enuresis: An etiologic and therapeutic study. *J. Pediatr.* 67:423, 1965.
66. Werry J.A.: The conditioning treatment of enuresis. *Am. J. Psychiatry* 123:226, 1966.
67. Werry J.: Enuresis: A psychosomatic entity? *Can. Med. Assoc. J.* 97:319, 1967.
68. Young G.C., Morgan R.T.T.: Conditioning technics and enuresis. *Med. J. Aust.* 2:329, 1973.
69. Zaleski A., Shokeir M.K., Gerrard J.W.: Enuresis: Familial incidence and relationship to allergic disorders. *Can. Med. Assoc. J.* 106:30, 1972.

128 ROBERT D. JEFFS
Exstrophy of the Urinary Bladder

HISTORY.—The first description of exstrophy of the bladder is on an Assyrian tablet from 2000 B.C. preserved in the British Museum in London. No other written reference occurs until Scheuke von Grafenberg describes it in 1597,[28] which may indicate a rather drastic treatment of newborn anomalies in ancient times. In 1849, MacKay and Syme[59] advocated the application of an external urinary receptacle. Syme[90] performed the first successful ureterosigmoid anastomosis in 1852, but 9 months later the patient died of ascending pyelonephritis. Carl Thiersch[92] covered the bladder with lateral flaps obtaining a bladder capacity of 100 ml. Successful urinary diversion began with Karl Maydl,[65] who transplanted the trigone into the rectum. Ureterosigmoidostomy began with Coffey's[12] method, but infection and acidosis caused severe complications until the introduction of mucosa-to-mucosa anastomosis by Nesbit[72] in 1949 and the combined tunnel and mucosa technique of Leadbetter.[53]

The anatomical reconstruction of the bony pelvis in exstrophy was first attempted by Trendelenburg[94] in 1906, but the first sporadic successes were reported by Burns[6] in 1924 and Janssen[37] in 1933. H. H. Young[98] in 1942 reported the first female with urinary continence after closure of exstrophy and, Michon[67] in 1948 reported success in a male.

Since 1950, many methods have been applied both in reconstruction and diversion. In diversion, emphasis has been on preventing reflux of infected urine to the kidneys. In reconstruction, increasing success has been achieved and can be attributed to staging of the repair, employing separate procedures for osteotomy, closure of bladder, repair of genitalia, and correction of continence at the bladder neck, which includes relocation of the ureters.

Embryology

The variance of the exstrophy-epispadias complex results from abnormal development during the 4th to the 10th week of gestation. Initially, the common cloaca is separated from the amniotic space by the bilayered cloacal membrane, which occupies the infraumbilical abdominal wall. Mesenchymal ingrowth between the ectodermal and endodermal layers of the cloacal membrane results in formation of the lower abdominal muscles and the pelvic bones. The simultaneous downgrowth of the urorectal septum divides the cloaca into a bladder anteriorly and a rectum posteriorly. Distally, this septum meets the posterior remnant of the cloacal membrane, which eventually perforates, forming anal and urogenital openings. The paired genital tubercles migrate medially and fuse in the midline cephalad to the cloacal membrane before perforation.

The present theory of embryologic maldevelopment in extrophy, held by Marshall and Muecke,[63, 70] is that the basic defect is an abnormal overdevelopment of the cloacal membrane, preventing migration of mesenchymal tissue and proper lower abdominal wall development. The position and timing of the rupture in this cloacal membrane would determine the variant of the epispadias-exstrophy complex that would result (Figs 128–1 and 128–2). This theory is supported by Muecke's[71] work in the chick embryo and by the expected high incidence of central perforation resulting in the preponderance of classic exstrophy variants.[62] Pohlman's[74] observation of an abnormal embryo in which the cloacal membrane was unusually large lends support to the Marshall-Muecke theory of overdevelopment of this membrane.

The rate of occurrence of the exstrophy complex in other mammals may be explained by the close association of the cloacal membrane to the allantois, which is a vital structure in obtaining nutriment from the uterine wall in animals, but is unimportant

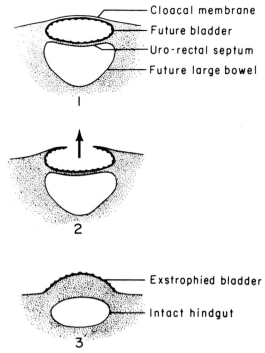

Cloacal membrane
Future bladder
Uro-rectal septum
Future large bowel

1

2

Exstrophied bladder
Intact hindgut

3

Fig 128–1.—Diagram of embryologic events leading to classic exstrophy. (From Muecke E.C.[70] Used by permission).

in man. Abnormalities of the cloacal membrane might be expected to interfere with the allantois, causing early demise of the animal embryo before exstrophy variants could develop.

Exstrophy of the bladder is part of a spectrum of conditions resulting from abnormal development of the cloacal membrane. The spectrum ranges from glandular epispadias to cloacal exstrophy, but classic exstrophy accounts for 50% of the patients in the group.[62]

Incidence and Inheritance

The incidence of exstrophy of the bladder has been estimated at between 1:10,000[77] to 1:50,000[49] live births. The male-to-female sex ratio of exstrophy of the bladder derived from the combined series of Higgins,[35] Gross and Cresson,[27] Jeffs et al.,[40] Bennett,[3] and Harvard and Thompson[31] is 2.3:1.0.

The risk of recurrence of exstrophy of the bladder in a given family is approximately 1:100.[36] Shapiro et al.[81] surveyed pediatric urologists and surgeons in North America and Europe by questionnaire and identified recurrence of exstrophy and epispadias in only nine of approximately 2,500 indexed cases. Lattimer and Smith[50] cited a set of identical twins with exstrophy of the bladder and another set of twins in which only one child had the condition. Higgins[35] observed two sets of twins and two sets of siblings in the same family with exstrophy of the bladder. From Shapiro's data, five sets of male and female nonidentical twins were identified in which only one twin was affected; five sets of male identical twins were identified in which both twins were affected; one set of identical male twins was identified in which only one twin was affected; and three sets of female identical twins were identified in which only one twin had the exstrophy anomaly.

The inheritance pattern of exstrophy of the bladder has not been established. Clemetson's[11] literature review identified 45 females with exstrophy of the bladder who produced 49 offspring, and in no instance did any of their offspring demonstrate features of the exstrophy-epispadias complex. Until recently, exstrophy of the bladder or epispadias had not been reported in offspring of parents with the exstrophy-epispadias complex. Shapiro et al.[81] reported two females with complete epispadias who each gave birth to a son with exstrophy of the bladder, and another female with exstrophy of the bladder who produced a son with exstrophy of the bladder. The inheritance of these three cases of exstrophy of the bladder was identified in a total of 225 offspring (75 males and 150 females) produced by individuals with exstrophy of the bladder and epispadias. Shapiro determined that the risk of exstrophy of the bladder in offspring of individuals with exstrophy of the bladder and epispadias is 1:70 live births, a 500+-fold greater incidence than that in the general population.

Anatomy, Pathology, and Clinical Features

In patients with classic exstrophy of the bladder, anomalous development in other systems is seldom seen. In the total group of patients with exstrophy-epispadias complex, multiple anomalies do occur. In patients with superior vesical fissure or with cloacal exstrophy, cardiac, vascular, and neural tube defects and skeletal anomalies have been seen. In 1952, Gross and Cresson[27] described seven cases of spina bifida, five omphaloceles, and three rectovesical fistulae among other anomalies in their series of 80 cases. It was not determined whether some of these patients' conditions would be classed as cloacal exstrophy. In general, children presenting with classic exstrophy of the bladder are usually robust, full-term babies with anomalous development

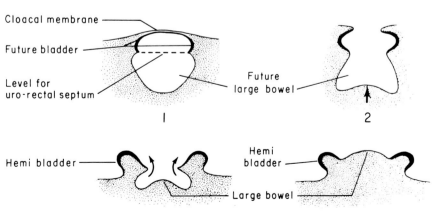

Cloacal membrane
Future bladder
Level for uro-rectal septum

Future large bowel

1

2

Hemi bladder

Hemi bladder

Large bowel

3

4

Fig 128–2.—Diagram of eventration of cloaca to form cloacal exstrophy. (From Muecke E.C.[70] Used by permission.)

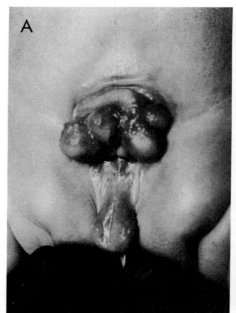
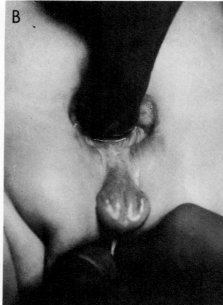
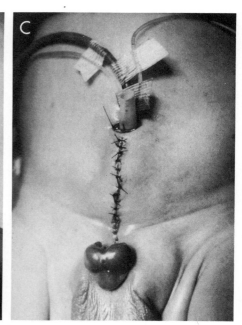

Fig 128–3.—Classic exstrophy in otherwise normal male. **A,** at presentation. **B,** with bladder indented. **C,** following primary closure. (From Jeffs R.D.: Epispadias, exstrophy, and other bladder anomalies, in Walsh P.C., Gittes R.F., Perlmutter A.D., et al. (eds.): *Campbell's Textbook of Urology.* Philadelphia, W.B. Saunders Co., 1985. Used by permission.)

confined to the structures adjacent to the open bladder and urethra (Fig 128–3).

Abnormal development and clinical problems will be discussed under the headings used by Williams,[96] namely musculoskeletal, anorectal, male and female genital, and urinary defects.

Musculoskeletal Defects

All cases of exstrophy have the characteristic widening of the symphysis pubis caused by outward rotation of the innominate bones in relation to the sagittal plane of the body along both sacroiliac joints. Second, there is an outward rotation or eversion of the pubic rami at their junction with the ischial and iliac bones. A third component is present in more severe cases of exstrophy, namely a lateral separation of the innominate bones inferiorly with the fulcrum at the ilial sacral joint (Fig 128–4).[70] The bony defect causes little or no long-term orthopedic problem.[15] The child may have a waddling gait secondary to external rotation of the lower extremities when he first begins to walk; but internal rotation of the long bones of the leg soon corrects this problem, leaving no orthopedic problem or defect in locomotion. Attempted reapproximation of the pubic rami anteriorly may, however, have advantages in initial bladder closure, in molding the pelvis to more normal dimensions, in bringing penile attachments closer together, and in making continence more easily achieved following reconstruction.

In exstrophy, the distance between the umbilicus and the anus is always foreshortened because of the poor development adjacent to the abnormal cloacal membrane, leaving an unusual expanse of uninterrupted upper abdominal skin. Rupture of the cloacal membrane allows bladder mucosa to fuse to adjacent abdominal skin through a triangular fascial defect. This fascial defect is limited laterally by the divergent rectus muscles and overlying rectus sheath and inferiorly by the open urogenital diaphragm stretched between the separated pubic bones. Tendon and tendon sheath of the rectus muscle, seeking midline attachment, have a fan-like extension behind the urethra and

bladder neck that inserts into the intersymphyseal band or urogenital diaphragm (see Fig 128–11,G).

At the upper end of the triangular defect, a small umbilical hernia is always seen during dissection, but it is usually of insignificant size. Omphaloceles, seen frequently with cloacal exstrophy, are rarely seen in exstrophy of the bladder or, if present, are easily dealt with at the time of closure of the bladder. The frequent occurrence of indirect inguinal hernias is attributed to a persistent processus vaginalis, large internal and external inguinal rings, and a lack of obliquity of the inguinal canal. An inguinal hernia should be treated when it presents, and requires both excision of the hernia sac and repair of the transversalis fascia and muscle defect to prevent recurrence in a direct herniation.

Anorectal Defects

The perineum is short and broad. The anus, situated directly behind the urogenital diaphragm, is displaced anteriorly and corresponds to the posterior limit of the triangular fascial defect. The anal canal may be stenotic, and, rarely, it ends ectopically in a rectovaginal or perineal fistula. Anal stenosis is usually treated by dilatation; however, anoplasty is required for the rare rectovaginal fistula. The anal sphincter mechanism is also anteriorly displaced and should be preserved intact in case internal urinary diversion should be required in future management of that patient.

The divergent levator ani and puborectalis muscles, and the distorted anatomy of the external sphincter, contribute to varying degrees of anal incontinence and rectal prolapse. Anal continence is usually imperfect at an early age, and in some patients the rectal sphincter mechanism may never be adequate to control liquid stools. Anorectal control should be assessed prior to ureterosigmoidostomy or other forms of internal urinary diversion. Rectal prolapse frequently occurs in untreated patients with widely separated symphyses, is usually transient, and is easily reduced. Rectal prolapse is frequently exacerbated by the child's

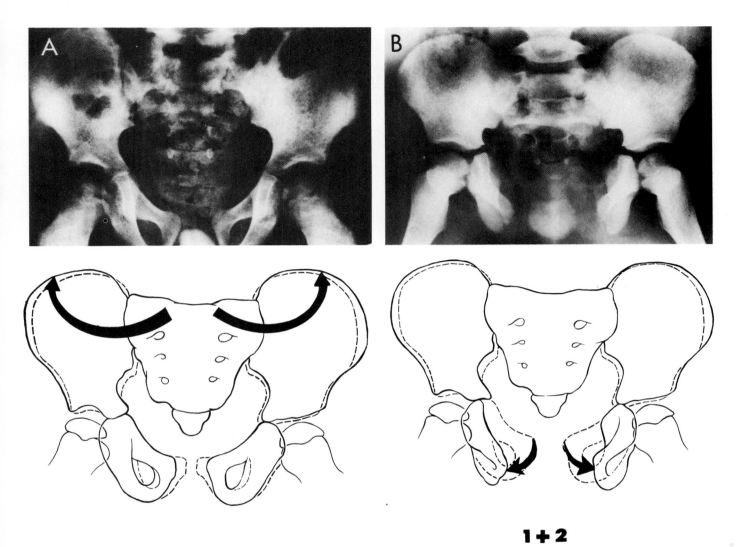

Fig 128–4.—Rotational and lateral deformities of the pelvic girdle in cases of exstrophy. **A,** widening of the symphysis caused by outward rotation of the innominate bones. This is usually the only skeletal abnormality present in epispa-dias. **B,** additional external rotation of the pubic bones: the characteristic skeletal changes in classic forms of exstrophy. *(Continued.)*

straining and crying, caused by the discomfort of the irritated exposed bladder. Prolapse virtually always disappears after closure of the bladder, or cystectomy and urinary diversion. The appearance of prolapse is an indication to proceed with definitive management of the exstrophied bladder.

Male Genital Defect

The male genital defect is severe and may be the most troublesome aspect of the surgical reconstruction, independent of whether the decision is made to treat by functional closure or by urinary diversion (Fig 128–5). The individual corpora cavernosa in exstrophy of the bladder are usually of normal caliber; however, the penis appears foreshortened because of the wide separation of the crural attachments, the prominent dorsal chordee, and the shortened urethral groove. The urethral groove may be so short and the dorsal chordee so severe that the glans becomes located adjacent to the verumontanum. A functional and cosmetically acceptable penis can be achieved when the dorsal chordee is released, the urethral groove is lengthened, and the penis is

lengthened by mobilizing and reanastomosing the crura in the midline. Duplication of the penis and unilateral hypoplasia of the glans and corpus are rare variants that may further complicate operative management. Patients with a very small or dystrophic penis should be considered for sex reassignment (Fig 128–6). In our experience, the need for sex reassignment in classic exstrophy occurs in only 1:50–100 cases.

The vas deferens and ejaculatory ducts are normal, providing they have not been iatrogenically injured.[30] Testicular function has not been comprehensively studied in a large series of postpubertal males with exstrophy; however, it is generally believed that fertility is not impaired. The autonomic innervation of the corpora cavernosa is provided by the cavernous nerves. The cavernous nerves normally course along the posterolateral surfaces of the prostate, traversing the urogenital diaphragm along or within the membranous urethra.[94] These autonomic nerves must be displaced laterally in patients with exstrophy, because potency is preserved following functional bladder closure, lengthening of the penis, and release of the dorsal chordee. Retrograde ejaculation may occur following functional bladder closure, be-

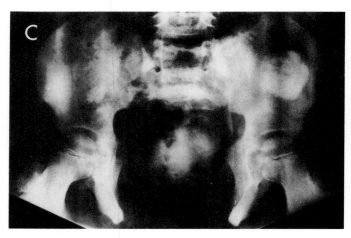

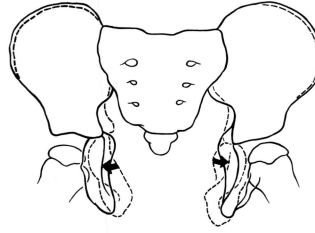

1 + 2 + 3

Fig 128–4 Cont.—C, the final addition of lateral inferior separation of the innominate bones, present in the extreme manifestation of the complex, namely, cloacal exstrophy. (From Muecke E.C.[70] Used by permission.)

cause the internal sphincter remains patent. The testicles frequently appear undescended in their course from the widely separated pubic tubercle to the flat, wide scrotum. Most testicles are retractile and have an adequate length of spermatic cord to reach the scrotum without the need for orchiopexy.

Female Genital Defect

Reconstruction of the female genitalia presents a less complex problem than reconstruction of the male phallus (Fig 128–7). The urethra and vagina are short, the vaginal orifice is frequently stenotic and displaced anteriorly, the clitoris is bifid, and the labia, mons pubis, and clitoris are divergent. The uterus, fallopian tubes, and ovaries are normal except for occasional uterine duplication. Approximation of the clitoral halves and the hair-bearing skin of the mons pubis provides satisfactory cosmetic restoration of the external genitalia.[17] Vaginal dilatation or episiotomy may be required to allow satisfactory intercourse in the mature female. The defective pelvic floor may predispose mature females to develop uterine prolapse, making uterine suspension necessary. Uterine prolapse does not appear to occur when osteotomy and closure of the anterior defect are performed early in life.

Urinary Defect

At birth, the bladder mucosa may appear normal; however, ectopic bowel mucosa or an isolated bowel loop may be present on the bladder surface. Abnormal histologic indications of the bladder were observed in each of 23 bladder specimens obtained from individuals with exstrophy of the bladder between the ages of 1 month to 52 years. Squamous metaplasia, cystitis cystica, cystitis glandularis, and acute and chronic inflammation were commonly identified in these exstrophic bladder specimens.[16] Scanning and transmission electron microscopy of human exstrophic bladders have demonstrated microvilli and the absence of surface ridges on the uroepithelial cells.[10] The abnormal histologic features demonstrated by both light and electron microscopy may represent chronic mucosal changes secondary to persistent infection.

The size, distensibility, and neuromuscular function of the exstrophied bladder, and the size of the triangular fascial defect to which the bladder muscle is attached, affect the decision to attempt functional closure. When the bladder is small, fibrosed, and inelastic, functional closure may be impossible. The more normal bladder may be invaginated or may bulge through a small fascial defect, indicating the potential for satisfactory capacity.

It has been suggested that the exstrophic bladder may be incapable of normal detrusor function, because normal bladder function was achieved in only 22% of closed exstrophies.[73] Persistent reflux and chronic infection may account for the apparent detrusor insufficiency observed in this series. When bladder function was assessed in continent closed exstrophy patients, normally reflexive bladders and normal plug electromyograms were demonstrated in 70% and 90% of cases respectively.[93] Muscarinic cholinergic drugs, such as probantheline bromide (Pro-Banthine) and bethanechol chloride (Urecholine), clinically and experimentally affect bladder muscle function. Lepor and Kuhar[55] have used radioligand receptor-binding techniques to identify the muscarinic cholinergic receptor in the bladder. With these techniques, Shapiro et al.[82] have demonstrated that exstrophied and control bladders contain similar levels of muscarinic cholinergic receptors.

The upper urinary tract is usually normal, but anomalous development does occur. We have seen horseshoe kidney, pelvic kidney, hypoplastic kidney, solitary kidney, and dysplastic megaureter. The peritoneal pouch of Douglas between the bladder and rectum is enlarged and unusually deep, forcing the ureter down and laterally in its course across the true pelvis. The distal segment of the ureter approaches the bladder from a point inferior and lateral to the orifice and enters the bladder with little or no obliquity. Therefore, reflux in the closed exstrophic bladder occurs in nearly 100% of cases and requires subsequent operative management.

Terminal ureteral dilatation frequently appears in pyelograms and is usually the result of edema, infection, and fibrosis of terminal ureter, acquired after birth. Prenatal ureterovesical obstruction also occurs and may represent the simultaneous occurrence of an adynamic ureteral segment.

Operative Management

The primary objectives of operative management of exstrophy of the bladder are to obtain secure abdominal wall closure, urinary continence with preservation of renal function, and reconstruction of a functional and cosmetically acceptable penis in the male. These objectives can be achieved following primary closure of the bladder; reconstruction of the bladder neck; and repair of epispadias; or following urinary diversion, internal or external; cystectomy; and epispadias repair. Historically, both

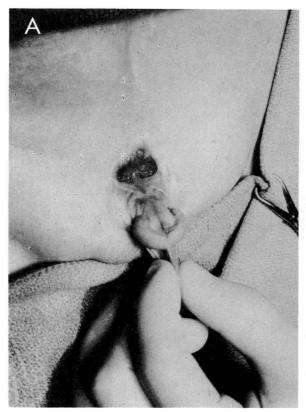

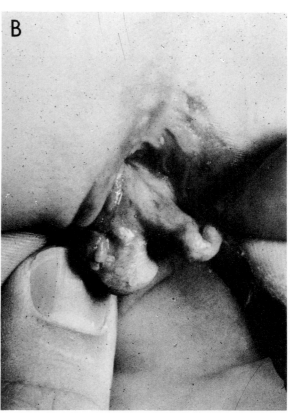

Fig 128–5.—Exstrophy of the bladder in the male. Difficult problems in genital reconstruction. **A,** short penis and very small bladder. **B,** duplex penis. (From Jeffs R.D.: Epispadias, exstrophy, and other bladder anomalies, in Walsh P.C., Gittes R.F., Perlmutter A.D., et al. (eds.): *Campbell's Textbook of Urology.* Philadelphia, W.B. Saunders Co., 1985. Used by permission.)

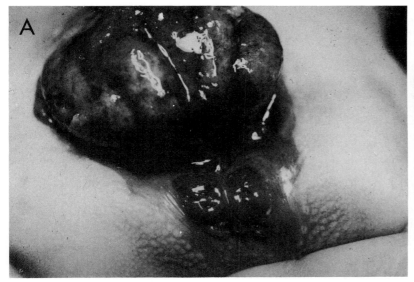

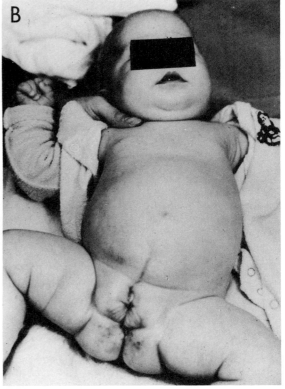

Fig 128–6.—Exstrophy of the bladder in the male. **A,** rudimentary penis. **B,** reconstructed and raised as a female. In males with hopelessly inadequate phallic material, this option should be taken as early as the decision can be made. (From Jeffs R.D.: Epispadias, exstrophy, and other bladder anomalies, in Walsh P.C., Gittes R.F., Perlmutter A.D., et al. (eds.): *Campbell's Textbook of Urology.* Philadelphia, W.B. Saunders Co., 1985. Used by permission.)

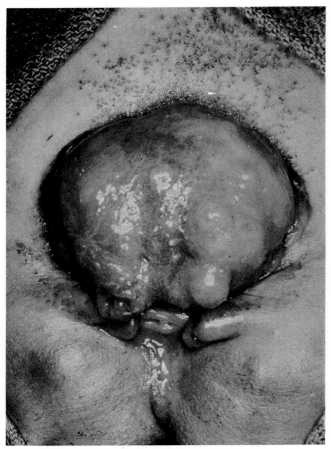

Fig 128–7.—Female with exstrophy showing right ureteral orifice and the vaginal orifice between the two parts of the bifid clitoris. (From Jeffs R.D.: Epispadias, exstrophy, and other bladder anomalies, in Walsh P.C., Gittes R.F., Perlmutter A.D., et al. (eds.): *Campbell's Textbook of Urology*. Philadelphia, W.B. Saunders Co., 1985. Used by permission.)

urinary diversion and functional bladder closure have been fraught with complications, and a consensus for the surgical management of exstrophy of the bladder has not been established. Advocates of urinary diversion concede that functional bladder closure provides the most ideal restoration of the genitourinary tract; however, they argue that the theoretical advantages of primary closure are seldom achieved.[3, 87] Castro and Martinez-Pineiro[7] have stated that urinary diversion for exstrophy of the bladder simply transforms a congenital anomaly into an iatrogenic anomaly. However, urinary continence in their series of functional bladder closures was achieved in only 22% of cases. The ideal surgical management of each individual patient with exstrophy of the bladder requires detailed study and investigation, knowledge of all possible surgical solutions and their results, and a creative team approach to the overall management of the individual patient.

Urinary Diversion

The first ureterosigmoidostomy was performed for exstrophy in 1852 by Simon.[84] The patient died 1 year later. Early experiences with ureterosigmoidostomy for exstrophy of the bladder were fraught with complications that included peritonitis; anastomotic strictures; acute and chronic pyelonephritis; stones; intestinal obstruction; anal incontinence; and hyperchloremic, hy-

pokalemic acidosis. The postoperative mortality in a large series of ureterosigmoidostomies performed between 1912–1946 was 12.5%.[31] The magnitude of early and late complications following ureterosigmoidostomy for exstrophy of the bladder was reported in Higgins'[35] personal series of 132 ureterosigmoidostomies. Two modifications in operative technique markedly diminished the morbidity of ureterosigmoidostomy. Coffey[13] described a mucosa-to-mucosa ureterointestinal anastomosis, and Leadbetter[53] described an antirefluxing ureterointestinal anastomosis that diminished subsequent chronic pyelonephritis and renal failure. The impact of these technical modifications is reflected in the series that compared the surgical results in ureterosigmoidostomies performed prior to 1954 (Group A) and after 1954 (Group B).[3] The renal units assessed by excretory urography were normal in 59% and 89% of individuals in Groups A and B respectively. The availability of broad-spectrum antibiotics and regimens for preoperative bowel sterilization are additional factors contributing to decreasing the morbidity of ureterosigmoidostomy.

In a recent long-term assessment of 31 ureterosigmoidostomies,[87] there were no immediate postoperative deaths and three subsequent deaths, attributed to ureterosigmoidostomy. Eleven (35%) patients required 13 additional operative procedures for stones, anastomotic strictures, and recurrent pyelonephritis. Sixty renal units were assessed by intravenous pyelography; 41 (67%) of the renal units were considered good (no or minimal dilatation of the collecting system, prompt and adequate excretion, and no stones); 5 units were fair; and 15 units were poor. Major infection developed in 14 (45%) cases; and nine (29%) individuals had absolutely no problems with infection. Half of the patients developed hyperchloremic acidosis; however, chronic alkalinization was required infrequently. Overall, 50% of patients in this series had no complications as measured by excretory pyelograms, infection, blood chemistries, and clinical assessment.

It is imperative that individuals be followed up carefully after ureterosigmoidostomy, because anastomotic strictures, chronic pyelonephritis, urinary calculi, and metabolic abnormalities may develop insidiously. The late occurrence of carcinoma of the bowel adjacent to the ureterocolic anastomosis must also be appreciated. A recommended follow-up protocol includes intravenous pyelograms (IVP) and blood chemistry analyses every 6 months for the first 2 years, annual appraisal for the subsequent 5 years, and biannual evaluation thereafter.[87]

Owing to the many complications associated with ureterosigmoidostomy, several alternative techniques of urinary diversion for exstrophy of the bladder have been described. In 1894, Maydl[65] described the trigonosigmoidostomy. Boyce and Vest[5] reviewed 23 trigonosigmoidostomies followed for a mean interval of 10 years. Renal function, assessed by excretory urography, was normal in 21 (91%) cases; stones formed in two (9%) cases; hyperchloremic acidosis developed in approximately 50% of cases. However, only a few individuals required chronic alkalinization; and reoperation was performed in two (9%) cases. All of the children achieved daytime continence, and overall 18 (78%) cases were considered good results.

The Heitz-Boyer and Hovelacque procedure[32] included diverting the ureters into an isolated rectal segment and pulling the sigmoid colon through the anal sphincter muscle just posterior to the rectum. Taccinoli et al.[91] reviewed 21 staged Heitz-Boyer and Hovelacque procedures for exstrophy of the bladder that were followed between 1–16 years. They reported 95% fecal and urinary continence; there were no cases of urinary calculi, electrolyte abnormalities, or postoperative mortality; and three (14%) patients developed ureterorectal strictures requiring surgical revision. Isolated cases treated in North America have been subject to multiple and severe complications. Boyce[4] described a technique that also diverted the ureters into a rectal bladder; however, a proximal colostomy was constructed rather than a pull-through procedure.

The early good results following ileal conduit urinary diversion suggested that this technique might be ideal for urinary drainage in patients with exstrophy of the bladder, because fecal contamination and acidosis resulting from reabsorption were avoided. Unfortunately, significant long-term complications have developed in children 10–15 years following ileal conduit diversion.[41, 83] Ileal conduit urinary diversion is not acceptable for children with exstrophy who may have a normal life expectancy.[58]

Hendren[33] described using colon urinary conduits in cases of exstrophy of the bladder. The nonrefluxing ureterointestinal anastomosis represents the primary advantage of colon conduits. The colon conduit is constructed at 1 year of age. If anal continence is achieved, the ureterocolonic anastomosis is nonrefluxing, and there is no upper-tract deterioration, the colon conduit is undiverted into the colon at age 4–5 years. Sixteen colon conduits and 11 subsequent colocoloplasties have been performed by Hendren, and the only reported postoperative complications were intestinal obstruction in three (19%) cases and ureteral obstruction in one (6%) case. There have been no cases of stomal complications, persistent reflux, pyelonephritis, or upper-tract deterioration in Hendren's series. The long-term assessment of renal function and continence following colon conduit diversion and subsequent colocoloplasty requires further investigation. Despite our preference for primary functional bladder closure for exstrophy of the bladder, colon conduit urinary diversion represents the most attractive alternative, because a nonrefluxing anastomosis is achieved and undiversion can be performed when clinically indicated. Careful assessment of anal control of fluid content must be made prior to urinary diversion to the rectum, and the possibility of night-time incontinence persisting must be understood.

Functional Bladder Closure (Primary Bladder Closure and Bladder Neck Reconstruction)

In 1869, Thiersch[92] raised neighboring skin flaps in order to enclose a narrow space in front of the everted bladder. Urine was retained by an external appliance that occluded the internal sphincter. In 1906, Trendelenburg[94] attempted to achieve urinary continence by sacroiliac osteotomy and bladder closures with narrowing of the patulous urethra. Trendelenburg attributed the lack of success with this procedure to subsequent displacement of the pubis.

Young[98] reported the first successful functional closure for exstrophy of the bladder. A narrow strip of posterior urethral mucosa was selected, the mucosa lateral to the posterior urethral strip was excised, the posterior urethral strip was tubularized, and the neourethra was reinforced with the denuded detrusor muscle. The bladder was inverted and closed, and the abdominal wall defect closed with fascial flaps. The patient eventually developed a 3-hour continent interval; however, no mention was made regarding renal function. Marshall and Muecke[64] reviewed 329 functional bladder closures reported in the literature between 1906–1966 and determined that urinary continence with preservation of renal function was achieved in only 16 (5%) cases. Dehiscence of the abdominal wall and bladder, urinary fistulae, incontinence, persistent reflux, and pyelonephritis frequently resulted in subsequent urinary diversion. Over the past 20 years, modifications in the management of functional bladder closure have contributed to a dramatic increase in the success rate following this procedure. The four most significant changes in man-

agement of exstrophy of the bladder were reconstructing a competent bladder neck, performing bilateral iliac osteotomies, staging the reconstruction procedures, and defining criteria for the selection of cases suitable for functional closure.

BLADDER NECK RECONSTRUCTION.—Dees[17] modified the Young technique for reconstructing the bladder neck for complete epispadias. A triangular wedge of tissue was removed from the roof and lateral aspect of the proximal urethra, and adjacent bladder wall that included a portion of each lateral lobe of the prostate. The remaining posterior urethral mucosal strip was tubularized, and the neourethra was reinforced with the adjacent denuded muscle. Leadbetter[52] considered that the length and the tone of the muscular reinforcement of the neourethra contributed to the achievement of urinary continence. The Dees procedure was modified by tubularizing a 3.5-cm long posterior urethral strip that included trigonal mucosa. The neourethra was reinforced with trigonal muscle, and bilateral ureteroneocystotomies were performed. A posterior urethral strip 3.5 cm long may be excessive, because urethral pressure profilometry, in a series of exstrophy patients with continent bladders, demonstrated that continence can be achieved with a functional closure pressure as low as 20 cm of water pressure and with a continence length as low as 0.6 cm.[93] The median functional closure pressure and continence length in this group of continent exstrophies was 40 cm of water pressure and 1.35 cm, respectively.

OSTEOTOMY.—Schultz[78] combined primary bladder closure with bilateral iliac osteotomies. The efficacy of iliac osteotomies is controversial. The primary arguments against osteotomies are that the pubis eventually pulls apart, that the penis further retracts, and that continence can be achieved without osteotomies.[64] The advantages of bilateral iliac osteotomies are that (1) reapproximation of the pubic symphysis diminishes the tension of the abdominal closure and eliminates the need for fascial flaps; (2) placement of the urethra within the pelvic ring reduces the excessive urethrovesical angle and permits urethral suspension after bladder neck reconstruction; and (3) reapproximation of the urogenital diaphragm and approximation of the levator ani may aid in voluntary urinary control.[40] Ezwell and Carlson[25] observed that urinary diversion was subsequently performed in 20% of functional closures without osteotomy, whereas urinary diversion was eventually required by 75% of individuals who had not undergone prior osteotomies during bladder closure. Ninety percent of children referred to our institution, following partial or complete bladder dehiscence, had not undergone a prior osteotomy.[57] It is our recommendation to perform bilateral iliac osteotomies when primary bladder closure is performed after 72 hours of life.

STAGED SURGICAL RECONSTRUCTION.—The disadvantage of performing the entire surgical reconstruction of exstrophy of the bladder as a single stage is that a single complication jeopardizes the entire repair. Sweetser et al.[89] first described a staged surgical approach for exstrophy of the bladder. Bladder closure was performed 4–6 days following bilateral iliac osteotomies, and epispadias repair was performed as a separate procedure. The continence procedure was limited to freeing the fibrous intersymphyseal band and wrapping this band around the urethra at the time of bladder closure. A staged approach to functional bladder closure that includes three separate stages—bladder closure, bladder neck reconstruction with an antireflux procedure, and epispadias repair—has been recommended by us for most cases of exstrophy reconstruction.[39]

PATIENT SELECTION.—Successful treatment of exstrophy by functional closure demands that the potential for success in each child be considered at birth (Fig 128–8).

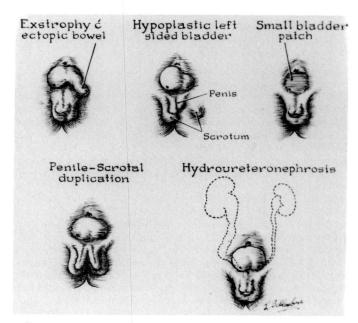

Fig 128–8.—Exstrophic bladders that may not be suitable for functional closure. (From Jeffs R.D.: Epispadias, exstrophy, and other bladder anomalies, in Walsh P.C., Gittes R.F., Perlmutter A.D., et al. (eds.): *Campbell's Textbook of Urology*. Philadelphia, W.B. Saunders Co., 1985. Used by permission.)

Bladder size and functional capacity of the detrusor muscle are important considerations in the eventual success of functional closure. The correlation between apparent bladder size and the potential bladder capacity must not be confused. In minor grades of exstrophy that approach the condition of complete epispadias with incontinence, the bladder may appear small, yet may demonstrate acceptable capacity by bulging when the baby cries or by indenting easily when touched by a gloved finger.[8] Stimulation of the bladder by a stream of cold water will indicate the ability of the detrusor muscle to contract and relax, proving its functional integrity. Once removed from surface irritation and repeated trauma, the small bladder will enlarge and will gradually increase its capacity, even in the absence of continence or of outlet resistance. The exstrophic bladder that is estimated at birth to have a capacity of 5 ml or more, and that demonstrates elasticity and contractility, can be expected to develop useful size and capacity following successful closure. A small fibrotic bladder patch that is stretched between the edges of a small triangular fascial defect without either elasticity or contractility should not be selected for the usual closure procedure. Bladder augmentation using bowel segments may be required in order to achieve closure,[75] and bladder augmentation using bowel at a later time may be required to achieve adequate capacity.[2] Examination under anesthesia may at times be required for adequate assessment of the bladder, particularly if considerable edema and excoriation have developed. The elasticity of the bladder can be demonstrated in this way, and the size of the triangular abdominal fascial defect can be appreciated by simultaneous abdominal and rectal examination. Neonatal closure of the abdominal defect, even when the bladder is small, allows for later assessment of bladder potential and provides an initial step in genital reconstruction, helpful in gaining acceptance by the family.

Genital Reconstruction

The techniques for reconstructing the male genitalia in exstrophy of the bladder are similar for patients managed by urinary diversion or functional bladder closure. Because male adolescents consider their odd-looking genitalia a greater psychosocial problem than their incontinence, every effort must be made to restore the penis to a normal appearance.[26] A well-planned program of surgical reconstruction must be designed at the initiation of treatment in order to avoid ineffective use of the limited penile skin.

The reconstruction of the male genitalia includes lengthening the penis, release of the dorsal chordee, and urethroplasty. Owing to the extent of the penile deformity and the limited availability of penile skin in patients with exstrophy of the bladder, a functionally and cosmetically acceptable penis can rarely be achieved in a single operative procedure. Many of the techniques used for reconstructing the male genitalia in exstrophy of the bladder were described initially for repair of hypospadias and epispadias.

Kelly and Eraklis[45] lengthened the penis by nearly totally mobilizing the crura from their inferior pubic attachments to the level of the ischial tubercles and joining the freed crura in the midline. The dorsal chordee was released by dividing the suspensory ligaments and the attachments of the crura to the skin. Johnston[42] described a more limited dissection of the corpora that achieved substantial penile length and minimized the potential risk of injuring the neurovascular bundle. The corpora were exposed by elevating a V-flap that extended from the pubic bones to the urethral meatus. The exposed corpora were only partially mobilized from the pubis and were joined in the midline. Skin coverage was provided by preputial flaps, and by closing the V-incision in a Y fashion. Six months following penile lengthening and release of the chordee, the dorsal penile skin was tubularized into the neourethra.

The number of stages for genital reconstruction can be reduced by performing penile lengthening and release of the dorsal chordee at the time of primary bladder closure.[20]

Construction of the urethra using full-thickness skin grafts obtained from the thigh[34] and prepuce[18] have been described for penile reconstruction in complete epispadias. These techniques can be used for urethral reconstruction in exstrophy of the bladder when there is insufficient penile skin available for tubularization to form a new urethra.

Staged Functional Reconstruction for Classic Exstrophy of the Bladder

The primary objective in functional closure of classic exstrophy of the bladder is to convert the exstrophy to complete epispadias with incontinence while preserving renal function. Secondarily, the best management for the incontinence and epispadias will be determined in a later stage or stages.

The Delivery Room and Nursery

At birth, the bladder mucosa is usually smooth, thin, and intact; it is sensitive and easily denuded. In the delivery room, the umbilical cord should be tied with nylon or polyglycolic acid (Dexon) sutures relatively close to the abdominal wall so that the umbilical clamp or long cord does not add to the trauma and excoriation of the bladder surface. The bladder may be covered with a nonadherent film of plastic wrap (Saran or Gladwrap) to prevent the mucosa from sticking to clothing or diapers. Standard varieties of petrolatum gauze become dry and lift up the delicate epithelium when removed. The counseling of the parents and the decisions about eventual therapy should be by surgeons with special interest and experience in managing cases of exstrophy of the bladder.

The distraught parents, at this stage, need reassurance. An awareness that renal function, locomotion, sexual function, and fertility can approach normal in patients with exstrophy of the bladder will restore hope. They will also be relieved to learn that the expectation of exstrophy of the bladder recurring in their future offspring is low and that parents with exstrophy rarely produce children with the exstrophy-epispadias complex.[81]

The social services offered by the hospital can be of great help to the parents in facing the family problems resulting from prolonged hospitalization and the financial strain of unexpected medical care, family separation, and home-to-hospital travel.

Early Management

Cardiopulmonary and general physical assessment can be carried out in the first few hours of life. Immediate intravenous pyelographic assessment of the kidneys in the newborn may lack clarity and detail, but useful information can usually be obtained between 24–48 hours of age. Radionuclide scans and ultrasound can provide evidence of renal function and drainage even in the first few hours of life. There is an advantage to being able to make a decision about bladder closure within the first 48 hours of life.[1] The ease with which the pelvis can be molded at this time allows approximation of the pubic diastasis and the rectus muscles without osteotomies.

Circumstances may be less than ideal at birth, however, and neonatal assessment may have to be deferred until transportation to a children's medical center can be arranged. In these days of air travel and fast motor transportation, no child should be more than a few hours away from a neonatal center with full diagnostic and consultative services. During travel, the bladder should be protected by a plastic membrane (not petrolatum gauze) to prevent contact of dressing or clothing with the delicate mucosa.

The Operative Procedure

OSTEOTOMY.—Suitable patients seen within 48 hours of life may not require osteotomy owing to the malleability of the pelvic ring. However, when the separation is unduly wide, or there is delay in referral and the patient is not seen until several days of age or older, osteotomy will be required to achieve closure of the pelvic ring. Osteotomy may be carried out at the same time as closure of the bladder, or it may be done a few days to a week in advance. A well-coordinated surgical and anesthesiology team can carry out osteotomy and proceed to closure of the bladder without undue loss of blood or risk to the child from prolonged anesthesia. The osteotomy is performed through bilateral incisions over the sacroiliac region. A vertical iliac osteotomy is performed close to the midline to allow the two wings of the pelvis to hinge and come together without anterior-to-posterior flattening of the true pelvic ring (Fig 128–9). The closure of the pelvic ring not only allows midline approximation of the abdominal wall structures, but also allows the levator ani and puborectalis muscles to lend potential support to the bladder outlet, thereby adding resistance to urinary outflow. Furthermore, the incontinence procedures can be carried out on the bladder neck and urethra within the closed pelvic ring at a distance from the surface and free from independent movement of the two halves of the pubis. When the urethra and bladder neck are set more normally within the true pelvis, they present a normal relationship with the vertical axis of the bladder, rather than an acute angulation. The fibrocartilage of the pubic symphysis is united by a horizontal mattress suture tied anterior to the pubic closure using no. 2 nylon. This horizontal mattress suture is placed directly through the calcified portion of the pubis on each side to provide good anchorage and maintain apposition after the suture is tied. Should the suture work loose or cut through the tissues during subsequent healing, the anterior placement of the knot in the horizontal mattress suture insures that it will not erode into the urethra and interfere with the bladder or urethral lumen. Postoperatively, the patient, whether the bladder was closed without osteotomy in the first 48 hours of life, or with osteotomy, is immobilized by modified Bryant's traction with adhesive skin traction to a position in which the hips have 90 degrees of flexion

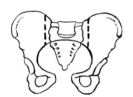
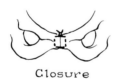

Closure

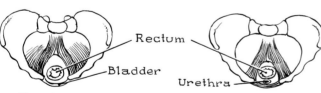

Preclosure · Rectum · Bladder · Urethra · Closure without osteotomy

(a) Approximation of levators and puborectalis sling

(b) Inclusion of bladder neck and urethra within pelvic ring

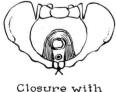

Closure with osteotomy

Fig 128–9.—The technique and advantages of bilateral iliac osteotomy. (From Jeffs R.D.: Epispadias, exstrophy, and other bladder anomalies, in Walsh P.C., Gittes R.F., Perlmutter A.D., et al. (eds.): *Campbell's Textbook of Urology.* Philadelphia, W.B. Saunders Co., 1985. Used by permission.)

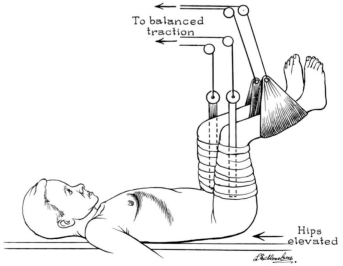

Fig 128–10.—Modification of Bryant's traction used for postoperative immobilization after initial bladder closure with or without osteotomy. (From Jeffs R.D.: Epispadias, exstrophy, and other bladder anomalies, in Walsh P.C., Gittes R.F., Perlmutter A.D., et al. (eds.): *Campbell's Textbook of Urology.* Philadelphia, W.B. Saunders Co., 1985. Used by permission.)

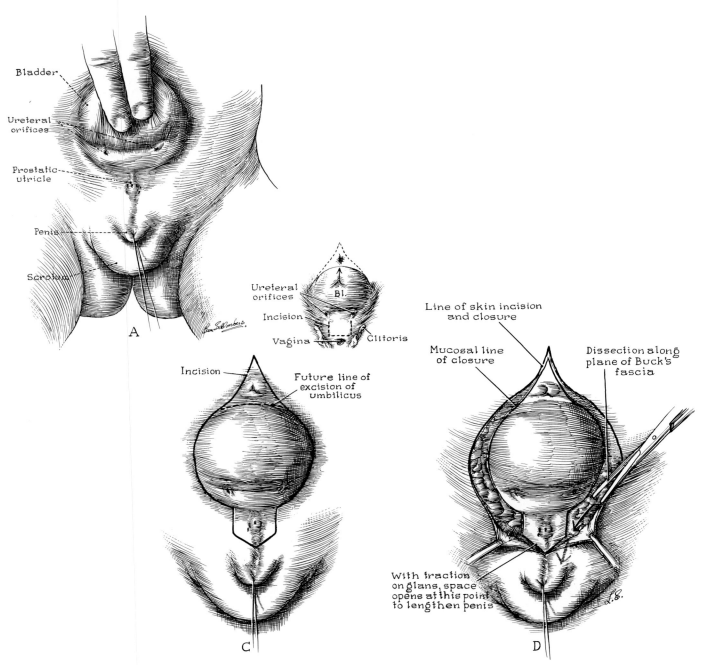

Fig 128–11.—Exstrophy of the bladder—primary bladder closure following osteotomy, or without osteotomy in newborns less than 72 hours of age. **A,** the deformity. **B, C, D,** circumferential incision around bladder and 2-cm posterior urethral flap to below verumontanum. *(Continued.)*

and the knees are slightly bent to protect the arterial tree (Fig 128–10). Traction is maintained for a period of 3–4 weeks, allowing firm fibrous healing of the pelvic ring anteriorly.

Bladder and Prostatic Urethral Closure

The various steps in primary bladder closure are illustrated in Figure 128–11. A 2-cm wide strip of mucosa extending from the distal trigone to below the verumontanum in the male, and to the vaginal orifice in the female, is outlined for reconstruction of the prostatic and posterior urethra. When the length of the urethral groove that extends from the verumontanum to the glans is

so short that it interferes with eventual length of the penis, the urethral groove is lengthened after the manner of Johnston[43] and Duckett.[21] The diagrams indicate that an incision is made outlining the bladder mucosa and the prostatic plate and that the urethral groove is transected distal to the veru; but continuity is maintained between the thin, mucosa-like, non–hair-bearing skin adjacent to the posterior urethra and bladder neck, and the skin and mucosa of the penile shaft and glans. Flaps from the area of thin skin are subsequently moved distally and rotated to reconstitute the urethral groove, which may be lengthened by 2 to 4 cm.

Penile lengthening is achieved by exposing the corpus caver-

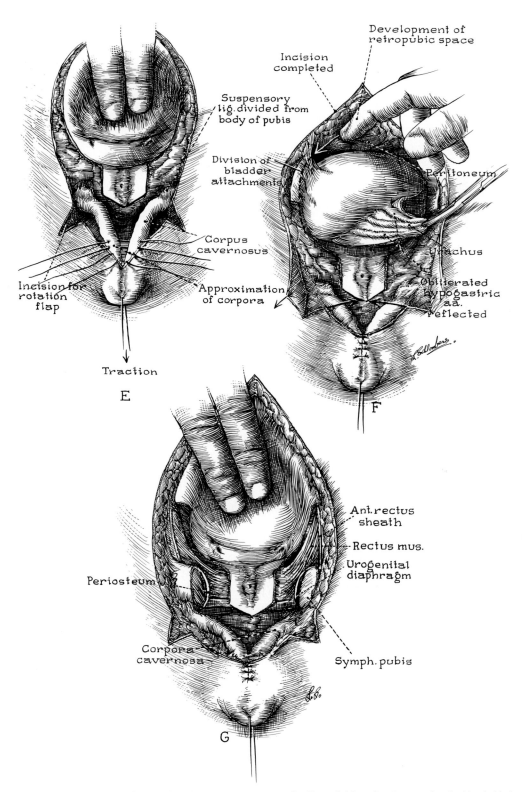

Fig 128–11 Cont.—**E,** lateral skin incision to allow rotation of paraexstrophy skin to cover elongated penis. **F,** development of retropubic space from area of umbilical dissection to facilitate separation of bladder from the rectus sheath and muscle. **G,** medial fan of rectus muscle attaching behind prostate to urogenital diaphragm. Diaphragm and anterior corpora freed from pubis in subperiosteal plane. *(Continued.)*

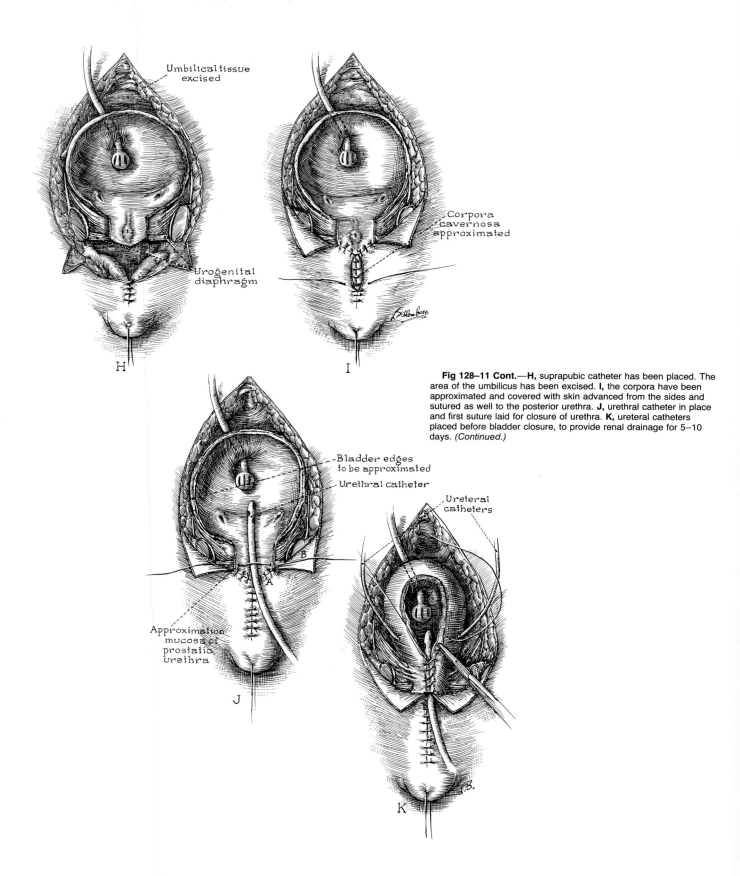

Fig 128–11 Cont.—H, suprapubic catheter has been placed. The area of the umbilicus has been excised. **I,** the corpora have been approximated and covered with skin advanced from the sides and sutured as well to the posterior urethra. **J,** urethral catheter in place and first suture laid for closure of urethra. **K,** ureteral catheters placed before bladder closure, to provide renal drainage for 5–10 days. *(Continued.)*

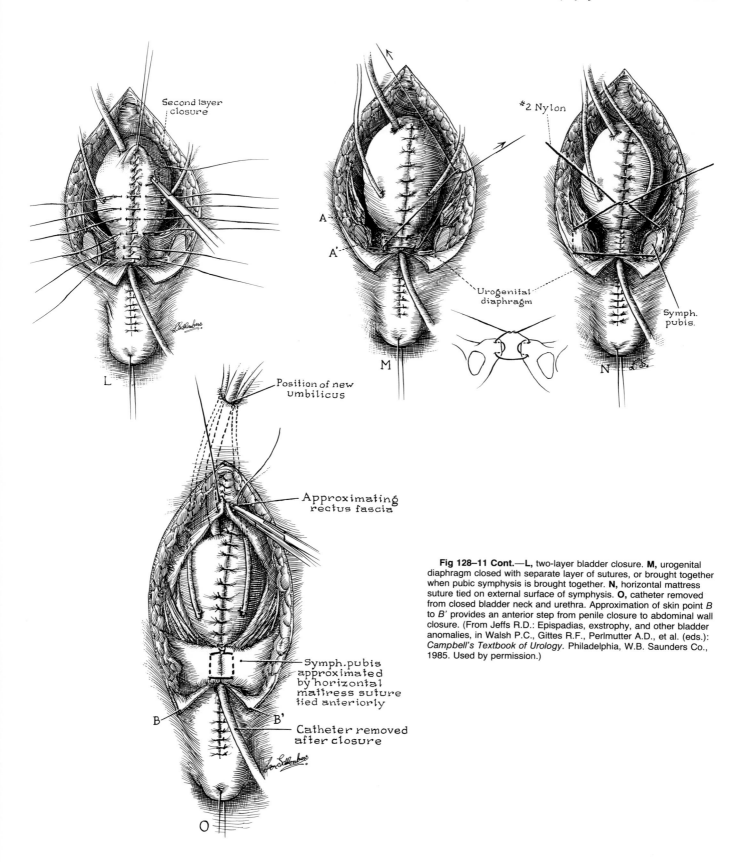

Fig 128–11 Cont.—L, two-layer bladder closure. **M,** urogenital diaphragm closed with separate layer of sutures, or brought together when pubic symphysis is brought together. **N,** horizontal mattress suture tied on external surface of symphysis. **O,** catheter removed from closed bladder neck and urethra. Approximation of skin point *B* to *B'* provides an anterior step from penile closure to abdominal wall closure. (From Jeffs R.D.: Epispadias, exstrophy, and other bladder anomalies, in Walsh P.C., Gittes R.F., Perlmutter A.D., et al. (eds.): *Campbell's Textbook of Urology.* Philadelphia, W.B. Saunders Co., 1985. Used by permission.)

nosum bilaterally and freeing the corpora from their attachments to the suspensory ligaments and anterior part of the inferior pubic rami. The partially freed corpora are joined in the midline, and the bare corpora are then covered with flaps of the thin paraexstrophy skin (mentioned previously), which are rotated medially to be attached to the distal mucosa of the posterior plate. These same flaps may also be used to lengthen the urethra in the female by detaching the urethral groove distally and suturing the flap to the urethra in a tubular fashion.

Closure of the bladder then proceeds by excision of the umbilical area, discarding the redundant skin adjacent to the superior aspect of the bladder mucosa, and freeing the bladder muscle from the fused rectus sheaths on each side. This dissection is facilitated by exposing the peritoneum above the umbilicus and then carefully dissecting extraperitoneally to enter the retropubic space on each side from above. The wide band of fibrous and muscular tissue representing the urogenital diaphragm is detached subperiosteally from the pubis, bilaterally. The dissection is extended for 5–10 mm in a subperiosteal plane onto the inferior ramus of the pubis, allowing the bladder neck and posterior urethra to fall back and achieve a position within the pelvic ring. The mucosa and muscle of the bladder and posterior urethra are then closed in the midline anteriorly. The posterior urethra and bladder neck are buttressed by the tissues of the urogenital diaphragm, which are closed as a second layer. The bladder is drained by a suprapubic Malecot catheter for a period of 4 weeks. The urethra is not stented, to avoid pressure necrosis or the accumulation of infected secretions in the urethra. Ureteral stents provide ureteral drainage during the first 5–7 days, when swelling or the pressure of the bladder closure may obstruct the ureters and give rise to obstruction and transient hypertension.

When the bladder and urethra have been closed, pressure over the greater trochanters allows the pubic bones to be approximated in the midline. The mattress suture is placed and tied, and the rectus sheath is closed in the midline. The suprapubic tube and ureteral stents emerge from the abdominal skin above the midline skin closure at a point corresponding to the normal position of the umbilicus.

During this procedure, the patient is given broad-spectrum antibiotics in an attempt to convert a contaminated field into a clean surgical wound. Nonreactive sutures of Dexon and nylon are used to avoid undesirable stitch reaction or stitch abscesses.

Interim Management After Initial Closure

The procedure just described converts a child with exstrophy into one with complete epispadias with incontinence. Prior to removing the suprapubic tube, 4 weeks postoperatively, the bladder outlet is calibrated by a urethral catheter or by cystoscopy to insure free outlet drainage. An intravenous pyelogram is obtained to record the status of the pelvis and ureters, and urinary antibiotics are administered, appropriate to treat any bladder contamination that may be present after removal of the suprapubic tube. Residual urine is estimated by straight catheterization, and cultures are obtained before the patient leaves the hospital and at subsequent intervals to detect infection and ensure adequate drainage. The intravenous pyelogram is repeated 3 months after discharge from the hospital and will be repeated at intervals of 6 months to a year during the next 2–3 years to detect any upper-tract change caused by reflux or infection. Urinary antibiotics should be continued at least through the first 6 months, and thereafter as necessary. Should bladder outlet resistance be such that urine is retained within the bladder, and reflux and ureteral dilatation develop with infected urine, it may be necessary to dilate the urethra or, occasionally, to resort to intermittent catheterization. If bladder outlet resistance persists, an antireflux procedure may be required as early as 6 months to 1 year after the initial bladder closure (Fig 128–12). If a useful continent interval has resulted unexpectedly from the initial closure, no further operation for incontinence may be required.

In the patient converted from exstrophy to complete epispadias with incontinence, the bladder gradually increases in capacity, and inflammatory changes in the mucosa resolve. Cystograms at 2–3 years will indicate bilateral reflux in nearly 100% of the patients and will provide an estimate of bladder capacity. Even in the completely incontinent patient, bladder capacity gradually increases to the point where it can be distended at cystography to a capacity of 50–60 ml. In some patients with very small bladders, the bladders may require 4–5 years to achieve this capacity.

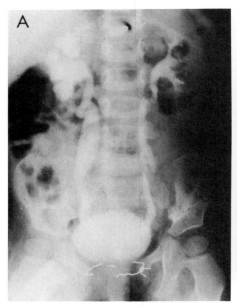 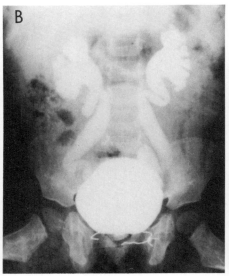 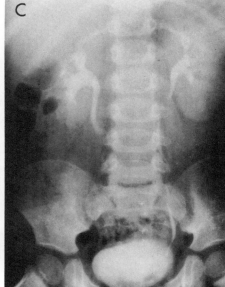

Fig 128–12.—Closed exstrophy. **A,** retention and hydroureter after initial closure. **B,** cystogram showing grade 4-B reflux. **C,** after reimplantation. Continence without bladder neck reconstruction.

A tight bladder closure, uncontrolled urinary infection, and reflux may cause uncontrollable ureteral dilatation. Judgment is required to know when to abort attempts at functional closure and turn to urinary diversion as a means of preserving renal function. This change of plan is seldom necessary if a wide outlet has been constructed at initial closure and if careful attention to the details of follow-up have been observed.

At the age of 3–5 years, providing the bladder has achieved a capacity of 50–60 ml when distended, treatment of the incontinence and reflux are undertaken. Cultures and radiologic studies should indicate sterile urine and good ureteral drainage in the undistended bladder. The rationale for performing bladder neck reconstruction prior to urethral reconstruction is that iatrogenic injury to a reconstructed urethra may result if instrumentation is required for urinary retention immediately following the bladder neck reconstruction. However, if by age 2½–3 years the bladder capacity in boys has not reached 50 ml, we proceed directly to epispadias repair; and bladder neck reconstruction is deferred until bladder capacity increases. The formation of the neourethra may produce additional resistance to urine outflow and, therefore, contribute to increasing bladder capacity.

Incontinence and Antireflux Procedures

The incontinence and antireflux procedures are illustrated in Fig 128–13. This illustration depicts a Cohen[14] type of transtrigonal advancement procedure for correcting reflux, in which a new hiatus lateral to the original orifice was selected prior to advancing the ureter across the bladder above the trigone. The bladder was originally opened through a V-incision at the bladder neck, but a vertical extension was used. The midline closure of this incision enlarges the vertical dimension of the bladder, which, in exstrophy, is often short.

The incontinence procedure is begun by selecting a posterior strip of mucosa 18–20 mm wide by 30 mm long that extends distally from the midtrigone to the prostate or posterior urethra. The bladder muscle lateral to this mucosal strip is denuded of mucosa. The edges of the mucosa and the underlying muscle are formed into a tube by interrupted sutures, and the adjacent denuded muscle flaps are overlapped and sutured firmly in place in order to provide reinforcement of the bladder neck and urethral reconstruction. Wide dissection of the bladder, bladder neck, and urethra is required within the pelvis to provide mobility both for this urethral reconstruction and for subsequent anterior suspension of the newly created urethra and bladder neck. Tailoring of the denuded lateral triangles of bladder muscle is aided by multiple small incisions in the free edges bilaterally.

Urethral profiles are obtained intraoperatively to measure continence length, and urethral closure pressure (Fig 128–14). Retrospective comparison of these values with subsequent success or failure in producing continence serve as guidelines for reconstructing the bladder neck. Preliminary results suggest that an intraoperative continence length of 2.5–3.5 cm is desirable, and that intraoperative closure pressures ranging between 70–100 ml of water required to prevent leakage when the bladder pressure is raised to 50 cm of water intraoperatively. Undoubtedly, the measurements of continence length and closure pressure will be considerably less in eventual follow-up, when stretching occurs and swelling and edema disappear. At the end of the procedure, the bladder neck reconstruction is further enhanced by suspending the urethra and the bladder neck to the structures of the pubis and anterior rectus sheath in the manner of Marshall et al.[61] Profiles taken after this stage of the procedure indicate that additional continence length and additional closure pressure are achieved.

In the small bladder, ureteral stents are placed in the reimplanted ureters, and the bladder is drained once again by suprapubic catheter, which is left indwelling for a 3-week period. Suprapubic catheter drainage avoids stretching or pressure on the reconstructed bladder neck. No urethral stent is used, and catheterization or instrumentation through the urethra is avoided for at least a 3-week period. The adequacy of bladder neck reconstruction is tested by a water manometer at the end of the procedure. The bladder neck should support 50 cm of water pressure without leakage if the bladder neck reconstruction and suspension are adequate. Immediate revision is advisable when this degree of resistance is not obtained. Attempts are made to reduce the postoperative frequency and severity of bladder spasms by the use of Pro-Banthine, oxybutynin hydrochloride (Ditropan), diazepam (Valium), or imipramine hydrochloride (Tofranil). The patients are given urinary antibiotics to prevent infection, and little or no leakage through the urethra should occur during the 3 weeks of suprapubic drainage. Prior to removing the suprapubic catheter, a clamp is applied to initiate voiding; and if necessary the urethra is calibrated using a soft catheter. Cultures are taken so that medication may be given to clear any bacterial colonization. In some patients, a period of intermittent catheterization may be required if reasonable bladder emptying does not occur.

When the catheter is removed, we expect a short, dry interval to occur, but bladder size and operative reaction may allow a capacity of no more than a few milliliters initially. The patient has to learn to recognize bladder filling and to initiate detrusor contraction, which he may not previously have experienced. A readjustment period that may extend for many months or, in some patients, for years, is required before a useful bladder volume and a long, dry interval develop. Initially, the absence of stress incontinence or continuous urethral dribbling suggests that urethral resistance has been produced and that an increasing dry interval will occur. The patient can learn to use this interval profitably for daytime and nighttime continence.

Urethroplasty

Construction of the neourethra and further penile lengthening and dorsal chordee release are usually performed approximately 1 year following reconstruction of the bladder neck. We recommend that a modified Young urethroplasty be performed when there is sufficient penile skin both for construction of the urethra and for coverage of the neourethra and when the dorsal urethral groove has sufficient length. The techniques for constructing the urethra from full-thickness skin grafts[18, 34] have been previously described. These procedures are utilized when penile skin is unavailable to perform a modified Young urethroplasty. A pedicle tube constructed from ventral preputial tissue may also be used to bridge a defect between prostatic and glandular urethra.[22]

The modified Young urethroplasty, illustrated in Figure 128–15, is begun by placing a nylon suture through the glans to provide for traction of the penis. Incisions are made on two parallel lines, previously marked on the dorsum of the penis, to outline an 18-mm strip of penile skin extending from the prostatic urethral meatus to the tip of the glans. Triangular areas of the dorsal glans are excised adjacent to the urethral strip, and flaps of glans are constructed. The lateral skin flaps are mobilized and a Z-incision over the subpubic area permits exposure and division of suspensory ligaments and old scar tissue. The urethral strip is then closed linearly with a 6-0 polyglycolic acid suture from the prostatic opening to the glans over a no. 10 pediatric feeding tube. The subcutaneous tissue is closed with two separate continuous layers of 6-0 polyglycolic acid suture. The skin is reapproximated with interrupted 5-0 polyglycolic acid sutures. The glans is reconstructed with vertical mattress sutures of 4-0 poly-

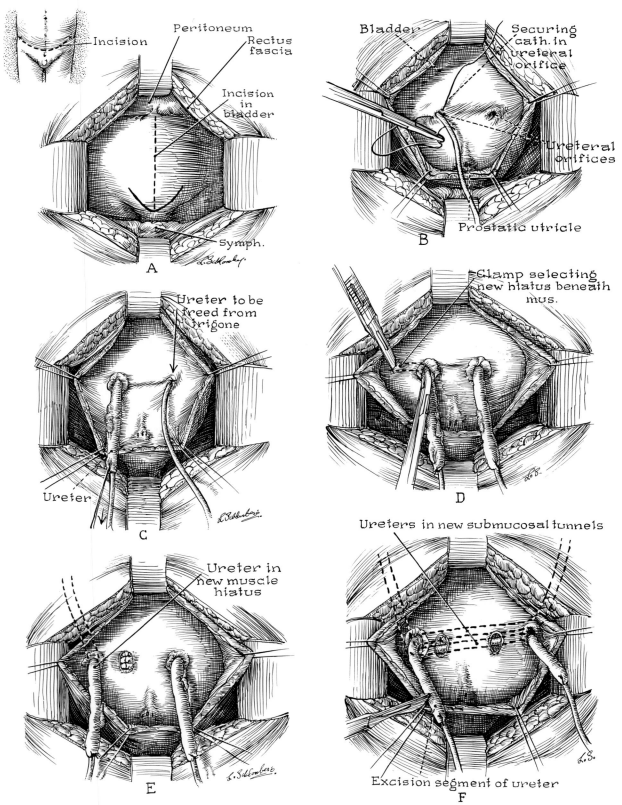

Fig 128–13.—Cohen transtrigonal crossed reimplantation of ureters, and bladder neck reconstruction for continence. **A,** transverse bladder incision with vertical extension, to be closed in midline so as to narrow bladder near bladder neck. **B,** catheter sutured to bladder at ureteral orifice. **C,** ureteral orifice circum- scribed and ureter drawn into bladder. **D** and **E,** left ureter brought down as well, submucosal tunnel created to new point of entry for right ureter, bladder muscle closed at native entrance of ureter. *(Continued.)*

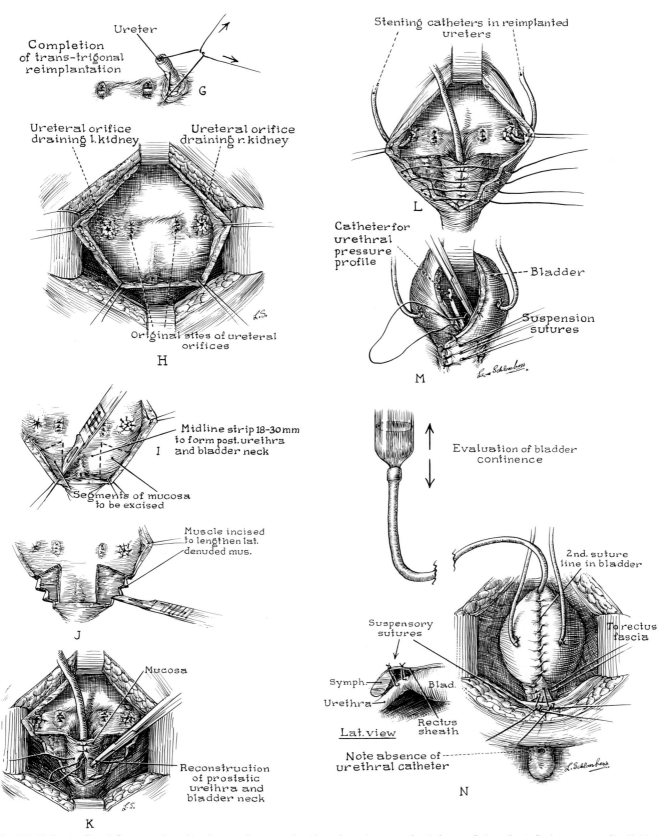

Fig 128–13 Cont.—**F** and **G**, ureters brought submucosally across the trigone, right ureter to left, and vice versa. **H**, native ureteral orifices closed. Mucosa-to-mucosa suture of ureteroneocystostomies. **I–L**, mucosal strip of trigone to form bladder neck and prostatic urethra. Lateral denuded muscle triangles are lengthened by several small incisions to allow easy tailoring of double-breasted muscle closure of bladder neck. **M**, pressure profile (see Fig 128–14) of closed bladder neck and urethra is obtained before closure of bladder dome. Suspension sutures are elevated manually to estimate final pressure profile. **N**, bladder neck and urethra are unstented, drainage by ureteral catheters and suprapubic tube. Bladder outlet resistance measured by water manometer. (From Jeffs R.D.: Epispadias, exstrophy, and other bladder anomalies, in Walsh P.C., Gittes R.F., Perlmutter A.D., et al. (eds.): *Campbell's Textbook of Urology*. Philadelphia, W.B. Saunders Co., 1985. Used by permission.)

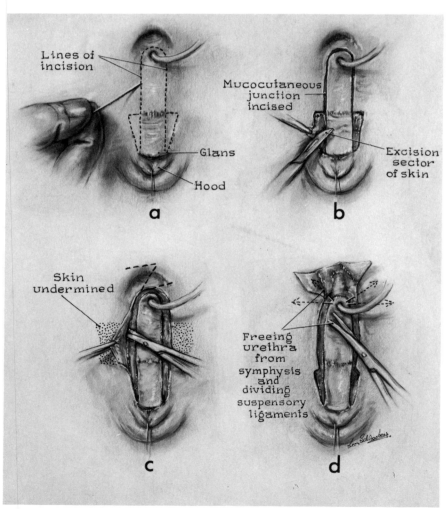

Fig 128–14.—Urethral pressure profile measured with bladder open, before bladder neck reconstruction, after reconstruction, and with addition of bladder neck suspension. Each increases continence length and closure pressure. (From Jeffs R.D.: Epispadias, exstrophy, and other bladder anomalies, in Walsh P.C., Gittes R.F., Perlmutter A.D., et al. (eds.): *Campbell's Textbook of Urology.* Philadelphia, W.B. Saunders Co., 1985. Used by permission.)

Fig 128–15.—a–k, modified Young urethroplasty for repair of epispadias when urethral groove is of sufficient length naturally or following prior lengthening procedures. (From Jeffs R.D.: Epispadias, exstrophy, and other bladder anomalies, in Walsh P.C., Gittes R.F., Perlmutter A.D., et al. (eds.): *Campbell's Textbook of Urology.* Philadelphia, W.B. Saunders Co., 1985. Used by permission.) *(Continued.)*

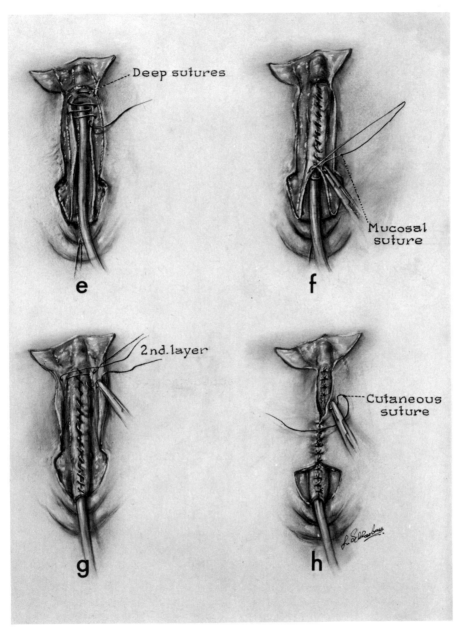

Fig 128–15 Cont.—e–h.

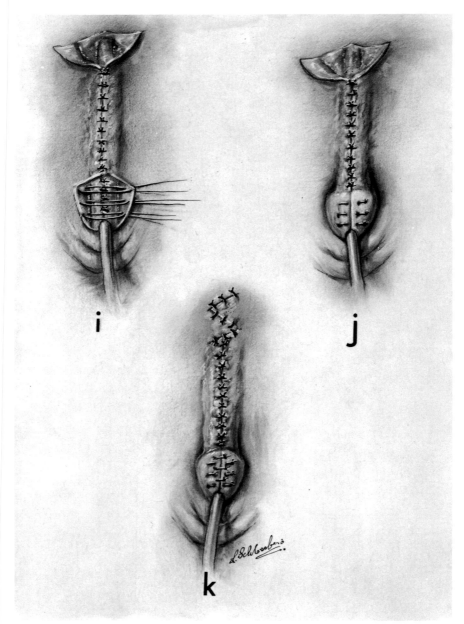

Fig 128–15 Cont.—i–k.

propylene (Prolene), and these sutures are removed in 10 days. The Z-plasty is closed with interrupted 6-0 polyglycolic acid suture. Several 6-0 polyglycolic acid sutures are inserted between the Prolene sutures in the glans. A pediatric feeding tube is left indwelling in the neourethra as a stent. Urinary drainage occurs through the stent or may be further insured by a percutaneous suprapubic tube.

Variable Presentation: Time and Pathologic Anatomy

It is possible to outline a program at birth for an ideal case with a large bladder, with relatively little pubic separation and with a long urethral groove. A plan of treatment for those with different anatomical features and for those who may present late or with partial previous treatment must also be formulated.

The ideal situation may allow for early bladder closure without osteotomy with a subsequent satisfactory incontinence interval, without infection, with good drainage, and with no hydronephrosis. At the end of 2½–3 years there is found a bladder with a capacity of 50–60 ml or more. It may then be possible, in one operation, to do a bladder neck reconstruction, possibly to do the epispadias repair at the same time, reimplant the ureters, and end with a patient who has outlet resistance, a dry interval, a satisfactory penis, and who requires little or no further additional treatment.

Table 128–1 indicates age of presentation and the variable problems which may be seen at the initial presentation, during the incontinent period after initial closure, or at the time when it is desirable to obtain continence and to perform the epispadias repair.

TABLE 128–1.—INITIAL PRESENTATION OF PATIENTS WITH EXSTROPHY OF BLADDER

AGE	PROBLEM	POSSIBLE SOLUTION
0–72 hr	Classic exstrophy with reasonable capacity and moderate symphyseal separation; long urethral groove; mild dorsal chordee	I. Midline closure of bladder, fascia and symphysis to level of posterior urethra, no osteotomy
0–72 hr	The above findings with short urethra and severe dorsal chordee	II. Close as above, adding lengthening of dorsal urethral groove by para-exstrophy skin
0–72 hr or late presentation	The above with very wide separation of symphysis or late presentation of patient (beyond 72 hours to 1–3 years) for initial treatment	Iliac osteotomy and closure as in I or II
0–2 wk	Male, penis duplex or extremely short	Consider female sex of rearing and closure as in I or II
0–2 wk	Very small nondistensible bladder patch	Prove by examination under anesthesia, then nonoperative expectant treatment awaiting internal or external diversion (experimental early augmentation by bowel and other material has been tried)
	THE INCONTINENT PERIOD AFTER INITIAL CLOSURE	
1 mo–3 yr	Infection with residual resulting from outlet stenosis	Urethral dilatation, occasional meatotomy or bladder neck revision
	Infection, grade III reflux with pliable outlet resistance	Continuous antibiotic suppression with plan for early ureteroneocystostomy
	Partial dehiscence at bladder neck or partial prolapse of bladder (both prevent bladder capacity increase)	Reclosure of bladder neck with or without osteotomy
	CONTINENCE AND EPISPADIAS REPAIR	
2½–5 yr	Closed bladder with incontinence, normal intravenous pyelogram, bladder capacity 60 ml or more, bilateral reflux, good penile size and length of urethral groove	Plan bilateral ureteroneocystostomy, bladder neck reconstruction, epispadias repair followed by 3 weeks of suprapubic drainage; prepare 5 weeks and 2 weeks before operation with two injections of testosterone in oil, 2 mg/kg
2½–5 yr	As above with small bladder capacity, less than 60 ml	Epispadias repair only after preparation with testosterone; bladder capacity will improve postoperatively
	Epispadias repaired, capacity greater than 60 ml	Proceed to bladder neck plasty and ureteroneocystostomy
	Epispadiac penis short with severe chordee before or after bladder neck reconstruction	Correction of chordee, lengthening of urethral groove and epispadias repair; prepare with testosterone (consider osteotomy to aid in achieving increased penile length)
3 yr plus	Completed repair of bladder, bladder neck and epispadias with dry interval but wet pants	Patience, biofeedback, Ditropan, imipramine, and time
	Above with marked stress incontinence	Wait—may require bladder neck revision or Teflon injection
	Small-capacity bladder unchanged by time, epispadias repair or attempted bladder neck reconstruction	Consider augmentation cystoplasty and bladder neck reconstruction; acceptance of intermittent catheterization may be necessary
3–7 yr	Small bladder unsuitable for bladder neck plasty	Consider temporary diversion by colon conduit with plan to undivert to bladder using bladder to form urethra and conduit for augmentation; in patients over 7 years, artificial sphincter can be considered
3–7 yr	Small closed exstrophy unsuitable for bladder neck reconstruction or augmentation, or late presentation of untreated exstrophy, unsuitable for closure	Consider permanent external or internal diversion; internal diversion direct by ureterosigmoidostomy or indirect by colocolostomy. Evaluate day continence of anal sphincter and night time seepage
5–15 yr	Closed exstrophy with epispadias repaired with uncontrolled stress or dribbling incontinence	Consider (1) revision; (2) Teflon injection; (3) augmentation and revision; (4) artificial sphincter with omental wrap
10–20 yr	Closed or diverted exstrophy with inadequate penis	Consider penile lengthening, urethral reconstruction with augmentation using free graft, pedicle grafts and tissue transfer

Many of the possible solutions are indicated in the right-hand column. These possible solutions simply indicate some of the many ways the more complicated presentations have been handled to arrive at that eventual solution of a satisfactory external appearance, preservation of renal function, continent dry interval, and a functional and cosmetically acceptable penis or external genitalia.

Results of Staged Functional Closure

Functional closure of bladders, both large and small, has been successful cosmetically and functionally in recent years. Small bladders that seem to suggest little promise have developed adequate capacity. Continence has been achieved without compromising renal function. With few exceptions, it is, therefore, recommended that all neonates with classic exstrophy of the bladder should be considered for staged functional reconstruction consisting of initial closure with or without osteotomy and careful follow-up during the incontinent period and subsequent stage or stages to correct the epispadias, the incontinence, and the bilateral reflux.

Recent reviews of functional closure indicate the improved frequency of success. In greater than 40% of cases reported by Mollard,[69] Chisholm,[9] Ansell,[1] and Jeffs[38] (Table 128–2), secure closure, urinary continence, and preservation of renal function have been achieved.

The author's recent experience (1975–1982) with functional bladder closure is reviewed in the following paragraphs.

Primary Bladder Closure

Twenty-eight of 29 (97%) consecutive patients with exstrophy of the bladder referred to our pediatric urology service prior to any surgical reconstruction between 1975–1982 underwent primary bladder closure.[54] Urinary diversion was initially performed in one child with a very small bladder patch. The postoperative complications following primary bladder closure and the additional surgical procedures required to correct these postoperative complications are presented in Table 128–3.

Bladder Neck Reconstruction (BNR)

Twenty-five patients have undergone initial BNR at our institution between 1975–1982.[54]

Urinary retention developed postoperatively in eight cases and resolved following dilatation or prolonged suprapubic catheter drainage in all cases.

The two measurements used to assess urinary continence were the average daytime dry interval and the frequency of incontinent episodes. An average daytime dry interval exceeding 3 hours represented an excellent surgical result, a dry interval of greater than 1 hour and less than 3 hours a satisfactory result,

TABLE 128–2.—Urinary Continence Following Functional Bladder Closure

SERIES*	NO. OF CLOSURES EVALUATED	NO. CONTINENT	% CONTINENT
Chisholm (1979)[9]	95	43	45
Mollard (1981)[69]	16	11	69
Jeffs (1982)[40]	55	33	60
Ansell (1983)[1]	23	10	43
Lepor & Jeffs (1983)[54]	22	19	86

*Only personal series reporting continence rates >40% are included. (From *Campbell's Textbook of Urology*, Chap. 43. Philadelphia, W.B. Saunders Co., 1985. Used by permission.)

TABLE 128–3.—Complications in 28 Primary Bladder Closures*

COMPLICATIONS	NO.
Bladder prolapse	2
Outlet obstruction	2
Bladder calculi	3
Renal calculi	1
Wound dehiscence	0
CORRECTIVE SURGICAL PROCEDURES	
Repair of bladder prolapse	2
Cystolithopaxy	3
Urethrotomy	1

*From Lepor H., Jeffs R.D.[54] Used by permission.

and a dry interval of less than 1 hour a poor result. Another measurement used to assess urinary continence was the number of times the underclothes were soiled during the day. Soiling of underclothes less than once per day was considered an excellent surgical result, soiling one to two times a day a satisfactory result, and soiling more than two times per day a poor result. Urinary continence according to average daytime dry interval and soiling of underclothing was achieved in 86% and 80% of cases respectively (Table 128–4).

Forty-two renal units from 21 patients were evaluated by intravenous pyelography between 6 months to 6 years following BNR in order to assess the preservation of renal function following functional bladder closure. Only 10% of these renal units showed significant hydronephrosis and deterioration of function.

Urethroplasty

Twenty-four patients with exstrophy of the bladder have undergone initial urethral reconstruction at the Johns Hopkins Hospital between 1975 and 1982.[56] A modified Young urethroplasty was performed in 22 patients, a distal urethral free graft in one patient, and a ventral preputial pedicle graft in one patient. The average age at the time of urethral reconstruction was 4 years.

Fistulae developed in nine patients following epispadias repair. Four of the fistulae spontaneously closed, and five required operative closure. Four of these five fistulae occurred near the corona, and one occurred at the midshaft. The corona is the area most deficient in circumferential penile skin, and multiple layered closure at this point over the tubularized urethra is difficult to achieve. Proximally, the skin is more redundant, and distally the glandar flaps cover the neourethra and heal quickly without fistulae. The coronal sulcus is, however, a weak spot in the repair.

The fistulae were closed by excising a small rim of penile skin and urethra adjacent to the fistulae and closing the defect with 6-0 Vicryl suture in three layers. No persistent fistulae occurred.

All 24 patients who have undergone epispadias repair are preadolescent, and a definitive assessment of their genital function cannot be determined. An attempt was made to evaluate the current status of the genital reconstruction from parental interviews. Eighteen parents were interviewed, four parents could not be contacted, and it is too early to evaluate the results of two children operated on within the last 3 months. The angulation of the flaccid penis when standing was directed downward to horizontally in 83% of the boys. Erections were witnessed in 83% of the youngsters; and in these individuals the penis was directed upward in 47%, horizontally in 47%, and downward in 6%. Every parent was extremely satisfied with the appearance of the penis,

TABLE 128–4.—URINARY CONTINENCE FOLLOWING 22 INITIAL
BLADDER NECK RECONSTRUCTIONS*

RESULT	AVERAGE DAYTIME DRY INTERVAL (hr)	PATIENTS NO.	%	INCONTINENT EPISODES/DAY	PATIENTS NO.	%
Excellent	>3	19	86	<1	16	80
Satisfactory	1–3	1†	5	1–2	1	5
Poor	<1	2†	9	>3	3†	15

*From Lepor H., Jeffs R.D.[54] Used by permission.
†Includes patients' continence level prior to secondary reconstructive surgery.

although some expressed concern regarding whether the penis would attain adequate size for sexual intercourse after puberty.

Management of Failed Bladder Closures

Urinary continence, defined as a 3-hour dry interval, is usually achieved within 1 year following bladder neck reconstruction. Delayed achievement of urinary continence has come with puberty in the male.[46] The increase in urethral length associated with prostatic enlargement provides additional resistance to urinary outflow. In our experience, patients who do not achieve a 1-hour dry interval within 2 years following bladder neck reconstruction seldom develop a sufficient continence mechanism. These unfortunate individuals may be treated by repeat Young-Dees-Leadbetter bladder neck reconstruction; tubularization of the remaining bladder into a neourethra and bladder augmentation by colocystoplasty;[2] anti-incontinence devices;[79] or urinary diversion. If failed reconstructive efforts are associated with the development of renal insufficiency, renal transplantation into an intestinal segment[60] or closed exstrophic bladder[88] may be considered. A patulous bladder neck with an adequate bladder capacity is managed by revising the Young-Dees-Leadbetter bladder neck reconstruction. Arap et al.[2] manages exstrophy of the bladder by initially constructing a colon urinary conduit. The entire bladder is subsequently tubularized into a 5–6-cm neourethra, and the colon conduit is anastomosed to this urethrovesical tube. This technique is useful for the failed Young-Dees-Leadbetter bladder neck reconstructions with small contracted bladders, or for the initial treatment of exstrophy of the bladder when the bladder capacity is less than 5 ml. Hanna[29] has inserted anti-incontinence devices to achieve continence in exstrophy of the bladder. The compromised blood supply to urethral and periurethral tissues from previous surgical manipulations increases the likelihood of erosion by these devices. We have inserted only one anti-incontinence device in a patient with exstrophy of the bladder referred to our institution following failed bladder neck reconstruction. Despite inserting and activating the device in two stages, erosion into the urethra occurred. Similar experiences with anti-incontinence devices in complete epispadias have been reported by others.[29, 46] The artificial sphincter may be useful in the older child with well-vascularized bladder neck tissues or in those in whom the mature omentum can be interposed between the cuff and the reconstructed bladder neck.

Malignancy

In the 1920s, it was estimated that 50% of individuals with exstrophy of the bladder were dead by 10 years of age.[66] The development of operative techniques that preserved renal function, the availability of broad-spectrum antibiotics, and the understanding of the metabolic disorders associated with urinary diversion have resulted in 91% of patients with this disorder surviving to age 30 years.[51] This extended survival has uncovered two latent malignant processes associated with bladder exstrophy. Eighty percent (45/57) of carcinomas identified in exstrophic bladders are adenocarcinomas.[44] The incidence of adenocarcinoma in the exstrophic bladder is approximately 400-fold greater than in the normal population.[24] According to Mostofi,[68] chronic irritation, infection, and obstruction can induce a metaplastic transformation of the urothelium to cystitis glandularis, a premalignant lesion. Adenocarcinoma may also develop from the malignant degeneration of embryonic rests of gastrointestinal tissue that are incorporated in the exstrophic bladder.[24] The inherent malignant potential of the closed exstrophic bladder has not been determined, because long-term follow-up of a large number of exstrophy cases without urinary tract infection, obstruction, and chronic irritation has not been evaluated. Bladder abnormalities, including squamous metaplasia, acute inflammation, fibrosis, and epithelial submucosal inclusions, were observed in a 2-week-old infant with exstrophic bladder,[16] suggesting that exstrophic bladders are inherently abnormal. On the other hand, a 17-year-old male, who underwent bladder closure at 1 year of age and developed normal urinary control with preservation of the upper urinary tract, was killed in an automobile accident; serial sectioning of this bladder revealed no evidence of malignant or premalignant changes.[38] Until the malignant potential of the noninfected, nonobstructed, closed exstrophic bladder is determined, a high index of suspicion must be maintained for potential malignant degeneration. Only two epithelial malignancies have been reported in closed exstrophy patients, and these bladders were not closed at birth. Exstrophic bladders that are left everted are predisposed to develop squamous cell carcinoma secondary to repeated trauma. Squamous cell carcinoma accounts for only four of 57 (7%) of the carcinomas reported in exstrophic bladders.[44] According to an unpublished case report by Jeffs, and other sources,[33, 80] rhabdomyosarcoma has been observed in three individuals with exstrophy.

Adenocarcinoma of the colon adjacent to the ureterointestinal anastomosis in an exstrophy patient was initially described in 1948.[19] The risk of adenocarcinoma of the colon following ureterosigmoidostomy in exstrophy patients is 100-fold that of the general population.[85] Spence et al.[86] recently surveyed the literature to identify patients with exstrophy who developed tumors following ureterosigmoid diversion. The mean latency interval from the time of ureterointestinal anastomosis to the diagnosis of intestinal tumor in these cases was 10 years, and the longest latent interval was 46 years. Twenty-eight of the 35 compiled tumors were malignant, 24 were adenocarcinomas, and approximately half of the adenocarcinomas had metastasized at the time of diagnosis. Individuals with ureterosigmoidostomy, therefore, should undergo periodic barium enema and/or sigmoidostomy.

Fertility

Reconstruction of the male genitalia and preservation of fertility were not primary objectives of the early surgical management of exstrophy of the bladder. Sporadic accounts of pregnancy or the initiation of pregnancy by males with exstrophy of the bladder have been reported. In two large exstrophy series, male fertility is rarely documented. Three of 68 men,[3] and four of 72 men[97] successfully fathered children. Six of 26 and seven of 27 women with exstrophy of the bladder in these respective studies successfully delivered offspring. Shapiro's survey of 2,500 exstrophy and epispadias patients[83] identified 38 males who had fathered children and 131 female patients who had borne offspring.

Hanna and Williams[30] studied semen analyses of men who had undergone primary bladder closure or ureterosigmoidostomy. A normal sperm count was found in only one of eight men following functional bladder closures and in four of eight men with urinary diversion. The difference in the observed fertility potential is most likely attributed to iatrogenic injury of the verumontanum during functional closure. Retrograde ejaculation may also account for the low sperm counts observed following functional bladder closure.

Libido in exstrophy patients is very high.[97] The erectile mechanism in patients who have undergone epispadias repair appears intact, because 87% of young boys in our series have had witnessed erections following epispadias repair.[54]

Pregnancy

Clemetson's[11] review of the literature identified 45 women with exstrophy of the bladder who successfully delivered 49 normal offspring. The main complications following pregnancy were cervical and uterine prolapse, which occurred in six of seven women.[47] Women must be informed of the likelihood that uterine prolapse will probably develop following pregnancy. Spontaneous vaginal deliveries were performed in women who had undergone prior urinary diversion, and cesarian sections were performed for women with functional bladder closure, to avoid stress on the pelvic floor and to avoid traumatic injury to the delicate urinary sphincter mechanism.[47]

Social Adjustment

Lattimer et al.[48] assessed the social adjustment of 11 men and six women with bladder exstrophy who were more than 17 years of age. Sexual experiences were reported in 12 individuals; marriage in six; attendance of college in 13; and employment in seven. Overall, 13 of the patients were considered well adjusted. A similar review by Woodhouse et al.[97] observed that 55 of 64 of their exstrophy patients under personal review were strikingly normal and well adjusted.

The objectives of surgical intervention for exstrophy of the bladder are designed to enable the individuals with this disorder to achieve normal social interactions with their community. It is gratifying that great progress has been achieved toward the realization of this goal.

REFERENCES

1. Ansell J.E.: Exstrophy and epispadias, in Glenn J.F. (ed.): *Urologic Surgery.* Philadelphia, J.B. Lippincott Co., 1983, p. 647.
2. Arap S., Giron A., Degoes G.M.: Complete reconstruction of bladder exstrophy. *Urology* 7:413, 1976.
3. Bennett A.H.: Exstrophy of the bladder treated by ureterosigmoidostomies. *Urology* 2:165, 1973.
4. Boyce W.H.: A new concept concerning treatment of exstrophy of the bladder 20 years later. *J. Urol.* 107:476, 1972.
5. Boyce W.H., Vest S.A.: A new concept concerning treatment of exstrophy of the bladder. *J. Urol.* 67:503, 1952.
6. Burns J.E.: A new operation for exstrophy of the bladder. *JAMA* 82:1587, 1924.
7. Castro E.P., Martinez-Pineiro J.A.: Entero-trigono urethroplasty—surgical technique for correction of bladder exstrophy. *Urol. Int.* 23:158, 1968.
8. Chisholm T.C.: *Pediatric Surgery.* Chicago, Year Book Medical Publishers, 1962, vol. 2, p. 933.
9. Chisholm T.C.: Exstrophy of the urinary bladder, in Kiesewetter W.B. (ed.): *Long-Term Follow-up in Congenital Anomalies: Pediatric Surgical Symposium.* Pittsburgh, Pittsburgh Children's Hospital, 1979, p. 31.
10. Clark M., O'Connell K.J.: Scanning and transmission electron microscopic studies of an exstrophic human bladder. *J. Urol.* 110:481, 1973.
11. Clemetson C.A.B.: Ectopia vesicae and split pelvis. *Br. J. Obstet. Gynaecol.* 65:973, 1958.
12. Coffey R.C.: Physiological implantation of the severed ureter as common bile duct into intestine. *JAMA* 56:397, 1911.
13. Coffey R.C.: Transplantation of the ureter into the large intestine in the absence of a functioning bladder. *Surg. Gynecol. Obstet.* 32:383, 1921.
14. Cohen S.J.: Ureterozystoneostomie, eine neue Antirefluxtechnik. *Aktuel. Urol.* 6:24, 1975.
15. Cracchiolo A. III, Hall C.B.: Bilateral iliac osteotomy. *Clin. Orthop.* 68:156, 1970.
16. Culp D.A.: The histology of the exstrophied bladder. *J. Urol.* 91:538, 1964.
17. Dees J.E.: Congenital epispadias with incontinence. *J. Urol.* 62:513, 1949.
18. Devine C.J. Jr., Horton C.E., Scarff J.E. Jr.: Epispadias: Symposium on pediatric urology. *Urol. Clin. North Am.* 7:465, 1980.
19. Dixon C.F., Weisman R.E.: Polyps of the sigmoid occurring 30 years after bilateral ureterosigmoidostomies for exstrophy of the bladder. *Surgery* 24:6, 1948.
20. Duckett J.W.: Use of paraexstrophy skin pedicle grafts for correction of exstrophy and epispadias repair. *Birth Defects* 13:171, 1977.
21. Duckett J.W.: Epispadias: Symposium on congenital anomalies of the lower genitourinary tract. *Urol. Clin. North Am.* 5:107, 1978.
22. Duckett J.W.: The island flap technique for hypospadias repair. *Urol. Clin. North Am.* 8:503, 1981.
23. Engel R.M.: Bladder exstrophy: Vesicoplasty or urinary diversion. *Urology* 2:29, 1973.
24. Engel R.M., Wilkinson H.A.: Bladder exstrophy. *J. Urol.* 104:699, 1970.
25. Ezwell W.W., Carlson H.E.: A realistic look at exstrophy of the bladder. *Br. J. Urol.* 42:197, 1970.
26. Feinberg T., Lattimer J.K., Jetir K., et al.: Questions that worry children with exstrophy. *Pediatrics* 53:242, 1974.
27. Gross R.E., Cresson S.L.: Treatment of epispadias: A report of 18 cases. *J. Urol.* 68:477, 1952.
28. Hall E.G., McCandless A.D., Rickham P.P.: Vesicointestinal fissure with diphallus. *Br. J. Urol.* 25:219, 1953.
29. Hanna M.K.: Artificial urinary sphincter for incontinent children. *Urology* 18:370, 1981.
30. Hanna M.K., Williams D.J.: Genital function in males with vesical exstrophy and epispadias. *Br. J. Urol.* 44:1969, 1972.
31. Harvard B.M., Thompson G.J.: Congenital exstrophy of the urinary bladder: Late results of treatment by the Coffey-Mayo method of uretero-intestinal anastomosis. *J. Urol.* 65:223, 1951.
32. Heitz-Boyer M., Hovelacque A.: Creation d'une nouvelle vessie et d'un nouvel uretre. *J. d'Urologie* 1:237, 1912.
33. Hendren W.H.: Exstrophy of the bladder: An alternative method of management. *J. Urol.* 115:195, 1976.
34. Hendren W.H.: Penile lengthening after previous repair of epispadias. *J. Urol.* 121:527, 1979.
35. Higgins C.C.: Exstrophy of the bladder: Report of 158 cases. *Am. Surg.* 28:99, 1962.
36. Ives E., Coffey R., Carter C.O.: A family study of bladder exstrophy. *J. Med. Genet.* 17:139, 1980.
37. Janssen P.: Die Operation der Blasenektopie ohne Inanspruchnahme des Intestinums. *Zentralbl. Chir.* 60:2657, 1933.
38. Jeffs R.D.: Exstrophy, in Harrison J.H., Gittes R.F., Perlmutter A.D., et al. (eds.): *Campbell's Textbook of Urology.* Philadelphia, W.B. Saunders Co., 1978, p. 1672.
39. Jeffs R.D., Charrios R., Many M., et al.: Primary closure of the exstrophied bladder, in Scott R. (ed.): *Current Controversies in Urologic Management.* Philadelphia, W.B. Saunders Co., 1972, p. 235.
40. Jeffs R.D., Guice S.L., Oesch I.: The factors in successful exstrophy closure. *J. Urol.* 127:974, 1982.
41. Jeffs R.D., Schwarz G.R.: Ileal conduit urinary diversion in children: Computer analysis follow-up from 2 to 16 years. *J. Urol.* 114:285, 1975.
42. Johnston J.H.: Lengthening of the congenital or acquired short penis. *Br. J. Urol.* 46:685, 1974.
43. Johnston J.H.: The genital aspects of exstrophy. *J. Urol.* 113:701, 1975.
44. Kandazari S.J., Majid A., Ortega A.M., et al.: Exstrophy of the uri-

nary bladder complicated by adenocarcinoma. *Urology* 3:496, 1974.

45. Kelly J.H., Eraklis A.J.: A procedure for lengthening the phallus in boys with exstrophy of the bladder. *J. Pediatr. Surg.* 6:165, 1971.
46. Kramer S.A., Kelalis P.: Assessment of urinary continence in epispadias: A review of 94 patients. *J. Urol.* 128:290, 1982.
47. Krisiloff M., Puchner P.J., Tretter W., et al.: Pregnancy in women with bladder exstrophy. *J. Urol.* 119:478, 1978.
48. Lattimer J.K., Beck L., Yeaw S., et al.: Long-term follow-up after exstrophy closure—late improvement and good quality of life. *J. Urol.* 119:664, 1978.
49. Lattimer J.K., Smith M.J.K.: Exstrophy closure: A follow-up on 70 cases. *J. Urol.* 95:356, 1966.
50. Lattimer J.K., Smith M.J.K.: The management of bladder exstrophy. *Surg. Gynecol. Obstet.* 123:1015, 1966.
51. Lattimer J.K., Hensle T.W., MacFarlane M.T., et al.: The exstrophy support team: A new concept in the care of the exstrophy patient. *J. Urol.* 121:472, 1979.
52. Leadbetter G.W. Jr.: Surgical correction of total urinary incontinence. *J. Urol.* 91:261, 1964.
53. Leadbetter W.F.: Consideration of problems incident to performance of uretero-enterostomy: Report of a technique. *J. Urol.* 73:67, 1955.
54. Lepor H., Jeffs R.D.: Primary bladder closure and bladder neck reconstruction in classical bladder exstrophy. *J. Urol.* 130:1142, 1983.
55. Lepor H., Kuhar M.J.: Characterization of muscarinic cholinergic receptor in genitourinary tissues of the rabbit. *J. Urol.* 132:392, 1984.
56. Lepor H., Shapiro E., Jeffs R.D.: Urethral reconstruction in males with classical bladder exstrophy. *J. Urol.* 131:512, 1984.
57. Lowe F.C., Jeffs R.D.: Wound dehiscence in bladder exstrophy: An examination of the etiologies and factors for initial failure and subsequent closure. *J. Urol.* 130:312, 1983.
58. MacFarlane M.T., Lattimer J.K., Hensle T.W.: Improved life expectancy for children with exstrophy of the bladder. *JAMA* 242:442, 1979.
59. MacKay J., Syme J.: Congenital exstrophy of the urinary bladder. *Month. J. Med. Sci.* 9:934, 1849.
60. Marchioro T.L., Tremann J.A.: Ureteroileostomy in renal transplant patients. *Urology* 3:171, 1974.
61. Marshall V.F., Marchetti A.A., Krantz K.E.: The correction of stress incontinence by simple vesicourethral suspension. *Surg. Gynecol. Obstet.* 88:509, 1949.
62. Marshall V.F., Muecke E.C.: Variations in exstrophy of the bladder. *J. Urol.* 88:766, 1962.
63. Marshall V.R., Muecke E.C.: Congenital abnormalities of the bladder, in Alken C.E., Dix V.W., Goodwin W.E. (eds.): *Handbuch der Urologie.* Berlin, Springer-Verlag, 1968.
64. Marshall V.F., Muecke E.C.: Functional closure of typical exstrophy of the bladder. *J. Urol.* 104:205, 1970.
65. Maydl K.: Über die radikaltherapie der Blasenectopie. *Wien. Med. Wochenschr.* 44:25, 1894.
66. Mayo C.H., Hendricks W.A.: Exstrophy of the bladder. *Surg. Gynecol. Obstet.* 43:129, 1926.
67. Michon L.: Conservative operations for exstrophy of the bladder, with particular references to urinary incontinence. *Br. J. Urol.* 20:167, 1948.
68. Mostofi R.K.: Potentialities of bladder epithelium. *J. Urol.* 71:705, 1954.
69. Mollard P.: Bladder reconstruction in exstrophy. *J. Urol.* 124:523, 1980.
70. Muecke E.C.: Exstrophy, epispadias and other anomalies of the bladder, in Harrison J.H., Gittes R.F., Perlmutter A.D., et al. (eds.): *Campbell's Textbook or Urology.* Philadelphia, W.B. Saunders Co., 1978, vol. 2, p. 1443.

71. Muecke E.C.: The role of the cloacal membrane in exstrophy: The first successful experimental study. *J. Urol.* 92:659, 1964.
72. Nesbit R.M.: Ureterosigmoid anastomosis by direct elliptical connection: A preliminary report. *J. Urol.* 61:728, 1949.
73. Nisonson I., Lattimer J.K.: How well can the exstrophied bladder work? *J. Urol.* 107:668, 1972.
74. Pohlman A.G.: The development of the cloaca in human embryos. *Am. J. Anat.* 21:1, 1911.
75. Ransley P.G.: Personal communication, 1984.
76. Remigalo R.V., Woodard J.R., Andrews H.G., et al.: Cloacal exstrophy: 18 year survival of an untreated case. *J. Urol.* 116:811, 1976.
77. Rickham P.P.: Vesico-intestinal fissure. *Arch. Dis. Child.* 35:97, 1960.
78. Schultz W.G.: Plastic repair of exstrophy of the bladder combined with bilateral osteotomy of the ilia. *J. Urol.* 92:659, 1964.
79. Scott F.B., Bradley W.E., Timm G.W.: Treatment of urinary incontinence by an implantable prosthetic urinary sphincter. *J. Urol.* 112:75, 1974.
80. Semerdjian H.S., Texter J.H., Yawn D.H.: Rhabdomyosarcoma occurring in repaired exstrophic bladder: Case report. *J. Urol.* 108:354, 1972.
81. Shapiro E., Lepor H., Jeffs R.D.: The inheritance of classical bladder exstrophy. *J. Urol.* 132:308, 1984.
82. Shapiro E., Jeffs R.D., Lepor H.: Muscarinic cholinergic receptors in closed exstrophied bladders. *J. Urol.* 1985.
83. Shapiro S.R., Lebowitz R., Colodny A.H.: Fate of 90 children with ileal conduit urinary diversion a decade later. *J. Urol.* 114:133, 1975.
84. Simon J.: Ectopia vesicae. *Lancet* 2:568, 1852.
85. Sooriyaarchchi G.S., Johnson R.O., Carbone P.P.: Neoplasms of the large bowel following ureterosigmoidostomy. *Arch. Surg.* 112:1174, 1979.
86. Spence H.M., Hoffman W.W., Fosmire P.P.: Tumors of the colon as a later complication of ureterosigmoidostomy for exstrophy of the bladder. *Br. J. Urol.* 51:466, 1979.
87. Spence H.C., Hoffman W.N., Pate V.A.: Exstrophy of the bladder: Long term results in a series of 37 cases treated by ureterosigmoidostomy. *J. Urol.* 114:133, 1975.
88. Spees E., Marshall F., Lepor H., et al.: Successful renal transplantation in closed bladder exstrophy, (abstracted). *J. Urol.* 131:935, 1984.
89. Sweetser T.H., Chisholm T.C., Thompson W.H.: Exstrophy of the urinary bladder: Discussion of anatomic principles applicable to its repair with a preliminary report of a case. *Minn. Med.* 35:654, 1952.
90. Syme J.: Ectopia vesicae. *Lancet* 2:568, 1852.
91. Taccinoli M., Laurenti C., Racheli T.: Sixteen years experience with the Heitz-Boyer Hovelacque procedure for exstrophy of the bladder. *Br. J. Urol.* 49:385, 1977.
92. Thiersch C.: Ueber die entstehungsweise und operative Behandlung der Epispadie. *Arch. der Heilkunde* 10:20, 1869.
93. Toguri A.G., Churchill B.M., Schillinger J.F., et al.: Gas cystometry in cases of continent bladder exstrophy. *J. Urol.* 119:536, 1978.
94. Trendelenburg R.: The treatment of ectopia vesicae. *Ann. Surg.* 44:281, 1906.
95. Walsh P.C., Donker P.J.: Impotence following radical prostatectomy: Insight into etiology and prevention. *J. Urol.* 119:538, 1978.
96. Williams D.I.: Urology in clinical childhood, in *Handbuch der Urologie.* New York, Springer-Verlag, 1974, p. 268.
97. Woodhouse C.R.J., Ransley P.C., Williams D.I.: The exstrophy patient in adult life. *Br. J. Urol.* 55:632, 1983.
98. Young H.H.: Exstrophy of the bladder: The first case in which a normal bladder and urinary control have been obtained by plastic operation. *Surg. Gynecol. Obstet.* 74:729, 1942.

129 ALAN B. RETIK
Urinary Diversion

HISTORY.—Attempts to divert the urine into various portions of the intestinal tract were described in the mid- to late 19th century. Urine was diverted to most segments of the intestinal tract, including the vermiform appendix. Electrolyte abnormalities resulting from diversion of urine into the intact intestinal tract resulted in abandonment of all internal diversions with the exception of that to the sigmoid colon. Ureterosigmoidostomy was reported by Syme in 1852. Coffey,[16] in 1921, introduced the use of the submucosal tunnel for anastomosis of the ureter to the colon. Nesbit,[86] in 1949, described a direct, elliptic mucosa-to-mucosa anastomosis of the ureter to the bowel, which was designed to prevent strictures. Subsequently, Cordonnier and Nicolai[19] described an end-to-side mucosal anastomosis. These procedures, although decreasing the incidence of ureteral obstruction, did not prevent reflux. In 1955, Leadbetter[74] reported his experience with ureteroenterostomy by a technique that combined the Coffey tunnel and direct mucosal anastomosis. This technique was designed to prevent obstruction and reflux. At approximately the same time, Goodwin and associates[46] described an open, transcolonic ureterosigmoidostomy with tunnel and direct mucosal anastomosis that accomplished the same purpose.

Electrolyte imbalance following ureterosigmoidostomy, as described by Ferris and Odel in 1950,[36] revived the concept of urinary diversion to an isolated segment of ileum, originally proposed by Tizzoni and Foggi in 1888. The ileal conduit (cutaneous ureteroileostomy) was popularized by Bricker[11] in 1950 and has been the procedure most commonly used for permanent urinary diversion. During the past few years, however, as long-term results of ileal conduit diversion in children have been reported, it has become apparent that a significant number of children suffer progressive renal deterioration. This has been thought to be due to reflux with infection, and methods of diversion were sought that might prevent reflux. Currently in vogue is the nonrefluxing colon conduit, advocated by Mogg,[82] Skinner,[111] Kelalis,[64] and Hendren.[52]

Interest in direct ureterocutaneous anastomosis has been sporadic throughout the years. Cutaneous ureterostomy is still advocated as a method of permanent diversion for the massively dilated ureter. Cutaneous pyelostomy,[59] loop cutaneous ureterostomy,[62, 91, 93] and cutaneous vesicostomy[14, 28, 63] have been recommended by a number of authors as temporary tubeless methods of diversion for infants with severe obstructive uropathy or neurogenic vesical dysfunction.

During the past several years, urinary diversion has been mentioned less frequently as a method of management for many conditions in which it had previously been used. Considerable emphasis has been placed on reconstructive surgery of the urinary tract, especially in infants and children. However, there are still a number of conditions for which diversion of urine is indicated on a temporary basis, and there are even occasions when the urine must be diverted permanently.

Temporary Urinary Diversion

Considerable controversy surrounds the management of the severely decompensated upper urinary tract in the infant or child. With increasing experience in the surgical techniques of remodeling ureters, recent advances in the medical management of the critically ill infant and improved pediatric anesthesia, primary reconstruction of the abnormal urinary tract has been advocated and is being performed successfully in a number of institutions. However, temporary urinary diversion should still be carefully considered in the baby with severe hydronephrosis and hydroureter and may be desirable in a number of other specific situations, primarily in the severely ill newborn with uremia and sepsis.

Intubated Procedures

Intubated diversions in children should be used infrequently and for short periods because of the complications and hazards of indwelling catheters in children. Any method of tubed drainage in infants and children obligates the surgeon to develop a rational plan of overall management, which must include a specific limitation on the duration of tube drainage.

PERCUTANEOUS CYSTOSTOMY.—Trocar or percutaneous cystostomy has replaced the formal suprapubic cystostomy as the most commonly used method of short-term tubed vesical diversion. It is particularly useful in infants with large, distended bladders as a method of diversion for hypospadias repairs and in children with severe urethral inflammatory disease or stricture.

It is important that the bladder be distended at the time of cystotomy. Either a straight or balloon-type catheter may be used; it should be made of Silastic or plastic. The catheter tip should lie in the dome of the bladder to avoid bladder spasm from trigonal irritation.

PERCUTANEOUS NEPHROSTOMY.—Percutaneous nephrostomy is most often done in children to promote immediate drainage of an acutely obstructed kidney. In many respects, it has replaced formal nephrostomy. We also use this technique to drain a kidney whose function is marginal in an effort to determine whether reconstruction rather than nephrectomy will be indicated. Pressure-flow relationships (Whitaker test) across ureteropelvic junctions or ureterovesical junctions as well as prograde pyelography can also be performed. The percutaneous nephrostomy tubes may be left in place for several months.

OPEN NEPHROSTOMY.—When tubeless methods of diversion are contraindicated for technical reasons, open nephrostomy placement is useful, but the tube should only be in place for a relatively short period of time. It is usually difficult to keep the tube in place for longer than 2–3 weeks in an infant. Leakage around the tube may be bothersome, and chronic bacilluria eventually occurs and is difficult to eradicate. Calculus formation and obstruction at the ureteropelvic junction have also been reported following long-term nephrostomy drainage.

Technique.—The technique is shown in Figure 129–1. Through a standard flank incision, the lower pole of the kidney is mobilized, exposing the renal pelvis. A radial pyelotomy incision is made and a right-angle clamp passed into a dilated lower calix until it can be palpated on the lateral aspect of the kidney. The clamp is then cut down on; a heavy silk suture is grasped by the clamp and drawn into the pelvis. The suture is tied to the beveled end of a Malecot catheter and then used to guide the catheter through the nephrotomy. The incision in the pelvis is closed with fine chromic catgut. The Malecot catheter and a small Penrose drain are brought out through a stab wound.

Nonintubated Procedures

Nonintubated methods for temporary diversion are especially suited to infants and young children still in diapers. They pro-

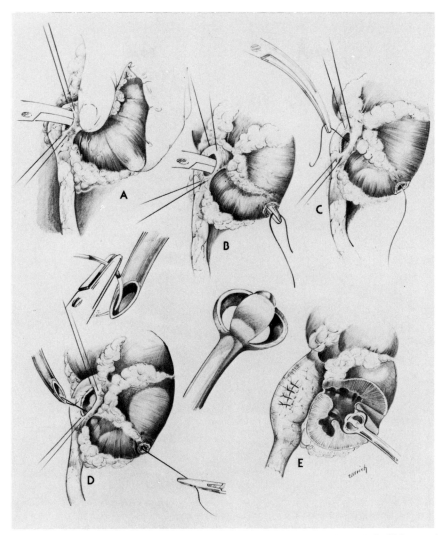

Fig 129–1.—Technique of nephrostomy. **A,** through a pyelotomy incision a right-angle clamp is passed into a dilated lower calix. **B,** the clamp is then cut down on, and a heavy silk suture **(C)** grasped and drawn into the pelvis. **D,** the suture is tied to the beveled end of a Malecot catheter and **(E)** used to guide the catheter through the nephrotomy.

vide maximal decompression of the urinary tract, allowing for optimal renal function, renal growth and reassessment of the entire urinary tract, both radiologically and physiologically, at a later date. Symptomatic urinary infections and stomal care have in general not been problems. Appliances are not needed in diaper-age infants, and peristomal skin inflammation rarely occurs.

CUTANEOUS VESICOSTOMY.—Cutaneous vesicostomy was popularized by Blocksom[10] in 1957 and Lapides et al.[71] in 1960. Vesicostomy is considered to be a very satisfactory method of temporary tubeless diversion in the infant with chronic bladder distention, especially when the etiology is uncertain. This procedure is ideally suited to the infant with neurogenic bladder dysfunction who has significant hydronephrosis and hydroureter with a large bladder that does not empty completely. It is also suitable for the premature newborn with posterior urethral valves and a very narrow urethra in whom transurethral fulguration of the valves would not be feasible. The diversion is a temporary measure only. When the true status of bladder involvement, renal function and growth of the child has been ascertained, some type of reconstruction or permanent diversion

may be desirable or necessary. The procedure is obviously contraindicated in the baby with supravesical obstruction. Vesicostomy is also an alternative to upper tract diversion if ureteral emptying improves after a brief period of urethral catheter drainage.

Vesicostomy has also been employed as a permanent method of urinary diversion, especially in older children and adults. Complications include poor vesical emptying with a large residual urine, chronic bacilluria, stone formation, and difficulty in fitting a stomal appliance.

Blocksom technique.—The technique is shown in Figure 129–2. A 2-cm transverse skin incision is made halfway between the symphysis pubis and umbilicus. The rectus fascia is incised transversely and a small triangle of fascia excised. The rectus muscles are then separated in the midline, exposing the bladder. The bladder is mobilized superiorly with the aid of traction sutures and the peritoneum peeled off the dome, which is mobilized well out into the incision. The wall of the bladder is sutured to the fascia with interrupted chromic catgut and the dome of the bladder incised. The edges of the bladder are sutured to the skin with interrupted chromic catgut or Dexon. It is important to ex-

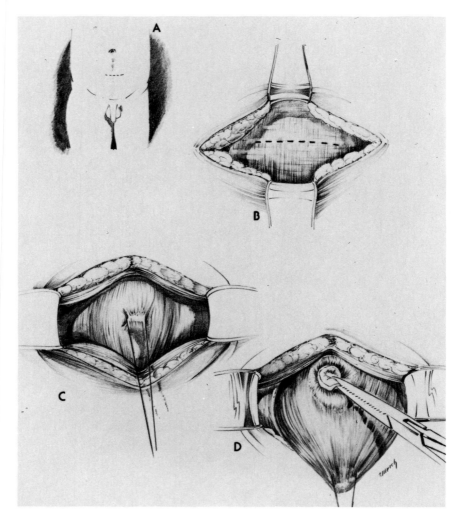

Fig 129–2.—Blocksom technique of cutaneous vesicostomy. **A,** a small transverse incision is made halfway between the symphysis pubis and umbilicus. **B,** the rectus fascia is incised transversely and the rectus muscles are divided in the midline, exposing the bladder. **C** and **D,** the bladder is mobilized superiorly with the aid of traction sutures and the peritoneum peeled off the dome, which is mobilized into the incision. *(Continued.)*

teriorize the dome rather than the anterior wall of the bladder, to avoid prolapse.

The main complications of this procedure have been prolapse and stenosis of the stoma. Revision of the stoma is occasionally necessary. It is sometimes difficult to do a vesicostomy in a small, thick-walled bladder. In neonates, Perlmutter has used a 1.5–2.0-cm U flap based inferiorly, midway between the umbilicus and symphysis pubis, extending to the bladder dome without using a counter incision.

Vesicostomy closure is simple and usually performed in conjunction with a program of management of the child with neurogenic bladder dysfunction (pharmacologic agents, intermittent catheterization, artificial sphincter, etc.) or following definitive treatment of the condition causing urinary retention (e.g., fulguration of posterior urethral valves).

Lapides' technique.—Lapides' technique of vesicostomy (Fig 129–3) was initially used in spinal cord injury patients and was adapted for use in older children. After the bladder is filled, a transverse incision is made two fingerbreadths above the symphysis pubis. The anterior rectus sheath is incised transversely and mobilized superiorly to the umbilicus. A skin flap 3.25 cm wide by 2.25 cm long is outlined on the abdominal wall. The flap

is then dissected free from the underlying rectus sheath and an opening made in the rectus fascia immediately underneath the skin flap by excising a portion of the sheath. This opening should not be made too large, to avoid herniation of bladder or bowel.

With the bladder distended to a volume of approximately 300 ml, a bladder flap measuring 4 × 4 cm is created. The base of the flap is cephalad in the region of the bladder dome and is created 2–3 cm wider than the apex. The bladder flap is then sutured to the skin flap with interrupted fine nonabsorbable sutures. The remainder of the defect in the bladder is closed with interrupted absorbable sutures.

This procedure, more extensive than the one described by Blocksom, is particularly suited to the older or obese child. Immediate complications of Lapides' procedure have been fistula formation and sloughs of the skin or bladder flap. However, these have not been common. Later complications have included severe stomal inflammation, increased residual urine, chronic bacilluria, calculus formation, and difficulty in wearing a suitable urinary collecting device.

LOOP CUTANEOUS URETEROSTOMY.—Several authors have employed loop cutaneous ureterostomy—the creation of a cuta-

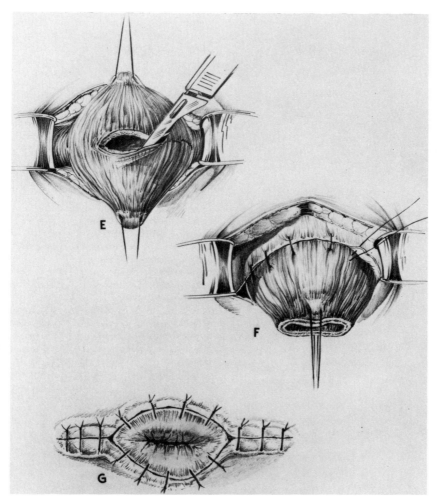

Fig 129–2 (cont.).—E, an incision is made in the dome of the bladder. **F,** the bladder wall is sutured to the fascia with interrupted chromic catgut. **G,** the edges of the bladder are sutured to the skin with interrupted chromic catgut or Dexon.

neous stoma along the lateral wall of a dilated and tortuous ureter, maintaining ureteral continuity—as the initial treatment in infants with massively dilated urinary tracts. This technique was popularized by Johnston[62] in a series of 10 children whose ureterostomies were subsequently closed. Several other reports of children who have had urinary tract reconstruction following loop cutaneous ureterostomies have appeared.[77, 91, 98] The majority of authors have concluded that a carefully performed loop cutaneous ureterostomy is well tolerated, with minimal stomal complications, and that in most cases the urinary tract can be successfully reconstructed.

Loop cutaneous ureterostomy is ideally suited to the septic and/or uremic infant with severe upper urinary tract dilatation. It quickly provides excellent drainage with minimal morbidity. The operation is appropriate *only* for the dilated, tortuous ureter that can easily be mobilized to the skin level with minimal dissection and without tension. It should not be used for the mildly dilated ureter.

Technique.—The technique is shown in Figure 129–4. With the infant in the lateral decubitus position, a posterolateral oblique skin incision is made in the upper or mid-flank region. The muscle layers are *divided* (if they are split, shifting of the layers postoperatively may create obstruction), and the retroperitoneum is entered. The upper ureter is mobilized minimally to preserve the blood supply. Bands from the proximal ureteral limb to the ureteropelvic junction are lysed to ensure that areas of relative obstruction are not present or created by the procedure. Enough ureter is mobilized to reach the skin without tension. Between fine stay sutures, a 1.0–1.5-cm incision is made along the lateral aspect of the ureter and a fine infant feeding tube passed proximally to ensure that there is no angulation. The ureteral adventitia is then sutured to the external oblique fascia anteriorly and posteriorly with fine chromic catgut. Muscle and fascial layers are not sutured under the loop of ureter, as this may cause obstruction. Stomal hernias have not been a problem. Muscle and fascial layers are reapproximated on both sides of the exteriorized ureter, which is then sutured flush at the skin level with interrupted fine Dexon or nylon. Intubation of the ureter is not necessary. The stomas are relatively easy to care for. The infant is put into large diapers, which require somewhat more frequent changing than usual.

Closure.—Although ureteral continuity can be restored by simple stomal closure, most surgeons prefer to resect the limbs of the ureterostomy and reanastomose the ureter, as the exteriorized segment may be adynamic. We prefer to wait at least 4 months after corrective operation on the lower tract before closing loop cutaneous ureterostomies, although some[29] have done both procedures simultaneously.

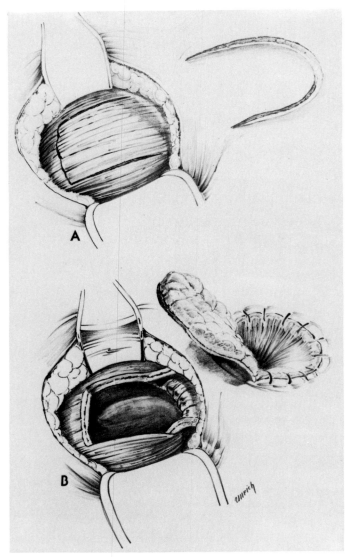

Fig 129–3.—Lapides' technique of cutaneous vesicostomy. After the bladder is filled, a transverse incision is made 2 fingerbreadths above the symphysis pubis. The anterior rectus sheath is incised transversely and mobilized to the umbilicus. **A,** the skin flap, 3.25 cm wide by 2.25 cm long, is outlined on the abdominal wall. The flap is mobilized and an opening made in the rectus fascia immediately underneath the flap. With the bladder distended to a volume of approximately 300 ml, a bladder flap measuring 4 × 4 cm is created. **B,** the bladder flap is sutured to the edges of the skin flap defect with interrupted fine nonabsorbable sutures. *(Continued.)*

The technique is shown in Figure 129–5. A circumferential incision is made around the stoma, the proximal and distal ureteral limbs are mobilized, and the stoma and redundant ureter are obliquely excised. The ureteral edges are spatulated, and the ureter anastomosed with a continuous fine chromic catgut suture. The urine is diverted for 7–10 days with a nephrostomy tube or a fine infant nasogastric tube emerging through a stab ureterotomy, distal to the anastomosis.

Y-URETEROSTOMY.—Y, or side-limb, ureterostomy, popularized by Sober[114] in 1972, permits ureteral reconstruction at the time of diversion and also allows some urine to drain to the bladder, thus preventing bladder contracture. This procedure is a modification of loop cutaneous ureterostomy and is used for sim-

ilar indications. However, the procedure is more extensive and should not be attempted in the critically ill infant.

Technique.—The surgical approach is identical to that employed for loop cutaneous ureterostomy (Fig 129–6). After a proximal end ureterostomy is established, the transected distal ureter is anastomosed to the renal pelvis, at which time it may be shortened and tailored. Most of the urine will drain to the skin, although some drains into the bladder. Closure of the Y-ureterostomy involves excising the segment of ureter draining to the skin up to the level of the renal pelvis.

END CUTANEOUS URETEROSTOMY.—This is used infrequently and should only be performed on a markedly dilated ureter. It is used as a temporary diversionary procedure chiefly in two specific instances: (1) in the child with severe uremia who requires supravesical diversion and who will be a candidate for renal transplantation; (2) to divert the upper pole ureter associated with an ectopic ureterocele at the time of excision of the ureterocele and reconstruction of the trigone. This allows a delay before deciding on the definitive procedure for the upper pole, i.e., anastomosis of the upper pole ureter to the lower pole pelvis or nephrectomy. End cutaneous ureterostomy has also been used as a temporary diversion with the option of ureteroneocystostomy at a later date.

As a permanent method of diversion, cutaneous ureterostomy offers a simple method of supravesical urinary diversion, most applicable to the rare child with markedly dilated ureters[15] who is perhaps azotemic and who does not have a reconstructable urinary tract. In the reasonably healthy child with severe bilateral hydroureter, most surgeons prefer one of the nonrefluxing colon conduits as a method of permanent diversion, perhaps tapering one or both ureters if necessary. Cutaneous ureterostomy must only be employed with ureters that are dilated (greater than 1 cm) and thick-walled. The basic advantages of cutaneous ureterostomy over nonrefluxing colon conduits are that it is simpler to perform, it may be done through a retroperitoneal approach, electrolyte reabsorption does not occur,[131] and the incidence of stomal stenosis has been reported to be lower.[39, 103]

Technique.—Through a low transverse incision, the ureters are isolated in the retroperitoneum, freed proximally, and straightened. A single stoma may be made in either the lower quadrant (Fig 129–7) or the midline below the umbilicus (Fig 129–8). If a midline stoma is desired, a full core of abdominal wall is excised and the ureters brought out through the opening in a gentle curve, avoiding angulation. After redundant ureter is excised, the ureters are spatulated medially and anastomosed to form a single stoma. They are then sutured to the skin with fine nylon or Dexon. An approximately 0.5-cm nipple is created. If the stoma is to be in one of the lower quadrants, the contralateral ureter may be tunneled retroperitoneally and sutured to the ipsilateral ureter at the skin level, as described above, or anastomosed to it retroperitoneally, thus creating a transureteroureterostomy. End cutaneous ureterostomies, in general, should be intubated for 5–7 days to ensure satisfactory drainage.

Lapides'[70] butterfly technique (Fig 129–9) provides another satisfactory method for joining two ureters at the skin level. A transverse skin incision is made, with formation of superior and inferior flaps. After both ureters are spatulated, the skin flaps are sutured between the ureters to prevent stricture.

When end cutaneous ureterostomy is used to divert the upper pole ureter associated with an ectopic ureterocele, the stoma may be placed through the lower transverse incision and should be everted slightly.

CUTANEOUS PYELOSTOMY.—The indications for cutaneous pyelostomy are similar to those for loop cutaneous ureterostomy. However, the renal pelvis must be very large, otherwise mobi-

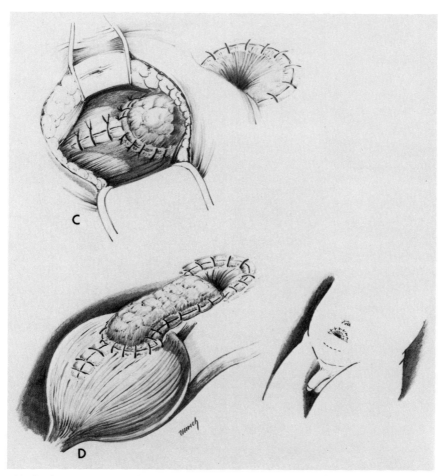

Fig 129–3 (cont.).—C, the skin flap is turned under the bridge of skin and sutured skin side down, with absorbable sutures, to the remaining edges in the defect in the bladder completing the closure. **D,** the completed closure (shown on the left as it appears with the overlying structures omitted).

lization could distort and obstruct the ureteropelvic junction, thus compromising the later closure. This procedure has also been advocated in neonates with giant hydronephrosis from ureteropelvic obstruction to promote drainage and maximal renal function before deciding whether pyeloplasty or nephrectomy is indicated.

Technique.—The technique is shown in Figure 129–10. The incision and approach are similar to those used in loop cutaneous ureterostomy. The retroperitoneum is entered and the renal pelvis mobilized sufficiently to be exteriorized. It is important to exteriorize the renal pelvis posteriorly and not to distort or angulate the ureteropelvic junction.

Closure.—Cutaneous pyelostomy is closed by mobilizing the pelvis and closing it with a running fine chromic catgut stitch. The ureteropelvic junction must not be disturbed during closure.

DISCUSSION.—The nonintubated temporary urinary diversionary procedures described above are rapid, technically easy forms of diversion that can be lifesaving for the newborn with severe dilatation of the upper urinary tract, sepsis, and uremia. These procedures have a low morbidity rate and allow for a period of growth and development of the child, with opportunities for periodic assessment of renal, ureteral, and bladder function. They also permit reconstruction of the urinary tract to be performed electively when the child is in good health. Unlike the situation with intubated diversions, there is no urgency in completing the repair. Problems encountered with these various forms of diver-

sion have usually resulted from faulty patient selection and less than meticulous dissection.

Failure of subsequent operation on the lower ureter for reflux or obstruction has not been a problem, even with a defunctionalized distal ureter. In addition, we have not found a defunctionalized bladder incapable of re-expansion, even after years of remaining "dry." However, a small capacity in a chronically infected bladder is still a possibility and may be a problem. Careful preservation of ureteral blood supply during ureteral reconstruction and reimplantation is critical, and cycling the bladder with saline to simulate normal urinary filling and voiding over a period of 5–10 days in the early postoperative period is sometimes helpful.

Bacilluria, present in many of the infants with tubeless forms of diversion, generally has not led to symptomatic infection or progressive renal damage. It is important to treat infection vigorously when continuity of the urinary tract is restored.

Other tubeless diversions, such as ileal, ileocecal, and sigmoid conduits, formerly considered to be permanent, are sometimes reconnected to the urinary tract or intact bowel and in that sense can also be temporary. These methods of diversion are discussed below.

Permanent Urinary Diversion

Despite increasing experience and facility with extensive reconstruction of the urinary tract, the use of pharmacologic

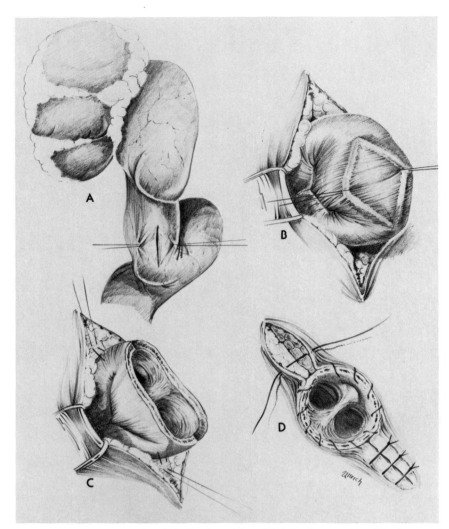

Fig 129–4.—Technique of loop cutaneous ureterostomy. **A** and **B,** after the upper ureter is mobilized to reach the skin without tension, a 1.0–1.5-cm incision is made along the lateral aspect of the ureter. **C,** the ureteral adventitia is sutured to the external oblique fascia anteriorly and posteriorly with fine chromic catgut. To avoid obstruction, muscle and fascia are not sutured under the loop of the ureter but are reapproximated on both sides of the exteriorized ureter, which is then **(D)** sutured flush at the skin level with interrupted fine Dexon or nylon.

agents, intermittent catheterization, artificial mechanical devices for urinary continence and decompression, and increasing emphasis on "undiversion," there are still several conditions that require the urine to be diverted permanently. The most common conditions requiring permanent diversion in children are exstrophy of the bladder, neurogenic bladder dysfunction, and tumors of the lower urinary tract. In addition, children with uremia and very severe dilatation of the urinary tract unresponsive to reconstructive surgical procedures may also require diversion. Many children who underwent "permanent" diversion in the past for conditions amenable to rehabilitative efforts have subsequently been "undiverted." Very careful selection is demanded before deciding on permanent diversion in a child. In some children, diversion should be used only after other modes of therapy have been exhausted.

Ureterosigmoidostomy

Ureterosigmoidostomy is an internal method of diversion that has been primarily used in children with exstrophy of the blad-der and lower urinary tract malignancies. Before the popularization of the submucosal tunnel technique of Leadbetter with accurate mucosa-to-mucosa anastomosis, ureterosigmoidostomy frequently led to pyelonephritis, stone formation, and eventual renal deterioration. However, long-term results[6, 115] with the antireflux technique have been good, and certainly this method of urinary diversion deserves prime consideration, especially in the child with exstrophy who is not a candidate for primary closure.

This operation is contraindicated in children with significant bilateral ureterectasis or in the child with a lax anal sphincter. This obviously precludes its usage in children with neurogenic vesical dysfunction. Spence[115] recommended that ureterosigmoidostomy be done in the patient with exstrophy between the ages of 3 and 6 months. Hendren[52] advocated a two-stage ureterosigmoidostomy. The first stage is the formation of a nonrefluxing sigmoid conduit (see below); subsequent anastomosis of the conduit to the intact sigmoid colon is done at a later date if there is no evidence of reflux or obstruction and anal sphincter tone is satisfactory. Because a few children with exstrophy of the bladder have deficient anal sphincter tone, we usually delay opera-

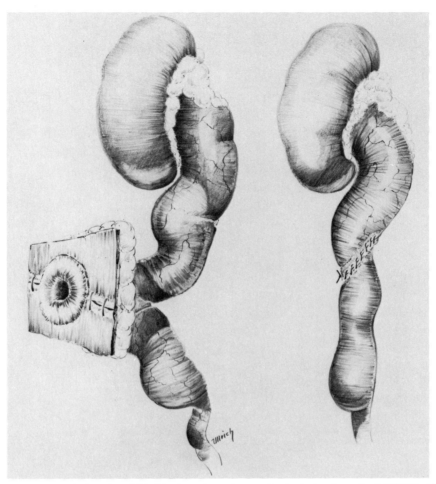

Fig 129–5.—Closure of loop ureterostomy. A circumferential incision is made around the stoma, the proximal and distal ureteral limbs are mobilized, and the stoma and redundant ureter excised obliquely. After the ureteral edges are spatulated, the ureter is anastomosed with a continuous fine chromic catgut suture.

tion until the child is approximately 18 months old, when rectal control can be better evaluated. Sphincter control is also tested preoperatively by the use of an oatmeal enema.

Technique.—The technique is shown in Figure 129–11. After the bowel is prepared mechanically and with neomycin, the abdomen is opened through a left paramedian incision. Both ureters are identified as they cross the iliac vessels. They are isolated, traced inferiorly and divided close to the bladder. The sigmoid colon is grasped between Babcock clamps, and the site for the right anastomosis is prepared first. With a fine-gauge needle, a 4–5-cm area along the tenia is infiltrated submucosally with a dilute epinephrine solution. This aids hemostasis and the development of the proper plane. An incision is then made along the tenia until the submucosa pouts up. The muscle is separated from the submucosa with scissors. It is important to reflect the muscle widely to ensure an adequate tunnel. An incision is made at the distalmost portion of the exposed submucosa, and the spatulated ureter is anastomosed to the mucosa with interrupted 5-0 chromic catgut. The seromuscular layer is then reapproximated over the ureter with interrupted 4-0 silk. The most proximal portion of the tunnel should allow passage of a right-angle clamp, to avoid constricting the ureter. The ureteral adventitia is then sutured to the serosa of the sigmoid just proximal to the tunnel with one or two 5-0 silk sutures to take tension off the anastomosis. The left ureteral anastomosis is performed at a slightly higher level on the sigmoid. It is important that both ureters have a smooth course without angulation. The anastomoses are retroperitonealized if at all possible. A Penrose drain is placed in the pelvis for 48 hours. Stents are not employed. A large-caliber rectal tube is taped in place and left indwelling for several days following the procedure.

Others have recommended different types of ureteral-sigmoid anastomoses. Goodwin[46] uses a transcolonic anastomosis. Mathisen[80] devised a nipple-valve technique, which is useful when sufficient length of ureter is not available.

Complications and Results

One of the major complications of ureterosigmoidostomy has been a reported 15% incidence of ureterosigmoid anastomotic obstruction, sometimes occurring rather late. Because the lower colon is highly absorptive, electrolyte imbalance is a common postoperative complication of ureterosigmoidostomy. Hyperchloremic acidosis with potassium depletion has been consistently observed. These findings are accentuated in children with marginal renal function. It is often desirable to use regular bicarbonate and potassium supplementation.

The major long-term complication of ureterosigmoidostomy is the increased risk for the development of adenocarcinoma at the site of the ureterocolic anastomosis. There is a several

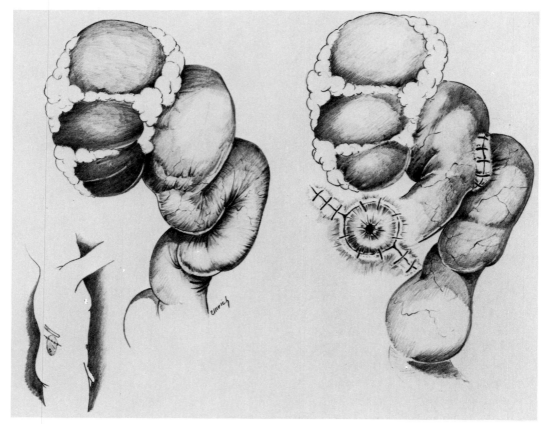

Fig 129–6.—Technique of Y-ureterostomy. After a proximal end ureterostomy is constructed, the transected distal ureter is anastomosed to the renal pelvis. For undiversion, the limit leading from the pelvis to the skin is excised.

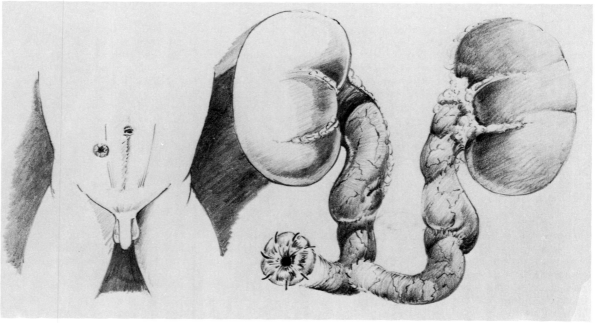

Fig 129–7.—Technique of single-stoma end cutaneous ureterostomy with transureteroureterostomy.

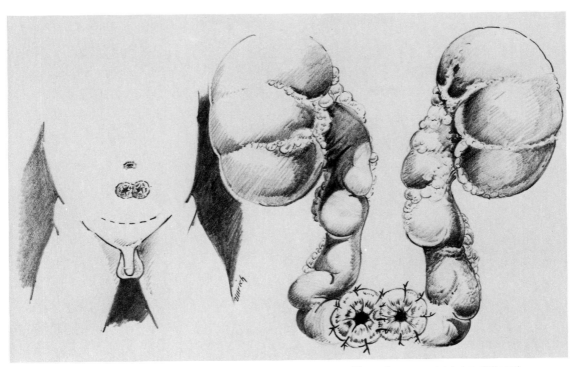

Fig 129–8.—Technique of double stoma end cutaneous ureterostomy. The ureters are spatulated medially and united to form a single stoma, and an approximately 0.5-cm nipple is created.

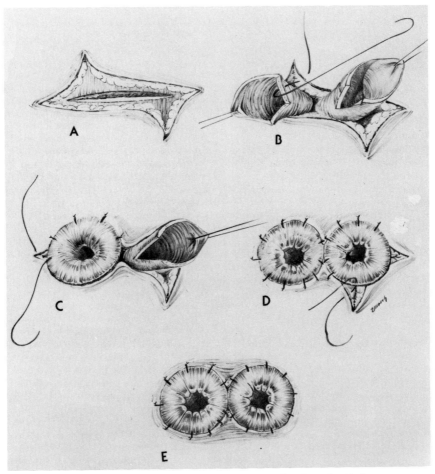

Fig 129–9.—Technique of butterfly cutaneous ureterostomy (Lapides).

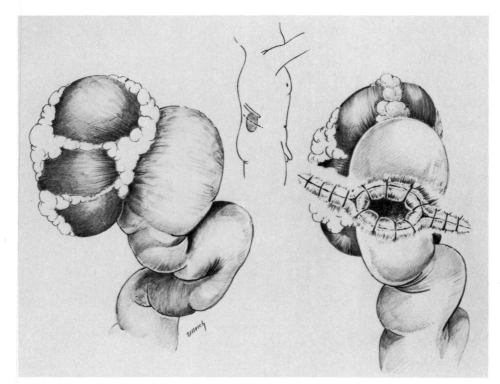

Fig 129–10.—Technique of cutaneous pyelostomy. The renal pelvis should be exteriorized posteriorly and care taken not to distort or angulate the ureteropelvic junction.

hundred-fold increased risk of carcinoma in these patients; these colon cancers generally appear at a much earlier age than usual.[6, 34, 73, 83, 89, 94, 109, 116, 117, 125, 133] For this reason, ureterosigmoidostomy has been rejected by some for urinary diversion in benign disease of children.[94] Excretory urograms must therefore be obtained annually for the life of the individual who has ureterosigmoidostomies. The finding of hydronephrosis in a child with a previously undilated upper urinary tract should suggest tumor at the anastomosis. We have also been performing colonoscopy routinely, starting at the seventh postoperative year.

The etiology of the adenocarcinoma is unknown. Tumors have occurred at the ureterosigmoid junction left in situ many years after diversion of the urine to an ileal conduit[34, 89, 109, 116] or after nephrectomy. It has been shown in rats that adenocarcinoma does not develop at the bladder-bowel junction if the fecal stream is diverted.[21] The staged ureterosigmoidostomy,[52] using a nonrefluxing colon conduit initially with later reanastomosis to the intact colon, may reduce the incidence of tumor by excluding the ureterocolic anastomosis from the fecal stream.

Cutaneous Diversions

THE STOMA.—Perhaps the most important consideration in the construction of the various cutaneous diversions to be discussed is the site and construction of the stoma.[25] Certainly, it is the most important to the patient and to a great extent determines the patient's acceptance of the procedure. Poorly constructed stomas predispose to leakage around the appliance, local inflammation and encrustation, bleeding, and stenosis.

The stomal site should not be near the umbilicus or abdominal scars and should not be close to any adjacent bony structure. The site should be flat and should be chosen with the child in both erect and supine positions. It is advisable to have children wear

an appliance on the proposed stomal location for a few days prior to operation to ascertain that the placement is correct. Although the conventional location for a urinary stoma is usually described as just below the center of a line connecting the anterior superior iliac spine to the umbilicus, in practice stomal locations are usually higher, especially in the child with myelodysplasia. The best stomal locations in many of these children are in the upper quadrant or even in the epigastrium.

Creation of the Stoma.—In most instances it is possible and desirable to prepare the stomal site before making the abdominal incision. This avoids the baffle effect of the abdominal wall, which can cause relative obstruction.

The technique for creation of the stoma is shown in Figure 129–12. A segment of skin that is somewhat larger than a quarter is excised. A core of subcutaneous tissue, fascia, and muscle is also removed. The posterior fascia and peritoneum are incised in cruciate fashion. In this manner, the opening from skin into the abdominal cavity should be straight and allow two fingers to be snugly inserted.

To prevent herniation around the stoma, fascia should be sutured to the serosa of the bowel with interrupted 3-0 chromic catgut. When it is not feasible to create the stoma before making the abdominal incision, all layers of the abdomen should be grasped in alignment during the creation of the stoma.

It is desirable to have a stomal bud of 1–2 cm to allow proper application of the permanent appliance. The bud is created by first placing quadrant sutures of 4-0 Dexon through the skin, the seromuscular layer of the bowel just above the fixation of the bowel to the fascia, and the full thickness of the bowel edge. Tying these sutures creates a very adequate bud, and the anastomosis can be completed by suturing skin to the edge of bowel.

A particular problem has been encountered with stomas created from large intestine. This has been the undesirable increase

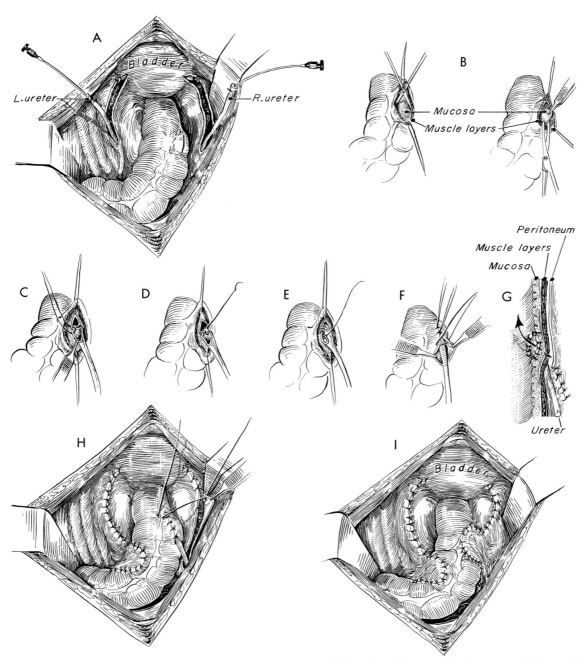

Fig 129–11.—Technique of ureterosigmoidostomy. Both ureters are identified as they cross the iliac vessels. They are isolated and divided close to the bladder **(A).** Not shown in the illustration, the sigmoid colon is grasped between Babcock clamps and the tenia infiltrated submucosally with a dilute epinephrine solution. **B,** an incision is made along the tenia, and the seromuscular layer separated from the submucosa with sharp and blunt dissection. **C–E,** an incision is made at the distal portion of the exposed submucosa, and the spatulated ureter is anastomosed to the mucosa with interrupted 5-0 chromic catgut. **F,** the seromuscular layer is reapproximated over the ureter with interrupted 4-0 silk. **G,** tunnel length should be approximately 4 cm. **H, I,** the anastomoses are retroperitonealized if at all possible.

in the diameter and bulkiness of the stoma, especially when compared with the small delicate ileal stomas that many of these children had previously. This can be circumvented by tapering the stoma. A triangular wedge is excised from the antimesenteric wall of the large bowel with the base distally and closed with two layers of chromic catgut. This decreases the diameter of the stoma without significantly reducing the capacity of the conduit.

THE ILEAL CONDUIT.—Although no form of urinary diversion is ideal, for many years the ileal conduit was considered to offer the best possibility of stable renal function, absence of electrolyte problems, and a decent stoma. Recently, however, several authors[106, 108, 110, 112] have reported major long-term complications of this form of diversion. Stomal stenosis has always been recognized as a problem, and revisions may be necessary in at least 40% of children. Some children have required two or even more stomal revisions.

Of greater concern are the observations of ureteroileal or in-

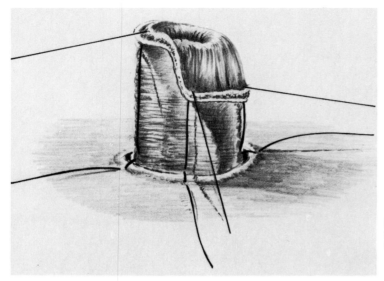

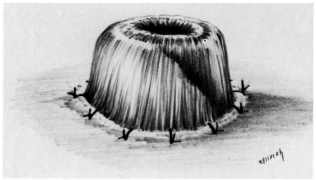

Fig 129–12.—Cutaneous ureterostomy—creation of the stoma. Sutures are placed through the skin and seromuscular layer of the bowel and bowel edge to create an adequate bud; the bowel edge is additionally sutured to the skin.

trinsic loop strictures occurring as late as 10–15 years postoperatively. It is also believed that a combination of reflux and infection has caused chronic pyelonephritis in many of these children. Increasing concern with the aforementioned problems has led to an increased utilization of nonrefluxing colon conduits. In our institution, since 1974, no ileal conduit has been performed as a method of permanent urinary diversion. It remains to be seen whether the nonrefluxing types of diversion will ultimately prove to be better.

Technique.—The technique is shown in Figure 129–13. After the stomal site has been prepared, the abdomen is opened through a left paramedian incision. Both ureters are isolated as they cross the iliac vessels, traced distally for a few centimeters, ligated, and divided. The proximal ends of the ureters are mobilized superiorly, the left ureter being mobilized somewhat more than the right, and then brought under the sigmoid mesentery to lie in a nice, gentle curve. A segment of ileum is chosen approximately 15–20 cm from the ileocecal valve; the segment should be 12–15 cm in length and supplied by two radial arteries. The distal mesentery is incised 5–6 cm to ensure adequate mobility of the isolated segment. The proximal mesentery need only be incised 2–3 cm. The bowel is divided, the ileal segment falling inferiorly, and continuity of the intestine is restored.

The proximal end of the ileal segment is turned in with a Parker-Kerr continuous catgut stitch reinforced by fine silk Lembert sutures. This end of the ileum is tacked down to the small-bowel mesentery with two fine catgut sutures. Both ureteroileal anastomoses are made on the antimesenteric surface of the ileum, the left one 2.5 cm from the turned-in upper end of the loop. Fine chromic catgut is used to tack the ureter to the bowel serosa to eliminate tension on the anastomosis. An incision is made in the bowel and a small portion of mucosa excised. With 4-0 and 5-0 chromic catgut, the right ureter is anastomosed to the ileum approximately 2 cm from the left. Wallace[124] advocated joining both ureters together in gun-barrel fashion and anastomosing them to the end of the loop. The isolated ileal segment is then brought through the opening previously made in the abdominal wall and any excess of the loop resected. Any bowstring effect of the mesentery or the loop may be corrected by incising the mesentery further. The external oblique aponeurosis is sutured to the ileal serosa in several places to prevent a parastomal hernia. The stoma is then fashioned to ensure an adequate nipple. A finger should easily pass into the ileal segment without compression by the abdominal wall. After the abdomen is closed, a temporary appliance is placed over the stoma. We ordinarily do not recommend stenting the ureteroileal anastomoses or placing a catheter in the loop for temporary drainage.

PYELOILEALCUTANEOUS OR PYELOJEJUNOCUTANEOUS ANASTOMOSIS.—During the early 1960s, pyeloilealcutaneous diversion was advocated by Holland, King, and associates[57, 58, 66] as a method of stabilizing renal function in children with large, adynamic ureters. With increasing emphasis on reconstructive surgery of the large ureter, the initial enthusiasm for this procedure has waned. We have employed this method of high diversion in only one child during the past 10 years. In the child who continues to form stones it should be considered to permit easy passage of these calculi to the exterior.

Technique.—This type of diversion is somewhat more of a procedure than the ileal conduit (Fig 129–14). A rather long segment (20–25 cm) of high ileum is isolated and is placed above the intestinal anastomosis rather than below it, as in the ileal conduit. The proximal and distal incisions in the mesentery should be at least 5–6 cm long to ensure adequate mobility of the segment. This is more easily accomplished with the proximal ileum or jejunum than with the distal ileum. The hepatic and splenic flexures are mobilized medially to expose both renal pelves. The segment of intestine is passed through a retroperitoneal tunnel behind the duodenum and pancreas and anterior to the aorta and vena cava and anastomosed to both renal pelves.

The procedure has been modified by employing two smaller segments of bowel, anastomosing each to a renal pelvis, and then anastomosing one segment to the other in a Roux-en-Y fashion. This procedure may allow a straighter course of the intestine from kidneys to skin.

Nonrefluxing Colon Conduits

The increasing number of late complications with ileal conduit diversion has prompted the use of the colon as a urinary conduit. The occurrence of chronic pyelonephritis following ileal conduit diversion has been attributed to reflux with infection. Richie et al.[100] have also shown in animal experiments the increased incidence of histologic pyelonephritis in freely refluxing ileal con-

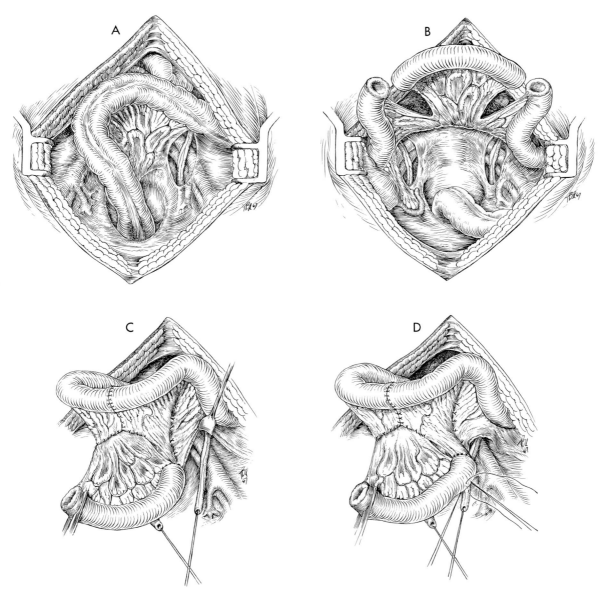

Fig 129–13.—Technique of ileal conduit formation. **A,** the sigmoid colon is reflected medially and the left ureter exposed as it crosses the iliac vessels. The right ureter is exposed in similar fashion. **B,** a segment of ileum is chosen approximately 15–20 cm from the ileocecal valve. It should be 12–15 cm in length and supplied by two radial arteries. The distal mesentery is incised 5–6 cm to ensure adequate mobility of the isolated segment. Proximally the mesentery need only be incised 2–3 cm. **C,** the ileal segment is dropped inferiorly and the bowel reconstructed. The proximal end of the ileal segment is closed and sutured to the posterior peritoneum. The left ureter is brought under the sigmoid mesentery to lie in a gentle curve and anastomosed to the ileum. **D,** the adventitia of the ureter is approximated to the serosa of the ileum to eliminate tension on the anastomosis. *(Continued.)*

duits when compared with nonrefluxing colon conduits. In addition, the incidence of stomal stenosis appears lower with the colon than with the small intestine. The following two methods of diversion are being employed in children with increasing frequency as methods of permanent or, in some instances, temporary urinary diversion. The initial results with both procedures have been excellent. The incidence of reflux, ureteral obstruction, and stomal stenosis has been low. However, enthusiasm for these methods of diversion should be reserved until long-term results become available.

THE SIGMOID CONDUIT.—The sigmoid conduit is the method of permanent urinary diversion that I currently use in children.

The indications for diversion are similar to those for ileal conduit diversion, i.e., neurogenic bladder dysfunction with repeated attacks of pyelonephritis and some tumors of the lower urinary tract. We have also used it in a number of children to convert failing ileal conduits to sigmoid conduits. Hendren[51, 52] has recommended the use of the sigmoid conduit as a temporary method of urinary diversion in infants with exstrophy of the bladder, to be later reconnected to the sigmoid colon after it is ascertained that the conduit is functioning well without reflux and the child has acceptable rectal control.

Technique.—The technique is shown in Figure 129–15. Stomal considerations are analogous to those for the ileal conduit, except that the stoma is usually located on the left side of the

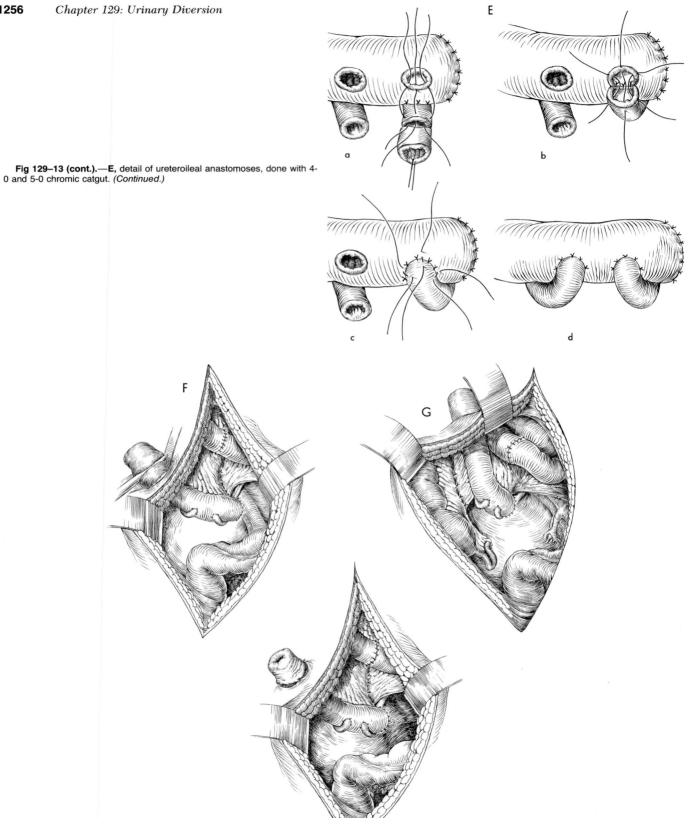

Fig 129–13 (cont.).—E, detail of ureteroileal anastomoses, done with 4-0 and 5-0 chromic catgut. *(Continued.)*

Fig 129–13 (cont.).—F, the conduit is brought through the previously created defect in the abdominal wall and excess ileum resected. **G,** closure of the right lateral gutter is optional. The appendix, seen here, in most situations would have been removed at the beginning of the operation. **H,** the completed ileal conduit with a 1–2-cm everted bud.

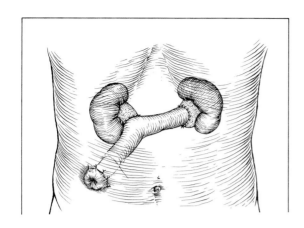

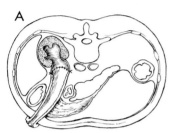
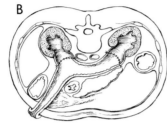

Fig 129–14.—Pyeloilealcutaneous or pyelojejunocutaneous conduit. A long segment of high ileum or jejunum measuring 20–25 cm is isolated and bowel continuity reestablished below the mesentery of the isolated segment. **A,** the intestine is anastomosed to the renal pelvis of the solitary kidney. **B,** the segment of intestine, passed through a retroperitoneal tunnel behind the duodenum and pancreas and anterior to the aorta and vena cava, has been anastomosed to both renal pelves.

abdomen. In children with ileal conduits being converted to sigmoid conduits, we prefer to use the previously located stomal site. The mobility of the sigmoid colon in children readily allows this.

The abdomen is opened through a paramedian incision and the ureters isolated and divided over the pelvic brim. The lateral attachments of the sigmoid colon are incised and a 15-cm segment chosen, with due care to ensure a broad blood supply. The isolated segment may be placed lateral or medial to the bowel anastomosis. The conduit is rotated 180 degrees to make it isoperistaltic and the proximal end closed with a Parker-Kerr stitch of chromic catgut and interrupted fine silk Lembert sutures. The ureteral anastomoses, done by a submucosal tunnel technique, should provide a tunnel length of 3–4 cm. The tunnels are staggered along the teniae, which are infiltrated with a dilute epinephrine solution to minimize bleeding and help define the correct plane. The teniae are incised and the seromuscular wall reflected from the submucosa. Most of the undermining is done laterally to avoid devitalizing the medial portion between the two ureteral tunnels. It is important to provide a tunnel adequate in width as well as length. The mucosa is incised at the distal portion of the tunnel, and the ureters are spatulated slightly and anastomosed to the mucosa with interrupted 5-0 chromic catgut. The seromuscular layer is then closed over the ureter with interrupted 4-0 silk. It is important to be able to insert a right-angle clamp easily into the entrance of the tunnel to ensure that the ureter is not constricted. The ureteral wall is also sutured to the serosa of the bowel just proximal to the tunnel with one or two fine chromic catgut sutures to take tension off the anastomosis. The stoma is constructed in a manner similar to that used for the ileal conduit stoma.

Large ureters may be implanted in the sigmoid conduit after being tapered. In this situation, no. 5 infant feeding tubes are left indwelling to protect the suture lines.

Results of Sigmoid Conduit Diversion.—A number of authors have reported encouraging results with sigmoid conduit diversion.[2, 84, 85] Althausen and associates[1] found no cases of stomal stenosis, a 10% incidence of ureterocolic stenosis, and a 14% incidence of low-pressure reflux in 40 children with sigmoid conduits followed from 1 to 8 years. However, a recent long-term follow-up report[31] on 41 children with the sigmoid conduit contrasted with the initial encouraging findings. In this series from Wales, with an average follow-up of 13.2 years, there was a 61% incidence of stomal stenosis, a 22% incidence of ureterocolic obstruction, a 58% incidence of coloureteral reflux, and a 48% incidence of upper urinary tract deterioration. Enthusiasm for any of the nonrefluxing colon conduits must be reserved until further long-term results become available.[22]

THE ILEOCECAL CONDUIT.—Although ileocecocystoplasty has often been employed for a variety of conditions during the past few years, the use of this segment of bowel as a urinary conduit has not received much attention. Zinman and Libertino[134] emphasized the effectiveness of the ileocecal valve as an antirefluxing mechanism. This intestinal segment has certain anatomical advantages as a conduit over other colonic segments. The ileocolic vessels supplying it are constant and are easily mobilized on a long mesentery. In obese patients with thick mesenteric attachments, they can be isolated accurately by palpation of the ileocolic and right colic arteries.

Other advantages of ileocecocystoplasty: (1) subsequent undiversion is easy; (2) stomal problems are minimal; (3) the segments can be added on to a pre-existing ileal segment if the ureteroileal anastomoses are well-functioning; (4) it is probably the procedure of choice for absent, short, or dilated ureters; and (5) incidence of tumor development may be lowered if internal diversion (ureterosigmoidostomy) is to be performed.

In our series of more than 60 children with ileocecal segment diversions, approximately 80% had failed ileal conduits. Most of these were patients with myelodysplasia. We have also employed this method of diversion in the few children with neurogenic bladder dysfunction not successfully managed by intermittent catheterization, pharmacologic means, bladder neck operation, or implantation of an artificial sphincter. It has also been used in children with malignant tumors of the bladder or prostate, and as a temporary method of urinary diversion as part of a series of operations to reconstruct complex anomalies such as exstrophy of the bladder or cloaca, severe female epispadias with maldevelopment of the bladder, or bilateral single ectopic ureters.

The ileocecal segment can be anastomosed to the sigmoid. If an ileocecal conduit with a well-functioning antireflux mechanism is anastomosed to the colon, contact between the uroepithelium and fecal stream will be minimized.

Technique.—The technique is shown in Figure 129–16. Through a midline incision the cecum, right colon and hepatic flexure are mobilized. The right ureter is isolated below the pelvic brim. The constant ileocolic vessels are identified and the ileum divided 10 cm proximal to the ileocecal valve. The ascending colon is divided proximal to the right colic artery and the mesentery incised appropriately. A 30 F catheter is introduced into the ileum, through the ileocecal valve, to emerge through the colonic stoma. The antireflux mechanism is obtained by plicating the cecum around the terminal ileum in a collarlike fashion. The use of a catheter avoids too much narrowing of the distal ileum during this process.

The ileum is then intussuscepted into the cecum for two to three cm with several sero-muscular sutures of 3-0 Tevdek. The anterior and posterior walls of the cecum are then wrapped like

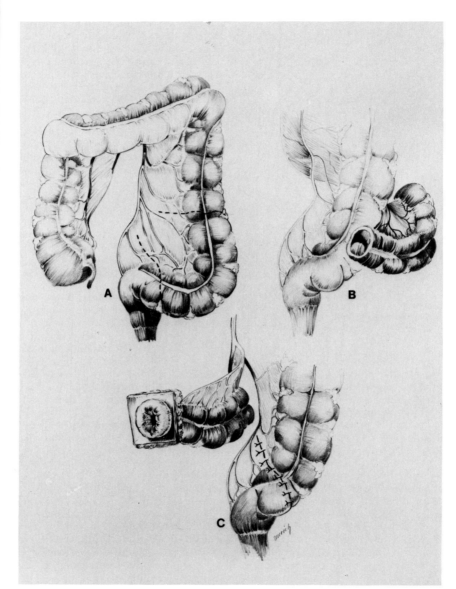

Fig 129–15.—Technique for the sigmoid conduit. **A,** a segment of sigmoid colon approximately 15 cm long is chosen. Incisions are made in the mesentery to ensure a broad blood supply. **B** and **C,** the isolated segment may be placed lateral or medial to the reconstructed bowel. The conduit is rotated 180 degrees to make it isoperistaltic and the proximal end closed. *(Continued.)*

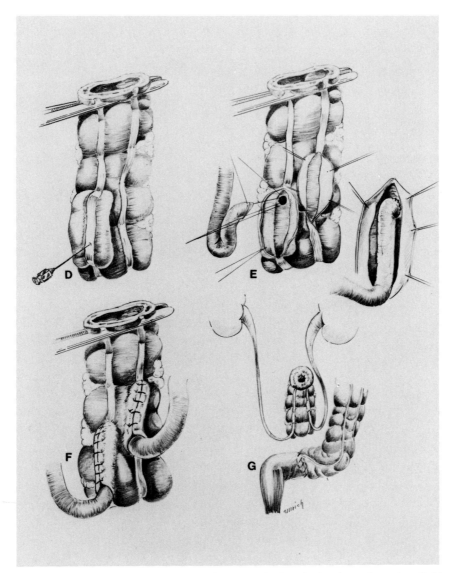

Fig 129–15 (cont.).—D, a dilute epinephrine solution injected along the tenia minimizes bleeding and defines the correct plane. **E,** the teniae are incised and the seromuscular wall reflected from the submucosa. Most of the undermining is done laterally to avoid devitalizing the area between the two tunnels. The mucosa is incised at the distal portion of the tunnel; the ureters are spatulated slightly and anastomosed to the mucosa with interrupted 5-0 chromic catgut. **F,** the sero-muscular layer is closed over the ureter with interrupted 4-0 silk. The proximal portion of the tunnel should allow the insertion of a right-angle clamp to ensure that the ureter is not constricted. **G,** the completed sigmoid conduit, after the stoma has been constructed in a manner similar to that for the ideal conduit stoma.

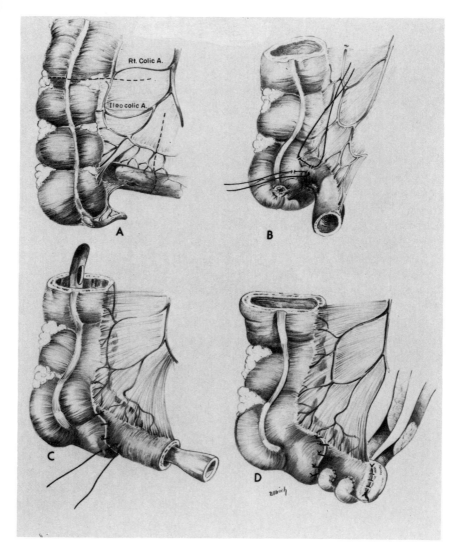

Fig 129–16.—Technique for the ileocecal conduit. **A,** the isolated ileocecal segment is based on the ileocolic vascular pedicle. **B,** the ileum is intussuscepted into the cecum for 2 cm with three seromuscular sutures of 3-0 Tevdek. **C** and **D,** the anterior and posterior walls of the cecum are wrapped like a collar around the terminal 4 cm of ileum in a 200-degree encircling fashion with seromuscular nonabsorbable sutures incorporating ileum and cecum on either side of the mesentery. The ureteroileal anastomoses may be performed separately, or a conjoint ureteroureterostomy may be constructed and sutured to the open proximal end of the conduit. *(Continued.)*

a collar around the terminal 4 cm of ileum in a 270 degree encircling fashion with interrupted sero-muscular Tevdek incorporating ileum and cecum on either side of the mesentery.

Hendren[53] has outlined an alternate technique for reflux prevention in which 6–8 cm of terminal ileum that has been scarified is intussuscepted into the cecum. The antireflux mechanism is tested by inflating the ascending colon and measuring pressures. The valve mechanism should be continent to at least 50 cm of water. It is advisable to make absolutely certain that the intussusception has not obstructed the flow of fluid from the ileum to the cecum.

The left ureter is then isolated lateral to the sigmoid colon and brought under the sigmoid mesentery through the peritoneal opening on the right side. The ureteral-ileal anastomoses are performed in a manner similar to that described for the ileal conduit after the proximal ileum is closed. Alternatively, I prefer a conjoint uretero-ureterostomy (Wallace technique), which is constructed by incising the ureters medially for 3 cm, suturing their walls with interrupted 5-0 chromic catgut and anastomosing the resultant single opening to the open proximal ileum.

Results of Ileocecal Conduit Diversion.—In adults, the results of ileocecal conduit diversion have been excellent.[111] Zinman has reported almost uniform success with the antireflux mechanism that he described.[134] The incidence of obstruction is minimal.

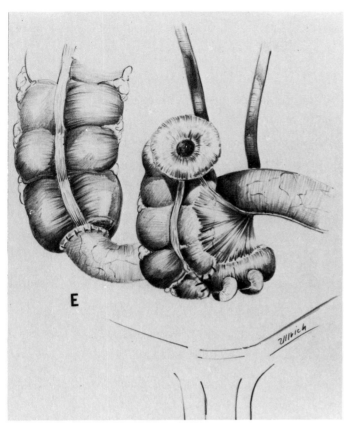

Fig 129–16 (cont.).—**E,** the completed ileocecal conduit is brought out through a previously constructed right lower quadrant defect.

Fig 129–17.—Technique for continent urinary ileostomy. **A,** distal ileum is scarified to encourage permanent adhesion of the intussuscepted ileum. **B,** ureters are tunneled into the ascending colon. **C,** completed continent ileostomy.

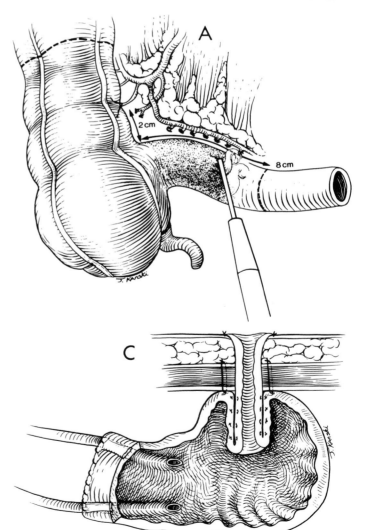

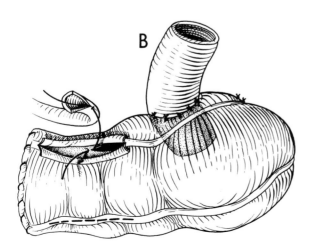

Long-term results of the ileocecal conduit in children are not yet available, although the short-term results are encouraging. The incidence of obstruction is negligible and the incidence of low pressure reflux is minimal. Reflux at higher pressures is seen more often, and this, in general, is not a problem when the ileocecal segment is used as a conduit. However, if the conduit is subsequently anastomosed to the bladder and subjected to higher intravesical pressures, the nipple often is completely reduced and free reflux has been observed.

The other major complication of the ileocecal conduit has been prolapse of the stoma. This is best prevented and treated by tapering the stoma and making the opening in the abdominal wall smaller.

TRANSVERSE COLON CONDUIT.—The transverse colon conduit is infrequently used as a method of diversion in children. It is almost exclusively employed in children with pelvic rhabdomyosarcoma undergoing cystectomy and extensive pelvic radiation requiring high cutaneous diversion. It is an excellent method of diversion and uses nonirradiated bowel.[85] Long tunnels to prevent reflux are easily constructed, as with the sigmoid conduit. Some of the long-term survivors of malignancy merit consideration for internal diversion by anastomosis of the transverse colon conduit to the sigmoid colon.

CONTINENT URINARY DIVERSIONS.—There has been some emphasis in recent years on continent urinary diversions. These have been most appealing to adolescents and young adults who cannot tolerate wearing an appliance. Certainly the concept of a continent urinary diversion is quite attractive, especially to a young person who has a benign condition and a normal life expectancy.

Schneider et al.[107] reported their technique for a continent vesicostomy. The mechanism relies on an intussuscepted bladder flap. This procedure has had some success in adults, but in general has been unsuccessful in children. In a teenager, S.B. Bauer bridged the gap between the bladder and abdominal wall with an isolated segment of ileum whose proximal end was intussuscepted into the bladder providing total continence. The bladder neck in such patients must be surgically closed.

A more popular form of continent urinary diversion involves the use of the ileum or ileocecal segment. In 1973, Sullivan et al.[119] reported their results with the continent ureterocecocutaneous ileostomy developed by Gilchrist[44] in 1950. The success rate was 94% in 40 patients followed at least 10 years. This technique was never really pursued and never really caught on. It involves the isolation of an ileocecal segment in which the ureters are tunneled in antireflux fashion along the tenia in the cecum. The ileum is intussuscepted into the cecum to provide continence and the proximal portion of the ileum brought out as the stoma (Fig 129–17).

Kock[68, 69] described his experiences with urinary diversion via a continent ileal reservoir, which he employed in 12 patients. An isolated ileal reservoir was constructed, using the techniques described for patients with a continent fecal ileostomy. The ureters were implanted into an afferent segment provided with a reflux-preventing nipple valve. Reoperation was necessary in seven of the 12 patients because of malfunction of the continence-producing valve. Follow-up in this group of patients ranged between 9 months and 6½ years. All patients were continent without reflux. The reservoir generally was emptied by intermittent catheterization, between three and six times per day. The volume capacity of the reservoir was more than 500 ml.

Methods of diversion, with continence, seem attractive. Encouraging long-term results would allow broader usage of these techniques.

REFERENCES

1. Althausen A.F., Hagen-Cook K., Hendren W.H.: Non-refluxing colon conduit: Experience with 70 cases. *J. Urol.* 130:35, 1978.
2. Altwein J.E., Jonas U., Hohenfellner R.: Long-term follow-up of children with colon conduit urinary diversion and ureterosigmoidostomy. *J. Urol.* 118:832, 1977.
3. Beland G.A., Weiss R.M.: Cutaneous vesicostomy in children. *J. Urol.* 94:128, 1965.
4. Bell T.E., Hoodin A.O., Evans A.T.: Tubeless cystostomy in children. *J. Urol.* 100:459, 1968.
5. Belman A.B., King L.R.: Vesicostomy: Useful means of reversible urinary diversion in selected infants. *Urology* 1:208, 1973.
6. Bennett A.H.: Exstrophy of the bladder treated by ureterosigmoidostomies: Long-term evaluation. *Urology* 2:165, 1973.
7. Binder C., Gonick P., Ciavarra V.: Experience with silastic U-tube nephrostomy. *J. Urol.* 106:499, 1971.
8. Bissada N.K., Cole A.T., Fried F.A.: Renal diversion with silicone circle catheters. *Urology* 2:238, 1973.
9. Blanchard T.W., Rinker J.R., McLendon R.L.: Cutaneous ureterostomy following blockage of the ureteral vasculature: An experimental study. *J. Urol.* 96:39, 1966.
10. Blocksom B.H. Jr.: Bladder pouch for prolonged tubeless cystotomy. *J. Urol.* 78:398, 1957.
11. Bricker E.M.: Bladder substitution after pelvic evisceration. *Surg. Clin. North Am.* 30:1511, 1950.
12. Brueziere J., Beurton D.: Traitement des mega-uretères de l'enfant et du nourrison par l'urèterostomie cutanée. 1re partie. *Ann. Urol.* 3:189, 1969.
13. Brueziere J., Beurton D.: Traitement des mega-uretères de l'enfant et du nourrison par l'urèterostomie cutanée. 2e partie. *Ann. Urol.* 4:41, 1970.
14. Carlson H.E.: Tubeless cystostomy in childhood. *J. Urol.* 83:669, 1960.
15. Claman M., Shapiro A.E., Orecklin J.R.: Cutaneous ureterostomy, the preferred diversion of the solitary functioning kidney. *Br. J. Urol.* 51:352, 1979.
16. Coffey R.C.: Transplantation of the ureters into the large intestine in the absence of a functioning urinary bladder. *Surg. Gynecol. Obstet.* 32:383, 1921.
17. Comarr A.E.: Experience with the U-tube for renal drainage among patients with spinal cord injury. *J. Urol.* 95:741, 1966.
18. Conger K.B., Toub L.: Obstruction of the bladder neck in the male infant and child: Present concepts of diagnostic methods and management, and a report of 14 cases. *J. Pediatr.* 57:855, 1960.
19. Cordonnier J.J., Nicolai C.H.: An evaluation of the use of an isolated segment of ileum as a means of urinary diversion. *J. Urol.* 83:834–838, 1960.
20. Cordonnier J.J.: Ureterosigmoid anastomosis. *Surg. Gynecol. Obstet.* 88:441, 1949.
21. Crissey M.M., Steele G.D., Gittes R.F.: Rat model for carcinogenesis in ureterosigmoidostomy. *Science* 207:1079, 1980.
22. Dagen J.E., Sanford E.J., Rohner T.J. Jr.: Complications of the non-refluxing colon conduit. *J. Urol.* 123:585, 1980.
23. Delgado G.E., Muecke E.C.: Evaluation of 80 cases of ileal conduit in children: Indications, complications, and results. *J. Urol.* 109:311, 1973.
24. Derrick W.A. Jr., Hodges C.V.: Ileal conduit stasis: Recognition, treatment and prevention. *J. Urol.* 107:747, 1972.
25. Dicus D.R.: New perspectives in the construction of the ileal stoma. *J. Urol.* 112:591, 1974.
26. Dretler S.P.: The pathogenesis of urinary tract calculi occurring after ileal conduit diversion. I. Clinical study. II. Conduit study. III. Prevention. *J. Urol.* 109:204, 1973.
27. Dretler S.P., Hendren W.H., Leadbetter W.F.: Urinary tract reconstruction following ileal conduit diversion. *J. Urol.* 109:217, 1973.
28. Duckett J.W. Jr.: Cutaneous vesicostomy in childhood: The Blocksom technique. *Urol. Clin. North Am.* 1:485, 1974.
29. Dwoskin J.Y.: Management of the massively dilated urinary tract in infants by temporary diversion and single-stage reconstruction. *Urol. Clin. North Am.* 1:515, 1974.
30. Eckstein H.B.: Cutaneous ureterostomy. *Proc. R. Soc. Med.* 56:749, 1963.
31. Elder D.D., Moisey C.U., Rees R.W.M.: A long-term follow-up of the colonic conduit operation in children. *Br. J. Urol.* 51:462, 1979.
32. Ellis D.G., Fonkalsrud E.W., Smith J.P.: Congenital posterior urethral valves. *J. Urol.* 95:549, 1966.
33. Ellis L.R., Udall D.A., Hodges C.V.: Further clinical experiences with intestinal segments for urinary diversion. *J. Urol.* 105:354, 1971.

34. Eraklis A.J., Folkman J.: Adenocarcinoma at the site of ureterosigmoidostomies for exstrophy of the bladder. *J. Pediatr. Surg.* 13:730, 1978.
35. Fein R.L., Young J.G., Van Buskirk K.E.: The case for loop ureterostomy in the infant with advanced lower urinary tract obstruction *J. Urol.* 101:513, 1969.
36. Ferris D.O., Odel H.M.: Electrolyte pattern of the blood after bilateral ureterosigmoidostomy. *JAMA* 142:634, 1950.
37. Felderhof J., Van Essen A.G., Oosterhof P.G.: Bilaterale lus-ureterostomie bij jonge kinderen als tijdelijke maatregel bij ernstige obstructie van de urinewegen. *Ned. Tijdschr. Geneeskd.* 112:1947, 1968.
38. Feminella J.G. Jr., Lattimer J.K.: A retrospective analysis of 70 cases of cutaneous ureterostomy. *J. Urol.* 106:538, 1971.
39. Filmer R.B., Honesty H.: Problems with urinary conduit stomas in children. *Urol. Clin. North Am.* 1:531, 1974.
40. Flinn R.A., King L.R., McDonald J.H., et al.: Cutaneous ureterostomy: An alternative urinary diversion. *J. Urol.* 105:358, 1971.
41. Fowler J.E., Meares E.M., Goldin A.R.: Percutaneous nephrostomy: Techniques, indications and results. *Urology* 6:428, 1975.
42. Francis D.R., Bucy J.G.: Inside-out kidney: An unusual complication of cutaneous pyelostomy. *J. Urol.* 112:514, 1974.
43. Giesy J.D., Hodges C.V.: Flaccid paralysis associated with hyperchloremic acidosis and hypokalemia following ileal loop urinary diversion. *J. Urol.* 94:243, 1965.
44. Gilchrist R.K., Merricks J.W., Hamlin H.H., et al.: Construction of a substitute bladder and urethra. *Surg. Gynecol. Obstet.* 90:752, 1950.
45. Goodwin W.E., Casey W.C., Woolf W.: Percutaneous trocar (needle) nephrostomy in hydronephrosis. *JAMA* 157:891, 1955.
46. Goodwin W.E., Harris A.P., Kaufman J.J., et al.: Open, transcolonic ureterintestinal anastomosis: A new approach. *Surg. Gynecol. Obstet.* 97:295, 1953.
47. Goodwin W.E., Scardino P.T.: Ureterosigmoidostomy. *J. Urol.* 118:169, 1977.
48. Habib H.N., McDonald D.F.: A technique for prevention of intramural obstruction of Bricker's ileal loop. *J. Urol.* 88:211, 1962.
49. Halpern G.N., King L.R., Belman A.B.: Transureteroureterostomy in children. *J. Urol.* 109:504, 1973.
50. Hendren W.H.: A new approach to infants with severe obstructive uropathy: Early complete reconstruction. *J. Pediatr. Surg.* 5:184, 1970.
51. Hendren W.H.: Exstrophy of the bladder—an alternative method of management. *J. Urol.* 115:195, 1976.
52. Hendren W.H.: Nonrefluxing colon conduit for temporary or permanent urinary diversion in children. *J. Pediatr. Surg.* 10:381, 1975.
53. Hendren W.H.: Reoperative ureteral reimplantation: Management of the difficult case. *J. Pediatr. Surg.* 15:770, 1980.
54. Hendren W.H.: Restoration of function in the severely decompensated ureter, in Johnston J.H., Scholtmeijer R.J. (eds.): *Problems in Pediatric Urology.* Amsterdam, Excerpta Medica, 1972, p. 1.
55. Hendren W.H.: Urinary tract refunctionalization after prior diversion in children. *Ann. Surg.* 180:494, 1974.
56. Hendren W.H., Hensle T.W.: Transureteroureterostomy: Experience with 75 cases. *J. Urol.* 123:826, 1980.
57. Holland J.M., King L.R., Schirmer H.K.A., et al.: High urinary diversion with an ileal conduit in children. *Pediatrics* 40:816, 1967.
58. Holland J.M., Schirmer H.K.A., King L.R., et al.: Pyeloileal urinary conduit: An 8-year experience in 37 patients. *J. Urol.* 99:427, 1969.
59. Immergut M.A., Jacobson J.J., Culp D.A., et al.: Cutaneous pyelostomy. *J. Urol.* 101:276, 1969.
60. Ireland G.W., Geist R.W.: Difficulties with vesicostomies in 15 children with meningomyelocele. *J. Urol.* 103:341, 1970.
61. Jeter K., Bloom S.: Management of stomal complications following ileal or colonic conduit operations in children. *J. Urol.* 106:425, 1971.
62. Johnston J.H.: Temporary cutaneous ureterostomy in the management of advanced congenital urinary obstruction. *Arch. Dis. Child.* 38:161, 1963.
63. Karafin L., Kendall A.R.: Vesicostomy in the management of neurogenic bladder disease secondary to meningomyelocele in children. *J. Urol.* 96:723, 1966.
64. Kelalis P.P.: Urinary diversion in children by the sigmoid conduit: Its advantages and limitations. *J. Urol.* 112:666, 1974.
65. King L.R., Belman A.B.: A technique for nephrostomy in the absence of caliectasis. *J. Urol.* 108:518, 1972.
66. King L.R., Scott W.W.: Ileal urinary diversion: Success of pyeloileocutaneous anastomosis in correction of hydroureteronephrosis

67. King L.R., Scott W.W.: Pyeloileocutaneous anastomosis. *Surg. Gynecol. Obstet.* 119:281, 1964.
68. Kock N.G., Myrvold H.E., Nilsson L.O., et al.: Continent ileostomy: An account of 314 patients. *Acta Chir. Scand.* 147:67, 1981.
69. Kock N.G., Nilson A.E., Nilsson L.O., et al.: Urinary diversion via continent ileal reservoir: Clinical results in 12 patients. *J. Urol.* 128:469, 1982.
70. Lapides J.: Butterfly cutaneous ureterostomy. *J. Urol.* 88:735, 1962.
71. Lapides J., Ajemian E.P., Lichtwardt J.R.: Cutaneous vesicostomy. *J. Urol.* 84:609, 1960.
72. Leadbetter G.W.: Skin ureterostomy with subsequent ureteral reconstruction. *J. Urol.* 107:462, 1972.
73. Leadbetter G.W. Jr., Zickermin P., Pierce E.: Ureterosigmoidostomy and carcinoma of the colon. *J. Urol.* 121:732, 1979.
74. Leadbetter W.F.: Consideration of problems incident to performance of ureteroenterostomy: Report of a technique. *J. Urol.* 65:818, 1951.
75. Leape L.L., Holder T.M.: Temporary tubeless urinary diversion in children. *J. Pediatr. Surg.* 5:288, 1970.
76. Lome L.G., Howat J.M., Williams D.I.: The temporarily defunctionalized bladder in children. *J. Urol.* 107:469, 1972.
77. Lome L.G., Williams D.I.: Urinary reconstruction following temporary cutaneous ureterostomy diversion in children. *J. Urol.* 108:162, 1972.
78. Lytton B., Weiss R.M.: Cutaneous vesicostomy for temporary urinary diversion in infants. *J. Urol.* 105:888, 1971.
79. Maloney J.D., Smith J.P.: Temporary cutaneous loop ureterostomy. *J. Urol.* 103:790, 1970.
80. Mathisen W.: A new method for ureterointestinal anastomosis: A preliminary report. *Surg. Gynecol. Obstet.* 96:255, 1953.
81. McGovern J.H.: Urinary diversion by nephrostomy, in Scott R. (ed.): *Current Controversies in Urologic Management.* Philadelphia, W.B. Saunders Company, 1972.
82. Mogg R.A.: Urinary diversion using the colonic conduit. *Br. J. Urol.* 39:687, 1967.
83. Mogg R.A.: Neoplasms at the site of ureterocolic anastomosis. *Br. J. Surg.* 64:758, 1977.
84. Mogg R.A., Syme R.R.A.: The results of urinary diversion using the colonic conduit. *Br. J. Urol.* 41:434, 1969.
85. Morales P., Golimbu M.: Colonic urinary diversion: Ten years of experience. *J. Urol.* 113:302, 1975.
86. Nesbit R.M.: Ureterosigmoid anastomosis by direct elliptical connection: A preliminary report. *J. Urol.* 61:728, 1949.
87. Ogg C.S., Saxton H.M., Cameron J.S.: Percutaneous needle nephrostomy. *Br. Med. J.* 4:657, 1969.
88. Parker R.M., Perlmutter A.D.: Upper urinary tract obstruction in infants. *J. Urol.* 102:355, 1969.
89. Parsons C.D., Thomas M.H., Garrett R.A.: Colonic adenocarcinoma: A delayed complication of ureterosigmoidostomy. *J. Urol.* 118:31, 1977.
90. Perlmutter A.D.: Temporary urinary diversion in the management of the chronically dilated urinary tract in childhood, in Johnston J.H., Goodwin W.E. (eds.): *Reviews in Paediatric Urology.* Amsterdam, Excerpta Medica, 1974.
91. Perlmutter A.D., Patil J.: Loop cutaneous ureterostomy in infants and young children: Late results in 32 cases. *J. Urol.* 107:655, 1972.
92. Perlmutter A.D., Tank E.S.: Ileal conduit stasis in children: Recognition and treatment. *J. Urol.* 101:688, 1969.
93. Perlmutter A.D., Tank E.S.: Loop cutaneous ureterostomy in infancy. *J. Urol.* 99:559, 1968.
94. Rabinovitch H.H.: Ureterosigmoidostomy in children: Revival or demise? *J. Urol.* 124:552, 1980.
95. Raney A.M., Zimskind P.D.: Replacement of loop cutaneous ureterostomy without excision of ureteral segment: An experimental study. *J. Urol.* 107:39, 1972.
96. Raper F.P.: The recognition and treatment of congenital urethral valves. *Br. J. Urol.* 25:136, 1953.
97. Rattner W.H., Meyer R., Bernstein J.: Congenital abnormalities of the urinary system. IV. Valvular obstruction of the posterior urethra. *J. Pediatr.* 63:84, 1963.
98. Retik A.B., Ontell R.: Temporary urinary diversion in infants and children, in *Reconstructive Urological Surgery.* Baltimore, Williams & Wilkins Co., 1977, pp. 135–142.
99. Retik A.B., Perlmutter A.D., Gross R.E.: Cutaneous ureteroileostomy in children. *N. Engl. J. Med.* 277:217, 1967.
100. Richie J.P., Skinner D.G., Waisman J.: The effect of reflux in the development of pyelonephritis in urinary diversion: An experimental study. *J. Surg. Res.* 16:256, 1974.

persisting after ureteroileocutaneous anastomosis. *JAMA* 181:831, 1962.

101. Rickham P.P.: Advanced lower urinary obstruction in childhood. *Arch. Dis. Child.* 37:122, 1962.

102. Rinker J.R., Blanchard T.W.: Improvement of the circulation of the ureter prior to cutaneous ureterostomy: A clinical study. *J. Urol.* 96:44, 1966.

103. Sadlowski R.W., Belman A.B., Filmer R.B., et al.: Follow-up of cutaneous ureterostomy in children. *J. Urol.* 119:116, 1978.

104. Schmaelze J.F., Cass A.S., Hinman F. Jr.: Effect of disease and restoration of function on vesical capacity. *J. Urol.* 101:700, 1969.

105. Schmidt J.D., Hawtrey C.E., Culp D.A., et al.: Experience with cutaneous pyelostomy diversion. *J. Urol.* 109:990, 1973.

106. Schmidt J.D., Hawtrey C.E., Flocks R.H., et al.: Complications, results, and problems of ileal conduit diversions. *J. Urol.* 109:210, 1973.

107. Schneider K.M., Reid R.E., Fruchtman B., et al.: Continent vesicostomy: Surgical technique. *Urology* 6:741, 1975.

108. Schwarz G.R., Jeffs R.D.: Ileal conduit urinary diversion in children: Computer analysis of follow-up from 2–16 years. *J. Urol.* 114:285, 1975.

109. Shapiro S.R., Biaz A., Colodny A.H., et al.: Adenocarcinoma of the colon at ureterosigmoidostomy site 14 years after conversion to ileal loop. *Urology* 3:229, 1974.

110. Shapiro S.R., Lebowitz R., Colodny A.H.: Fate of 90 children with ileal conduit urinary diversion a decade later: Analysis of complications, pyelography, renal function and bacteriology. *J. Urol.* 114:289, 1975.

111. Skinner D.G.: Further experience with the ileo-cecal segment in urinary reconstruction. *J. Urol.* 128:252, 1982.

112. Smith E.D.: Follow-up studies on 150 ileal conduits in children. *J. Pediatr. Surg.* 7:1, 1972.

113. Smith E.D.: Ileo-cutaneous ureterostomy in children: Operative technique and complications. *Aust. N.Z. J. Surg.* 34:89, 1974.

114. Sober I.: Pelviureterostomy-en-Y. *J. Urol.* 107:473, 1973.

115. Spence H.N.: Ureterosigmoidostomy for exstrophy of the bladder: Results in a personal series of thirty-one cases. *Br. J. Urol.* 38:36, 1966.

116. Spence H.M., Hoffman W.W., Fosmire G.P.: Tumor of the colon as a late complication of ureterosigmoidostomy for exstrophy of the bladder. *Br. J. Urol.* 51:466, 1979.

117. Spence H.M., Hoffman W.W., Pate V.A.: Exstrophy of the bladder: Long-term results in a series of 37 cases treated by ureterosigmoidostomy. *J. Urol.* 114:133, 1975.

118. Stamey T.A.: The pathogenesis and implications of the electrolyte imbalance in ureterosigmoidostomy. *Surg. Gynecol. Obstet.* 103:736, 1956.

119. Sullivan H., Gilchrist R.K., Merricks J.W.: Ileo-cecal substitution bladder: Long-term follow-up. *J. Urol.* 109:43, 1973.

120. Swenson O., Smyth B.T.: Aperistaltic megaloureter: Treatment by bilateral cutaneous ureterostomy using a new technique: Preliminary communication. *J. Urol.* 82:62, 1959.

121. Tanagho E.A.: Congenitally obstructed bladders: Fate after prolonged defunctionalization. *J. Urol.* 111:102, 1974.

122. Udall D.A., Hodges C.V., Pearse H.M., et al.: Transureteroureterostomy: A neglected procedure. *J. Urol.* 109:817, 1973.

123. Waldbaum R.S., Marshall V.F.: Posterior urethral valves: Evaluation and surgical management. *J. Urol.* 103:801, 1970.

124. Wallace D.M.: Ureteric diversion using a conduit: A simplified technique. *Br. J. Urol.* 38:522, 1966.

125. Warren R.B., Warner T.F., Hafez G.R.: Late development of colonic adenocarcinoma 49 years after ureterosigmoidostomy for exstrophy of the bladder. *J. Urol.* 124:550, 1980.

126. Wasserman D.H., Garrett R.A.: Cutaneous ureterostomy: Indications in children. *J. Urol.* 94:380, 1965.

127. Weiss R.M., Beland J.A., Lattimer J.K.: Transureteroureterostomy and cutaneous ureterostomy as a form of urinary diversion in children. *J. Urol.* 96:155, 1966.

128. Weyrauch H.M., Rous S.N.: U-tube nephrostomy. *J. Urol.* 97:225, 1967.

129. Williams D.F., Burkholder G.V., Goodwin W.E.: Ureterosigmoidostomy: A 15-year experience. *J. Urol.* 101:168, 1969.

130. Williams D.I., Eckstein H.B.: Obstructive valves in the posterior urethra. *J. Urol.* 93:236, 1965.

131. Williams D.I., Rabinovitch H.H.: Cutaneous ureterostomy for the grossly dilated ureter of childhood. *Br. J. Urol.* 39:696, 1967.

132. Wosnitzer M., Lattimer J.K.: Comparison of permanent nephrostomy and permanent cutaneous ureterostomy. *J. Urol.* 83:553, 1960.

133. Zincke H., Segura J.W.: Ureterosigmoidostomy: Critical review of 173 cases. *J. Urol.* 113:324, 1975.

134. Zinman L., Libertino J.A.: Ileocecal conduit for temporary and permanent urinary diversion. *J. Urol.* 113:317, 1975.

130 W. Hardy Hendren
Urinary Tract Undiversion

THE URINARY TRACT accounts for a large share of surgically correctable problems of infants and children. Techniques of managing these disorders have changed greatly in the past two decades. For example, ureteral reimplantation was rarely performed until the 1960s; however, today it is readily accepted as the best means of managing many cases of vesicoureteral reflux, the most common cause of pyelonephritis in children. Megaureter, which was formerly considered not amenable to repair, has recently become another problem that the surgeon can correct with a high rate of success. Before current techniques were developed for managing some of these problems, many youngsters were treated by urinary diversion. In some, it was believed that renal function was too poor to allow any other means of treatment than permanent urinary diversion. In other children, urinary diversion was done after an operation that failed to correct the problem. Diversion methods have included ileal conduit, cutaneous vesicostomy, various types of cutaneous ureterostomy, and tube nephrostomy. Although diversion may give striking initial improvement in a child with obstructive uropathy, or recurrent pyelonephritis from a nonobstructive uropathy such as massive reflux, all too often the long-term follow-up shows a dismal result.

Improved results in various types of urinary reconstructive surgery in children prompted us to attempt urinary tract refunctionalization in children who had undergone prior diversion, some of them many years previously. Since 1969, "undiversion" operations have been performed in 145 patients, as shown in Table 130–1. Ten of these patients had undergone diversion procedures on our own service many years previously; the remaining 135 had their diversions elsewhere and had been referred later for a reconstructive procedure.

Preoperative Assessment of Bladder Function

It would be reassuring to be able to assess bladder function completely before performing an undiversion procedure, but that is not possible in some cases. In most patients, a long-un-

TABLE 130–1.—Urinary
Diversion, 1969–1984

Ileal loop (12 pyeloileal)	56
Colon conduit (3 ileal loops)	10
Loop ureterostomy or pyelostomy	34
End ureterostomy	17
Cystostomy	21
Nephrostomy	7
Total	145*
Permanent diversions	109
Temporary diversions	36
Females	49
Males	96
Patients with one kidney	36

*Ten personal diversions; 135 had been diverted elsewhere.

used bladder proves to be quite satisfactory when urine flow is redirected to it. Most bladders that have not been used for many years are small and thin-walled, but in some the capacity is satisfactory. Also in some cases the bladder wall may remain thick, especially in boys with urethral valves. Neurogenic bladder should be assessed by looking for spinal abnormality and by neurologic examination of the perineum. Some patients with neurogenic bladder can be treated by undiversion, with the ultimate goal of management by intermittent self-catheterization and/or pharmacologic control of the bladder, which has become better understood in recent years. I have not favored use of an artificial sphincter[49] in these cases because these devices, even on short term follow-up, can lead to serious problems when there is erosion of soft tissue, infection, or mechanical malfunction. Cystometrography has not proved especially helpful because pressures are hard to evaluate when the bladder capacity is small, and the patient experiences pain when it is filled. Sensation can be tested by filling the bladder slowly with saline or radiopaque contrast medium. Pain and the sensation of fullness are usually evoked when a relatively small amount is instilled. Curiously, some patients are able to void on command without any difficulty, although the majority have been unable to do so.

Preoperative testing of bladder sensation, size, compliance, and continence has been used in candidates for undiversion in the last 10 years. This is accomplished by inserting a soft Silastic catheter percutaneously, during cystoscopy under anesthesia. Through this catheter sterile saline is instilled as many times per day as the patient can manage. Some long-diverted, but basically normal, bladders will stretch their capacity from 2–3 ounces to 300–400 ml in 1–2 weeks. These have usually been children with failed ureteral reimplants leading to diversion despite basically good bladders. In some patients, the bladder remains small and noncompliant, despite several weeks or months of attempted hydrostatic stretching. An augmentation procedure should be considered,[9, 10, 32, 51, 58] using colon or intestine during undiversion of such cases. If the patient who has a neurogenic bladder or who has had bladder outlet surgery cannot retain a reasonable volume of instilled saline, it is likely that undiversion should include narrowing the bladder neck and proximal urethra, and in females sometimes subsequent lengthening of the distal urethra to gain more outlet resistance.[28] Total urethral obstruction must obviously be corrected before undiversion. For example, we have treated several boys who had urethral valves fulgurated when urine flow had been diverted. This will often result in stricture. It is satisfactory to repair the stricture before undiversion, provided bladder physiotherapy, i.e., saline irrigation, is begun soon after the stricture is repaired.

It is tempting to overstretch the long-diverted bladder hydro-

statically under anesthesia, but this can prove impractical. On two occasions we ruptured the dome of the bladder by this maneuver, although the rupture was recognized and caused no serious complications.

Illustrative Undiversion Cases

The following cases, some of which have been reported elsewhere,[3, 13, 14, 16, 19, 22, 23] illustrate certain aspects of undiversion surgery. It should be emphasized that this is very difficult surgery that should be attempted only by those with ample experience in all phases of reconstructive urinary surgery. A technical misadventure can result in disaster, although fortunately this has not occurred in any of our patients. These procedures have taken from 5 to 12 hours, occasionally even longer. Many involved operating on all levels of the urinary tract in a single procedure, which can be risky with respect to blood supply of the ureter. Expert anesthesia and postoperative care are demanded, particularly in a patient with limited renal function. There is no margin for tolerating obstruction, extravasation, or pyonephrosis.

Each of these cases differs substantially from the others, and so it is usually not possible to predict preoperatively exactly what will be required.

The surgeon must be prepared to improvise and must be thoroughly familiar with all available techniques to accomplish satisfactory redirection of the urine to the bladder, so that it will drain well without vesicorenal reflux. Tortuosity of a ureteropelvic junction may require resection. It may be necessary to mobilize the kidney and its ureter widely to gain sufficient length. Anastomotic tension is never permissible. Transureterostomy is sometimes needed.

Undiversion from an Ileal Loop

When Bricker[2] introduced the ileal conduit in 1950, it represented a major advance over previous methods for managing many problems in both children and adults. Nevertheless, long-term follow-up of patients with ileal loops showed a significant rate of upper tract deterioration.[4, 39, 46, 48, 50] Bacteria enter a conduit at the stoma and can travel from there to the kidney through the mechanism of reflux. Certainly any patient today who has an ileal conduit should be reassessed as a possible candidate for undiversion if the bladder has a reasonable likelihood of satisfactory function. Furthermore, there is ample evidence that, in patients who require diversion, a nonrefluxing conduit is better than an ileal conduit.[1, 18, 35, 40, 41]

In Figure 130–1 are shown the techniques that can be employed in reconstructing the urinary tract of a patient with an ileal loop conduit. Of the 56 patients with ileal loops, in the undiversion, the bowel was tapered and implanted into the bladder in 28; 19 were completely successful; six had reflux and required reoperation to make a longer tunnel to stop the reflux; three had poor bladders in which tapering and tunneling had been, in retrospect, a poor choice and, to correct this, cecal augmentation was used. In two patients, the bowel was used as the mid- or upper ureter, joining it to a usable ureter stump. In 26 patients, the ileal loop was discarded. Their reconstructions included: joining at least one ureter to the bladder in 12 patients, two by autotransplanting a kidney downward; or cecal augmentation, joining the ureters to a nonrefluxing nipple made from the terminal ileum in all but one case.

CASE 1.—A 6-year-old girl was evaluated in 1969 for possible reconstruction. Pyeloileal conduit had been performed at age 4 months for severe bilateral hydronephrosis secondary to a large ureterocele (Fig 130–2, *A* and *B*). The shrunken, tiny, functionless left kidney was removed, together with that part of the ileal segment. The remaining ileal conduit was tapered and joined end to end to the remaining right lower ureteral segment (*C* and *D*). In 15 years since undiversion, this young-

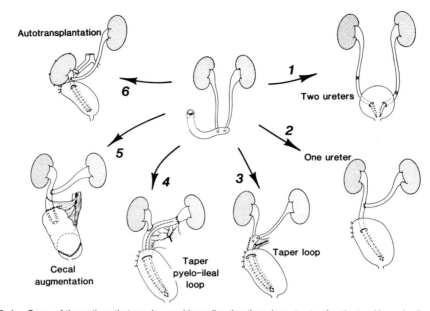

Fig 130–1.—Some of the options that can be used in undiverting the urinary tracts of patients with a prior ileal conduit. The method to use depends on the anatomy of the ureters in an individual case.

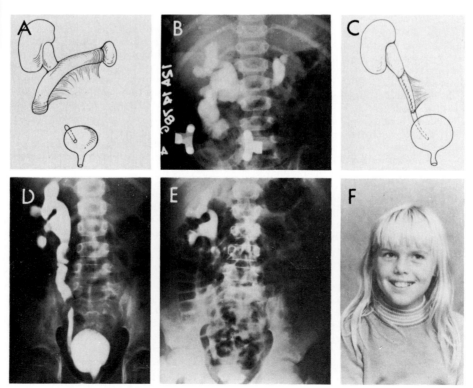

Fig 130–2.—Case 1: a pyeloileal conduit for ureterocele and hydronephrosis had been done at age 4 months in this 6-year-old girl. **A,** anatomy before reconstruction. **B,** intravenous pyelogram (IVP) before reconstruction, showing conduit, moderate right hydronephrosis and shrunken left kidney. "Function" in the left kidney was probably dye refluxing into it from the right. **C,** anatomy after reconstruction. **D,** nephrostogram 2 weeks after repair showing tapered bowel conduit substituting for upper half of ureter. **E,** an IVP 5 years postoperatively, showing stable upper tract. **F,** the patient at age 11 years.

ster has led a normal life and has had consistently sterile urine without antimicrobial therapy. During the years with an ileal conduit, although she thrived, the urine was continuously infected despite continuous antimicrobial therapy. In 1978, 9 years after undiversion, a stricture in the bowel segment was excised, reanastomosing the ends of the "ileal ureter." The patient, now aged 18 years, is completely well.

Comment.—The possibility was considered that mucus from the bowel conduit might produce obstruction in passing through a nondilated lower ureter, but that has not been a problem in this case. If a satisfactory lower ureter is present, we prefer to use it instead of implanting the ileal conduit itself into the bladder. The likelihood of averting reflux is better with a ureter than with a tapered bowel segment, especially if the bladder is of small capacity, in which it may be difficult to attain a long tunnel implantation of tapered bowel.

We have used a bowel segment for mid-ureter in one other patient, although this is not a frequently needed option. Late stricture of an ileal loop is a well-recognized complication, possibly secondary to lymphocyte depletion in bowel mucosa exposed to urine. We have encountered the complication of later stricture of bowel used as ureter in three of our own cases and in two referred from elsewhere.[30] Thus it is mandatory to follow indefinitely any patient with bowel in the urinary tract to detect this late and sometimes clinically silent complication.

CASE 2.—A 12-year-old boy was referred with an ileal loop constructed 3½ years previously for continuing urinary incontinence. At age 1 month, he had been treated elsewhere for hydronephrosis from urethral valves by nephrostomies and suprapubic cystostomy and later *open* resection of the valves. Subsequently the bladder neck had been resected. When urinary incontinence persisted, despite additional operations at ages 7 and 8 years, he underwent ileal loop diversion (Fig 130–3, *A*).

An extensive reconstruction was performed, lasting 11 hours. The ileal conduit was removed, and the left half of his horseshoe kidney was joined to the right half by transureteropyelostomy, dividing the left colic artery so that it would not compress the left ureter. Continuity of the right ureter was reestablished by mobilizing the right half of the horseshoe kidney and "pexing" it downward. The symphysis pubis was opened, narrowing the urethra as much as possible from the bulb up through the bladder neck. A temporary suprapubic cystostomy tube was removed 2 weeks later (Fig 130–3, *B*). Although the bladder had held only 25 ml preoperatively under anesthesia, 1 month later its capacity had increased to 100 ml; it gradually enlarged further to normal (Fig 130–3, *C* and *D*). The patient voids without reflux or residual. Urinary wetting was a problem initially, but it disappeared over the next 2 years. He is now 20 years old, and it has been 9 years since this extensive reconstruction. More than 6 feet tall, he enjoys good health.

Comment.—This illustrates a frequent complication of open resection of urethral valves, namely urinary incontinence. Resection of valves by open technique is today entirely outmoded.[11, 12, 21, 56] With modern pediatric fiberoptic endoscopes, urethral valves can be removed endoscopically, even in tiny infants. A patient with urinary incontinence presents a serious social and psychological problem; we believe it is better to direct additional efforts toward repair of the incontinence than to turn to a permanent urinary diversion. In the patient's view, having an ileal loop merely substituted one serious problem for another. His outlook on life improved substantially after getting rid of both his incontinence and the urinary appliance.

Today, a small bladder like this would be "cycled" for a time preoperatively to stretch it to a larger size, possible in the majority if they were normal bladders before diversion. Scarred, noncompliant bladders, or neurologically impaired bladders, may require augmentation at the outset if reconstruction is to succeed.

CASE 3.—A 13-year-old boy was referred for possible undiversion of an ileal loop. Multiple operations had been performed during infancy for Hirschsprung's disease, including colostomy, closure of a wound dehiscence, and a Duhamel pull-through procedure. Reimplantation of the left ureter was performed, and later bilateral ureteral reimplantation was

done at a second institution. Finally, 5 years previously, ileal loop urinary diversion had been carried out in a third hospital for "neurogenic bladder" (Fig 130–4, *A*). The patient had a bladder capacity of 100 ml, normal sensation and the ability to empty the bladder when it was filled. Review of previous films from early childhood showed anterior displacement of the bladder. This appeared to have been caused by an overdistended rectosigmoid, which was now of normal size. The proximal ileal loop was redundant, and the lower end of the left ureter was fibrous. Both of these structures were resected, together with left-to-right transureteroureterostomy. The bowel conduit was tapered and implanted into the bladder with a 6-cm tunnel to prevent reflux. Psoas hitch was performed, partially immobilizing the bladder to prevent angulation of the conduit at its point of entry and effectively increasing the tunnel length.[45, 54] The procedure lasted 9 hours (Fig 130–4, *B*).

Postoperatively the patient soon exhibited normal bladder size and control. He is free of urinary infection and on no medication now, over 8 years later. Because he is allergic to IVP contrast medium, anatomical evaluation of his urinary tract was accomplished by prograde perfusion through a percutaneous needle inserted into the left renal pelvis,[44] simultaneously measuring pressures, which were normal (Fig 130–4, *D*).

Comment.—This patient's urinary diversion was performed after two failures of ureteral reimplantation, on the assumption that a third reimplantation would fail also. It is important to recognize that for most failures of ureteral reimplantation there is a better solution than permanent urinary diversion.[15, 17, 25, 26] Several technical procedures can help avert a urinary diversion in these circumstances. In some cases both ureters can be mobilized for a third time, reimplanting the better one with a very long tunnel and draining the other ureter by transureteroureterostomy. When a ureter is somewhat short, tacking the bladder to the psoas muscle just lateral to the new point of entry of the ureter through the bladder muscle, the so-called psoas hitch, can improve the results of ureteral reimplantation.[45, 54] Extensive mobilization of the kidney and its ureter, taking great care to leave all the periureteral tissues with the ureter for blood supply, can provide additional length for a difficult ureteral reimplantation. To augment the blood supply of the ureter, the spermatic or ovarian vessels can be divided low to leave them with the ureter for collateral blood supply if the ureter is to be mobilized extensively. If the ureter is still too short, a tapered small bowel segment can be employed in much the same fashion as a previously established ileal conduit for the distal ureter.[25]

As a second line of defense against reflux, when using a tapered bowel segment implanted into the bladder as a substitute ureter, I formerly made a nipple anastomosis between the short upper ureter and the proximal end of the bowel segment. In my experience, however, these nipples cannot be relied on because, if there is any back pressure, they tend to become undone and allow reflux (see Fig 123–21).

Figure 130–5 shows the steps for converting an ileal conduit to a satisfactory "ureter." The stoma should be mobilized with great care, for the entire length of the loop may be needed to reach the bladder. A finger inserted into the stoma during its mobilization reduces the likelihood of injury to the bowel wall. Often the bowel will not reach the bladder unless its mesentery is incised, which must be done with care to preserve enough arcades to nourish the distal loop. The conduit should be tapered for several reasons. First, a satisfactory nonrefluxing anastomosis to the bladder is more easily accomplished if the caliber of the loop is made smaller. Second, fluoroscopic observation of the tapered loop shows more effective propulsion of urine, for the bowel wall coapts better, which enhances peristaltic emptying. An untapered conduit shows churning back and forth of the bolus. Third, tapering reduces the bowel surface area and potential resorption of electrolytes, an important consideration in patients with reduced renal function. Although for patients with recurrent stone disease it can be useful to join the renal pelvis directly to the bladder with an untapered segment of bowel, making no attempt to prevent reflux, the circumstances are dif-

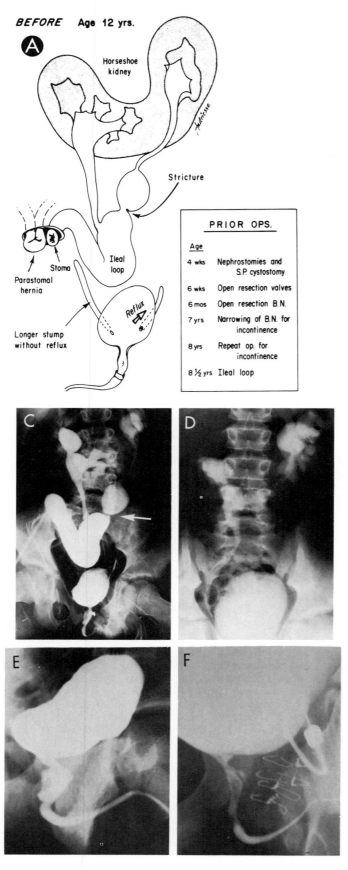

BEFORE Age 12 yrs.

Ⓐ

Horseshoe kidney

Stricture

Ileal loop

Stoma

Parastomal hernia

Longer stump without reflux

Reflux

PRIOR OPS.	
Age	
4 wks	Nephrostomies and S.P. cystostomy
6 wks	Open resection valves
6 mos	Open resection B.N.
7 yrs	Narrowing of B.N. for incontinence
8 yrs	Repeat op. for incontinence
8½ yrs	Ileal loop

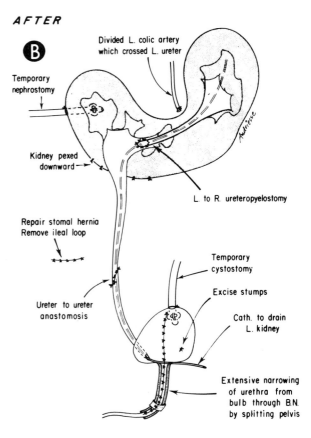

AFTER

Ⓑ

Divided L. colic artery which crossed L. ureter

Temporary nephrostomy

Kidney pexed downward →

L. to R. ureteropyelostomy

Repair stomal hernia Remove ileal loop

Temporary cystostomy

Excise stumps

Cath. to drain L. kidney

Ureter to ureter anastomosis

Extensive narrowing of urethra from bulb through B.N. by splitting pelvis

Fig 130–3.—Case 2: boy aged 12 years with horseshoe kidney and incontinence from open resection of urethral valves; subsequent ileal loop. **A** and **B**, anatomy before and after undiversion. **C**, simultaneous loopogram and cystogram done preoperatively to outline anatomy. Note stricture of loop *(arrow)* and small bladder. **D**, an IVP 7 months postoperatively. Note normal-sized bladder. **E**, preoperative cystogram. Note dilated prostatic urethra. Two incontinence procedures had been performed several years previously without success. **F**, voiding cystourethrogram study 7 months after undiversion with simultaneous reoperation for incontinence by splitting symphysis and resecting and narrowing outlet from bulbous urethra up through the bladder neck. Cystogram being performed by suprapubic needle filling of the bladder. Note wire closure of pubic symphysis (all four wires broken!).

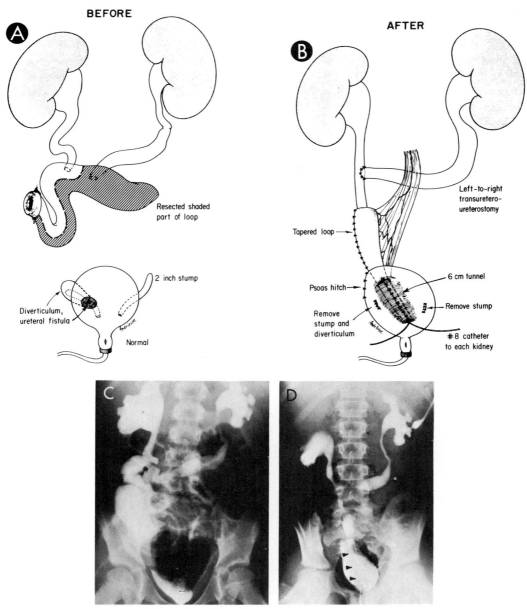

Fig 130–4.—Case 3: a 13-year-old boy with failed ureteral implantations and finally a ureteral loop for some complications of operation for Hirschsprung's disease. **A** and **B**, anatomy before and after undiversion. **C**, preoperative simultaneous cystogram and loopogram to outline the anatomy. **D**, study 8 months postoperatively via percutaneous needle in left renal pelvis to infuse dye and measure pressure, which were normal (patient allergic to IVP dye). Note left-to-right transureteroureterostomy, tapered ileal conduit substituting for right lower ureter, right psoas hitch of the bladder and long-tunneled implantation of bowel conduit to prevent reflux *(arrows)*.

ferent in most pediatric patients. They often have a damaged upper tract, and it is important to prevent reflux, which can cause and perpetuate urinary infection.

It should be possible to achieve a nonrefluxing and nonobstructed implantation of tapered small bowel into the bladder if (1) the bladder is relatively normal; (2) a very long (7–10 cm) tunnel is made; (3) there is no bladder outlet obstruction; (4) the bowel is narrowed in caliber sufficient to give a tunnel-length-to-"ureter"-diameter ratio of about 5:1. In 28 such implantations, our initial failure in nine seems excessive. In retrospect, attempting the procedure in three small, scarred bladders was a mistake. This was remedied by augmenting the bladders with colon. In six cases, reoperation was done to make a longer tunnel and higher psoas hitch, which we do at the outset today, having learned that a short tunnel will not prevent reflux.

CASE 4.—A 15-year-old boy with the prune belly syndrome was referred for possible undiversion (Fig 130–6). Severe urinary infection had occurred at age 2 weeks; bilateral nephrostomies were performed, and later an ileal loop; the loop did not drain well, so the nephrostomies were maintained. One year previously a second conduit had been constructed, but that also did not drain well.

There was ureteropelvic junction obstruction on the right and obstruction of the left ureter by the left colic artery. An extensive operation was performed, lasting 11 hours. First, diaphragmatic narrowing of the prostatic urethra was incised endoscopically. The bladder held only 100 ml when filled to capacity under anesthesia. Reconstruction included partial resection of both renal pelves and ureters, tapering of the conduit and implantation into the bladder by nonrefluxing technique. The bladder

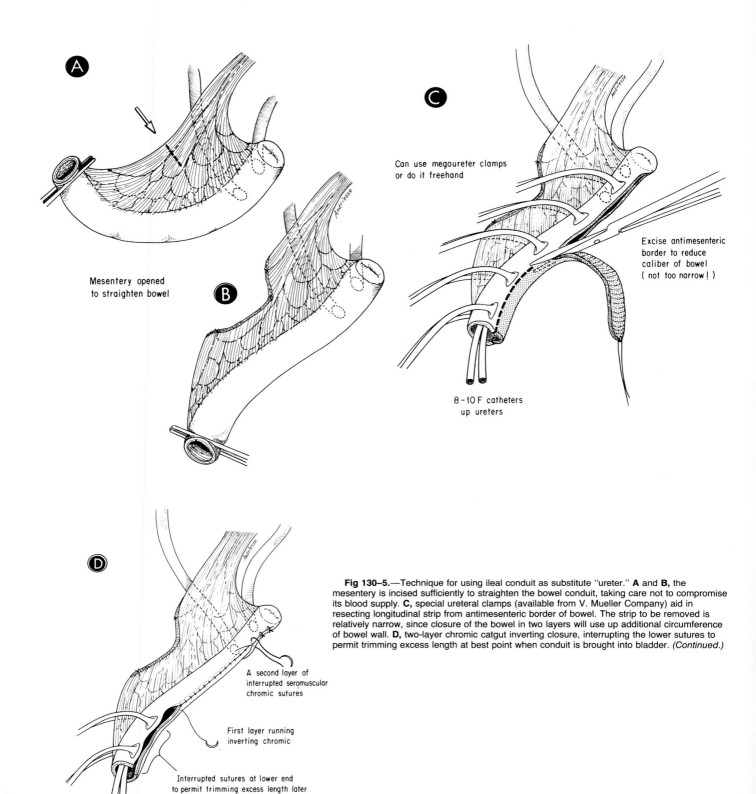

Mesentery opened
to straighten bowel

Can use megaureter clamps
or do it freehand

Excise antimesenteric
border to reduce
caliber of bowel
(not too narrow !)

8 - 10 F catheters
up ureters

A second layer of
interrupted seromuscular
chromic sutures

First layer running
inverting chromic

Interrupted sutures at lower end
to permit trimming excess length later

Fig 130–5.—Technique for using ileal conduit as substitute "ureter." **A** and **B,** the mesentery is incised sufficiently to straighten the bowel conduit, taking care not to compromise its blood supply. **C,** special ureteral clamps (available from V. Mueller Company) aid in resecting longitudinal strip from antimesenteric border of bowel. The strip to be removed is relatively narrow, since closure of the bowel in two layers will use up additional circumference of bowel wall. **D,** two-layer chromic catgut inverting closure, interrupting the lower sutures to permit trimming excess length at best point when conduit is brought into bladder. *(Continued.)*

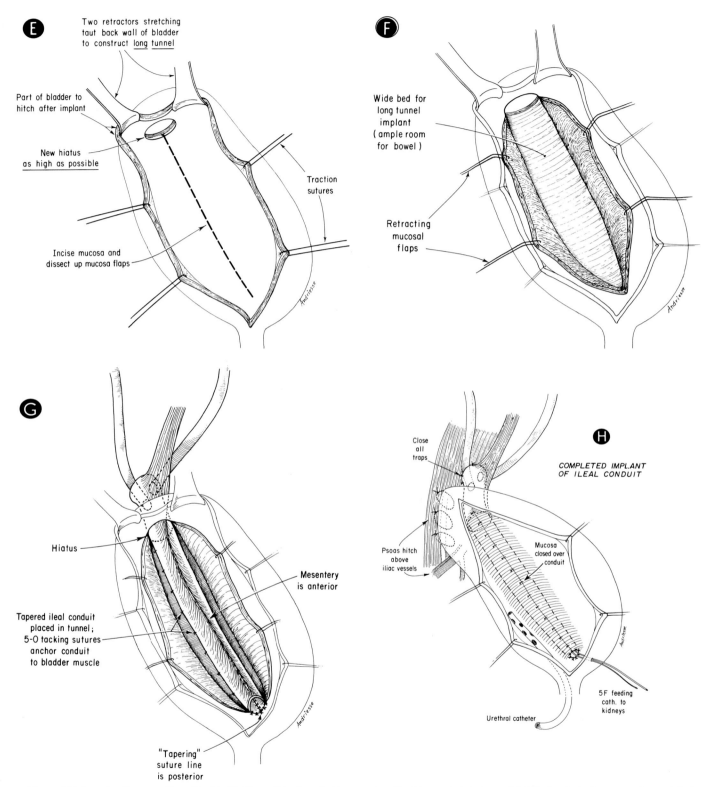

E

Two retractors stretching taut back wall of bladder to construct <u>long tunnel</u>

Part of bladder to hitch after implant

New hiatus as high as possible

Incise mucosa and dissect up mucosa flaps

Traction sutures

F

Wide bed for long tunnel implant (ample room for bowel)

Retracting mucosal flaps

G

Hiatus

Mesentery is anterior

Tapered ileal conduit placed in tunnel; 5-0 tacking sutures anchor conduit to bladder muscle

"Tapering" suture line is posterior

H

Close all traps

COMPLETED IMPLANT OF ILEAL CONDUIT

Psoas hitch above iliac vessels

Mucosa closed over conduit

5F feeding cath. to kidneys

Urethral catheter

Figure 130–5 cont.—E, preparation of bed in bladder wall for tunneled implantation. Hiatus should be selected to be as high as possible, but on the back wall of the bladder. Mucosa is incised diagonally to gain maximum length. **F,** mucosa flaps are dissected widely to create ample room for implantation of conduit. Making a submucosal tunnel by blunt dissection is usually not feasible in these previously diverted bladders. **G,** bowel conduit is placed in tunnel with its suture line lying posteriorly to avert fistulization through mucosa closure anterior to it. Redundant mesentery can be trimmed from conduit, but not so much as to devascularize it. **H,** completed 7–10-cm tunnel. Feeding catheter passed to each kidney for drainage. Psoas hitch immobilizes bladder wall on side of hiatus, which also gives additional tunnel length by stretching trigone upward.

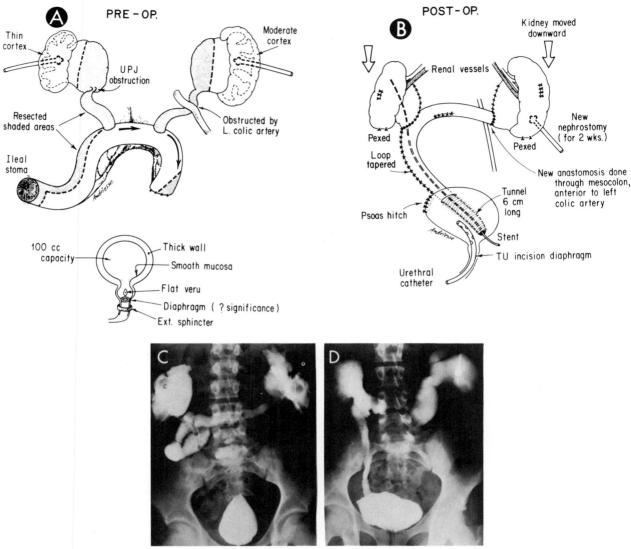

Fig 130–6.—Case 4: a 15-year-old boy with prune belly syndrome, bilateral ureterostomies, and nonfunctioning ileal loop. **A** and **B**, anatomy before and after undiversion. **C,** preoperative film shows simultaneous filling through both nephrostomy tubes and a catheter in the ileal loop stoma. There was no flow through either renal pelvis into the bowel conduit. Simultaneous cystogram also shows a small bladder. **D,** left percutaneous antegrade infusion 18 months postoperatively. Note tapered bowel conduit from left kidney to right, and from right kidney into the bladder. Bladder capacity and function are satisfactory; no reflux. Normal infusion pressures.

capacity became normal within several weeks, with normal stream and control. Since early infancy, the patient had known a life complicated by multiple tubes and appliances and chronic urinary infection. He led an essentially normal life for 10 years after undiversion, with relatively stable renal function of about 30% of normal. Although then a 25-year-old adult in good general health, his creatinine rose suddenly to very high levels (over 20 mg%). It is believed that this was acute interstitial nephritis occurring from ingestion of cimetidine, which has been reported as causing this rare complication. Renal transplantation with his brother's kidney was recently performed.

Comment.—High pyeloileal diversion is not a contraindication to undiversion. Additionally, diminished renal function is not a contraindication to undiversion. Reconstruction may provide many years of life of better quality for a diverted patient before transplantation is necessary. Further, that day may be forestalled by getting rid of the urinary infection so common in patients with diversions and rare when the urinary tract has been successfully repaired. Of particular importance, the patient with a function-

ing bladder is a much better candidate for renal transplantation than one with a diversion. Ten of our patients have had transplantation 1–10 years after their undiversion. In none was the transplant date advanced by the undiversion procedure. The level of renal function in about 25 more patients is low enough that they may ultimately require transplantation, as did the patient in case 4.

Case 5.—A 13-year-old boy with the prune belly syndrome was referred for reconstruction (Fig 130–7). At age 3 weeks he was found to have urinary infection and bilateral massive hydronephrosis. A suprapubic tube was inserted and had remained. At age 5 years left megaureter repair was attempted, but the ureter became obstructed and the kidney ceased functioning. At age 6 years the right ureter was tapered and implanted but became obstructed. Additionally there were multiple strictures of the urethra, possibly secondary to endoscopy. Creatinine clearance remained excellent, 80 L absolute.

Preoperative cystography showed an enormous bladder capacity, although the bladder had been defunctionalized for 13 years via tube cys-

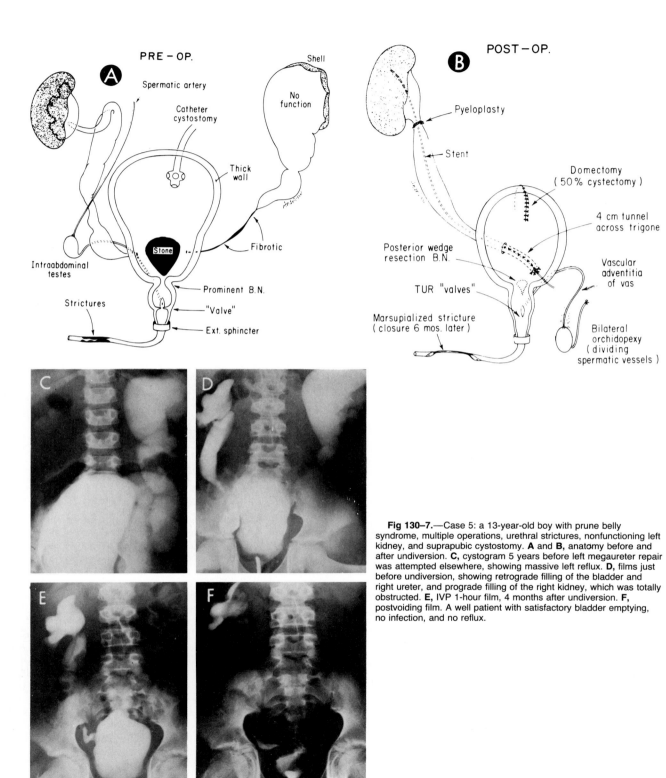

Fig 130–7.—Case 5: a 13-year-old boy with prune belly syndrome, multiple operations, urethral strictures, nonfunctioning left kidney, and suprapubic cystostomy. **A** and **B**, anatomy before and after undiversion. **C**, cystogram 5 years before left megaureter repair was attempted elsewhere, showing massive left reflux. **D**, films just before undiversion, showing retrograde filling of the bladder and right ureter, and prograde filling of the right kidney, which was totally obstructed. **E**, IVP 1-hour film, 4 months after undiversion. **F**, postvoiding film. A well patient with satisfactory bladder emptying, no infection, and no reflux.

tostomy. Prograde pyelography showed total obstruction on the left and partial obstruction on the right. An extensive reconstructive operation was performed, lasting 12 hours. A first-stage Johanson urethroplasty was performed to relieve urethral obstruction. Folds of tissue narrowing the prostatic urethra at the level of the veru were incised endoscopically. Left nephroureterectomy was performed. The right ureter was tapered, shortened, and reimplanted; and a kinked ureteropelvic junction that appeared partially obstructed was removed. The dome of the bladder was removed, together with the suprapubic cystostomy site. Bilateral orchiopexy was accomplished. The very short spermatic vessels were divided, bringing the testes down as far as possible with a pedicle of vas deferens and surrounding tissue for blood supply. It was possible to get them down to the level of the pubic tubercle but not into the scrotum. Eleven months later the second-stage urethroplasty was accomplished. Eighteen months later at a secondary orchiopexy each testis was brought the additional distance down into the scrotum. Each was noted to have acquired additional collateral circulation. Now aged 23 years, the patient is a robust college graduate who leads a normal life.

Comment.—Many boys with the prune belly syndrome, like this patient and the one in case 4, have lived most of their lives with urinary diversion. They should be reevaluated for possible undiversion. Not only can there be great improvement in the quality of life, but quite likely longevity will be increased by reducing the incidence of bacilluria. Many of the patients have chronic low-grade urinary infection, which causes gradual and progressive loss of renal function with various types of diversion. Following undiversion, infection has proved less troublesome.

This patient prefers to wear an elastic corset for abdominal support, although in our experience most of these patients will get some spontaneous improvement in the laxity of the abdominal wall as they grow older. In general we do not think that reefing procedures are required for the abdominal walls, although in a few at the time of laparotomy for urinary reconstruction we have excised some of the flabby abdominal wall, which has improved their appearance (see Chap. 125).

Undiversion from Ureterostomy

Cutaneous ureterostomy has been used extensively in the past 15 years as temporary or permanent urinary diversion in children with various types of obstructive uropathy, as well as those with myelodysplasia.[2, 5-8, 34, 36-38, 42, 43, 47, 52, 53, 55, 57] Although ureterostomy is an easy operation, it is not without complications. We have rarely resorted to cutaneous ureterostomy, but we have had an opportunity to care for 51 young patients referred for reconstructive procedures after ureterostomies elsewhere. The following cases illustrate some of the diverse problems encountered in these patients; no two were entirely similar.

CASE 6.—A 5-year-old boy was referred for possible undiversion (Fig 130–8). At age 5 days the bladder was found to be distended; suprapubic cystostomy was performed. He did poorly and was transferred to a second hospital; a cystogram showed marked reflux, hydronephrosis and poor ureteral peristalsis. At age 5 weeks bilateral end ureterostomies were performed. The right ureter became ischemic, and this caused stenosis. Pyonephrosis resulted, and a repeat right end cutaneous ureterostomy was performed at a higher level.

Preoperatively creatinine clearance was 11 L/sq m of body surface area on the right and 60 L on the left. A cystogram showed a bladder capacity of 50 ml and a diverticulum on the right. Filling the bladder with only modest pressure resulted in some extravasation of the dye. At operation, type I urethral valves were resected. There was great hypertrophy of the bladder neck, despite 5 years of nonuse of the bladder, and it was incised a little at 6 and 12 o'clock to prevent possible obstruction. There was enough length of the left ureter to reimplant it into the bladder with an adequate tunnel to prevent reflux, utilizing the psoas hitch. The implantation was performed obliquely across the trigone to attain maximal length for the tunnel. The right ureter was very short; therefore, the right kidney was drained into the left ureter. This was accomplished by mobilizing it widely, preserving all perirenal fat and Gerota's capsule so that its only remaining attachment was at the hilar vessels. The lower pole was tacked medially next to the vena cava. This gave sufficient length to join the right ureter to the left ureter. Postoperatively the patient had an impressive gain in height and weight. The urine has remained consistently sterile without the suppressive antimicrobial therapy

he had taken continuously for 5 years. Laboratory values 6 years post reconstruction included BUN 21 mg/100 ml, creatinine 0.9 mg/100 ml, and creatinine clearance 110 L absolute!

Comment.—Sloughing of the right ureter due to ischemia in this patient serves to emphasize that when a ureter is mobilized extensively, even if only to bring it to the surface, all possible periureteral tissue should remain with it. This created a difficult problem in reconstruction, which was solved by transureteroureterostomy. Although the right kidney was small, it was spared because it contributed about 20% of the renal function. Extravasation during cystography emphasizes that a long-defunctionalized bladder may not be able to stand much pressure. Interestingly, it was a thin-walled bladder, although the original pathology was urethral valves; in some cases, however, the bladder wall remains thick. This boy's quality of life was greatly improved by getting rid of his two urinary appliances. Preoperatively his medical costs included frequent physician visits for cultures, continuous antimicrobial therapy, and $500 per year for disposable ureterostomy bags. Current health care costs are a fraction of those previous to undiversion. He is well 10 years after operation.

CASE 7.—A 12-year-old boy was referred with bilateral end cutaneous ureterostomies for possible undiversion. At age 9 months he was found to have bilateral hydronephrosis, duplex collecting systems, and a large ureterocele. The ureterocele was incised, and suprapubic cystostomy was performed. Y-V plasty of the bladder neck was done at age 2 years. He did poorly; at age 3 years bilateral end ureterostomies were performed. Despite continuous antimicrobial therapy, periodic cultures usually showed bacilluria in the drainage from both stomas. The right side gradually drained progressively less and had no remaining function at age 12 years (Fig 130–9, *A*). The patient was combative, ill-adjusted, did poorly in school, and spoke of suicide if his urinary collecting bag could not be removed.

An extensive reconstructive procedure was performed (Fig 130–9, *B*). The right kidney and ureter were removed. Chronic urosepsis had caused extensive periureteral and perinephric inflammatory tissue. This tissue could be dissected only by knife technique, for scissors would not cut through it. On the left, the upper pole ureter was satisfactory for reimplantation, but the lower pole ureter was dilated (*C*) and was therefore removed; the lower pole was drained by pyeloureterostomy.

Laboratory values 2 years postoperatively were amazingly good despite loss of the right kidney and a poor lower pole of the left kidney. They were: BUN 16 mg/100 ml, creatinine 0.9 mg/100 ml, and creatinine clearance 129 L absolute.

Comment.—Ureterostomy in this patient apparently did not provide satisfactory drainage, resulting in eventual nonfunction of the right kidney, chronic bacilluria, and a poor quality of life. The high rate of stomal stenosis precludes using end ureterostomy for ureters that are relatively normal in size. Dilated ureters have shown a lower rate of stomal obstruction, but even these can later retract and become stenotic. Bacilluria in this case was not caused by stenosis, for a large catheter could be passed easily through each stoma.

In assessing patients with end ureterostomy by simultaneously filling the bladder and ureters, it is not always possible to judge whether a ureter will be long enough to reach the bladder. A ureter may appear shorter than it actually is, because of the additional length as it goes from the posterior gutter forward to the skin. In taking down ureterostomies, dissection should be done well away from the ureteral wall, leaving attached all possible periureteral tissue and even a strip of overlying peritoneum in some cases, because the ureter will depend on the collateral blood supply. Skeletonizing a ureter out of this investing tissue carries a high risk of ischemic necrosis.

In reconstructive pediatric urology a duplex collecting system is a common finding. Often one ureter is relatively normal in size and the other very dilated. It is best to remove the dilated ureter, concentrating on satisfactory reimplantation of the better one (Fig 130–9, *D*). In order not to jeopardize the blood supply of

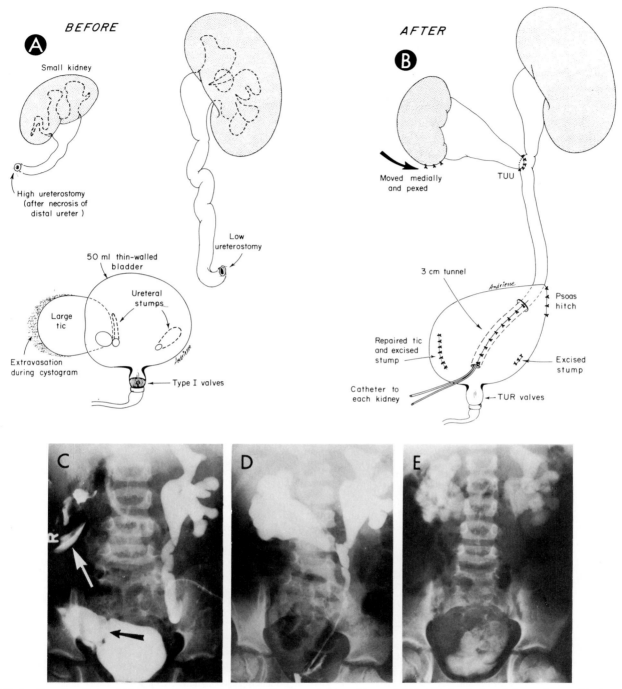

Fig 130–8.—Case 6: a 5-year-old boy with bilateral end ureterostomies for untreated urethral valves. **A** and **B,** anatomy before and after undiversion. **C,** simultaneous preoperative ureterograms and cystograms to outline anatomy. Note short right upper ureter, which had originally sloughed *(white arrow),* and extravasation around bladder diverticulum during cystogram *(black arrow).* **D,** injection of stent catheters draining upper tracts 12 days postoperatively, outlining high transureteroureterostomy. **E,** IVP 2 years and 3 months after undiversion. Note how bladder veers to left secondary to psoas hitch procedure.

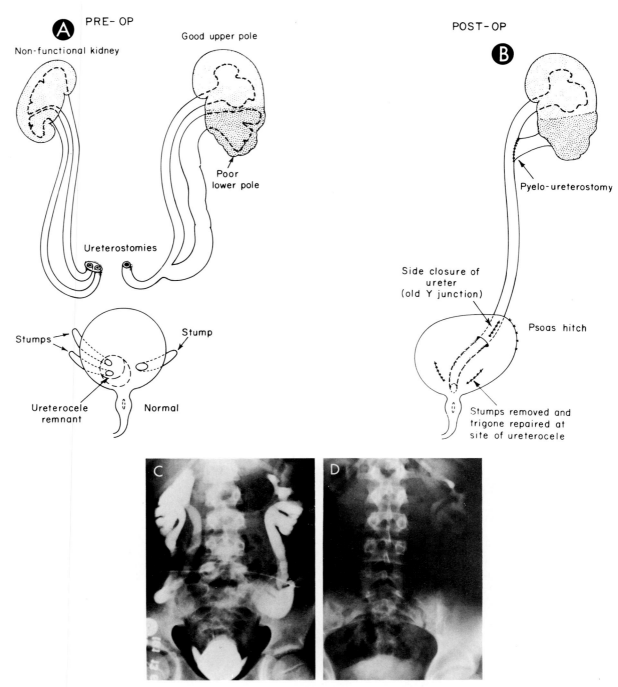

Fig 130–9.—Case 7: a 12-year-old boy with bilateral end ureterostomies for hydronephrosis, double collecting systems, and ureterocele. **A** and **B,** anatomy before and after undiversion. **C,** preoperative simultaneous ureterograms and cystogram to outline anatomy. Note small bladder, refluxing stumps. Right side was nonfunctional. Left side shows good upper pole with a satisfactory ureter, and poor lower pole with a very dilated ureter. **D,** and IVP 4 years postoperatively. Note normal bladder size and collecting system of remaining kidney con-

verted into a single one to drain through the better ureter, which had originally drained the upper pole. When there are two ureters with a duplex collecting system, one relatively normal in size and the other very dilated, it is preferable to remove the very dilated ureter to achieve drainage through the better one. We have seen many failures after attempts to reimplant the duplex collecting systems with a dilated ureter, especially when tapering was attempted.

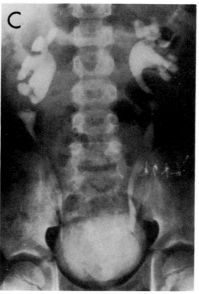
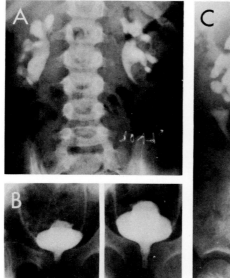
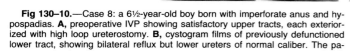

Fig 130–10.—Case 8: a 6½-year-old boy born with imperforate anus and hypospadias. **A,** preoperative IVP showing satisfactory upper tracts, each exteriorized with high loop ureterostomy. **B,** cystogram films of previously defunctioned lower tract, showing bilateral reflux but lower ureters of normal caliber. The patient was treated initially by simple closure or ureterostomies. **C,** IVP 6 months after closure of ureterostomies. Upper tract stable. Bladder now of normal size. No reflux on cystogram after bladder was refunctionalized.

the ureter to be spared, the following technique should be used. The dilated ureter is dissected close to its wall for a length of 2 or 3 inches; all of its adventitia is left with the ureter to be saved. A small incision is made in the periureteral adventitia at a higher point and the specimen pulled through to that level, again dissecting an additional segment of the ureter close to its wall. This procedure is repeated until the entire ureter is dissected out, leaving all of the periureteral adventitia intact except for the three or four "stair-step" incisions made to pull the ureter through progressively to a higher level. These reconstructions are generally long and tedious; this operation lasted for 9 hours. However, it produced a sterile urinary tract and a normal quality of life, reflected in a complete change for the better in the patient's personality. Now 12 years after undiversion, the patient has completed school and works full time in good health.

CASE 8.—A 6½-year-old boy with bilateral ureterostomies was referred for possible reconstruction. He was born with imperforate anus, treated initially by colostomy. Later at another institution he was found to have bilateral hydronephrosis, treated at age 10 months with bilateral ureterostomies. At age 3 years abdominoperineal pull-through of the rectum was performed. At age 4 years the first-stage repair of a hypospadias was carried out.

A preoperative IVP (Fig 130–10, A) showed satisfactory upper tracts; a cystogram (B) showed a small bladder. There was moderate reflux on the right. The patient was able to empty the bladder satisfactorily. Cystoscopy showed a normal ureteral orifice on the left, and a slightly dilated one on the right. There were no urethral valves, but there was a 3-cm diverticulum from the prostatic urethra, the stump of rectum remaining from his abdominoperineal pull-through procedure. (The rectum had not been transected flush with the urethra.)

It was elected merely to close the ureterostomies as an initial procedure in this boy, because endoscopically the lower ureters looked reasonably normal. Following this, the bladder function was satisfactory; a cystogram 4 months later showed no reflux (Fig 130–10, C). The stump of the congenital rectourethral communication was removed via perineal approach 1 year later, and after this the hypospadias repair was completed.

The patient was last seen at 5 years after undiversion. He had satisfactory urine control, no reflux, stable IVP, and no urinary infection.

Comment.—The reason for this patient's hydronephrosis in the first place is not entirely clear, for his previous records were not available. There may have once been urethral valves that were eroded by an inlying urethral catheter during some of the previous procedures. In some patients a defunctionalized bladder will show reflux, which will disappear when ureterostomies are closed. As the bladder increases its capacity, presumably this lengthens relatively short submucosal tunnels. That proved to be the case in this instance, and it was to some extent predictable because endoscopy showed relatively normal-appearing lower ureters. In many cases, however, endoscopy will show the lower ureter to be grossly abnormal, often with a large paraureteral diverticulum, when the patient's original problem was urethral valves. In these cases it may be better to reimplant the lower ureter at the same time that the ureterostomy closure is performed.

CASE 9.—A 9-year-old boy was referred for possible reconstruction (Fig 130–11). At age 3 years severe bilateral hydronephrosis was discovered and treated with bilateral loop cutaneous ureterostomy. The diagnosis of urethral valves was made radiographically, but during cystoscopy, at age 5½, valves were thought not to be present. At age 6 years the left ureterostomy was closed, and 1 month later the left ureter was reimplanted to correct massive reflux. A suprapubic tube was left in place, because the patient was never able to void. Many previous urethral dilatations were performed; open resection of "a stricture of the membranous urethra" was considered, but the parents refused.

Investigation showed a loop ureterostomy on the right, suprapubic cystostomy and free reflux bilaterally on the cystogram. At cystoscopy, only a pinpoint opening could be seen at the level of the "stricture," too small to admit even an 8 F infant panendoscope. After dilatation with a filiform and small follower, the anatomy could be visualized. It was consistent with type I urethral valves, although the diaphragm formed by confluence of the valve leaflets was thicker than usual. It was felt that this might represent secondary stricture from prior instrumentation of valves. The diaphragm was resected with a wire electrode. To reconstruct the urinary tract, a long midline incision was made from pubis to xiphoid to afford simultaneous exposure of the entire urinary tract. The left ureter was mobilized widely to gain sufficient length for its repeat reimplantation in the trigone. The segment previously exteriorized and closed was widely mobilized. The right ureterostomy was taken down and closed, and the right lower ureter was reimplanted. A small plastic catheter was placed in the urethra, whose valves had been resected, for 2 weeks postoperatively. When it was removed the patient had difficulty voiding. This was managed by the use of intermittent catheterization,

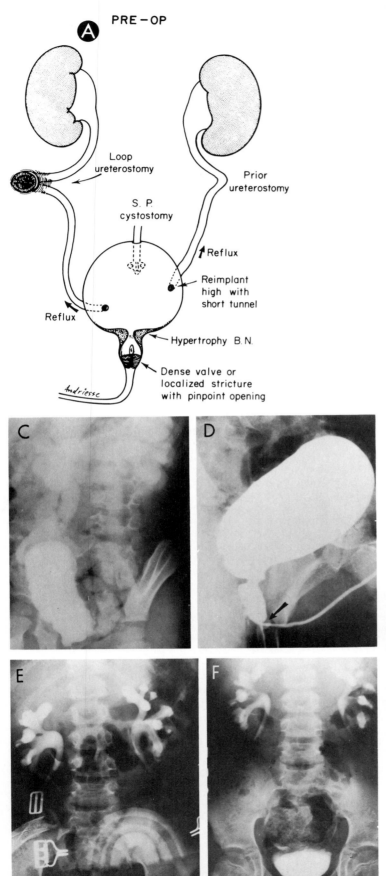

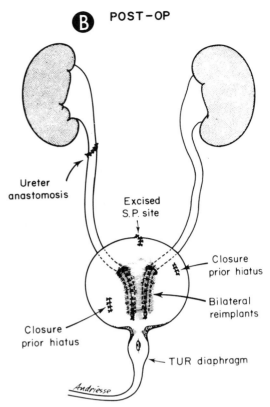

Fig 130–11.—Case 9: a 9-year-old boy with urethral valves, right loop ureterostomy, suprapubic cystostomy, reimplanted left ureter, and almost complete urethral obstruction. **A** and **B,** anatomy before and after undiversion. **C,** IVP at age 3 years before loop ureterostomy, showing massive hydroureteronephrosis. **D,** voiding cystourethrogram at age 5½ years showing contour typical for type I urethral valves *(arrow)*. **E,** IVP before operation. Right kidney drains into the loop ureterostomy, left kidney into bladder through refluxing previous ureteral reimplantation; bladder draining via suprapubic cystostomy. **F,** IVP 4 months after undiversion. Upper tracts stable. Ureters normal.

phenoxybenzamine, and urocholine. During the next week he began to void normally. Cystogram showed satisfactory bladder emptying. There was a trace of reflux into the lower 2 inches of the ureter on the left. Cystoscopy 4 months later showed slight narrowing of the urethra at the level where the atypical valve had been. Decadron, 3 ml, was injected through the panendoscope into this area, and it was dilated to size 20 F. Eight years after undiversion, the patient's renal function and general health are both normal.

Comment.—Several important points are illustrated here. First, the diagnosis of urethral valves was overlooked, although that is the primary problem in most males with bilateral hydroureteronephrosis. An open operation for "stricture" would have been ill advised. We have seen many boys with severe valves that have escaped diagnosis. Second, the previous reimplantation of the left ureter was doomed to failure because the ureter had been originally implanted without adequate mobilization to gain sufficient length to replace it in the posterior part of the trigone with a long enough tunnel. If preoperative studies show a straight ureter from the site of ureterostomy to the bladder, this can be managed in two ways. First, the ureterostomy can be closed, reestablishing the flow of urine to the bladder, and then several weeks later the ureter can be reimplanted; it is mobilized at that time usually all the way up to the recent ureterostomy closure to gain sufficient length. A ureter can be mobilized rather extensively if all the periureteral tissue is maintained with it for collateral blood supply. A second approach, which we favor when it is clear that the lower ureter needs operation, is simultaneously to take down the ureterostomy, reanastomose the ureter ends and reimplant the ureter in a single procedure, as was done on the right side in this patient. Third, this patient required several days to learn how to void. This was managed by a combination of pharmacologic stimulation of the bladder and intermittent catheterization to prevent its overdistention.

CASE 10.—A 4-year-old girl was referred for reconstruction of the genitourinary tract (Fig 130–12). She was one of female twins, the other of whom was normal. At birth, marked abdominal distention, imperforate anus, and genital ambiguity were noted. End colostomy was performed, at which time internal female structures were noted. Because of increasing hydronephrosis, at age 10 months bilateral loop ureterostomies were performed. Although the upper tracts improved considerably, at age 4 years ileal conduit urinary diversion was advised. The family declined this suggestion, and the child was referred for possible restoration of urinary tract continuity.

Evaluation disclosed a long male-type "urethra" with an apparently normal sphincter at the level of the pubic symphysis. This urogenital sinus ended superiorly in a patulous bladder neck; adjacent to that was the entry to double vaginas, each with a separate cervix. An extensive lower genitourinary operation was performed. The laterally placed, gaping, and refluxing ureters were reimplanted by cross-trigone technique. The enlarged vagina was separated from its communication with the urogenital sinus; flaps were constructed of its lateral walls and tubularized to pull through to the perineum. This tedious reconstruction took 12 hours. It was thought inadvisable to add ureterostomy closure, particularly since there was enough length of both ureters distal to the ureterostomies to accomplish reimplantation without disturbing the ureterostomies. Two weeks later, the ureterostomies were closed. Gradually during the next 3 months satisfactory bladder emptying was achieved.

Comment.—In this patient, unlike the two previous cases, lower ureter operation was best performed first, with subsequent closure of the ureterostomies. A word of caution is in order, however, when a "dry implantation" is performed, i.e., the lower ureter is reimplanted while still defunctionalized. A completely satisfactory reimplantation can seal over postoperatively if there is no urine flow through it. We, and others, have noted this in several instances. It is therefore best to leave in place a small, soft Silastic stent until closure of the ureterostomies is performed.

We have reported previously the surgical management of urogenital sinus abnormalities.[24, 31] They occur in a spectrum from mild cases, which can be repaired from below, to complex ones like this one, which require abdominoperineal repair.

This youngster is now over 9 years past this extensive reconstruction. She has normal urinary control. Her mother empties the patient's colon every other day with an enema, which prevents fecal soiling. It is necessary to revise the vaginal introitus at an older age in most girls who have had an extensive vaginoplasty at a young age. In my opinion, however, that is not a valid reason to defer the initial reconstruction until the patient is older.

CASE 11.—A 24-year-old woman, born with myelomeningocele, was referred for possible undiversion. After various orthopedic operations, when she was 14 years old, ileal loop urinary diversion was performed for urinary incontinence and infection (Fig 130–13, *A*).

A Silastic suprapubic tube was passed percutaneously to test bladder function. During the next 3 months, which the patient spent at home, it was clear that her maximum bladder volume was less than 100 ml. Saline instilled through the tube ran freely from the urethra. An extensive reconstruction was performed. The urethra and bladder neck were narrowed as much as possible to create more outlet resistance. The bladder was small and thick-walled. It was thought unwise to attempt reimplantation of even one ureter into this bladder, which was, therefore, augmented using the cecum, creating a nonrefluxing mechanism with the ileocecal junction. The dilated right ureter was joined to the terminal ileum of the ileocecal cystoplasty. The left ureter was drained into the right via transureteroureterostomy[29] (Fig 130–13, *B*).

Convalescence following this extensive reconstruction was uneventful. Postoperative radiographic study showed satisfactory drainage of the upper tract into her augmented bladder, and no reflux on cystographic examination. The patient returned to college, emptying her bladder by intermittent self-catheterization. Although socially continent, she was not absolutely dry for the first 4 postoperative months. It was thought that she would probably require a urethral extension procedure to gain more resistance.[28] However, by 8 months postoperatively, she was completely dry on the program of intermittent self-catheterization. Now, two years following undiversion, the patient is doing well. She greatly prefers intermittent self-catheterization to wearing an abdominal appliance.

Comment.—There are many young adults like this who had ileal loop urinary diversion for neuropathic bladder during the heyday of the ileal loop, from about 1955 to 1975. Although some patients with long-standing ileal loops are free from infection and have stable, normal upper tracts, there is overall, in these patients, an unacceptable rate of upper tract deterioration. I have not performed ileal loops on young patients since 1969. If bowel conduit diversion is needed, we use a nonrefluxing colon conduit or nonrefluxing ileocecal conduit. Recently, based on a large series done by the late Richard Mogg, the suggestion was made that the nonrefluxing colon conduit does not protect against upper tract deterioration. In my opinion, this is not valid, because those colon conduits were not made with long ureterocolic tunnels to prevent reflux. We are firmly convinced by both clinical follow-up and laboratory studies that an effective tunneling ureterocolic implantation will usually prevent reflux and upper tract deterioration.

It is fruitless to rejoin the upper tract to a bladder that was once incontinent unless some measure is taken to create outlet resistance. To be effective, the Young-Dees narrowing of the proximal urethra and bladder neck must be made very small in caliber. When the mucosa adjacent to that segment is resected and the muscle is closed over it, it should be snug to the passage of a 10 F catheter. After return of function, the remaining bladder will expand. In a small-capacity bladder like this, augmentation must also be used to avoid having the upper tract empty into a small-volume, high-pressure bladder. The ureters in this case were actually long enough to justify consideration of ureteral reimplantation. It was decided against, however, because the bladder was small and thick-walled, reducing the likelihood of successful reimplantation. We thought that it would be safer to rely on a nipple of terminal ileum intussuscepted into the cecum.

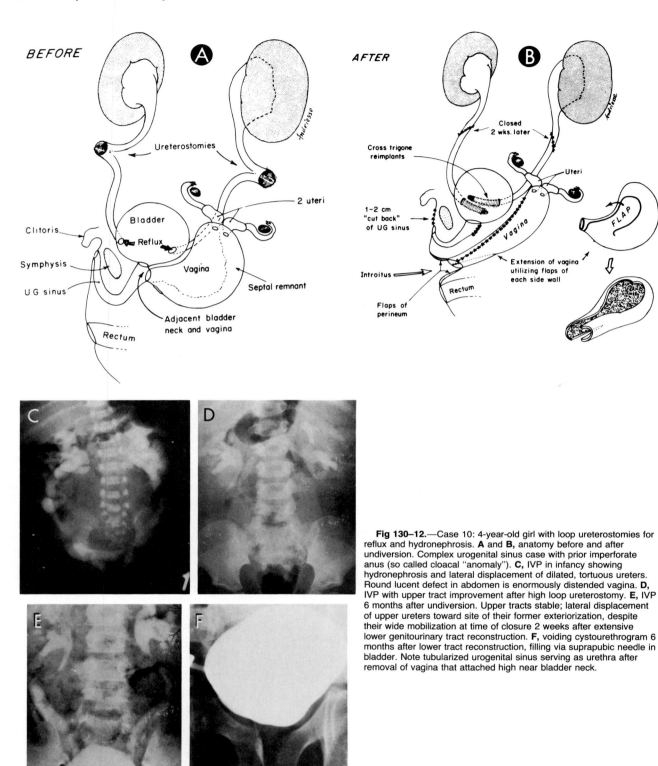

Fig 130–12.—Case 10: 4-year-old girl with loop ureterostomies for reflux and hydronephrosis. **A** and **B**, anatomy before and after undiversion. Complex urogenital sinus case with prior imperforate anus (so called cloacal "anomaly"). **C**, IVP in infancy showing hydronephrosis and lateral displacement of dilated, tortuous ureters. Round lucent defect in abdomen is enormously distended vagina. **D**, IVP with upper tract improvement after high loop ureterostomy. **E**, IVP 6 months after undiversion. Upper tracts stable; lateral displacement of upper ureters toward site of their former exteriorization, despite their wide mobilization at time of closure 2 weeks after extensive lower genitourinary tract reconstruction. **F**, voiding cystourethrogram 6 months after lower tract reconstruction, filling via suprapubic needle in bladder. Note tubularized urogenital sinus serving as urethra after removal of vagina that attached high near bladder neck.

BEFORE

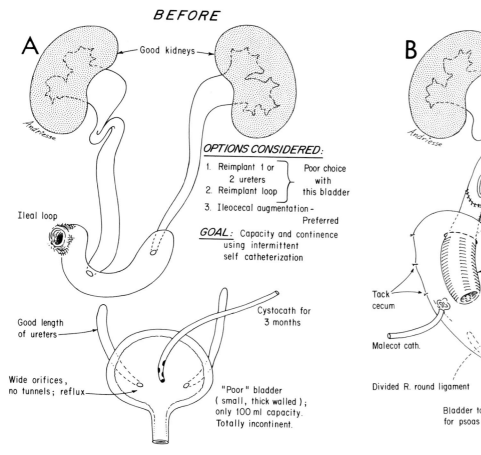

AFTER

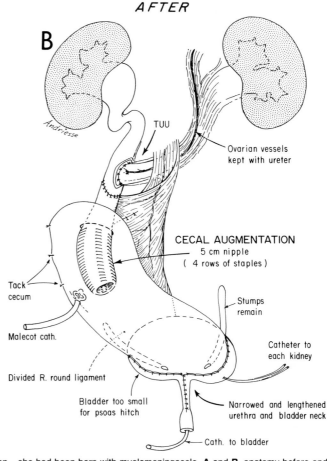

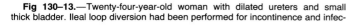

Fig 130–13.—Twenty-four-year-old woman with dilated ureters and small thick bladder. Ileal loop diversion had been performed for incontinence and infec-tion—she had been born with myelomeningocele. **A** and **B**, anatomy before and after undiversion. *(Continued.)*

Special mention should be made of altering the ileocecal valve to prevent reflux. In testing the ileocecal segment for reflux at the operating table, we learned that most will resist reflux until the pressure exceeds 15 cm of water. The ileocecal junction can be reinforced by the technique described by Zinman and Liber-tino,[58] plicating cecal wall in several layers over the terminal ileum, except on its mesenteric side. At the operating table, this will be competent to withstand pressures of 60 cm of water or greater. If the segment is used as an isolated conduit to the sur-face, this nonrefluxing mechanism continues to be competent. However, in our experience, when the ileocecal segment is joined to the bladder, thereby intermittently filling and empty-ing, this antireflux mechanism breaks down. For this reason we began creating a 4–5-cm nipple by intussuscepting 8–10 cm of terminal ileum. Some of these nipples held up and continued to protect against reflux when joined to the bladder. However, oth-ers broke down. Therefore, subsequently, the bowel was scari-fied and its mesentery was removed before it was intussus-cepted, in an effort to maintain the nipple.[27] Some of these also broke down. Still later, we placed many tacking sutures into the nipple; this also proved unreliable. Finally, three to four rows of staples were placed because it was thought that this would surely maintain the nipple. Even this measure proved unreliable. Nip-ples that early postoperatively could be seen hanging down into the cecum and that did not show reflux on early follow-up cys-tograms, later popped out of the cecum and refluxed. The cur-

rently employed technique consists of creating the nipple as be-fore, using staples, but then incising the back wall the full length of nipple through the ileocecal valve and down a corresponding distance along the adjacent wall of the cecum. The nipple is then sewn to the adjacent cecal wall to hold it in place. Early follow-up of this method during the past year has shown it to be effec-tive. It maintains the nipple within the cecum. It also is an ef-fective way to revise a nipple that becomes undone. Most staples become covered with bowel mucosa. In three cases, however, small stones were seen on exposed staples at follow-up cystos-copy. These were easily plucked out with alligator forceps. We have employed cecal augmentation of the bladder in 41 young patients. In 28, the ileocecal junction was used to prevent reflux. I believe it is better to implant a ureter into the bladder or into the cecal wall to prevent reflux, if the length and quality of ure-ter will permit. Only if this is not feasible do we use the ileocecal junction to prevent reflux.

There were 14 cases of neurogenic bladder in this group of 145 patients, most of them seen within the past 2 years. All but one were similar to this case, needing bladder augmentation and more outlet resistance. Most of these patients prefer intermittent self-catheterization as a way of life rather than drainage of the ordinary tract through an abdominal stoma. If and when mechan-ical artificial sphincters become perfected in the future, it may be possible to resect the narrowed bladder neck endoscopically, reducing the resistance created and allowing the bladder to

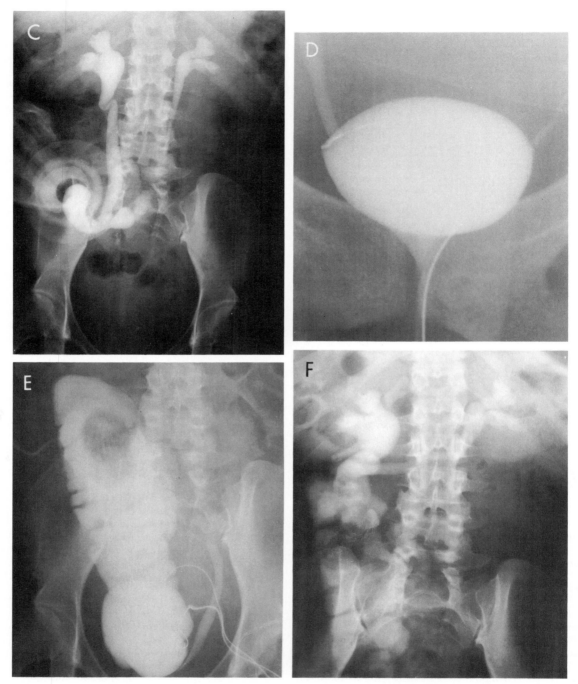

Fig 130–13 Cont.—C, preoperative loopogram with moderate upper tract dilatation. Note strictures of ileal loop. **D,** preoperative cystogram showing small-capacity, completely incontinent bladder with refluxing ureteral stumps. **E,** cystogram 10 days following reconstructive procedure. Various postoperative catheters still in place. Note cecum and ascending colon added to the small bladder. The intussuscepted ileum is evident as a filling defect in the cecum. Staples are visible. **F,** excretory urogram 9 months postoperatively. Stable upper tracts. Cystogram shows no reflux. Patient is dry, and manages very well with intermittent clean catheterization.

empty without catheterization. Continence could then be attained with the artificial sphincter. Mechanical sphincters are not yet sufficiently reliable to warrant this approach.

Other Horizons for Undiversion

Another group of patients who should be considered for removal of urinary bags are the many children who have had permanent ileal conduit urinary diversion for exstrophy of the bladder. Many have undergone this form of urinary diversion either as a primary procedure or after failure of attempted functional closure of the bladder. Some can be treated with success by a staged method of ureterosigmoidostomy.[20] The following case will illustrate.

CASE 12.—An 8-year-old girl born with a rudimentary exstrophied bladder had undergone ileal conduit diversion at age 1 year and later cystectomy and epispadias repair (Fig 130–14, *A*). There were moderate dilatation of the right side and intermittent bacilluria, often seen with ileal conduit diversions. The ileal conduit was removed, and in its place a nonrefluxing colon conduit was constructed (*B*). Subsequently the IVP became normal. Loopogram (*C*) showed no reflux even at pressures up to 60 cm of water. One year later, the conduit was taken down from the abdominal wall and anastomosed to the rectosigmoid (*E*).

The patient, now aged 21 years, is 12 years following anastomosis of the nonrefluxing colon conduit to the rectosigmoid. She is a senior in nursing school, leading a normal life; her IVP is stable. Two years ago, she suffered a febrile illness with flank pain, but needle aspiration of urine percutaneously from each kidney showed no bacterial growth.

Comment.—This method of "internal urinary diversion" to the rectosigmoid has been used in exstrophy patients who have had a previous "permanent" urinary diversion by an ileal loop, as well as in some new patients whose bladders were not suited for primary closure. We believe this staged method of ureterosigmoid diversion may be somewhat safer than primary ureterosig-

moid anastomosis in both new patients and patients with a previous ileal conduit. It allows healing of the ureter-to-colon anastomoses in a clean environment, and then long-term observation for satisfactory drainage and absence of low-pressure reflux before joining the conduit to the fecal stream filled with bacteria, which can rapidly destroy the upper tract if there is either obstruction or free reflux at a ureterocolic anastomosis. This staged approach can also be used in young patients requiring anterior pelvic exenteration for sarcomas of the lower genitourinary tract.

In some patients with good ureters and normal upper tracts, conversion from ileal loop to ureterosigmoidostomy has been performed in one stage, shown in Figure 130–15. Different approaches to this have been described recently.[33] There is an increased incidence of colon carcinoma in patients with ureterocolic diversion of the urine. Therefore, we advise periodic endoscopic evaluation for all of these patients, having seen several develop carcinoma.

Conclusion

Experience with 145 young patients who had undergone previous urinary diversion, most of them "permanent," underscores the fact that many deserve a second look that may permit them to live much more normal lives. Closing the urinary tract and getting rid of an external appliance can greatly improve the quality of life. It can also facilitate maintenance of a sterile urinary tract. There is another group of patients who should be considered for removal of external appliances, namely, patients who do not have a bladder but who have normal anorectal control and satisfactory upper tracts. Some of these are suitable candidates for a different type of "undiversion," i.e., staged ureterosigmoid internal diversion.

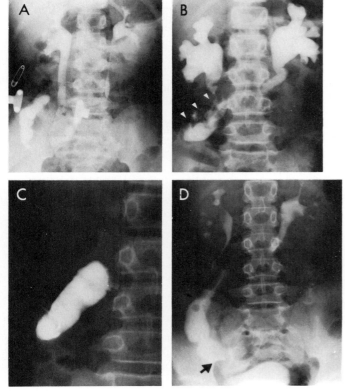

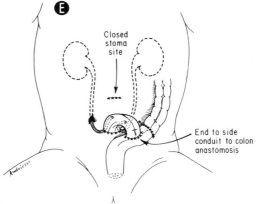

Fig 130–14.—Case 12: an 8-year-old girl with an ileal loop and cystectomy done in infancy for exstrophy of the bladder. **A,** IVP at age 7 years, 6 years after ileal loop was constructed. **B,** IVP 10 days after discarding ileal loop and constructing nonrefluxing colon conduit. Note edema around tunneled right ureter (*arrows*) and bilateral hydronephrosis, often present for several weeks postoperatively. If these tunneled implantations were in colon filled with feces, this temporary obstruction could result in pyelonephritis. It has not caused a problem in defunctioned conduits. The IVP 1 month later looked normal. **C,** loopogram 6 months after colon conduit, showing no reflux even at pressures over 60 cm of water. **D,** IVP 2 years after anastomosis of conduit to colon. Note delicate upper tracts, right ureter of normal size, and anastomosis of conduit to rectosigmoid (*arrow*). **E,** scheme of anatomy after eventual anastomosis of nonrefluxing colon conduit to rectosigmoid, with satisfactory drainage of upper tracts and absence of low-pressure reflux are observed.

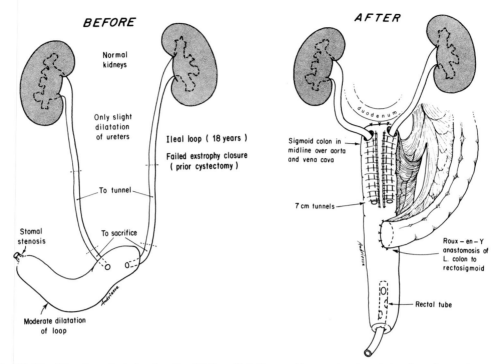

Fig 130–15.—Alternate method of ureterosigmoidostomy that allows making very long-tunneled ureterocolic anastomoses. This is vital to prevent colorenal reflux.

REFERENCES

1. Altwein J.E., Hohenfellner R.: Use of the colon as a conduit for urinary diversion. *Surg. Gynecol. Obstet.* 140:33, 1975.
2. Bricker E.M.: Bladder substitution after pelvic evisceration. *Surg. Clin. North Am.* 30:1511, 1950.
3. Dretler S.P., Hendren W.H., Leadbetter W.F.: Urinary tract reconstruction following ileal conduit diversion. *J. Urol.* 109:217, 1973.
4. Durham-Smith E.: Follow-up studies on 150 ileal conduits in children. *J. Pediatr. Surg.* 7:1, 1972.
5. Dwoskin J.Y.: Management of the massively dilated urinary tract in infants by temporary diversion and single-stage reconstruction. *Urol. Clin. North Am.* 1:515, 1974.
6. Eckstein H.B., Kapila L.: Cutaneous ureterostomy. *Br. J. Urol.* 42:306, 1970.
7. Feminella J.G. Jr., Lattimer J.K.: A retrospective analysis of 70 cases of cutaneous ureterostomy. *J. Urol.* 106:538, 1971.
8. Ghazali S.: Experience with the Sober ureterostomy. *J. Urol.* 112:142, 1974.
9. Gil-Vernet J.M.: The ileocolic segment in urologic surgery. *J. Urol.* 94:418, 1965.
10. Gittes R.F.: Bladder augmentation procedures, in Libertino J., Zinman L. (eds.): *Reconstructive Surgery in Urology.* Philadelphia, W.B. Saunders Co., 1977.
11. Hendren W.H.: A new approach to infants with severe obstructive uropathy: Early complete reconstruction. *J. Pediatr. Surg.* 5:184, 1970.
12. Hendren W.H.: Posterior urethral valves in boys: A broad clinical spectrum. *J. Urol.* 106:298, 1971.
13. Hendren W.H.: Restoration of function in the severely decompensated ureter, in Johnston J.H., Scholtmeijer R.J. (eds.): *Problems in Paediatric Urology.* Amsterdam, Excerpta Medica, 1972.
14. Hendren W.H.: Reconstruction of previously diverted urinary tracts in children. *J. Pediatr. Surg.* 8:135, 1973.
15. Hendren W.H.: Reoperation for the failed ureteral reimplantation. *J. Urol.* 111:403, 1974.
16. Hendren W.H.: Urinary tract refunctionalization after prior diversion in children. *Ann. Surg.* 180:494, 1974.
17. Hendren W.H.: Complications of megaureter repair in children. *J. Urol.* 113:238, 1975.
18. Hendren W.H.: Non-refluxing colon conduit for temporary or permanent urinary diversion in children. *J. Pediatr. Surg.* 10:381, 1975.
19. Hendren W.H.: Refunctionalizing the urinary tract after prior diversion. *Contemp. Surg.* 7:63, 1975.
20. Hendren W.H.: Exstrophy of the bladder: An alternative method of management. *J. Urol.* 115:195, 1976.
21. Hendren W.H.: Complications of urethral valve surgery, in Smith R.B., Skinner D.G. (eds.): *Complications of Urologic Surgery.* Philadelphia, W.B. Saunders Company, 1976.
22. Hendren W.H.: Urinary diversion and undiversion in children. *Surg. Clin. North Am.* 56:425, 1976.
23. Hendren W.H.: Reconstruction ("undiversion") of the diverted urinary tract. *Hosp. Practice* 11:70, 1976.
24. Hendren W.H.: Surgical management of urogenital sinus abnormalities. *J. Pediatr. Surg.* 12:339, 1977.
25. Hendren W.H.: Reconstructive surgery of the urinary tract in children. *Curr. Probl. Surg.* May 1977.
26. Hendren W.H.: Some alternatives to urinary diversion. *J. Urol.* 119:652, 1978.
27. Hendren W.H.: Reoperative ureteral reimplantation: Management of the difficult case. *J. Pediatr. Surg.* 15:770, 1980.
28. Hendren W.H.: Construction of female urethra from vaginal wall and a perineal flap. *J. Urol.* 123:657, 1980.
29. Hendren W.H., Hensle T.W.: Transureteroureterostomy: Experience with 75 cases. *J. Urol.* 123:826, 1980.
30. Hendren W.H., McLorie G.A.: Later stricture of intestinal ureter. *J. Urol.* 129:584, 1983.
31. Hendren W.H.: Further experience in reconstructive surgery for cloacal anomalies. *J. Pediatr. Surg.* 17:695, 1982.
32. Hendren W.H., Radopoulos D.: Complications of ileal loop and colon conduit urinary diversion. *Urol. Clin. North Am.* 10:451, 1983.
33. Hendren W.H.: Ureterocolic diversion of urine: Management of some difficult problems. *J. Urol.* 129:719, 1983.
34. Johnston J.H.: Temporary cutaneous ureterostomy in the management of advanced congenital urinary obstruction. *Arch. Dis. Child.* 38:161, 1963.
35. Kelalis P.: Urinary diversion in children by sigmoid conduits: Its advantages and limitations. *J. Urol.* 112:666, 1974.
36. Leape L.L., Holder T.M.: Temporary tubeless urinary diversion in children. *J. Pediatr. Surg.* 5:288, 1970.
37. Lome L.G., Howat J.M., Williams D.I.: The temporary defunctionalized bladder in children. *J. Urol.* 107:469, 1972.
38. Lome L.G., Williams D.I.: Urinary reconstruction following temporary cutaneous diversion in children. *J. Urol.* 108:162, 1972.

39. Middleton A.W. Jr., Hendren W.H.: Ileal conduits in children at the Massachusetts General Hospital from 1955 to 1970. *J. Urol.* 115:591, 1976.
40. Mogg R.A., Syme R.R.A.: The results of urinary diversion using the colonic conduit. *Br. J. Urol.* 41:434, 1969.
41. Morales P., Golimbu M.: Colonic urinary diversion: 10 years of experience. *J. Urol.* 113:302, 1975.
42. Perlmutter A.D., Tank E.S.: Loop cutaneous ureterostomy in infancy. *J. Urol.* 99:559, 1968.
43. Perlmutter A.D., Patil J.: Loop cutaneous ureterostomy in infants and young children: Late results in 32 cases. *J. Urol.* 107:655, 1972.
44. Pfister R.C., Newhouse J.H., Hendren W.H.: Percutaneous pyeloureteral urodynamics. *Urol. Clin. North Am.* 9:41, 1982.
45. Prout G.R. Jr., Koontz W.W. Jr.: Partial vesical immobilization: An important adjunct to ureteroneocystostomy. *J. Urol.* 103:147, 1970.
46. Richie J.P., Skinner D.G.: Urinary diversion: The physiological rationale for non-refluxing colonic conduits. *Br. J. Urol.* 47:269, 1975.
47. Schmidt J.D., Hawtrey C.E., Culp D.A., et al.: Experience with cutaneous pyelostomy diversion. *J. Urol.* 109:990, 1973.
48. Schwarz G.R., Jeffs R.D.: Ileal conduit urinary diversion in children: Computer analysis of follow-up from 2–16 years. *J. Urol.* 114:285, 1975.
49. Scott F.B., Bradley W.E., Timm G.W.: Treatment of urinary incontinence by an implantable prosthetic urinary sphincter, *J. Urol.* 112:75, 1974.
50. Shapiro S.R., Lebowitz R., Colodny A.H.: Fate of 90 children with ileal conduit urinary diversion a decade later: Analysis of complications, pyelography, renal function and bacteriology. *J. Urol.* 114:289, 1975.
51. Skinner D.G.: Secondary urinary reconstruction: Use of the ileocecal segment. *J. Urol.* 112:48, 1974.
52. Sober I.: Pelviureterostomy-en-Y. *J. Urol.* 107:473, 1972.
53. Straffon R.A., Kyle K., Corvalan J.: Technique of cutaneous ureterostomy and results in 51 patients. *J. Urol.* 103:138, 1970.
54. Turner-Warwick R.T., Worth P.H.C.: The psoas hitch procedure for replacement of the lower third of the ureter. *Br. J. Urol.* 41:701, 1969.
55. Wasserman D.H., Garrett R.A.: Cutaneous ureterostomy: Indications in children. *J. Urol.* 94:380, 1965.
56. Williams D.I., Whitaker R.H., Barratt T.M., et al.: Urethral valves. *Br. J. Urol.* 45:200, 1973.
57. Williams D.I., Cromie W.J.: Ring ureterostomy. *Br. J. Urol.* 47:789, 1975.
58. Zinman L., Libertino J.A.: Ileocecal conduit for temporary and permanent urinary diversion. *J. Urol.* 113:317, 1975.

131 A. BARRY BELMAN

Hypospadias

THE INCIDENCE of hypospadias is about 8.2 per 1,000 male births. The glanular and coronal varieties are most common, representing 87% of total cases. Ten percent of patients reviewed by Sweet et al. had penile hypospadias (0.8 per 1,000 births), and 3% had penoscrotal hypospadias (0.3 per 1,000 births).[66] The term *hypospadias* is derived from the Greek prefix *hypo*, meaning below, and the stem *spadon*, meaning rent or defect.[26]

The classification of hypospadias is based on the position of the urethral meatus. Anatomical description of meatal position instead of "degree of hypospadias" would improve understanding, i.e., glanular, coronal, distal, mid, and proximal shaft, penoscrotal, scrotal, and perineal (Fig 131–1). To best ascertain the position of the urethral meatus, the outstretched penis is held with the left hand while the ventral parameatal skin is pulled outward by the right hand (Fig 131–2). The meatus, firmly attached to the skin, will open, and its position becomes obvious. In addition to the meatal position, the severity of chordee is noted. Chordee is referred to as mild, moderate, or severe. The severity of chordee correlates with meatal position. In cases of severe chordee, however, the meatus may be located at the coronal sulcus (Fig 131–3).

Embryology[3]

The genital tubercle appears at about the fifth week of fetal life, determining the site of the phallus. On the undersurface of the rudimentary genital tubercle, urogenital folds form, between which lies the urethral groove. The genital (labioscrotal) swellings are found on either side of these folds. By the fourteenth week, following growth of the phallus, the urethral folds have united, completing formation of the penile urethra. The glanular meatus is formed from an epithelial ingrowth which then meets the urethral groove at the fossa navicularis. By the end of the first trimester, the external genitalia are completely formed. Hypospadias is the result of failure of fusion of the urethral folds on the ventral aspect of the penis. The concomitant chordee is caused by foreshortened ventral skin devoid of dartos fascia, along with splaying and fibrosis of the incompletely formed corpus spongiosum.

Etiology

Genetic factors appear to be the underlying cause of hypospadias. Inheritance is multifactorial. In a review of the family histories of 307 children with hypospadias, Bauer et al. found 21% had some family member affected.[6] Fourteen percent of families had two sons with hypospadias, and in 7% of affected children, the father also had hypospadias. If a more distant family member (cousin or uncle) was affected with hypospadias, the chance of having a second child with hypospadias was 19%, while the risk for a family without a previous history of hypospadias is 12% for having a second child with hypospadias. If a father has hypospadias and has one son with hypospadias, the family's chance of having a second son with hypospadias rises to 26%. Although racial information is scanty at this time, there is a slight increase of hypospadias in Caucasians.[17]

Hormonal production from the fetal testis influences the development of the external male genitalia. Testicular Leydig cells, in response to stimulation by chorionic gonadotropin, begin producing hormone at about eight weeks gestational age. This rises to a peak at about 12 weeks. The development of the internal duct system (wolffian) is in response to the local effect of testicular testosterone. The external genitalia, however, are stimulated by the more potent dihydrotestosterone, which is converted from testosterone by 5α-reductase at the tissue level. Any failure of timely or adequate hormone production or inability to convert testosterone to dihydrotestosterone may result in genital abnormalities.

Because of the possibility of genital abnormalities developing secondary to maternal ingestion of progestational hormones during pregnancy,[1] a carefully obtained antenatal history is essential when confronted with a child with hypospadias. A family history is helpful in determining the likelihood of hypospadias in future siblings.

Sexual Ambiguity

Gender identity may be a serious problem in children with severe hypospadias. Most cases can be sorted out by simple physical examination, since the presence of palpable scrotal or inguinal testes strongly suggests that the patient is a genetic male. However, buccal smears and tissue karyotype become important in the newborn with a masculinized phallus and nonpalpable testes, to rule out the adrenogenital syndrome in a female. In extreme cases the "phallus" has been circumcised, only to have the diagnosis discovered later.

In the genetic male, the presence of an abnormally small phallus requires extensive evaluation in the newborn period to determine if the penis has the capacity to respond normally in the future. The normal penile stretched length in the newborn is 3.5 cm, with a range of 2.8 cm to 4.2 cm for the 3rd and 97th percentiles, respectively.[32] The parenteral administration of testosterone cypionate, 25 mg every 3 weeks, or testosterone enanthate in oil, 25 mg monthly, should reveal, by 8–12 weeks, whether the small penis has the capability for normal growth.[38]

Associated Abnormalities

Although there is a known correlation between hypospadias and undescended testes, there appears not to be any significantly increased incidence of internal urinary abnormalities. The incidence of undescended testes in boys with hypospadias is approximately 10%, and inguinal hernias also appear to be more common.[46] Genitography should be reserved for those children with truly ambiguous genitalia in whom internal female structures are suspected. Some authors report a minimally increased incidence of significant urinary anomalies in boys with hypospadias.[30, 43] Most would agree, however, that routine excretory urography would not appear to be justifiable.[61] Lutzker et al. recommend sonographic screening of the upper urinary tract in the course of evaluating these children, since it is noninvasive.[52]

Devine et al. have pointed out the enlarged utriculus mascu-

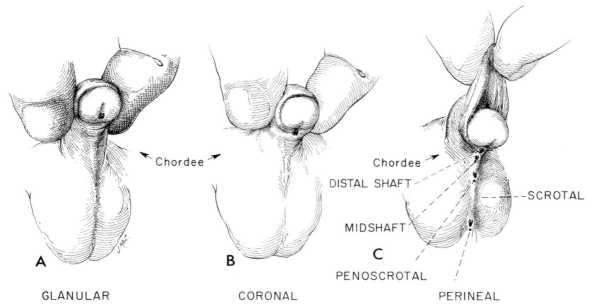

GLANULAR   CORONAL   PERINEAL

Fig 131–1.—Classification of hypospadias based on anatomical meatal position. (From Belman A.B., King L.R.: The urethra, in Kelalis P., et al. (eds.): *Clinical Pediatric Urology,* ed. 2. Philadelphia, W.B. Saunders Co., 1984. Reprinted with permission.)

linus in boys with severe hypospadias.[22] Ten percent with penoscrotal hypospadias and 57% with perineal hypospadias have significant utricular enlargement. The significance of an enlarged utricle is uncertain, and it generally is not a cause for concern. Practically speaking, it may interfere with urethral catheterization. Stasis with infection and stone formation in the utricle are potential problems to be dealt with only as they occur. Prophylactic removal of this utricle would not appear to be indicated.

Hypospadias in Females

True hypospadias, of course, does not occur. However, abnormal urethral meatal positioning can be found, suggesting a form of hypospadias. In all likelihood, those whose meatuses are proximal to the hymenal ring fall into the category of patients with urogenital sinus abnormalities.

Chordee

Significant degrees of chordee are present in about 35% of patients with hypospadias.[66] This correlates well with the greater incidence of the more mild rather than more severe forms of hypospadias. Chordee may be an arrested normal fetal phenomenon. Kaplan and Lamm found ventral penile curvature in 44% of fetuses through the sixth gestational month in their study of abortus specimens.[45]

In the late 1960s and early 1970s, there was a strong feeling that the ventral skin alone was responsible for chordee.[63] Correction of distal hypospadias by release of the ventral skin and transposition of the prepuce ventrally was introduced by Allen and Spence in 1968[2] and applied to a form of more distal hypospadias repair by King in 1970.[48] In many of these patients, however, a

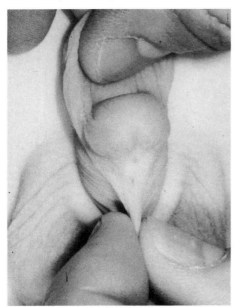

Fig 131–2.—Demonstration of hypospadiac meatus by retracting ventral skin. (From Belman A.B., Kaplan G.W.: *Genitourinary Problems in Pediatrics.* Philadelphia, W.B. Saunders Co., 1981. Reprinted with permission.)

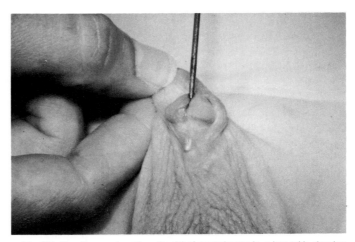

Fig 131–3.—Abnormal urethra devoid of spongiosum in a boy with chordee without hypospadias. Resection of urethra required to achieve straight penis.

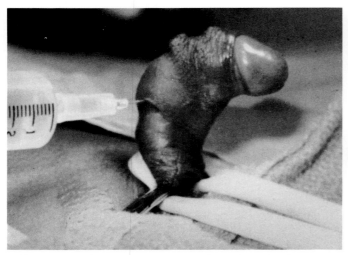

Fig 131–4.—Artificial erection test in boy with chordee without hypospadias. (From Belman A.B., Kaplan G.W.: *Genitourinary Problems in Pediatrics.* Philadelphia, W.B. Saunders Co., 1981. Reprinted with permission.)

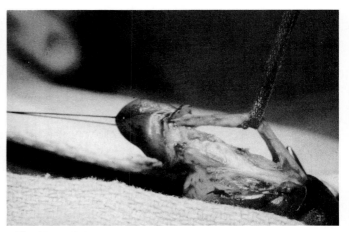

Fig 131–5.—Release of urethra from corpora; same patient as in Figure 131–4. (From Belman A.B., King L.R.: The urethra, in Kelalis P., et al. (eds.): *Clinical Pediatric Urology,* ed. 2. Philadelphia, W.B. Saunders Co., 1984. Reprinted with permission.)

meatus in the corona or proximal glans was accepted as satisfactory.

An important contribution by Gittes and McLaughlin was the introduction of the artificial erection test, which allowed for accurate assessment of chordee[36] (Fig 131–4). Utilization of this test suggests that skin alone is seldom a cause for significant chordee and, in children with true chordee, more extensive dissection of the ventral subcutaneous tissue and urethra itself may be required to achieve a straight penis. Excision of deep bands, which probably represent the remnant of corpus spongiosum associated with the uncanalized urethral groove, is usually necessary to correct chordee fully. The abnormal spongiosum tends to splay out distal to the hypospadiac meatus and may be associated with thickening of Buck's fascia (deep tunica albuginea).[19, 44] Release of chordee may not in all instances be achieved simply by dissection of skin and the deep tissue *distal* to the hypospadiac meatus. In children with more severe forms of hypospadias, mobilization of the urethra proximal to its abnormal position is often necessary.

Chordee Without Hypospadias

One occasionally sees children with chordee and a normally or near normally positioned urethral meatus. Three pathologic classes of "chordee without hypospadias" have been described by Devine and Horton.[23] In the most common type, the spongiosum is missing from the urethra for a variable distance. The often paper-thin distal urethra adheres to the ventral skin, making its preservation impossible. Cendron and Melin have labeled this "concealed hypospadias."[16] Dissection and excision of the abnormal urethra is required.

In the second class of chordee without hypospadias, Devine and Horton found that the urethra itself is completely developed,[23] but the Buck's and dartos layers are abnormal. Chordee may be corrected by mobilizing the intact urethra from the coronal sulcus to the penoscrotal junction, or even more proximally, followed by dissection of the deep tunics (Fig 131–5). Following complete dissection, an artificial erection test should be carried out to prove that the penis is totally straight. In some cases, urethral transection and simultaneous urethroplasty may be the only means of achieving full penile straightening.

The third class of chordee is caused by the ventral skin alone. Some now believe this is relatively rare. It is dealt with simply by releasing ventral skin and allowing it to retract, covering the resultant defect with transposed hooded prepuce.[2] If, with an artificial erection, the penis is then determined to be straight, deeper dissection and urethral mobilization are unnecessary.

Another approach to the problem of chordee without hypospadias is to avoid ventral dissection, and to excise wedges of fascia from the dorsal aspect of the penis. This is an application of the procedure introduced by Nesbit in 1965 for the management of lateral penile curvature.[56] Although this procedure has been applied to congenital glanular tilt (the SST deformity), the risk of damage to the dorsal neurovascular bundle, which splays laterally as it approaches the coronal sulcus, suggests that other means of managing glanular tilt would be more appropriate. Excision of wedges of deep fascia, however, can be appropriately applied to more proximal chordee. Kramer et al. reported successful penile straightening without the necessity for urethral transection in eight of nine children with penile curvature without hypospadias.[49] Cendron and Melin also reported success by this method.[16]

Hypospadias Repair

History

For a two-stage hypospadias repair to be effective, chordee must first be released. In the earliest types of repair, a transverse skin incision was closed longitudinally after release of chordee. The use of ventral penile skin rolled to form a tube during the second stage was introduced by Dieffenbach between 1837 and 1845.[25] Thiersch[67] and Duplay[29] recommended modifications to avoid overlapping suture lines. In many of these earliest trials of hypospadias repair, the new urethra was not initially attached to the hypospadiac meatus. This was left for a separate, third procedure, after the distal tube had healed and was demonstrated to be patent.

Scrotal skin was mobilized to form the urethra by Rochet in 1899[60] and Bucknall[13] in 1907. By and large, the use of hair-bearing scrotal skin has been discouraged because of later complications of encrustation, stone formation, and infection. Cecil, in a notable variation of this technique, also used ventral skin previously transposed from foreskin to form the urethra but buried the penis into the scrotum temporarily, to avoid complications.[15]

The use of a proximal ventral skin pedicle flapped over the hypospadiac meatus to form the new urethra was introduced by Ombrédanne in 1911.[59] That, along with the use of the dorsal prepuce to cover the ventral skin defect and the new urethra, has resulted in procedures currently in vogue today. Transposition of the foreskin by the buttonhole technique was modified and popularized by Nesbit.[57]

Free graft repairs were attempted as early as 1897 by Nové-Josserand.[58] Hairless skin of the upper arm tunneled subcutaneously from the hypospadiac meatus as a second-stage procedure met with limited success. Most of these procedures were not attempted as single-stage repairs, however, with the anastomosis of the hypospadiac meatus to the newly formed urethra being postponed until it was proved that the newly created urethra was intact

A significant contribution was that of Browne who, in 1949, demonstrated that a buried strip of ventral skin would roll up on itself to form a fully tubed urethra.[12] This procedure, still used in certain situations, was very widely used until a few years ago.

Reviews of the various procedures advanced over the years have been published.[5, 7, 21, 41, 71]

Age of Repair

There has been agreement for many years that hypospadias reconstruction should be completed before the child starts school. Recent technical advances support the concept that hypospadias repair can be carried out at almost any age. In 1981, Manley and Epstein reported a series of 17 children operated on between the ages of 10 and 18 months, with noted decrease in the emotional ramifications of genital surgery.[53] Belman and Kass published the results of a prospective study in 37 children ranging in age from 2 to 11 months (average 6.0 months), demonstrating both decreased anxiety and absence of increased technical complications in these infants.[9] A full range of hypospadias abnormalities was seen in that group of patients (Table 131–1). Further reviews by Belman and Kass suggest that there is no difference in complication rates for various procedures, regardless of the age of the patient at the time of operation.[10]

Surgical Procedures

Release of Chordee

For the majority of patients undergoing hypospadias repair, release of chordee will either be the first step in a planned multistaged repair or the initial step in a single-stage repair. In children who have an intrinsically abnormal urethra, release of chordee often requires some degree of excision of urethra. The chordee must be completely released before formal urethroplasty is undertaken.

Multistage Hypospadias Repairs

Certain situations still exist for the use of planned multistaged repairs, although single-stage hypospadias repair has become more popular and is applicable in almost all patients by those with significant surgical expertise. In patients with perineal hypospadias or those with penoscrotal transposition, a two-stage repair may be elected. It is feasible to perform the first stage when the patient is 4–6 months of age and complete the repair approx-

TABLE 131–1.—NUMBER
OF PATIENTS BY MEATAL
POSITION

Glanular	4
Coronal	5
Distal shaft	6
Midshaft	9
Proximal shaft	5
Penoscrotal	7
Perineal	1
Total	37

From Belman and Kass.[9] Reprinted with permission.

imately 6 months later. Reconstruction can thus be completed before the first birthday, obviating emotional problems related to genital surgery carried out at a later age.

BROWNE TECHNIQUE.—In 1949, Browne introduced his procedure, based on the concept of spontaneous tubularization of a buried skin strip.[12] Following release of chordee and healing of ventral tissue, a strip of skin half the width of the desired circumference is outlined from the meatus to the coronal sulcus. Lateral skin flaps are widely dissected and brought together in the midline to cover the undisturbed central skin strip. Horizontal nonabsorbable mattress sutures over a long strip of rubber tubing are used to approximate skin edges and prevent fistulae (Fig 131–6). This technique is now rarely utilized in this country.

BYARS PROCEDURE.—In 1955, Byars introduced a successful two- to three-stage hypospadias repair that allowed creation of a meatus in the glans.[14] At the time of release of chordee, the ventral glans was incised. Dorsal prepuce was mobilized, transposed ventrally after being split in the midline, and laid into the glans to provide skin for the formation of the future distal, glanular urethra. Splitting of the hooded prepuce allowed transposition of adequate skin ventrally, at the first stage, to form the urethra later and to be able to cover the urethral suture line with multiple layers during the second stage. To prevent fistulae, Byars initially postponed joining the new urethra to the hypospadiac meatus, saving that for a third procedure. Shortly after his original description, however, he modified the technique to include incorporation of the hypospadiac meatus during the second stage.

At the second stage, a strip of skin of adequate length is outlined from the hypospadiac meatus into the glans and turned into a tube. The width of the strip should equal in millimeters the caliber of the new urethra in French units, e.g., 12 French equals approximately 12 mm in tube circumference. The lateral skin edges are generously freed to allow complete coverage of the neourethral suture line (Fig 131–7).

CECIL MODIFICATION.—As noted earlier, Cecil added a third stage to hypospadias repair to prevent complications of fistulae.[15] Following creation of the urethra at the time of the second-stage repair, a skin incision is carried out along the midline scrotal raphe to create a trough into which the ventral surface of the

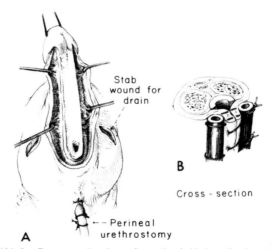

Fig 131–6.—Browne urethroplasty. **A,** a strip of skin is outlined ventrally and buried under skin flaps from the two sides. Lateral bolsters had been used historically to compress skin over the underlying strip. **B,** cross-section of the penis and buried skin strip that will tubulate to become the urethra. (From Belman A.B., King L.R.: The urethra, in Kelalis P., et al. (eds.): *Clinical Pediatric Urology*, ed. 1. Philadelphia, W.B. Saunders Co., 1976. Reprinted with permission.)

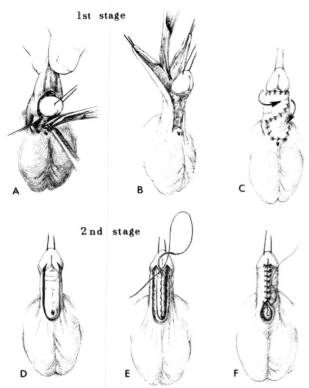

1st stage

A B C

2nd stage

D E F

Fig 131–7.—Two-stage Byars repair of penoscrotal hypospadias. **A–C,** chordee is released and the hooded prepuce split and brought ventrally to cover that surface. **D–F,** formation of the urethra rolling a midline tube. (From Belman A.B., King L.R.: The urethra, Kelalis P., et al. (eds.): *Clinical Pediatric Urology,* ed. 1. Philadelphia, W.B. Saunders Co., 1976. Reprinted with permission.)

penis is buried (Fig 131–8). Lateral edges of penile skin are sutured to lateral edges of scrotal skin, thereby completely eliminating overlapping suture lines. About 4 months after the second stage, the penis is freed from the scrotum, cautiously ensuring that adequate skin exists for closure of the ventral penile flaps.

Disadvantages of this procedure include the transference of hair-bearing scrotal skin to the ventral surface of the penis, pos-

sible outlining of inadequate skin to close the ventral aspect of the penis without tension, and failure to create the normal penoscrotal angle. A fourth problem inherent in this procedure was failure to create a glanular meatus. The coronal meatus that resulted was often patulous and frequently required surgical reduction and revision.

BELT-FUQUA PROCEDURE.—The Belt-Fuqua procedure is a planned two-stage repair that combines release of chordee with transposition of the hooded prepuce ventrally by the buttonhole technique as the first procedure (Fig 131–9). Fuqua reported this repair, which he apparently learned directly from Elmer Belt.[33] Six months following the first stage, the urethra is formed by creating a tube, from the hypospadiac meatus distally, using the previously transposed preputial skin. This tubularized skin is then freed sufficiently from the remaining prepuce and tunneled into the glans, maintaining its viability with a vascular pedicle. An advantage of this repair is the opportunity to create a glanular meatus; a disadvantage is the unsightly residual ventral skin, which may require trimming in a third procedure.

SMITH REPAIR.—A modification of the Byars two-stage technique was reported by Durham Smith in 1973.[64] As in the procedure described by Byars, the ventral aspect of the glans is de-epithelialized and the tips of the split, transposed preputial flaps are laid onto the de-epithelialized glans at the time of initial release of chordee. This preputial skin is fixed to the glans with delicate absorbable sutures and is used to create a meatus at the tip of the glans at the definitive second stage (Fig 131–10). After 3–4 months, the second stage is carried out, incorporating the hypospadiac meatus into the rolled midline skin tube. An ingenious means of preventing fistulae adds to the success of this procedure. After freeing the lateral skin flaps, the medial portion of one of these flaps is cautiously de-epithelialized. This de-epithelialized flap is then brought completely over the midline urethral suture line to the base of the opposite flap and fixed in place with absorbable suture material. The intact skin flap is then brought over this de-epithelialized portion and sutured to its new skin edge, thereby creating a double-layer closure completely covering the new urethra. Smith's exceedingly low fistula rate of 2.9%[65] is documentation of the success of this procedure. As will be noted later, a de-epithelialized flap can add to the successful repair of urethrocutaneous fistulae.

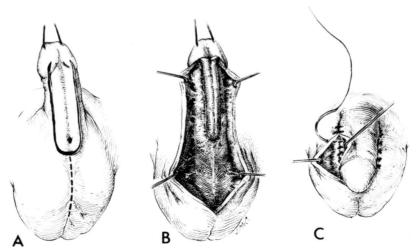

A B C

Fig 131–8.—Cecil urethroplasty. Following the first stage, shown in Figure 131–7, the second stage includes burying the newly formed urethra in the scrotum. A third stage is later required to release the penis. (From Belman A.B., King L.R.: The urethra, in Kelalis P., et al. (eds.): *Clinical Pediatric Urology,* ed. 1. Philadelphia, W.B. Saunders Co., 1976. Reprinted with permission.)

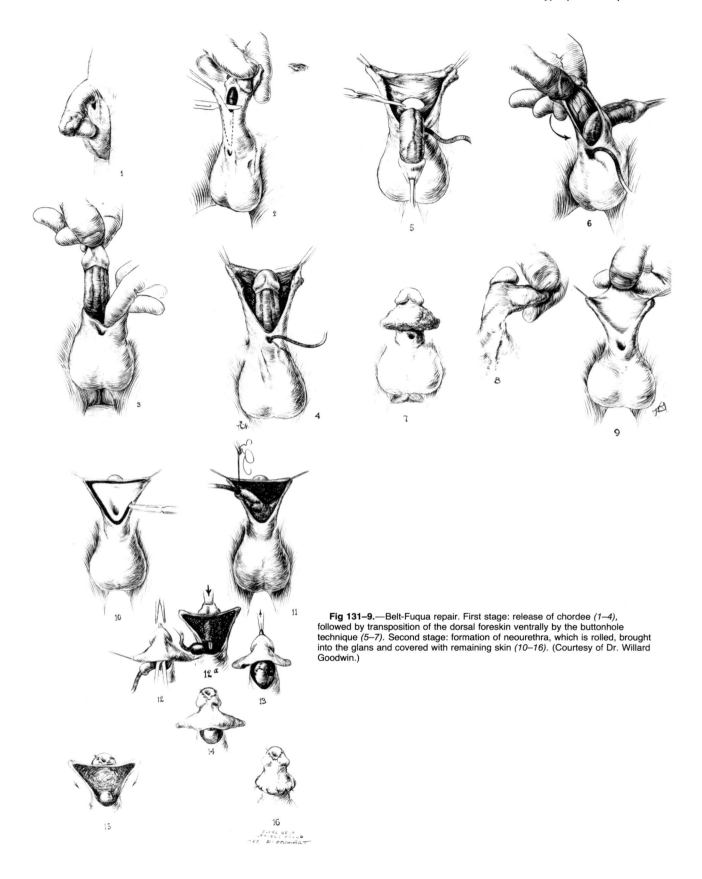

Fig 131–9.—Belt-Fuqua repair. First stage: release of chordee *(1–4)*, followed by transposition of the dorsal foreskin ventrally by the buttonhole technique *(5–7)*. Second stage: formation of neourethra, which is rolled, brought into the glans and covered with remaining skin *(10–16)*. (Courtesy of Dr. Willard Goodwin.)

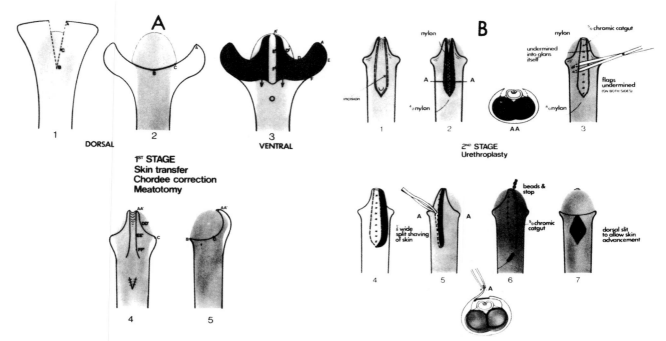

Fig 131–10.—Durham Smith two-stage repair. **A,** first stage. After release of chordee, the dorsal hood is split *(1)* and brought ventrally. The ventral glans is partially de-epithelialized (*dark area* in glans) and the raw surface of the transposed prepuce sutured to the glans *(4)*, thereby resurfacing that portion with redundant skin. *(5),* lateral view of resurfaced ventral penis and glans. **B,** second stage. A midline tube is rolled (including the previously transposed dorsal pre-

puce) to the tip of the glans *(1, 2)*. Lateral skin flaps are freed up *(3)* and one of these is de-epithelialized *(4)*. The de-epithelialized flap is brought *over* the urethral suture line and sutured to the base of the opposite flap *(5)*. The second flap then covers the de-epithelialized portion *(6)* thereby placing two layers over the suture line. (From Smith, E.D. in Holder T.M., Ashcraft K.W. (eds.): *Pediatric Surgery.* Philadelphia, W.B., Saunders Co., 1980. Reprinted with permission.)

Distal Hypospadias Without Chordee

MAGPI.—In individuals with a coronal or glanular hypospadiac meatus without chordee or with only "skin chordee," a normal penile appearance can be achieved by the meatal advancement-glanuloplasty (MAGPI) introduced by Duckett.[27] Following a distal meatotomy, the dorsal edge of urethral mucosa is advanced into the glans, using two to three 6–0 absorbable sutures (Fig 131–11). This tends not only to lengthen the urethra minimally but also to widen its aperture. Following a subcoronal circumcising incision, the ventral skin is carefully dissected off the shaft, avoiding the often thin urethra. Skin hooks and fine tenotomy scissors are helpful in preventing urethral injury. Success of the procedure entails bringing skin of the glans together ventrally, proximal to the advanced meatus, thereby giving the meatus the appearance of being more distal. The urethra itself is actually only minimally changed or unchanged in length. A single hook is applied to the transverse distal ventral skin in the midline and advanced distally. The ventral glanular edges are approximated with interrupted mattress sutures. If inadequate ventral penile skin was present preoperatively causing minimal chordee, dorsal preputial skin is transposed ventrally. This creates both the appearance of penile lengthening and a more normal penoscrotal angle.

The success in achieving a normal penis with this simple procedure has been extremely gratifying. Postoperatively, neither stents nor urinary diversion is necessary, and the patient is discharged the day of operation. However, all individuals with coronal hypospadias are not candidates for the MAGPI procedure.[35] A relatively fish-mouthed or wide urethral meatus or a distal urethra, which is relatively inflexible and cannot be advanced into the glans, precludes this procedure (Fig 131–12). In those circumstances, a meatus based repair is recommended.

Meatus Based Flap Urethroplasty

Hypospadias of the distal shaft rather than of the corona, or a fixed meatus that precludes the MAGPI procedure, can best be repaired with a single-stage meatus based flap. These procedures are not applicable for midshaft hypospadias since the meatal based flap is created from skin proximal to the hypospadiac meatus. If a relatively long urethra must be formed, this would result in the use of hair-bearing scrotal skin and risk the development of a "urethral beard" at adolescence. These procedures are based on the proximal skin flap repair introduced by Ombrédanne.[59]

MATHIEU.[54]—This procedure is particularly applicable to patients with distal shaft or coronal hypospadias with a wide glanular groove. Because it does not involve transection of skin distal to the hypospadiac meatus, it cannot resolve distal glandal tilt. Parallel flaps of sufficient width to create an adequate urethra are outlined from the skin proximal to the meatus extending distally into the glans (Fig 131–13). The combined width of the two flaps, in millimeters, should equal the desired urethral circumference in French catheter units. The incisions are carried into the glans along the entire width to free the lateral glanular wings completely. Two suture lines then result; these are covered by approximating the glanular wings, achieving a normally placed urethral meatus. Excellent results from this procedure have been reported.[37, 69]

Distal Hypospadias With Deep Chordee

In the presence of tilt of the glans, transection of the skin distal to the hypospadiac meatus may be necessary to achieve a straight penis. Two procedures applicable to this circumstance have had excellent results.

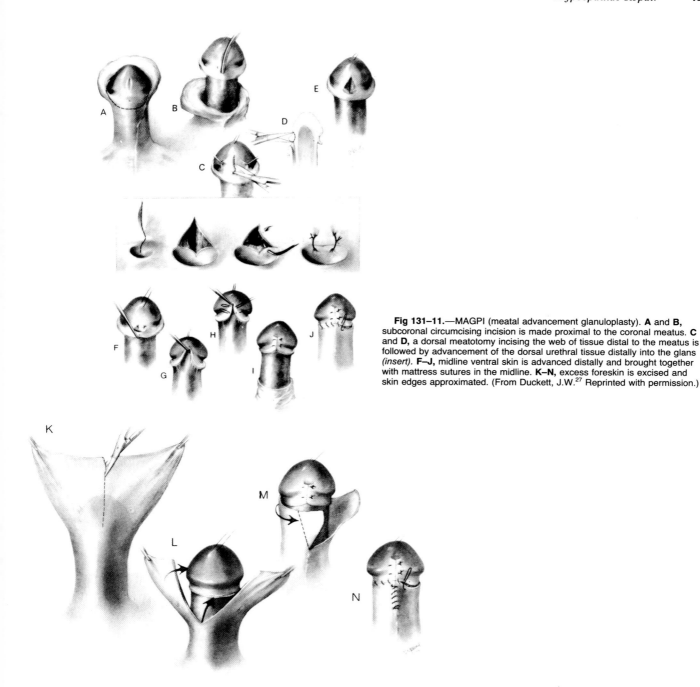

Fig 131–11.—MAGPI (meatal advancement glanuloplasty). **A** and **B,** subcoronal circumcising incision is made proximal to the coronal meatus. **C** and **D,** a dorsal meatotomy incising the web of tissue distal to the meatus is followed by advancement of the dorsal urethral tissue distally into the glans *(insert).* **F–J,** midline ventral skin is advanced distally and brought together with mattress sutures in the midline. **K–N,** excess foreskin is excised and skin edges approximated. (From Duckett, J.W.[27] Reprinted with permission.)

FLIP-FLAP.—In 1973, Horton and Devine[42] introduced their meatal-based flap combining contributions by Bevan[11] and Mustardé.[55] A distal meatus in the glans is achieved, as well as release of any distal chordee (Fig 131–14). A triangular flap of skin proximal to the hypospadiac meatus is created of sufficient length to reach the tip of the glans when the chordee is released. The glans itself is also triangulated, interdigitating the midline flap of the glans into the partially tubularized proximal skin. The glans wings are then either interdigitated or approximated in the midline to cover the new urethra. As in the Mathieu procedure, the ventral skin defect which results from creation of the urethral flap is covered by transposed hooded prepuce.

MUSTARDÉ.—This procedure is similar to the two previously discussed meatal based flaps in that skin proximal to the hypospadiac meatus is employed to create the new urethra.[8] However, compared with both the Mathieu and the flip-flap procedure, a single urethral suture line results and the urethra is brought into the glans by the glans tunnel technique (Fig 131–15).

A flap of proximal tissue of sufficient length and width to create the new urethra, based on the formula previously mentioned, is outlined. Skin distal to the hypospadiac meatus is also transected, thereby freeing any distal chordee. The tube is rolled and the new urethra flipped distal to the hypospadiac meatus,

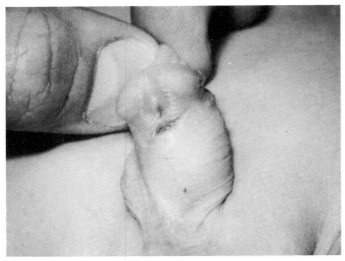

Fig 131–12.—Patient with wide distal shaft meatus, *not* a candidate for MAGPI.

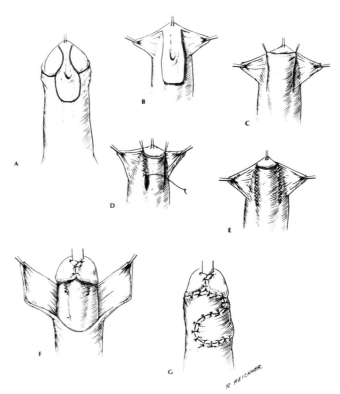

Fig 131–13.—Mathieu repair (flip-flap without urethral mobilization). A flap of tissue proximal to the meatus is marked out, the incisions extending into the glans **(A, B)**. The proximal skin flap is flipped distally and the lateral edges approximated **(C, D)**. Lateral tissue of the glans is freed up and closed in the midline **(E, F)**. Hooded prepuce is split and brought ventrally **(F, G)**. (From Glenn J.F. (ed.): *Urologic Surgery,* ed. 3. Philadelphia, J.B. Lippincott, 1983. Reprinted with permission.)

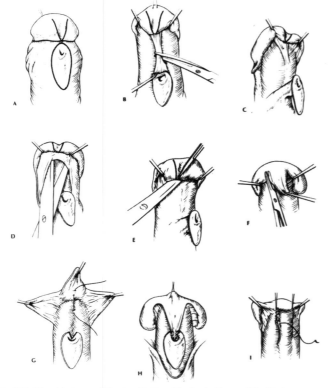

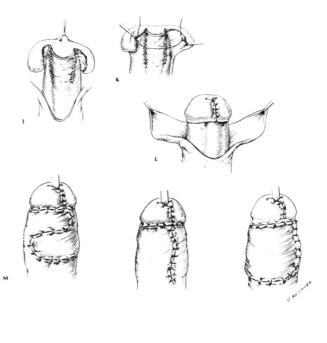

Fig 131–14.—Horton and Devine flip-flap. Similar to Figure 131–13; however, skin distal to the urethra is transected, thereby a tilt of the glans can be relieved. The glans is triangulated **(E–G)** and a spatulated anastomosis carried out **(G–I)**. Lateral wings of glans are brought together **(J–L)** and the hooded prepuce split and brought ventrally to cover the resultant skin defect (a variety of methods of skin coverage are illustrated). (From Glenn J.F. (ed.): *Urologic Surgery,* ed. 3. Philadelphia, J.B. Lippincott, 1983. Reprinted with permission.)

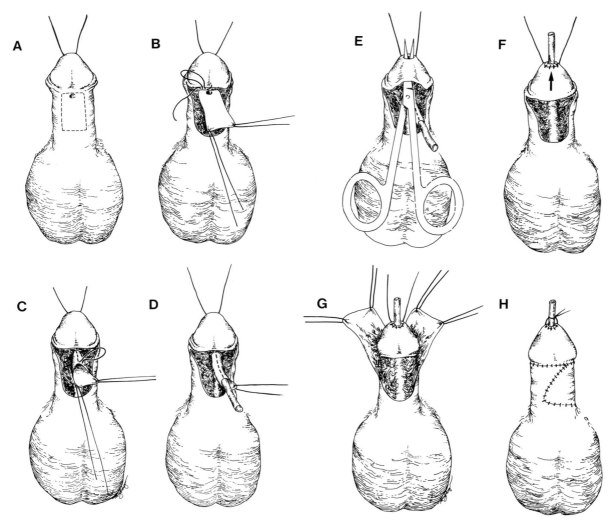

Fig 131–15.—The Mustardé repair. A flap of tissue is outlined proximal to the meatus and freed from the adjacent skin, leaving as much subcutaneous tissue attached as possible **(A, B)**. This flap is rolled into a tube, using a subcuticular running stitch of fine absorbable suture **(C, D)**. The neourethra is brought through a glans tunnel and sutured to the glans **(E, F)**. Dorsal skin is split and transposed ventrally to close the skin defect **(G, H)**. (From Belman A.B., King, L.R.: The urethra, in Kelalis P., et al. (eds.): *Clinical Pediatric Urology,* ed. 2. Philadelphia, W.B. Saunders Co., 1984. Reprinted with permission.)

thereby abutting the single ventral suture line against the corpora. A tunnel is created between the skin of the glans and the glandal erectile tissue and a divot of glans excised at the new meatal site. In all of these procedures, a 5–7-day period of urinary diversion is recommended.

Island Flap Techniques

Between 1969 and 1970, Hamilton,[39] Hodgson,[40] and Toksu[68] each introduced island flap techniques for formation of the urethra. A vascularized tube is formed from preputial skin that remains attached to its underlying subcutaneous tissue. The entire pedicle is transferred ventrally to the site of the new urethra and the tubularized epithelial island anastomosed to the hypospadiac meatus after release of the chordee. Remaining penile skin is then used to resurface that portion of the penis.

HODGSON I.—In 1970, Hodgson introduced a single-stage hypospadias repair using a longitudinal island flap (Fig 131–16).[40] After release of chordee, on the undersurface of the foreskin an island is outlined longitudinally, which will be rolled into a tube. The epithelial island remains attached to the remainder of the dorsal skin and is transposed ventrally by the buttonhole technique. It is rolled into a tube, carefully avoiding devascularization, and anastomosed to the hypospadiac meatus proximally and the glans distally. This procedure is applicable to patients with proximal and midshaft hypospadias.

HODGSON II.—This is a variation of the Hodgson I urethroplasty combined with the procedure advocated by King. It also shares some similarity with the Mathieu procedure. An island of dorsal foreskin is transposed ventrally and then attached to a strip of skin left intact from the meatus into the glans (Fig 131–17). This procedure is applicable only to those patients with hypospadias and no chordee.

HODGSON III.—The Hodgson III procedure uses the dorsal aspect of the penile skin and is applied to more severe forms of hypospadias. The buttonhole is made at the penile base with transposition of the entire penile skin ventrally (Fig 131–18). The island is then formed from the dorsal aspect of the penis and the penis is then resurfaced with lateral flaps brought dorsally. The skin closure is then on the dorsal aspect of the penis, completely avoiding crossing suture lines. A modification of this operation

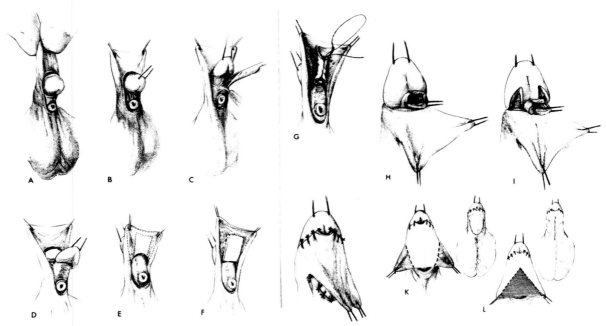

Fig 131–16.—Hodgson I repair. Following release of chordee **(A–C),** the hooded prepuce is transposed ventrally by the buttonhole technique. An island of epithelium is outlined on the undersurface of the prepuce **(E, F)** and rolled into a tube **(G).** Anastomosis to the hypospadiac meatus proximally and glans distally is followed by approximation of the foreskin ventrally **(H–L).** Excessive skin can be removed, but care must be taken not to devascularize the new urethra. (From Belman A.B., King L.R.: The urethra, Kelalis P., et al. (eds.): *Clinical Pediatric Urology,* ed. 1. Philadelphia, W.B. Saunders Co., 1976. Reprinted with permission.)

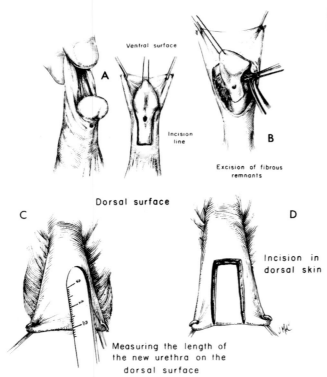

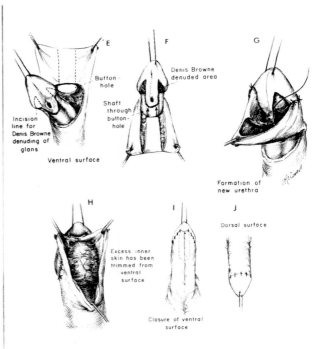

Fig 131–17.—Hodgson II repair (for hypospadias without *chordee*). Skin distal to the meatus is outlined and the subcorona circumscribed **(A, B).** A dorsal island flap is formed and the foreskin transposed ventrally by the buttonhole technique to the meatus and onto the glans, which may be partially de-epithelialized **(G, H).** Excessive skin is trimmed and edges approximated. (From Harrison J.H., et al. (eds.): *Campbell's Urology,* ed. 4. Philadelphia, W.B. Saunders Co., 1979. Reprinted with permission.)

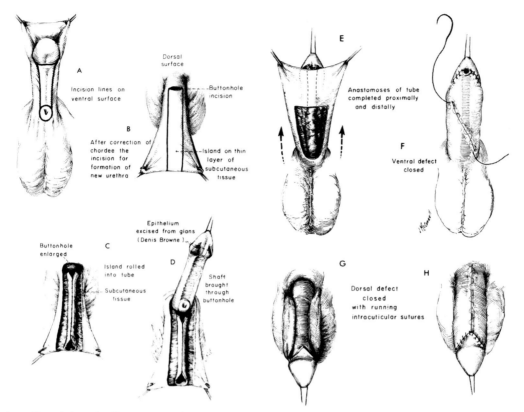

Fig 131–18.—Hodgson III repair (see also Figs 131–16 and 131–17). Immediately following release of the chordee, a long dorsal island is constructed and rolled into a skin tube **(A–C)**. Through a buttonhole at the base of the penis, all penile skin is transposed and the new urethra anastomosed to the hypospadiac meatus **(D)**. Lateral skin is brought dorsal and skin edges approximated **(E–H)**. From Harrison J.H., et al. (eds.): *Campbell's Urology,* ed. 4. Philadelphia, W.B. Saunders Co., 1979. Reprinted with permission.)

has been reported by Kroovand and Perlmutter;[50] however, one must be concerned about the use of dorsal hair-bearing skin for the proximal portion of the urethra.

A concern with flaps of all these types is that the distal urethra is not truly placed within the glans but is attached to it and covered by remaining foreskin. Although the risk of meatal stenosis must be very low, these procedures inherently produce a floppy meatus.

TRANSVERSE PREPUTIAL ISLAND FLAP.—In 1980, Duckett introduced a variation on the island flap technique, using the undersurface of the prepuce transversely.[28] This is a variation of the theme introduced in 1971 by Asopa.[4] The procedure is a single-stage repair that can be applied to virtually all forms of hypospadias with meatuses from the penoscrotal junction to the distal shaft.

After release of chordee, the dorsal skin, including all its deep subcutaneous tissue, is dissected from the shaft (Fig 131–19). The length of urethra required is measured and marked out on the undersurface of the foreskin. An incision is made transversely at the junction between the undersurface of the foreskin and the remainder of the dorsal skin. The success of this operation is based on the existence of a separate blood supply to the undersurface of the foreskin, from the remainder of the dorsal skin. This pedicle must be carefully teased from the deep subcutaneous tissue of the dorsal skin, maintaining its vascularity. The residual dorsal skin is then split in the midline to the base of the pedicle. The skin flap can then be tubularized with secondary anastomosis to the dissected hypospadiac meatus, or tubularization can follow the anastomosis of this flap to the hypospadiac

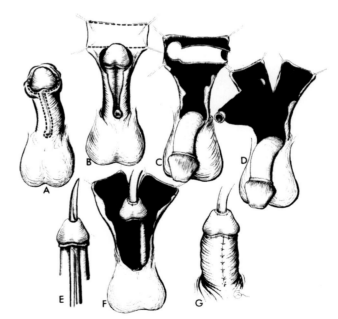

Fig 131–19.—Duckett transverse preputial island flap hypospadias repair. Following release of chordee and mobilization of the dorsal penile skin **(A)**, the undersurface of the hooded prepuce with its blood supply is separated from the remainder of the dorsal skin **(B–D)**, rolled into a tube **(D)**, swung ventrally, anastomosed to the hypospadiac meatus, and tunneled through the glans to create a normally positioned urethral meatus **(E, F)**. Dorsal skin covers the resultant ventral defect **(F, G)**. (From Duckett J.W.[27] Reprinted with permission.)

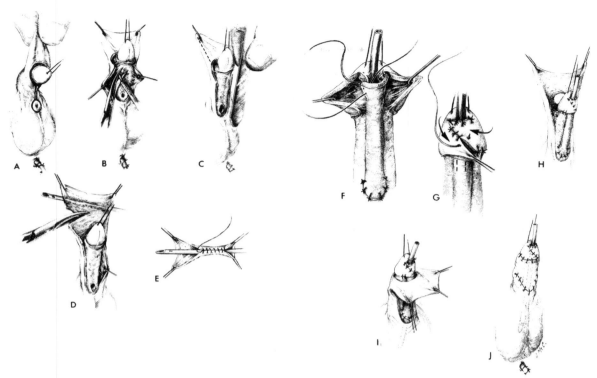

Fig 131–20.—Devine and Horton free graft hypospadias repair. Following correction of chordee **(A, B),** an appropriate amount of undersurface of the foreskin is removed, defatted, and rolled into a tube **(C–E).** Proximal and distal anastomosis, including triangulation of the glans **(F–H),** is followed by transposition of dorsal skin to cover the resultant ventral defect. (From Belman A.B., King L.R.: The urethra, in Kelalis P., et al. (eds.): *Clinical Pediatric Urology,* ed. 1. Philadelphia, W.B. Saunders Co., 1976. Reprinted with permission.)

meatus. Because the new tube is free of any surrounding skin, it can either be laid into the split glans or tunneled through it to create a meatus at the tip of the glans. The remaining dorsal skin that was previously split in the midline is swung around laterally to cover the ventral skin defect.

Free Graft Techniques

Free graft techniques, using skin from a variety of locations, have been used in hypospadias repair for many decades. However, it was not until 1961, when Devine and Horton applied full-thickness skin grafts rather than split-thickness skin, that significant success with this approach was achieved.[24] Ideally, foreskin should be utilized since it is thin and non–hair-bearing; however, other non–hair-bearing skin, such as that from the region of the iliac crest, inner arm, and neck may also be used. Tissue other than skin has also been utilized for the creation of the urethra, including bladder mucosa.[18, 51] The advantage of the free graft technique is that single-stage repairs can be universally applied and this method can be freely utilized for complicated reoperations. The greatest disadvantage is the risk of loss of the graft with stenosis and fibrosis of the new urethra rather than a simple fistula, which is more common with the pedicle graft techniques.

Following release of chordee, the skin graft is defatted and rolled into a tube over a catheter (Fig 131–20). Spatulation of the urethra is desirable to prevent stenosis, and the construction of the meatus in the glans can be individualized, based on the technique preferred by the surgeon. Classically, Horton and Devine have spatulated the glans, forming a triangularized anastomosis with a pedicle of well-vascularized glans tissue inserted into the distal graft. Dorsal skin is then closed over the ventral skin defect in as many layers as possible.

Perineal Hypospadias

There are many approaches to the child with perineal hypospadias, including application of the various procedures described above, either as single-stage or multistage repairs. Most surgeons prefer a staged approach to this more severe problem. Recent combining of two different procedures has met with some success. Following release of chordee, the midline perineal skin is rolled to extend the urethra into the region of the penoscrotal junction, followed by application of the transverse preputial island flap. Repair completed before 1 year of age allows these children to grow up without the emotional stigma of abnormal genitalia or having to adjust to multiple procedures.

Technical Factors

The advances in hypospadias surgery over the past decade are attributable to numerous sources. Innovations, improvements in suture material, and optical magnification all play an important role. However, the use of fine skin hooks and traction sutures, multiple layered closure, and fine hemostatic technique may be principally responsible for improvements in results and our ability to perform the procedures in younger children and infants.

Urinary Diversion

Most urethroplasties require some form of postoperative urinary diversion. The choices range from an indwelling urethral catheter to formal perineal urethrostomy or suprapubic diversion. In the past few years, several forms of disposable percutaneous trochar cystostomy sets, which are easily inserted and function satisfactorily, have been introduced. Our own practice is to use the Stamey (UPI) cystostomy set along with a silicone urethral stent. The suprapubic tube is maintained for 7–10 days, depending on the extent of the surgical procedure. For a meatal-based flap, a 7-day diversion is employed. For a more complicated hypospadias requiring an island flap urethroplasty, urinary diversion is maintained for 10 days. Nevertheless, perineal urethrostomy is still reported to be successful.[47] The use of a silicone catheter without other forms of urinary diversion is favored by others.[31] Cromie and Bellinger, in a report based on a questionnaire sent to a group of pediatric urologists, found that 64% of the responders used either some form of urethral stent in conjunction with cystostomy or a catheter for a variable period of time after operation.[20] Urethral intubation prevents meatal encrustation, which can cause proximal blowout and a fistula when the child begins to void. The stent also serves as a route for egress of urine if the patient should have bladder spasms secondary to the cystostomy.

Hemostasis

Since both bleeding and swelling are not always entirely controllable after hypospadias repair, most surgeons choose some form of compression dressing postoperatively. The use of 1:100,000 epinephrine in a local anesthetic base has been recommended by some as a means of minimizing intraoperative bleeding. Of the many forms of hypospadias dressings, I use the Elastoplast dressing introduced by Falkowski and Firlit.[31] The dressing is maintained for a variable period of time but generally no more than 2–3 days. In addition to the compression dressing, the penis is initially wrapped with a layer of Owens gauze, which is maintained intact throughout the postoperative period. The gauze is then soaked off the day before the urinary diversion is removed. A disadvantage noted by many is the inability to inspect the penis during the postoperative period; however, that has not been a problem in my practice.

By and large, preoperative antibiotics are probably not necessary. If, however, a child has a history of urinary tract infections and/or has had multiple previous procedures, specific or prophylactic antibiotics should be considered. The child who has had urinary tract infection should be evaluated before definitive genital surgery to rule out any urinary abnormality. A urine culture is done 5 days before the procedure to ascertain urine sterility. For those having the second stage of a planned two-stage procedure, or those who are having correction of complications of previous attempts at hypospadias repair, preoperative antibiotic prophylaxis is probably indicated. The combination of an aminoglycoside and penicillin has been effective in preventing wound infection following hypospadias repair. I use preoperative antibiotics routinely in the child with pubic hair; they are usually given twice prior to operation, i.e., the evening before and the morning of the planned procedure.

In a report by Shohet et al.,[62] those patients on postoperative sulfa prophylaxis had significantly reduced bacilluria. We use trimethoprim-sulfa postoperatively in all these patients and maintain that regimen for 2 or 3 days following removal of tubes. Additionally, these children are kept on oxybutynin chloride to minimize bladder spasms throughout the postoperative period and often are given diazepam for sedation during the first 2 or 3 postoperative days, when the compression dressing is being used.

Complications

One of the most severe and disconcerting problems following hypospadias repair is persistent chordee. Every effort must be made to ensure that chordee is completely released before the formation of the neourethra.

Meatal Stenosis

A more common but less disconcerting complication is meatal stenosis. With the current effort to place the meatus in the normal position at the tip of the glans, the risk of meatal stenosis increases. Devine and Horton's triangularization of the glans, minimizing meatal stenosis, has been adopted by many. Another approach is to create a glans tunnel of sufficient width to accept readily the new urethra, excising a divot of distal glans at the meatal site. Although some make it a practice to dilate the urethra postoperatively, we do not do it routinely. Meatal stenosis is also one of the causes for disruption of the proximal urethra, or formation of a diverticulum. The caliber of the meatus and distal urethra should be closely evaluated in all individuals who develop a fistula.

Meatotomy can be simply carried out by performing a dorsal or ventral incision into the meatal ring and advancing the urethra distally. In patients with more extensive distal urethral stenosis, conversion to a more proximal meatus and simultaneous MAGPI procedure may resolve the stenotic problem, maintaining the meatus in an adequate position.

Fistula

The most common complication of hypospadias repair is urethrocutaneous fistula. The incidence of fistulae ranges from virtually zero to 50%, depending on the extent of the surgical procedure. The incidence of fistulae with a meatal-based flap ranges about 5% to 10%. In the more severe forms of hypospadias treated by a single-stage repair, either the free graft technique or the transverse island flap, fistula incidence ranges between 6% and 30% (Table 131–2). Many small fistulae will close spontaneously, and a period of observation is recommended before closure is attempted. Induration following operation must have resolved completely before attempted closure. By applying the technical considerations previously referred to, a high success rate has been achieved in closure of fistulae. Either pedicle flaps or a modification of the de-epithelialized flap technique of Smith for fistulae on the penile shaft will virtually assure successful closure without the necessity for urinary diversion.[34,70] Closure of distal urethral fistulae, particularly in the region of the corona, has been more challenging. Skin advancement into the de-epithelialized proximal glans has met with considerable success, again without the need for urinary diversion.[34]

Urethral Diverticula

Another complication secondary to distal obstruction or infection is a pseudodiverticulum. A blowout of the urethra may result in a urine leak that does not reach the skin level but instead forms a contained urinoma. Epithelialization of this area may result in a narrow-mouthed diverticulum, which can be troublesome. Postvoiding urinary dribbling is the primary sign of this complication. Excision of the diverticulum, closure of its mouth, and a multilayered skin approximation, using either a pedicle flap or a de-epithelialized skin flap, is curative.

Urethral Stricture and Urethral Stenosis

Those procedures which involve an abutted end-to-end anastomosis (i.e., the free graft technique or transverse preputial flap technique) may lead to stenosis at the hypospadiac meatus. Spatulation or triangulation of this anastomosis will minimize this complication. These procedures may result in devascularization, scarring, and stenosis of any portion of the urethra. Late stenosis manifests itself by voiding difficulties, urinary tract infection, or

TABLE 131–2.—PROCEDURES FOR HYPOSPADIAS REPAIR

PROCEDURE	AUTHOR	EXPERIENCE	FISTULAE (%)	STENOSES (%)
Single-Stage Techniques				
Glanular-Coronal				
MAGPI	Duckett (1981)	200	1 (0.5)	0
Urethral	Mills et al. (1981)[1]	8	0	0
advancement	Koff (1981)[2]	10	0	1 (10)
Distal shaft without chordee				
Mathieu	Wacksman (1981)	20	1 (5)	1 (5)
	Gonzales et al. (1983)	63	3 (5)	1 (1.5)
Distal shaft with or without chordee				
Flip flap	Devine and Horton (1976)	55	6 (10.9)	?
	Shubailat and Ajlumi (1978)[3]	62	1 (1.6)	1 (1.6)
	Woodard and Cleveland (1982)[4]	76	8 (10.5)	9 (12)
Mustardé	Kim and Hendren (1981)	50	0	2 (4)
	Belman (1981)[5]	30	1 (3.3)	3 (10)
Midshaft with skin chordee				
King	Sadlowsky et al. (1974)[6]	85	3 (3.5)	1 (1.2)
	Marshall et al. (1978)[7]	102	3 (3.0)	2 (2.0)
Island flap techniques				
Hodgson I	Hodgson (1975)[8]	38	3 (7.8)	4 (10.5)
Hodgson II	Hodgson (1975)	93	0	1 (1.1)
Hodgson III	Kroovand and Perlmutter (1980)[9]	47	3 (6.0)	10 (22.7)
Duckett	Duckett (1980)	100	10%*	
Free graft techniques				
Devine and Horton	Devine and Horton (1977)[10]	20	4 (20)	?
	Woodard and Cleveland (1982)	28	8 (29)	5 (17.9)
Bladder mucosa	Li et al. (1981)	64	12 (18.8)	7 (10.9)
Multistage Techniques				
Denis Browne	Kelalis et al. (1977)[11]	23	(25)	?
	Gearhart and Witherington (1979)[12]	64	11 (17.1)	4 (6.2)
	Bailen and Howerton (1980)[13]	40	2 (50)	1 (2.5)
	Donnelly and Prenderville (1981)[14]	72	4 (5.5)	5 (6.9)
Crawford (modified)	Marberger and Paner (1981)[15]	183	34 (18.6)	?
	Yarbrough and Johnston (1977)[16]	96	9 (9.3)	3 (3.1)
Byars	Wray et al. (1976)[17]	253	54 (21.3)	17 (6.7)
Cecil	Kelalis (1981)[18]	135	4 (3.0)	9 (6.6)
Belt-Fuqua	Hensle and Mollitt (1981)[19]	30	2 (6.6)	1 (3.3)
	Hendren (1981)[20]	140	2 (1.4)	4 (2.8)
Smith	Smith (1980)[21]	210	6 (2.9)	7 (3.3)

Modified from Kelalis P. et al. (eds): *Clinical Pediatric Urology*, Philadelphia, W.B. Saunders Co., 1976.

*Specific details not given regarding fistulae, stenoses, flap breakdown.

[1]Mills C., McGovern J., Mininberg D., et al.: *J. Urol.* 125:701, 1981
[2]Koff S.A.: *J. Urol.* 125:394, 1981.
[3]Shubailat G.F., Ajlumi N.J.: *Plast. Reconstr. Surg.* 62:546, 1978.
[4]Woodard J.R., Cleveland R.: *J. Urol.* 127:1155, 1982.
[5]Belman A.B.: *Urol. Clin. North Am.* 8:483, 1981.
[6]Sadlowski R.W., Belman A.B., King L.R.: *J. Urol.* 112:677, 1974.
[7]Marshall M., Jr., Beh W.P., Johnson S.H. III, et al.: *J. Urol.* 120:229, 1978.
[8]Hodgson N.B.: In Glenn J.F. (ed.): *Urologic Surgery*, ed. 2. Hagerstown, Md., Harper & Row, 1975.
[9]Kroovand R.C., Perlmutter A.D.: *J. Urol.* 124:530, 1980.
[10]Devine C.J., Jr., Horton C.E.: *J. Urol.* 118:188, 1977.
[11]Kelalis P.P., Benson R.C. Jr., Culp O.S.: *J. Urol.* 118:657, 1977.
[12]Gearhart J.P., Witherington R.: *J. Urol.* 127:66, 1979.
[13]Bailen J., Howerton L.W.: *J. Urol.* 123:754, 1980.
[14]Donnelly B.J., Prenderville J.B.: *J. Urol.* 125:706, 1981.
[15]Marberger H., Paner W.: *J. Urol.* 125:698, 1981.
[16]Yarbrough W.J., Johnston J.H.: *J. Urol.* 117:782, 1977.
[17]Wray R.C., Ribando J.M., Weeks P.M.: *Plast. Reconstr. Surg.* 58:329, 1976.
[18]Kelalis P.P.: *J. Urol. (Paris)* 87:93, 1981.
[19]Hensle T.W., Mollitt D.C.: *J. Urol.* 125:703, 1981.
[20]Hendren W.H.: *Urol. Clin. North Am.* 8:431, 1981.
[21]Smith E.D.: In Holder T.M., K.W. Ashcraft (eds.): *Pediatric Surgery*. Philadelphia, W.B. Saunders Co., 1980.

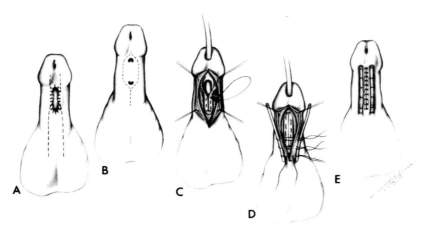

Fig 131–21.—Repair of urethral stricture utilizing the two-stage Johanson technique. The stricture is incised, opened, and the edges sutured to the lateral skin edges **(A)**. Following healing (6 months), a tube of skin is rolled to form the urethra and multiple layers closed over the new urethra **(B, C)**. Lateral bolsters **(D, E)** are now seldom used. (From Belman A.B., King L.R.: The urethra, in Kelalis P., et al. (eds.): *Clinical Pediatric Urology,* ed. 1. Philadelphia, W.B. Saunders Co., 1976. Reprinted with permission.)

both. Some surgeons carry out routine postoperative urethral dilatations or calibrations hoping to prevent this complication or to recognize it early. It is unlikely that periodic urethral dilatation will prevent problems secondary to poor blood supply of the neourethra.

Urethral stricture or stenosis may be initially treated by either dilatation or by direct urethrotomy. Ultimately, some will require a two-staged procedure based on the Johanson technique (Fig 131–21) or with a free or pedicle patch graft as a single-stage procedure.

REFERENCES

1. Aarskog D.: Maternal progestins as a possible cause of hypospadias. *N. Engl. J. Med.* 300:75, 1979.
2. Allen T.D., Spence H.M.: The surgical treatment of coronal hypospadias and related problems. *J. Urol.* 100:504, 1968.
3. Arey L.B.: *Developmental Anatomy: A Textbook and Laboratory Manual of Embryology,* ed. 7. Philadelphia, W.B. Saunders Co., 1974.
4. Asopa H.S., Elhence E.P., Atria S.P., et al.: One stage correction of penile hypospadias using a foreskin tube: A preliminary report. *Int. Surg.* 55:435, 1971.
5. Backus H.L., DeFelice C.A.: Hypospadias—then and now. *Plast. Reconstr. Surg.* 25:147, 1960.
6. Bauer S.B., Retik A.B., Colodny A.H.: Genetic aspects of hypospadias. *Urol. Clin. North Am.* 8:559, 1981.
7. Beck C.: Hypospadias and its treatment. *Surg. Gynecol. Obstet.* 24:511, 1917.
8. Belman A.B.: The modified Mustardé hypospadias repair. *J. Urol.* 127:88, 1982.
9. Belman A.B., Kass E.J.: Hypospadias repair in children less than one year old. *J. Urol.* 128:1273, 1982.
10. Belman A.B., Kass E.J.: Unpublished data.
11. Bevan A.D.: A new operation for hypospadias. *JAMA* 68:1032, 1917.
12. Browne D.: An operation for hypospadias. *Proc. R. Soc. Med.* 42:466, 1949.
13. Bucknall R.T.H.: A new operation for penile hypospadias. *Lancet* 2:887, 1907.
14. Byars L.T.: A technique for consistently satisfactory repair of hypospadias. *Surg. Gynecol. Obstet.* 100:184, 1955.
15. Cecil A.B.: Repair of hypospadias and urethral fistula. *J. Urol.* 56:237, 1946.
16. Cendron J., Melin Y.: Congenital curvature of the penis without hypospadias. *Urol. Clin. North Am.* 8:389, 1981.
17. Chung C.S., Myrianthopoulos N.C.: Racial and prenatal factors in major congenital malformations. *Am. J. Hum. Genet.* 20:44, 1968.
18. Coleman J.W.: The bladder mucosal graft technique for hypospadias repair. *J. Urol.* 125:708, 1981.
19. Creevy C.D.: The correction of hypospadias: A review. *Urol. Surg.* 8:2, 1958.
20. Cromie W.J., Bellinger M.F.: Hypospadias dressings and diversions. *Urol. Clin. North Am.* 8:545, 1981.
21. Culp O.S., McRoberts J.W.: Hypospadias, in Alken C.E., et al. (eds.): *Encyclopedia of Urology.* Berlin, Springer-Verlag, 1968.
22. Devine C.J. Jr., Gonzalez-Serva L., Stecker J.F. Jr., et al.: Utricular configuration in hypospadias and intersex. *J. Urol.* 123:407, 1980.
23. Devine C.J. Jr., Horton C.E.: Chordee without hypospadias. *J. Urol.* 110:264, 1973.
24. Devine C.J. Jr., Horton C.E.: A one-stage hypospadias repair. *J. Urol.* 85:166, 1961.
25. Dieffenbach J.F.: The simple canalization method, in *Dictionnaire encyclopédique de médicine,* Paris, Bibliothèque National, 1838.
26. *Dorland's Illustrated Medical Dictionary,* ed. 26. Philadelphia, W.B. Saunders Co., 1981.
27. Duckett J.W. Jr.: MAGPI (meatoplasty and glanuloplasty): A procedure for subcoronal hypospadias. *Urol. Clin. North Am.* 8:513, 1981.
28. Duckett J.W. Jr.: Transverse preputial island flap technique for repair of severe hypospadias. *Urol. Clin. North Am.* 7:423, 1980.
29. Duplay S.: Perineal hypospadias. *Arch. Gen. Med.* (Paris) 1:513, 1874.
30. Fallon B., Devine C.J. Jr., Horton C.E.: Congenital anomalies associated with hypospadias. *J. Urol.* 116:585, 1976.
31. Falkowski W.S., Firlit C.F.: Hypospadias surgery: The X-shaped elastic dressing. *J. Urol.* 123:904, 1980.
32. Feldman K.W., Smith D.W.: Fetal phallic growth and penile standards for newborn male infants. *J. Pediatr.* 86:395, 1975.
33. Fuqua F.: Renaissance of urethroplasty: The Belt technique of hypospadias repair. *J. Urol.* 106:782, 1971.
34. Geltzeiler J., Belman A.B.: Results of closure of urethrocutaneous fistulae in children. *J. Urol.* 132:734, 1984.
35. Gibbons M.D., Gonzales E.T. Jr.: The subcoronal meatus. *J. Urol.* 130:739, 1983.
36. Gittes R.F., McLaughlin A.P.: Injection technique to induce penile erection. *Urology* 4:473, 1974.
37. Gonzales E.T. Jr., Veeraraghavan K.A., Delaune J.: The management of distal hypospadias with meatal-based vascularized flaps. *J. Urol.* 129:119, 1983.
38. Guthrie R.D., Smith D.W., Graham C.B.: Testosterone treatment for micropenis during early childhood. *J. Pediatr.* 83:247, 1973.
39. Hamilton J.M.: Island flap repair of hypospadias. *South. Med. J.* 62:881, 1969.
40. Hodgson N.B.: One-stage hypospadias repair. *J. Urol.* 104:281, 1970.
41. Horton C.E. (ed.): *Plastic and Reconstructive Surgery of the Genital Area.* Boston, Little, Brown & Co., 1973.
42. Horton C.E., Devine C.J. Jr.: One stage repair, in Horton C.E. (ed.): *Plastic and Reconstructive Surgery of the Genital Area.* Boston, Little, Brown & Co., 1973, p. 278.
43. Ikoma H.S., Terakawa T., Satoh Y., et al.: Developmental anomalies associated with hypospadias. *J. Urol.* 122:619, 1979.
44. Jones H.W. Jr., Scott W.W.: *Hermaphroditism, Genital Anomalies and Related Endocrine Disorders,* ed. 2. Baltimore, Williams & Wilkins Co., 1971.
45. Kaplan G.W., Lamm D.L.: Embryogenesis of chordee. *J. Urol.* 114:769, 1975.
46. Khuri F.J., Hardy B.E., Churchill B.M.: Urologic anomalies associated with hypospadias. *Urol. Clin. North Am.* 8:565, 1981.

47. Kim S.H., Hendren W.H.: Repair of mild hypospadias. *J. Pediatr. Surg.* 16:806, 1981.
48. King L.R.: Hypospadias—a one-stage repair without skin graft based on a new principle: Chordee is sometimes produced by the skin alone. *J. Urol.* 103:660, 1970.
49. Kramer S.A., Aydin G., Kelalis P.P.: Chordee without hypospadias in children. *J. Urol.* 128:539, 1982.
50. Kroovand R.L., Perlmutter A.D.: Reverse tumble flap with tubed island-flap urethroplasty or chordee without hypospadias. *J. Urol.* 124:530, 1981.
51. Li C., Zheng Y.H., Sheh Y.X., et al.: One stage urethroplasty for hypospadias using a tube constructed with bladder mucosa—a new procedure. *Urol. Clin. North Am.* 8:463, 1981.
52. Lutzker L.G., Kogan S.J., Levitt S.S.: Is routine intravenous urography indicated in patients with hypospadias? *Pediatrics* 59:630, 1977.
53. Manley C.B., Epstein E.S.: Early hypospadias repair. *J. Urol.* 125:698, 1981.
54. Mathieu P.: Traitement en un temps de l'hypospadias balanique et juxtabalanique. *J. Chir.* 39:481, 1932.
55. Mustardé J.C.: One-stage correction of distal hypospadias and other people's fistulae. *Br. J. Plast. Surg.* 18:413, 1965.
56. Nesbit R.M.: Operation for correction of distal penile ventral curvature with or without hypospadias. *J. Urol.* 97:720, 1967.
57. Nesbit R.M.: Plastic procedure of correction of hypospadias. *J. Urol.* 45:699, 1941.
58. Nové-Josserand G.: Résultats éloignés de l'urethroplastie par la tunnelisation et la greffe dermo-épidermique dans les formes graves de l'hypospadias et de l'épispadias. *J. Urol. Méd. Chir.* 5:393, 1914.
59. Ombrédanne L.: Précis clinique et opération de chirurgie infantile. Paris, Masson, 1932, p. 851.
60. Rochet W.: Noveau procédé pour refaire le canal pénien dans l'hypospadias. *Gaz. Hebd. Méd. Chir.* 46:673, 1899.
61. Rozenman J., Hertz M., Boichis H.: Radiological findings of the urinary tract in hypospadias: A report of 110 cases. *Clin. Radiol.* 30:471, 1979.
62. Shohet I., Alagam M., Shafir R., et al.: Postoperative catheterization and prophylactic antimicrobials in children with hypospadias. *Urology* 22:391, 1983.
63. Smith D.R.: Repair of hypospadias in the preschool child: A report of 150 cases. *J. Urol.* 97:723, 1967.
64. Smith E.D.: A de-epithelialized overlap flap technique in the repair of hypospadias. *Br. J. Plast. Surg.* 26:106, 1973.
65. Smith E.D.: Malformations of the bladder, urethra and hypospadias, in Holder T.M., Ashcraft K.W. (eds.): *Pediatric Surgery.* Philadelphia, W.B. Saunders Co., 1980, p. 785.
66. Sweet R.A., Schrott H.G., Kurland R., et al.: Study of the incidence of hypospadias in Rochester, Minn., 1940–1970, and a case control comparison of possible etiologic factors. *Mayo Clin. Proc.* 49:52, 1974.
67. Thiersch C.: Uber die Entstehungsweise und operative Behandlung der Epispadie. *Arch. Heilkunde.* 10:20, 1869.
68. Toksu E.: Hypospadias: One-stage repair. *J. Plast. Reconstr. Surg.* 45:365, 1970.
69. Wacksman J.: Modification of the one-stage flip-flap procedure to repair distal penile hypospadias. *Urol. Clin. North Am.* 8:527, 1981.
70. Walker R.D.: Outpatient repair of urethral fistulae. *Urol. Clin. North Am.* 8:582, 1981.
71. Young F., Benjamin J.A.: Preschool age repair of hypospadias with free inlay graft. *Surgery* 26:384, 1949.

132   Robert D. Jeffs / John S. T. Masterson

Epispadias

HISTORY.—In 1769, Morgagni[43] first described epispadias in a patient who had been declared unfit for matrimony by a court of law. The patient committed suicide and was examined postmortem by Morgagni.[43] The earliest operations were concerned with creation of a neourethra in male patients and were carried out in 1845 by Dieffenbach[15] and in 1869 by Thiersch.[53] Duplay in 1880 and Boiffin in 1895 recognized a deficiency of bladder neck fibers. This was postulated to be the cause of urinary incontinence, and both authors described isolated cases cured by excision of bladder neck tissue with reapproximation of the bladder neck. However, the overall results from such anti-incontinence procedures were so poor that Stiles[51] in 1911 recommended internal urinary diversion even though ureterosigmoidostomy was associated with a mortality rate of 55%. In 1895, Cantwell[6] described a method of tubularizing the dorsal urethral strip, which was totally detached from the glans and corpora. The mobilized neourethra was then transposed to a more anatomical position on the ventral aspect of the penis. An improved procedure was described by Young[59] in 1918, who preserved the blood supply to the neourethra by preserving its attachment to one corpus cavernosum. The corpora were then rotated to produce ventral displacement of the neourethra.

In 1922, Young[60, 61] described his "double sphincter" reconstruction in a male epispadiac. Using a combined suprapubic and subpubic approach, he excised the anterior tissues of the bladder neck and urethra, and reapproximated the edges, bladder neck, and urethra over a silver probe. Complete urinary continence in patients treated by this method was reported in 12 of 13 patients in 1937.[62] In 1942, Dees[11] tubularized the trigone to produce a longer neourethra. This concept was extended by Leadbetter,[33] who reimplanted the ureters to allow longer tubularization of the trigone with reinforcement by overlapping buttress flaps of denuded detrusor muscle.

Epispadias in isolation may be defined as a dorsally deficient urethra with the urinary meatus opening at the bladder neck or on the dorsum of the penis. It may not be an isolated defect and is associated most commonly with the bladder exstrophy complex. Rarely, epispadias is associated with urethral duplication.[7, 19, 21, 55] A classification of epispadias is as follows:

I. Epispadias
   A. Male
      1. Glandular
      2. Penile
      3. Subsymphyseal
   B. Female
      1. Bifid clitoris
      2. Subsymphyseal
II. Epispadias with exstrophy
III. Epispadias with urethral duplication

Dees[12] found an incidence of one in 117,604 of male epispadias patients with incontinence, and one in 487,110 of female epispadias patients with incontinence among 5,292,212 hospital admissions. Campbell,[5] in an autopsy series of 10,712 males, found an incidence of one in 3,570 cases of epispadias and one in 936 cases of exstrophy. Classic exstrophy would appear to occur three to four times more frequently than epispadias.

No familial cases of epispadias have been described, although

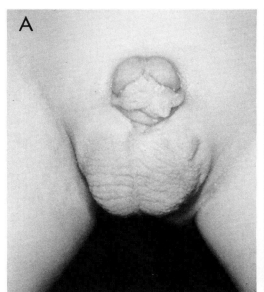
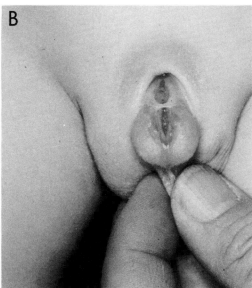

Fig 132–1.—Penile epispadias. **A,** ventral view with prepuce.
B, dorsal view of defect localized to penile shaft.

an epispadiac mother has given birth to a child with exstrophy.[24] Epispadias has also been described in association with multiple anomalies and abnormal karyotypes. Of six male patients with the chromosome 13q − syndrome, one was born with epispadias, three were born with hypospadias, and five were born with cryptorchid testes.[1] Epispadias has also been reported in the trisomy 9 − P + syndrome,[9] and in Klinefelter's (XXY) syndrome.[48]

In both sexes, the patients have a deficient prepubic fat pad and, following puberty, deficient midline pubic hair. In the severe forms of epispadias, there is diastasis of the symphysis pubis; in the milder forms of epispadias, the separation of the pubic bones is variable. The distance from the umbilicus to the anus is foreshortened.

In male patients, the crura are widely separated at the base of the penis because of their attachment to the separated pubic bones. The corpora cavernosa meet in the midline more distally than is normal, producing a stubby, foreshortened penis (Fig 132–1). Erectile tissue representing the corpus spongiosum underlies the urethral groove.[46] A short, dorsal urethral plate and ventral fibrous tissue uniting the corpora cavernosa to the pubic bones combine to produce a dorsal chordee. On occasion, the underlying corpora may be concave dorsally, further exaggerating the dorsal chordee. The dorsal urethral groove runs into a deep, dorsal cleft in the glans penis, producing a "spade-like" penis (Fig 132–2). The prepuce is deficient dorsally, but is otherwise in the normal subcoronal position.

In female patients, the clitoris and the clitoral hood are bifid, and the urethra short or nonexistent (Fig 132–3). The labia minora run posteriorly from the lateral aspects of the bifid clitoris. They are of reduced length because of anterior displacement of the introitus. In contrast to the condition in girls with bladder exstrophy, these females have normal internal genital structures.[50]

Radiologic examination of the upper urinary tracts reveals a small incidence of anomalies. In one series, three of 77 (4%) patients had abnormalities, including one case each of renal agenesis, multicystic kidney, and renal calculus.[8] Radiologic exami-

nation of the lower urinary tract demonstrates a significant incidence of vesicoureteral reflux.[3] Cendron and Melin[8] found vesicoureteral reflux in one of 10 continent epispadiac patients, and in 26 of 67 (40%) incontinent epispadias patients.

The premalignant potential of the bladder mucosa in epispadias is unknown. A single case of adenocarcinoma of the bladder in an adult male epispadiac has been reported.[2] In that instance, chronic inflammation, focal cystitis glandularis, and colonic metaplasia were present in the adjacent bladder mucosa.

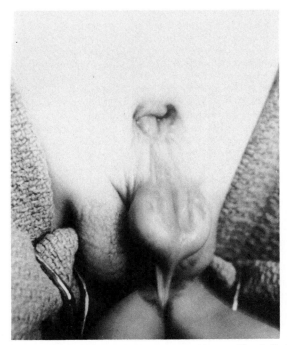

Fig 132–2.—Subsymphysial epispadias with incontinence. "Spade-like" glans with deep dorsal cleft.

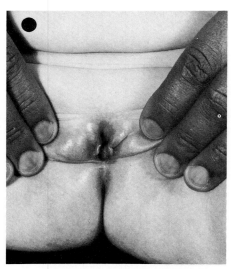

Fig 132–3.—Epispadias in the female. Complete epispadias in a girl, showing absence of dorsal urethra extending through the bladder sphincter.

Embryology

Epispadias represents not an arrest of normal development, but an abnormal embryonic event.[25] The normal embryo does not pass through a phase in which the amniotic cavity and the cloaca communicate. Normally, they are separated by a fused layer of endoderm and ectoderm, the cloacal membrane. At 4 weeks gestation, the cloacal membrane extends cephalad as far as the body stalk. The paired genital tubercles are identifiable by the 4th week lateral to the cephalic border of the cloacal membrane. By the 5th week, the paired genital tubercles have fused in the midline in the cephalic border of the cloacal membrane. Progressive growth of the infraumbilical body wall allows normal formation of the body wall, displacing the paired genital tubercles caudally. Subsequently, the urorectal septum divides the cloaca into the urogenital sinus and rectum.[47, 58]

Abnormal persistence of the cloacal membrane cephalad to the genital tubercles produces an unstable fusion of endoderm and ectoderm. Elsewhere in the body, such as the oral cavity and nasal choanae, this combination of endoderm and ectoderm is unstable and disintegrates. Rupture of this portion of the membrane results in the abnormal communication between the urogenital portion of the cloaca and the amniotic cavity (Fig 132–4). Two theories exist to explain the persistent cloacal membrane cephalad to the genital tubercles. Patten and Barry[46] theorize that the paired genital tubercles are displaced caudally. Subsequent fusion of the tubercles would then isolate a portion of the cloacal membrane cephalad to the tubercles. Marshall and Muecke[38, 44] theorize that an abnormal overdevelopment and cephalic extension of the cloacal membrane prevents the paired genital tubercles from fusing in the midline on the cephalic rim of the cloacal membrane. The paired genital tubercles and their associated mesenchyme would, therefore, fail to fuse in the midline as evidenced by separation of the pubic symphysis, a bifid clitoris, separated corpora cavernosa, and a cleft glans penis.

The rupture of a small cloacal membrane persisting cephalad to the genital tubercles would produce an epispadiac communication between the urogenital portion of the cloaca and the amniotic cavity.

NORMAL

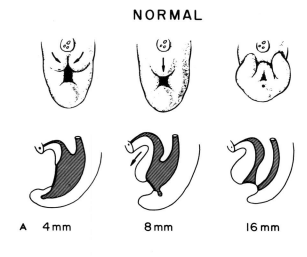

A   4mm   8mm   16mm

EXSTROPHY

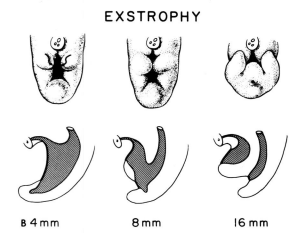

B 4mm   8mm   16mm

Fig 132–4.—Schematic view of regression of cloacal membrane and formation of the primitive phallus. **A,** normal sequential events. **B,** genesis of the exstrophy group of anomalies by a persistent cloacal membrane impeding mesodermal flow. The paired genital folds fuse inferiorly carrying the thin cloacal membrane along the anterior surface of the enlarging phallus. A weak, membranous anterior body wall persists, leading to the eventual catastrophic event of exstrophy. (From Muecke E.D.: *Campbell's Textbook of Urology.* Philadelphia, W.B. Saunders Co., 1979, Chap. 40. Used by permission.)

Clinical Assessment

Although epispadias is almost always a sporadic condition, history of familial cases, antenatal drug exposure, or other possible etiologic factors should be sought. Parents should be asked about the appearance of the penis during erection, about continuous urinary dribbling, or dry intervals signifying some degree of urinary continence.

Epispadiac children are otherwise generally normal, because they appear to have a low incidence of associated anomalies. If associated anomalies are present, or the genetic sex of the child is in doubt, karyotyping should be performed. Examination of the penis should include documentation of stretched penile length, chordee, and pubic separation. These observations may be augmented by photography of the erect penis. Urethral plate length should be documented and measured from the verumontanum to the end of the urethral groove.

Radiologic examination should include an intravenous pyelo-

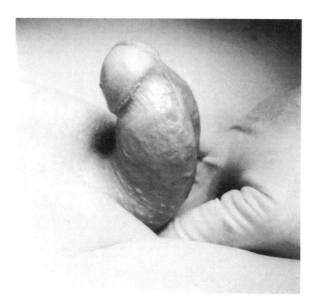

Fig 132–5.—Epispadias with severe dorsal chordee demonstrated by compression of the crura.

gram and a voiding cystourethrogram to document upper urinary tract status, presence of vesicoureteral reflux, bladder neck closure, and bladder capacity.

Cystoscopic examination will allow assessment of ureteral orifices and examination of the bladder neck. Examination under anesthesia will allow assessment of chordee by artificial erection, employing a modified technique that substitutes digital compression of the crura (Fig 132–5) for the elastic tourniquet. It may be necessary to infuse saline into each corpus cavernosum, because in the epispadiac penis the corpora may not communicate.[14] However, saline infusion into the glans is usually satisfactory, producing turgidity of both corpora cavernosa.

Urodynamic assessment is indicated in the 3–4-year-old epispadiac child who remains incontinent. An assessment of bladder capacity and contractility, and functional urethral length and resistance, should be obtained for baselines, prior to surgical or pharmacologic manipulation.[30]

Surgical Treatment

The surgical correction of epispadias must be individualized according to the sex, severity of epispadias, and degree of urinary control. In this section, the treatment of the most severe problem will be discussed: the male with subsymphyseal epispadias, chordee, and total urinary incontinence. Staged reconstruction is planned. The first stage includes penile lengthening, elongation of the urethral strip, and correction of the chordee.

The second stage consists of urethral reconstruction. The third stage includes bladder neck reconstruction and suspension, with ureteral reimplantation and/or augmentation cystoplasty as required.

Timing

The first stage, penile reconstruction, is undertaken after the first birthday. By this age, some genital growth has occurred, and anesthetic difficulties have decreased to more acceptable levels. The second stage, urethral reconstruction, is carried out at least 6 months after the successful completion of the first stage. The final stage, bladder neck reconstruction, is under-

taken after the third birthday, by which time the lack of urinary control will be obvious clinically and urodynamically. Ideally, reconstruction should be complete by school age.

First Stage: Penile Reconstruction

Factors to be considered in the first stage of reconstruction include penile length, chordee, urethral strip length, and degree of pubic separation. Testosterone enanthate, 2 mg/kg, may be given 6 weeks and 2 weeks prior to operation to increase the size, vascularity, and thickness of the penile tissues. In some patients, there is little or no chordee, and urethral length is in keeping with overall penile length, making a first stage unnecessary.

A subcoronal circumferential skin incision is made distal to the ventral prepuce. The urethral strip is divided transversely, and dissection is carried down to Buck's fascia. The urethral strip is detached from the corpora by sharp dissection. All dorsal fibrous attachments are lysed, allowing retraction of the urethral strip toward the bladder. The dissection is carried to the level of the verumontanum, at which point injury to the ejaculatory ducts must be avoided. The urethral plate may be tubularized once all dorsal chordee has been corrected (Fig 132–6). An artificial erection is produced by infusing saline into either the glans or both corpora, and by digitally compressing the crura. Any intrinsic curvature of the corpora is corrected by plication or by excising transverse ellipses from the convex aspect of the tunica albuginea and closing the defect as described by Nesbit.[45] Alternatively, a dermal patch graft may be placed in the concave aspect of the tunica albuginea.

Any tilting of the glans penis may be corrected by suturing the subcoronal tissues to the ventral aspect of the corpora cavernosa.

At this point, lysis of the rudimentary suspensory ligament (Fig 132–7) and detachment of the crura from the inferior pubic rami is considered if the penis is short, if the corpora cavernosa are widely divergent, or if the symphysis pubis is widely separated. Iliac osteotomies may be considered, but may cause foreshortening and retraction of the penis if the anterior-posterior diameter is flattened by bilateral or oblique osteotomy. Detachment of the crura is accomplished by sharp dissection or by subperiosteal elevation and detachment. Dissection should stay very close to the periosteum to avoid injury to the nervi erigentes. The neurovascular pedicles to the crura are preserved as described by Johnston and Kogan.[25] The corpora cavernosa are approximated in the midline to increase the length of the penile

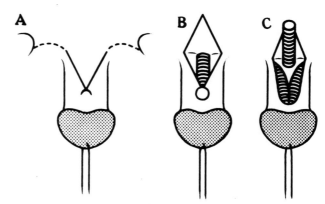

Fig 132–6.—Correction of chordee in epispadias. **A,** V-incision from urethral meatus to pubic bones. **B,** skin flap elevated from urethra. **C,** urethra detached from corpora cavernosa. (From Johnston J.H.: *J. Urol.* 113:701, 1975. Used by permission.)

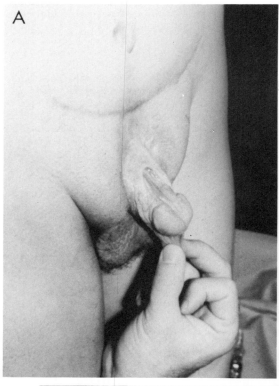

Fig 132–7.—Subsymphysial epispadias following operation for incontinence. **A,** appearance. **B,** wide diversion of suspensory ligaments. **C,** repaired epispadias with mattress sutures in glans, chordee released. **D,** early postoperative result with normal appearance of glans. Patient subsequently had functional erections.

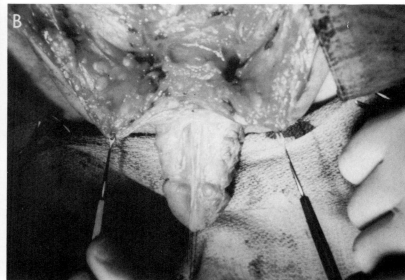

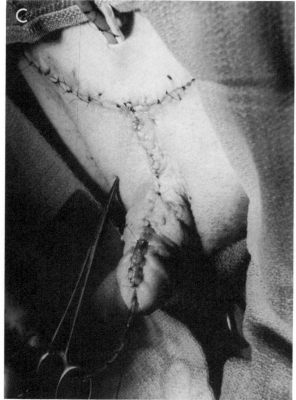

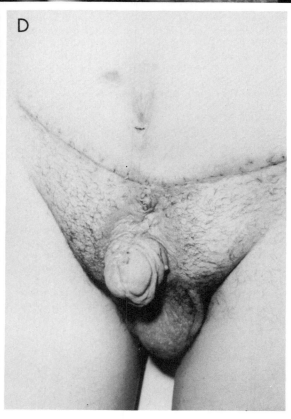

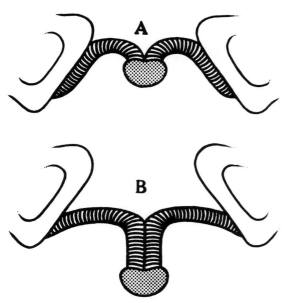

Fig 132–8.—Penis lengthening procedure. **A,** shortness of penis caused by separation of pubes. **B,** lengthening obtained by partial detachment of crura from bony rami. (From Johnston J.H.: *J. Urol.* 113:701, 1975. Used by permission.)

shaft (Fig 132–8). (See also penile lengthening in epispadias with classic exstrophy, Fig 128–11.)

Skin coverage is required to bridge the gap in the urethral plate, which was created by lysis of the ventral chordee. As the skin used to bridge this defect will be incorporated into the neourethra at the second stage, non–hair-bearing skin should be used. Ventral preputial skin may be rotated by using Byar's flaps or by the Nesbit buttonhole method. Alternatively, split- or full-thickness skin grafts may be applied. Only as a last resort should scrotal skin be used to cover the defect in the urethral strip.

Should a generous portion of ventral preputial skin be present, urethral reconstruction may be undertaken at this stage by the use of a "reverse" Duckett transverse island flap (Fig 132–9).[16, 17]

Because postoperative edema is a frequent and dramatic problem, we have recently been using a compression dressing of Op Site (3M) and Microfoam (3M) tape. This dressing controls edema well and is easily removed without anesthetic.

Second Stage: Urethral Reconstruction

Urethral reconstruction is undertaken a minimum of 6 months after successful completion of the first stage. Factors to be considered include urine flow, urethral strip, and ventral cleft through the glans penis. In patients who have undergone urinary diversion, the accumulation of debris and subsequent infection can lead to the complications of stricture and fistula more commonly than in children passing urine through the urethra.

A modification of Young's procedure for urethral closure is utilized.[59] A 3-0 nylon monofilament suture is placed through the glans for traction and immobilization. A 14-mm strip is outlined on the ventral aspect of the penis from the urinary meatus to the corona of the glans penis. Triangular areas on the glans penis lateral to the urethral skin strip are denuded to facilitate the formation of glandular flaps. The skin strip is mobilized laterally to allow tubularization and closure with running and interrupted 6-0 polyglycolic acid suture. Detachment from the underlying corpora is minimal so as to preserve maximal blood supply to the neourethra. As the corpora cavernosa were approximated during the first stage repair, no attempt is made to displace the urethra ventrally. A Z-plasty incision may facilitate the lysis of any residual suspensory ligament or scar tissue (Fig 132–10,A–D). The neourethra is closed along the length of the penile shaft in 2 or 3 layers (Fig 132–10,E–H). The urethral cleft in the glans penis is usually deep enough to provide sufficient skin for tubularization and coverage with flaps from the glans. The flaps are closed over the neourethra with 4-0 nylon monofilament ventrical mattress sutures placed over the silicone rubber buttresses. The skin of the glans is approximated between the nylon sutures with 6-0 polyglycolic acid sutures. Closure of the Z-plasty portion of the incision will serve to minimize the effects of scar contracture during wound healing (Fig 132–10,I–K).

The nylon sutures are removed from the glans penis on the tenth postoperative day.

Should the urethral groove be too shallow, individualized techniques of reconstruction are employed. Penile shaft coverage is accomplished by local rotation flaps with or without a ventral relaxing incision. Alternatively, the penis may be buried in the scrotum.[22] Devine et al.[14] advocate the use of a free graft from the prepuce or non–hair-bearing skin to augment urethral tissues; their free grafts may allow a combination of chordee correction with urethral reconstruction (Fig 132–11). Following this stage, bladder capacity frequently will increase, facilitating the third-stage repair.

Third Stage: Bladder Neck Reconstruction

Factors to be considered in the third stage reconstruction include any spontaneous continence, bladder capacity, and vesicoureteral reflux. At 3–4 years of age, bladder neck reconstruction may be undertaken if the bladder capacity is greater than 50 ml, the bladder mucosa is not inflamed, and no sign of urinary continence has appeared.

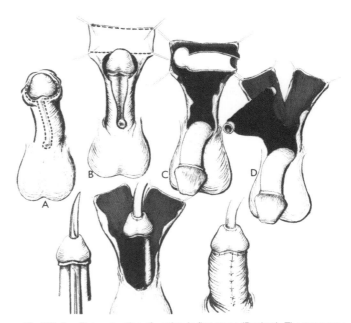

Fig 132–9.—Reconstruction of urethra in first stage (Duckett). The transverse island flap, depicted here in treatment of hypospadias, may be constructed from the ventral prepuce in epispadias and used to construct urethra after chordee correction and before covering dorsum of penis. (From Duckett J.W.: *Urol. Clin.* 8(3):503, 1981. Used by permission.)

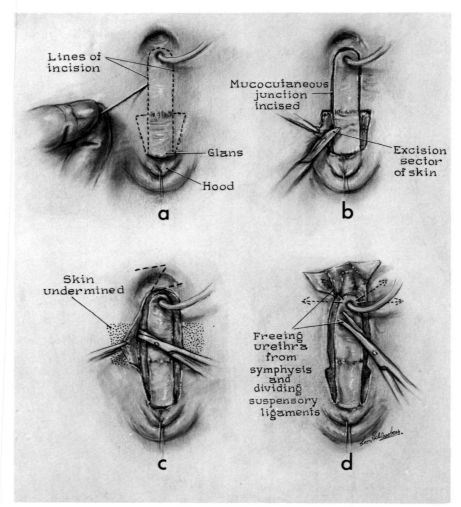

Fig 132–10.—Urethral closure in second stage. **a,** urethral strip outlined. **b,** excision of triangular area of lateral glans tissue to prepare glandular flaps. **c** and **d,** mobilization of lateral skin and residual suspensory ligament tissue. *(Continued.)*

Bilateral ureteral reimplantation is indicated for any grade of reflux, and in the absence of reflux when space is required for bladder neck reconstruction. When the capacity of the bladder continues to be less than 50 ml despite prior urethral reconstruction, bladder augmentation with bowel may have to be considered. This decision should be delayed until the child is 6 or 7 years of age, because emptying of the bladder may require intermittent catheterization and the cooperation of the child. The augmentation colocystoplasty may be staged in the Arap[4] manner, creating a sigmoid conduit for later undiversion to the bladder, which has been used to fashion a bladder neck and posterior urethra.

The majority of epispadias patients at age 3 years will have a capacity greater than 50 ml, and bladder neck reconstruction can proceed. Exposure is gained via a Pfannenstiel incision; the intersymphysial band is left intact to maintain stability of the pelvic ring.

An inverted T-incision in the anterior bladder gives access to the bladder floor, and longitudinal closure of the bladder neck area in a straight line elongates the small, shallow bladder (Fig 132–12,A). Bilateral ureteral reimplantation is carried out using the cross trigonal method of Cohen[10] if vesicoureteral reflux is present or if the ureteral orifices are less than 3.0 cm from the bladder neck.

A 16 mm × 30 mm strip of bladder mucosa extending from the trigone into the proximal urethra is outlined. The triangular mucosal segments lateral to the bladder strip are denuded, and the bladder strip is closed over a temporary French no. 10 stent (Fig 132–12,B&C). The mucosal tube is buttressed and reinforced by overlapping denuded detrusor flaps.[23] (See also Chap. 128.) An intraoperative urethral pressure profile is then performed (Fig 132–12,D&E) to ensure that closure pressures are above 70 cm of water; lower closure pressures may not result in desired urinary control. The bladder is then closed, leaving in place ureteral catheters and a suprapubic Malecot catheter. The reconstructed bladder neck and urethra are then suspended to the intersymphysial fibrous bar and rectus fascia. A stent in the urethra is contraindicated, because pressure or infection may interfere with healing, with resultant shortening of the new bladder neck producing a shortened continence zone, increased caliber of the bladder neck lumen, and a decreased closure pressure (Fig 132–12,F).

Discussion

Probably the most important new facet in epispadias surgery is the preliminary penile reconstruction. Early reconstructive procedures as described by Cantwell[6] and modified by

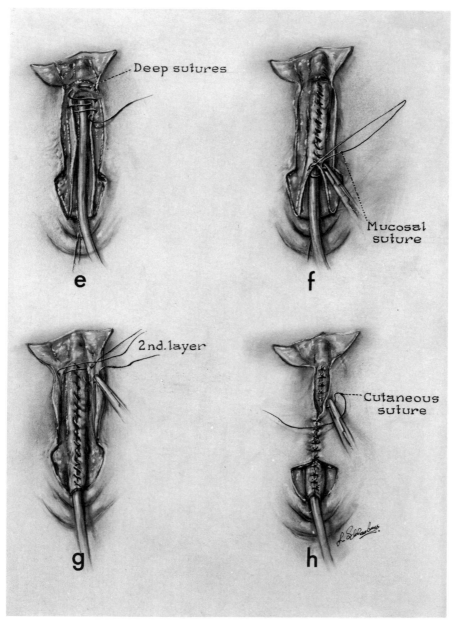

Fig 132–10 Cont.—e–h, closure of the urethral strip on penile
shaft and on glans in multiple layers. *(Continued.)*

Young[59, 60] emphasized urethral reconstruction while ignoring
the penile deformity. Lysis and resection of the dorsal fibrous
chordee was first described in 1948 by Mays,[40] and reiterated for
exstrophy by Hinman[22] in 1958. Kelley and Eraklis[26] advocated
complete separation of the crura and associated cartilage or periosteum from the inferior pubic rami. The neurovascular bundles
were then dissected from Alcock's canal. The cartilage or periosteum was then sutured to the intersymphysial fibrous bar, and
the corpora approximated in the midline. Johnston and Kogan's[25]
partial detachment of the crura and midline approximation represents a much safer procedure. In the long-term follow-up by
Hanna and Williams[20] of 15 epispadiac patients treated by release of chordee and staged reconstruction, 15 of 15 had good
erections, 11 of 15 had satisfactory intercourse, and 14 of 15 had
normal ejaculation. Cendron and Melin[8] reported that four patients in his series were able to father children after staged surgical reconstruction.

Many methods have been described for covering the dorsal
skin defect produced by release of the dorsal chordee, with or
without plication of the tunica albuginea for intrinsic curvature
of the corpora. These include V-Y plasty,[55] transposition of ventral preputial skin,[22, 25] full-thickness skin graft,[13] and burying the
penile shaft in the scrotum.[54] The method of choice for skin coverage varies from individual to individual, but should not compromise the exposure necessary during preliminary dissection for
release of the chordee. The use of scrotal skin should be avoided
if possible to prevent hair-bearing skin from being incorporated
into the neourethra.

An alternate method for elongation of the urethral strip by Z-
shaped incision of the strip has been described by Michalowski

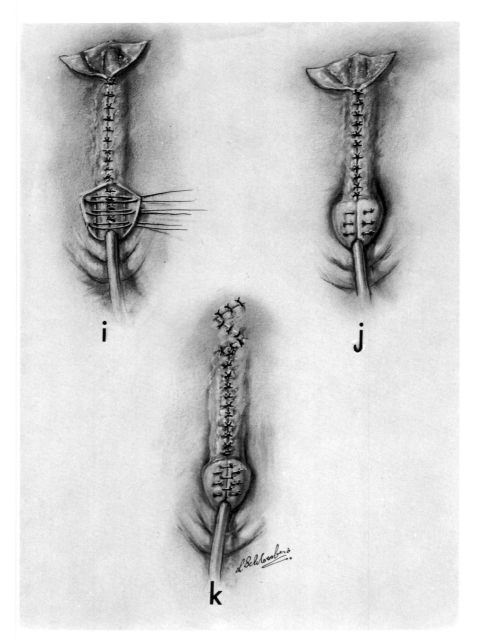

Fig 132–10 Cont.—i–k, closure of glandular tissue with nylon vertical mattress sutures. (Silicone rubber protection under mattress suture loops not shown.) Proximal Z-plasty skin closure to reduce scar contraction.

and Modelski.[42] The parallel strips thus formed are then sutured end-to-end to elongate the urethral strip.

The classic method of urethral reconstruction described by Cantwell[6] involved distal detachment of the skin strip and complete dissection. This frequently produced a tube of insufficient length and poor vascularity. Young's[59] modification preserved the attachment of the urethral strip to one corpus cavernosum, preserving the vascularity and reducing the rate of stricture and fistula formation. In 1937, Young[62] reported successful urethral reconstruction in 11 of 12 patients. With preliminary penile lengthening, chordee correction, and approximation of the corpora in the midline, it is no longer possible to transpose the neourethra to the ventral aspect of the penis.

Reconstruction of the glandular urethra is greatly facilitated by the deep urethral groove present in most patients. Tubularization of the groove provides a urethra of adequate caliber, and reapproximation of the glandular flaps as described by Devine and Horton[13] provides an excellent cosmetic result.

A modification of the Cantwell-Young technique of urethral reconstruction has been applied to a consecutive series of 22 bladder exstrophy patients from 1975–1982.[36] Preliminary penile lengthening had been done at the time of exstrophy closure. Urethral fistulae occurred postoperatively in nine patients. Four of these patients had spontaneous healing of their fistulae, and five patients underwent successful surgical closure.

Many operations for the correction of urinary incontinence have been devised. These may be classified as follows into transvesical and extravesical procedures:

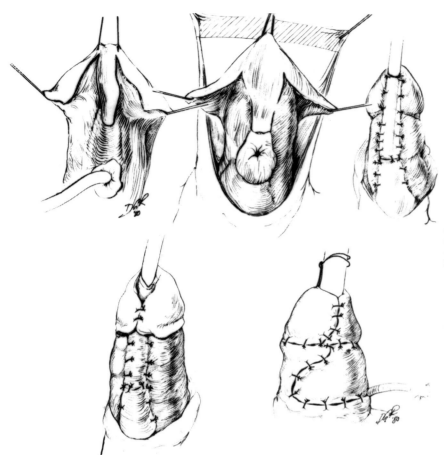

Fig 132–11.—Epispadias repair. Correction of chordee and free graft of prepuce to augment urethral tissues. (From Devine C.J., Horton C.E., in Stewart B.H. (ed.): *Epispadias Repair in Operative Urology.* Baltimore, Williams & Wilkins Co., 1982, p. 291. Used by permission.)

I. Transvesical
  A. Young[61]
  B. Dees[11, 12]
  C. Leadbetter[33]
  D. Anterior detrusor tube
II. Extravesical
  A. Transvaginal plication
  B. Marshall-Marchetti suspension
  C. Muscle autotransplantation
  D. Artificial urinary sphincter

Young's double sphincter operation, described in 1922,[61] consisted of excision of anterior urethral tissue from the bladder neck and the epispadiac urinary meatus. The urethra was then reapproximated over a silver probe. The majority of these procedures were carried out in postpubertal males, with complete success in 10 of 13, mild incontinence in 1 of 13, fistula in 1 of 13, and failure in 1 of 13. Dees'[11] modification, which extended the length of the urethra by tubularizing the trigone, produced good urinary control in five of six patients.[12] Reimplantation of the ureters to allow an even longer trigonal tube, as described by Leadbetter,[33] produced perfect results in eight of 15 patients.[34]

Kramer and Kelalis[32] reviewed the results of the Young-Dees or Leadbetter techniques in 53 male and 12 female incontinent epispadias patients. In the male patients, a 34% postoperative continence rate was found; and, with the onset of puberty, the overall success rate rose to 70%. An 83% continence rate obtained in the female patients was not influenced by puberty. An adequate bladder capacity, defined as 50 ml per year of age, was associated with a 79% success rate, while an inadequate bladder capacity was associated with a 42% success rate. In 22 exstrophy patients converted to incontinent epispadias and undergoing a Young-Dees-Leadbetter reconstruction with suprapubic suspension, a continence rate of 80% is reported by Lepor and Jeffs[35] (see Chap. 128).

Six patients with complete epispadias and incontinence treated by bladder neck reconstruction and tested intraoperatively by profilometry, had closure pressures over 60 cm of water pressure before suspension. Each of these children achieves a dry interval of 3 hours and is either continent 24 hours per day or is expected to achieve this at grade school age.

For patients with inadequate bladder capacity despite closure of the urethra to increase outlet resistance, augmentation of the bladder with a segment of colon combined with either conventional bladder neck reconstruction or with whole bladder tubularization as described by Arap[4] is preferred over ureterosigmoidostomy or external diversion.

The anterior bladder tube has been used successfully in two male patients without epispadias by Tanagho.[52] Williams and Snyder[56] believe that the anterior detrusor tube is contraindicated in epispadias, because the primary urethral defect is in the anterior bladder neck.

The transvaginal plication technique originally described by Kelly[27, 28] was modified by King and Wendel[29] in six incontinent female epispadiac patients. A successful result was obtained in three of four patients in whom satisfactory plication was demon-

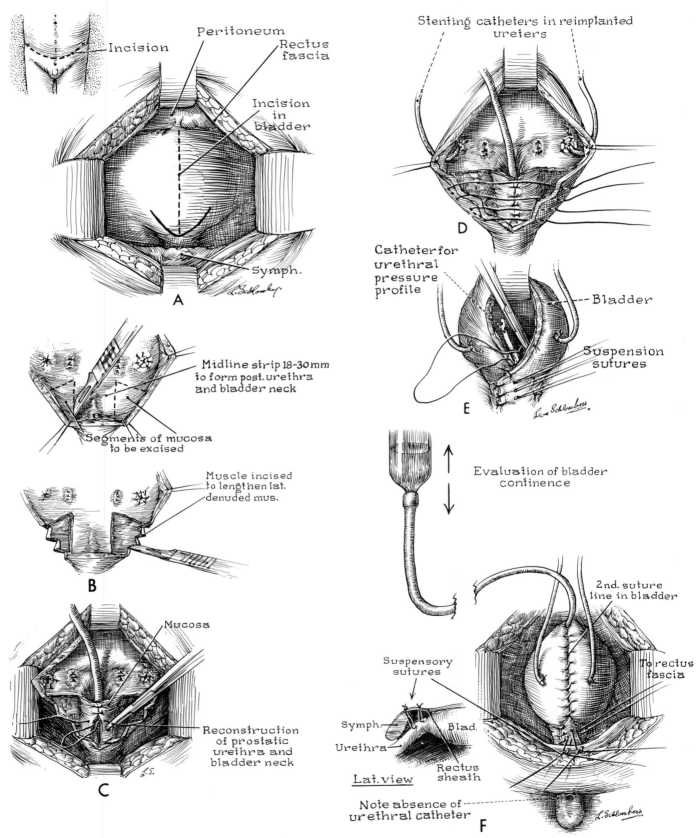

Fig 132–12.—See legend on facing page.

strated by intraoperative endoscopy. An isolated Marshall-Marchetti repair has not been reported in any series to date.

No series has been reported utilizing the artificial urinary sphincter in epispadias. However, Light and Scott[37] have recently obtained a 91% success rate in a series of ten exstrophy and one epispadias patients. The age at time of treatment ranged from 11–19 years, follow-up ranging from 15–42 months (mean 25.5 months). The rate of reoperation was 36%. Six patients with failed bladder neck procedures were successfully treated with the artificial sphincter. This preliminary report is encouraging, but the role of the artificial sphincter in the treatment of epispadias remains to be defined.

An interesting concept involving autotransplantation of denervated skeletal muscles has been reported recently by Gierup and Hakelius.[18] A U-shaped graft of muscle, denervated 2–3 weeks previously, was placed around the posterior urethra in patients with failed bladder neck reconstruction. Postoperative ciné studies revealed activity of the transplant, and "good" results were obtained in four of eight patients.

Conclusions

Neither internal nor external diversion can be considered as the primary treatment of choice for incontinent patients with epispadias. The long-term upper urinary tract complications and the malignant potential encountered with ureterosigmoidostomy are unacceptable unless all other reconstructive options have been exhausted. With attention to penile reconstruction, better cosmetic and functional results may be obtained. The reproductive potential for both male and female epispadiacs has been established. Fortunately, the risk of offspring being affected in the epispadias-exstrophy complex appears to be small (Shapiro et al.[49]).

Urethral reconstruction by the modified Cantwell-Young procedure is still complicated by fistula formation, but surgical techniques now exist for reliable closure of such fistulae.[39] The results of bladder neck reconstruction are good, but not perfect. An 80% successful result may be expected in females; and, with passage through puberty, an overall success rate of 75%–80% may be expected in males. Intraoperative measurement of bladder neck closure pressures may continue to prove valuable in predicting the resulting continence and allow immediate revision if pressures are below 60 cm of water. A preoperative search for vesicoureteral reflux is important to allow correction of reflux concomitantly with bladder neck reconstruction. Repeated reconstructive attempts, Teflon injection, or artificial sphincter placement may salvage some of the failed bladder reconstructions. Bladder capacity should be carefully assessed, because an adequate bladder capacity greatly improves the chances of successful reconstruction. The minimal incidence of associated anomalies in epispadias ensures good general health and reproductive potential, thus justifying an aggressive surgical attempt at reconstruction. Strict attention must be paid to preserving renal function, and only as a last resort should urinary diversion be performed.

Fig 132–12.—Third stage—bladder neck reconstruction. **A,** Pfannenstiel incision, intersymphysial band left intact. Inverted T bladder incision. **B** and **C,** following-cross trigonal ureteral implantation, a 16 mm × 30 mm strip is outlined for construction of the posterior urethra and bladder neck. The muscle on either side is denuded of mucosa and incised to lengthen flaps. **D** and **E,** double-breasted closure of bladder muscle over tubularized mucosa, closing bladder neck and posterior urethra. Urethral pressure profile determined with bladder open with and without similar suspension of bladder neck. **F,** completion of bladder neck reconstruction by suspension to pubic tissues and rectus fascia. Bladder and ureteral drainage by suprapubic tube and ureteral catheters. No urethral stent or catheter. Further testing of outlet resistance to leakage by suprapubic filling and pressure measurement.

REFERENCES

1. Allerdice P.W.: Chromosome Thirteen q-Syndrome, in Bergsma D. (ed.): *Birth Defects Atlas and Compendium.* Baltimore, Williams & Wilkins Co., 1973, p. 250.
2. Altamura M.J., Gonick P., Brooks J.J.: Adenocarcinoma of the bladder associated with epispadias: Case report and update. *J. Urol.* 127:322, 1982.
3. Ambrose S.S.: Epispadias and vesicoureteral reflux. *South. Med. J.* 63:1193, 1970.
4. Arap S.A.: Complete reconstruction of bladder exstrophy. *Urology* 7:413, 1976.
5. Campbell M.: Epispadias: A report of fifteen cases. *J. Urol.* 67:988, 1952.
6. Cantwell F.V.: Operative treatment of epispadias by transplantation of the urethra. *Ann. Surg.* 22:689, 1895.
7. Cendron J., Desgrez J.P.: Urethres surnumeraires chez le garcon à propos de 12 cas personnels. *J. D'Urol. Nephrol.* 81:11, 1975.
8. Cendron J., Melin Y.: L' epispadias. *Ann. Pediatr.* 27:463, 1980.
9. Chipail A., Constantinescu V., Covic M., et al.: Phenotypical and cytogenetic analysis of a particular malformative syndrome (Trisomia 9 p +). *Rev. Pediatr. Obstet. Ginecol.* 25:201, 1976.
10. Cohen S.J.: Ureterozystoneostomie: Eine neue Antirefluxtechnik. *Aktuel. Urol.* 6:24, 1975.
11. Dees J.E.: Epispadias with incontinence in the male. *Surgery* 12:621, 1942.
12. Dees J.E.: Congenital epispadias with incontinence. *J. Urol.* 62:513, 1949.
13. Devine C.J., Horton C.E.: Hypospadias and epispadias. *Clin. Symp.* 20:24, 1972.
14. Devine C.J., Horton C.E., Scarff J.E.: Epispadias. *Urol. Clin. North Am.* 7:465, 1980.
15. Dieffenbach J.F.: *Plastiche Operationen an den Harnwegen in die operative Chirurgie.* Leipzig, Germany, F.A. Brockhaus, 1845, p. 526.
16. Duckett J.W.: Epispadias. *Urol. Clin. North Am.* 5:107, 1978.
17. Duckett J.W.: Transverse preputial island flap technique for repair of severe hypospadias. *Urol. Clin. North Am.* 7:423, 1980.
18. Gierup H.J.W., Hakelius L.: Further experience of free muscle transplantation in children with urinary incontinence. *Br. J. Urol.* 55:211, 1983.
19. Gross R.E., Moore T.C.: Duplication of the urethra. *Arch. Surg.* 60:749, 1950.
20. Hanna M.K., Williams D.I.: Genital function in males with vesical exstrophy and epispadias. *Br. J. Urol.* 44:169, 1972.
21. Hermann G., Goldman H.: Double urethra with vertebral anomaly. *Int. Surg.* 58:574, 1973.
22. Hinman F. Jr.: A method of lengthening and repairing penis in exstrophy of the bladder. *J. Urol.* 79:237, 1958.
23. Jeffs R.D.: Exstrophy and cloacal exstrophy. *Urol. Clin. North Am.* 5:127, 1978.
24. Jeffs R.D.: Unpublished material.
25. Johnston J.H., Kogan S.J.: The exstrophic anomalies and their surgical reconstruction. *Current Problems in Surgery.* Chicago, Year Book Medical Publishers, August, 1974.
26. Kelley J.H., Eraklis A.J.: A procedure for lengthening the phallus in boys with exstrophy of the bladder. *J. Pediatr. Surg.* 6:645, 1971.
27. Kelly H.A.: Incontinence of urine in women. *Urol. Cut. Rev.* 17:291, 1913.
28. Kelly H.A., Dumm W.M.: Urinary incontinence in women, without manifest injury to the bladder. *Surg. Gynecol. Obstet.* 18:444, 1914.
29. King L.R., Wendel R.M.: A new application for transvaginal plication in the treatment of girls with total urinary incontinence due to epispadias or hypospadias. *J. Urol.* 102:778, 1969.
30. Kramer S.A.: Epispadias management. *Dialogues in Pediatric Urology* 5:10, 1982.
31. Kramer S.A., Kelalis P.P.: Surgical correction of female epispadias. *Eur. Urol.* 8:321, 1982.
32. Kramer S.A., Kelalis P.P.: Assessment of urinary continence in epispadias: A review of 94 patients. *J. Urol.* 128:290, 1982.
33. Leadbetter G.W.: Surgical correction of total urinary incontinence. *J. Urol.* 91:261, 1964.
34. Leadbetter G.W., Fraley E.E.: Surgical correction for total urinary incontinence: 5 years after. *J. Urol.* 97:869, 1967.
35. Lepor H., Jeffs R.D.: Primary bladder closure and bladder neck reconstruction in classical bladder exstrophy. *J. Urol.* 130:1142, 1983.
36. Lepor H., Shapiro E., Jeffs R.D.: Urethral reconstruction in males with classical bladder exstrophy. *J. Urol.* 131:512, 1984.
37. Light J.K., Scott F.B.: Treatment of the epispadias-exstrophy complex with the AS 792 artificial urinary sphincter. *J. Urol.* 129:738, 1983.
38. Marshall V.F., Muecke E.C.: Variations in exstrophy of the bladder. *J. Urol.* 88:766, 1962.

39. Masterson J.S.T., Johnson H.W., Coleman G.U., et al.: Development of microsurgical techniques in experimental and clinical repair of urethrocutaneous fistulae. *J. Urol.* 128:285, 1982.
40. Mays H.B.: Epispadias with incontinence: A method of treatment. *J. Urol.* 60:749, 1948.
41. Mays H.B.: Epispadias—II, in Horton C.E. (ed.): *Plastic and Reconstructive Surgery of the Genital Area.* Boston, Little, Brown & Co., 1973, p. 229.
42. Michalowski E., Modelski W.: The surgical treatment of epispadias. *Surg. Gynecol. Obstet.* 117:465, 1963.
43. Morgagni J.B.: *The Seats and Causes of Disease Investigated by Anatomy* (1769), Alexander B. (trans.). New York, Hafner Publishing Co., 1980.
44. Muecke E.C.: The role of the cloacal membrane in exstrophy: The first successful experimental study. *J. Urol.* 92:659, 1964.
45. Nesbit R.M.: Operation for correction of distal penile ventral curvature with or without hypospadias. *J. Urol.* 97:720, 1967.
46. Patten B.M., Barry A.: The genesis of exstrophy of the bladder and epispadias. *Am. J. Anat.* 90:35, 1952.
47. Pohlman A.G.: The development of the cloaca in human embryos. *Am. J. Anat.* 12:1, 1911.
48. Raboch J.: Incidence of hypospadias and epispadias in chromatin-positive men. *Andrologia* 7:237, 1975.
49. Shapiro E., Lepor H., Jeffs R.D.: The inheritance of the exstrophy-epispadias complex. *J. Urol.* 132:308, 1984.
50. Stanton S.L.: Gynecologic complications of epispadias and bladder exstrophy. *Am. J. Obstet. Gynecol.* 119:749, 1974.
51. Stiles H.J.: Epispadias in the female and its surgical treatment. *Surg. Gynecol. Obstet.* 13:127, 1911.
52. Tanagho E.A.: Bladder neck reconstruction for total urinary incontinence: 10 years of experience. *J. Urol.* 125:321, 1981.
53. Thiersch K.: Ueber die Entstehungsweise und operative Behandlung der Epispadie. *Arch. Heildk.* 10:20, 1869.
54. Williams D.I.: Epispadias—I, in Horton C.E. (ed.): *Plastic and Reconstructive Surgery of the Genital Area.* Boston, Little, Brown & Co., 1973, p. 223.
55. Williams D.I., Keeton J.E.: Further progress with reconstruction of the exstrophied bladder. *Br. J. Surg.* 60:2:3, 1973.
56. Williams D.I., Snyder H.: Anterior detrusor tube repair for urinary incontinence in children. *Br. J. Urol.* 48:671, 1976.
57. Wilson A.N.: Complete dorsal duplication of the male urethra as an isolated deformity presenting as glandular epispadias. *Br. J. Urol.* 43:338, 1971.
58. Wyburr G.M.: The development of the infra-umbilical portion of the abdominal wall, with remarks on the aetiology of ectopia vesicae. *J. Anat.* 71:201, 1937.
59. Young H.H.: A new operation for epispadias. *J. Urol.* 2:237, 1918.
60. Young H.H.: An operation for the cure of incontinence of urine. *Surg. Gynecol. Obstet.* 28:84, 1919.
61. Young H.H.: An operation for the cure of incontinence associated with epispadias. *J. Urol.* 7:1, 1922.
62. Young H.H.: Epispadias, in *Genital Abnormalities, Hermaphroditism and Related Adrenal Diseases.* Baltimore, Williams & Wilkins Co., 1937, p. 440.

133 Francis F. Bartone / Lowell R. King

Abnormalities of the Urethra, Penis, and Scrotum

Many developmental and acquired abnormalities of the urethra result in bladder outlet obstruction with or without secondary upper tract dilatation. Urine formation begins during the 12th week of gestation and adds to amniotic fluid volume shortly thereafter.[5] By maternal ultrasonography of the fetus, 90% of the malformations of the urinary tract can be tentatively diagnosed between the 17th and the 20th weeks of gestation.[85] Production of fetal urine is essential to the formation of adequate amounts of amniotic fluid. With oligohydramnios the fetus is molded, and maturation of the lung is retarded. The volume of amniotic fluid must be reconstituted before 20 weeks' gestation for the lung to develop normally.[5] Yet, no urologic anomaly detectable in utero as yet warrants fetal intervention,[32] because severe oligohydramnios is often the result of renal dysgenesis (often associated with hydronephrosis), and decompression may not then increase amniotic fluid significantly. Early induction of labor or cesarean section is not often justified to facilitate early treatment.[32] Prenatal diagnosis with spontaneous delivery does permit early surgical treatment of viable infants.[85] Fetal intervention does not appear to salvage infants with dysgenetic kidneys. Early diagnosis does permit early decompression of obstructed kidneys in the first days or week or so of life, with greater improvement in function and less opportunity for infection than when corrective operation is delayed.

Despite the availability of fetal ultrasonography, many babies with severe obstruction are still diagnosed only after birth, because of an abnormal abdominal mass, inability to void, hematuria, or poor feeding, usually associated with a rising blood creatinine. Patients with milder degrees of obstruction and residual urine are predisposed to early infection. Failure to thrive should alone initiate diagnostic studies. A perceptive parent may note that voiding is frequent, dribbling, or intermittent, suggesting bladder obstruction, infection, or faulty innervation. Observation of voiding, prograde and/or retrograde urethrography,[5] cystography, ultrasonography, renal scintigraphy, urethral and meatal calibration, and cystoscopy, the most pertinent studies, will diagnose urethral, bladder, and upper tract pathology.[49, 88]

Trabeculation of the bladder indicates obstruction or neurogenic bladder and has a characteristic appearance on cystography. Mild degrees of trabeculation are not reliably diagnosed by cystography. At cystoscopy, the bladder of the normal child usually exhibits a pattern of fine ridges formed by interlacing detrusor fibers.

When gross trabeculation, cellules, and diverticula are present, the urethra should be visualized radiographically and further evaluated by calibration and urethroscopy. Congenital focal absence of bladder muscle (local dysgenesis) and occult neurologic disease may also cause such changes.

The congenitally obstructed bladder, with an increase in muscle fibers and cholinergic nerve endings, rarely has the large capacity of bladders that become obstructed later in life. The congenitally obstructed bladder is also more often spastic and hyperreflexic. Trigonal hypertrophy, increased detrusor tone, spasticity, and high intraluminal pressure increase resistance to flow in the distal ureter, leading to persistent ureteral dilatation and hydronephrosis.[116]

Phimosis

Extreme phimosis may impede urinary flow. The voiding orifice is tiny, and the foreskin balloons out during voiding. The diagnosis is made by inspection, and the treatment is circumcision. Most obstetricians advocate routine neonatal circumcision, while some pediatricians consider routine circumcision a form of sadistic mutilation with benefits that are purely financial.[61] An ad hoc committee on circumcision of the American Academy of Pediatrics (1975) stated: "There is no absolute medical indication for the routine circumcision of the newborn. A program of good penile hygiene—simply retracting the foreskin to wash away accumulated smegma on a daily basis—would appear to offer all the advantages of circumcision without the attendant surgical risks or the increased risk of meatal stenosis."[11] Despite these differences in viewpoints, circumcision is widely practiced for reasons of culture and tradition.

The most compelling reason given for routine circumcision is that it prevents penile cancer. However, annual deaths from circumcision in this country quite possibly outnumber those due to carcinoma of the penis.[81] The low incidence of cervical carcinoma in Scandinavia and in Israel refutes statistics often cited in favor of routine circumcision. Circumcision of males is universal in Israel but rarely performed in Scandinavia.

One or 2% of males may require circumcision later in life for phimosis, paraphimosis, or balanitis. It does not seem unreasonable to recommend circumcision if the foreskin seems excessively long or the hiatus is small, 1 or 2 mm in diameter at birth.[82]

Whenever circumcision is contemplated, the parents should be fully informed of the indications, advantages, disadvantages, and possible complications. Circumcision should be supervised by a trained surgeon, with informed consent, as with any operation.

Technique of Circumcision

An encircling skin incision is made 0.8 cm proximal to the corona (Fig 133–1). Subcutaneous vessels are ligated with an absorbable suture. A hemostat is applied to the preputial opening on each side of the dorsal midline. When the foreskin is free of the glans, the prepuce is divided along the dorsal midline with scissors. The foreskin is then retracted proximally and an encircling incision is made through the skin of the inner aspect of the foreskin. The frenular artery is ligated and divided, and the freed prepuce is now excised by dividing its thin fascial attachments to the penis. The skin edges are united with interrupted absorbable sutures.[73] A greater amount of shaft skin is left on the ventrum to avoid "tightening" during erection.

In an attempt to correct phimosis and yet retain a normal-appearing foreskin, several authors recommend a form of foreskinplasty.[39, 106]

Meatal Stenosis

Meatal stenosis is commonly diagnosed, and often overdiagnosed, by inspection alone. Signs of obstruction, such as a trabeculated bladder, are usually absent.[97, 101] Meatal webs may deflect the urinary stream and flow rate may be reduced. The meatus may be enlarged by gentle dilatation, or a formal meatotomy may be required. This is performed by crushing about ¼ inch of glans in the ventral midline and then dividing the

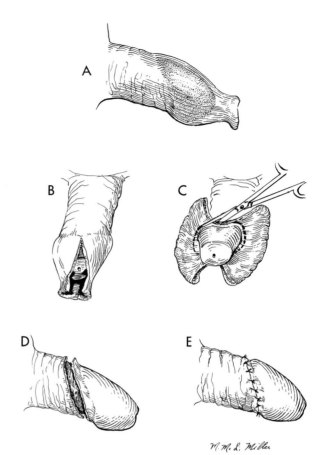

Fig 133–1.—Circumcision: technique. Care should be taken to leave a narrow cuff of mucosa adjacent to the coronal sulcus, to which the skin of the shaft can be sutured neatly. Tendency to leave the skin of the shaft too long should be avoided, lest adhesions form between any redundant prepuce and the glans.

crushed tissue. The parents are instructed to separate and lubricate the wound edges twice a day for a week, while healing occurs. An alternate technique is the Y-V meatoplasty described by Scott.[109]

Most severe meatal strictures are found in boys who have undergone neonatal circumcision. This suggests that the secretions of the deep layer of the foreskin really do lubricate and protect the meatus and prevent meatitis. Circumcision performed in infancy may predispose to such inflammation and the risk of meatal stenosis, and is one of the strongest arguments against routine neonatal circumcision.[97, 101]

Lacuna Magna (Valve of Guerin)

Any discussion of the lesions of the urethral meatus should include the "lacuna magna."[114] Its presence is often manifested by recurrent dysuria or hematuria. It is a common embryologic remnant consisting of a small diverticulum in the fossa navicularis. The diagnosis is best made by antegrade urethrography during voiding, although retrograde urethrography may occasionally suffice. The lacuna magna or valve of Guerin may cause no symptoms, or the symptoms may subside spontaneously. If symptoms persist, transmeatal incision of the valve leaflet to open the diverticulum into the urethra is usually curative.[114] The incision can be made with an infant urethrotome[13] or a "hook" electrode if the lesion is too proximal to grasp with hemostats or to engage transmeatally with scissor tips.

Distal Urethral Stenosis in Girls

Meatal stenosis and distal urethral stenosis have been implicated in girls as causes of intermittent or incomplete voiding and predisposition to urinary infection.[91] When calibrated with urethral bougies, the narrowest points in the female child's urethra are at the meatus in approximately one third and in the remainder at the distal urethral ring, where the smooth muscle of the urethra meets fibrous tissue near the level of the external sphincter. Both the meatus and the distal ring obstructions respond permanently to enlargement by gentle, progressive, one-time dilation to 26 F or more.

The distal urethral ring is a normal structure in prepubescent girls and disappears at puberty. The diameter of the narrowest portion of the urethra is the same in urologically normal controls and in girls undergoing cystoscopic evaluation because of recurrent urinary tract infection.[66, 67] Meatal stenosis or distal urethral stenosis is not now thought to play a significant role in the etiology of urinary tract infections except in rare instances. The infection rate is not reduced after urethral dilatation or urethrotomy.[42, 55, 76]

Labial Fusion

Labial fusion occurs in otherwise normal girls. It is treated simply by separating the labia under sedation or anesthesia. Alternatively, application of estrogen cream over a few weeks usually dissolves the fusion.

Urethral Masses in Girls

Interlabial masses include cysts of Skene's duct, Gärtner's cysts, congenital epithelial inclusion cysts, a prolapsed urethra, hydro(metro)colpos, a prolapsed ectopic ureterocele, and rhabdomyosarcoma of the urethra or vagina. Cysts of Skene's duct are paraurethral, lined by squamous epithelium, and treated by simple marsupialization if they do not respond to manual decompression.[53] Gärtner's cysts, vestigial mesonephric duct remnants usually found along the anterolateral wall of the vagina, are lined by mucus-secreting cuboidal or low columnar epithelium.[24] Marsupialization is again the treatment of choice. Urethral prolapse is encountered almost exclusively in black girls and usually presents as "vaginal" bleeding.[40, 84] A doughnut-shaped lesion of engorged dark mucosa around the meatus is characteristic, but it must be differentiated from a prolapsing ureterocele or sarcoma botryoides. Biopsy and cystoscopy may be necessary for proper identification. Urethral prolapse is treated by excising the prolapsed mucosa and reapproximating the normal urethral mucosa to the vestibule with interrupted absorbable sutures.[84]

Diverticula of the Female Urethra

Diverticula of the female urethra, not uncommon in parous adults, are rarely encountered in girls.[3, 23, 69] They may be congenital or the result of trauma. Excision is generally required, although a distal diverticulum may be treated by a generous meatotomy extending into the diverticulum.

Urethral Strictures

Strictures of the urethra may be congenital in boys and acquired in either sex. The etiology differs from that in adults in that fewer are inflammatory; most are traumatic-iatrogenic (79%)[77] and are therefore preventable. Congenital strictures are uncommon.[22] Strictures secondary to catheterization may be inflammatory rather than iatrogenic, since urethritis seems to be the inciting factor.[77] The consensus is that a single urethral dilatation should be tried first, but this seldom affords permanent cure.[57, 77] The failures of dilatation are sometimes not apparent for 8 or 9 years, which makes reports of the efficacy of the procedure, or the cause attributed for the stricture, suspect.[25] Repeated dilatations in children require anesthesia and are generally undesirable.[77] Urethrotomy may be efficacious in the management of congenital diaphragmatic strictures and for iatrogenic strictures, but the follow-up period is not yet long enough to be certain that in the long run urethrotomy will be more effective than dilatation.[77, 102] Open repair, mostly simple excision of the stricture and reanastomosis of the urethra, or single-stage island flap or patch graft procedures, seems superior to staged repair as long as active inflammation is not present at operation.[57, 77, 102, 103] Transpubic urethroplasty for membranous urethral strictures following pelvic fractures has given good results[57, 77, 117] and has become almost standard treatment for such strictures. It should be remembered that infants with "congenital strictures" may be best treated with a temporizing cutaneous vesicostomy, especially when they are ill or infected.[29, 77] The usefulness of flow rate determinations in the diagnosis and follow-up of strictures is now established, and these should be obtained routinely to follow the patient after repair.[58, 77]

Anterior Urethral Valves

Anterior urethral valves are a rare cause of urethral obstruction. Obstructive symptoms are more severe in infants and young children, while in older children the chief symptoms consist of diurnal enuresis or urinary infection.[46, 89, 120] The diagnosis is made by urethrography, but the entire urinary tract should be investigated to detect secondary hydronephrosis. Such valves may be treated by transurethral resection[104] or incision. The valve may be cusp-like, iris-like, or semilunar.[52] Anterior valves may arise from congenital cystic dilatation of normal or accessory periurethral glands. Another theory is that they represent an abortive attempt at urethral duplication.[120] There is often an association with a urethral diverticulum.[120] It is sometimes difficult to differentiate between an anterior valve with a diverticulum immediately proximal to it and a congenital diverticulum in which the anterior "lip" acts as a flap valve to cause obstruction.

Anterior Urethral Diverticula

Anterior urethral diverticula in the male child are located in the bulbous or pendulous urethra, are saccular or globular, lack supporting corpus spongiosum, and are lined by urethral mucosa[96] (Fig 133–2). Globular diverticula are usually located in the bulbous urethra, are pedunculated, and communicate with the urethra by a discrete narrow opening. Obstruction of this small orifice and stone formation may result.[105] Saccular diverticula lack a true neck and are located on the ventral surface of the bulbous or proximal pendulous urethra[83] (Fig 133–3).

The etiology of such diverticula is argued. Some believe they form because of obstruction secondary to a congenital urethral valve. When a valve is present there is always some proximal urethral dilatation, sometimes with formation of a diverticulum.[105] Others believe that congenital urethral diverticula form because of a lack of supportive corpus spongiosum.[18, 44] Normal-appearing corpus spongiosum covering the mucosa of the diverticulum has, however, been reported.[16, 105]

The symptoms are palpable penile swelling (noted only while voiding), terminal dribbling, or urinary infection.[16, 44, 83, 96] Upper urinary tract dilatation may also be present.

Early treatment is recommended by some,[87] but, in the infected male infant, a temporizing tubeless cystostomy with secondary operation on the urethra when the child is healthy and stable may be safest. Generally, the diverticulum is opened longitudinally in the ventral midline. The opened urethra is care-

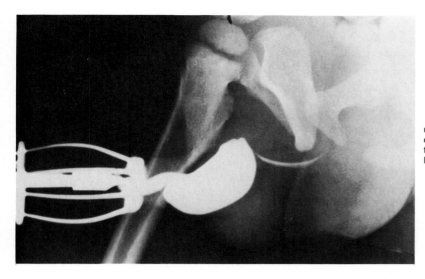

Fig 133–2.—Urethral diverticulum. A retrograde urethrogram in a boy with bladder outlet obstruction due to a large urethral diverticulum. As the diverticulum fills, the distal roof exerts a valve-like effect and encroaches on the urethral lumen.

fully inspected and a distal valve, if present, is excised. The proximal and distal portions of the diverticulum should be carefully dissected from the underlying urethra and removed. The lateral walls of the diverticulum are resected, making certain that enough tissue is left to re-form a urethra of slightly greater than normal caliber. Overlying tissues are closed in as many layers as possible, and the urine should be diverted.[16, 80]

Megalourethra

Megalourethra may be scaphoid or fusiform. The scaphoid type is more common and less severe. The fusiform type is associated with a marked deficiency of the corpora cavernosa and absence of the corpus spongiosum.[112] The scaphoid type often accompanies the prune belly syndrome. The fusiform type is usually accompanied by severe malformations leading to early death. Renal hypoplasia or dysplasia is common to both types and largely determines the prognosis.[27, 112]

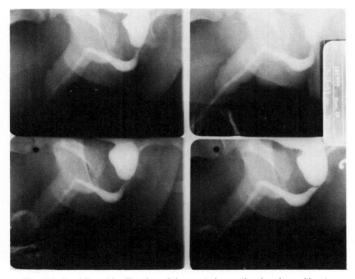

Fig 133–3.—Idiopathic dilatation of the posterior urethra in a boy without urethral valves or any discernible obstruction. Note the relatively good urinary stream and the absence of secondary bladder neck contraction. No tretment is indicated.

Megalourethra results from failure of mesodermal columns of the urethral folds to differentiate and provide support for the urethral epithelium.[115] Some postulate that megalourethra is part of a spectrum of developmental mesenchymal defects, including the prune belly syndrome, posterior urethral valves, and, possibly, anterior urethral valves secondary to a congenital urethral diverticulum.[100]

Shrom et al. recommend study by excretory urography alone, with a voiding film.[112] If prograde urography is necessary, percutaneous puncture of the bladder is recommended rather than urethral catheterization because of the danger of sepsis. Early repair of scaphoid megalourethra is strongly advocated by some.[90] An alternate approach consists of temporary ventral marsupialization of the megalourethra. The operation described by Nesbitt[100] consists of making a collar incision around the corona, dissecting the penile skin back to the penoscrotal junction, and excising redundant urethral tissue. A new urethral tube is formed around a catheter, which serves as a stent. The penile skin is tailored, reapproximating it as a cylinder to the coronal cuff. Proximal diversion is optional.

Cowper's Gland Anomalies

Cowper's gland cysts were first described radiographically in 1953 by Edling.[37] Maizels et al., in 1983,[92] grouped the lesions by their urethrographic appearance. There may be dilatation of the entire Cowper's gland duct or an imperforate orifice resulting in a cyst that encroaches on the urethral lumen (Fig 133–4). Perforate Cowper's cyst or syringocele represents the dilated portion of the distal duct open into the bulbar urethra through a wide orifice. In imperforate Cowper's syringocele the cyst intrudes into the urethra as a rounded filling defect without communication with the urethral lumen.

A simple Cowper's syringocele is the commonest variety and is often found in adults with urethral strictures of inflammatory etiology.

Urinary infections, hematuria, initial or terminal, and difficult voiding are common.[92] The lesion is best demonstrated by voiding or retrograde urethrogram[4] and by urethroscopy.

Urethral extravasation can mimic a Cowper's duct cyst, but the outlines are sharper with the latter. Congenital urethral membranes in the membranous urethra[43] and anterior urethral valves in the penile urethra are differentiated from Cowper's duct cysts by their location and appearance.

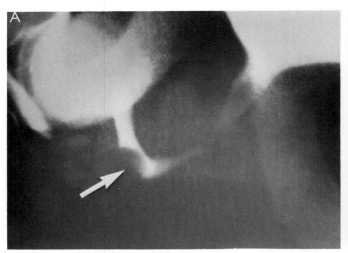
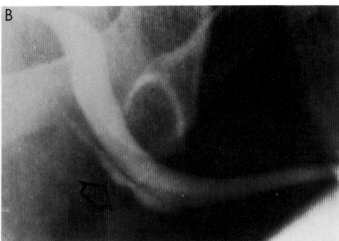

Fig 133–4.—Cowper's duct anomalies in the male. **A,** a Cowper's duct cyst is seen as a consistent urethral filling defect in the bulbar urethra *(arrow).* Such cysts are easily unroofed by transurethral resection. **B,** reflux into Cowper's duct on voiding cystourethrography. No treatment is required. (Courtesy of Drs. Arnold H. Colodny and Robert L. Lebowitz.)

Treatment consists of endoscopic resection, marsupializing the syringocele into the urethra. Maizels reported excellent results in 8 cases.[92]

Posterior Urethral Valves

In the normal male, folds arise from the distal portion of the veru, the cristae urethralis, also called plicae colliculi, which course inferolaterally and disappear into the lateral wall near the membranous urethra. When these folds are deeper than normal and fused anteriorly, they cause outlet obstruction and the characteristic secondary dilatation of the posterior urethra, apparent contracture of the bladder neck, and severe trabeculation.[116] Varying degrees of upper tract damage often result from ureteral obstruction and/or reflux, with or without renal dysplasia. The kidneys and ureters may be further injured by infection secondary to obstruction and/or reflux.

Stephens' studies indicate that the renal dysplasia associated with urethral valves is often a primary phenomenon and correlates best with ureteral orifice position and reflux. Renal dysplasia is a primary developmental failure in the nephrogenic mesenchyma of the metanephric blastema. Kidneys with near-normal ureteral orifice positions were near-normal in structure, while those with extremely lateral ureteral orifices were quite dysplastic. Those with intermediate grades of lateral orifice displacement exhibited thin parenchyma, minimal dysplasia, and fewer nephrons than normal.[59] Obstruction alone does not, to any marked extent, impair nephron development in the fetus.[59] Urethral ligation in chick embryos 2 days after fertilization caused only hydronephrosis without dysplasia.[15] Renal dysplasia, posterior urethral valves, and unilateral reflux have been noted in 15–20% of boys with urethral valves.[64]

Neonates with posterior urethral valves present with a distended bladder, poor stream, dribbling, flank masses, urinary infection, renal failure, or failure to thrive.[7, 33] Many are now detected prenatally by maternal ultrasound. Premature delivery or fetal intervention has not yet been demonstrated to improve treatment results.[32] Wetting, both day and night, is the most common symptom in older children.[33] Very rarely an older child may present only with nocturnal enuresis.[33] Occasionally, the infant may present with urinary ascites due to urinary extravasation.[94]

A voiding cystourethrogram shows a dilated and elongated posterior urethra "squared off" at the site of the valve[56] and a poor stream distal to the obstruction. The bladder neck appears narrow relative to the dilated posterior urethra (Fig 133–5,A). Secondary signs of obstruction, such as bladder trabeculation, hydroureteronephrosis, and/or reflux must be present or the diagnosis becomes suspect. The diagnosis should be confirmed by urethroscopy.

After the diagnosis is made, the sick infant often requires a period of initial bladder drainage per urethram or by percutaneous placement of a suprapubic polyethylene tube.[33, 125] There is almost complete agreement that suprapubic intubated cystostomy should be used for a very short period and should never be used for long-term drainage as it causes chronic infection, and increased fibrosis of the bladder wall, which may exacerbate ureteral obstruction and render the bladder useless in the future. In the uremic infant, the assistance of a pediatric nephrologist is desirable.[33, 125] Bladder drainage may not result in adequate upper tract decompression, and bilateral temporary percutaneous nephrostomies may be required, especially when infection is present.[3, 34, 125] Many would proceed to temporary high-loop skin ureterostomies.[70]

There are four choices of management after the stabilization period. The simplest is primary ablation of the valves, transurethrally or through a perineal urethrostomy.[125] The second is cutaneous vesicostomy;[1, 20, 30, 58] the third is loop ureterostomy[94, 126] or cutaneous pyelostomy;[68] and the fourth is total reconstruction with tapering and reimplantation of the dilated ureters along with ablation of the valves.[50] The availability of superb infant fiberoptic resectoscopes of very small caliber (8–10 F) makes valve ablation safe and effective in the great majority of cases (Fig 133–5,B). Primary "total" reconstruction is generally being abandoned because of the high risk of obstruction associated with ureteral reimplantation into a thick and obstructed bladder.[33, 125] We prefer to use the infant resectoscope, incising the valves at the inferolateral margins near the attachment to the veru and cutting toward the sphincter. Cutting the apex of the valve at the ventral midline has been advocated by some as the only incision needed,[30] and by others, following the posterolateral cuts.[127] A hook or Bugbee electrode may also be used.[30] Others favor a ureteral catheter with fulgurating wire protruding beyond the tip.[50] All these methods seem effective.

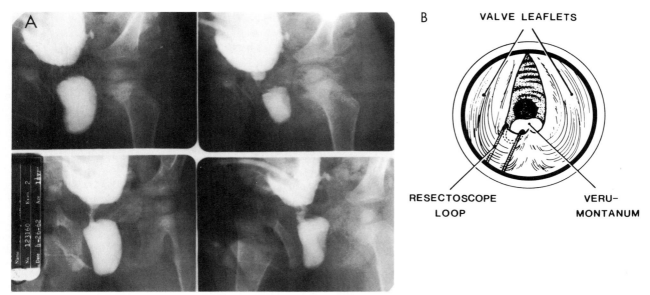

Fig 133–5.—Posterior urethral valve. **A,** voiding cystourethrogram in a male infant with severe obstruction due to posterior urethral valves (type I). Note the bladder irregularity (trabeculation), the characteristic marked dilatation and elongation of the posterior urethra, the poor urinary stream distal to the valve, and the marked thickening of smooth muscle at the neck of the bladder. **B,** endo-scopic resection of the paired valve cusps was all that was necessary to relieve obstruction, and the secondary hypertrophy of the bladder neck then subsided. (**B** from Kelalis P., et al. (eds.): *Clinical Pediatric Urology.* Philadelphia, W.B. Saunders Co., 1976.)

Cutaneous ureterostomy was the primary treatment of valves for many years.[70, 107] Krueger et al.[86] found somatic growth to be much better in patients who underwent primary diversion, compared with those who had valves resected in infancy; renal function was also better preserved. Duckett, reviewing a similar group of patients and using similar parameters, did not reach this conclusion.[33] He did note that, if the creatinine level falls below 1.0 mg/dl during the initial hospitalization, prognosis for growth and near-normal renal development remains good. If the postoperative creatinine remains above 1.0 mg/dl, there is some likelihood of chronic renal failure as the child grows.[31,33]

The major disadvantage of high diversion is that it may compromise the blood supply of the ureter and hamper total reconstruction for the correction of ureteral obstruction or reflux.[33, 50, 125] However, in the infant who is septic and/or gravely uremic, or in those whose upper tracts fail to drain well after valve resection, high diversion is still the safest method of management and allows the maximum degree of recovery.

The technique of loop ureterostomy consists of isolating the highest loop of ureter, mobilizing it, and bringing it through the wound to skin level on the abdominal wall.[70] Williams and Cromie believe that a ring ureterostomy technique should be used. This consists of anastomosing the ureter so that a ring is created. The most lateral portion of the ring is opened onto the skin. Urine can also flow from the pelvis through the anastomosis to the bladder, thus avoiding complete defunctionalization and the risk of permanent bladder contracture.[123]

Cutaneous pyelostomy is an excellent alternative, but its usefulness is limited to that low proportion of cases in which the pelvis is both extrarenal and quite dilated.[68]

Cutaneous vesicostomy for temporary diversion has been strongly advocated,[1, 20, 29] especially when the small size of the urethra of the male newborn precludes primary fulguration. The procedure is easy to perform and to reverse and does not require an appliance, awkward for infants in diapers. Others have advocated vesicostomy in the neonate with bilateral reflux[33] when follow-up may be difficult, or occasionally when the valves are inadequately resected on a first attempt.

Most employ the Blocksom technique of vesicostomy,[20, 33, 125] while others have used Lapides' technique.[1] Unfortunately, when the ureters are obstructed at the ureterovesical junction, vesicostomy may not adequately decompress the upper tracts. To determine whether the ureters are obstructed at bladder level, a furosemide renogram or a Whitaker test may be necessary before deciding on the level of diversion.

In brief, the management of the infant with urethral valves after stabilization can be said today to be primary valve ablation in almost all instances. In the case of a septic and/or severely uremic neonate who does not respond to initial stabilization by catheter drainage or who continues to do poorly after adequate valve ablation, temporary ureterostomies are required. The chief role of vesicostomy is in the interim management of the infant with severe bilateral reflux or a high-pressure, small-capacity bladder.

Roughly half of the boys with valves have unilateral or bilateral reflux. In one series of 83 patients, 39 (47%) had reflux. Of these, 21 were unilateral. Reflux persisted after valve ablation in 18. Of these, 13 had a nonfunctioning kidney, usually with dysplasia, and a nephroureterectomy was eventually done.[33] In another series of 100 patients, 21% had unilateral reflux while in 27% the reflux was bilateral. Of the 21 cases of unilateral reflux, five ceased after valve resection. Ten patients underwent nephroureterectomy for nonfunction, four are being followed, one had cessation of reflux, nine required bilateral reimplantation, six underwent unilateral reimplantation and required contralateral nephrectomy for nonfunction. Nine had ureterostomies to improve drainage.[124] Results were similar in a third group.[75] Bilateral reflux is more apt to be associated with eventual renal failure (because of associated dysplasia) than unilateral reflux. With the latter, the refluxing unit is often functionless and requires nephroureterectomy.[34, 125] In general, if the urinary tract is uninfected, the patient can be placed on antibacterial prophylaxis and followed. Reimplantation of a dilated ureter into a thickened trabeculated bladder does not carry a great chance of immediate success. Complication rates are reported between 15% and 60%. If reflux is severe and renal function poor, temporary diversion is the safest method of management, as superimposed infection is prevented.[125] The consensus is to delay reimplantation until the upper tracts are decompressed and optimal bladder function is restored.[33, 125] Renal function should be assessed by a renogram or an intravenous pyelogram with a catheter in the bladder to be sure a functionless kidney has not been opacified by reflux.[34, 64]

Brief mention should be made of the obstructed ureter secondary to urethral valves. Reimplantation should be delayed unless there is proof by diuresis renogram, or pressure flow studies, that severe obstruction continues after resection of the valve. Such obstruction is often less common than the degree of hydroureteronephrosis might suggest.[35, 125] Before any surgical attempt to reimplant a ureter for reflux or obstruction, the bladder must be assessed for its ability to empty, and pressure volume relationships ascertained. Reimplanting a ureter into a noncompliant bladder with high pressures at low volumes, or with residual urine, is likely to fail. Indeed, the symptoms and mechanism of this type of bladder have been called the "valve bladder syndrome."[95]

To diagnose the noncompliant bladder, urodynamic evaluations should be performed. If a "valve bladder" is noted, the problem must be treated. Anticholinergic drugs have been useful in some cases.[95, 116] Bladder augmentation with resection of most of the abnormal bladder ("bladder substitution") is necessary in the majority.[95]

Incontinence secondary to posterior urethral valves or valve resection has been reported to vary from 15% to 30%. In one recent series, 13%, and in another, 11 of 76 children, followed for a sufficient time after resection, were incontinent.[41] Most boys dribble for some time after valve ablation but eventually gain control, especially at puberty when the prostate develops. Wetting is thought to be a consequence of prolonged dilatation of the sphincters around the distended posterior urethra, which improves slowly as the urethra shrinks in size. Recovery is by no means certain, especially if the external sphincter has been damaged by extensive fulguration or incisions carried into the sphincter. If the bladder neck has been resected or a Y-V plasty performed, incontinence and retrograde ejaculation are likely. In one review, 88% of children with bladder neck resection were incontinent.[119] The radiologic and endoscopic findings at the bladder neck in valve patients often suggest obstruction at this level but represent only hypertrophy of detrusor muscle, which will subside with time after ablation of the valve. Preservation of the bladder neck is important in the maintenance of urinary control.[71] The risk of incontinence seems greater in patients treated in early infancy, as they have the most severe degrees of obstruction. The greater the degree of obstruction and dilatation, the greater the deformity of the urethral sphincters.[41]

Eight boys with incontinence after valve resection were studied urodynamically by Bauer.[10] He found that persistent voiding difficulty was caused by myogenic detrusor failure in three and high voiding pressures in one. Uninhibited bladder contractions were responsible in two, a small capacity in one, and severe reflux in another. At times, anticholinergics, intermittent catheterization, correction of severe reflux,[10] resection of the intereureteric ridge,[116] and subtotal cystectomy with bladder augmentation[95] are each necessary.

The long-term prognosis in the majority of patients with valves is satisfactory. Even of those with severe hydronephrosis, 60% ultimately achieved normal renal function. The mortality rate is now only about 5%. The deaths tend to occur in infants with renal dysplasia whose renal function fails to improve following valve ablation or high-loop ureterostomy. When serum creatinine levels return to normal within 2 years, the prognosis is good. When they remain moderately elevated there is considerable risk of eventual renal failure in adolescence or in early adult life. Deterioration is manifested by proteinuria, hypertension, and a rising creatinine level. Ultimately, dialysis or transplantation is required.[125]

Cysts of the Utricle

Cysts of the utricle may be present in intersex patients, or in association with hypospadias or the prune belly syndrome. The utricle is derived from the müllerian ducts and is enlarged when the müllerian structures are incompletely suppressed by the fetal testes. The cyst may be very large, form a mass in the pelvis, and cause pain, recurrent infection, postvoiding incontinence, or epididymitis when the vas enters the cyst. Large cysts may not be demonstrated radiologically unless the communication with the urethra is widely patent. Cystourethrography provided the diagnosis in 11 of 12 cases in one series. In most patients, the opening can be seen in the floor of the posterior urethra in the region of the veru. Occasionally, a calculus in the cyst is seen on a plain roentgenogram. Excision of the cyst is required only in symptomatic cases. A transperitoneal approach with mobilization of the bladder provides access in most babies, while in older children it may be preferable to make a midline incision across the trigone.[98] A posterior parasacral approach, with resection of the coccyx and lateral retraction of the rectum, has also been employed.[98]

Polyps of the Urethra

Polyps of the posterior urethra in males are quite rare, only 50 cases reported to date. The signs are obstruction, hematuria, retention, and infection.[98] The diagnosis is usually not apparent on intravenous pyelography. Voiding cystourethrography shows a polypoid nonopaque filling defect arising from the area of the verumontanum and prolapsing into the prostatic urethra with voiding, diagnostic of a benign fibrovascular polyp. The majority of such polyps have been removed transvesically, but several instances of transurethral excision have also been reported, one in a child of 3 weeks.[26] There have been reports of inadequate removal of polyps via suprapubic excision.[28, 78] A more recent technique consists of passing grasping forceps through a suprapubic Cystocath, removing the resected polyp under cystoscopic visualization. The endoscopic technique affords the most complete removal with the least possible risk to the ejaculatory ducts.[78] If the base is not removed completely the polyp may recur.[28] It has been postulated that mesonephric derivatives form urethral polyps in boys; just as in girls they form polyps in the vagina and cervix but seldom in the urethra.[65, 78, 110]

Bladder Neck Obstruction

Primary or congenital bladder neck obstruction is a rare clinical entity, which in the past was overdiagnosed and overtreated.[2, 21, 128] The diagnosis, now seldom made, must be one of exclusion. Internal sphincter spasm or dyssynergia may mimic primary bladder neck contracture (Fig 133–6). Criteria for diagnosis, as promulgated by Allen, are as follows:[2]

1. A history of obstructed voiding that can be traced back to infancy or early childhood.

2. Objective evidence of obstruction, trabeculation of the bladder, often with hydronephrosis.

3. Urodynamic studies that show elevated intravesical pressures on voiding, with poor flow rates, despite adequate perineal and external sphincter relaxation, indicating a true mechanical obstruction.

4. Voiding cystourethrograms that show a persistent narrowing of bladder neck with restricted flow distally.

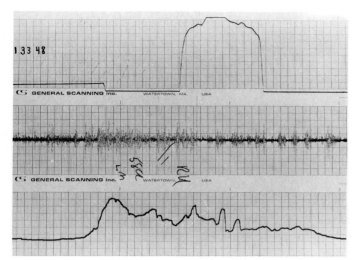

Fig 133–6.—Failure of the external sphincter to relax during voiding in a child with spasm of the external urinary sphincter, causing daytime incontinence and hydronephrosis. As the bladder pressure rises *(lower register)*, the striated sphincter not only fails to relax but exhibits increased electrical activity *(middle register)*. Voiding eventually occurs—the top graph records urine flow—but against the increased resistance of a closed "voluntary" sphincter, which has not learned to work in synergy with the detrusor. After 3 months of diazepam (Valium) therapy, urinary control is normal and hydronephrosis is diminishing.

5. No other neurologic, dyssynergic, or mechanical abnormalities that could account for the obstruction.

6. Unequivocal clinical, urodynamic, radiographic, and biochemical improvement following emptying by intermittent catheterization or operation to enlarge the bladder neck.

Some consider bladder neck contracture and internal sphincter dyssynergia to be the same disease, best treated by continuing intermittent clean catheterization while instituting pharmacotherapy, usually with Dibenzyline.

Sphincter Dyssynergia

Voiding dysfunctions in children are most often caused by inappropriate detrusor and/or sphincter activity. Such children present with an unexplained propensity for infection or with day-time wetting. Obstructive urologic or neurologic problems, such as occult spinal dysraphism, must not be overlooked.[93] A good classification for sphincter dyssynergia is that proposed by Bauer.[11] He divides patients into those with a small-capacity hypertonic bladder, a hyperreflexic bladder, a large-capacity hypotonic bladder, or a non-neurogenic neurogenic bladder often with diverticulum formation, hydronephrosis, and/or reflux. One or both sphincters may be "dyssynergic" in that they fail to relax as the bladder contracts.

Isolated internal sphincter dyssynergia is occasionally encountered. The diagnosis is made by exclusion or by therapeutic trial. These patients have a poor flow rate with intermittent flow, can generate normal or elevated bladder pressures, and have normal external sphincter electromyographic activity. Response to an adrenergic blocker confirms the diagnosis.[113]

Smey et al. recommend that no instrumentation be performed before urodynamic evaluation. Electromyographic activity is recorded with perineal electrodes.[113] However, the placement of suprapubic Cystocaths and wire electrodes in the external sphincter the day before the examination allows repeated bladder filling for repetitive voiding studies.[45] Familiarity with the latest advances in bladder physiology, patience, and experience are necessary to perform these studies correctly.

Penile Agenesis

Penile agenesis is an extremely rare anomaly; approximately 50 cases have been reported.[6, 14, 36, 62] The urethral meatus is just anterior to the rectum in the perineum, adjacent to a small tag of perianal skin that may contain erectile tissue, or actually in the rectum (Fig 133–7). Occasionally, the urethral opening is anterior to the scrotum or even above the pubic symphysis. The testes and scrotum are usually well developed and normal in size and position.

Associated genitourinary anomalies are common and include cryptorchidism, hypoplasia or agenesis of the prostate, polycystic kidneys, abnormalities of renal position and location, and even agenesis of the urinary tract. Concomitant abnormalities of the anus, rectum, and lower colon are often present as well.

None of the several techniques to reconstruct the penis has been satisfactory for infants. The psychological problems inherent in a male growing up without a penis dictate that these patients be castrated and reared as girls. This is all the more nec-

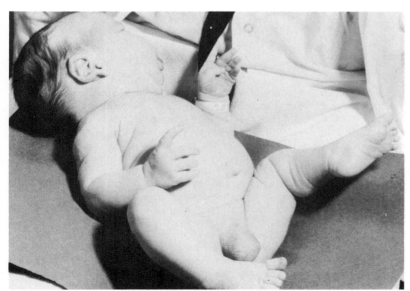

Fig 133–7.—Agenesis of the penis. Two-week-old male infant with normal testes and scrotum and no penis. A tiny red spot just below the pubis, appearing like a freshly healed scar, suggests the site of the penis. The child voided intermittently through the anus, the opening of the urethra being in rectal mucosa. The child was castrated, birth certificate changed, and the child reared as a female. Vaginoplasty was planned for puberty. (Courtesy of Dr. Mark M. Ravitch.)

essary in these patients, given the ectopic position of the urethral stump. The vesical sphincters are intact, and the patients can be continent. The condition is compatible with survival into adult life. Testes should be removed in infancy and the scrotal skin infolded. Formal vaginoplasty is postponed until puberty. Estrogen therapy is begun at 10–12 years of age to promote near-normal puberty and mammary development.

Male Urethral Duplications

Urethral duplications are rare, approximately 50 cases having been reported.[99] Most commonly, the duplication is in the sagittal plane. In some, this represents a variant of the exstrophy-epispadias complex (see Chap. 128). In others, there is a failure in the closure of the urethral folds.[121] Urethral duplications have been classified according to the position of the ectopic urethra:[121]

Sagittal duplication
    Y-duplication: preanal or perineal accessory channel
    Spindle urethra: urethra splits into two and then reunites
    Epispadias: dorsal penile accessory urethra
    Hypospadias: both urethrae ventral to corpora
        Complete: two channels leave the bladder separately
        Bifid or incomplete: urethra divides below the bladder
        Abortive: accessory urethra is a blind sinus
Collateral duplication
    Complete with diphallus
    Abortive: one urethra is a blind sinus

The aim of treatment is to restore normal anatomy. This is most easily accomplished by excising the more incomplete urethra, called the accessory urethra.[121]

In cases of complete duplication a combined penile and retropubic transvesical approach may be necessary.[99, 121] When the urethra is bifid, dividing below a single bladder neck, the septum between the urethra of normal caliber and the atretic urethra may be divided endoscopically utilizing a "cold knife."[51] With Y duplications and a perineal accessory tract, the best solution is to form a neourethra of adequate caliber to reach the tip of the penis. The operation is performed in two stages. The first stage consists of transferring the larger urethral opening from the anal verge to a point in the anterior perineum. The atretic, more dorsal urethra is excised. In some instances, colostomy has been advised to promote healing. The second stage consists of tubularizing a strip of ventral skin, burying the tube much as in a hypospadias repair. Alternatively, a scrotal flap urethroplasty may be performed without preliminary colostomy.

Penile Duplication

Diphallus is a rare anomaly, which occurs in about 1 in 5,000,000 live births[63] (Fig 133–8). In a review of diphallus, Hollowel et al. noted that, in 46 cases, all but four fell into two major groups. The first group, with complete duplication of the shaft and glans, comprised 29 cases, with a high proportion of duplicated bladders. There were 15 intestinal anomalies in this group with imperforate anus in 12 and bifid scrotum in 12 instances also. In the second group of 15 cases, the anomaly was incomplete. Four had bladder exstrophy and epispadias, and nine exhibited symphyseal separations without exstrophy. Urethral duplications were present in the majority of both groups, with one urethra in each phallus.

The anomalies involving complete duplication of the shaft of the penis appear to arise posteriorly and caudally in the young embryo, before the fourth week, perhaps because of partial twinning of the hindgut. Group 1 duplications are associated with anomalies of the lumbosacral spine, imperforate anus, bifid scro-

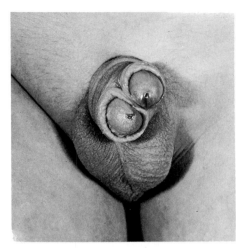

Fig 133–8.—Diphallus in which each glans was separated for about half the length of the shaft. Each urethra communicated with a separate bladder, the left being much larger. One kidney emptied into each bladder, but the right kidney was hypoplastic and finally was removed.

tum, and duplication of the bladder. In Group 2, the defect seems more likely to involve the cephalic portion of the cloacal membrane and midline growth of extraembryonic mesoderm. This could account for the higher incidence of isolated vesical exstrophy in this group (Fig 133–9).

In general, with complete diphallus, one must excise the phallus with the less well developed corpora cavernosa and urethra. Correction of chordee and penile lengthening may be required, as described by Johnston.[72, 118] Two complete sagittal trifurcations have been described.[108, 127]

Female Urethral Duplications

Accessory urethras in the female are even more rare than in the male. These are of two types: A, those in which the major urethra is perineal and the accessory urethra is subcorporeal, or B, those in which both urethras are perineal or vaginal.[17, 19] Type A duplications are more common and are not associated with virilization. Abnormal descent of the müllerian ducts, causing posterior displacement of the vaginal introitus, may allow the accessory phallic urethra to form. Genitoplasty with or without ablation of the accessory urethra is recommended.[12]

Torsion of the Penis

Penile torsion is a rare anomaly believed to be caused by abnormal skin attachment and not by any structural abnormality of the corpora (Fig 133–10). The rotation is almost always to the left (counterclockwise). The urethral meatus is often obliquely positioned, and the median raphe makes a spiral curve as it passes from the base of the penis toward the tip.[8] Two procedures have been described to correct this anomaly. The first, described by Johnston,[74] employs a circumferential incision at the base of the penis with the subcutaneous tissues divided all around, down to the corpora; derotation is accomplished and the skin is sutured in a slightly overcorrected position. In the reverse of this technique, the incision is made behind the corona, and correction is then effected when the penis is "degloved." The latter technique seems the more reliable of the two, for it avoids devascularization and impaired lymphatic drainage of the skin of the shaft.

If a two-stage operation is deemed necessary, 6 months should

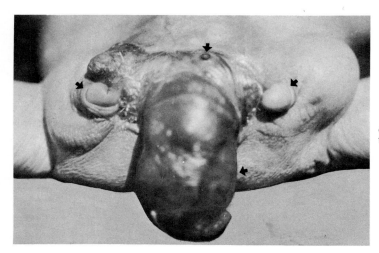

Fig 133–9.—Complete diphallus in a 2-day-old infant born with exstrophy of the cloaca, complete rectal prolapse and vesicointestinal fistula *(upper arrow)*. (From *Pediatrics* 23:927, 1959.)

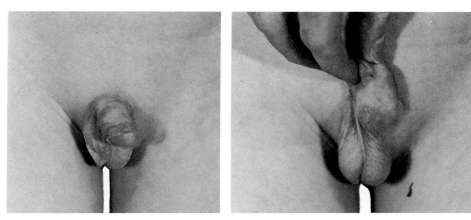

Fig 133–10.—Torsion of the penis with 90-degree rotation, associated pinhole meatus and glandular hypospadias. The rotation caused no impairment of function.

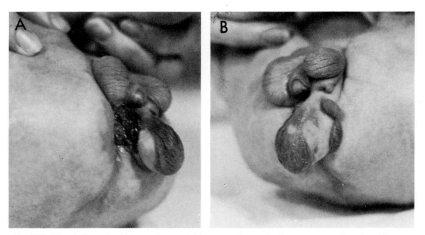

Fig 133–11.—A 5-week-old boy with scrotal transposition, ectopic scrotum, and perineal lipoma. The patient also had perineal hypospadias and imperforate anus.

elapse between stages to allow complete healing and revascularization of the skin.[74]

Penoscrotal Webs

Webbed penis is a congenital anomaly in which the penile and scrotal skin are fused. The fusion may be complete, with a total absence of separation of the penis from the scrotum, or incomplete, with a web of varying length connecting the proximal penis and scrotum. It has been reported to occur in 3.5% of cases of hypospadias.[111] The condition is repaired by utilizing W-plasty flaps along the shaft of the penis, with a rectangular scrotal flap to prevent webbing at the penoscrotal junction. A simpler technique is to incise the skin of the penoscrotal junction transversely and suture it longitudinally after the penile shaft is freed from underlying connective tissue.

Penoscrotal Transposition and Ectopic Scrotum

Scrotal transposition can appear in several forms, ranging from the bifid scrotum associated with the more proximal and severe forms of hypospadias to the more unusual severe malpositions, including the prepenile scrotum (Fig 133–11), the webbed scrotum (incomplete transposition), and the ectopic scrotum. The necessity for surgical correction depends on the degree of displacement and the presence or absence of associated abnormalities. The rarest form of malposition, prepenile scrotum, is often associated with perineal hypospadias, absence of the urinary tract, polycystic kidneys, and imperforate anus.[79]

Correction of penile scrotal transposition with perineal hypospadias consists of mobilizing the two scrotal halves as rotational advancement flaps, relocating and reapproximating them beneath the penis. Ehrlich and Scardino stress the desirability of leaving a wide skin bridge connecting the midline dorsal penile skin with the suprapubic skin. A proximal incision behind the urethral meatus allows formation of a Thiersch-Duplay skin tube.[38] In one case, the same authors achieved a good result employing an island flap, transposing the scrotum, correcting the chordee, and constructing the neourethra in a single operation.

Patches of ectopic scrotum in the inguinal area or on the thigh should be excised. An ectopic testis can usually be transposed subcutaneously into the hemiscrotum, which is in or near the normal site.

REFERENCES

1. Allen T.D.: Vesicostomy for the temporary diversion of the urine in small children. *J. Urol.* 123:929, 1980.
2. Allen T.D.: Congenital bladder neck obstruction: Criteria for diagnosis. Presented at International Society of Urology, 1982.
3. Anderson M.J.T.: The incidence of diverticula in the female urethra. *J. Urol.* 98:96, 1967.
4. Ansell J.S.: Cysts of the ducts of Cowper's glands. *J. Urol.* 115:390, 1976.
5. Arant B.S.: Nonrenal factors influencing renal function during the perinatal period. *Clin. Perinatol.* 8:225, 1981.
6. Attie J.: Congenital absence of penis: Report of case with congenital concealed penile agenesis and congenital absence of the left kidney and ureter. *J. Urol.* 83:343, 1961.
7. Atwell J.D.: Posterior urethral valves in the British Isles: A multicenter BAPS review. *J. Pediatr. Surg.* 18:70, 1983.
8. Azmy A., Eckstein H.B.: Surgical correction of torsion of the penis. *Br. J. Urol.* 53:378, 1981.
9. Bartone F.F., et al.: Diagnosis and treatment of fluid-filled renal structures in children, with ultrasonography and percutaneous puncture. *Urology* 16:432, 1980.
10. Bauer S.B., Dieppa R.A., Habib K.K., et al.: The bladder in boys with posterior urethral valves: A urodynamic assessment. *J. Urol.* 121:769, 1979.
11. Bauer S.B., et al.: The unstable bladder of childhood. *Urol. Clin. North Am.* 7:321, 1980.
12. Bellinger M.F., Duckett J.W.: Accessory phallic urethra in the female patient. *J. Urol.* 127:1159, 1982.
13. Bellinger M.T., Purohit G.S., Duckett J.W., et al.: Lacuna magna: A hidden cause of dysuria and bloody spotting in boys. *J. Pediatr. Surg.* 28:163, 1983.
14. Benirschke K.: Penile agenesis: Report of a case, review of the world literature and discussion of pertinent embryology. *Arch. Pathol.* 70:252, 1960.
15. Berman D.J., Maizels M.: Role of urinary obstruction in the genesis of renal dysplasia: A model in the chick embryo. *J. Urol.* 128:1091, 1982.
16. Bissada N.K., Hanash K.A.: Obstructive urethral diverticula in children. *Urology* 20:281, 1982.
17. Boissonnat P.: Two cases of complete double functional urethra with a single bladder. *Br. J. Urol.* 33:453, 1961.
18. Boissonnat P., Duhamel B.: Congenital diverticulum of the anterior urethra associated with aplasia of the abdominal muscles in a male infant. *Br. J. Urol.* 34:59, 1962.
19. Bonney W.W., et al.: Complete duplication of the urethra with vaginal stenosis. *J. Urol.* 112:132, 1975.
20. Bruce R.B., Gonzales E.T.: Cutaneous vesicostomy: A useful form of urinary diversion in children. *J. Urol.* 123:927, 1980.
21. Burns E., Shasky D.: Problems in the management of bladder neck obstruction in children. *Ohio Med. J.* 52:170, 1957.
22. Currarino G., Stephens F.D.: An uncommon type of bulbar urethral stricture, sometimes familial, of unknown cause: Congenital versus acquired. *J. Urol.* 126:658, 1981.
23. Davis H.J., Telinde R.W.: Urethral diverticula: An assay of 121 cases. *J. Urol.* 80:34–39, 1958.
24. Depisch L.M.: Cysts of the vagina: Classification and clinical correlations. *Obstet. Gynecol.* 45:632, 1975.
25. Devereux M.H., Burfield G.D.: Prolonged follow-up of urethral strictures treated by intermittent dilatation. *Br. J. Urol.* 42:321, 1970.
26. DeWolf W.C., Fraley E.E.: Congenital urethral polyp in the infant: Case report and review of the literature. *J. Urol.* 109:515, 1973.
27. Dorairajan T.: Defects of spongy tissue and congenital diverticula of the penile urethra. *Aust. N.Z. J. Surg.* 32:209, 1963.
28. Downs R.: Congenital polyps of the prostatic urethra: Review of literature and report of two cases. *Br. J. Urol.* 42:76, 1970.
29. Duckett J.W.: Cutaneous vesicostomy in childhood: The Blocksom technique. *Urol. Clin. North Am.* 1:485, 1974.
30. Duckett J.W.: Current management of posterior urethral valves. *Urol. Clin. North Am.* 1:471, 1974.
31. Duckett J.W.: Editorial comments on Rabinowitz R.T. et al.: Upper tract management when posterior urethral valve ablation is insufficient. *J. Urol.* 122:370, 1979.
32. Duckett J.W.: Fetal intervention for obstructive uropathy. *Dialogues Ped. Urol.* 5:8, 1982.
33. Duckett J.W.: Management of posterior urethral valves. *AUA Update Series* 38:3, 1983.
34. Duckett J.W.: Management of posterior urethral valves. *AUA Update Series* 38:5, 1983.
35. Duckett J.W.: Management of posterior urethral valves. *AUA Update Series* 38:6, 1983.
36. Edgerton M.T., Gillenwater J.Y., Kenney J.G., et al.: The bladder flap for urethral reconstruction in total phalloplasty. *Plast. Reconstr. Surg.* 74:259, 1984.
37. Edling N.F.: The radiologic appearance of diverticula of the male cavernosus urethra. *Acta Radiol.* 40:1, 1953.
38. Ehrlich R.M., Scardino P.T.: Scrotal transposition and correction of perineal hypospadias. *Urol. Clin. North Am.* 8:531, 1981.
39. Emmett A.J.J.: Four V-flap repair of preputial stenosis: An alternative to circumcision. *Plast. Reconstr. Surg.* 55:687, 1975.
40. Esposito J.M.: Circular prolapse of the urethra in children: A cause of vaginal bleeding. *Obstet. Gynecol.* 31:363, 1968.
41. Eyami K., Smith D.E.: A study of the sequelae of posterior urethral valves. *J. Urol.* 127:84, 1982.
42. Fair W.R., et al.: Urinary tract infections in children. *West. J. Med.* 121:366, 1974.
43. Field P.L., Stephens F.D.: Congenital urethral membranes causing urethral obstruction. *J. Urol.* 111:250, 1974.
44. Firlit C.F.: Urethral abnormalities. *Urol. Clin. North Am.* 5:31, 1978.
45. Firlit C.F., Smey P., King L.R.: Micturition urodynamic flow studies in children. *J. Urol.* 119:250, 1978.
46. Firlit R.S., Firlit C.F., King L.R.: Anterior urethral valves in children. *J. Urol.* 108:972, 1972.
47. Frates R., DeLuca T.G.: Urethral polyps in male children. *Radiology* 89:289, 1967.
48. Fuqua F.: Utilization of full thickness skin grafts for the management of urethral strictures in the male child. *Birth Defects* 13:223, 1977.

49. Gates G.F.: *Atlas of Abdominal Ultrasonography in Children.* New York, Churchill-Livingstone, 1978, pp. 191–283.
50. Ginsburg H.B., Hendren W.H.: Severe urethral valves: Experience with 120 cases. Abstracts, American Urological Association Program, 1980, p. 65.
51. Goldstein H.R., Hensle T.W.: Visual urethrotomy in management of male urethral duplication. *Urology* 18:374, 1981.
52. Golimbu M., et al.: Anterior urethral valves. *Urology* 12:343, 1978.
53. Gottesman J.E., Sparkuhl A.: Bilateral Skene duct cysts. *J. Pediatr.* 94:945, 1979.
54. Graham D.S., Krueger R.P., Glenn J.F.: Anterior urethral diverticulum associated with posterior urethral valves. *J. Urol.* 128:376, 1982.
55. Graham J., et al.: The significance of distal urethral obstruction in little girls. *J. Urol.* 97:1045, 1967.
56. Griesbach W.A., Waterhouse R.K., Mellins H.Z.: Voiding cystourethrography in the diagnosis of posterior urethral valves. *Am. J. Roentgenol.* 82:521, 1959.
57. Harshman M.W., et al.: Urethral stricture disease in children. *J. Urol.* 126:650, 1981.
58. Hedenberg C., Ericsson N.O., Gierup J.: Urodynamic studies in boys with disorders of the lower urinary tract. Urethral strictures: A pre- and postoperative study. *Scan. J. Urol. Nephrol.* 11:111, 1977.
59. Hennelberry M.O., Stephens F.D.: Renal hypoplasia and dysplasia in infants with posterior urethral valves. *J. Urol.* 123:912, 1980.
60. Hennig K.R.: The history and physical examination in neurogenic bladder disease. *Urol. Clin. North Am.* 1:29, 1974.
61. Herrera A.J., et al.: The role of parental information in the incidence of circumcision. *Pediatrics* 70:597–612, 1982.
62. Hester T.R., Hill H.L., Jurkiewica M.J.: One-stage reconstruction of the penis. *Br. J. Plast. Surg.* 31:279, 1978.
63. Hollowel J.G., et al.: Embryologic considerations of diphallus and associated anomalies. *J. Urol.* 117:728, 1977.
64. Hoover D.L., Duckett J.W.: Posterior urethral valves, unilateral reflux and renal dysplasia: A syndrome. *J. Urol.* 128:994, 1982.
65. Huffman J.W.: Mesonephric remnants in the cervix. *Am. J. Obstet. Gynecol.* 56:23, 1948.
66. Immergut M.A., et al: Urethral caliber in normal female children. *J. Urol.* 97:693, 1967.
67. Immergut M.A., Wahman G.E.: The urethral caliber of female children with recurrent urinary tract infections. *J. Urol.* 99:189, 1968.
68. Immergut M.A., et al.: Cutaneous pyelostomy. *J. Urol.* 101:276, 1969.
69. Johnson D.M.: Diverticula and cyst of female urethra. *J. Urol.* 39:506, 1938.
70. Johnston J.H.: Temporary cutaneous ureterostomy in the management of advanced congenital urinary obstruction. *Arch. Dis. Child.* 38:161, 1963.
71. Johnston J.H., Kulatilake A.E.: The sequelae of posterior urethral valves. *Br. J. Urol.* 43:743, 1971.
72. Johnston J.H.: The genital aspects of exstrophy. *J. Urol.* 113:701, 1975.
73. Johnston J.H.: Phimosis, in *Surgical Pediatric Urology.* Philadelphia, W.B. Saunders Co., 1977, p. 414.
74. Johnston J.H.: Other penile abnormalities, in *Surgical Pediatric Urology.* Philadelphia, W.B. Saunders Co., 1977, p. 413.
75. Johnston J.H.: Vesicoureteric reflux with urethral valves. *Br. J. Urol.* 51:100, 1979.
76. Kaplan G.W., Sammons T.A., King L.R.: A blind comparison of dilatation, urethrotomy and medication alone in the treatment of urinary tract infections in girls. *J. Urol.* 109:917, 1973.
77. Kaplan G.W., Brock W.A.: Urethral strictures in children. *J. Urol.* 129:1200, 1983.
78. Kearney J.P., Lebowitz R.L., Retik A.B.: Obstructive polyps of the posterior urethra in boys: Embryology and management. *J. Urol.* 122:802, 1979.
79. Kernaban D.A.: Congenital abnormalities of the scrotum, in Horton C.E. (ed.): *Plastic and Reconstructive Surgery of the Genital Area.* Boston, Little, Brown & Co., 1973, pp. 175–181.
80. King L.R.: Abnormalities of the urethra, in Ravitch M.M., et al. (eds.): *Pediatric Surgery*, ed. 3. Chicago, Year Book Medical Publishers, 1979, p. 1349.
81. King L.R.: Neonatal circumcision. *Dialogues Ped. Urol.* 5:12, 1982.
82. King L.R.: Neonatal circumcision. *Dialogues Ped. Urol.* 5:6, 1982.
83. Kirks D.R., Grossman H.: Congenital saccular anterior urethral diverticula. *Radiology* 140:367, 1981.
84. Klaus H., Stein R.T.: Urethral prolapse in young girls. *Pediatrics* 52:645, 1973.
85. Kroovand R.L.: Fetal intervention for obstructive uropathy. *Dialogues Ped. Urol.* 5:7, 1982.
86. Krueger R.P., Hardy B.E., Churchill B.M.: Growth in boys with posterior urethral valves. *Urol. Clin. North Am.* 7:265, 1980.
87. Law J.T., Ong G.B.: Congenital diverticulum of the anterior urethra. *Aust. N.Z. J. Surg.* 51:305, 1981.
88. Lebowitz R.L.: *Postoperative Pediatric Uroradiology.* New York, Appleton-Century-Crofts, 1981, pp. 43–58.
89. Lewis E.L., Palmer J.M.: Anterior urethral valves. *Urology* 18:494, 1981.
90. Lindner A., et al.: Scaphoid megalourethra: A report of two cases. *Br. J. Urol.* 52:143, 1980.
91. Lyon R.P., Tanagho E.A.: Distal urethral stenosis in little girls. *J. Urol.* 93:379, 1965.
92. Maizels M., et al.: Cowper's syringocele: A classification of dilatations of Cowper's gland duct based upon clinical characteristics of 8 boys. *J. Urol.* 129:111, 1983.
93. Mandell J., et al.: Occult spinal dysraphism: A rare but detectable cause of voiding dysfunction. *Urol. Clin. North Am.* 7:349, 1980.
94. Mitchell M.E., Garrett R.A.: Perirenal urinary extravasation associated with urethral valves in infants. *J. Urol.* 124:688, 1980.
95. Mitchell M.: Persistent ureteral dilatation following valve resection. *Dialogues Ped. Urol.* 5:8, 1982.
96. Mohan V., et al.: Urethral diverticulum in male subjects: Report of 5 cases. *J. Urol.* 123:592, 1980.
97. Morton H.G.: Meatus size in 1000 circumcised boys from two weeks to sixteen years of age. *J. Fla. Med. Assoc.* 50:137, 1963.
98. Moyan R.J., Williams D.I., Pryor J.P.: Müllerian duct remnants in the male. *Br. J. Urol.* 51:488, 1979.
99. Naparstek S., et al.: Complete duplication of male urethra in children. *Urology* 16:391, 1980.
100. Nesbitt T.E.: Congenital megalourethra. *J. Urol.* 73:839, 1955.
101. Noe H.N., Dale G.A.: Evaluation of children with meatal stenosis. *J. Urol.* 114:455, 1975.
102. Noe H.N.: Endoscopic management of urethral strictures in children. *J. Urol.* 125:712, 1981.
103. Olsson C.A., Krane R.J.: The controversy of simple vs. multistaged urethroplasty. *J. Urol.* 120:414, 1978.
104. Ono Y., et al.: Anterior urethral valve. *Urology* 20:538, 1982.
105. Ortlip S.A., Gonzales R., Williams R.D.: Diverticula of the male urethra. *J. Urol.* 114:350, 1980.
106. Parkash S., Rao B.R.: Preputial stenosis: Its site and correction. *Plast. Reconstr. Surg.* 66:281, 1980.
107. Rabinowitz R.T., et al.: Upper tract management when posterior urethral valve ablation is insufficient. *J. Urol.* 122:370, 1979.
108. Schmeller N.T., Scherrmer H.K.: Trifurcation of the urethra: A case report. *J. Urol.* 127:545, 1982.
109. Scott L.E.: YV meatoplasty for hypospadias repair. *Urol. Clin. North Am.* 8:581, 1981.
110. Selzer I., Nelson H.M.: Benign papilloma (polypoid tumor) of the cervix uteri in children: Report of 2 cases. *Am. J. Obstet. Gynecol.* 84:165–169, 1962.
111. Shepard J.H., Wilson C.S., Sallade R.L.: Webbed penis. *Plast. Reconstr. Surg.* 66:453, 1980.
112. Shrom S.H., Cromie W.J., Duckett J.W.: Megalourethra. *Urology* 17:152, 1981.
113. Smey P., King L.R., Firlit C.T.: Dysfunctional voiding in children secondary to internal sphincter dyssynergia: Treatment with phenoxybenzamine. *Urol. Clin. North Am.* 7:337, 1980.
114. Sommer J.T., Stevens F.D.: Dorsal urethral diverticulum of the fossa navicularis: Symptoms, diagnosis and treatment. *J. Urol.* 124:94, 1980.
115. Stephens F.D.: *Congenital Malformations of the Rectum, Anus, and Genitourinary Tract.* London, Churchill-Livingstone, 1963, p. 226.
116. Tanagho E.A.: Persistent ureteral dilatation following valve resection. *Dialogues Ped. Urol.* 5:4, 1982.
117. Waterhouse K.: The surgical repair of membranous urethral strictures in children. *Birth Defects* 13:227, 1977.
118. Westenfelder M.: Diphallus and bladder exstrophy: A case report. *Monogr. Pediatr.* 12:50, 1981.
119. Whitaker R.H., Keeton J.E., Williams D.I.: Posterior urethral valves: A study of urinary control after operation. *J. Urol.* 108:167, 1972.
120. Williams D.I., Retik A.B.: Congenital valves: Diverticula of the anterior urethra. *Br. J. Urol.* 41:228, 1969.
121. Williams D.I., Kenawi M.M.: Urethral duplication in the male. *Eur. Urol.* 1:209, 1975.
122. Williams D.I., Cromie W.J.: Ring ureterostomy. *Br. J. Urol.* 47:789, 1976.
123. Williams D.I., Bloomberg S.: Bifid urethra with preanal accessory tract (Y duplication). *Br. J. Urol.* 47:877, 1976.
124. Williams D.I.: Urethral valves: 100 cases with hydronephrosis. *Birth Defects* 13:55, 1977.

125. Williams D.I.: Male urethral obstructions, in Williams D.I., Johnston J.H. (eds.): *Pediatric Urology*, ed. 2. London, Butterworth & Co., 1982 pp. 259–262.
126. Williams D.J., Cromie J.W.: Ring ureterostomy. *Br. J. Urol.* 47:787, 1976.
127. Wirtshafter A., et al.: Complete trifurcation of the urethra. *J. Urol.* 123:431, 1980.
128. Young B.W., Niebel J.D.: Vesicourethroplasty for congenital vesical neck obstruction in children. *J. Urol.* 79:838, 1958.

134 ROBERT M. FILLER

Testicular Tumors

TESTICULAR TUMORS are the seventh most common pediatric neoplasm and represent approximately 1% of the malignant neoplasms in children.[21] Two to five percent of all testicular tumors occur in children,[23] and most of the children affected are under 3 years of age at presentation.[4, 6]

Types of Tumors

Approximately 75% of testicular tumors seen in childhood are of germinal origin and most of these are malignant. The most common type is endodermal sinus tumor (yolk sac tumor). Other names that have been applied to this tumor include: clear cell adenocarcinoma, orchioblastoma, infantile embryonal carcinoma, and embryonal adenocarcinoma. Before endodermal sinus tumor was recognized as a distinct entity, this tumor was classified as "embryonal carcinoma." As a result, the older literature may be unreliable and confusing because the diagnosis of "embryonal carcinoma" also included germ cell tumors that occur in adults. Although the adult and childhood variants both arise from totipotential germ cells, more recent evidence indicates that the endodermal sinus tumor is derived from extra embryonic tissues of the yolk sac, whereas the embryonal carcinoma seen in the adult arises from embryonal cells in the testis. This distinction is important because the patterns of incidence and behavior of the adult and childhood variants are different. Theories of the histogenesis of germ cell tumors have been discussed by Mostofi.[13]

The relative frequency of the different types of childhood testicular tumors seen over a 30-year period at the Hospital for Sick Children, Toronto, is shown in Table 134–1. A similar distribution has been noted in other reports.[6] Teratoma is the most common benign tumor. Seminomas are exceedingly rare in patients under 16 years of age. Rhabdomyosarcoma is the commonest sarcoma seen and usually originates from paratesticular tissues.

Clinical Features and Initial Diagnostic Steps

Most boys with a testicular tumor present with a painless mass that has been present for one to several months. Most children affected are less than 6 years of age; those with endodermal sinus tumors are usually under age 3; those with paratesticular sarcoma are several years older. Testicular tumors occur rarely in adolescents. Physical examination usually reveals a hard, painless testicular mass 2 or more cm in diameter, not involving the scrotal wall or spermatic cord. Transillumination may be misleading because translucency may be noted with cystic teratomas and in endodermal sinus tumor or other solid masses when hydrocele is associated with the tumor. Initial physical examination should assess the possibility of distant spread, particularly to lymph nodes in the inguinal and supraclavicular regions and retroperitoneum. The scrotum should be carefully examined for evidence of direct extension to the scrotal skin and to determine if the mass is in the testis or is paratesticular.

After a suspicious mass is discovered, the next step is to establish the exact histologic diagnosis. Needle biopsy or biopsy from a scrotal incision for diagnosis is contraindicated because, if a neoplasm is present, seeding of the scrotum is likely. If a testicular tumor is suspected, an inguinal incision should be made. At operation, the spermatic cord is exposed and occluded at the internal abdominal ring with a noncrushing vascular clamp before manipulation of the testis. If a gross diagnosis of neoplasm can be made when the testis is delivered into the wound, radical orchiectomy is performed by ligating and dividing the spermatic cord at the internal ring and removing the mass with the entire cord. If the testicular mass is obviously benign (e.g., hydrocele), appropriate treatment is provided and the testis is returned to the scrotum. When the diagnosis is uncertain, the testis is walled off with sponges and an incisional biopsy is performed. The frozen-section diagnosis determines further treatment. It is unnecessary to excise a portion of the scrotum unless the tumor has been previously biopsied in situ or the extragonadal tissues are grossly involved. If retroperitoneal lymph node dissection is contemplated, placement of a nonabsorbable suture on the ligated spermatic cord aids in defining the distal end of the inguinal dissection during lymphadenectomy.

When a biopsy of a testicular malignancy has been done previously through the scrotum and/or the lesion treated by less than radical inguinal orchiectomy, immediate and aggressive

TABLE 134–1.—30-YEAR EXPERIENCE
WITH TESTICULAR TUMORS, HOSPITAL FOR
SICK CHILDREN, TORONTO

TUMORS	NO. OF PATIENTS
Tumors of Germinal Origin	
Endodermal sinus tumor	26
Teratocarcinoma	3
Choriocarcinoma	1
Teratoma	11
Tumors of Nongerminal Origin	
Sarcomas	8
Interstitial cell tumor	1
Sertoli cell tumor	1

steps should be taken to remove the potentially contaminated field. This should include wide local excision of the scrotal wound, the scrotal contents, and the cord structures, to the internal ring.

Staging of the Neoplasm

After completing radical orchiectomy, it is important to assess the extent of the disease (staging) before deciding on the need for further therapy.

A variety of staging systems are used. Most are modifications of the system proposed by Boden and Gibb.[1]

Stage I (A)
Tumor confined to the scrotum
No evidence of tumor in retroperitoneum or chest by standard and special diagnostic tests
No nodes positive on retroperitoneal lymph node dissection
Stage II (B)
Tumor metastases below the diaphragm
No evidence of tumor in chest or mediastinum
Stage III (C)
Metastases above the diaphragm

In the evaluation of reports from different centers, the distinction between clinical staging (evaluation by all diagnostic techniques except retroperitoneal node dissection) and pathologic staging must be recognized. Retroperitoneal node involvement by endodermal sinus tumor is not common. Therefore, pathologic stage and clinical stage are nearly always the same in boys with this neoplasm.

Since testicular neoplasms spread both hematogenously and via lymphatics, the imaging techniques used for clinical staging are aimed at detecting tumor in the retroperitoneal lymph nodes and lungs.

Although standard chest radiographs show most lung metastases, we employ computer tomography of the lungs for staging, since it can reveal much smaller lesions. Since lymphangiography is technically difficult in children under 3 years of age (the usual age of occurrence of most testicular tumors), ultrasonography and/or computed tomography (CT) are used to evaluate the retroperitoneal lymph nodes.

Most germ cell tumors of the testis produce α-fetoprotein (AFP) and/or the beta subunit of human chorionic gonadotropin (HCG). As a result, tumor can be detected by measuring these markers in the serum. Levels of HCG and AFP are used to improve the accuracy of clinical staging of patients after the primary tumor has been excised.[9] For example, persistently elevated serum markers after orchiectomy indicate stage II or stage III disease; and elevated markers after retroperitoneal lymphadenectomy indicate stage III disease. Similarly, in patients with AFP- or HCG-secreting tumors, serial measurement of these markers in the serum can be used to detect recurrent disease and to evaluate response to treatment.

AFP, the most useful marker in childhood testicular tumors, has been found in abnormal amounts in approximately 90% of patients of all ages with nonseminomatous testicular tumors.[9] AFP is produced in the normal fetus by cells in the liver, yolk sac, and gastrointestinal tract. After birth it can be produced by germ cell tumors, regenerating liver, and hepatocellular carcinoma. The normal serum level of AFP in the fetus is about 3 mg/dl. The concentration of AFP drops to below 20 ng/ml by 1 year of age. It has a half-life of 5 days so that 25 days (5 half-lives) after operation, an elevated level of AFP should return to normal if no tumor is present.

TABLE 134–2.—ENDODERMAL SINUS TUMOR OF TESTIS*

SERIES	NO. OF PATIENTS HAVING LYMPHADENECTOMY	NO. OF PATIENTS WITH POSITIVE NODES
HSC	8	0
Hopkins[6]	11	0
Young[23]	8	0
Quintana[16]	5	0
Kaplan[10]	10	4
Gangai[5]	11	0
Totals	53	4 (7.4%)

*Results of lymphadenectomy in children with clinical stage I disease.

HCG is produced by syncytiotrophoblastic giant cells of the placenta and choriocarcinoma. The presence of giant cells scattered among neoplastic cells in other germ cell tumors explains the HCG elevations in these cases. HCG has a half-life of only 24 hours so that in 5 days, an elevated level should drop to normal if all tumor has been removed. Since HCG is produced by only a small fraction of endodermal sinus tumors, it has limited usefulness as a marker in testicular tumors of childhood.

Retroperitoneal node dissection has been recommended for accurate pathologic staging of testicular tumors. For example, in a series of adults with clinical stage I embryonal carcinoma, Whitmore[22] found that 53% were proved by retroperitoneal lymphadenectomy to have stage II disease. For endodermal sinus tumor, the results of node dissection have been quite different. In the experience of six centers[5, 6, 10, 16, 23] (Table 134–2) positive nodes were found in only four of 53 node dissections in clinical stage I patients, and all four positive dissections were reported from the same institution.[10] Therefore, on the basis of current data, retroperitoneal node dissection for staging purposes appears useful only for children with suspected retroperitoneal node involvement on ultrasound or CT scan, and for those without lung metastases in whom AFP or HCG remains elevated after orchiectomy.

Management of Endodermal Sinus Tumor

After radical orchiectomy and clinical staging are completed, further therapy may include retroperitoneal node dissection, chemotherapy, and irradiation. Approximately 80% of the children will have stage I disease and 20% stage II or III.

Retroperitoneal Node Dissection

The value of node dissection in the treatment of endodermal sinus tumor is not clear. Since most node dissections have been negative, one would expect that radical orchiectomy would cure as many patients with stage I disease as orchiectomy plus retroperitoneal node dissection. Data from this institution and others[6, 10, 23] suggest that this is indeed the case for children under 36 months of age with a diagnosis of "embryonal carcinoma" or endodermal sinus tumor (Table 134–3). Older data compiled by Sabio[18] indicate that, for children of all ages with stage I "embryonal carcinoma," the cure rate after orchiectomy and node dissection is nearly twice that after orchiectomy alone (84% vs. 48%). These discrepancies may be due in part to: inclusion in the older studies of patients over 36 months of age, some of whom may not have had endodermal sinus tumor; more accurate staging in recent years; less radical orchiectomy in the past. Data from studies like that of Hopkins,[6] which reports that five of nine

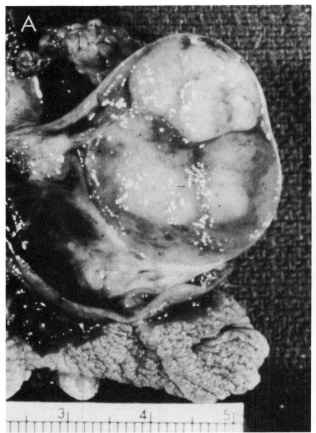

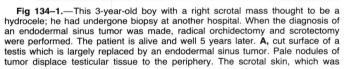

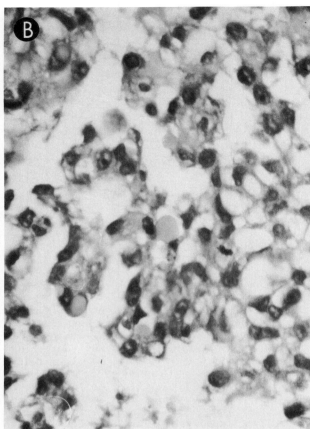

Fig 134–1.—This 3-year-old boy with a right scrotal mass thought to be a hydrocele; he had undergone biopsy at another hospital. When the diagnosis of an endodermal sinus tumor was made, radical orchidectomy and scrotectomy were performed. The patient is alive and well 5 years later. **A,** cut surface of a testis which is largely replaced by an endodermal sinus tumor. Pale nodules of tumor displace testicular tissue to the periphery. The scrotal skin, which was excised in continuity, is at the bottom of the specimen. **B,** endodermal sinus tumor made up of papillary formations of pleomorphic epithelial cells which have clear cytoplasmic vacuoles and rounded homogeneous cytoplasmic inclusions of protein that can be identified as alpha-fetoprotein. (Hematoxylin and eosin stain; ×740.)

boys developed metastases when the testicular tumor was treated by scrotal but not radical orchiectomy, suggest that the extent of orchiectomy may be the major factor responsible for these differences. Furthermore, since the older reports did not accurately describe sites of recurrence in those who relapsed, it is difficult to determine if node dissection would indeed have prevented them. On the basis of current data, we do not perform

TABLE 134–3.—ENDODERMAL SINUS TUMOR*

	ORCHIECTOMY		ORCHIECTOMY AND NODE DISSECTION	
Series	No. of Patients	1-yr Disease-Free Survivors	No. of Patients	1-yr Disease-Free Survivors
HSC	15†	15†	8	7
Hopkins[6]	5	4	9‡	9‡
Kaplan[10]	0	0	8§	6‖
Young[23]	6	5	8	6
Totals	26	24 (92%)	33	28 (85%)

*Results of radical orchiectomy and radical orchiectomy plus node dissection for stage I disease in patients under 36 months of age.
†2 patients had chemotherapy.
‡9 patients had chemotherapy.
§6 patients had chemotherapy.
‖4 patients had chemotherapy.

retroperitoneal lymphadenectomy for stage I disease, although some centers disagree[10] (Fig 134–1).

When retroperitoneal lymph nodes are the site of metastatic disease (stage II disease) lymphadenectomy appears to increase survival. Kaplan and Firlit[10] salvaged three of four boys with stage II endodermal sinus tumor with radical orchiectomy, retroperitoneal lymphadenectomy, and chemotherapy. McCullough's cumulative review[14] included two boys with positive nodes who were long-term survivors after orchiectomy and node dissection.

Considerable controversy surrounds the advantage of bilateral over unilateral lymphadenectomy. The classic work of Jamieson and Dobson[8] demonstrating cross-communications between the lymphatic channels of the testes has given support to the need for bilateral retroperitoneal node dissection. However, in an extensive review of 283 postlymphadenectomy surgical specimens in patients with testicular tumors, Ray[17] found only one patient with negative ipsilateral nodes and positive contralateral nodes. Skinner[19] found positive contralateral nodes in only two of 59 patients with negative ipsilateral nodes, and one of these patients had a contralateral primary tumor. Similarly, Maier[11] and his associates were unable to demonstrate improved survival figures when the results of unilateral and bilateral adenectomies were compared in 213 patients with germ cell neoplasms. On the basis of these data and our own experience in children, unilateral dissection is recommended if lymphadenectomy is undertaken and no gross tumor is discovered. When ipsilateral nodes are grossly positive, bilateral adenectomy is advisable. A modified node dissection on the contralateral side, as described by Whitmore,[22] minimizes the possibility of retrograde ejaculation, a disturbing complication of bilateral adenectomy in which both second lumbar sympathetic ganglia are excised. Although some reports raise doubts about the safety of this procedure in small children, our experience and that of others indicate that retroperitoneal node dissection is well tolerated by children. A simple midline, paramedian, or transverse abdominal incision gives adequate exposure and we have not found it necessary to enter the chest. Only rare complications have been noted, and these have not been serious.

Radiation Therapy

The indication for prophylactic irradiation of the retroperitoneum in clinical stage I disease is open to debate. Matsumoto et al.[12] reported that 19 boys with stage I disease treated by orchiectomy and retroperitoneal irradiation (2,000–3,000 rad in 4–7 weeks) were alive and well 1–5 years later. This compared with a survival rate of five of nine boys treated by orchiectomy alone, a rate similar to that noted in the older literature.[18] However, as already noted, our data and that of others (see Table 134–3) indicate that survival rate in stage I endodermal sinus tumor treated only by radical orchiectomy is greater than 90%, far greater than previously thought. Because of this low rate of relapse, and the effects of radiation on growth and the production of second neoplasms, retroperitoneal irradiation is not recommended for stage I disease.

The place of radiation therapy for stages II and III has not been completely settled. Reports of Tefft,[20] Hopkins,[6] and others[18] indicate that irradiation, usually in conjunction with chemotherapy, can lead to lasting survival in patients with nodal and pulmonary metastases. However, no controlled studies are available to indicate whether lymphadenectomy, radiation therapy, or a combination of both, is best for children with endodermal sinus tumor with retroperitoneal nodal metastases. At present, we favor not irradiating the retroperitoneum in those in whom all gross retroperitoneal disease has been removed surgically. For those with pulmonary metastases, irradiation of the lungs (with chemotherapy) appears indicated.

Chemotherapy

Chemotherapeutic agents that have been used with apparent beneficial effect include dactinomycin, vincristine, cyclophosphamide,[6, 10, 18] and, more recently, Adriamycin.[3] Often, these agents have been used in conjunction with radiation so that the individual effect of chemotherapy and irradiation on the growing metastasis is uncertain. However, most oncologists recognize the importance of chemotherapy and radiation for the treatment of those who present with stage II and III disease and for those who develop metastases later. Tefft et al.[20] salvaged two children with pulmonary metastases with whole lung irradiation and dactinomycin. Other survivors with metastatic disease treated with chemotherapy have been reported by Sabio,[18] Young,[23] and Kaplan.[10]

The value of chemotherapy in stage I disease has not been established. However, since fatal pulmonary metastases occur in about 10% of boys with stage I disease, adjunctive chemotherapy may have some validity. In the report of Kaplan and Firlit,[10] the majority of children with stage I disease were given chemotherapy. Similarly, Hopkins et al.[6] recommended chemotherapy (as well as irradiation and operation) for all patients regardless of stage. In children with stage I disease, our current recommen-

TABLE 134–4.—ENDODERMAL SINUS TUMOR: RECOMMENDATIONS FOR TREATMENT, BY STAGE OF DISEASE

STAGE	TREATMENT
Clinical stage I	Follow-up only
Clinical stage I— histologic evidence of vascular invasion	Adjuvant chemotherapy
Apparent clinical stage I and elevated AFP	Retroperitoneal lymphadenectomy, chemotherapy
Clinical Stages II and III	Retroperitoneal lymphadenectomy when nodes involved, chemotherapy, radiation for pulmonary metastases

dation is to reserve chemotherapy for those in whom there is histologic evidence of vascular invasion. In our series, two stage I patients with vascular invasion were given vincristine, 0.05 mg/kg; dactinomycin, 30 mcg/kg; cyclophosphamide, 20 mg/kg; and Adriamycin, 1.3 mg/kg (total dose 14 mg/kg) every 3 weeks for 18 months. Both are long-term survivors. This protocol was similar to the T2 program described by Exelby.[3] More recent experience with this regimen for germ cell tumors at other sites and in older patients suggests that it may not be effective in eradicating bulk disease. A more aggressive drug protocol in use for other germ cell neoplasms at this institution and others[3] is under trial in children with stage II and III endodermal sinus tumors. The drugs employed include vinblastine, cisplatin, bleomycin, dactinomycin, and cyclophosphamide.

A summary of the recommendations for the treatment of different stages of endodermal sinus tumor of the testis in childhood is given in Table 134–4.

Management of Other Testicular Tumors

Teratoma

Almost all teratomas of the testis are benign. Most boys affected are under 3 years of age. Houser et al.[7] collected 30 cases from the literature, and in our series an additional 11 cases were noted (see Table 134–1). Radical orchiectomy has been curative in all cases.

Sarcoma of the Distal Spermatic Cord

Of the paratesticular sarcomas, embryonal rhabdomyosarcoma is the most common variant[19] and was noted in five of seven sarcomas in Hopkins' series[6] and in six of eight in our experience. These tumors metastasize early to regional lymph glands and lungs. Although cures have been reported with orchiectomy alone, the best results have been obtained with orchiectomy, pelvic and retroperitoneal node dissection, and radiotherapy,[3, 4, 6, 20] even for stage I disease. Radiation therapy of 3,500–4,000 rad should be given to areas of gross or microscopic disease after lymphadenectomy. Chemotherapy protocols that have been effective are identical to those used for rhabdomyosarcoma at other sites. They include combinations of vincristine, dactinomycin, and cyclophosphamide. A chemotherapy program that has been used in patients with large nonresectable rhabdomyosarcomas is recommended by Exelby.[3] With multimodality therapy, the cure rate for these tumors is approximately 75%.[3, 6]

Gonadal Stromal Tumors

Tumors of gonadal stroma occur rarely, and none were seen in our series. In 1965, Houser[7] reviewed 21 cases that could be found reported in the literature. All but four occurred in the first year of life, and none were considered malignant. Orchiectomy should be curative.

Interstitial Cell Tumors

The treatment of choice is orchiectomy. Houser[7] collected over 40 cases, all of which appeared benign although Dalgaard[2] reported a case with metastases. These tumors cause a rise in blood and urinary 17-ketosteroid levels, which should fall to normal when the tumor is completely excised.

Teratocarcinoma and Choriocarcinoma

These malignant tumors are very rare in children and are usually seen in the older teenager. Often, they occur in association with embryonal carcinoma or teratoma of the testis. Management of these tumors should be identical to the management of adult germ cell testis cancers. Stage I tumors are treated by radical orchiectomy, followed by retroperitoneal lymph node dissection for staging, as described by Whitmore.[22] Pathologic stage I tumors receive no further therapy. For stage II and stage III tumors, chemotherapy and radiation therapy are utilized. The various radiation and chemotherapy protocols have been thoroughly reviewed by Paulson et al.[15]

REFERENCES

1. Boden G., Gibb R.: Radiotherapy and testicular neoplasms. *Lancet* 2:1195–1197, 1951.
2. Dalgaard J.B., Hesselberg F.: Interstitial cell tumors of the testis: Two cases and survey. *Acta Pathol. Microbiol. Scand.* 41:219, 1957.
3. Exelby P.R.: Testicular cancer in children. *Cancer* 45:1803–1809, 1980.
4. Filler R.M., Hardy B.E.: Testicular tumors in children. *World J. Surg.* 4:63–70, 1980.
5. Gangai M.P.: Testicular neoplasms in an infant. *Cancer* 22:658–662, 1968.
6. Hopkins T.B., Jaffe N., Colodny A., et al.: The management of testicular tumors in children. *J. Urol.* 120:96–102, 1978.
7. Houser R., Izant R.J., Persky L.: Testicular tumors in children. *Am. J. Surg.* 110:876–892, 1965.
8. Jamieson J.K., Dobson J.F.: The lymphatics of the testicle. *Lancet* 1:493, 1910.
9. Javadpour N.: The role of biologic tumor markers in testicular cancer. *Cancer* 45:1755–1761, 1980.
10. Kaplan W.E., Firlit C.F.: Treatment of testicular yolk sac carcinoma in the young child. *J. Urol.* 126:663–664, 1981.
11. Maier J.G., VanBuskirk K.E., Sulak M.H., et al.: An evaluation of lymphadenectomy in the treatment of malignant testicular germ cell neoplasms. *J. Urol.* 104:778–780, 1970.
12. Matsumoto K., Nakauchi K., Fujita K.: Radiation therapy for the embryonal carcinoma of testis in childhood. *J. Urol.* 104:778–780, 1970.
13. Mostofi F.K.: Pathology of germ cell tumors to testis. *Cancer* 45:1735–1754, 1980.
14. McCullough D.L., Carlton C.E., Seybold H.M.: Testicular tumors in infants and children: Report of 5 cases and evaluation of different modes of therapy. *J. Urol.* 105:140–148, 1971.
15. Paulson D.F., Einhorn L., Peckham M., et al.: Cancer of the testis, chapter 24 in DeVito V.T. Jr., Hellman S., Rosenberg S.A. (eds.): *Cancer.* Philadelphia, J.B. Lippincott Co., 1982, pp. 786–822.
16. Quintana J., Beresi V., Latorre J.J., et al.: Infantile embryonal carcinoma of testis. *J. Urol.* 128:785–787, 1982.
17. Ray B., Hajdu S.I., Whitmore W.F. Jr.: Distribution of retroperitoneal lymph node metastases in testicular germinal tumors. *Cancer* 33:340, 1974.
18. Sabio H., Burgert E.O. Jr., Farrow G.M., et al.: Embryonal carcinoma of the testis in childhood. *Cancer* 34:2118–2121, 1974.
19. Skinner D.G., Leadbetter W.F.: The surgical management of testis tumor. *J. Urol.* 106:84, 1971.
20. Tefft M., Vawter G.F., Mitus A.: Radiotherapeutic management of testicular neoplasms in children. *Radiology* 88:457–465, 1967.
21. The Third National Cancer Study. Advanced 3 Year Report, 1969–1971 Incidence. DHEW Publication No. (NIH) 74–637.
22. Whitmore W.F. Jr.: Cancer management: The treatment of germinal tumors of the testis. A special graduate course on cancer sponsored by the American Cancer Society, Inc. Philadelphia, J.B. Lippincott Co., September 1966, pp. 347–355.
23. Young P.G., Balfour M., Foote F.W. Jr., et al.: Embryonal adenocarcinoma in the prepubertal testis: A clinicopathologic study of 18 cases. *Cancer* 26:1970.

135 L. L. Leape
Torsion of the Testis

History.—Torsion of the testis was first described in 1840 by Delasiauve.[6] Taylor[33] first reported the condition in the newborn in 1897, and Colt[5] first reported torsion of the testicular appendage in 1922. That lesion was probably first reported in 1913 by Ombrédanne,[22] although he failed to recognize its true nature.

Pathogenesis and Definitions

Twisting of the testis results in occlusion of the blood supply, which if unrelieved, results in necrosis of the organ. Under normal circumstances, posterior fixation of the epididymis, its close apposition to the testis, and incomplete investment by the tunica vaginalis ensure both mobility and relative stability of the testis. If the tunica vaginalis has a high investment on the spermatic cord (the so-called bell-clapper deformity), the testis is not fixed, and *intravaginal* torsion may occur (Fig 135–1A). This is the most common form of testicular torsion. Torsion may also occur

between the epididymis and the testis if the two are separated by an elongated mesorchium (Fig 135–1,C). The testes in the newborn, and undescended testes, are not fixed in the scrotum, and the entire cord may twist—*extravaginal* torsion (Fig 135–1,B). The term *torsion of the spermatic cord* is used by some to refer to testicular torsion.

After the newborn period, testicular torsion is almost always associated with the bell-clapper abnormality of fixation. Trauma to the scrotum may cause the testicle to twist, and testicular torsion is a far more common cause of persistent testicular pain after injury than is testicular contusion or hematoma. Ambient temperature may be relevant. In one study, it was observed that 40 of 46 patients developed torsion when the temperature was less than 2 C.[30] This observation, plus the well-known phenomenon of spontaneous reduction of torsion with the administration of anesthesia, suggest that contraction of the cremaster muscle or

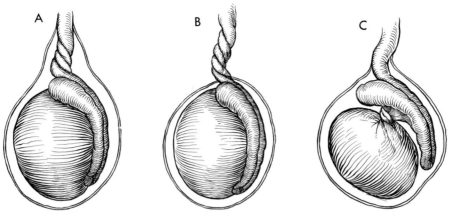

Fig 135–1.—Torsion of the testis. **A,** torsion below the attachment of the tunica vaginalis (intravaginal). **B,** torsion above the attachment (extravaginal). **C,** torsion between the epididymis and the testis.

the dartos may play a significant role in initiating or perpetuating torsion.

The preponderant occurrence of torsion at puberty points to a relation to the sexual response cycle. Longo[15] has suggested that increased testosterone levels and the elevation and rotation of the testes during the nocturnal sex response cycle initiates the rotation. Testicular torsion is commonly discovered upon awakening in the morning. The left testicle is affected twice as often as the right, perhaps related to the fact that the left cord is normally longer. Although neonatal torsion is presumably due to a different mechanism, since it is extravaginal, it is of interest that testosterone levels are higher at this time than at any other time during childhood until puberty. Antenatal torsion has been proposed as a cause of the absent testis when a "blind vas" is found at exploration in a patient with cryptorchidism.[8] Contralateral orchiopexy has been recommended in these patients because of a high incidence of bell-clapper deformity on the contralateral side.

Minor degrees of torsion tend to produce venous occlusion, which leads to testicular edema and pain. With more complete and prolonged occlusion, venous thrombosis, and later arterial thrombosis occur, leading to testicular infarction. Damage to the testis varies with the degree of torsion, its tightness, and duration. Sonda and Lapides[32] demonstrated experimentally in dogs that four complete turns (1,440 degrees) of the spermatic cord produced irreversible changes within 2 hours, whereas one turn (360 degrees) produced no changes up to 12 hours. In man, clinical evidence suggests much greater variability, and some patients have intermittent and self-resolving torsion, while others have early complete vascular occlusion. However, few testes have survived 24 hours of symptomatic torsion (see Fig 135–4) and a necrotic testis has been found at exploration as early as two hours after the onset of symptoms.[12]

The appendix testis, described by Morgagni in 1761,[17] also known as the hydatid, is embryologically a remnant of the upper end of the müllerian (paramesonephric) duct. It is present in about 90% of males, and varies in size from 1 to 10 mm in diameter. It is the most frequently (90%) twisted of the four testicular appendages. The others are the appendix epididymidis (vestige of the wölffian tubercle), the paradidymis of Waldeyer, and the vas aberrans (Fig 135–2). These vestigial structures are histologically similar, composed of gelatinous vascular connective tissue lined with columnar epithelium.[19] The appendix testis is usually pedunculated, perhaps accounting for its greater frequency of torsion.

Clinical Findings

Torsion of the testis is not rare, occurring in 1 in 160 males by the age of 65.[10] It may occur at any age from the first day of life and has been reported in a patient of 68 years. Two thirds of patients are adolescents,[37] and the peak incidence is at 14 years. A second peak is in the newborn period.

Pain in the testis is the first symptom in 80% of patients.[14] The pain is usually gradual in onset and increases in severity. Less commonly, its onset is sudden and may be dramatic. About 20% of patients have a history of trauma, but in most there is no apparent antecedent cause. Over a third of patients have had prior episodes of transient testicular pain,[3] probably due to self-reducing episodes of torsion. The severity of pain varies and is not clearly related to the extent or the duration of the torsion. In a small percentage of patients, the pain originates in the right lower quadrant rather than in the testis. Swelling of the scrotum gradually develops, followed by erythema and edema. Nausea, anorexia, and vomiting may occur. A low-grade fever is occasionally seen.

Physical examination typically shows a swollen hemiscrotum with local edema and erythema. After 24 hours, reddish-dark discoloration of the scrotum may ensue and extend into the groin or to the other side. The testis is usually exquisitely tender. In

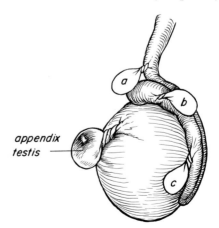

Fig 135–2.—Torsion of the appendages of the testis: *a,* torsion of the appendix of the cord (organ of Giraldés); *b,* torsion of the appendix of the epididymis; *c,* torsion of the appendix of the vas (vas aberrans of Haller). The commonest type involves the appendix testis (hydatid of Morgagni).

early cases, a "transverse lie" of the testis may be noted. There is considerable variability in clinical findings. Approximately 10% of patients have no pain; in some there is little erythema; others may demonstrate marked discoloration and exquisite tenderness. Torsion of the testis in the newborn infant is usually noted at birth and is asymptomatic. The scrotum is enlarged and red, a finding that is often passed off as from hemorrhage due to a traumatic delivery. The torsion usually occurs in utero so that the testis is already necrotic at birth, and torsion may be bilateral.[14] Rarely, torsion may develop after birth, in which case prompt treatment may result in testicular salvage.[7, 11]

Undescended testes are more likely to undergo torsion because they lack fixation. Delay in diagnosis is common, markedly reducing the testicular salvage rate. Typically, the patient has a hot, red, tender mass in the groin. The diagnosis of torsion of an undescended testis should be considered in any patient with lower quadrant pain and absence of an intrascrotal testis. Paraplegics are particularly susceptible to torsion of an ectopic interstitial undescended testis.[23] Torsion of an intra-abdominal testis may present at any age, either as an "acute abdomen" or as a palpable abdominal mass.[26]

Torsion of the appendix testis is a disease of young boys and is rarely seen after puberty. Pain is the typical symptom, but it is less striking than that seen with torsion of the testis, resulting in many cases in considerable delay in presentation to the physician. A few have severe pain. Scrotal swelling and erythema eventually develop but are typically less severe than with testicular torsion. Approximately 25% of patients have a history of trauma or vigorous activity.[31] If the patient is examined early, the "blue dot" sign may be noted, evidence of a necrotic appendix testis beneath the skin. An exquisitely tender, pea-sized nodule may be palpated separate from a nontender testis. If the patient is seen somewhat later, the tenderness and swelling are more diffuse and differentiation from testicular torsion may be impossible.

Diagnosis

Successful treatment of testicular torsion requires early diagnosis and prompt operation. Delay in diagnosis, all too common, results in loss of the testis. The patient may not initially recognize the seriousness of his symptoms, but more commonly it is the physician who errs. The most common error is the diagnosis of epididymitis or epididymo-orchitis. The age of the patient is the clue. Acute epididymitis is almost never seen in prepubertal males and is rare even in late adolescence. In epididymitis, pain develops gradually, accompanied by fever, urinary symptoms, and pyuria. Scrotal swelling, redness, and tenderness may be quite similar to that seen in testicular torsion (Fig 135–3). Because epididymitis is rare in childhood, any male under the age of 20 years with an acute scrotal swelling should be presumed to have testicular torsion until the diagnosis has been excluded.

Other causes of acute scrotal swelling to be considered in the differential diagnosis include strangulated hernia, acute hydrocele, torsion of a hernia sac within the scrotum, idiopathic scrotal edema (usually a bacterial cellulitis and bilateral),[21, 24] traumatic hematoma or hematocele, fat necrosis of the scrotum, acute varicocele, testicular tumor, Schönlein-Henoch purpura, leukemic infiltration of the scrotum, and scrotal abscess.

Radioisotope scans, using ^{99m}Tc pertechnetate and gamma-camera imaging, may be of great assistance in the diagnosis of testicular torsion.[20] Five to ten millicuries of the isotope are injected intravenously as a bolus, followed by serial images at 4-second intervals for 1 minute to record the angiographic phase, then at 5, 10, and 15 minutes for the tissue phase. Diminished blood flow and avascularity in the testis indicate torsion, whereas epididymo-orchitis typically shows increased vascularity. Since

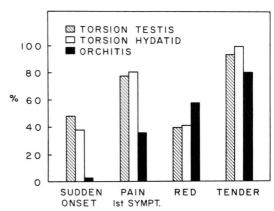

Fig 135–3.—Comparison of signs and symptoms in 120 children with orchitis, torsion of testis, and torsion of hydatid.

ischemic necrosis eventually results in inflammation in the scrotum, the scan is less accurate late in the course of the disease. Errors also occur in patients with partial or resolving torsion (who still require operation) and in young children, and those with small testes. Thus, results of the scan must be interpreted in the clinical context and correlated with the physical findings. Overall, a 95% level of accuracy has been reported.[10, 27]

A Doppler stethoscope has been recommended in the diagnosis of testicular torsion, since with it one can detect blood flow to the testis. Unfortunately, a high error rate (up to 30%) has rendered this modality unreliable, and it cannot be recommended.[28] Other imaging techniques, such as ultrasound and CT, have not proved of consistent value in differentiating testicular torsion from epididymo-orchitis.

Treatment

The treatment of torsion of the testis is immediate emergency scrotal exploration, detorsion, and bilateral fixation orchiopexy. Because of the difficulty of being certain that torsion is not present, the policy of urgent exploration of all patients with acute scrotal pain and swelling will result in the highest rate of success.[2] Since there is significant variation in the degree of torsion and in individual response to ischemia, operation should never be delayed for the purpose of obtaining laboratory tests, isotope scans, etc. The best results are obtained when the patient is operated on within 6 hours after the onset of symptoms, and there

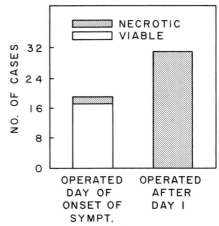

Fig 135–4.—Torsion of the testis: salvage versus necrosis with respect to delay in operation in 50 children.

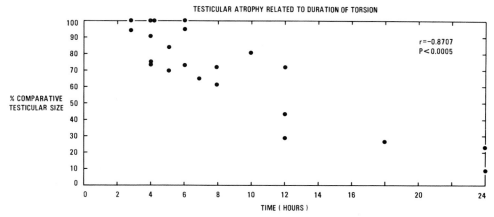

Fig 135–5.—The relationship of atrophy to duration of torsion. (From Thomas.[34] Used by permission.)

are few successes after 24 hours (Fig 135–4). Sometimes, with the aid of sedation, it is possible to reduce the torsion manually before operation, significantly reducing the testicular ischemia time.

The scrotal approach is recommended. It reveals the pathology directly, eliminates difficulties in delivering a swollen testis out of the scrotum into a groin incision, and is necessary in any case for the fixation orchiopexy that must be carried out. Once the tunica vaginalis is opened, the testis is untwisted and observed as necessary for return of normal color. If viability is in question, the testis should be covered with a warm, wet cloth and re-evaluated 20 minutes later, after fixation orchiopexy has been carried out on the opposite side (where a defect of fixation will almost always be found).

The purpose of the bilateral fixation orchiopexy is to prevent recurrent torsion. It is not sufficient merely to place a few sutures between the testis and the scrotal wall. A window of tunica vaginalis must be excised to permit apposition of a broad area of tunica albuginea (2–3 cm^2) to the dartos fascia with multiple non-absorbable sutures.[18] The objective is to achieve permanent fusion. Recurrent torsion has been reported following orchiopexy. In every case, it was associated with inadequate fixation with absorbable sutures.[16, 35]

Should orchiectomy be performed if the viability of the testis is in question? In the past, while most surgeons would remove a frankly necrotic testis, if there was any possibility of survival of even part of the testicular tissue, it was usually left in the scrotum. The hope was that it would at least provide hormone func-

tion, since Leydig cells are more resistant to ischemia and may survive. Recent long-term follow-up reports indicate that retention of the compromised testis inhibits spermatogenesis in the normal *contralateral* testis (see Outcome, below). For this reason, the testis should be removed if its viability is not reasonably certain. Incision of the tunica albuginea may help in this determination. Rapid section histological examination is not helpful.

Should the neonate with an obviously infarcted testis be explored? Since the only neonates in whom the testis has been salvaged are those in whom torsion developed *after* birth, many surgeons have believed that operative treatment was useless in an infant born with torsion of the testis. It now appears that removal of an infarcted testis may be beneficial to the remaining normal testis, so a unilateral necrotic testis should be excised. If both testes are involved, they should be retained in the hope of preserving hormone production.

Bilateral orchiopexy should be carried out on patients with a history of recurrent episodes of testicular pain or swelling.[3] These patients have the best possible opportunity for testicular salvage. Since they represent one third of patients who subsequently undergo operation for acute symptomatic torsion of the testis, earlier operation could increase overall testicular salvage by one third.

Torsion of the appendix testis is best treated by emergency surgical excision. The necrotic tissue is removed, with instant relief of pain, which otherwise may persist for 1–2 weeks. If symptoms are mild and the diagnosis is certain, analgesics are a reasonable alternative.

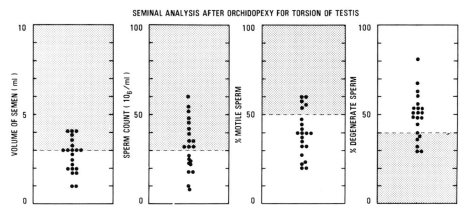

Fig 135–6.—Analysis of semen after orchiopexy for torsion of the testis. *Cross-hatched areas* show the normal range. Overall, only three of 21 patients studied had normal analyses. (From Thomas.[34] Used by permission.)

Outcome

Testicular salvage rates have increased in the past decade with increasing awareness of the condition and earlier surgical treatment. Initial salvage rates of 54–81% have been reported.[2, 4, 25, 29, 36] Long-term follow-up results are not nearly so good, however. Up to two thirds of the testes examined 2 or more years later show significant atrophy[1, 13, 34] The degree of atrophy is usually proportional to the duration of torsion at the time of operation (Fig 135–5). Of far greater concern, semen analyses show that 80–95% of these patients have abnormalities in volume, sperm count, motility, and percentage of degenerated sperm, indicating *bilateral* dysfunction[13, 34] (Fig 135–6). This is true even when the contralateral testis has been explored at the time of orchiopexy and found to be normal. Hormone analyses usually show normal levels of testosterone and prolactin, but LH and FSH levels may be elevated, especially if there is a low sperm count. If the previously twisted testis is atrophied, testicular biopsy of the other side will show hypospermatogenesis as well.[1]

In contrast, semen analysis and testicular biopsy of the contralateral testis are normal in patients who have had the twisted testis removed.[1] It is apparent that retention of an ischemic testis may result in damage to the other, normal testis. Experiments in rats have shown that an ischemic testis leads to autoimmunization, with destruction of spermatogonia on the opposite side.[9] It may be that the mechanism of contralateral injury in man is also autoimmunization from ischemic testicular damage.

These findings necessitate a revision in surgical decision-making at the time of testicular exploration: if the viability of the testis is questionable, it should be removed to prevent impairment of spermatogenesis in the contralateral testis. Retention for possible testosterone production alone is unnecessary, since a single testis is more than adequate for that purpose. Because of individual differences in the degree of torsion, intermittency, pain threshold, and tissue response to ischemia, it is unlikely that a specific duration of symptoms can be established beyond which testicular salvage should not be attempted. However, it now appears that most twisted testes should be removed if operation is performed more than 12 hours after the onset of acute symptoms. Wishful thinking may convert the misfortune of loss of a testis from torsion to the tragedy of permanent sterility.

REFERENCES

1. Bartsch G., et al.: Testicular torsion: Late results with special regard to fertility and endocrine function. *J. Urol.* 124:375, 1980.
2. Cass A.S., et al.: Immediate exploration of the unilateral acute scrotum in young male subjects. *J. Urol.* 124:829, 1980.
3. Cass A.S.: Elective orchiopexy for recurrent testicular torsion. *J. Urol.* 127:253, 1982.
4. Cattolica E.V.: High testicular salvage rate in torsion of the spermatic cord. *J. Urol.* 128:66, 1982.
5. Colt G.H.: Torsion of the hydatid of Morgagni. *Br. J. Surg.* 9:464, 1922.
6. Delasiauve L.J.F.: Descente tardive du testicule gauche, prise pour une hernie étranglée. *Rév. Méd. Fr. Etrang.* 1:363, 1840.
7. Guiney E.J., McGlinchey J.: Torsion of the testes and the spermatic cord in the newborn. *Surg. Gynecol. Obstet.* 152:273, 1981.
8. Harris B.H., et al.: Protection of the solitary testis. *J. Pediatr. Surg.* 17:950, 1982.
9. Harrison R.G., et al.: Mechanism of damage to the contralateral testis in rats with an ischemic testis. *Lancet* 2:723, 1981.
10. Haynes B., et al.: The diagnosis of testicular torsion. *JAMA* 249:2522, 1983.
11. Jerkins G.R., et al.: Spermatic cord torsion in the neonate. *J. Urol.* 129:121, 1983.
12. Kaplan G.W., King L.R.: Acute scrotal swelling in children. *J. Urol.* 104:219, 1970.
13. Krarup T.: The testis after torsion. *Br. J. Urol.* 50:43, 1978.
14. Leape L.L.: Torsion of the testis. *JAMA* 200:93, 1967.
15. Longo V.J.: Torsion of the testis: A new twist. *Urology* 12:743, 1978.
16. May R.E., Thomas W.E.G.: Recurrent torsion of the testis following previous surgical fixation. *Br. J. Surg.* 67:129, 1980.
17. Morgagni G.B., quoted by Jones P.: Torsion of the testis and its appendages during childhood. *Arch. Dis. Child.* 37:214, 1962.
18. Morse T.S., Hollabaugh R.S.: The "window" orchidopexy for prevention of testicular torsion. *J. Pediatr. Surg.* 12:237, 1977.
19. Murnaghan G.F.: The appendages of the testis and epididymis: A short review with case reports. *Br. J. Urol.* 31:190, 1959.
20. Nadel N.S., et al.: Preoperative diagnosis of testicular torsion. *Urology* 1:478, 1973.
21. Nicholas J.L., et al.: Idiopathic edema of scrotum in young boys. *Surgery* 67:847, 1970.
22. Ombrédanne L.: Torsions testiculaires chez les enfants. *Bull. Mem. Soc. Chir. Paris* 38:799, 1913.
23. Phillips N.B., Holmes T.W. Jr.: Torsion infarction in ectopic cryptorchidism. *Surgery* 71:335, 1972.
24. Quist O.: Swelling of the scrotum in infants and children. *Acta Chir. Scand.* 110:417, 1955.
25. Ransler C.W., Allen T.D.: Torsion of the spermatic cord. *Urol. Clin. North Am.* 9:245, 1982.
26. Riegler H.C.: Torsion of intra-abdominal testis. *Surg. Clin. North Am.* 52:371, 1972.
27. Riley T.W., et al.: Use of radioisotope scan in evaluation of intrascrotal lesions. *J. Urol.* 116:472, 1976.
28. Rodríguez, D.D., et al.: Doppler ultrasound versus testicular scanning in the evaluation of the acute scrotum. *J. Urol.* 125:343, 1981.
29. Scott J.H., et al.: The management of testicular torsion in the acute pediatric scrotum. *J. Urol.* 129:558, 1983.
30. Shukla R.B., et al.: Association of cold weather with testicular torsion. *Br. Med. J.* 285:1459, 1982.
31. Skoglund R.W., et al.: Torsion of testicular appendages: Presentation of 43 new cases and a collective review. *J. Urol.* 104:598, 1970.
32. Sonda L.P., Lapides J.: Experimental torsion of the spermatic cord. *Surg. Forum* 12:502, 1961.
33. Taylor M.R.: A case of testicle strangulated at birth: Castration: Recovery. *Br. Med. J.* 1:458, 1897.
34. Thomas W.E.G., Williamson R.C.N.: Diagnosis and outcome of testicular torsion. *Br. J. Surg.* 70:213, 1983.
35. Thurston A., Whitaker R.: Torsion of testis after previous testicular surgery. *Br. J. Surg.* 70:217, 1983.
36. Williams J.D., Hodgson N.B.: Another look at torsion of testis. *Urology* 14:36, 1979.
37. Williamson R.C.N.: Torsion of the testis and allied conditions. *Br. J. Surg.* 63:465, 1976.

136 William J. Cromie

Varicocele and Other Abnormalities of the Testis

Varicocele as a potentially reversible cause of male subfertility was first suggested in Tulloch's report in 1952. He noted an improved semen analysis following operative correction of bilateral varicoceles in a man who subsequently impregnated his wife.[46] Since this report, numerous investigators have reviewed the incidence of varicocele in the healthy male population. According to a mean value calculated from Saypol's review of reports on varicocele, its incidence is 15% in the general male population and from 21% to 41% in males presenting to an infertility clinic.[37] There are only sporadic reports of cases in children less than 10 years old; however, by the age of 19 years, the incidence in Caucasians is 16.2%, and is equivalent to that of the general healthy male population.[33] Of more importance is that the incidence at 10 years of age is 6%, compared with 15% by age 13. A recent study of black adolescents showed no difference from the white population, with an incidence of 13.7%.[35] Most commonly, varicocele occurs as a unilateral left-sided lesion (78%–93% of cases), less commonly as a bilateral lesion (2%–20% of cases), and least commonly as a unilateral right-sided lesion (1%–7% of cases).[37]

The above data suggest that changes at puberty are responsible for varicocele formation in susceptible individuals. With this in mind, several investigators have taken an interest in the early evaluation of selective treatment of the adolescent with varicocele at a time when deleterious effects upon fertility are minimal and might be reversible.[27, 28, 33, 35, 41] Ipsilateral testicular deficiency in size and consistency[27, 35, 41] and ipsilateral testicular histologic changes identical to those in adults with varicocele and infertility[20, 32, 35] have been noted in adolescents with varicocele. Abnormal FSH (follicle-stimulating hormone) and LH (luteinizing hormone) response to GnRH (gonadotropin-releasing hormone) infusion in adolescents with varicocele have been reported. These responses are identical to those seen in oligospermic adults with varicocele.[18, 22, 32] Histologic changes in the contralateral testicle in adults[5, 34, 45] and in experimental animals with varicocele[25] have been cited as further evidence of the deleterious effect of childhood varicocele.

The predominant clinical finding in a varicocele patient is a unilateral left-sided lesion. It is seldom painful and is usually recognized as a scrotal enlargement during or after adolescence (Fig 136–1). The primary etiologic factor appears to be the right-angle entry of the left spermatic vein into the high-pressure venous system of the left renal vein. Anatomically this provides, in the upright position, a long pressure column against which the pampiniform plexus must operate in order to effect testicular venous outflow. Ahlberg and associates demonstrated the absence of valves in 40% of left spermatic veins examined postmortem as compared with the absence of valves in 23% of right spermatic veins.[3] Venography in the upright position demonstrated that some of the left spermatic vein valves when present were actually incompetent.[4] Saypol et al. created experimental varicoceles in dogs by surgical destruction of the left spermatic venous

valves.[38] Coolsaet, employing venography in varicocele patients, found compression of the left renal vein between the aorta and the superior mesenteric artery in 17 of 67 cases reviewed.[9] Shafik et al. proposed cremasteric muscle atrophy, with loss of the muscular pump of the pampiniform plexus, as a contributing factor to venous dilatation in varicocele patients.[40]

Although the clinical lesion in varicocele is often unilateral, many studies have noted the histologic lesions to be bilateral, based on testicular biopsy specimens from children,[18, 20, 32] adults,[2, 5, 11, 12, 34, 39, 45] and experimental animals with varicocele.[25, 38] Other authors have observed microscopic findings of atrophy, or growth arrest of the varicocele testis, compared with testes in the normal population.[27, 28, 41]

Microscopic studies have examined the histologic alterations of the interstitium, Sertoli cells, and the germinal epithelium, with particular emphasis on Leydig cells and the "blood-testis barrier." Early observations by Scott[39] in 1958 and by Entriby et al.[12] in 1967 showed bilateral sloughing of immature germinal epithelium. Cameron and Snydle[5] and Terquem and Dadoune[45] demonstrated progressive degeneration of adluminal compartments and thus of the Sertoli cells support function, resulting in "sloughing" of immature germ cells. The morphology of the basal Sertoli-Sertoli compartments and, therefore, presumably of the blood-testis barrier, was well preserved. Alternatively, Hadzis-elimovic noted the frequent presence of mast cells in this area, and cites this and adluminal changes as evidence for an altered blood-testis barrier.[18] He observed interstitial changes, including Leydig cell hyperplasia, Leydig cell atrophy and normal Leydig cells. Leydig cell hyperplasia was noted earlier in reports by Dubin and Hotchkiss[10] in 1969 and by Agger and Johnsen[2] in 1978. A quantitative analysis of Leydig cells in the latter study yielded an incidence of hyperplasia of 39%. In other studies, Leydig cell hyperplasia varies from 23% to 67%, while sloughing of immature germ cells ranges from 68% to 83%.[34, 45]

Any theory of the pathophysiology of varicocele and associated infertility must explain the contralateral testicular effect. The most acceptable theories include an increase in testicular temperature, reflux of toxic metabolites through collateral venous circulation to the contralateral testis, and a modification of the normal hypothalamic-pituitary-gonadal axis. Increased scrotal and testicular temperature have been proved to decrease spermatogenesis.[37] As early as 1954, Russell proposed the theory that varicocele affected the normal thermoregulatory mechanisms of the testis.[36] In 1962, Hanley and Harrison documented scrotal temperature to be 2.5 C lower than rectal temperature in normal men, whereas the difference was as small as 0.1 C in patients with a large varicocele.[19] Recent efforts to improve evaluation of testicular temperature in patients with varicocele have been stimulated through human studies[50] and through studies of experimental animals with varicocele.[16, 25, 38] In the animal models cited, significant bilateral increase in blood flow and testicular temperature were noted, associated with decreased quality of

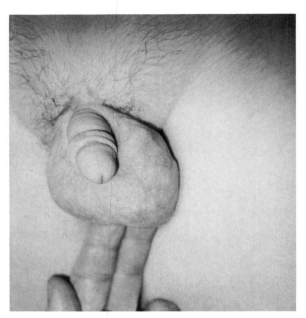

Fig 136–1.—Varicocele in preadolescent boy.

spermatograms and the histologic testicular changes previously presented. Green et al. noted complete reversal of these changes in testicular blood flow and temperature in nine of 11 experimental animals undergoing varicocelectomy (internal spermatic vein ligation).[16]

Many venographic studies have demonstrated retrograde flow down the spermatic vein since the original report of its existence by MacLeod in 1965.[29] This phenomenon was said to cause infertility as a result of refluxed renal and/or adrenal metabolites with decreased spermatogenesis. Other studies have refuted this theory.[23, 37, 47] Ito et al. observed reflux of renal metabolites (prostaglandins E and F) in varicocele patients.[23] A transfer of small amounts of vasoactive substances, among them prostaglandins, from the testicular vein to the testicular artery has been reported.[14, 15, 24] In addition to their vasoactive properties, prostaglandins have been noted to have direct antispermatogenic effects in rat and mouse testes.[1, 31] Any contralateral effect of refluxed metabolites would presumably require collateral testicular venous circulation. Evidence of such collaterals has been presented;[7, 21] however, the degree of collateral flow based on review of these venographic studies appears to be insufficient to effect a significant contralateral concentration of such refluxed metabolites.[47]

A more popular theory of varicocele induced infertility is that of a progressive subclinical deficiency of the hypothalamic-pituitary-gonadal axis. Peripheral serum testosterone values in varicocele patients are usually within the normal range.[6] Furthermore, according to studies by Swerdloff and Walsh in 1975, which compared FSH, LH, T (testosterone), and E_2 (estradiol) levels in peripheral and testicular venous blood of men with varicocele and those of normal men, no significant differences were noted.[43] Several studies have demonstrated increased local venous E_2 levels in experimental animals with varicocele,[25] as well as increased peripheral venous E_2 levels[34] and increased basal FSH levels[18] in varicocele patients. Pujol et al. correlated an increased Leydig cell index (histologic Leydig cell hyperplasia) with significantly increased peripheral venous E_2 levels in 10 of 11 varicocele patients, compared with normal controls.[34] Hadziselimovic correlated childhood varicoceles manifesting Leydig cell hyperplasia with an exceedingly high basal FSH level, compared

with FSH levels in normal controls.[18] GnRH (gonadotropin-releasing hormone) infusion as a stimulatory test in varicocele patients and in normal men while monitoring changes in FSH, LH, T, E_2 and prolactin has been reported by Hudson et al.[22] Responses of T and E_2 levels to GnRH infusion were equivalent in both groups. Varicocele patients with sperm counts between 10 and 30 $\times$ 10^6 per milliliter demonstrated significantly increased FSH and LH response in comparison with normal men and varicocele patients with counts greater than 30 $\times$ 10^6 sperm per milliliter. Varicocele patients with sperm counts less than 10 $\times$ 10^6 sperm per milliliter had an even greater increase in FSH and LH levels. Abnormal GnRH stimulation testing has already been proposed as one criterion for varicocele treatment.[18]

The effects of varicocele are often progressive. This realization has led to early diagnosis and the search for the "subclinical" varicocele. Original attempts were based on testicular temperature studies. In 1976, Comhaire et al. compared infrared scrotal thermography with venography in studies of 36 patients suspected of subclinical varicocele.[8] In 19 patients, an abnormal left-sided thermogram, with increased heat, was noted. Subsequent venography documented left spermatic vein reflux in 16 of these 19 patients. Additionally, 37 of 39 patients with palpable varicocele had an abnormal thermogram on the ipsilateral side. The two patients with normal thermograms had ipsilateral gross testicular atrophy. Lewis and Harrison used contact scrotal thermography, a much less expensive procedure, with identical findings.[26] Equal success has been reported with the Doppler ultrasonic stethoscope by Greenberg et al.[17] and with a radionuclide varicocele scan by Wheatley et al.[49] Fogh-Andersen et al. performed left spermatic vein ligation in 22 infertile men without a clinically palpable varicocele.[13] Subsequently, the pregnancy rate was 32% during 16 months of follow-up, compared with 5% for 22 similar but unoperated-on controls. Greenberg et al. performed left internal spermatic vein ligation on five patients with Doppler positive subclinical varicocele and infertility.[17] Postoperative spermatograms showed improvement in two of five patients, with subsequent pregnancies in both instances.

A system in general use for classifying the degree of varicocele appears to have stemmed from systems proposed by Uehling[48] in 1968 and by Dubin and Amelar[11] in 1970 (Table 136–1). Varicoceles are classified as small (grade I), moderate (grade II), or large (grade III). As a result of their 1970 study, Dubin and Amelar concluded that the degree of varicocele bears no relation to infertility. However, a recent retrospective analysis of treated varicocele patients by McClure and Robaire revealed a high degree of correlation between the grade of varicocele, effect on testicular volume, and results following varicocelectomy.[30] Volume differentials between right and left testes revealed no difference among grade I varicocele patients, a mean volume differential of 8% for grade II patients, and a mean differential of 19% in grade III patients. Postvaricocelectomy spermatograms showed significant improvement in grade I and grade II patients in 86–100% of cases, while only 50% of patients with grade III lesions had improved spermatograms. The authors concluded that grade III lesions have a deleterious effect upon ipsilateral

TABLE 136–1.—CLASSIFICATION
OF VARICOCELES

Grade I (small)	Palpably enlarged peritesticular vein(s) increased by Valsalva maneuver
Grade II (moderate)	Scrotal mass of veins identified easily upon palpation without Valsalva maneuver
Grade III (large)	Visible scrotal mass before palpation

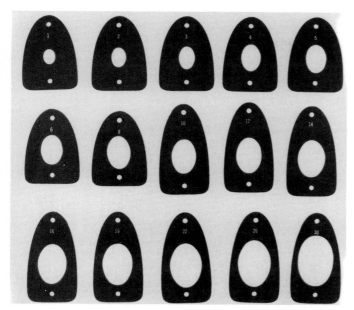

Fig 136–2.—Takihara orchidometer, showing variation in milliliter volumes.

testicular size and carry a poor varicolectomy prognosis after operative treatment of the varicocele.

Other authors stressed the importance of recognizing testicular atrophy and encouraged earlier treatment of adults[27] and children.[18, 28, 41] Objective measurement of testicular size in varicocele and normal patients was reported by Lipshultz and Corriere in 1977.[27] Testicular calipers were employed to record the long axis of the testis. More recently, Takihara et al. report that their orchidometer has a better correlation with testicular volume ($r = 0.81$) than testicular calipers ($r = 0.58$).[44] Their orchidometer consists of a series of elliptical rings with a number indicating the millimeter volume of each ellipsoid (testis) (Figs 136–2 and 136–3). They recommend the orchidometer as an accurate device for objective follow-up of varicocele patients both preoperatively and postoperatively. Testicular size was noted to increase bilaterally in the postvaricocelectomy group.

Varicocele is the most common surgically correctable cause of male infertility.[44] In adult patients with varicocele and infertility,

pregnancy rates following varicocelectomy were 55%, compared with 7% in unoperated controls.[44] The initial presentation of varicocele occurs during puberty, and the incidence in 13-year-old boys is equivalent to that in the general male population.[33] This occurrence has been referred to as the childhood or adolescent varicocele. Varicocele is a progressive disorder in many, if not all, cases. It is not possible to predict accurately the time course of progression in individual cases. However, significant prognostic features in adolescent varicocele are: (1) testicular atrophy or arrested testicular growth, (2) high-grade varicocele (grade II or III), (3) bilateral lesions, (4) pathologic GnRH stimulation test, and (5) a histologic picture of Leydig cell hyperplasia. The presence of these features either alone or in combination is an indication for surgical treatment.

While scrotal and retroperitoneal approaches to varicocele have been proposed, my own preference is for the high inguinal procedure. A standard inguinal skin-crease incision is made in the area of the internal ring, the external oblique incised, and a self-retaining retractor placed within the wound. The spermatic cord is identified, dissected free, and a Penrose drain placed beneath the spermatic cord. Following this, the external spermatic fascia is incised and the dilated veins are carefully dissected free while trying to preserve lymphatic channels. The internal spermatic veins are then ligated and partially excised at the internal inguinal ring (Fig 136–4). Usually two or three branches of the internal spermatic vein are located in this area. An optional maneuver is to inject contrast in the vein distal to the ligature followed by a roentgenogram to see if any patent veins persist; if so, they should be found and ligated. The spermatic cord is returned to the normal position; the external oblique fascia and skin is closed in a routine fashion without drains. In many cases, the patient may be discharged on the same day.

Unlike adults, children and adolescents with varicocele are not followed with spermatograms. Alternatively, they may be followed easily and objectively both preoperatively and postoperatively with the use of ellipsoid orchidometer measurements and endocrine profiles (basal LH, FSH, T, prolactin levels and GnRH stimulation tests). In certain instances, serial scrotal thermography and/or radionuclide varicocele scans may be of benefit.

As a progressive disorder with distinct individual variation, the childhood varicocele requires at least annual follow-up through puberty. A left testis 5 ml or more smaller than the right testis at initial presentation indicates a difference greater than expected by standard deviation. Failure of testicular growth occurs

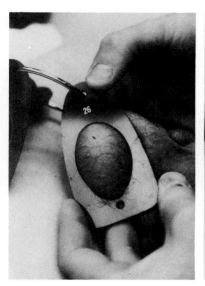
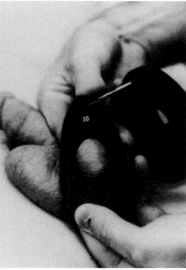

Fig 136–3.—Comparison of right and left testicular volumes in preadolescent with a clinically detectable varicocele.

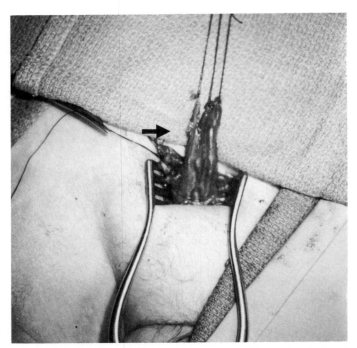

Fig 136–4.—Ligated varices *(arrow)* pictured during a high inguinal ligation of the incompetent internal spermatic veins.

despite normal development of adult pubic hair distribution and phallus growth, and the lagging growth of the testis is a key to decision to perform internal spermatic vein ligation. As GnRH and its analogues become more readily available, hormonal stimulation tests with intravenous infusion of these agents may provide further data in support of surgical intervention.

Children and adolescents with otherwise unexplained testicular atrophy or growth arrest should be suspected of having a subclinical varicocele. Contralateral subclinical varicocele may exist in postvaricocelectomy patients who fail to improve their orchidometer readings or endocrine profiles in follow-up.

REFERENCES

1. Abbatiello E.R., Kaminskm M., Weisbroth S.: The effect of prostaglandins F$_1$ and F$_2$ on spermatogenesis. *Int. J. Fertil.* 21:82–88, 1976.
2. Agger P., Johnsen S.G.: Quantitative evaluation of testicular biopsies in varicocele. *Fertil. Steril.* 19:52, 1968.
3. Ahlberg N.E., Bartley O., Chidekel N.: Right and left gonadal veins: An anatomical and statistical study. *Acta Radiol. (Diagn.)* 4:517–528, 1966.
4. Ahlberg N.E., Bartley O., Chidekel N., et al.: Phlebography in varicocele scroti. *Acta Radiol. (Diagn.)* 4:593–601, 1966.
5. Cameron D.F., Snydle F.E.: Ultrastructural surface characteristics of seminiferous tubules from men with varicocele. *Andrologia* 14:425–433, 1982.
6. Comhaire F., Vermeulen A.: Plasma testosterone in patients with varicocele and sexual inadequacy. *J. Clin. Endocrinol. Metab.* 40:824–829, 1975.
7. Comhaire F., Kunnen M.: Selective retrograde venography of the internal spermatic vein: A conclusive approach to the diagnosis of varicocele. *Andrologia* 8:11, 1976.
8. Comhaire F., Monteyne R., Kunnen M.: The value of scrotal thermography as compared with selective retrograde venography in the internal spermatic vein for the diagnosis of "subclinical" varicocele. *Fertil. Steril.* 27:694–698, 1976.
9. Coolsaet B.L.R.A.: The varicocele syndrome: Venography determining the optimal level for surgical management. *J. Urol.* 124:833–839, 1980.
10. Dubin L., Hotchkiss R.S.: Testis biopsy in subfertile men with varicocele. *Fertil. Steril.* 20:50–57, 1969.
11. Dubin L., Amelar R.D.: Varicocele size and results of varicocelectomy in selected subfertile men with varicocele. *Fertil. Steril.* 21:606–609, 1970.
12. Entriby A.A., Girgis S.M., Hernawy H., et al.: Testicular changes in subfertile males with varicocele. *Fertil. Steril.* 18:666–671, 1967.
13. Fogh-Andersen P., Nielsen N.C., Rebbe H., et al.: The effect on fertility of ligation of the left spermatic vein in men without clinical signs of varicocele. *Acta Obstet. Gynecol. Scand.* 54:29–32, 1975.
14. Free M.L., Jaffe R.A.: Dynamics of circulation in the testis of the conscious rat. *Am. J. Physiol* 223:241–248, 1972.
15. Free M.L., Jaffe R.A.: Effect of prostaglandins on blood flow and pressure in the conscious rat. *Prostaglandins* 1:483–498, 1972.
16. Green K.F., Turner T.T., Howards S.S.: Varicocele: Reversal of testicular blood flow and temperature changes by varicocelectomy. Presented at annual meeting, American Urological Association, Las Vegas, 1983 (abstract 502).
17. Greenberg S.H., Lipshultz L.I., Wein A.J.: A preliminary report on "subclinical varicocele": Diagnosis by Doppler ultrasonic stethoscope. *J. Reprod. Med.* 22:77–81, 1979.
18. Hadziselimovic F.: Im kindesalter erkenbare ursachen der männlichen sterilität. *Schweiz. Rundschau Med. (Praxis)* 72(10):316–323, 1983.
19. Hanley H.G., Harrison R.G.: The nature and surgical treatment of varicocele. *Br. J. Surg.* 50:64–67, 1962.
20. Hienz H.A., Voggenthaler J., Weissbach L.: Histologic findings in testes with varicocele during childhood and their therapeutic consequences. *Eur. J. Pediatr.* 133:139–146, 1980.
21. Hill H.T., Hirsh A.V., Pryor J.P., et al.: Changes in the appearance of venography after ligation of a varicocele. *J. Anat.* 135:47–52, 1982.
22. Hudson R.W., Crawford V.A., McKay D.E.: The gonadotropin reponse of men with varicoceles to a four-hour infusion of gonadotropin releasing hormone. *Fertil. Steril.* 36:633–637, 1981.
23. Ito H., Fuse H., Minagawa H., et al.: Internal spermatic vein prostaglandins in varicocele patients. *Fertil. Steril.* 37:218–222, 1982.
24. Jacks F., Setchell B.N.: A technique for studying the transfer of substances from venous to arterial blood in the spermatic cord of wallabies and rams. *J. Physiol.* (London) 233:17p–18p, 1973.
25. Kay R., Alexander N.J., Baugham W.L.: Induced varicoceles in rhesus monkeys. *Fertil. Steril.* 31(2):195–199, 1979.
26. Lewis R.W., Harrison R.M.: Contact scrotal thermography: Application to problems of infertility. *J. Urol.* 122:40–42, 1979.
27. Lipshultz L.I., Corriere J.N. Jr.: Progressive testicular atrophy in the varicocele patient. *J. Urol.* 117:175–176, 1977.
28. Lyon R.P., Marshall S., Scott M.P.: Varicocele in childhood and adolescence: Implication in adulthood fertility? *Urology* 19:641–644, 1982.
29. MacLeod J.: Seminal cytology in the presence of varicocele. *Fertil. Steril.* 16:735–757, 1965.
30. McClure R.D., Robaire B.: Relationship of varicocele size to testicular volume and to the effect on varicocelectomy outcome. Presented at annual meeting, American Urological Association, Las Vegas, 1983 (abstract 504).
31. Memon G.N.: Effects of intratesticular injections of prostaglandins on the testis and accessory sex glands of rats. *Contraception* 8:361–370, 1973.
32. Okuyama A., Koide T., Itatani H., et al.: Pituitary-gonadal function in schoolboys with varicocele and indications for varicocelectomy. *Eur. Urol.* 7:92–96, 1981.
33. Oster J.: Varicocele in children and adolescents. *Scand. J. Urol. Nephrol.* 5:27–32, 1971.
34. Pujol A., Rodriguez Tolra M.A., Navarro R., et al.: The hormonal pattern in varicocele and its relationship with the findings of testicular biopsy. Preliminary results. *Br. J. Urol.* 54:300–304, 1982.
35. Risser W.L., Lipschultz L.I.: The frequency of varicocele in black adolescents. *J. Adolescent Health Care* New York, Elsevier Science Publishing Co., 1983.
36. Russell J.K.: Varicocele in groups of fertile and subfertile males. *Br. Med. J.* 1:1231–1233, 1954.
37. Saypol D.C.: Varicocele. *Int. J. Androl.* 2:61–71, 1981.
38. Saypol D.C., Howards S.S., Turner T.T., et al.: Influence of surgically induced varicocele in testicular blood flow, temperature, and histology in adult rats and dogs. *J. Clin. Invest.* 68:39–45, 1981.
39. Scott L.S.: Report of Glasgow Obstetrical and Gynecological Society. *J. Obstet. Gynecol. Brit. Emp.* 65:504, 1958.
40. Shafik A., Khalil A.M., Saleh M.: The fascio muscular tube of the spermatic cord: A study of its surgical anatomy and relation to varicocele. A new concept for the pathogenesis of varicocele. *Br. J. Urol.* 44:147–151, 1972.
41. Steeno O., Knops J., DeClerck L., et al.: Prevention of fertility disorders by detection and treatment of varicocele at school and college age. *Andrologia* 8:47–53, 1976.
42. Stewart B.H.: Varicocele in infertility: Incidence and results of surgical therapy. *J. Urol.* 112:222–223, 1974.

43. Swerdloff R.S., Walsh P.C.: Pituitary and gonadal hormones in patients with varicocele. *Fertil. Steril.* 26:1006–1012, 1975.
44. Takihara H., Cosentino M.J., Cockett A.T.K., et al.: Significance of a new orchidometer in andrology clinic: Testicular atrophy in the varicocele patient and recovery after varicocelectomy. Presented at annual meeting, American Urological Association, Las Vegas, 1983 (abstract 503).
45. Terquem A., Dadoune J.P.: Morphological findings in varicocele: An ultrastructural study of 30 bilateral testicular biopsies. *Int. J. Androl.* 4:515–531, 1981.
46. Tulloch W.S.: A consideration of sterility factors in the light of subsequent pregnancies: Subfertility in the male. *Trans. Edinburgh Obstet. Soc.* 59:29–34, 1952.
47. Turner T.T.: Varicocele: Still an enigma. *J. Urol.* 129:695–699, 1983.
48. Uehling D.T.: Fertility in men with varicocele. *Int. J. Fert.* 13:58–60, 1968.
49. Wheatley J.K., Fajman W.A., Witten F.R.: Clinical experience with the radioisotope varicocele scan as a screening method for the detection of subclinical varicoceles. *J. Urol.* 128:57–59, 1982.
50. Zorgniotti A.W., MacLeod J.: Studies in temperature, human semen quality, and varicocele. *Fertil. Steril.* 24:854–863, 1973.

Other Abnormalities of the Testis

Polyorchidism or Triorchidism

This unusual anomaly involves the presence of a supernumerary testis, and results from transverse division of the embryonic genital ridge. In most reported cases, the patients are asymptomatic and have painless groin or testicular masses. Approximately 50% are associated with cryptorchidism, and about 30% are associated with an indirect hernia. The remainder are discovered in association with hydrocele, epididymitis, torsion, varicocele, or infertility.[3]

A slightly higher percentage of supernumerary testes occurs on the left side. This trend may be related to the reported larger size of the left testicle, which may subdivide more readily.[1] Usually the spermatic vessels bifurcate to supply each duplicated testis. However, one testis of the duplicated gonad may or may not have an attached epididymis or ductal connection. Some may appear dysplastic. Occasionally, these supernumerary testes may develop normally and even function well from both the spermatogenic and endocrine standpoints. Therapeutically, the duplicated testis may be best left alone if it has normal ductal apparatus and appears normal morphologically. Orchiectomy may be necessary in cases of torsion, infarction, dysplasia, or cryptorchidism where the duplicated testis interferes with the orchidopexy of the functional isotopic testis. Finally, a possible consequence of such a functioning supernumerary testis may be unexpected fertility, after a bilateral vasectomy has been performed in an adult.[2]

REFERENCES

1. Butz R.E., Croushore J.H.: Polyorchidism. *J. Urol.* 119:289, 1978.
2. Hakami M., Mosavy S.H.: Triorchidism with normal spermatogenesis: An unusual cause for failure of vasectomy. *Br. J. Surg.* 62:633, 1975.
3. Jichlinski D., Ward-McQuaid N.: Duplication of the testis and infertility. *J. Urol.* 90:583, 1963.

Splenogonadal Fusion

This rare malformation results from an abnormal connection between the splenic and gonadal anlagen in utero. There are two forms of this abnormality, continuous and discontinuous. In continuous splenogonadal fusion, the spleen remains connected to the left gonad by a continuous strand of tissue. This cord may be completely splenic, fibrous, or beaded with multiple nodules of splenic tissue. It usually arises from the upper pole of the spleen, and in most cases in which a cord is present, it runs transperitoneally. With discontinuous splenogonadal fusion, there is no connecting cord between the spleen proper and the left gonad. The ectopic splenic tissue is usually a distinct encapsulated mass.

Splenogonadal fusion is most often encountered incidentally in the course of operations for inguinal hernia or cryptorchidism.[3] When presenting as a primary problem, the patient frequently reports long-standing, painless swelling of the "testis."[1] Occasionally, the swelling may be aggravated and accompanied by pain, tenderness, and discoloration. These symptoms usually occur in conjunction with vigorous exercise. Most cases are found in adults, but the lesion has been reported in children.[1] The frequency is nine times greater in males than in females, and virtually all lesions are left-sided. Most cases are discovered clinically because of a left intrascrotal mass. A smaller percentage are discovered at operation for undescended testis or hernia. A preoperative diagnosis of left testicular tumor is often entertained in cases discovered clinically. If the possibility of splenogonadal fusion is considered preoperatively, radionuclide imaging with ^{99m}Tc sulfur colloid may demonstrate the unusual pattern of activity consistent with this abnormality.[2]

Removal of the splenic tissue is usually uncomplicated, since there is seldom true fusion with the gonad. There may be fibrous adhesions to the tunica albuginea.[3] As there is usually no abnormality of the orthotopic spleen, exploratory laparotomy is not needed to confirm the diagnosis of splenogonadal fusion. Diagnosis of the discontinuous variety may prevent unnecessary orchiectomy. Once the splenic component of this abnormality is removed, the gonad can be safely replaced within the scrotum.

REFERENCES

1. Lynch J.B., Kareim O.A.: Aberrant splenic tissue in the scrotum. *Br. J. Surg.* 49:546–548, 1962.
2. McLean G., Alavi A., Ziegler M., et al.: Splenic-gonadal fusion: Identification by radionuclide scanning. *J. Pediatr. Surg.* 16:649–651, 1981.
3. Putschar W.G.J., Manion W.C.: Splenic-gonadal fusion. *Am. J. Pathol.* 32:15–33, 1956.

Absence of the Vas and Cystic Fibrosis

The question of fertility in both males and females with cystic fibrosis may frequently be raised as their life expectancy continues to improve. The finding of aspermia in adult males with cystic fibrosis by Blanc[1] and by Denning[2] prompted a more detailed look into the etiology of this problem. Kaplan[3] studied 25 male patients with cystic fibrosis over 17 years of age. All were found to have aspermia, and reduced semen volume composed primarily of fructose, citric acid, and acid phosphatase, indicating that the ejaculate was derived mainly from prostatic secretion. In six of these patients undergoing herniorrhaphy or orchidopexy, no vas deferens could be identified. Ten males over 17 years of age were found at postmortem examination to have no vas deferens and marked abnormalities of the epididymis and seminal vesicles. It thus appears that abnormalities of the wolffian or mesonephric duct are common in males with cystic fibrosis. In spite of this, not all males with cystic fibrosis are sterile (Taussig).[4] In a review of 105 cystic fibrosis centers, fertility data were reported for 117 males; two were fertile and another six were believed to have fathered children, but their semen was not studied. Thus, normal fertility may occur in a very small, but appreciable, number of males (2–3%). The finding of fertile males has genetic, social, and psychological implications and makes it mandatory in all postpubescent males with this disease to evaluate the semen for appropriate counseling.

REFERENCES

1. Blanc W.A., Franciosi R., and Wigger H.J.: Pathology of organs of reproduction in cystic fibrosis: Testis and prostate in prepubertal and early pubertal cases. Presented at Sixth Annual Meeting of the Cystic Fibrosis Club, Atlantic City, New Jersey, May 3, 1965.

2. Denning C.R., Sommers S.C., Quigley H.J. Jr.: Infertility in male patients with cystic fibrosis. *Pediatrics* 41:7–17, 1968.
3. Kaplan E., Shwachman H., Perlmutter A., et al.: Reproductive failures in males with cystic fibrosis. *N. Engl. J. Med.* 279:65–69, 1968.
4. Taussig L., Lobeck C., DeSant'Agnese P., et al.: Fertility in males with cystic fibrosis. *N. Engl. J. Med.* 287:586–589, 1972.

Blind-Ending Vas Deferens in Testicular Agenesis

Differentiation of the wolffian ductal system is usually completed by the 13th week of gestation.[1] Loss of the wolffian duct before this time results in absence, not only of the epididymis and vas deferens but the kidney as well.[3] Mercer[2] made some additional observations on 237 cases of undescended testis. Nine patients (3.4%) had ipsilateral agenesis of the vas deferens and testis. In three of the nine cases, renal agenesis was found: two ipsilateral and one contralateral. Three patients had testicular agenesis alone, three patients had testicular atrophy presumably due to in utero torsion, and neither group had renal agenesis or upper urinary tract abnormalities. It thus appears that a renal ultrasound or intravenous pyelogram is indicated to determine the presence or absence of a kidney in cases of monorchia with vasal agenesis. This will occur rarely, as the incidence of monorchism in the general population is reported as being 0.02% to 0.1%.

REFERENCES

1. Lukash F., Zwiren G.T., Andrews H.G.: Significance of absent vas deferens at hernia repair in infants and children. *J. Pediatr. Surg.* 10:765, 1975.
2. Mercer S.: Agenesis or atrophy of the testis and vas deferens. *Can. J. Surg.* 22:245–246, 1979.
3. Ochsner M.G., Brannan W., Goodier E.H.: Absent vas deferens associated with renal agenesis. *JAMA* 222:1055, 1972.

Testicular Abnormalities in Diethylstilbestrol-Exposed Males

Diethylstilbestrol (DES) was given to about 2 million pregnant women in the United States from the early 1940s through 1971. Attention was first brought to the effects of DES by the occurrence of vaginal adenosis in female offspring.[4] Subsequent screening of male children similarly exposed to DES has revealed effects consequent upon DES exposure.[3] Some of the genitourinary conditions reported to occur with increased frequency in men exposed to DES in utero include epididymal cysts, testicular hypoplasia, cryptorchidism, capsular induration of the testis, decreased penile length, hypospadias, varicoceles, and abnormal semen (decreased sperm density, decreased sperm motility, and abnormal sperm morphology).[2] The epididymal cysts may be observed clinically. The hypoplastic testis should be monitored by patient self-examination because of the rare possibility of the development of neoplasia. Cryptorchid boys in most cases require orchidopexy. Three cases of testicular neoplasm were reported by Conley[1] in DES-exposed men. In spite of this report, no published control studies have demonstrated a relation in the human male between exposure to DES in utero and carcinogenesis.

REFERENCES

1. Conley G., Sant G., Ucci A., et al.: Seminoma and epididymal cysts in a young man with DES exposure in utero. *JAMA* 249:1325–1326, 1983.
2. Cosgrove M.D., Benton B., Henderson B.E.: Male genitourinary abnormalities and maternal diethylstilbestrol. *J. Urol.* 117:220, 1977.
3. Gill W.B., Schumacher G.F.B., Bibbo M., et al.: Association of diethylstilbestrol exposure in utero with cryptorchidism, testicular hypoplasia and semen abnormalities. *J. Urol.* 122:36, 1979.
4. Herbst A.L., Ulfelder H., Poskanzer D.C.: Adenocarcinoma of the vagina: Association of maternal stilbestrol therapy with tumor appearance in young women. *N. Engl. J. Med.* 284:878, 1971.

137 Denis R. King

Ovarian Cysts and Tumors

OVARIAN CYSTS and tumors are diagnosed infrequently during infancy and childhood. Of the 2,680 ovarian lesions reviewed by Gagner and Sjovall,[17] only 1.5% were observed in children. Lindfors[29] has estimated that the incidence of ovarian neoplasms (both benign and malignant) in Scandinavian girls from birth to 14 years of age is 2.6 cases per 100,000 per year.[29] Reports from the United States and Great Britain have confirmed the relative rarity of ovarian lesions in childhood. Forshall,[16] in Liverpool, and Thatcher,[46] in Milwaukee, have indicated that, overall, one ovarian tumor can be expected for every 3,000–5,000 children's hospital admissions. Adelman et al.[2] reported an incidence rate of 27 per 100,000 admissions at the Children's Hospital of Michigan.

Although ovarian tumors are observed throughout infancy and childhood, there is very clearly an increased incidence with advancing age. In Groeber's[21] survey, 17% of ovarian tumors occurred between birth and 4 years of age, 28% in the 5–9-year age group, and 55% during adolescence. This was confirmed by Norris and Jensen[32] who reported a doubling of the incidence during successive 5-year periods (Fig 137–1).[32] The risk of malignancy varies inversely with age, the highest incidence being observed in very young patients and the lowest in adolescents, approaching in them the 15% incidence of malignancy in adult ovarian tumors.

A substantial proportion of the ovarian masses presenting in infancy and childhood are not neoplastic. These lesions are incorporated in the World Health Organization's histologic classification of ovarian pathology as tumor-like conditions including simple cysts, follicular cysts, corpus luteum cysts, endometriosis, and a variety of other malformations and inflammatory conditions.[43] In a collected series of 2,567 patients under 16 years of age with ovarian cysts and tumors, there was a 23% incidence of nonneoplastic lesions.[23]

The relative frequency of benign vs. malignant tumors varies with the reporting institution. Fifty-five percent of the 353 tumors reviewed by Norris and Jensen[32] at the Armed Forces Institute of Pathology were malignant. Lindfors'[29] report from Scandinavia presented a 67% incidence of malignancy, and 32% of Huffman's[23] collected series from the world literature were cancer. It would appear that, overall, approximately one half of the neoplastic ovarian tumors diagnosed in childhood will be malignant.

Symptoms and Signs

The most common presenting symptom in children with ovarian tumors is abdominal pain. Two thirds of the 99 patients reported by Towne et al.,[48] presented for evaluation of abdominal discomfort. In 40%, an acute onset of symptoms was observed as a result of torsion, hemorrhage, or perforation; in the remaining patients, the abdominal discomfort was chronic, frequently of 3–6 months' duration. A palpable abdominal mass is second in frequency. Other complaints include urinary tract infection or dysuria as a result of compression of the bladder, or ureteral obstruction, nausea, vomiting, and abdominal distention.

Endocrinopathies occur in 5–10% of the children with ovarian tumors. Isosexual precocious pubertal development may be observed with estrogen-producing sex cord-stromal tumors containing granulosa-theca cells, with human chorionic gonadotropin (HCG)-producing germ cell neoplasms, and with hormonally active nonneoplastic follicular and luteal cysts. Heterosexual development—virilization—is most commonly noted in association with androblastoma, but may occasionally be seen in patients with dysgerminoma, choriocarcinoma, lipoid cell tumors, or polycystic ovaries.

Pertinent physical findings are restricted to the abdomen in the majority of patients. Evidence of distant metastasis is infrequent even with advanced ovarian malignancies. Careful abdominal and bimanual rectoabdominal palpation is mandatory. Vaginal examination may be helpful in adolescent girls, but rarely adds any substantial clinical information in younger children. The ovaries are abdominal organs throughout childhood, and ovarian tumors are usually palpable above the pelvic inlet. The physical characteristics of the tumor with regard to size, shape, fixation, tenderness, topography (smooth vs. nodular), and consistency (cystic vs. solid) should be recorded. The voice, face, axillae, breasts, and vulvar structures should be evaluated for evidence of hormonal effects. Somatic growth measurements should be charted.

Diagnostic Studies

A pregnancy test should be performed initially on all postmenarchal girls with pelvic masses to rule out intrauterine or ectopic pregnancy. False-positive pregnancy tests may be obtained in patients with HCG-producing germ cell tumors. Chest radiographs are obtained to rule out parenchymal metastasis or mediastinal lymphadenopathy. Abdominal x-ray films may show the tumor and demonstrate calcifications. Ultrasonography provides an accurate assessment of pelvic anatomy. Tumor size, consistency (cystic vs. solid) and internal wall characteristics can often be defined. An intravenous pyelogram may be important to identify ureteral obstruction or displacement if malignancy is suspected. Computerized axial tomography with oral and intravenous contrast can provide graphic information about hepatic metastasis; ascites; para-aortic lymphadenopathy; omental implants; and the status of the kidneys, ureters, and pelvic viscera. Barium contrast studies and angiography are of less importance and need not be obtained. Radiographic determination of bone age should be obtained in all children with evidence of endocrine effects. Lymphangiography has been utilized to demonstrate unsuspected para-aortic lymph node metastases in adults, but intraoperative examination and open biopsy are preferred for precise clinical staging. Radionuclide scans of the liver and/or bone may be indicated for staging purposes. Laparoscopy is not as useful in pediatric patients with ovarian masses as it is in adults, because the increased incidence of neoplastic tumors and the relatively high risk of malignancy in childhood dictate formal laparotomy for the vast majority of patients. The requirement for general anesthesia further diminishes the practicality of this technique in children.

Laboratory studies of importance include HCG and α-fetopro-

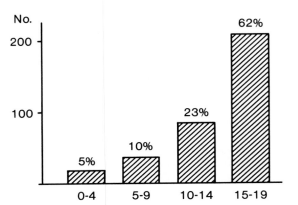

Fig 137–1.—The incidence of ovarian tumors increases throughout childhood and adolescence.

tein (AFP) determinations in patients with germ cell tumors, vaginal cytology, and urine and serum biochemical hormone profiles for those with apparent endocrine dysfunction. These levels are important biologic indicators of tumor activity and useful for serial monitoring of the remote results of therapy.

Embryology

Gonadal differentiation is controlled by the genetic information on the sex chromosomes. In the absence of a Y chromosome and the presence of two X chromosomes, the gonadal anlagen develop into ovaries. During the process of gonadal development, three primordia combine to form the ovary: (1) mesenchymal elements of the urogenital ridge, (2) coelomic epithelium (germinal epithelium) covering the urogenital ridge, and (3) germ cells that arise from the caudal portion of the yolk sac.

By the 4th week of fetal life, an undifferentiated gonad is recognizable in the human embryo. The gonad initially appears as a thickening of the coelomic epithelium overlying the mesenchyme of the urogenital ridge. At this time the germ cells, which are extragonadal in origin, arise within the yolk sac adjacent to the hindgut. The germ cells undergo proliferation, and by the 6th week of fetal life they migrate to, and can be recognized within, the mesenchymal tissue of the urogenital ridge. Subsequently, the coelomic epithelium grows into the mesenchyme and the germ cells (oogonia) undergo mitotic division, rapidly increasing in number to approximately 5 million. Once the oogonia initiate meiotic division, they are considered oocytes and enter a resting stage of development that is not completed until ovulation 10–50 years later. The oocytes become enclosed by granulosa cells derived from the germinal epithelium; and these in turn are surrounded by a layer of theca cells derived from the mesenchymal blastema, thus forming a follicle. At the time of birth, the ovaries have their full complement of primary follicles (400,000) comprising all three embryologic components of the gonad. Only 400 or so of these oocytes will be utilized during the standard 30–40 year period of human fertility.

Classification

A clinical classification system should provide some understanding of ovarian cysts and tumors based upon their developmental embryology, endocrine activity, and malignant potential. The following is adapted from the International Histologic Classification of Tumors proposed by the World Health Organization in 1973[43]:

I. Nonneoplastic lesions
  A. Luteinoma of pregnancy
  B. Hyperthecosis
  C. Simple cyst
  D. Follicular cyst
  E. Corpus luteum cyst
  F. Endometriosis
  G. Inflammatory lesions
  H. Parovarian cysts
  I. Polycystic ovaries
  J. Inclusion cysts
II. Neoplastic lesions
  A. Epithelial tumors
    1. Serous
    2. Mucinous
    3. Endometrioid
    4. Clear cell
    5. Brenner
    6. Mixed
    7. Undifferentiated
  B. Sex cord-stromal tumors
    1. Granulosa-stroma
      a. Granulosa
      b. Theca-fibroma
    2. Androblastoma
    3. Gynandroblastoma
  C. Lipoid cell tumors
  D. Germ cell tumors
    1. Dysgerminoma
    2. Endodermal sinus
    3. Embryonal cancer
    4. Polyembryoma
    5. Choriocarcinoma
    6. Teratoma
    7. Mixed Forms
  E. Gonadoblastoma
  F. Soft tissue tumors
  G. Unclassified tumors
  H. Metastatic tumors

Nonneoplastic Ovarian Tumors

Normal ovarian function is dependent upon the reproducible cyclic production of cystic structures within the gonadal tissue. During each menstrual cycle, the ovary develops structural changes analogous to the majority of nonneoplastic ovarian tumors observed in clinical practice. The cyclic anatomical changes that occur in the ovary are under the control of a complex series of hormonal interactions, collectively referred to as the hypothalamic-pituitary-ovarian axis. This process is initiated at the outset of each cycle under the influence of follicle-stimulating hormone (FSH) (Fig 137–2). Typically, a group of five to ten primary follicles increase in size, developing many layers of granulosa cells about the enlarging oocyte. Only one of these graafian follicles will mature during each cycle, while the others become atretic and are resorbed.

As the preovulatory follicle develops, the granulosa cells produce large amounts of estrogenic hormones; and serum estrogen levels increase. At approximately midcycle, a surge of luteinizing hormone (LH) and FSH is noted, and ovulation occurs. The follicle is then transformed into a functioning corpus luteum under the influence of LH, and progesterone production is initiated. Subsequently, LH and FSH levels return to baseline; and, if fertilization and implantation fail to occur and placental HCG is not produced, the corpus luteum regresses, estrogen and progesterone levels fall, and the entire process begins again.

Nonneoplastic ovarian lesions represent 25–35% of the ovarian tumors reported in the pediatric age group.[23] Recognition of the benign nature of these tumors is important and quite possible in the majority of cases. Preferred surgical management of nonneo-

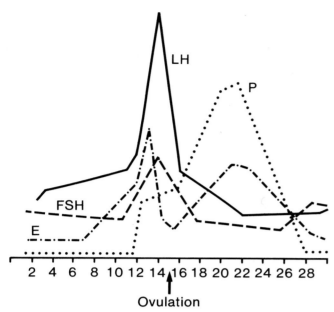

Fig 137–2.—The relationships between the various pituitary and ovarian hormones during a normal menstrual cycle. (*LH* indicates luteinizing hormone; *FSH*, follicle-stimulating hormone; *E*, estrogen; and *P*, progesterone.)

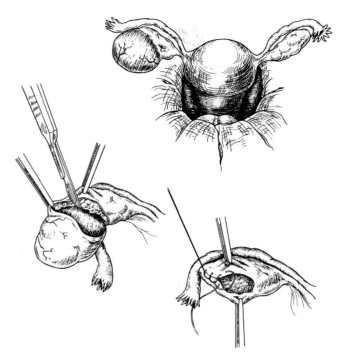

Fig 137–3.—Removal of non-neoplastic ovarian cyst. With careful dissection, it is usually possible to remove completely a nonneoplastic ovarian cyst and preserve the adjacent normal gonadal tissue.

plastic lesions includes removal of the tumor with careful preservation of as much ovarian tissue as possible (Fig 137–3). This will maximize the child's opportunity for subsequent normal endocrine and reproductive function.

Follicular Cysts

Follicular cysts are the most common of the nonneoplastic ovarian tumors, representing up to 50% of the total. It is not unusual to observe many small follicular cysts (0.5–10 mm) protruding from the surface of the ovary at the time of laparotomy. These lesions are asymptomatic and are the result of physiologic hormonal fluctuations. Follicular cysts have a smooth, glistening, grayish-blue surface that bulges through the cortex of the ovary. They are unilocular, 3–12 cm in diameter, thin-walled, and usually filled with clear, watery, yellow fluid. Histologically, the cysts are lined by a layer of granulosa cells and surrounded by a connective tissue capsule.

From an endocrinologic standpoint, follicular cysts would be expected to be uncommon in premenarchal girls because of the low output of pituitary gonadotropins. The majority of these lesions occur in adolescence. As a corollary, it may be important to evaluate the premenarchal patient with a follicular cyst for evidence of abnormal sources of gonadotropins. Isosexual precocious puberty is occasionally observed in young girls with follicular cysts that produce large amounts of estrogenic hormones. Follicular cysts are the single most common ovarian tumor observed during the neonatal period, presumably as a result of maternal placental HCG production.

In the prepubertal child with a palpable ovarian cyst or tumor, laparotomy is indicated because of the low incidence of nonneoplastic gonadal lesions and the relatively high risk of malignancy. In the postmenarchal girl, the presence of a unilocular ovarian cyst is not an absolute indication for operation. Laparotomy in them is recommended only for (1) cysts greater than 5 cm in diameter; (2) symptoms of abdominal pain when torsion, hemorrhage, or perforation are suspected; and (3) lesions that fail to decrease in size during a 2–3-month period of observation. The administration of exogenous hormones may be suggested during the observation period to minimize the patient's endogenous pituitary gonadotropin production.

At the time of operation, if the appearance of the lesion is characteristic of a nonneoplastic cyst, conservative surgical management with preservation of normal ovarian tissue is indicated. By incising the surface of the ovary adjacent to the thickened plaque of gonadal tissue, it is usually possible to develop a plane of dissection that provides complete removal of the cyst with the capsule intact (see Fig 137–3). Unroofing with excision of the major portion of the cyst wall is perhaps less desirable, but appears to be equally efficacious. Occasionally, there will be no apparent residual ovarian tissue to salvage or reconstruct; and, under these circumstances, oophorectomy is appropriate. If there is suspicion that the ovarian cyst represents a neoplastic lesion, oophorectomy or unilateral salpingo-oophorectomy is indicated.

Simple Cysts

It is impossible to differentiate simple cysts from their follicular counterparts on the basis of any gross anatomical criteria. On microscopic examination, these lesions are lined by a nondescript, flattened epithelium with no distinguishing characteristics. They are not endocrinologically active, and treatment guidelines are identical to those for follicular cysts.

Corpus Luteum Cysts

Functioning corpora lutea do not develop until after ovulation has occurred; and, as a result, cysts of corpus luteum origin are usually not observed until adolescence. These lesions may appear hemorrhagic and are filled with amber blood-stained fluid. The cyst lining is composed of luteinized granulosa and theca cells and has a characteristic golden yellow color. These cysts are capable of producing both estrogen and progesterone. Corpus luteum cysts may be associated with amenorrhea, irregular menses, or dysfunctional uterine bleeding. Clinical management of patients with cysts of corpus luteum origin is similar to that for follicular lesions.

Endometriosis

The natural history of endometriosis as proposed by Sampson,[36] with obstruction of menstrual outflow and subsequent regurgitation and implantation of endometrial elements on the peritoneal surfaces, indicates that this diagnosis should be made very infrequently in the premenarchal patient. With the onset of menses, however, symptomatic endometriosis may develop rapidly. Goldstein et al.[19] documented a 47% incidence of endometriosis in a cohort of 140 adolescent females between 10–19 years of age who underwent laparoscopy and biopsy for evaluation of chronic pelvic pain. Twenty-eight of the 66 patients (43%) had implants on the ovaries, and 18 (27%) presented with an adnexal mass on physical examination.

Endometriosis classically produces dysmenorrhea, cyclic pelvic pain, and dyspareunia. The implants in the earliest stages of the disease may appear as small petechiae, but more typically the peritoneal surfaces are studded with nodules. Within the ovaries, endometrial cysts are variable in size (3–10 cm) and dark brown in color (chocolate cysts). Endometrial cysts are filled with the breakdown products of blood and endometrial debris and characteristically produce a substantial local inflammatory reaction. Because of tissue implantation on adjacent peritoneal surfaces and fixation secondary to the local inflammatory response in advanced cases, differentiation from ovarian malignancy may be difficult on the basis of gross appearance. Fortunately, this rarely occurs in children.

Treatment of endometriosis is primarily nonoperative and includes prolonged suppression of ovulation with the continuous use of oral progestogens or the administration of danazol, a mild androgenic steroid that blocks the effect of estrogen on endometrial tissue. Operative intervention may be required for diagnosis or for treatment of local complications. Conservative surgical management with fulguration or resection of symptomatic endometrial tissue is recommended.

Neoplastic Ovarian Tumors

Because the relative incidence of malignancy in childhood ovarian tumors is quite high (35%), and because it is frequently difficult to differentiate benign ovarian neoplasms from localized malignant tumors simply on the basis of clinical characteristics, a rational approach to these lesions must be grounded on well-defined surgical principles. Familiarity with the following current staging system of the International Federation of Gynecology and Obstetrics is mandatory, because appropriate utilization of the various elements of modern multimodal treatment requires precise surgical staging:

I. Growth limited to the ovaries
   Ia. Limited to one ovary; no ascites
   Ib. Limited to both ovaries; no ascites
   Ic. Limited to one or both ovaries; ascites present containing malignant cells
II. Growth involving one or both ovaries with pelvic extension
   IIa. Extension or metastases to uterus and tubes only
   IIb. Extension to other pelvic tissues
III. Growth involving one or both ovaries with widespread intraperitoneal metastasis to the abdomen (omentum, small intestines, and mesentery)
IV. Growth involving one or both ovaries with widespread metastases outside the peritoneal cavity
Note: The presence of ascites does not influence classification of stages II, III, IV.

Recently, it has been recognized that ovarian cancer patients with apparently localized tumors have a significant incidence of occult intraperitoneal metastasis. Piver et al.[34] have documented unsuspected metastases on the undersurface of the diaphragm (11%), in the omentum (3%), para-aortic lymph nodes (10%), pelvic lymph nodes (8%), and in cytologic washings of the peritoneal cavity (33%) in a series of suspected stage I ovarian cancer patients. Young and coauthors[53] reported a 24% incidence of unrecognized residual tumor in a group of supposedly tumor-free patients referred for adjuvant chemotherapy. At the present time, standard surgical staging for neoplastic ovarian tumors should include (1) collection of ascitic fluid and/or peritoneal washings for cytologic study (prior to operative manipulation of the tumor), (2) careful inspection of the liver and the undersurfaces of both diaphragms, (3) omentectomy, (4) biopsy of para-aortic and pelvic lymph nodes, (5) appropriate management of the primary ovarian tumor, and (6) careful inspection and often biopsy or bisection of the contralateral gonad.

Other surgical principles applicable to patients with either benign or malignant disease are as follows: (1) The abdominal incision must be large enough to permit removal of the tumor without excessive manipulation and possible rupture of the tumor. (2) The peritoneal cavity should be well walled off to prevent diffuse peritoneal contamination if tumor contents are spilled. (3) Cyst puncture and aspiration is not appropriate if there is any suspicion that the tumor is neoplastic. (4) All solid tumors should be considered malignant. (5) All cystic lesions with papillary excrescences or local adherence should be considered malignant. (6) If bilateral oophorectomy is required for benign tumors, preservation of the uterus may be desirable in childhood in order to provide the psychological advantages of induced cyclic menstruation in adolescence and the potential for "in vitro" fertilization, embryo transfer, and subsequent pregnancy in later life.

Ovarian cancer amounts to 1% or less of all malignancies in the childhood population.[5] The incidence of ovarian cancer is estimated to be 2.5 cases per million children per year, which represents a total of perhaps 100–150 new cases nationwide annually. Because no single institution could possibly accumulate a sizable series of cases for evaluation of changing treatment modalities in any reasonable period of time, collaborative studies have evolved.

Precise surgical guidelines for management of children with ovarian cancer are difficult to outline. This remains an area of controversy; and, as more successful adjuvant therapies are developed, there is a continuous redefinition of the role of operation. Radical ablative operations are less frequently performed in children with ovarian cancer, and every reasonable effort should be made to conserve endocrine and reproductive function.

Patients with localized disease (stage Ia or Ic) are in many cases candidates for unilateral salpingo-oophorectomy. Bilateral ovarian cancer, of course, suggests the advisability of panhysterectomy. In children with more extensive tumors (stage II, III, or IV), hysterectomy and bilateral salpingo-oophorectomy have been routinely recommended in the past, but the role of these ablative procedures may be reevaluated in light of recent advances in adjuvant chemotherapy. Current surgical management must be individualized, depending on the natural history of the tumor and its predicted response to both radiation and chemotherapy.

Epithelial Tumors

These tumors arise from the surface epithelium of the ovary, which is an embryologic derivative of the coelomic epithelium overlying the urogenital ridge. Overall, epithelial tumors account for approximately two thirds of all primary ovarian neoplasms and almost 85% of ovarian cancers, but they are relatively infrequent in children. Of the 353 ovarian tumors in children reported by Norris and Jensen,[32] 19% were epithelial in origin; and only eight of the 67 (12%) were malignant. Bilateral tumors were observed on ten occasions (15%). Lindfors'[29] review documented a 15% incidence of epithelial tumors, of which almost one half were cancerous. Welch reported only 18 tumors (8%) of epithelial origin in a group of 216 children with ovarian malignancy.[49]

Tumors in this category may be described as benign, malignant, or of low malignant potential. Unilateral oophorectomy or salpingo-oophorectomy are adequate surgical treatment for benign lesions, those of low malignant potential and Stage Ia cancers. The opposite ovary should be bivalved and a biopsy obtained of any suspicious areas. In the face of more advanced intra-abdominal disease with ascites, matted intestinal loops, or peritoneal seeding, aggressive cytoreductive surgery should be undertaken. This has provided significant palliation and improved survival in adult patients.[20] Panhysterectomy, omentectomy, and excision of large peritoneal implants are indicated. Radiation and/or chemotherapy have been found to be useful in certain patients with advanced clinical staging.[30]

Sex Cord-Stromal Tumors

Sex cord-stromal tumors are derived from the specialized blastemal mesenchyme that makes up the urogenital ridge. During fetal development, this tissue has the potential to differentiate into either the stromal tissue (granulosa-theca cells) of the ovary, or the interstitial tissue (Leydig and Sertoli cells) of the testis.[54]

Of the 353 childhood ovarian tumors reported by Norris and Jensen,[32] 18% were of sex cord-stromal origin. Stromal tumors are the most common type of ovarian neoplasm to produce endocrine effects. The majority of these tumors elaborate physiologically significant amounts of estrogenic or androgenic hormones. Sex cord-stromal tumors are typically indolent, slow-growing lesions of relatively low malignant potential. Only 10% of patients have evidence of tumor invasion or dissemination at the time of presentation. Long-term survival cannot be accurately assessed at 5 years in patients with stromal tumors because of the well-documented incidence of remote postoperative recurrence.

Granulosa-Theca Cell Tumors

Granulosa-theca cell tumors constitute the vast majority of the sex cord-stromal neoplasms, accounting for 84% of the 233 cases reviewed by Huffman.[23] These tumors have the highest incidence of symptomatic hormone production of all pediatric ovarian neoplasms, the overwhelming majority elaborating estrogenic compounds (Fig 137–4). Clinical evidence of isosexual precocious pseudopuberty was observed in 15 of the 20 prepubertal patients in Zaloudek and Norris'[55] series. Lack et al.[28] reported a 70% incidence of precocious feminization in ten premenarchal patients. Virilization has been described in an occasional patient. Common clinical manifestations in prepubertal patients include breast enlargement, vaginal bleeding, development of pubic hair, genital maturation, and an increase in velocity of somatic growth. After menarche, clinical signs of a feminizing tumor are more difficult to detect, and adolescent patients frequently present with nonspecific complaints such as abdominal pain or distention and menstrual irregularities. Overall, ovarian tumors are the cause of less than 10% of all cases of isosexual precocious pubertal development. The differential diagnosis includes (1) true sexual precocity, (2) exogenous administration of estrogenic hormones, (3) gonadotropin-secreting tumors, (4) feminizing adrenal tumors, and (5) other ovarian cysts and neoplasms.

The typical hormonal profile of patients with granulosa-theca

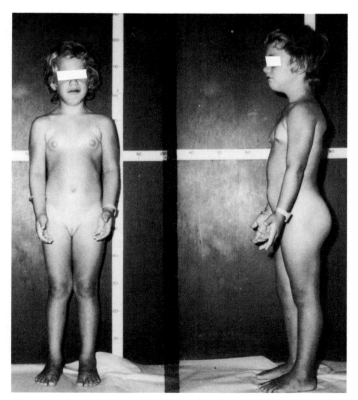

Fig 137–4.—Granulosa cell tumor-sexual precocity. Front and side views of a 3-year-old girl who presented for evaluation of isosexual precocious pubertal development caused by a malignant granulosa-theca cell tumor. Tall stature, breast development, and somatic maturity are apparent.

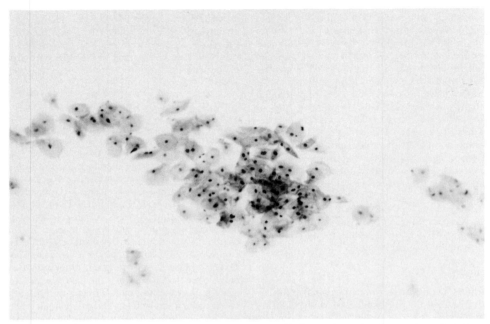

Fig 137–5.—Cytosmear demonstrating the mature squamous epithelium and cytoplasmic granules typical of an estrogen effect on the vaginal epithelium, taken from a normal 13-year-old girl.

cell tumors includes elevated serum and urine estrogen levels in conjunction with low gonadotropin output. The vaginal cytosmear characteristically reveals a significant estrogen effect, and the bone age is advanced (Fig 137–5). A palpable abdominal or pelvic mass was appreciated in 28 of the 32 patients reported by Zaloudek and Norris.[55] In their series, the tumors varied in size from 5.5–30 cm, with a median diameter of 11.5 cm. All of the tumors had a smooth surface with no evidence of external tumor growth. Thirteen of the 32 lesions were predominantly solid masses, while the remaining 19 had major cystic components. Bilaterality has been uncommon (less than 5%) in children, but has been observed in up to 30% of adults.[37] All 32 patients had stage Ia tumors, and 30 were treated by unilateral salpingo-oophorectomy. Only two of the patients developed tumor recurrence during the follow-up period (median, 6 years). In the series of Lack et al.,[28] ten children presented with stage I tumors, and all were successfully treated by unilateral salpingo-oophorectomy. Of the 198 adult patients reported by Bjorkholm and Sifversward,[4] 91% had stage I disease at presentation, but 25% (42 patients) ultimately died as a result of tumor progression. Advanced clinical staging (greater than stage I), tumor rupture, and evidence of nuclear atypia were associated with poor prognosis. Granulosa cell tumors appear to have a more favorable outlook in childhood.

On the basis of the aforementioned clinical reports, conservative surgical management seems to be entirely appropriate. Because most of these tumors are benign or well-localized cancers (stage I) at presentation, unilateral salpingo-oophorectomy is recommended. Panhysterectomy is suggested only for malignant tumors with more advanced clinical staging. Radiotherapy is advised for patients with advanced local disease (greater than stage I) or recurrent tumor. The role of chemotherapy in clinical management remains entirely speculative.

Androblastoma

Androblastoma (rather than arrhenoblastoma) is the proper current terminology for the Sertoli-Leydig cell tumors of the ovary. They are among the most interesting and rarest of all ovarian tumors, representing less than 10% of the sex cord-stromal neoplasms. Androblastomas are analogous to granulosa-theca cell tumors in every respect, except that they produce androgenic hormones.

Masculinizing ovarian tumors are distinctly uncommon prior to puberty. Young children with functioning androblastomas typically develop evidence of virilization with hirsutism, coarsening of the voice, clitoral hypertrophy, and an accelerated somatic growth pattern. Postmenarchal girls present with complaints of oligomenorrhea or amenorrhea, hirsutism, acne, and a masculinizing change in body habitus. The differential diagnosis of such virilization includes (1) exogenous androgen administration, (2) adrenal tumor or hyperplasia, (3) intersex anomalies with gonadal dysgenesis or true hermaphroditism, (4) polycystic ovaries, and (5) other ovarian neoplasms.

The expected hormonal profile includes normal excretion of urinary 17-ketosteroids and pregnanetriol, with low levels of gonadotropins and an elevated serum testosterone. The bone age is usually advanced. Management principles are identical to the recommendations outlined for granulosa-theca cell tumors. Most of the symptoms of virilization should regress after tumor removal. Serum testosterone level is an excellent biologic marker for this tumor.

Lipoid Cell Tumors

The term lipoid cell tumor is used to describe a small group of ovarian neoplasms composed exclusively of lipid-laden, hormone-producing cells that possess no other identifying histologic features. Lipoid cell tumors originate within the ovary, or in extraovarian sites, and may be designated by the pathologist as adrenal rest tumors, hilus cell tumors, Leydig cell tumors, or stromal luteinomas. The precise embryologic derivation of these lesions remains uncertain.

Lipoid cell tumors usually produce symptoms and signs of virilization. The typical biochemical profile of hormone secretion includes increased urinary 17-ketosteroid excretion, elevated serum testosterone and androstenedione levels, with low normal LH and FSH values. These tumors are autonomous, demonstrating little or no response to dexamethasone suppression.

Lipoid cell tumors are well-encapsulated solid masses with a characteristic bright yellow color on cross section. These lesions almost always follow a benign clinical course. Surgical management is unilateral salpingo-oophorectomy only. Substantial resolution of the virilizing symptoms should be expected following tumor removal. Radiation and chemotherapy are not indicated because of the very low incidence of malignancy.

Germ Cell Tumors

The primordial germ cells arise initially in an extragonadal position at the base of the yolk sac and migrate to the urogenital ridge for incorporation into the developing gonad. During migration, nests of these totipotential cells may be left along the route of migration in the midline of the developing embryo. As a result, germ cell tumors arise anywhere along the migratory pathway and have been described in the brain, mediastinum, and retroperitoneum, as well as the gonads. The totipotential nature of these cells explains the tremendous diversity of tissue types categorized as germ cell tumors. The classification proposed by Teilum[45] graphically demonstrates the interrelationships of the germ cell tumors (Fig 137–6).

Neoplasms of germ cell origin are the most common of the pediatric ovarian tumors, representing 62% of the 1974 ovarian neoplasms reported in the world's literature between 1936 and 1979.[23] Of the 353 cases reviewed by Norris and Jensen,[32] 205 were of germ cell origin. Tumors representing the entire clinical spectrum, from completely benign to the most aggressive malignant lesions, are included in this category. The malignant potential of germ cell tumors appears to vary inversely to age. Breem et al.[5] cite "a 33 percent malignancy rate in germ cell tumors of patients less than 18 years of age, compared to an incidence of 2 to 6 percent in patients older than 18." Because of the tremendous variety of germ cell tumors, and the fact that the various tumor types are often intermixed, Scully[41] has emphasized that "careful gross examination and judicious sampling for microscopic study are necessary to achieve the complete diagnosis. . . . Quantitation of the various components of a mixed germ cell tumor is important in the determination of treatment and prognosis." A minimum of one tissue block per centimeter of tumor diameter has been considered adequate tissue sampling. Historically, malignant germ cell tumors other than dysgerminoma have had a relatively poor prognosis, and the outlook

for patients with disease beyond the ovary was bleak. Only recently has effective multimodal therapy begun to improve the outcome for children with germ cell cancer. In 1975, Smith and Rutledge[42] reported a substantial prolongation of survival in 15 of 20 patients treated with vincristine, actinomycin D, and cyclophosphamide (Cytoxan) (VAC). Wollner et al.[52] reviewed the Memorial Hospital experience with pediatric ovarian cancer in 1976 and confirmed the efficacy of their four-drug chemotherapy regimen (VAC plus doxorubicin hydrochloride [Adriamycin]), which had prevented tumor recurrence in six of nine patients with extensive intra-abdominal disease.[52] In 1981, Brodeur et al.[6] reported a 60% long-term survival (greater than 24 months) in 20 girls with ovarian germ cell cancer and affirmed the utility of multiple-agent chemotherapy for extragonadal germ cell tumors as well. Most recently, bleomycin and cisplatin have been utilized successfully in the treatment of ovarian germ cell malignancy.[7] If the results achieved with chemotherapeutic management of testicular germ cell tumors can be duplicated in childhood ovarian cancer, we could anticipate a 75% survival even in those patients with disease disseminated at presentation.[12] The current Children's Cancer Study Group protocol for patients with malignant germ cell tumors utilizes repeated cycles of a six-drug combination of vinblastine, actinomycin D, cyclophosphamide, doxorubicin hydrochloride (Adriamycin), bleomycin, and cisplatin.[10] Results of this study, which was initiated in 1978, should be available in the near future.

Dysgerminoma

Dysgerminoma ranks as the second-most-frequent ovarian neoplasm in childhood (16%), but is the single most common type of ovarian malignancy.[23] The tumor arises from undifferentiated primordial germ cells and is histologically indistinguishable from seminoma, its counterpart in the testicle (Fig 137–7). Dysgerminoma characteristically presents in young women, 72% of all cases being reported during the second and third decades of life.[11]

Complaints at presentation are quite nonspecific and are usually related to local discomfort or symptoms of pelvic pressure from the bulky ovarian mass. Occasionally, torsion or hemorrhage may produce an acute abdominal crisis. Pure dysgerminomas are hormonally inactive. If patients display any evidence of remote endocrine effects, a mixed germ cell tumor must be suspected and HCG and AFP determinations obtained. Lymphangiography has been useful in assessing extent of disease.[11] Pathologic features associated with poor prognosis include (1) tumor diameter greater than 10 cm, (2) high mitotic index, (3) minimal lymphocytic or granulomatous reaction, (4) tumor necrosis, and (5) microscopic foci of other germ cell elements.[18]

At laparotomy, dysgerminomas are typically bulky, solid, encapsulated tumors that are yellowish-white in color. Bilaterality may be observed in up to 20% of cases and is frequently microscopic (50%).[11] Bisection and *biopsy* of the opposite ovary are therefore strongly recommended. Dysgerminoma spreads primarily by the lymphatic route and para-aortic node metastases are commonly observed. Peritoneal dissemination is a less frequent but clearly ominous observation.

Dysgerminoma is known to be a very radiosensitive tumor, and the combination of operation and radiation has provided enviable relapse-free survival rates. Krepart et al.[26] reviewed 36 patients treated at the M. D. Anderson Hospital, with an overall survival of 86%. Of the 16 patients with clinical stage I or II disease, 100% survived. Fifteen of the 20 women who were stage III or IV at presentation also were cured. All of the patients who developed tumor recurrence had bulky primary lesions greater than 10 cm in diameter (average = 18 cm), a well-known high-

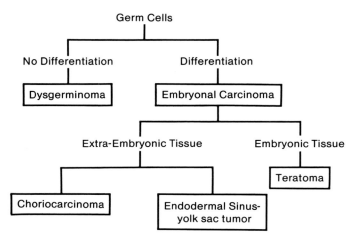

Fig 137–6.—The developmental relationships of the various germ cell neoplasms (schema initially proposed by Teilum[45]).

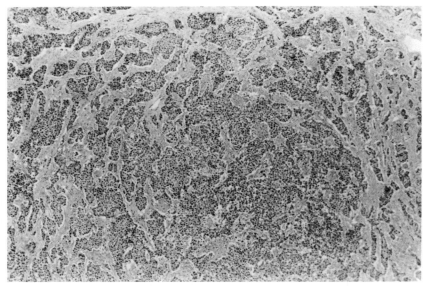

Fig 137-7.—Dysgerminoma showing the typical nests of tumor cells with uniform round nuclei separated by thick fibrous bands (hematoxylin-eosin, ×132).

risk characteristic. The vast majority (82%) of tumor recurrences were observed within 2 years of initial diagnosis, and most presented in the abdomen and pelvis.

Cyclic combination chemotherapy (VAC) has been reported by Weinblatt and Ortega[50] to be effective in children with extensive intraperitoneal dysgerminoma, and this treatment modality may deserve a more significant role in the clinical management of patients with dysgerminoma in the future. Current treatment guidelines continue to emphasize the well-recognized utility of operation and radiation.

Unilateral salpingo-oophorectomy is suggested for children with stage Ia dysgerminoma. Bisection *and biopsy* of the opposite ovary should be performed. Additional postoperative radiation therapy, limited to the involved hemipelvis, is advised with shielding of the contralateral ovary. Using this technique, Brody[8] has reported a 95% survival rate with preservation of contralateral ovarian function. Any dysgerminoma beyond clinical stage Ia is best managed by total abdominal hysterectomy, bilateral salpingo-oophorectomy, and excision biopsy of suspicious para-aortic lymph nodes. Postoperatively, radiotherapy should be administered to the entire abdomen and pelvis.

If para-aortic nodal metastases are documented, the radiation field should be extended to include both the mediastinum and the left supraclavicular fossa. De Palo et al.[11] have reported an actuarial 5-year survival of 91% in 31 patients with stage I dysgerminoma and 74% for 18 women with stage III disease.[11] Multiagent chemotherapy (VAC) may be advised for the treatment of children with distant metastases and for those who have tumor recurrence within the radiation portal.

Endodermal Sinus Tumor

Endodermal sinus tumors (yolk sac tumors) are aggressively malignant germ cell neoplasms that had an extremely poor prognosis prior to the development of effective multiagent chemotherapy.[24] Morphologically, the tumor simulates the endodermal sinuses and structures of yolk sac origin within the rodent placenta. Endodermal sinus tumors elaborate the oncofetal antigen AFP, a glycoprotein with a metabolic half-life of 5 days, which is normally produced in the fetal yolk sac, liver, and intestine. A reliable biologic marker of tumor activity, AFP is quite useful as

an indicator of the adequacy of operation and the response to chemotherapy.[14] Serum AFP activity falls to normal adult values (less than 16 ng) by 1 year of age, and elevated serum levels are observed only in patients with hepatoma, germ cell neoplasia, hepatitis, or cirrhosis.

Endodermal sinus tumors characteristically present with symptoms related to rapid growth of the intra-abdominal mass. At operation, the tumor is a bulky, friable mass filled with grayish mucoid material. Histologically, Schiller-Duval bodies and periodic acid-Schiff–positive granules are observed in the majority of cases (Fig 137-8). Kurman and Norris reviewed 71 cases, confirming the highly malignant nature of this tumor.[27] In their series, an 84% recurrence rate was observed, even in patients with stage Ia disease at presentation; and the overwhelming majority of the recurrences (90%) became apparent within 12 months of diagnosis. Sixteen of the 18 patients reported by Huntington and Bullock[24] died within a year of diagnosis. Radical ablative surgery does not appear to improve the survival of children with localized unilateral tumors, and they may be treated by ipsilateral salpingo-oophorectomy. Bilateral tumors are uncommon. More extensive primary lesions demand panhysterectomy with removal of all bulk tumor. Because of the aggressive nature of this lesion, adjuvant chemotherapy is mandatory regardless of the clinical stage at presentation, or the apparent completeness of tumor removal. Intensive multiagent cyclic chemotherapy utilizing a combination of vincristine, bleomycin, cisplatin, actinomycin, Adriamycin, and Cytoxan, as recommended by the Children's Cancer Study Group, has produced an initial 80% complete tumor remission in 17 evaluable patients.[1] Seven of the eight patients reported by Wiltshaw et al.[51] survived with no evidence of disease following cyclic chemotherapy administration.

Embryonal Carcinoma

Embryonal carcinoma is an aggressive malignancy that fortunately is relatively uncommon, representing only 2.8% of the 1,217 germ cell tumors reviewed by Huffman[23] and 32 of the 353 ovarian tumors (8%) reported by Norris and Jensen.[32] This tumor may produce both AFP and HCG, a glycoprotein hormone that is a normal product of placental syncytiotrophoblast. As a result

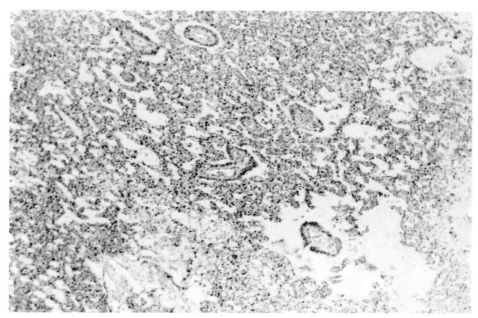

Fig 137–8.—Endodermal sinus tumor demonstrating characteristic Schiller-Duval bodies (hematoxylin-eosin ×132).

of the hormonal stimulation of HCG, patients frequently present with clinical endocrinopathies manifested by precocious pseudo-puberty and menstrual irregularities. In the adolescent female, the combination of a mass on pelvic examination and positive test results for urinary HCG may simulate an early pregnancy.

Surgical management of children with embryonal carcinoma is similar to that for endodermal sinus tumors. Both lesions are highly malignant and infrequently bilateral. Stage Ia and Ic tumors require only unilateral salpingo-oophorectomy, but advanced local disease demands panhysterectomy. Adjuvant multiagent chemotherapy should be administered to all patients regardless of stage. Embryonal carcinoma is a radiosensitive lesion. Serial HCG and AFP determinations are useful for monitoring tumor activity.

Choriocarcinoma

Choriocarcinoma is the rarest of all ovarian malignancies in childhood, representing less than 1% of the 1974 tumors reported in the literature from 1936–1979.[23] This is fortunate, in view of the highly malignant nature of this tumor and its resistance to both radiation and chemotherapy. Most choriocarcinomas are endocrinologically active lesions that elaborate HCG. The elevated HCG levels typically produce isosexual precocious pubertal development in premenarchal girls by stimulating ovarian estrogen production. After menarche, menstrual irregularities are frequently produced that, in conjunction with high HCG levels and a pelvic mass, may simulate pregnancy.

Surgical management of patients with choriocarcinoma may be complicated by the friability of the tumor and its proclivity for early invasion of contiguous organs and structures. Unilateral salpingo-oophorectomy is appropriate for localized lesions, but the majority of patients will require panhysterectomy because of local tumor extension. Aggressive surgical management is required because of the relative radioresistance of this lesion. Postoperative chemotherapy with actinomycin D, chlorambucil, and high-dose methotrexate with folic acid rescue is recommended. Of the germ cell tumors, ovarian choriocarcinoma remains the least responsive to multiagent chemotherapy. Serum HCG levels will provide an accurate biologic marker of tumor activity in most cases.[14]

Teratomas

Teratomas represent approximately two thirds of childhood ovarian germ cell tumors and perhaps 40% of all ovarian neoplasms in children.[23] Teratomas typically remain asymptomatic until they become large enough to produce pressure on adjacent pelvic and abdominal organs or acutely develop torsion, hemorrhage, or perforation. Physical findings of significance are primarily related to the presence of the mass, which characteristically presents on abdominal examination in young girls or as a pelvic tumor in adolescents. Routine abdominal radiographs will demonstrate calcification within the tumor in 40% of patients (Fig 137–9).

At operation, the majority of teratomas are encapsulated, predominantly cystic lesions with a thick, dull gray capsule. There are no surface characteristics to reliably distinguish teratomas from other cystic ovarian tumors. On cut section, the hair, teeth, and sebaceous material are easily recognized in mature tumors (Fig 137–10). By definition, tissues derived from endoderm, mesoderm, and ectoderm should be recognized within the tumor to sustain a diagnosis of teratoma (Fig 137–11). From the pathologist's viewpoint, teratomas are divided into three categories: (1) mature, (2) immature, and (3) monodermal. The prognosis for patients with teratomas depends upon the clinical stage at presentation and the degree of differentiation of the various tissues within the tumor.

Mature Teratomas

The vast majority of teratomas in pediatric patients are mature tumors with little or no propensity to develop malignant degeneration. Of the 786 ovarian teratomas reviewed by Huffman,[23] 75% were initially considered benign; and only ten tumors (1.6%) subsequently underwent malignant transformation. Mature teratomas are composed of well-differentiated tissues representing all three embryologic germ layers. These tumors were

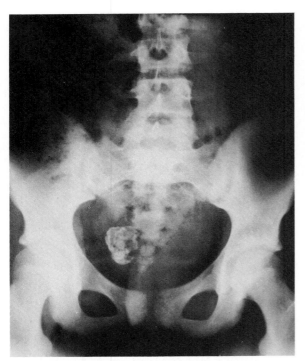

Fig 137–9.—Ovarian teratoma. Abdominal radiograph of an adolescent girl who presented with abdominal pain and tenderness demonstrates a calcified pelvic mass typical of teratoma.

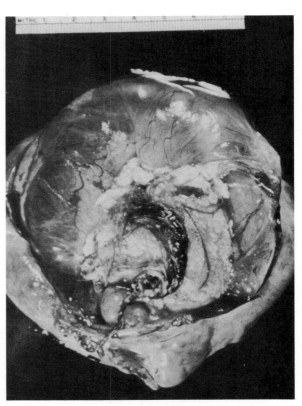

Fig 137–10.—Ovarian teratoma. Gross surgical specimen of a mixed cystic and solid teratoma. The mature tissue elements (hair and sebaceous material) are easily recognized.

previously classified as benign cystic teratomas and known generically as dermoid cysts of the ovary. Surgical management includes only removal of the affected gonad with preservation of the ipsilateral fallopian tube if possible. Bilateral tumors may be observed in up to 20% of adult patients, but are infrequent (less than 10%) in childhood. If the contralateral ovary is of normal size and consistency, blind biopsy or bisection is not mandatory.

One unusual and alarming-appearing variant of the mature teratoma is the occurrence of diffuse intraperitoneal gliomatosis,

first reported by Robboy and Scully in 1970.[35] If the glial implants consist of well-differentiated mature tissue, they require no treatment. Conservative surgical management of the primary ovarian tumor is recommended. Despite the apparent widespread tumor dissemination, the overall prognosis for such patients is quite good.[3, 15, 31]

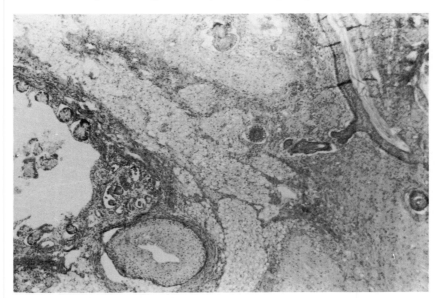

Fig 137–11.—Mature ovarian teratoma demonstrating all three germ layers, with mature nervous tissue, keratinizing squamous cells, and a segment of intestinal epithelium (hematoxylin-eosin ×132).

Immature Teratomas

A teratoma is classified as immature when any of its components are undifferentiated, resembling embryonal tissue. Mature, well-differentiated elements are also present in the majority of cases. Tapper and Lack reported 94 patients with ovarian teratoma, in whom 16 tumors had immature tissue components.[44] Overall, approximately 10% of ovarian teratomas in childhood fall into this classification.

The prognosis for patients with immature teratoma is best correlated with the clinical stage of disease and the histologic grade as proposed by Thurlbeck and Scully:[47]

Grade 0: All tissues mature; no mitotic activity

Grade I: Minor foci of abnormally cellular or embryonal tissue mixed with mature elements; rare mitoses

Grade II: Moderate quantities of embryonal tissue mixed with mature elements; moderate mitotic activity

Grade III: Large quantities of embryonal tissue present

Survival is directly related to the histologic grade of the tumor, grade I lesions having a better prognosis and grade III tumors having the worst. In the series of Norris et al.[33] from the Armed Forces Institute of Pathology, all patients with immature stage I teratomas that were histologically grade I survived with no evidence of recurrence.[33] Overall, grades I, II, and III were associated with 82%, 62%, and 30% survival respectively (Fig 137–12).

Surgical management of children with immature teratomas remains an area of considerable controversy. Kosloske et al.[25] and others[13, 22] have advocated conservative operations, whereas Cham et al.[9] have been proponents of more extensive procedures. A reasonable approach to the immature teratoma of ovarian origin may well be analogous to the management of their clinical counterparts in the testicle. The goals of surgical management should include (1) complete excision of the primary lesion, (2) accurate clinical staging, (3) removal of all bulk tumor in patients with intra-abdominal metastasis, (4) second-look procedures to assess the results of therapy, and (5) preservation of normal urogenital organs. On the basis of these guidelines, unilateral salpingo-oophorectomy alone (stages Ia–Ic) or in combination with cytoreductive procedures such as retroperitoneal lymphadenectomy, omentectomy, and excision of peritoneal implants should be sufficient for the majority of patients.

Bilateral ovarian tumors, or local extension to include the uterus, would indicate the advisability of panhysterectomy. Cyclic chemotherapy, using a combination of agents with demonstrated efficacy in patients with germ cell tumors, should be administered to all children with lesions beyond a stage I, grade I classification. Radiation therapy is efficacious in children with intra-abdominal dissemination.

In the current Children's Cancer Study Group protocol, radiotherapy is reserved for patients with residual tumor at the time of second-look laparotomy.[10] These recommendations seem entirely reasonable, because preservation of the functional integrity of the contralateral gonad is an important consideration.

Gonadoblastomas

Gonadoblastomas, first described by Scully[39, 40] in 1953, are tumors that can exhibit either benign or malignant clinical features. These tumors characteristically are found in phenotypic females with intersex anomalies who have an XY sex chromatin pattern. This may include patients with pure gonadal dysgenesis, mixed gonadal dysgenesis, or male pseudohermaphroditism. The incidence of tumor development in these patients may be as high as 50%.[38] Gonadoblastomas typically arise in streak or dysgenetic gonads. They are well encapsulated, noninvasive, and unilateral in the majority of cases. Because of the potential for asynchronous bilaterality, the contralateral gonad should be removed. If there is evidence of malignant degeneration, subsequent therapy should be guided by the histologic characteristics of the invasive germ cell elements. Prophylactic removal of nonfunctional streak gonads in girls with identifiable intersex anomalies and an XY karyotype has been recommended.

Summary

Because of the relative rarity of ovarian tumors in childhood and the tremendous variety of lesions that arise in gonadal tissue, even very senior clinicians seldom achieve a vast personal experience with all types of ovarian lesions. Surgeons caring for children with ovarian pathologic conditions have a serious responsibility to consider carefully the potential for preservation of both endocrine and procreative function. If ablative surgery fails to offer clear advantages, conservative management is recommended. With the recent progress in the chemotherapeutic management of pediatric ovarian malignancies, prolonged survival and cure may be achievable in many instances.[10] Wise clinical decisions must be based upon a foundation of accurate diagnosis, familiarity with current classification and staging systems, and a thorough understanding of the natural history of the various lesions encountered and the opportunities for successful nonoperative management.

REFERENCES

1. Ablin A.: Malignant germ cell tumors in children. *Front. Radiat. Ther. Oncol.* 16:141, 1982.
2. Adelman S., Benson C.D., Hertzler J.H.: Surgical lesions of the ovary in infancy and childhood. *Surg. Gynecol. Obstet.* 141:219, 1975.
3. Albites V.: Solid teratoma of the ovary with malignant gliomatosis peritonei. *Int. J. Gynaecol. Obstet.* 12:59, 1974.
4. Bjorkholm E., Sifversward C.: Prognostic factors in granulosa cell tumors. *Gynecol. Oncol.* 11:261, 1981.
5. Breem J.L., Bonamo J.F., Maxson W.S.: Genital tract tumors in children. *Pediatr. Clin. North Am.* 28:355, 1981.
6. Brodeur G.M., Howarth C.B., Pratt C.B., et al.: Malignant germ cell tumors in 57 children and adolescents. *Cancer* 48:1890, 1981.
7. Bradof J.E., Hakes T.B., Ochoa M., et al.: Germ cell malignancies of the ovary. *Cancer* 50:1070, 1982.
8. Brody S.: Clinical aspects of dysgerminoma of the ovary. *Acta Radiol.* 56:209, 1961.
9. Cham W.C., Wollner N., Exelby P., et al.: Patterns of extension as a guide to radiation therapy in the management of ovarian neoplasms in children. *Cancer* 37:1443, 1976.
10. Children's Cancer Study Group, Protocol CCG-861: The treatment of malignant germ cell tumors, primary and metastatic, of children, February, 1978.
11. De Palo G., Pilotti S., Kenda R., et al.: Natural history of dysgerminoma. *Am. J. Obstet. Gynecol.* 143:799, 1982.
12. Donohue J.P., Einhorn L.H., Williams S.D.: Cytoreductive surgery for metastatic testis cancer: Considerations of timing and extent. *J. Urol.* 123:876, 1980.
13. Ein S.: Malignant ovarian tumors in children. *J. Pediatr. Surg.* 8:539, 1973.

	STAGE I	STAGE II	STAGE III	SURVIVED
GRADE				
1	14	4	4	82%
2	20	2	2	62%
3	6	2	2	30%

Fig 137–12.—The prognosis of patients with immature teratoma is clearly related to the histologic grade at diagnosis.

14. Ewing H.P., Newsom B.D., Hardy J.D.: Tumor markers. *Curr. Probl. Surg.* 19:2, 1982.

15. Favara B.E., Franciosi R.A.: Ovarian teratoma and neurological implants on the peritoneum. *Cancer* 31:678, 1973.

16. Forshall I.: Ovarian neoplasms in children. *Arch. Dis. Child.* 35:17, 1960.

17. Gagner S., Sjovall A.: Ovarian and parovarian tumors in children; report on 43 cases. *Acta Obstet. Gynecol. Scand.* 28:10, 1949.

18. Gillespie J.J., Arnold L.K.: Anaplastic dysgerminoma. *Cancer* 42:1886, 1978.

19. Goldstein D.P., De Cholnoky C., Emans S.J.: Adolescent endometriosis. *J. Adolesc. Health Care* 1:37, 1980.

20. Griffiths C.T., Fuller A.F.: Intensive surgical and chemotherapeutic management of advanced ovarian cancer. *Surg. Clin. North Am.* 58:131, 1978.

21. Groeber W.R.: Ovarian tumors during infancy and childhood. *Am. J. Obstet. Gynecol.* 86:1027, 1963.

22. Harris B.H., Boles E.T. Jr.: Rational surgery for tumors of the ovary in children. *J. Pediatr. Surg.* 9:289, 1974.

23. Huffman J.W.: Ovarian tumors in children and adolescents, in Huffman J.W., et al. (eds.): *The Gynecology of Childhood and Adolescence,* ed. 2. Philadelphia, W.B. Saunders Co., 1981.

24. Huntington R.W., Bullock W.K.: Yolk sac tumors of the ovary. *Cancer* 25:1357, 1970.

25. Kosloske A.M., Favara B.E., Hays T., et al.: Management of immature teratoma of the ovary in children by conservative resection and chemotherapy. *J. Pediatr. Surg.* 11:839, 1976.

26. Krepart G., Smith J.P., Rutledge F., et al.: The treatment for dysgerminoma of the ovary. *Cancer* 41:986, 1978.

27. Kurman R.J., Norris H.J.: Endodermal sinus tumor of the ovary: A clinical and pathological analysis of 71 cases. *Cancer* 38:2404, 1976.

28. Lack E.E., Perez-Atayde A.R., Murthy A.S.K., et al.: Granulosa theca cell tumors in premenarchal girls. *Cancer* 48:1846, 1981.

29. Lindfors O.: Primary ovarian neoplasms in infants and children: A study of 81 cases diagnosed in Finland and Sweden. *Ann. Chir. Gynaecol.* (suppl.) 177:1, 1971.

30. Longo D.L., Young R.C.: The natural history and treatment of ovarian cancer. *Ann. Rev. Med.* 32:475, 1981.

31. Nogales F.F., Oliva H.A.: Peritoneal gliomatosis produced by ovarian teratomas. *Obstet. Gynecol.* 43:915, 1974.

32. Norris H.J., Jensen R.D.: Relative frequency of ovarian neoplasms in children and adolescents. *Cancer* 30:713, 1972.

33. Norris H.J., Zirkin H.J., Benson W.L.: Immature (malignant) teratoma of the ovary. *Cancer* 37:2359, 1976.

34. Piver M.S., Barlow J.J., Lele S.B.: Incidence of subclinical metastasis in Stage I and Stage II ovarian carcinoma. *Obstet. Gynecol.* 52:100, 1978.

35. Robboy S.J., Scully R.E.: Ovarian teratoma with glial implants on the peritoneum. *Hum. Pathol.* 1:643, 1970.

36. Sampson J.A.: Development of the implantation theory for the origin of peritoneal endometriosis. *Am. J. Obstet. Gynecol.* 40:549, 1940.

37. Schweppe K.W., Beller F.K.: Clinical data of granulosa cell tumors. *J. Cancer Res. Clin. Oncol.* 104:161, 1982.

38. Scott J.S.: Intersex and sex chromosome abnormalities, in Macdonald R.R. (ed.): *Scientific Basis of Obstetrics and Gynecology.* Edinburgh, Churchill Livingstone, 1978, p. 301.

39. Scully R.E.: Gonadoblastoma: A gonadal tumor related to the dysgerminoma (seminoma) and capable of sex hormone production. *Cancer* 6:455, 1953.

40. Scully R.E.: Gonadoblastoma: A review of 74 cases. *Cancer* 25:1340, 1970.

41. Scully R.E.: Ovarian tumors—a review. *Am. J. Pathol.* 87:686, 1977.

42. Smith J.Q., Rutledge F.: Advances in chemotherapy for gynecologic cancer. *Cancer* 36:669, 1975.

43. Serov S.F., Scully R.E., Sobin L.H.: Histologic typing of ovarian tumors, in *International Histologic Classification of Tumors No. 9.* Geneva, World Health Organization, 1973.

44. Tapper D., Lack E.E.: Teratomas in infancy and childhood. *Ann. Surg.* 198:398, 1983.

45. Teilum G.: Classification of endodermal sinus tumor (meloblastoma vitellinum) and so-called embryonal carcinoma of the ovary. *Acta. Pathol. Microbiol. Scand.* 64:407, 1965.

46. Thatcher D.: Ovarian cysts and tumors in children. *Surg. Gynecol. Obstet.* 117:477, 1963.

47. Thurlbeck W., Scully R.E.: Solid teratomas of the ovary—a clinicopathological analysis of 9 cases. *Cancer* 13:804, 1960.

48. Towne B.H., Mahour G.H., Woolley M.M., et al.: Ovarian cysts and tumors in infancy and childhood. *J. Pediatr. Surg.* 10:311, 1975.

49. Welch K.J.: Ovarian Cysts and Tumors, in Ravitch M., et al. (eds.): *Pediatric Surgery,* ed. 3. Chicago, Year Book Medical Publishers, 1979, p. 1437.

50. Weinblatt M.E., Ortega J.A.: Treatment of children with dysgerminoma of the ovary. *Cancer* 49:2608, 1982.

51. Wiltshaw E., Stuart-Harris R., Barker G.H., et al.: Chemotherapy of endodermal sinus tumor (yolk sac tumor) of the ovary: Preliminary communication. *J. R. Soc. Med.* 75:888, 1982.

52. Wollner N., Exelby P.R., Woodruff J.M., et al.: Malignant ovarian tumors in childhood. *Cancer* 37:1953, 1976.

53. Young R.C., Wharton J.T., Decker D.G., et al.: Staging laparotomy in early ovarian cancer. *J. Am. Soc. Clin. Oncol.* 20:399, 1979.

54. Young R.H., Scully R.E.: Ovarian sex cord-stromal tumors: Recent progress. *Int. J. Gynecol. Pathol.* 1:101, 1982.

55. Zaloudek C., Norris H.J.: Granulosa tumors of the ovary in children. *Am. J. Surg. Pathol.* 6:503, 1982.

---

138 PATRICIA K. DONAHOE / ALBERTO PENA
Abnormalities of the Female Genital Tract

VAGINAL ABNORMALITIES occur because of (1) isolated absence of the vagina, (2) cloacal or urogenital abnormalities, or (3) intersex disorders. Intersex problems are dealt with in Chapter 139.

Müllerian Embryology

The development of the müllerian duct—the anlage of the uterus, fallopian tubes, and upper vagina—occurs within the milieu of the developing hindgut and the urogenital ridge, which contain the gonadal and mesonephric structures. If the müllerian duct is to undergo regression, as occurs in the male, the gonad must differentiate as a testis. In the absence of a gonad or in the presence of an ovary, the müllerian ducts will develop autono-mously as an invagination of the coelomic epithelium. More caudally, the paired ducts form in close approximation to the wolffian or mesonephric duct, first as a cord of cells and then with a lumen, so close, in fact, that initially no basement membrane separates the one epithelium from the other.[10, 12–15] The growth vector is cephalad to caudad. Each end may, in fact, be influenced or induced separately. While it is clear that the cephalic portion of the duct invaginates from the coelomic epithelium, it is not certain whether the distal, or caudal, end migrates down from the newly formed tubular structure from above, or itself invaginates from the coelomic structures. It is known, however, that müllerian duct development cannot take place in the absence of the wolffian duct. Gruenwald[12] has shown that experimental interruption of the wolffian or mesonephric duct results in failure of müllerian duct development. As a result of these studies and many "experiments in nature," we have proposed that the mesonephros may act as an inducer of müllerian duct development.[5]

Koff[24] described the müllerian ducts conjoining and descending caudally to end in a hillock called the müllerian tubercle at the posterior wall of the urogenital sinus. Sinovaginal bulbs in the urogenital sinus fuse with the müllerian tubercle to form the vaginal plate, which then grossly enlarges and foreshortens the urogenital sinus. The widened vaginal plate tends to pull the urethra down toward the perineum;[37, 39] and both the urethra and vagina widen caudally and turn outward in an exstrophic, trumpet fashion to form the vestibule. As the fused müllerian ducts migrate caudally as the müllerian tubercle, the separating septum is lost; and the vaginal plate canalizes.[41] The demarcation between the lower vagina of urogenital origin and the upper vagina of müllerian origin is not clear. Ulfelder and Robboy[42, 43] propose that the müllerian duct fusion site at the vaginal plate descends caudally to the level of the future hymen, and that, subsequently, squamous cells from the urogenital sinus migrate upward and epithelialize over an indeterminate portion of the müllerian vagina.

The wolffian duct and the mesonephric system are seen at 4 weeks (3–5 mm)[31, 32] in the human embryo. The duct connects the mesonephros to the urogenital sinus and provides the anlagen for the vas, seminal vesicles, and epididymis. At 10 mm (5 weeks),[3, 24, 32] the müllerian duct begins to invaginate proximally and tubularize distally, guided by the wolffian duct. Fusion of the caudal end of the müllerian duct with the urogenital sinus occurs at about 30 mm (8 weeks)[24, 32] of development. Canalization of the vaginal plate occurs at the 150-mm (17 weeks)[24, 30] stage.

Fetal inducers, probably originating from mesenchymal sources, may play an important role in the normal development of the urogenital ridge and hindgut. The frequent coincidence of vaginal atresia and caudal regression anomalies, with pelvic kidneys and with renal agenesis, as well as vertebral anomalies, led us to suspect that a mesenchymal defect centering around the mesonephros may be a common denominator in all of these defects. We propose that the mesonephros and its duct are obligate

inducers for (1) metanephros development and ascent and (2) müllerian duct development.[5] The metanephric duct forms as an outpouching of the lower mesonephric duct, from which it ascends to meet the metanephric blastema, whose excretory duct it then provides. The kidney ectopically located in the pelvis has failed to undergo the normal course of embryonic ascent from its early position as the metanephric blastema, posterior and lateral to the urogenital sinus, where the mesonephros provides a scaffold for its ascent. The mesonephros, in addition, is critical to development of the müllerian duct (Fig 138–1). The wolffian or mesonephric duct appears to serve as a buttress for the müllerian duct.[2] If the wolffian duct does not form, the müllerian ducts may not invaginate and grow.

If mesonephric resorption occurs prematurely in the *male* (Fig 138–2), the resulting phenotype will have an absent kidney as well as associated absent or abnormal vas and epididymis. If mesonephric resorption occurs after the metanephric blastema and ureteric bud have appeared, epididymal and vas anomalies will occur; and the kidney, rather than being absent, will be in a pelvic position, because there is no mesonephros to provide the course for its ascent. If mesonephric and wolffian duct resorption occur early in the *female*, absence of the kidney and müllerian duct agenesis result. If mesonephric and wolffian duct agenesis occur later, i.e., after the ureteric bud has joined the metanephros, but before the müllerian duct development is complete at about 50 days, the kidney will be in the pelvis; and lower müllerian duct agenesis, i.e., vaginal atresia, will occur.

The importance of the early role of the mesonephros and the wolffian duct in müllerian duct formation and renal ascent may not be apparent in the female, because the wolffian duct eventually resorbs. The pivotal role of the wolffian duct in the male also may not be apparent, because abnormalities are not appreciated unless they are bilateral and cause infertility. The association of vaginal atresia with renal agenesis or pelvic kidney can be explained by this as yet-unproved hypothesis. The association of vertebral anomalies supports the concept of an obligate mesenchymal inducer. Grobstein[11] demonstrated that the dorsal spine, for example, can act as an in vitro inducer, causing isolated metanephric mesenchyme to differentiate in tubular form. Maizels and Stephens,[25] in a series of elegant chick embryo experiments, created vertebral anomalies at an early stage of em-

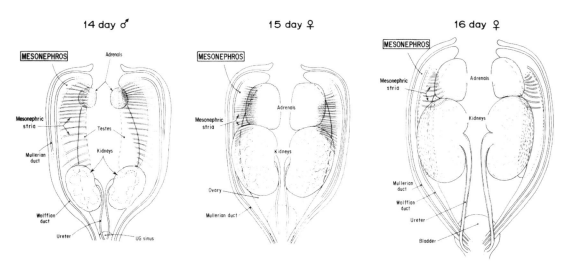

14 day ♂   15 day ♀   16 day ♀

Fig 138–1.—The mesonephros is a posterior structure that provides a retroperitoneal backing for the adrenal superiorly, gonad and the müllerian and wolffian ducts laterally, and the kidney inferiorly. Its extent is seen in the 14-day rat embryo, two thirds of the way through gestation, before renal ascent accelerates. The mesonephros resorbs as the kidney ascends and differentiates, as seen in the 15-day and the 16-day rat embryos. We propose that the mesonephros serves as an obligate inducer (1) to renal differentiation and ascent and (2) to the paramesonephric duct, either through or in conjunction with the mesonephric duct. (From Donahoe P.K., Hendren W.H.[5] Used by permission.)

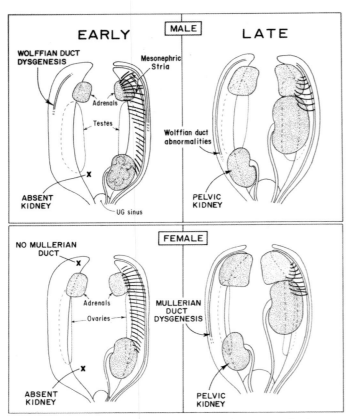

Fig 138–2.—If, in the *male*, mesonephric resorption occurs earlier than normal, renal agenesis and wolffian agenesis will occur. Later resorption can lead to pelvic kidney with less severe wolffian anomalies. Early resorption in the *female* leads to renal agenesis and müllerian duct atresia. Later resorption in the female can cause pelvic kidney and vaginal atresia. (From Donahoe P.K., Hendren W.H.[5] Used by permission.)

bryonic development; the surviving chicks developed not only kidney and ureteric anomalies characterized by ectopia, agenesis, or hypoplasia, but also had arrested caudal growth of the müllerian duct. Similar relationships have been seen in a strain of tailless mice with absent kidneys.[9] The developmental anomalies of the urinary tract, skeleton, and genital tract may be related by a common mesenchymal defect.[10]

Embryology of Cloacal and Urogenital Defects

Urogenital sinus and cloacal abnormalities, including cloacal exstrophy, fall into the category of hindgut anomalies or caudal regression syndromes,[6] presenting as a wide variety of vaginal, bladder, kidney, and rectal anomalies. In urogenital sinus anomalies, the vagina and the urethra are conjoined. In cloacal anomalies, the urethra, vagina, and rectum are conjoined. The formation of a *cloaca* may result from failure of descent of the urorectal septum, a mesenchymal mass that migrates between the urogenital sinus and the rectum. Mesenchyme apparently is needed to induce descent and to support development of the epithelium-lined structures, partition of which is complete by 16 mm (6 weeks). If mesenchyme does not provide a support between the epithelial layers for future induction, they break down. If the müllerian ducts do not fuse to form the müllerian tubercle, the vaginal plate does not form and join with the sinovaginal bulbs, and the vagina will not migrate down to and open on the perineum.[41] Thus, the urogenital sinus remains a long, narrow tube.[38] Arrest of migration of the müllerian tubercles to

the vestibule may occur at any stage, to produce the complex of *urogenital sinus* defects.[17, 18, 21, 22] *Cloacal exstrophy*, the most severe hindgut anomaly, occurs as a result of (1) failure of migration of the urorectal septum and (2) failure of migration of mesenchymal elements between the anterior abdominal wall and the bladder, resulting in exstrophy of the bladder with fusion of the cecum in the posterior midwall of the bladder. The approximation of abdominal wall skin and bladder epithelium breaks down without mesenchymal support. Because the mesenchymal defects occur so early, there are many associated cardiovascular, CNS, and respiratory abnormalities. Some cases of müllerian aplasia and dysgenesis are compatible with recessive inheritance.[1] An example is Winter's syndrome of middle ear anomalies, renal and vaginal agenesis.[45] Transverse vaginal septum can also have autosomal recessive inheritance in certain cases,[27, 28] and at least one heritable form is associated with polydactyly.[23] The dominant inheritance of a longitudinal vaginal septum has been associated with hand anomalies.[7]

Vaginal Atresia

Less severe forms of vaginal atresia or simple obstruction can occur because of imperforate hymen or a low transverse septum. The defect also may be unilateral,[36, 46] resulting from incomplete resorption or failure of fusion of the medial walls of the müllerian ducts, which produces a blind uterine horn. Vaginal atresia itself may be *complete*, *proximal*, or *distal*. All müllerian structures may regress and be absent if Müllerian Inhibiting Substance is secreted from a testis (46 XY), as in patients with male pseudohermaphrodism caused by androgen receptor abnormalities. When the *complete* müllerian atresia is due to some mesenchymal defect, it results in failure of the müllerian ducts to reach the urogenital sinus. The more cephalad Fallopian tubes may appear normal, but the proximal and bicornuate uterus is rudimentary. The ovaries are invariably normal. *Proximal* vaginal atresia is thought to result[38] from müllerian ducts that do not fuse to form the müllerian tubercle. In these cases, the uterus and tubes are normal, but the cervix is abnormal. If the sinovaginal bulbs do not proliferate, *distal* vaginal atresia results, with normal proximal cervix, uterus, and Fallopian tubes.

Diagnosis and Surgical Repair

Patients with vaginal atresia usually have a normal female 46 XX karyotype and a buccal smear that tests positive for chromatin bodies. Hydrocolpos, or hydrometrocolpos, may occur early in life if the vagina, or the vagina and uterus, fill with mucinous secretions because of maternal estrogen stimulation of uterine and vaginal glands. At menarche, hematocolpos or hematometrocolpos can occur dramatically when the obstructed vagina is filled with menstrual discharge. Either can present as a large abdominal mass that displaces the bladder and the rectum. If vaginal atresia is distal, and proximal müllerian structures are normal, cyclic abdominal pain will occur at menarche, with an enlarging abdominal mass. If cyclic pain is absent, then agenesis of both vagina and uterus is likely. In such cases, ultrasound is diagnostic and avoids unnecessary laparotomy. Intravenous pyelograms (IVP) may show kidney abnormalities such as atresia, ectopia, or hypoplasia or ureteral displacement resulting from a distended vagina. Vertebral anomalies, including scoliosis, duplications, or agenesis must be sought. Voiding cystourethrogram and cystoscopy will show displacement and, in some cases, may reveal an elongated "urogenital sinus" urethra, with anterior angulation. Laparoscopy might be helpful. Laparotomy may be needed to evacuate a hematometrocolpos that cannot be reached from below, and to mobilize a dilated vagina from above to reach perineal flaps.[44]

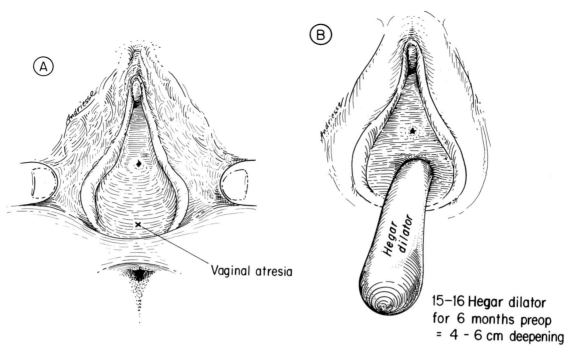

Fig 138–3.—Vaginal atresia. **A,** appearance of perineum of patient with vaginal atresia. The introitus may be flat or slightly deeper. **B,** Hegar dilators, daily applied with pressure for 6 months prior to repair, deepen, and toughen the introitus. *(Continued.)*

Vaginal Reconstruction

SEPTUM.—The perineal approach can be used to correct a low transverse septum or an imperforate hymen. These can be easily excised and the raw edges of vaginal mucosa oversewn.

AGENESIS.—Surgical repair of true vaginal atresia is more complex. Because the lower vagina derives from the urogenital sinus, an introitus (Fig 138–3,A) may be present and should be incorporated into the vaginal reconstruction. We often begin a dilatation program after menarche, when endogenous estrogens have toughened the introitus, to prepare the patient for vaginal reconstruction. Selection for dilatation depends upon the patient's readiness. Preservation of the hormonally responsive introital skin, we believe, is important to insure function that is satisfying and not unpleasant for the patient. The vaginal introitus may be shallow or as deep as 5 cm. We use a Hegar dilator (Fig 138–3,B) and progress to a Young's dilator to increase the diameter of the vaginal opening. In some cases, as Frank[8] has suggested, dilatations will provide an adequate depth and width of vagina, without additional intervention. Even if the dilatation program does not provide adequate depth, a natural introitus is created.

The commonly used "McIndoe technique"[26] creates a neovagina using a split-thickness skin graft. The entire lower body is prepared for the operative field and draped so that the perineum can be opened and the buttock exposed. It is important to prepare the patient carefully with a full-bowel clean-out for several days prior to the procedure, both to avoid contamination by stool during the procedure and to delay bowel movement during the early phases of healing. The bladder is catheterized and a finger placed in the rectum to avoid the serious complications of rectovesical or rectovaginal fistula. The perineum is entered through a transverse incision between the urethral orifice and the rectum (Fig 138–3,C). A plane can be readily developed by blunt dissection between the rectum and the urethra to achieve a depth of 12 cm. Care, of course, must be taken not to enter either the rectum posteriorly or the urethra and bladder anteriorly. Absolute hemostasis must be achieved to permit the split-thickness skin graft to adhere to the surrounding tissues.

A pack is then placed in the new tunnel and the patient turned over for the skin graft. We prefer to use the Reese dermatome to harvest one or two full skin patches of 18/1,000-in. thickness. These are then fashioned over a soft inflatable Heyer-Schulte vaginal prosthesis (Fig 138–3,D). The proximal end of the prosthesis is left open and drained to the outside by an internal catheter. The degree and security of inflation must be tested under water prior to use of the prosthesis, and again after the graft has been loosely sutured over the prosthesis. The optimal degree of inflation is chosen, and the integrity of the ball valve is again tested. The buttock wound is dressed and the patient turned back into the lithotomy position for placement (Fig 138–3,E) of the prosthesis in the previously created perineal vault, which by this time should be dry. Heavy nylon sutures are used to close the labia minora and majora over the inserted prosthesis. The prosthesis is then inflated to the previously selected pressure and the ball valve fixed in place to prevent leak (Fig 138–3,F). After 7–10 days of bed rest, the prosthesis is removed, the skin graft loosely sutured (Fig 138–3,G) to the previously stretched introitus, and the new vault irrigated. Use of the soft prosthesis avoids pressure on the urethra and reduces the risk of a urethrovaginal fistula.

Postoperatively, the patient is asked to insert a mold at night, first using the soft inflatable mold and later a firmer model, to prevent foreshortening of the graft until sexual activity can provide natural dilatation. Long-term results have indicated satisfaction with the procedure.[40] Severely masculinized patients with male pseudohermaphroditism will have a flat perineum. In these cases, U-flaps can be raised, in two or even four quadrants on the perineum, and turned in to meet the skin graft neovagina. Some surgeons prefer to use a colon segment as a neovagina, because the colon provides its own lubrication and does not re-

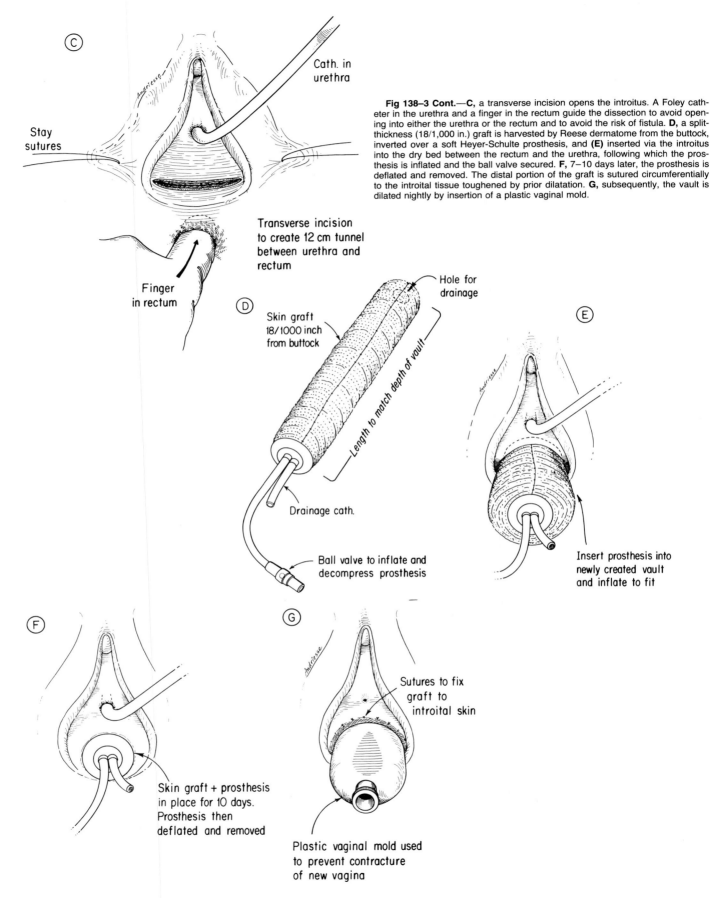

C

Cath. in urethra

Stay sutures

Fig 138–3 Cont.—C, a transverse incision opens the introitus. A Foley catheter in the urethra and a finger in the rectum guide the dissection to avoid opening into either the urethra or the rectum and to avoid the risk of fistula. **D,** a split-thickness (18/1,000 in.) graft is harvested by Reese dermatome from the buttock, inverted over a soft Heyer-Schulte prosthesis, and **(E)** inserted via the introitus into the dry bed between the rectum and the urethra, following which the prosthesis is inflated and the ball valve secured. **F,** 7–10 days later, the prosthesis is deflated and removed. The distal portion of the graft is sutured circumferentially to the introital tissue toughened by prior dilatation. **G,** subsequently, the vault is dilated nightly by insertion of a plastic vaginal mold.

Transverse incision to create 12 cm tunnel between urethra and rectum

Finger in rectum

D

Hole for drainage

Skin graft 18/1000 inch from buttock

Length to match depth of vault

Drainage cath.

Ball valve to inflate and decompress prosthesis

E

Insert prosthesis into newly created vault and inflate to fit

F

Skin graft + prosthesis in place for 10 days. Prosthesis then deflated and removed

G

Sutures to fix graft to introital skin

Plastic vaginal mold used to prevent contracture of new vagina

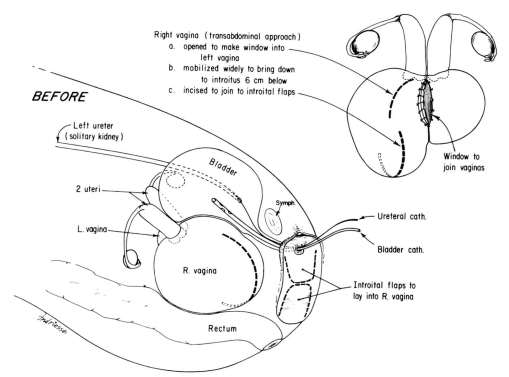

Fig 138–4.—A case of vaginal atresia with two vaginas with hydrometrocolpos, managed by abdominoperineal pull-through after tubularization of the dilated vagina. Perineal flaps were also used. (From Hendren W.H., Donahoe P.K.: *J. Pediatr. Surg.* 15:751–763, 1980. Used by permission.)

quire dilatation; but this, of course, requires an abdominal approach.[35] In the event of a hematometrocolpos, the extensively dilated vagina can be used if necessary to create tubularized flaps that can be brought down to the perineum (Fig 138–4). It is important to note that the vagina is often septate, and the septum must be removed.[22]

Urogenital Sinus Defects

The urogenital sinus deformity occurs in 46 XX females when the urethra and vagina are conjoined but the rectum is separate and has reached the perineum. High confluence of these structures can be associated with other severe genitourinary anomalies and often results in dribbling incontinence. The uterus is often bicornuate. The anomaly, resulting from a failure of fusion of the müllerian ducts as they form the müllerian tubercle and the vaginal plate, takes place after the urorectal septum has descended to separate the rectum from the urogenital sinus. Vaginal plate formation and downward migration halting at various stages can result in a wide variety of urogenital sinus defects. The techniques chosen to repair these anomalies depend upon the level at which the structures join and upon the related anomalies. If the child is continent, flaps from the perineum can be mobilized to meet a high vagina. If the patient is incontinent, urethral lengthening must be performed using a portion of the vagina to create the neourethra. Under these circumstances, tissue for mobilization is often limited. Progress in the care of these patients was made with Hendren's introduction of the buttock flap, which can be created with the patient in the prone or "sky diver" position.[19, 20, 29] The legs are suspended, with the patient prone and supported beneath the pubis to avoid hyperextending the lumbar spine (Fig 138–5,A). A lateral relaxing incision across the labia minora and majora may be done at four or eight o'clock

to facilitate exposure of the introitus. A mucosal incision is made around the bladder or urethral opening into the vagina, and extended caudally (Fig 138–5,B and C) so that the neourethra is constructed from tissue of the vaginal wall in two layers (Fig 138–5,D). The flap of vagina should be several centimeters lateral and cephalad to the urethral tube closure to prevent stricture of the tube and formation of a fistula. A broad-based full-thickness anteriorly based buttock and perineal skin flap (Fig 138–5,E) is then swung into the vagina through the labial relaxing incisions to cover the two-layer closure used to lengthen the urethra (Fig 138–5,F). The buttock flap must be both sufficiently long and broad at its base to insure good blood supply. A catheter stent should be left in the neourethra for about 2 weeks. Two months later, the flap can be divided from its base, and the labia can be reapproximated to give a more normal perineal appearance (Fig 138–5,G). These techniques have for the first time afforded consistent success in the repair of these previously frustrating lesions.[17, 18, 21]

Vaginal Atresia Associated with Cloacal Deformity

Patients with cloacal deformities have a single opening on the anterior perineum (Fig 138–6); i.e., there is no separate external vaginal or rectal opening. The labia are flat, and a small phallic structure is present with a small opening at its base. Although the karyotype may be 46 XX or 46 XY, the sex of rearing depends solely on the size of the phallus. If inadequate, the 46 XY child should be raised as a female. If near normal, sex-rearing should be concordant with the karyotype. In the female, an abdominal mass may develop if the vaginal orifice is partially obstructed and the vagina collects either backwash of urine or secretions resulting from stimulation by maternal hormones.

The combination of arrest of descent of the urorectal septum

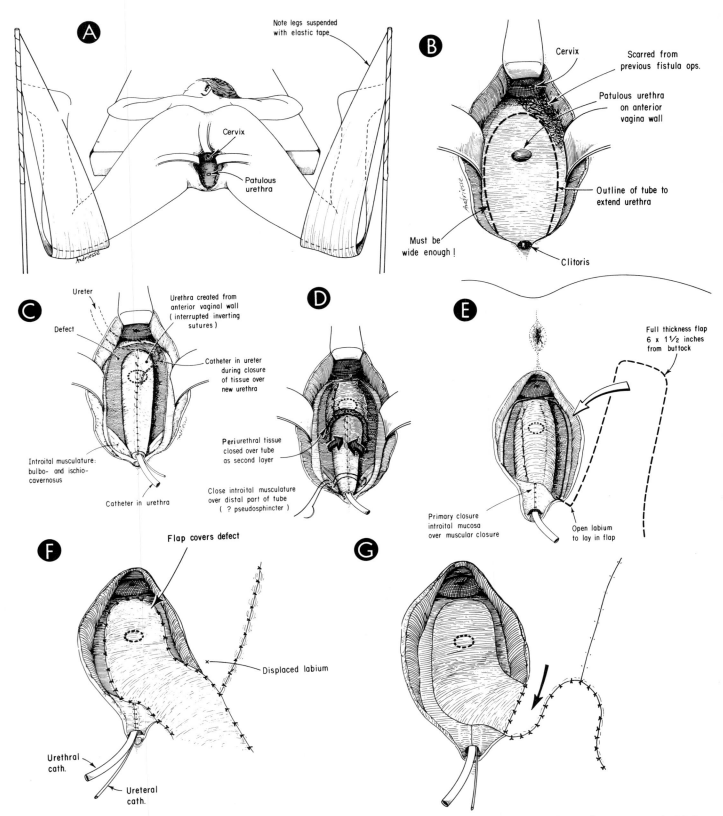

Fig 138–5.—Urogenital sinus repair. The distal urethra is created from the anterior vaginal wall and covered with a buttock flap. **A,** the patient is placed in the "sky diver" or prone position to facilitate access; the labia may be opened at 4 or 8 o'clock to facilitate exposure and for later swinging in the buttock flap. **B,** a U-flap outlined on the anterior vagina wall generously circumscribes the urethral orifice. **C,** the mobilized flap is rolled around the bladder catheter. **D,** peri- urethral and introital tissue provide a second layer of coverage over the tubularized neourethra, but this is usually not adequate to prevent fistula formation. **E,** a broad, appropriately thick, anteriorly based flap is outlined on the perineum and swung in through the opened labia to **(F)** cover the newly tubularized urethra and the vaginal wall. **G,** the pedicle is later (>2–3 weeks) divided, and the labia repaired. (From Hendren W.H.[20] Used by permission.)

1358

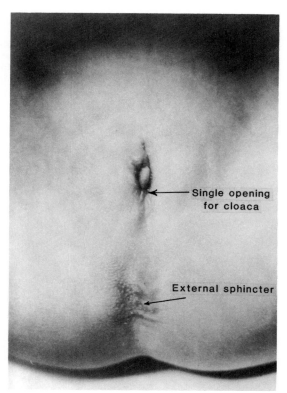

Fig 138–6.—Appearance of the perineum of a patient with a cloacal deformity. A single opening, flat labia, and a dimple marking the midpoint of the external rectal sphincter are characteristic.

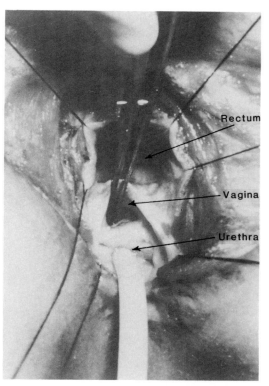

Fig 138–8.—View of the cloaca opened via the posterior sagittal approach. The Foley catheter is in the urethra; the forceps are in the vagina. The opening above is the rectum.

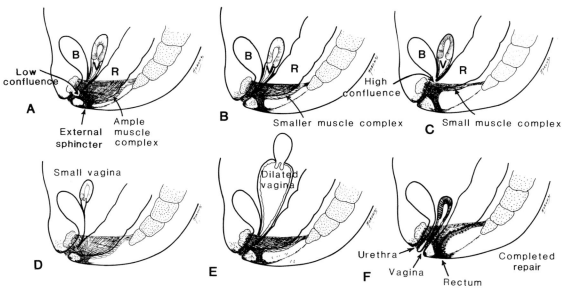

Fig 138–7.—Cloacal defect. **A,** low cloacal defect. The muscle complex is ample. **B,** intermediate defect. The muscle complex is located higher above the external sphincter. The rectum joins the urethra higher. **C,** high defect. The external sphincter and muscle complex are narrow, and the latter joins the levator very high. A good deal of tapering will have to be done to bring the rectum through the center of the muscle complex and posteriorly angulated external sphincter. **D,** the rare variant of the small high vagina. A segment of colon may be needed to connect the vagina to the exterior. **E,** the obstructed vagina can become markedly dilated. This, however, provides ample vaginal tissue to meet the perineum. **F,** completed repair showing the tubularized urethra, vagina, and rectum. The rectum courses through the center of the muscle complex and external sphincter, while the vagina exits anterior to the external sphincter, but within the levator.

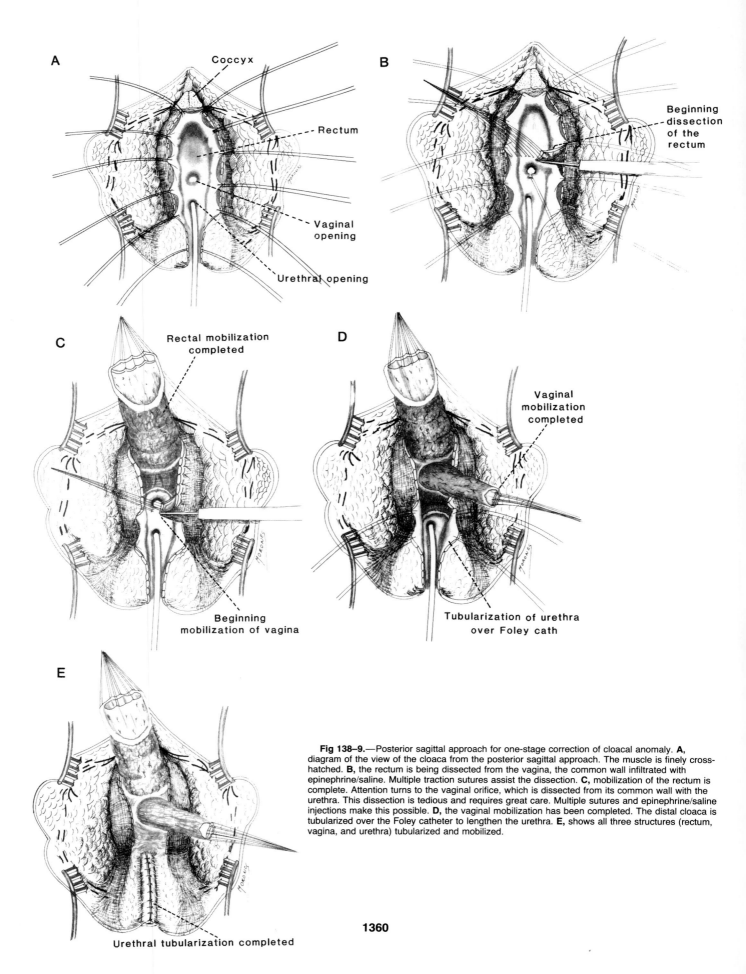

A Coccyx

Rectum

Vaginal opening

Urethral opening

B Beginning dissection of the rectum

C Rectal mobilization completed

Beginning mobilization of vagina

D Vaginal mobilization completed

Tubularization of urethra over Foley cath

E Urethral tubularization completed

Fig 138–9.—Posterior sagittal approach for one-stage correction of cloacal anomaly. **A,** diagram of the view of the cloaca from the posterior sagittal approach. The muscle is finely cross-hatched. **B,** the rectum is being dissected from the vagina, the common wall infiltrated with epinephrine/saline. Multiple traction sutures assist the dissection. **C,** mobilization of the rectum is complete. Attention turns to the vaginal orifice, which is dissected from its common wall with the urethra. This dissection is tedious and requires great care. Multiple sutures and epinephrine/saline injections make this possible. **D,** the vaginal mobilization has been completed. The distal cloaca is tubularized over the Foley catheter to lengthen the urethra. **E,** shows all three structures (rectum, vagina, and urethra) tubularized and mobilized.

and failure of fusion of the müllerian ducts at the müllerian tubercle leads to this complex anomaly. The five major types described by Raffensperger and Ramenofsky,[37, 39] indicate the broad spectrum of these abnormalities, depicted in Figure 138–7. The severity of the anomaly depends upon the height of the conjoined fistula above the perineum, i.e., more proximal lesions (see Fig 138–7,*C*) are more severe than the more distal lesions (see Fig 138–7,*A* and *B*). These children have been operated on at birth by the methods of Ramenofsky and Raffensperger[37, 39] to take advantage of the enlarged vagina (see Fig 138–7,*E*). The vagina is entered transabdominally, and the vagina and rectum are both separated from the urogenital sinus and pulled through to the perineum. We prefer to treat these infants first with a divided sigmoid colostomy, at a level sufficiently proximal to allow mobilization of the rectum down to the perineum. More recently, we have repaired the three defects simultaneously, using the posterior sagittal approach (see Fig 138–7,*F*).[4, 33, 34]

Definitive operation is performed when the patient weighs 8 kg if other major associated malformations do not interfere. Cystoscopy helps to define the anatomy, as does a careful retrograde sinogram and a prograde distal colostomy cologram. The skin is prepared circumferentially from the nipples down, and the infant placed on a sterile field to allow sacral, perineal, and abdominal approaches. Introduction of a Foley catheter is not attempted, because it is often difficult to enter the bladder as a result of severe anterior urethral angulation. An electrical transcutaneous stimulator defines the external sphincter (Fig 138–6). The point of maximum contraction marks the center of the external sphincter while the cephalic component pulls the anal dimple upward along the midline to the coccyx, deepening the midline intergluteal groove.

A midline skin incision is carried from the midsacrum down the cloacal orifice (Fig 138–8). It is important to observe symmetric contractions. Herniation of fat through the thin sagittal fascia signals departure of the dissection from the midline. One must carefully define the center of the external sphincter and the more proximal muscle complex and levator ani, and then cut carefully through all of the muscles, posteriorly and anteriorly, to reach the anterior cloacal orifice. The size of the entire muscle tract determines the extent of bowel tapering that is necessary to provide an appropriate fit in the muscle funnel (see Fig 138–7,*A*,*B*, and *C*). It is generally true that the higher the malformation, the narrower the muscular funnel; the lower the malformation, the wider the funnel with more foreshortening of the muscle complex.

The coccyx is split, the cloaca opened posteriorly in the midline. Only then is a Foley catheter inserted into the urethral opening (Fig 138–9,*A*). Separation of the rectum from the vagina is tedious and difficult (Fig 138–10,*B*). Numerous 6-0 silk sutures are placed in the mucosa of the conjoined anterior rectal wall. A plane of dissection is established by injecting epinephrine/saline 1/100,000. The rectal mucosa is carefully dissected from the common wall (see Fig 138–9,*B*) it shares with the vagina. After the common wall has been passed (1–4 cm), the rectum can be mobilized anteriorly. A series of longitudinal creases, thicker than the proximal bowel, resembling the pectinate line, and containing smooth muscle layers may represent an internal sphincter. All attempts are made to preserve this very distal portion of the bowel as it joins the cloaca. To mobilize sufficient length to deliver the rectum to the perineum, circumferential branches of the hemorrhoidal vessels must be divided. This dissection must often be carried as high as the peritoneal reflection and, in some cases, even higher.

The next step entails separation of the vagina and the urethra. Again, a number of traction sutures are placed in the mucosa of the vaginal orifice as it communicates with the urethra (see Fig

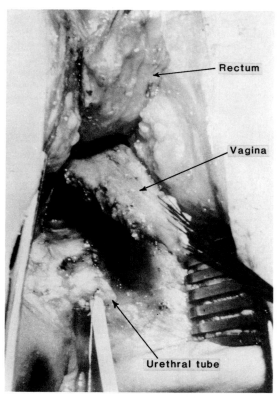

Fig 138–10.—Rectum, vagina, and urethra have been tubularized and mobilized. The extent of trimming of the rectum is determined by the size of the muscle complex. Creation of perineal flaps may be required to externalize the vagina.

138–9,*C*), allowing submucosal dissection and separation from the common wall between the vagina and urethra. After separation from the common wall, the vagina must be sufficiently mobilized above to gain enough length to reach the perineal skin. Occasionally, perineal flaps must be created to reach the vagina, or a dilated vagina can be tubularized to reach the perineum.[4, 33, 34] The urethra is then rolled over the Foley catheter using a U-flap from the wall of the cloaca to provide an adequate lumen (see Fig 138–9,*D* and *E*). A second layer is provided by periurethral tissue, which is closed over the tubularized neourethra. One must then estimate and tailor both the width and the length of the vagina and rectum (see Fig 138–10). Close to the posterior urethra, the bowel may angulate as much as 90 degrees posteriorly to follow the muscle tract represented by the levator muscle complex and the external sphincter (see Fig 138–7,*F*). The vagina must be in front of the complex to reach the perineum, and the rectum must go through the exact center of the external sphincter and muscle complex, which is then sutured to the outside of the bowel and vagina to prevent prolapse. The vagina is brought out, the anterior portions of the external sphincter and muscle complex are sutured, the bowel is laid in, and the posterior portions of the muscle are closed. Electrical stimulation assists accurate placement. In the event that a very small vagina cannot be mobilized sufficiently to reach the perineum, an extrapolated segment of colon[16] can be brought down to bridge the gap between the vagina and the perineum.[21] This segment must also be tapered to fit anterior to the sphincter complex. Mesentery can provide a welcome tissue barrier between the suture line of the tubularized urethra and the neovagina.

Two weeks after operation, the anus is calibrated and the

Foley catheter removed. After 3 weeks, rectal dilatations can begin. If a suprapubic cystostomy has been placed, a clamping schedule can begin. The colostomy can be closed in about 3 months if dilatations are progressing well. The younger the child, the easier the dilatations.

Nineteen cases have been operated on for cloacal abnormalities by this posterior sagittal approach. Nine who have undergone closure of colostomy and are old enough were evaluated for fecal continence. Excellent results, i.e., toilet-trained with no soiling, have been achieved in five; good results, i.e., children younger than 3 years having one to two bowel movements per day with no soiling, in two. Two others are still soiling and await reevaluation.

REFERENCES

1. Bercu B.B., Donahoe P.K., Schulman J.D.: Clinical implications of Müllerian duct anomalies. *Contemp. Obstet. Gynecol.* 16:145, 1980.
2. Boyden E.: Experimental obstruction of the mesonephric ducts. *Proc. Soc. Exp. Biol. Med.* 24:572, 1927.
3. Davis J., Kusama H.: Developmental aspects of the human cervix. *Ann. N.Y. Acad. Sci.* 97:534–550, 1962.
4. deVries P., Pena A.: Posterior sagittal anorectoplasty. *J. Pediatr. Surg.* 17:638–643, 1982.
5. Donahoe P.K., Hendren W.H.: Pelvic kidney in infants and children: Experience with 16 cases. *J. Pediatr. Surg.* 15:486–495, 1980.
6. Duhamal B.: From the mermaid to anal imperforation: The syndrome of caudal regression. *Arch. Dis. Child.* 36:152–155, 1961.
7. Edwards J.A., Gale R.F.: Camptobrachydactyly: A new autosomal dominant trait with two probable homozygotes. *Am. J. Hum. Genet.* 24:464–474, 1972.
8. Frank R.T.: The formation of an artificial vagina without operation. *Am. J. Obstet. Gynecol.* 35:1053–1055, 1938.
9. Gluechsohn-Schoenheimer S.: Causal analysis of mouse development by the study of mutational effects. *Growth* (suppl.) 9:163–176, 1949.
10. Griffin J.E., Edwards C., Madden J.D., et al.: Congenital absence of the vagina: The Mayer-Rokitansky-Kuster-Hauser syndrome. *Ann. Intern. Med.* 85:224–236, 1976.
11. Grobstein C.: Transfilter section of tubules in mouse metanephrogenic mesenchyme. *Exp. Cell Res.* 10:424–440, 1956.
12. Gruenwald P.: The relation of the growing Müllerian duct to the Wolffian duct and its importance for the genesis of malformations. *Anat. Rec.* 81:1–19, 1941.
13. Gruenwald P.: Developmental basis of regenerative and pathologic growth in the uterus. *Arch. Pathol.* 35:53–65, 1943.
14. Gruenwald P.: Mechanisms of abnormal development: II. Embryonic development of malformations. *Arch. Pathol.* 44:495–543, 1947.
15. Gruenwald P.: Growth and development of the uterus: The relationship of epithelium of mesenchyme. *Ann. N.Y. Acad. Sci.* 75:436–440, 1959.
16. Harrison M., Glick P., Nakayama D., et al.: Loop colon rectovaginoplasty for high cloacal anomaly. *J. Pediatr. Surg.* 18:885–886, 1983.
17. Hendren W.H.: Surgical management of urogenital sinus abnormalities. *J. Pediatr. Surg.* 12:339–357, 1977.
18. Hendren W.H.: Urogenital sinus and anorectal malformations: Experience with 22 cases. *J. Pediatr. Surg.* 15:628–641, 1980.
19. Hendren W.H.: Reconstructive problems of the vagina and the female urethra. *Clin. Plast. Surg.* 7:207–234, 1980.
20. Hendren W.H.: Construction of female urethra from vaginal wall and perineal flap. *J. Urol.* 123:657–664, 1980.
21. Hendren W.H.: Further experience in reconstructive surgery for cloacal anomalies. *J. Pediatr. Surg.* 17:695–717, 1982.
22. Hendren W.H., Donahoe P.K.: Correction of congenital abnormalities of the vagina and perineum. *J. Pediatr. Surg.* 15:751–763, 1980.
23. Kaufman R.L., Hartmann A.F., McAlister W.H.: Family studies in congenital heart disease: II. A syndrome of hydrometrocolpos, postaxial polydactyly and congenital heart disease. *Birth Defects* 8:85–87, 1972.
24. Koff A.: Development of the vagina and the human fetus. *Contrib. Embryol.* 140:61–90, 1933.
25. Maizels M., Stephens F.D.: The induction of urological malformations: Understanding the relationship of renal ectopia and congenital scoliosis. *Invest. Urol.* 17:209–217, 1979.
26. McIndoe A.: Treatment of congenital absences and obliterative conditions of the vagina. *Br. J. Plast. Surg.* 2:254–267, 1950.
27. McKusick V.A., Bauer R.L., Koop C.E., et al.: Hydrometrocolpos as a simple inherited malformation. *J. Am. Med. Assoc.* 189:813–816, 1964.
28. McKusick V.A., Weibalcher R.G., Gragg G.W.: Recessive inheritance of a congenital malformation syndrome. *JAMA* 204:113–118, 1968.
29. Mitchell M., Hensle T., Crooks K.: Urethral reconstruction of the young female using a perineal pedicle flap. *J. Pediatr. Surg.* 17:687–694, 1982.
30. O'Rahilly R.: The embryology and anatomy of the uterus, in *The Uterus.* Baltimore, Wilkins & Wilkins Co., 1973, p. 17.
31. O'Rahilly R., Muecke E.C.: The timing and sequence of events in the development of the human urinary system during the embryonic period proper. *Z. Anat. Entwickl-Gesch.* 138:99–109, 1972.
32. O'Rahilly R.: Prenatal human development, in Wynn R.M. (ed.): *Biology of the Uterus.* New York, Plenum Press, 1977, p. 35.
33. Pena A.: Posterior sagittal anorectoplasty as a secondary operation for the treatment of fecal incontinence. *J. Pediatr. Surg.* 18:762–773, 1983.
34. Pena A., deVries P.: Posterior sagittal anorectoplasty: Important technical considerations and new applications. *J. Pediatr. Surg.* 17:796–811, 1982.
35. Pratt J., Smith G.: Vaginal reconstruction with sigmoid loop. *Am. J. Obstet. Gynecol.* 96:31–40, 1966.
36. Radhakrishnan J., Reyes H.: Unilateral renal agenesis with hematometrocolpos: Report of two cases. *J. Pediatr. Surg.* 17:749–750, 1982.
37. Raffensperger J., Ramenofsky M.: The management of a cloaca. *J. Pediatr. Surg.* 8:647–657, 1973.
38. Ramenofsky M.: Vaginal lesions, in Holder T., Ashcraft K. (eds.): *Pediatric Surgery.* Philadelphia, W. B. Saunders Co., 1980, pp. 891–908.
39. Ramenofsky M.L., Raffensperger J.G.: An abdomino-perineal-vaginal pull-through for definitive treatment of hydrometrocolpos. *J. Pediatr. Surg.* 6:381–387, 1971.
40. Salvatore C., Lodovicci O.: Vaginal agenesis: An analysis of 90 cases. *Acta Obstet. Gynecol. Scand.* 57:89–94, 1978.
41. Stephens F.D.: *Congenital Malformations of the Urinary Tract.* New York, Praeger Publishers, 1983.
42. Ulfelder H.: Agenesis of the vagina. *Am. J. Obstet. Gynecol.* 100:745–751, 1968.
43. Ulfelder H., Robboy S.J.: The embryonic development of the human vagina. *Am. J. Obstet. Gynecol.* 126:769–776, 1976.
44. Welch K.J.: Abnormalities and neoplasms of the vagina and uterus, in Ravitch M.M., Welch K.J., Benson C.D. (eds.): *Pediatric Surgery,* ed. 3. Chicago, Year Book Medical Publishers, 1979, pp. 1452–1464.
45. Winter J.D., Kohn G., Mellinan W.J., et al.: A familial syndrome of renal, genital, and middle ear anomalies. *J. Pediatr.* 72:88–93, 1968.
46. Yoder I.C., Pfister R.C.: Unilateral hematocolpos and ipsilateral renal agenesis: Report of two cases and review of the literature. *Am. J. Roentgenol.* 127:303–308, 1976.

139

PATRICIA K. DONAHOE / JOHN D. CRAWFORD

Ambiguous Genitalia in the Newborn

THE INFANT with ambiguous genitalia must be dealt with expeditiously so that gender assignment appropriate to the anatomy of the infant can be made. "Is it a boy or a girl?" is often the first question asked of new parents. They must be able to give an answer that is commensurate with the most satisfying eventual functional result for the child. Gender assignment and surgical correction must be done as early as possible to assure unambiguous bonding between the parents and the child and to allow the child to develop a body image that will lead to self-esteem. The complexity of intersex disorders has often overwhelmed physicians. The object here is to present an orderly approach to patients with ambiguous genitalia, stressing the logic leading to diagnosis, surgical correction, and long-term care. The major categories of causes for gender ambiguities at birth, the diagnostic maneuvers necessary to differentiate them, and the causes speculated or established for each are shown in Fig 139–1.

Initial Evaluation and Gender Assignment

Four major categories of abnormality can cause gender confusion at birth: *female pseudohermaphroditism, male pseudohermaphroditism, true hermaphroditism,* and *mixed gonadal dysgenesis.* Problems of genital development that present later in life, when gender is already fixed, will not be discussed. Using two criteria, gonadal symmetry and cytology (chromatin mass and/or Y fluorescent staining), one can establish a working diagnosis of one of the four categories with 90% accuracy before the results of other diagnostic measures have returned (Fig 139–2). Symmetry refers to the position of one gonad relative to the other, above or below the external inguinal ring. Both gonads will be symmetrically placed, either above or below the inguinal ring, if the etiologic influence causing the abnormality is applied equally to both sides. Gonadal symmetry occurs in the androgenized female with female pseudohermaphroditism, and in the incompletely virilized male with male pseudohermaphroditism. Asymmetry will occur if one gonad has differentiated predominantly as a testis and the other as an ovary, as in mixed gonadal dysgenesis or true hermaphroditism.

With these criteria, one can make a preliminary diagnosis in the first 24 hours of life with a high degree of accuracy. Genetic females recognized in the neonatal period should be reared as females, no matter how severely virilized. In genetic males, the gender assignment must be based on the infant's anatomy, that is, the size of the phallus, and not on the karyotype; 46 XY does not ensure proper functioning as a male. If the phallus is inadequate, it will be unwise to rear the child as a male; and one should recommend assignment to the female gender. The average penile length for a 30-week gestation male is 2.5 ± 0.4 cm, and of the 34-week gestation male, 3.0 ± 0.4 cm.[36, 109] The average phallic size of a term infant is 3.5 ± 0.4 cm.[39] A penis 2½ standard deviations below the mean measures 1.5 cm in the 30-week premature, 2.0 cm in the 34-week premature, and 2.5 cm in the term infant.[59, 62] It is important that these measurements be made along the dorsum, from the pubic symphysis to the tip of the stretched glans. In the presence of severe chordee, two

additive measurements must be made. The average penile diameter of the full-term male is 1–1.5 cm. We become concerned if the length and width measurements fall below 2 cm × 0.9 cm, and alarmed if below 1.5 × 0.7 cm. A thin phallus that is also less than 1.5 cm in length would cause us to recommend female gender assignment, particularly if the remainder of the findings, i.e., dysgenetic gonads as in mixed gonadal dysgenesis, or defective androgen receptors as in male pseudohermaphroditism, support this decision. Exception must always be made if the patient presents late and has become firmly committed to one or the other gender role. Successful management depends upon the endocrinologic and surgical skill available to the baby.

Normal Development in the Embryo

In order for the infant to develop as a phenotypically complete male or female, a cascade of events must occur in the proper sequence and at the proper times. The embryo must have the correct chromosomal endowment. The germ cells must migrate from the endoderm of the yolk sac to the urogenital ridge, and there initiate induction of the gonad. The gonad, in turn must produce hormones, and the receptor tissues must respond appropriately to the secreted hormones. Should any of these events fail, or occur too late, the result is an infant with an abnormal phenotype.

Primitive germ cells are first found in the yolk sac entoderm. They migrate to the urogenital or mesonephric ridge through a series of ameboid movements, combined with growth and folding of the caudal end of the embryo (Fig 139–3).[46, 73, 108] There, they play a critical but unknown role in further differentiation of the gonad (Figs 139–4 and 139–5).

The difference between the normal male and female somatic karyotype is that the male has a Y chromosome and only one X, whereas the female lacks a Y and possesses two Xs. It was not known until recently whether the double X, or the Y, chromosome was the determining factor in gonadal differentiation. The discovery of XXY male mice[123] and the finding that humans with as many as four X chromosomes, and a Y, expressed testicular gonadal histology[4] provided impressive evidence that the Y chromosome leads to the formation of a testis. Exactly what it is on the Y chromosome that initiates testicular differentiation is not entirely understood. One of the current theories is that H-Y antigen initiates differentiation of the primitive gonad into a testis. H-Y antigen is a cell surface protein coded for by a region on chromosome 6 in close proximity to the histocompatibility (HL-A) antigen or major histocompatibility complex. The antigen is bound to the cell surface through the smaller surface molecule, β_2-microglobulin; H-Y antigen can be found on all male cells, hence can be measured on cells of all types, including blood cells. The only cells thought to have receptors for H-Y antigen, however, are those of the genital ridge. H-Y antigen binding to these receptors of the genital ridge tissue is thought to lead to its differentiation as a testis. Somatic elements assemble from rapidly proliferating epithelial cells that have migrated from the involuting mesonephros.[53, 115] Under the influence of a testis-

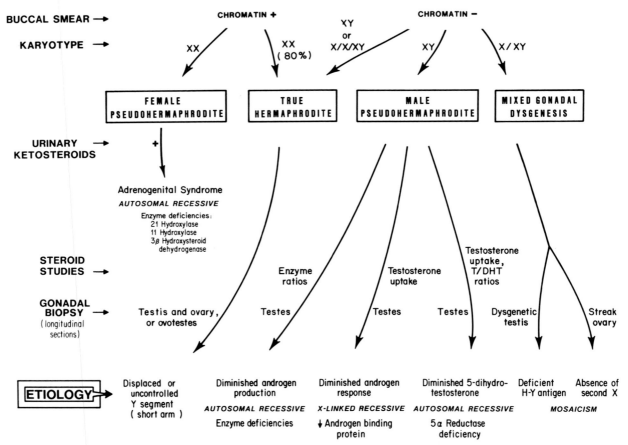

Fig 139–1.—Four major intersex abnormalities causing gender ambiguity in the newborn, the diagnostic modalities necessary to establish each diagnosis, and the etiologies proposed.

directing factor, the medullary cords of the primitive gonad differentiate as seminiferous tubules.[84, 85] Subsequently in normal testicular development (4–12 weeks), Sertoli cells of the seminiferous tubules begin to produce müllerian inhibiting substance,[51, 54, 55, 56, 81, 110] which causes regression of the müllerian duct. This substance,[9, 10] a large molecular-weight glycoprotein, affects the mesenchymal/epithelial component of the müllerian duct, leading to morphological changes in the mesenchyme and to death of some of the epithelial cells, as well as migration of others of the cells into the surrounding mesenchyme.[47, 113] Soon thereafter, interstitial cells differentiate as Leydig cells and begin to produce testosterone. This hormone stimulates the development of the wolffian duct system to form the ductus deferens, seminal vesicles, and epididymides; after local reduction to di-

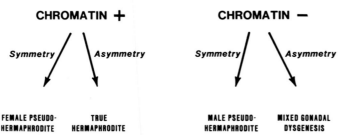

Fig 139–2.—Chromatin mass (Barr body). Symmetry or asymmetry of the gonads and buccal smear for chromatin mass can be used to establish an early working diagnosis in newborns with ambiguous genitalia.

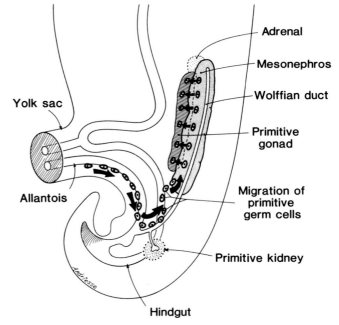

Fig 139–3.—Germ cell migration during early embryonic development, lateral view. Primitive germ cells migrate from the yolk sac along the allantois to the hindgut. They subsequently travel via the retroperitoneum to the mesonephros and then take residence in the primitive gonad.

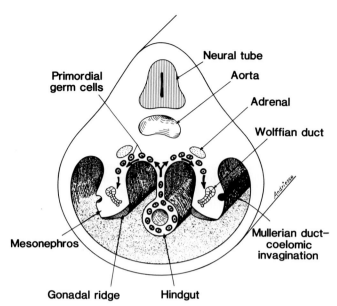

Fig 139–4.—Germ cells migrate from the hindgut to the retroperitoneum and mesonephros as seen in the transverse section.

hydrotestosterone, it mediates the development of the external genitalia into penis and scrotum.[122, 125]

Local concentrations of these substances, the timing of their production, as well as the ontogeny and concentration of their receptors, are important in mediating the development of the perfect male phenotype. Concentrations of testosterone are under the influence of placental human chorionic gonadotropin

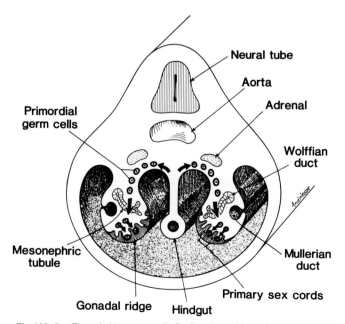

Fig 139–5.—The primitive germ cells finally take residence in the mesial portion of the mesonephros as seen in transverse section. If the gonad is induced to form a testis, and seminiferous tubules develop from the primary sex cords, müllerian inhibiting substance is produced, causing regression of the müllerian duct. Subsequently, testosterone causes stimulation of the wolffian duct. If the primitive gonad is induced to form an ovary in the absence of müllerian inhibiting substance, the müllerian duct develops. The wolffian duct or mesonephric tubules regress in the absence of testosterone.

(HCG). Receptors may appear during only a limited window of development. The müllerian duct in the rat,[88] for instance, is measurably responsive to müllerian inhibiting substance only between days 14 and 16 of gestation; and regression is complete by day 17. In the human,[28] müllerian regression begins at least as early as day 51[110] and is complete by day 77. Receptor sensitivity to müllerian inhibiting substance is maximum during the early phase of that interval. The peak of embryonic responsiveness to testosterone has not been precisely determined, but probably lies between the beginning of testosterone synthesis on day 65 and urethral groove closure, which is accomplished by day 74.[28] Maximum concentrations of a mediator substance such as H-Y antigen, müllerian inhibiting substance, or testosterone, if delayed so as to appear after the normal period of receptivity, may result in development as defective as does an appropriately timed but subnormal concentration of mediating substance.[68] Receptor abnormalities can also produce mishaps in embryogenesis, as seen in the X-linked type of male pseudohermaphroditism, often referred to as testicular feminization. H-Y antigen receptor deficiencies may be the cause of testicular dysgenesis, as in mixed gonadal dysgenesis or 46 XY pure gonadal dysgenesis.[75, 117, 120, 121, 124]

The factors responsible for differentiation of an ovary are not entirely clear. Byskov and Grinsted[12] speculate that, irrespective of the sex of the embryo, a substance produced by the mesonephros, through which the germ cells migrate to reach the primitive gonad, may be responsible for differentiation of the ovary. On the other hand, the Moscona-type reaggregation experiments of Ohno[83] using gonadal tissue suggest that ovarian differentiation is autonomous. When testes of newborn mice are treated with trypsin and the individual cells allowed to reaggregate, those that have been exposed to antibody that binds or inactivates H-Y antigen will reorganize in ovarian follicle-like aggregates; those not exposed to antibody, in which the H-Y antigen continues to be expressed, will re-form in seminiferous tubule-like clusters. Whether, like the H-Y antigen in the testis, there is an H-X antigen required for ovarian differentiation is not yet known. The presumptive H-X may be a gene product that requires for expression the second X chromosomal complement. This second X is usually dormant, except in the very early female embryo,[34, 48] during which time it could conceivably exert an ovarian differentiating function. An as-yet-undetected H-X antigen or receptor deficiency may be a pathogenetic factor in 45 X gonadal dysgenesis (Turner syndrome). The germ cell, with its full complement of genetic material and the second X fully expressed in female somatic cells, may be required in order for the urogenital ridge to differentiate with normal ovarian morphology. Study of these patients' ovaries, which are normal in early fetal development,[105] indicates that the X, and products it may code for, appear necessary to "stabilize" the primitive follicles and prevent premature senescence or nonresponse.

Female development of the müllerian duct system and external genitalia is an autonomous process. To what extent the usual ovarian steroid hormones are produced during fetal life is unclear; it is apparent, however, that they have little effect on early female morphogenesis, because in the absence of the ovaries this proceeds normally. Differentiation of the female sex ducts is completed before 11 or 12 weeks. When müllerian inhibiting substance is absent, as in the normal female or in males with early embryonic testicular regression, the müllerian ducts persist to form the Fallopian tubes, uterus, cervix, and upper portion of the vagina. In the absence of testosterone, the wolffian duct regresses passively. In the absence of 5α-dihydrotestosterone, the genital tubercle, genital folds, genital swellings, and urogenital sinus develop into clitoris, labia minora, labia majora, and lower vagina. After 11 weeks, the ovary enlarges, the cortical germ cells become surrounded by granulosa cells, and the stroma proliferates.

The role of placental and fetal gonadotropins in sexual organogenesis is not fully known. Placental HCG is probably important in boosting the androgens made by the fetal testis. A significant number of mothers of patients with male pseudohermaphroditism, for which there is no documented cause, give the history of one or two failed pregnancy tests before their pregnancies were confirmed. This observation, suggestive of diminished HCG production, may also explain the deficient masculinization seen so frequently in placental insufficiency and the "twin B" syndrome. Internal and external genital morphogenetic events in the male coincide with peak fetal levels of chorionic gonadotropin, which is presumed to exert the principal trophic influence on the testes. The subsequent events are basically growth of the external genitalia and descent of the testes. During the time of these occurrences, fetal levels of chorionic gonadotropin are declining and those of the pituitary gonadotropins are rising, suggesting that the fetal pituitary gonadotropin, luteinizing hormone (LH), may be the important mediator of these later events. The frequency of micropenis but not of hypospadias in such conditions as Kallmann syndrome of luteinizing hormone-releasing hormone (LHRH) deficiency, and in males with anencephaly, reinforces this speculation.

Preoperative Diagnostic Evaluation: An Orderly Approach (Fig 139–6)

Evaluation of the newborn infant with ambiguous genitalia begins in the delivery room or soon thereafter with a careful history and physical examination. History should include inquiries regarding contraception, maternal illnesses during pregnancy, and ingestion of drugs, alcohol, or androgenic or progestational substances. Dates and extent of exposure should be ascertained as closely as possible. A detailed pedigree is obtained, with particular investigation into the occurrence of genital abnormalities in relatives, unexplained death of young infants during the first week or two of life, and existence of infertile family members, or maternal aunts with sterility, amenorrhea, or inguinal hernia with "prolapsed ovary."

Examination of the infant can often be done to mutual advantage with both parents present. Frequently, this enables the parents to see the problem for the first time with the physician, who can explain fetal genital development. The examiner should look first for symmetry. Is one gonad above, the other below, the inguinal ring? Is one hemiscrotum much larger than the other, or is the scrotum bifid? Is the scrotum positioned normally be-

hind the penis, or are the anterior attachments draped over the base of the penis as in the "shawl" or "prepenile" scrotal anomaly? Are the labioscrotal folds rugose? Is there hypospadias and/or chordee, and what exactly are the dimensions of the phallus? Can one be certain of the presence of an epididymis embracing the gonad? On rectal examination, can one feel a midline uterus? Be prepared to make a smear of any urethral discharge obtained by milking the vagina during rectal examination. The discharge should be stained and examined microscopically for the presence of vaginal epithelial cells. Excessive pigmentation or signs of dehydration support the possibility of one of the salt-losing congenital adrenal hyperplasia syndromes. Dysmorphic features should alert the examiner to the possibility of a chromosomal disorder and other major associated congenital anomalies.

Immediately after history and physical examination, laboratory examination should be initiated, choosing first those procedures that will yield results rapidly. Buccal smears should be obtained to determine the frequency of cells showing Barr chromatin bodies, indicative of the presence of a second X chromosome. Blood smears should be made to determine the percentage of leukocytes showing the bright spot of fluorescence characteristic of the Y chromosome. The same specimen can be used to initiate leukocyte culture for karyotyping and to provide serum for sodium, potassium, and glucose determinations as well as for gonadotropin and steroid analyses.

A bag is placed for collection of urine. We avoid asking for 24-hour collections. To do so invokes delay and maceration of an area likely to be involved by imminent surgical procedures. The urine creatinine content can be used as a timer, calculating 12.5 mg/kg of body weight as the daily output of the neonate. Ten to twenty milliliters of urine is quite sufficient for measurement of creatinine, and 17-ketosteroids. Both of these are determinations done accurately and expeditiously in virtually all hospital laboratories. Radioimmunoassay or high-pressure gas liquid chromatography of serum and/or urine to determine specific steroids and substrate-product ratios in the steroid biosynthetic pathways are done well in only a few laboratories, thus do not constitute part of the first-line information. These tests are rather done later, frequently after stimulation with HCG.

Information concerning the internal anatomy can be obtained promptly by the pediatric radiologist. The skillful retrograde injection of contrast media into the perineal openings can demonstrate the vagina and determine the position of its outlet, and whether it opens via a cervix to a uterine cavity. Panendoscopy and/or laparotomy may be needed for gender assignment or planning of definitive surgical repair. At the same time, biopsies of genital area skin, prepuce, scrotum or labia majora, and/or of each gonad may be obtained. The skin biopsies will be useful to provide cultured fibroblasts for later determination of androgen receptor number, whole cell and nuclear binding affinities, and 5α-steroid reductase activity. Histologic sections of the gonadal biopsies can be prepared promptly and help to discriminate between mixed gonadal dysgenesis, true hermaphroditism, and dysgenetic male pseudohermaphroditism. The patient with true hermaphroditism has normal ovarian and testicular tissue, either in separated gonads or in an ovotestis in which the testicular tissue is central and the ovarian tissue is polar. In a patient with mixed gonadal dysgenesis, typically one sees a streak ovary characterized by increased fibrosis and progressive follicular degeneration on one side. The testis is dysgenetic with thickened basement membranes and immature seminiferous tubules. Bilateral dysgenetic testes characterize the gonads of patients with dysgenetic male pseudohermaphroditism.[92] Immunohistochemical methods have been used to identify individuals with Leydig cell aplasia, as well as those with specific errors in testosterone biosynthesis.[6, 8, 30, 99]

EVALUATION OF "INTERSEX INFANT"

Examination	hCG stimulation and enzyme ratios
Family pedigree	
Drug ingestion Hx	Urethrogram or sinogram
Buccal smear, Y fluorescence	Cystoscopy
Urinary steroids	Laparotomy
Chromosomes	Gonadal biopsy (longitudinal)
Electrolytes	Androgen receptors (genital skin)

Fig 139–6.—The expeditious work-up of the newborn with ambiguous genitalia. The column on the left indicates what can be done immediately. The column on the right lists those studies that can be undertaken in a somewhat more leisurely fashion. Urethrograms can be scheduled electively.

Gender assignment can usually be made in the first 48 hours. Later information is important to the precise diagnosis and definition of the specific cause of the disorder.

Tests to Determine Genetic Sex and to Assess Steroid Production

Chromatin Mass

In 1949, a mass of chromatin, thought to represent the "inactivated" biochemically inert second X chromosome, was found in a high percentage of female nuclei. The second X is randomly inactivated.[66, 67] This "Barr" body is identifiable in 20% or more of the nuclei of normal females and is absent from the cells of normal males, although artifact may lead to counts of up to 2%. Cells from any human tissue can be used for the study of sex chromatin; but buccal cells, usually harvested by scraping the inside of the cheek with a tongue depressor, are readily available, and have large oval nuclei in which the characteristic chromatin mass closely applied to the nuclear membrane is particularly well seen.

Y Fluorescence

Buccal mucosal cells or blood cells can be stained with quinacrine dyes and examined by fluorescent microscopy. Because buccal cells are always associated with bacteria, some of which fluoresce with great intensity, most cytologists prefer to work with leukocytes, where the fluorescence more certainly identifies a segment of the long arm of the Y chromosome. Normally, about 50% of leukocytes from a normal male examined under ultraviolet light will show this uniquely bright spot of fluorescence. Results of this study, like the Barr chromatin mass, can be obtained in 24 hours.

Karyotype

In 1956, it was found that the human chromosome number was 46 and that the female had two X chromosomes and the male an X and a Y.[112] For karyotyping, cells are fixed in metaphase and then placed in hypotonic solution. The nuclear chromosomes are then stained, photographed, enlarged, and mapped. Abnormalities such as aneuploidy (incorrect number of chromosomes due to nondisjunction), deletion, breakage and rearrangement, and structural abnormalities such as translocation can be detected. Nondisjunction refers to incomplete division of chromosomes after metaphase, when each normally divides into two, which then migrate to opposite poles of the dividing cell. If nondisjunction occurs in meiosis, the zygote will be monosomic or trisomic for the affected chromosome. If nondisjunction occurs in an early mitotic division after fertilization, two or more genetically different cell lines can result, a phenomenon called mosaicism. Banding studies, or focused prophase analysis, are necessary to show the small interstitial deletions, such as that of chromosome 11, associated with hypospadias, aniridia, and Wilms tumor.

Although highly informative, karyotyping generally requires 1–2 weeks for completion and is not available in the early period when gender must be assigned. Of all the chromosomal anomalies, however, only true hermaphroditism and mixed gonadal dysgenesis are likely to cause serious gender confusion in the newborn period. Eighty percent or more of true hermaphrodites

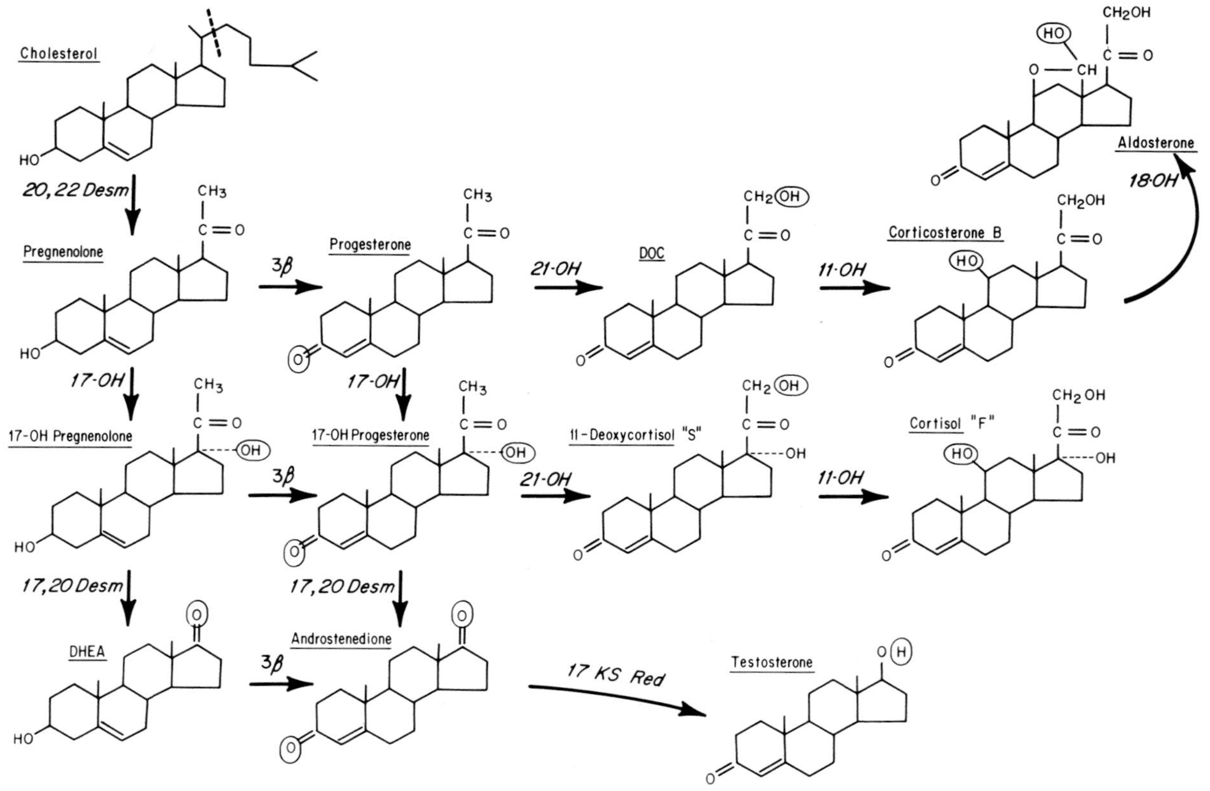

Fig 139–7.—Metabolism of cholesterol to corticosterones or androgenic steroids. Enzymatic defects of 21-hydroxylase, 11-hydroxylase, and 3β-hydroxysteroid dehydrogenase can lead to congenital adrenal hyperplasia and, in genetic females, result in female pseudohermaphroditism. Deficiencies in testosterone production can, in the genetic male, lead to male pseudohermaphroditism as a result of deficiency in 20,22-desmolase, 17-hydroxylase, 17,20-desmolase, 3β-hydroxysteroid dehydrogenase, and 17-ketosteroid reductase.

have a 46 XX karyotype. Most patients with mixed gonadal dysgenesis have a 45 X/46 XY mosaic karyotype.

Steroid Hormones (Fig 139–7)

The amount of intermediary metabolites and end products produced in conversion of cholesterol in the adrenal cortex to cortisol, aldosterone, and androgen, and in the ovary and testis, to estrogens and testosterone, can be used to assess the efficiency of the steroid biosynthetic machinery. The congenital adrenal hyperplasia syndromes depend upon subnormal activity of one of five enzymes. These are the 20,22-desmolase, the 17α-hydroxylase, the 3β-ol-dehydrogenase, the 11-hydroxylase, and the 21-hydroxylase. With deficiency of the 20,22-desmolase, all three classes of hormones—glucocorticoid, mineralocorticoid, and sex steroids—will be produced in subnormal quantities so that neonates of either sex will promptly manifest life-threatening symptoms of adrenal insufficiency while the males will show pseudohermaphroditism. The 17α-hydroxylase deficiency also interferes with production of cortisol, aldosterone, and sex steroids; but production of corticosterone, an adequate glucocorticoid and potent mineralocorticoid, prevents symptoms of adrenal insufficiency. Because the enzyme defect is common to both the adrenals and gonads, the deficiency of testosterone production results in male pseudohermaphroditism in the newborn; and in both sexes there is failure of secondary sexual differentiation at adolescence. The 3β-ol-dehydrogenase deficiency results in both male and female pseudohermaphroditism because the level of androgens produced is excessive for normal in utero development of the female, but insufficient for normal male development. Infants with deficiency of the 3β-ol-dehydrogenase enzyme complex are subject to collapse resulting from salt loss or cortisol insufficiency. Like the 17α-hydroxysteroid dehydrogenase deficiency, the 11β-hydroxylase deficiency results in overproduction of mineralocorticoid, in this instance 11-deoxycortisol, or compound S. In adults, both of these deficiencies are associated with hypertension. This is seldom a problem through the first decade. The 11-hydroxylase deficiency gives rise to female pseudohermaphroditism in infancy. Vomiting, suggestive of pyloric stenosis, is a common presentation. Three of the five affected males cared for in our unit have had Ramstedt procedures, one in England, one in Atlanta, and one done locally. A fourth infant was referred here with the provisional diagnosis of pyloric stenosis. The cause of vomiting and failure to thrive in the fifth infant posed no diagnostic difficulty, inasmuch as his older sister had been affected. Severe hyponatremia and hyperkalemia should suggest the diagnosis, which can be confirmed by elevated plasma levels of 11-deoxycortisol.

The commonest of all the adrenal hyperplasia syndromes, accounting for above 90% of cases, is the 21-hydroxylase deficiency. This results in female pseudohermaphroditism. In both sexes, the infants are at risk of sudden collapse caused by salt loss, which generally manifests at about a week of age. While in females ambiguities of the genitalia warn of the possibility, there are few symptoms in the males other than poor feeding. Hyperpigmentation of the nipple-areolar complex and genitalia caused by the high levels of melanocytic-stimulating hormone (MSH) associated with overproduction of adrenocorticotropic hormone (ACTH) may provide a clue to diagnosis. The impending salt loss crisis can be circumvented in the neonate by monitoring serum sodium and potassium concentrations once or twice daily. A presumptive diagnosis is readily made from the elevation of serum 17-ketosteroids in a random urine sample. Stimulation with ACTH can accentuate the enzyme defect by priming the substrate to measurable levels. Where the determination is available, the marked elevation of serum 17α-hydroxyprogesterone is similarly helpful. It should be recalled[101] that pregnanetriol, the usual urinary metabolite of plasma 17α-hydroxyprogesterone, is not a reliable indicator of 21-hydroxylase deficiency in the first month of life, because the neonate uses the 16-hydroxylase pathway.

Male pseudohermaphroditism may result from failure of testosterone production caused by testicular deficiency of 17, 20-desmolase or 17-ketosteroid reductase. Stimulation with HCG can accentuate the defect.

Protein Hormones

Pituitary gonadotropins are measured during neonatal evaluations. Early elevated LH levels reflect placental gonadotropins. After 2 weeks, however, elevated levels reflect deficiency of gonadal function or receptor defects. Low gonadotropins can be detected in Kallmann syndrome.

Research Tools

Androgen Receptors

Fibroblast cultures can be established from genital skin specimens within 4–6 weeks, and whole cell[32] and nuclear[114] uptake of dihydrotestosterone (DHT) determined. Androgen receptors are depressed or absent in patients with classic testicular feminization and certain other variants of male pseudohermaphroditism. Abnormalities, however, have not been detected in patients with isolated cryptorchidism or hypospadias,[31] nor in patients thought clinically to represent variants of androgen resistance. It may be that these patients represent postreceptor defects or some as-yet-undetected receptor abnormality rather than receptor absence. A few laboratories are now equipped to report reliably or consistently on androgen receptor levels.

H-Y Antigen

This cell surface antigen was first appreciated when it was noted that female inbred mice grafted with skin from males of the same strain rejected the male tissue.[29] Because differences did not exist between the genes of other chromosomes, the rejection was presumably due to the development of antibodies against a Y-directed substance. This substance has been termed H-Y antigen, and techniques have been developed for its measurement[44, 58] and purification.[46, 76] Daudi lymphoma cells, which lack the required HL-A and β2-microglobulin anchorage site and hence shed H-Y antigen, have been used as a source for purification. Conventional serologic methods detect H-Y antigen by the ability of an unknown sample to diminish cytotoxicity against sperm target cells of serum raised in female mice previously challenged with male spleen cells. Wachtel[33] and Koo[77] and colleagues have developed immunoassays using monoclonal antibodies to H-Y antigen, which will allow measurement of the substance in clinical intersex states.

The antigen has been found in the heterogametic sex of almost all animals so far studied. In addition, it was noted that H-Y antigen was present in both XX true hermaphrodites and XX males,[119] despite the apparent absence of the Y chromosome. It has been suggested that in those instances the coding region of the Y has become translocated to another chromosome, where it directs production of H-Y antigen.[22, 44, 46, 70, 85, 118] While the Y chromosome may immediately code for the substance directing male gonadal differentiation, it appears that functional expression of the critical genes may be secondarily controlled by a site on either an autosome or the X chromosome.

Luteinizing Hormone-Releasing Hormone

Although studied extensively and clinically applied to the treatment of older patients with Kallmann syndrome[48] and precocious puberty,[15, 70] LHRH has been little used either diagnostically or therapeutically in the newborn infant. It may, however, find an important place in the diagnosis and treatment of micropenis and undescended testes.

Sex Chromosomal DNA Sequences

Studies of the sex-determining satellite DNA of snakes show that it comprises highly reiterated tetranucleotide sequences.[103, 104] Homologies between the snake satellite DNA and sequences from the mouse Y chromosome have been shown, suggesting that these characteristic sequences may be used as probes to locate sex-determining genes from human gene libraries. In the future, correlations may be made with intersex abnormalities. Experimentally, these Y chromosome sequences can be transferred into recipient cells and the effect of donor sequences on host cell function determined. Such techniques may eventually allow analysis of the effects of cloned sex chromosomal sequences on embryonic sexual development.

Major Classifications of Intersex Abnormalities

The four major categories of conditions resulting in genital ambiguity in the newborn infant occur either because of hormonal influences or structural defects. Hormonal influences, by affecting the fetus as a whole, impart a symmetric abnormality. The hormonal abnormalities occurring with a normal male karyotype and producing male pseudohermaphroditism are due to enzyme or to receptor deficiencies and result in deficient masculinization. Hormonal abnormalities that occur with the normal female karyotype and produce female pseudohermaphroditism result from enzyme defects that cause androgenization of the female fetus. Whatever the cause, including transplacental passage of androgens or antiandrogens from the mother, the effect on the fetus is symmetric.

The structural abnormalities affecting external genital development are usually associated with chromosomal anomalies and result in asymmetry in the phenotype. This is usually because one gonad develops predominantly as a testis, which mediates the formation of a scrotum and its descent into that structure. The other gonad develops as an ovary or a streak, which remains higher or in the abdominal cavity. Detailed descriptions of the four major categories of intersex abnormalities that cause gender confusion in the newborn period follow.

Male Pseudohermaphroditism

Male pseudohermaphroditism is a generic term connoting patients who are genetically 46 XY, but who have deficient masculinization of the external genitalia. In our series of over 90 patients with male pseudohermaphroditism, in only about 50% can a definite cause be determined.[31] When ascertainable, it is found that heritable single-gene disorders characterize this group. Among these are the males whose genital anomalies occur because of (1) insufficient testosterone production caused by defects in its biosynthesis; (2) target organ inability to convert testosterone to dihydrotestosterone; and (3) deficiencies in androgen receptors so that testosterone cannot be bound to its receptor to engender typical male responses of the cell (Fig 139–8).

Enzyme defects leading to deficient biosynthesis of testosterone are inherited as autosomal recessive traits (Fig 139–9). The first three enzymes (20,22-desmolase, 3β-hydroxysteroid dehydrogenase, and 17α-hydroxylase) are necessary to the elaboration

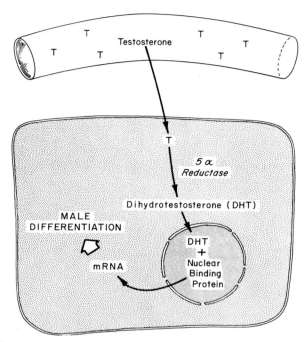

Fig 139–8.—Etiology of male pseudohermaphroditism. Insufficient testosterone production, caused by deficiencies in enzymes responsible for the biosynthesis of testosterone, failure of conversion of testosterone to dihydrotestosterone, or defect or deficiency of androgen receptors, so that the cell machinery is not converted to male differentiation, can lead to incomplete masculinization in 46 XY males.

of cortisol; male infants affected with the first two, but not the 17α-hydroxylase deficiency, will have adrenal insufficiency. Each of these three biosynthetic errors results in a variable degree of deficient masculinization. Deficiencies of 17,20-desmolase or 17-ketosteroid reductase block only steps required for testosterone elaboration and therefore are not critical to the survival of the affected infant. All of these defects can be detected by comparing substrate/product ratios in the steroid biosynthetic pathways.

5α-Reductase deficiency (see Fig 139–9), also an autosomal recessive trait, causes defective metabolism of testosterone to dihydrotestosterone. This results in deficient masculinization of the external male genitalia. The syndrome has been called pseudovaginal perineoscrotal hypospadias by Opitz et al.[86] Walsh and his colleagues[122] termed this entity familial incomplete male pseudohermaphroditism, type II. A large cohort of patients from

DIMINISHED ANDROGEN PRODUCTION	DIMINISHED ANDROGEN RESPONSE	DIMINISHED 5-DIHYDRO-TESTOSTERONE
Autosomal recessive	*X-Linked recessive*	*Autosomal recessive*
Enzyme deficiencies:	Abnormal androgen binding receptor	5α Reductase deficiency
20, 22 Desmolase		Familial Incomplete ♂ pseudohermaphroditism
3β Hydroxysteroid dehydrogenase	Testicular feminization (complete expression)	(type II)
17α Hydroxylase		Pseudovaginal perineoscrotal hypospadias
17, 20 Desmolase	Familial Incomplete ♂ pseudohermaphroditism	
17β Ketosteroid reductase	(type I)	
	Lubs', Reifenstein, Gilbert-Dreyfus, and Rosewater syndromes	

Fig 139–9.—Various mechanisms responsible for—and commonly used names to describe—diminished androgen production, diminished androgen response, or diminished 5-dihydrotestosterone.

the Dominican Republic has been studied by Peterson et al.[87] Deficiencies in androgen receptor function are usually inherited as X-linked recessive traits (see Fig 139–9).[69] The complete expression of this disorder is seen in patients with classic testicular feminization. Absence of receptors leads to a feminine genital appearance in the newborn and often an exquisite feminine phenotype at maturity, with fully developed breasts, little pubic or axillary hair, and unblemished skin. At birth, testes may be found in the labioscrotal folds. Incomplete forms of androgen receptor malfunction produce a broad spectrum of genital ambiguities. Because virtually the whole spectrum of anatomical abnormality may be seen in a single family, the disorder exemplifying how multiple factors may impinge on the expression of a single gene, Wilson and his colleagues[125] proposed the term familial incomplete male pseudohermaphroditism, type I. Hitherto, these patients had been grouped anatomically and assigned to syndromes associated with the eponyms of Lubs, Reifenstein, Gilbert-Dreyfus, and Rosewater.

A large number of male pseudohermaphrodites remain etiologic enigmas. Maternal ingestion of drugs can be responsible. Barbiturates[40] and hydantoins are thought to hasten the degradation of steroids by microsomal induction,[57, 102] and the hydantoins[89] to inhibit 5α-reductase; experimentally, cyproterone acetate, a competitive antagonist of testosterone given during pregnancy, can produce male pseudohermaphroditism;[78] medroxyprogesterone[1] has been thought to induce hypospadias; cimetidine and spironolactone are competitive inhibitors of DHT at its intracellular receptor,[41] an inhibitor of 17,20-desmolase.[98] Thus, a number of drugs in relatively common use could be the cause of incomplete masculinization in the male fetus.

Placental insufficiency[14, 93] presumably caused by insufficient chorionic gonadotropin production, may be a more common cause of genital undevelopment than we had formerly thought. This has been speculated to be the basis of the "twin-B syndrome." The androgen produced by the fetal testis may require a boost from the placental gonadotropin in order to be fully expressed at appropriate levels and at an appropriate time. The fetal pituitary contributes little to this except to complete growth, because anencephalic individuals develop small but normal genitalia, as is the case in males with Kallmann syndrome of congenital gonadotropin-releasing hormone deficiency.[48]

Dysgenetic male pseudohermaphroditism[34, 90] describes 46 XY males with bilateral severely dysgenetic testes. In addition, there is almost complete retention of the müllerian ducts. This group of patients may represent a variant of mixed gonadal dysgenesis.[92] Congenital anorchia results from bilateral in utero torsion in some patients, complete failure of induction of the gonads in others. Testes may form and then disappear as a result of circulatory, inflammatory, or toxic insults.[16] If the "vanishing" testes syndrome occurs early, then a feminine phenotype results. If it occurs later, for example in the critical period between the beginning of testosterone production at day 65 and closure of the urethral groove on day 77 of gestation, less severe forms such as hypospadias may result.[28]

Many patients with the incomplete androgen receptor function have been raised as males. We prefer to rear them as females if they present in the newborn period and the phallus is very small. It must be remembered that these children may respond imperfectly to testosterone either in utero or in adolescence. The gonads with normal testicular morphology may be found in the scrotal folds and may be inguinal or abdominal. Uteri cannot be detected by rectal examination, but the urethrogram may show an enlarged prostatic utricle, which can be the source of recurrent infection from urinary backwash. Normal levels of serum electrolytes and urinary 17-ketosteroids are found, the leukocytes will show Y-body fluorescence, and the buccal smear will be chromatin negative. The karyotype is 46 XY. Testosterone and dihydrotestosterone levels are normal or elevated. At the time of operation, the gonads may show normal testis histologically. Genital skin is harvested and grown in tissue culture. After fibroblasts reach confluency, they can be studied for (1) their ability to bind androgen, (2) their 5α-reductase activity, and (3) their yield of H-Y antigen.

If female gender is assigned, the child undergoes clitoral recession, labioscrotal reduction, and gonadectomy at 3–6 months of age, or earlier if necessary. Vaginal reconstruction is performed in late adolescence. At this same time, or sooner if necessary, an enlarged prostatic utricle, if symptomatic, may have to be removed, either transabdominally or through a posterior vertical cystostomy. If a vaginal introitus is present, even if it ends only 1–2 cm from the surface, it can be stretched and dilated at adolescence over a period of 6–12 months to provide either a complete vagina or to serve as an introitus to which a skin graft or tube of colon can be sutured more proximally.

Young infants with testicular feminization can present with incarceration of an inguinal hernia containing a gonad. Some physicians recommend leaving the testis in place so that it can provide the substrate for normal adolescent breast development. In classic testicular feminization, inasmuch as testosterone receptors are absent, the hormone has no direct effect. However, testosterone is aromatized to estradiol peripherally, particularly in adipose tissue, so that its influence is as an estrogen. We suggest removing the gonads in infancy at the time of hernia repair, to avoid the psychological consequences of this type of operation in the older child. Extraglandular conversion of adrenal androgens will probably bring about satisfactory breast development at adolescence.[2] If necessary, small doses of exogenous estrogen can be used to augment the endogenous output. Pubertal androgen effects, such as acne and growth of pubic and axillary hair, are classically absent and are refractory to administered androgen. After puberty, the incidence of gonadoblastoma rises sharply,[70] making the removal of retained testes almost mandatory.

Female Pseudohermaphroditism

When a chromatin-positive genetic female (46 XX) is exposed to exogenous or endogenous androgens in utero, female pseudohermaphroditism results. The congenital adrenal hyperplasia syndromes, autosomal recessive deficiencies of the adrenal enzymes of cortisol synthesis,[7, 79] result in overproduction of endogenous intermediary metabolites, proximal in the chain to the deficient enzyme. A number of these metabolites are androgens. The faulty biosynthetic machinery, incapable of normal cortisol production, is constantly goaded by compensatory overproduction of pituitary ACTH. Excessive androgens masculinize the female fetus; excessive mineralocorticoids can lead to hypertension, while diminished aldosterone or high levels of aldosterone antagonists such as 17α-hydroxytestosterone can cause excessive salt loss.[7, 45, 126]

In the virilizing forms of congenital adrenocortical hyperplasia, the müllerian derivatives (uterus, Fallopian tubes, upper vagina) and ovaries are normal; but the prostate and external genitalia are masculinized as a result of adrenal overproduction of androgenic steroids after the 10th week of gestation, when the adrenal differentiates. The defects of the external genitalia and urogenital sinus can range (Fig 139–10) from clitoral enlargement alone, sometimes of such minor degree as to escape attention, to complete labioscrotal fusion, formation of a perfect scrotum, and severe clitoromegaly with urethral tubularization completed to the tip of the phallus. Although masculinization is variable in each of the three virilizing biosynthetic defects, it is fairly constant in a given sibship. The three virilizing defects, the 21-hydroxylase,

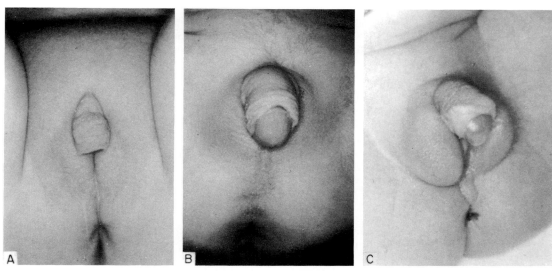

Fig 139–10.—Masculinization of the external genitalia in patients with female pseudohermaphroditism or adrenogenital syndrome. Phenotypic expression varies from **(A)**, mild clitoral hypertrophy, **(B)**, severe clitoral hypertrophy, to **(C)**, clitoral hypertrophy and formation of labioscrotal folds.

11-hydroxylase and 3β-hydroxysteroid dehydrogenase deficiencies (see Fig 139–7)[63] can be differentiated by relatively simple tests. Levels of urinary ketosteroids are greatly elevated in the first two and modestly increased in the 3β-hydroxysteroid dehydrogenase deficiency. Serum levels of 17-hydroxyprogesterone are characteristically elevated in the 21-hydroxylase deficiency. Elevated serum 11-deoxycortisol is the hallmark of the 11-hydroxylase deficiency, whereas elevation of the ratio of the plasma δ^5(17-hydroxypregnenolone) steroids to δ^4(17-hydroxyprogesterone) is pathognomonic of the 3β-hydroxysteroid dehydrogenase deficiency. All three of these disorders can be associated with salt wasting as well as virilization.[126]

Of the conditions responsible for ambiguous genital development, only the adrenal hyperplasia syndromes are likely to be life-threatening. Cardiovascular collapse and vomiting can occur in the first week of life in a neonate of either sex. Prior to such a crisis, hyperpigmentation may provide a clue to diagnosis. The history of early death in an apparent male sibling reinforces the suspicion. To avoid calamity, monitoring for salt loss should be initiated immediately. Progressive hyponatremia and hyperkalemia are characteristic. Electrocardiographic changes may suggest the diagnosis even before serum electrolyte levels are available to confirm the imbalance of sodium and potassium and long before urinary steroid determinations are returned. Treatment consists of rehydration, with a glucose-enriched saline solution, and administration of glucocorticoid (cortisol) and mineralocorticoid (fluorocortisone, 9α-fluorohydrocortisone, Florinef). Steroid replacement must be given immediately in large doses for crisis needs, and in smaller doses for maintenance. The 11-hydroxylase defect can cause hypertension resulting from the accumulation of 11-deoxycortisol and 11-deoxycorticosterone proximal to the enzyme defect, but this is never a problem in the neonate.

All neonates with female pseudohermaphroditism should be raised as females. Exploratory laparotomy is almost never necessary. The external genitalia can be reconstructed successfully in all of these females. Repair should be done as early as possible. Regardless of how severely virilized the patient may be, she can be self-confident, fertile, and healthy if the perineum is appropriately reconstructed and, in those with virilizing adrenal hyperplasia, if glucocorticoid replacement is given early, in adequate doses, and is well maintained.

The malformations are corrected by clitoral recession (see Fig 139–16), vaginoplasty (see Fig 139–17), or vaginal pull-through (see Fig 139–18). Present-day clitoral reconstruction entails preservation of the clitoral glans with reanastomosis of the clitoral corpora and preservation of the neurovascular bundles. The choice of vaginoplasty or vaginal pull-through depends upon the degree of masculinization of the urogenital sinus, i.e., whether the vagina enters the urogenital sinus proximal (high) or distal

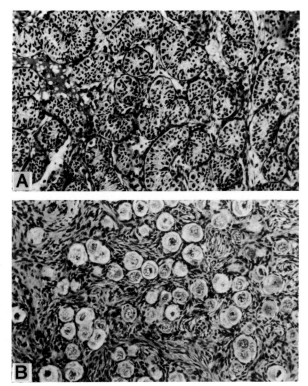

Fig 139–11.—Gonadal histology in true hermaphroditism. This can be surprisingly normal in separate areas. The seminiferous tubules of the testicular gonad **(A)** are normal, showing good basement membrane formation and normal Sertoli, germ cell, as well as interstitial Leydig cell development. The ovarian moiety **(B)** is also nondysgenetic, showing good primary follicle formation.

(low) to the external sphincter (see Fig 139–15). The age at which these surgical procedures are undertaken depends on (1) the severity of the virilization and (2) the stability of the home environment. Clitoral recession should be done as early as possible if the defect is severe. A cutback or flap vaginoplasty (see Fig 139–17) can be done either in the newborn period or preferably at 3–6 months of age. The pull-through vaginoplasty should be delayed until about 2 years of age (see Fig 139–18).

True Hermaphroditism

Except among the Bantus of Africa, true hermaphroditism is one of the rarest causes of sexual ambiguity. Only three cases have been seen at the Massachusetts General Hospital, while Van Niekerk[116] has reported over 300 from Africa. True hermaphrodites have well-developed, nondysgenetic male and female gonadal tissue (Fig 139–11);[25] there may be a testis on one side and an ovary on the other. The two tissues may be combined in ovotestes, or there may be a normal gonad on one side and an ovotestis on the other. Over 80% of these patients have a 46 XX karyotype; most of the remainder have either mosaic (46 XX/46 XY) or male (46 XY) karyotypes. Thus, a Barr chromatin mass is generally present in the buccal smear. Furthermore, despite the fact that most true hermaphrodites have a 46 XX karyotype, they have uniformly manifested H-Y antigen.[119] Because H-Y antigen is thought to be the product of one or more genes on the short arm or centromeric portion of the Y, it must be presumed that a gene-bearing fragment of the short arm is present somewhere in the karyotype, resulting not only in expression of H-Y antigen, but in initiation of testicular differentiation and male development.

Four major hypotheses have been proposed to explain the cause of true hermaphroditism and the phenomenon of testicular differentiation occurring, despite the fact that the majority of these individuals have 46 XX karyotypes and lack the Y chromosome:

1. Mosaicism with loss of the Y-containing cell line, which had earlier initiated gonadal differentiation.[11, 20, 43, 50, 119]

2. Translocation of the short arm of the Y chromosome to an autosome.[11, 19, 20, 43, 72, 119] A high familial incidence would be expected if this were the case, but few families have been described.[3, 42, 65]

3. Mutation of an autosomal gene that normally represses male expression. This phenomenon occurs in Saanen goats, homozygous for the "polled" gene (Po/Po),[107] and in sex-reversed mice with the autosomal dominant mutation of the Sxr gene.[13, 74] One would expect among relatives of true hermaphrodites a predominance of males or XX human males were this hypothesis correct. This has not been reported.[15]

4. The most likely explanation for true hermaphroditism is translocation of a fragment of the short arm of the Y to the X chromosome.[37, 38, 65, 119] This hypothesis is supported by the observation that XX males, thought to be the result of exchange of the genes of the short arm of the Y chromosome coding for H-Y antigen for those of the short arm of the X coding for the red cell antigen, Xga,[80, 97] do not follow the rules of X-linked inheritance.[18, 19, 94] For example, XX sons fail to inherit Xga from their Xga+ fathers.

If genes on the short arm of the Y adjacent to its pericentric region code for H-Y antigen, and these in turn mediate testicular differentiation and male development, what is the function of the genes of the long arm of the Y (Fig 139–12)? Electron microscopic studies of testicular tissue of a 2-year-old 46 XX true hermaphrodite reveal the presence of Sertoli and interstitial cells, but germ cells are absent.[95] It may be that the genes of the long arm of the Y are required for germ cells to mature beyond the spermatogonia stage.[19] If so, it would follow that the full comple-

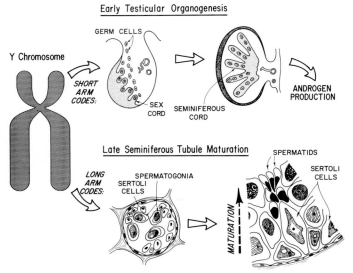

Fig 139–12.—The mechanism of true hermaphroditism. True hermaphroditism patients have taught us the importance of the short arm of the Y in directing early testicular differentiation. This portion of the Y is probably translocated to the X chromosome. The long arm of the Y is lost. Because maturation of the testis fails to occur, one can speculate that the long arm may code for later seminiferous tubule maturation.

ment of the genes of the Y chromosome is required for sperm to develop.

The patient with true hermaphroditism who presents early in the neonatal period and has a small phallus should be raised as a female. At abdominal exploration (Fig 139–13), the gonads can be bivalved, all testicular tissue removed, and the ovarian tissue, which occupies the poles of the ovotestis can be preserved.[35] This dissection should, of course, be monitored by both frozen and permanent sections. The clitoris should be recessed. All müllerian elements should be preserved and the vagina exteriorized. Wolffian structures should be excised and the scrotum reduced. If the phallus is of adequate size and the patient is committed to the male role, then ovarian and müllerian structures should be removed. Again, dissection of the bivalved gonad can be done with frozen-section monitoring. Hypospadias should be repaired and testicular prostheses inserted. The gonads in these patients should be followed carefully for the appearance of gonadoblastoma, although this may be less likely than in dysgenetic gonads.

Mixed Gonadal Dysgenesis

Characteristically, patients with mixed gonadal dysgenesis have dysgenetic gonads; retained müllerian structures; asymmetry, both internal and external; and mosaicism of the karyotype, often 45 X/46 XY. Unlike the gonads of the true hermaphrodite, the gonads in mixed gonadal dysgenesis exhibit increased fibrosis with sparse follicles or tubules. Although a dysgenetic testis on one side and a streak ovary on the other are the most characteristic gonadal findings,[99, 106] one can also find (1) unilateral gonadal agenesis or tumor, (2) bilateral streak gonads with rudimentary tubular elements, usually in the medullary area, or (3) a gonad on one side and a gonadal tumor on the other. Although 45 X/46 XY is the common karyotype, and mosaics of greater complexity are sometimes encountered, a euploid 46 XY karyotype was found in 40% of our series of 21 patients.[92] An aggressive but vain effort has been made to detect mosaicism in a variety of tissues, including the gonads of those with 46 XY. The mosaicism with two distinct cell lines, one aneuploid, is thought to result

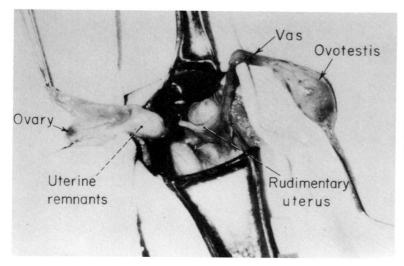

Fig 139–13.—Intra-abdominal anatomy of a patient with true hermaphroditism. The testicular tissue on the right produces sufficient müllerian inhibiting substance to cause ipsilateral regression, and adequate androgens to stimulate the development of the vas. On the left, the side of the ovary, the müllerian duct persists.

from postmeiotic nondisjunction. Lateralization of the 45 X line to the side of the streak or the 46 XY line to the side of the testis has not been found. Asymmetry of the gonads remains one of the mysteries of both mixed gonadal dysgenesis and true hermaphroditism.

The anomalies of mixed gonadal dysgenesis probably relate to improper gonadal induction. The strength of the testicular inducer, H-Y antigen, is roughly correlated with the representation of the Y chromosomal material in the karyotype.[119] In these syndromes, H-Y antigen may be limited or delayed, or its receptor may be defective or absent (Fig 139–14). As a consequence of reduced expression of the H-Y antigen, induction of seminiferous tubule differentiation may be weakened, so that müllerian inhibiting substance is produced in poorer concentration or late, when receptivity of the target issue has begun to wane. Truncation and

obliteration of the fimbriated end of the Fallopian tube, often seen on the side of the dysgenetic testis, is indicative of subnormal or late production of müllerian inhibiting substance.[23, 26] Leydig cell differentiation may also be deficient or delayed, leading to subnormal production of testosterone or a delay in its elaboration until receptor responsiveness has begun to decline. Such phenomena could explain the poor development of the wolffian system and external genitalia.

Proper differentiation and maturation of the ovary may require influence of the second X chromosome. In the early fertilized oocyte,[34, 46] the second X is not inactivated. Barr bodies can be detected at 12 days and are no longer present at 16 days. Functionally, this second X may lead to a timely expression of an X-related surface antigen, similar to that of the H-Y antigen; and this may be required to initiate differentiation of the urogenital

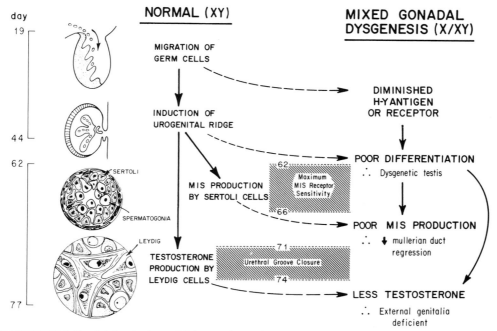

Fig 139–14.—Cause of testicular dysfunction in mixed gonadal dysgenesis. Failure of induction by a substance such as H-Y antigen appears to be responsible for the composite anomalies. If the inductive agent or its receptor is abnormal, then the urogenital ridge differentiates poorly, producing reduced amounts of müllerian inhibiting substance *(MIS)* leading to retained müllerian ducts, and producing reduced amounts of testosterone, leading to deficient masculinization of the external genitalia.

ridge to an ovary.[24, 34] Based on the absence of germinal elements in the adult streak, it was initially thought that the streak gonad developed because of the absence of primitive germ cells.[49] However, if the gonad of the 45 X embryo before 3 months of gestation is compared with that of the 46 XX embryo, there is no deficiency of germ cells.[105] Later gonads of 46 XX embryos develop primary follicles, whereas gonads in 45 X monosomy show an increase in connective tissue elements; and primary follicles diminish in number. These changes become more manifest with further maturation of the gonads of the 45X embryo. This process of premature senescence accelerates in the newborn infant, so that by 4–6 years of age the characteristic streak morphology is apparent. The two X chromosomes may be necessary to code for maturation of granulosa and persistence of ova, in a fashion analogous to the requirement we speculated for the presence of both the short and long arms of the Y for normal tubule and sperm maturation in the male. Primitive germ cells unnurtured by granulosa cells may degenerate.

The streak gonad observed in the patient with mixed gonadal dysgenesis differs from the streak ovaries of the patient with Turner syndrome, suggesting that the contralateral testis may exert an additional influence on the already altered gonad.[92] If normal ovaries are transplanted simultaneously with testes, in either the rat[68] or the rabbit, ovarian development is inhibited. Similar observations have been made in the freemartin,[64] the sterile female of heterosexual twin calves. The ovaries in these cases are dysplastic, showing the formation of seminiferous tubules. The tubularization of the ovary of the freemartin led Jost et al.[52] to predict that it would produce functional H-Y antigen, a speculation later proved correct.[82, 118] Dysgenesis of the freemartin ovary was directly proportional to the extent of cross-circulation between the twin pairs. In the human, H-Y antigen disseminated from the contralateral testis may be the cause of the tubularization in the streak gonad of patients with mixed gonadal dysgenesis, not seen in the streak ovaries of patients with Turner syndrome.

The dysgenetic gonads of mixed gonadal dysgenesis are prone to neoplastic transformation. Gonadoblastoma, an embryonal lesion composed of germ, Sertoli, and interstitial cell forms,[100] is

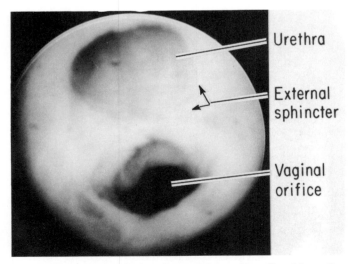

Fig 139–15.—Endoscopic view of urogenital sinus. The orifice of the urethra, above, and the vagina, below, are clearly seen when the bladder is full. The external sphincter contracts around the urethra. It is obvious in this case that the vagina enters the urogenital sinus just distal to the external urethral sphincter, thereby allowing repair of this anomaly by a low vaginoplasty, which can be done early, with a direct cutback from the meatus of the urogenital orifice into the vagina posteriorly as described in Figure 139–17.

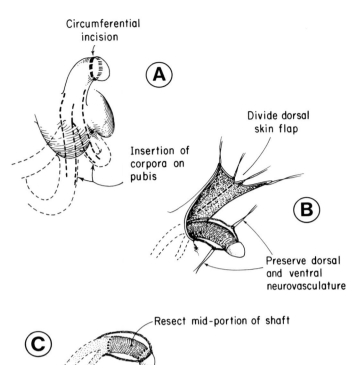

Fig 139–16.—Clitoral recession. **A,** the appearance of the enlarged clitoris, too large for the female phenotype and often too small for the male phenotype. The corpora cavernosa join, taking their origin from the pubic rami. The dissection is started by circumscribing the clitoris 2 mm below the glans. The dorsal flap is usually generous and the ventral flap marginal. The dorsal skin flap is divided cephalad **(B)** in the midline. On either side of the midline, both the prominent dorsal neurovascular bundles, consisting of two lateral arteries and a central vein, and the smaller ventral neurovascular bundle are carefully dissected out of Buck's fascia and retracted away from the corpora cavernosa. Dissection is carried back to the bifurcation of the corpora **(C),** which are then resected between that point and the glans, preserving neurovascular bundles. Hemostasis is secured gently with cautery, taking care not to cause undue fibrosis that would prevent eventual clitoral erection. The near and far ends of the corpora **(D)** are circumferentially approximated with very fine interrupted suture. The glans is positioned cephalad between the divided dorsal flaps and sutured in dorsally to the mons, and ventrally to the urogenital sinus mucosa. *(Continued.)*

the tumor most often seen. Although the dysgenetic testis is more often affected, the streak may also be involved. The seminoma-dysgerminoma, which cytologically simulates the medullary cord,[96] is more commonly seen in the streak. Virilization or breast development in a patient with mixed gonadal dysgenesis, if it occurs apart from the normal period of adolescence, usually indicates the presence of a tumor. At any time, however, the tumor can present as an asymptomatic mass or because of acute torsion of the gonad.[111] Tumor expectancy has been calculated at 3% by 10 years, 10% by 13 years, 20% by 15 years and 75% at 26 years.[71] We have seen a gonadoblastoma in the newborn period. Another patient at age 26 developed a gonadoblastoma with an outgrowth of dysgerminoma in a retained streak.[24] Apparently, the primordial germ cells, localized in an unphysiologic environment, may themselves be mitogenic. Likewise, the Sertoli cells in the dysgenetic testes of mixed gonadal dysgene-

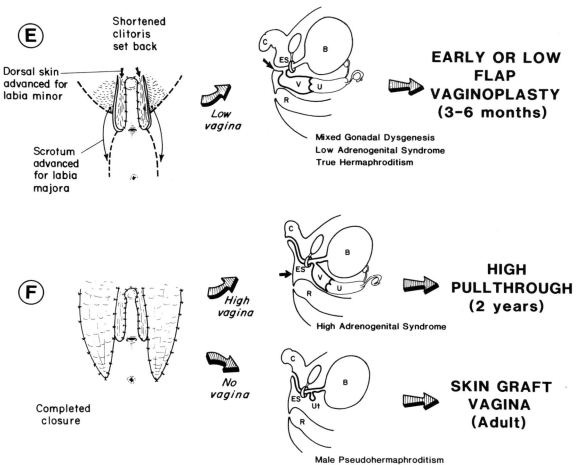

Fig 139–16 Cont.—The excess skin from the dorsal flap of the clitoral shaft **(E)** is then wrapped downward as a shawl to recreate the labia minora, as they both derive from the same genital fold anlage. The decision to proceed with vaginoplasty at this stage is made cystoscopically by determining whether the vagina enters the urogenital sinus proximal or distal to the external urethral sphincter. In most patients, i.e., those with "low" adrenogenital syndrome, mixed gonadal dysgenesis, or true hermaphroditism, **(E)** the vagina will be found to enter the urogenital sinus distal to the external urethral sphincter; and therefore a "low" flap vaginoplasty (see Fig 139–17) may be performed early. In the event that the vagina enters the urethra proximal to the external sphincter as occurs in the patient with "high" adrenogenital syndrome, then pull-through vaginoplasty (see Fig 139–18) should be deferred until the structures are larger, at age 2 years. If vaginoplasty is to be deferred, only the clitoral recession and the recreation of the labia minora should be done **(F)**. If the labioscrotal folds are grossly enlarged, some trimming may be done at this time. However, the complete labioscrotal reduction should be reserved until the "high" vaginal pull-through is done. Patients with male pseudohermaphroditism usually have only a rudimentary vagina. The labioscrotal folds should be reduced during the first procedure, as in **F**, and dilatation and a substitute vaginoplasty planned for the late adolescent, early adult years. Patients with testicular feminization in whom an introitus is often present may be dilated with bougies at a later age to enlarge the introitus as the functional vagina. (*C* indicates clitoris; *ES*, external sphincter; *B*, bladder; *V*, vagina; *U*, ureter; and *R*, rectum.)

sis often occur in a syncytium that does not organize into seminiferous tubules and may be the site of tumor development.

A further consideration is that aplasia and dysgenesis may lead to reduced hormone production, reduced negative pituitary feedback, and elevated production of follicle-stimulating and luteinizing hormones. Prolonged hyperstimulation by gonadotropins may be a factor in neoplastic transformation of the gonad analogous to the neoplasia that occurs in the thyroid subjected to increased thyrotropin stimulation.[21] Elevated gonadotropin levels, dystrophic gonadal spermatic cells, and persistent germ cells in an unphysiologic milieu may all be factors contributing to the neoplasia of these abnormal gonads. In addition, endometrial carcinoma has been found in the persistent müllerian duct derivatives.[17] Whether it is more prone than normal endometrium to neoplastic degeneration as a result of the chromosomal anomaly is not yet clear, but the endometrium in mixed gonadal dysgenesis, as in Turner syndrome, may be another site

of neoplastic transformation, particularly if stimulated by unopposed estrogen replacement therapy.

We recommend that the patients with mixed gonadal dysgenesis who present early usually be raised as females, even if the phallus is ample. The dysgenetic gonads should be removed, considering the risks of neoplasia just discussed and the fact that the reproductive capability, whichever the sex of rearing, is essentially nil. The external genitalia must be repaired by clitoral recession, flap vaginoplasty, and labioscrotal reduction. Estrogen and progesterone replacement should be commenced near the normal age of puberty. From that time on, cervical smears should be followed at yearly intervals and on indication of, for example, intermenstrual bleeding, for early detection of endometrial carcinoma. In all probability, the risk of this neoplasm can be greatly reduced or avoided by combined estrogen-progesterone replacement.

In infants with the more fully expressed male phenotype, rearing in the male gender role may be considered. This will require correction of the hypospadias and removal of the müllerian duct derivatives and streak gonad. In a patient referred late, no choice may exist but to support the child as a male. If needed, androgen replacement should be given during and after adolescence, although we have been struck by the tendency of individuals with this condition to react to low levels of testosterone with extreme hirsutism. Even before this time, these boys should be taught self-examination in order that tumors of the testis can be discovered early. The gonads should be removed before the third decade.

Operative Repair

The essential components of perineal reconstruction in infants to be reared as females, either because of grossly incomplete male genital development or predominantly female anatomy, are clitoral recession, vaginoplasty, and labioscrotal reduction. Management is similar whether the diagnosis is mixed gonadal dysgenesis, true hermaphroditism, or male or female pseudohermaphroditism. The first and most important determination, made cystoscopically, is the position of entry of the vagina into the urethra or urogenital sinus (Fig 139–15). If the vagina enters distal to the external sphincter, as in patients with mixed gonadal dysgenesis, "low" adrenogenital or congenital adrenal hyperplasia syndrome, or most of those with true hermaphroditism, the opening can be exteriorized using a flap vaginoplasty (Fig 139–16,E). If the vagina enters the urethra proximal to the external sphincter, as in patients with "high" adrenogenital or congenital hyperplasia syndrome, then a more complicated pull-through vaginoplasty will be required (see Fig 139–16,F). If no vagina is found (see Fig 139–16,F), as in patients with male pseudohermaphroditism, vaginal replacement can be planned for late adolescence. Miniaturized fiberoptic cytoscopes (Storz) are available in no. 8, 10, 13, and 14 F, a size range appropriate for assessment of prematures, newborns or older infants. The external urethral sphincter can be defined accurately only when the bladder is filled, a maneuver that accentuates the rounded nature of the structure. In the severely masculinized child ("high" adrenogenital syndrome), the vagina will enter the urethra proximal to the external sphincter, in the area where the verumontanum usually resides. In these cases, the base of the veru is flattened and the abnormal opening is narrow. More often, however, the vaginal opening is seen just distal to the external sphincter. If a low entry is detected, repair (Fig 139–17) can be undertaken at 3–6 months of age, or even in the newborn period if the social circumstances are such that the baby might otherwise be rejected.

Clitoral recession is the first procedure carried out. A circumferential incision is made just proximal to the glans (see Fig 139–16,A), and dorsally created Byars' flaps are divided in the midline (see Fig 139–16,B). Severe associated chordee makes the dorsal flap much more generous than its ventral counterpart. Two incisions, giving generous lateral berth, are then made into Buck's fascia to both sides of the dorsal and ventral neurovascular bundles, which are held aside with a soft Silastic holder (see Fig 139–16,B). The corpora are divided and removed from a point just below the glans, proximal to the entry of the neurovascular bundle, to a point just distal to where the corporal extensions from the pubic rami join in the midline (Fig 139–16,C). Hemostasis is secured and a meticulous microvascular end-to-end interrupted anastomosis performed between the ends of the corpora (see Fig 139–16,D), using a very fine suture, 6-0 in newborns and 5-0 in the slightly larger infant. The dorsal Byars' clitoral skin flap is then further divided to a point cephalad to the clitoris, and the latter is set back by approximating the circumscribed glans to the skin of the mons. The divided skin flaps

are then draped around the sides of the clitoris to create "labia minora" (see Fig 139–16,E), remembering that both the penile shaft skin and the labia minora derive from the same genital fold anlage.[34] If the clitoris is much enlarged, there may be a copious amount of skin that can be used more caudally to augment the lateral suture line between the opened urogenital sinus and vagina.

In the majority of cases, the vagina enters the urethra distal to the external sphincter, and thus a low vaginoplasty can be performed. This is true in patients with mixed gonadal dysgenesis, "low" adrenogenital syndrome, and in patients with true hermaphroditism (see Figs 139–16,E and 139–17). The urogenital sinus can be opened posteriorly in the midline until the posterior wall of the vagina is reached. Categorically, this must *not* be done if the vagina enters the urogenital sinus proximal to the external sphincter, as in severely masculinized patients with "high" adrenogenital or congenital adrenal hyperplasia syndrome, as the sphincter would be severed by this maneuver, leaving the patient incontinent. Vaginoplasty in these specialized cases must be deferred until 2 years of age, at which time a pull-through procedure can be performed (see Figs 139–16,F and 139–18). In the patient with male pseudohermaphroditism, the vagina is completely absent. The perineal repair is completed with labioscrotal posterior advancements (see Fig 139–16,F) and creation of a neovagina deferred until young adult or late adolescent years (see Chap. 138).

The largest number of patients (mixed gonadal dysgenesis, "low" female pseudohermaphroditism, and true hermaphroditism) can have the vagina exteriorized by low vaginoplasty done early in infancy (see Fig 139–17,A). An inverted U-flap based on the anus is raised on the perineum (see Fig 139–17,B). It is important to keep the base of this flap as generous as possible to assure the blood supply of its tip. Labioscrotal U-flaps are raised for posterior advancement. A finger is then placed in the rectum and the tissue entered between the elevated flap and the rectum. Dissection is carried to the back wall of the vagina, which is then mobilized (see Fig 139–17,C), taking care not to enter the rectum posteriorly. The vagina may have a long thin neck as it enters the urethra. The more proximal vagina may be bulbous, extending back toward the perineum and coming precariously close to the rectum. The back wall of the vagina is opened in its posterior midline and the apex of the vaginal opening sutured to the top of the inverted U-shaped perineal flap, inserted so as to externalize the vagina.

More cephalad, the distal urogenital mucosa is sutured laterally to the labioscrotal folds, which are advanced posteriorly to form labia majora (see Fig 139–17,D). U-flaps are created on the often copious scrotum. These are advanced posteriorly and fit snugly into the V created by the limb of the inverted U-flap raised to create the back wall of the vagina, thus simultaneously completing the closure while reducing the scrotum (see Fig 139–17,D). In the event of a female hypospadias, limited urethral lengthening can be achieved by tubularizing the urogenital sinus skin. This can then be covered by the elongated labia minora from the clitoral skin or the more lateral labioscrotal flaps (see Fig 139–17,E). A urethral catheter is fixed upward over the mons to prevent pressure on the suture line if one has done a urethral lengthening (see Fig 139–17,F). It is important to note that the maximum amount of pliable, nonscarred tissue is available during the first operative procedure, so as much as possible should be accomplished at this time.

Thus, the combination of flap vaginoplasty, clitoral recession with corporectomy and preservation of the dorsal and ventral neurovascular bundles, use of the clitoral skin to create labia minora and/or to amplify the lateral-vaginal opening, and posterior advancement of the labioscrotal folds to create labia majora, con-

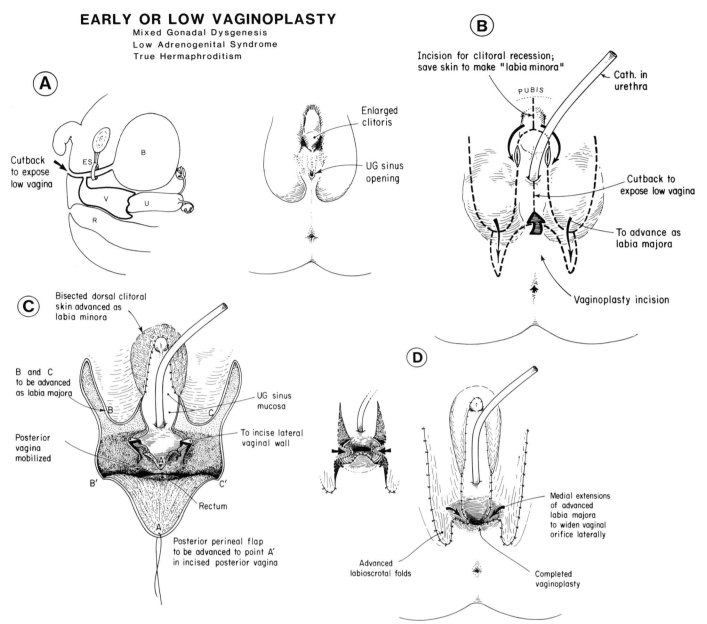

EARLY OR LOW VAGINOPLASTY

Mixed Gonadal Dysgenesis
Low Adrenogenital Syndrome
True Hermaphroditism

A

Cutback to expose low vagina

ES
B
V
U
R

Enlarged clitoris

UG sinus opening

B

Incision for clitoral recession; save skin to make "labia minora"

PUBIS

Cath. in urethra

Cutback to expose low vagina

To advance as labia majora

Vaginoplasty incision

C

Bisected dorsal clitoral skin advanced as labia minora

B and C to be advanced as labia majora

Posterior vagina mobilized

B

C

B'

C'

UG sinus mucosa

To incise lateral vaginal wall

A'

Rectum

A

Posterior perineal flap to be advanced to point A' in incised posterior vagina

D

Advanced labioscrotal folds

Medial extensions of advanced labia majora to widen vaginal orifice laterally

Completed vaginoplasty

Fig 139–17.—Low vaginoplasty. **(A)** if the vagina enters the urogenital sinus distal to the external urethral sphincter, vaginoplasty may be done ideally at 3–6 months of age, or even as early as the newborn period if there is a suspicion that the child risks rejection by the family. (*ES* indicates external sphincter; *B,* bladder; *V,* vagina; *U,* uterus; and *R,* rectum.) After the clitoris is recessed and the bisected shaft skin rotated around the repositioned glans **(B),** U-flaps are outlined on the labioscrotal folds, their extent depending upon the degree of enlargement. An inverted U-flap, outlined on the perineum and broadly based at the level of the anus, is raised. A catheter is placed in the urethra and the cutback done in the midline with one blade slipped into the vaginal orifice after the vagina has been dissected from the rectum. The labioscrotal flaps are raised **(C)** and the shawl of the labia minora sutured in place. The urogenital sinus mucosa is preserved. The inverted U-flap based on the rectum is dissected back toward the anus. At this point, a finger is placed in the rectum, which is dissected away from the back wall of the vagina, often up to the peritoneal cul-de-sac. Care must be taken to avoid creating a rectovaginal fistula. It is preferable to err on the side of opening into the vagina, rather than the rectum. The vagina is opened in the midline posteriorly and flap *A* laid into *A'* with interrupted Vicryl sutures, preferred because they slide so well. Two small incisions are made in the lateral wall of the vagina. The labioscrotal flaps are then advanced into the sidearms of the inverted U-flap created on the perineum (*B* to *B'* and *C* to *C'*). This gives an elongated appearance to the refashioned labia majora **(D).** The medial portions of the often copious labioscrotal folds are advanced into the lateral incisions on the vaginal wall so as to enhance the vaginal opening, **(D,** *lefthand insert),* stenosis of which is one of the commonest long-term complications. If the clitoral skin is particularly long, it can be further advanced between the mucosa of the urogenital sinus and the labioscrotal folds. In some cases, it may even tuck into the lateral incision on the vaginal wall. One must be careful, however, to assess the vascular supply to the distal end of this shaft skin. Posterior and lateral flaps from the scrotal folds can augment the vaginal orifice **(D).** On the right, suturing of the inverted labioscrotal flaps is completed; the clitoris is recessed; a labium minus is recreated from clitoral skin; a labium majus has been fashioned from labioscrotal folds; and the vagina has been exteriorized. Dilatations with a Hegar dilator are begun 2 weeks after operation and continue daily for 6 months.

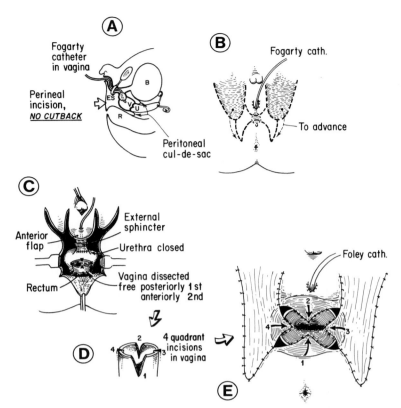

Fig 139–18.—High vaginal pull-through. **A,** in the event that the vagina *(V)* is found to enter the urogenital sinus proximal to the external sphincter *(ES)*, exteriorization should be delayed until the child is older and larger, usually age 2 years. The vaginal opening is catheterized with a small Fogarty balloon and a sound passed into the bladder *(B)*. A cutback of the urogenital sinus is *not* done as in the low vaginoplasty. This maneuver would divide the external sphincter and most probably make the child incontinent. *(U* = uterus, *R* = rectum) **B,** a posterior inverted U-flap is raised. Labioscrotal U-flaps are raised, as in an anterior U-flap, based on the urogenital sinus mucosa. *No* cutback is done. **C,** dissection comes in from behind the urethra until the Fogarty balloon is felt. Firm prostatic tissue may be encountered at this point. Care is taken to avoid the external sphincter, which may be identified with a nerve stimulator. The vagina is then divided from the urethra, which is closed transversely after pulling back the Fogarty balloon. The urethra is closed neither too tightly, avoiding a stricture, nor too loosely, avoiding creation of a diverticulum. The urethral sound is then removed and a Foley catheter placed in the bladder. The vagina is mobilized first posteriorly, a finger placed in the rectum to prevent entering that structure. Dissection must often continue back to the peritoneal cul-de-sac. The vagina is then mobilized from the back wall of the bladder, again dissecting to the peritoneal cul-de-sac. The orifice of the vagina is usually exceptionally narrow. It is therefore opened, if possible, in four quadrants **(D).** The posterior perineal flap is advanced **(E)** posteriorly to point *1,* the anterior flap of the urogenital sinus to point *2,* and the labioscrotal folds into the lateral arms of the perineal flap and into the lateral incisions of the vagina (points *3* and *4*). Even with all these precautions, stenosis of the vaginal orifice can be a late complication. We therefore recommend that daily dilatations with a Hegar dilator begin 2 weeks after operation and continue for 6 months to maintain pliability of the orifice during healing.

stitutes the complex of procedures that may be required for perineoplasty with the most efficient use of available tissue. This can be done at age 3–6 months or in the newborn infant who is at risk for rejection, in all true hermaphrodites and mixed gonadal dysgenesis patients, and in female pseudohermaphrodites with the low entry of the vagina distal to the external sphincter. Various methods have been devised for diminishing the clitoris. The most widely used is recession as described by Lattimer[61] and Randolph and Hung,[91] who sutured the corpora back to the symphysis pubis. Because the buried clitoris can respond with painful erections in adrenogenital patients exposed to endogenous androgens released if the patient neglects medication, we have preferred the technique herein described. Partial corporectomy with reanastomosis preserves erectile function, and careful dissection of the neurovascular bundles preserves sensation to the glans.

In the event of a high entry of the vagina into the urethra, as in some patients with congenital adrenal hyperplasia or adrenogenital syndrome, vaginoplasty is delayed until 2 years of age. The psychologically important clitoroplasty, however, can still be done at 3–6 months or in the newborn period. Under these circumstances, the clitoral skin is preserved as labia minora; and the labioscrotal folds are only partially reduced so that they can be used later to augment the vaginal opening.

At 2 years of age, in patients with the vagina entering the urethra proximal to the voluntary sphincter, anterior- and posterior-based U-flaps are raised (Fig 139–18,*B*). A Fogarty balloon is placed in the vagina, which is then dissected from below so as carefully to preserve the external urethra sphincter. *Under no circumstances should a cutback of the urogenital sinus be done.* A finger in the rectum is helpful. Dissection is carried up from beneath the posterior U-flap toward the vaginal opening into the urethra. The external sphincter must be assiduously protected; it can be seen and functionally defined by nerve stimulation. The vagina is divided from the urethra, and the latter is sutured transversely, taking care neither to narrow the urethra nor to leave a diverticulum (see Fig 139–18,*C*). The Fogarty catheter is removed; a Foley catheter is placed in the bladder, and the vagina is carefully cleared from the posterior bladder wall. Catheters in the ureters may protect them from harm in the event of a very high dissection, which often must be carried up to the peritoneal cul-de-sac.

After mobilization, the narrowed neck of the vagina is opened in four quadrants (see Fig 139–18,*D*) and U-flaps from posterior,

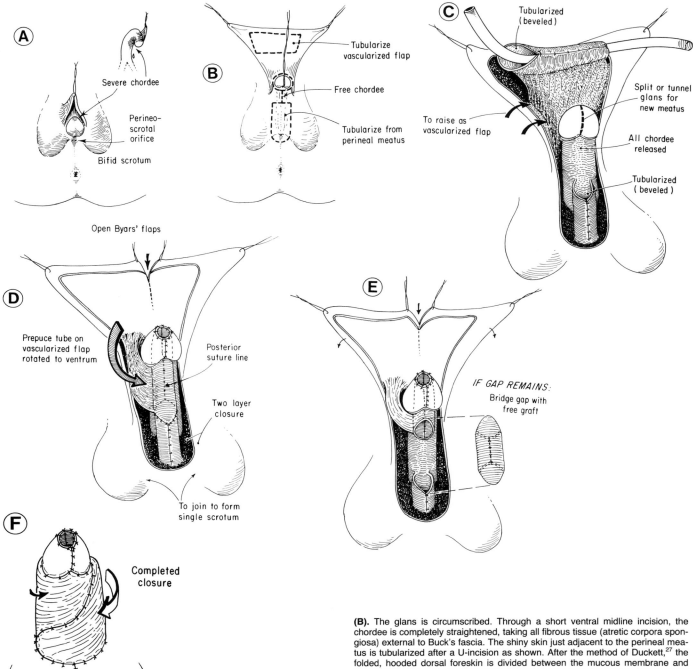

Fig 139–19.—Hypospadias. The hypospadias in intersex babies committed to the male gender is often quite severe (**A**). Its meatal opening is usually perineoscrotal, the chordee is marked, and there is often associated micropenis, making the repair particularly difficult. Preliminary testosterone treatment, if done within the first 6 months of life, can enhance the size of a microphallus. In the older child, the testosterone effect may not be as rewarding. Also, the child may be made hyperactive, making difficult the enforced bedrest necessary in the immediate postoperative period. The anomaly is often associated with the prepenile ("shawl") and bifid scrotum, to be repaired at a later date if it is severe. Repair of severe micropenis with hypospadias may have to be staged if the hooded foreskin is small. At the first stage, the chordee should be straightened and the dorsal flaps rotated to cover the ventral surface. If the dorsal foreskin is more ample, hypospadias repair may be accomplished in a single procedure as shown

(**B**). The glans is circumscribed. Through a short ventral midline incision, the chordee is completely straightened, taking all fibrous tissue (atretic corpora spongiosa) external to Buck's fascia. The shiny skin just adjacent to the perineal meatus is tubularized after a U-incision as shown. After the method of Duckett,[27] the folded, hooded dorsal foreskin is divided between the mucous membrane and the foreskin (**C**). The mucous membrane is outlined to create a patch that can be rolled into a tube. This patch is dissected away from the dorsal foreskin, preserving its vasculature, and rolled into a tube with a running Dexon or Vicryl suture. The tubularized graft is then rotated ventrally (**D**), so that its suture line faces inward toward the shaft of the penis, and anastomosed to the tubularized graft from the midscrotum. The suture line between the two tubes must be beveled, to avoid stricture. The distal end of the vascularized graft may be tunneled through the glans to the meatus. Otherwise, the glans is opened, the graft laid in, and the glans closed around the distal portion of the graft to create a new meatus, as in **D**. The remaining dorsal foreskin is divided in the midline and rotated ventrally over the neourethra, which has already been covered with a layer of adventitia. The proximal part of the scrotum is brought together in the midline to correct the bifid scrotum. In the event that the proximal tubularized graft cannot meet the distal tubularized graft (**E**), the defect can be bridged with a free skin graft taken with a Reese dermatome from the inside of the upper arm, or a free bladder mucosa graft. As before, it is extremely important to bevel the grafts at the anastomoses. Stricture will invariably occur if this is not done. It is important to close the tissue in multiple layers over the neourethra. This often consists of the dartos proximally in the area of the scrotum and shaft, and subcutaneous tissue distally over the vascularized graft. The dorsal foreskin is divided as Byar's flaps (**F**) and swung ventrally to cover all defects.

anterior, and the two sides, using tissue brought posteriorly from the labioscrotal folds, are turned in to enhance as well as to externalize the vaginal opening (see Fig 139–18,*E*).

Two weeks after either early (3–6 months) or delayed (2 years) operation, we suggest dilatation of the vaginal orifice, once a day for 6 months with progressively wider Hegar dilators. Dilatations keep the introitus supple and prevent stenosis, the most common long-term complication encountered after this type of procedure.

In the event of an absent vagina, as in the male pseudohermaphrodite, clitoral recession and labioscrotal reduction are done at 3–6 months and vaginal reconstruction undertaken in late adolescence (see Fig 139–16,*F*). If an introitus is present, dilatations to enlarge and deepen the introitus are undertaken, first with Hegar dilators, and later with Young's dilators. Dilatations alone may provide an adequate vagina; or they may provide a widened, less fragile, estrogen-responsive vaginal opening to which a skin graft or colon can be anastomosed more proximally (see Chap. 138).

Patients with male pseudohermaphroditism who are to be supported in the male gender must usually undergo a difficult hypospadias repair, often of the perineoscrotal variety (see Fig 139–19,*A*). This can often be done in a single stage with a neourethra constructed proximally from the midportion of a bifid scrotum (see Fig 139–19,*B*) meeting a distal rotated vascularized skin graft from the hooded foreskin (see Fig 139–19,*C* and *D*).[27] If necessary, a thick, split-thickness graft can be taken from the medial surface of the upper arm or from the bladder mucosa to bridge a gap of any length (see Fig 139–19,*E*). It is important to note that the proximal anastomosis of these grafts must be bevelled in order to prevent stricture. The neourethra should be brought out to the tip of the glans and the glans re-created ventrally to give a normal appearance.

At a later stage, a prepenile or "shawl" scrotum that drapes around the base of the penis can be brought distally, often coordinated with repair of a bifid scrotum. Testicular prostheses may have to be inserted. We suggest the soft Silastic variety of Heyer-Schulte. These must be changed as the male approaches adolescence. A mastectomy may be necessary in a male developing gynecomastia as puberty approaches.

REFERENCES

1. Aarskog D.: Clinical and cytogenetic studies in hypospadias. *Acta. Pediatr. Scand.* (suppl.) 203:1, 1970.
2. Andler W., Zachmann M.: Spontaneous breast development in an adolescent girl with testicular feminization after castration in early childhood. *J. Pediatr.* 94:304, 1979.
3. Armendares S., Salamanca F., Cantu J., et al.: Familial true hermaphroditism in three siblings: Clinical, cytogenetic, histological and hormonal studies. *Hum. Genet.* 29:99, 1975.
4. Atkins L., Book J.A., Gustavson K.H., et al.: A case of XXXXY sex chromosome anomaly with autoradiographic studies. *Cytogenetics* 2:208, 1963.
5. Barr M.L., Bertram E.G.: A morphological distinction between neurons of the male and female and the behavior of the nucleolar satellite during accelerated nuclear protein synthesis. *Nature* 163:676, 1949.
6. Berthezene L., Forest M.G., Grimaud J.A., et al.: Leydig cell agenesis: A cause of male pseudohermaphroditism. *N. Engl. J. Med.* 295:969, 1976.
7. Bongiovanni A.M., Root A.W.: Adrenogenital syndrome. *N. Engl. J. Med.* 268:1283, 1963.
8. Brown D.M., Markland C., Dehner L.P.: Leydig cell hypoplasia: A cause of male pseudohermaphroditism. *J. Clin. Endocrinol. Metab.* 46:1, 1978.
9. Budzik G.P., Powell S.M., Kamagata S., et al.: Müllerian inhibiting substance fractionation by dye affinity chromatography. *Cell* 34:307, 1983.
10. Budzik G.P., Swann D.A., Hayashi A., et al.: Enhanced purification of müllerian inhibiting substance by lectin affinity chromatography. *Cell* 21:909, 1980.
11. Buyse M., Fordney-Settbage D., Towner J., et al.: 46XX/47XYY mosaicism in a true hermaphrodite. *Lancet* 1:1300, 1975.
12. Byskov A., Grinsted J.: Feminizing effect of mesonephros on cultured differentiating mouse gonads and ducts. *Science* 212:817, 1981.
13. Cattanach B., Pollard C., Hawkes S.: Sex reversed mice: XX and XO males. *Cytogenetics* 10:318, 1971.
14. Chen Y.C., Woolley P.V.: Genetic studies on hypospadias in males. *J. Med. Genet.* 8:153, 1971.
15. Comite F., Cutler G., Rivier J., et al.: Short-term treatment of idiopathic precocious puberty with a long-acting analog of luteinizing hormone-releasing hormone. *N. Engl. J. Med.* 305:1546, 1981.
16. Coulom C.: Testicular regression syndrome. *Obstet. Gynecol.* 53:44, 1979.
17. Cutler B., Forbes A., Ingersoll G., et al.: Endometrial carcinoma after stilbestrol therapy in gonadal dysgenesis. *N. Engl. J. Med.* 287:628, 1972.
18. de la Chapelle A., Hortling H., Wennstrom M., et al.: Two males with female chromosomes. *Acta. Endocrinol.* (suppl.) 100:90, 1965.
19. de la Chapelle A.: Analytic review: Nature and origin of males with XX sex chromosomes. *Am. J. Hum. Genet.* 24:71, 1972.
20. De Marchi M., Carbonara A., Carozzi F., et al.: True hermaphroditism with XX/XY sex chromosome mosaicism: Report of a case. *Clin. Genet.* 10:265, 1976.
21. DeGroot L.V., Stanbury J.B.: *The Thyroid and Its Disease.* New York, John Wiley & Sons, 1975.
22. DeVictor-Vuillet M., Luciani J., Carlon N., et al.: Abnormalities de structure et role du chromosome Y chez l'homme. *Pathol. Biol.* 19:231, 1971.
23. Donahoe P.K., Budzik G.P., Trelstad R., et al.: Müllerian-Inhibiting Substance: An update, in Greep R.O. (ed.): *Recent Progress in Hormone Research.* New York, Academic Press, 1982, vol. 38, p. 279.
24. Donahoe P.K., Crawford J.D., Hendren W.H.: Mixed gonadal dysgenesis, pathogenesis and management. *J. Pediatr. Surg.* 14:287, 1979.
25. Donahoe P.K., Crawford J.D., Hendren W.H.: True hermaphroditism: A clinical description and a proposed function for the long arm of the Y chromosome. *J. Pediatr. Surg.* 13:293, 1978.
26. Donahoe P.K., Ito Y., Morikawa Y., et al.: Müllerian inhibiting substance in human testes after birth. *J. Pediatr. Surg.* 7:323, 1977.
27. Duckett J.W.: Hypospadias. *Clin. Plast. Surg.* 7:149, 1980.
28. Edman C.D., Winters A.J., Porter J.D., et al.: Embryonic testicular agenesis: A clinical spectrum of agonadal individuals. *Am. J. Obstet. Gynecol.* 49:208, 1977.
29. Eichwald E., Silmser C.: Skin. *Transplant. Bull.* 2:148, 1955.
30. Eil C., Austin R.M., Sesterhenn I., et al.: Leydig cell hypoplasia causing male pseudohermaphroditism: Diagnosis 13 years after prepubertal castration. *J. Clin. Endocrinol. Metab.* 58:441, 1984.
31. Eil C., Crawford J.D., Donahoe P.K., et al.: Fibroblast androgen receptors in patients with genitourinary anomalies. *J. Androl.* 5:313–320, 1984.
32. Eil C., Lippman M., Loriaux D.: A dispersed whole cell method for the determination of androgen receptors in human skin fibroblasts. *Steroids* 35:389, 1980.
33. Farba C., Liebenthal D., Wachtel S., et al.: Detection of H-Y antigen in the ELISA. *Hum. Genet.* 65:278–279, 1984.
34. Federman D.D.: *Abnormal Sexual Development.* Philadelphia, W.B. Saunders Co., 1967.
35. Fékété C., Lortat-Jacob S., Cachin O., et al.: Preservation of gonadal function in true hermaphroditism. *J. Pediatr. Surg.* 19:50, 1984.
36. Feldman K.W., Smith E.W.: Fetal phallic growth and penile standards for newborn male infants. *J. Pediatr.* 86:395, 1975.
37. Ferguson-Smith M.: Abnormal gonadal differentiation in XY females and XX males. *Birth Defects* 7:204, 1971.
38. Ferguson-Smith M.: X-Y chromosomal interchange in the aetiology of true hermaphroditism and of XX Klinefelter's syndrome. *Lancet* 2:475, 1966.
39. Flateau E., Josefsberg Z., Reiner S.H., et al.: Penile size of the newborn male infant. *J. Pediatr.* 87:663, 1975.
40. Forest M.G., Lecoq A., Salle B., et al.: Does neonatal phenobarbital treatment affect testicular and adrenal functions and steroid binding in plasma in infancy? *J. Clin. Endocrinol. Metab.* 52:103, 1981.
41. Funder J.W., Mercer J.E.: Cimetidine, a histamine H2 receptor antagonist, occupies androgen receptors. *J. Clin. Endocrinol. Metab.* 48:189, 1979.
42. Gallegos A., Guizar E., Armendares S., et al.: Familial true hermaphroditism in three siblings: Plasma hormonal profile and in vitro steroid biosynthesis in gonadal structures. *J. Clin. Endocrinol. Metab.* 42:653, 1976.

43. Gerli M., Biagioni G., Bruschelli G.M., et al.: A case of true hermaphroditism with 45X/46XY mosaicism. *Hum. Genet.* 34:93, 1976.

44. Goldberg E., Boyse E., Bennett D.: Serological demonstration of H-Y (male) antigen on mouse sperm. *Nature* 232:478, 1971.

45. Grumbach M.D., VanWyk J.J.: Disorders of sex differentiation, in Williams R.H. (ed.): *Textbook of Endocrinology.* Philadelphia, W.B. Saunders Co., 1974, p. 480.

46. Haseltine F.P., Ohno S.: Mechanisms of gonadal differentiation. *Science* 211:1272, 1981.

47. Hayashi A., Donahoe P.K., Budzik G.P., et al.: Periductal and matrix glycosaminoglycans in rat müllerian duct development and regression. *Dev. Biol.* 92:16, 1982.

48. Hoffman A., Crowley W.: Induction of puberty in men by long-term pulsatile administration of low-dose gonadotropin-releasing hormone. *N. Engl. J. Med.* 307:1237, 1982.

49. Jones W.H., Ferguson-Smith M.A., Heller R.H.: The pathology and cytogenetics of gonadal agenesis. *Am. J. Obstet. Gynecol.* 87:578, 1963.

50. Josso N., DeGrouchy J., Auvert J., et al.: True hermaphroditism with XX/XY mosaicism, probably due to double fertilization of the ovum. *J. Clin. Endocrinol. Metab.* 25:114, 1965.

51. Josso N.: Interspecific character of mullerian inhibiting substance: Action of the human fetal testis, ovary, and adrenal on the fetal rat mullerian duct in organ culture. *J. Clin. Endocrinol. Metab.* 32:404, 1971.

52. Jost A., Vigier B., Prepin J.: Freemartins in cattle: The first steps of sexual organogenesis. *J. Reprod. Fertil.* 29:349, 1972.

53. Jost A.: Données preliminaires sur les stages initiaux de la différenciation du testicule chez le rat. *Arch. Anat. Microsc. Morphol. Exp.* 61:415, 1972.

54. Jost A.: Sur la différenciation sexuelle de l'embryon de lapin. Expériences de parabiose. *C.R. Soc. Biol.* 140:463, 1946.

55. Jost A.: Sur la différenciation sexuelle de l'embryon de lapin: Remarques au sujet de certaines operations chirurgicales, sur l'embryon. *C.R. Soc. Biol.* 140:461, 1946.

56. Jost A.: Sur les dérivés mulleriens d'embryons de lapin des deux sexes castres a 21 jours. *C.R. Soc. Biol.* 141:135, 1946.

57. Jubiz W., Meikle A.W., Levinson R.A., et al.: Effect of diphenylhydantoin on metabolism of dexamethasone. *N. Engl. J. Med.* 283:11, 1970.

58. Kasdan R., Nankin H., Troen P., et al.: Paternal transmission of maleness in XX human beings. *N. Engl. J. Med.* 288:539, 1973.

59. Kogan S.: Micropenis: Etiologies and management considerations. *Clin. Androl.* 7:197, 1981.

60. Koo G., Wachtel S., Breg W., et al.: Mapping the locus of the H-Y antigen. *Birth Defects* 12:151, 1976.

61. Lattimer J.K.: Relocation and recession of the enlarged clitoris with preservation of the glans: An alternative to amputation. *J. Urol.* 86:113, 1961.

62. Lee P.A., Mazur T., Danish R., et al.: Micropenis: I. Criteria, etiologies, and classification. *Johns Hopkins Med. J.* 146:156, 1980.

63. Liddle G.W.: The adrenal cortex, in Williams R.H. (ed.): *Textbook of Endocrinology.* Philadelphia, W.B. Saunders Co., 1974, p. 276.

64. Lillie G.: The theory of freemartin. *Science* 43:611, 1916.

65. Lowry R., Honore L., Arnold W., et al.: Familial true hermaphroditism. *Birth Defects* 11:105, 1975.

66. Lyon M.F.: X-chromosome inactivation and developmental patterns in mammals. *Biol. Rev.* 47:1, 1972.

67. Lyon M.F.: Mechanisms and evolutionary origins of variable X-chromosome activity in mammals. *Proc. R. Soc. Lon.* 187B:243, 1974.

68. MacIntyre M.: Effect of the testis on ovarian differentiation in heterosexual embryonic rat gonad transplant. *Anat. Rec.* 124:27, 1956.

69. Madden J.D., Walsh P.C., MacDonald P.C., et al.: Characterization of a patient with the syndrome of incomplete testicular feminization. *J. Clin. Endocrinol. Metab.* 41:751, 1975.

70. Mansfield M., Beardsworth D., Loughlin J., et al.: Long-term treatment of central precocious puberty with a long-acting analog of luteinizing hormone-releasing hormone. *N. Engl. J. Med.* 309:1286, 1983.

71. Manuel M., Katayama K.P., Jones H.W.: The age of occurrence of gonadal tumors in intersex patients with a Y chromosome. *Am. J. Obstet. Gynecol.* 124:205, 1976.

72. Milunsky A.: Sex-determining genes and the Y chromosome. *N. Engl. J. Med.* 288:577, 1973.

73. Mintz B., Russell E.: Gene induced embryological modifications of primordial germ cells in the mouse. *J. Exp. Zool.* 134:207, 1957.

74. Mittwoch U., Buehr M.: Gonadal growth in embryos of sex reversed mice. *Differentiation* 1:219, 1973.

75. Muller U., Aschmoneit I., Zenzes M.T., et al.: Binding studies of H-Y antigen in rat tissue indicative of a gonad specific receptor. *Hum. Genet.* 43:151, 1978.

76. Nagai Y., Ciccarese S., Ohno S.: Identification of human H-Y antigen and testicular transformation induced by its interaction with the receptor site of bovine fetal ovarian cells. *Differentiation* 13:155, 1979.

77. Nagamine C., Reidy J., Koo G.: A radiobinding assay for human H-Y antigen using monoclonal antibodies. *Transplantation* 37:13, 1984.

78. Neuman F., BonBorswordt-Wallrobe R., Elger W., et al.: Aspects of androgen dependent events as studies by antiandrogens, in Greep R.O. (ed.): *Recent Progress in Hormone Research.* New York, Academic Press, 1970, vol. 26, p. 337.

79. New M.I., Dupont B., Pang S., et al.: An update of congenital adrenal hyperplasia, in Greep R.O. (ed.): *Recent Progress in Hormone Research.* New York, Academic Press, 1981, vol. 37, p. 105.

80. Noades J., Gavin J., Tippett P., et al.: The X-linked blood group system Xg tests on British, Northern American, and Northern European unrelated people and families. *J. Med. Genet.* 3:162, 1966.

81. O'Rahilly R.: Prenatal human development, in Wynn R.M. (ed.): *Biology of the Uterus.* New York, Plenum Press, 1977, p. 35.

82. Ohno S., Christian L.D., Wachtel S., et al.: A hormone-like role of H-Y antigen in the bovine freemartin gonad. *Nature* 261:597, 1976.

83. Ohno S.: The role of H-Y antigen in primary sex determination. *JAMA* 239:217, 1978.

84. Ohno S., Nagai Y., Ciccarese S.: Testicular cells lysostripped of H-Y antigen organize ovarian follicle-like aggregates. *Cytogenet. Cell Genet.* 20:351, 1978.

85. Ohno S.: Major regulatory genes for mammalian sexual development. *Cell* 1976.

86. Opitz J.M., Simpson J.L., Sario G.E., et al.: Pseudovaginal perineoscrotal hypospadias. *Clin. Genet.* 3:1, 1972.

87. Peterson R.E., Imperato-McGinley J., Gautier T., et al.: Male pseudohermaphroditism due to steroid 5a reductase deficiency. *Am. J. Med.* 62:170, 1977.

88. Picon R.: Action du testicule foetal sur le development in vitro des canaux de Muller chez le rat. *Arch. Anat. Microsc. Morphol. Exp.* 58:1, 1969.

89. Pinto W., Gardner L.I., Rosenbaum D.: Abnormal genitalia are presenting sign of two male infants with hydantoin embryopathy syndrome. *Am. J. Dis. Child.* 62:170, 1977.

90. Rajfer J., Mendelsohn G., Arnheim J., et al.: Dysgenetic male pseudohermaphroditism. *J. Urol.* 119:525, 1978.

91. Randolph J.G., Hung W.: Relocation clitoroplasty in females with hypertrophied clitoris. *J. Pediatr. Surg.* 5:224, 1970.

92. Robboy S.J., Miller T., Donahoe P.K., et al.: Dysgenesis of testicular and streak gonads in the syndrome of mixed gonadal dysgenesis: Perspective derived from a clinicopathologic analysis of twenty-one cases. *Hum. Pathol.* 12:700, 1982.

93. Roberts C.J., Lloyd S.: Observations on the epidemiology of simple hypospadias. *Br. Med. J.* 1:768, 1973.

94. Roe T., Alfi O.: Ambiguous genitalia in XX male children: Report of two infants. *Pediatrics* 60:55, 1977.

95. Roth L., Cleary R., Hokum F.: Case reports: Ultrastructure of an ovotestis in a case of true hermaphroditism. *Obstet. Gynecol.* 48:619, 1976.

96. Salle B., Hedinger C.: Gonadal histology in children with male pseudohermaphroditism and mixed gonadal dysgenesis. *Acta Endocrinol.* 64:211, 1970.

97. Sanger R., Tippett P., Gavin J., et al.: Xg groups and sex chromosome abnormalities in people of northern European ancestry: An addendum. *J. Med. Genet.* 14:210, 1977.

98. Santen R.J., Van den Bossche J., Symoens J., et al.: Site of action of low dose ketoconazole on androgen biosynthesis in men. *J. Clin. Endocrinol. Metab.* 57:732, 1983.

99. Schwartz M., Imperato-McGinley J., Peterson R.E., et al.: Male pseudohermaphroditism secondary to an abnormality in Leydig cell differentiation. *J. Clin. Endocrinol. Metab.* 53:123, 1981.

100. Scully R.E.: Gonadoblastoma: A review of 74 cases. *Cancer* 25:1340, 1970.

101. Shackleton C.H., Mitchell F.L., Farquhar J.W.: Difficulties in the diagnosis of the adrenogenital syndrome in infancy. *Pediatrics* 49:198, 1972.

102. Sijernholm M.R., Katz F.H.: Effects of diphenylhydantoin, phenobarbital and Diazepam on the metabolism of methylprednisolone and its sodium succinate. *J. Clin. Endocrinol. Metab.* 41:887, 1975.

103. Singh L., Jones K.: Sex reversal in the mouse (mus musculus) is caused by a recurrent nonreciprocal crossover involving the X and an aberrant Y chromosome. *Cell* 28:205, 1982.

104. Singh L., Phillips C., Jones K.: The conserved nucleotide sequences of Bkm, which define Sxr in the mouse, are transcribed. *Cell* 36:111, 1984.

105. Singh R.P., Carr D.H.: The anatomy and histology of XO human embryos and fetuses. *Anat. Rec.* 155:369, 1966.
106. Sohval A.: Hermaphroditism with "atypical" or "mixed" gonadal dysgenesis. *Am. J. Med.* 36:281, 1964.
107. Soller M., Padeh B., Wysoli M., et al.: Cytogenetics of Saanen goats showing abnormal development of the reproductive tracts associated with the dominant gene for polledness. *Cytogenetics* 8:51, 1969.
108. Spigelman M., Bennett D.: A light and electron microscopic study of primordial germ cells in the early mouse embryo. *J. Embryol. Exp. Morphol.* 30:97, 1973.
109. Stephens F.D.: *Congenital Malformations of the Urinary Tract.* New York, Praeger, 1983.
110. Taguchi O., Cunha G.R., Lawrence W.D., et al.: Timing and irreversibility of müllerian duct inhibition in the embryonic reproductive tract of the human male. *Dev. Biol.* 106:394–398, 1984.
111. Teter J.: A new concept of classification of gonadal tumors arising from germ cells (gonocytoma) and their histogenesis. *Gynecologia* 150:84, 1960.
112. Tijo J.H., Levan A.: The chromosome number of man. *Hereditas* 42:1, 1956.
113. Trelstad R.L., Hayashi A., Hayashi K., et al.: The epithelial-mesenchymal interface of the male rat müllerian duct: Loss of basement membrane integrity and ductal regression. *Dev. Biol.* 92:27, 1982.
114. Tsai J., Samuels H.: Thyroid hormone action: Demonstration of putative nuclear receptors in human lymphocytes. *J. Clin. Endocrinol. Metab.* 38:919, 1974.
115. Upadhyay S., Luciani J., Zamboni L.: *Ann. Biol. Anim. Biochem. Biophys.* 19:1179, 1919.

116. Van Niekerk W.: True hermaphroditism. *Am. J. Obstet. Gynecol.* 126:898, 1976.
117. Wachtel S., Koo G.C.: H-Y antigen and abnormal sex differentiation. *Birth Defects* 14:1–7, 1978.
118. Wachtel S., Koo G.C., Breg W., et al.: Expression of H-Y antigen in human males with two Y chromosomes. *N. Engl. J. Med.* 293:1070, 1975.
119. Wachtel S., Koo G.C., Breg W., et al.: Serologic detection of a Y-linked gene in XX males and XX true hermaphrodites. *N. Engl. J. Med.* 295:750, 1976.
120. Wachtel S.: Immunogenetic aspects of abnormal sexual differentiation. *Cell* 16:691, 1979.
121. Wachtel S.S., Ohno S.: The immunogenetics of sexual development. *Prog. Med. Genet.* 3:109, 1979.
122. Walsh P.C., Madden J.D., Harrod M.J., et al.: Familial incomplete male pseudohermaphroditism, type 2: Decreased dihydrotestosterone formation in pseudovaginal perineoscrotal hypospadias. *N. Engl. J. Med.* 291:944, 1974.
123. Welshons W.J., Russell L.B.: The Y-chromosome as the bearer of male determining factors in the mouse. *Proc. Natl. Acad. Sci. U.S.A.* 45:560, 1959.
124. Wilson J.D., George F.W., Griffin J.E.: The hormonal control of sexual development. *Science* 212:1278, 1982.
125. Wilson J.D., Harrod M.J., Goldstein J.L., et al.: Familial incomplete male pseudohermaphroditism, type 1: Evidence for androgen resistance and variable clinical manifestations in a family with the Reifenstein syndrome. *N. Engl. J. Med.* 290:1098, 1974.
126. Zadik A., Kahana L., Kauffman H., et al.: Salt loss in hypertensive form of congenital adrenohyperplasia (11-Beta hydroxylase deficiency). *J. Clin. Endocrinol. Metab.* 58:384, 1984.

PART IX

Special Areas of Pediatric Surgery

140

Thomas M. Holder / Keith W. Ashcraft

Cardiac Disease

ALTHOUGH MANY of the early developments in the surgical treatment of congenital heart disease were made by pediatric surgeons, there are few whose practice now includes extensive experience with cardiac surgery. Still, it is important that the surgeon who is called upon to correct esophageal atresia, for instance, have at least a working knowledge of how and when an associated cardiac malformation should be treated. It is important that the pediatric surgeon coordinate his management of gastroesophageal reflux with the cardiac surgeon's treatment for ventricular septal defect. Similarly, an associated coarctation of the aorta in the small baby who has necrotizing enterocolitis requires an understanding of both conditions in order to make intelligent decisions regarding the management of either lesion.

In this chapter, we shall discuss the treatment options for congenital heart disease in the pediatric surgical patient. Our experience with combined cardiac and other surgical lesions has been compiled from the last 1,000 consecutive patients we have operated upon for congenital heart disease at The Children's Mercy Hospital in Kansas City, Mo. (Table 140–1).

HISTORY.—The first successful corrective procedure of a congenital heart defect was performed in 1938 by Robert E. Gross[34] when he ligated a patent ductus arteriosus.[16] Crafoord,[24] in early 1944, successfully resected a coarctation of the aorta, a feat which Gross[35] also accomplished about the same time. In 1945, Blalock and Taussig[9] reported the successful shunting of blood from the systemic to the pulmonary artery circuit for relief of cyanosis caused by Fallot's tetralogy. In 1946, Potts et al.[60] described the anastomosis of the descending aorta to the pulmonary artery, and in 1962 Waterston[76] described the intrapericardial anastomosis of the right pulmonary artery to the ascending aorta. Among the other milestones in the palliation of congenital heart defects was the atrial septectomy of Blalock and Hanlon[8] to allow better atrial venous mixing in patients with transposition of the great arteries; the introduction of pulmonary artery banding for reduction of excessive pulmonary flow in patients with large left-to-right shunts by Muller and Dammann[53] in 1952; and the cava-to-pulmonary artery anastomosis by Glenn[32] and Patino in 1954 as a treatment for the hypoplastic right heart syndrome.

The era of corrective intracardiac operations for congenital heart defects began in 1952 with successful suture of an atrial septal defect by Gross and associates using the well technique. In 1953, Gibbon[31] introduced the use of the mechanical heart-lung device to clinical surgery for the repair of an atrial septal defect and made practical the whole field of intracardiac surgery. In 1954, Lillehei et al.[46] corrected Fallot's tetralogy using a cross-circulated donor as the oxygenator. Vast simplifications and improvements in equipment and techniques have been incorporated over the ensuing 30 years, perhaps the most significant advance being the introduction of deep hypothermia and circulatory arrest for the correction of all sorts of congenital heart disease in infants and young children.[4]

Extracardiac Lesions: Patent Ductus Arteriosus and Coarctation of the Aorta

Patent Ductus Arteriosus in the Older Child (see Chap. 141)

The indication for closure of a patent ductus arteriosus (PDA) is its presence. Although the shunt may be hemodynamically insignificant, the turbulence created by a PDA is thought to be an etiologic factor in the late development of subacute bacterial endocarditis.

Closure of the ductus in a child can be accomplished either by ligation or division (Fig 140–1). Ligation of the ductus is practiced at the Great Ormond Street Hospital For Sick Children in London, where three and sometimes four heavy ligatures are used to occlude the ductal lumen.[70] The technique described by Blalock[7] consists of purse-string ligatures at either end of the ductus, with a transfixion ligature in the center portion to obliterate the ductus. The results of ductus ligation very nearly approximate those of division and suture, with perhaps a little less risk of bleeding. Our preference, however, is for division and suture in order to obviate the very small but real incidence of recanalization of the ductus. Mortality rates in the otherwise healthy child should be well under 1%.

Patent Ductus Arteriosus in the Neonate

The most dramatic manifestation of the patent ductus arteriosus is that seen in the premature infant with IRDS. Adequate

TABLE 140–1.—1,000 CONSECUTIVE PATIENTS OPERATED UPON FOR CONGENITAL HEART DISEASE*

CARDIAC LESION	TOTAL PATIENTS
PDA	
Premature–IRDS	30
Older	121
Coarctation	112
TGA	67
Tetralogy of Fallot	111
Truncus arteriosus	7
Hypoplastic right heart	41
TAPVD	12
ASD, primum	25
ASD, secundum	97
ASD, sinus venosus	9
VSD	152
Complete AV canal	48
Pulmonic stenosis	
Critical newborn	9
Older	57
Aortic stenosis	39
Vascular ring	14
Miscellaneous	49

*Abbreviations used in this and other tables: PDA indicates patent ductus arteriosus; UPJ, ureteropelvic junction; GER, gastroesophageal reflux; fundo, fundoplication; LIH, left inguinal herniorrhaphy; RIH, right inguinal herniorrhaphy; BIH, bilateral inguinal herniorrhaphy; TEF, tracheoesophageal fistula; EA, esophageal atresia; A-V fistula, arteriovenous fistula; NB, newborn; IRDS, infant respiratory distress syndrome; SBO, small bowel obstruction; COA, coarctation of aorta; NEC, necrotizing enterocolitis; AG, adrenogenital; TGA, transposition of great arteries; PS, pulmonic stenosis; BH, Blalock-Hanlon atrial septectomy; ASD, atrial septal defect; TET, tetralogy of Fallot; VSD, ventricular septal defect; AV canal, atrioventricular canal; AS, aortic stenosis; and TAPVD, total anomalous pulmonary venous drainage.

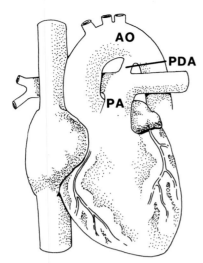

Fig 140–1.—The patent ductus arteriosus *(PDA)* connects the under side of the aortic arch *(AO)* with the superior aspect of the pulmonary artery at its bifurcation *(PA)*. In the older child, purse-string ligatures, transfixion ligatures, or simple surrounding ligatures of heavy silk may be used to ligate and obliterate an undivided ductus. Our preference is for division and suture. In this way, the possibility of recanalization is considerably reduced. We have not seen infection with the division and suture technique as we have with the heavy silk ligatures. In the exceedingly ill neonate with idiopathic respiratory distress syndrome (IRDS), ligation with a single no. 5 silk suture is our preference for obliterating the ductus. This is done through a standard thoracotomy, which in our experience is no more difficult for the child than is an extrapleural, anterior, or posterior approach. We likewise prefer doing this under the more certain sterile conditions and optimum lighting provided in an operating room, rather than under an infant warmer in the neonatal intensive care unit as advocated by some. The mortality rate with elective division and suture in the older child should be under 1%. The mortality rate will be higher in the premature infant with IRDS because of the respiratory complications.

arterial oxygen saturation, which is the stimulus for the ductus to close, is prevented by the IRDS. The large left-to-right shunt through the ductus produces congestion, which further interferes with oxygenation. The condition is diagnosed by the presence of a systolic murmur, bounding femoral pulses, and an enlarged left atrium on echocardiography. Unless there are special circumstances, cardiac catheterization is not necessary for confirmation of the diagnosis.[11, 33, 64]

The controversy over indomethacin therapy vs. operative ligation continues. Indomethacin prevents synthesis of naturally occurring prostaglandins, which have the effect of preventing ductal closure. Most neonatologists recognize jaundice and renal impairment as contraindications to administration of indomethacin. In addition to the occasional development of necrotizing enterocolitis believed to be due to indomethacin, there may be long-term CNS complications of the drug. Additionally, the patent ductus arteriosus may appear clinically to close, only to re-open as the indomethacin is slowly excreted.[29]

Indomethacin in a dose of 0.1 mg/kg may be used to close or reduce the size of the ductus. The drug is given every 8 hours for a total of three doses. Should distinct improvement not be seen, ligation of the PDA is indicated. Successful shrinkage of the PDA without complete closure may still relieve the cardiac failure. Surgical closure of the ductus arteriosus can then be accomplished electively between 6–18 months.

Some have urged emergency ligation or clipping[75] of the PDA in the nursery, under local anesthesia and morphine.[49] We prefer ligation in the operating theater using muscle relaxants and light general anesthesia. Sterility and lighting are two important advantages of the operating room. We prefer the standard posterolateral transpleural approach. The chest tube is removed af-

ter 12–24 hours. The mortality rate has been reported to be up to 40%,[56] which is due primarily to late complications and not to the operation. In our experience with 30 premature babies, the only perioperative death occurred in a patient who had unrecognized septicemia at the time of ligation of the ductus arteriosus.

In the group of 151 patients having ligation or division and suture of their PDA, 14 required other general pediatric surgical procedures. Table 140–2 indicates the nature of the other procedure and its relation to the cardiac procedure.

Coarctation of the Aorta (see Chap. 141)

Coarctation is often associated with patent ductus arteriosus. With a preductal coarctation or with an interrupted aortic arch (the most severe form of coarctation), the lower portion of the body is perfused with desaturated blood from the pulmonary artery via a PDA. Most often, the coarctation is located at or below the ductus arteriosus so that the shunt is left to right from aorta to pulmonary artery, resulting in pulmonary vascular congestion and pressure overload of the right ventricle. With an associated ventricular septal defect (VSD), there is both pressure and volume overload on the right ventricle.

Diagnosis

The diagnosis of coarctation is made by diminished femoral pulses, coupled with relative hypertension in the upper body. Catheterization is worthwhile unless one has good echocardiographic evidence of an otherwise normal heart.[26] Commonly associated defects are a bicuspid aortic valve, VSD, and patent ductus arteriosus.

Treatment

Elective resection of coarctation in the asymptomatic child is usually best done between 12 and 36 months. At this age and with proper technique, the incidence of recurrent coarctation should be about 1%.

Congestive heart failure resulting from coarctation is often manageable by digoxin, diuretics, and fluid restriction. Continued failure or the diagnosis on ECG of left ventricular strain are indications for urgent operation. Long-standing left ventricular strain detected by ECG may indicate that subendocardial fibrosis

TABLE 140–2.—GENERAL SURGICAL PROCEDURES IN 151 PATIENTS WITH PATENT DUCTUS ARTERIOSUS

PDA (4 mo.) VSD untreated → 1st stage urethroplasty 4 yr.
PDA (6 mo.) → UPJ (7 mo.)
PDA, prune-belly syndrome, lobectomy for emphysema (1 mo.) → GER fundo (3 mo.)
PDA (5 mo.) → feeding gastrostomy (8 mo.) → cheiloplasty (12 mo. & 15 mo.)
PDA (7 mo.) → LIH (12 mo.)
PDA (NB) → BIH (2 mo.) → eyes (4 mo.)
PDA (3 wk.) → BIH (7 wk.)
PDA, TEF ligated with division and suture (NB) → repair EA (1 mo.) → fundo (2 mo.)
PDA (1 mo.) → BIH (2 mo.)
BIH (1 mo.) → PDA (13 mo.)
PDA (13 mo.) → costocervical A-V fistula (17 mo.)
PDA (NB) → BIH (4 mo.)
Closure gastric perforation (NB) → PDA (NB) → circumcision (6 wk.)
PDA, IRDS (4 mo.) → fundo, Ladd's bands (4.2 mo.) → SBO (intussusception) (4.5 mo.) *died*

For key to abbreviations see Table 140–1.

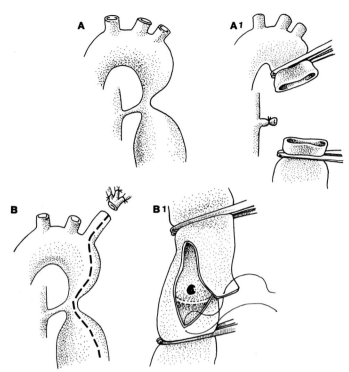

Fig 140–2.—Coarctation of the aorta is most often located at the level of the ligamentum arteriosum or ductus. **A,** the time-honored repair entails excision of the narrowed, thickened segment of aorta, ligation of the ductus, and end-to-end aortic anastomosis, as shown in *A1*. Unless all the abnormal aortic tissue is removed, the coarctation is likely to recur. Fortunately, the smaller the child, the easier the mobilization of the aorta above and below to allow approximation of the two ends. Anastomosis entirely with interrupted sutures and eversion of the aortic ends was believed to be necessary to insure growth of the anastomosis. We now know that growth will occur if a running proline suture is used, interrupted at one or two places. If abnormal aortic tissue is the cause of recoarctation, then this repair should theoretically be preferable to the one illustrated in *B* and *B1*, in which none of the aorta is removed. End-to-end repair also has the advantage of leaving the subclavian circulation intact. **B,** the subclavian flap technique has been popular in the neonate who needs urgent relief of the coarctation. The coarcted area is widened by an onlay flap of subclavian vessel. It was originally believed that there was little or no chance of recoarctation, but de Leval[26] has reported an 8% incidence of recoarctation after this technique. Theoretical disadvantages of this procedure include interruption of the major blood supply to the left arm. "Invasive cardiologists" have recently begun dilating coarctations by the balloon angioplasty technique and are enthusiastic about their early results. It should have all the recoarctation potential, and more, of every operative procedure described, in that all the abnormal aortic tissue remains in continuity. Clinical experience with this technique is limited, and the incidence of recoarctation is not known.

has occurred. Infarction thus caused, once the proximal aortic pressure is reduced,[73] will reduce operative survival.

The operative approach is by left thoracotomy unless the arch and descending aorta are on the right. In the neonate, the technique of subclavian flap angioplasty is probably the least likely to result in recoarctation of the aorta. The subclavian artery is ligated and transected near its trifurcation at the apex of the left chest. With control of the aorta, both above the origin of the left subclavian and below the coarctation, the subclavian artery is opened on its lateral aspect and the incision continued downward to well below the coarctation (Fig 140–2,*B, B1*). The rim of coarcted tissue is excised from within the aorta. The flap of subclavian artery is then sutured to the U-shaped opening in the aorta, across the area of coarctation. It is possible that another shelf of aortic intima and media may result, but because the flap of subclavian artery is not involved, a hemodynamically significant stenosis is unlikely. The obvious disadvantage of this tech-

nique is the loss of some portion of blood flow to the left arm. Collateral vessels almost always suffice, and the risk of limb loss is exceedingly remote. Growth of the subclavian flap has been documented.[51] Resection of the coarcted segment with end-to-end anastomosis is the time-honored method of treatment of coarctation of the aorta and is usually employed in the older infants and in children (see Fig 140–2,*A, A1*). In smaller infants, it has the disadvantage of having a higher incidence of recoarctation. This is probably due to incomplete resection of all abnormal aortic tissue and anastomotic narrowing or failure of growth of the anastomosis.[26] After the age of 6 months, the incidence of recoarctation is probably the same with either technique.[73] Prosthetic patch angioplasty, a third surgical method of treatment of coarctation, is not often used in infants and small children. Its most common application is for recurrent coarctation, to avoid the hazardous mobilization of the two ends. Balloon dilatation of the coarctation has recently gained attention.[44] Long-term results are not known, but prompt relief of failure has been impressive.

Results of operation are directly related to the presence or absence of associated intracardiac defects and/or other life-threatening complications such as necrotizing enterocolitis. For infants from Great Ormond Street, de Leval reports a 6% mortality with isolated coarctation and 20% mortality with complicated coarctation.[26] He reports an 8% incidence of recoarctation with the subclavian flap angioplasty.[26] Mortality rates in children over the age of 1 year should probably be less than 2%. Postoperative hypertension requiring medication is the most common complication following coarctation. The institution of pulsatile blood flow to the kidneys probably results in an activation of the renin angiotensin system, which produces hypertension postoperatively.[74] Postoperative pain and ileus may be due to vasculitis, which presumably results from the sudden institution of pulsatile blood flow to the mesenteric vessels; and intestinal infarction may occur.[40, 45] Spinal cord damage from prolonged cross-clamping or interference with collaterals may occur in up to 1.5% of patients.[13, 45]

Associated Lesions

Table 140–3 outlines the associated pediatric surgical lesions that we have seen with coarctation.

Cyanotic Congenital Heart Disease

Intracardiac defects that allow or obligate shunting of blood from the right ventricle to the left side of the heart will result in peripheral desaturation and cyanosis of varying degrees. There are basically six lesions that will produce cyanosis. These include transposition of the great arteries (TGA), tetralogy of Fallot (TET), tricuspid atresia (TA), and pulmonary atresia (PA), which can produce intense cyanosis even in the neonate. Truncus arteriosus (truncus) and the total anomalous pulmonary venous drainage (TAPVD) tend to produce less severe cyanosis.

TABLE 140–3.—GENERAL SURGICAL PROCEDURES IN 112 PATIENTS WITH COARCTATION OF THE AORTA

COA (4 mo.) → fundo (4.5 mo.)
NEC–no operation → COA (10 days)
COA (14 mo.) → RIH (3 yr.)
COA (NB) → AG syndrome (NB)
NEC–no operation → COA (died 5 days)
COA (4 yr.) → suture duodenal ulcer (3 wk. later)
COA, PDA (5 days) → fundo (3 wk.)
COA, PDA (3 yr.) → bronchoscopy (3.5 yr.)
Urethral valves (8 yr.) → COA (9 yr.) → ureteral reimplant (9.5 yr.)

For key to abbreviations see Table 140–1.

Transposition of the Great Arteries

Transposition of the great arteries causes cyanosis in the newborn period. Postnatal survival requires an intracardiac shunt at atrial or ventricular levels. Most commonly, a stretched foramen ovale in the atrial septum allows some mixing of pulmonary and systemic venous return, but often this is inadequate to support the oxygen demand. Intense cyanosis and acidosis are seen shortly after birth. The lesion is usually diagnosed by echocardiography and confirmed by cardiac catheterization; usually, at the time of catheterization, a balloon atrial septostomy is performed.[63] Improved peripheral oxygen saturation generally results. Although still cyanotic, the patient can grow without further palliation to a size at which operative correction of the defect is least risky. Lack of improvement in arterial oxygen saturation after ballooning will require an operative atrial septectomy as described by Blalock and Hanlon.[8]

Correction

The first successful procedure used to correct transposition of the great arteries was that described by Senning[67] in 1959. This

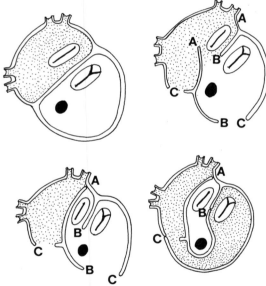

Fig 140–3.—Transposition of the great vessels. The Senning venous switch operation for correction of transposition of the great vessels. As shown in transverse section through the atria, the pulmonary veins with oxygenated blood *(stippled area)* drain into the mitral valve; and the cavae (represented by *black dot*) in the lower atrium drain unoxygenated *(clear area)* blood to the tricuspid valve. Three incisions are made in the atria—*BC* in the right atrial wall, *AB* in the atrial septum, and *C* in the left atrium behind the interatrial groove. The posterior atrial septum *(A)* is sutured to point *A* between the pulmonary veins and the mitral valve. The atrial septum *B* is then sutured to the right atrial wall *B,* directing caval blood to the mitral valve. The pulmonary venous return is then directed around the outside of the heart to the tricuspid valve by suturing the right atrial wall *C* to the left atrial wall *C.* The venous return is thus transposed, functionally correcting the transposition. Mustard's repair places a convoluted patch over the orifice of the superior and inferior venae cavae, directing blood through the atrial septal defect to the mitral valve. Pulmonary venous blood must also traverse the atrial septal defect to reach the tricuspid valve. It is because of the close relation of these pathways that obstruction to venous return, either from the lungs or from the cavae, occurs and complicates the postoperative course of patients with the Mustard operation. Anatomical correction by transposing the arteries is gaining popularity and may very well replace venous switch corrections of transposition in the future. For the present, however, and for the surgeon who is quite familiar with Senning's procedure and the care of the patient after repair by this technique, the Senning operation appears to carry the lowest mortality and have the best long-term outlook. We use the arterial switch operation for those patients having transposition and VSD with an unobstructed left ventricular outflow tract. These are not common lesions.

is a rather complicated intra-atrial *redirection of venous return,* so that the systemic caval return is shunted through the mitral valve to the left-sided ventricle, from which it is pumped to the lungs (Fig 140–3). The pulmonary venous return is brought through a tunnel around the outside of the newly constructed systemic venous atrium through the tricuspid valve to the right ventricle, and hence to the aorta. The complexity of the Senning procedure created a climate ripe for acceptance of the simpler Mustard[54] intra-atrial pericardial baffle, which was described in 1964. A majority of cardiac surgeons elected to use Mustard's technique. It was presumed that the pericardial patch would grow, because it was bathed in blood. It is now well established that such a pericardial graft does not grow, but indeed shrinks over a period of time. Refinement in the geometry of the patch described by Brom[14] has resulted in fewer complications from shrinkage. Nonetheless, both caval and pulmonary venous obstruction seen with the Mustard procedure brought about a widespread resurgence of interest in the Senning procedure in 1977.[62] Correction is usually carried out at 6–12 months of age by either procedure. The early and long-term results of Senning's procedure have been superior to those of the Mustard procedure.[23] Obstruction to caval and pulmonary venous return is rare with the Senning procedure. Intra-atrial leaks with shunting have likewise not been common. Dysrhythmias, which often complicate the late follow-up of patients after the Mustard procedure, have been minimal with the Senning procedure. The mortality for uncomplicated TGA should be under 5%.

Correction of transposition by *arterial retransposition* actually was the first technique attempted by Mustard,[55] but without success. It was not successful until 1975 when Jatene et al.[41] reported the first survivor. The theoretical appeal is that the ventricle designed for a specific function is thereby attached to the appropriate great vessel. The current high mortality and the need for balanced ventricular pressure and an unobstructed left ventricular outflow tract limit the applicability of the arterial switch. Castaneda[17] has recently reported neonatal Jatene procedures with a very low mortality. Although arterial retransposition still carries an overall mortality of at least 25% in most series, it is a useful technique to be kept in mind for those patients who have a large VSD that will require a right ventriculotomy for patching.

Complex transposition, i.e. with VSD (of any type) and left ventricular outflow tract obstruction, carries a significantly increased mortality or morbidity.[58] Some are best repaired using the Senning approach, transatrial patching of the VSD and transvalve resection of the outflow obstruction. The complexities of some others are best treated by a Rastelli repair, in which the VSD is repaired by a patch that directs all the left ventricular blood through the VSD to the aorta. The proximal pulmonary artery is sewn over and the right ventricular blood directed to the distal pulmonary artery by a valved conduit.[47, 48]

Associated Lesions

Table 140–4 lists the associated lesions that we have seen in patients with TGA.

TABLE 140–4.—GENERAL SURGICAL PROCEDURES IN 67 PATIENTS WITH TRANSPOSITION OF GREAT ARTERIES

TGA—Waterston (2 wk.) → redo (2 wk.) → fundo (6 wk.) → ASD (5 yr.)
TGA, PS–Blalock shunt (NB) → fundo (6 wk.) → Gore-Tex shunt (7 wk.) *died*
Circumcision with BH (15 mo.) → Mustard repair (3 yr.) *died 2 days*
TGA, PS–Blalock shunt (NB) → Waterston (NB) → fundo (3 wk.) *died 2 mo.*

For key to abbreviations see Table 140–1.

Tetralogy of Fallot

Fallot's tetralogy consists of right ventricular outflow tract stenosis. associated with a VSD, dextroposition of the aorta, and right ventricular hypertrophy (Fig 140–4). The 1981 concept of Anderson et al.,[2] that the VSD and outflow obstruction result from "misplacement" of the infundibular septum (crista supraventricularis), seems plausible and helps explain the extreme variability in individual anatomy. Cyanosis may be present in the neonatal period, but may not be clinically apparent before 6 weeks of age. The degree of right-to-left shunting depends upon the degree of outflow tract obstruction. Progressive hypertrophy of the septal insertion of the infundibular septum (septal band) leads to increased cyanosis. The demands of increased cardiac output necessitated by exercise may result in further constriction of the right ventricular outflow tract and more shunting of blood from right to left. When this becomes severe, deep cyanotic spells may occur—the so-called TET spells. Hypoxia further contributes to infundibular muscle spasm and accounts for rapid acidosis, which may cause a TET spell to be fatal. Correction of tetralogy of Fallot, while reasonably elective, may need to be done urgently if spells are frequent or severe or if the hemoglobin count is increasing. A systemic-to-pulmonary shunt may be called for if the patient is not deemed a satisfactory risk for total correction.

In at least 25% of patients with tetralogy of Fallot, the aortic arch will be on the right side—a significant factor that has a bearing upon the approach for the repair of associated esophageal atresia.

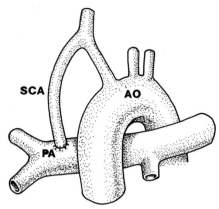

Fig 140–5.—The Blalock-Taussig shunt is illustrated with the end of the right subclavian artery *(SCA)* sewn to the pulmonary artery *(PA)* to increase pulmonary blood flow. This is the most desirable of the systemic-pulmonary shunts. Such shunts are necessary for patients not at the time suited for correction of tetralogy of Fallot and for other right-sided obstructive lesions. The inherent diameter of the subclavian artery limits the amount of flow that will occur, so that congestive heart failure rarely results from this anastomosis. It is much the easiest of the shunts to take down at the time of total correction of the defect. In the very small infant, this shunt is a little more likely to thrombose than other shunts. A variation of this shunt is performed by placing a tubular prosthesis (usually 4 or 6 size Gore-Tex) from the side of the subclavian to the side of the pulmonary artery. The Waterston aortopulmonary anastomosis is created behind the ascending aorta *(AO)* where it touches the front of the right pulmonary artery. The size of the anastomosis is somewhat difficult to control. If it is too large, congestive heart failure results. Closing the Waterston shunt is usually done by cross-clamping the aorta (with cardiopulmonary bypass), and suturing the anastomosis shut through an anterior aortotomy. Distortion by the differing vectors of growth of the aorta and pulmonary artery sometimes necessitates actually taking the two vessels apart; closing the aortic side; and then performing an extensive repair of the pulmonary artery, is a difficult thing to do, given the position of the pulmonary artery. Potts' shunt is made from the descending aorta to the left pulmonary artery where the aorta passes behind it. This anastomosis is even more difficult to manage at the time of open heart correction. It is most often used in those situations in which it is expected to be a permanent palliative procedure or where all other avenues of systemic-to-pulmonary shunting have been exhausted.

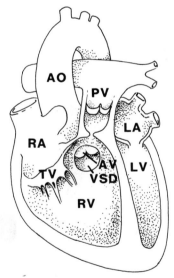

Fig 140–4.—The tetralogy of Fallot has four components—right ventricular outflow obstruction with infundibular or valvar pulmonic stenosis, ventricular septal defect *(VSD)* of the membranous septum, overriding of the *VSD* by the aorta *(AO)*, and right ventricular hypertrophy secondary to the outflow obstruction. The most significant variables in tetralogy are the degree of right ventricular outflow tract obstruction and the development of the pulmonary arterial trunks. Excising or incising the infundibular stenosis will allow opening of the outflow tract. In our experience, however, most often a patch is required to open the outflow tract adequately. This patch extends from about the lower edge of the ventriculotomy for a variable distance out onto the pulmonary artery. Usually, the patch must be carried out at least to the end of the main pulmonary artery. Pulmonary insufficiency results from the incision of the pulmonary annulus for the patch. This pulmonary valve *(PV)* insufficiency usually is not a big problem unless further obstructions are present in the pulmonary arteries, which elevate the pulmonary vascular resistance. For the same reason, an outflow patch of pericardium may become aneurysmal over the course of months or years. Gore-Tex material is therefore frequently used for the outflow tract patch. We continue to use Dacron or Teflon fabric patches for the VSD because of their quick and complete incorporation in endocardial tissue. (*RA* = right atrium; *LA* = left atrium; *AV* = aortic valve; *TV* = tricuspid valve; *LV* = left ventricle; *RV* = right ventricle.)

Elective correction of tetralogy of Fallot is probably best carried out sometime after the age of 18 months. Although repair of tetralogy in the neonate or infant has been accomplished successfully a number of times,[18,59] in most hands it carries an unacceptable mortality rate.[22] Faced with a small infant who has an increasing hemoglobin count or is having cyanotic spells, a systemic-to-pulmonary artery shunt is safer than total correction.[3,15] The most commonly used shunts are the Blalock-Taussig (Fig 140–5) and the Waterston. The Blalock-Taussig shunt is best performed on the side opposite the aortic arch. The subclavian artery is divided at the apex of the chest and sutured end-to-end onto the pulmonary artery. Interruption of the anterior suture line allows the anastomosis to grow as the diameter of the subclavian artery enlarges. A variation of the Blalock-Taussig shunt that is gaining popularity utilizes a 5–6-mm Gore-Tex graft inserted between the underside of the subclavian artery and the pulmonary artery without interruption of the subclavian artery.[65] The Blalock-Taussig shunt in the neonate is a technically demanding procedure. Its advantages, however, far outweigh the disadvantages because of the protection against overloading, provided by the fact that the amount of blood that shunts through this communication is limited by the inherent diameter of the subclavian artery. Too large a shunt, which might put the child into congestive heart failure, is much less likely than with Potts or Waterston shunts, which are from the aorta. Another distinct advantage of the Blalock-Taussig shunt is that, at the time of correction, the subclavian artery simply needs to be ligated.[66] Waterston's ascending aorta to right pulmonary artery anastomosis is useful when the anatomy, or exceedingly small size, precludes the use of the Blalock shunt. It is difficult to control the size of this shunt. It must be constructed properly with a continuous suture, or excessive flow may be fatal. Closure of Waterston's shunt at time of correction is sometimes a matter of simple transaortic suture, but it may require extensive reconstruction of the pulmonary artery in a very difficult location posterior to the ascending aorta.[66]

The Potts shunt between descending aorta and ipsilateral pulmonary artery is one resorted to when other possibilities have been exhausted or when the shunt will be permanent rather than a temporary palliative procedure.

Total Correction

We prefer to correct the tetralogy defect under the age of 2 years and preferably under the weight of about 10–12 kg so that correction can be accomplished under deep hypothermia and circulatory arrest.[18] Although the concern has been that in the younger child an outflow patch will more often be required, in our experience the need for outflow tract patches is probably not determined by the age of the patient, but rather by the individual anatomy. Correction of Fallot's tetralogy requires exposure of the infundibular septum through a right ventriculotomy. Excision or incision of the septal or parietal limbs of the septum allows the main body of the right ventricle to be entered and the ventricular septal defect to be visualized. Interrupted mattress sutures are placed around the ventricular septal defect, avoiding the area of the conduction bundle. These sutures are carried through an appropriately sized Dacron or Teflon patch to close the ventricular septal defect. An outflow tract patch may also be necessary. If there is annular or supravalvar narrowing, this patch may be extended across the annulus and onto either branch pulmonary artery. Pure pulmonary valvar stenosis may be relieved by pulmonary valvotomy without disturbing the annulus.

Results

Correction of Fallot's tetralogy probably should carry with it a less than 5% mortality.[19] The result depends largely upon the completeness of relief of the right ventricular outflow obstruction, which is reflected in the postoperative ratio of right ventricular and left ventricular pressures. Intraoperative pressures may be disconcerting, yet improve considerably over time.[6] An indwelling PA catheter for the first few days is useful in the postoperative management.[19]

Residual ventricular septal defects, right ventricular outflow obstruction, or aneurysmal dilatation of an outflow patch are all well-known complications of correction of Fallot's tetralogy. Sec-

TABLE 140–5.—GENERAL SURGICAL PROCEDURES IN 111 PATIENTS WITH TETRALOGY OF FALLOT

Esophageal atresia, distal TEF (NB) → Waterston, TEF division (12 days) → EA repair (21 mo.) → TET repair (39 mo.) died
GER with pneumonitis, bronchomalacia, absent left pulmonary artery → fundo (5 mo.) → TET repair (7 mo.) → bronchial stents (8 mo.) → right upper lobectomy (9 mo.)
Cantrell's pentalogy → Waterston, omphalocele closure (NB) → awaiting TET repair & closure ectopia cordis
Inguinal hernias → BIH (infant) → Blalock-Taussig shunt (8 mo.) → TET repair (2.5 yr.)
RIH → TET repair (3 yr.) → RIH (3.5 yr.)
BIH → Blalock-Taussig (infant) → TET repair (2 yr.) → BIH (4 yr.)
Testicular torsion → Blalock-Taussig (infant) → TET repair (2 yr.) → orchiectomy for torsion (6 yr.)

For key to abbreviations see Table 140–1.

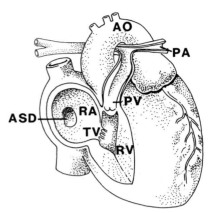

Fig 140–6.—The hypoplastic right heart syndrome consists of stenosis or atresia of the tricuspid valve *(TV)*, the right ventricle *(RV)*, and the pulmonic valve *(PV)*, associated with atrial septal defect *(ASD)* and sometimes with ventricular septal defect. Usually, a patent ductus is present. Pulmonary blood flow is from right atrium *(RA)* to left atrium through the atrial septal defect to the aorta *(AO)* and through the ductus to the pulmonary artery *(PA)*. There are many variations and combinations of these lesions, so that one patient is difficult to compare with another. The principles involved, however, require that the atrial septal defect be nonrestrictive and that the systemic-to-pulmonary artery flow be adequate for physiologic requirements and for a stimulus of growth to the branch pulmonary arteries. The degree of pulmonary vascular resistance is probably the most important determinant of the long-term survival of these patients. Our preference for palliation in the neonate is a balloon atrial septostomy and a left-sided Blalock-Taussig or Gore-Tex shunt to be followed a few years later by the Fontan anastomosis of the right atrium to pulmonary artery (see Fig 140–7).

ondary procedures for correction of these disorders carry about the same risk as the original procedure.[20, 69]

Associated Lesions

Table 140–5 outlines the associated pediatric surgical lesions that we have seen in patients with tetralogy.

Hypoplastic Right Heart

The hypoplastic right heart syndrome includes isolated tricuspid atresia or PA or a combination of both. Right ventricular hypoplasia may be associated with an intact or defective ventricular septum (Fig 140–6). The ductus arteriosus is usually patent.

Tricuspid Atresia

Intense cyanosis is the rule in the delivery room. Cardiac catheterization is usually necessary to delineate the precise anatomy in order to select the best-suited type of palliative procedure. At catheterization, an atrial septal defect may be enlarged by the balloon technique to achieve some palliation. Additionally, the patency of the ductus arteriosus may be maintained with prostaglandin E1 in a dose of 0.05–0.10 μg/kg/min. This usually is effective for periods of under 48 hours, by which time arrangements can be made for operative augmentation of pulmonary blood flow, by one shunt or another. Many times the right ventricle is severely hypoplastic and of little functional use to the patient. The "corrective" operation may consist only of variations upon the technique described by Fontan (Figs 140–7 and 140–8). These procedures consist of venous bypass of the right side of the heart directing caval blood to the pulmonary arteries, either by means of a valved conduit or by direct anastomosis of the right atrium to the pulmonary artery. The risk of such a corrective procedure in infants and even young children has been prohibitive. Prior to the age of 6 or 7 years, a systemic-to-pulmonary artery shunt is usually done for palliation.

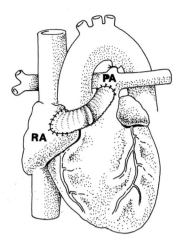

Fig 140–7.—The Fontan concept of correction of right heart hypoplasia is illustrated here with a Dacron graft, containing a porcine valve, which extends from the right atrium *(RA)* to the pulmonary artery *(PA)*. Any number of modifications of this concept can be used, including that shown in Figure 140–8. The use of a valve in this position remains controversial. In the child, the rapid metabolism of calcium results in the calcification and destruction of porcine valves. This presently necessitates replacement of the valve because of obstruction. It may be wise to eliminate valves entirely.

Pulmonary Atresia

In some patients with PA and an intact ventricular septum, the right ventricle is of adequate size; and the tricuspid valve is relatively normal, so that reconstruction of the outflow tract with a valved conduit may be possible. If forward flow is not established through the right ventricle soon after birth, underdevel-

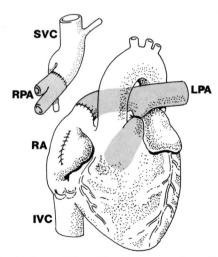

Fig 140–8.—Another variation of the Fontan procedure utilizing the Glenn shunt from the superior vena cava *(SVC)* to the right pulmonary artery *(RPA)* and the stump of superior vena cava to the proximal end of the right pulmonary artery, as shown, will separate the two circulations. The disadvantage here is that 70% of the venous return to the body comes from the inferior vena cava *(IVC)* and 30% from the superior vena cava. Thus, an inordinate amount of blood is shunted to the left or smaller lung, while the right, or larger lung, receives only 30% of the systemic venous return. Further variations on this theme have been proposed, utilizing an anastomosis of the superior vena cava to the right pulmonary artery without interruption of the pulmonary artery (thus the superior caval flow can go to either side) and an anastomosis of the right atrium *(RA)* to the underside of the pulmonary artery, allowing the inferior caval blood flow to be distributed to either lung. The optimal time for doing any of the Fontan procedures probably is after the age of 3 years, although the Glenn anastomosis may be safely accomplished in children of 1 year or older as a preliminary or partial Fontan correction. *(LPA = left pulmonary artery)*.

opment of the ventricular cavity will result; and a correction of this kind will later be impossible. These are exceedingly difficult patients to manage. Immediate valvotomy by the transventricular or pulmonary artery approach coupled with a systemic-pulmonary artery shunt allows the best chance of survival.[52] At a much later date, outflow reconstruction is possible. The overall mortality rate is high.

The most severe form of tetralogy of Fallot is represented by PA with VSD, which has sometimes been called a "pseudo-truncus." Treatment in the neonatal period is by a systemic pulmonary shunt. The lesion is reparable by outflow tract patching or by a valved conduit if there is sufficient pulmonary artery into which the right ventricular outflow can be directed.[50] Oftentimes, enlarged bronchial arteries are the only pulmonary supply, and they may not be amenable to such reconstruction. A major determinant of survival is the degree of pulmonary vascular resistance present after correction, as reflected in the right ventricular pressure.[1] Mortality of correction will probably be at least 15% in most hands, although a recent report would suggest a more favorable outlook.[61]

Associated Lesions

Our only patient requiring further general surgical treatment in 41 patients having right heart hyperplasia was a newborn with persistent pneumonitis who underwent successful fundoplication 1 month after a Blalock-Taussig shunt for TA. He has not as yet had further correction of his cardiac anomaly.

Critical Pulmonic Stenosis

Severe valvar pulmonic stenosis may present in the newborn period, much as does TA or PA. Suprasystemic pressures in the right ventricle are a result of near-total obstruction at the pulmonary valve. Right-to-left shunting through a patent foramen ovale, which reduces systemic venous congestion, may be enhanced by balloon atrial septostomy. Patency of the ductus arteriosus should be maintained by prostaglandin infusion until the pulmonary valvotomy can be accomplished. Valvotomy is performed by prograde, closed, cutting or dilating of the pulmonary valve or by an approach from the main pulmonary artery. The latter may be done open using the method of Stark and de Leval,[52a] but without cardiopulmonary bypass. Infundibular muscle spasm may complicate the postoperative course. Shunting remains an alternative to a direct attack upon the valve. One of our two survivors (out of nine patients) was shunted, and much later repaired.

Truncus Arteriosus

Truncus arteriosus is a conotruncal malformation in which both ventricles empty into a single vessel from which the aorta and pulmonary arteries arise (Fig 140–9). The truncal valve often has four cusps and is incompetent. The type 1 truncus has a single main pulmonary artery coming off the truncal vessel. In the type 2 truncus malformation, the vessels come off the back of the truncus at or near the same place. In the type 3 deformity, the right pulmonary artery comes off the right side of the truncal vessel and the left pulmonary artery off the left side; and in type 4, the pulmonary arteries arise from the descending aorta.

Truncus arteriosus produces cyanosis, because the mixture of desaturated and saturated blood coming out of the truncal vessel is distributed both to the lungs and to the body. A large pulmonary flow may result in little cyanosis, but can lead to congestive heart failure. High pressure and unrestricted flow to the pulmonary arteries may produce fixed pulmonary hypertension by 6–12

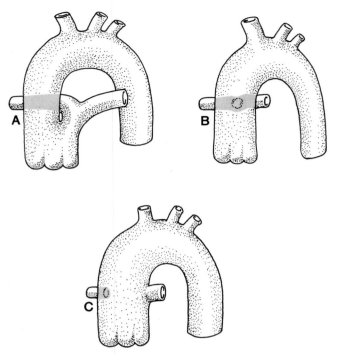

Fig 140–9.—Truncus arteriosus. **A,** type 1. **B,** type 2. **C,** type 3.

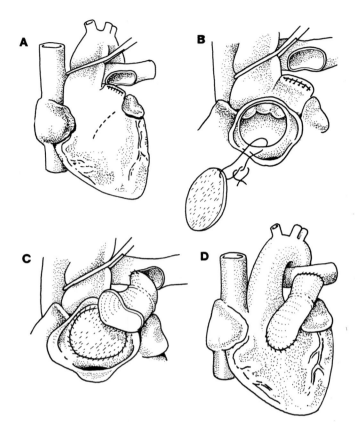

Fig 140–10.—The truncus arteriosus type 1 is corrected in infancy under profound hypothermia and circulatory arrest. This is obviously the easiest of the truncus deformities to correct because it requires only the simple closure of the communication between aorta and the pulmonary artery. Types 2 and 3 truncus malformations involve much more ingenuity, much more sewing, and much more chance of obstruction and postoperative hemorrhage. **A,** the pulmonary artery is divided, and the proximal end is closed. **B,** the ventricular septal defect is exposed and patched through the right ventricular outflow tract, thus directing all left ventricular flow to the truncal vessel, which now supplies only the aorta. **C, D,** a valved conduit is sutured to the pulmonary artery distally and to the right ventricle proximally, directing systemic venous caval blood flow to the lungs.

months of age.[71] Banding of the pulmonary arteries in infancy provides some protection and may allow delay in performing corrective operation, but the mortality of banding added to the risk of ultimate correction probably makes a two-stage operative procedure more risky than a one-stage total correction. Most uncorrected patients die within the first year of life.

Correction consists of closure of the ventricular septal defect to direct left ventricular output to the truncal vessel, and insertion of a valved conduit from the right ventricle to the pulmonary artery (Fig 140–10).[27] Under the age of 12 months, it is unlikely that a graft larger than 14 mm should be used as a conduit. Even if the mechanical or tissue valve in this prosthesis functions without degeneration over the course of several years, it will be necessary, because of growth of the child, to replace the conduit at 3 or 4 years of age. We have not found this to be a particularly difficult procedure in our limited experience.

Results of operation depend most upon the competency of the truncal valve and the pulmonary vascular resistance. If there is a competent valve and the pulmonary vessels are not too seriously damaged, a mortality rate in the range of 15% can be anticipated. Overall, however, mortality probably will run 25–30%.[27]

There were no associated surgical lesions in our seven patients with truncus arteriosus.

Total Anomalous Pulmonary Venous Drainage

Total anomalous pulmonary venous drainage may be of three types (Fig 140–11). The right and left pulmonary veins join together behind the heart and drain into it by way of an ascending vein on the side opposite the superior vena cava (supracardiac type), by way of the coronary sinus to the right atrium (cardiac type), or by way of a descending vein that usually enters into the portal venous system (infracardiac type). The interposed hepatic venous system results in pulmonary venous hypertension, leading to severe hypoxia and a very high mortality rate. Because the coronary sinus is often of limited size, pulmonary venous hypertension is likewise seen in the cardiac type of total anomalous

pulmonary venous drainage. The supracardiac type is the least often associated with pulmonary venous hypertension. In all three forms, all oxygenated venous blood drains to mix with the systemic venous blood in the right atrium. An atrial septal defect is necessary for survival. The atrial septal defect can be enlarged by the balloon technique at the time of diagnostic catheterization.

Recognition that there is a cardiac defect may be difficult in these patients, because the heart size is normal and there is no murmur. Chest roentgenograms will show pulmonary venous obstruction.

Correction should be delayed only to allow adequate resuscitation. The use of deep hypothermia and circulatory arrest has been a great advantage in the surgical treatment of children with total anomalous pulmonary venous drainage, because many of them would not tolerate manipulation of the heart for cannulation and repair using the standard perfusion technique. Retrocardiac open anastomosis[12] or transatrial open anastomosis[38] both allow satisfactory repair (Fig 140–12). The mortality in the neonate relates to the degree of acidosis present at time of maximal preoperative correction and will probably approach 25–30%.[10] Correction in the older infant or child carries a much lower mortality of about 2%.

We have treated 12 patients with total anomalous pulmonary venous drainage, and none have required other procedures.

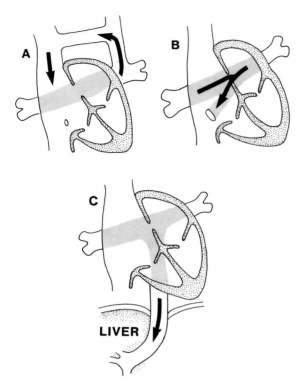

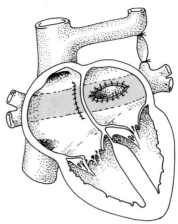

Fig 140–12.—Correction of the supracardiac total anomalous pulmonary venous drainage. This entails closure of the atrial septal defect and anastomosis of the common pulmonary vein to the back side of the left atrium. Obliteration of the abnormal ascending vein is then necessary, so that retrograde flow of systemic venous blood to the left atrium will not occur. Corresponding techniques are used for correction of cardiac level or infracardiac total anomalous pulmonary venous drainage as well. Obstruction of the anastomosis between the pulmonary vein and left atrium is the most common and sometimes fatal of the complications of this corrective procedure. The left atrium usually is underdeveloped; and this anastomosis, although initially large, will sometimes narrow down to the point of severe obstruction. Pulmonary venous hypertension thus results, with attendant right heart failure. Reoperation on these patients is not pleasant and sometimes is not successful.

Fig 140–11.—Total anomalous pulmonary venous drainage is classified according to the route by which blood from the common pulmonary vein drains to the right atrium. In addition to the three pictured are varieties of mixed drainage, wherein pulmonary drainage may reach the heart by different routes. **A,** supracardiac total anomalous pulmonary venous drainage is the most common type. The blood flow from the common pulmonary veins reaches the heart by way of an ascending vein, across the innominate vein, and down through the superior vena cava. Mixed caval blood is then distributed, partly to the right and partly to the left ventricle through the atrial septal defect, so that oxygen saturation in the aorta and pulmonary artery are very nearly equal. **B,** the cardiac level drainage from the confluent pulmonary veins is by way of the coronary sinus. **C,** the infracardiac type drains through the diaphragm and usually into the portal system below the liver. Because of the interposed hepatic vascular bed, the venous pressure is considerably increased, making this the most lethal of the types of total anomalous pulmonary venous drainage. Oxygenated blood in this instance reaches the right atrium by way of the inferior vena cava.

Congestive Lesions

There is a group of lesions that produce congestive heart failure without cyanosis because of left-to-right shunting of blood within the heart. These include atrial septal defects, VSD, and atrioventricular canal defects.

Secundum and sinus venosus atrial septal defects rarely produce symptoms in the neonate or in early childhood. Oftentimes, the diagnosis is not established until 2 or 3 years of age when the amount of blood shunting at the atrial level from left to right produces a flow rumble. Atrial septal defects produce little recognizable physiologic disturbance in the neonate and small child. With a large ASD, the pulmonary blood flow may reach four times systemic. Direct suture closure of the secundum defects is usually undertaken after the age of at least 18 months and frequently not until 3 or 4 years of age. Untreated, an atrial septal defect will produce cardiac failure or arrhythmia in adult life, and pulmonary hypertension may make correction, at that time, fatal.[25] Sinus venosus atrial septal defects usually require patching or construction of a tunnel to direct pulmonary venous blood to the left atrium.

Because atrial septal defects are often undiagnosed in the neonate or young infant, they rarely complicate the treatment of other disorders.

Ostium primum atrial septal defect is one end of the spectrum of anomalies resulting from an endocardial cushion defect. The other end of the spectrum is the complete atrioventricular canal defect. The primum atrial septal defect is located low in the atrial septum just above the atrioventricular valves. It is more likely to cause symptoms early in life than other atrial defects. Its repair requires a patch. Results are dependent on the character of any involvement of the mitral valve. Heart block is a potential complication of repair.

Associated Lesions

Associated lesions that we have seen with atrial septal defect are listed (Table 140–6).

Ventricular Septal Defect

An isolated VSD most often results from incomplete development of the membranous portion of the ventricular septum. It is to be distinguished from the septal defect associated with Fallot's tetralogy or the defect of the atrioventricular canal (see below) (Fig 140–13). A majority of membranous VSD will close spontaneously by the age of 6 years, having produced no physiologic disturbance. In the child, those associated with large left-to-right

TABLE 140–6.—GENERAL SURGICAL PROCEDURES IN 131
PATIENTS WITH ATRIAL SEPTAL DEFECT

Pyloromyotomy (1 mo.) → ostium secundum ASD (9 mo.)
Fundo (12 mo.) → sinus venosus ASD (3 yr.)
Sinus venosus ASD (3 yr.) → BIH (37 mo.)
Omphalocele (NB) → ostium secundum ASD (7 mo.)
Duodenal atresia (NB) → sinus venosus ASD (2 yr.)
Ostium secundum ASD (3 yr.) → umbilical hernia (4 yr.)
Ostium primum ASD (3 mo.) with fundo
Ostium primum ASD (11 mo.) → sigmoidoscopy with removal rectal
 polyp (3 yr.)

For key to abbreviations see Table 140–1.

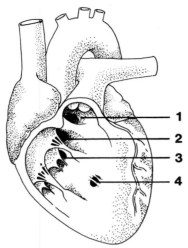

Fig 140–13.—Ventricular septal defects occur in four basic locations: *(1)* supracristal, *(2)* membranous (most common), *(3)* beneath the atrioventricular valves (the common endocardial cushion defect abnormality), and *(4)* within the muscular septum. The muscular septal defects often are closed by direct suture over pledgets. Unfortunately, the defects are often multiple, sometimes impressively so. The swiss-cheese sort of ventricular septum is a difficult lesion to correct completely. With the exception of the supracristal-type VSD, all are fraught with the hazard of conduction disturbances, because the bundle of His very closely approximates the defect posteriorly and inferiorly. Sutures for the closing of these VSD may, though rarely, interfere permanently with the conduction pathways, necessitating placement of a permanent pacemaker, with its attendant problems. The defects in positions *1, 2,* and *3* usually require patching, because attempts at direct suture result in tearing out of the stitches and recurrence of the defect.

shunts or with elevated right heart pressures may require patch closure. Multiple muscular VSD do not often close spontaneously and are also difficult to close surgically. Supracristal VSD is uncommon.

In the young infant, VSD can produce rather severe congestive heart failure. The amount of shunt increases as pulmonary vascular resistance drops in the neonate; and so a very insignificant murmur, early, may be followed within days or weeks by severe congestive heart failure. Fortunately, many infants with VSD respond to decongestive measures using digoxin and diuretics. If after an intensive period of medical therapy the congestive failure is unchanged or the infant fails to thrive, surgical closure of the VSD is indicated.

Cardiac catheterization is necessary to determine the precise anatomy and the relationship of the great vessels to the VSD. Pulmonary artery banding formerly was used as palliative therapy,[39, 68] but since the advent of deep hypothermia and circulatory arrest, the mortality of banding far exceeds that of patching the defect even in a very small child.[28, 72] Currently, about two thirds of these patients come to operation during the first year of life. Residual leak about the patch or damage to the conduction bundle are the major complications of VSD repair. Transatrial patch closure via the tricuspid valve is our preference. The mortality should be less than 2%.

Associated Lesions

Ventricular septal defect is one of the more common congenital heart defects recognizable early in life. Table 140–7 lists the associated malformations that we have seen with VSD.

Atrioventricular Canal Defects

The complete atrioventricular canal defect consists of an absence of the lower portion of the atrial septum and the upper

TABLE 140–7.—General Surgical Procedures in 151 Patients With Ventricular Septal Defect

VSD with fundo (4 mo.)
VSD with fundo (2 wk.)
VSD (2.5 yr.) → sternoplasty for deformity (3.5 yr.)
VSD with fundo (2 yr.)
VSD (9 mo.) → fundo (17 mo.)
VSD (3 mo.) → trach. for subglottic stenosis (4 mo.)
BIH (13 mo.) → VSD (25 mo.)
VSD (18 mo.) → LIH (33 mo.)
VSD (4 mo.) → tongue lesion (12 mo.)
Fundo (13 mo.) → Hypertensive VSD (16 mo.)
Fundo (3 mo.) → VSD (4 mo.)
VSD, PS (12 mo.) → ventral hernia (6.5 yr.)
VSD (7 mo.) → recurrent VSD (25 mo.) → BIH (5 yr.)
VSD (4 yr.) → dental (5 yr.) → urethral dilatation (8 yr.)
Pull-through imperforate anus (4 mo.) → vascular ring (6 mo.) → VSD (6.5 mo.)

For key to abbreviations see Table 140–1.

portion of the ventricular septum. The septal leaflets of the mitral and tricuspid valves are cleft, their anterior portions and posterior portions fused across the septal defects. These valves are often incompetent. Partial atrioventricular canal defect may occur with only the atrial or the ventricular defects being present. The complete canal is a complicated lesion to understand and combines all of the physiological disadvantages of both atrial septal defect and VSD. Manifestations of cardiac failure, usually seen early, are severe. Function of the atrioventricular valves is of prime importance to successful medical or surgical therapy.

The diagnosis of atrioventricular canal defects is made by echocardiography and ECG. Left axis deviation on ECG is seen in almost all patients with either partial or complete atrioventricular canal. Cardiac catheterization is necessary to delineate the function of the atrioventricular valves and to determine the extent of the atrial septal defects and VSD.

If untreated, complete atrioventricular canal defects will cause death in 65% by age 12 months and in 96% of patients by age 5 years.[5] Pulmonary vascular disease is likely to preclude repair in the child who is over 2 years of age. Early correction is therefore indicated. Pulmonary artery banding is not usually helpful in these patients.

Surgical correction requires placement of a patch to close the septal defect. Separate patches below and above the atrioventricular valve leaflets may be used.[57] We use a single patch method that requires division of the fused anterior and posterior common atrioventricular valve leaflets, directly over the ventricular septum. The atrial and ventricular septa are reconstructed. This repair requires attachment of the respective septal leaflets to the patch (Fig 140–14). If satisfactory reconstruction of the mitral valve can be done at the time of operation, so that there is little or no mitral incompetence, the child is very likely to survive and do well. Mitral incompetence cannot be treated by valve replacement in the small infant heart. These defects are among the most complicated of cardiac defects to correct satisfactorily. The mortality rate of repair of total atrioventricular canal defects runs in the range of 25–30% in most hands. Among the factors involved in this high mortality rate are the atrioventricular valve incompetence pre- and postoperatively, the severity of congestive failure preoperatively, pulmonary vascular resistance, and the association of Down syndrome. Down syndrome is associated with atrioventricular canal defects in about 50% of our patients.

Table 140–8 shows the associated lesions that we have seen with complete atrioventricular canal defects.

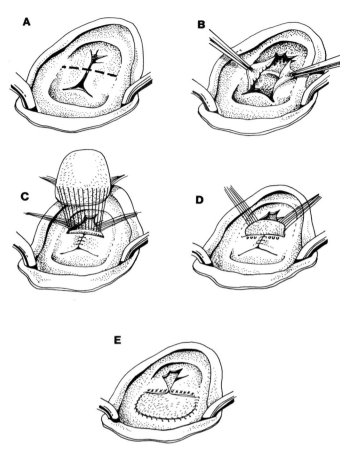

Fig 140–14.—Complete atrioventricular canal is a complex anomaly. Viewed in these diagrams as seen at operation, through a right atriotomy, there is a defect in the lower atrial and upper ventricular septa. A cleft in the septal leaflets of the mitral and tricuspid valves, coupled with the vertical defect in the heart, usually results in fusion of the mitral and tricuspid leaflets across the septal defects. **A,** the common atrioventricular valves are incised out to the common valve annulus along the dashed line. **B,** prior to the incision of these fused valves, they are lifted so that the upper rim of the VSD can be visualized. **C,** after incision of the fused valve leaflets, interrupted sutures are placed along the upper edge of ventricular septal defect; and a patch of appropriate size is pulled down into the ventricular chamber. **D,** the mitral valve cleft has been sutured, and the cut edge of the mitral valve is sewn to the septal patch using interrupted fine sutures. The upper edge of the patch then is used to close the atrial septal portion of the defect, thus completely isolating the repaired mitral valve and the left side of the heart. **E,** the tricuspid leaflets are attached to this inserted patch, completing the repair. The success of this repair depends almost entirely on the function of the mitral valve. If adequate tissue is present, and if the sutures in the mitral cleft and the sutures attaching the mitral edge to the septal patch all hold, then the patients often do well. If there is inadequate function of this valve because of pulling out of any of the above sutures or because of inadequate tissue, the patient very often succumbs to the stress and strain of the operative correction. An initial good result may be followed in some weeks by deterioration resulting from failure of the mitral valve. Mitral valve replacement may then be necessary.

Obstructive Lesions

Isolated obstructive lesions amenable to correction include pulmonic valve stenosis, subvalvar aortic stenosis, valvar aortic stenosis, and supravalvar aortic stenosis. These patients are acyanotic and often have few symptoms. All have a harsh systolic ejection murmur at the base of the heart.

Pulmonic Stenosis

Pulmonic valve stenosis is uncommon as a cause of physiologic disturbance in the infant and often produces only ECG and pres-

TABLE 140–8.—GENERAL SURGICAL PROCEDURES IN 48 PATIENTS WITH ATRIOVENTRICULAR CANAL DEFECT

AV canal and fundo (2.5 mo.)
Fundo (5 mo.) → AV canal (7 mo.) → pacer (9 mo.) → lead (12 mo.)
AV canal and fundo (3 mo.)

For key to abbreviations see Table 140–1.

sure disturbances in older children. Some develop decreased exercise tolerance, and a rare patient will become cyanotic secondary to right ventricular failure and right-to-left shunting through a patent foramen ovale. Treatment is a pulmonary valvotomy through the pulmonary artery. Mortality is about 1%. Critical pulmonic stenosis in an infant is physiologically similar to pulmonary valve atresia (see above).

Table 140–9 lists the associated lesions that we have seen in patients with pulmonic stenosis.

Aortic Stenosis

More common and more dangerous in infancy are the left ventricular outflow obstructions. Valvar aortic stenosis may produce severe cardiac failure in the neonate. Decongestive measures are of no help, because the pump failure results from left ventricular muscle decompensation working against a fixed resistance—not as a result of volume overload.

The diagnosis is established by auscultation and echocardiography. Catheterization is necessary to delineate pressure relationships, to define precisely the area of obstruction, and to search for associated cardiac lesions. It is not uncommon to find normal systemic arterial blood pressure, but a left ventricular pressure may be twice as high.

Surgical "correction" of critical aortic stenosis in infancy is an urgent and risky procedure. If the obstruction is at the valve level and the anatomy favorable, the results may be dramatic. If the annulus is very small, or if there is a unicuspid valve, the outlook is dismal. Subvalvar aortic stenosis rarely produces symptoms in infancy. This is fortunate, because in them satisfactory treatment is difficult (Fig 140–15). Excision of the obstruction may result in damage to the mitral valve or the ventricular conduction system. Incomplete relief of either subvalvar or valvar aortic stenosis is the rule rather than the exception. The aortic valve is usually bicuspid, and the commissural fusion is only partially correctable (Fig 140–16). Insertion of a prosthetic aortic valve may be necessary even in small children, and is made possible by the incision in the annulus described by Konno et al.[43] The mortality of correcting these obstructions is probably 50%.[21] Very satisfactory palliation may be achieved in older patients, but some still require valve replacement once growth is completed.

Table 140–10 lists the associated lesions that we have seen in patients with aortic stenosis.

TABLE 140–9.—GENERAL SURGICAL PROCEDURES IN 66 PATIENTS WITH PULMONIC STENOSIS

PS–Waterston with repair of EA/TEF (NB)
PS, ASD (11 mo.) → appendectomy (4 yr.)
PS (2 yr.) → BIH (4 yr.)
PS (12 mo.) → BIH (12 mo.) → meatotomy (36 mo.)
PS (8 mo.) → orchiopexy (24 mo.)
LIH (1 yr.) → PS (4 yr.) → testicular implant (11 yr.)

For key to abbreviations see Table 140–1.

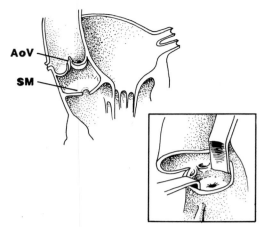

Fig 140–15.—Subvalvular aortic stenosis may occur as a diaphragm *(SM)* or a more diffuse fibrosis located just beneath a normal aortic valve *(AoV)*. Through a transverse aortic incision in the aorta, the narrowed area is approached by retracting the aortic leaflets. Usually this discrete diaphragm is easily resected, but the more diffuse lesion unfortunately has a propensity for recurrence.

Miscellaneous Cardiac Lesions

In addition to the above patients, there were 14 who had vascular ring abnormalities and 49 who had miscellaneous lesions, including double-outlet right ventricle and single ventricle; aortopulmonary window; intracardiac tumors; aortic, mitral, and tricuspid insufficiency; and mitral stenosis. There were few patients with any single lesion in this group. Those in whom additional associated surgical lesions are seen are found in Table 140–11.

Noncardiac Operations in Patients With Congenital Heart Disease

For most of the patients listed above, the congenital heart defect did not alter the usual care of patients undergoing noncardiac procedures, save the need in some for prophylaxis against bacterial endocarditis.

Patients with congenital heart disease are susceptible to bacterial endocarditis; and because some operations are associated with bacteremia, antibiotic prophylaxis should be employed at time of risk. Dental procedures (particularly extractions), tonsillectomy, adenoidectomy, bronchoscopy, nasotracheal intubation, difficult oral tracheal intubation, and other procedures of the upper respiratory tract involving disruption of the mucosa place the patient at risk from alpha-hemolytic streptococci. Generally, parenteral antibiotics are preferred. The American Heart Associa-

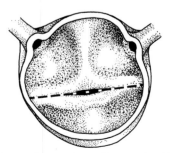

Fig 140–16.—Valvar aortic stenosis usually occurs in a bicuspid valve. Treatment consists of incising the fused commissure well out to the valve annulus. Attempts at making this valve tricuspid, even though a ridge may be seen where the commissure should be, are likely to produce insufficiency. Frequently, these valvotomies need to be repeated, and occasionally valve replacement must be carried out in a teenager.

TABLE 140–10.—GENERAL SURGICAL PROCEDURES IN 39 PATIENTS WITH AORTIC STENOSIS

AS (NB) → fundo (6 wk.) → valve replacement (4 yr.)
AS (2.5 mo.) → RIH (6 mo.)
AS (4 yr.) → ureteroplasty (5 yr.)
LIH (1 yr.) → AS (3 yr.)

For key to abbreviations see Table 140–1.

tion recommends aqueous penicillin G, 30,000 units/kg, mixed with procaine penicillin G, 600,000 units intramuscularly 30–60 minutes preoperatively, followed by penicillin V, 250 mg every 6 hours for 8 doses (not to exceed the adult dose). For patients allergic to penicillin, erythromycin orally or vancomycin parenterally can be employed.[43]

Enterococci are the common cause of endocarditis following genitourinary and lower gastrointestinal procedures. Patients undergoing cystoscopy and even bladder catheterization are at risk, as are patients having rectal biopsy, polypectomy, fistulectomy, and, of course, all patients having major colonic and genitourinary procedures. For these patients, penicillin or ampicillin plus gentamicin intravenously or intramuscularly for 24 hours is recommended.[43]

Any patient with congenital heart disease who has an incision and drainage of an abscess, or an operation through infected tissue, should have antibiotic protection. Indwelling vascular catheters in patients with congenital heart disease should receive special care and be removed as soon as possible.

A cardiac lesion is most likely to alter the care of the pediatric surgical patient in the neonatal period. Because both the cardiac and the surgical problems may require urgent repair, it is necessary to determine priorities.

The cyanotic cardiac lesions are most likely to pose an immediate threat to life. Cardiac catheterization is necessary for diagnosis. Should the patient have transposition of the great vessels, a balloon septostomy done at the time of catheterization will probably provide sufficient palliation to allow correction of the pediatric surgical anomaly. If the patient has a right-to-left shunt with inadequate pulmonary flow (tetralogy of Fallot, pulmonic atresia, and tricuspid atresia), prostaglandin will probably maintain patency of the ductus arteriosus for several hours, until a systemic pulmonary shunt can be constructed. Most pediatric surgical procedures can be postponed for this length of time.

Acyanotic congenital heart disease less frequently poses an immediate risk in the newborn period. Lesions producing left-to-right intracardiac shunts are usually not symptomatic at birth, because the high pulmonary vascular resistance, which requires several days before resolution, minimizes the shunting. Obstructive lesions may be symptomatic and require prompt surgical intervention. The most serious is critical aortic stenosis. An occasional patient will be found at catheterization to have an irreparable lesion such as a hypoplastic left heart. In these patients, there is obviously no need to repair the pediatric surgical lesion. Coarctation producing symptoms in the neonate is likely to have an associated intracardiac lesion such as a VSD. Correction of the coarctation alone may control the congestive failure and improve the blood flow to the gut and kidneys.

TABLE 140–11.—GENERAL SURGICAL PROCEDURES IN 60 PATIENTS WITH MISCELLANEOUS CARDIAC DEFECTS

Ebstein's anomaly (8.5 yr.) → appendectomy (10 yr.)
Vascular ring and fundoplication (10 wk.)
Vascular ring (21 mo.) → urethroplasty (36 mo.)

Esophageal atresia and tracheoesophageal fistula are frequently associated with congenital heart disease. A recent report from the Los Angeles Children's Hospital listed the incidence of associated cardiovascular anomalies as 54%. The lesions were VSD, patent ductus arteriosus, right-sided aortic arch, single umbilical artery, patent foramen ovale, left superior vena cava, atrial septal defect, dextrocardia, and vascular ring, in that order.[30] This is an interesting group of anomalies, but most are of no clinical significance so far as the immediate care of the patient with esophageal atresia is concerned.

An anomaly that in itself causes no symptoms, but may present technical problems in the repair of esophageal atresia, is a right-sided aortic arch.[37] It is present in 25% of patients with tetralogy of Fallot. While it is possible to repair esophageal atresia through a thoracotomy on the side of the arch, it is much easier through the opposite chest. A right aortic arch can be detected by the position of an umbilical artery catheter, if one has been inserted, or by computerized axial tomography. We have been disappointed in locating the side of the arch by sonography. This distinction need only be of concern in the patient having clinical evidence of congenital heart disease.

In our own experience with the last 100 consecutive patients with esophageal atresia and tracheoesophageal fistula treated in the past 10 years (about twice the time span for the 1,000 cardiac procedures reported above), there were 14 patients with significant congenital heart disease. Six died of severe congenital heart disease: four prior to repair of the esophageal atresia (one related to a shunt procedure) and two after repair of the esophageal anomaly. Eight patients survived. Two patients with tetralogy of Fallot had a shunt procedure prior to repair of the esophagus. One patient with patent ductus arteriosus had ductus ligation prior to the esophageal repair, and one had the ductus ligated 10 days after repair of the esophageal atresia. Two with ventricular septal defect required no therapy for the heart disease during the initial hospitalization. One patient with double-outlet right ventricle and pulmonary stenosis did well following repair of esophageal atresia, but died following cardiac repair performed 2 years later. One patient with mild tetralogy of Fallot did well during esophageal repair and did not require operative intervention for the tetralogy until later elective repair.

EXAMPLE 1.—A 1,320-gm male was admitted with esophageal atresia, distal tracheoesophageal fistula, and IRDS. Shortly after admission, a gastrostomy was done to prevent reflux, and a central venous catheter was positioned for nutrition. Ventilator support was required. Congestive heart failure developed, which was due to a patent ductus arteriosus. At age 10 days, the PDA was ligated and the tracheoesophageal fistula divided and closed through the left chest to improve ventilatory support and allow feeding per gastrostomy. At 3 weeks of age, the esophageal atresia was repaired through the right chest. This infant's major threat was first IRDS. Ventilatory support was hampered by the tracheoesophageal fistula. With development of congestive heart failure, the PDA became the major risk. After the ductus was ligated, cardiac failure was improved. Ligation of the tracheoesophageal fistula improved ventilation, which allowed repair of the esophageal atresia.

EXAMPLE 2.—A 2,920-gm male with esophageal atresia and distal tracheoesophageal fistula was admitted at age 1 day. He was markedly cyanotic with a PaO$_2$ of 25. Chest x-ray films showed a boot-shaped heart with decreased pulmonary vasculature. Cardiac catheterization demonstrated a severe tetralogy of Fallot with right arch. Shortly thereafter, a Waterston shunt was done through the right chest, and a gastrostomy was done for decompression. One week later, the esophageal atresia and tracheoesophageal fistula were repaired through the left chest. At age 3 years, the tetralogy was repaired. The cyanotic heart disease posed the greatest initial risk and was therefore treated first. Care of the esophageal atresia could be safely postponed.

In two infants critically ill with necrotizing enterocolitis, severe congestive failure developed secondary to coarctation of the aorta. Both were treated intensively for several hours prior to repair of the coarctation. The necrotizing enterocolitis improved

in both patients. One survived, and the other died of acute renal tubular necrosis.

In both cardiac and noncardiac surgical conditions occurring beyond the neonatal period, there is usually less urgency and the conditions are less serious. There is therefore more leeway in deciding which lesion should be repaired first or if both can be repaired under the same anesthetic.

There have been 24 patients with congenital heart disease and significant gastroesophageal reflux that resulted in recurrent pneumonia and/or failure to thrive. In seven patients, fundoplication was carried out prior to the corrective or palliative cardiac procedure. Eight patients had the cardiac procedure combined with fundoplication. In nine patients, fundoplication was undertaken following correction of the heart defect, because the cardiac procedure did not significantly improve the symptoms. The patients who underwent concomitant correction of the heart lesion and fundoplication were patients with gross reflux, unresponsive to positional therapy, who were nutritional failures. The fundoplication was done through the lower portion of the midline chest incision during the period of cooling prior to hypothermic arrest or during warming following arrest. Anticoagulants caused no bleeding problems with the fundoplication.

In addition to the general surgical procedures listed above, there were 15 patients who underwent various otorhinolaryngologic procedures, 8 patients who had ophthalmologic procedures, 6 who had dental procedures, and 2 each who had orthopedic or neurosurgical procedures.

REFERENCES

1. Alfieri O.,Blackstone E.H., Kirklin J.W., et al.: Surgical treatment of tetralogy of Fallot with pulmonary atresia. *J. Thorac. Cardiovasc. Surg.* 76:321, 1978.
2. Anderson R.H., Allwork S.P., Ho S.Y., et al.: Surgical anatomy of tetralogy of Fallot. *J. Thorac. Cardiovasc. Surg.* 81:887, 1981.
3. Arciniegas E., Blackstone E.H., Pacifico A.D., et al.: Classic shunting operations as part of two-stage repair of tetralogy of Fallot. *Ann. Thorac. Surg.* 27:514–518, 1979.
4. Barratt-Boyes B.G., Simpson M., Neutze J.M.: Intracardiac surgery in neonates and infants using deep hypothermia with surface cooling and limited cardiopulmonary bypass. *Circulation* 43, 44 (suppl.1):25–30, 1971.
5. Berger T.J., Blackstone E.H., Kirklin J.W., et al.: Survival and probability of cure without and with operation in complete atrioventricular canal. *Ann. Thorac. Surg.* 27:104–111,1979.
6. Bertranou E.G., Thibert M., Aiguperse J.: Short-term variations of the right ventricular/left ventricular pressure ratio following repair of tetralogy of Fallot. *Ann. Thorac. Surg.* 35:427–429, 1983.
7. Blalock A.: Operative closure of the patent ductus arteriosus. *Surg. Gynecol. Obstet.* 82:113–114, 1946.
8. Blalock A., Hanlon C.R.: The surgical treatment of complete transposition of the aorta and pulmonary artery. *Surg. Gynecol. Obstet.* 90:1, 1950.
9. Blalock A., Taussig H.B.: The surgical treatment of malformations of the heart in which there is pulmonary stenosis or pulmonary atresia. *JAMA* 128:189, 1945.
10. Bove E.L., de Leval M.R., Taylor J.F.N., et al.: Infradiaphragmatic total anomalous pulmonary venous drainage: Surgical treatment and long-term results. *Ann. Thorac. Surg.* 31:544–550, 1981.
11. Brandt B., Marvin W.J., Ehrenhaft J.L., et al.: Ligation of patent ductus arteriosus in premature infants. *Ann. Thorac. Surg.* 32:167–172, 1981.
12. Breckenridge I.M., de Leval M., Stark J., et al.: Correction of total anomalous pulmonary venous drainage in infancy. *J. Thorac. Cardiovasc. Surg.* 66:447–453, 1973.
13. Brewer L.A. III, Fosburg R.G., Mulder G.A., et al.: Spinal cord complications following surgery for coarctation of the aorta. *J. Thorac. Cardiovasc. Surg.* 64:368–381, 1972.
14. Brom G.A.: Technique of Mustard operation, in Hahn C. (ed.): *Thorax Chirurgie.* Leiden, The Netherlands, Drukkerij Bedrijf, 1975, p. 194.
15. Browdie D.A., Norberg W., Agnew R., et al.: The use of prostaglandin E1 and Blalock-Taussig shunts in neonates with cyanotic congenital heart disease. *Ann. Thorac. Surg.* 27:508–513, 1979.
16. Castaneda A.R.: Patent ductus arteriosus: A commentary. *Ann. Thorac. Surg.* 31:92–96, 1981.

17. Castaneda A.R., Norwood W., Jonas R.A., et al.: Transportation of the great arteries with intact ventricular septum: Anatomical repair in the neonate. *Ann. Throac. Surg.* 38:438–443, 1984.
18. Castaneda A.R., Freed M.D., Williams R.G., et al.: Repair of tetralogy of Fallot in infancy: Early and late results. *J. Thorac. Cardiovasc. Surg.* 74:372–381, 1977.
19. Castaneda A.R., Norwood W.I.: Fallot's tetralogy, in Stark J., de Leval M. (eds.): *Surgery for Congenital Heart Defects.* New York, Grune & Stratton, 1983, pp. 321–329.
20. Castaneda A.R., Sade R.M., Lamberti J., et al.: Reoperation for residual defects after repair of tetralogy of Fallot. *Surgery* 76:1010–1017, 1974.
21. Chiariello L., Agosti J., Vlad P., et al.: Congenital aortic stenosis: Experience with 43 patients. *J. Thorac. Cardiovasc. Surg.* 72:182–193, 1976.
22. Chiariello L., Meyer J., Wukasch D.C., et al.: Intracardiac repair of tetralogy of Fallot: Five-year review of 403 patients. *J. Thorac. Cardiovasc. Surg.* 70:529–535, 1975.
23. Coto E.O., Norwood W.I., Lang P., et al.: Modified Senning operation for treatment of transposition of the great arteries. *J. Thorac. Cardiovasc. Surg.* 78:721–729, 1979.
24. Crafoord C., Nylin G.: Congenital coarctation of the aorta and its surgical treatment. *J. Thorac. Surg.* 14:347, 1945.
25. Craig R.J., Selzer A.: Natural history and prognosis of atrial septal defect. *Circulation* 37:805, 1968.
26. de Leval M.: Coarctation of the aorta and interruption of the aortic arch, in Stark J., de Leval M. (eds.): *Surgery for Congenital Heart Defects.* New York, Grune & Stratton, 1983, pp. 213–225.
27. de Leval M.: Persistent truncus arteriosus, in Stark J., de Leval M. (eds.): *Surgery for Congenital Heart Defects.* New York, Grune & Stratton, 1983, pp. 417–425.
28. de Leval M.: Ventricular septal defects, in Stark J., de Leval M. (eds.): *Surgery for Congenital Heart Defects.* New York, Grune & Stratton, 1983, pp. 271–284.
29. Edmunds L.H.: Operation or indomethacin for the premature ductus? *Ann. Thorac. Surg.* 26:586–589, 1978.
30. German J.C., Mahour G.H., Woolley M.M.: Esophageal atresia and associated anomalies. *J. Pediatr. Surg.* 11:299–306, 1976.
31. Gibbon J.H.: Application of a mechanical heart lung apparatus to cardiac surgery. *Minn. Med.* 37:171, 1954.
32. Glenn W.W.L.: Circulatory bypass of the right side of the heart. Shunt between the superior vena cava and distal right pulmonary artery: Report of clinical application. *N. Engl. J. Med.* 259:117, 1958.
33. Graham T.P. Jr., Bender H.W. Jr.: Preoperative diagnosis and management of infants with critical congenital heart disease. *Ann. Thorac. Surg.* 29:272–288, 1980.
34. Gross R.E., Hubbard J.P.: Surgical ligation of a patent ductus arteriosus: Report of first successful case. *JAMA* 112:729, 1939.
35. Gross R.E., Hufnagel C.A.: Coarctation of the aorta: Experimental studies regarding its surgical correction. *N. Engl. J. Med.* 233:287, 1945.
36. Gross R.E., Watkins E. Jr., Pomeranz A.A., et al.: Method for surgical closure of interauricular septal defects. *Surg. Gynecol. Obstet.* 96:1, 1953.
37. Harrison M.R., Hanson B.A., Takahashi M., et al.: The significance of right aortic arch in repair of esophageal atresia and tracheoesophageal fistula. *J. Pediatr. Surg.* 12:861–869, 1977.
38. Hawkins J.A., Clark E.B., Doty D.B.: Total anomalous pulmonary venous connection. *Ann. Thorac. Surg.* 36:548–560, 1983.
39. Henry J., Kaplan S., Helmsworth J.A., et al.: Management of infants with large ventricular septal defects. *Ann. Thorac. Surg.* 15:109–119, 1973.
40. Ho E.C., Moss A.J.: The syndrome of "mesenteric arteritis" following surgical repair of aortic coarctation: Report of nine cases and review of the literature. *Pediatrics* 49:40–45, 1972.
41. Jatene A.D., Fontes V.F., Paulista P.P., et al.: Successful anatomic correction of transposition of the great vessels: A preliminary report. *Separata. Arq. Card.* 28:461, 1975.
42. Kaplan E.L., Anthony B.F., Bisno A., et al.: Prevention of bacterial endocarditis. *Circulation* 56:139A–143A, 1977.
43. Konno S., Imai Y., Iida Y., et al.: A new method of prosthetic valve replacement in congenital aortic stenosis associated with hypoplasia of the aortic valve ring. *J. Thorac. Cardiovasc. Surg.* 70:909–917, 1975.
44. Lababidi Z.: Neonatal transluminal balloon coarctation angioplasty. *Am. Heart J.* 106:752, 1983.
45. Lerberg D.B., Hardesty R.L., Siewers R.D., et al.: Coarctation of the aorta in infants and children: 25 years of experience. *Ann. Thorac. Surg.* 33:159–170, 1982.
46. Lillehei C.W., Cohen M., Warden H.E., et al.: Direct vision intracardiac surgical correction of the tetralogy of Fallot, pentalogy of Fallot, and pulmonary atresia defects: Report of first ten cases. *Ann. Surg.* 142:418, 1955.
47. Marcelletti C., Mair D.D., McGoon D.C., et al.: Complete repair of transposition of the great arteries with pulmonary atresia. *J. Thorac. Cardiovasc. Surg.* 72:215–220, 1976.
48. Marcelletti C., Mair D.D., McGoon D.C., et al.: The Rastelli operation for transposition of the great arteries. *J. Thorac. Cardiovasc. Surg.* 72:427–434, 1976.
49. Mavroudis C., Cook L.N., Fleischaker B.A., et al.: Management of patent ductus arteriosus in the premature infant: Indomethacin versus ligation. *Ann. Thorac. Surg.* 36:561–566, 1983.
50. McGoon D.C., Baird D.K., Davis G.D.: Surgical management of large bronchial collateral arteries with pulmonary stenosis or atresia. *Circulation* 52:109, 1975.
51. Moulton A.L., Brenner J.I., Roberts G., et al.: Subclavian flap repair of coarctation of the aorta in neonates. *J. Thorac. Cardiovasc. Surg.* 87:220–235, 1984.
52. Moulton A.L., Bowman F.O., Edie R.N., et al.: Pulmonary atresia with intact ventricular septum: A sixteen-year experience. *J. Thorac. Cardiovasc. Surg.* 78:527, 1979.
52a. Moulton A.L., Malm J.R.: Right ventricular outflow tract obstruction, in Stark, J., de Leval M. (eds): *Surgery for Congenital Heart Defects.* New York, Grune and Stratton, 1983, chap. 22.
53. Muller W.H., Dammann J.F. Jr.: The treatment of certain congenital malformations of the heart by the creation of pulmonic stenosis to reduce pulmonary hypertension and excessive pulmonary blood flow. *Surg. Gynecol. Obstet.* 95:213, 1952.
54. Mustard W.T.: Successful two-stage correction of transposition of the great vessels. *Surgery* 55:469, 1964.
55. Mustard W.T., Chute A.L., Keith J.D., et al.: A surgical approach to transposition of the great vessels with extracorporeal circuit. *Surgery* 36:39, 1954.
56. Nelson R.J., Thibeault D.W., Emmanouilides G.C., et al.: Improving the results of ligation of patent ductus arteriosus in small preterm infants. *J. Thorac. Cardiovasc. Surg.* 71:169–178, 1976.
57. Pacifico A.D.: Atrioventricular septal defects, in Stark J., de Leval M. (eds.): *Surgery for Congenital Heart Defects.* New York, Grune & Stratton, 1983, pp. 285–300.
58. Penkoske P.A., Westerman G., Marx G.R., et al.: Transposition of the great arteries and ventricular septal defect: Results with the Senning operation and closure of the ventricular septal defect in infants. *Ann. Thorac. Surg.* 36:281–288, 1983.
59. Piccoli G.P., Dickinson D.F., Musumeci F., et al.: A changing policy for the surgical treatment of tetralogy of Fallot: Early and late results in 235 consecutive patients. *Ann. Thorac. Surg.* 33:365–372, 1982.
60. Potts W., Smith S., Gibson S.: Anastomosis of aorta to pulmonary artery: Certain types in congenital heart disease. *JAMA* 132:627, 1946.
61. Puga F.J., McGoon D.C., Julsrud P.R., et al.: Complete repair of pulmonary atresia with nonconfluent pulmonary arteries. *Ann. Thorac. Surg.* 35:36–44, 1983.
62. Quaegebeur J.M., Rohmer J., Brom A.G.: Revival of the Senning operation in the treatment of transposition of the great arteries. *Thorax* 32:517–524, 1977.
63. Rashkind W.J., Miller W.W.: Creation of an atrial septal defect without thoracotomy: A palliative approach to complete transposition of the great arteries. *JAMA* 196:173, 1966.
64. Rittenhouse E.A., Doty D.B., Lauer R., et al.: Patent ductus arteriosus in premature infants: Indications for surgery. *J. Thorac. Cardiovasc. Surg.* 71:187–194, 1976.
65. Sade R.M., in discussion, Azzolina G., Russo P.A., Maffei G., et al.: Waterston anastomosis in two-stage correction of severe tetralogy of Fallot: Ten years of experience. *Ann. Thorac. Surg.* 34:420–421, 1982.
66. Sade R.M., Sloss L., Treves S., et al.: Repair of tetralogy of Fallot after aortopulmonary anastomosis. *Ann. Thorac. Surg.* 23:32–38, 1977.
67. Senning A.: Surgical correction of transposition of the great vessels. *Surgery* 45:966, 1959.
68. Seybold-Epting W., Reul G.J. Jr., Hallman G.L., et al.: Repair of ventricular septal defect after pulmonary artery banding. *J. Thorac. Cardiovasc. Surg.* 71:392–397, 1976.
69. Shaher R.M., Foster E., Farina M., et al.: Right heart reconstruction following repair of tetralogy of Fallot. *Ann. Thorac. Surg.* 35:421–426, 1983.
70. Stark J.: Persistent ductus arteriosus, in Stark J., de Leval M. (eds.): *Surgery for Congenital Heart Defects.* New York, Grune & Stratton, 1983, pp. 203–211.
71. Stark J., Gandhi D., de Leval M., et al.: Surgical treatment of persistent truncus arteriosus in the first year of life. *Br. Heart J.* 40:1280, 1978.

72. Suzuki Y., Ishizawa E., Tanaka S., et al.: Surgical treatment of large ventricular septal defect with pulmonary hypertension in the first 24 months of life. *Ann. Thorac. Surg.* 22:228–234, 1976.
73. Tawes R.L. Jr., Aberdeen E., Waterston D.J., et al.: Coarctation of aorta in infants and children: A review of 333 operative cases, including 179 infants. *Circulation* 39, 40 (suppl. 1):173–184, 1969.
74. Tawes R.L. Jr., Bull J.C., Roe B.B.: Hypertension and abdominal pain after resection of aortic coarctation. *Ann. Surg.* 171:409–412, 1970.
75. Traugott R.C., Will R.J., Schuchmann G.F., et al.: A simplified method of ligation of patent ductus arteriosus in premature infants. *Ann. Thorac. Surg.* 29:263, 1980.
76. Waterston D.: Treatment of Fallot's tetralogy in children under one year of age. *Rozhl. Chir.* 41:181, 1962.

141 John A. Waldhausen / Walter E. Pae, Jr.
Thoracic Great Vessels

Patent Ductus Arteriosus

Galen,[27] in the second century, described the anatomy and closure of the patent ductus arteriosus. Although it became well known that in patients living to puberty a common sequel of patent ductus arteriosus was subacute bacterial endarteritis, it was not until 1907 that Munro suggested an operation for its closure.[54, 61] Thirty years passed before Strieder accomplished the partial closure of a patent ductus arteriosus in a patient with subacute bacterial endarteritis, who expired 4 days later secondary to gastric dilatation.[29] One year later, Gross[32] ligated a patent ductus arteriosus successfully and opened the door to modern cardiovascular surgery.

Anatomy and Physiology

The ductus arteriosus is an embryologic remnant of the distal portion of the left sixth aortic arch and connects the main or left pulmonary artery with the descending thoracic aorta about 5–10 mm distal to the origin of the left subclavian artery. In most instances, it is located on the left; but, in the case of a right aortic arch, it may be on the left or on the right. Very rarely is it bilateral. It varies in length and diameter. During fetal life, the patent ductus arteriosus is equal in diameter to the descending aorta and diverts blood from the nonventilated lungs, with their high pulmonary vascular resistance into the descending thoracic aorta, where blood then goes into the placenta for gas exchange. The media of the ductus is thick with smooth muscle, which is biochemically highly responsive. Hypoxia and prostaglandin E_1 and E_2 induce its dilatation. At birth with ventilation, the pulmonary vascular resistance falls, flow reverses in the ductus, and the partial pressure of oxygen in the arterial blood rises. In response to these events, there is functional closure of the ductus secondary to contraction of its muscle, usually within hours after birth. The infolding of the endothelium and subintimal proliferation that causes permanent closure may take up to 12 weeks, but usually ranges between 2–3 weeks. Delayed closure in premature infants is recognized. Complete failure to close is believed to be secondary to the immaturity of the histologic structures of the patent ductus coupled with some lack of biochemical responsiveness.[28] Nevertheless, the degree of left-to-right shunting, which is the result of a persistent ductus arteriosus, is directly related to the pulmonary vascular resistance. The well-recognized sequelae of the shunt include subacute bacterial endarteritis, congestive heart failure, and pulmonary hypertension.[13, 89]

Diagnosis and Management

The incidence of patent ductus arteriosus depends upon whether or not one includes premature infants in the cohort.[56, 57] Its causes include maternal rubella, prematurity, and neonatal respiratory distress. It occurs predominantly in females at a ratio of approximately two females to one male. Many patients with a patent ductus arteriosus are asymptomatic, and clinical features depend on the magnitude of the left-to-right shunt. Growth and development may be normal or retarded, but frequent respiratory infections and distress are common.

In the premature infant, the murmur is usually systolic; but as the pulmonary vascular resistance falls, the shunt becomes larger, and the murmur extends into diastole. Femoral pulses may be water-hammer. The classic continuous machinery murmur at the left upper border of the sternum is usually heard in older children with large shunts and is accompanied by bounding peripheral pulses.

With a small patent ductus arteriosus, the ECG is normal. With larger shunts it demonstrates left ventricular hypertrophy. The chest roentgenogram may be normal or may demonstrate moderate cardiomegaly and pulmonary vascular congestion. The need for cardiac catheterization to diagnose an uncomplicated patent ductus arteriosus is disputed. Catheterization is essential, however, to confirm the diagnosis if there are any atypical features present, or in small infants where the incidence of associated cardiac abnormalities is high, particularly if the two-dimensional echocardiographic examination is not completely diagnostic. On the other hand, it is rarely indicated for premature infants in whom a patent ductus is common and intracardiac lesions less so.

Hypoxia prevents closure of the ductus and increases pulmonary blood flow, thereby aggravating the clinical situation. Closure of the patent ductus arteriosus can be stimulated by administration of an inhibitor of prostaglandin E_1 synthesis, in the form of indomethacin. The effectiveness of this in premature infants has been well documented.[26, 39] Ligation in the hands of most experts causes a nearly zero operative and perioperative mortality.[48, 52, 55] We perform surgical ligation in a premature infant with respiratory distress syndrome and patent ductus arteriosus if there is a contraindication to the administration of indomethacin or if indomethacin therapy has failed.

Congestive heart failure in infancy is a clear indication for surgical closure. For all others with a patent ductus arteriosus, elective operative interruption is recommended when the patent ductus arteriosus is discovered.[64] This is particularly true after

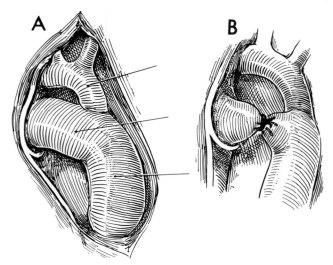

Fig 141–1.—Ligation of ductus arteriosus in the neonate. **A,** operative exposure after the pleura is incised. **B,** the ductus is encircled and tied with a heavy silk ligature. (From Waldhausen J.A., Pierce W.S.[110] Used by permission.)

the age of 1 year when spontaneous closure is less likely. Elective closure in the absence of symptoms is based on studies that have demonstrated decreased life expectancy because of the development of pulmonary hypertension and its sequelae, as well as the risk of subacute bacterial endarteritis, while the operative mortality is less than 1%.[13, 71, 106] In our series of well over 300 infants and children with patent ductus arteriosus, the operative mortality is 0. Only in children whose pulmonary vascular resistance is greater than 8 units/m^2 and in adults with pulmonary hypertension and Eisenmenger's syndrome should the ductus not be obliterated.[7, 98]

In neonates, the ductus is exposed through a left posterolateral thoracotomy in the fourth intercostal space. (We prefer to do this in the controlled and sterile environment of the operating room rather than in the neonatal intensive care unit.) The lungs are

retracted anteriorly. A heavy silk ligature is passed around the ductus and tied (Fig 141–1).

In older infants and children, the ductus is approached also through a standard left fourth interspace posterolateral thoracotomy. The mediastinal pleura is opened over the aortic isthmus, and the incision is continued up along the left subclavian artery. The highest intercostal vein must be divided. Dissection is carried out over the anterior surface of the aorta to the patent ductus and across the ductus toward the pulmonary artery. In this fashion, the patent ductus will be exposed without injury to the recurrent laryngeal nerve. As the pulmonary artery adjacent to the ductus is approached, the vagus nerve comes into view. Usually, this nerve can be seen clearly through the pleura. The recurrent laryngeal nerve leaves the vagus nerve just below the ductus and curves posteriorly around the ductus and aorta. The pericardial sac usually extends over the anterior surface of the patent ductus. This pericardial extension is mobilized and reflected medially. Dissection of the posterior wall of the ductus is the most critical part of the operation and should be attempted only after preparation has been made to occlude the aorta in the event of hemorrhage. Tapes are placed around the aorta, both above and below the ductus arteriosus, and around the left subclavian artery. Exposure of the posterior wall of the ductus may be obtained by retracting the aorta upward and anteriorly and dissecting out the isthmus as well as the posterior wall. Tissue behind the ductus may be relatively dense. The recurrent laryngeal nerve is not likely to be injured if it is adequately visualized and maintained on the pulmonary artery side. In infants under 1 year, the ductus is ligated with a purse-string suture on the aortic side, and a second ligature on the pulmonary side (Fig 141–2). In older children, when the patent ductus arteriosus is dissected and tapes have been placed around the aorta above and below the ductus, vascular clamps are applied as close to the aorta and pulmonary artery as possible so that an adequate cuff will be available for suture when the ductus is divided (Fig 141–3,*A*). As a precaution against the clamps slipping, the ductus is divided half-way and partially sutured by beginning anteriorly with a continuous horizontal mattress suture of polypropylene at the pulmonary and aortic ends (see Fig 141–3,*B*). The ductus is

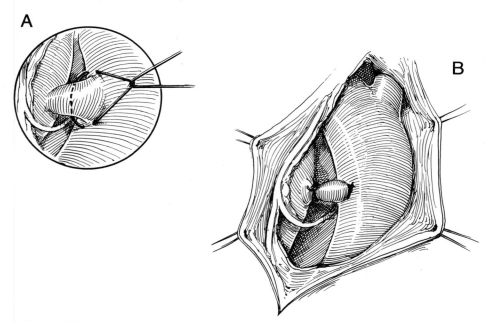

Fig 141–2.—Technique of ligation of the ductus in infancy. **A,** a purse-string suture is inserted about the ductus and tied. **B,** an additional ligature of heavy silk is tied about the pulmonary end of the ductus. (From Waldhausen J.A., Pierce W.S.[110] Used by permission.)

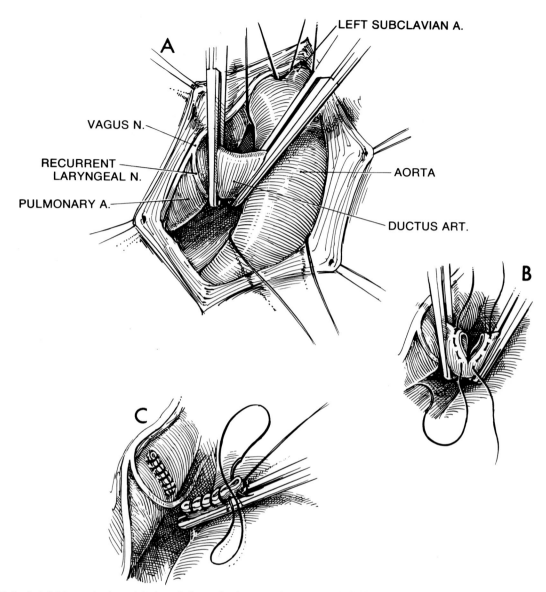

LEFT SUBCLAVIAN A.

VAGUS N.

RECURRENT
LARYNGEAL N.

PULMONARY A.

AORTA

DUCTUS ART.

A

B

C

Fig 141–3.—Method of division and suture of ductus arteriosus. **A,** after exposure of the ductus and proximal and distal control of the aorta, vascular clamps are applied to the ductus. **B,** the ductus is partially divided and a basting suture begun on each divided edge. **C,** division is finished; and, after the basting suture is completed, each divided end is oversewn continuously before removal of the clamps. (From Waldhausen J.A., Pierce W.S.[110] Used by permission.)

then divided, and the continuous mattress suture adjacent to the clamps is completed and the free edge oversewn as a continuous layer (see Fig 141–3,C). The pulmonary clamp is released first, followed by release of the aortic clamp.[67]

Considerable success with nonoperative, mechanical closure of the patent ductus arteriosus using either a transvenous or arterial approach has been described by Portsmann. This experimental approach must be shown to carry a lower mortality and morbidity than current surgical techniques before its widespread use is advocated.[77]

Excellent long- and short-term results for repair of patent ductus arteriosus are often reported. The risk of operation for children without associated anomalies is less than 0.5%.[71] The operative risk increases in the face of associated cardiac defects and increased pulmonary vascular resistance, and in adults when the ductus is calcified and aneurysmal. However, once the patent ductus arteriosus is divided, there is no long-term morbidity.

Coarctation of the Aorta

Introduction

Coarctation of the aorta is defined as an abrupt constriction of a section of the aorta. It may occur anywhere from the arch to the bifurcation of the aorta, but in 98% of cases it is situated in the aortic isthmus between the origin of the left subclavian artery proximally and the junction of the aorta and ductus arteriosus distally. The anomaly comprises 5–8% of all congenital cardiac malformations.[44, 84]

History

Coarctation of the aorta was first described by Morgagni[59] in 1760. In 1903, Bonnet[8] attempted to establish a clinical pathologic classification by dividing coarctations into infantile and adult types. The infantile type was usually preductal, with tubular narrowing of the aortic isthmus proximal to a usually patent ductus arteriosus through which blood flowed to the descending thoracic aorta. The adult type was characterized by a localized sharp constriction of the aorta in the area of the aortic insertion of the ductus arteriosus or ligamentum arteriosum. Additionally, shelf-like narrowing was often noted within the lumen. In 1951, Johnson et al.[42] based a classification on the position of the ductus and its relation to the coarctation, thus recognizing preductal and postductal patterns. Recently, it has been shown that the infantile or preductal type can be detected in older children and vice versa.[84] Current classification is based on the location and type of narrowing. Thus, there is hypoplasia of the isthmus and coarctation seen in preductal coarctation, and there is juxtaductal coarctation. Postductal coarctation was probably initially a juxtaductal type with subsequent downward displacement caused by hemodynamic molding. It is seen only in older children and adults. Associated cardiac abnormalities are common in infants with preductal coarctation; this is not true with localized juxtaductal coarctation.[84] Surgical therapy for coarctation of the aorta has improved in immediate and late results since the first successful surgical corrections of the lesion were reported independently in 1945 by Crafoord and Nylin[17] and Gross.[30]

Cause

Coarctation of the aorta is thought to be the result of a fetal imbalance of aortic and pulmonary artery blood flows. In the normal fetus, left and right ventricular stroke volume are equal, and the pulmonary and systemic circulation are in parallel rather than in series, as they become after birth (Fig 141–4,A). The effect of "hemodynamic molding" on the volume of flow through the cardiac chambers and great arteries is thought to determine their size at birth. Therefore, a significant decrease in aortic blood flow relative to pulmonary artery flow decreases flow through the isthmus, which results in narrowing or obliteration of the isthmus (see Fig 141–4,B). A resistive foramen ovale, aortic stenosis or hypoplasia, mitral valve abnormality, or large ventricular septal defect all cause increased pulmonary flow and decreased aortic flow, and result in failure of the isthmus to grow. The eventual location of a coarctation is dependent on both the volume and direction of the fetal isthmic flow. The presence of ductus-like tissue in the aortic wall at the insertion of the ductus has been demonstrated, and this tissue probably causes the contraction of the coarctation membrane.

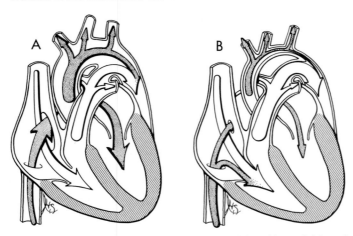

Fig 141–4.—Fetal circulation. **A,** normal fetal circulation with equal right and left ventricular outputs. **B,** a resistive foramen ovale results in increased pulmonary flow and decreased aortic flow. Hypoplasia of the isthmus results. (From Waldhausen J.A., Parr G.V.S.[109] Used by permission.)

Anatomical and Physiologic Considerations

Invariably, examination of the aorta in infants with coarctation and hypoplasia of the isthmus demonstrates diffuse narrowing of the aorta distal to the left common carotid artery and especially below the left subclavian artery. The pulmonary artery is connected to the descending thoracic aorta by a large similarly sized patent ductus. A coarctation membrane is seen proximal to the entrance of the ductus at the junction of the isthmus and the descending thoracic aorta. Enlargement of intercostal arteries is minimal in comparison to juxtaductal coarctation, and there is minimal poststenotic dilatation of the descending thoracic aorta.

On the other hand, gross examination of the juxtaductal coarctation shows localized narrowing in the region of the ductus or ligamentum arteriosum. The extent of narrowing is variable. With age, because of unequal growth of the aortic wall, the coarctation appears more distal than its juxtaductal position in the neonate and is termed a postductal coarctation. Poststenotic dilatation of the descending aorta is marked, as is the enlargement of the intercostal arteries. In older patients, saccular aneurysms of the intercostal arteries are often present just proximal to their entrance into the aorta. There is shelf-like narrowing of the aorta at the ligamentum; at times, this may completely obliterate the lumen. In these cases, the arch is truly interrupted. The aortic wall may be quite thin in the region of poststenotic dilatation.

The development of symptoms in neonates with obstructive lesions of the aortic arch is related to the postnatal constriction of the ductus. Talner and Berman[99] demonstrated that constriction of the ductus begins at the pulmonary artery end of the ductus and thereby allows continued flow around the coarctation shelf. After complete ductal closure at approximately 2 weeks of age, obstruction to flow in the distal aorta becomes evident. With inadequate collateral flow in cases of narrowing of the isthmus, interrupted arch, or juxtaductal coarctation, closure of the ductus results in ischemia of the lower body (Fig 141–5). Renal failure, acidosis, and congestive heart failure may, therefore, be the first signs of these lesions.

Collateral flow around coarctation of the aorta develops from the subclavian arteries and their branches. The internal mammary, intercostal, musculophrenic, transverse cervical, scapular, lateral thoracic, superior epigastric, and spinal arteries all provide flow to the lower body and have been angiographically demonstrated to be dilated during the first weeks of life.[14, 22] From the age of 8 years on, roentgenograms show notching on the inferior and posterior border of the ribs caused by the continuous pressure of dilated and tortuous collateral arteries. Scapular collateral arteries may be palpated, and their pulsations may be evident on physical examination. Pedal pulses may be present, but femoral pulses are either absent or diminished.

Although not a predominant sign in infants with isthmic narrowing and associated cardiac defects, hypertension is a common sequel of simple coarctation and is seen in older patients. Its cause is unclear. Mechanical, renal, adrenal, and baroreceptor mechanisms have been espoused. It was shown by Gupta and Wiggers[34] that narrowing the aorta in animals by 50% produces proximal systolic hypertension and a distal decrease in pressure. They suggest that the ascending aorta has reduced distensibility and capacity. Renal mechanisms suggested by Page,[70] who expanded on the work of Goldblatt, have been supported by the experiments of Scott and Bahnson.[86] They demonstrated that by transplanting one kidney in the neck of a dog and then creating a coarctation, upper extremity hypertension resulted.[70, 86] Removing the abdominal kidney abolished the hypertension. Renin assays have not been uniformly elevated, although there appears

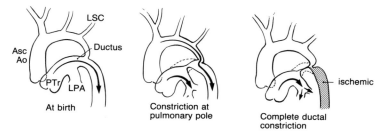

A. Coarctation

LSC

Asc Ao

Ductus

PTr LPA

At birth

Constriction at pulmonary pole

Complete ductal constriction

— ischemic

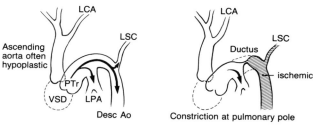

B. Interrupted arch

LCA

LSC

Ascending aorta often hypoplastic

PTr

VSD LPA

Desc Ao

LCA

LSC

Ductus

— ischemic

Constriction at pulmonary pole

Fig 141–5.—Importance of postnatal constriction of the ductus arteriosus on development of symptoms in neonates with obstructive lesions of the aortic arch. **A,** flow through the aortic isthmus continues even after the ductus begins to constrict at the pulmonary end; flow to the lower body is reduced when the constriction of the ductus progresses toward the aorta. **B,** interrupted aortic arch.

Constriction of the ductus at the pulmonary pole immediately interferes with flow to the lower body. *Asc Ao* indicates ascending aorta; *LSC,* left subclavian artery; *PTr,* pulmonary trunk; *LPA,* left pulmonary artery; *LCA,* left carotid artery; *VSD,* ventricular septal defect; and *Desc Ao,* ascending aorta. (Modified from Fishman N.H., et al.: *J. Cardiovasc. Surg.* 71:35, 1976. Used by permission.)

to be diurnal variation.[113] Furthermore, hypertension may persist after a satisfactory repair of the coarctation.[51] Accordingly, abnormal baroreceptors in the ascending aorta and abnormal adrenal function have been postulated as factors.[87, 96] Indeed, measurement of adrenal medullary hormones has supported the latter.[5]

Although infant mortality has been closely related to the presence or absence of associated cardiac anomalies, adult patients with untreated coarctation usually die of the sequelae of prolonged hypertension. Necropsy series show frequent aortic dissection and aortic rupture, as well as either intracranial hemorrhage or thrombosis.[47, 79, 90] Increased incidence of coronary artery disease has been demonstrated, and turbulent flow at the coarctation site may lead to infective endarteritis and mycotic aneurysm with rupture.[16]

Diagnosis and Management

Symptomatic Infants (under 1 year of age)

Nearly one half of all patients with coarctation of the aorta have symptoms during the first months of life.[44] These patients, frequently neonates, are seen with medically refractory and life-threatening congestive heart failure. Tachypnea, poor feeding, hepatomegaly, and cardiomegaly are the most common early signs of congestive heart failure. Cyanosis is not uncommon, even in the absence of associated severe cardiac defects, and may be present especially in preterminal or in very low-output states. Auscultatory findings, although absent in 50% of patients, are influenced by associated anomalies, which are present in 75% of cases in the neonatal period.[100] When present in infants with either coarctation alone or coarctation with a patent ductus arteriosus, the soft systolic murmur is best heard at the left sternal border. Louder murmurs are usually due to associated malformations, the most common ones being ventricular septal defects and mitral valve abnormalities.[100] Peripheral pulses are, classi-

cally, easily palpable and prominent in the upper extremities and diminished or weak in the lower extremities, but may be weak in both. After adequate therapy for congestive heart failure, it becomes apparent that a pulse pressure differential exists between the upper and lower extremities.

The chest roentgenogram shows cardiomegaly, congestion, and increased pulmonary vascularity in the lung fields. Invariably, ECG shows right ventricular hypertrophy during the first few months of life and shows left ventricular hypertrophy in patients who have survived 6 months to 1 year. Left ventricular hypertrophy is common in older patients.

Nonoperative therapy for symptomatic infants with coarctation of the aorta has resulted in mortality rates as high as 86%,[92, 107, 109] and 66% if the coarctation is not associated with highly complex lesions.[107] Management of these patients begins with Doppler measurement of blood pressure and two-dimensional echocardiography. If a 30-mm Hg gradient between the upper and lower extremities is recorded and the two-dimensional echocardiogram shows continuity between the ascending and descending aorta, the diagnosis of coarctation of the aorta is accepted. Furthermore, some investigators believe that if a two-dimensional echocardiogram rules out associated cardiac abnormalities, no further investigation is necessary. On the other hand, should the clinical diagnosis not be evident and should two-dimensional echocardiography demonstrate either associated cardiac anomalies or discontinuity of the ascending and descending aorta, cardiac catheterization is carried out. These investigations and operation are undertaken after the patient becomes clinically stable and has no evidence of low cardiac output, metabolic acidosis, or renal failure. If any of these are present, intensive medical therapy is begun with prostaglandin E_1 (0.1 µg/kg/min), to dilate the ductus temporarily and improve descending aortic flow, coupled with digitalis and diuretics.[38] In the sickest patients, mechanical ventilation and inotropic support with dopamine are necessary. Operation is then undertaken in all symptomatic infants as soon as they are clinically stable. For pa-

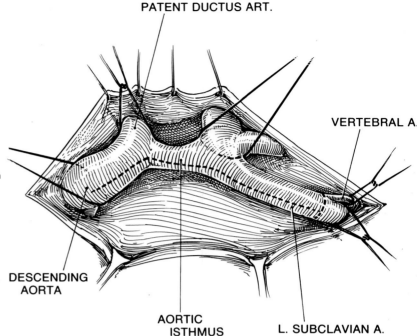

PATENT DUCTUS ART.

VERTEBRAL A.

DESCENDING AORTA

AORTIC ISTHMUS

L. SUBCLAVIAN A.

Fig 141–6.—Subclavian flap angioplasty for coarctation of aorta in infants. The aorta and left subclavian arteries are mobilized. The ductus, and the left subclavian, and vertebral arteries are ligated. The *dotted line* represents proposed incision for fashioning subclavian flap. (From Waldhausen J.A., Pierce W.S.[110] Used by permission.)

tients who are not critically ill, or who are asymptomatic but who manifest cardiomegaly or severe hypertension, elective repair should be considered in later infancy.[10]

Coarctectomy followed by end-to-end anastomosis performed during the first year of life results in restenosis in 16%–50% of patients.[23, 37, 41, 45, 49, 74, 92, 100, 109] The subclavian flap angioplasty, first described by Waldhausen and Nahrwold[108] in 1966, has virtually eliminated recurrent stenosis and is the preferred method of repair in infancy.[3, 10, 36, 60, 76, 101, 109, 111] Through a fourth interspace thoracotomy, the aorta and left subclavian arteries are mobilized and the ductus is ligated (Fig 141–6). The left subclavian and vertebral vessels are then ligated (the latter to prevent subclavian steal). The aorta is clamped proximally and distally, and the subclavian artery is transected (Fig 141–7). The aorta is then incised from below the coarctation, across the narrowed segment, through the isthmus, and along the lateral border of the subclavian artery (Fig 141–7). The frequently found coarctation shelf is excised (Fig 141–8). The subclavian flap is then turned down into the aortic incision and sutured into place with interrupted polypropylene sutures (Fig 141–9).[10] Experimental studies in growing piglets have shown that a continuous suture technique with nonabsorbable suture is less satisfactory than an

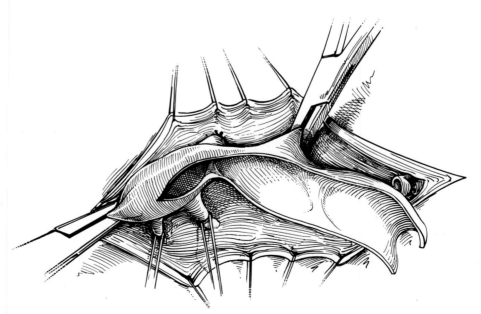

Fig 141–7.—Subclavian flap angioplasty (cont.). The aorta is clamped proximally and distally and the subclavian ligated and transected distally. The aorta has been incised from below and across coarctation through the isthmus and then along the lateral border of the subclavian. (From Waldhausen J.A., Pierce W.S.[110] Used by permission.)

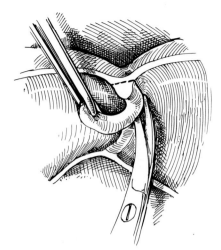

Fig 141–8.—Subclavian flap angioplasty (cont.). Endoaortic excision of the coarctation shelf. (From Waldhausen J.A., Pierce W.S.[110] Used by permission.)

TABLE 141–1.—COARCTATION
OF THE AORTA: AGE AT
OPERATION AND MORTALITY

AGE	PATIENTS	DEATHS
1–7 days	13	2
8–30 days	22	0
31–365 days	18	0
Total	53	2 (4%)

*From Campbell D.B., et al.[10]

interrupted technique and may result in a bowstring formation in the lumen, a rough intima, and thrombus formation.[68] More recently, continuous sutures of absorbable polydioxanone have been used to secure the angioplasty. We have excellent results with this technique, and it has eliminated the need for using interrupted sutures of nonabsorbable material. This technique, in addition to the intensive medical therapy described, has been used in 53 infants less than 12 months of age (Table 141–1), with two deaths (4.0%). No patient more than 7 days old has died. Associated defects in 34 patients under 1 month of age at operation included patent ductus arteriosus in all but two, and intracardiac anomalies such as ventricular septal defect, mitral stenosis, and double-outlet right ventricle in 22 (65%). At a mean follow-up period of 42 months, only two patients had significant gradients (15 and 20 mm Hg); and both gradients were in patients done early in the series with continuous sutures of polypropylene. All patients repaired with interrupted suture were free of gradients. Initial follow-up for the group with absorbable suture suggests no gradients, and angiography has demonstrated growth of the aorta in the repaired area. Similar results have been reported by other groups of investigators.[3, 10, 36, 60, 76, 101, 111]

Whether or not pulmonary artery banding is necessary in patients with an unrestricted ventricular septal defect is controversial, because repair of the coarctation is often followed by spontaneous closure of the ventricular septal defect or by the ventricular septal defect becoming restrictive with a subsequent decrease in pulmonary artery pressure.[53, 66] Early operative closure of the ventricular septal defect is indicated only in those infants with persistent congestive heart failure or pulmonary artery hypertension.

Asymptomatic Patients Over 1 Year of Age

In the previous discussion, the clinical findings and the natural history of coarctation of the aorta were shown to be quite variable. Nearly half of all patients remain asymptomatic. In older children, coarctation is often first recognized at routine physical examination by weak or absent femoral pulses, a heart murmur, or the presence of upper extremity hypertension. About 5% of patients over 1 year of age will have dyspnea on exertion, headache, or nose bleeds.[44] Pulsations may be visible in the sternal notch, and pulsations over the scapula may be felt. A systolic heart murmur is almost always present at the left sternal border; it is rarely loud or harsh and is often transmitted to the back or apex.

The chest roentgenogram may be either normal or show car-

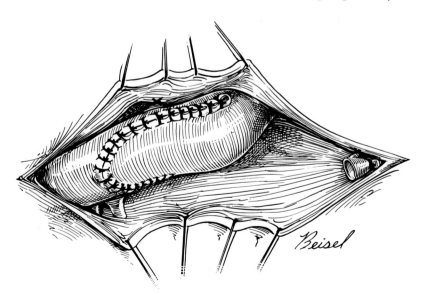

Fig 141–9.—Subclavian flap angioplasty (cont.). The completed angioplasty after turning the flap down into the aortic incision and suturing in place with an interrupted technique. (From Waldhausen J.A., Pierce W.S.[110] Used by permission.)

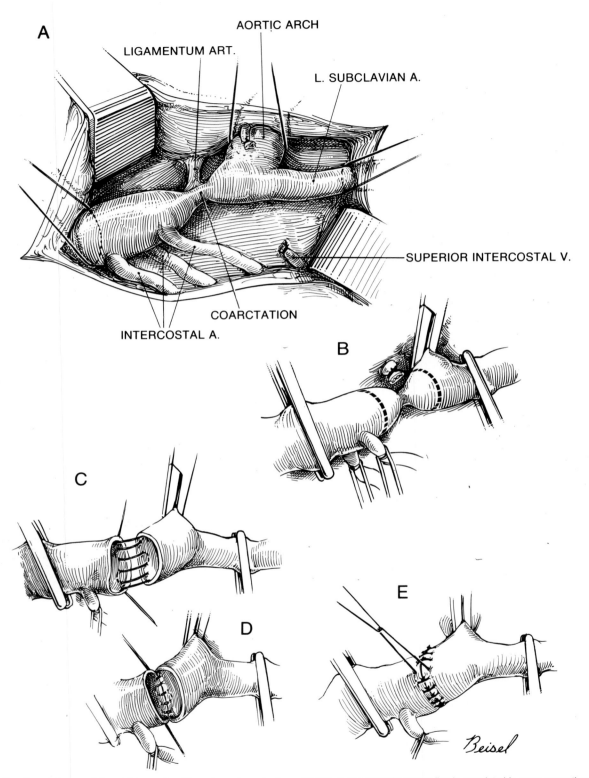

Fig 141–10.—Coarctation repair by excision and end-to-end anastomosis. **A,** operative exposure and proximal and distal control. Note large collaterals. **B,** the ductus is ligated after vascular clamps are applied. The area of coarctation is excised. **C,** the posterior suture line is completed in an open continuous fashion and **(D)** tightened. **E,** repair is finished anteriorly in an interrupted fashion to allow for future growth. (From Waldhausen J.A., Pierce W.S.[110] Used by permission.)

diomegaly. Rib notching may be present, and an indentation may be seen over the left border of the heart in the area of the coarctation, especially in the left anterior oblique view—the so-called 3 sign. The ECG generally demonstrates left ventricular hypertrophy and is normal in only 12% of patients.[44] Combination of coarctation with other lesions may result in combined ventricular hypertrophy in approximately 14% of patients and right ventricular hypertrophy in only 3%.

Cardiac catheterization and angiocardiography are carried out if the clinical diagnosis is not sufficiently clear or typical, or if associated cardiac anomalies are suspected. Associated malformations are less frequent than in symptomatic infants. Untreated coarctation of the aorta results in premature death in over 80% of patients, nearly 20% dying before the age of 10 years.[11] Death in older patients commonly results from intracranial hemorrhage, aortic rupture or dissection, and bacterial endarteritis complicated by rupture.[47, 79, 90]

Excision and direct end-to-end anastomosis of the coarctation, as originally described in the mid 1940s by Crafoord and Nylin[17] and by Gross,[30] are preferred to any other technical variation. The chest is entered through a posterolateral fourth interspace thoracotomy, and dissection and mobilization of the aorta are carried out paying particular attention to the well-developed collateral circulation (Fig 141–10,A). Great care is taken not to injure the intercostal vessels, which may be dilated and thin-walled. These are gently occluded. The proximal aorta and the subclavian artery, and then the distal aorta, are clamped with vascular clamps (see Fig 141–10,B). Following this, the coarctation is excised, and the aortic clamps are approximated. The posterior walls are joined either with a continuous over-and-over suture or a continuous everting mattress suture of polypropylene (see Fig 141–10,C–D). The anterior walls are approximated with similar but interrupted sutures, allowing for future growth (see Fig 141–10,E).[43, 93] Recently, it has been proposed that the entire anastomosis be performed using an absorbable polydioxanone technique. This avoids the hazard of the continuous nonabsorbable suture which has been shown, in growing animals, to result in bowstring formation, intraluminal suture material, and thrombus formation, as well as anastomotic stricture.[62, 63, 69] In approximately 5% of cases, excessive tension may result when the aortic ends are approximated. The interposition of a vascular tube prosthesis solves this problem (Fig 141–11).[93] An alternative approach is the patch-graft aortoplasty, as described by Vosschulte in 1957[105] and readvocated by Reul et al. (Fig 141–12).[80]

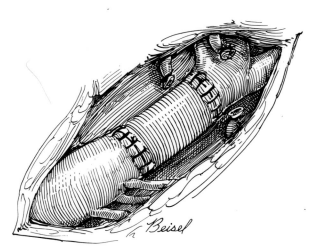

Fig 141–11.—Coarctation repair by excision of a long narrowed segment and interposition of a Dacron graft. (From Waldhausen J.A., Pierce W.S.[110] Used by permission.)

This consists of the insertion of a large diamond-shaped prosthetic patch.

Operative mortality for coarctation repair in this age group has been less than 2% or 3%. In our series of 110 children operated upon between the ages of 3 and 15 years, the mortality has been 0.9% (one death).

A recurrent coarctation is mainly a complication after surgical repair of coarctation in infancy utilizing an end-to-end anastomosis and is often best treated with a prosthetic tube bypass.[93, 110] This can be done with partial occlusion of the aorta, allowing for distal perfusion and protection of the spinal cord. If complete occlusion of the aorta is necessary, a temporary Gott shunt may be used.[18] An extra-anatomical bypass graft from the ascending aorta to the abdominal aorta has been employed in complicated cases.

The most common postoperative complication following repair of coarctation of the aorta in patients over 1 year of age is paradoxical hypertension, which occurred in 56% of our patients.[24] In most cases, this hypertension occurs rapidly and peaks within 24–36 hours of the surgical repair.[97] The initial systolic hypertension is probably related to excessive secretion of norepinephrine in response to increased baroreceptor activity, as well as to the surgical manipulation of the aorta at the isthmus where numerous sympathetic nerve fibers are located.[82] An increase in renin activity, which occurs 24–72 hours after operation, results in a rise in the diastolic pressure. This rise is frequently associated with abdominal pain resulting from mesenteric arteritis and spasm.[88] Reserpine and hydralazine are the drugs of choice in treating this condition, which, when neglected, can allow the arteritis to progress and result in necrotizing lesions of the bowel, necessitating bowel resection.[40] Spinal cord ischemia is a rare but disastrous complication of surgical repair of aortic coarctation and may result in paraplegia.[4, 31] The overall incidence is approximately 0.4%.[9] This complication appears to be related to the anatomy of the anterior spinal artery and to the magnitude of the collateral circulation, as well as to the presence of severe operative hypotension.

Relief of hypertension in both children and adults has been excellent in terms of early follow-up. At hospital discharge, approximately one third of the patients are normotensive, and 74% of all patients are normotensive 1–9 years after operation.[50] Unfortunately, the long-term follow-up of patients treated surgically for aortic coarctation has suggested persistent cardiovascular disease. Maron and his colleagues[51] have noted a 12% increase in premature death from cardiovascular disease, primarily from arterial rupture. Persistent systolic or diastolic hypertension was noted in 40% of the cases. In a large study of 190 patients operated on between the ages of 1 and 15 years, nearly 25% had persistent hypertension; many had hypertension even in the absence of a gradient across the repair.[65] A correlation was demonstrated—excluding patients with residual gradients—that the earlier the age at operation, the greater the likelihood of normal postoperative blood pressure. The cause of postoperative hypertension in successful repair of aortic coarctation, like the cause of preoperative hypertension, is not clear.

The age at which elective surgical repair of a coarctation is undertaken must be balanced to avoid recoarctation, operative mortality, and persistent late postoperative hypertension and early cardiovascular death. In the past, it was believed that the optimal age for repair was between 3 and 5 years old. Because recoarctation and mortality are so low in infants who are repaired with the subclavian flap procedure and who received modern perioperative management, we have proposed elective repair at the end of the first year of life to avoid the devastating late mortality and morbidity of patients whose repair is done in later childhood.[10]

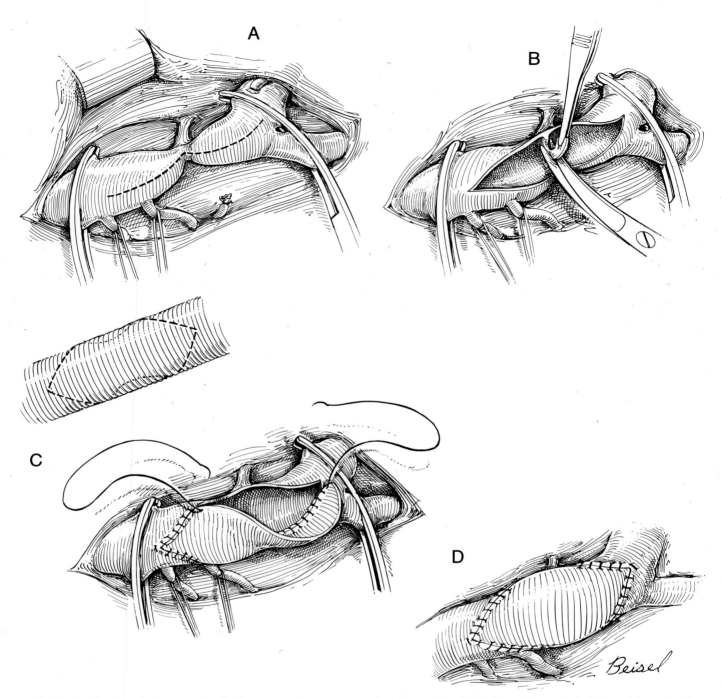

Fig 141–12.—Patch repair of a coarctation. **A,** after vascular clamps are applied, the aorta is incised from below, across the coarctation, to above the area. *Dashed line* represents proposed incision. **B,** the coarctation membrane is excised. **C,** a patch graft is fashioned from a standard Dacron tube graft and sutured into the aortic incision. **D,** the completed repair. (From Waldhausen J.A., Pierce W.S.[110] Used by permission.)

Interrupted Aortic Arch

Anatomy

This rare cardiovascular defect is defined as the absence of luminal continuity between the ascending and descending aorta. The aortic segments may or may not be entirely separated; and when they are connected, the length of the atretic segment is variable. Interrupted aortic arch is divided into three types: type A (42%) refers to interruption distal to the left subclavian artery; type B (53%) is interruption between the left subclavian and left common carotid arteries; type C (4%) is interruption between the innominate and left common carotid arteries (Fig 141–13).[15] At birth, a large patent ductus arteriosus is present between the pulmonary artery and the descending aorta. Associated cardiac anomalies are present in the majority of cases, and the cause of all types is easily understood on the basis of hemodynamic molding. Type A resembles a preductal coarctation; and types B and

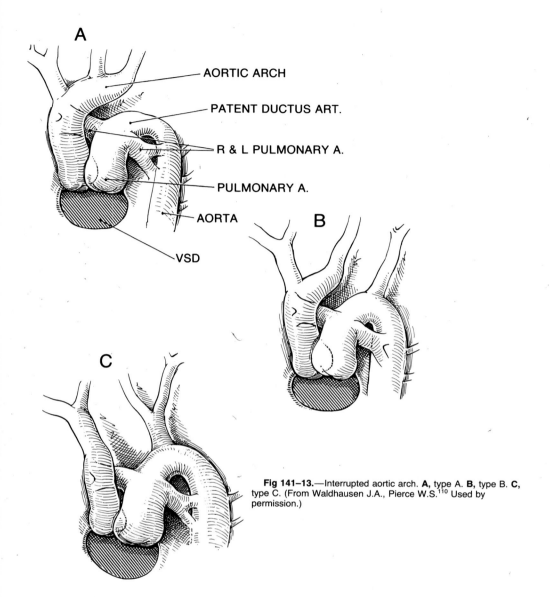

A

AORTIC ARCH

PATENT DUCTUS ART.

R & L PULMONARY A.

PULMONARY A.

AORTA

VSD

B

C

Fig 141–13.—Interrupted aortic arch. **A,** type A. **B,** type B. **C,** type C. (From Waldhausen J.A., Pierce W.S.[110] Used by permission.)

C can be explained by this concept if fetal blood flow to the brachiocephalic vessels is derived from the ductus, with retrograde flow through the isthmus. Ventricular septal defect, associated 80% of the time with aortic interruption, is consistent with this explanation.[104] The ventricular septal defect is commonly infundibular and often associated with left ventricular outflow tract obstruction.[25, 104]

Diagnosis and Management

At the time of birth, a large patent ductus arteriosus provides blood supply to the lower half of the body. As the ductus closes, pulmonary congestion and hypoperfusion of the lower body develop (see Fig 141–5,*B*). Severe congestive heart failure, oliguria, and acidosis are present. The presence of a ventricular septal defect often complicates the picture. Differential cyanosis between the upper and lower extremities in type A, or between the right arm and the remainder of the body in types B and C, is diagnostic but seldom overt. Pulse differentials may exist. Echocardiography and cardiac catheterization define the precise anatomy of the aorta and associated cardiac defects. Prostaglan-

din E₁ infusion will maintain the patency of the ductus and relieve lower body hypoperfusion, acidosis, and oliguria.[38] Inotropic support with dopamine and mechanical ventilation are essential in the sickest infants. After medical stabilization, operation is undertaken without delay.

Numerous palliative and corrective techniques have been employed in the treatment of neonates and small infants with interrupted aortic arch. Selection of the technique to be used in an individual case is based on the particular anatomy and associated cardiac abnormalities. When the atretic segment is short, a direct anastomosis is performed in a manner similar to that for coarctation.[93] This is particularly applicable in type A lesions. If the distance between the two segments does not permit direct anastomosis in spite of ample mobilization, an anastomosis of the left subclavian artery to the distal aorta is performed while recognizing that a residual pressure gradient may exist. In type B anomalies, the left common carotid artery may be anastomosed to the distal aorta, or the left subclavian artery anastomosed to the proximal aortic segment. Again, a residual gradient may occur. An alternative technique that eliminates this problem is the use of the left common carotid and subclavian arteries to fashion

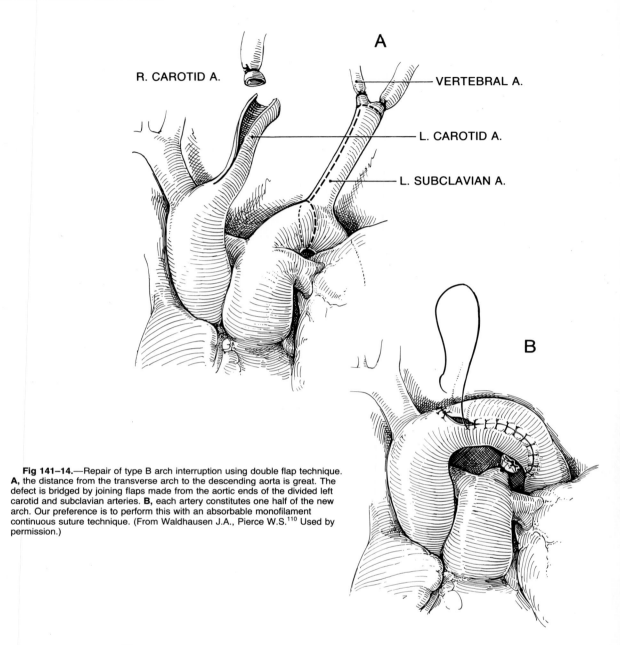

R. CAROTID A.

VERTEBRAL A.

L. CAROTID A.

L. SUBCLAVIAN A.

A

B

Fig 141–14.—Repair of type B arch interruption using double flap technique. **A,** the distance from the transverse arch to the descending aorta is great. The defect is bridged by joining flaps made from the aortic ends of the divided left carotid and subclavian arteries. **B,** each artery constitutes one half of the new arch. Our preference is to perform this with an absorbable monofilament continuous suture technique. (From Waldhausen J.A., Pierce W.S.[110] Used by permission.)

a "tube" of larger caliber (Fig 141–14).[110] Prosthetic grafts have been used, although their inability to grow will ultimately lead to restenosis and decreased patency. Some patients have a slow, gradual closure of the ductus arteriosus and have time to develop sufficient collaterals to survive to childhood. In these, prosthetic grafting is quite satisfactory.

The natural history of aortic interruption is bleak; 80% of patients die in early infancy.[104] The mortality for correction remains high regardless of the technique, but successful repairs are reported.[102] In the past, most surgeons have first repaired the interrupted arch and banded the pulmonary artery. At a second operation, the ventricular septal defect was closed, and the band was removed. Few patients have survived the two-stage procedure. More recently, a single-stage approach has been advocated. Through a median sternotomy under deep hypothermia, the aortic arch is repaired followed by closure of the ventricular septal defect. Successful repair of type C abnormalities is

virtually unknown. Approximately 20 cases of successful management of neonates with an interrupted aortic arch have been reported.[103] With the introduction of prostaglandin E_1 infusion for preoperative stabilization, and an understanding of the development as well as the treatment of associated left ventricular outflow tract obstruction, this dismal prognosis will improve.

Vascular Rings

Vascular rings are a group of relatively rare congenital cardiovascular lesions that result from faulty embryologic development of the aortic arch.[21] Although some of the lesions do not constitute a complete ring, they nevertheless may result in compression of the trachea, the esophagus, or both. Anatomically, these are most easily understood in terms of complete and incomplete rings with or without other vascular lesions.

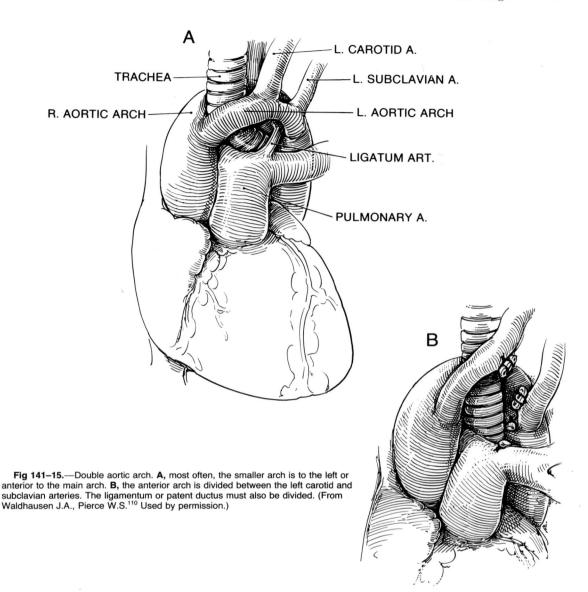

A

TRACHEA

R. AORTIC ARCH

L. CAROTID A.

L. SUBCLAVIAN A.

L. AORTIC ARCH

LIGATUM ART.

PULMONARY A.

B

Fig 141–15.—Double aortic arch. **A,** most often, the smaller arch is to the left or anterior to the main arch. **B,** the anterior arch is divided between the left carotid and subclavian arteries. The ligamentum or patent ductus must also be divided. (From Waldhausen J.A., Pierce W.S.[110] Used by permission.)

Anatomy

Complete Rings

DOUBLE AORTIC ARCH.—The most common type of complete vascular ring is the double aortic arch. It represents persistence of both the right and the left embryologic aortic arches. The double aortic arch arises from the ascending aorta and bifurcates, one branch going to the right and behind the trachea and esophagus, the other going to the left and in front of the trachea. The branches then join posteriorly to form the descending thoracic aorta (Fig 141–15,A). Each arch gives rise to a common carotid and a subclavian artery. Usually, an innominate artery is absent; all vessels arise as separate branches. The ductus arteriosus may be bilateral, on the left or on the right. Although the relative size of the lumen, the patency of each arch, and the involved portion of the upper descending aorta are variable, the smaller of the two arches is usually to the left and anterior.

RIGHT AORTIC ARCH RINGS.—Right aortic arch with retroesophageal left subclavian artery and left ligamentum arte-

riosum or ductus arteriosus represents the next most frequent vascular ring. It results from regression of the left fourth aortic arch. The right aortic arch arises from the ascending aorta and passes behind and to the right of the trachea and esophagus to join the descending aorta. Commonly, the left common carotid artery is the first branch off the aortic arch, followed by the right common carotid and subclavian arteries and, lastly, the left subclavian artery, which passes to the left and behind the esophagus. Alternatively, the innominate, left common carotid, and left subclavian artery may arise in this order, the left subclavian passing to the left and behind the esophagus. A complete ring is formed by the ascending aorta and pulmonary artery anteriorly, the aortic arch on the right, and either the ductus arteriosus or ligamentum arteriosum and the left subclavian artery on the left (Fig 141–16,A,B).

The least common type of complete ring is represented by the right aortic arch with mirror-image branching and left ligamentum arteriosum or ductus arteriosus. The right aortic arch arises and passes behind as previously described; however, regression between the left ductus and the descending aorta produces mirror-image branching of the aorta, i.e., the left innominate, right

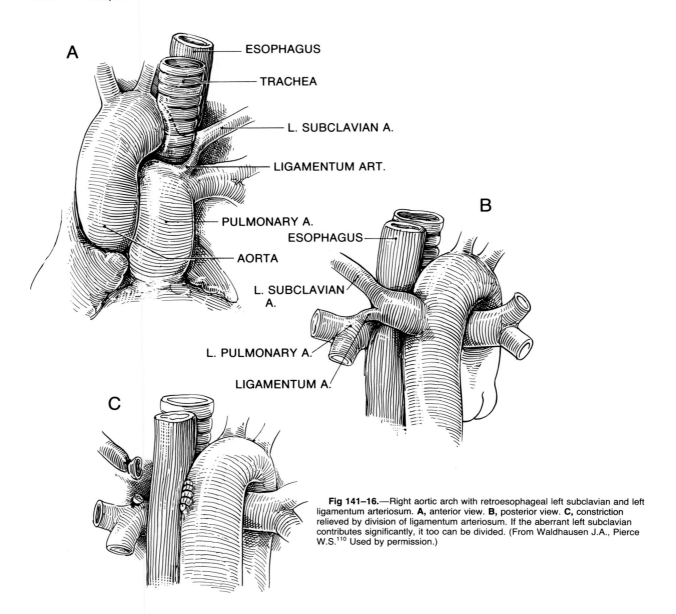

ESOPHAGUS

TRACHEA

L. SUBCLAVIAN A.

LIGAMENTUM ART.

PULMONARY A.

ESOPHAGUS

AORTA

L. SUBCLAVIAN A.

L. PULMONARY A.

LIGAMENTUM A.

Fig 141–16.—Right aortic arch with retroesophageal left subclavian and left ligamentum arteriosum. **A,** anterior view. **B,** posterior view. **C,** constriction relieved by division of ligamentum arteriosum. If the aberrant left subclavian contributes significantly, it too can be divided. (From Waldhausen J.A., Pierce W.S.[110] Used by permission.)

carotid, and right subclavian arteries arise in that order. If the left ductus connects the left pulmonary artery to the upper descending aorta, a complete vascular ring is made. Most commonly, however, the ligamentum originates anteriorly from the subclavian portion of the innominate artery, and there is no ring at all. Associated congenital heart anomalies are frequent.

LEFT AORTIC ARCH RING.—A rare anomaly exists in which a left aortic arch passes upwards and arches above the trachea to proceed behind and to the right of the esophagus, then continues to a right-sided descent. The right ligamentum arteriosum or ductus arteriosus connects the right pulmonary artery either to the upper right-sided descending aorta or to the origin of an aberrant right subclavian artery, thereby forming a complete ring. Such an anomaly results from an interruption of the right aortic arch between the right subclavian artery and the right ductus arteriosus. In addition, it is associated with intracardiac defects.[73]

Incomplete Rings/Other Vascular Lesions

ABERRANT RIGHT SUBCLAVIAN ARTERY.—An aberrant right subclavian artery, the most common vascular anomaly of the aorta, occurs in 0.5% of the population. It develops when the segment of the right fourth arch between the right carotid and subclavian arteries regresses. The right subclavian artery arises as the last branch of the aortic arch and passes obliquely from the left to reach the right arm. Most often, the vessel passes behind the esophagus. However, it may pass between the esophagus and trachea or, rarely, in front of the trachea. The patients infrequently have dysphagia (dysphagia lusoria).

PULMONARY ARTERY SLING.—An aberrant left pulmonary artery arises from the right pulmonary artery posteriorly, passes over the right mainstem bronchus, turns left, and traverses the mediastinum between the trachea and esophagus to reach the hilus of the left lung at a level lower than normal (Fig 141–17,A).

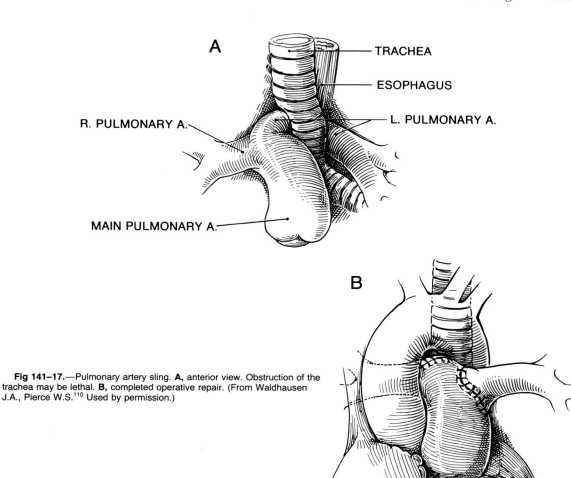

A

TRACHEA

ESOPHAGUS

R. PULMONARY A.

L. PULMONARY A.

MAIN PULMONARY A.

B

Fig 141–17.—Pulmonary artery sling. **A,** anterior view. Obstruction of the trachea may be lethal. **B,** completed operative repair. (From Waldhausen J.A., Pierce W.S.[110] Used by permission.)

The sling compresses the right mainstem bronchus and the distal end of the trachea. Hypoplasia of these structures and their cartilaginous rings is usual, as are associated cardiovascular anomalies, seen in at least 50% of the cases.[72, 85]

ANOMALOUS INNOMINATE ARTERY.—Although not a true ring, compression of the trachea may result from an innominate artery, which arises more distally than normal or is congenitally short (Fig 141–18,A). The anatomical correlates, in terms of tracheal compression, are controversial; and, in many cases, the anatomy of the great vessels is normal.[33]

DIAGNOSIS.—A vascular ring may be an incidental finding on chest roentgenograms, gastrointestinal series, arteriography, or at postmortem examination. If symptoms are present, they are due to compression of the trachea, or the esophagus, or both. The severity of symptoms and the age of the patient at their onset reflect the degree of tracheoesophageal compression. The double aortic arch is generally the most symptomatic, and the majority of the patients have symptoms at birth.[2] The patient may exhibit coughing, inspiratory wheezing, or noisy breathing. A history of wheezing, stridor, shortness of breath, or frequent pneumonia may be elicited. Feeding problems become apparent when solid foods are begun, and feeding in itself may either exaggerate stridor and wheezing or initiate apnea. Quite similar

symptoms may be seen in patients with a right aortic arch ring or the left aortic arch ring and right descending aorta. An anomalous innominate artery may cause tracheal obstruction and lead to symptoms of respiratory distress, recurrent pneumonia, or apnea secondary to compression of the trachea posteriorly by a bolus of food. In the pulmonary artery sling, at least one half of the patients are symptomatic at birth, and two thirds of the others are symptomatic by 1 month of age. Nearly 90% have respiratory obstruction, manifested by expiratory stridor and wheezing. Repeated upper respiratory tract infections are common, but esophageal symptoms are uncommon.

Physical findings in infants with vascular rings are dependent upon the degree of tracheal obstruction, which may be exacerbated by flexion of the neck and relieved by an almost opisthotonic hyperextension.

Plain chest roentgenograms and a barium swallow are the most important diagnostic tests.[72] Angiography is generally superfluous; and endoscopic procedures, although informative, generally do not alter management and may be considered meddlesome in sick infants. An overpenetrated chest roentgenogram most often shows the laterality of the aortic arch and often shows tracheal compression. Anteroposterior and lateral esophagograms demonstrate the characteristic indentation produced by the specific type of vascular anomaly.

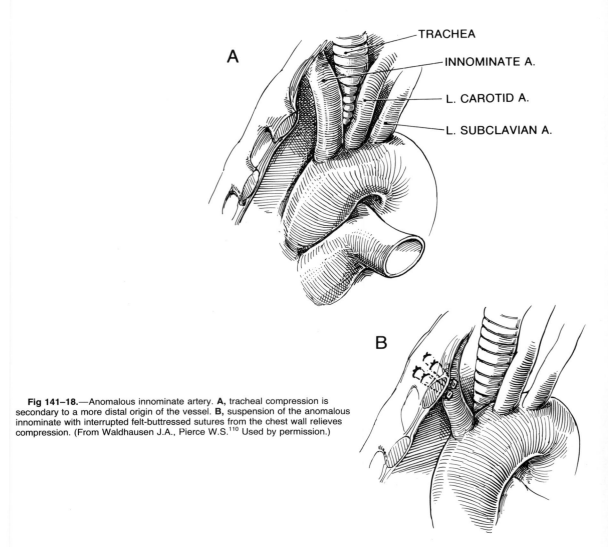

Fig 141–18.—Anomalous innominate artery. **A,** tracheal compression is secondary to a more distal origin of the vessel. **B,** suspension of the anomalous innominate with interrupted felt-buttressed sutures from the chest wall relieves compression. (From Waldhausen J.A., Pierce W.S.[110] Used by permission.)

In double aortic arch, the chest roentgenogram shows a right-sided aortic arch; and the esophagogram discloses two unequal indentations, one on each side (Fig 141–19). The right arch is usually higher and larger than the left arch, which is lower and smaller. In cases of right aortic arch with retroesophageal left subclavian artery and left ligamentum arteriosum or ductus arteriosus, in addition to the chest roentgenogram demonstrating a right aortic arch, the anteroposterior esophagogram shows a small left indentation (representing the subclavian artery) and small right indentation (representing the right aortic arch) (Fig 141–20). The lateral esophagogram shows a pronounced posterior impression caused by the bulbous origin of the left subclavian artery (Fig 141–20). In patients with a right aortic arch with mirror-image branching and left ligamentum arteriosum or ductus arteriosus, the chest roentgenogram shows a right aortic arch and esophagographic findings that are similar to those with the double aortic arch. In the left aortic arch with right-sided upper descending segment, the chest roentgenogram shows the left arch with a right descending aorta. Bilateral posterior esophageal indentations are seen. Generally, arteriography is performed to be sure of this defect, because correction is through a right thoracotomy. An aberrant right subclavian artery produces a normal chest roentgenogram. In asymptomatic patients, an oblique linear indentation in the anteroposterior projection and a shallow

linear defect just below the level of the aortic arch in the lateral projection are seen on barium studies (Fig 141–21). The anomalous innominate artery causes anterior tracheal compression, best seen on the lateral chest roentgenogram; the esophagogram is normal. Generally, bronchoscopy is performed to confirm that there is a significant tracheal compression.

Lastly, careful examination of the chest roentgenogram of a pulmonary artery sling often shows hyperinflation of the right lung, abnormally low branching of the left pulmonary artery in the left hilum, and a mass effect representing the anomalous vessel located at the carinal level between the esophagus and trachea. Anterior indentation of the esophagus and posterior indentation of the trachea are apparent on the lateral esophagogram (Fig 141–22). Angiography confirms the diagnosis (Fig 141–23).

Management

In general, surgical treatment is indicated in all symptomatic patients. The goals of therapy are to identify the components of the vascular ring and to divide the constricting bands without compromising the blood flow to the carotids or to the descending thoracic aorta.[115] A left lateral thoracotomy incision in the fourth interspace provides good exposure for the majority of these anomalies.

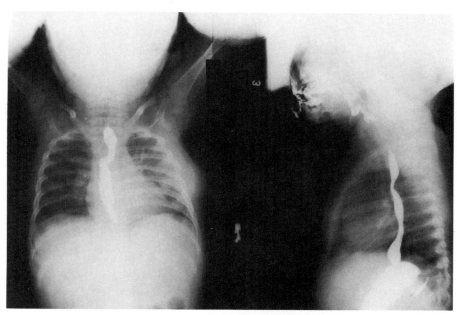

Fig 141–19.—Anteroposterior *(left)* and lateral *(right)* views of the chest with barium swallow in a patient with a double aortic arch. (From Park C.D., Waldhau- sen J.A., Friedman S., et al.: *Arch. Surg.* 103:626–632, 1971. Copyright 1971, American Medical Association. Used by permission.)

Double Aortic Arch

Through a left fourth interspace posterolateral thoracotomy, the two arches are thoroughly dissected; the ductus arteriosus or ligamentum arteriosum is divided for mobility (see Fig 141– 15,*B*). The smaller ring is divided distal to the origin of the left subclavian artery when the anterior (left) arch is hypoplastic, and near its junction with the descending aorta when the posterior (right) arch is hypoplastic. If the arches are equal in size, the right or posterior arch is preferentially divided. In all cases, the esophagus and trachea are dissected thoroughly and any fibrous bands divided. Care must be taken to protect the vagus, recur- rent laryngeal, and phrenic nerves as well as the thoracic duct.

Right Aortic Arch Rings

The surgical approach is via a left fourth interspace thoracot- omy, and division of the ductus arteriosus or ligamentum arterio- sum coupled with appropriate lysis about the esophagus and tra- chea is performed (see Fig 141–16,*C*). At times, it is necessary to divide the left subclavian artery.

Left Aortic Arch Rings

The surgical approach in the symptomatic patient with a left aortic arch and a right-sided upper descending aorta and right

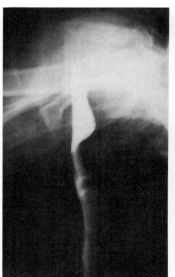
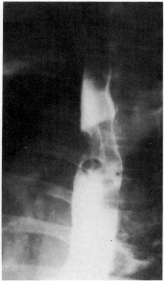

Fig 141–20.—Anteroposterior *(right)* and lateral *(left)* barium esophagogram of a patient with a right aortic arch, aberrant left subclavian artery, and left liga- mentum arteriosum.

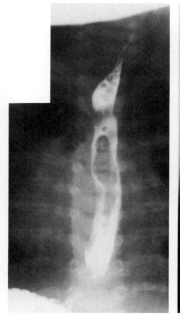
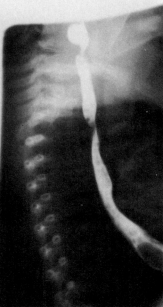

Fig 141–21.—Anteroposterior *(left)* and lateral *(right)* barium esophagograms of a patient with an aberrant left subclavian artery.

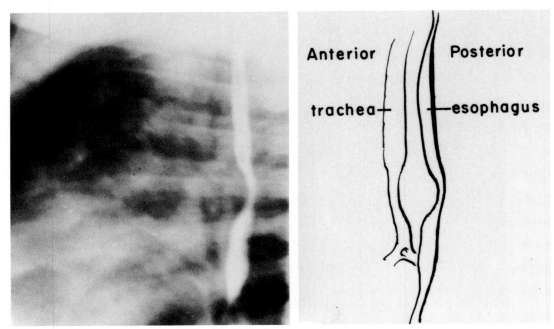

Fig 141–22.—Lateral view of roentgenogram of the chest with barium swallow in a patient with a pulmonary artery sling. Posterior compression of the distal trachea and anterior compression of the esophagus are apparent. (From Park C.D., Waldhausen J.A., Friedman S., et al.: *Arch. Surg.* 103:626–632, 1971. Copyright 1971, American Medical Association. Used by permission.)

ductus arteriosus or ligamentum arteriosum is via a right fourth interspace posterolateral thoracotomy. The ductus or ligamentum is divided, and structures are freed as before.

Aberrant Right Subclavian Artery

If it is responsible for symptoms, the aberrant right retroesophageal subclavian artery in infants is usually divided through a left fourth interspace posterolateral thoracotomy. Division of the ductus arteriosus or ligamentum arteriosum is also per-

formed. In older children and adults, right thoracotomy with division and reimplantation of the subclavian artery may be considered to prevent subclavian steal syndrome.[35, 95]

Anomalous Innominate Artery

The repair consists of suspending the innominate artery from the sternum and thus elevating it away from the trachea (see Fig 141–18,*B*).[33, 58] The procedure can be performed from either side. After opening the pericardium anterior to the phrenic

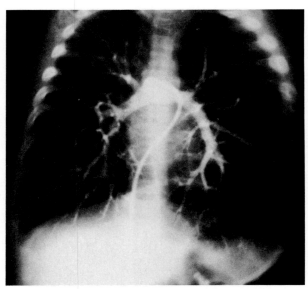

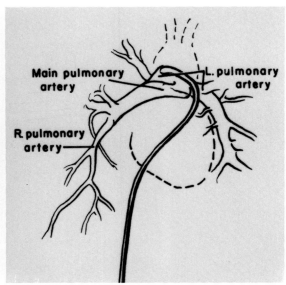

Fig 141–23.—Pulmonary angiogram of a patient with a pulmonary artery sling. (From Park C.D., Waldhausen J.A., Friedman S., et al.: *Arch. Surg.* 103:626–632, 1971. Copyright 1971, American Medical Association. Used by permission.)

nerve, two or three Teflon felt-buttressed interrupted sutures are used to approximate the adventitia of the aorta or innominate artery to the posterior aspect of the manubrium.

Pulmonary Artery Sling

The most common surgical treatment for this anomaly is division and reimplantation of the left pulmonary artery, as originally described by Potts et al. in 1954.[78] The standard approach is through a median sternotomy. The ductus or ligamentum arteriosum is divided, and the left pulmonary artery is dissected from between the trachea and the esophagus. Using cardiopulmonary bypass, the left pulmonary artery is divided at its origin from the right pulmonary artery; and the proximal end is oversewn. The left pulmonary artery is then anastomosed to the main pulmonary artery (see Fig 141–17,*B*).

Results

With prompt diagnosis and surgical treatment aimed at avoidance of intraoperative damage to the tracheobronchial tree and nerve structures, and with proper postoperative care, division of vascular rings carries a low mortality.[2, 6, 81, 83] Postoperative death is rare when there are no associated cardiac lesions; and the long-term results are quite satisfactory, even though complete resolution of symptoms may take many months because of residual tracheomalacia. In most series, early mortality has been approximately 4%.

In contrast, the overall mortality for operative treatment of the pulmonary sling is in the range of 50%, closely related to the associated anomalies of the tracheobronchial tree.[19, 72] Immediate deaths are usually related to severe tracheobronchial stenosis.

Common Thoracic Systemic Venous Anomalies

Anomalous systemic venous return occurs via drainage into the right or left atrium. When drainage is into the right atrium, no functional disturbance is produced. Drainage into the left atrium produces a right-to-left shunt at the atrial level, and cerebral embolism or brain abscess is common. Additional surgical importance lies in the techniques used for venous cannulation for cardiopulmonary bypass, repair of associated cardiac defects, and recognition of the consequences of planned or inadvertent ligation of the anomalous veins.

Anomalous Return to the Right Atrium

Left Superior Vena Cava Connected to the Coronary Sinus

This anomaly results when the left anterior cardinal vein does not obliterate during fetal life. It is the most common of all anomalous systemic venous connections and occurs in 2%–4% of patients with congenital heart disease.[12] In 75% of the cases, the left innominate vein is absent or hypoplastic.[114] The left superior vena cava arises at the junction of the left subclavian and internal jugular veins and descends anterior to the aorta and the left hilum. It then penetrates the pericardium and joins the coronary sinus in the posterior atrioventricular groove. The vessel may be ligated if the pressure above the occlusion of the anomalous vessel does not exceed 15–20 mm Hg. Sometimes this is possible, even in the absence of a left innominate vein.

Interrupted Inferior Vena Cava

In this anomaly, the hepatic and prerenal segments of the developing inferior vena cava failed to fuse. Most commonly, the prerenal segment of the interrupted inferior vena cava joins the azygos vein, which continues to drain normally into the right

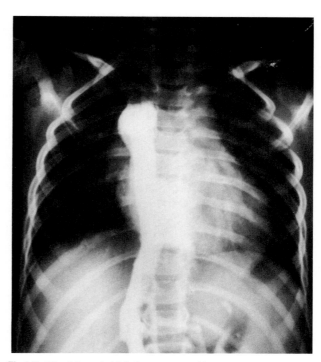

Fig 141–24.—Interrupted inferior vena cava. Venogram in a patient showing azygos continuation draining normally into the superior vena cava.

superior vena cava (Fig 141–24).[20] The hepatic veins drain directly into the right atrium. This azygos extension of the interrupted inferior vena cava is associated often with complex cyanotic heart disease and has been seen in 0.6% of patients with congenital heart defects.

Anomalous Return to the Left Atrium

The most common malformation is a left superior vena cava that drains into the left atrium, whose orifice is situated in its left upper corner. Typically, the coronary sinus is absent, and there is a coronary sinus-type atrial septal defect. The innominate vein is often absent. Surgical correction is indicated to prevent the long-term sequelae of cyanosis and paradoxical emboli in the presence of a right-to-left shunt. Correction has been achieved by ligation (using the aforementioned criteria), reimplantation, or intra-atrial redirection.[91]

REFERENCES

1. Anderson R.C., Adams P. Jr., Burke B.: Anomalous inferior vena cava with azygos continuation (intra-hepatic interruption of the inferior vena cava). *J. Pediatr.* 59:370, 1961.
2. Arciniegas E., Hahemi M., Hertzler J.H., et al.: Surgical management of congenital vascular ring. *J. Thorac. Cardiovasc. Surg.* 77:721, 1979.
3. Barbero-Marcial M., Verginelli G., Sirera J.C., et al.: Surgical treatment of coarctation of the aorta in the first year of life: Immediate and late results in 35 patients. *Thorac. Cardiovasc. Surg.* 30:75, 1982.
4. Beattie E.J., Nolan J., Howe J.S.: Paralysis following surgical correction of coarctation of the aorta. *Surgery* 33:754, 1953.
5. Benedict C.R., Grahame-Smith D.A., Fisher A.: Changes in plasma catecholamines and dopamine beta-hydroxylase after corrective surgery for coarctation of the aorta. *Circulation* 57:598, 1978.
6. Binet J.P., Langlois J.: Aortic arch anomalies in children and infants. *J. Thorac. Cardiovasc. Surg.* 73:248, 1977.
7. Black L., Goldman B.S.: Surgical treatment of the patent ductus arteriosus in the adult. *Ann. Surg.* 175:290, 1972.

8. Bonnet L.M.: Sur la lesion dite sténose congénitale de l'aorte dans la region de l'isthme. *Rev. Med. Paris* 23:108, 1903.
9. Brewer L.A., Fosburg R.G., Mulder G.A., et al.: Spinal cord complications following surgery for coarctation of the aorta. *J. Thorac. Cardiovasc. Surg.* 64:368, 1972.
10. Campbell D.B., Waldhausen J.A., Pierce W.S. et al.: Should elective repair of coarctation of the aorta be done in infancy? *J. Thorac. Cardiovasc. Surg.* 88:929–938, 1984.
11. Campbell M., Baylis J.H.: Course and prognosis of coarctation of the aorta. *Br. Heart J.* 18:475, 1956.
12. Campbell M., Deuchar D.C.: The left-sided superior vena cava. *Br. Heart J.* 16:423, 1954.
13. Campbell N.: Natural history of persistent ductus arteriosus. *Br. Heart J.* 30:4, 1968.
14. Clagett O.T., Kirklin J.W., Edwards J.E.: Anatomic variations and pathologic changes in coarctation of the aorta: A study of 124 cases. *Surg. Gynecol. Obstet.* 98:103, 1954.
15. Cleoria G.C., Patton R.B.: Congenital absence of the aortic arch. *Am. Heart J.* 58:407, 1959.
16. Cokkinos D.V., Leachman R.D., Cooley D.A.: Increased mortality rate from coronary artery disease following operation for coarctation of the aorta at a late age. *J. Thorac. Cardiovasc. Surg.* 77:315, 1979.
17. Crafoord C., Nylin G.; Congenital coarctation of the aorta and its surgical treatment. *J. Thorac. Cardiovasc. Surg.* 14:347, 1945.
18. Donahoo J.S., Brawley R.K., Gott V.L.: The heparin coated vascular shunt for thoracic aortic and great vessel procedures: A ten-year experience. *Ann. Thorac. Surg.* 23:507, 1977.
19. Dunn J.M., Gordon I., Chrispin A.R., et al.: Early and late results of surgical correction of pulmonary artery sling. *Ann. Thorac. Surg.* 28:230, 1979.
20. Edwards E.A.: Clinical anatomy of lesser variations of the inferior vena cava; and a proposal for classifying the anomalies of this vessel. *Angiology* 2:85, 1951.
21. Edwards J.E.: Anomalies of the derivatives of aortic arch system. *Med. Clin. North Am.* 32:925, 1948.
22. Edwards J.E.: Congenital malformations of the heart: Malformations of the thoracic aorta, in Gould S.E. (ed.): *Pathology of the Heart and Blood Vessels*, ed. 4. Springfield, Ill., Charles C Thomas, Publisher, 1968.
23. Eshaghpour E., Olley P.M.: Recoarctation of the aorta following coarctectomy in the first year of life: A follow-up study. *J. Pediatr.* 80:809, 1972.
24. Fox S., Pierce W.S., Waldhausen J.A.: Pathogenesis of paradoxical hypertension after coarctation repair. *Ann. Thorac. Surg.* 29:135, 1980.
25. Freedom R.M., Barn H.H., Esplugas E., et al.: Ventricular septal defect in interruption of aortic arch. *Am. J. Cardiol.* 39:572, 1977.
26. Friedman W.F., Hirschklau M.J., Printz M.P., et al.: Pharmacologic closure of patent ductus arteriosus in the premature infant. *N. Engl. J. Med.* 295:526, 1976.
27. Galen C.: Opera Omnia IV:243, Kuhn edition. Dalton J.C. (trans.): *Doctrines of the Circulation*. Philadelphia, Lea's Son & Co., 1884, p. 68. Translated from the Greek with an Introduction and Commentary, Mary Tallmadge May. Ithaca, N.Y., Cornell University Press, 1968, vol. 1, p. 333.
28. Gittenberger De-Grott A.C.: Ductus arteriosus: Histologic observations, in Goodman M.D., Marquis R.M. (eds.): *Paediatric Cardiology: Heart Disease in the Newborn*. London, Churchill Livingstone, 1979, vol 2, p. 2.
29. Graybiel A., Strieder J.W., Boyer N.H.: An attempt to obliterate the patent ductus arteriosus in a patient with subacute bacterial endarteritis. *Am. Heart J.* 15:621, 1938.
30. Gross R.E.: Surgical correction for coarctation of the aorta. *Surgery* 18:673, 1945.
31. Gross R.E.: Coarctation of the aorta. *Circulation* 7:757, 1953.
32. Gross R.E., Hubbard J.P.: Surgical ligation of a patent ductus arteriosus. *JAMA* 8:729, 1939.
33. Gross R.E., Neuhauser E.B.D.: Compression of the trachea by an anomalous innominate artery: An operation for its relief. *Am. J. Dis. Child.* 75:570, 1948.
34. Gupta T.C., Wiggers C.J.: Basic hemodynamic changes produced by aortic coarctation of different degrees. *Circulation* 3:17, 1951.
35. Hallman G.L., Cooley D.A.: Congenital aortic vascular ring: Surgical considerations. *Arch. Surg.* 88:666, 1964.
36. Hamilton D.I., DiEusano G., Sandrasagra F.A., et al.: Early and late results of aortoplasty with a left subclavian flap for coarctation of the aorta in infancy. *J. Thorac. Cardiovasc. Surg.* 75:699, 1978.
37. Hartman A.F. Jr., Goldring D., Hernandez A., et al.: Recurrent coarctation of the aorta after successful repair in infancy. *Am. J. Cardiol.* 25:405, 1970.
38. Heymann M.A., Berman W. Jr., Rudolph A.M., et al.: Dilatation of the ductus arteriosus by prostaglandin E1 in aortic arch abnormalities. *Circulation* 59:169, 1979.
39. Heymann M.A., Rudolph A.M., Silverman N.H.: Closure of the ductus arteriosus in premature infants by inhibition of prostaglandin synthesis. *N. Engl. J. Med.* 295:530, 1974.
40. Ho E.C.K., Moss A.J.: The syndrome of "mesenteric arteritis" following repair of aortic coarctation. *Pediatrics* 49:40, 1972.
41. Ibarra-Pérez C., Cataneda A.R., Varco R.L., et al.: Recoarctation of the aorta: Nineteen year clinical experience. *Am. J. Cardiol.* 23:778, 1969.
42. Johnson A.L., Ferencz C., Wiglesworth F.W., et al.: Coarctation of the aorta complicated by patency of the ductus arteriosus: Physiologic considerations in the classification of coarctation of the aorta. *Circulation* 4:242, 1951.
43. Johnson J., Kirby C.K.: The relationship of the method of suture to the growth of end-to-end arterial anastomoses. *Surgery* 27:17, 1950.
44. Keith J.D.: Coarctation of the aorta, in Keith J.D., Rowe R.D., Vlad P. (eds.): *Heart Disease in Infancy and Childhood*, ed. 3. New York, MacMillan Publishing Co., 1978, pp. 736–760.
45. Khoury G.H., Hawes C.R.: Recurrent coarctation of the aorta in infancy and childhood. *J. Pediatr.* 72:801, 1968.
46. Kitterman J.A., Edmunds L.H., Gregory G.A., et al.: Patent ductus arteriosus in premature infants: Incidence, relation to pulmonary disease and management. *N. Engl. J. Med.* 287:473, 1972.
47. Landtman B., Tuuteri L.: Vascular complications in coarctation of the aorta. *Acta Paediatr.* 48:329, 1959.
48. Levitsky S., Fisher E., Vidyasagar D., et al.: Interruption of patent ductus arteriosus in premature infants with respiratory distress syndrome. *Ann. Thorac. Surg.* 22:131, 1976.
49. Lindesmith G.G., Stanton R.E., Stiles Q.R., et al.: Coarctation of the thoracic aorta. *Ann. Thorac. Surg.* 11:482, 1971.
50. March H.W., Hultgren H.N., Gerbode F.: Immediate and remote effects of resection on the hypertension in coarctation of the aorta. *Br. Heart J.* 22:361, 1960.
51. Maron B.J., Humphries J.O., Rowe R.D., et al.: Prognosis of surgically corrected coarctation of the aorta: A 20 year postoperative appraisal. *Circulation* 47:119, 1973.
52. Mavroudis C., Cook L.N., Fleischaker J.W., et al.: Management of patent ductus arteriosus in the premature infant: Indomethacin versus ligation. *Ann. Thorac. Surg.* 36:561, 1983.
53. McNicholas K., Stratford M., Hayes C., et al.: Management of the infant with ventricular septal defect, and coarctation of the aorta, abstracted. *World Congr. Cardiol.* 128, 1980.
54. Meade R.H.: The story of the development of surgery for the patent ductus arteriosus. *Surgery* 40:807, 1956.
55. Merritt T.A., DiSessa T.G., Feldman B.H., et al.: Closure of the patent ductus arteriosus with ligation and indomethacin: A consecutive experience. *J. Pediatr.* 93:639, 1978.
56. Mikhail M., Lee W., Toews W., et al.: Surgical and medical experience with 734 premature infants with patent ductus arteriosus. *J. Thorac. Cardiovasc. Surg.* 83:349, 1982.
57. Mitchell S.C., Korones S.B., Berendes H.W.: Congenital heart disease in 56,105 births: Incidence and natural history. *Circulation* 43:323, 1971.
58. Moes C.A.F., Izukawa T., Trusler G.A.: Innominate artery compression of the trachea. *Arch. Otolaryngol.* 101:733, 1975.
59. Morgagni J.B.: De sedibus et causis morborum. Epist. XVIII: Article 6, 1760.
60. Moulton A.L., Brenner J.I., Roberts G., et al.: Subclavian flap repair of coarctation of the aorta in neonate: Realization of growth potential? *J. Thorac. Cardiovasc. Surg.* 87:220, 1984.
61. Munro J.C.: Ligation of the patent ductus arteriosus. *Am. J. Surg.* 46:335, 1907.
62. Myers J.L., Pae W.E. Jr., Waldhausen J.A., et al.: Vascular anastomosis in growing vessels: Comparison of absorbable polydioxanone and nonabsorbable polypropylene monofilament suture materials. *Surg. Forum* 32:399, 1981.
63. Myers J.L., Waldhausen J.A., Pae W.E. Jr., et al.: Vascular anastomosis in growing vessels: The use of absorbable sutures. *Ann. Thorac. Surg.* 34(5):529, 1982.
64. Nadas A.S., Fyler D.C.: *Pediatric Cardiology*. Philadelphia, W.B. Saunders Co., 1972, pp. 405–426.
65. Nanton M.A., Olley P.M.: Residual hypertension after coarctectomy in children. *Am. J. Cardiol.* 37:769, 1976.
66. Neches W.H., Park S.C., Lennox C.C.: Coarctation of the aorta with ventricular septal defect. *Circulation* 55:189, 1977.
67. O'Neill M.J. Jr., Waldhausen J.A.: The use of TDMAC-heparin shunt in the closure of a calcified patent ductus arteriosus. *J. Cardiovasc. Surg.* 22:569, 1981.

68. Pae W.E. Jr., Myers J.L., Waldhausen J.A., et al.: Subclavian flap angioplasty: Experimental study in growing piglets. *J. Thorac. Cardiovasc. Surg.* 82:922, 1981.
69. Pae W.E. Jr., Waldhausen J.A., Prophet G.A., et al.: Primary vascular anastomosis in growing pigs: A comparison of polypropylene and polyglycolic acid sutures. *J. Thorac. Cardiovasc. Surg.* 81:921, 1981.
70. Page I.H.: The effect of chronic constriction of the aorta on arterial blood pressure in dogs: An attempt to produce coarctation of the aorta. *Am. Heart J.* 19:218, 1940.
71. Panagopoulos P.H.G., Tatooles C.J., Aberdeen E., et al.: Patent ductus arteriosus in infants and children: A review of 936 operations. *Thorax* 26:137, 1971.
72. Park C.D., Waldhausen J.A., Friedman S., et al.: Tracheal compression by the great arteries in the mediastinum. *Arch. Surg.* 103:626, 1971.
73. Park S.C., Siewers R.D., Neches W.H., et al.: Left aortic arch with right descending aorta and right ligamentum arteriosum. *J. Thorac. Cardiovasc. Surg.* 71:779, 1976.
74. Parsons C.G., Ashley R.: Recurrence of aortic coarctation after operation in childhood. *Br. Med. J.* 1:573, 1966.
75. Pelletier C., Davignon A., Ethier M.F., et al.: Coarctation of the aorta in infancy: Postoperative follow-up. *J. Thorac. Cardiovasc. Surg.* 57:171, 1969.
76. Pierce W.S., Waldhausen J.A., Berman W.B. Jr., et al.: Late results of subclavian flap procedure in infants with coarctation of the thoracic aorta. *Circulation* 58 (suppl. 1):78, 1978.
77. Portstmann W., Wierny L.: Percutaneous transfemoral closure of the patent ductus arteriosus—an alternative to surgery. *Semin. Roentgenol.* 16:95, 1981.
78. Potts W.L., Holinger P.H., Rosenblum A.M.: Anomalous left pulmonary artery causing obstruction to right main bronchus. *JAMA* 155:1409, 1954.
79. Reifenstein G.H., Levine S.A., Gross R.E.: Coarctation of the aorta: A review of 104 autopsied cases of the "adult type," 2 years old or older. *Am. Heart J.* 33:146, 1947.
80. Reul G., Kabbani S., Sandiford F., et al.: Repair of coarctation of the thoracic aorta by patch graft aortoplasty. *J. Thorac. Cardiovasc. Surg.* 68:696, 1974.
81. Richardson J.V., Doty D.B., Rossi N.P., et al.: Operation for aortic arch anomalies. *Ann. Thorac. Surg.* 31:426, 1981.
82. Rocchini A.P., Rosenthal A., Barger A.C., et al.: Pathogenesis of paradoxical hypertension after coarctation resection. *Circulation* 54:382, 1976.
83. Roesler M., deLeval M., Grispan A., et al.: Surgical managment of vascular ring. *Ann. Surg.* 197:139, 1983.
84. Rudolph A.M.: *Congenital Disease of the Heart.* Chicago, Year Book Medical Publishers, 1974.
85. Sade R.H., Rosenthal A., Fellows K., et al.: Pulmonary artery sling. *J. Thorac. Cardiovasc. Surg.* 69:333, 1975.
86. Scott H.W. Jr., Bahnson H.T.: Evidence for renal factor in the hypertension of experimental coarctation of the aorta. *Surgery* 30:206, 1951.
87. Sealy W.C.: Coarctation of the aorta and hypertension. *Ann. Thorac. Surg.* 3:15, 1967.
88. Sealy W.C.: Indications for surgical treatment of coarctation of the aorta. *Surg. Gynecol. Obstet.* 97:301, 1953.
89. Shapiro M.J., Keys A.: Prognosis of untreated patent ductus arteriosus and results of surgical intervention: Clinical series of 50 cases and analysis of 139 operations. *Am. J. Med. Sci.* 206:174, 1943.
90. Shearer W.T., Rutman J.Y., Weinberg W.A., et al.: Coarctation of the aorta and cerebrovascular accident: A proposal for early corrective surgery. *J. Pediatr.* 77:1004, 1970.
91. Sherafat M., Friedman S., Waldhausen J.A.: Persistent left superior vena cava draining into the left atrium with absent right superior vena cava. *Ann. Thorac. Surg.* 11:160, 1971.
92. Shinebourne E.A., Tam A.S.Y., Elseed A.M., et al.: Coarctation of the aorta in infancy and childhood. *Br. Heart J.* 38:375, 1976.
93. Shumacker H.B., King H., Nahrwold D.L., et al.: Coarctation of the aorta. *Curr. Probl. Surg.*, February 1968.
94. Siassi B., Blanca C., Cabal L.A., et al.: Incidence and clinical features of patent ductus arteriosus in low weight infants: A prospective analysis of 150 consecutively born infants. *Pediatrics* 57:347, 1976.
95. Siderys H.: A new operation for symptomatic aberrant right subclavian artery in the adult. *J. Thorac. Cardiovasc. Surg.* 57:269, 1969.
96. Srouji M.N., Trusler G.A.: Paradoxical hypertension and the abdominal pain syndrome following resection of coarctation of the aorta. *Can. Med. Assoc. J.* 92:412, 1965.
97. Stansel H.C., Tabry I.F., Poirier R.A., et al.: One hundred consecutive coarctation resections followed from one to thirteen years. *J. Pediatr. Surg.* 12:279, 1977.
98. Stark J.: Persistent ductus arteriosus, in Stark J., de Leval M. (eds.): *Surgery for Congenital Heart Defects.* New York, Grune & Stratton, 1983, p. 203.
99. Talner N.S., Berman M.A.: Postnatal development of obstruction of the ductus arteriosus: Role of the ductus arteriosus. *Pediatrics* 56:562, 1975.
100. Tawes R.L., Aberdeen E., Waterston D.J., et al.: Coarctation of the aorta in infants and children: A review of 333 operative cases including 179 infants. *Circulation* 39,40 (suppl. 1):1–173, 1969.
101. Thibault W.N., Sperling D.R., Gazzaniga A.B.: Subclavian patch angioplasty: Treatment of infants and young children with aortic coarctation. *Arch. Surg.* 110:1095, 1975.
102. Tyson K.R.T., Harris L.C., Nghiem Q.X.: Repair of aortic arch interruption in the neonate. *Surgery* 67:1006, 1970.
103. Van der Horst R., Hastreiter A.R., Levitsky S., et al.: Interrupted aortic arch operation in the first week of life: Hemodynamic and angiographic evaluation one year later. *Ann. Thorac. Surg.* 27:112, 1979.
104. Van Praagh R., Bernhard W.F., Rosenthal A., et al.: Interrupted aortic arch: Surgical treatment. *Am. J. Cardiol.* 27:200, 1971.
105. Vosschulte K.: Isthmusplastik zur behandlung der Aorten Isthmusstenose. *Thoraxchirurgie* 4:443, 1957.
106. Wagner H.R., Ellison R.C., Zierler S., et al.: Surgical closure of patent ductus arteriosus in 268 preterm infants. *J. Thorac. Cardiovasc. Surg.* 87:870, 1984.
107. Waldhausen J.A., King H., Nahrwold D.L., et al.: Management of coarctation in infancy. *JAMA* 187:270, 1964.
108. Waldhausen J.A., Nahrwold D.L.: Repair of coarctation of the aorta with a subclavian flap. *J. Thorac. Cardiovasc. Surg.* 51:532, 1966.
109. Waldhausen J.A., Parr G.V.S.: Coarctation of the aorta, in Glenn W.L. (ed.): *Thoracic and Cardiovascular Surgery.* Norwalk, Conn., Appleton-Century-Crofts, 1983.
110. Waldhausen J.A., Pierce W.S. (eds.): *Johnson's Surgery of the Chest,* ed. 5. Chicago, Year Book Medical Publishers, 1985, Chap. 16.
111. Waldhausen J.A., Whitman V., Werner J.C., et al.: Surgical intervention in infants with coarctation of the aorta. *J. Thorac. Cardiovasc. Surg.* 81:323, 1981.
112. Weldon C.S.: Coarctation of the aorta, in Cohn, L.H. (ed.): *Modern Techniques in Surgery, Cardiac/Thoracic Surgery,* Mt. Kisco, N.Y., Futura Pub. Co., 1979.
113. Werning C., Schonbeck M., Weidman P., et al.: Plasma renin activity in patients with coarctation of the aorta. *Circulation* 47:119, 1973.
114. Winter F.S.: Persistent left superior vena cava: Survey of world literature and report of thirty additional cases. *Angiology* 5:90, 1954.
115. Wychulis A.R., Kincaid D.W., Weidman W.H., et al.: Congenital vascular ring: Surgical considerations and the results of operations. *Mayo Clin. Proc.* 46:182, 1971.

142
Neurosurgery

General Considerations
Donlin M. Long

PEDIATRIC NEUROSURGERY is now a clearly defined subspecialty. The surgery of the nervous system of children differs in many ways from neurosurgery in the adult. Congenital malformations are more important, and hydrocephalus is the most frequent condition treated. Management of fluid and electrolytes is critical in the child, and more difficult than in the adult. The immature nervous system has a greater capacity for recovery. An injury that might be permanently devastating in the adult may be followed by an excellent recovery in the child. This is fortunate, because palliation is a less viable alternative in the child with a neurosurgical problem. A 10-year survival in an elderly adult may be an excellent therapeutic alternative. In children, cure must be the goal whenever possible.

The Diagnosis of Neurosurgical Conditions

Perhaps no field in medicine has been so dramatically changed by new diagnostic techniques as has neurosurgery. It has always been an axiom that accurate localization of the lesion before operation is mandatory for the best possible results. Until the recent past, localization depended upon a skilled neurologic examination and a group of diagnostic procedures, many of which were interventional and nonspecific. Even so, localization was imperfect, and true explorations were still required when only the general localization of the lesion could be demonstrated. Lumbar puncture, subdural puncture, ventricular puncture, EEG, radioactive brain scanning, plain x-ray films, and air encephalography and ventriculography supplemented by the more specific angiography represented the diagnostic possibilities (Figs 142–1 and 142–2). The advent of computed axial tomographic (CAT) scanning has completely changed this and virtually eliminated the nonspecific and most of the interventional procedures in diagnosis in neurosurgery.[3]

Computed Axial Tomography

The CAT scan is the basis for most neurosurgical diagnosis.[14, 16] The equipment for high-quality scans is now widely disseminated, and this technique has eliminated most of the complicated combinations of tests previously required. A single examination allows careful investigation of the skull, in general as accurately as with routine skull x-ray films. The subdural space can be visualized. The brain is seen, and its status can be accurately assessed. Mass lesions of all kinds are well seen, as are congenital anomalies and traumatic injuries. The ventricular system can be seen in its entirety, and reconstructions can be carried out to visualize the intracranial contents in virtually every plane. The CAT scan is now the most important diagnostic aid in neurosurgery (Fig 142–3).[3, 4]

Children present a special problem with CAT scans, because they so often require general anesthetic. The scans require a long period of time, often 45 minutes to 1 hour, during which the patient must be quite still. To obtain satisfactory scans in all but the most cooperative children, a light general endotracheal anesthetic is required. In younger children where information need not be so detailed, as with scans for the assessment of hydrocephalus, sedation alone may be satisfactory. This decision must be based upon the age of the patient, the degree of cooperativeness, how effective restraint can be, and the information that is to be obtained.

Nuclear Magnetic Resonance Scanning

The newest technique now available is the nuclear magnetic resonance scan, also called magnetic resonance imaging (MRI). This images the brain with great accuracy and provides close-to-photographic assessment of the intracranial contents. The MRI technique is in its infancy and not yet widely available, and its eventual place in diagnosis remains to be determined. At present, this form of scanning is most accurate in the sagittal plane, allowing complete assessment of lesions in the pineal area, in the brain stem, at the cervical medullary junction, in the third ventricle, and in the region of the optic chiasm. There is every indication that this will become steadily more useful as instrumentation improves and the scans become more widely available. Spectroscopy with MRI provides functional assessment of the brain. By this technique it is possible to gain accurate information concerning the energy metabolism of the brain. As yet, these functional images have not achieved clinical significance, but offer the first practical opportunity for a way to assess brain function.

Positron Emission Tomography (PET)

The positron emitting techniques, thus far limited to a few centers, have been more valuable in research than in clinical medicine. Nevertheless, there are already well-recognized clinical applications. The use of a glucose analogue to assess glucose metabolism in the brain has proved to be of great value in assessing the patient with intractable epilepsy. The region of abnormality can be effectively demonstrated by this functional imaging. Gallium scans have been utilized to localize brain tumors and assess focal disruption of the blood-brain barrier. Blood flow can be measured, and glucose metabolism may be important in the evaluation of a variety of conditions other than epilepsy. However, because PET scanning is not widely available, it is utilized only in very specific clinical situations.

Angiography

Angiography remains an important part of neurosurgical diagnosis,[10] but its role has changed significantly. The angiogram is

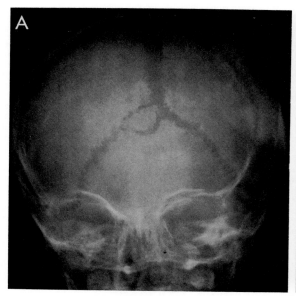
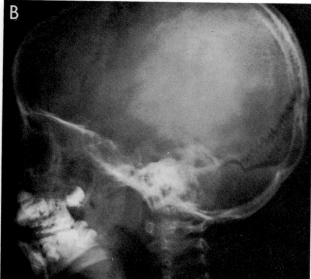

Fig 142–1.—Sutural diastasis. Intracranial leukemic infiltrations caused enough pressure in the head of this 2-year-old child to cause the suture lines to separate, as seen in anteroposterior (A) and lateral (B) roentgenograms of the skull. Treatment of the systemic disease relieved the intracranial pressure. Sutural diastasis occurs in any condition of chronic increase of intracranial pressure, usually in children under age 8 years.

now utilized primarily for vascular problems or to assess the blood supply of tumors. Diagnostic angiography is rarely indicated. The carotid, vertebral, and brachial angiograms have been virtually eliminated. At the present time, almost all angiography, even in small children, is carried out by selective catheters introduced through the femoral artery. Many technical advances have been made in the recent past. Magnification is now routine. Stereoscopic angiography may be useful in localizing some kinds of vascular lesions, and subtraction of bone from the film accentuates the vascular pattern. Digital angiographic techniques utilizing intravenous injection now offer simpler alternatives to the intra-arterial procedures. Interventional radiography is now utilized to occlude the arterial supply of tumors or of vascular malformations, even in children.[8]

Cisternography

The use of dilute intrathecal contrast material with CT scanning has virtually replaced myelography and all air encephalography. The CT cisternogram may be carried out with contrast material injected into the lumbar region or into the cervical subarachnoid space by lateral C-2 puncture.[7, 12] The spinal CT with intrathecal contrast is carried out in a fashion similar to myelography.[1] Both allow CT scans with contrast material completely outlining the nervous system. Cisternography with CT is particularly helpful with small lesions in the cerebellopontine angle and ill-defined lesions around the optic chiasm. Myelography with CT will demonstrate the spinal cord and intrathecal contents more effectively than traditional myelography and is now

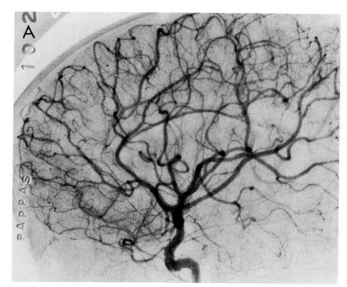
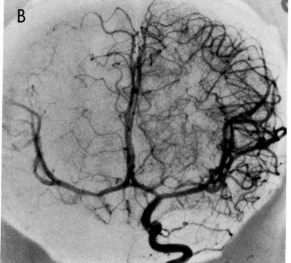

Fig 142–2.—A, lateral carotid angiogram in a child. Note the relative elevation and straightening of the middle cerebral artery, normal in an infant. B, anterior posterior view carotid angiogram. Intracranial vessels are in normal position In general, the use of angiography is limited today to investigation of vascular lesions or evaluation of the blood supply of tumors.

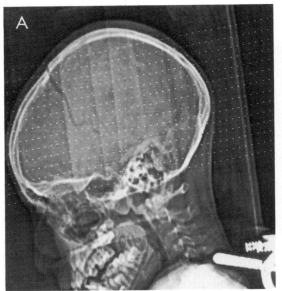

Fig 142–3.—**A,** the tomogram taken for the CT scan done on an emergency basis in this 9-year-old boy who had suffered a serious head injury demonstrates a diastatic fracture involving the coronal suture. The view of the skull obtained by this technique is satisfactory, and additional skull x-ray films were not necessary. **B,** this 9-year-old boy sustained a severe head injury in an automobile accident. At the time of admission, he was comatose and demonstrated decerebrate posturing. The CT scan demonstrated diffuse cerebral swelling and marked compression of the ventricles, but no focal abnormality for which intervention would be useful. **C,** this 11-year-old girl was struck by an automobile and was in coma with decerebrate posturing. The CT scan shows a small right-sided extracerebral collection and a focal hemorrhage on the left side of the third ventricle at the junction of midbrain and thalamus. No interventional procedures were indicated. **D, E,** this 8-year-old child suffered a prolonged period of hypoxia secondary to drowning. These scans illustrate the value of sequential studies in assessing a pathologic process. The initial scan **(D)** demonstrated only significant brain edema. Approximately 2 weeks later, ventricular enlargement was apparent with hemorrhages in basal ganglia, thalamus, and occipital lobes. **E,** 5 weeks later, the scan demonstrated marked hydrocephalus ex vacuo, sulcal enlargement and loss of brain parenchyma. The child remained in a coma, with no sign of neurologic improvement. **F,** this 1-year-old child presented with a history of steady increase in head size and failure to thrive. The differential diagnosis included hydrocephalus or chronic subdural hematoma. CT scan immediately revealed slight hydrocephalus, but the principal pathologic process was a large extracerebral subdural collection, which proved to be a chronic subdural hematoma. **G,** this 4-day-old child was seen because of a large head, bulging fontanel, and feeding difficulties. The CT scan clearly defines the large posterior fossa cyst typical of the Dandy-Walker syndrome with mild associated hydrocephalus. Intraventricular contrast demonstrated patency of the aqueduct, and a shunt of the posterior fossa cyst relieved the symptoms.

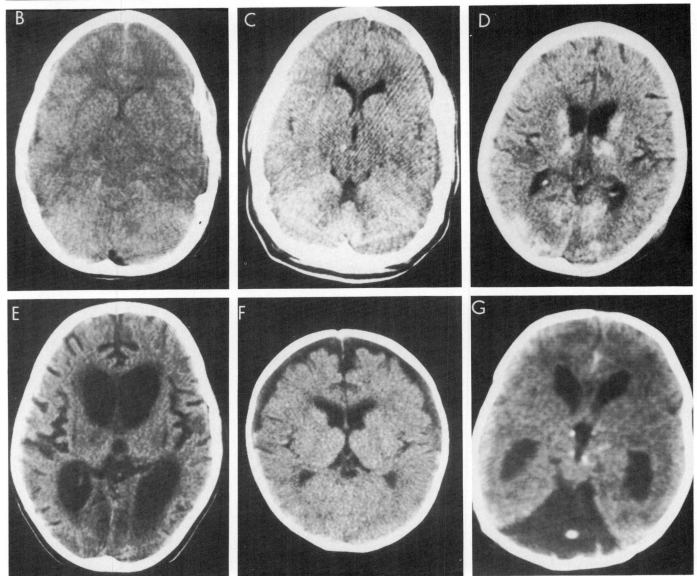

utilized for the examination of all intraspinal problems. In addition to the information gained from scanning immediately after injection of the dye, delayed scans may show contrast material in cysts within the spinal cord. Both these forms of CT scan have the same disadvantage that routine CT scanning has, that is, they do require sedation or general anesthesia for children; but the advantages are great enough that the risk of the anesthetic is well worth taking.

There is a variety of procedures used much less frequently than formerly in neurosurgical practice. The CT scan and newer diagnostic techniques have been responsible for the reduction in utilization of the diagnostic needle punctures, which formed an important diagnostic base for neurosurgical practice for many years.[2]

Lumbar Puncture

Lumbar puncture now is utilized primarily as a diagnostic tool in infectious disease and to substantiate subarachnoid hemorrhage. Even in the latter case, it is rarely necessary now, because the CT scan will much more effectively demonstrate the subarachnoid blood, and often its source. There is a real risk with lumbar puncture in the face of a space-occupying lesion, and the procedure should not be considered in patients with evidence of increased intracranial pressure where a mass lesion is suspected.

The subarachnoid space is entered with a small needle, preferably a 22–25 gauge, at the L2-3 space or below. Sedation and restraint should be adequate to allow the test to be carried out. The skin is prepared sterilely, as for a surgical procedure, and anesthetized. The needle is introduced between the spinous processes, with the child in the lateral position, and passed through the intraspinous ligaments exactly in the midline. In most situations, it is wise to measure the pressure; and then the fluid is removed for inspection, cell count, and determination of protein and sugar. When infection is a possibility, enough fluid should be removed for all appropriate cultures. Gram stain of the centrifuge residuum of the spinal fluid is helpful in the rapid diagnosis of meningitis. Lumbar puncture is rarely indicated in trauma; and its use on the neurosurgical service has virtually disappeared, except in the diagnosis and therapy of infection.

Cisternal or Second Cervical Lateral Puncture

These techniques are not commonly employed in the child, but they may be useful for CT cisternography or when, for some reason, it is not possible to carry out lumbar puncture at a lower level. The midline posterior cisternal puncture has been virtually replaced by fluoroscopically controlled puncture of the subarachnoid space through the second cervical foramen. It is most important that the child be restrained so that movement is impossible. Injury to the spinal cord at this level may be catastrophic. For this reason, anesthesia may be required. Excellent sedation and careful restraint can substitute. The fluoroscope is utilized to demonstrate the correct position of the puncture; then, using fluoroscopic control, a small needle, 25 or 22 gauge, can be inserted easily into the cervical subarachnoid space.

Subdural and Ventricular Punctures

Diagnostic subdural taps, virtually eliminated by the CT scan, which effectively shows the subdural hematoma, are still utilized for therapy of subdural fluid collection; but the procedure is required much less commonly than in the past. The incidence of recalcitrant subdural hematoma has declined significantly in the past decade; and the subdural puncture, once so common, has become a rarity. When subdural puncture is required in the

small child, it can now be carried out with great accuracy, because the location of the hematoma is known. In most instances, if the hematoma is localized in an area not easily accessible, the simplest thing is to place a burr hole over it and drain the fluid this way, providing access for subsequent needles through the burr hole. When the hematoma is accessible, a standard subdural puncture technique may be carried out through a convenient suture. The hair must be shaved and the skin prepared as for any surgical procedure. A short beveled 22-gauge spinal needle is inserted perpendicularly through the coronal suture at the lateral angle of the anterior fontanelle. The needle is advanced perpendicularly, millimeter by millimeter, until the surgeon feels the needle pop through the dura. As soon as this is felt, the stylet is withdrawn and the fluid allowed to drain out slowly. It is important not to remove large amounts of fluid at one time. A good general rule is not to remove more than 15 ml from each side at the time of first tapping. Complicated rules utilized in the past for the amount of fluid to be removed have now been replaced by reassessment with CT scan.

Ventricular puncture in the young child is carried out by inserting the needle at the lateral margin of the fontanelle, directing it toward the medial canthus of the eye. The ventricle should be easily encountered as the needle is slowly passed into the depths. As with subdural puncture, the CT scan gives an excellent puncture of the ventricular system; and the blind taps formerly based upon usual locations of the ventricles are no longer necessary. Occasionally, ventricular puncture may be complicated by hemorrhage. When this occurs, the needle should be left in place and the bleeding allowed to stop. The dye studies and multiple punctures that used to be necessary for the evaluation of hydrocephalus are no longer done and are no longer important. Ventricular puncture is now most commonly employed in trauma for the placement of a ventricular drain or, postoperatively, when ventricular drainage is necessary. In such a situation, one uses, instead of the 22-gauge spinal needle, a larger needle through which a soft plastic catheter can be inserted.

Roentgenographic Procedures

Standard x-ray films have also greatly decreased in importance. The CT scan of the head gives all the necessary information concerning the skull. Routine skull x-ray films add little to the evaluation of the patient in whom an intracranial mass is strongly suspected. Even though abnormalities do occur, the recognition of these abnormalities has been greatly reduced in importance by the definitive information provided in the CT scan.

Spinal x-ray films remain important, especially to guide the areas to be scanned more definitively. In most situations, anteroposterior and lateral films are required. Tomograms are no longer utilized extensively, because the CT scan through areas of suspected abnormalities will provide more important information.

There are a number of diagnostic studies that have been virtually eliminated in routine neurosurgical practice. The EEG has little to offer in patients suspected of harboring mass lesions. It is primarily utilized now in the diagnosis and treatment of epilepsy or in the assessment of brain function following severe injury.

Radioisotope Brain Scanning

The radioisotope brain scan has been eliminated as a diagnostic tool, because CT scanning is so much more effective.

Echoencephalography

The echoencephalogram has disappeared as well. The information to be gained from CT scan is much greater and much more specific.

Air-Contrast Cerebral Radiography

Ventriculography and pneumoencephalography are not done, nor is contrast ventriculography. There are rare exceptions to this in specific circumstances; but, for diagnostic use, these procedures have been supplanted by the newer techniques available.

Venography

The venograms, which at one time were carried out to assess sinus patency, have also been made unnecessary by advances in angiography. No neurosurgical patient has undergone venography in our hospital in the past 10 years.

Myelography

The standard myelogram, particularly when carried out with iodinated contrast material, has also been virtually eliminated. The CT scan with intrathecal contrast has replaced myelography. The uses remain the same. The new techniques are utilized to visualize the spinal cord, spinal subarachnoid space, cervical medullary junction, and cerebellopontine angle.

General Conditions in Perioperative Management

Preoperative Care

Several specialized situations in pediatrics require the surgeon to make important decisions in the timing of surgical management. Marked intracranial hypertension, secondary to hydrocephalus, still occurs in tumors of all kinds and in hydrocephalus.[5] A decision for management by ventricular drainage, as contrasted to the placement of an internal shunt, is still under discussion in pediatric neurosurgery. Some advocate control of hydrocephalus by a shunt before definitive operation for tumor. Others prefer to manage intracranial pressure by ventricular drainage for a short period of time and to attempt to restore normal fluid pathways by successful operation.[6] Ventricular drains are placed in the same way that a ventricular puncture is performed, but a larger needle is employed. A soft plastic catheter is inserted into the ventricle through the needle. The needle is removed and the catheter firmly sutured into position at the scalp. A careful dressing must be applied to be certain the catheter cannot be dislodged. The catheter is then connected to a closed drainage system. The greatest risk of ventricular drainage is infection, and the drain should not be left in place for a long period of time. The current techniques of measurement allow the pressure in the ventricular system to be normalized slowly over several hours, utilizing direct pressure readings, rather than depending upon any predetermined formula. When it appears that the patient may require prolonged postoperative drainage, an internal shunt is a better choice, but adds the risk of a major surgical procedure in the face of an intracranial neoplasm.

Intracranial lesions in children, which occur in the posterior fossa, hypothalamus, and third ventricle, may be associated with prolonged vomiting and serious disturbance of water and electrolyte balance. These clearly must be corrected in the preoperative period and any hormonal imbalances corrected as well.[6]

In general, preoperative management in the child is not significantly different from that in the adult.[15] Most patients undergoing craniotomy for tumor will receive preoperative glucosteroids, usually dexamethasone. A dose of 0.2–0.3 mg/kg/24 hours administered in four divided doses is standard, but much higher doses may be utilized safely when necessary. This is most common in trauma and with recurrent neoplasms. The intracranial pressure may be reduced quickly by the administration of a concentrated infusion of mannitol, 1 gm/kg, administered intravenously over 15–20 minutes. An appropriate dose of furosemide (Lasix), given shortly after, will potentiate the action of mannitol beyond the expected 3 hours. The use of osmotic diuretics provides rapid reduction of intracranial pressure by shrinking normal brain. It is useful for the long-term support of the traumatized patient, but now this situation has changed significantly because of newer monitoring techniques. Hypothermia is a serious problem in these children, and infrared lamps and warming blankets are routinely employed. The general techniques of good anesthesia practice, smooth induction, careful rapid intubation, and constant adequate ventilation with monitoring of blood gases are important to be sure that oxygen and CO_2 remain normal. Intravenous fluids must be given at controlled rates and strictly monitored. The injured brain can be markedly swollen by the injudicious overuse of fluids. It is much better to be on the dry side than to provide excess fluid. In general, it is quite satisfactory to maintain fluid administration as necessary for the child's age, weight, and body habitus. Only rarely are any specific manipulations required.[9, 13]

Blood loss may be a serious problem as well. Scalp incisions, particularly, tend to be long, and a significant amount of blood may be lost from the operative incision. The need for blood replacement may be rapid. These patients require constant monitoring in the operating room.[17]

Monitoring During Anesthesia

Utilizing the new electrophysiologic techniques available, it is now possible to monitor many kinds of neurologic function. From a practical standpoint, assessments of spinal evoked potentials and brain stem auditory evoked potentials have been most useful. Assessment of visual evoked potentials has been utilized less commonly. Constant monitoring of spinal evoked potentials allows assessment of spinal cord function during operations upon the spinal cord, and can give a measure of transmission through the brain stem and in peripheral nerves. Assessment of the brain stem auditory evoked potentials during an operation in which the brain stem must be manipulated is very helpful in determining if some injury may be occurring. These techniques now allow constant assessment of vital functions without the need for the extremely light anesthesia and spontaneous respirations that once were the hallmark of pediatric neurosurgical anesthesia.

Postoperative Care

Children require greater care to prevent laryngeal and tracheal complications. Moist air should be available, and the children must be watched carefully for laryngeal or tracheal irritation in the immediate period after extubation. The hematocrit level and fluid and electrolyte balance are monitored. As in so many areas, the previously utilized empirical rules once applied to all postoperative patients can now be eliminated because of the easily obtained regular determinations of electrolyte balance, blood volume, and hematocrit levels. It is best to monitor these on a regular basis and to judge therapy according to the abnormalities actually found, rather than to follow a formula that may or may not be applicable to a specific patient.

Some lesions of the brain do have their own set of specific problems. Diseases of the hypothalamus are often complicated by diabetes insipidus, with excessive water loss and at times inappropriate antidiuresis. The child's hematocrit level may change rapidly, and rapid changes in temperature are more common than in the adult.

Children generally are out of bed more rapidly than are adults. However, when hydrocephalus is excessive, children should be mobilized carefully, with gradual elevation over several days.

Surgical Incisions and Operative Techniques

Incisions in children are virtually the same as in adults. They must be planned so that whenever possible they are hidden by hair growth, and they must be large enough to expose the lesion. An adequate base is required so that the blood supply of the flap will not be compromised. This is virtually never a problem in children, but is it wise to base most flaps upon major arteries. The large horseshoe flap incisions always utilized in the past are increasingly being replaced by linear and S-incisions as the accuracy of localization of intracranial lesions improves.

The posterior fossa is still exposed through a midline incision unless the approach is to be unilateral, when a linear mastoid incision is satisfactory.

Spinal incisions are virtually always midline or paramedian. The removal of large amounts of bone in the spine of a young child may have serious orthopedic consequences, and bony removal should be limited to the minimum. Children undergoing spinal procedure must be carefully followed for the development of orthopedic deformities.

Operative techniques are little different than in the adult. Blood loss and tissue trauma must be minimized in small children, and the same meticulous procedures always required in the nervous system are employed in the pediatric patient.[11, 17]

REFERENCES

1. Anand A.K., et al.: Plain and metrizamide CT of lumbar disc disease: Comparison with myelography. *AJNR* 3(5):567–571, 1983.
2. Apuzzo M.L., et al.: Computed tomographic guidance stereotaxis in the management of intracranial mass lesions. *Neurosurgery* 12(3):377–385, 1983.
3. Davis D.O., Kobrine A.: Computed tomography, in Youmans J.R. (ed.): *Neurological Surgery*, ed. 2. Philadelphia, W.B. Saunders Co., 1982, vol. 1, pp. 111–142.
4. Fileni A., et al.: Dandy-Walker syndrome: Diagnosis in utero by means of ultrasound and CT correlations. *Neuroradiology* 24(4):233–235, 1983.
5. Hoffman H.J.: Supratentorial brain tumors in children, in Youmans J.R. (ed.): *Neurological Surgery*, ed. 2. Philadelphia, W.B. Saunders Co., 1982, vol. 1, p. 2702.
6. Humphreys R.P.: Posterior cranial fossa brain tumors in children, in Youmans J.R. (ed.): *Neurological Surgery*, ed. 2. Philadelphia, W.B. Saunders Co., 1982, vol. 1, p. 2733.
7. Mawad M.E., et al.: Computerized tomography of the brainstem with intrathecal metrizamide: II. Lesions in and around the brainstem. *Am. J. Radiol.* 140(3):556–571, 1983.
8. Michelsen W.J., Hilal S.K.: Interventional neuroradiology, in Youmans J.R. (ed.): *Neurological Surgery*, ed. 2. Philadelphia, W.B. Saunders Co., 1982, vol. 1, p. 1194.
9. Michenfelder J.D., Gronert G.A., Rehder K.: Anesthesia, in Youmans J.R. (ed.): *Neurological Surgery*, ed. 2. Philadelphia, W.B. Saunders Co., 1982, vol. 1, p. 1119.
10. Raimondi A.J.: Angiographic diagnosis of hydrocephalus in the newborn. *J. Neurosurg.* 31:550, 1969.
11. Rhoton A.L.: Micro-operative technique, in Youmans J.R. (ed.): *Neurological Surgery*, ed. 2. Philadelphia, W.B. Saunders Co., 1982, vol. 1, p. 1160.
12. Scott R.M., Wolpert S.M.: Metrizamide CT cisternography in cranial arachnoid cysts, in *Concepts in Pediatric Neurosurgery*. Basel, Switzerland, Karger, 1981, pp. 69–78.
13. Smith R.M.: *Anesthesia for Infants and Children*, ed. 2. St. Louis, C.V. Mosby Co., 1963.
14. Snead O.C., Acker J.D., Morowetz R.W., et al.: High resolution computerized tomography with coronal and sagittal reconstruction in the diagnosis of brain tumors in children. *Childs Brain* 9:1–9, 1982.
15. Stern W.E.: Preoperative evaluation: Complications, their prevention and treatment, in Youmans J.R. (ed.): *Neurological Surgery*, ed. 2. Philadelphia, W.B. Saunders Co., 1982, vol. 1, p. 1051.
16. Thompson M.G., Eisenberg H.M., Levin H.S.: Hydrocephalic infants: Developmental assessment and computed tomography. *Childs Brain* 9:400–410, 1982.
17. Wilkins R.H., Odom G.L.: General operative technique, in Youmans J.R. (ed.): *Neurological Surgery*, ed. 2. Philadelphia, W.B. Saunders Co., 1982, vol. 1, p. 1136.

Spina Bifida and Hydrocephalus
Melvin H. Epstein / George B. Udvarhelyi

Hydrocephalus

HYDROCEPHALUS, by strict definition, implies an increase in the volume of cerebrospinal fluid (CSF) producing enlargement of any fluid cavity within the head. It is not a disease entity. It is a term descriptive of a pathologic condition with many presentations and causes. Although clinically the term is used loosely to characterize abnormal fluid accumulations within large ventricles under pressure, it also includes hydrocephalus as a result of cerebral agenesis or decreased cerebral substance (hydrocephalus ex vacuo), low-pressure hydrocephalus, and porencephalic cysts. As far as can be determined, Hippocrates[101] (460–377 B.C.) was the first to recognize that water accumulation in the head could cause it to enlarge. Herophilus and Erasistratus were aware of the ventricular cavities within the brain. The first clear description of internal hydrocephalus was by Vesalius, who described the condition in a child.

Pathophysiology

Increased Fluid Production

Hydrocephalus is a result of increased production or decreased absorption of fluid, with blockage anywhere from the point of production in the ventricular system to the venous circulation of the brain. Documentation of increased fluid production is extremely rare, except in the case of choroid plexus adenoma. Most cases of hydrocephalus are a result of decreased absorption. Occasionally, a condition called arrested hydrocephalus occurs, in which enough alternate routes of outflow develop so that the hydrocephalus stays under control without treatment. In these cases, any increase in fluid production takes on importance. An increase in body temperature, as with a simple fever, can increase production and upset equilibrium, as can infections of the nervous system.

Impeded Fluid Absorption

CONGENITAL MALFORMATIONS.—Many congenital malformations can obstruct CSF flow. In aqueductal stenosis (Figs 142–4 and 142–5), the diameter of the aqueduct is reduced to such a point that it impedes the outflow of fluid from the lateral ventricular system, producing internal obstructive hydrocephalus with dilatation of the lateral and third ventricles.[96] This may occur in association with additional anomalies of the brain and other organs. In its severest form, it is incompatible with life unless a shunting procedure is performed. In aqueductal atresia, the aqueduct is subdivided into tiny forked channels. At times, a septum of fibrillary glia covered irregularly by ependymal cells may be found obstructing the aqueduct. This malformation has occasionally been associated with a granular ependymitis, so it is uncertain whether the septum is congenital or postinflammatory. Aqueductal atresia may be familial. In a family with 15 affected

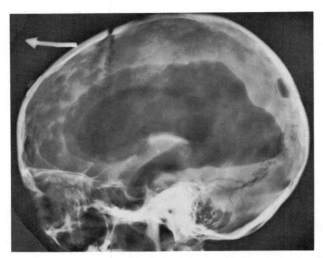

Fig 142–4.—Obstructive hydrocephalus. Lateral ventriculogram showing dilatation of lateral and third ventricles and lack of filling of the aqueducts and fourth ventricles in a 12-year-old child with aqueductal stenosis probably caused by periaqueductal gliosis. Note the beaten silver appearance of the skull and separation of the coronal suture secondary to prolonged increased intracranial pressure. The pressure was relieved by a Torkildsen procedure.

members, the pattern of appearance indicated a probable recessive sex-linked inheritance.[22]

A greatly enlarged fourth ventricle produces a posterior fossa cyst with an interior ependymal lining and a thin external arachnoidal membrane, thought to be caused by an absence of the foramina of Luschka and Magendie. This condition, Dandy-Walker syndrome,[91] frequently does not produce a rapidly advancing hydrocephalus; and it is quite possible that the congenital membrane is thin enough to allow for diffusion of a certain amount of ventricular fluid into the subarachnoid pathways. The condition is associated with a large posterior fossa and upward displacement of the torcular Herophili, lateral sinuses, and inion, creating a diagnostic radiographic appearance (Figs 142–6 and 142–7).

The Arnold-Chiari malformation is associated with spinal meningomyelocele and hydrocephalus (Fig 142–8).[10, 31] At the end of the last century, Arnold[6] and Chiari[18] separately described malformations of the hind end of the brain and upper spinal cord that were frequently associated with spinal meningomyelocele. The type of malformation that causes hydrocephalus consists of a deformed fused cerebellar prolongation entirely adherent to the underlying brain stem,[19] extending into the spinal canal to the level of the second or even third cervical vertebra. The medulla oblongata, with the fourth ventricle, is displaced into the spinal canal with reversal of the angles of the upper cervical nerve roots leaving the cord. The spinal cord just below the upper cervical region is frequently hydromyelic. Polygyria and microgyria of the cerebral cortex, stenosis of the aqueduct of Sylvius, and enlargement of the inferior commissure are frequent associated findings.

It is thought by some that this anomaly is a result of traction on the brain stem and cerebellum by spinal cord tethering within a meningomyelocele. However, this condition occurs without meningomyelocele. Barry et al.[8] have advanced the theory that in this condition there is an associated hyperplasia of the contents of the posterior fossa, forcing some of its contents through the foramen magnum.

Decompression of the foramen magnum by suboccipital craniectomy and excision of the dysplastic cerebellar tongue have not been uniformly successful in alleviating hydrocephalus, espe-cially in young infants in whom there usually are also defective subarachnoid pathways at the base of the brain. Quite frequently, it is noticed that hydrocephalus appears after the excision of the meningocele sac. Many factors account for this phenomenon. The sac may serve as a vent for the loss by evaporation of CSF, allowing the ventricular system to remain compensated. After the operation, there is probably an inflammatory reaction, as well as a blockage by blood in the CSF, which may overtax the absorption mechanism. Also, the loss of CSF space in the sac may cause slight shifting of the brain and further herniation of the cerebellar tongue, tamponading the foramen magnum.[78, 79]

In the deformity called platybasia, the angle formed by the basisphenoid and the clivus, normally 130–140 degrees is increased. There is associated shortening of the basioccipital bone and a variety of bony malformations around the foramen magnum and the cervical spine, such as the Klippel-Feil malformation. The shortening and concavity of the base of the skull in this condition produce a situation in which the medulla oblongata and cerebellar tonsils may be herniated into the upper cervical canal, much as in the Arnold-Chiari malformation. Deformity of the base of the skull in achondroplasia may contribute to the development of hydrocephalus in those patients.

Hydrocephalus may be caused by congenital cysts, either porencephalic cysts within the substance of the brain or arachnoid cysts outside the brain. Congenital porencephalic cysts, although normally communicating with the ventricular system, frequently enlarge, deform the overlying skull, and act as space-occupying lesions to produce increased intracranial pressure. The only reasonable explanation for this phenomenon is that the communication with the ventricle is intermittently occluded by a ball-valve phenomenon.

The explanation for the space-taking and pressure-producing phenomena of both porencephalic and arachnoid cysts is unsatisfactory. However, there is no evidence that the arachnoidal membrane forming the arachnoid cyst is capable of producing CSF on its own. It is basically an avascular structure and has been shown to be deficient in the enzymes found in active transport systems.

In hydranencephaly, despite the absence of large amounts of supratentorial brain tissue, the CSF-producing choroid plexus is frequently intact. Presumably, the absorptive mechanism is impaired by decomposed brain products obstructing the arachnoid villi. Fluid accumulation within the cranial cavity and abnormal growth of the head occur frequently.

Neoplasms

Obstructive hydrocephalus can be produced by tumors if they block the CSF pathway, or if they secrete sufficient protein or cause enough hemorrhage within the CSF to block the absorptive mechanism.[5, 11] In children, gliomas or craniopharyngiomas often occlude the foramen of Monro. Posterior fossa tumors such as cerebellar astrocytomas, medulloblastomas, or ependymomas occlude the fourth ventricle or the caudad aspect of the aqueduct of Sylvius. Tumors in the superior aspect of the aqueduct most commonly arise from the pineal area.

Infection

Infection within the ventricular system with subsequent ependymitis may result in mechanical obstruction of the aqueduct or the outlets of the fourth ventricle, giving rise to obstructive hydrocephalus. Viral and other in utero infections may cause aqueductal stenosis. There are well-documented cases of toxoplasmosis, cytomegalic inclusion disease, mumps, and congenital syphilis causing hydrocephalus. Bacterial meningitis produces

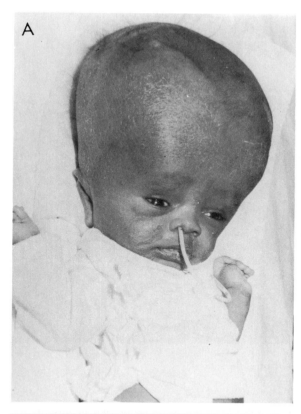

Fig 142–5.—**A,** hydrocephalus. Two-month-old infant with congenital aqueductal stenosis. The large head caused dystocia at birth, necessitating ventricular puncture to permit delivery. Hydrocephalus developing in utero resulted in brain damage by the time of birth. **B,** CAT (computed axial tomographic) scan of infant showing greatly thinned cortical mantle and massive internal hydrocephalus. **C,** CAT scan of normal baby for comparison showing lateral ventricles of normal size.

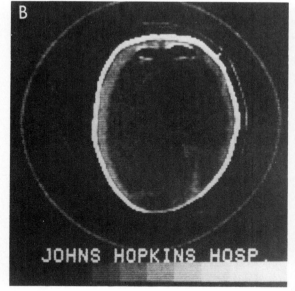

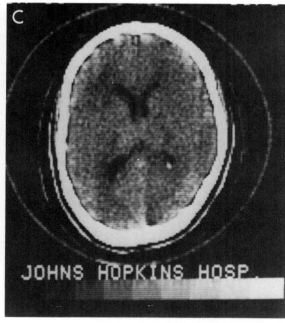

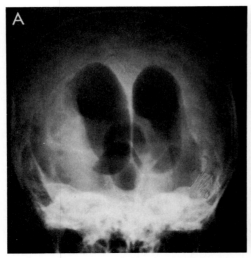
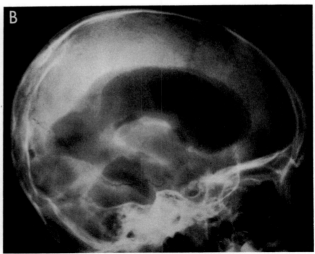

Fig 142–6.—Membranous occlusion of outlet of the fourth ventricle (Dandy-Walker syndrome). **A,** anteroposterior, and **B,** lateral ventriculogram of a 4-year-old child who had insidious onset of headache, vomiting, and enlargement of the head. Note symmetric hydrocephalus, hugely dilated fourth ventricle, and unusually large posterior fossa. Suboccipital craniectomy and resection of the membrane resulted in cure.

marked adhesions of the basal meninges, with arachnoidal adhesions of the external surface of the brain obliterating the subarachnoid pathways. The most common organisms in children are *Hemophilus influenzae*, pneumococcus, meningococcus, *Staphylococcus*, and tuberculosis (Fig 142–9). Yeast and fungi— *Monilia* and *Torula*—may produce hydrocephalus. Rarely, *Taenia solium* may produce granulomatous meningitis with inflammatory adhesions. The parasite also tends to become en-

cysted within the fourth ventricle, producing obstruction. Since the introduction of antibiotics, the bacterial forms of meningitis are more readily treatable; and the incidence of hydrocephalus after meningitis has decreased.

Sterile Inflammations

Hydrocephalus has been produced experimentally by the instillation of lamp black or silicone rubber into the ventricles or subarachnoid spaces. These substances either stimulate the arachnoid cells to marked proliferation or result in adhesions or fibrosis blocking the normal routes of CSF flow and absorption. Hydrocephalus has resulted in man from injections of such substances as antibiotics and Thorotrast into the ventricles or sub-

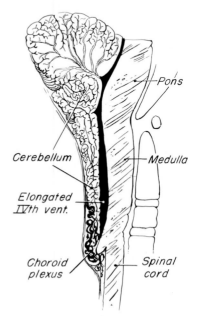

Fig 142–7.—Dandy-Walker cyst. A CAT scan demonstrating a large Dandy-Walker cyst and associated hydrocephalus in a 4-year-old child. The child was eventually treated with double shunting, one shunt in the right lateral ventricle and the second shunt in the posterior fossa cyst. Children with Dandy-Walker syndrome frequently do not have marked cerebellar findings despite the striking loss of cerebellar tissue and frequently have a good prognosis in terms of neurologic development.

Fig 142–8.—Arnold-Chiari malformation. Note caudal displacement of the dysplastic cerebellar tonsils, medulla oblongata, and fourth ventricle into the spinal canal. It may lead to mechanical obstruction of CSF circulation with resultant hydrocephalus.

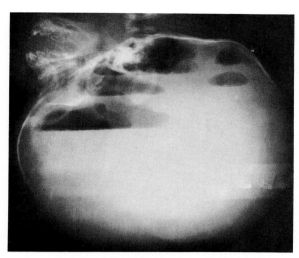

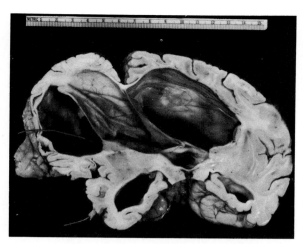

Fig 142–11.—Hydrocephalus; cross-section of brain at level of basal ganglia. The lateral ventricles are enormous, and the overlying cortex, thinned, flattened, and unsupported, has fallen over to the left. The huge third ventricle is just above the cleft between the temporal lobes. The temporal horns of the lateral ventricles show at this level. A straw has been passed through the site of a perforation of the temporal horn.

Fig 142–9.—Communicating hydrocephalus, advanced. Ventriculogram, lateral, inverted (hanging-head) view of an infant of 2 months shows large head, marked thinning of the occipital cortex, and air in the posterior fossa and cervical spinal canal. Air outside the ventricular system verifies the communicating nature of the process. Lack of air over the cerebral convexities is probably due to obstruction of basal subarachnoid channels. A ventricular-atrial shunt was successful.

arachnoid pathways. Infiltration of the meninges, such as occurs in the lipoidoses, leukemia, and carcinomatous meningitis, may result in obliteration of the subarachnoid pathways or blockage of the arachnoid villi and so lead to hydrocephalus.

Vascular Malformations

A number of vascular problems can cause hydrocephalus. In infancy and childhood, arteriovenous malformations involving the distribution of the posterior cerebral artery can greatly dilate the vein of Galen with a resultant occlusion of the aqueduct. Also, large posterior fossa malformations may obstruct the fourth ventricle, creating obstructive hydrocephalus. There is some evi-

dence that thrombosis of the dural sinuses may be followed by hydrocephalus, although this has not been reproducible experimentally. The condition, called "otitic hydrocephalus" by Symonds,[82] is seen in children following middle ear infection with thrombosis of the lateral sinus adjacent to the infected temporal bone. Sagittal sinus thrombosis occurs as a result of direct extension of infection usually from mastoiditis, or severe dehydration in infants. In these conditions with an acute increase in intracranial pressure, the brain swells and the ventricles may not dilate. There is also an excess accumulation of fluid in the subarachnoid spaces and in the basilar cistern.

The condition caused by venous thrombosis is not clearly distinguished from a disease entity known as "pseudotumor," where there appears to be an excess accumulation of CSF and extracellular fluid, both within and outside the brain. Pseudotumor cer-

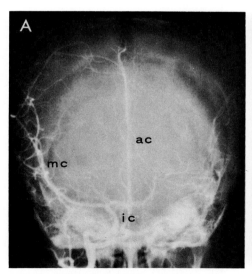

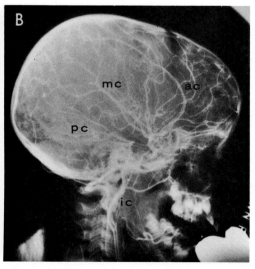

Fig 142–10.—Communicating hydrocephalus. Right retrograde brachial angiogram. **A,** anteroposterior, and **B,** lateral views. Anterior cerebral artery is stretched and attenuated as a result of ventricular dilatation, which results in stretching and elevation of the corpus callosum and pericallosal branch of *ac,* which hugs its circumference, best seen in **B.** In **A** is also seen the flattening of

the carotid siphon and *mc* against the inner table of the skull, also a result of ventricular dilatation. Had the hydrocephalus resulted from a vascular lesion, it might also be demonstrated by this study. *ic,* internal carotid artery; *ac,* anterior cerebral artery; *mc,* middle cerebral artery; *pc,* posterior cerebral artery.

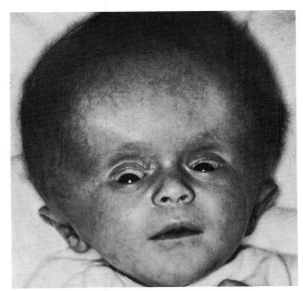

Fig 142–12.—Typical appearance of a child with advanced hydrocephalus, showing enlarged head, dilated scalp veins, and early downturning of the eyes.

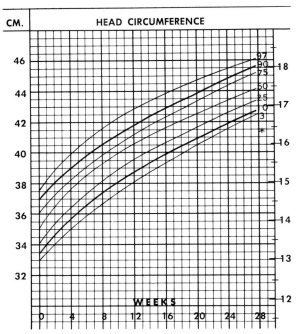

Fig 142–13.—Growth chart for recording head circumference. The head circumference is plotted every week. Perusal of the graph allows the examiner to know whether the head is large or small for a given age and whether it is growing more or less rapidly than normal for age. This is of particular value in deciding whether hydrocephalus is active or arrested.

ebri is a poorly understood entity that can be caused by long-term steroid administration and may actually represent an over-production syndrome. Obstruction of the superior vena cava by a mediastinal mass may cause hydrocephalus or brain swelling and papilledema.[35] Collateral venous channels over the upper chest, a ruddy complexion, and attacks of cyanosis and shortness of breath are characteristic of caval obstruction.

The extravasated blood from a subarachnoid hemorrhage in early life, as from a ruptured berry aneurysm, can cause a communicating hydrocephalus (Figs 142–10 to 142–12).[32]

Trauma

Trauma of various types can cause hydrocephalus by producing subarachnoid hemorrhage or ventricular bleeding with obstruction of the aqueduct by blood clot. Trauma can also cause subdural hematomas that, if severe and long-standing, can obstruct the absorptive mechanism over the convexity of the brain. Trauma severe enough to cause breakdown of brain tissue can lead to porencephaly or hydrocephalus ex vacuo. The rare posterior fossa subdural, or intracerebellar hematoma, can cause hydrocephalus.

Clinical Symptoms

Signs and Symptoms

In infancy, the most prominent presenting sign of hydrocephalus is an enlarged head, with enlargement continuing[54] beyond the normal growth percentiles. Although hydrocephalus frequently may present in utero, the large fetal head producing dystocia, these cases represent a minority of the hydrocephalic patients who come to medical attention. Most frequently, hydrocephalus appears to develop insidiously some time after birth. It cannot be overemphasized that a single head-size observation is not nearly so important as repeated measurements, which indicate the increasing growth of the head (Fig 142–13). During the initial examination of newborn infants, the head should be routinely transilluminated with a bright light (Fig 142–14). This helps in early detection of hydranencephaly and chronic subdural hematomas and should be part of every ordinary pediatric ex-

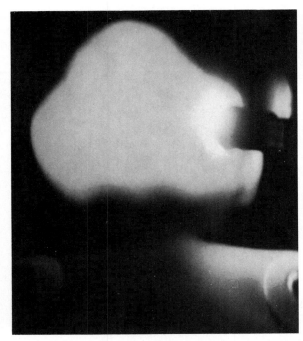

Fig 142–14.—Transillumination. A large posterior fossa cyst is demonstrated in a 2-year-old child, using a high intensity light beam in a darkened room. Transillumination is a valuable technique especially in children whose skulls are so thin that light rays can penetrate into the intracranial space.

amination. The adequacy of neurologic specialists is inverse to the delay in diagnosing developmental nervous system disorders.

Comparison between head and chest circumference and total body weight is useful, but less important than the rate of head growth. An abnormally enlarging head can occur in the absence of hydrocephalus. Achondroplasia,[20] cranioskeletal dysplasia, craniosynostosis, and neurocutaneous syndromes can all cause megaencephaly. It can also occur in Alexander's disease, Canavan's spongy degeneration, generalized gangliosidosis, maple syrup urine disease, metachromatic leukodystrophy, Tay-Sachs disease, mucopolysaccharidosis, lead poisoning, vitamin A toxicity, tetracyline toxicity, leptomeningeal cysts, and subdural hygromas.

The hydrocephalic skull usually enlarges equally in all directions, with a prominent forehead and a discrepancy between cranial and facial proportions. Prominent dilated veins are seen in the thin scalp. The fontanelle is usually bulging, tense, and enlarged and frequently is without visible pulsations. The crackpot sound when the head is percussed is Macewen's sign. A clear margin of sclera is seen beneath the upper lid, the so-called setting-sun sign. This has been thought to be a result of paralysis of downward gaze from pressure on the tectal plate of the mesencephalon and possibly also from pressure over the thin orbital plates in the anterior fossa depressing the globe. Sixth nerve palsies are frequently present as the posterior shift of the brain stem stretches the abducens nerve to the lateral rectus muscles. The sutures are usually widely, often palpably, patent. Nystagmus is common. Papilledema is unusual in infants with open sutures.

As the cerebral mantle thins, transillumination is more dramatic, the patient becomes more irritable, eats poorly, and shows poor control of the head, mostly because of its heavy weight. Intellectual development is retarded; the child may vomit and in advanced cases becomes somnolent. The deep tendon reflexes are hyperactive. Terminally, disturbances of respiration with irregular breathing and frequent apneic spells end in respiratory arrest. The more rapidly hydrocephalus progresses, the more prominent the symptoms. The more slowly it progresses, the better compensation can occur; and change in head size may be the only detectable clinical sign.

In hydrocephalus beginning beyond infancy, the fused sutures prevent enlargement of the head. Headaches, vomiting, and papilledema are manifestations of rapidly developing hydrocephalus in children. Internal hydrocephalus with slow dilatation of the ventricles and few symptoms may occur if the condition has progressed over a long period of time.[105] The posterior fossa is small in aqueductal stenosis and large when there is a posterior fossa cyst. The entire skull is enlarged in communicating hydrocephalus. Although the neurologic changes that can occur in hydrocephalus are very real, the diagnosis should be made well before any of them can occur, especially in infancy when transillumination and measurement of the head circumference are so informative. At the first suspicion of an abnormality, a child should be referred for diagnostic studies.

Diagnostic Procedures

Head circumference is measured with a metal tape from the prominence of the forehead to the prominence in the occipital area at the inion.[51, 90] Transillumination performed with a rubber-shielded, high-intensity light source in a darkened room is useful in detecting hydranencephaly and very thin cortical mantles (see Fig 142–14). The plain skull film, which should precede major diagnostic techniques, may show increased size of the cranial vault, separation of the sutures, demineralization of the sphenoid wings and clinoid processes, and, occasionally, intracranial calcifications.

In the past, evaluations consisted of subdural taps, echoencephalography, and ventriculography, occasionally preceded by cerebral angiography. Diagnosis has now been greatly simplified by the advent of computerized axial tomography (CAT scan) (Fig 142–15), which yields an image of the infant's brain and demonstrates abnormal fluid accumulations, enlarged ventricles, and tumor masses or developmental abnormalities. Air studies are now used much less frequently than formerly. Occasionally, iophendylate (Pantopaque) is instilled into the ventricles[66] to determine the patency of the aqueduct.

Angiography can be a formidable procedure in infants and should be used only when the blood supply must be further defined in a tumor or arteriovenous malformation or to clarify the blood supply to an infarcted area of the brain. Usually, CT scan shows subdural effusions, although there is a time in the development of the subdural hematoma when it can be isodense and not visible on the CT scan, so that the clinical problems may indicate the need for subdural tap or angiography. Infants must be sedated for CT scanning, because motion artifacts interfere with imaging. In hydrocephalic children, anesthetics that raise intracranial pressure, such as ketamine, may cause respiratory arrest from the sudden decompensation.

In more complex cases, when the CT scan does not clearly show communication between cysts and other compartments within the brain, pneumoencephalography or ventriculoencephalography must be performed. Electroencephalography frequently shows no abnormality even in very advanced cases of hydrocephalus, but in hydranencephaly there are characteristic flat waves in all leads. Isotope bound to protein[7] may be injected into the ventricular system and its course followed over 24 hours by image scanning to show the flow of CSF. In infants with increased intracranial pressure, bulging fontanelles, and hydrocephalus, lumbar puncture is never done as a primary study. If lumbar puncture must be performed, it is done only following a ventricular tap and after the determination that there is no mass in the posterior fossa that can herniate through the foramen magnum.

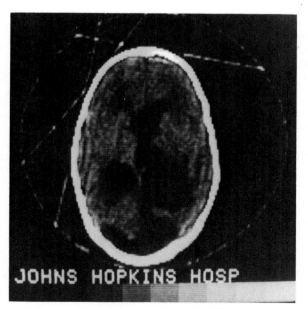

Fig 142–15.—Communicating hydrocephalus. The CAT scan demonstrates a communicating hydrocephalus with an enlarged cisterna magna as a result of *Hemophilus* meningitis. The basal cisterns in this child have been obliterated by the arachnoidal reaction, which blocked the passage of CSF to the convexity of the skull.

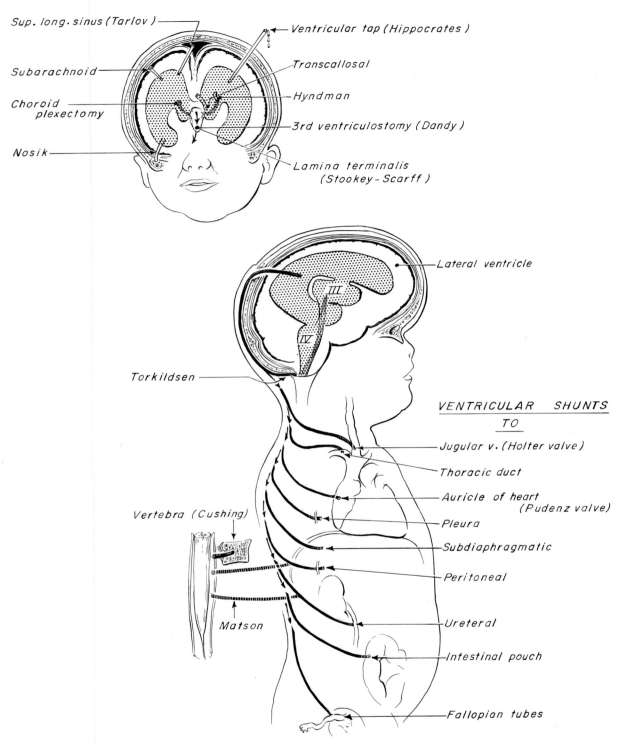

Sup. long. sinus (Tarlov)

Ventricular tap (Hippocrates)

Subarachnoid

Transcallosal

Choroid plexectomy

Hyndman

3rd ventriculostomy (Dandy)

Nosik

Lamina terminalis (Stookey-Scarff)

Lateral ventricle

Torkildsen

VENTRICULAR SHUNTS TO

Jugular v. (Holter valve)

Thoracic duct

Auricle of heart (Pudenz valve)

Vertebra (Cushing)

Pleura

Subdiaphragmatic

Peritoneal

Matson

Ureteral

Intestinal pouch

Fallopian tubes

Fig 142–16.—Methods of ventricular drainage. Some of the procedures used in treatment of hydrocephalus. (From Ransohoff and Hiatt.[74] Used by permission.)

Treatment

Operation

The most common currently employed surgical treatment of hydrocephalus involves shunting from the ventricle to the right atrium or to the peritoneal cavity. In the past, shunt tubes were placed into the distal ureter.[12, 60] However, this required sacrificing a kidney as well as a continuous loss of CSF. Shunts have also been placed in the Fallopian tube, the pleural cavity,[32, 73] the gallbladder, and the stomach (Fig 142–16).[2, 23, 61] None of these methods has become established. With the advent of a variety of shunting devices[93, 94, 104] made by numerous manufacturers,[21] the surgeon has gained a tremendous armamentarium of equipment useful for varying needs. Since the development of the slit-valve catheter, the ventriculoperitoneal[38, 70, 74] shunt has slowly advanced to a position of leadership. The slit valve at the end of the catheter opens at a predetermined pressure and may protect the end of the catheter from being invaded by scar tissue or omentum. The catheter is connected to a flushing device or a one-way pump mounted on the skull and connected by tubing to the ventricular system.[75]

In the ventriculoatrial shunt,[58] the distal end in the right atrium has either a slit valve or an open end with a one-way valve in the midsection of the shunt tubing. In general, the peritoneal shunt is more likely to be obstructed, but less likely to become infected, than the atrial shunt, and does not cause pulmonary hypertension. The advantages of the peritoneal shunt with the new technical modifications make it the procedure of choice for young infants. The catheter can be so placed that an extra coil of catheter in the peritoneal cavity provides length as the child grows. This, coupled with the lower incidence of bloodstream infection, offsets the greater revision rate. External ventricular drainage is a temporary measure to control hydrocephalus during resolution of infection, when it is not possible to place an internal shunt.[36, 37] Such a catheter placed through the skull into the brain creates its own possible avenue for infection.

On the theory that the choroid plexus is the site of active secretion of spinal fluid, Lespinasse many years ago attempted coagulation of the plexus; and Hildebrand resected it.[80] Because the procedure involves a major operation and because complete removal of the plexus is difficult and does not assure that CSF will not be formed from extra choroid plexus sites, choroid plexectomy is no longer performed.[89]

Nonoperative Treatment

There has recently been increasing interest in medical management of some patients with hydrocephalus. It has been known for many years that acetazolamide (Diamox) has a specific effect on the CSF production mechanism and can decrease CSF production by more than 40%. Because few hydrocephalic states result from CSF overproduction, clinical success with Diamox has been only modest. In spite of decreased production of CSF, a net imbalance remains; and shunting is necessary. Diamox is effective in some situations, such as in the period following subarachnoid or intraventricular hemorrhage, when it would appear that the normal subarachnoid pathways need time for development or have temporary interference.

The dose of Diamox can be as high as 100 mg/kg, because more than 99% of carbonic anhydrase must be blocked before CSF production decreases. Diamox causes a metabolic acidosis by increasing the excretion of bicarbonate (a direct effect on the kidney) and also decreases the hydrolysis of carbon dioxide, leaving an excess of carbon dioxide in the blood. Patients frequently show hyperventilation and a decrease in serum bicarbonate. This can be treated quite adequately by oral administration of sodium bicarbonate.

More recently, it has been found that furosemide and ethacrynic acid have a specific effect of decreasing CSF production that is not related to the biochemical site of action of acetazolamide. The use of gross dehydrating agents such as urea or isosorbide, a mannitol derivative, only transiently decreases CSF production.

Renewed interest has been shown in head wrapping, first described in medieval times. The concept is that head wrapping forces an increase in pressure that opens absorptive pathways and diminishes the need for shunts. Thus far, it seems more reasonable to attempt to decrease fluid production by taking the load off the absorptive mechanism rather than by increasing pressure on the young growing brain.

Spontaneous Arrest

Hydrocephalus occasionally arrests spontaneously during early childhood. The children appear to do well over a period of years, but then a discrepancy is manifested between mental and motor development, the motor development lagging progressively. As time goes on, ataxia and spasticity progress; and eventually there is intellectual deterioration. Such children cannot be truly defined as arrested hydrocephalics, because, although they do not require immediate shunting, there is a progressive insult to the brain and progressive accumulation of fluid within the ventricular space. It is difficult to know how many cases of hydrocephalus are borderline or low grade and then arrest spontaneously. It is the opinion of Laurence[41–43] that as many as 45% of all cases of hydrocephalus may arrest spontaneously. The patient with successfully treated hydrocephalus has a relatively good outlook for ultimate intellectual development, provided the shunt has been put in early in the development of hydrocephalus and is kept working properly.

A child with hydrocephalus that arrests spontaneously must be

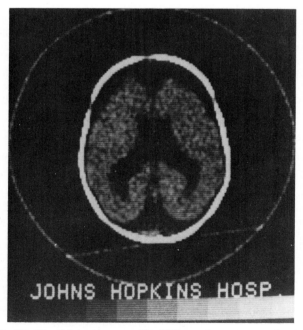

Fig 142–17.—Subdural hygroma. The CAT scan demonstrates a chronic collection of fluid following shunting in patient with arrested hydrocephalus. This is a 7-year-old child with an enlarged skull, who was shunted because of progressive neurologic problems resulting from decompensating hydrocephalus. This fluid collection was successfully treated by a subdural peritoneal shunt.

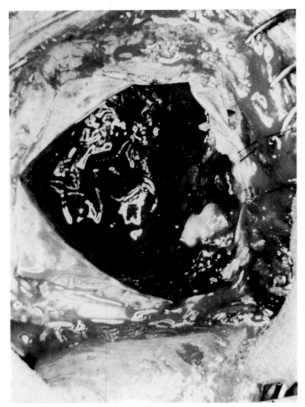

Fig 142–18.—Subdural hematoma. This is a 20-year-old white man with arrested hydrocephalus and an enlarged head, who developed an acute subdural hematoma after the ventricles were shunted. The collapse of the brain, tearing of communicating veins, and mild head trauma after discharge were the reasons for this complication. The subdural hematoma was removed, and the patient eventually made a good recovery.

followed carefully for evidence of progressive deterioration of intellectual function and by periodic scans to monitor ventricular size. Beyond the age of 8 or 9 years, when the head can reach relatively large size with huge fluid accumulations, the discrepancy between head circumference and ventricular size makes a subdural effusion or hematoma a significant probability following shunting (Figs 142–17 and 142–18).

Complications

Silicone rubber tubes, while less irritating than some other substances, are still foreign bodies. The overall incidence of infection in ventriculoperitoneal shunts can be as low as 5%. The ventricular catheter tip can be obstructed by cell debris, protein, blood, and choroid plexus. The peritoneal tips can be obstructed by omental wrapping or peritoneal entrapment of the distal end of the catheter. Tubes can come apart as the patient grows.

Reservoirs are incorporated into shunts so that the shunt can be tested by the depression of a one-way valve or punctured with a small-gauge needle for the injection of antibiotics or for pressure measurements. It has become our practice to put patients on prophylactic cephalothin in a dosage of 40 mg/kg for 24 hours prior to shunting, intraoperatively, and for 2 days postoperatively. Each treatment day involves a 40-mg intrashunt dose of cephalothin. Superinfection with a resistant bacterial strain has not been a problem in our 3 years of experience with this regimen.

Lumbar subarachnoid shunts are feasible, but can cause ad-

hesive arachnoiditis with painful involvement of the cauda equina. The hemilaminectomy required to place lumbar shunts can cause a significant scoliosis in children.[81] In older patients with more rigid skulls and a large cerebrocranial discrepancy, rapid decompression of the hydrocephalic brain may cause a collapse of the cerebral tissue with tearing of the bridging veins and subdural hematomas (see Fig 142–18). Even when the veins are not torn, an arachnoid tear may lead to an accumulation of CSF in the subdural space. Subdural peritoneal shunting is effective in treatment of such subdural hygromas. Before ventriculoureteral and lumboureteral shunting were abandoned, it was found that fluid loss, as the CSF was passed with the urine, resulted in a tremendous salt depletion and death unless electrolytes and fluid were regularly replaced.[55, 57]

Ventriculoatrial shunting (Fig 142–19) has been widely used,[17] and a good deal is known about its complications. Infection—bacteremia, septicemia, endocarditis—represents the single largest problem.[85] Anderson,[4] using a slit-valve atrial catheter, observed 48 patients for short periods: 28 were doing well; plugging of the catheter required revision in 3; 7 died of septicemia; 3 suffered the complication of thrombus formation around the catheter in the atrium.

The incidence of infection in the reported series is at least 10%. It has been maintained that, once infection develops, systemic antibiotics in high dosage or a combination of systemic or intraventricular antibiotics can be curative. However, most neurosurgeons prefer to remove the shunt with all foreign material and replace it when the infection is cured. Endocarditis may be particularly stubborn, and valvular damage may be permanent. Overton et al.[63, 64] reported a 7.7% incidence in 65 infants of

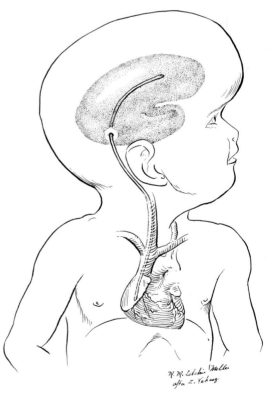

Fig 142–19.—Ventricular-atrial anastomosis. The catheter is carried subcutaneously from the occipital trephine to the neck, then passed from the common facial vein via the internal jugular and superior vena cava to the atrium. The lower end of the catheter is guarded by a valve. (From Pudenz et al.[72] Used by permission.)

partial or complete superior vena cava or innominate obstruction following ventriculoatrial shunt. This results in the superior vena cava syndrome, characterized by cyanosis, swelling of the face and hands, shortness of breath, somnolence, dilated superficial veins over the head and chest, and papilledema. Attempts to revise such a shunt may result in pulmonary embolism, which has occurred spontaneously as well (see Chap. 59).

Overton and his colleagues[63, 64] believe that proper placement of the tube in the atrium, but not in the vena cava, will prevent thrombosis. They have advocated placement of the tube in the atrium via the inferior vena cava when the superior venous inflow to the heart becomes occluded. It would seem more attractive to think in terms of extravascular shunting in such circumstances.[50, 72]

Sperling et al.[87] found pathologic changes characteristic of cor pulmonale in all of 12 children studied at autopsy after ventriculoatrial shunt. In each, a firm thrombus had formed around the cardiac end of the tube. In many of these cases, there was no history of infection; but, presumably, showers of emboli into the lungs from this thrombus caused pulmonary hypertension. Among 30 children surviving ventriculoatrial shunt, two had this complication.

Black et al.[13] described two cases of nephrotic syndrome with severe hematuria associated with long-standing bacteremia from colonization of coagulase-positive staphylococci in a pressure valve. Bacterial infection can occur with minimal symptoms—irritability, intermittent fever, anemia, and splenomegaly. Low-grade fever is an indication for serial blood cultures. A rare complication is migration of the cardiac end of the catheter into the right ventricle or pulmonary artery, possibly because of over-zealous manipulation of the flushing device. Among 50 patients treated with ventriculoatrial shunts, Pertuiset et al.[69] noted the following complications: empyema, fistulae (2); thromboses (5); infections (12); septicemia (10); and meningitis (2). There were 21 deaths.

Nulsen and Becker,[62] in their 10-year experience with 140 patients requiring 433 operations, had an overall infection rate of 10%. The commonest organism was usually the saprophytic *Staphylococcus albus*. They believe that the most frequent cause of endocarditis, valvular damage and bacteremia, is too low placement of the cardiac catheter. According to them, it should never be placed below the seventh thoracic segment; and its position should be checked by injection of contrast material into the shunting tube. Intraoperative and postoperative chemotherapy is considered essential. There were five cases of superior vena cava thrombosis in their series and four cases of increasing pulmonary difficulties suggestive of thromboembolic phenomena. Nine deaths were attributed to infection. Erosion over the flushing device, and wound disruption, were rare problems. Nulsen and Becker[62] carefully studied migration of the cardiac end of the catheter, the tip of which is radiopaque, and concluded that an initial shunt performed on an infant aged 3 months will require revision when the child reaches the age of 16 months. Their average shunt remained functional for 1–3½ years. Second revisions after age 2 years usually remained patent until adolescence. The authors stressed the importance of placing the proximal end of the catheter into the frontal horn of the lateral ventricle to avoid ingrowth of the choroid plexus.

Because of the long list of complications of ventriculoatrial shunting in young children, ventriculoperitoneal shunting has become more popular. It is not without complications; and because of the reaction of the omentum to a foreign body, obstruction is somewhat more common than with ventriculoatrial shunts. Septicemia is rare, although the incidence of shunt infection from the primary surgical procedure does not markedly differ. Ventriculoperitoneal shunts have large amounts of extra tub-

ing placed in the peritoneal cavity to provide length as the child grows. Peritonitis, subdiaphragmatic abscesses, and peritoneal pseudocysts have all been reported. Catheters have perforated intestine. This complication may be more common with stiff tubing or spring-reinforced tubing. Intestinal obstruction and progressive scarring of the peritoneal cavity, with resultant inadequate absorption of fluid, are rare complications.

Prognosis and Future Developments

The outlook for the child developing hydrocephalus early in life has dramatically improved over the last decade, primarily because of more sophisticated diagnostic techniques that make early detection possible and because of technological innovations that have resulted in better treatment. When hydrocephalus occurs in utero, usually because of aqueductal stenosis or atresia, even with the best postnatal treatment the outlook for intellectual development is relatively poor. Extreme dilatation of the head during development has already destroyed much functional brain tissue. Fortunately, these represent a minority of cases seen clinically. To provide the best opportunity for a normally developing brain, the physician must detect hydrocephalus as soon as it begins and treat it promptly. In pediatric practice, routine head circumference measurements are made, and computerized scanning is used to determine ventricular size when percentile lines are crossed. A slit-valve pressure catheter made of silicone rubber, placed from the ventricular system to the peritoneal cavity, offers a simple, safe, and effective means of treating and immediately relieving hydrocephalus. When properly placed, these shunts can last for several years without need for revision. Once they are in place and the wound has healed, infection is unusual.

With follow-up of large groups of children who have been successfully shunted for many years, additional complications are being recognized. Foltz and Shurtleff[24] reported 12 patients with communicating hydrocephalus who had ventriculoatrial shunts and later showed evidence of aqueductal stenosis or occlusion. This was thought to be related partially to bleeding or infection leading to ependymitis. A second factor might be aqueductal col-

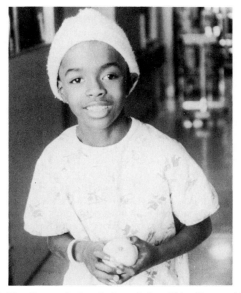

Fig 142–20.—Communicating hydrocephalus. This 10-year-old child has been successfully shunted for her entire life for communicating hydrocephalus resulting from meningitis in infancy. She has a good school record, has a normal IQ, and represents the excellent potential of many children with hydrocephalus.

lapse associated with prolonged ventricular drainage. The so-called syndrome of shunt dependency may be partially related to secondary closure of the aqueduct from reversal of flow or non-flow of fluid through this channel. It is also well known that children who have been shunted for long periods of time develop gliotic ventricles with loss of elasticity. Subsequent shunt failure then leads to what appears to be passage of fluid into the brain substance, cerebral edema, and moderately small ventricles with extremely high intracranial pressure (slit ventricle syndrome). The replacement of shunts in these individuals can be particularly difficult and treacherous.[92] As children grow older, psychiatric problems play a larger role. Headaches are clearly psychogenic in some children, but in others are related to the varying pressures in different postures. A number of devices are coming into use to measure intracranial pressure telemetrically without penetrating the scalp. These offer promise in terms of monitoring the effectiveness of shunts. Many children with treated hydrocephalus lead close to normal lives (Fig 142–20) and have normal or above average IQs.[27, 30] Better understanding of CSF biochemistry and continued technological development in shunting devices offer hope for improved treatment in the future.

Spina Bifida

The term spina bifida was introduced by Nicolaas Tulp in 1641 to define certain congenital malformations of the spine associated with overt cystic protrusions of some of the contents of the vertebral canal. Tulp ("Tulip," the topical pseudonym of Claes Pieterszoon, whose anatomical pursuits were immortalized by Rembrandt) described three cases with cystic lesions and provided two striking plates on which were clearly indicated the prime gross abnormalities. The dire results that followed operation in all three led to his condemnation of the operative approach. He presented the first precise description of the lesion, which had been noted earlier in the same century and was also known in ancient times.

Morgagni[59] recognized the common association with such abnormalities as hydromyelia and hydrocephalus and believed that the bifid spine arose as the result of an erosion by the CSF under increased pressure. This theory is not without its supporters even today, although most would side with Cruveilhier, who in 1832 attributed the process to a frank maldevelopmental error.[101] In 1875, Virchow[98] first defined the syndrome of spina bifida occulta and introduced the term. The report of the London Clinical Society of 1885[76] includes a series of unrivaled plates. These, rather than therapeutic considerations, constitute the main contribution of this classic investigation. Various classifications of the many forms of spina bifida cystica have been proposed, most of them based on the pathologic studies of von Recklinghausen.[100] Local neural concomitants were discussed under the heading of myelodysplasia by Fuchs[29] in 1909.

The surgical results during the 18th century and most of the 19th century were almost entirely catastrophic, although an occasional successful use of snaring, ligation, or aspiration was reported. The attitude of physicians as late as 1885 may be noted in the report of the London Clinical Society,[76] which recommended the use of a local injection technique, such as the application of Dr. Morton's iodoglycerin solution in preference to other techniques (ligation, aspiration, excision) in spite of the fact that 27 of 71 patients died following the use of Morton's method. Present-day techniques evolved through the efforts of such men as Bayer[9] in 1892, von Bergmann[99] in 1899, Brodmann[16] in 1911, and Frazier[26] in 1918. Many needless osteoplastic repairs were fashioned in this same period by Albee[1] and others.

The concept of "status dysraphicus" was introduced by Bremer.[15] The closure defects along the neuraxis were further systematically explored (Tridon[95]) and the neurosurgical approaches analyzed (Lepintre et al.[49]).

Spinal and Cranial Dysraphism

Spina Bifida Cystica

Operable lesions may be subdivided basically into two groups: meningoceles and meningomyeloceles. In either instance, an epithelium-lined sac filled with CSF in free communication with the spinal subarachnoid space is apparent at birth. Nerve roots, and perhaps cord, are incorporated within the walls of the sac in a meningomyelocele, but not in a meningocele. The frequency of overt spina bifida is difficult to ascertain. The classic report of the London Clinical Society[76] of 1885 indicates from two sources a frequency of about one per 1,000 births. More recent reports based on birth records[65, 71] tend to substantiate this figure, although Wallace et al.[103] suggested a lower frequency of about one per 1,500. Two reports[83, 88] covering the neonatal period as well confirm this same general range. Increased incidence has been reported in specific ethnic groups in certain geographic areas. The natural history and the survival of untreated vs. operatively corrected spina bifida cystica patients have been extensively reported by Laurence.[44–47]

Unfortunately, the term spina bifida is variously defined, or not defined at all; and many listings contain separate headings for spina bifida, meningocele, and meningomyelocele. Many occurrences of the clinically occult group are obviously not recorded in any of these studies. Meningoceles may be included under the heading of myelodysplasia because the methods of surgical management are in common and because of the occasional association of remote neural lesions.

CLINICAL PICTURE.—In spina bifida cystica, the newborn child presents with an obvious posterior midline mass containing fluid and usually covered with a thin integument (Fig 142–21,A). This has been classically described as the zona epithelioserosa of von Recklinghausen or, more commonly, the parchment-like membrane. It extends to the base to meet an area of skin (zona dermatica), which frequently is thickened and may be hypertrichotic. The junction is irregular, but usually well defined. The spinal membranes pass into the sac, form its inner lining, and join the epithelial cover in such a way that the layers, readily separable near the neck, are fused at the summit. These large, rubicund, sessile swellings are the common forms; but many other varieties are found. The sacs may be pedunculated, and they may be covered with a layer of full-thickness skin or sometimes with thickened corrugated skin. A considerable quantity of unusual fat may be contained in or beneath the layers of the sac. Occasionally, the serous membrane may lie flush, without a protrusion. About 85% of the total group occur in the lumbar or sacral region. Very rarely, a meningocele protrudes anteriorly and causes symptoms of a mass in the thorax, abdomen, or pelvis. The frequency of such protrusions cannot be accurately estimated. They appear to constitute much less than 1% of the total. Anterior meningoceles are most frequently found in the thoracic and sacral regions. In the thoracic area, they are of particular interest, because they may protrude through an enlarged intervertebral foramen or may be associated with von Recklinghausen's disease. Symptoms of anterior meningoceles may not appear until well into adult life. Anterior sacral meningoceles are more common in girls than in boys.

In most instances, the early attention of the pediatrician is divided between the mass and the manifest neurologic defect. The deficiency is usually in the form of a gross deficit in the functions subserved by the roots of the cauda equina. The preponderance of low spinal lesions and direct local involvement accounts for

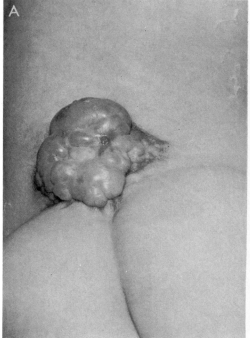

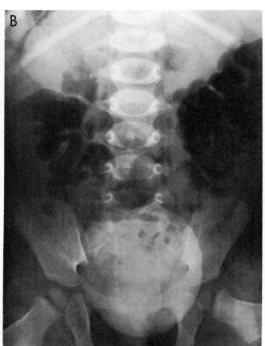

Fig 142–21.—Meningomyeloceles. **A,** lesion in the usual low lumbar position in an infant with virtually complete denervation of the lower limbs and bladder. Note blebs covered with a parchment-like membrane and thickened hypertrichotic skin at the base. Surgery was not indicated because of the neurologic deficit. **B,** roentgenogram showing a large soft tissue mass centered over the sacrum and fusiform dilatation of the spinal canal extending from the third lumbar to first sacral level. Disordered vertebral segmentation is not marked. The only neurologic deficit noted in examination of this infant was mild paraparesis, despite the fact that the cord was drawn into the sac. Operative results were excellent.

this common syndrome. Long tract signs may accompany higher lesions. Preoperative differentiation between the meningocele and the meningomyelocele cannot be based on the size of the lesion or the character of its covering. Occasionally, intramural neural structures may be identified directly or with the aid of transillumination. More often, the proper diagnosis is suggested by the presence or absence of overt neurologic signs. If the lesion is covered with normal full-thickness skin or if it is in the upper thoracic or cervical portion of the spine, it is probably a simple meningocele. A neurologic deficit in association with a simple meningocele points to dysplasia elsewhere in the neural axis. The practical management has been reported in detail elsewhere.[27]

The infant with a meningomyelocele characteristically presents complete or marked lack of motor and sensory function at birth. In general, myelodysraphism in the high lumbar or thoracocervical segments produces a spastic type of motor involvement. The lumbosacral myelomeningoceles manifest themselves with a flaccid type of paraplegia, abolished reflexes, and amyotrophy. Improvement that may appear in the ensuing days or weeks is best explained on the basis of recovery from birth trauma.

Sensory deficits are apparent from the absent or meager response to light pinprick. The lax anal sphincter is recognizable from its gaping appearance and the response to digital examination; in more severe forms, the rectum is prolapsed. Loss of tone in the urethral and vesical sphincters is difficult to discern in the newborn. Such impairment may be suggested in later weeks by dribbling of urine. With major dysraphic states, associated congenital lesions are particularly common. These include clubfoot and hydrocephalus (the most common), dislocation of the hip, absent ribs, exstrophy of the bladder and other anomalies of the genitourinary tract, prolapsed uterus, the Klippel-Feil deformity, congenital heart disease, and umbilical hernia.

The high incidence of clubfoot in association with overt and occult forms of spina bifida strongly suggests a specific relation, although local neural derangements may not be demonstrable. Hydrocephalic states are regularly associated with well-evolved meningomyeloceles, and an associated Arnold-Chiari malformation is the rule. This fact profoundly affects any decision regarding operability. The neural changes associated with spinal dysraphism usually are inaugurated at or before the time of closure of the neural tube between the third and fourth fetal weeks. The results of the early inception of attendant skeletal defects are clearly shown on the roentgenograms.

The most common radiographic finding is a fusiform dilatation of the spinal canal centered at the site of the posterior mass (see Fig 142–21,*B*). The interpeduncular distances are increased over several segments, the pedicles thinned and tilted. Coupled with this are diverse forms of disordered vertebral segmentation. The occult laminar defects so common in older children and adults are not usually apparent in infants. Centers of ossification in the vertebral arches appear between the second and fifth fetal months, but do not fuse to the point of radiographic visibility until the sixth to twenty-fourth month after birth. This fusion is delayed to the fifth year in the upper two cervical segments and upper sacral segments. The diagnosis of an anterior thoracic meningocele may be suggested by the presence of defects in the posterior arches or by kyphoscoliosis. Sacral meningoceles frequently are associated with complete or partial agenesis of the sacrum, at times presenting the roentgenographic picture of the so-called scimitar sacrum (Fig 142–22). The diagnosis of posterior spina bifida cystica is almost never uncertain, although the literature contains references to sacrococcygeal teratomata initially interpreted as meningoceles. Anteriorly situated protrusions must be differentiated from other masses. They may sometimes be demonstrated with myelography.

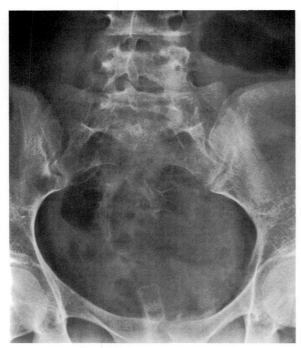

Fig 142–22.—Meningomyelocele showing extensive sacral hypoplasia and widening of the interpeduncular distances.

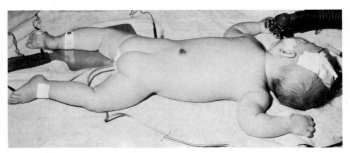

Fig 142–23.—Position on the operating table of a child with diastematomyelia and a small "atretic" meningocele with underlying lipoma.

OPERATIVE TREATMENT.—The operative management of these lesions is quite simple in the sense that the basic surgical principles are plain. These are obliteration of the sac, firm closure of the spinal membranes at the level of the laminae, and adequate skin coverage. However, the indications for such interventions and the selection of the best time for the repairs present problems in many cases.

The approach to a simple, small-based meningocele is quite direct. The operation is carried out in the first days of life.

The tendency now is to carry out many more procedures than previously because of the availability of shunts for hydrocephalus and of potent antibiotic agents. Delayed operation may allow more certain skin closure. Delay is occasionally the appropriate course in the case of meningomyeloceles.

There is now a consensus (Sharard et al.,[84] Rickham and Mawdsley,[77] Hide et al.,[33] Lorber[52, 53]) in regard to an immediate repair of these lesions. It is claimed that, in many cases, axonal conduction was present a few hours after birth, but disappeared during the following days. Aggressive emergency repair was recommended. No valid control series was published. Operation should be postponed in the presence of infection.

Many meningomyeloceles with thin-walled sacs present at birth with impending or actual rupture. In this situation, prompt judgment must be made regarding operative repair. If operation is deferred, the sac should be covered with petrolatum gauze or thin plastic film and protected by circumferential padding and a binder. The importance of the total care of these patients has been stressed by Smith.[86]

Operative Technique.—Repair is carried out with the child prone and the head of the table depressed at least 30 degrees to minimize loss of CSF at the time of incision into the sac (Fig 142–23). A wide operative field, which may include part of the buttocks should skin grafting be anticipated, is prepared and draped. The sac is meticulously cleansed and aspirated with a 22-gauge needle to evacuate the fluid contents slowly until the

sac collapses. Slow aspiration is particularly important in cases of meningomyelocele, in which one may assume some form of the Arnold-Chiari malformation to be present. It seems likely in these circumstances that minor shifts in the neuraxis at the level of the foramen magnum may block a narrow fluid channel and precipitate acute hydrocephalus. If hydrocephalus of significant degree is recognized prior to the planned repair of the myelomeningocele, a prior ventriculoperitoneal shunt may reduce the size of the sac.

A transverse elliptical incision is used for low lumbar masses; a longitudinal incision may be more suitable at higher levels. The incision is made through normal skin at the base, although occasionally portions of the zona dermatica have to be transversed to make closure possible. One may minimize trauma to adherent nerve roots by refraining from the application of manual or other forms of traction to the sac during dissection. The operative microscope and microsurgical instrumentation provide great precision for the surgeon to deal atraumatically with these delicate structures.

The incision is carried down through the subcutaneous tissues to the deep fascia, and the neck of the sac defined with blunt dissection. The defect at the fascial level usually is relatively small and easily exposed. The sac is then freed over all aspects and opened over the dome. The incision, so placed as to avoid neural elements, is extended to expose the contents widely. In the absence of adherent neural filaments, the sac is amputated at the base and a watertight closure obtained with fine silk sutures. The sac is less easily discarded during the repair of a meningomyelocele.

In 1932, Penfield and Cone[68] studied the histology of these membranes and followed the local dispersion of particles of India ink that had been injected into the lumbar subarachnoid space. They assigned a significant proportion of the reabsorptive mechanism for CSF to these membranes and recommended that they be retained. This theory has not gained wide acceptance and remains controversial. However, the application of their operative technique with reference to the reposition of nerve roots within the spinal canal has definite merit. Occasionally, one may find the neurologic status of infants worsened after repair. This may be explained by trauma in nerve root dissection and the manipulation entailed in returning the roots to their usual position. Accordingly, the gentlest dissection is used to free nerve filaments. The use of a stimulating electrical current and the operative microscope helps the surgeon identify the roots. If they are adherent, it is preferable to retain the attached portion of the membrane. If there has been preoperative infection, the potential danger of sepsis from buried portions of contaminated membrane forbids this practice.

The repair is completed with an imbrication of leaves of the lumbodorsal fascia and by an adequate skin closure. The latter repair may be formidable in the presence of a large skin defect

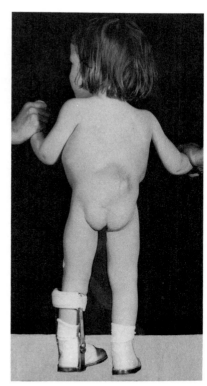

Fig 142–24.—Spina bifida occulta. This 2-year-old child presents many of the common features of the occult group: a mound of bone and zone of hypertrichosis in the lumbar region, atrophy of all muscle groups in the left leg and buttocks, and clubfoot. Of particular interest is the low sacral scar, marking an incision through which an anteriorly protruding sacral meningocele was repaired soon after birth.

ings such as a subcutaneous lipoid tumor, an area of cutaneous telangiectasia, hypertrichosis, an anomalous midline bony prominence or a midline dimple (excluding the common fovea sacralis of the young child) (Fig 142–24). Neural involvement may be manifested by sphincter impairment causing enuresis or persistent urinary tract infection or by motor deficits with pedal deformity, limp, pelvic tilt, or frank muscle palsy. Trophic disturbances may be present, usually in the form of ulcerations on the toes or buttocks.

Roentgenograms of the full spine should be obtained. Myelography is indicated if there is any neurologic deficit or sphincter disturbance (Fig 142–25). A contrast study should also be made

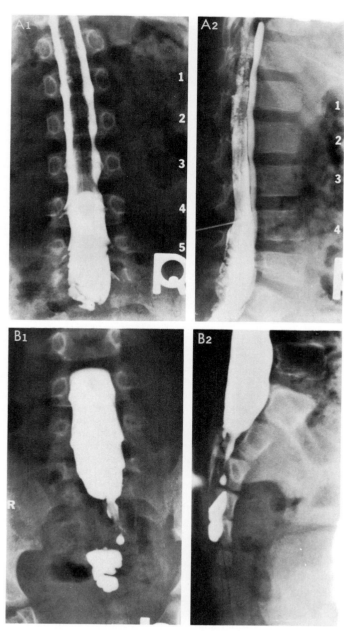

Fig 142–25.—Myelodysplasia. **A,** myelogram through lumbar puncture at L3-4. Posteroanterior **(1)** and lateral view **(2)** showing the presence of a tethered cord and terminal lipoma. **B,** lumbar myelogram supine **(1)** and lateral **(2)**. Note the extremely low position of the dural sac (at S4-5), the presence of tethered cord, enlarged filum terminale, and an irregular, constricting mass (lipoma).

and should be so managed as to allow the skin edges to be brought together without tension. Frequently, large skin flaps may be apposed by the use of relaxing incisions and extensive undermining of the skin. One may use a low dorsal transverse relaxing incision or double-pedicle sliding grafts for larger defects. The latter procedures require the use of split-thickness grafts to cover the denuded areas. The wound is meticulously sealed to avoid contamination. The child is nursed in the prone position on a Bradford frame with the head lowered until the wound has healed. Daily head measurements are mandatory in the postoperative period.

Spina Bifida Occulta

Defects of the laminae, which may be classified as spina bifida occulta, are seen in roentgenograms of the spines of a significant proportion of the general population. Walker and Bucy[102] found these defects to be most common in the low lumbar and sacral regions, where the following incidences were noted: first sacral vertebra, 1.62%; second sacral vertebra, 0.65%; third sacral vertebra, 0.51%; fifth lumbar vertebra, 0.37%.

Myelography and operative intervention are not indicated in the absence of clinical findings. The term spina bifida occulta has a second connotation that refers to the mild forms of dysraphism not accompanied by extrusions of the contents of the vertebral canal. These forms may be recognized in the newborn period or may become apparent only as the child learns to walk or reaches puberty.

The manifestations are similar to, but much less severe than, those accompanying the cystic forms. There may be local find-

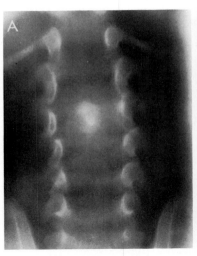
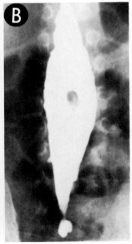
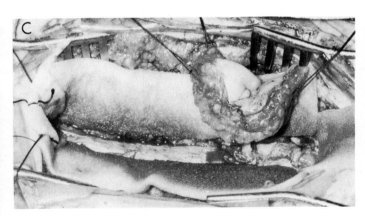
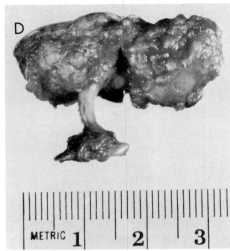

Fig 142–26.—Diastematomyelia in a 6-month-old child. **A,** tomographic cut in anteroposterior projection showing the presence of a midline bony spur at L-2. **B,** myelographic confirmation of diastematomyelia with duplication of cord shadow. **C,** at operation the subcutaneous lipoma is seen to extend through the dura, and the bony spur is located between the two halves of the split cord. **D,** the specimen after the *total* removal of the lesion.

if the diagnosis of diastematomyelia is suggested by the presence of a midline bony spur in the plain films. Hoare[34] has stressed the importance of careful neuroradiologic evaluation to differentiate incomplete, false, and true diastematomyelia (Fig 142–26).

Decision for or against exploratory laminectomy in this so-called occult group is greatly influenced by the results of myelography. Exploration is generally indicated in those cases in which filling defects are found resulting from such space-occupying masses as lipomas, congenital tumors, or intraspinal meningoceles. In certain instances, the normally disproportionate growth of the cord and vertebral axis may be impeded because the cord has been penetrated by or is adherent to a bony spicule (diastematomyelia) (Fig 142–26) or because of a taut filum terminale or previous adhesions (tethered cord). In these circumstances, the bony spur may be removed, the filum sectioned, or the adhesions freed, with a good chance of relief as the cord is untethered. The late results from surgical treatment of the spina bifida occulta group are difficult to evaluate. One of us summarized the importance of early recognition and neurosurgical management of this particular group of children (Udvarhelyi[97]). Long-term follow-up studies (up to 10 years) seem to indicate significant improvement or at least arrest of the previously progressing neurologic, urologic, and orthopedic deficits (Tables 142–1 and 142–2).

The congenital dermal sinus[3] is a form of fusion defect that may or may not be associated with a bifid spine. These tracts, lined with stratified epithelium, may be found at or near the midline at any point along the spinal axis and posterior fossa. They are of particular importance because they may serve as conduits for bacterial contamination to or beneath the dural membrane.

Although complete communication with the CNS is not very frequent (Lepintre and Labrune[48]), careful differentiation between the superficial sacrococcygeal forms, which do not constitute a site of propagated infection, and the penetrating fistulae is of great importance. Children with penetrating fistulae commonly have a history of repeated episodes of unexplained meningitis or findings suggesting a space-occupying intraspinal or intracranial mass such as a subdural abscess or dermoid cyst. It is most important that the dimple associated with the ostium of such a sinus be recognized and that probing and injection techniques *not* be used. The presence of these lesions is an unequivocal indication for early exploration with extirpation of the tract and all of its deep ramifications.

REFERENCES

1. Albee F.H.: Original surgical uses of the bone graft. *Surg. Gynecol. Obstet.* 18:699, 1914.

TABLE 142–1.—SPINAL DYSRAPHISM (LIPOMENINGOCELE): 11 CASES BELOW AGE 5 YEARS

	5 WM	5 WF	5 WM	4½ WM	3½ WM	3 WM	3 WM	1½ WM	¾ WF	½ WF	½ WF	TOTALS (7M:4F)
"Sacral mass" positive cutaneous signs	+	+	+	+	+	+	+	+	+	+	+	11/11
Spina bifida occulta or sacral dysplasia	+	+	+	+	+	+	+	+	+	+	+	11/11
Onset, yr	½	4½	3½	4	3	2½	2	1½	¾	1 mo	1 mo	–
Rectal incontinence	+	±	–	+	–	–	–	+	–	–	–	4/11
Urinary incontinence	±	+	+	+	±	+	–	+	±	+	±	10/11
Motor—upper and lower limbs	–	+	–	–	–	+	–	±	–	–	–	3/11
Motor—lower limbs	+	–	+	+	+	+	±	–	+	+	+	9/11
Sensory deficit	±	+	+	+	+	+	+	+	+	±	±	11/11
Previous surgery	–	+	–	+	–	–	–	–	–	–	–	2/11
Postoperative results and follow-up												
Excellent	4½					4½				7½	4	4
Good			4½				4					2
No change				5½	5½			5½	5			4
Worse		4½										1
Total												11

TABLE 142–2.—SPINAL DYSRAPHISM (LIPOMENINGOCELE): 13 CASES ABOVE AGE 5 YEARS

	21 CF	19 WF	19 WM	16 WM	13 WF	12 WM	11 WF	10 WF	9½ WM	8 WM	7 WM	6½ WM	5½ WM	TOTALS (8M:5F)
"Sacral mass" positive cutaneous signs	+	+	+	+	+	+	+	+	+	+	+	+	+	13/13
Spina bifida occulta or sacral dysplasia	+	+	+	+	+	+	+	+	+	+	+	+	+	13/13
Onset, yr	14	18	16	12	5	9	9	8	3½	7	5½	5½	5½	–
Rectal incontinence	–	+	+	–	–	+	–	–	+	–	–	–	±	5/13
Urinary incontinence	±	+	+	+	+	+	±	+	+	+	±	+	+	13/13
Motor-upper and lower limbs	–	–	±	–	–	+	–	–	+	+	–	±	–	5/13
Motor-lower limbs	+	+	–	+	+	–	±	+	–	+	+	+	+	10/13
Sensory deficit	+	+	+	+	+	+	±	+	+	+	±	+	+	13/13
Previous surgery	+	+	+	+	+	+	–	+	–	+	–	–	–	8/13
Postoperative results and follow-up														
Excellent	6½			5		9½		9			4½			5
Good		7			10		4½					5		4
No change			6						10	3½			8	4
Worse														–
Total														13

2. Alther E.: Die ventriculo-ventriculare Liquor Drainage in der Behandlung des Hydrocephalus. *Acta Neurochir.* 12:26, 1964.

3. Amador L.V.: Congenital spinal dermal sinuses. *J. Pediatr.* 47:300, 1955.

4. Anderson F.M.: Ventriculoauriculostomy in treatment of hydrocephalus. *J. Neurosurg.* 16:551, 1959.

5. Anton and von Bramann: Balkenstich bei Hydrozephalien, Tumoren und bei Epilepsie. *Munch. Med. Wochenschr.* 55:1673, 1908.

6. Arnold J.: Myelocyste: Transposition von Gewebskeimen und Sympodie. *Beitr. Pathol. Anat.* 16:1, 1894.

7. Atkinson J.R., Foltz E.L.: Intraventricular "Risa" as a diagnostic aid in pre- and post-operative hydrocephalus. *J. Neurosurg.* 19:159, 1962.

8. Barry A., et al.: Possible factors in the development of the Arnold-Chiari malformation. *J. Neurosurg.* 14:285, 1957.

9. Bayer C.: Zur-technik der Operation der Spina bifida und Encephalocele. *Prag. Med. Wochenschr.* 17:317, 1892.

10. Bensman A., et al.: Myelomeningocele birth defect: Habilitation of the child. *Minn. Med.* 54:599, 1971.

11. Bhagwati S.: A case of unilateral hydrocephalus secondary to occlusion of one foramen of Monro. *J. Neurosurg.* 21:226, 1964.

12. Biddle A.: Lumbar arachnoid-ureterostomy combining the Matson technique and the Pudenz-Heyer valve: Report of a case. *J. Neurosurg.* 24:760, 1966.

13. Black J.A., et al.: Nephrotic syndrome associated with bacteraemia after shunt operations for hydrocephalus. *Lancet* 2:921, 1965.

14. Bowsher D.: Pathways of absorption of protein from the cerebrospinal fluid. *Anat. Rec.* 218:25, 1957.

15. Bremer F.N.: Die pathologisch-anatomische Begrundung des Status dysraphicus. *Dtsch. Ztschr. Nervenheilk.* 99:104, 1927.

16. Brodmann W.: Ein Beitrag zur Behandlung der Spina bifida. *Beitr. Klin. Chir. Tub.* 76:297, 1911.

17. Carrington K.W.: Ventriculovenous shunt using the Holter valve as a treatment of hydrocephalus. *J. Mich. Med. Soc.* 58:373, 1959.

18. Chiari H.: Ueber Veränderungen des Kleinhirns, des Pons und der medulla oblongata in folge von congenitaler Hydrocephalie des grosshirns (Vienna: F. Tempsky, 1895), in *Clinical Neurosurgery.* Baltimore, Williams & Wilkins Co., 1958, vol. 5.

19. DeLong W.B., Schneider R.C.: Surgical management of congenital spinal lesions associated with abnormalities of the cranio-spinal junction. *J. Neurol. Neurosurg. Psychiatry* 29:319, 1966.

20. Dennis J.P., et al.: Megalencephaly, internal hydrocephalus and other neurological aspects of achondroplasia. *Brain* 84:427, 1961.

21. Dijksterhuis D.F., et al.: Behandeling van hydrocefalie volgens de methode van Pudenz-Heyer (voorlopige mededeling). *Ned. Tijdschr. Geneeskd.* 109:168, 1965.

22. Edwards J.H., et al.: Sex-linked hydrocephalus: Report of a family with 15 affected members. *Arch. Dis. Child.* 36:481, 1961.

23. Ferguson A.H.: Intraperitoneal diversion of the cerebrospinal fluid in cases of hydrocephalus. *N. Y. Med. J.* 67:902, 1898.

24. Foltz E.L., Shurtleff D.B.: Conversion of communicating hydrocephalus to stenosis or occlusion of the aqueduct during ventricular shunt. *J. Neurosurg.* 24:520, 1966.

25. Foltz E.L., Ward A.A. Jr.: Communicating hydrocephalus from subarachnoid bleeding. *J. Neurosurg.* 13:546, 1956.

26. Frazier C.H.: *Surgery of the Spine and Spinal Cord.* New York, D. Appleton & Co., 1918.

27. Freeman J.M.: The shortsighted treatment of myelomeningocele: A long term case report. *Pediatrics* 54:311, 1974.

28. Freeman J.M. (ed.): *Practical Management of Meningomyelocele.* Baltimore, University Park Press, 1974.

29. Fuchs A.: Uber den Klinischen Nachweis kongenitaler Defektbildungen in den unteren Ruckenmarksabschnitten (Myelodysplasie). *Wien. Med. Wochenschr.* 59:2141, 1909.

30. Heffelfinger J.C.: Progressive hydrocephalus: Should it be surgically corrected in institutions for the mentally retarded? *Am. J. Dis. Child.* 103:139, 1962.

31. Heile B.: Zur chirurgischen Behandlung der Spina bifida mit Hydrocephalus. *Berl. Klin. Wehnschr.* 47:2298, 1910.

32. Heile B.: Zur Chirurgischen Behandlung des Hydrocephalus internus durch Ableitung der cerebrospinal flussigkeit nach der Bauchhohle und nach der Pleurakuppe. *Arch. Klin. Chir.* 105:501, 1914.

33. Hide D.W., Williams H.P., Ellis A.L.: The outlook for the child with a meningomyelocele for whom early surgery was considered inadvisable. *Dev. Med. Child. Neurol.* 14:304, 1972.

34. Hoare R.: Incomplete, false and true diastematomyelia: Radiological evaluation by air myelography and tomography. *Radiology* 116(02):349, 1975.

35. Hooper F.: Hydrocephalus and obstruction of the superior vena cava in infancy: Clinical study of the relationship between cerebrospinal fluid pressure and venous pressure. *Pediatrics* 28:792, 1961.

36. Ingraham F.D., Campbell J.D.: An apparatus for closed drainage of the ventricular system. *Ann. Surg.* 114:1096, 1941.

37. Ingraham F.D., Matson D.D.: *Neurosurgery of Infancy and Childhood.* Springfield, Ill.: Charles C Thomas, Publisher, 1954.

38. Jackson I.J., Snodgrass W.: Peritoneal shunts in the treatment of hydrocephalus: 4-year study of 62 patients. *J. Neurosurg.* 12:216, 1955.

39. Kaloss W., Kuhnlein E.: Hydranencephaly. *Am. J. Dis. Child.* 103:99, 1962.

40. Lannelongue M.: De la craniectomie dans la microcephalie. *C. R. Acad. Sci.* 110:1382, 1890.

41. Laurence K.M.: The natural history of hydrocephalus. *Lancet* 2:1152, 1958.

42. Laurence K.M., Coates S.: The natural history of hydrocephalus: Detailed analysis of 182 unoperated cases. *Arch. Dis. Child.* 37:345, 1962.

43. Laurence K.M., Coates S.: Further thoughts on the natural history of hydrocephalus. *Dev. Med. Child Neurol.* 4:263, 1962.

44. Laurence K.M.: The natural history of spina bifida cystica. *Proc. R. Soc. Med.* 53:1005, 1960.

45. Laurence K.M.: The natural history of spina bifida cystica: Detailed analysis of 407 cases. *Arch. Dis. Child.* 39:41, 1964.

46. Laurence K.M.: The survival of untreated spina bifida cystica. *Dev. Med. Child. Neurol.* (suppl.) 11:10, 1966.

47. Laurence K.M.: Effect of surgery for spina bifida cystica on survival and quality of life. *Lancet* 2:301, 1974.

48. Lepintre J., Labrune M.: Fistules dermiques congenitales communiquant avec le systéme nerveux central. *Neurochirurgie* 16:335, 1970.

49. Lepintre J., Pierre-Kahn A., Renier D., et al.: Les dyraphies en neurochirurgie pediatrique. *Med. Infant.* 83(4):415, 1976.

50. Long D.M., et al.: Unusual complication of ventriculo-auriculostomy: Report of two cases. *J. Neurosurg.* 21:233, 1964.

51. Lorber J.: The diagnosis and management of hydrocephalus in infancy. *N.Z. Med. J.* 60:416, 1961.

52. Lorber J.: Results of treatment of meningomyelocele: An analysis of 524 unselected cases with special reference to possible selection for treatment. *Rev. Med. Child. Neurol.* 13:279, 1971.

53. Lorber J.: Early results of selective treatment of spina bifida cystica. *Br. Med. J.* 2:201, 1973.

54. Marburg A.: *Hydrocephalus: Its Symptomatology, Pathology, Pathogenesis and Treatment.* New York, Oskar Piest, 1940.

55. Matson D.D.: A new operation for the treatment of communicating hydrocephalus: Report of a case secondary to generalized meningitis. *J. Neurosurg.* 6:238, 1949.

56. Matson D.D.: Symposium on neurological surgery: Treatment of hydrocephalus. *Surg. Clin. North Am.* 34:1021, 1954.

57. Matson D.: *Neurosurgery of Infancy and Childhood.* Springfield, Ill., Charles C Thomas, Publisher, 1969.

58. McClure R.D.: Hydrocephalus treated by drainage into a vein in the neck. *Bull. Johns Hopkins Hosp.* 20:110, 1909.

59. Morgagni J.B.: *The Seats and Causes of Diseases Investigated by Anatomy: in Five Books, Containing a Great Variety of Dissections, With Remarks.* Alexander B. (trans. ed.). London, A. Miller and T. Cadell, Johnson and Payne, 1769, vol. 1.

60. Nashold B.S. Jr., Mannarino E.: Treatment of hydrocephalus by ureteral-subarachnoid shunt: A 14 year follow-up. *South. Med. J.* 57:270, 1964.

61. Neumann C.G., Hoen T.I., Davis D.A.: The adaptation of ileoentectrophy to the control of congenital communicating hydrocephalus. *Plast. Reconstr. Surg.* 23:159, 1959.

62. Nulsen F.E., Becker D.P.: Control of hydrocephalus by valve-regulated shunt: Infections and their prevention. *Clin. Neurosurg.* 14:256, 1966.

63. Overton M.C. III, et al.: Surgical management of superior vena cava obstruction complicating ventriculoatrial shunts. *J. Neurosurg.* 25:164, 1966.

64. Overton M.C. III, Snodgrass S.R.: Ventriculovenous shunts for infantile hydrocephalus: A review of five years' experience with this method. *J. Neurosurg.* 23:517, 1965.

65. Owens G.: Review of spina bifida and cranium bifidum with follow-up studies of 81 cases. *Am. J. Surg.* 86:410, 1953.

66. Papatheodorou C.A., Teng P.: Air-Pantopague ventriculography in congenital hydrocephalus and myelomeningocele. *Am. J. Roentgenol.* 91:647, 1964.

67. Payr E.: Bemerkungen uber Hydrocephalus. *Arch. Klin. Chir.* 87:801, 1908.

68. Penfield W., Cone W.: Spina bifida and cranium bifidum. *JAMA* 98:454, 1932.

69. Pertuiset B., et al.: Indications, complications et resultats de la ventriculo-auriculostomie dans l'hydrocephalie non tumorale de l'enfant (d'aprés 50 cas). *Neurochirurgie* 10:43, 1964.

70. Picaza J.A.: Posterior-peritoneal shunt technique for treatment of internal hydrocephalus. *J. Neurosurg.* 13:289, 1956.
71. Poole T.R.: Congenital malformations in West Virginia. *W.Va. Med. J.* 56:16, 1960.
72. Pudenz R.A., et al.: Ventriculoauriculostomy: A technique for shunting cerebrospinal fluid into the right auricle; preliminary report. *J. Neurosurg.* 14:171, 1957.
73. Ransohoff J.: Ventriculopleural anastomosis in treatment of midline obstructional neoplasms. *J. Neurosurg.* 11:295, 1954.
74. Ransohoff J., Hiatt R.: Ventriculoperitoneal anastomosis in the treatment of hydrocephalus: Utilization of the suprahepatic space: A preliminary report. *Trans. Am. Neurol. Assoc.* 77:147, 1952.
75. Ransohoff J., Shulman K., Fishman R.A.: Hydrocephalus. *J. Pediatr.* 56:399, 1960.
76. Report of a committee of the London Clinical Society nominated November 10, 1882 to investigate spina bifida and its treatment by injection of Dr. Morton's iodoglycerin solution. *Trans. Clin. Soc. London* 18:339, 1885.
77. Rickham P.P., Mawdsley T.: The effect of early operation on the survival of spina bifida cystica. *Dev. Med. Child. Neurol.* (suppl.) 11:20, 1966.
78. Russell D.S.: Observations on the Pathology of Hydrocephalus, M. Med. Res. Council Spec. Rep. Series. London, His Majesty's Stationery Office, 1949.
79. Russell D.S., Donald C.: The mechanism of internal hydrocephalus in spina bifida. *Brain* 58:203, 1935.
80. Scarff J.E.: Nonobstructive hydrocephalus: Treatment by endoscopic cauterization of the choroid plexus. *J. Neurosurg.* 9:164, 1952.
81. Scott J., et al.: Observations on ventricular and lumbar subarachnoid peritoneal shunts in hydrocephalus in infants. *J. Neurosurg.* 12:65, 1955.
82. Symonds C.P.: Thrombophlebitis of the dural sinuses and cerebral veins. *Brain* 60:531, 1937.
83. Shapiro R.N., et al.: The incidence of congenital anomalies discovered in the neonatal period. *Am. J. Surg.* 96:396, 1958.
84. Sharard W.J.W., Zachary R.B., Lorber J., et al.: A controlled trial of immediate and delayed closure of spina bifida cystica. *Arch. Dis. Child.* 38:18, 1963.
85. Sharkey P.C.: Ventriculosagittal-sinus shunt. *J. Neurosurg.* 22:362, 1965.
86. Smith E.D.: *Spina Bifida and the Total Care of Spinal Myelomeningocele.* Springfield, Charles C Thomas, Publisher, 1965.
87. Sperling D.R., et al.: Cor pulmonale secondary to ventriculoauriculostomy. *Am. J. Dis. Child.* 107:308, 1964.
88. Stevenson S.S., Worchester J., Rice R.G.: 677 congenitally malformed infants and associated gestational characteristics. *Pediatrics* 6:37, 1950.
89. Stookey B., Scarff J.E.: Occlusion of the aqueduct of Sylvius by neoplastic and non-neoplastic processes with a rational surgical treatment for relief of the resultant obstructive hydrocephalus. *Bull. Neurol. Inst.* 5:348, 1936.
90. Swaiman K.W. Wright F.S.: *The Practice of Pediatric Neurology.* St. Louis, C.V. Mosby Co., 1975.
91. Taggart J.K. Jr., Walker A.E.: Congenital stenosis of the foramina of Luschka and Magendie. *Arch. Neurol. Psychiatry* 48:583, 1942.
92. Taylor A.R., et al.: Long-term follow-up of hydrocephalic infants treated by operation. *Br. Med J.* 2:1356, 1960.
93. Torkildsen A.: A new palliative operation in cases of inoperable occlusion of the Sylvian aqueduct. *Acta Chir. Scand.* 82:117, 1939.
94. Torkildsen A.: *Ventriculocisternostomy.* Oslo, Johan Grunndt Tanum Forlag, 1947.
95. Tridon P.: *Les Dysraphies de L'axe Nerveux et de Ses Enveloppes Craniorachidiennes.* Paris, Doin & Co., 1959.
96. Turnbull I.M., Drake C.G.: Membranous occlusion of the aqueduct of Sylvius. *J. Neurosurg.* 24:24, 1966.
97. Udvarhelyi G.B.: Mild forms of spinal dysraphism and associated conditions, in Freeman J.M. (ed.): *Practical Management of Meningomyelocele.* Baltimore, University Park Press, 1974.
98. Virchow R.: Ein fall von Hypertrichosis circumscripta mediana, kombiniert mit Spina bifida occulta. *Ztschr. Ethnol.* 7:279, 1875.
99. von Bergmann E.: Spina bifida. *Int. Clin. Philadelphia* 2:160, 1899.
100. von Recklinghausen F.D.: Untersuchungen über die Spina bifida. *Arch. Pathol. Anat.* 105:243, 1886.
101. Walker A.E.: *A History of Neurological Surgery.* Baltimore, Williams & Wilkins Co., 1951.
102. Walker A.E., Bucy P.C.: Congenital dermal sinuses: A source of spinal meningeal infection and subdural abcesses. *Brain* 57:401, 1934.
103. Wallace H.M., Hoenig L., Rich H.: Newborn infants with congenital malformations or birth injuries. *Am. J. Dis. Child.* 91:529, 1956.
104. Wullenweber R., Kaufer C.: Ergebnisse der Ventrikulocisternostomie nach Torkildsen. *Acta Neurochir.* 9:595, 1961.
105. Yashon D., et al.: The course of severe untreated infantile hydrocephalus: Prognostic significance of the cerebral mantle. *J. Neurosurg.* 23:509, 1965.

Infections of the Nervous System
Donlin M. Long

THE SURGEON'S INVOLVEMENT with infections of the nervous system has been changed dramatically by the computed tomographic (CT) scan. The diagnosis can be made and verified by simple needle aspiration. More and more, this progression, followed by appropriate antibiotic therapy, replaces major operation.

Osteomyelitis of the Skull and Epidural Abscess

Spontaneous infection of the skull is now virtually unknown. It occasionally will complicate frontal, mastoid, or maxillary sinusitis. It is most commonly a complication of systemic infection. Rarely, trauma that has been inadequately treated will also result in osteomyelitis. Infection can be suspected by the presence of tenderness, swelling of the scalp, or sinus drainage, associated with fever and leukocytosis. It is possible to have an infection without systemic effects. The CT scan will demonstrate the presence or absence of epidural or subdural abscess and define areas of bone destruction. Bone destruction will usually appear within 2–3 weeks after the onset of a serious infection. The local area may be aspirated to culture the organism involved. Lumbar puncture is unnecessary unless the patient has clear-cut evidence for meningitis.

In most cases without a bone flap or fracture fragments, antibiotic therapy alone will be adequate. Infected bone flap or infected fragments will usually have to be removed. At operation, the area is irrigated thoroughly. Intravenous antibiotics are administered until the infection is healed. When the bone is seriously infected, debridement followed by antibiotics is usually adequate therapy. The choice of antibiotics and to some extent the duration of treatment depend upon the organism and should be based upon culture and sensitivity results, with an assessment of the virulence of the organism involved in the infection.

Extradural Abscess

When osteomyelitis occurs, it is not unusual to have an extradural collection of pus. The CT scan demonstrates this very clearly. Headache is the most common symptom. There may be fever and leukocytosis. If the abscess becomes large, the patient may exhibit signs and symptoms of increased intracranial pressure. The treatment is surgical evacuation, irrigation, and subsequent therapy with antibiotics.[4]

Subdural Abscess

The subdural abscess is a much more serious problem. In the past, the mortality rate was extremely high; but it has fallen because of improvements in diagnosis and in antibiotic therapy. Infants and children are more likely to develop subdural abscess than adults. Purulent meningitis (chiefly in infants) and paranasal sinusitis or otitis media are the most common causes. The symptoms begin with severe headache and fever; but focal seizures, the development of focal neurologic deficits, and declining level

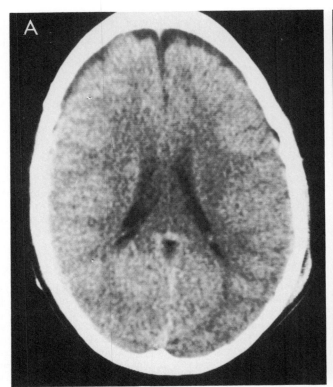

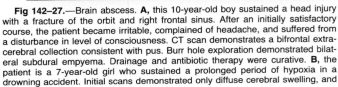

Fig 142–27.—Brain abscess. **A,** this 10-year-old boy sustained a head injury with a fracture of the orbit and right frontal sinus. After an initially satisfactory course, the patient became irritable, complained of headache, and suffered from a disturbance in level of consciousness. CT scan demonstrates a bifrontal extracerebral collection consistent with pus. Burr hole exploration demonstrated bilateral subdural empyema. Drainage and antibiotic therapy were curative. **B,** the patient is a 7-year-old girl who sustained a prolonged period of hypoxia in a drowning accident. Initial scans demonstrated only diffuse cerebral swelling, and the patient remained comatose. Intracranial pressure was monitored by means of an indwelling catheter for approximately 5 days. Two months later, the patient's neurologic status deteriorated. CT scan demonstrates a left frontal cystic lesion with an enhancing ring-like capsule consistent with brain abscess. The *dotted line* and *x* represent the CT-controlled trajectory of the tap for biopsy of the lesion. Aspiration proved this to be an abscess, and antibiotic therapy brought satisfactory resolution.

of consciousness follow quickly. This is a serious disease, and the patients are ill. The CT scan is the definitive way to make the presumptive diagnosis. Therapy requires immediate drainage. In infants, needle puncture of the subdural space may be satisfactory. In older children, burr holes are made to drain the fluid (Fig 142–27,A). When adequate drainage is not possible with a few well-placed burr holes, extensive craniotomy with removal of the infection is the best therapy. Intravenous antibiotics are then continued. The duration of antibiotic therapy will again depend upon the type of organism and the patient's response. Fortunately, the recurrence of pockets of infection can now be reliably assessed with CT scan.[4]

Brain Abscess

The sources of brain abscess are many. Most commonly in children, they are hematogenous, having spread from another infection. Direct extension, with or without venous thrombosis, commonly complicates chronic ear infection and paranasal sinusitis. Open trauma, particularly that inflicted by gunshot wound, is also a common cause. Brain abscesses rarely complicate osteomyelitis and meningitis. In a significant number of cases, no source of infection can be found.[5]

Brain abscesses occur throughout the brain, more or less in relation to the blood supply and the anatomy of the petrous bone and paranasal sinuses. Abscesses that arise from these focal areas tend to be in the immediate proximity of the bony infection. Hematogenous abscesses spread in the distribution of the major vessels, the majority in the middle cerebral complex. Multiple abscesses are common. Symptoms may occur from the mass, from edema of the brain, and from associated venous thrombophlebitis.

The most common presenting symptom is headache. Other nonspecific signs of increased intracranial pressure such as nausea, vomiting, and lethargy are common. Seizures may be associated. Fever is not typical. Neurologic deficits may occur, but a declining level of consciousness is more common than focal signs. Leukocytosis is not consistently present. The CT scan has removed most of the concern in the diagnosis of abscess (see Fig 142–27,B). Multiple lesions are identified. The localization of the major lesion is accurate. Brain edema can be assessed, and the effect upon underlying brain anatomy is clearly demonstrated. Lumbar puncture is not commonly necessary now, and the need for other diagnostic aids is quite uncommon.[3]

Surgical Management

In the past, three basic techniques have been advocated for the management of brain abscess. (1) Total removal by craniotomy had many advocates. (2) Needle aspiration and irrigation with antibiotics through a catheter left in the abscess cavity was a common technique. Needle aspiration through a burr hole utilizing EEG control was advocated as well.[2] The CT scan has now become the determining therapeutic technique. (3) It is currently our policy to utilize, whenever possible, needle puncture and drainage, using the CT scan to be certain that adequate resolution of the abscess occurs. The technique is as follows. The abscess is visualized on CT scan. The child is taken to the operating room; under general anesthesia, a needle through a burr hole is directed into the abscess. The contents are at least partially aspirated, and cultures are taken. Gram stain will give an immediate indication of the type of organism. It is important to remember that anaerobic and aerobic cultures both should be carried out and that fungal and tuberculosis cultures are also important. Appropriate intravenous antibiotic therapy begins. Unless the patient has meningitis, there is no need to consider intrathecal therapy. Regular CT scans based upon the patient's apparent response to therapy will demonstrate gradual resolution of the abscess cavity. Occasionally, a rapidly expanding mass may require more direct therapy, and craniotomy still can be indicated; but it is most unusual now to have to perform a craniotomy in the management of abscess.

The choice of antibiotics is based upon the identification of the organism and the reports of culture and antibiotic sensitivities. The period of time required for antibiotic use has not been established. Most recommend a course of at least 3 weeks of intravenous antibiotics and 3 additional weeks of oral antibiotics if the CT scan shows adequate resolution of the abscess.[1]

In the period of time before the abscess organism is identified, it is necessary to give general coverage. The antibiotics currently employed most commonly are penicillin and metronidazole. The change to specifically appropriate antibiotics should be utilized as quickly as they are identified.

Infections of the Spinal Epidural Space

Spinal epidural infection is rare in children and is commonly secondary to disc space infection, vertebral bacterial osteomyelitis, or tuberculosis. Spinal infections, uncommon in the very young child, usually have spread from elsewhere in the body.[6]

Most spinal epidural infections occur in the thoracic or lumbar space. The patients usually have fever and leukocytosis. Pain and tenderness may be present, but it is more common that the patient has a febrile illness followed by the development of a progressive neurologic deficit without other symptoms. X-ray films may be entirely normal. A soft tissue mass is more likely to be present than is a bony abnormality. The CT scan will demonstrate any bony changes, disc changes, and the soft tissue abnormalities more reliably than plain films. A large paravertebral soft tissue mass is highly suggestive of tuberculosis. Diagnosis and therapy depend upon the patient's situation. A rapidly progressive neurologic deficit demands urgent care. A CT scan with intrathecal contrast may be carried out to demonstrate the level of spinal cord compression. The CT scan allows the location of the abscess and the direction of compression of the spinal cord to be accurately assessed. The surgical procedure may then be undertaken to provide maximum access and decompression. The mass discovered may be pus, in which case drainage and irrigation will be adequate. However, even with bacterial infections, a kind of granulomatous mass may occur, which must be removed virtually like a tumor. Whether or not to drain the wound will depend upon the amount of pus present. In general, primary closure is satisfactory, and treatment with appropriate antibiotics should then continue. Antibiotic therapy should begin empirically, using the same antibiotics as for brain abscess until the infecting organism is identified. Therapy of 4–6 weeks is required.

The role of operation in infection of the nervous system has declined significantly, and the magnitude of the procedures required for diagnosis and therapy has also decreased. The neurosurgeon should retain primary charge, but the best results are achieved by collaborative efforts between neurosurgery and consultants in infectious disease.

REFERENCES

1. Black P., Graybill J.R., Charache P.: Penetration of brain abscess by systemically administered antibiotics. *J. Neurosurg.* 38:705, 1973.
2. Carey M.E., Chou S.N., French L.A.: Experience with brain abscess. *J. Neurosurg.* 36:1, 1972.
3. Cheek W.R.: Brain abscess: Diagnosis and treatment, in *Concepts in Pediatric Neurosurgery.* Basel, Switzerland, Karger, 1982, pp. 205–215.
4. Farmer T.W., Wise G.R.: Subdural empyema in infants, children and adults. *Neurology* 23:254, 1973.
5. Idriss Z.H., Gutman L.T., Kranfol N.M.: Brain abscesses in infants and children. *Clin. Pediatr.* 17:738–746, 1978.
6. McLaurin R.L.: Spinal suppuration. *Clin. Neurosurg.* 14:314, 1967.

Aneurysms and Arteriovenous Malformations
Donlin M. Long

THE MAJOR neurologic vascular problems in children are arteriovenous malformations, aneurysms, and occlusive diseases of the major intracranial vessels. Arteriovenous malformations are the most common.[1,8] Surgical therapy of these malformations has improved dramatically in the recent past. Particularly in older children, successful obliteration of malformations has become the rule.[3,9,10,11] The addition of catheter embolization techniques and intraoperative occlusion using adhesives are important advances.[3] Vascular reconstruction is an uncommon need in children. However, the improvement in microvascular surgical technique now makes it possible to carry out bypass operations to provide additional blood to the brain even in children. Even so, the arteriovenous malformation remains the major focus for pediatric vascular surgery.

Intracranial Arterial Aneurysms

Aneurysms are much less common in children than in adults. Laitinen[7] reported that 1.3% of all patients with aneurysms were less than 15 years old. Only one was less than 10 years old. It is clear that the ruptured aneurysm in the child has the same grim prognosis as it does in the adult. However, it is equally clear that aneurysms are much less common in children and represent only about 1% of all aneurysms.

Clinical Features

The clinical features of subarachnoid hemorrhage and intracranial arterial aneurysms are well recognized. There appear to be no special characteristics of these lesions in children. The distribution around the circle of Willis is also approximately the same as for adults. The reported series suggest that aneurysms in children are often accompanied by massive subarachnoid hemorrhage, that there is increased incidence of intracerebral hematoma, and that recovery from a precarious state is more likely to occur.

Diagnosis and Treatment

Diagnosis of subarachnoid hemorrhage is quite straightforward. The clinical combination of signs and symptoms, including severe headache, a stiff neck, cranial nerve abnormalities, evidence of increased intracranial pressure, and focal neurologic deficit, is similar to the syndrome seen in adults. Subarachnoid hemorrhage is verified by lumbar puncture. If there is any question concerning the validity of the puncture, it is profitable to collect multiple tubes of fluid. In a true subarachnoid hemorrhage, the blood remains mixed with the fluid throughout the

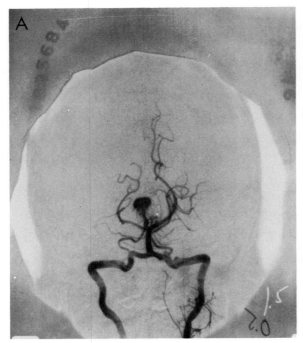

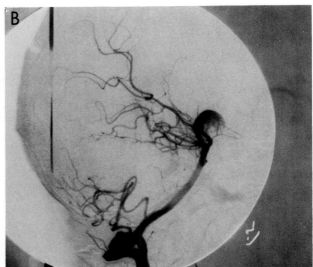

Fig 142–28.—Basilar apex aneurysm presenting in a 13-year-old child. **A,** anterior posterior and **B,** lateral vertebral angiogram. The child suffered a spontaneous subarachnoid hemorrhage and recovered. At operation, the aneurysm was found to arise from the basilar apex and from the origin of the left posterior cerebral artery. The aneurysm was clipped, and the child recovered without deficit.

collecting tubes. If a traumatic tap has occurred, there will be progressive clearing of the fluid. It is also possible to spin down the fluid and investigate the supernatant for xanthochromia, a sign of earlier hemorrhage. Definitive evaluation requires angiography (Fig 142–28). Patients in whom a ruptured aneurysm is suspected should undergo four-vessel angiography, preferably by the femoral route. Direct carotid or brachial angiography may also be acceptable.

Operative Therapy

Definitive treatment of aneurysms in childhood is particularly important. The expected long lifespan in these patients makes it imperative to obliterate the aneurysm permanently if at all possible.

Standard craniotomy with intracranial clipping of the aneurysms is the procedure of choice. The results of operation appear to be approximately the same as with the more common aneurysm in the adult population. Children have a greater capability for recovery from serious neurologic injury, but aside from this capability no improved prognosis occurs in children as contrasted with adults.

Timing of the operation is important. That children tend to present with serious neurologic deficits and tend to have a greater incidence of intracerebral hematomas influences the decision for operation. It is generally wise for the surgeon to wait a few days after hemorrhage to allow recovery to a significant extent before operating on patients who do not harbor intracerebral hematomas or have acute hydrocephalus. If an intracerebral hematoma is present, emergency operation is often necessary. A definitive attack upon the aneurysm may or may not be carried out when the hematoma is evacuated.

Children exhibit an increased tendency to develop hydrocephalus at least for a short time following massive subarachnoid hemorrhage. Ventriculoatrial shunting may be necessary as an additional procedure to provide the greatest degree of improvement for these patients.

Arteriovenous Malformations

The most common intracranial vascular lesion is the arteriovenous malformation. This abnormality is more common in adults, but improved angiographic techniques and greater awareness of the problem are increasing the number of these lesions discovered in children.

Arteriovenous malformations are complex vascular lesions composed of many abnormal vessels. There are large feeding arteries, a tangled mass of abnormal interconnecting vessels, which gradually merge into tortuous thin-walled venous channels that tend to collect for drainage into huge veins, which drain either to the deep midline system or, superficially, into the great venous sinuses.

Symptoms and Signs

In the newborn child, a giant arteriovenous malformation presents with a specific triad of symptoms. Cardiac failure is the single most common finding. When this is associated with a large or enlarging head and an intracranial bruit, the diagnosis of a giant intracranial arteriovenous malformation is almost certain. These huge malformations, which become symptomatic in early infancy and childhood, may be of two types. The first is located in the midline, usually draining into the great vein of Galen. The second is lateral, usually in the distribution of the middle cerebral artery or in the posterior fossa, and drains into large lateral venous channels.[2, 8]

In older children, the majority of lesions are detected following spontaneous subarachnoid hemorrhage. The hemorrhage may be of any degree; intracerebral hematomas regularly complicate the rupture of the arteriovenous malformation. The next-most-common presentation is the epileptic seizure. A third im-

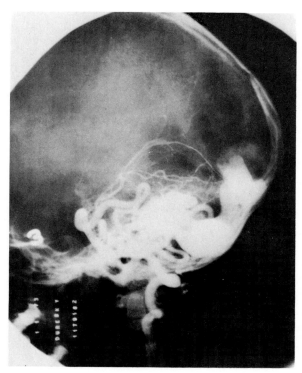

Fig 142–29.—Arteriovenous malformation; lateral vertebral angiogram. Large laterally placed arteriovenous malformation involving the left cerebellar hemisphere of a 6-year-old girl. The patient presented with a subarachnoid hemorrhage. At operation, extirpation of the malformation was possible even though the brain stem was partially involved. The child had a stormy postoperative course, but recovered completely and is now without neurologic deficit.

portant symptom is recurrent or persistent headache, often severe. Children with progressive mental deterioration in the absence of some other cause should be examined for the possibility of an arteriovenous malformation producing progressive ischemia of the cortex.

Diagnosis

The diagnosis of subarachnoid hemorrhage or seizures is straightforward and has already been discussed. Plain skull x-ray films are unlikely to be of value. Computerized axial tomography or a brain scan may show a mass, but this is certainly not definitive. Cerebral angiography is the definitive diagnostic method. Four-vessel angiography, preferably by the femoral route, should be carried out, with special emphasis upon identification of all major feeding and draining vessels.

Operative Treatment

Improvement in operative techniques for arteriovenous malformations continues. The operating microscope has proved to be the major factor in permitting definitive treatment of these lesions.[9] Recently, there have been dramatic improvements in other forms of therapy. It is now possible, using flow-directed catheters, to direct emboli accurately into the feeding vessels of many malformations. Small intravascular balloons may be so utilized to occlude large feeding vessels. Techniques of intravascular adhesive injection are just being developed, and the method is feasible for some lesions. Intraoperative embolization or occlusion of major vessels with vascular adhesive under direct vision is an important new technique.[3] Nevertheless, improved understanding of the surgical anatomy of the arteriovenous malformation and refinements in microsurgical operative technique are responsible for the greatest advances in the management of these lesions.[14, 15]

The primary indications for operation are serious or recurrent spontaneous subarachnoid hemorrhage, particularly with the presence of a significant intracerebral blood clot, incapacitating headache, evidence of increased intracranial pressure, focal seizures, the development of focal neurologic deficit, and intellec-

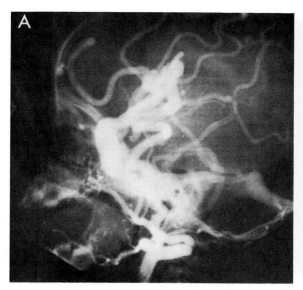

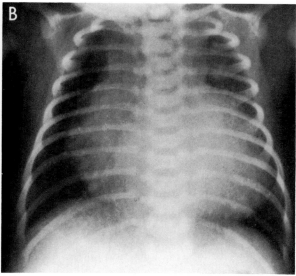

Fig 142–30.—Huge middle cerebral arteriovenous malformation in a 7-month-old child. The patient had a large head and intracranial bruit and had suffered chronic congestive heart failure since birth. **A,** carotid angiogram. At operation, the malformation was found to be separate from intrinsic brain vasculature and was easily removed. The child recovered without difficulty and suffered no neu-rologic deficit. **B,** the chest x-ray film of the same child demonstrates massive enlargement of the heart. The child had been in congestive heart failure since birth. Postoperatively, the heart failure was controlled easily, and the heart has since returned to normal size.

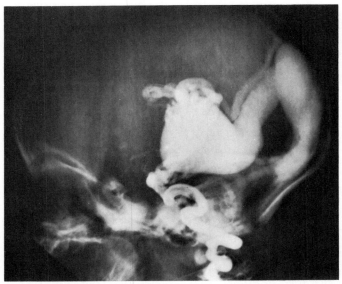

Fig 142–31.—Vein of Galen malformation—lateral vertebral angiogram. This newborn child presented with intractable cardiac failure. The cardiac angiographer noted enlarged vessels leaving the aortic arch and studied both carotid and vertebral circulations. The arteriovenous malformation is characterized by the large feeding vessels that enter the dilated great vein of Galen on its dorsal surface. Feeding vessels from both anterior cerebrals and both middle cerebral arteries were demonstrated by carotid angiography. At operation, the feeding vessels were carefully divided, and the blood volume was lowered simultaneously. The patient tolerated the procedure well. Unfortunately, approximately 18 hours after surgery, intractable cardiac failure developed, the patient suffered a cardiac arrest and could not be resuscitated. When cardiac failure is present at birth, the prognosis with or without operation is very poor.

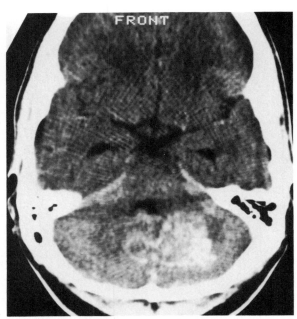

Fig 142–32.—The CT scan demonstrates an enhancing mass in the left cerebellar hemisphere. The serpiginous enhancements around it clearly suggest an arteriovenous malformation. This 16-year-old patient suffered the acute onset of a severe headache and disequilibrium while skiing. She was rushed to the hospital, where she was found to have marked cerebellar ataxia, a stiff neck, and paralysis of gaze. The CT scan suggested hematoma from arteriovenous malformation. An angiogram was confirmative. The patient was operated on and the lesion totally removed without difficulty.

tual or behavioral deterioration. The assessability and configuration of the malformation are the most important factors.[11, 12] It is important to obliterate completely the arteriovenous connections. It is rarely worthwhile merely to ligate feeding vessels. Recurrence of malformations following partial treatment is well documented; and, whenever possible, complete obliteration is the surgical method of choice. The goal of operation is total excision of the malformation with minimal sacrifice of normal brain tissue (Fig 142–29 and 142–30). This is usually possible with the malformations that are lobar in nature and with the giant malformations of childhood that are laterally placed, particularly those deep in the Sylvian fissure and in the posterior fossa. Deeply placed malformations that occupy critical positions in the brain and giant malformations that drain to the great vein of Galen may not be amenable to total excision (Fig 142–31).[4, 13] In these locations, obliteration of the arteriovenous connections may be all that is possible. The embolic techniques are usually not curative alone, but they have been utilized with great advantage as an adjunct to operation.

The surgical technique utilized for the excision of arteriovenous malformations does not differ from that employed in most vascular surgical procedures. It is now recognized that the malformations can be treated virtually as extracerebral collections, and it is relatively easy to remove them without serious injury to surrounding brain (Fig 142–32). Of course, this is not always possible, and the critical factor is the configuration of the malformation. The giant malformations of childhood present special difficulties. The circulating blood volume is increased,[6] and in newborns cardiac failure is common. It is important that the malformation be obliterated slowly so that the stressed heart will not be overburdened with a suddenly increased load to pump against an increased peripheral resistance when the shunt is

obliterated.[5] This is particularly important in lesions that drain posteriorly into the great vein of Galen. The operating microscope, microsurgical techniques, bipolar coagulation, and the preoperative and intraoperative techniques of embolic or intravascular adhesive occlusion have greatly improved the outlook for all these children. However, newborns with aneurysms of the great vein of Galen, in whom the need for operation is precipitated by cardiac failure, are rarely salvaged; and their operative management remains a challenge.[4, 13]

REFERENCES

1. Brunelle F.O., Harwood-Nash D.C., Fitz C.R., et al.: Intracranial vascular malformations in children: Computed tomographic and angiographic evaluation. *Radiology* 149(2):455–461, 1983.
2. Drake C.C.: Surgical removal of arteriovenous malformations from the brain stem and cerebellopontine angle. *J. Neurosurg.* 43:661, 1975.
3. Epstein F., Beranstein A.: Pediatric vascular anomalies: Combined neurosurgical and neuroradiological intervention, in *Concepts in Pediatric Neurosurgery*. Basel, Switzerland, Karger, 1981, pp. 49–68.
4. Hoffman H.J., Chuang S., Hendrick E.B., et al.: Aneurysms of the great vein of Galen, in *Concepts in Pediatric Neurosurgery 3*. Basel, Switzerland, Karger, 1983, pp. 52–74.
5. Jedeikin R., Rowe R.D., Freedom R.M., et al: Cerebral arteriovenous malformation in neonates: The role of myocardial ischemia. *Pediatr. Cardiol.* 4(1):29–35, 1983.
6. Lakier J.B., Milner S., Cohen M., et al.: Intracranial arteriovenous fistulas in infancy—haemodynamic considerations. *S. Afr. Med. J.* 61(7):242–245, 1982.
7. Laitinen L.: Arteriella aneurysm med subarachnoidalblödning hos barn. *Nord. Med.* 71:329, 1964.
8. Long D.M., Seljeskog E.L., Chou S.N., et al.: Giant arteriovenous malformations of infancy and childhood. *J. Neurosurg.* 40:304, 1974.
9. Malis L.I.: Arteriovenous malformations of the brain, in Youmans J.R. (ed.): *Neurological Surgery*, ed. 2. Philadelphia, W.B. Saunders Co., 1982, vol. 1, p. 1786.
10. Martin N.A., Edwards M.S.B., Wilson C.I.B.: Management of in-

tracranial vascular malformations in children and adolescents, in *Concepts in Pediatric Neurosurgery 4*. Basel, Switzerland, Karger, 1983, pp. 264–290.

11. Mazza C., Pasqualin A., Scienza R., et al.: Intracranial arteriovenous malformations in the pediatric age: Experience with 24 cases. *Childs Brain* 10(6):369–380, 1983.

12. Mori K., Murata T., Hashimoto N., et al.: Clinical analysis of arteriovenous malformations in children. *Childs Brain* 6(1):13–25, 1980.

13. Pasqualin A., Mazza C., Da Pian R., et al.: Midline giant arteriovenous malformations in infants. *Acta Neurochir.* 64(3-4):259–271, 1982.

14. Schauseil-Zipf U., Thun F., Kellermann K., et al.: Intracranial arteriovenous malformations and aneurysms in childhood and adolescents. *Eur. J. Pediatr.* 140(3):260–267, 1983.

15. Takashima S., Becker L.E.: Neuropathology of cerebral arteriovenous malformations in children. *J. Neurol. Neurosurg. Psychiatry* 43(5):380–385, 1980.

Miscellaneous Neurosurgical Conditions
Donlin M. Long

Conditions of Increased Intracranial Pressure That Require Neurosurgical Intervention

HERPES SIMPLEX ENCEPHALITIS occurs in all age groups, but certainly may be seen in children. There usually has been a febrile illness, followed by the slow development of mental obtundation that may or may not be associated with focal neurologic deficit. The temporal lobe is the most common site of the lesion, but other lobes may be involved as well. Computerized axial tomography makes the diagnosis relatively simple.[5] In such a situation, the child is found to have lucency in the temporal lobe, and the diagnosis is then highly suspect (Fig 142–33). The diagnosis is confirmed by brain biopsy, which will demonstrate characteristic inflammatory changes of acute encephalitis in association with Cowdry type A intranuclear inclusion bodies. Culture of the virus is definitive. A greater than fourfold rise in serum titer of herpes simplex virus antibodies is diagnostic, but of no therapeutic use, because treatment must be started early. The newer antiviral agents show great promise in salvaging these patients. At one time, there was no treatment, and the disease was virtually uniformly fatal or at least catastrophic. Now successfully treated cases have been reported. Spontaneous recovery is virtually unknown in any patient who has become comatose. It is important to start immediate therapy with an antiviral agent. Biopsy can follow if done within 24 hours. The treatment may be supplemented with the use of osmotic diuretics to reduce brain swelling and intracranial pressure. In most patients, the intracranial pressure should be monitored before and following biopsy, and throughout early therapy when the patient remains seriously ill. An osmotic diuretic such as mannitol, 1 gm/kg given intravenously on a regular basis to reduce swelling, will be advantageous. The duration of action of the mannitol may be increased by the judicious use of furosemide. In the past, decompressive craniotomy has been recommended. However, this is rarely done now. When the patient's intracranial pressure cannot be controlled easily, it is much more common to carry out temporal lobectomy early in the course of the disease.

Reye Syndrome

Reye syndrome is an acute encephalopathy, characteristically associated with dramatically increased intracranial pressure.[13]

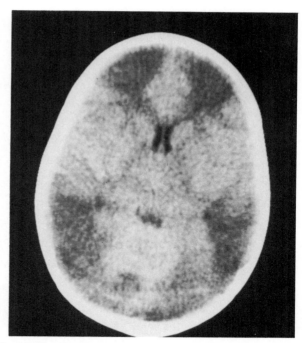

Fig 142–33.—Herpes encephalitis. This 1-year-old boy presented to the Johns Hopkins Hospital with a suspected diagnosis of meningitis. However, lumbar puncture yielded clear fluid under high pressure without the expected cellular changes. CT scan demonstrated multiple areas of lucency of both frontal lobes, the inferior temporal lobes, occipital lobes, and cerebellum bilaterally. Biopsy of right frontal lobe demonstrated changes consistent with herpes encephalitis. The diagnosis was proved by subsequent culture of the organism. Antiviral therapy, begun immediately, was ineffective in this far advanced case.

The problem usually complicates a flu-like viral respiratory illness in a previously well child. Typically, there is a history of several days of vomiting, following which the child develops agitation, confusion, and progressive deterioration of mental function, culminating in coma. There is a significant rise in pressure, and internal herniations are common. The cause of the intracranial pressure is massive brain edema, and the focal neurologic deficits are primarily related to internal herniations from brain edema. The syndrome is associated with a panlobar microfascicular hepatic deterioration, which is in turn associated with a significant increase in blood ammonia.[12] Encephalopathy is progressive, and the liver enlarges. Abnormalities of liver function and elevated blood ammonia will usually lead to liver biopsy, which confirms the diagnosis. Treatment consists of control of intracranial pressure and all necessary supportive care. A pressure monitor should be placed, preferably subdural, because the massive brain swelling makes the placement of a ventricular drain difficult, and the duration of the disease further complicates the use of ventricular drainage. Patients require intubation and respiratory care. Brain swelling may be reduced by the use of osmotic diuretics. Steroids are not known to be effective. Supportive care includes intravenous infusion of 10–15% glucose solutions, peritoneal dialysis, and exchange transfusion when indicated. Overhydration and excess sodium worsen the brain edema. Strict control of intracranial pressure is the key to survival. When the neurologic picture progresses in spite of all appropriate medical therapy, decompressive craniectomy can be carried out on an emergency basis. Extensive bifrontal craniotomy has been used successfully in treating patients with Reye syndrome, but medical therapy has improved sufficiently that it is now unusual to employ a surgical procedure.

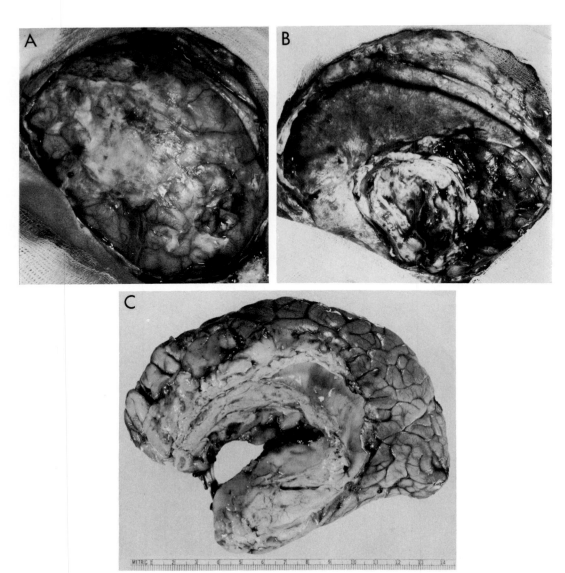

Fig 142–34.—Hemispherectomy for hemicranial hypoplasia. At about age 2 years, the patient was comatose for 5 days, and soon thereafter an operation was done to remove a blood clot on the brain. Since then, the patient has had left hemiplegia and a convulsion beginning in the left arm every day. **A,** appearance of the cerebral cortex. **B,** the empty supratentorial region after hemispher- ectomy showing the falx, medial surface of the left frontal lobe and central nubbin representing the remaining basal ganglions. **C,** medial surface of the ablated hemisphere. In the years since hemispherectomy, the patient has had no attacks while awake and only a few nocturnal seizures. Hemiparesis is no more pronounced than before the operation, and behavior has improved greatly.

Lead Poisoning

The neurosurgeon is occasionally involved in the therapy of lead poisoning because of the severe degree of brain edema, increased intracranial pressure, and severe encephalopathy. Lead poisoning is most common in disadvantaged children and usually is ingested from paint or inhaled when battery casings are burned as fuel. Lethargy, weakness, seizures, and acute encephalopathy are the principal symptoms. A definitive diagnosis is verified by an increased lead content in the blood and urine. Coproporphyrins are usually increased in the urine and provide an early clue to the diagnosis. Study of the peripheral blood will demonstrate a reduced hemoglobin concentration and basophilic stippling of red cells. There may be a lead line on the gums, and lead lines at the epiphysis are seen in some chronic cases.

The treatment now is usually medical. Control of seizures is necessary. Intravenous diphenylhydantoin (Dilantin) is most commonly employed, but phenobarbital or diazepam (Valium)

are reasonable choices as well. Treatment of the increased intracranial pressure is next in importance. Glucosteroids (dexamethasone) are given intravenously for the control of brain edema. The loading and maintenance doses depend upon the size of the child, but a loading dose of 3–10 mg and maintenance doses of 1–4 mg intravenously every 6 hours are typical. Steroids may be supplemented with osmotic diuretics for short-term control of intracranial pressure. The decompressive craniectomies employed in the past have been virtually eliminated by improvements in medical therapy. The definitive treatment is chelation and removal of the lead. As the lead is eliminated, the brain edema will gradually relent, and the outcome for these children is now excellent.[10]

Operations for Epilepsy

There is an increasing interest in the surgical therapy of seizures in younger children. At one time, it was believed that op-

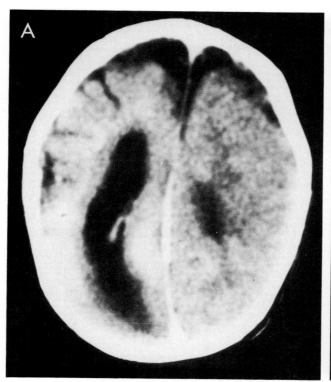
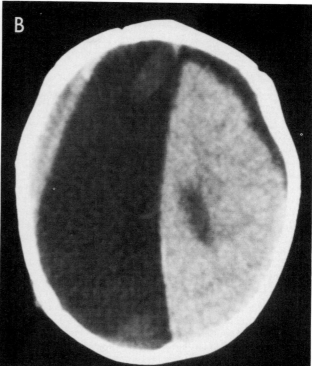

Fig 142–35.—This 1-year-old child had suffered from intractable seizures since birth. Intensive medical treatment failed to control her almost continuous seizure activity. Hemispherectomy was elected in the hope of preserving some function in the most normal-appearing frontal lobe. **A,** the CT scan demonstrates the enormous loss of substance of the left hemisphere with hydrocephalus. **B,** the CT scan illustrates the total removal of the abnormal hemisphere. No neurologic deficit attended this removal.

erations for seizures should not be carried out in children, because many outgrow the problem. It is now recognized that a small number of patients are good candidates for early operative control of seizures, and there is reasonable evidence that this early control of seizures will prevent some brain deterioration.

Infantile Hemiplegia and Hemispherectomy

A number of children undergo massive injury to one hemisphere in utero; significant injury to the brain may also follow perinatal trauma or hypoxia. An acute febrile illness, carotid arteritis or occlusion, and head injury are causes. Many of these patients suffer from intractable seizures and show progressive personality disturbances in addition to the expected hemiplegia and sensory loss.[14]

Characteristically, computed tomography (CT) scan demonstrates one shrunken deformed hemisphere with a large ventricle. Frequently there is an associated porencephalic cyst. Middle cerebral artery occlusion is commonly demonstrated on angiogram. The middle cerebral artery occlusion is seen most commonly in those who have apparently suffered an in utero or perinatal event. When the syndrome follows an acute febrile illness, it more commonly is associated with diffuse vascular abnormalities; porencephaly is rare.

Obviously, medical control of seizures is preferable to any surgical intervention; however, many of these patients are difficult to control or may show a progressive neurologic deficit secondary to a chronic encephalitis. In such instances, removal of the damaged cerebral hemisphere may be curative (Figs 142–34 and 142–35). The neurologic deficit is rarely increased; when it is worsened, slow recovery is the rule. Seizure control is excellent, and the personality disturbance usually improves as well. The

most common postoperative complication has been the development of hydrocephalus.[7]

Section of the Corpus Callosum

Some children with a less seriously damaged hemisphere, for whom hemispherectomy is not feasible, may benefit from disconnection of the two hemispheres by division of the corpus callosum. Again, medical therapy is always indicated and must be exhausted before operative therapy is contemplated. Patients with a strikingly abnormal hemispheral electrical abnormality and secondary generation of seizures across the corpus callosum are reasonable candidates for this procedure. The operative technique is much simpler than hemispherectomy, and division of the corpus callosum rarely produces a neurologic deficit in these children. Control of seizures may be excellent.[9]

Temporal Lobe Epilepsy

Some young children suffer from intractable psychomotor seizures that seriously interfere with their function and education. It has been unusual to treat these patients with surgical excision, because many will improve with time. However, there is an occasional patient whose incapacity is so great that early removal of the temporal lobe is indicated. The clinical situation should be desperate and the localization of the temporal lobe lesion accurate before any such surgical approach is contemplated.[6]

Focal Cortical Excision for the Control of Seizures

Seizures generated from any abnormal area of the brain may be controlled through focal cortical excisions. The same principles obtain as in adults. The abnormality must be well defined electrically and must be in an area in which removal will not produce an unacceptable neurologic deficit. Medical therapy must have failed, and the seizures must be incapacitating enough to warrant the surgical procedure. In such situations, careful excision of abnormal tissue may be very beneficial.

Stereotactic Surgery for Movement Disorders

Until quite recently, stereotactic surgery for movement disorders, particularly in children, had steadily reduced in importance. The advent of computed axial tomographic control of stereotaxis and the introduction of new physiologic monitoring techniques have reawakened some interest in this field. Stereotactic lesions in the basal ganglia, thalamus, and subthalamus have been utilized to provide symptomatic relief from rigidity, spasticity, and dyskinesia in cerebral palsy victims. Stereotactic destructive procedures have been utilized most commonly for dystonia musculorum deformans. There has been significant experimental work with electrical stimulation of the cerebellum and upper spinal cord for these same disorders, but these remain investigational techniques at the present time.[2, 11]

The Herniated Lumbar Intervertebral Disc and Related Problems

Low back pain is not a common complaint in childhood. When disk herniation occurs in teenagers, it is commonly associated with trauma. The spontaneous complaint of low back pain is frequently associated with an underlying congenital abnormality, particularly spondylolisthesis. Several large series reporting diskectomy in patients of all age groups illustrate the rarity of the syndrome in children. The disc herniation is virtually unknown below teenage years. The symptoms are identical to those of adults, but radicular leg pain appears to be even more striking than is usual in the adult. With spondylolisthesis, the herniation occurs characteristically at L-5, S-1 and may involve either root. Conservative care should always be undertaken, but is unlikely to be beneficial when true radicular pain is present. Treatment consists of removal of the herniated disc. These patients do extremely well, and recurrences are rare. Intradiscal therapy with chymopapain may be utilized, but the results of chymopapain injection in children are not yet known.[3, 4]

REFERENCES

1. Ausman J.I., Rogers C., Sharp H.L.: Decompressive craniectomy for the encephalopathy of Reye's syndrome. *Surg. Neurol.* 6:97, 1976.
2. Balasutramaniam V., Kanaka T.S., Ramanujam P.M.: Stereotaxic surgery for cerebral palsy. *J. Neurosurg.* 40:577, 1974.
3. Barghoom J., Hensell V.: Surgical treatment of herniation of a lumbar intervertebral disc in young people. *Dtsch. Med. Wochenschr.* 101:1185, 1976.
4. Beks J.W.F., ter Weeme C.A.: Herniated lumbar discs in teenagers. *Acta Neurochir.* 31:195, 1975.
5. Brodtkorb E., et al.: Diagnosis of herpes simplex encephalitis: A comparison between electroencephalography and computed tomography findings. *Acta Neurol. Scand.* 66(4):462–471, 1983.
6. Fisher R.S.: Surgical therapy of complex partial epilepsy. *Johns Hopkins Med. J.* 151(6):332–343, 1982.
7. French L.A., Johnson D.R., Brown I.A., et al.: Cerebral hemispherectomy for control of intractable convulsive seizures. *J. Neurosurg.* 12:154, 1955.
8. Green J.R., Sidell A.D.: Neurosurgical aspects of epilepsy in children and adolescents, in Youmans J.R. (ed.): *Neurological Surgery*, ed. 2. Philadelphia, W.B. Saunders Co., 1982, vol. 1, p. 3858.
9. Luessenhop A.J.: Interhemispheric commissurotomy: As an alternate to hemispherectomy for control of intractable seizures. *Am. Surg.* 36:265, 1970.
10. McLaurin R.L., Nichols J.B.: Extensive cranial decompression in the treatment of severe head encephalopathy. *Pediatrics* 20:653, 1957.
11. Ojemann G.A., Ward A.A.: Abnormal movement disorders, in Youmans J.R. (ed.): *Neurological Surgery*, ed. 2. Philadelphia, W.B. Saunders Co., 1982, vol. 1, p. 3821.
12. Partin J.C.: Reye's syndrome (encephalopathy and fatty liver). *Gastroenterology* 69:511, 1975.
13. Sarnaik A.P.: Diagnosis and management of Reye's syndrome. *Compr. Ther.* 8(10):47–53, 1982.
14. Shillito J.: Carotid arteritis: A cause of hemiplegia in childhood. *J. Neurosurg.* 21:540, 1964.

143 Paul P. Griffin
Congenital Deformities

Congenital Dislocation of the Hip

CONGENITAL DISLOCATION of the hip (CDH) is a multifaceted problem in which there are unresolved issues concerning the cause and the most effective technique of treatment, as well as inadequate explanation for a certain incidence of poor results, regardless of how well the child is thought to have been treated.

The incidence given for the United States is 1.5/1,000 live births, but it is greater in other countries and is recorded as 1.7/1,000 live births in Sweden[10] and 1.55/1,000 live births in England, although certain sections of England seem to have a higher incidence.[1] There is a problem with reporting the incidence of CDH, because one out of 60 newborns has an unstable hip, according to Barlow.[1] However, 60% of these hips become stable in the first week without any treatment, and 88% are stable by the end of 2 months without treatment. One could look upon this as an indication that the incidence is higher than 1.5/1,000, but that most infants recover spontaneously from their dislocatable hips, reflecting some differences in the capsular structure in these children, or in their environment, from those in whom the hip remains dislocated. Incidence of CDH is very rare in Africans, perhaps related to the historical way the African infant has been carried on the mother's back or side with the hips abducted. This may have some influence on the incidence of dislocations; but in black Americans the incidence is also extremely low, and it is rare indeed to find a dislocated hip in a black male. Girls are more frequently affected than boys at a ratio of about 4:1. The cause of CDH has not been completely worked out, but it is apparently multifactorial. There is a genetic aspect, and 20–30% of children with dislocated hip have a positive family history. The incidence in siblings of patients with a dislocated hip or in children of a mother with a dislocated hip is much greater than that in the general population. Beyond the genetic aspects, hormonal and mechanical factors come into play. Ligamentous and capsular laxity must play a part in the stability of the hip. This laxity may be temporary, from the influence of high levels of estrogen or relaxin in the mother. Both of these substances may affect the capsule's ability to resist the mechanical forces that tend to dislocate the hip. The mechanical forces are exerted in several ways. The left hip rests in adduction in the typical in utero position and is the most frequently dislocated. Babies delivered in the breech position have a higher incidence of dislocation than do those in the vertex presentation. The incidence of dislocation in the breech position is 16%. The first-born children and pregnancies with oligohydramnios have a higher incidence of dislocated hips. There is, therefore, a group of babies who are at risk and who should receive exceptionally close scrutiny at birth and for several months afterwards to make certain the hips are stable. This group includes infants with a positive family history, breech presentations, firstborn females, and those with oligohydramnios. Infants with several of these high-risk factors should not only have very close physical examination, but radiographic evaluation as well.

Diagnosis

The diagnosis of congenital dislocation can, in most instances, be made at birth.[10] However, MacKenzie and Wilson[6] reported a 0.11 incidence of late diagnosis. It is my belief that there are hips that dislocate later as a result of an acetabular dysplasia with asymmetry of adduction-abduction of the two hips, and a pelvic obliquity produced by an abduction contracture on the contralateral side. At birth, and in the first few weeks after birth, the diagnosis can generally be detected by close examination of the hips, and specifically by the Ortolani maneuver. This maneuver is performed with the examiner facing the baby, the hips flexed 90 degrees, with the examiner's hands on the thighs so that the fingers rest on the trochanter and the thumb on the medial side of the thigh (Fig 143–1). If the hip is dislocated, it can be felt to reduce as the hip is abducted and can be seen and felt to dislocate as the hip is adducted. The instability of the hip may be so great that there is little sensation of reduction on abduction or of dislocation on adduction, and in such instances the examiner may have difficulty in making the diagnosis. At the time of the examination of the hip, the baby must be relaxed and not crying, because the resistance of the child to being manipulated can make it impossible to feel the femoral head enter and leave the acetabulum.

The so-called teratologic dislocated hip, a hip in which the dislocation occurred very early in fetal life, may not reduce on the Ortolani maneuver and can only be diagnosed on x-ray film. Teratologic dislocations are usually associated with other generalized musculoskeletal conditions, and in such infants x-ray films of the hips should be considered.

The radiograph of a dislocated hip in the newborn may appear normal. The hip, which has the ability to go in and out of the acetabulum, may be resting in the reduced position at the time the x-ray film is made and therefore appear normal. However, in some, the proximal metaphysis is seen to be displaced laterally and, on occasion, even slightly superior to the acetabulum (Fig 143–2).

From the above, it is apparent that in the newborn the diagnosis is made on physical examination simply by testing the stability of the hip. There is no asymmetry of folds, nor limitation of motion, in the typical dislocated hip in the newborn. The diagnosis should be confirmed by radiographs if possible. After several weeks, the diagnosis becomes easier in the unilateral dislocations, because the asymmetry of the gluteal folds associated with a pelvic obliquity and an apparent leg length discrepancy are usually present (Fig 143–3). The asymmetry of gluteal folds is not diagnostic of dislocation, because it is also present in congenital abduction contractures, with or without acetabular dysplasia.[4] The frequency of a positive Ortolani sign decreases with time, but the test is positive for the first 3 months in over 50%. In older infants in whom the Ortolani is negative, the diagnosis is suggested by the asymmetry of abduction-adduction, prominence of the trochanter, asymmetric gluteal folds, and an abductor lurch gait if the child walks.

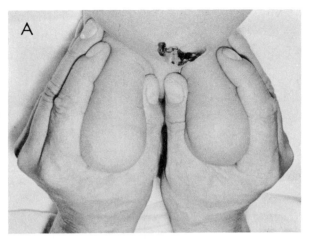

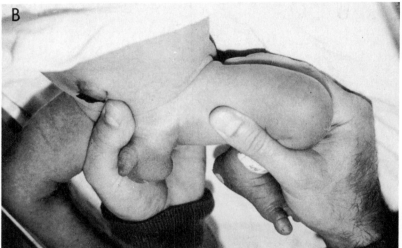

Fig 143–1.—Congenital dislocation of the hip (CDH). **A,** the correct positioning of the hands on the thigh and the hip to initiate Ortolani's maneuver. From this position, the thighs are abducted. If the hip is dislocated, it can be felt to relocate upon abduction. After abducting the hip, return to the adducted position and the hip can be felt to dislocate. As it does a "clunk" can be heard. **B,** some prefer to test one hip at a time. One hand is used to hold the pelvis and the other to abduct and adduct the hip.

Treatment

The treatment of CDH depends upon the reducibility, the degree of instability, and the age of the child. In the armamentarium of the orthopedic surgeon are the Pavlic harness or other types of abduction orthoses, traction, cast, and operative treat-

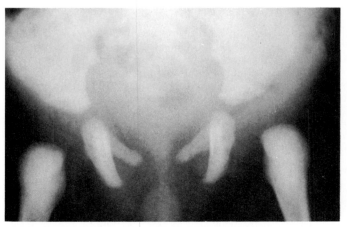

Fig 143–2.—CDH. This anterior-posterior roentgenogram of a newborn shows the left hip to be wide. Ortolani's test was positive.

ment. The simplest method of treatment that has a reasonable likelihood of being effective should be the treatment of choice. The most effective and most satisfactory treatment is in the newborn infant, in whom most of the hips will reduce and be stable with the Pavlic harness.[5] In infants less than 6 months of age, with a positive Ortolani sign, the Pavlic harness has a success rate of better than 80%, in our experience. If, in this age group, 0–6 months, the dislocated hip cannot be reduced by simple flexion and abduction (that is, the Ortolani test is negative), it is still reasonable to try the Pavlic harness. If in such patients the hip has not reduced by 3–4 weeks, the harness should be discontinued. If the hip is reduced by the Pavlic harness, but remains unstable after 5 or 6 weeks in spite of wearing the Pavlic harness full-time, the hip should be immobilized in a spica cast. In the treatment of a dislocated hip, it is important that the Pavlic harness be applied appropriately and that it be worn full-time until the hip is stable (Fig 143–4). Most hips are stable after 5 or 6 weeks, and when they are stable the Pavlic harness can be removed for baths and other care; but it should be worn essentially full-time for 3 months. If at 3 months the x-ray films show the development of the acetabulum is approaching normal and, by clinical examination, the hip is stable, the Pavlic harness can be discontinued during the day and worn only at night for another few weeks.

In the correct application of the Pavlic harness, the straps are tightened to pull the hip into flexion of 80–90 degrees for the

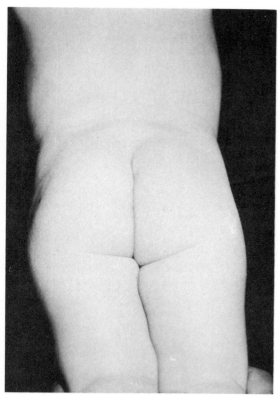

Fig 143–3.—CDH. The gluteal clefts are asymmetric, with the left higher (the dislocated side). This same clinical feature is present in the unilateral dysplastic hip.

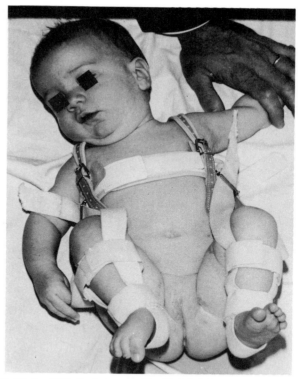

Fig 143–4.—CDH. Pavlic harness. The hip is held flexed above 90 degrees, but not above 110 degrees. The medial and lateral straps should be held together near the knee, because if they separate too far distally the effect will be to flex the knee acutely and externally rotate the hip.

first week. After the first week, the strap should be adjusted to hold the hips flexed around 100–110 degrees. The posterior strap should always be loose enough so that the hips can adduct almost to neutral. Great care should be taken in adjusting the posterior straps, because, if they hold the hip in excessive abduction, the blood supply to the femoral head can be compromised sufficiently to cause avascular necrosis.

The Pavlic harness should not be a part of the treatment in children whose diagnosis is made at 6 months or later. Children under 6 months of age who have a negative Ortolani sign, and all other children with congenital dislocation of the hip who are under 18 months of age, should have an initial period of traction prior to undergoing closed reduction. In the young infant, traction of the Bryant type is preferred because of the ease with which the position is maintained. The legs initially are suspended at 90% flexion and 10–20 degrees abduction and then gradually abducted to 60 degrees over the next 7 days. Two weeks of this type of traction are usually sufficient to reduce most hips. In the older child, or in the child whose femoral head is riding cephalad to the acetabulum, longitudinal traction of the split Russell type is preferred. This traction should be used for 2–3 weeks, or at least until the femoral head has been pulled distally and is level to or below the triradiate cartilage.[3] The incidence of avascular necrosis following reduction without prior traction approaches 40–50%.

Closed reduction is done under general anesthesia and should require little more than flexion of the hips to 100% with abduction while lifting the femur forward with finger pressure behind the trochanter. At this point, the very critical decision has to be made as to whether or not the hip is stable in a safe position that does not compromise circulation of the femoral epiphysis. If the

hip requires maximum abduction to be stable, closed reduction cannot be accepted, because maximum abduction will obstruct blood supply to the femoral head. The hip must be stable at 90 degrees of flexion, and if it becomes dislocated when flexion is reduced to 90 degrees while held abducted 45–50 degrees, the stability of the reduction is insufficient. The hip must then be immobilized in a position of stability, which, in general, is 100 degrees of flexion, and abduction somewhere between the maximum abduction and the point of adduction at which the hip dislocates. Should more than 45–55 degrees of abduction be required to maintain the reduction, the reduction cannot be accepted. If, at 45–55 degrees of abduction, the adductor muscles are tight, a subcutaneous release of the adductor longus is advisable to reduce the pressure on the head. With the hip flexed 100 degrees and abducted 45–55 degrees, there should be neither deleterious compression of the head of the femur against the infolded labrum and the acetabulum, nor occlusion of the circumflex vessels supplying the femoral head. After the reduction is accepted as being in a safe position, a cast is applied. The hip is held in the desired position as a spica cast is applied from the nipple line to just above the ankles. If, at the time of closed reduction, the surgeon believes the hip is too unstable to remain reduced at the desired position as described above, he has the choice of returning the child to traction for a short period of time and of closed reduction later, or of proceeding to an open reduction. It is vital that the reduction not be lost after the cast is applied, because immobilization with the femoral head dislocated is deleterious to the femoral head and to the hip joint in general. An AP film of the hip is usually not sufficient to determine with accuracy the position of the femoral head in the acetabulum. A computerized tomographic evaluation is probably the

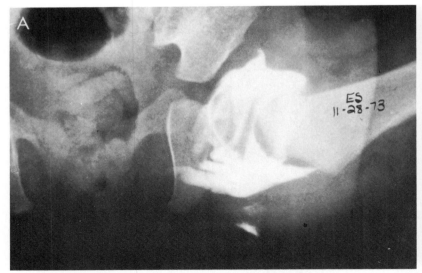
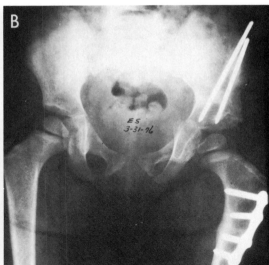

Fig 143–5.—CDH. **A,** arthrogram on 14-month-old patient with CDH. Labrum deformed into joint; isthmus narrow. Hip was stable in a safe degree of abduction and flexion. Patient was held in cast 6 months. **B,** 3 years later, innominate os- teotomy and femoral osteotomy were required because of failure of acetabulum to improve.

most accurate way of determining the position of the femoral head in the acetabulum after the cast has been applied.

The major obstruction to reduction and stability of the hips is the isthmus in the capsule and the infolded labrum. If the labrum is deformed and prevents the femoral head from proper contact with the triradiate cartilage, the acetabulum will not develop as it should.[8] Because a hip may feel adequately reduced and sufficiently stable to accept the femoral head at the time of reduction and still have the infolded labrum between the head and the acetabulum, an arthrogram is required before accepting the reduction and applying a cast (Fig 143–5). If the femoral head does not rest beneath the labrum, the author does not accept the closed reduction as adequate and proceeds to an open reduction.

After 18 months of age, there is small likelihood of successful closed reduction without an inordinately long period of immobilization and additional operation upon either the proximal femur or the acetabulum. In these patients, open reduction is generally the procedure of choice. In children under 3 years of age, the open reduction should be preceded by a period of traction, to facilitate the reduction at operation. The stretching of the pericapsular structures and tendons also reduces pressure across the femoral head. Open reduction of a dislocated hip is a very demanding operation. There is no opportunity like the first to obtain a concentric and stable reduction that has the potential for progressively improving until the hip approaches normal.

In the open reduction, a transverse anterior incision just below the superior iliac spine is an excellent approach as the incision heals, so that one can barely detect a scar. The incision is made as follows. Develop the interval between the tensor fasciae latae and sartorius in the usual way for the anterior approach. Split the apophysis of the ilium along the center and pull each half away from the bone. Strip the muscles subperiosteally from the inner table and outer surfaces of the ilium. Divide the reflected head of the rectus and retract the rectus, exposing the capsule. After the superior, anterior, and inferior portions of the capsule are well exposed and the inferior portion of the acetabulum can be felt, open the capsule anteriorly in T fashion along the neck and along the edge of the acetabulum, about 1 cm lateral to the labrum. Further expose the joint by removing the ligamentum teres from the head of the femur and from its inferior attach-

ment. All of the pulvinar except a small portion in the center of the acetabulum is removed.

It is important that the labrum be reflected so that the articular cartilage posteriorly, superiorly, and anteriorly can be visualized. The transverse acetabular ligament is always tight and should be divided. Once the acetabular ligament is divided and the articular cartilage visualized in its entirety, the acetabulum is ready to accept the femoral head. The head is reduced into the acetabulum and should be stable and seat well. If, with the hip abducted 15–20 degrees and slightly internally rotated, the head is not well covered, additional measures should be taken to improve the stability. One may choose to operate on the femur and perform a varus osteotomy with some external rotation of the distal fragment, or to operate upon the acetabulum. When the contour of the acetabulum matches the femoral head, but is maldirected, an innominate osteotomy, as described by Salter,[9] is the procedure of choice. If the acetabulum is long and oblique so that, in spite of the head being down in the center of the acetabulum, there is a space superior and lateral, it is apparent that redirecting the acetabulum would still leave a lateral recess into which the femoral head could migrate. In such cases, a Pemberton osteotomy of the ilium would be preferable,[2,7] whether on the pelvic side or on the femoral side. If, with the hip abducted and internally rotated, the hip is stable and the femoral head is well covered, femoral osteotomy is the procedure to increase stability. When, after reduction of the head into the acetabulum, the head is not adequately covered by reasonable abduction and rotation, the coverage and stability should be improved by an innominate osteotomy.

In children who are over 3 years of age, the period of traction required to bring the hip distally is such that the osteoporosis that occurs in the interval of traction may very well compromise the results; and in them, for this reason, traction is not used. The open reduction is done without traction, and to decompress the hip an osteotomy is performed at the level of the lesser trochanter. The acetabulum should be managed the same way as described above. With the femoral head reduced into the acetabulum, that portion of the femoral shaft that overlies the proximal fragment is excised, so that the proximal fragment is medially rotated on the distal fragment and placed in some varus. The degree of varus should never be more than 115–120 degrees.

At the completion of the reduction, the capsule is closed in a pants-over-vest technique, with the superior lateral flap sutured to the medial rim of the capsule distally and medially so as to keep the femoral head pulled distally, and medially rotated. This also obliterates the capsular space over the false acetabulum where the head had been prior to the open reduction.

The hip should be immobilized with a spica cast for 6 weeks. The position of immobilization, determined before the capsule is closed, is the position in which the reduction is stable. A night splint to keep the hip in abduction, for several months after the cast is removed, may be beneficial to the development of the acetabulum.

In children diagnosed early and treated with a Pavlic harness, prognosis is excellent, 80% being successful. Those who fail with the Pavlic harness still have a good chance of obtaining a good result by further immobilization in plaster. If the diagnosis is late, most children still do well with accurate reduction, whether closed or open, and with the additional osteotomies as needed. The postimmobilization follow-up is most important. After the reduction, the acetabulum very rapidly improves for the first year in almost all cases where the reduction has been concentric. After 1 year, in certain patients, the development of the acetabulum appears to cease. In these children, additional operation is indicated to improve the coverage of the femoral head, the relationship of the femoral head to the triradiate cartilage, and the direction of the acetabulum. Procrastination, once it has been determined that the acetabulum has shown no improvement for a year, will lead only to a femoral head-acetabulum relation inadequate to prevent further difficulties in adult life.

REFERENCES

1. Barlow T.G.: Early diagnosis and treatment of congenital dislocation of the hip. *J. Bone Joint Surg.* 44B:292–301, 1962.
2. Eyre-Brook A.L., Jones D.A., Harris F.C.: Pemberton's acetaluloplasty for congenital dislocation or subluxation of the hip. *J. Bone Joint Surg.* 60B:18–24, 1978.
3. Gage J.R., Winter R.B.: Avascular necrosis of the capital femoral epiphysis as a complication of closed reduction of congenital dislocation of the hip: A critical review of twenty years experience at Gillette Children's Hospital. *J. Bone Joint Surg.* 54A:373, 1972.
4. Green N.E., Griffin P.P.: Hip dysplasia associated with abduction contracture of the contralateral hip. *J. Bone Joint Surg.* 64A:1273–1281, 1982.
5. Kalamchi A., McFarlane R. III: The Pavlic harness: Results in patients over 3 months of age. *J. Pediatr. Orthop.* 2:3–8, 1982.
6. MacKenzie I.G., Wilson J.G.: Problems encountered in early diagnosis and management of congenital dislocation of the hip. *J. Bone Joint Surg.* 63B:38–42, 1981.
7. Pemberton P.A.: Pericapsular osteotomy of the ilium for treatment of congenital subluxation and dislocation of the hip. *J. Bone Joint Surg.* 47A:65–86, 1965.
8. Renshaw T.S.: Inadequate reduction of congenital dislocation of the hip. *J. Bone Joint Surg.* 63A:1114–1121, 1981.
9. Salter R.B.: Innominate osteotomy in the treatment of congenital dislocation and subluxation of the hip. *J. Bone Joint Surg.* 43B:518–539, 1961.
10. Rosen S. Von: Diagnosis and treatment of congenital dislocation in the newborn. *J. Bone Joint Surg.* 44B:284–291, 1982.

Proximal Focal Femoral Deficiency (PFFD) (see Chap. 145)

Focal deficiency of the proximal femur is an uncommon but severe abnormality. It is apparently the result of an unknown insult to the limb bud. The extent of the deficiency varies from a short femur to almost complete absence.[4]

Four problems are to be addressed in the child with focal deficiency of the proximal femur: discrepancy in limb length, stability of the hip, malrotation, and poor musculature.

The initial treatment should be limited to an appropriate shoe lift when the child begins to walk. In Type 1, a valgus osteotomy

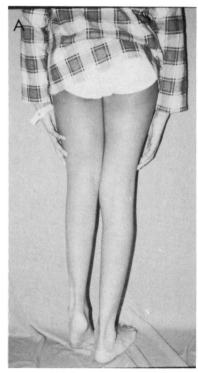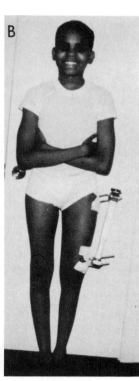

Fig 143–6.—PFFD. A, a teenage boy with a 7-cm discrepancy with type 1 PFFD. A good candidate for correction by lengthening. **B,** the patient had a 7-cm lengthening of the short femur by the Wagner technique. Here he is at the completion of the lengthening and just prior to removal of the lengthening apparatus.

to correct the coxa vara should be done around 3 years of age. It is important that the coxa vara be completely corrected, but it does not have to be overcorrected as in congenital coxa vara. Close observation of the rate of inhibition or deficiency in growth is needed to predict the expected discrepancy in limb length at maturity. Measurement of the length of the femur should be made yearly. If the discrepancy is predicted to be 2 inches or less, the length problem should be solved by an epiphysiodesis of the opposite femur at the appropriate skeletal age. With a prediction that the discrepancy will be greater than 2 inches, femoral lengthening should be considered. Multiple operations are required to lengthen a congenital short femur. It is a formidable experience for the patient, and the family must understand the many procedures and problems inherent in the leg lengthening operation. In type 1, the hip is stable, and the only issues to address are the coxa vara and shortness of the femur (Fig 143–6).

In types 2 and 3, correction of the coxa vara and pseudarthrosis can be obtained by valgus osteotomy, bone grafting, and internal fixation.[3] In the young child, the leg length discrepancy is managed by a prosthesis. In the 18-month or 2-year-old child, a below-the-knee prosthesis functions well. Later, an above-knee type prosthesis with a hinged knee is needed. The most satisfactory definitive management of the limb discrepancy in types 2 and 3 is arthrodesis of the knee with appropriate resection of bone and a Syme amputation of the foot, calculated to bring the end of the stump 2 inches above the opposite knee at maturity. An above-knee prosthesis is fitted after the knee fusion is solid. Better function can be obtained by a Van Ness procedure than by a Syme amputation.[1] If the Van Ness procedure is done (rotation osteotomy in which the foot and ankle are rotated 180 degrees so that the foot and ankle can extend the knee of the prosthesis), the ankle should be at the level of the opposite knee. With the Van Ness procedure, a below-the-knee prosthesis is used, and the gastrocnemius-soleus muscle becomes the extensor of the knee. If the Van Ness procedure is to be done, it should be the initial procedure at around 5–6 years of age, followed in a year by the proximal femoral osteotomy. After another year or two, the knee resection and arthrodesis should be done. The Van Ness will recur and have to be repeated.[1]

King[2] has described a technique that corrects the proximal deformity in types 2 and 3 and gives fixation to the resected knee until the proximal pseudarthrosis is healed and the arthrodesis of the knee is solid. When the intermedullary space of the femur and tibia are large enough to accept an 8-mm Küntscher rod, King's operation can be carried out. In this procedure, the knee is resected and the Küntscher rod passed down the tibia to exit the sole of the foot. The resected knee is reduced and the rod driven proximally into the femur. An intertrochanteric osteotomy is done to correct the varus of the proximal femur and the rod driven across the osteotomy and into the neck and head. No graft is used. After the osteotomy, the femoral neck ossifies rapidly. A Syme amputation is performed after the arthrodesis at the knee is solid, when the rod is removed. Following the King procedure, the flexion external rotation deformity of the hip disappears over a period of several months.

In Panting's types 4 and 5, procedures upon the proximal femur are not recommended. A one-segment extremity the length of the opposite thigh is the goal of treatment in these two types. After resection of the knee and arthrodesis, the flexion-external rotation deformity of the hip gradually corrects. A Syme amputation or Van Ness procedure can be done simultaneously with arthrodesis of the knee, which gives better control of the extremity and the prosthesis.

REFERENCES

1. Hall J.E.: Personal communication.
2. King R.E.: Surgical correction of proximal femoral focal deficiencies. *Inter-Clin. Info. Bull.* 4:1, 1965.
3. Lloyd-Roberts G.C., Stone K.H.: Congenital hypoplasia of the upper femur. *J. Bone Joint Surg.* 45B:557–560, 1963.
4. Panting A.L., Williams P.F.: Proximal femoral focal deficiency. *J. Bone Joint Surg.* 60B:46–52, 1978.

Foot Deformities

Clubfoot

Talipes equinocavovarus is a congenital deformity of the foot. Its cause and treatment have been the subject of controversies, which arise from the difficulties in nomenclature and in the variability of the severity of the deformity and its resistance to correction. The incidence of clubfoot varies in different geographic areas, but is somewhere between 1–2/1,000 births.

There are two types of clubfoot. One is an extrinsic clubfoot, with little or no structural deformity and a foot near normal in size. The circumference of the calf is almost equal to that of the opposite calf. In bilateral cases, the calves appear to be of normal size. These extrinsic clubfoot are readily corrected with standard nonoperative treatment. The second type is an intrinsic clubfoot. This is the "true" structural clubfoot, with deformities of bones, ligaments, tendons, and muscles. Nonoperative treatment will fail to correct most clubfeet of the intrinsic type.

Four causes of a clubfoot deformity are recognized.[1] Extrinsic factors, such as excessive in utero pressure in oligohydramnios, or constricting bands from early rupture of the amnion, may contribute to clubfoot deformities. Certain drugs are recognized to affect the limb bud, and these are a possible cause. A second known cause is a genetically transmitted trait seen in both mendelian dominant or recessive transmission. The recognizably mendelian transmissions are associated with syndromes such as the whistling face syndrome or diastrophic dwarfism. A third cause is a cytogenetic abnormality. Such defects are seen in some patients with clubfeet. The fourth and most common cause is multifactorial inheritance.

PATHOLOGY.—The most consistent abnormality is the small talus with a short, medially deviated neck.[3] There is a medial tilt to the talus and a flattened posterior medial surface. The navicular is wedge-shaped and displaced medially toward the medial malleolus.

The calcaneus has a medial bow, is tilted into varus, and is rotated medially so the anterior part lies beneath the talus. Both the talus and calcaneus are in equinus, and the cuboid is displaced medially on the calcaneus. The Achilles tendon, posterior tibialis tendon, and toe flexors are shortened (Fig 143–7).

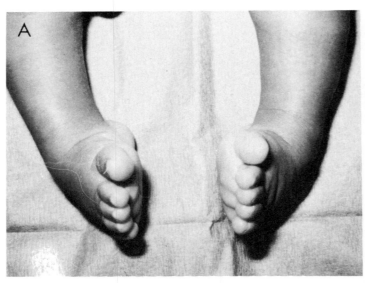
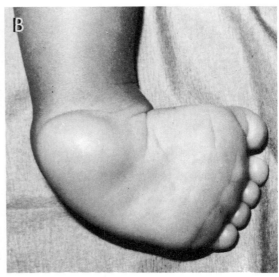

Fig 143–7.—Clubfoot. **A,** untreated clubfoot that shows the supination of the clubfoot. **B,** the varus of the heel. The deep transverse crease and the adduction of the forefoot are typical of a clubfoot.

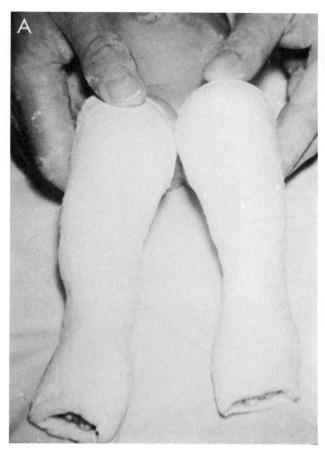

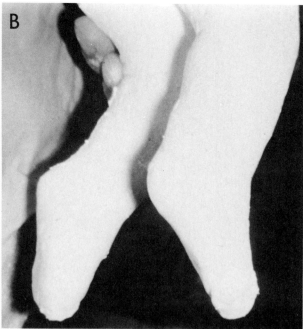

Fig 143–8.—Clubfoot. **A,** long leg cast. The attempt at correction of the medial rotation is apparent. The foot is externally rotated. **B,** the degree of equinus still present in the same foot is severe even if the medial rotation of the foot has been partially corrected.

TREATMENT.—Treatment should begin as soon as possible after birth. Treatment is directed at reducing the displaced navicular in relation to the distal end of the talus, rotating and tilting the calcaneus from beneath the talus, and correcting the equinus of the calcaneus and talus. The reduction of the navicular and varus of the hindfoot should be corrected before correction of the equinus is attempted.[4, 5] Gentle manipulation of the foot for several minutes, followed by the application of a plaster cast, or taping the foot in the corrected position repeated at least every 3 days for several weeks and then at weekly intervals until the foot is corrected, will be successful in most extrinsic clubfeet, but in less than a third of the intrinsic clubfeet. After each manipulation with the foot held in the corrected position, an assistant applies a snug-fitting cast. The cast may be a short leg cast or extend above the knee. There is no evidence that one is superior to the other, although McKay[6] advises a long leg cast (Fig 143–8).

For those feet not corrected by manipulation and casting, operative correction is required. Most orthopedists proceed to operative release as soon as the nonoperative treatment is seen to be inadequate. Others prefer to delay operation until the child is nearly 1 year old (Fig 143–9,A–C).[8, 9] There is some support for immediate operation in the neonate without going through a nonoperative treatment program.[7] The operative technique popularized by Turco[9] is a one-stage procedure that emphasizes the importance of subtalar release. Goldner,[2] to the contrary, places little importance on the subtalar joint, but rather sees the deltoid ligament as the major resistance to correction and advocates complete diversion of the superficial and deep deltoid. McKay[6] releases the subtalar joint medially, posteriorly, and laterally,

but emphasizes the importance of the peroneal retinaculum and sheath as well as the posterior fibulocalcaneal ligaments in hampering correction.

The surgical procedure has to be somewhat tailored for every clubfoot because of the differences in degree of deformity. In general, clubfeet associated with a musculoskeletal syndrome are more difficult to treat, they almost always require extensive surgical release, and functional results are least satisfying.

The various procedures for operative release of the restraining ligamentous contractures require good access to all sides of the ankle and to subtalar and talonavicular joints. A Z-plasty is usually required to lengthen the Achilles tendon. The flexor tendons are freed. The several joints are widely opened by division of capsule and overlying ligaments. The posterior tibial tendon may have to be lengthened. At this point, with abduction of the forefoot (if the dissection has been adequate), the navicular should slide laterally on the talus: and the os calcis should move laterally and posteriorly and rotate so that the anterior portion goes laterally and the posterior portion medially. The varus component of the os calcis should also be corrected by this maneuver. With dorsiflexion, the talus should move posteriorly into the ankle mortise sufficiently for one to see 1½ cm or so on the articular cartilage of the talus from the posterior view. If the talus does not come into this position, the posterior fibular ligament should be divided so that the fibula can spring out enough to allow the talus to slide posteriorly. If, after the talus is back into the mortise properly, the foot still does not rotate laterally, one approaches the foot laterally and frees the cuboid, os calcis, and navicular anterior laterally. At this point, if the foot is corrected, the toe flexors should be tight; and these can be managed by

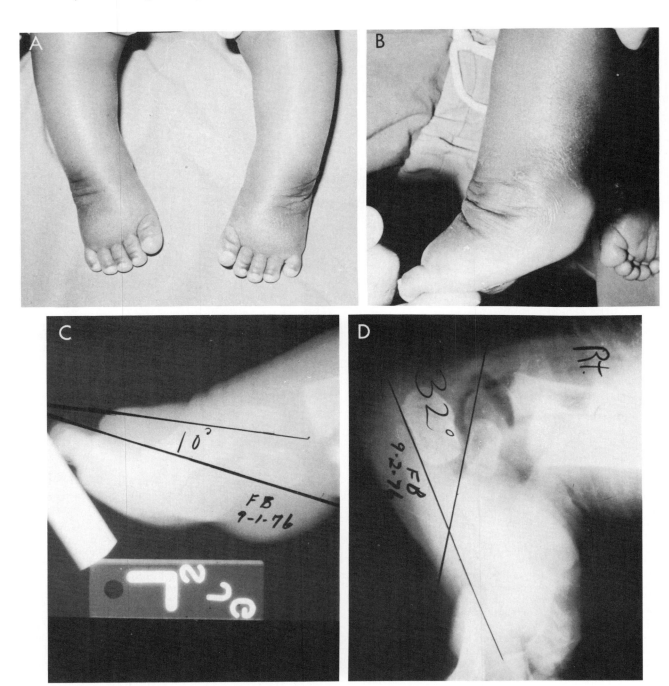

Fig 143–9.—Clubfoot. **A,** front view of a clubfoot after repeated manipulations and cast changes for 3 months. Partial correction of medial rotation, supination, and adduction of forefoot has been corrected. **B,** the equinus of the same foot remains severe. Surgical release of the foot is indicated by the lack of response to nonoperative treatment. **C,** the lateral roentgenogram shows the plantar-flexed metatarsals, which are caused by the tight plantar fascia that will have to be surgically released to obtain correction. More important is the minimal angle between a line along the long axis of the talus and calcaneus (Kite's angle) with the foot dorsiflexed. Parallelism of the talus and calcaneus indicates that the calcaneus remains medially rotated beneath the head of the talus. **D,** this lateral roentgenogram in dorsiflexion after correction shows the increase in Kite's angle, which can take place only after there is motion in the subtalar joint that allows the calcaneus to rotate laterally and from beneath the head of the talus. In this patient, the release includes the subtalar joint, except that the interosseous ligament between the talus and calcaneus was not divided.

lengthening the flexor hallucis proximally in Z-fashion and the common toe flexor lengthened at its muscular tendinous junction, allowing the tendon to slide distally. The plantar fascia should always be divided. This can be done anterior to the tubercle of the os calcis, and at the same time the short toe muscles are divided. One should check and make certain that the abductor hallucis has been freed from its origin on the os calcis. With the foot held corrected, a Kirschner wire is passed across the talonavicular joint and a second wire across the talocalcaneal joint from the plantar surface. With the foot held at neutral dorsiflexion, repair the Achilles tendon with slight tension. Overlengthening of the Achilles tendon permanently limits the range of plantar flexion. At this point in the procedure, x-ray the foot, and make certain that in the lateral view the talus and os calcis have a normal relationship and that the parallelism that existed preoperatively has been corrected (see Fig 143–9,*D*). If the talus is not plantar flexed in relation to the os calcis, the subtalar joint has not been adequately released.

After the wounds are closed, a long leg cast is applied with the degree of dorsiflexion that is allowable by the tightness of the skin. If the skin at the suture line blanches when the foot is held in maximum correction, it cannot be immobilized in this position, as the skin will necrose. The cast should be applied with the foot in a position that does not compromise the skin. After 10 days, the cast is removed under general anesthesia, and a new long leg cast is applied with the foot in the corrected position. This cast is worn for 4 weeks. At the end of that time, the Kirschner wires should be removed and a short leg cast applied. If the child is at walking age, he should be allowed to get up and walk on the cast after the Kirschner wires are out.

There is some controversy as to the timing of the operative correction. The author believes that waiting until the child is ready to start walking will give the correction a better chance of being satisfactory. This is possibly related to the fact that in the larger foot the correction can be adequately held in plaster, and walking may provide significant benefit. This is difficult to prove, but the author's opinion is that weight-bearing on the subtalar joint would make the joint move with each weight-bearing step, which is its function; this should be beneficial.

The surgical correction of a clubfoot is not a procedure that should be taken lightly, nor one to be approached with a "cookbook" philosophy. To achieve good results in surgical correction of clubfeet requires considerable experience, an understanding of the goals to be achieved, and a good concept of function of the hindfoot and midfoot. A well-done operation with adequate correction and appropriate postoperative management should, in 85–90% of the patients, give a satisfactory result. Additional procedures may be indicated in a few patients who have a tendency to go back into varus or into medial rotation. In these patients, a tightening of the peroneus brevis at its insertion and/or a transfer of the anterior tibialis to the middle of the foot will occasionally be required to correct the supination and inversion deformity that may tend to recur after the initial surgical correction.

REFERENCES

1. Cowell H.R., Wein B.K.: Current concepts review: Genetic aspects of clubfoot. *J. Bone Joint Surg.* 62A:1381–1384, 1980.
2. Goldner J.L.: Congenital talipes equinovarus: Fifteen years of surgical treatment. *Curr. Pract. Orthop. Surg.* 4:61–123, 1969.
3. Ippolito E., Ponseti I.V.: Congenital clubfoot in the human fetus. *J. Bone Joint Surg.* 62A:8–22, 1980.
4. Kite J.H.: Principles involved in the treatment of clubfoot. *J. Bone Joint Surg.* 21:595, 1939.
5. Lovell W.W., Hancock C.I.: Treatment of congenital talipes equinovarus. *Clin. Orthop.* 70:79, 1970.
6. McKay D.W.: New concept of and approach to clubfoot treatment: I. Principles and morbid anatomy. *J. Pediatr. Orthop.* 2:347–356, 1982.
7. Ryoppy S. Sairanen H.: Neonatal operative treatment of clubfoot. *J. Bone Joint Surg.* 65B:320–325, 1983.
8. Thompson G.H., Richardson A.B., Westin G.W.: Surgical management of resistant congenital talipes equinovarus deformities. *J. Bone Joint Surg.* 64A:652–655, 1982.
9. Turco V.J.: Resistant congenital clubfoot—one stage posteromedial releases with internal fixation. *J. Bone Joint Surg.* 61A:805–814, 1979.

Metatarsus Adductus

Metatarsus adductus is present at birth. Unfortunately, the gravity of the problem based upon the appearance of the newborn foot is difficult to define. Most such feet will correct spontaneously, and these are postural deformities resulting from the in utero position. The task in diagnosis is to distinguish the postural from the structural metatarsus adductus, which will not correct without treatment.

Clinical Features

The metatarsals are adducted, and the heel is in valgus. The base of the fifth metatarsal and the cuboid form a lateral prominence. The medial border of the foot is concave and the lateral border convex. There is a transverse crease on the medial and plantar surface in the tarsal-metatarsal area, with an increased arch (Fig 143–10). Plantar flexion of the foot is somewhat limited because of a contracture of the anterior tibial muscle. The abductor hallucis is tight and frequently hyperactive. Attempts to stimulate the peroneal muscles by stroking the dorsolateral surface of the foot does not elicit the abduction movement seen in normal infants. Radiographs of the foot will show the hindfoot to be in valgus and the metatarsals adducted.[3]

Treatment

Ponseti and Becker[3] describe gentle manipulation to stretch the forefoot into abduction without increasing the valgus of the hindfoot, and retaining this position with a long leg cast. The technique of manipulation and casting is to place the foot into slight equinus and varus, so as not to increase the valgus of the hindfoot. With the hindfoot held in this position, abduct the forefoot while applying counterpressure over the cuboid. Hold the foot in this corrected position for several seconds; then release the forefoot momentarily and repeat the abduction motion. Do this exercise for 5 minutes or so; then apply a plaster cast to hold the new position. The cast is applied first to the foot and ankle and then extended above the knee to hold the knee flexed 60–70 degrees.

Operation may be necessary to correct persistent deformity in children 3 years of age and older. The procedure described by Hegman et al.[2] to release the tarsal-metatarsal capsules and the intertarsal ligaments is effective. In children over 4 or 5 years of age, the soft tissue release is not as satisfactory as it is in the 2- or 3-year age group; and, in the older age group, osteotomies at the base of the metatarsal are required.

To treat or not to treat is not always an easy decision. Bleck[1] looked at the parameters that affect the results of plaster treatment. The only significant factor that he found was the age at the time of treatment. Severity of deformity and flexibility do not correlate with the results of treatment.[1] Deformities in children over 8 months of age are not corrected as readily with plaster treatment as in children under 8 months old. It is therefore important that treatment of the structural metatarsus deformity be undertaken as early as possible.

REFERENCES

1. Bleck E.E.: Metatarsus adductus classification and relationship to outcome of treatment. *J. Pediatr. Orthop.* 3:2–9, 1983.
2. Hegman C.H., Herudin C.H., Strong J.M.: Mobilization of the tarsometatarsal and intermetatarsal joints for the correction of resistant adduction of the forepart of the foot in congenital clubfoot or congenital metatarsus varus. *J. Bone Joint Surg.* 40A:299, 1958.

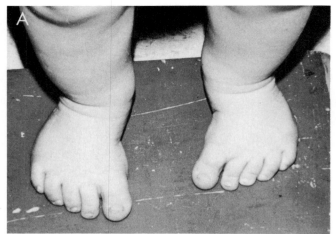

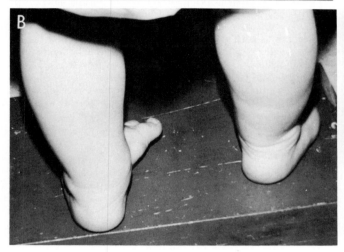

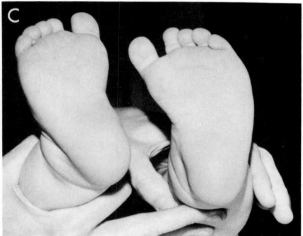

Fig 143–10.—Metatarsus adductus. **A,** a metatarsus adductus deformity in a 13-month-old child that has not been treated. The convex lateral border of the foot, the medial crease at the midfoot, and the adduction of the metatarsals are typical. **B,** the heel is in valgus, as can be seen in this view. The valgus may be even more than in this patient. **C,** the plantar view of the foot shows the deep transverse crease on the medial and plantar surfaces, the convex lateral border, and the adduction of the metatarsals.

3. Ponseti I.V., Becker J.R.: Congenital metatarsus adductus: the results of treatment. *J. Bone Joint Surg.* 48A:702–711, 1966.

Congenital Recurvatum, Subluxation, and Dislocation of the Knee

Congenital genu recurvatum, or hyperextension of the knee, is a relatively easy abnormality to recognize and to treat. In the newborn, however, hyperextension of the knee may present in association with a congenital subluxation or dislocation of the knee—two more serious abnormalities requiring more extensive treatment.

The congenital recurvatum is secondary to in utero position with hyperextension of the knee. It can be successfully treated by repeated cast changes with progressive flexion of the knee until it reaches 90% of flexion. Minor degrees of recurvature can be treated with passive stretching exercise.

In all knees with recurvatum, roentgenograms are required to determine the relationship of the tibia to the femur. In the hyperextended knee, the tibia and femur are in proper alignment except for the hyperextension. In the subluxated knee, the tibia is forward on the femur; in the dislocated knee, it is anterior, lateral, and rotated in relation to the femur. The treatment of subluxation is by traction to reduce the subluxation, followed by progressive cast applications to obtain flexion. With the dislocated knee, there is frequently a congenital fibrosis of a part of the quadriceps. In the open reduction of the knee, the fibrous mass must be excised. It is essential that the simple recurvatum knee be differentiated from the subluxated or dislocated knee. Treating the dislocated knee by stretching, or by repeated cast changes, is hazardous and may result in damage to the epiphyseal plate, and fracture.

Congenital Pseudarthrosis of the Clavicle

Pseudarthrosis of the clavicle is a congenital anomaly that apparently results from the lack of union between the medial and lateral centers of ossification. It is painless and occurs almost always on the right side.

The diagnosis is made usually in early childhood when the bulbous ends of the pseudarthrosis are recognized as a mass over the clavicular area. Unlike the pseudarthroses of other bones, the ends are not tapered. Growth leads to an increasing asymmetry of the shoulder girdle and winging of the scapula, but functional disability is minimal.

Surgical correction in childhood improves the symmetry of the shoulders and eliminates the bulbous mass of the pseudarthrosis. The bulbous ends should be modified by partial resection to give good apposition and held reduced by a smooth Kirschner wire. Cortical-cancellous grafts should always be placed around the pseudarthrosis fixation. The fixation is important to correct the alignment and to immobilize the clavicle so that healing occurs. Results are very satisfactory in almost all patients.

Sprengel's Deformity

In 1891, Sprengel[3] described four patients with undescended scapulae. Although the deformity had been previously described, Sprengel's name has become the eponym for this deformity. The scapula begins its development at the level of the 4th, 5th, and 6th cervical vertebrae. During the 9th–12th week, it descends to its usual level and undergoes a change both in its vertical orientation and its shape. Early in its development, the transverse width of the scapula is greater than the vertical length; and the scapula gradually rotates counterclockwise as seen from the back. The arrest of the development results in the halt of the descent of the scapula and in the vertical orientation, so that the inferior angle is nearer the midline. In addition to the deformity of the scapula, there are anomalies of the muscles attached to the scapula. The middle and lower trapezius muscle is frequently deficient, and in some patients the rhomboids are also abnormal. Most patients with this deformity have other anomalies. Congenital scoliosis occurs in over half these patients. Other associated anomalies uncommonly present are diastematomyelia, tethered cord, and visceral anomalies such as absence of a lung. The associated deformities may cause serious problems, and it is important that they be identified and addressed.

The diagnosis of Sprengel's deformity is usually not difficult. There is elevation of the scapula with limited abduction of the shoulder. Rotation of the shoulder internally and externally may be limited. The shape and size of the scapula varies considerably, but usually the scapula is shorter in its vertical length and rotated so that the inferior angle rests nearer the midline.

Operation to improve cosmetic appearance and function may be indicated in selected patients. If the restriction of abduction is sufficient to limit a functional range of abduction of the shoulder, or if the appearance is objectionable to the patient, both can, in most cases, be improved by surgical correction.

In 1957, Green[1] reported his technique for the correction of the Sprengel deformity. His operation is extensive and requires thorough knowledge of the anatomy and function of the shoulder and scapula. He removed the insertion of all muscles attaching to the scapula except the subscapularis and resected the supraspinatus portion of the scapula. He then lowered the scapula to the desired position and held it in the new position with a wire attached to the spine of the scapula and connected to a spring, which was attached to a spica cast. The results reported by Green were very good, averaging 40-degree improvement in shoulder abduction.

In 1961 Woodward,[4] reported a new technique for correction of this deformity. He removed the origin of the muscles from the spinous processes, divided the trapezius transversely high in the neck, removed the supraspinous portion of the scapula, displaced the scapula caudally to the desired level, and reattached the muscle to a vertebral spinous process at a lower level. In my experience, the operation described by Woodward is less difficult than the Green procedure. The results of the Green and the Woodward procedures are similar, although in older patients the Green procedure may give better correction.

Klisic et al.[2] have described a procedure similar to the Green procedure, but with additional features. In addition to removing the muscles from the spine and vertebral border of the scapula, he performed an incomplete osteotomy of the clavicle and divided the coracoclavicular ligament. The two steps increase the distance that the scapula can be lowered without compressing the brachial plexus. Klisic tethered the spine of the scapula to a spinous process with a large nonabsorbable suture. He held the scapula in its new position with an absorbable suture through the inferior angle and around a rib. Neither Klisic nor Woodward removed the serratus anterior muscle from the scapula. Green thought it was important to do so.

The osteotomy of the clavicle and the release of the coracoclavicular ligaments protect the brachial plexus when the scapula has to be displaced a great distance. This should probably be a routine part of both the Woodward and Green procedure when the scapula has to be displaced a great distance.

Exercises to strengthen the muscles about the scapula and to increase the range of motion of the shoulder are important to the final result. All of the above procedures can give satisfactory results. The Klisic procedure appears to give the most correction of the elevation, and is equal to the others in improvement of motion. Operative correction is ideally performed at ages 5 or 6 years, but can be done up until the late teens. It should not be done in children under 4 years of age.

REFERENCES

1. Green W.T.: The surgical correction of congenital elevation of the scapula (Sprengel's Deformity). *J. Bone Joint Surg.* 39A:1439, 1957.
2. Klisic P., Filiporic M., Uzelac O., et al. Relocation of congenitally elevated scapula. *J. Pediatr. Orthop.* 1:43–45, 1981.
3. Sprengel O.G.H.: Die angeborene Verschiebung des Schulterblattes nach oben. *Arch. f. Klin. Chir.* 42:545–549, 1891.
4. Woodward J.W.: Congenital elevation of the scapula correction by release and transplantation of muscle origins: A preliminary report. *J. Bone Joint Surg.* 43A:219–228, 1961.

144 Paul P. Griffin

Bone and Joint Infections

Acute Hematogenous Osteomyelitis

ACUTE HEMATOGENOUS OSTEOMYELITIS is more common in infancy and early childhood than in any other age. It most frequently affects the metaphysis of long bones, but may involve any part of the skeleton. Features of the skeleton characteristic of the age influence the sequelae of the infection. Boys are affected about twice as often as girls.

The most common sites involved in osteomyelitis are the femur, tibia, humerus, fibula, and radius, in descending order of frequency. In the debilitated neonate, osteomyelitis not uncommonly involves several bones; and, unlike the situation in older

TABLE 144–1.—OSTEOMYELITIS: 276 CASES*

	NEWBORN (%) (N = 13)	1 MO.–5 YR (%) (N = 142)	OVER 5 YR (%) (N = 121)
Staphylococcus	54	49	71
Hemophilus influenzae	8	5	0
Streptococcus			
Group A	0	11	7
Group B	0	2	0
Pneumococcus	0	4	0
Salmonella	8	1	0
Other	8	9	4
Unknown	23	17	17

*Adapted from Jackson and Nelson.[9]

infants, neonates show a significant incidence of osteomyelitis of the facial bones. Direct infections of the skull, and osteomyelitis of the calcaneus from scalp vein infusions and heel pricks for blood studies, are seen in the neonate and young infant.

The most common pathogen cultured from sites of osteomyelitis in all age groups is *Staphylococcus aureus* (Table 144–1). *Salmonella* or *Hemophilus influenzae* are found in 8% of osteomyelitis in the newborn, but much less commonly in older children. The second most common organism in older infants and children is *Streptococcus*.

Clinical Features

The clinical presentation is influenced by the bone involved and by the age of the child.

In general, the child with acute osteomyelitis is ill with high fever, anorexia, and general malaise. The affected part is painful. Young children may refuse to move the affected limb. This pseudoparalysis often causes initial concern that the basic problem may be neurologic. Patients of walking age may refuse to walk or may walk with a limp.

Local swelling over the affected metaphysis is present very early in the disease. In infants, the swelling rapidly affects the entire limb (Fig 144–1). Tenderness on pressure over the metaphysis is usually severe. Increased heat and redness may be present. There is frequently some limitation of motion, with or without effusion in the joint adjacent to the infected bone.

Pathophysiology

An antecedent infection, such as a boil, may or may not be known. There is general acceptance that osteomyelitis begins in the metaphysis, from hematologic dissemination. The sluggish blood flow and the deficient lymphocytes in the sinusoids at the physeal and metaphyseal junction provide a favorable environment for bacteria to settle out and multiply. Morrissy[11] has developed a model for hematogenous osteomyelitis in rabbits. He found that the colonization of bacteria sufficient to invoke an inflammatory reaction was in the metaphysis and in juxtaposition to the physis.

Age influences the course and sequelae. In the infant, vessels extend across the physis. These vessels allow the passage of the infection from the metaphysis to the epiphysis with destruction of the physis and the epiphysis, and secondary infection of the joint. In the neonate, it is common for the epiphysis and physis to be partially or completely destroyed by the infection, usually with combined septic arthritis and osteomyelitis.[6] The destruction of the physis and epiphysis leaves the patient with deformity of the bone, deficiency in limb length, and limited motion.

It is uncommon to have physeal involvement after 18 months of age, because there are no longer vascular spaces across the physis. Two important features of osteomyelitis in the young child are the severity of the toxic symptoms and the rarity with which chronic osteomyelitis develops. The reason for the sparing of the infant from chronic osteomyelitis is not clear, but a cortical sequestrum seldom occurs in children under 2 or 3 years of age. The porosity of the cortex in the young child may allow the purulent exudate to escape into the subperiosteal space without involving the diaphyseal medullary space and the nutrient vessels to the cortex. In older children, the cortex is less porous, delaying the spontaneous decompression into the subperiosteal space. The pus and inflammatory reaction then spreads into the diaphysis and destroys the nutrient vessels. With the subsequent disruption of the periosteal vessels by the subperiosteal pus, the cortex is made avascular, and a sequestrum is produced, the hallmark of osteomyelitis (Fig 144–2). Since the introduction of antibiotics, serious chronic osteomyelitis requiring multiple sequestrectomies is not common. Host resistance to the bacteria, with or without treatment, may be sufficient to contain and wall

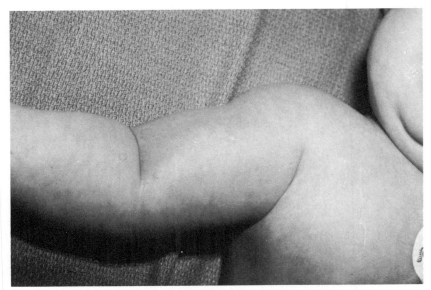

Fig 144–1.—Swelling of entire limb, which is typical of osteomyelitis in an infant.

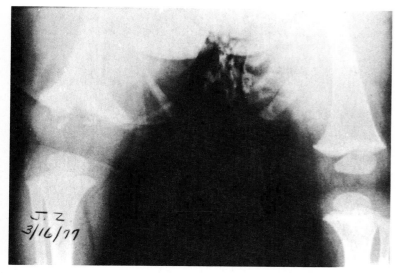

Fig 144–2.—Physeal and epiphyseal damage from neonatal osteomyelitis of the distal femur. Growth in the femur has been compromised, and the femur is short.

off the inflammation and produce an abscess that may persist asymptomatically for some period of time.

Trauma influences the onset and location of osteomyelitis. In approximately one third of patients with osteomyelitis, there is a history of an antecedent injury. It is difficult to cause consistent osteomyelitis in animals by injection of bacteria unless the part is injured prior to the injection.[1, 11]

Diagnosis

The diagnosis of acute osteomyelitis is made by a careful history of the onset of localized bone pain with swelling and tenderness over the affected part. In acute osteomyelitis, an elevated temperature, increased white cell count with a shift to the left, and an elevated sedimentation rate support the diagnosis. The earliest roentgenographic finding is deep soft tissue swelling (Fig 144–3). Lytic areas and subperiosteal new bone (the involucrum) are not seen on the radiograph until 10 days or more after the onset. Aspiration in the area of maximum tenderness should always be done as part of the diagnostic evaluation of a patient with appropriate signs and symptoms. If there is subperiosteal pus, the diagnosis is confirmed. Where pus is not found subperiosteally, the needle should be pushed into the metaphysis, if possible. The subperiosteal pus and/or the aspirate from the metaphysis should be gram-stained and cultured. When pus is not obtained on aspiration, a bone scan should be done if there is doubt about the diagnosis. A simple needle aspiration will not cause sufficient response in the bone to confuse the scan. Cultures should be made of the nose, throat, blood, and any cutaneous lesions.

Special Locations

Osteomyelitis of the vertebral column or of the pelvis is frequently a problem in diagnosis. The usual symptoms of vertebral body osteomyelitis are back pain and an antalgic gait. The back pain may radiate into the thigh and is not unlike sciatica. The patient sits or stands with the spine in extension. Flexion of the spine is painful. Pressure or percussion over the affected vertebra reproduces the pain. Patients with osteomyelitis of the spine are not generally as ill as those with osteomyelitis of a long bone. The white blood cell count and sedimentation rate are usually moderately elevated. Radiographs may be normal early in the disease, or a disc space may be narrowed—the first radiographic

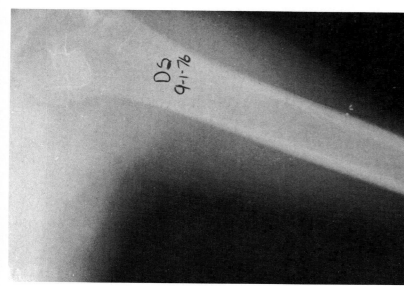

Fig 144–3.—Osteomyelitis of proximal humerus with soft tissue swelling that obliterates muscle planes. This is the earliest radiographic sign of osteomyelitis.

change. When the radiograph is negative, a bone scan will localize the vertebrae involved. Tomography of the area will usually show a lytic area in two adjacent vertebrae. Osteomyelitis of the spine should be treated with antibiotics and immobilization.

In osteomyelitis of the ilium, the symptoms and physical findings are similar to those of vertebral body osteomyelitis. A noticeable difference, however, is that with vertebral osteomyelitis the patient resists flexion of the spine, whereas the patient with iliac osteomyelitis prefers flexion of the spine and hips. There are three distinct presentations of iliac osteomyelitis.[2] One of these is easily mistaken for osteomyelitis of the spine, because the symptoms are similar to those of a lumbar disc—low back pain and pain in the thigh. The patient walks with a limp and has limited straight-leg raising and atrophy of the painful leg. In a second type, the patient presents with buttock pain. Swelling and tenderness are found over the buttock. The third group present with abdominal pain and few or no other complaints. This may be mistaken for an acute intra-abdominal infection. Careful physical examination will localize the tenderness over the ilium and buttock. Antibiotic treatment and bed rest are usually successful. If an abscess has developed, it must be drained. Rarely, the iliac wing may need debridement if there is significant bone destruction.

A special type of hematogenous osteomyelitis is seen in closed fractures.[4, 17] The incidence of infection in closed fractures is low, but infection must be suspected in a patient who has recurrence of pain several days or weeks after the fracture. Examination of the extremity out of plaster should reveal unusual swelling and tenderness at the fracture. The diagnosis can be established by aspiration about the fracture.

An unusual but particularly severe osteomyelitis may be secondary to a septic thrombophlebitis. Jupiter et al.[10] reported four such cases. The bone involvement was mostly subperiosteal abscess. One of their four patients developed chronic osteomyelitis.

Treatment

Early diagnosis and the administration of appropriate antibiotics is the most important aspect of the management of acute osteomyelitis.[5, 6, 12] The bacteria most commonly found in osteomyelitis are sensitive to synthetic penicillin. In older infants and children, a penicillin should be the initial antimicrobial agent administered. In children under 6 months, an aminoglycoside should be given along with the synthetic penicillin. The dosage should be in the highest range for the age and weight of the child; and, at the onset, the drug should be given parenterally. The antibiotic can be changed as indicated by the organism cultured. The antibiotic can be given orally in selected patients after the patient has shown improvement. Oral antibiotics should not be used unless there is a known causative organism and there are facilities for testing the drug level in the blood. The patient must be reliable and must be able to tolerate the large oral dose of antibiotic necessary to obtain a peak bactericidal level at a 1–8 serum dilution and a trough level at 1–2. The antibiotic should be given for at least 4 weeks. In children with bone destruction, 6–12 weeks may be necessary.[5, 6, 8, 13, 14] Gillespie and Mayo[6] reported no difference in the recurrence rate in patients treated for 3 weeks and those treated for longer periods of time.

Surgical drainage is indicated if pus is found on aspiration.[5, 10] This should include making an adequate window in the metaphysis and evacuation of the pus, granulation, and necrotic bone, even when there is subperiosteal pus. If pus is not obtained at aspiration and the patient does not respond to the antibiotic treatment, exploration of the affected area is indicated. A positive bone scan is helpful in such patients to support the diagnosis and locate the site for drainage. A drain should be left in the

wound and the skin closed, with removal of the drain after 48–72 hours.

Immobilization of the extremity by traction, splints, or cast gives comfort to the patient with acute osteomyelitis. Infection weakens the bone structure, and fractures are not uncommon during recovery from severe infection. This complication can be avoided by protection with a cast until the bone healing, as seen radiographically, suggests the strength of the bone is sufficient for the cast to be discontinued. In the child over 6 years of age, further protection by the use of crutches is advisable for several weeks until muscle strength and motion of the joints returns toward normal.

Subacute Osteomyelitis

All children with hematogenous osteomyelitis are not ill. Some apparently have sufficient resistance to avoid the severe bone destruction that is typical. These patients do not appear ill, and their major complaint is pain. Temperature and white blood cell count are mildly elevated. The sedimentation rate may be normal or moderately elevated. On physical examination, the skin over the affected part is warm, and the area is tender to pressure. Swelling may or may not be present. Radiographs show sclerosis of the cortex. Tomography may show small lytic lesions in the cortex. Needle biopsy of the sclerotic area will show the bone changes of osteomyelitis, and cultures are usually positive. Antibiotic therapy with protection of the limb for 8 weeks appears to be adequate treatment.

Primary subacute osteomyelitis of the epiphysis has been reported, but is rare.[7] The symptoms of osteomyelitis of an epiphysis are joint pain and a limp, with minimal decrease in motion. Joint effusion is usually slight. Radiographs show a lytic area in the epiphysis. Antibiotic treatment with a synthetic penicillin and rest may be sufficient treatment, although the author has curetted these lesions in addition to giving antibiotics.[7]

Chronic Osteomyelitis

Chronic osteomyelitis occurs when treatment is delayed or is ineffective (Fig 144–4). If treatment is started before there is suppuration and destruction of blood supply to the cortex, chronic osteomyelitis does not occur. Small sequestra may become incorporated into the adjacent bone by creeping substitution. Larger sequestra will eventually have to be removed. When removing a sequestrum, as little bone as possible should be sacrificed, because osteogenesis in chronically infected bone may be severely impaired and the bone may remain fragile for years.

Where large bone defects are created, cancellous bone grafts, muscle transposition with secondary skin graft, or the use of vascularized composite grafts may be helpful in solving the problems of reconstruction. These once-common problems have become rare in the antibiotic era.

Septic Arthritis

Acute septic arthritis is seen primarily in young children, although it can occur at any age. The peak incidence is between 1 and 2 years of age.[8] In infants and young children, the hip is the most frequent joint affected. However, the knee is more frequently affected in older children.

The most common pathogen found in patients with acute septic arthritis is *S. aureus*, but its dominance is not as great as in osteomyelitis. The pathogens and their frequency of involvement vary in different age groups (Table 144–2). *Staphylococcus* is the most common pathogen in the neonate and in older children; but, in patients between 1 month and 5 years of age, *S. aureus*

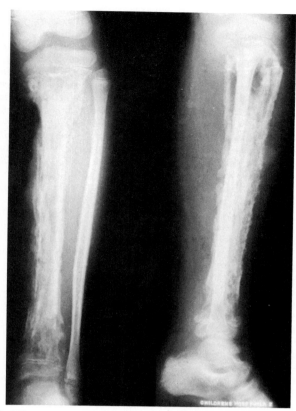

Fig 144–4.—Chronic osteomyelitis with sequestra. Such severe changes are now rare, but still occur when diagnosis is delayed. The strength of this bone is severely compromised.

was cultured from only 11%, while 31% had *H. influenzae* as the causative organism. *Neisseria gonorrhoeae* may be found in all age groups, including the newborn, and is found in 7% of both newborns and older children with acute septic arthritis.

Pathogenesis

There are three pathways for bacteria to invade a joint. The most common in children is direct hematogenous involvement of the synovium. A second pathway is by spontaneous decompression of a metaphyseal or epiphyseal osteomyelitis into the joint

cavity. The hip joint is commonly infected secondary to osteomyelitis, because the proximal metaphysis of the femur is partially intracapsular.[8] The shoulder is occasionally infected secondary to osteomyelitis of the humerus, and osteomyelitis of the distal femur or proximal tibia may secondarily infect the knee. In infants, infection of the metaphysis can spread to the epiphysis and joint through vascular spaces traversing the physis. The third route for infection of the joint is entry as a result of penetrating injury.

Pathology

The inflammatory response rapidly spreads through the synovium. There is an outpouring of purulent exudate into the joint cavity with progressive destruction of the articular cartilage. The precise mechanism of the cartilage destruction is not known beyond the fact that collagenases degrade the collagen. The collagenase may be produced by synovial cells, bacteria, and the inflammatory cells. When treatment is delayed, the cartilage undergoes vascular invasion. Hyaline cartilage is an avascular structure, which therefore acts as a foreign protein following the vascular erosion; and an autoimmune response is initiated, which causes further chondrolysis.[3]

Clinical Features

The onset of acute septic arthritis is usually rapid, with all of the signs and symptoms of septicemia. The clinical response of the newborn and young infant to acute septic arthritis is different from that of the older child.

The infant presents with features of septicemia plus local signs and symptoms. Fever may be mild or absent; the infant is listless and irritable when handled. Leukocytosis and elevation of the sedimentation may not be marked, but anemia is usually present. The severe pain on motion seen in the older child is seldom present in the infant; but the infant will not move the infected limb, which may suggest a paralytic disorder. It is important that septic arthritis be suspected in all infants who have the general symptoms of septicemia. Prior to the antibiotic era, the morbidity in infants with septic arthritis was very high.

The older infant and child rapidly becomes ill after the onset of acute pyarthrosis. Fever is always present, generally in the range of 102–104F. Pain is a prominent feature of the infected joint, and motion is severely limited. Early in the disease, the patient walks with an antalgic gait; but within 24–48 hours, even the older child will refuse to bear weight. The joint is swollen, warm, and tender to palpation; the overlying skin may be red.

Differential Diagnosis

Monoarticular juvenile rheumatoid arthritis, when acute, severe, and accompanied by fever, poses the most difficult differential diagnosis. The pain in this condition is seldom severe enough to be confused with pyarthrosis; but, on occasion, the two can be differentiated only by careful analysis of the joint fluid. Osteomyelitis, with or without a sympathetic effusion, may present a problem if the child is acutely ill. Motion of the joint adjacent to the osteomyelitis is generally only moderately limited. The most significant difference is that the swelling of osteomyelitis is extensive, whereas the swelling in septic arthritis is limited to the region of the joint capsule. In osteōmyelitis, the point of maximal tenderness is over the metaphysis rather than over the joint, as in septic arthritis. The pain associated with acute rheumatic fever may be severe, but its migratory nature and the paucity of physical findings about the joint easily differentiate it from acute pyarthrosis. The patient with nonspecific or

TABLE 144–2.—SUPPURATIVE ARTHRITIS: 471 CASES*

	NEWBORN (%) (N = 14)	1 MO.–5 YR (%) (N = 337)	OVER 5 YR (%) (N = 120)
Bacteria			
Staphylococcus aureus	36%	11%	33%
Hemophilus influenzae	7%	31%	1%
Streptococcus			
Group A	0	6%	18%
Group B	21%	2%	0
Pneumococcus	0	4%	1%
Neisseria gonorrhoeae	7%	2%	7%
Neisseria meningitis	0	3%	1%
Pseudomonas aeruginosa	7%	2%	3%
Escherichia coli/Klebsiella Enterobacteriaceae	14%	2%	3%
Other	7%	4%	5%
Unknown	0	35%	34%

*Adapted from Jackson and Nelson.[9]

toxic synovitis will rarely be difficult to diagnose. These children are not ill, have little or no fever, and have pain only at the extremes of motion. The range of motion is seldom limited more than 15–20 degrees in any direction.

Diagnosis

The diagnosis of septic arthritis is made from the clinical presentation of a sick child with a painful swollen joint that has very little active motion and severe pain on passive motion. It is confirmed by joint aspiration and careful analysis of the fluid. The joint fluid in septic arthritis is usually cloudy. The inflammatory process destroys the hyaluronic acid in the joint fluid, loss of which makes the fluid thin and watery. The joint fluid will not string between thumb and finger, as does normal joint fluid. The white blood cell count, with few exceptions, is between 50,000 and 200,000/cu mm, and the differential cell count is above 90% polymorphonuclear leukocytes. It is important that the fluid be used for white blood cell count be immediately anticoagulated. Cultures for aerobic and anaerobic organisms should be done. If there is sufficient fluid, the content of mucin and sugar should be measured. The mucin is always poor and the joint sugar usually 50 mg/dl or so less than the peripheral blood sugar. A well-done Gram stain can also be helpful in diagnosis and in selection of the appropriate initial antibiotic. Radiographs of the joint will show the effusion. These films are indirectly helpful and should always be made. In young children, the joint space in an infected hip is usually wide and may be subluxated or dislocated.

Treatment

The principles of treatment for septic arthritis include sterilization, thorough cleansing of the joint, and protection of the articular cartilage from stress until recovery. The essential feature for success is early, adequate treatment. Delay in the onset of treatment is associated with poor results, whereas the results of early treatment are uniformly good, unless there is associated osteomyelitis or if the hip has dislocated. Most poor results are in the neonate and young infant. This is most likely a result of delay in diagnosis and treatment.

The appropriate antibiotics should be started immediately after the joint is aspirated. They should be given parenterally from the start. If an organism is cultured and there are facilities to do assay serum drug levels, oral antibiotics can be successfully used in children. If the patient has shown a good clinical response, a regimen of parenteral antibiotics with a switch to oral antibiotics after 3–4 days has been our recent routine. The problem of oral antibiotics and the large dosage necessary to obtain the desired bactericidal level (1–8 serum dilution at peak and a 1–2 dilution at trough) may not be tolerated by small children. Compliance has to be assured, and some patients may need to remain hospitalized throughout the course of treatment. Antibiotics should be continued for 2–4 weeks, depending upon the rapidity of response.

Age and the expected organism dictate the choice of the initial antibiotics. The most common organisms in septic arthritis are *Staphylococcus* and *Streptococcus*, except in patients between 1 month and 5 years of age, in whom *H. influenzae* is the responsible pathogen in 31% of cases. A synthetic penicillin, plus an aminoglycoside, should be the antibiotic of choice in the patient under 6 months of age. Between 6–24 months, Chloramphenicol (Chloromycetin) should be given, along with a synthetic penicillin. After 24 months, a synthetic penicillin alone is the drug of choice until culture and sensitivities prove otherwise.

Cleansing of the joint is a necessary part of treatment. The joint must be cleansed of the purulent fluid, destructive enzymes, fibrin, and debris brought by the inflammatory process. This is best accomplished by surgical drainage with a thorough cleansing of the joint. There has been a controversy as to whether or not repeated aspiration is equally capable of adequate cleansing of the joint.[12] There are no reports in the literature to prove this, and it is unlikely that there will ever be. The variables are great, and a randomized study of similar patients would be difficult to perform. Certainly, surgical cleansing produces no deleterious effects; it is over and done with at one event; and the surgeon can see the cartilage, synovium, and joint contents and know that the joint has been thoroughly cleaned. The synovium and capsule are kept open by suturing them to the adjacent tissue. A drain is placed at the joint margin and the skin closed. The drain should be removed in 3 days.

Historically, immobilization of the joint after drainage has been used with success.[8, 14] More recently, Salter et al.[15] have advocated the use of continuous, machine-guided, passive motion in septic arthritis. The benefit of continuous passive motion has not yet had sufficient clinical trials for it to be generally accepted. There is little evidence that immobilization after debridement of the joint and the institution of antibiotics is harmful. Certainly, when the hip of a child has been dislocated by the pyarthrosis, immobilization is necessary to maintain reduction of the hip. The author's experience has been with protection of the joint after drainage, by traction with range-of-motion exercises for 9–10 days, followed by immobilization in a bivalved cast that is removed three or four times a day for active assisted motion. Crutches are used in the older patient until the joint motion is normal, there is no pain, good muscle strength is present, and radiographs show good subchondral bone.

The results in treatment of septic arthritis in children are generally good, and significant sequelae are rare. Age under 6 months, the presence of osteomyelitis, and a delay of 4 or more days before diagnosis and treatment all contribute to a poor prognosis.

REFERENCES

1. Andriole V.T., Nagel D.A., Southwick W.: A paradigm for human chronic osteomyelitis. *J. Bone Joint Surg.* 55A:1511–1515, 1973.
2. Beaupre A., Carroll N.: The three syndromes of iliac osteomyelitis in children. *J. Bone Joint Surg.* 61A:1087–1092, 1979.
3. Bobechko W.P., Madel L.: Immunology of cartilage in septic arthritis. *Clin. Orthop.* 108:84–89, 1975.
4. Canale S.T., Puhl J., Watson F.M., et al.: Acute osteomyelitis following closed fractures. *J. Bone Joint Surg.* 57A:415, 1975.
5. Cole W.G., Dalziel R.E., Lerth S.: Treatment of acute osteomyelitis in children. *J. Bone Joint Surg.* 64B:218–223, 1982.
6. Gillespie W.J., Mayo K.M.: The management of acute osteomyelitis in the antibiotic era: A study of the outcome. *J. Bone Joint Surg.* 63B:126–131, 1981.
7. Green N.E., Griffin P.P.: Primary subacute epiphyseal osteomyelitis. *J. Bone Joint Surg.* 63A:107–114, 1981.
8. Griffin P.P.: Bone and joint infections in children. *Pediatr. Clin. North Am.* 14:533–548, 1967.
9. Jackson M.S., Nelson J.D.: Etiology and medical management of acute suppurative bone and joint infections in pediatric patients. *J. Pediatr. Orthop.* 2:313, 1982.
10. Jupiter J.B., Ehrlich M.G., Novelline R.A., et al.: The association of septic thrombophlebitis with subperiosteal abscess in children. *J. Pediatr.* 101:690–695, 1982.
11. Morrissy R.T.: An experimental model for osteomyelitis. American Academy of Orthopaedic Surgeons Annual Meeting, 1984.
12. Nelson J.D.: The bacterial etiology and antibiotic management of septic arthritis in infants and children. *Pediatrics* 50:437–448, 1972.
13. O'Brien T., McManus F., MacAuley P.H., et al.: Acute haematogenous osteomyelitis. *J. Bone Joint Surg.* 64B:450–453, 1982.
14. Paterson D.A.: Acute suppurative arthritis. *J. Bone Joint Surg.* 52B:474–482, 1970.
15. Salter R.B., Bell R.S., Keeley F.W.: The protective effect of contin-

uous passive motion on living cartilage in acute septic arthritis: An experimental investigation in the rabbit. *Clin. Orthop.* 159:223–247, 1981.
16. Wall J.J.: Acute hematogenous synarthrosis caused by hemophiliac influenza. *J. Bone Joint Surg.* 50A:1657–1662, 1968.

17. Watson F.M., Whitesides T.E. Jr.: Acute hematogenous osteomyelitis complicating a closed fracture. *Clin. Orthop.* 117:296–302, 1976.

145   Curtis D. Edholm

Amputations

AMPUTATIONS IN CHILDREN may be performed for trauma, disease, or conversion of congenitally malformed limbs. The incidence of amputation in children is unknown. It has been reported that congenital limb deficiencies occur twice as often as do acquired amputations.[10]

General Considerations

The child amputee is a skeletally immature individual who has either an acquired amputation or congenital absence of all or a portion of one or more limbs. The philosophy of management of the child differs from that for the adult.[8] Physically, the child is dynamically growing longitudinally and circumferentially, whereas the adult is mature and adynamic, with only circumferential growth, related to dietary habit. The child's circulation and tissue tolerance are apt to be ideal. That of the adult may vary with age and health. These physical factors will influence surgical indications, sites of amputation, and training goals. Socially, the child is a member of a family group and has few independent responsibilities, whereas the adult is socially independent with variable responsibilities related to age and marital and parental status. Economically, the child is dependent upon family, whereas the adult's economic level has been self-established and may be altered as the result of amputation, affecting not only self, but the family. The child's vocation has not been established, and education can be oriented around the handicap; the adult usually will have an established vocation that may require reorientation because of the amputation, and age often makes reeducation and retraining difficult or perhaps impossible. The adult's psychological response to amputation may vary from profound psychoneurosis to reasonable and mature acceptance of the disability. The child's emotional response may be influenced by the congenital or acquired nature of the limb loss and the age at which loss occurs, and will be determined by parental and peer attitudes.[7]

Treatment

Acquired Amputations

TRAUMA.—Acquired amputations in children[5] may be performed for trauma or disease. The frequency of specific causations is age-related.[11] Traumatic acquired amputations are more frequent in males. Vehicular injuries leading to amputation increase steadily from birth on and peak with the midteen years and licensing to drive. Amputations resulting from gunshot and explosions increase in frequency at adolescence. Railroad injuries

causing amputation rise from ages 8–16 years. Injuries from household accidents, childhood recreation, and thermal insults are seen at all ages, as are a great number of amputations resulting from powered tools and farm equipment. Vascular and neurogenic impairments frequently result in amputation in the first 5 years of life. In the past, disease-related amputations have been due mostly to sarcomas, with a predominance in the second decade of life.

DISEASE (OSTEOSARCOMA).—In recent years, the management of osteosarcomas has become increasingly controversial. Some optimism seemed warranted because of earlier diagnosis, patients presenting with tumors smaller than usually discovered previously, and reported benefits of adjuvant chemotherapy. Analysis of reports raises new questions regarding any seeming improvement in results of treatment.[13, 15] Standard past treatment for osteosarcoma has been amputation. Forequarter levels were performed for those with proximal humeral sarcoma sites, hip disarticulations, or high above-knee level amputations for those with lower femoral primary sites, and low femoral above-knee amputations for those with sites in the proximal tibia or below. Computed tomography may be of assistance in determining degree of intramedullary extension, but it must be remembered that skip lesions may exist within a bone and should be sought. Unfortunately, there is no completely reliable means of detecting skip lesions. Many chemotherapy protocols have been used. Adjuvant chemotherapy has been used prior to or following amputation and also in association with limb salvage procedures. Confusion still exists regarding the optimal protocol because of the limited numbers of patients and limited follow-up reports. More precise staging of the tumor or inclusion of variants with a more favorable inherent prognosis also may influence results obtained with chemotherapy. Limb salvage techniques have been devised to avoid amputation. Their efficacy obviously depends upon careful selection of the candidates. It remains to be determined whether cost benefits justify this degree of extensive operating and prolonged recovery/rehabilitation, compared with more standard management. Surgeons treating children with sarcomas should be aware of centers specializing in the study and management of musculoskeletal tumors under chemotherapy protocols, with or without limb salvage efforts.

The most important basic principles in amputation surgery in children[14] are to save all length of bone, and preservation of epiphyses by disarticulation rather than diaphyseal amputations. Surgeons should be aware of contributions to length resulting from epiphyseal growth. Even very short stumps created in small children will grow epiphyseally and be suitable for prosthetic fitting. Conversion of a very short stump by disarticulation at the next most distal joint is not indicated, and conversion of a very short stump by amputation through the more proximal bone is contraindicated. The skin of children usually will have good vascularity and elasticity. The techniques of amputation particularly devised for dysvascular adults are less important in childhood amputations. One hopes to avoid scars at the end of weight-bearing surfaces, but it is preferable, in a child, to accept such a scar rather than to amputate at a higher level. Prosthetic techniques will allow for adequate modifications of sockets so that such scars will not be troublesome. A skin-grafted stump in an adult does not tolerate weight-bearing. However, such skin-grafted stumps in children will tolerate weight-bearing, though appropriate adjustment of the socket interface may require a prosthetist experienced in fitting children.

COMPLICATIONS.—If amputation has occurred through the metaphysis or diaphysis of a child's bone, one may expect the complication of bone overgrowth.[3] The humerus, fibula, tibia, and femur, in that order, are the bones most frequently involved in overgrowth. Such overgrowth is due to appositional bone production and not to more proximal epiphyseal growth. Bone overgrowth manifests itself by bone production at the distal end of the stump, the bone tapering to a point. Such points may become very sharp and cause the skin to be tented or penetrated. A bursa may develop between the end of the bone and the skin. Pain may be present because of stretch of skin, pressure on skin between the end of bone and the socket interface, or distention of or pressure on an accompanying bursa. Bursitis is not unknown. Management of the overgrowth phenomenon may include relief of prosthetic sockets. Eventually, revision of the stump, including excision of bursa, will be necessary. One can anticipate repeated revisions for overgrowth until skeletal maturity of the bone. The number of revisions cannot be predicted. Prevention of overgrowth has been attempted by capping the end of the bone with cartilage-covered autografts or with inert synthetics such as Silastics. These efforts usually have not been successful. Marquardt[12] has devised a technique for capping bones using articular cartilage and subjacent bone when an indicated surgical procedure is to be performed elsewhere in a patient with multiple deficiencies, in whom overgrowth may occur. In instances of fibular overgrowth, in addition to standard shortening revision, a number of techniques have been used, such as angulation osteotomy of the fibula imbedding its end into the tibia, imbedding the distal fibula without osteotomy, and total extirpation of the fibula. No technique has been predictably successful.

Other complications of acquired amputations include bursa formation (without overgrowth), neuromata, and bone spurs. Bursae may form between bony prominences and prostheses, most often over the fibular head, tibial tuberosity, and distal tibia. They may be managed by relief of the sockets. Surgical intervention is rarely required. Neuromata always form in acquired amputations. Techniques standard in adults are used in children to place neuromata in nontroublesome locations away from end-bearing surfaces or from closely approximating socket walls. It is not recommended that sectioned nerves be injected with alcohol or phenol or cauterized. Large nerves with accompanying significant vascular supply may need ligation for control of bleeding. These and all other nerves should be simply pulled down, transected sharply, and allowed to retract. In spite of good amputation technique, excision of neuromata may be needed when prosthetic socket revision fails to relieve symptoms of local pain. Bone spurs are rarely a problem. They can be distinguished from bone overgrowth in that spurs are eccentrically located on a cortex near the end of bone and do not involve the

entire bone end. They may be prevented by minimizing periosteal stripping during amputation. Socket relief possibly may be needed for pressure symptoms. Revision of stumps is not required for spurs.

Phenomena that may be concomitant with acquired amputations in children include burn scars, phantom limb, and painful phantom. Burn scars on stumps may require special care in prosthetic fitting, and scars proximal to stumps may require altered harnessing techniques, especially in upper limb amputations, and altered suspension mechanisms in lower limb amputations. Phantom limb sensation is present in all adults who undergo amputation. Phantom limb is seldom experienced in the child in whom amputation occurs before the age of 5 years. Children who undergo amputation between ages 5–10 years may possibly admit to phantom sensation if questioned about it. Over age 10 years, phantom limb occurs as in adults. Painful phantom occurs in those who experience amputation over age 12 years in the same proportion that painful phantom occurs in adults. Children under age 10 years do not experience painful phantom.

The time of fitting of acquired amputations in children varies. In lower limbs, immediate prosthetic fitting can be done, but there is little functional benefit to the child. Immediate postoperative fitting should be distinguished from a rigid postoperative dressing to control edema and pain. Rigid postoperative dressings are indicated in children. If a below-knee stump is casted, the cast should cover the extended knee to prevent flexion contractures. Nonimmobilized joints should have full range of motion maintained at all times. In those whose amputation is performed because of tumor (usually adolescents), in light of their prognosis fitting should be considered immediately after operation, at least to alleviate the loss of body image. Immediate fitting may be considered for any whose emotional stability is in question. In most patients, fitting of definitive lower limb prostheses will be possible in 6–8 weeks. Fitting of upper limbs will be possible in 4 weeks. In any instance, fitting of upper or lower prostheses for amputation should be accomplished as soon as possible to avoid development of substitution patterns.

Congenital Deficiencies

Children with congenital limb deficiencies may require surgical intervention. The true incidence of such deficiency is unknown. Over 30% of children with congenital limb deficiency will have more than one limb involved. Nearly 10% will have some involvement of all four limbs. The incidence is almost equally divided between males and females.

The first complete detailed classification of congenital limb deficiency was that of Frantz and O'Rahilly[9] in 1961, and this is used in this chapter. The system relies upon naming the absent part of the limb, divided into terminal and intercalary deficiencies, each in turn divided into transverse and longitudinal types (Fig 145–1). Terminal transverse deficiencies are homologues of acquired amputation levels.

Most congenital limb deficiencies are sporadic. Some have known genetic implications such as tibial hemimelia, partial adactylia, and partial aphalangia. Patients with these diagnoses and their families, at least, should have genetic counseling. Some congenital deficiencies have been related to maternal drug use (e.g., thalidomide), but it should be noted that no new deficiency has been related to a specific drug, in that all types of deficiency existed prior to any single drug discovery.

Biomechanical losses may exist in those with congenital limb deficiency.[6] The major problems in the lower limb are severe leg length inequality, gross instability at one or more proximal joints that seriously impairs weight-bearing, total or partial malrotation of the limb, and inadequacy of proximal musculature. In the upper limb, the problems are primarily those of loss of varying de-

TERMINAL

TRANSVERSE

LONGITUDINAL

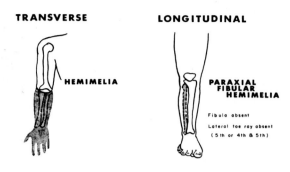

HEMIMELIA

PARAXIAL
FIBULAR
HEMIMELIA

Fibula absent

Lateral toe ray absent
(5 th or 4th & 5th)

INTERCALARY

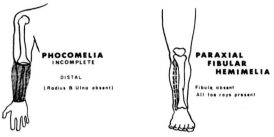

PHOCOMELIA
INCOMPLETE

DISTAL

(Radius & Ulna absent)

PARAXIAL
FIBULAR
HEMIMELIA

Fibula absent
All toe rays present

Fig 145–1.—Basic schema of classification of congenital skeletal limb deficiencies. (From Frantz and O'Rahilly.[9])

grees of prehension; lack of power to, and instability of, the proximal joints; limitation of motion in proximal joints, which hinders placement of the hand; malrotation; and severe length inequality.

The management of congenital skeletal deficiencies often requires prosthetic fitting. In order to provide satisfactory prosthetic substitutions, one must identify the "key joint."[6] The "key joint" is the most stable distal joint having the most nearly normal range of motion and adequate motors to actuate a prosthesis. Once this joint is defined, everything distal to it should be considered stump. Thus, the deficiency is translated to a prosthetic type, albeit one that requires nonstandard techniques. A great deal of ingenuity is required on the part of the prosthetist to fabricate satisfactorily these nonstandard prostheses.

In congenital limb deficiency, surgical intervention may be indicated in certain well-defined circumstances: when stability may be improved, when cosmesis may be enhanced, or when better prosthetic fit may be obtained. Surgical conversion of an anomalous limb to produce a stump more amenable to prosthetic fitting is indicated in approximately 50% of lower limb deficiencies.[6] In the upper limb, however, it has been reported that less than 10% have undergone conversion procedures. Conversion amputation is rarely indicated in congenital upper limb deficiency. Surgical reconstruction to improve hand function should follow well-established guidelines. Skin tags and nubbins rarely interfere with prosthetic fitting or function unless pedunculated, and their removal is not recommended. Anomalous digits, regardless of their location, should be preserved either for motoring portions of a prosthesis or for sensory feedback, and whenever possible in prosthetic fitting should be left uncovered.

For every child with congenital limb deficiency(ies), a plan for long-term management must be devised as early as possible. This plan should be based upon the combination of deficiency diagnoses, available function, and the need to produce maximum

functional independence. Surgical intervention should be governed by these principles. The plan of management should be discussed with family when the patient is in infancy, recognizing that the timing of some surgical interventions may not be precisely identified at that time. The life histories of certain lower limb anomalies are known and well documented.[2, 4] In those cases in which conversion amputation is the preferred treatment, the timing of the conversion is dependent upon agreement between the surgeon and family/patient. It is recommended that conversion amputation be carried out at the latest 1 year prior to beginning school, in order to allow a child to adapt to a new prosthetic prescription.

COMPLETE FIBULAR HEMIMELIA.—The most frequent lower limb deficiency is complete fibular hemimelia (Fig 145–2A,B). The fibula is absent. The tibia is present, but shorter than normal, often thicker than normal, frequently possesses an anterior bow, and may be anteromedially bowed. There is a dimple in the skin over the apex of the bowed tibia. This finding alone is nearly diagnostic of fibular hemimelia. The foot in this condition usually will have three or four toes, although there may be five. The foot may be in a plantigrade attitude or in varying degrees of equinus or equinovalgus. There are frequently tarsal coalitions, especially of the talus and calcaneus, in abnormal relation to one another, limiting foot mobility. Lacking a lateral malleolus, there may be lateral ankle instability. The major problem is the degree of leg length discrepancy that will develop. The percentage of shortening extant will persist throughout life. With growth, therefore, increasing length discrepancy occurs. Eventual length discrepancy at skeletal maturity is predictable, and is usually in the range of 5–8 inches. The treatment of choice will be foot ablation and prosthetic substitution. Efforts toward correcting equinus or equinovalgus deformities are meddlesome and should be avoided. No treatment is needed until the child stands. At that time, equalization of leg lengths may be accomplished by shoe lifts with ankle stabilization, if needed, by means of a simple orthosis (see Fig 145–2,C). Foot ablation is carried out, usually after independent ambulation occurs. However, this conversion amputation may be performed at any time that family and surgeon agree.

The technique of foot ablation is that of a modified Syme-type disarticulation (see Fig 145–2,D). The articular surface of the distal tibia must not be violated or removed. The distal tibial epiphysis will be deficient (contributing to the length discrepancy), but should not be damaged operatively. Careful extraperiosteal dissection of the heel pad from the os calcis is often difficult, but is needed to preserve an optimal weight-bearing stump. The Achilles tendon may be carefully transected to prevent later migration of the heel pad posteriorly and proximally. The medial malleolus is not trimmed, because it will not grow in the absence of normal stimuli and will not interfere with prosthetic fitting, either cosmetically or functionally (see Fig 145–2,E). Careful skin closure with drainage of the stump is desired. If proper incision is planned, the scar will lie anterior to the "ankle" level. Fixation of the heel pad to the tibia should be assured by means of one or two small Kirschner pins drilled through the heel pad into the intramedullary tibial canal. A rigid dressing should be used, carried above the flexed knee for stability of the cast and comfort in a very young child. Pins can be removed at about 3 weeks under a brief general anesthetic, at which time the cast can be taken for the prosthetic mold. Rigid dressings continue until 4–5 postoperative weeks, at which time prosthetic fitting is undertaken. If the degree of tibial kyphosis is sufficiently severe to threaten future plantar positioning of the stump pad in a prosthesis, or to interfere with prosthetic cosmesis, correction of the tibial bowing by closed-wedge osteotomy can be performed at

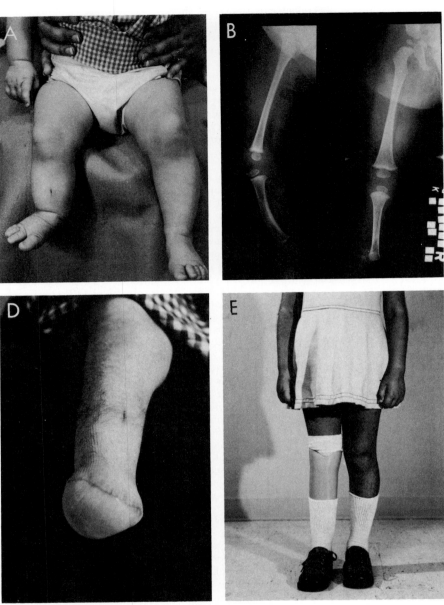

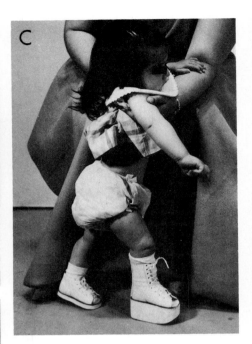

Fig 145–2.—Fibular hemimelia: terminal, longitudinal, complete. This is the most frequent lower limb deformity. **A** and **B,** the fibula is entirely absent. The tibia is shorter than normal, often thicker, and, as here, bowed anteriorly. The diagnostic dimple in the skin over the apex of the bow does not show up in this photograph. **C,** preconversion limb length equalization by a lift. Stabilization of the ankle is necessary because of lack of the external malleolus. **D,** fibular hemimelia following foot ablation. Note position of scar and heel pad in this Syme-type amputation. **E,** prosthetic fitting of fibular hemimelia after foot ablation.

the time of foot ablation, the pin for heel pad fixation being used to provide intramedullary fixation of the tibia. Fibular hemimelia often accompanies more proximal ipsilateral skeletal deficiencies such as congenital short femur or proximal femoral focal deficiency.

PROXIMAL FEMORAL FOCAL DEFICIENCY.—Proximal femoral focal deficiency (PFFD) presents with a very short thigh held in flexion, abduction, and external rotation.[1, 2] There will be variable degrees of clinical "hip" instability. The ankle on the affected side will be at the level of the knee on the normal side. The clinical appearance is nearly diagnostic of the entity. Aitken[1, 2] classified PFFD into four types (Fig 145–3). In type A

PFFD, there is an acetabulum containing a femoral head, a femoral neck, greater trochanter, and short femoral shaft. In the subtrochanteric region, a lateral angulation will be present, usually resulting from a pseudarthrosis, the angulation contributing to functional shortening. In type B PFFD, there is an acetabulum, a femoral head, no apparent femoral neck or connection to the remainder of the femur, a trochanteric tuft, and a short femoral shaft. Motion of the shaft is not transmitted directly to the femoral head. The head may or may not be mobile in the acetabulum. In type C PFFD, there is no acetabulum; no femoral head, neck, or trochanter; and the proximal end of the femoral shaft ends in a tuft. In type D PFFD, there is no acetabulum; no femoral head, neck, or trochanter; and the femoral shaft is

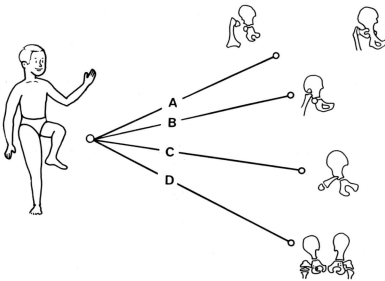

Fig 145–3.—Aitken classification of PFFD, types *A, B, C, D.*

exceedingly short and usually directed horizontally. Eventually, the proximal end of the femur in types A, B, and C will lie above the level of the acetabulum. In infancy, lack of ossification of the cartilaginous femoral neck in type A PFFD will create the radiologic appearance of a "space," making differentiation from type B PFFD difficult. Ossification of the neck in type A may be delayed for years. Computed tomography may assist in early differentiation of type A from type B PFFD. Hip arthrography with examination under an image intensifier may be helpful. Initially, all patients with PFFD are provided nonstandard prostheses fitted around the presenting limb (Fig 145–4,*A,B*).

Surgical intervention in PFFD is limited to repair of the pseudarthrosis of the proximal femur in type A; knee arthrodesis in types A, B, and C; and foot ablation only in the unilateral PFFD. As in fibular hemimelia, foot ablation in the unilateral PFFD may be carried out at any time (see Fig 145–4,*C,D*). Osteosynthesis to repair type A pseudarthrosis improves hip stability, prosthetic alignment, comfort, and gait. Timing of osteosynthesis is determined by the presence of sufficient ossified femur on both sides of the pseudarthrosis to permit resection of the angulation with internal fixation. Knee arthrodesis may be desired to produce a longer, more stable, stump-lever arm, converting the deformity to a long above-knee amputation type.

Patients with bilateral PFFD should not have foot ablation, because they will have the ability to ambulate in their homes without prostheses (Fig 145–5,*A,B*).

TIBIAL HEMIMELIA.—In tibial hemimelia,[4] there is complete absence of the tibia, a fibula of variable length and contour extending proximal to the distal end of the femur, and a foot positioned in severe inversion and equinus, the sole of the foot facing the perineum (Fig 145–6,*A*). There may be a severe popliteal pterygium. If there is insufficient quadriceps activity to produce active extension of the knee, the treatment of choice is a knee disarticulation type of amputation followed by prosthetic fitting (see Fig 145–6,*B*). This procedure may be done at any age. If there is no pterygium and if good quadriceps activity exists, one has the option of performing fibular transposition beneath the femur with resultant transformation of the shape of the proximal fibula into that of the proximal tibia, foot ablation, and fitting

with a modified Syme-type prosthesis with rigid knee hinges and thigh support. In incomplete tibial hemimelia, there is a proximal tibial segment of variable length, absence of the distal tibia, a foot positioned as in complete tibial hemimelia, and an unstable proximal tibiofibular joint. Management is by means of synostosis of the fibula to the tibia, ablation of the foot, and fitting with a below-knee prosthesis.

Fitting with Prostheses

Age of fitting of children should be geared to their level of neuromuscular development. The child should not be expected to function at a level above the norm for his chronological age. Unimembral upper limb deficiency can be fitted as early as 3 months of age in order to establish bimanual gross prehension and begin production of prosthetic tolerance. Unilateral lower limb deficiency should be fitted at about the time the child indicates a desire to stand by attempting to pull to a standing position. Time of fitting of bilateral upper limb deficiency will be governed by the need to maintain sensory feedback, the level of amputation, and general trunk stability. In those with severe bilateral upper limb loss (e.g., amelia, complete phocomelia), foot function will be automatic unless discouraged by the treating team or family. Foot function should always be encouraged and retained. In those with bilateral lower limb deficiency, age of fitting is governed by level of loss. In those unable to achieve sitting balance without prostheses, fitting is initiated at about 5 months of age, when independent sitting balance would be expected, using a prosthetic bucket. In those able to sit independently, age of fitting is at the time of initiation of pull to stand. In those with both upper and lower limb involvement, upper limb function needs take precedence. Fitting for ambulation can be expected to be delayed.

In training children fitted with prostheses, it must be remembered that attention span will limit treatment time. In general in patients up to 6 years of age, attention time in minutes equals age in years. In upper limb prosthetic training, activation of terminal devices may occur accidentally at any age. Purposeful activation will occur at 18–24 months of age, but not before it occurs in the normal hand. Control of elbow locks will not occur

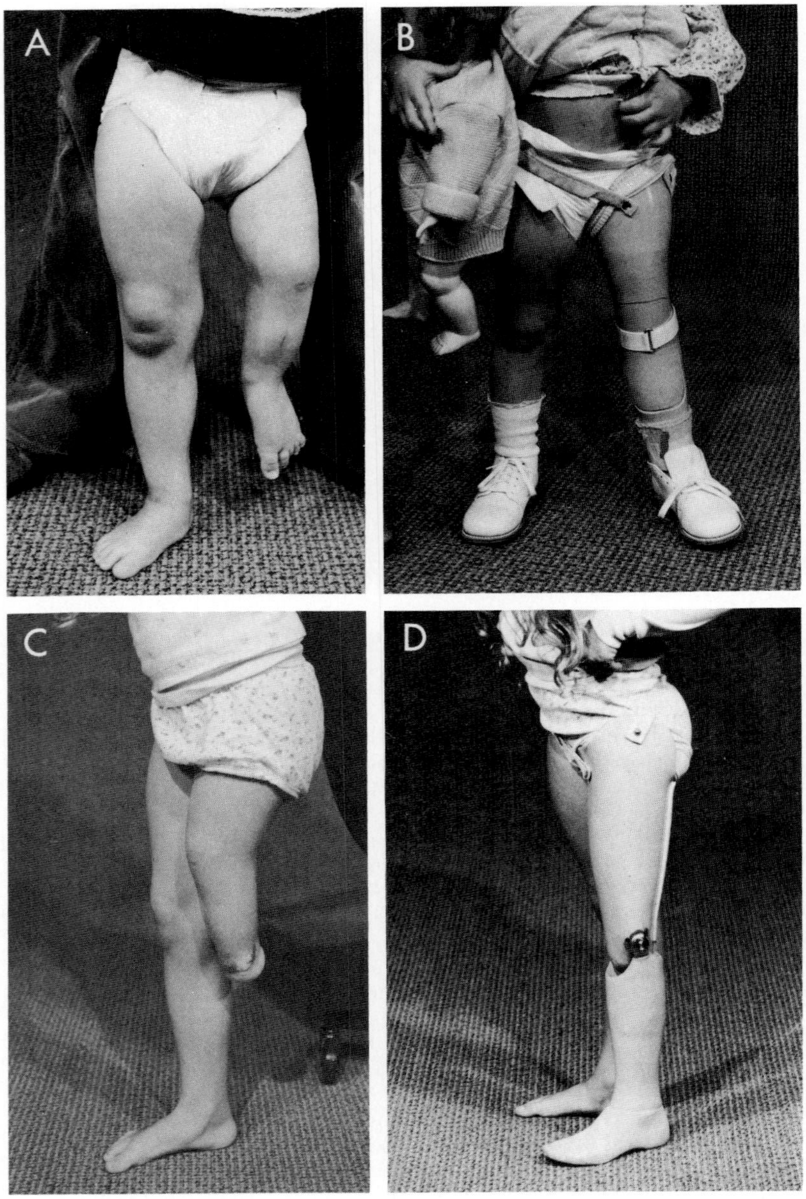

Fig 145–4.—PFFD, type A, with accompanying fibular hemimelia. **A,** and **B,** the initial prosthesis is fitted around the foot to equalize leg lengths. The proximal femoral pseudarthrosis has been repaired. **C** and **D,** the result following foot ablation and fitting with an above-knee type of prosthesis. In addition to repair of the femoral pseudarthrosis, arthrodesis of the knee is required for the obvious reasons.

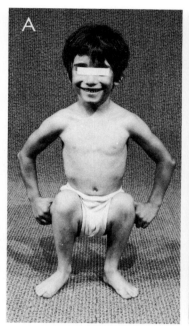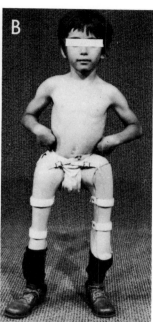

Fig 145–5.—Bilateral femoral focal deficiencies. **A** and **B,** the child can walk at home without the prosthesis. Therefore, the feet are preserved, and a non-standard prosthesis is fashioned.

REFERENCES

1. Aitken G.T. (ed.): *Proximal Femoral Focal Deficiency: A Congenital Anomaly.* Washington, D.C., National Academy of Sciences, 1969.
2. Aitken G.T.: Proximal femoral focal deficiency, in Swinyard C.W. (ed.): *Limb Development and Deformity: Problems of Evaluation and Rehabilitation.* Springfield, Ill, Charles C Thomas, Publisher, 1969, pp. 456–476.
3. Aitken G.T.: Osseous overgrowth in amputations in children, in Swinyard C.W. (ed.): *Limb Development and Deformity: Problems of Evaluation and Rehabilitation.* Springfield, Ill., Charles C Thomas, Publisher, 1969, pp. 448–456.
4. Aitken G.T. (ed.): *Selected Lower-Limb Anomalies: Surgical and Prosthetic Management.* Washington, D.C., National Academy of Sciences, 1971.
5. Aitken G.T. (ed.): *The Child with an Acquired Amputation: A Symposium.* Washington, D.C., National Academy of Sciences, 1972.
6. Aitken G.T.: The Child Amputee: An Overview. *Orthop. Clin. North Am.* 3:447–472, 1972.
7. Aitken G.T., Frantz C.H.: Management of the child amputee, in *Instructional Course Lectures.* St. Louis, American Academy of Orthopaedic Surgeons, 1960, vol. 17, pp. 246–295.
8. American Academy of Orthopaedic Surgeons: *Atlas of Limb Prosthetics: Surgical and Prosthetic Principles.* St. Louis, C.V. Mosby Co., 1981.
9. Frantz C.H., O'Rahilly R.: Congenital skeletal limb deficiencies. *J. Bone Joint Surg.* 43A:1202–1224, 1961.
10. Krebs D.E., Fishman S.: Characteristics of the child amputee population. *J. Pediatr. Orthop.* 4:89–95, 1984.
11. Lambert C.N.: Etiology, in Aitken G.T. (ed.): *The Child with an Acquired Amputation: A Symposium.* Washington, D.C., National Academy of Sciences, 1972, pp. 1–5.
12. Marquardt E.: The Multiple Limb-Deficient Child, in *Atlas of Limb Prosthetics: Surgical and Prosthetic Principles.* American Academy of Orthopaedic Surgeons, St. Louis, C.V. Mosby Co., 1981, pp. 595–641.
13. Simon M.A.: Causes of increased survival of patients with osteosarcoma: Current controversies. *J. Bone Joint Surg.* 66A:306–310, 1984.
14. Tooms R.E.: Acquired amputations in children, in *Atlas of Limb Prosthetics: Surgical and Prosthetic Principles.* American Academy of Orthopaedic Surgeons, St. Louis, C.V. Mosby Co., 1981, pp. 553–559.
15. Watts H.G.: Special considerations in amputations for malignancies, in *Atlas of Limb Prosthetics: Surgical and Prosthetic Principles.* American Academy of Orthopaedic Surgeons, St. Louis, C.V. Mosby Co., 1981, pp. 459–463.

purposefully before 36 months of age. Most children with lower limb prostheses do not require extensive therapy for gait training. It should be remembered that small children do not have a gait similar to adults, and gait expectation should be geared to their age and neuromuscular development.

In all instances, the goal of treatment of the juvenile amputee is that of maximum independence in activities of daily living in adulthood.

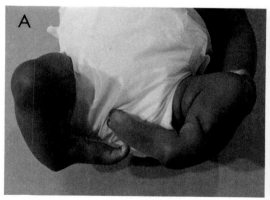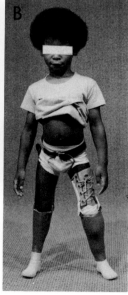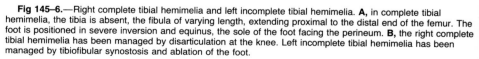

Fig 145–6.—Right complete tibial hemimelia and left incomplete tibial hemimelia. **A,** in complete tibial hemimelia, the tibia is absent, the fibula of varying length, extending proximal to the distal end of the femur. The foot is positioned in severe inversion and equinus, the sole of the foot facing the perineum. **B,** the right complete tibial hemimelia has been managed by disarticulation at the knee. Left incomplete tibial hemimelia has been managed by tibiofibular synostosis and ablation of the foot.

Skin, Soft Tissues, and Blood Vessels

PLATE VI

A. Port-wine stain. A 10-year-old boy with a capillary hemangioma, or port-wine stain, which was present at birth. The lesion has not, and will not change appreciably. It has been necessary to tell the parents that little worthwhile can be done to improve this condition. Excision and resurfacing procedures would leave marks or defects as obvious as the lesion. Some centers attempt surgical tattoo procedures, and others use staged excision with a laser.

B. Complicated syndactylism. A 6-month-old baby with mitten hands, as part of Crouzon's deformity. The baby also had craniostenosis, a high-arched palate and partial choanal atresia, and absence of some proximal interphalangeal joints, hypoplasia of phalanges and tendons, and soft-tissue webbing. The fingers were individualized by using dorsal rotation flaps for the base of the interdigital web spaces and free partial-thickness skin grafts for the sides of the fingers. The fingers, although cosmetically more acceptable, will always be relatively stiff.

C. Wringer injury. A 5-year-old boy with a wringer injury had an area of contused, abraded, and ecchymotic skin above the elbow and a friction burn with full-thickness skin necrosis below the shoulder. The skin between these two areas was avulsed from the subcutaneous fascia and was the site of an expanding hematoma containing crumbled avascular fat. Because there was one large definite area of full-thickness skin loss, primary excision of both this area and that of questionable viability above the elbow was carried out. After evacuation of the hematoma and the avascular fat from the avulsed zone, the two raw areas were resurfaced with partial-thickness skin grafts.

D. Hemangioma. This photograph of a superficial and deep cavernous hemangioma of the ulnar region of the hand in a 3-month-old baby illustrates the controversy of spontaneous regression vs. operative intervention. The fingers involved were becoming spread as the infant grew, indicating that regression of the lesion should be hastened by operation.

E. Congenital lymphedema. A 4-year-old boy with congenital lymphedema, or Milroy's disease. The involvement in this child was restricted to one upper extremity and showed no significant improvement either spontaneously or after elastic occlusive bandaging. Both the parents and the child encountered increasing difficulty with the sleeves of the child's winter clothing. The lymphedematous tissue on the dorsum of the hand and the wrist was excised down to paratenon. Partial-thickness skin was removed from the excised tissue and returned as a free graft. The result, although not spectacular, was appreciated by the parents and the child. An alternative preferred by many is excision of all subcutaneous tissue from beneath elevated skin flaps and closure over suction drains. Long-term compression therapy is still required.

F. Giant, hairy pigmented nevi. Photograph of a 2½-year-old girl for whom a plan was outlined to make the exposed regions of the body—the face, hands, and arms below the level of short sleeves, and the legs below the level of short skirts—more acceptable. The smaller lesions were electrocoagulated in stages; slightly larger and suitably placed lesions were removed by multiple excision. Still other lesions were removed and resurfaced by free skin grafts. The parents were encouraged to report any rapid changes in residual lesions. Cosmetically, the result was satisfactory.

PLATE VI

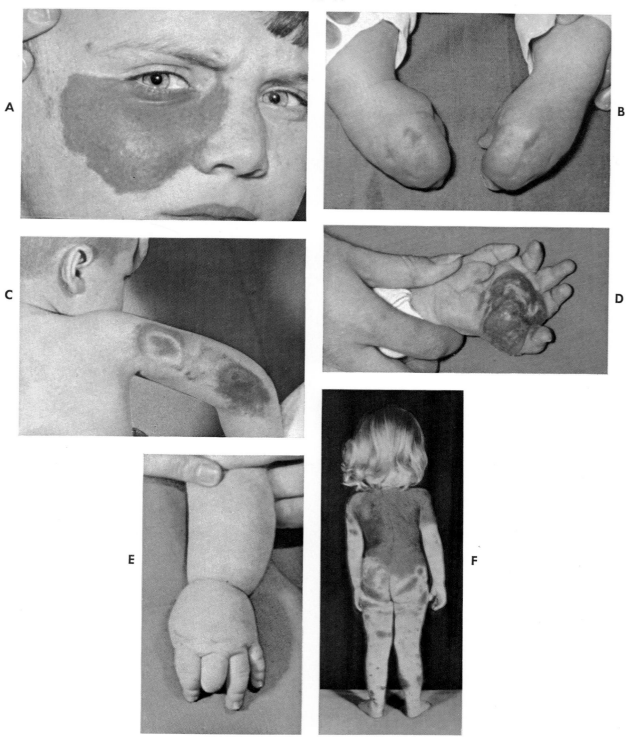

Congenital Defects of the Skin, Muscles, Connective Tissues, Tendons, and Hands

Incidence

WITH SO MANY and varied anomalies to be considered, it is impossible to give detailed incidence data. For comparative purposes, the general distribution of congenital anomalies in a segment of Canada, as obtained from medical information given by physicians within 48 hours of the infant's birth, is outlined in Table 146–1[46] using, where possible, the International Classification of Diseases (ICD).

The congenital lesions of somatic soft tissues are found within ICD nos. 228, 758, and 759 and under the heading All Other Abnormalities. They comprise only a portion of the totals, however, and any one of the anomalies to be considered has a low incidence in comparison with clubfoot, spina bifida, and meningocele, and with cleft palate or cleft lip. This low incidence makes it difficult to obtain significant data for epidemiologic studies. The incidence in the area reporting has remained the same over the years. It is common to find anomalies of the somatic soft tissues occurring in combination with those of other tissues, as in Apert's disease[28] and the Ellis-van Creveld syndrome.[12] It is generally agreed that heredity plays a role in the production of congenital limb defects, but to what degree and in what way are controversial. Certain conditions, e.g., brachydactyly, may represent dominant genes and are transmitted through generations. Polydactyly, however, does not appear as regularly in families because of a genetic phenomenon called incomplete penetrance. The term is used to explain an abnormal genetic constitution not visible in the immediate offspring, but present in later generations. The achondroplastic dwarf in whom the gene is dominant and fully penetrant may be born of normal parents; the gene in this case has undergone mutation.

Many environmental factors during gestation have been shown in animal experiments to have a direct influence on the production of anomalies. The embryos of radiation-mutant strains of rats have had lymph sacs and hematomas lying on limb buds where deformities were later found.[1] Anoxia during the 2d to 7th weeks of gestation can produce controlled extremity anomalies.[21, 25] Metabolic trauma in the form of insulin injection[10] and cortisone injection can cause extremity deformities. Dietary deprivation[56] and radiation exposure of the mother will do likewise. Experimental embryologists can produce extremity defects in lower vertebrates by notochordal interference and other stimuli, suggesting an early neural influence on the developing embryo. Series of anomalies have been produced by arterial interference with the pregnant uterus.[21]

Classification and Nomenclature

Congenital defects of the somatic soft tissues may be classified in a number of different ways: (1) Segmental—most defects have either a basic longitudinal distribution (radial ray and ulnar ray defects) or a basic transverse distribution (congenital bands and congenital amputations). Many anomalies present combinations of both. (2) Tissue—here again, an anomaly rarely involves a sin-

TABLE 146–1.—CONGENITAL ABNORMALITIES REPORTED IN INFANTS BORN ALIVE (1959)

CONGENITAL ABNORMALITY	ICD* NO.	NO. OF PTS.	% OF TOTAL	RATE†	% UNDER 2,501 gm
Hemangioma and lymphangioma	228	85	4.6	0.54	3.5
Mongolism	325.4	45	2.4	0.29	17.8
Hernia of abdominal cavity	560	41	1.7	0.20	12.9
Clubfoot	748	221	11.9	1.41	15.4
Monstrosity	750	46	2.5	0.29	71.7
Spina bifida and meningocele	751	192	10.4	1.22	15.6
Hydrocephalus	752	76	4.1	0.48	14.5
Other CNS lesions	753	40	2.2	0.25	32.5
Circulatory system	754	30	1.6	0.19	13.3
Cleft palate and/or harelip	755	170	9.2	1.08	17.7
Digestive system	756	55	3.0	0.35	30.9
Genitourinary system	757	154	8.3	0.98	9.7
Bone and joint	758	152	8.2	0.97	18.4
Other malformations	759	449	24.2	2.86	13.4
Erythroblastosis	770	52	2.8	0.34	21.2
All other abnormalities	–	56	2.9	0.36	7.3
		1,854	100.0	11.81	16.4

*International Classification of Diseases, 1955.
†Per 1,000 live births (tentatively 156,982).

gle tissue. Multiple tissue or multiple segmental involvement makes precise classification difficult. (3) Degree of involvement—most anomalies present primarily as excesses (accessory parts; hyperplasias) or deficiencies (partial or complete absence of parts; hypoplasias). The planning and results of treatment are closely related to this consideration. The value of the classification method is restricted, because many anomalies contain combinations of excesses and deficiencies; for instance, an accessory thumb usually is associated with some hypoplasia of the main thumb. (4) Generic—a complete return to this detailed descriptive method of classification is necessary if reporting of epidemiologic and technical advances is to be successful. Table 146–2 contains such a classification of the basic extremity defects.

It is impossible to consider the soft tissue anomalies without considering those of tendons, joints, and bone because of the frequency of multiple tissue involvement.

Congenital Defects of Skin

Congenital absence of the skin (aplasia cutis congenita) is less common on the extremities and trunk than on the scalp, but generally it is more extensive, often being multiple, bilateral, and symmetric.[18, 40, 54, 55] The lesion may involve in varying degrees the skin, subcutaneous tissue, muscle, and bone. Infants may be born with areas of granulation tissue on the surface; with areas in which the skin has a dark, recently necrosed appearance; or with areas that are covered by thin, tight scar skin (Fig 146–1). The very small areas of involvement will epithelialize spontaneously and rapidly, but larger areas require appropriate resurfacing, usually by partial-thickness skin grafts. Unstable scar skin should be excised and resurfaced because of the possibility of malignant change many years later.

CONGENITAL AGENESIS OF THE SCALP.—This is a rare condition.[18, 40, 54, 55] Various areas of the scalp may be involved, but when the involvement is severe, the region of the vertex is commonly the site of the maldevelopment. At birth there is a non-hair-bearing patch covered by a thin transparent membrane or by a dry scabbed area, which eventually granulates. This is followed by an ingrowth of epithelium so that a scarred area is formed (Fig 146–2). It is possible to skin-graft the large areas and to treat the small areas by rotation flaps of hair-bearing ad-

TABLE 146–2.—CLASSIFICATION OF BASIC EXTREMITY DEFECTS

DEFORMITIES OF ARM
 Melomelia: supernumerary limbs, normal or rudimentary
 Peromelia: deformed limbs
 Ectromelia: grossly defective or absent limbs
 Hemimelia: absence of forearm and hand
 Brachymelia: short limb
 Micromelia: diminished size of limb
 Phocomelia: absence of limbs
 Abrachia: absence of arms
 Amelia: absence of limbs
 Cubitus valgus and varus: angulation at elbow

DEFORMITIES OF HAND
 Radial ray defect: clubhand
 Ulnar ray defect: clubhand
 Central ray defect: split hand or lobster claw
 Perochiria: deformed hand
 Ectrochiria: absence of hand
 Microchiria: hypoplasia of all parts of hand
 Brachymetacarpia: abnormal shortness of metacarpal bones
 Ectrometacarpia: absence of metacarpal bones
 Polymetacarpia: more than normal number of metacarpal bones

DEFORMITIES OF FINGERS
 Ectrophalangia: absence of one or more phalanges
 Hyperphalangia: more than normal number of phalanges in longitudinal axes
 Polyphalangia: more than normal number of phalanges in transverse direction
 Symphalangia: end-to-end fusion of phalanges
 Acrosyndactyly: fusion of terminal portion of digits; sometimes proximal clefts or sinuses
 Brachydactyly: abnormal shortness of fingers
 Ectrodactyly: partial absence of digit; absence of digit or portion of digit
 Polydactyly: more than normal number of fingers
 Syndactyly: fused digits (webbed fingers)
 Synostosis: bony fusion of transversely placed bone
 Synonychia: fusion of finger nail common to two or more digits
 Clinarthrosis: oblique or lateral angular deviation in alignment of joints
 Arachnodactyly: digital abnormally long phalanges
 Adactyly: absence of fingers
 Megalodactyly: giant digits

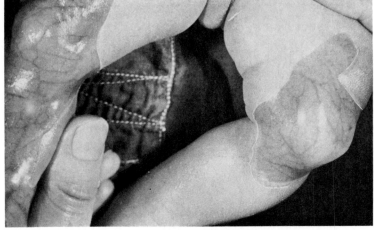

Fig 146–1.—Hypoplasia cutis congenita. A newborn infant with large areas of thin, tight hypoplastic skin lacking in elastic fibers. The patient also had some marginal vesicles (not shown) that may be considered an example of the dystrophic form of epidermolysis bullosa. Contractures developed around the knee that required elective resurfacing with free partial-thickness skin grafts. Noncontracted areas of hypoplastic skin become stable and mature, which rarely happens with epidermolysis bullosa.

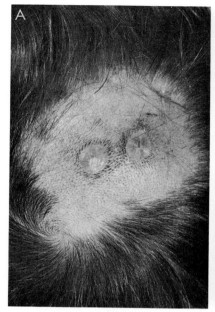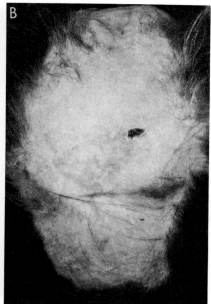

Fig 146–2.—Agenesis of the scalp. **A,** small areas with a thin, easily traumatized, hairless surface, most commonly involving the parietal area of the scalp. **B,** large hairless areas occur occasionally. When the dry eschar separates or is removed, there is danger of hemorrhage from the sagittal sinus. Such areas granulate slowly and may be surfaced with free grafts, already accomplished in this patient.

jacent scalp or by elliptic excision with direct suture. The small defects are probably best left untreated until the patient is of such an age that with the growth of scalp hair the ultimate appearance can be accurately assessed. The ability of the surface covering to withstand trauma improves within a few months. In a few cases, there may be an underlying bone defect. The death

rate with large defects is high. Associated congenital anomalies are frequent with this condition.

Epidermolysis bullosa is characterized by vesicles and bullae in the skin together with a defect in the elastic fibers. The congenital variety either is present at birth or appears shortly after birth. There may be a familial history. The spontaneous form

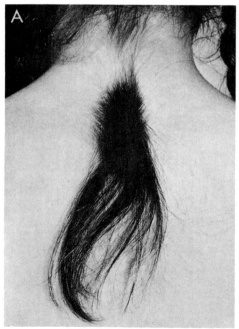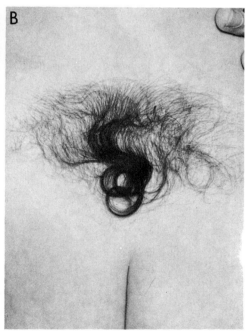

Fig 146–3.—Aberrant hair. **A,** resemblance to a horse's mane is striking. Local excision is indicated. **B,** meningocele frequently accompanies this lesion, although this patient had only spina bifida, demonstrated on x-ray study. Surgical removal by multiple excision is often worthwhile, but the residual scarring to be expected must be explained in detail to parents.

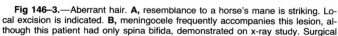

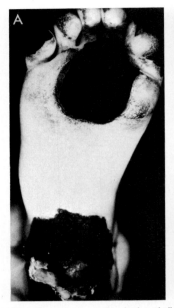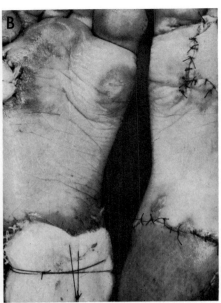

Fig 146–4.—Keratodermia plantaris. The patient's mother had a similar involvement. **A,** lesions at age 3 years, having progressed since birth. They were hard, black, tender, and prevented weight-bearing. Keratolytics, cortisone, and vitamin A therapy were not effective. **B,** immediately after excision and a free partial-thickness skin graft. Narrow marginal recurrences required further excision and additional grafts.

occurs later in childhood, usually after mild trauma or exposure to the sun's rays. The condition may be simple or complex. Simple lesions are relatively small and usually situated on the extensor aspect of the extremities, but they also may occur on the trunk. They almost always resolve spontaneously. The complex form (see Fig 146–1) as a rule is associated with considerable dystrophy of the skin and even of the underlying soft tissues and bone. This form frequently requires replacement with more stable soft tissue. There may be involvement of oral, pharyngeal, and even tracheal mucosa, making oral and dental hygiene and endotracheal anesthesia a problem. Parents must develop atraumatic skin care techniques. Patients with extensive involvement develop epidermoid carcinoma changes over the years.

The condition is to be differentiated from Ritter's disease (dermatitis exfoliativa infantum or keratolysis neonatorum), Leiner's disease (erythroderma desquamativum), impetigo neonatorum, and congenital syphilis.

Congenitally fragile skin may occur by itself or as a manifesta-

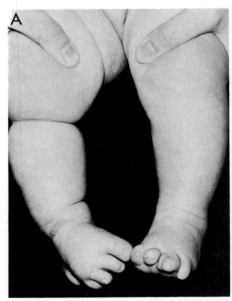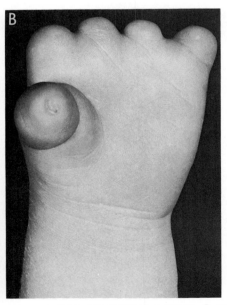

Fig 146–5.—**A,** congenital annular bands. The most severe lesion is immediately below the knee and requires lengthening by two paired Z-plasty operations; the first on the anterior and posterior surfaces, the second on the medial and lateral surfaces by 3 months of age. There is a partial band more distal on the medial aspect of the same leg, which should be corrected by a single Z-plasty during one of the aforementioned operations. **B,** congenital amputations of all digits through the proximal phalanges, with a secondary annular band on the thumb proximal to the amputation. Deepening of the thumb-index finger web is indicated to allow as much coarse pinch as possible. Deepening of the other interdigital web spaces will be of more limited value.

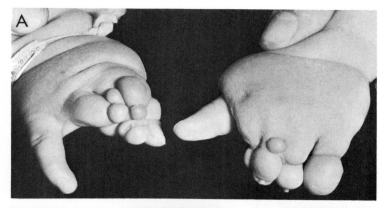

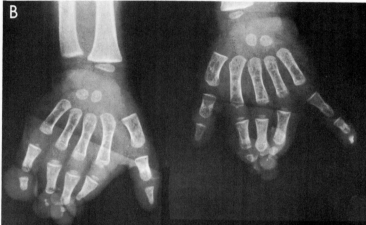

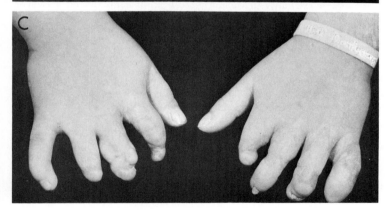

Fig 146–6.—Jumbled fingers, congenital bands, congenital amputation, acrosyndactyly. **A,** the preoperative condition at 3 months of age. Note lymphedema distal to some of the bands. **B,** preoperative radiographs to show absence of phalanges and varying degrees of hypoplasia. **C,** at 9 months of age, after correction of the bands by Z-plasties and the syndactyly, as shown in Figure 146–19. The patient still requires excision of the lymphedematous areas and lengthening by free full-thickness grafts of the more shortened areas.

tion of ectodermal dysplasia, Ehlers-Danlos syndrome.[30] The condition requires careful protection against skin trauma, including the wearing of a helmet and shin guards. It is important to avoid the usual therapeutic radiation doses in such patients because of the possibility of skin breakdown. Lacerations and elective incisions heal with marked scar spread.

Ectopic or misplaced hair (Fig 146–3) usually occurs in the midline of the back with or without spina bifida, dermal sinuses, and dermoid cysts. Treatment is by excision, due consideration being given to the possibility of an underlying myelomeningocele.

Keratodermia palmaris et plantaris (Fig 146–4) is a severe specific form of callus formation or tylosis. It frequently is familial and is caused by progressive thickening of the horny layer of the epidermis to such a degree that it may prevent weight-bearing.

There may be associated dystrophy of the nails, leukoplakia of the oral mucosa, and vitamin A deficiency. Use of keratolytics, vitamin A, and cortisone and radiation therapy have offered improvement in isolated case reports. More recently, excision of the lesions and replacement with suitable skin grafts have proved more satisfactory.

Congenital bands were formerly thought to be due to exogenous complications such as amniotic bands (Simonart's bands), hydramnios, umbilical cord slings, other uterine space-narrowing processes, and various maternal constitutional deficiencies. Extensive reviews of the theories related to these forms of exogenous causes are available[3] and are still worthy of consideration, although they have been abandoned to a large extent, to be replaced by the theory of endogenous germ cell deficit or defectively developed tissues.[40, 52]

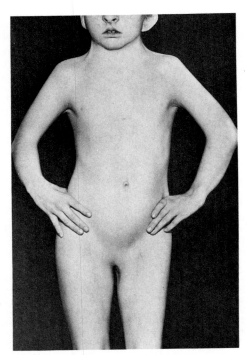

Fig 146–7.—Webbing of neck and crural region. The patient, with ovarian agenesis, also had axillary and columellar-labial webbing and required paired crural Z-plasties, in order to uncover the introitus, and large bilateral neck Z-plasties. The posterior axillary webs became more obvious with time and later required correction.

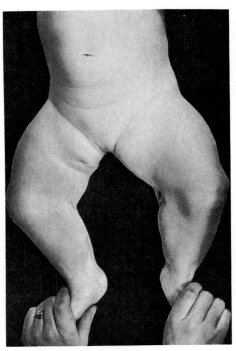

Fig 146–8.—Webbing of popliteal space. Bilateral involvement was worse on the left, where the hamstring muscles were abnormally inserted on the os calcis. Staged lengthening by large Z-plasties, together with careful splinting, avoided undue stretching of the sciatic nerve. The hamstrings were detached and replaced more normally.

Transverse or circular, partial or complete soft tissue defects of varying depth and tightness may involve any or all layers of the skin and the soft tissues beneath them (Fig 146–5,*A*). The most severe degrees of congenital bands may involve bone or present as a congenital amputation (Fig 146–5,*B*). There may be edema of the tissue distal to the band—to be distinguished from congenital lymphedema. Treatment is started at 3 months of age and consists of circumferential lengthening of the bands by means of serial Z-plasty maneuvers (Fig 146–6). If edema persists after correction of the band, excision of the edematous area may be necessary, with direct closure or conversion of the overlying skin to thick, free partial-thickness skin grafts. If there is a gross motor or sensory deficit in the extremity distal to the band, early amputation and fitting of a prosthesis are the treatments of choice.

Congenital webs or pterygia are commonest in the neck (pterygium colli), but similar webbing may occur in the anterior axillary folds and in the crural region (Fig 146–7). In the neck, the webbing is frequently a manifestation of Turner syndrome.

If the webs produce a significant cosmetic or functional disability, they should be lengthened at 1–6 years of age by means of Z-plasties. Congenital webs may also occur across the cubital and popliteal fossae (Fig 146–8). Such webs usually contain misplaced or aberrant tendons and nerves. Treatment is by serial Z-plasties. On occasion, aberrant muscles or tendons may require lengthening or even excision. Extensive soft tissue, tendon, and nerve lengthening by free nerve grafting has been reported.[53]

Congenital Defects of Muscle

Individual muscles or muscle groups may be totally or partially absent. Perhaps the most clear-cut example of this is congenital absence of the pectoralis major muscle (Fig 146–9). The condition may be present by itself; with more distal lesions of the upper extremity, particularly those of ulnar ray defect, known as Poland syndrome; or with absence of breast and costal cartilage (see Chap. 57). The lesion causes no significant functional disability, although it produces obvious deformity. Hypoplastic muscles may be short and tight and difficult to tell from muscle contracture.[38]

Generalized hypertrophy or overdevelopment of the whole body musculature (wrestler's syndrome) may occur.[33] Such infants are strong and accomplish unusual physical feats. Mucopolysaccharide disorders must be ruled out. Associated hypertrophy of the tongue frequently occurs, and mental retardation may be present. In almost all of these children, the tongue becomes proportionate with time, and no treatment is necessary. The tongue is accepted inside the mouth in 2–3 years. A degree of prognathism may or may not result. Endocrine disorders must be ruled out. Localized muscle hypertrophy (Fig 146–10) may require partial or complete excision of the involved muscle. Misplaced origins and insertions of muscles usually are associated with congenital webs or congenital contractures. Treatment is by lengthening or excision.

Congenital Defects of Tendons and Sheaths

Tendons may be short, thin, misplaced, abnormally inserted, or absent.[7] The resultant deformity may be confused with more generalized myodystrophia fetalis. The abductor pollicis longus tendon may be absent or misplaced as part of a radial ray defect. The flexor digitorum sublimis tendon may be short or abnormally inserted and may be the cause of a congenital flexion contracture of the proximal interphalangeal joint. The flexor digitorum profundus tendon may be short, causing flexion of the interphalangeal and metacarpophalangeal joints, with the wrist extended. Lengthening of the tendon at the wrist will give satisfactory im-

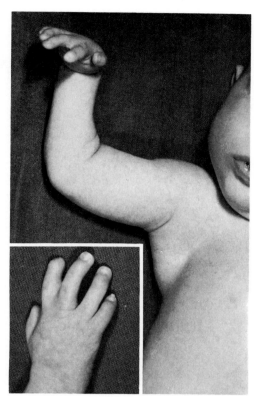

Fig 146–9.—Congenital absence of pectoralis major muscle, associated with hypoplasia of arm, forearm, hand, and fingers (micromelia and brachymelia) and syndactyly—Poland syndrome (see Chap. 57). Only the syndactyly was treated.

provement. Absence of the central band of the extensor expansion of the extensor digitorum longus tendon will cause flexion deformity of the proximal interphalangeal joint with or without hyperextension of the distal interphalangeal joint, or boutonniere deformity. Treatment requires reconstruction of this portion of the extensor expansion by means of free fascial grafts or shifting of the lateral bands dorsally. The lateral bands of the extensor expansion may be short, causing a similar deformity, and lengthening of these bands by partially transecting them at the sides of the proximal phalanges will improve the deformity.

Stenosing tenovaginitis (trigger finger or thumb), if not congenital, frequently occurs spontaneously in children. The flexor

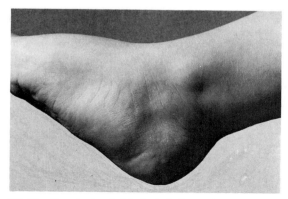

Fig 146–10.—Hypertrophy of abductor hallucis muscle present at birth as an isolated lesion. Wedge excision of some overlying skin and most of the muscle was carried out to facilitate the fitting of shoes.

pollicis longus tendon and sheath are most commonly involved, but any of the fingers may be the site. The digit assumes a fixed flexion deformity, although it may occasionally actively or passively extend with a painful clunk (trigger action). The lesion is due to a narrowing of the digital flexor sheath overlying the metacarpal head. Swelling and chronic inflammation of the tendon distal to the constriction are common. Treatment consists of exposing the tendon sheath through a transverse incision in a skin crease close to the metacarpal head, and opening the sheath and fibrous tunnel longitudinally and laterally over a length sufficient to allow sliding of the secondarily thickened zone of the tendon. This should be carried out after allowing about 3 months for the possibility of spontaneous improvement.

Congenital flexion contractures commonly involve the proximal interphalangeal joints of the little finger. Similar involvement of the ring and middle fingers occurs less commonly. The deformity may have a number of causes: deficit of volar subcutaneous tissue in the region, shortening of volar capsule and collateral ligaments, anomaly of flexor digitorum sublimis with abnormal insertion or shortening of that tendon, or absence of the central band of the extensor expansion. It is important to be certain that the defect is not a more generalized case of myodystrophia fetalis. The lesion tends to correct itself in certain instances, but manipulation and plaster splinting may be of value in the very young. If there is no improvement by 6 months of age, it is necessary to divide all the involved tissues transversely just proximal to the region of the proximal interphalangeal skin crease and resurface the resulting defect appropriately with either a free full-thickness skin graft or a cross finger pedicle skin-fat flap. A capsulotomy and freeing of the volar plate may be necessary. Examining the palm for an anomalous lumbrical muscle is occasionally rewarding.

Congenital Defects of the Hand

Most hand defects[5, 8] are associated with forearm or finger anomalies (Figs 146–11 and 146–12). The radial side of the hand and forearm is commonly involved with a radial ray defect (Fig 146–13). The severity of the anomaly may vary from a deficit in some portion of the structures affecting opposition of the thumb to a carpal anomaly, to absence of elbow joint, radius, thumb, and index finger. The remaining hand is pronated on the forearm as a flipper. Treatment is controversial.[5, 13, 17] Patients always have a useful little finger, particularly when the hand is pronated on the forearm. Some patients are better if left untreated. They may be able to use the hand amazingly well, although in a bizarre manner, but may have difficulty with sleeves of clothing.

Ideal treatment consists of obtaining a normal relationship between the hand remnant and the forearm. This should be initiated by neonatal manipulation, splinting, and occasionally plaster casting. Centralization of the hand on the ulna is completed by excising a central proximal row carpal bone, setting the ulna into it, and maintaining it there for a long time with a longitudinal Kirschner wire. Soft tissue lengthening procedures such as Z-plasty, local rotation flaps or free full-thickness grafts, capsulotomy, and tendon lengthenings at the radial side of the wrist may be necessary by 6 months of age. Pollicization of the index finger with opponens strengthening may be carried out at about 18 months of age.[5] Wrist stabilization by longitudinal splitting of the lower end of the ulna and blocking with an iliac crest bone graft at age 3 years will then give maximal surgical correction.

Madelung's deformity, produced by abnormalities of the radial epiphysis, is more often acquired than congenital. The ulnar side of the forearm and hand is less commonly involved (ulnar ray defect) (Fig 146–14). This lesion may vary from mild ulnar deviation of the wrist to partial or complete absence of the little and/

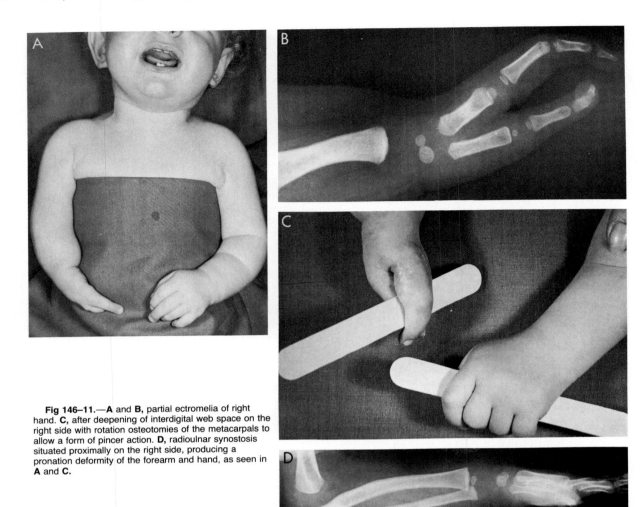

Fig 146–11.—**A** and **B,** partial ectromelia of right hand. **C,** after deepening of interdigital web space on the right side with rotation osteotomies of the metacarpals to allow a form of pincer action. **D,** radioulnar synostosis situated proximally on the right side, producing a pronation deformity of the forearm and hand, as seen in **A** and **C.**

or ring finger to total absence of the ulna.[16] Correcting and maintaining the position of the hand and the forearm shortly after birth are important. Radial osteotomy may be helpful. Reconstructive work on hypoplastic fingers may be indicated, but is not as worthwhile on the ulnar as on the radial side of the hand.

Central hand defects (Fig 146–15) are often referred to as split, lobster claw, or pincer hand. Such a hand is ungainly in appearance, but amazingly useful. Fortunately, the remainder of the arm usually grows well. Function may be improved by such procedures as deepening the web in the center of the hand and straightening and mobilizing or stabilizing the digits.

Split foot (Fig 146–16) requires treatment only if the fitting of shoes becomes a problem. The forefoot is narrowed by closing the central defect directly, with or without osteotomies of the metatarsal bones.

Congenital Defects of Fingers

Ectrophalangia or absence of one or more phalanges commonly involves the middle phalanges as an isolated anomaly or is combined with other finger anomalies such as generalized digital hypoplasia or syndactyly. Treatment, when indicated, is di-

rected at the associated deformities. Patients tend to have poker or stiff fingers, but this should be accepted, because it is not a great disability functionally or aesthetically.

Hyperphalangia refers to an excessive number of phalanges in the longitudinal axis. Simple excision followed by plaster immobilization for 3 weeks in the position of function produces an improvement. In polyphalangia, an increased number of phalanges is present in the transverse direction, often associated with an extra metacarpal. Excision of the extra element is indicated.[20] Symphalangia refers to end-to-end fusion of the phalanges and usually is associated with very gross deformities of the phalanges. Surgical separation will give a degree of improvement. Acrosyndactyly (see Fig 146–6) refers to fusion of the terminal portion of digits. Proximal clefts or sinuses may be present. Treatment is by separation of the phalanges and resurfacing of the raw areas.

Adactyly or absence of the fingers requires no treatment unless the digit involved is the thumb. In such cases, pollicization of the index finger is indicated.[11, 31, 32] Ectrodactyly or partial absence of a digit, or portion of fingers, and brachydactyly, or abnormal shortness of fingers, usually require no treatment unless the abnormal digit is obstructing the action of contiguous digits;

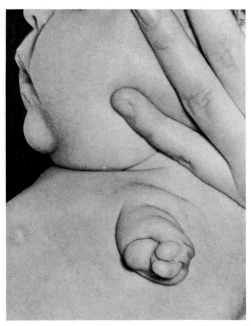

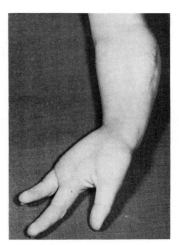

Fig 146–14.—Ulnar ray defect (clubhand). Shortening of the forearm and deformed radius have already been straightened by osteotomy. Note ulnar deviation of the hand and forearm and absence of the little and ring fingers. The condition was later improved by soft tissue lengthening of the ulnar side of the wrist. Ulnar ray defects usually have good function, because the thumb is usually well developed.

Fig 146–12.—Phocomelia, the anomaly associated with thalidomide ingestion. There is severe involvement, which for all practical purposes represents amelia. Early fitting of an upper extremity prosthesis is indicated.

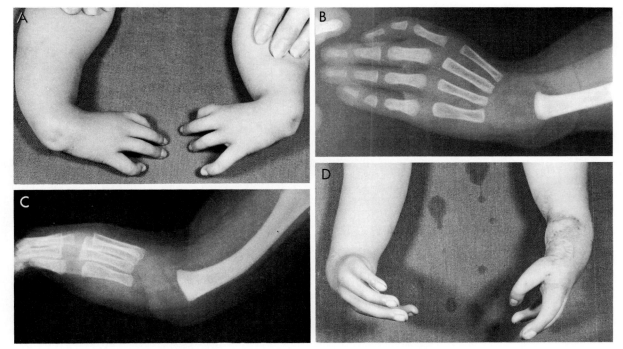

Fig 146–13.—Radial ray defect (clubhand). **A,** bilateral involvement, with short forearms, radial deviation and dorsal displacement of the hand on the forearm, and congenital absence of thumbs. **B** and **C,** anteroposterior and lateral radiographs of the left side show absence of radius and thumb and shortening and bowing of the ulna. **D,** the patient's mother, who had an identical deformity, requested treatment of the child. The more seriously involved side was treated first by lengthening all soft tissues on the radial side of the wrist, followed by pollicization of the index finger. The mother considered the result a significant improvement and requested reconstruction of the opposite side.

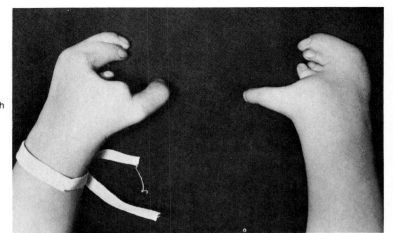

Fig 146–15.—Central hand defect. A variety of this anomaly, in which the lateral elements are more developed and longer, is termed lobster-claw hand. The pincer action of the hand was later improved by individualizing and osteotomizing the ulnar elements.

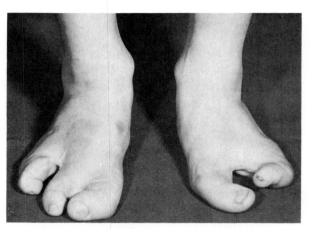

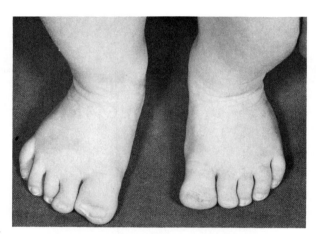

Fig 146–16.—Central foot defect, also known as split foot. This boy of 12 years had the cleft on the left narrowed in infancy. Shoe fitting and foot function were satisfactory.

Fig 146–17.—Polydactyly, synonychia, and synostosis, with reduplication of the great toes. The less well-developed digit will be removed to keep the forefoot narrow.

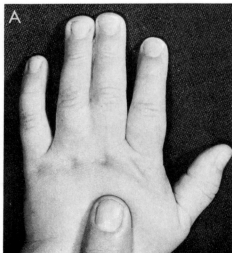

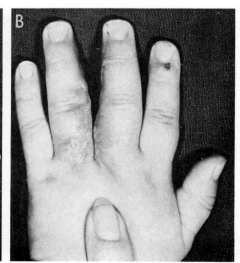

Fig 146–18.—**A,** syndactyly with mild degree of involvement without regional deformities such as hypoplasia of the phalanges or flexion deformities. **B,** syndactyly after operation, as shown in Figure 146–19.

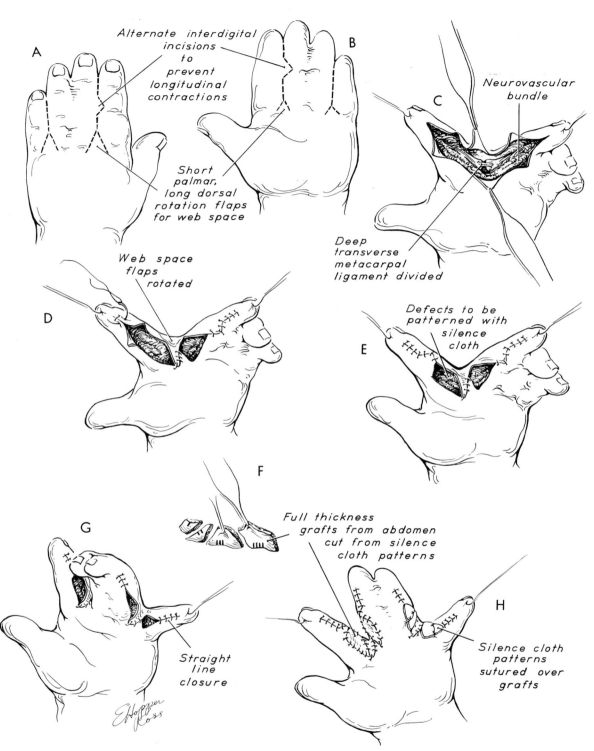

Fig 146–19.—Syndactyly: operative repair **(A–H)**. Both straight-line and zig-zag interdigital incisions are shown in **A** and **B.** Zigzag incisions reduce the tendency to postoperative formation of flexion contractures, because the lines of closure will be broken up. Long dorsal and short volar triangular rotation flaps are shown. Some surgeons prefer a single, large, dorsal-only rotation flap for the web space reconstruction.

(Labels within figure:)

A **B** Alternate interdigital incisions to prevent longitudinal contractions

Short palmar, long dorsal rotation flaps for web space

C Neurovascular bundle

Deep transverse metacarpal ligament divided

D Web space flaps rotated

E Defects to be patterned with silence cloth

F

G Straight line closure

Full thickness grafts from abdomen cut from silence cloth patterns

H Silence cloth patterns sutured over grafts

amputation is then indicated. Polydactyly (Fig 146–17) refers to more than the normal number of fingers or toes. Rudimentary or well-formed extra parts may be present. The accessory thumb is the most common such lesion. Treatment is excisional, but must not be taken lightly, because positional deformities of the major remaining digit, resulting from hypoplasia of ligaments, joints, and phalanges, as well as misplaced tendons, may be severe. Deboning of the digit to be removed, with search for and replacement of aberrant tendons, is worthwhile. Longitudinal Kirschner wire fixation and plaster immobilization for 3–6 weeks, and later osteotomy, may be necessary. Megalodactyly refers to giant digits and may occur as an isolated anomaly or associated with a soft tissue tumor, as in neurofibromatosis, lipomatosis, or hemangiomatosis. Surgical reduction of milder cases is worthwhile, but, if the digit is grossly enlarged, it should be amputated. Arachnodactyly refers to abnormally long digits and in itself is not a disability. Such lesions may be associated with congenital heart disease (Marfan syndrome).[39]

Syndactyly (Fig 146–18) refers to fused digits.[5] Commonly, only skin is involved, but any of the above-mentioned digital anomalies may be present, as well as synostosis, bony fusion of transversely placed bone, and synonychia or fusion of fingernails. The basic operation for syndactyly is shown in Figure 146–19 and is best performed at 6 months of age if there are other associated anomalies of the fingers. If the anomaly exists as uncomplicated webbing, the operation may be deferred to 2 years of age or even later, at which time postoperative dressings will be easier. Great care should be taken to avoid longitudinal midline scars, because these will form secondary flexion contractures. Every effort should be made to reconstruct the normal web spaces at the base of the fingers to prevent secondary tenting of this region. If the webbing involves many digits, as seen in Apert's deformity (Fig 146–20), partial-thickness skin may be used. Otherwise, free full-thickness skin grafts produce a better surface.

Syndactyly of the thumb requires special consideration, because even the very hypoplastic thumb is worth reconstructing.

Short thumb-index finger webs and even moderate degrees of syndactyly, phalangization, and hypoplasia of the thumb can be corrected by the use of a long dorsal rotation flap with free full-thickness grafts on either side. Subsequent rotation osteotomy of the thumb metacarpal may be necessary. The most severe degrees of involvement (Fig 146–21) may require web reconstruction by a jump pedicle flap, osteotomy, and reanimation by modified opponens transfer.

Syndactyly of the toes is a common anomaly that does not require correction. Clinodactyly, clinarthrosis, or oblique or lateral angulation deviation in alignment of joints may be due to abnormalities of articular surfaces and may occur as an isolated anomaly or as a portion of a more complex lesion. There frequently is a deficit of soft tissue on the concave side that requires lengthening by either local rotation flaps or free full-thickness grafts. Wedge osteotomy of the phalanx may be indicated (Fig 146–22).

Congenital hallux varus may present as an isolated lesion or in combination with polydactyly.[15] The soft tissues on the medial side of the metatarsophalangeal region almost always need lengthening. This can best be done by local rotation flaps obtained from the extra digit or from the space between the first and second toes.

Congenital Tumors

Tumors of the somatic soft tissues in children present a variegated picture and yet show certain general trends. Tumors of mesodermal origin are much more common than tumors of epidermal origin. Benign lesions are much more common than malignant ones. Malignant lesions may be present at birth, but usually develop later in childhood or adolescence, either spontaneously or through changes in previously existing benign lesions. Histologic malignancy does not always parallel clinical malignancy. The low-grade malignancies present difficulties to pathologist and surgeon, because both the normal tissues and benign lesions of childhood contain numbers of large active young cells, stain hypochromatically, and exhibit mitoses (Fig 146–23).

It is perhaps necessary to develop a new concept of malignancy when dealing with some of the histologically benign lesions in childhood, because they tend to be deforming and destructive. A classification is presented in Table 146–3.

Ectopic Tissue

Ectopic or misplaced tissue may present far from its intended site and should be considered in the differential diagnosis of soft tissue tumors. Skin tags and rudimentary appendages are common on the extremities. External ear tissue commonly presents on the face or along the line of the sternocleidomastoid muscle. Aberrant salivary gland tissue presents on the lower face and neck.

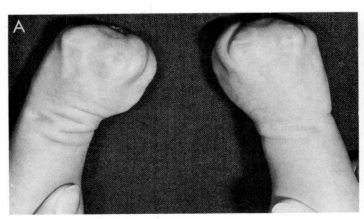

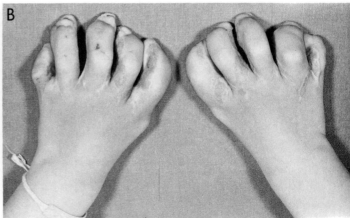

Fig 146–20.—**A,** severe syndactylism, synostosis, and ectrophalangia. The anomaly is seen frequently as part of Apert's deformity. **B,** postoperative appearance. Individualization was accomplished in stages. The operation shown in Figure 146–19 was modified in that free partial-thickness skin grafts were used because of the large amount of tissue required. Pollicization of the most radial of the five digits is still required.

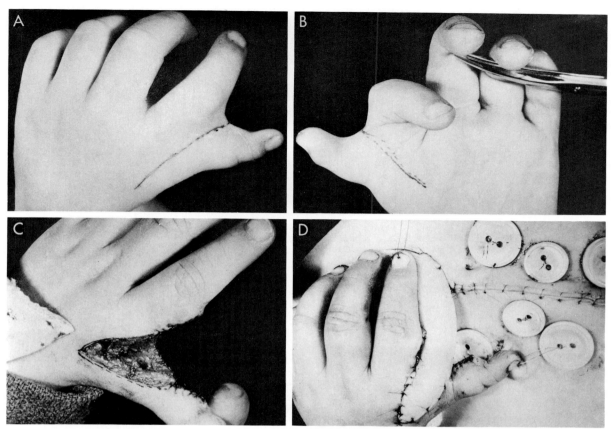

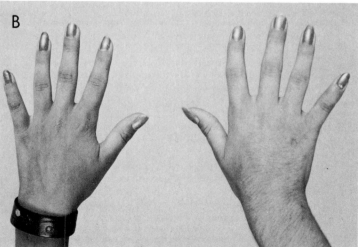

Fig 146–21.—**A** and **B,** hypoplasia, phalangization, and syndactyly of thumb. The thumb is so severely involved that use of a skin-fat pedicle graft is justified. **C,** at operation following division of the web. **D,** at operation following transfer of an inferior epigastric circumflex iliac artery jump pedicle flap to the dorsum of the hand. The pedicle will be separated in 3 weeks. Further procedures to make the thumb as functional as possible are carried out later. Less severe degrees of involvement would be reconstructed by some form of local rotation flaps with or without free skin graft.

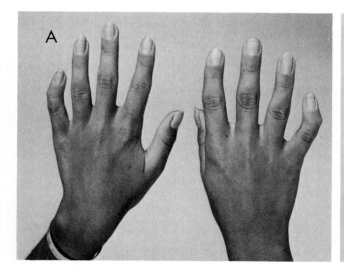

Fig 146–22.—Clinodactyly. **A,** preoperative view of radial curvature and angulation of the little finger caused by hypoplasia of the middle phalanx and its articular surfaces. **B,** postoperative view. A closing wedge osteotomy of the ulnar side of the middle phalanx has been done, keeping the radial cortex intact, except for a greenstick fracture. Any shortening that the closing osteotomy produces is compensated for by the straightening obtained. It is difficult to obtain soft tissue healing with opening osteotomies and bone grafts.

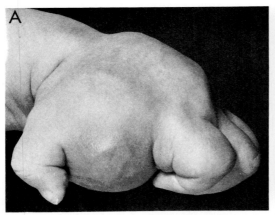

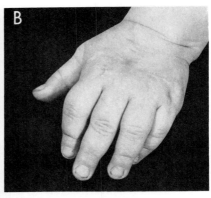

Fig 146–23.—A, fibrosarcoma of hand present at birth, with diagnosis confirmed by an international panel of pediatric pathologists. **B,** 1 year after excision in two stages at 3 weeks. The patient was free from tumor 10 years later with an essentially normal hand. The original pathology was reviewed and rediagnosed hemangioma!

Teratoid Lesions

It is often difficult to differentiate twinning attempts, reduplications, and teratoid lesions. The last are less completely formed, but contain elements of all tissue layers: ectoderm, mesoderm, and endoderm. Epignathus (Fig 146–24) is an example of a teratoid lesion. Excision of the lesion must be followed by any necessary reconstructive work.

Hamartomatous Lesions

A hamartoma may be defined as a malformed growth of normal tissues normally found in an organ. This concept differentiates the majority of the benign somatic soft tissue tumors from teratomas and ectopic lesions, but is primarily of academic interest. The choristoma or persistent lateral cervical cystic thymus[19] is a variant of the hamartoma concept.

Epithelial Tissue Lesions

Each constituent of the skin can be involved in a tumor process.

EPIDERMAL (DERMOID) CYSTS.—These lesions occur most frequently in regions of embryologic fusion. Thus, they are common at the corners of the eye; over the midline of the nose; along the line of the sternocleidomastoid muscle, where they are to be differentiated from branchial cysts; and in the midline of the neck, where they are to be differentiated from thyroglossal duct tract abnormalities. As a rule, they are freely mobile in the subcutaneous tissues or are attached to skin. Occasionally, they arise from the midline of the roof of the mouth, where they produce, or are associated with, a cleft of the palate (Fig 146–25). They contain keratin and occasionally hair within a well-circumscribed but thin wall that contains epidermal elements. The preauricular epidermal cyst almost always has a deep attachment to the origin of the helix cartilage. Similarly, the mucous cyst may be present at birth or occur later during childhood and is commonly seen in the labial mucosa. Treatment is excision.

PAPILLOMAS.—Papillomas resemble skin tags of mucous membrane. When more sessile, they are termed verrucae. They may be present at birth or appear at any time in childhood. Simple excision is indicated.

WARTS.—Warts are common from age 4 years throughout childhood. They are most common on the hands, but may occur around the mouth and genitalia. They are caused by a virus and tend to spread to other sites as well as throughout the family. Electric or chemical cauterization, or excision of the larger lesions, is indicated primarily for aesthetic reasons, although the lesions tend to recur until they eventually disappear spontaneously. The plantar wart characteristically occurs as a solitary lesion in the region of the transverse arch of the foot. It may occur elsewhere on the sole of the foot or even very rarely in the palmar skin. It is also considered to be mildly infectious. It is situated in or immediately deep to the dermis, has a dark central nidus surrounded by callus, and is exquisitely tender. Treatment is cauterization with fine tip electrocautery or by chemical agents such as trichloracetic acid crystals followed by curettage. Recurrences may require excision. Radiation therapy is effective, but the risk of radiation damage is unjustifiable for these viral lesions.

ABERRANT SKIN GLANDS.—Small patches of plaque-like roughened yellow or brownish skin may be present at birth and closely resemble xanthomas or pigmented nevi. Microscopically, the picture may be that of adenoid hyperplasia or adenoma sebaceum. Complete excision is indicated because of the possibility of malignant change.

MALIGNANT EPITHELIAL TUMORS.—Basal cell and squamous cell carcinoma are extremely rare in young children. A well-documented series in predominantly older children has been recorded.[24, 35] There are only two cases of basal cell carcinoma in the records of the Toronto Hospital for Sick Children, the patients surviving for 10 and 20 years, respectively, without recurrence. Carcinosarcoma occurred in the subcutaneous tissues of the face of one child, with fatal outcome after radical operation and radiation therapy. In general, malignant epithelial tumors require wide excision and careful follow-up. Radiation therapy should be considered immediately following the excision of a recurrence.

Nerve Tissue Lesions

NEUROFIBROMA.—Overgrowth of all nerve elements may follow complete or incomplete division of a nerve and is usually called a neuroma. Isolated overgrowth of all nerve elements not associated with nerve division is termed neurofibroma.

TABLE 146–3.—CLASSIFICATION OF SOMATIC SOFT TISSUE
TUMORS IN CHILDREN

TISSUE	BENIGN	MALIGNANT
Ectopic tissue		
Teratoid lesions		
Hamartomatous tissue		
Epithelial tissue		
Epidermis	Papilloma, verruca, wart, epidermoid (dermoid) cyst, calcifying epithelioma	Basal cell and epidermoid carcinoma
Sweat gland	Spiradenoma, hidradenoma	Adenocarcinoma
Sebaceous gland	Sebaceous cyst	Epidermoid carcinoma
Nerve tissue	Neurofibroma, neurilemmoma	Neurofibrosarcoma, malignant schwannoma
Pigmented tissue	Nevus: epidermal, intradermal, junctional, compound, blue, juvenile (pubertal) melanoma, xanthoma	Malignant melanoma, melanotic sarcoma
Mesenchymal tissue		
Undifferentiated mesenchyma	Mesenchymoma, myxoma	Malignant mesenchymoma
Fibrous tissue	Fibroma: hard, soft, calcifying, ossifying Epulis Fibromatosis Keloid	Fibrosarcoma
Vascular tissue	Hemangioma Lymphangioma (cystic hygroma) Glomus	Hemangioendothelioma or sarcoma
Adipose tissue	Lipoma Lipomatosis	Liposarcoma
Muscle tissue	Rhabdomyoma, myofibromatosis	Rhabdomyosarcoma
Synovial tissue	Giant cell synovioma	Malignant synovioma

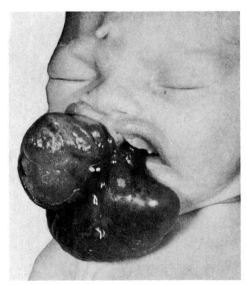

Fig 146–24.—Teratoma of palate (epignathus) in newborn infant. The lesion arises from anterior hard palate, producing a median cleft lip and alveolus. There is also accessory nose tissue. (Courtesy of late Dr. J.T. Mills, Dallas.)

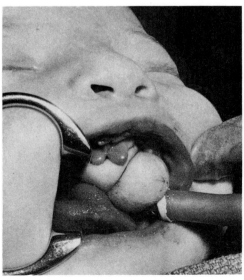

Fig 146–25.—Dermoid cyst of palate arising from vomerine bone and associated with cleft palate.

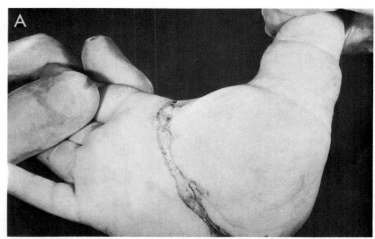

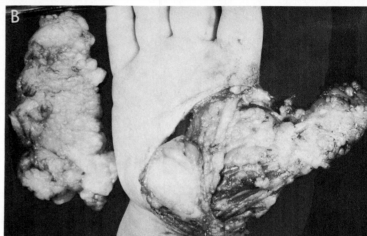

Fig 146–26.—Neurofibromatosis of thumb and hand. **A,** photograph taken at start of operation to decrease bulk of the area. **B,** hypertrophy of all regional tissues—in particular, enlargement of the median nerve and digital nerve to the index finger.

The most common nerve tissue tumor in childhood is neurofibromatosis or von Recklinghausen's disease[44] (see Chap. 147). The lesions may be present at birth, but commonly appear sometime later. Any anatomical region and any tissue of the body may be involved. Café-au-lait spots in the region of the lesion or elsewhere usually are diagnosed at birth. Neurologic signs are unusual, but pain may be present from pressure on a nerve in an enclosed space, as with the ulnar nerve at the elbow.

Marked enlargement involves many of the nerves in the affected region (Fig 146–26), together with overgrowth of fibrous tissue, fatty tissue, and bone. Regional gigantism (elephantiasis nervorum) results—grotesque and deforming.[54] The nerves are thickened throughout their long axes in the area of involvement, but, in addition, have massive elliptic bulges. The epineurium generally is unchanged and is not abnormally attached to the surrounding tissues. Histologically, the cells of the sheath of Schwann are found to have undergone proliferation and are often arranged in rows or in palisade formation. Large or small nerves may be involved. There may be areas of degeneration and cystic change within the nerve.

It is often impossible to excise the lesion totally, but large surgical excisions may be done to decrease mass and grotesqueness. Rapidly growing, changing or painful tumors should be excised for fear of sarcomatous degeneration.

NEURILEMMOMA (NEURINOMA: SCHWANNOMA).—When the process of neurofibromatosis occurs as an isolated tumor of a peripheral nerve, it may be referred to as a neurilemmoma, although it is difficult to differentiate from neurofibroma. The only sign usually is a mass with or without local pressure symptoms. Tumors producing pressure signs may be treated operatively, although the actual nerve affected will have an important bearing on treatment, because the anesthesia or motor disability resulting from resection may be more serious than the tumor.

NEUROFIBROSARCOMA.—Sarcomatous change may occur in any of the above benign lesions.[4, 36] Such change usually is manifested by rapid growth and development of pain in the region, paresthesia, or anesthesia in the nerve distribution. This is uncommon in childhood. The reported incidence of malignant change in adult life varies from 5–30%.[8] Neurofibrosarcoma may occur spontaneously as a solitary lesion, but is rare in childhood. It must be treated by radical excision of the involved nerve and surrounding tissues.

Pigmented Tissue Lesions

The term nevus is a general, often unsatisfactory term meaning a mole or birthmark or a circumscribed lesion of the skin of congenital origin. These lesions may be shades of red when they are hemangiomatous, or of brown when they are melanoblastic. The term benign melanoma would be preferable for the latter group of lesions, although melanoma connotes malignancy to some. The term nevus is here restricted to the various types of brown pigment spots seen frequently in childhood. It is helpful to think in terms of three types of nevi.

EPIDERMAL OR MARGINAL NEVUS.—The characteristic nevus of childhood is flat and moderately brown. It varies greatly in size and may cover large areas of the body. There is an overproduction of melanoblasts and melanin in the basal layers of the epidermis, which may separate the malpighian cells from the basement membrane. The lesions that maintain junctional activity are most likely to undergo change at puberty.

COMPOUND NEVUS.—Many nevi become slightly more raised and rougher as time goes by. Microscopically, groups of melanoblasts are seen to penetrate the basement membrane into the dermis. As long as the migration of melanoblasts goes on, the lesion is known as a compound nevus.

INTRADERMAL NEVUS.—The intradermal nevus is the typical mole or nevus of adult life, often present during childhood. It is more raised and is frequently hairy. Microscopically, all connection with the epidermis has disappeared, and the melanoblasts are situated entirely in the dermis. The lesion remains benign.

JUVENILE (PUBERTAL) MELANOMA.—It has been necessary to create this classification, because certain nevi in children appear malignant clinically and histologically and yet usually remain localized at least until puberty. Local excision is indicated.

BLUE NEVUS.—This lesion, frequently the blackest of all nevi, may have a bluish hue. It is entirely different from the others, perhaps being related to the mongolian spot. It consists of interlacing fasciculae of fibroblasts in which pigment cells are interspersed. It does not become malignant.

Treatment

Nevi may be removed because of the possibility of malignant change or for aesthetic considerations. Nevi on exposed areas and those subject to trauma from clothing, belts, or straps probably should be removed, although this statement is controversial. There is no controversy about whether nevi that have appeared recently or that have undergone recent change (e.g., increase of size and development of irregular margins or satellite areas, increased pigmentation, friable areas, or itchiness) should be removed. Excision is preferable to electrocoagulation and should be wide and complete.

Many patients seek treatment for aesthetic reasons. Large lesions may be removed by multiple excision (Fig 146–27), or excision and resurfacing may be done by means of local rotation flaps or free partial-thickness skin grafts. Anticipated scarring must be explained to these patients. The giant[2, 42] and bathing trunk[49] lesions present severe aesthetic and social problems. Massive excision of the more exposed and more grotesque portions of the lesions followed by partial-thickness skin grafting may be rewarding, provided donor sites in conspicuous areas are avoided. There is much controversy about the incidence of malignant change in giant and bathing trunk nevi. Risks as high as 35% have been reported. The Hospital for Sick Children incidence of malignant change in such lesions is very low[2]—not sufficient of itself to warrant total surgical excision of such lesions.

MALIGNANT MELANOMA.—Malignant melanoma is rare in childhood. It is often difficult to know whether the lesion is a juvenile or malignant melanoma.[49] In dealing with malignant melanoma, it is helpful to carry out an additional wider local excision to be absolutely certain that no tumor has been left lo-

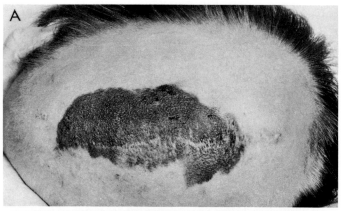

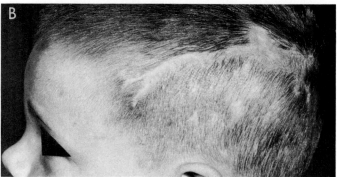

Fig 146–27.—Pigmented nevus. **A,** deeply pigmented area, which originally measured 4 × 2 × ½ in. Hair over this area was considerably darker than that of the normal scalp. A single partial excision has already been performed within pigmented area. **B,** result after four procedures. The scar "spread," common after suture under tension, may be excised later to produce a narrower scar.

cally. If the lesion is adjacent to regional lymph nodes, this wide, deep local reexcision may be combined with en bloc excision of the intervening lymph channels, together with the regional nodes. If the lesion is far removed from intervening lymph channels, the wide local excision should be combined with a radical block dissection of the regional lymph nodes. Radiation has no place in treatment of this tumor. The roles of chemotherapy and immunotherapy for this lesion in childhood have not been worked out.

Radical excision is not so important for lesions appearing before puberty.

XANTHOMA.—Children may develop yellow plaque-like patches or nodules on the skin with or without an associated disturbance of cholesterol metabolism. Similar nodules or areas are found also in extensor tendon sheaths and over the extensor surfaces of joints. The lesions are characterized by areas of tissue destruction with pathognomonic pale, swollen "foam cells" and giant cells. Local recurrence is common unless excision is complete. In the widely generalized xanthomatosis, only the symptomatic or disfiguring lesions are excised.

Mesenchymal Tissue Lesions

Undifferentiated Mesenchyma

MESENCHYMOMA AND MYXOMA.—These two lesions are considered together, because they are both tumors of primitive mesenchyma and because they cannot be given more specific histologic labels. They occur in the somatic soft tissues in childhood as firm subcutaneous masses fixed both to overlying skin and underlying structures. Their margins are poorly defined. At operation, they have either the appearance of young flesh or a gelatinous appearance; they frequently invade muscle.

The true myxoma has a gelatinous mucinous consistency and contains fibroblasts widely separated by pale mucoid material that stains positively with mucicarmine. The mesenchymoma is firmer and contains a variable stroma that is loose in some regions, dense in others. It is composed primarily of primitive mesenchymal cells with some admixture of mature connective tissue cells. Local excision usually is adequate.

MALIGNANT MESENCHYMOMA.—Some mesenchymal cell tumors show a more bizarre, more hyperchromatic, and actively mitotic histologic picture.[48] If there is doubt about the adequacy of excision of such a lesion, additional wider surgical excision should be carried out. Experience with radiation therapy has been inadequate for this type of lesion, but its possible use should be considered.

Fibrous Tissue Lesions

Fibrous tissue replacements or excesses may occur in the hand or the foot: palmar or plantar fibromatosis.[41, 43] They are not as common in childhood as in adult life. Wide excision is necessary, because the lesions are prone to recur. Other congenital conditions such as annular bands, flexion contractures, chordee of the penis, and myodystrophia fetalis are associated with excessive amounts of fibrous tissue, but can be differentiated from the fibromatoses, because the fibrous tissue does not tend to recur and proliferate after excision.

KELOID.—Keloids are characterized by massive formation of scar tissue in and deep to skin after any trauma, often trivial. The condition is to be differentiated from hypertrophic scar, which tends to resolve with time and as a rule is not associated with prolonged itchiness. Keloid tissue tends to recur after excision. Children have a greater tendency to form and re-form keloid than do adults, and sometimes the keloid tendency diminishes after puberty. The fibrous tissue tends to lie in bundles parallel to the surface. Keloids warrant one attempt at excision, every effort being made to avoid the unnecessary addition of extending incision lines. Sometimes it is worthwhile to carry out a trial excision, staying within the confines of the lesion to see what response is obtained. If the lesion recurs, it may be reexcised and appropriately closed, either directly or by free skin graft (Fig 146–28). This should be followed in 2–10 days by surface irradiation except over the face or neck, lest the thyroid be irradiated. Intralesional triamcinolone—20 mg for 1–2-year-olds, 40 mg for 3–5-year olds, 80 mg for 6–10-year-olds—will produce some keloid resolution. Injection is painful, and the dose must be dispersed evenly throughout the lesion. Both hemorrhage and excessive resolution with crater formation have been produced.

FIBROMA.—The fibroma may present anywhere in the somatic soft tissue[23] (Fig 146–29). It may be hard or soft and is usually small, but may vary in size. The soft fibroma contains more young fibrous tissue and less collagen. It may be present at birth or appear later in life. Calcification and ossification may be present. Occasional lesions contain giant cells. The epulis that occurs on the gingiva is an example of such a lesion. A fibromatous lesion occurring on synovial tissue may be termed a giant cell tumor. The dermatofibroma is a hard, nonencapsulated lesion of the corium, which usually occurs after surface break and contains dense masses of fibrous tissue.

FIBROSARCOMA.—Fibrous tissue tumors may exhibit all degrees of histologic malignancy.[14, 27, 29, 47, 50] Such lesions are highly invasive locally (Fig 146–30). They also tend to metastasize to regional lymph nodes and lung. They may be present at birth but can occur in any age group. Incomplete surgical excision is almost always associated with local recurrence. Local recurrences may be slow in manifesting themselves. In general, the less well-differentiated types offer a poor prognosis, and yet the clinical correlation between the histologic and the clinical picture is not absolute. Carefully planned and executed radiation therapy is providing better early results as experience is gained with new sources of radiation (Fig 146–31). Experience with

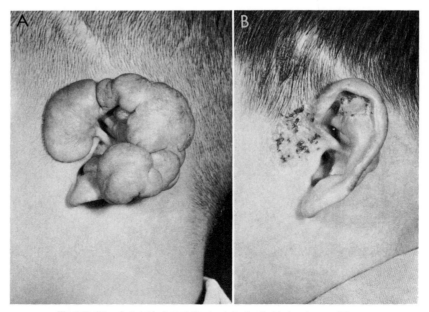

Fig 146–28.—A, keloid of ear following infection behind and around the ear.
B, postoperative view following excision in two stages and partial-thickness skin grafting.

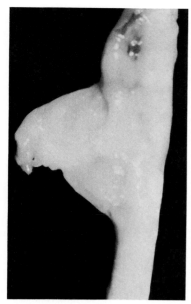

Fig 146–29.—Fibroma of tendon. Recurrent fibroma of flexor digitorum sublimis tendon in palm of a 5-year-old child. Following this recurrence, the sublimis tendon was excised.

these methods in children has been insufficient. Wide local excision, together with radical block dissection of the involved lymph nodes, is indicated. The role of quarter amputation has been discussed by Pack and Ariel.[37]

Many fibrosarcomas contain other mesenchymal tissues. Still others are so poorly differentiated that they must be called sarcoma of undetermined origin. In fact, most studies of malignant soft tissue tumors in childhood report a large group of undifferentiated sarcomas.[50] Recently, it has been possible to separate the rhabdomyosarcoma from this group, and the results of chemotherapy, radiation, and surgical excision are so promising that they are covered in a separate chapter (Chap. 32).

Vascular Tissue Lesions

Hemangiomas are manifested in so many different ways that they are difficult to classify. A useful, although not all-inclusive,

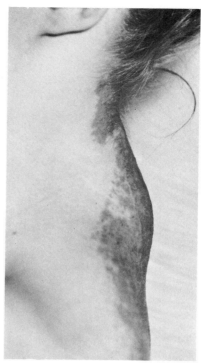

Fig 146–31.—Fibromyxosarcoma of neck and back. The patient survived 3 years after excision and radiation therapy.

method of classification is as follows: (1) capillary hemangioma (port-wine stain); (2) cavernous hemangioma (a) superficial (strawberry mark), deep or mixed, and (b) involuting or noninvoluting; and (3) other hemangiomas, venous or arterial.

Other classifications and treatment methods are presented in Chapter 149. Lymphangioma is discussed in Chapter 148.

Adipose Tissue Lesions

An isolated tumor of fatty tissue, the lipoma, is not as common in childhood as in adult life.[23] Liposarcoma rarely occurs by itself, being seen more often in combination with mesenchymal tissues.

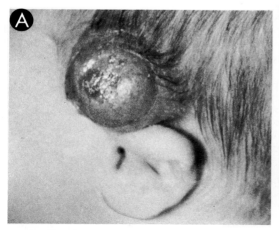

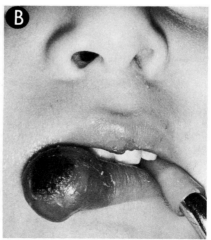

Fig 146–30.—**A,** fibrosarcoma of scalp excised at age 3 years. The patient was well 20 years later. **B,** fibrosarcoma of lip that appeared rapidly at age 4 years. Following wedge resection, disease developed in a lymph node, which required suprahyoid block dissection. The patient was well 10 years later.

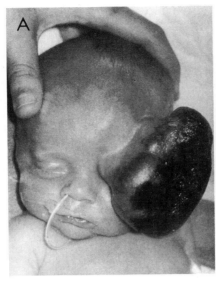
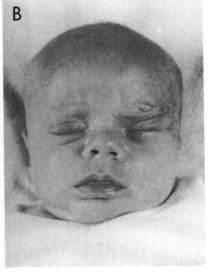

Fig 146–32.—A, infantile myofibromatosis. The lesion was present at birth, involving eyelids, forehead, and temporal scalp. **B,** 1 month after excision, at 6 weeks of age. Lid and eye functions are normal. The small skin excess will be excised when the eyebrow level can be determined reliably.

Tumors of Muscle Tissue Origin

Leiomyoma[51] and leiomyosarcoma are exceedingly rare in the somatic soft tissues.

RHABDOMYOMA.—With improved histologic techniques and criteria, there has been a steady increase in the diagnosis of tumors of primitive muscle cell origin. The rhabdomyoma and the granular cell myoblastoma are extremely rare in the somatic soft tissues, the latter tumor having a curious predilection for the upper respiratory and digestive passages. Treatment is complete surgical excision with careful follow-up.

INFANTILE MYOFIBROMATOSIS.—This relatively new entity[6] is one of the fibrous proliferations of childhood consisting of highly vascular spindle cells with a heterogeneous appearance with ultrastructure features compatible with myofibroblastic origin. It is benign when occurring as a single lesion (Fig 146–32). Treatment is by complete local excision.

Synovial Tissue Lesions

The ganglion is the most common subcutaneous lesion occurring on fingers, hand, and wrist and may be present on the foot as well. It is a true tumor, rather than a synovial cyst or bursa, such as occurs in preexisting or adventitious bursae. It is a cystic lesion associated with a tendon sheath or joint synovium. Certain movements may cause pain or discomfort. The capsule consists of thin or dense fibrous tissue that is continuous with the surrounding connective tissue and contains clear jelly-like mucoid material rich in hyaluronic acid. Some lesions disappear spontaneously after direct trauma. A ganglion present for more than 3 months should be excised under tourniquet, with good exposure, to eradicate the lesion and to permit pathologic diagnosis.

GIANT CELL SYNOVIOMA.—The benign giant cell synovioma or xanthoma (Fig 146–33), although the second most common tumor of tendon sheath and synovium, is not as common in childhood as in adult life. It occurs on the dorsal and volar aspects of fingers and hand as a small firm lesion of the tendon sheath, grossly yellow or brown. Microscopically, it is fibrous or highly cellular and contains numerous lipid-filled histiocytes and giant cells. Careful wide excision is necessary, for local recurrence is common, although malignant change is rare.

MALIGNANT SYNOVIOMA.—By definition, this is a tumor arising from the synovial tissue of joints, tendon sheaths, and bursae with histologic features characteristic of synovial tissue. The knee, hand, and foot are the sites most commonly involved. It is a treacherous tumor both histologically and clinically—histologically, because synovial tissue contains an outer supporting fibrous layer and an inner specialized layer of secretory cells that make this tumor difficult to distinguish from other types of sarcoma, particularly fibrosarcoma and even carcinoma; and clinically, because it is prone to recur locally even in its more differentiated forms unless completely excised and is prone to metastasize widely in its less well-differentiated forms. Resection is the treatment of choice. Amputation is necessary to accomplish this in the case of deep-seated lesions. When feasible, the excision should include an in-continuity resection of the regional draining lymphatic area. Postoperative radiation therapy usually is advised, although the radiosensitivity of this lesion has not been well defined.

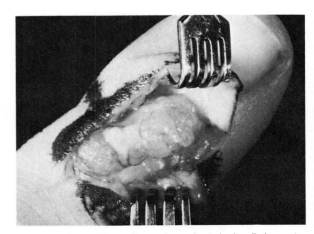

Fig 146–33.—Benign giant cell synovioma situated primarily in paratenon of a digital extensor tendon insertion.

REFERENCES

1. Bagg H.J.: Etiology of certain congenital structural deformities. *Am. J. Obstet. Gynecol.* 8:131, 1924.
2. Birch J.R., Anderson K.: *Giant Pigmented Nevi* (1975 study). The Hospital for Sick Children, Toronto. To be published.
3. Birch-Jensen A.: *Congenital Deformities of the Upper Extremities.* Copenhagen, Andelsbogtrykkereit i Odense, 1949.
4. Bodian M., Wilkinson A.W.: Congenital malignant neurilemmoma. *J. Clin. Pathol.* 17:130, 1964.
5. Buck-Gramcko D.: Congenital malformations of the hand: Indications, operative treatment and results. *Scand. J. Plast. Reconstr. Surg.* 9:190, 1975.
6. Chung E.B., Enzinger F.M.: Infantile myofibromatosis: A review of 59 cases with localized and generalized involvement. *Cancer* 48:1807, 1981.
7. Crawford H.H., Harton C.E., Adamson J.E.: Congenital aplasia or hypoplasia of the thumb and finger extensor tendons. *J. Bone Joint Surg.* 48A:82, 1966.
8. Davis R.G., Farmer A.W.: Mirror hand anomaly: A case presentation. *Plast. Reconstr. Surg.* 21:80, 1958.
9. Davis W.B., et al.: Neurofibromatosis of the head and neck. *Plast. Reconstr. Surg.* 14:186, 1954.
10. Duraiswami: Production Experimental de Deformités Congenitales. *Concours Med.* (Paris) 73:38, 1951.
11. Edgerton M.T., Snyden G.B., Webb W.L.: Surgical treatment of congenital thumb deformities (including psychological impact of correction). *J. Bone Joint Surg.* 47A:1453, 1965.
12. Ellis W.B., van Creveld S.: A syndrome characterized by ectodermal dysplasia, polydactyly, chondrodysplasia and congenital morbus cordus. *Arch. Dis. Child.* 15:65, 1940.
13. Entin M.A.: Reconstruction of congenital abnormalities of the upper extremities. *J. Bone Joint Surg.* 41A:681, 1959.
14. Evans J.P., Miller L.S.: Congenital sarcoma of the hand. *W. Va. Med. J.* 72:58, 1976.
15. Farmer A.W.: Congenital hallux varus. *Am. J. Surg.* 95:274, 1958.
16. Farmer A.W.: Congenital absence of ulna. *Can. J. Surg.* 2:204, 1959.
17. Farmer A.W.: Congenital absence of radius. *Can. J. Surg.* 1:301, 1958.
18. Farmer A.W., Maxman M.: Congenital absence of skin. *Plast. Reconstr. Surg.* 25:291, 1960.
19. Fielding J.F., et al.: Cystic degeneration in persistent cervical thymus: A report of 4 cases. *Can. J. Surg.* 6:178, 1963.
20. Flatt A.E.: Problems in Polydactyly, in Cramer L., Chase R., (eds.): *Symposium on the Hand.* St. Louis, C.V. Mosby Co., 1971, vol. 3, p. 150.
21. Franklin J.B., Brent R.L.: Cited by Murray J.E.: What's new in plastic surgery. *Surg. Gynecol. Obstet.* 112:246, 1961.
22. General principles of care of open wounds. *Bull. Am. Coll. Surgeons* 45:117, 1960.
23. Goslee L., Bernstein J.: Superficial connective tissue tumors in early infancy. *Pediatrics* 65:377, 1964.
24. Hernandez-Perez E.: Basal cell carcinoma in children. *Dermatologica* 150:311, 1975.
25. Ingalls G.H., Fillbrook F.R.: Monstrosities produced by hypoxia. *N. Engl. J. Med.* 259:558, 1958.
26. Ingalls N.W.: Congenital defects of the scalp. *Am. J. Obstet. Gynecol.* 25:861, 1933.
27. Jäger M.: Der Angeborene umschriebene Riesenwuel Hand und des Fussen. *Arch. Orthop. Unfallchir.* 61:151, 1967.
28. King J.E.J.: Oxycephaly. *Ann. Surg.* 115:488, 1942.
29. Lawrence W., Jegge G., Foote F.W.: Embryonal rhabdomyosarcoma. *CA* 17:361, 1964.
30. Lewitus Z.: Ehlers-Danlos syndrome. *Arch. Dermatol.* 73:158, 1956.
31. Littler J.W.: Neurovascular empirical method of digital transposition for reconstruction of thumb. *Plast. Reconstr. Surg.* 12:303, 1953.
32. Mathews D.: Congenital absence of functioning thumb. *Plast. Reconstr. Surg.* 26:487, 1960.
33. Marshall R., Hodes H.L.: De Lange's Disease: Congenital Muscular Hypertrophy with Mental Deficiency, in Gellis, S.S.: *Year Book of Pediatrics 1956–1957.* Chicago, Year Book Medical Publishers, 1957, p. 457.
34. Michaelson I.C., Hill J.: Von Hippel-Lindau disease. *Br. J. Ophthalmol.* 33:657, 1949.
35. Murray J.E., Cannon B.: Basal cell cancer in children and young adults. *N. Engl. J. Med.* 262:440, 1960.
36. Nesbitt K.A., Vidone R.A.: Primitive neuroectodermal tumour (neuroblastoma) arising in sciatic nerve of a child. *CA* 37:1562, 1976.
37. Pack G.P., Ariel I.M.: *Tumors of the Soft Somatic Tissues.* New York, Paul B. Hoeber, Inc., 1958, p. 681.
38. Pandey S.: Congenital bilateral contracture of gluteus maximus. *Int. Surg.* 61:49, 1976.
39. Parker A., Hare H.: Arachnodactyly. *Radiology* 45:220, 1945.
40. Pers M.: Congenital absence of skin: Pathogenesis and relation to ring constriction. *Acta Chir. Scand.* 126:388, 1963.
41. Phelan T.P., Grace J.T., Pickren J.W.: Juvenile fibromatosis. *Surgery* 64:492, 1968.
42. Pilney F.T., et al.: Giant pigmented nevi of the face: Surgical management. *Plast. Reconstr. Surg.* 40:469, 1967.
43. Rios-Dalenz J.L., Kim J.S., McDowell F.W.: The so-called "juvenile aponeurotic fibroma." *Am. J. Clin. Pathol.* 44:632, 1965.
44. Ross D.E.: Skin manifestations of von Recklinghausen's disease and associated tumors (neurofibromatosis). *Am. Surg.* 31:729, 1965.
45. Savage D.: Localized congenital defect of the scalp. *Br. J. Obstet. Gynaecol.* 63:351, 1956.
46. Sellers E.H.: Congenital abnormalities reported by physicians: Infants born alive; 1959. Spec. Rep. No. 9, Div. Med. Statistics, Ontario, Canada.
47. Shands W.C.: Soft tissue sarcomas in children and adults. *Am. Surg.* 29:811, 1963.
48. Shrivastava R.K., Shrivastava D.K., Tardon P.L.: Congenital malignant mesenchymoma. *Indian J. Surg.* 26:235, 1964.
49. Skov-Jensen T., Hastrup J., Lembrethsen E.: Malignant melanoma in children. *Cancer* 19:620, 1966.
50. Soule E.H.: Soft tissue sarcomas of infants and children: A clinicopathologic study of 135 cases. *Mayo Clin. Proc.* 43:313, 1968.
51. Stout A.P.: Solitary cutaneous and subcutaneous leiomyoma. *Am. J. Cancer* 29:435, 1937.
52. Streeter G.L.: Focal deficiencies in fetal tissues and their relation to intrauterine amputation. *Contrib. Embryol.* (Carnegie Inst., Washington) 22:1, 1930.
53. Tuerk D., Edgerton M.T.: The surgical treatment of congenital webbing (pterygium) of the popliteal area. *Plast. Reconstr. Surg.* 56:339, 1975.
54. Von L. Giley Z.: Aplasia cutis circumscripta congenita. *Kinderchir.* vol. 5, bk. 314, 1968.
55. Walker J.C., et al.: Congenital absence of skin (aplasia cutis congenita). *Plast. Reconstr. Surg.* 26:209, 1960.
56. Warkany J.: Production of congenital malformation by dietary measures: Experiments in mammals. *JAMA* 168:2020, 1958.

147 John C. Adkins / Mark M. Ravitch

Neurofibromatosis— Von Recklinghausen's Disease

HISTORY.—The 1882 monograph of Friedrich von Recklinghausen of Strassburg, "Multiplen Fibrome der Haut und ihre Beziehung zu den multiplen Neuromen,"[37] part of a Festschrift honoring Rudolph Virchow's 25th year at the Pathological Institute of Berlin, clearly established the nature of the disease. As with so many eponymic diseases, there was an extensive antecedent literature. Von Recklinghausen lists 123 references, the earliest being to Wilhelm G. Tilesius of Tilenau,[34] whose 1793 description was of a 52-year-old man with multiple cutaneous neurofibromas and café-au-lait spots. Von Recklinghausen cited Kraemer's 1847 case of a 15-year-old boy with pubic and genital involvement, the first known pediatric case. Smith (1849) of Dublin, Virchow, and Balzer all had presented detailed reports, and the catalogue of famous names in von Recklinghausen's bibliography includes Hesselbach, Hebra, Rokitansky, von Bergman, Hilton Fagge of Guy's Hospital, Billroth, Volkmann, Larrey, Valentine Mott, and numerous others. The little book published in 1956 by Crowe, Schull, and Neel[8] presents a detailed study of the clinical, pathologic, and genetic features of the disease and is the source for much of the data in the literature on genetic behavior, frequency, and distribution of the various forms of the disease.

A number of excellent reviews have been published. Holt's Neuhauser Lecture[21] covers beautifully the radiology of the disease in childhood. Wander and Das Gupta[38] have reviewed exhaustively the surgery of the disease in children and adults.

Introduction

Von Recklinghausen's neurofibromatosis is a familial disorder characterized by hamartomatous growths that may occur in virtually any part of the body. The characteristic stigmata of the disease are café-au-lait spots and neurofibromas that develop in the skin, along the nerve trunks, in the viscera, and in the CNS. Essentially every organ and region of the body can be affected. Hundreds of reports from all over the world attest to the extraordinary diversity of the manifestations of the disease and its worldwide occurrence. Unlike most of the other phakomatoses, neurofibromatosis carries a significant risk of sarcomatous degeneration of the tumors.[11, 23] There is also an increased incidence of nonfibromatous malignant tumors as well as leukemias. Boys are at a higher risk of developing malignancy than are girls.[6]

The disease occurs in one in 3,000 births and is transmitted as an autosomal dominant with variable penetrance. Among heritable syndromes, it has the highest known incidence of new mutations, and around 50% of patients represent these sporadic cases. There is no sex preference. Palmar and plantar neurofibromas and acoustic neurinomas tend to cluster within families.[14] With these exceptions, there seems to be little tendency for the disease to adopt a single pattern within families with regard to such features as extent and character of the manifestations, organ involvement, and development of malignancy.

Miller and Hall[24] have described 62 patients with neurofibromatosis whose symptoms began in childhood. The severity of the disease was greater in offspring of affected mothers than in children of affected fathers or in sporadic cases.

The disease is often discussed in two forms: a central form manifested by orbitofacial and CNS involvement, and a peripheral form displaying a preponderance of cutaneous, visceral, and musculoskeletal manifestations.

Von Recklinghausen demonstrated the origin of the tumors in the connective tissue sheaths of the nerves. It is now generally agreed that the tumors arise in the Schwann cells, originating in the neural crest. Lesions of bone associated with von Recklinghausen's disease and characteristic of it occur without any neurofibromatous elements. Salyer and Salyer[30] have submitted evidence that the arterial lesions are Schwannian in origin. Fabricant et al.[13] have demonstrated increased levels of nerve growth factor in several groups of patients with "central neurofibromatosis."

The presence of five or more café-au-lait spots larger than 1.5 cm is pathognomonic. About 45% of children with von Recklinghausen's disease will have had physical evidence of it from birth, and 65% will have manifested the disease by age 1 year.[14] The congenital giant bathing trunk nevus may occur in association with von Recklinghausen's disease. The size and number of café-au-lait spots tend to increase through puberty.

Clinical Forms

The forms of von Recklinghausen's disease may be separated for convenience of discussion into several groups: (1) fibroma molluscum; (2) plexiform neurofibroma; (3) elephantiasis nervorum and neurofibromas of the extremities; (4) mediastinal neurofibroma; (5) visceral involvement; (6) skeletal manifestation; (7) central neurofibromatosis; (8) endocrine manifestations; and (9) cardiovascular manifestations.

Fibroma Molluscum

This represents the classic pattern of neurofibromatosis in which hundreds or thousands of small sessile or pedunculated nodules occur in the skin and subcutaneous tissue, rubbery firm or so soft as to suggest lymphangiomas. These tumors appear in the second decade and increase in number and size throughout life. They usually are not a problem in childhood. Their sheer number makes cosmetic excision not feasible.

Plexiform Neurofibroma

The lesion, often seen around the face and scalp, particularly the parotid region, is characterized by thickened, frequently pigmented skin, beneath which runs a mass of racemose, curling, twisting, branching fibers and bundles of tumor nerve. Thirty-three of 85 patients with neurofibromatosis reported from the Children's Hospital of Pittsburgh (CHP)[1] had such tumors, 17 involving the head or neck. Cranial and facial bony deformity occurs by pressure erosion by tumor lesions (Fig 147–1). The disfiguring plexiform neurofibromas of the parotid region and of the scalp should be vigorously, and, if necessary, repeatedly attacked. These are often diffusely infiltrative tumors in which complete removal is neither feasible nor necessary. Each of the myriad plexiform extensions may be accompanied by vessels of

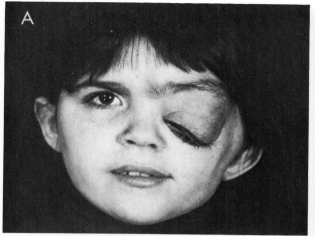

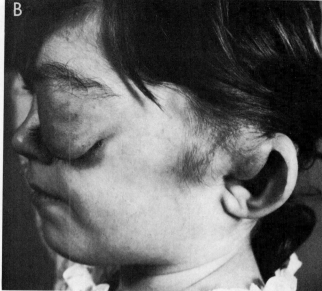

Fig 147–1.—Orbital neurofibroma in a 10-year-old girl with longstanding, progressive enlargement of the left orbit and proptosis from neurofibroma. At age 2 years, she underwent an ill-advised craniotomy for exploration of the optic nerve. No intracranial tumor was found. Operation on the intraorbital tumor had been repeatedly postponed in infancy and childhood. **A and B,** enormous enlargement of the orbit, proptosis, and huge plexiform tumor in the frontal, temporal, preauricular and postauricular regions extending down to the neck. The hair obscures the frontal and parietal swellings. **C,** skull. Enormous expansion of the orbit and erosion of the orbital rim, by communications between the orbital and frontal tumors. The wire sutures are from the craniotomy. In a series of operations, the orbital tumor has been removed, as well as the frontal extensions, pre- and postauricular masses, and cervical extension. The child's appearance has been vastly improved, and the prominence of the left orbital contents is substantially less, but there is no way in which the globe can be replaced and supported so as to prevent diplopia. A partial lower facial palsy resulting from excision of the massive tumor in the neck is scheduled for plastic correction. Operation years earlier would have been simpler and safer, have prevented the grotesque expansion of the orbit, and spared the child gross disfigurement. In the end, binocular vision could not be restored, and the eye was removed from its great orbit. The child wears a prosthesis attached to eyeglasses, and her appearance is remarkably normal.

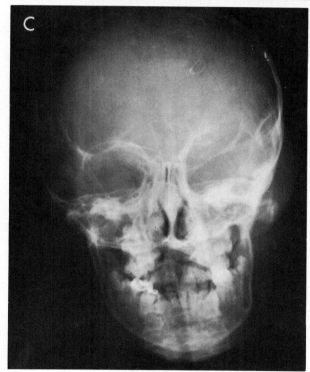

surprising size. Patient dissection and control of bleeding with electrocautery will permit removal of extensive tumors. When the bulky mass of tumor has been resected, it is usually found that much of the abnormal overlying skin is redundant and can be excised. Care must be exercised to avoid damage to functional nerves and major vessels with which the tumor projections intertwine. No child should be permitted to develop a grotesque deformity that can be prevented, even though it is known that the tumor cannot be totally extirpated.

Oral tumors can cause bleeding or difficulty with feeding. The tongue is the most frequently affected intraoral site. Partial glossectomy may be beneficial in improving speech and eating (Fig 147–2). Buccal or gingival lesions are disfiguring and destructive to dentition. Lesions of the palate or retropharynx can be troublesome. Tumors of the larynx cause obstruction[4] and present problems in anesthesia.[15] Removal of these tumors is recom-

mended before operation is made difficult by growth to large size or extension into awkward areas.

Neurofibromas of the soft tissues of the trunk, scrotum, or vulva can reach great size. Clitoral involvement with neurofibromatosis can simulate a penis[22] or precocious puberty.[9] Operation is recommended for tumors that are painful or excessively bulky, increase rapidly in size, or interfere with the child's self-concept.

Elephantiasis Nervorum and Neurofibroma of the Extremities

Elephantiasis nervorum is the term Cushing used to describe numerous large and small tumors that occur along the nerves of the scalp, together with large areas of thickened and involved skin (Figs 147–3 and 147–4). The term is now used to describe a similar appearance of the limb. The picture is often confused with hemi- or monohypertrophy.[17] Large tumors or those that

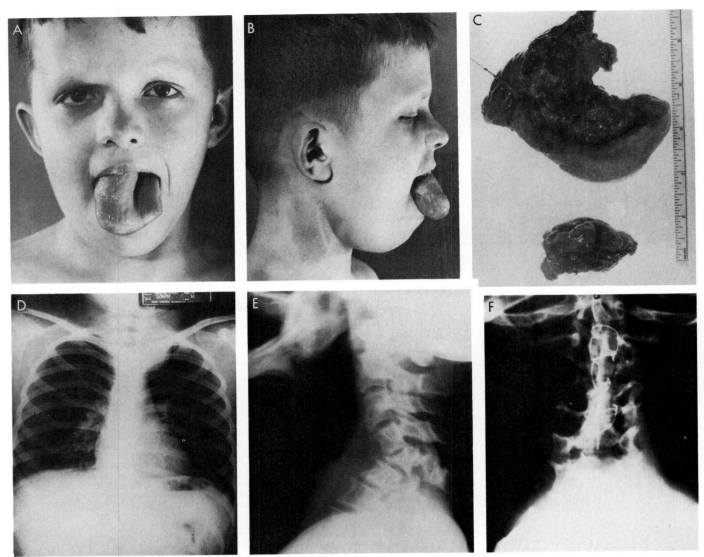

Fig 147–2.—Neurofibroma of tongue, mediastinum, and dumb-bell neurofibroma of the spine. **A** and **B**, the patient at age 7 years showing enlargement of the right half of the tongue and continuous masses running down into the neck, where large café-au-lait spot and scar of an earlier biopsy are seen. **C**, right hemiglossectomy and in-continuity resection of extension to the neck of this tumor from the hypoglossal nerve relieved him of the growing mass. There was no recurrence. **D**, at the same time, a spherical, discrete and dense left superior-posterior mediastinal tumor was noted, which proved to be a neurofibroma. There was no recurrence, despite the fact that there were a number of small tumor-nerve fibers going off in all directions. **E**, 7 years later, cervical spine showing extensive destruction and sharp gibbus. The boy presented then with incipient spastic paraplegia. There was no discrete cervical mass. **F**, decompression and cervical fusion provided temporary relief, but the tumor had eroded multiple intervertebral foramina and, both inside and outside the vertebral canal, was inextirpable. He ultimately succumbed to recurrent paraplegia.

impair function of the extremity should be resected to the extent compatible with preservation and improvement of function. In tumors that involve major nerves of the extremity, it can be difficult to tell which of the strands is the main trunk of the nerve and which constitutes tumor. Unless malignancy is suspected, every effort is made to spare the principal nerves. The bipolar nerve stimulator can be useful here.

Discrepancy in limb length may be difficult to manage. Procedures to arrest growth or lengthen bones are frequently required in order to minimize abnormalities in gait or posture (Fig 147–5).

Mediastinal and Thoracic Neurofibroma

Often detected incidentally on chest x-ray films (see Fig 147–2), these lesions arise from any of the intrathoracic nerves or from a spinal nerve root. The principal differential diagnosis is between neurofibroma and lateral (intrathoracic) meningocele. A dense, rounded, sharply demarcated posterior mediastinal tumor is a tumor of nerve origin until proved otherwise. The tumors frequently have an intraspinal extension (dumb-bell tumor). Computed tomography is useful in delineating the presence and extent of involvement within the canal. Myelography may be indicated if there are neurologic signs. Once more, the principal discrete mass often is found at operation to have innumerable tumor nerve processes growing from it. There is a substantial incidence of malignant degeneration, figures varying widely from 5–40%.[23, 25] For this reason, removal of the bulk of the tumor mass is recommended when it is first found. Six children have been operated upon for mediastinal neurofibromas at CHP in the past 25 years: one of these tumors was malignant, and the child died 2 weeks following the operation; another child

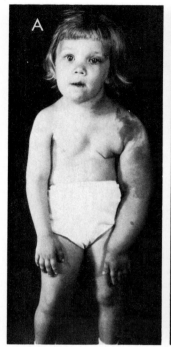
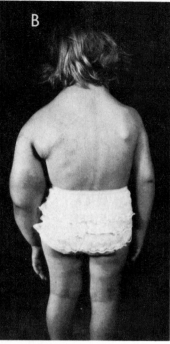
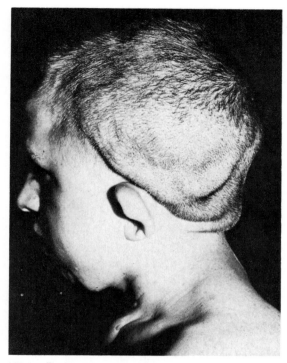

Fig 147–3.—Elephantiasis nervorum, mediastinal neurofibroma, vertebral lesions. Multiple lesions in a child age 3 years, demonstrating the rapidity with which multiple lesions can develop and progress. **A** and **B,** at age 3 years, showing the very large pigmented areas over the left arm and shoulder, as well as small ones, and enlargement of the entire arm (elephantiasis nervorum). At age 3 months, the girl had had a biopsy of a neurofibroma in the left axilla. At 8 months of age, a posterior mediastinal neurofibroma was removed (note Horner's syndrome), and at age 2 years a retropharyngeal mass was removed. At age 5 years, she required a cervical spine fusion for vertebral destruction and gibbus not unlike that seen in Figure 147–2, *E.* At age 14 years, the girl underwent wide excision of a rapidly growing neurofibroma over the left scapula; the lesion proved to be benign.

Fig 147–4.—Elephantiasis nervorum of scalp. This is the lesion usually referred to as a plexiform neurofibroma, but it is the type of lesion for which Cushing coined the term elephantiasis nervorum. Aside from this lesion, at the time of operation, this 13-year-old boy had only numerous café-au-lait spots and a few cutaneous nodules. Resection in two stages produced a gratifying improvement in his appearance.

had a destructive chest wall lesion that required repeated excision.

Visceral Involvement

Symptomatic involvement of the intestinal tract is not common in children. None of 85 patients seen over a 20-year period at CHP was so affected. These neurofibromas arise from neural elements in the bowel wall or mesentery and may cause chronic anemia,[5] acute bleeding, or intestinal obstruction. The small intestine is affected more often than is the colon. Sivak et al.[33] recommend endoscopic removal of accessible polyps of the small intestine or colon. Other abdominal masses should be removed when discovered. The larger tumors seem disposed to malignant degeneration. (See Neurofibrosarcoma, below.)

The kidney is rarely affected with von Recklinghausen's disease except for renovascular problems. Bladder involvement is more common than is involvement of the upper tract. Eleven of 32 such cases found by Torres and Bennett[35] were in children. Any area of the bladder may be involved. The symptoms are those of a mass, of decreased bladder capacity, or of obstruction. Resection and urinary diversion usually have been necessary and should be undertaken before significant upper tract damage occurs. At CHP, we have had three patients with bladder involvement: one required diversion; another had a localized bladder tumor that allowed partial cystectomy without diversion. The third child underwent partial cystectomy for a neurofibrosarcoma. This was followed by radiation therapy and chemotherapy

for microscopic residual tumor. He is alive and well with normal bladder function after 5 years.

Skeletal Manifestations

The kyphoscoliosis seen with von Recklinghausen's disease varies greatly in severity and is not well understood. Whereas the mechanism is clear enough in such instances as that illustrated in Figure 147–2, with bony erosion from the pressure of tumor masses, in other instances, severe scoliosis occurs in the absence of spinal or paraspinal tumors. Winter et al.[39] reviewed 102 patients with spinal deformities and outlined the care and follow-up of this group. Scoliosis is best approached early through use of straightening and fusion procedures, in an attempt to avoid further rapid progression and pulmonary insufficiency.

Unilateral bowing or pseudarthrosis of the tibia appears early, at times at birth, and represents a particularly difficult problem. The cause is unknown; the bone is not involved by tumor. The bowed tibia is best treated by successive castings,[27] but many go on to fracture and nonunion. Congenital pseudarthroses have been approached by resection and bone graft,[3] but the failure rate is high unless microsurgical techniques are emloyed, utilizing vascularized free grafts. Pseudarthrosis of the ulna seems to have a more favorable prognosis when treated early by removal of the dysplastic nonunion site and bone grafting.[32]

Central Neurofibromatosis

Meningiomas, gliomas of the cerebral substance, optic gliomas, and acoustic neurinomas all occur. Das Gupta and Brasfield[12] reported 26 patients with von Recklinghausen's dis-

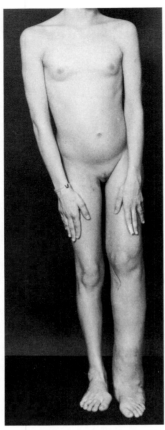

Fig 147–5.—Elephantiasis nervorum. This 15-year-old girl was inactively followed as numerous tender neurofibromas and monohypertrophy rendered the left leg progressively more useless. Removal of the tumors will now require many more procedures and greater risk of nerve injury. The choice must be made between epiphyseal arrest now on the long side, or postpubertal lengthening of the short side.

ease diagnosed at birth, in five of whom brain lesions developed before the age of 12 years; all died. Lesions that appear in the older children have a less dismal outlook. Assiduous follow-up and intensive neurosurgical investigation are called for in children with neurofibromatosis and neurologic signs or symptoms. Optic gliomas, sometimes bilateral, are distressingly common. Computed tomography is essential in the work-up of any of these patients with CNS symptoms. Intraocular neurofibroma has been reported, but blindness in von Recklinghausen's disease is usually due to optic nerve glioma. The presence of unilateral proptosis or visual loss in a patient with von Recklinghausen's disease should suggest orbital neurofibroma, meningioma, or optic glioma. Pulsating proptosis may result from erosion of the orbit with meningeal and cerebral herniation. The patient with a neurofibroma, rather than a glioma of the orbit, usually has other facial or cervical neurofibromas.[2]

Acoustic neurinomas, often bilateral, occur in the second decade and later. In some patients, erosion of the internal auditory canal may be seen on skull film. The annual evaluation of a child with von Recklinghausen's disease includes tests of hearing. The tumors do not differ from those seen independent of the disease.

An unusual CNS manifestation of neurofibromatosis involves diffuse or discrete cerebral arterial stenoses;[20] hemiplegias occur. Intrahemispheric vascular steal effects may be responsible for seizures or other symptoms.[36]

Certain children with neurofibromatosis develop gradual or

sudden paraplegia. This may be due to intraspinal tumor, but vertebral angulation with kyphosis is the most common cause. Those with neurofibromas of the neck or thorax frequently develop subsequent cord symptoms at the level of the cervical or thoracic tumor. Expeditious computed tomographic scanning and possibly myelography are imperative in any child who develops motor weakness or is considered a candidate for it. Laminectomy and fusion, although the best hope for improvement,[10] often fail (see Fig 147–2). The previously bleak outlook for these tumors should be improved by microneurosurgical techniques.

Mental retardation or low intelligence is common, whether as a result of the condition or because the cosmetic disadvantage has resulted in hereditarily unfavorable matings.

Endocrine Manifestations

The association of von Recklinghausen's disease with pheochromocytoma and with medullary carcinoma of the thyroid has been known for some time. Pheochromocytoma is the most common endocrine lesion seen in the adult with neurofibromatosis, but is rare in children.[31] A thyroid mass may be due either to a neurofibroma or to a thyroid carcinoma, and operation is undertaken for any thyroid nodule. Medullary thyroid carcinoma demands total thyroidectomy.

The relationship between von Recklinghausen's disease and the syndromes of multiple endocrine adenomatosis is not clear. A kinship is suggested by their common manifestations: a frequently familial occurrence of tumors of neurectodermal origin.

Disorders of sexual development constitute the most common endocrinologic derangement. Sexual precocity is common and seems to be due to hypothalamic involvement. Developmental retardation also is frequent in these children and is similarly central in origin.

Cardiovascular Manifestations

The heart is infrequently involved. Tumors may cause symptoms due to interference with contractility, outflow, valvular function, or electric conduction. Successful resection of localized cardiac neurofibromatosis using cardiopulmonary bypass has been reported.[18]

Serious arterial lesions are relatively common. Thoracic and abdominal coarctation is reported in all age groups. These tend to be long, involving segments that give off large branches. Collateral circulation around the coarctation is often poor. Shunts around the narrowed segment using autogenous vessels, e.g., splenic artery, or synthetic grafts have been preferred to resection and anastomosis.[18, 29] Hypertension is common in patients with von Recklinghausen's disease. Infants so affected are usually found to have coarctations. Older children are more likely to have one of a variety of renal arterial problems, ranging from a single stenosis of one renal artery to an increasingly complex spectrum of involvement of one or both renal arterial systems. Resection of the stenosis may be feasible, but total or subtotal nephrectomy may be required. Hardy et al.[19] report using localized in situ cooling to allow repair of an aneurysm distal to a stenosis in a solitary kidney in a man age 27 with von Recklinghausen's disease. Bilateral lesions too extensive for operative correction require pharmacologic treatment of the hypertension.

Neurofibrosarcoma

Although the frequency of malignancy of many types is increased in neurofibromatosis, neurofibrosarcoma deserves special mention. Larger neurofibromas have a propensity for malignant degeneration. Rapid growth of a tumor is an ominous signal of such degeneration. Recent reports have been encouraging in this previously lethal sarcoma. Raney et al.[26] have shown the value of chemotherapy and radiation therapy in this treatment.

The report of Chu et al.[7] is one of several that indicate a relationship between radiation and subsequent development of neurofibrosarcoma. This should wave a flag of caution for the surgeon treating Wilms or other tumors in the patient with neurofibromatosis.

Summary

The patient with diagnosed von Recklinghausen's disease, and his parents, must be enlisted in a lifetime systematic observation: periodic complete physical examinations, including blood pressure; examinations to detect optic or acoustic nerve tumors; and repeated chest films in the search for posterior mediastinal tumors and evaluation of spinal deformity.

Individual tumors that are large, cause pain or disfigurement, or seem to be growing should be removed. Immediate removal is undertaken for lesions in the mediastinum or in the abdomen where tumors of modest size can be dealt with, and very large tumors pose problems. If the principal tumor mass and many of its racemose extensions are removed, the remaining strands of tumor nerve may not form a new tumor of any consequence. Although the implications of the disease are always serious and the ultimate outcome uncertain, careful observation and judicious operation undertaken appropriately early may make a great difference to the patient in both the quality and duration of life.

REFERENCES

1. Adkins J.C., Ravitch M.M.: The operative management of von Recklinghausen's neurofibromatosis in children, with special reference to lesions of the head and neck. *Surgery* 82:342, 1977.
2. Baltzell J.W., Davis D.O., Condon V.R.: Unusual manifestations of neurofibromatosis. *Med. Radiogr. Photogr.* 50:2, 1974.
3. Battin J., Hehunstre J.P., Bondonny J.M., et al.: Les inflexions et les pseudarthroses congenitales du tibia dans la maladie de von Recklinghausen. *Ann. Chir. Infant* 16:385, 1975.
4. Buchman L.A., Kozhevnekova T.V.: Neurofibromatosis of larynx in connection with neurofibromatosis. *Vestn. Otorinolaringol.* 30:86, 1968.
5. Buntin P.T., Fitzgerald J.F.: Gastrointestinal neurofibromatosis. *Am. J. Dis. Child.* 119:521, 1970.
6. Chabalko J.J., Creagan E.T., Fraumeni J.F.: Epidemiology of selected sarcomas in children. *J. Natl. Cancer Inst.* 53:675, 1974.
7. Chu J.Y., O'Connor D.M., Danis R.K.: Neurofibrosarcoma at irradiation site in a patient with neurofibromatosis and Wilms' tumor. *CA* 31:333, 1981.
8. Crowe F.W., Schull W.J., Neel J.V.: *A Clinical, Pathological and Genetic Study of Multiple Neurofibromatosis.* Springfield, Ill., Charles C Thomas, Publisher, 1956.
9. Curran J.P., Coleman R.D.: Neurofibromata of the chest wall simulating prepubertal gynecomastia. *Clin. Pediatr.* 16:1064, 1977.
10. Curtis B.H., Fisher R.L., Butterfield W.L., et al.: Neurofibromatosis with paraplegia. *J. Bone Joint Surg.* 51A:843, 1969.
11. D'Agostino A.N., Soule E.H., Miller R.H.: Sarcomas of the peripheral nerves and somatic soft tissue associated with multiple neurofibromatosis (von Recklinghausen's disease). *CA* 16:1015, 1963.
12. Das Gupta T.K., Brasfield R.D.: von Recklinghausen's disease. *CA* 21:174, 1971.
13. Fabricant R.N., Todaro G.J., Eldridge R.: Increased levels of nerve-growth-factor cross-reacting protein in "central" neurofibromatosis. *Lancet* 1:4, 1979.
14. Fienman N.L., Yakovac W.C.: Neurofibromatosis in childhood. *J. Pediatr.* 76:339, 1970.
15. Fisher M.M.: Anaesthetic difficulties in neurofibromatosis. *Anaesthesia* 30:648, 1975.
16. Greene J.F., Fitzwater J.E., Burgess J.: Arterial lesions associated with neurofibromatosis. *Am. J. Clin. Pathol.* 62:481, 1974.
17. Haiken B.N.: Neurofibromatosis in childhood. *J. Pediatr.* 77:923, 1970.
18. Halpern M., Currarino G.: Vascular lesions causing hypertension in neurofibromatosis. *N. Engl. J. Med.* 273:248, 1965.
19. Hardy D.G., Hately W., Newton J.R., et al.: Hypertension and renal artery stenosis with aneurysm formation in a solitary kidney in a patient with neurofibromatosis. *Br. J. Urol.* 47:137, 1975.
20. Hilal S.K., Solomon G.E., Gold A.P., et al.: Primary cerebral arterial occlusive disease in children. *Radiology* 99:87, 1971.
21. Holt J.F.: Neurofibromatosis in children. *Am. J. Roentgenol.* 130:615, 1978.
22. Kenny F.M., Fetterman G.H., Preeyasombat C.: Neurofibromata simulating a penis and labioscrotal gonads in a girl with von Recklinghausen's disease. *Pediatrics* 37:456, 1966.
23. Lee C.W., Shulman K., Morecki R., et al.: Malignant degeneration of thoracic neurofibroma. *N.Y. State J. Med.* 75:347, 1975.
24. Miller M., Hall J.G.: Possible maternal effect on severity of neurofibromatosis. *Lancet* 2:1071, 1978.
25. Parish C.: Complications of mediastinal neural tumors. *Thorax* 26:392, 1971.
26. Raney R.B., Littman P., Jarrett P., et al.: Results of multimodal therapy for children with neurogenic sarcoma. *Med. Pediatr. Oncol.* 7:229, 1979.
27. Rose G.K.: Restraint in the treatment of a bowed tibia associated with neurofibromatosis. *Acta Orthop. Scand.* 46:704, 1975.
28. Rosenquist G.C., Krovetz L.J., Haller J.A., et al.: Acquired right ventricular outflow obstruction in a child with neurofibromatosis. *Am. Heart J.* 79:103, 1970.
29. Rowen M., Dorsey T.J., Kegel S.M., et al.: Thoracic coarctation associated with neurofibromatosis. *Am. J. Dis. Child.* 129:113, 1975.
30. Salyer W.R., Salyer D.C.: The vascular lesions of neurofibromatosis. *Angiology* 25:510, 1974.
31. Saxena K.M.: Endocrine manifestations of neurofibromatosis in children. *Am. J. Dis. Child.* 120:265, 1970.
32. Shertzer J.H., Bickel W.H., Stubbins S.G.: Congenital pseudarthrosis of the ulna. *Minn. Med.* 52:1061, 1969.
33. Sivak M.V., Sullivan B.H.: Neurogenic tumors of the small intestines. *Gastroenterology* 68:374, 1975.
34. Tilesius W.G.: *Historia Pathologica Singularis Cutis Turpitudinis.* Leipzig, Germany, 1793.
35. Torres H., Bennett M.J.: Neurofibromatosis of the bladder: Case report and review of the literature. *J. Urol.* 96:910, 1966.
36. Voigt K., Beck U.: Arterial developmental anomalies of one hemisphere with inter- and intrahemispheric steal effects in neurofibromatosis (Recklinghausen's disease). *Radiol. Clin. Biol.* 43:483, 1974.
37. Von Recklinghausen F.: *Ueber die Multiplen Fibrome der Haut und ihre Beziehung zu den multiplen Neuromen in Rudolph Virchow Festschrift,* Berlin, August Hirschwald, 1882.
38. Wander J.V., Das Gupta T.K.: Neurofibromatosis. *Curr. Probl. Surg.* February 1977.
39. Winter R.B., Moe J.H., Bradford D.S., et al.: Spine deformity in neurofibromatosis: A review of 102 patients. *J. Bone Joint Surg.* 61A:677, 1979.

148 Eric W. Fonkalsrud
Disorders of the Lymphatic System

MOST MALFORMATIONS of the lymphatic system have their origin during fetal development and are first noted at birth or shortly thereafter. Occasional anomalies such as lymphedema praecox may not become clinically evident until adolescence. Lymphatic obstruction is usually a common feature, resulting in dilated endothelium-lined spaces ranging in size from microscopic channels, as in lymphangiomas, to large cysts several centimeters in diameter, as with cystic hygromas.[2] Congenital lymphedema and intestinal or thoracic lymphangiectasia may represent variations of the same malformation caused by congenital lymphatic obstruction or partial absence of lymphatic channels.[7] More than one type of lymphatic malformation may be present in the same patient.

Lymphangiomas

Lymphangiomas are benign tumors of the lymphatic system, characterized by anastomosing lymphatic channels and cystic spaces varying in size, but generally less than 0.5 cm in diameter. They characteristically infiltrate surrounding structures by local extension and have the ability to produce new lesions by extension or by new growth.[13] The size of the lymphangioma appears directly related to the degree of obstruction of lymphaticovenous drainage as evidenced by histologic appearance[21] and by studies of the microvascular circulation of lymphangiomas with xenon[133] clearance. Lymphangiomas show a predilection for the tongue, cheek, thorax, extremities, and retroperitoneal tissues.[8] Usually more firm than hygromas, they are somewhat irregular and consist of tiny cysts with a rather dense stroma of connective and lymphoid tissue.[11]

Approximately 65% of lymphangiomas are apparent at birth, and 90% appear by the end of the second year.[10] Spontaneous regression is very rare; infection is the prevailing serious complication, potentially leading to sepsis or pressure on adjacent tissues. Lymphatic fluid weeping from small cutaneous vesicles overlying the deeper lymphangioma is not uncommon from tumors involving the trunk and extremities.

Lymphangiomas have been classified into the following three groups[16]: (1) lymphangioma simplex, composed of small capillary-sized lymphatic channels; (2) cavernous lymphangioma, comprising dilated lymphatic channels, often with fibrous adventitial covering; and (3) cystic lymphangioma, or hygroma (separately considered in Chap. 53). Different macroscopic and microscopic forms of lymphangioma may occur in different parts of the same lesions. Hyperplastic lymph nodes often exist in close proximity. Dilated capillaries and venous channels are occasionally interspersed with or adjacent to lymphangiomas, causing extensive vascularity; in such cases, the lesion may be called a "hemolymphangioma."

Disfigurement from the lymphangioma is the principal reason for seeking medical care. Pain and discomfort are rare, unless secondary infection or hemorrhage has developed. Lymphangiomas usually do not transilluminate, because the cysts are tiny and multiple, with fibrous stroma intervening. Malignant degeneration of the lymphangioma is unlikely.

Treatment

Radiation therapy and needle aspiration with insertion of sclerosing solution have been of no apparent benefit in the management of microcystic lymphangiomas. Surgical excision is the only consistently effective (albeit usually incomplete) method of management. Operation in small infants is avoided whenever possible to minimize the risk of injuring vital tissues. Cavernous lymphangiomas, in contrast to hemangiomas, do not expand appreciably during the first year of life and appear amenable to safe operative resection when the child is a few years old.

Whenever feasible, complete excision of the lymphangioma is performed; staged resection is necessary in approximately one third of cases. However, in occasional patients complete resection is not feasible, because the lesion extends too deeply into vital structures (Fig 148–1).[9] The most prominent, or grotesque, portion of the lymphangioma should be resected when feasible, realizing that recurrent growth and skin weeping from cutaneous vesicles is likely to occur and that multiple small resections may be required over the course of many years. Preservation of life and function must take precedence over the desire for complete excision of the lesion.

Lymphangioma of the Tongue

Lymphangiomas of the tongue usually extend into the floor of the mouth and are often accompanied by bilateral submandibular swelling from lymphangiomatous tissue, often including hygromas.[18] They are the most common cause of macroglossia in infancy (see Fig 53–5 and 62–4). Multiple tiny vesicles are present on the major portion of the surface of the distal tongue and tend to weep, often causing infection, and giving a "warty" appearance. Repeated episodes of inflammation owing to trauma to the tongue, protruding outward from the oral cavity, usually cause extensive lymphocytic infiltration and an increase in fibrous tissue. The posterior half of the tongue is rarely involved. Bleeding within the lesion or into the oral cavity is not uncommon. Atrophy of the striated muscle may occur in areas where the muscle is not compressed.

During the first years after birth, the tongue may enlarge substantially, from inflammation caused by trauma or an upper respiratory infection, or from hemorrhage. The enlarged tongue may protrude between the lips for 2–3 cm, preventing the child from closing his mouth and allowing saliva to drip. The exposed tongue becomes dry and swollen, leading to infection, edema, and bleeding. Deformity of the mandible is often produced by pressure from the size and weight of the large lymphangiomatous mass in the tongue and floor of the mouth.

Extirpation during the first year of life is the preferred treatment for most lingual lymphangiomas.[3] One should excise enough tumor to reshape the contour of the tongue and reduce its size sufficiently to permit it to fit comfortably within the oral cavity; radical resection is not necessary for a favorable result. Such resection of the tip of the tongue is performed by making bilateral marginal V-shaped wedge resections. Residual vesicles

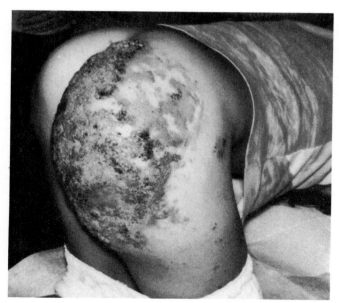

Fig 148–1.—Extensive lymphangioma involving buttocks, showing cutaneous vesicles and chronic inflammation, extending deeply into gluteal and thigh muscles. Repeated local resections were followed by prompt recurrence. A hip disarticulation was performed, achieving a satisfactory long-term result.

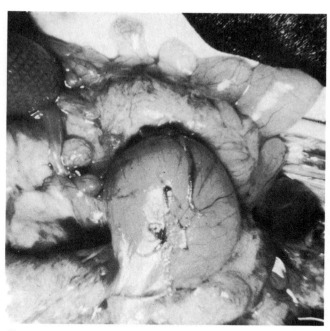

Fig 148–2.—Lymphangiomatosis of intestine and peritoneal surface, showing clusters of lymph-filled sacs extending from mesentery and bowel wall.

on the lingual surface may be temporarily destroyed by electrocoagulation. When patients with lingual lymphangiomas achieve adolescence, the lesion stabilizes and usually will not increase further in size. Courses of antibiotics are often helpful to reduce the severity of the inflammation during the months and years after operation. Extensions of the lymphangioma into the floor of the mouth and submental area can usually be resected in secondary procedures. Anesthetic management of patients with large lingual lymphangiomas is often difficult; after operation, several days of nasotracheal intubation may be required until edema recedes. Tracheostomy is generally avoided, if at all possible, because the lesions often extend into the lower anterior neck, but may be necessary in occasional patients to provide an adequate airway.

Lymphangiomas affect the parotid gland far less frequently than do hemangiomas and are rarely found in other salivary glands in childhood (see Chap. 49).

Mesenteric Cysts and Lymphangiomas

Lymphangiomatous cysts of varying size can occur in the mesentery of the small intestine or the omentum and extend diffusely into the retroperitoneal space (Fig 148–2).[12] Small intraperitoneal lymphangiomas usually do not produce symptoms, although small-to-moderate volumes of peritoneal fluid may develop. Larger lesions can cause increased abdominal girth, occasional abdominal pain, and intestinal obstruction by compression of adjacent bowel. Mesenteric cysts are somewhat similar to cystic hygromas, consisting of large unilocular or multilocular lymphatic cysts, which may become enormous.[17] Volvulus of the attached intestine can develop. Hemorrhage into the cyst following trauma or erosion may cause rapid expansion and pain. Rupture of mesenteric cysts is uncommon.

Large intra-abdominal cystic lymphangiomas localized to the mesentery or to one area of the retroperitoneal tissues may lend themselves to total resection. Localized intestinal resection with adjacent large mesenteric cysts is recommended by most authors,[17] but, if total excision is not possible, opening the cyst

widely into the peritoneal cavity is the next best method of drainage. As much of the cyst wall should be resected as possible without injuring vital structures; the abdomen should be drained with catheters until drainage has become sparse. Anastomosis of the incompletely removed cyst to the bowel, or external marsupialization, are not acceptable modes of treatment.

Chylous Ascites

Chylous fluid in the peritoneal cavity results from leakage of mesenteric, cisternal, or lower thoracic duct lymphatic fluid into the abdomen. The characteristic milky appearance of the fluid indicates its high lipid content, unless there had been scant ingestion of fat for a prolonged period.

The cause of chylous ascites is often undeterminable. A few patients have been found to have congenital anomalies such as chylous cysts of the small bowel mesentery, congenital bands constricting the root of the mesentery, or atresia of the thoracic duct.[23] In older children, chylous ascites may result from trauma or from neoplastic or inflammatory obstruction and secondary rupture of the intestinal lymphatics.[20]

Although chylous ascites is rarely a malignant condition, the clinical course is often unrelenting and may be fatal, particularly in infancy. Thirty percent of reported patients died from severe malnutrition, hypoproteinemia, and dehydration. Children with chylous ascites experience symptoms caused by increased intra-abdominal pressure and, when ascites becomes massive, scrotal edema, inguinal and umbilical hernias, pulmonary atelectasis, or edema of the lower extremities.

Plain roentgenograms of the abdomen and chest, skeletal bone survey, intravenous pyelogram, and barium studies of the gastrointestinal tract are recommended when attempting to determine whether the ascites results from an obstructing tumor, mesenteric cyst, or congenital malformation. Evaluation of vitamin A absorption shows that almost all of the vitamin enters the chyle rather than the bloodstream in patients with chylous ascites. The same phenomenon is seen in the protein-losing enteropathy of intestinal lymphangiectasia. Levels of carotene in the serum are quite low in these patients.

Initially, a conservative program of management is advised, consisting of a diet low in fat and high in protein, repeated paracenteses for relief of symptoms, and intravenous administration of plasma or albumin. Intravenous hyperalimentation may become necessary if caloric and fluid loss, together with poor dietary intake, portends malnutrition. Reducing the volume of chyle production by dietary restriction may be effective in many cases.[14] Diets containing short- and medium-chained fatty acids as the fat source can reduce the amount and concentration of fat and protein in the ascitic fluid. Intravenous infusion of the ascitic fluid has been undertaken in occasional patients without significant side reaction, although the technique is not practical for chronic use in infants and young children. Internal drainage by venoperitoneal shunt may be temporarily effective.[22]

Laparotomy is indicated for children with chylous ascites when there is (1) a known surgically correctable lesion, (2) persistence of symptomatic ascites unresponsive to low-fat diet, and (3) deterioration in the clinical status of the patient. Although some chylous leaks may be identified at operation and closed, and certain chyle-producing tumors may be dissected, diffuse lymphangiomatosis usually does not lend itself to surgical resection. Occasional patients may experience surprising improvement after exploration and external drainage.[22]

Intestinal Lymphangiectasia

Intestinal lymphangiectasia usually occurs in children under 3 years of age, commonly producing diarrhea and occasional vomiting. Protein loss into the intestinal lumen may be mild to severe; growth retardation is common. Some develop mental aberrations as well. Occasionally, there may be associated hypoproteinemic pitting lymphedema of the extremities, or a history of lymphedema in the family, or both. Lymphopenia, which is often present, is directly related to the degree of fluid loss. Biopsies of the small intestine may show a range from normal tissue to severe aberrations. The lymphatic block in lymphangiectasia can occur (1) in the lamina propria only; (2) as generalized involvement of the lamina propria, submucosa, serosa, and mesentery; or (3) in the mesentery alone, with minimal involvement of the lamina propria.

Treatment of intestinal lymphangiectasia is similar to that for chylous ascites: high-protein, fat-free diet, and added medium-chained triglycerides. This dietary regimen usually prevents or alleviates the diarrhea and hypoproteinemia.[13] In rare cases, when the lymphatic obstruction is localized to a small segment of the bowel, intestinal resection with anastomosis may be helpful.

Lymphangiomas and Lymphangiectasia of Solid Organs

Pulmonary lymphangiectasia is believed to be secondary to obstruction of major pulmonary lymphatics with obstruction of pulmonary venous flow or anomalous pulmonary development. The condition is usually bilateral and can produce severe respiratory distress shortly after birth, rapidly becoming fatal,[19] or it can resolve spontaneously within a few weeks. The treatment is supportive, frequently requiring endotracheal intubation and respirator support. Pulmonary lymphangiectasia has been seen in older patients with generalized lymphangiomas, generating excessive pulmonary secretions if such patients receive general anesthesia.[5]

Lymphangiomas of the lung and trachea are uncommon, but may produce hydrothorax. The lymphatic fluid accumulation is serous, in contrast to the chylous fluid associated with thoracic

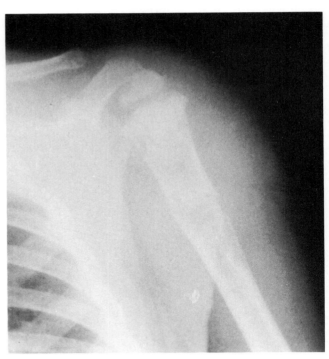

Fig 148–3.—Lymphangiomatosis of humerus in adolescent male with lymphangioma of chest wall as well.

duct injuries. Persistent fluid reaccumulation may require resection of the involved tissues if chest tube drainage does not relieve the condition. Repeated episodes of pulmonary infection and atelectasis, as well as the likelihood that closely associated organs will become involved, portend a poor outcome.

Lymphangiomatous involvement of the spleen and/or liver is unusual. These patients may have small asymptomatic solitary lymphangiomas, or diffuse cystic lymphangiomatous disease involving multiple organ systems, in which case the prognosis is unfavorable.[1]

Lymphangiomas may involve the skeletal system, frequently as a part of a generalized disorder with cystic involvement of various organs and tissues. A combination of osseous lymphangiomatosis with chylothorax, cystic hygromas, or lymphangiomas of the thoracic wall or trunk is occasionally seen. Lymphangiomatous involvement of bone may also occur as an isolated phenomenon. Roentgenograms of the skeleton may show diffuse involvement of many bones with well-circumscribed, small, destructive lesions that may have sclerotic borders (Fig 148–3). These lesions may occasionally cause pathologic fractures. Osseous lymphangiomas should be differentiated from histiocytosis X, from metastases, and sometimes from fibrous dysplasia and fibromatosis. No specific treatment is available for diffuse lymphangiomatous involvement of bone.

Lymphedema

Primary lymphedema is caused by an idiopathic maldevelopment of the subcutaneous lymphatic channels of the extremities. Based on the age of onset, Kinmonth et al.[15] have classified primary lymphedema into three categories: (1) congenital—present at birth; (2) praecox—usually appearing in early adolescence; and (3) tarda—occurring spontaneously in middle age. In our experience, primarily with children, congenital lymphedema was present in approximately 35% of patients. Hereditary congenital lymphedema is designated as Milroy's disease,[4] but true hereditary congenital lymphedema of this type is rare.

In the normal extremity, tissue fluid collected by the dermal lymphatic system drains into the subcutaneous lymphatics accompanying the main superficial veins to the regional lymph nodes in the groin or axilla. The superficial lymphatics are separated from the deep system by the deep fascia, except for small communications through the lymph nodes in the popliteal fossa, the adductor canal, and the epitrochlear nodes of the arm.

Primary lymphedema, which is usually confined to the tissues superficial to the deep fascia, has been classified as aplastic, hypoplastic, or hyperplastic. Although the precise pathophysiology of congenital lymphedema has not been clearly elucidated, it is believed that the superficial lymphatic network is hypoplastic or absent. The lymph, therefore, pools in the subcutaneous fat until the oncotic pressure of the tissue exceeds the superficial venous osmotic pressure, causing venous decompression. Whereas lymphedema praecox is almost invariably a disorder of the superficial lymphatics, congenital lymphedema may involve the subfascial lymphatics as well.

Congenital lymphedema most often involves the dorsum of the foot, occasionally the plantar surface, but rarely extends above the knees (Fig 148–4). It occasionally occurs in the upper extremities, although the other forms of primary lymphedema almost never involve the hand and arm (Fig 148–5). Congenital lymphedema affects females almost twice as often as males.[5] In approximately one third of patients, both lower extremities are affected. Children whose hands and arms are affected frequently appear to have lymphatic abnormalities in other areas of the body, particularly those involving the external genitalia, intestinal lymphangiectasia with protein-losing enteropathy, cervical cystic hygroma, and pulmonary lymphangiectasia (Fig 148–6).[5] Obesity appears to accelerate the limb swelling of congenital lymphedema as well as of lymphedema praecox; lymphangitis is rare in both conditions.

Lymphangiograms tend to be unsuccessful technically and are not helpful in evaluating children with primary lymphedema. Ar-

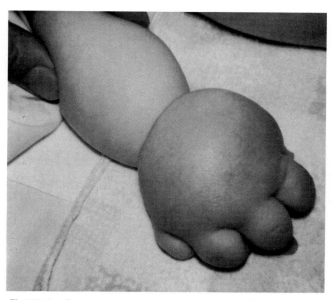

Fig 148–5.—Severe congenital lymphedema of hand and forearm in 3-month-old girl. The patient also had lymphedema of both lower extremities and of the genitalia. Staged subcutaneous lymphangiectomy was performed after the age of 2 years.

teriograms and venograms are rarely abnormal. Roentgenograms of the hands and feet may show wide separation of the metacarpal or metatarsal bones in severe cases. The overlying skin is usually normal, without the hypertrophic changes of lymphedema praecox.

Nonoperative measures are recommended for congenital lymphedema during the first 2 years of life, because the majority of children experience gradually less severe lymphedema compared with general body growth. Elastic stocking support or bandages are only minimally beneficial. When severe congenital lymphedema persists beyond the first 3 years of life, staged sub-

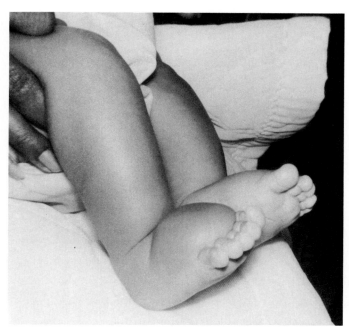

Fig 148–4.—Congenital lymphedema of both lower extremities in 2-month-old boy. No swelling was present in the thighs. The swelling became less prominent during the ensuing 3 years.

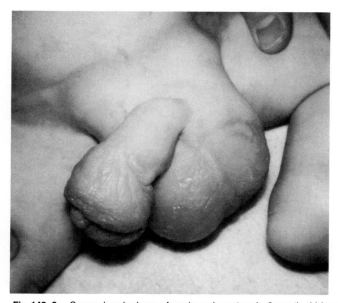

Fig 148–6.—Severe lymphedema of penis and scrotum in 2-month-old boy with lymphedema of both lower and upper extremities, and cystic hygroma. Note swelling in inguinal region caused by bilateral inguinal hernias, which contained ascitic fluid.

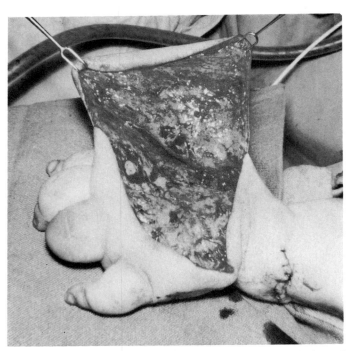

Fig 148–7.—Subcutaneous lymphangiectomy for congenital lymphedema of hand and forearm in 18-month-old infant. All subcutaneous tissue is resected between skin flap and fascia immediately overlying muscles and tendons.

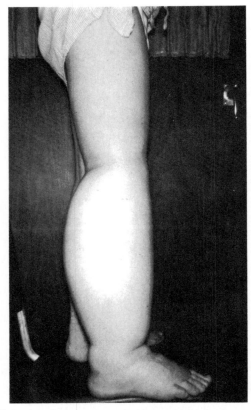

Fig 148–8.—Lymphedema praecox in 14-year-old girl showing marked swelling of right calf and dorsum of foot. There is minimal swelling of thigh. Left lower extremity was normal in size. Subcutaneous lymphangiectomy was performed, resulting in marked improvement.

cutaneous lymphangiectomy can significantly reduce the bulk of the extremity and improve its function.[6] The modified Kondoleon procedure, in which full-thickness skin flaps are constructed, generally provides an excellent functional and cosmetic result (Fig 148–7). Multiple staged procedures under tourniquet control are usually necessary. Free skin grafts have generally been unsatisfactory in managing childhood primary lymphedemas, because they produce hypertrophic scars and persistent weeping of lymphatic fluid. Surgical wounds in children with primary lymphedema appear to heal satisfactorily in most cases, and there is a low incidence of infection. Subcutaneous catheter drainage of wounds in combination with pressure dressings helps to diminish fluid accumulation beneath the skin flaps.

Lymphedema praecox generally involves one or both lower extremities, often extending up to the groin; it is three times more common in females (Fig 148–8). The extremity may look normal during the first several years of life; however, once the condition appears, there is usually a gradual progression until early adulthood. In contrast to patients with congenital lymphedema, considerable benefit may be achieved by using full-leg, form-fitting elastic stockings. Inflatable compression units for the entire extremity may reduce limb swelling for a few hours, but are not practical for most children. Exercise promotes lymphatic drainage from the extremities and should be encouraged. Diuretics have minimal effect on congenital lymphedema. Patients with lymphedema praecox are usually somewhat overweight, and this seems to accelerate the swelling of the extremity.

Staged subcutaneous lymphangiectomy with tourniquet control may significantly reduce the swelling of extremities with lymphedema praecox. Blood transfusion will very likely be required. It is well to plan for autologous blood transfusion. Prolonged postoperative elastic bandage support is recommended. Omental transposition operations have been unsuccessful in the management of childhood primary lymphedemas.

Acquired or secondary lymphedema may result from wide resection of inguinal or axillary tissues, or may occur subsequent to radiation of these areas. In contrast to primary lymphedema, the subcutaneous lymphatics are markedly distended, and recurrent lymphangitis is common. The condition can be readily identified by lymphangiographic studies. Whereas acquired lymphedema can be improved symptomatically by wearing elastic compression bandages, staged subcutaneous lymphangiectomy may provide significant functional and cosmetic improvement. Although primary lymphedema rarely becomes malignant, longstanding secondary lymphedema can progress to aggressive lymphangiosarcoma, particularly after radical mastectomy.[24]

REFERENCES

1. Asch M.J., Cohen A.H., Moore T.C.: Hepatic and splenic lymphangiomatosis with skeletal involvement: Report of a case and review of the literature. *Surgery* 76:334, 1974.
2. Bill A.H. Jr., Sumner D.S.: A unified concept of lymphangioma and cystic hygroma. *Surg. Gynecol. Obstet.* 120:79, 1965.
3. Dingman R.O., Grabb W.C.: Lymphangioma of the tongue. *Plast. Reconstr. Surg.* 27:214, 1961.
4. Milroy W.R.: An undescribed variety of hereditary oedema. *N.Y. Med. J.* 56:505, 1892.
5. Fonkalsrud E.W.: A syndrome of congenital lymphedema of the upper extremity and associated systemic lymphatic malformations. *Surg. Gynecol. Obstet.* 145:228, 1977.
6. Fonkalsrud E.W.: Congenital lymphedema of the extremities in infants and children. *J. Pediatr. Surg.* 4:231, 1969.
7. Fonkalsrud E.W.: Lymphangiomas in infancy and childhood. *Pediatr. Dig.* 11:29, 1969.
8. Fonkalsrud E.W.: Malformations of the lymphatic system, and hemangiomas, in Holder T., Ashcraft K. (eds.): *Pediatric Surgery.* Philadelphia, W.B. Saunders Co., 1980, pp. 1042.
9. Fonkalsrud E.W.: Surgical management of congenital malformations of the lymphatic system. *Am. J. Surg.* 128:152, 1974.
10. Gross R.E.: *The Surgery of Infancy and Childhood.* Philadelphia, W.B. Saunders Co., 1953.

11. Harkins G.A., Sabiston D.C.: Lymphangioma in infancy and childhood. *Surgery* 47:811, 1960.
12. Henzel J.H., Pories W.J., Burgett D.E., et al.: Intra-abdominal lymphangiomata. *Arch. Surg.* 93:304, 1966.
13. Hill J.T., Briggs J.D.: Lymphangioma. *West. J. Surg. Obstet. Gynecol.* 69:78, 1961.
14. Kessel I: Chylous ascites in infancy. *Arch. Dis. Child.* 27:79, 1952.
15. Kinmonth J.B., Taylor G.W., Tracy G.D., et al.: Primary lymphoedema: Clinical and lymphangiographic studies of a series of 107 patients in which the lower limbs were affected. *Br. J. Surg.* 45:1, 1957.
16. Landing B.H., Farber S.: Tumors of the cardiovascular system, in *Atlas of Tumor Pathology.* Washington, D.C., Armed Forces Institute of Pathology, 1956.
17. Mollitt D.L., Ballantine T.V.N., Grosfeld J.L.: Mesenteric cysts in infancy and childhood. *Surg. Gynecol. Obstet.* 147;182, 1978.
18. Morfit H.M.: Lymphangioma of the tongue. *Arch. Surg.* 81:761, 1960.
19. Rywlin A.M., Fojaco R.M.: Congenital pulmonary lymphangiectasis associated with a blind common pulmonary vein. *Pediatrics* 41:931, 1968.
20. Sanchez R.E., Mahour G.H., Brennan L.P., et al.: Chylous ascites in children. *Surgery* 69:183, 1971.
21. Touloukian R.J., Rickert R.R., Lange R.C., et al.: The microvascular circulation of lymphangioma: A study of Xenon[133] clearance and pathology. *Pediatrics* 48:36, 1971.
22. Vasko J.S., Tapper R.I.: The surgical significance of chylous ascites. *Arch. Surg.* 95:355, 1967.
23. Vollman R.W., Keenan W.J., Eraklis A.J.: Post-traumatic chylous ascites in infancy. *N. Engl. J. Med.* 275:875, 1966.
24. Woodward A.H., Ivins J.E., Soulf E.H.: Lymphangiosarcoma arising in chronic lymphedematous extremities. *Cancer* 30:562, 1972.

149   Milton T. Edgerton / Raymond F. Morgan

Hemangiomas: Congenital Hamartomas

HEMANGIOMAS are the most common of all human birth defects. The term hemangioma, however, has been used to describe a wide variety of vascular lesions. Hamartia (from the Greek "to sin") is defined as any developmental anomaly that involves several tissues. Albrecht introduced the term "hamartoma" to describe a proliferative anomaly of developmental origin that also produces a tumor-like swelling.[1] The term "hamartoma" alone is too comprehensive. It may be applied to any lesion that histologically shows a nonmalignant proliferation of cells which are normally present in a tissue. The term "hemangioma" is too specific and has been confused in the literature by combining it with terms like "strawberry," "capillary," "cavernous," "cellular," "juvenile," and "capillary-cavernous." The most common cutaneous tumor seen in a pediatric practice is the congenital vascular hamartoma. Each congenital lesion has a slightly different clinical course and prognosis. The parents and the physician must appreciate the natural history of each tumor in order to form a treatment plan. The term "congenital vascular hamartomas" would seem appropriate and specific to describe the entire family of congenital vascular anomalies.

Classification

This classification of congenital vascular hamartomas is based on the primary involvement of the afferent vs. the efferent sides of the fetal vascular tree. A correlation can be made with the postnatal growth potential of these vascular lesions. The prognosis of the vascular hamartomas and the possible treatment available for these lesions can also be based on this classification:[5]

I. Growing (afferent) with potential for involution ("Hemangiomas" of infancy)
II. Stationary or slowly enlarging (efferent)
  A. Venous
    Port-wine stain
    Verruca linearis
    Cirsoid (racemose)
  B. Lymphatic
    Lymphangioma
    Hygroma
  C. Mixed
    With regional giantism
    Without regional giantism
III. Progressively growing (afferent-efferent)
  A. Congenital arteriovenous fistula
  B. Arterial hemangioma
  C. Angiosarcoma

A vascular hamartoma may grow rapidly, slowly, or not at all. The lesions that grow most rapidly also have the greatest potential for spontaneous involution. These prognostic growth characteristics appear to be correlated with the particular anatomical part of the vascular tree from which they develop.

The treatment goals include the avoidance of cardiac enlargement or hemodynamic instability; the arrest of abnormal growth; the prevention of ulceration, infection, and scarring; the prevention of edema or ischemic necrosis; and the prevention or correction of deformity as soon as possible.

If the anomaly affects primarily the afferent capillary bed, the hamartoma has the characteristics of the typical hemangioma of infancy (Fig 149–1). This type of hemangioma is usually not present at birth. It frequently occurs within several weeks after birth. It is usually bright red, raised, and grows rapidly. The growth of the hemangioma is frequently more rapid than that of the child for several months. A plateau may be reached in which the growth parallels that of the infant. The head and neck region is a frequent location (65%) for the lesions, which may be single or multiple, small and innocent, or large and ulcerated. Spontaneous involution can be expected in virtually all of these "afferent limb" hemangiomas. The involution may, however, be incomplete and take many years to occur. The first sign of regression is usually the evidence of central gray spots. The spots then gradually coalesce and reduce the area of the raised red hemangioma. Trauma to the lesions may cause bleeding, usually

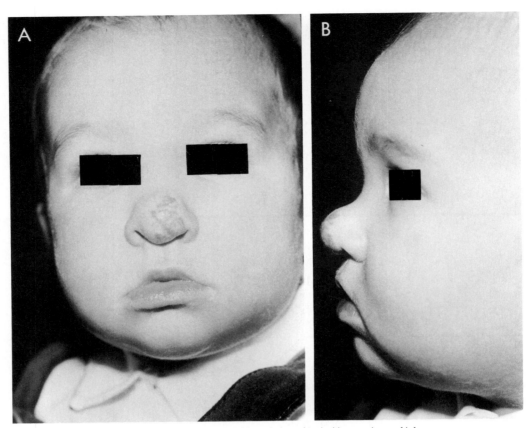

Fig 149–1.—**A** and **B,** anterior and lateral view of typical hemangioma of infancy. The lesion on the nasal tip became apparent during the second week of life.

easily controlled with local pressure. The vast majority (greater than 80%) of these hemangiomas of infancy may be induced to undergo premature involution by the use of systemic steroid therapy.

If the vascular hamartoma involves primarily the efferent limb of the vascular tree (efferent capillaries, veins, or lymphatics), it will be present and clinically visible at birth 90% of the time. These efferent lesions grow slowly, or not at all, do not spontaneously involute, and do not respond to steroid therapy.[6] They are similarly unresponsive to radiation therapy.[9]

The "efferent limb" vascular hamartomas include venous, lymphatic, and mixed lesions. Clinical conditions included in this group are port-wine stains (Fig 149–2), cirsoid venous angiomas, hygromas, and noncystic lymphangiomas. They may progressively enlarge or remain the same size. Efferent hamartomas are usually distributed along the patterns of cutaneous sensory nerves. This neurogenic influence is much less evident in the anatomical distribution patterns of afferent hamartomas, or of those involving both afferent and efferent limbs of the vascular tree.

The port-wine stain (nevus flammeus) usually is present at birth and is located primarily on the face in the areas supplied by the sensory branches of the fifth cranial nerve. It may also occur on an extremity. The lesion has no tendency for spontaneous regression. It usually becomes darker with age, and verrucous eruptions may occur in adulthood. Sturge-Weber syndrome may be, rarely, associated with the port-wine stain. Early clinical manifestations may be present secondary to the intracranial involvement of the pia mater and choroid with the hemangioma. The areas innervated by the ophthalmic and maxillary divisions of the fifth nerve are those most frequently affected with this syndrome. Epileptic seizures may be the presenting symptom. Glaucoma may also be an associated ipsilateral anomaly, especially with those port-wine stains that involve both the ophthalmic and maxillary divisions on the same side. In these situations, an early ophthalmology consultation should be obtained.

Verruca linearis hemangiomas occur much less frequently than the typical hemangiomas of infancy. These lesions are purplish-red, warty, irregular patches that occur superficially in the dermis and may be isolated or diffuse. Frequent small hemorrhages are common. Deeper dermal involvement is possible, and regional giantism may be associated.

When hamartomas involve both venous and lymphatic elements, they may be associated with regional giantism of the affected part. If giantism is present, as in Maffucci syndrome, the enlarged part will usually reflect the pattern of the regional sensory nerve distribution.[14] At times, a plexiform neurofibroma may be found in the tissues affected with giantism.[7] These lesions overlap with that group of hamartomas seen in patients with neurofibromatosis (von Recklinghausen's disease). This group of vascular-neural hamartomas carries a significant risk of malignant degeneration.

A third group of vascular hamartomas arises from *both* afferent and efferent limbs of the vascular tree. Congenital arterial hemangiomas and arteriovenous fistulae (Fig 149–3) are included. Congenital arterial hemangiomas are believed by some to represent "microshunting" arteriovenous fistulae with communica-

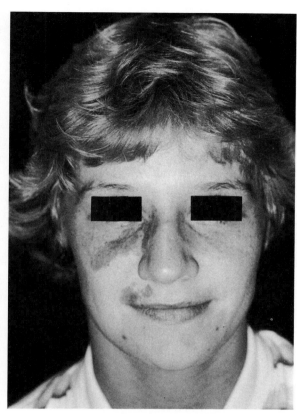

Fig 149–2.—Port-wine stain type of efferent limb vascular hamartoma present in the maxillary division area of the trigeminal distribution in this teenage girl.

tions too small to be seen on conventional arteriograms. Their natural history is, in fact, very similar to that of arteriovenous malformations. They are not present at birth, but may grow rapidly, once they appear. Growth may begin suddenly in the child or adult, or during pregnancy. The patient with a true macroshunting congenital arteriovenous malformation has a potentially lethal surgical problem. More than half of these lesions involve the head and neck region. A bruit is a constant physical finding in the macroshunting lesion. Angiosarcomas are highly malignant vascular hamartomas and are also included in this major group. These lesions are unresponsive to steroid therapy and radiation. Gross deformity, pain, bleeding, infection, and even cardiac failure and death may result from these lesions.

Many differences separate the three major groups of congenital vascular hamartomas. Both clinical and endothelial characteristics can be used to differentiate the "afferent," "efferent," and "afferent-efferent" groups. The recent work of Mulliken and Glowacki[13] would support our concept of the origin of these lesions.

Table 149–1 summarizes the clinical and laboratory features we use to diagnose and delineate these lesions.

Treatment

Early accurate diagnosis is critical for effective treatment of the patient with a congenital vascular hamartoma. The pediatrician or primary care physician should consult a plastic surgeon or pediatric surgeon early, so that they may work together with the family and the child. Pediatricians may often not have had clinical experience with the more unusual types of hamartomas. Appreciable deformity can result if "watchful waiting" is employed

with a rapidly expanding lesion that is not destined to undergo spontaneous involution. In such circumstances, "conservative" treatment may be damaging to the child.

Several modes of treatment are ineffective or even dangerous and should not be used. These include electrocautery, cryotherapy, and dermabrasion. Radiation therapy should not be used to treat any form of hemangioma. Fosh and Esterly[8] have reported, secondary to radiation, damage to epiphyses, breasts, gonads, skin, lens, and thyroid; and in a large series, it yielded no better results than were achieved in untreated controls. They also noted that the complications were ten times those in untreated patients. Li[11] et al. have also reported deaths from lymphosarcoma and testicular teratoma secondary to small doses of radiation of hemangiomas during infancy.

Steroid Therapy

Systemic steroid therapy has proved to be an effective treatment method for many vascular hamartomas.[4, 8, 16] Steroid therapy in the form of prednisolone has continued to be highly effective in causing premature involution of growing afferent hemangiomas of infancy. Initially, a daily dose of 20 mg for a 15-lb (6.8 kg) infant was given orally for 10 days. The dose was then cut in half each succeeding 10-day period, until 2.5 mg was reached. Although this usually produced a satisfactory result, the dosage schedule has been altered in recent years. In order to minimize the potential systemic effects of the steroids, an alternate day regimen has been adopted. The initial dose for a healthy newborn child is now 40 mg every other day for 20 days (ten doses). The dose is subsequently reduced 20 mg, 10 mg, 5 mg, and, finally, 2.5 mg. Each lower dose is given every other day for 20-day periods each.

When the steroid dose is reduced to the 10-mg level, about 30% of the hemangiomas that are initially responsive may display some rebound growth. When this occurs, the dose is elevated to the 20-mg level for an additional 20-day (ten-dose) course. Rarely, two or three full treatment courses may be needed for optimum effect. It is clear that hemangiomas of children under 6 months of age are substantially more responsive to steroids than those in children who are over 18 months of age. An early decision to use prednisolone is thus important for the best response. Fortunately, the effectiveness of steroid therapy is greatest in precisely those children who most need help, that is, in those with large, rapidly growing hemangiomas of the head and neck that spread to involve the major facial features. Steroids are less effective with smaller, circumscribed, monolocular cystic hemangiomas (Fig 149–4). For these lesions, observation or surgical excision is recommended.

In the majority of instances, effective steroid therapy may bring about sufficient involution that no surgery is required. In a smaller percentage (approximately 35%), common sense will dictate the need for a surgical procedure. This includes (1) patients who respond poorly or not at all to adequate doses of prednisolone, either because of the age of the patient or the presence within the tumor of significant numbers of microscopic arteriovenous shunts. Indeed, the failure to respond is suggestive of the presence of such shunting, even in the absence of a clinically detectable thrill or bruit. (2) Other lesions that are very bulky will regress and then stabilize, leaving a core of large vascular spaces that, on biopsy, turn out to contain much adult-type endothelium. Such patients may be greatly helped by surgery to remove the "core" portion of these vascular sinuses. (3) Patients who have had ulceration either before or during the period of steroid therapy may be left with sufficient scarring or contracture so that removal of the scars may be reasonably accompanied by further reduction in the bulk of deep tumor. Such procedures

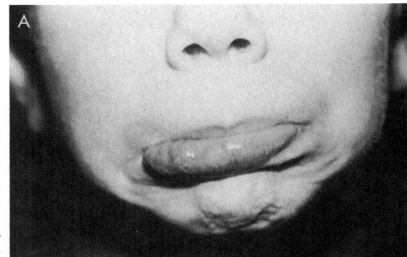

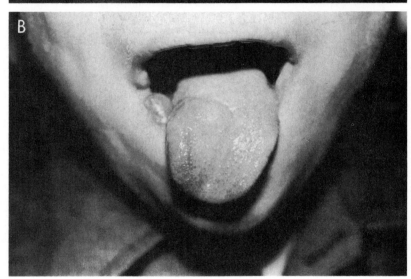

Fig 149–3.—A and B, congenital arteriovenous malformations, which began to expand rapidly in this 7-year-old boy. They are seen here on the right lower lip and right tongue. Four years after resection, this child has had no recurrence of the arteriovenous malformation. However, local recurrence is common in such tumors, and the families and patients should always be so advised. Females should be cautioned that any future pregnancy may rapidly reactivate the arteriovenous shunting.

often seem to further accelerate late involution of adjacent hemangioma. (4) The following may be appropriate indications for follow-up operations after effective steroid treatment: the aesthetic deformity of a residual facial hemangioma; the functional handicap imposed by remaining tumor, such as those on the free borders of the lips; or the simple liability to injury in certain locations, such as tumors on the tops of the shoulders. The timing for such surgical efforts, of course, will be individualized, depending on the particular problem presented. It is often advisable that the treatment be completed, when possible, before the child enters public school.

Complications associated with the use of steroids have been very limited. Because prednisolone is a glucocorticoid, potential side effects in children were carefully considered. Information was gained from the long-term use of large doses of steroids in the treatment of children with chronic diseases such as nephrosis, as well as from those involved in organ transplantation programs. Only occasional and temporary facial edema has been observed. There appears to be no experimental or clinical suggestion that permanent growth suppression develops in patients treated with this type of large-dose, short-term course of ste-

roids. Alternate-day therapy appears to minimize cushingoid effects, preserve hypophyseal activity, and facilitate the ultimate withdrawal from steroid therapy. Dluhy et al.[3] have reported that alternate-day therapy tends to be followed by normal growth patterns in children. The preservation of facial features or vision in a child with a large, fast-growing facial hemangioma certainly justifies the careful use of high-dose steroids. Small-dose steroid therapy has had no effect in bringing about early resolution of the hemangiomas. A response rate of over 80% has been observed in children under 1 year of age with growing hemangiomas. Steroids cannot be expected to improve lymphangiomas, venous anomalies, or arteriovenous fistulae.

Selective Embolization

Noninvoluting hemangiomas and arteriovenous malformations present difficult problems to the surgeon. Small hemangiomas may be simply excised to correct the deformity (Fig 149–5). Larger lesions may require more aggressive treatment. Embolism with an absorbable gelatin sponge (Gelfoam), silicone spheres, and other materials has been reported by many workers

TABLE 149–1.—Clinical-Histophysiologic Characteristics of Congenital Vascular Hamartomas*

I. GROWING-INVOLUTING HAMARTOMAS†	II. STATIONARY OR SLOWLY ENLARGING HAMARTOMAS‡	III. PROGRESSIVE VASCULAR HAMARTOMAS§
40% present at birth	90% recognizable at birth	Only 3% recognizable at birth
Bright red color-oxygenated blood	Colorless or *dark* red	Bright red color-skin temperature elevated
Female-to-male ratio, 5:1	Female-to-male ratio, 1:1	Female-to-male ratio, 4:1
Grow rapidly 1st year of life	Grow in relation to growth of child	Grow steadily or intermittently
High endothelial cell mitotic rates	Normal endothelial mitotic rates	Normal endothelial mitotic rates
Alkaline phosphatase activity as in all endothelium	Alkaline phosphatase activity in the abnormal endothelium	Alkaline phosphatase activity in the mature endothelium
Factor VIII antigen in proliferating and normal endothelium	Factor VIII antigen localized to abnormal endothelium	Factor VIII localization not known
Laminated subendothelial basement membranes	Single layer subendothelial basement membranes	Thrills and bruits often present
Active rough endoplasmic endothelial reticulum	Smooth endoplasmic endothelial reticulum	Venules and capillaries show "arterialization"
Fatty deposits and fibrosis during involution	No involuting phase occurs	No involution—pregnancy may enlarge
Increased thymidine incorporation with growth	Thymidine incorporation not elevated	Cardiac enlargement may result
Involution accelerated by prednisolone (80%)	No clinical response to prednisolone	No clinical response to prednisolone
Spontaneous involution may take years	Enlargement may reflect opening of occult vascular shunts	Enlargement may reflect opening of occult vascular shunts
Endothelial cells grow in tissue culture	Endothelial cells grow poorly in culture	Endothelial cells grow poorly in culture
Increased numbers of mast cells	Normal numbers of mast cells	Normal numbers of mast cells

*All show neurogenic distribution patterns.
†Involve afferent vessels.
‡Involve efferent vessels.
§Involve afferent-efferent communication.

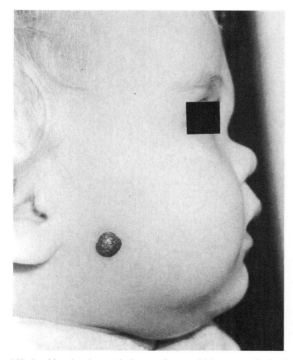

Fig 149–4.—Monolocular cystic hemangioma, which appeared shortly after birth. Such a lesion does not usually respond to steroids.

in their efforts to control the progression of arteriovenous fistulae.[10, 12, 15] Initial effects of such embolism are usually encouraging. However, the early response is usually followed in a few months by return of pulsations and further enlargement of the arteriovenous malformation.[4] Embolism alone is usually not adequate treatment. As an adjunctive procedure carried out 30 days before surgical resection, it may prove to be very helpful. Bleeding during operation is much easier to control if operation promptly follows embolism.

In the child with a large steroid-resistant hemangioma, or with an arteriovenous malformation, embolization and operation may afford a permanent cure. Superselective angiography may be performed with a trained radiologist and a surgeon in the angiography department, and then followed by operation a short time later.[10] Emboli of Gelfoam or polyvinyl alcohol foam (Ivalon) may be used. An operative approach may also be used to treat head and neck malformations. The external carotid artery is exposed and a small intracatheter cannula inserted deeply into each branch of the artery supplying the lesion. Gelfoam cubes (4 × 4 mm) are soaked in thrombin and placed in a tuberculin syringe. These emboli are packed hydrostatically into the artery until its lumen is filled back to the level of the arteriotomy. The artery is then sutured and ligated proximal to the arteriotomy. Each artery leading to the lesion is similarly embolized.[5] Simple ligation of the external carotid artery only encourages the lesion to be fed by surgically inaccessible collateral vessels and should not be performed.

Nonoperative embolism of the external carotid by radiographic techniques alone should be avoided. Severe hemiplegias and deaths have been reported as the catheters were withdrawn and emboli entered the internal carotid artery.

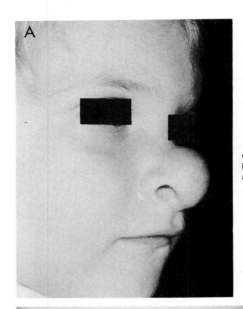

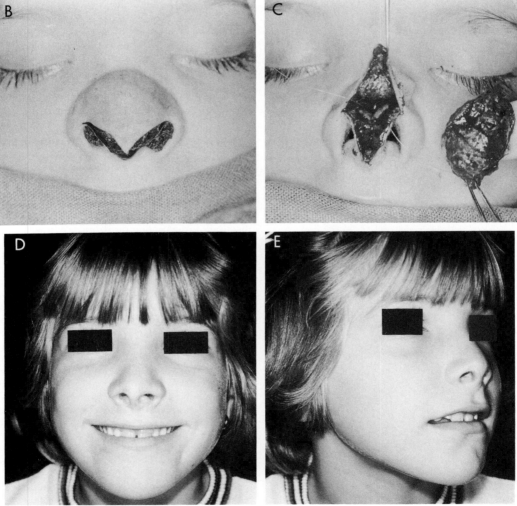

Fig 149–5.—Noninvoluting hemangioma of the nasal tip. **A,** lateral view, **B,** incisions designed to be hidden under the nasal rims. **C,** hemangioma excised. The normal lower lateral nasal cartilages are apparent. **D** and **E,** anterior and lateral view 1 year after excision.

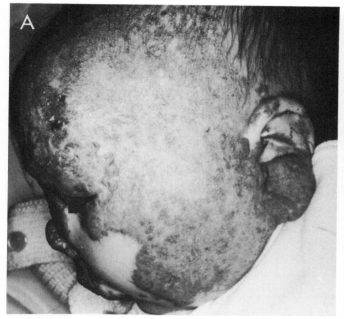

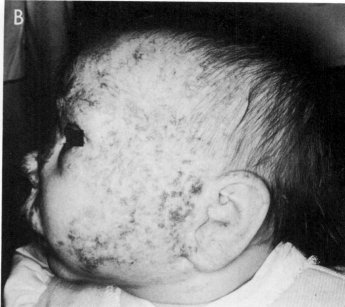

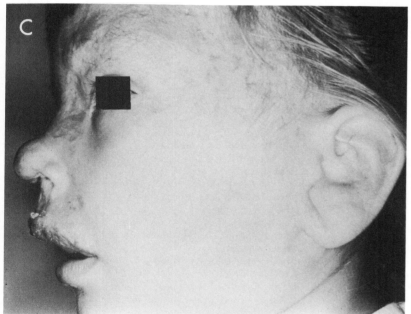

Fig 149–6.—A, the hemangioma seen in this child at 10 weeks of age was expanding so rapidly that it occluded the left nostril, eye, and external ear canal. **B,** a single course of steroids was used to hasten the involution of the hemangioma. At 15 weeks of age, the involution has proceeded, and the nostril, eye, and ear canal have opened. **C,** the involution continued until the age of 5 years.

Laser Therapy

The argon laser continues to interest surgeons for the treatment of vascular hamartomas. A beam of coherent light in the blue-green visible light range with a wave length of 5,000 A is emitted by the argon laser. The argon wavelength of light selectively damages pigmented cutaneous lesions with satisfactory healing of the laser wound and sparing of the overlying skin. The wavelength coincides with the maximum absorption of hemoglobin. The laser beam begins as visible light. It penetrates the intact dermis and is absorbed by the hemoglobin and converted to heat. This very localized beam causes selective coagulation without damaging adjacent skin appendages. Preliminary studies have shown the laser to be useful in the treatment of hemangiomas that do not involute completely or that warrant treatment prior to their involution phase.[2] It is also useful in treating the superficial port-wine hemangiomas. The principal drawback to the use of the laser continues to be the technical difficulties associated with the need to deliver a uniform dosage to the entire surface of the hemangioma. The pinpoint size of the laser beam has defied attempts to solve this limitation. It is of little or no value with hamartomas that lie below the skin dermis.

Summary

Early recognition and accurate diagnosis of the exact type of vascular hamartoma is critical. At the time of diagnosis, cooperation between the pediatrician, primary family physician, and surgeon proves most beneficial for the patient. Early high-dose, short-course steroid therapy has provided the best method for initiating early involution of afferent-type hemangiomas (Fig 149–6). Plastic surgery, with or without steroid therapy, is enormously helpful in reducing both morbidity and ultimate deformity for many types of hemangiomas and hamartomas.

REFERENCES

1. Albrecht E.: Die Grundprobleme der Geschwulstlehre: I. Teil. *Frank. Z. Pathol.* 1:221, 1907.
2. Apfelberg D.B., Greene R.A., Maser M.R., et al.: Results of argon laser exposure of capillary hemangiomas of infancy—preliminary report. *Plast. Reconstr. Surg.* 67:188, 1981.
3. Dluhy R.G., Lauler D.P., Thorn G.W.: Pharmacology and chemistry of adrenal glucocorticoids. *Med. Clin. North Am.* 57:1155, 1973.
4. Edgerton M.T.: Steroid therapy of hemangiomas, in Williams H.B.(ed.): *Symposium on Melanotic Lesions and Vascular Malformations.* St. Louis, C.V. Mosby Co., 1983.
5. Edgerton M.T.: Vascular hamartomas and hemangiomas: Classification and treatment. *South. Med. J.* 75:1541–1547, 1982.
6. Edgerton M.T., Hiebert J.M.: Vascular and lymphatic tumors in infancy, childhood and adulthood: Challenge of diagnosis and treatment. *Curr. Probl. Cancer* 2:2–44, 1978.
7. Edgerton M.T., Tuerk D.B.: Macrodactyly (digital giantism): Its nature and treatment, in Littler J.W., Cramer L.M., Smith J.W. (eds.): *Symposium on Reconstructive Hand Surgery.* St. Louis, C.V. Mosby Co., vol. 9, 1974.
8. Fosh N.C., Esterly N.B.: Successful treatment of juvenile hemangiomas with prednisone. *J. Pediatr.* 72:351, 1968.
9. Kolar J.: Radiation cancer following treatment for hemangioma. *Strahlentherapie* 117:147, 1962.
10. Leikensohn J.R., Epstein L.I., Vasconez L.O.: Superselective embolization and surgery of noninvoluting hemangiomas and A-V malformations. *Plast. Reconstr. Surg.* 68:143, 1981.
11. Li F.P., Cassady J.R., Barnett E.: Cancer mortality following irradiation in infancy for hemangioma. *Radiology* 113:177, 1974.
12. Luessenhop A.J.: Artificial embolization for cerebral arteriovenous malformations. *Prog. Neurol. Surg.* 3:320, 1969.
13. Mulliken J.B., Glowacki J.: Hemangiomas and vascular malformations in infants and children: A classification based on endothelial characteristics. *Plast. Reconstr. Surg.* 69:412, 1982.
14. Mullins J.F., Livingood C.S.: Maffucci's syndrome (dyschondroplasia with hemangiomas). *Arch. Dermatol.* 63:478, 1961.
15. Olcutt C., Newton T., Stoney R., et al.: Intra-arterial embolization in the management of arteriovenous malformations. *Surgery* 79:3, 1976.
16. Zarem H.A., Edgerton M.T.: Induced resolution of cavernous hemangiomas following prednisolone therapy. *Plast. Reconstr. Surg.* 39:76, 1967.

150 Bruce M. Smith

Venous Disease

VENOUS DISEASE in children encompasses congenital entities that produce significant illness or disability in childhood and, at a lower frequency, those acquired entities also recognized in adults.[43] These disorders can be categorized into congenital and acquired abnormalities of central veins, congenital and acquired abnormalities of peripheral veins, and the general category of thromboembolic disease, as follows:

Three paired embryonic subsystems contribute to the completed systemic venous circuit, which assumes its final configuration with division of the umbilical cord. *Anterior cardinal* (precardinal) veins become the superior vena cava and its tributaries, *posterior cardinal* (subcardinal and supracardinal) veins form the inferior vena cava and its tributaries, and the *vitelline veins* become the portal vein and its tributaries.

1. Congenital abnormalities of central veins
   A. Anomalies of the superior vena cava
      1. Duplication of the superior vena cava
      2. Left superior vena cava
      3. Anomalous systemic venous return to the heart
   B. Venous aneurysm
   C. Anomalies of the inferior vena cava
      1. Absence of the inferior vena cava
      2. Duplication of the inferior vena cava
      3. Left inferior vena cava
      4. Congenital obstruction of the inferior vena cava
   D. Portal vein anomalies
      1. Absence of the portal vein
      2. Preduodenal portal vein
      3. Congenital portosystemic connections
      4. Duplication of the portal vein

II. Acquired abnormalities of central veins
   A. Superior vena cava obstruction
   B. Inferior vena cava obstruction
   C. Renal vein thrombosis
III. Congenital abnormalities of the peripheral veins
   A. Varicose veins
   B. Absence of valves
   C. Familial thromboses—antithrombin III deficiency
   D. Congenital aplasia/hypoplasia of deep veins (Klippel-Trenaunay syndrome)
   E. Iliac compression syndrome
   F. Axillary vein obstruction
   G. Duplications and anomalies of course
IV. Acquired disorders of peripheral veins
   A. Effort thrombosis
   B. Catheter-related thrombophlebitis
   C. Spontaneous deep venous thrombosis
V. Pulmonary embolism

Congenital Anomalies of the Central Veins

Anomalies involving derivatives of the anterior cardinal system include *duplication of the superior vena cava, left superior vena cava,* and *anomalous systemic venous return of the heart.* Duplication of the superior vena cava with drainage of the left-sided element into the coronary sinus is of no clinical significance unless the child is to be placed on cardiopulmonary bypass for the not uncommonly associated congenital heart disease.[31, 39, 46] Left superior vena cava likewise is clinically silent in the absence of a requirement for cardiopulmonary bypass.[31] Anomalous systemic

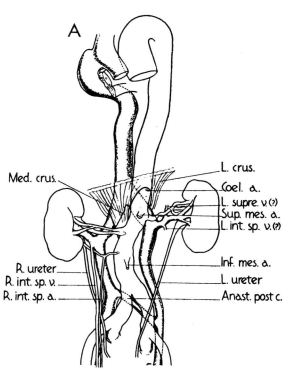

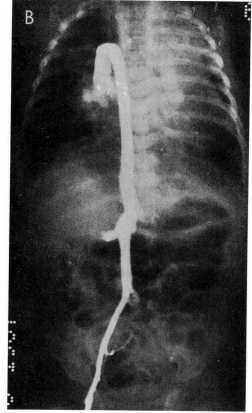

Fig 150–1.—Azygos continuation of inferior vena cava. **A,** schematic representation. (From *J. Pediatr.* 59:370, 1961. Used by permission.) **B,** inferior vena cavogram demonstrating interruption of the inferior vena cava at the level of the liver and drainage of the lower extremities via the azygos vein. (From Dean R.H., O'Neill J. (eds.): *Vascular Disorders of Childhood.* Philadelphia, Lea & Febiger, 1983. Used by permission.)

venous return to the heart, on the other hand, produces varying degrees of oxygen desaturation and may complicate management of children with other intracardiac anomalies.[22, 39, 46] The child's prognosis is often dependent on the severity of the associated anomalies, rather than on that of the anomalous venous return itself. An intracardiac baffle appears to be the most satisfactory way of returning the left atrial systemic blood to the right atrium (see Chaps. 140 and 141).

Congenital *venous aneurysms* have been described of the superior vena cava and jugular vein; and most, if not all, appear to have been asymptomatic. Rupture of these lesions is not a threat, and in the absence of symptoms, no treatment is necessary or desirable.[1, 15]

Abnormalities in course and union of the inferior vena cava are relatively common, perhaps present in 1–4% of the population.[12, 42] The majority of these present a threat only as a source of hemorrhage when injured by the incautious surgeon. Absence of the inferior vena cava (azygos continuation) is associated with the asplenia-polysplenia syndrome and congenital heart disease[9, 30] and may also present as an isolated anomaly.[2, 3] Confirmation of this anomaly is by its characteristic appearance on cavography (Fig 150–1).

Congenital obstruction of the inferior vena cava may occur secondary to a persistent eustachian valve in the right atrium[40] or from a suprahepatic web.[33, 47] While these lesions may remain asymptomatic for a variable period of time, symptoms of caval and hepatic vein obstruction eventually develop and cause the patient's death in young adulthood.[24] Successful treatment by ex-

cision of the web or cavocaval bypass has been reported.[5, 13, 25, 33]

Portal vein anomalies include absence, duplication, and malposition (preduodenal portal vein). The "absent" portal vein presumably results from failure of vitelline veins to communicate with the intrahepatic capillary plexus, resulting in a mesocaval or mesorenal connection.[6, 29] Duplication of the portal vein or a preduodenal portal vein (Fig 150–2) are hazards at the time of biliary or duodenal surgery, or liver transplantation.[26]

Acquired Abnormalities of the Central Veins

Superior vena cava obstruction in children is most frequently caused by thrombosis from indwelling catheters and pacemakers, although, as in adults, invasion or compression by malignant tumors or inflammatory nodes is also possible. In children, the full-blown picture of the superior vena cava syndrome may be absent, and its true incidence is therefore unknown. Emergency thrombectomy may be of use in rare cases, as, logically, would thrombolytic therapy. Improvement in the child's condition usually accompanies the appearance of venous collaterals, and symptoms of swelling and cyanosis may be helped by elevation of the head and anticoagulation. The long-term disability of this illness in children is unknown (see also Chap. 59).

Inferior vena caval thrombosis may propagate from the iliofemoral, renal, or hepatic veins. The cause of the primary process may be obscure, but is usually associated with severe concurrent illness or dehydration. The caval obstruction may present with dramatic symptoms, edema, cyanosis, ulceration,

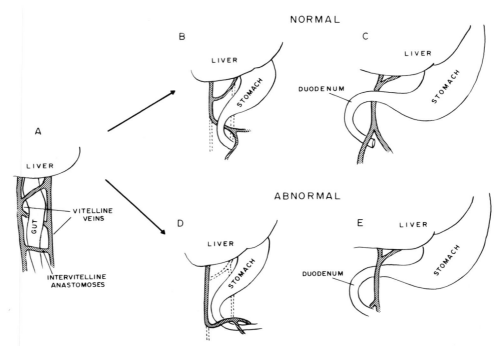

Fig 150–2.—Development of normally positioned and preduodenal portal vein. **A,** normal vitellovitelline anastomoses (4–6 week embryo). **B,** regression of vitelline and collateral veins (7-week embryo). **C,** evolution of normal retroduodenal portal veins. **D, E,** regression of the retroduodenal collaterals with development of the preduodenal portal vein. (Adapted from Marios D., VanHeerden J.A., Carpenter H.A. et al.: Congenital absence of the portal vein. *Mayo Clin. Proc.* 54:55, 1979. Used by permission.)

and priapism,[8] or may present only with lower extremity varicosities and collaterals. Inferior vena cavography is diagnostic (Fig 150–3). Fulminant acute cases should be treated with anticoagulants or, possibly, thrombolytic therapy. If the child survives, prognosis is largely of that of the underlying illness. Chronic venous insufficiency secondary to caval occlusion is managed with elevation, elastic stockings, and patient education. Varicose veins in this condition are important venous collaterals and should never be removed.

Renal vein thrombosis, like thrombosis of the inferior vena cava, almost always accompanies a severe, dehydrating illness, birth trauma, or anoxia, and is usually a primary process rather than extension of thrombus from the vena cava.[7, 11] The diagnosis should be suggested by proteinuria, hematuria, and unilateral or bilateral abdominal masses. Treatment and prognosis will depend on the severity of the renal involvement and the underlying disease process. If the child survives, return of renal function is the rule, although nephrectomy may be required for late hypertension or infection.[11] Heparinization should be employed to minimize propagation of thrombus and reduce the risk of pulmonary emboli (see also Chap. 120).

Congenital Anomalies of Peripheral Veins

The childhood presentation of *varicose veins* is rare, even though varicosities are thought to have a congenital predisposition. Adolescent members of families with a strong history of varicosities may demonstrate venous valvar incompetency,[4, 35] however, and children have been described with classic saphenous varicosities and chronic venous ulcers who were demonstrated to have absent valves in the femoral and iliac systems.[26]

Familial antithrombin III (AT III) deficiency predisposes to venous thrombosis in children and may produce a lifetime of morbidity from the sequelae of deep venous thrombosis and carry the threat of pulmonary embolism. The AT III deficiency is an autosomal dominant trait of variable penetrance, which results in a 25–50% deficiency in fibrinolytic activity in affected patients. Because AT III is identical with heparin cofactor, heparin alone is not maximally effective in treating thromboembolic episodes. Chronic or concurrent treatment with sodium warfarin (Coumadin) will lead to a striking increase in AT III levels and improve the efficacy of heparin anticoagulation.[20, 27]

Congenital aplasia or hypoplasia of the iliofemoral veins is found in approximately 20% of cases of the Klippel-Trenaunay syndrome (varicose veins, hemangioma, and extremity hypertrophy) (Fig 150–4).[16] This entity may be separated from the similar Parkes-Weber syndrome by the absence of arteriovenous fistulae on arteriograms. Resection of varices is not recommended in patients with aplasia or hypoplasia because of the danger of increasing the venous insufficiency. If venography demonstrates patent deep veins, vein stripping may be useful in permitting ulcers to heal and relieving symptoms. Most patients respond to compressive therapy. Venous bypass and repair have not been successful.[14, 30] The ultimate outlook, with ulcers, pain, edema, is unhappy.

Venous insufficiency in adolescence may be caused by the *iliac compression syndrome,* the compression of the iliac vein by the overlying iliac artery,[37] or by abnormal *intraluminal valves and bands.*[34, 36] These entities may present with acute venous thrombosis as well, often in settings that make spontaneous deep venous thrombosis more likely (pregnancy, surgery, bed rest) and that may mask the underlying congenital predisposition or render its existence debatable. It is likely, however, that this represents a true congenital anomaly.

Venous insufficiency or thrombosis of the upper extremity may be caused by thoracic outlet narrowing and subclavian vein compression[38] or by an anomalous axillopectoral muscle that compresses the axillary vein.[41, 45] Thoracic outlet decompression or simple excision of the constricting axillopectoral muscle has been curative in the few reported cases.

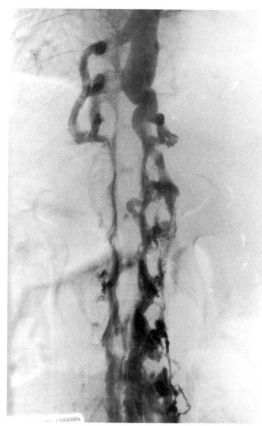

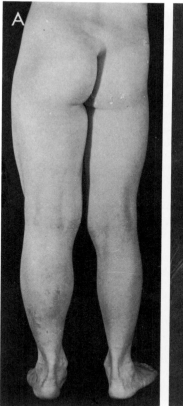

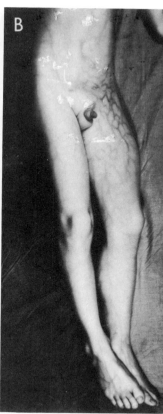

Fig 150–3.—Inferior vena cavogram demonstrating complete occlusion of the IVC with reconstitution by extensive retroperitoneal collaterals in a child with swelling of the leg. Bilateral saphenous vein cutdowns had been performed in infancy. (From Dean R.H., O'Neill J. (eds.): *Vascular Disorders of Childhood.* Philadelphia, Lea & Febiger, 1983. Used by permission.)

Fig 150–4.—**A,** hypertrophy of the left leg in an 8-year-old patient with Klippel-Trenaunay syndrome. The child complained of "heaviness" in the limb. **B,** infrared photograph of the patient at age 11 years, showing marked pattern of venous collateralization of the involved extremity. His symptoms had remained stable. (From Dean R.H., O'Neill J. (eds.): *Vascular Disorders of Childhood.* Philadelphia, Lea & Febiger, 1983. Used by permission.)

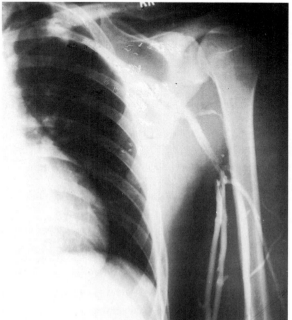

Fig 150–5.—Venogram demonstrating spontaneous thrombosis of basilic vein in an 18-year-old college student. He had noted mild pain, swelling, and cyanosis after vigorous weight-lifting. His symptoms rapidly resolved with anticoagulation and elevation. (From Dean R.H., O'Neill J. (eds.): *Vascular Disorders of Childhood.* Philadelphia; Lea & Febiger, 1983. Used by permission.)

Abnormalities in course and union of peripheral veins are common and of no clinical significance, although duplications of the greater or lesser saphenous systems may present in adulthood as recurrent superficial varicosities after apparently successful vein stripping.

Acquired Disorders of Peripheral Veins

Spontaneous "effort" thrombosis of the subclavian and brachial veins (Paget-Van Schrotter syndrome) usually occurs in the dominant arm of athletic males and is not uncommon in childhood or adolescence.[18, 45] The usual presentation is with swelling and pain in the arm associated with edema, cyanosis, and obvious venous collateralization. Venous Doppler examination and impedance plethysmography may suggest the diagnosis, which is confirmed by venography (Fig 150–5). Although conservative treatment in adults has been suggested to be associated with significant residual disability,[45] elevation of the arm and anticoagulation in younger patients have produced favorable results, especially when the involvement is of more peripheral veins. Thrombolytic therapy has not been reported in children with this problem.

Catheter-induced thrombophlebitis following peripheral or central venous cannulation is relatively common and may present either as unexplained fever when peripheral veins are involved, or as venous insufficiency with the thrombosis of more central veins. Percutaneously placed scalp vein or plastic catheters appear to produce thrombophlebitis less frequently than cannulae placed via cutdown. Treatment is the removal of the offending catheter and application of warm compressors. Antibiotics are generally *not* required, but may be indicated in infants with depressed immune competency.

Deep venous thrombosis in the lower extremity may also occur in the absence of trauma or intravenous cannulation, often in overweight children immobilized in casts[10, 28] or in the presence of malignancy or severe systemic illness.[17, 32] As in adults, silent deep venous thrombosis occurs with unknown frequency.

Pulmonary embolism in children may be more common than is recognized clinically and is often a secondary manifestation of congenital heart disease, systemic infection, dehydration, hydrocephalus, nephrotic syndrome, or burns. Symptoms may be falsely attributed to upper respiratory infections or pneumonia.[19] The deep veins of the legs and pelvis are less commonly a source of emboli than the dural sinuses, renal and hepatic veins, vena cava, jugular veins, pulmonary artery, and right heart.[21] The majority of cases appear to occur in children under the age of 1 year and are not temporally related to surgical procedures.[21, 44] Treatment of pulmonary embolism in children must be directed simultaneously at the primary disease process and the thromboembolic phenomenon.

REFERENCES

1. Abbott O.A.: Congenital aneurysm of the superior vena cava. *Ann. Surg.* 131(2):259, 1950.
2. Anderson R.C., Adams P. Jr., Burke B.: Anomalous inferior vena cava with azygos continuation. (Infra-hepatic interruption of the inferior vena cava): Report of 15 new cases. *J. Pediatr.* 59:370, 1961.
3. Anderson R.C., Heilig C.W., Novick R., et al.: Anomalous inferior vena cava. *Am. Heart. J.* 49:318, 1955.
4. Basmajian J.V.: The distribution of valves in the femoral, external iliac, and common iliac veins and their relationship to varicose veins. *Surg. Gynecol. Obstet.* 95:537, 1952.
5. Bennett I.L. Jr.: A unique case of obstruction of the inferior vena cava. *Bull. Johns Hopkins Hosp.* 87:290, 1950.
6. Braun P., Collin P.O., Ducharme J.C.: Preduodenal portal vein: A significant entity. Report of two cases and a review of the literature. *Can. J. Surg.* 17:316, 1974.
7. Bruns W.T.: Ascending thrombosis involving inferior vena cava and renal veins. *A. J. D. C.* 99:276, 1960.
8. Bunn W.H.: Report of a case of thrombosis of the inferior vena cava and extensive skin necrosis following scarlet fever. *Ohio State Med. J.* 29:485, 1933.
9. Campbell M., Deuchar D.C.: Absent inferior vena cava, symmetrical liver, splenic agenesis, and situs inversus and their embryology. *Br. Heart. J.* 29:268, 1967.
10. Coon W.W.: Epidemiology of venous thromboembolism. *Ann. Surg.* 186(2):149, 1977.
11. Duncan R.E., Evans A.T., Martin L.W.: Natural history and treatment of renal vein thrombosis in children. *J. Pediatr. Surg.* 12:639, 1977.
12. Effler D.B., Greer A.E., Sifers E.C.: Anomaly of the vena cava inferior: Report of fatality after ligation. *JAMA* 146:1321, 1951.
13. Eguchi S., Endo S., Yamaguchi A., et al.: Inferior caval occlusion associated with the Budd-Chiari Syndrome: Treatment with bypass operation. *J. Cardiovasc. Surg.* 7:490, 1966.
14. Foster J.H., Kirtley J.A.: Unilateral lower extremity hypertrophy. *Surg. Gynecol. Obstet.* 108:35, 1959.
15. Gallucci V., Sanger P.W., Robicsek F., et al.: Aneurysm of the superior caval vein. *Vasc. Surg.* 1:158, 1967.
16. Gloviczki P., Hollier L.H., Telander R.L.: Surgical implications of Klippel-Trenaunay Syndrome. *Ann. Surg.* 197(3):353, 1983.
17. Horwitz J., Shenker I.R.: Spontaneous deep vein thrombosis in adolescence: Clinical observations with 10 patients. *Clin. Pediatr.* 16(9):787, 1977.
18. Horwitz J., Schenker I.R.: Spontaneous deep vein thrombosis in adolescence. *Clin. Pediatr.* 16(9):787, 1977.
19. Joffe S.: Postoperative deep vein thrombosis in children. *J. Pediatr. Surg.* 10:539, 1975.
20. Jones D.R.B., MacIntyre I.M.C.: Venous thromboembolism in infancy and childhood. *Arch. Dis. Child.* 50:153, 1975.
21. Jones R.H., Sabiston D.C. Jr.: Pulmonary embolism in childhood. *Monogr. Surg. Sci.* 3:35, 1966.
22. Kabbani S., Feldman M., Angelini P.: Single left superior vena cava draining into the left atrium. *Ann. Thorac. Surg.* 16:518, 1973.
23. Kramer A.H., Cooperman A.M.: Thrombosis in a cavernous left-sided inferior vena cava. *Arch. Surg.* 111:1025, 1976.
24. Kimura C., Shirotani H., Hirooka M.: Membranous obliteration of the inferior vena cava in the hepatic portion. *J. Cardiovasc. Surg.* 4:87, 1963.
25. Kimura C., Shirotani H., Kuma M.: Transcardiac membranotomy for obliteration of the inferior vena cava in the hepatic portion. *J. Cardiovasc. Surg.* 3:393, 1962.
26. Lodin A., Lindvall N.: Congenital absence of valves in the deep veins of the leg: A factor in venous insufficiency. *Acta Dermatovener.* 41(suppl. 45): 1–83, 1961.
27. Marciniak E., Farley C.H., DeSimone P.A.: Familial thrombosis due to antithrombin III deficiency. *Blood* 43:219, 1974.
28. Marks C.: Developmental basis of the portal venous system. *Am. J. Surg.* 117:671, 1969.
29. Marois D., VanHeerden J.A., Carpenter H.A.: Congenital absence of the portal vein. *Mayo Clin. Proc.* 54:55, 1979.
30. May R.: Surgery of the veins of the leg and pelvis. *Major Problems in Clinical Surgery.* Philadelphia, W.B. Saunders Co., vol. 23, 1979.
31. Miller G., Inman T.W., Pollock B.E.: Persistent left superior vena cava. *Am. Heart J.* 49:267, 1955.
32. Nachbur B., Baumgartner G., Heuser H.J.: Deep thrombophlebitis of the lower extremities in children. *Vasa* 8:53, 1979.
33. Ohara I., Ouchi H., Takahashi K.: A bypass operation for occlusion of the hepatic inferior vena cava. *Surg. Gynecol. Obstet.* 117:151, 1963.
34. Peck M.E.: Obstructive anomalies of the iliac vein associated with growth shortening in the ipsilateral extremity. *Ann. Surg.* 146:619, 1956.
35. Plate G., Brudin L., Eklöf B.: Physiologic and therapeutic aspects in congenital vein valve aplasia of the lower limb. *Ann. Surg.* 198(2):229, 1983.
36. Raju S.: Venous insufficiency of the lower limb and stasis ulceration. *Ann. Surg.* 197(6):688, 1983.
37. Poulias G.E., Polemis L., Skoutas B., et al.: Acute venous occlusion within the scope of justified surgical aggresion (eight years experience with review of respective literature). *J. Cardiovasc. Surg.* 18:379, 1977.
38. Rob C., May G.: Neurovascular compression syndromes, in *Advances in Surgery.* Chicago, Year Book Medical Publishers, vol. 9, 1975.
39. Rojas R.H., Hipona A.: Anomalous systemic venous return. *J. Thorac. Surg.* 50:590, 1965.
40. Rossall R.E., Caldwell R.A.: Obstruction of inferior vena cava by a persistent Eustachian valve in a young adult. *J. Clin. Pathol.* 10:40, 1957.

41. Sachatello C.R.: The axillopectoral muscle (Langer's axillary arch): A cause of axillary vein obstruction. *Surgery* 81(5):610, 1977.

42. Sarma K.P.: Anomalous inferior vena cava—anatomical and clinical. *Br. J. Surg.* 53:600, 1966.

43. Smith B.M., Wolfe W.G.: Venous disease in childhoood, in Dean R.H., O'Neill J. (eds.): *Vascular Disorders of Childhood.* Philadelphia, Lea & Febiger, 1983, p. 120.

44. Stevenson G.F., Stevenson F.L.: Pulmonary embolism in childhood. *J. Pediatr.* 34:62, 1949.

45. Tilney N.L., Griffiths H.J.G., Edwards E.A.: Natural history of major venous thrombosis of the upper extremity. *Arch. Surg.* 101:792, 1970.

46. Viart P., LeClerc J.L., Pimo G.: Total anomalous systemic venous drainage. *A. J. D. C.* 131:195, 1977.

47. Watkins E., Fortin C.L.: Surgical correction of a congenital coarctation of the inferior vena cava. *Ann. Surg.* 159(4):536, 1964.

151 JAMES A. O'NEILL, JR.
Arterial Disorders

THE ARTERIAL TREE may be affected by connective tissue disorders; congenital malformations; acquired disorders including aneurysms, thrombosis, and embolism; and occlusive syndromes, most of which appear to be related to inflammatory or immunologic disorders. Individually, each of these entities is relatively unusual. Taken as a group, they affect large numbers of children, and treatment is challenging (Table 151–1).

Connective Tissue Disorders

In 1896, Marfan described an hereditary dominant disorder typified by a characteristic body habitus including a tall, slender frame, hyperextensibility of the joints with arachnodactyly, pectus carinatum, and dislocation of the lenses of the eye.[27] Sometime later, it was recognized that as these individuals got older they also had problems with inguinal hernias, spontaneous pneumothorax, and dissecting aneurysms of the ascending aorta. This vascular disorder is characterized by progressive degenerative changes that tend to reduce the lifespan of these individuals.[45] Marfan syndrome as it affects the vasculature would appear to produce cystic medial necrosis with intimal rupture and subsequent dissection within the vessel wall.

McKusick has summarized the similarities between Marfan syndrome and the Ehlers-Danlos syndrome, a hereditary disorder in which excessive elasticity and delicacy of the skin are associated.[30] The vascular malformations associated with the Ehlers-Danlos syndrome frequently lead to spontaneous rupture of arteries, because the collagen matrix of the vessel wall is defective. Suture and clamp occlusion of affected vessels may result in progressive disruption of the vessel wall, making operative management impossible in some instances. In the Ehlers-Danlos syndrome, aneurysms may develop in any artery, but progressive aneurysmal dilatation and rupture of the ascending or abdominal aorta or major branch vessels is usually fatal. Successful repair has been reported only very rarely. Fikar et al.[11] have collected a series of children with aortic aneurysms related to a variety of congenital degenerative disorders including Marfan syndrome, Ehlers-Danlos syndrome, familial cystic medial necrosis, Turner syndrome, and cystinosis. They point out that salvage of individuals with aneurysms related to these disorders depends upon prompt surgical correction once the aneurysm has been discovered and prior to the time of rupture.

Congenital Malformations

Arteriovenous Malformations (Fig 151–1)

Fortunately, most arteriovenous malformations are peripheral and localized. Szilagyi and co-workers[46] have classified arteriovenous malformations into microfistulous and macrofistulous types depending upon the degree of embryologic differentiation present. The microfistulous variety is difficult to demonstrate angiographically, and the symptoms and signs are less obvious, while the macrofistulous types are ordinarily easily demonstrable angiographically, and the clinical manifestations more obvious. Taken as a group, congenital arteriovenous malformations are relatively common, but the extensive life-threatening variety is rare. A review by Tice et al.[49] found that one half of congenital arteriovenous fistulae occur in the extremities, two thirds of those, in the lower limb. On the other hand, an arteriovenous malformation of the upper extremity is more likely to be physiologically active. Arteriovenous malformations may present as vascular nevi, hemangioma variants, or aneurysmal varices on an extremity, as originally described by Parkes-Weber[35] in 1907 when he reported the association of such malformations with hemihypertrophy of limbs. In the latter instance, limb overgrowth and microfistulous arteriovenous malformations are independent of one another. In other instances of isolated extremity arterio-

TABLE 1.—RECENT 3-YEAR INCIDENCE OF ARTERIAL DISORDERS AT CHILDREN'S HOSPITAL OF PHILADELPHIA

ARTERIAL DISORDER	NO. OF PATIENTS
Connective tissue disorders	
Aortic aneurysm (Marfan syndrome)	1
Congenital malformations	
Arteriovenous malformations	7
Renal artery aneurysm	2
Acquired disorders	
Coronary artery aneurysms	1
Thrombosis, spontaneous	4
Thrombosis caused by umbilical catheters	12
Mycotic aneurysms	5
Occlusive syndromes	
Intracranial arteries	0
Extracranial arteries	1
Midaortic syndrome	6
Peripheral arteries	9

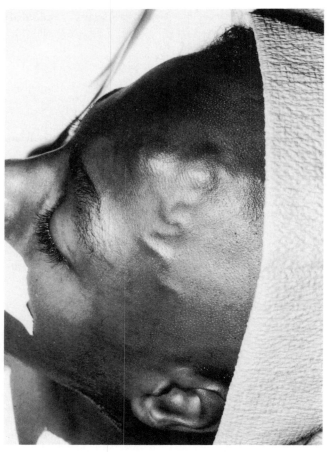

Fig 151–1.—Arteriovenous malformation of the scalp in a 12-year-old girl. In this instance, it was possible to excise completely the progressively enlarging vessels.

venous fistula, late overgrowth of the affected part is presumed to be the result of increased blood flow, and the increased core temperature would appear to lead to increased epiphyseal growth. Arteriovenous malformations may also be encountered in other parts of the body such as the head and neck, the gut, the liver, the lung, and the CNS.

The most frequent signs and symptoms related to arteriovenous malformations are skin disfigurement, limb swelling, and pain. Varicose veins associated with pulsation, skin ulceration, and bleeding, as well as overgrowth of the affected adjacent bones, are commonly seen in extremity lesions. The signs and symptoms related to arteriovenous malformations in other areas of the body are related to a number of factors. In the gut, bleeding is the most common manifestation, and lesions are frequently multiple. In the liver, congestive heart failure from a massive shunt is common, particularly in the newborn. Lung lesions may either be asymptomatic or associated with infectious complications. Arteriovenous malformations of the CNS produce symptoms by compression of associated vital structures or by intracranial hemorrhage.

Knudsen and Alden[25] recently described a variety of symptomatic arteriovenous malformations in infants less than 6 months of age and stressed the common occurrence of high-output congestive heart failure, often refractory to therapy.

The diagnosis of arteriovenous malformations is often clearly evident on physical examination—increased warmth of the part associated with pulsating varicosities under or within the skin.

Occasionally, major deep arteriovenous malformations will be associated with unimpressive small hemangiomatous skin lesions. Examination with the Doppler will ordinarily reveal a continuous signal characteristic of a macrofistulous communication. The classic angiographic features of congenital arteriovenous malformations are arterial dilatation and tortuosity, demonstration of arteriovenous connections, puddling of dye in arteriole-venule channels, early venous filling, and associated dilatation of venous channels. These classic findings are not present in all cases by any means; and in the report by Szilagyi and co-workers,[46] angiographic demonstration of the arteriovenous communication itself was made in only 60% of the patients. There was early venous filling in 68%, venous dilatation in 56%, arterial dilatation in 40%, and arterial tortuosity in 26%.[46] In patients with diffuse microfistulous malformations, skin and muscle blood flow determinations may need to be performed to establish a diagnosis; in other instances, comparative venous blood oxygen saturations from the affected and unaffected limbs may establish the existence of an arteriovenous shunt.

The approach to management of congenital arteriovenous fistulas depends upon the extent of the lesion, its location, whether or not there are associated physiologic derangements, and the expected prognosis.[8, 36] While a cure can only be obtained by total resection of the entire malformation, that is not always possible, and at times periodic surgical interventions are necessary in order to minimize intercurrent problems that limit the patient's life-style. At times, the disability that would be associated with total resection of an arteriovenous malformation outweighs the advantage that would be gained from it.

A large number of the arteriovenous malformations of the extremities can be treated nonoperatively with compression garments. It is of interest that in the series of Szilagyi and co-workers,[46] patients had better long-term follow-up results with nonoperative compression therapy of extremity lesions than with operative therapy.

There is a place for operative treatment in the management of arteriovenous malformations, however, particularly when lesions are so located that they can be completely excised without interfering with normal function. Partial excision may be indicated for the management of painful skin erosions and bleeding, as pointed out by Malan.[26] However, considering the usual diffuse nature of arteriovenous malformations in the extremity and elsewhere, aggressive removal of feeding vessels and ligation of multiple fistulous connections are likely to be of only temporary value and buy time while painful skin ulcerations heal and bleeding is controlled. Glovizcki et al.[15] show this very well in the series of patients with the Klippel-Trenaunay syndrome followed a number of years at the Mayo Clinic. Such operative therapy must always be followed by rigorous compression garment support. At other times, surgical therapy must be directed at altering limb growth as described by McCullough and Kenwright[29] in their study of prognosis in congenital lower limb hypertrophy. In some parts of the body, adjunctive compression dressings cannot be utilized, as in extensive arteriovenous fistulae of the head and neck, where a holding action is the best one can hope to achieve. In some instances, additional help can be obtained by means of angiographic embolism of extensive peripheral lesions.[22] An infant in our series, with a large pelvic arteriovenous malformation associated with congestive heart failure, was returned to an asymptomatic state by use of an embolization technique with coiled wire. She remains asymptomatic 3 years later. The majority of patients with congenital arteriovenous malformations will require multiple forms of therapy over a long period of time in the hope of maintaining adequate function. Occasional patients will require amputation, but generally that should be a last resort.

Visceral Artery Aneurysms

Congenital aneurysms of various visceral arteries occur rarely and in most instances are discovered incidentally. Rupture of such aneurysms is even more unusual, although hypertension is common when renal artery branches are involved, because of compression of adjacent renal arterial branches. Rare reports, such as the one by Schiller et al.,[37] describe multiple visceral aneurysms in the same patients, all of which must be managed by resection and primary repair or grafting. Histologic examination of such aneurysms usually demonstrates only ectasia related to medial dysplasia with no further indication of cause. As pointed out by Boijsen and Efsing,[4] the most common site of what is presumed to be congenital aneurysm is the splenic artery. Because these aneurysms are so uncommon and because rupture has rarely been reported, the indications for operative management are obscure. Generally speaking, repair is indicated for patients with aneurysms larger than 2 cm in diameter and that appear to be enlarging. There are no reports of splenic artery aneurysms in young children; they seem not to become evident until young adulthood, particularly in females of childbearing age. Aneurysms of the renal artery associated with hypertension require repair by excision and revascularization, while those of the splenic artery may simply be resected, preserving the spleen on its blood supply from the short gastric vessels. We have seen two renal artery aneurysms in children.

Acquired Disorders

Aneurysms

Kawasaki syndrome may produce single or multiple coronary artery aneurysms.[1, 18, 24] These are best diagnosed by echocardiography followed by coronary artery angiography. Kawasaki syndrome is a disorder of unknown cause, presumed to be caused either by a microorganism or some sort of environmental toxin. Host, environmental, and other factors may also be important, because Kawasaki syndrome does not seem to be transmissible from person to person, or related to a common source of exposure. Initially referred to as the mucocutaneous lymph node syndrome, Kawasaki disease is characterized by rash, erythema of the palms and soles, edema of the hands and feet, fissured lips, an injected pharynx, bilateral conjunctivitis, cervical lymphadenopathy, and arthritis. Approximately 14% of patients may develop coronary artery aneurysms, but up to a fourth of patients will have ECG abnormalities. The manifestations in children do not differ from those in young adults except for the frequency of hydrops of the gallbladder in affected children.

Thrombosis and Embolism

Occasional patients, primarily infants, develop spontaneous arterial thromboses (Fig 151–2).[17] The external iliac and various visceral arteries are the ones most commonly involved.[5] The infant, with a relatively small vascular volume, is particularly at risk when septic and subject to low-flow states. Newborn infants are relatively polycythemic and hyperviscous and, because of this, some infants, such as those of diabetic mothers, may demonstrate a severe hyperviscosity syndrome associated with various visceral artery or even major aortic tributary thromboses.[34] The management of infants with these complications may require plasmapheresis or even exchange transfusion in addition to vascular repair or thrombectomy. Infants such as this should also be treated with heparin.[34] The most common presentation of infants with visceral arterial thrombosis related to polycythemia is segmental intestinal necrosis. Thromboses related to low-flow states and sepsis tend to produce skin necrosis of the distal portions of extremities. In selected instances, intra-arterial infusion of streptokinase or urokinase might be in order if there is not excessive risk related to associated derangements of coagulation, which might predispose such infants to intracranial hemorrhage. We have not employed such enzyme therapy. Clotting disorders associated with thrombosis and embolism occur in sickle-cell disease, leukemia, bacterial endocarditis, and other disease states. The majority of these do not require operative intervention.[33, 43, 51] However, patients with bacterial endocarditis caused by *Staphylococcus aureus* are particularly at risk of embolic complications. We have treated five patients with staphylococcal endocarditis of the aortic or mitral valve who developed ruptured aneurysms of the aorta or iliac vessels, all of whom required staged repair (Fig 151–3). The majority of patients who have peripheral emboli from bacterial endocarditis caused by other organisms will usually require only embolectomy. The most common site of major peripheral embolism is usually the femoral artery, but occlusions of all major branch vessels have been reported. Patients with bacterial endocarditis should be followed with echocardiography. If a valvar vegetation is found to have disappeared, careful search is made for clinical evidence of re-

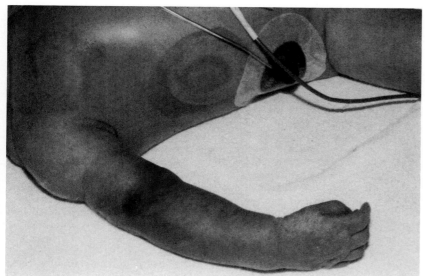

Fig 151–2.—Spontaneous thrombosis of subclavian artery. This newborn presented with obviously compromised circulation to the right arm. A cineangiogram demonstrated thrombosis of the right subclavian artery. The infant was polycythemic. The arm remained viable. A mild skin slough on the medial aspect of the arm required a small skin graft.

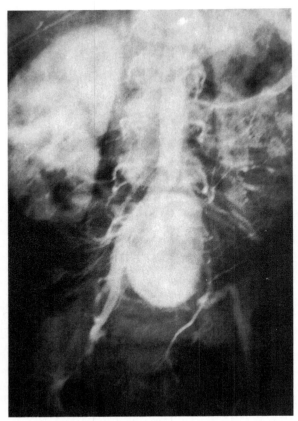

Fig 151–3.—Mycotic aneurysm of the aortoiliac region of the aorta in a 5-year-old boy with bacterial endocarditis on a diseased mitral valve. The aneurysm seen in the aortogram was resected, and later staged prosthetic repair successfully performed.

sultant embolism. Infected emboli should be extracted early in order to avoid vascular degeneration and aneurysm formation. Once an infected aneurysm is recognized it must be treated either by excision with staged repair or excision and extra-anatomical bypass.

It is not rare for patients to develop thrombotic or embolic complications related to umbilical artery catheters. Our group reported a series of 41 patients who sustained such complications, including one patient who developed an infected aneurysm of the aorta, four who developed aortoiliac thrombosis, and the remainder with embolic occlusion of extremity and visceral vessels.[7, 12, 34, 41, 42, 48] Thrombectomy is indicated whenever the aorta or a major tributary is occluded and the viability of a part threatened. There may be a place for streptokinase infusion and heparinization in cases such as this as well.

Occlusive Syndromes

Intracranial Arteries

A variety of causes of stroke have been reported in childhood, although the problem is rare. Such disorders as sickle-cell disease, neurofibromatosis, congenital heart disease, and arteritis of unknown cause have been mentioned most frequently.[14, 43] Moyamoya disease, described in the Japanese literature, probably includes a number of disorders that result in the production of multiple stenoses in the intracranial arteries.[21, 33, 44] The term moyamoya, a Japanese word descriptive of the angiographic pattern of the cerebral vasculature in children with this condition,

literally translated means something hazy, like a puff of cigarette smoke drifting in the air. The disorder produces major strokes, but may be alleviated by superficial temporal to middle cerebral artery anastomosis, provided the lesions involve the proximal middle cerebral or internal carotid artery within the cranium.[10]

Extracranial Arteries

In 1908, Takayasu[47] described a patient with occlusion of the branch vessels of the aorta associated with peculiar changes of the central retinal vessels. As with so-called moyamoya disease, Takayasu syndrome is progressive, as shown by Ishikawa,[21] Martorell and Fabre,[28] and others. While revascularization procedures are successful in some instances of Takayasu's disease, the long-term outlook is unfavorable in most instances as the disease continues to progress. Ordinarily, Takayasu's disease involves primarily the vessels of the aortic arch, but many patients have progressive occlusion of abdominal visceral vessels, particularly the renal arteries, and in other branches of the abdominal aorta as shown by Schire and Asherson.[38] The disorder is related to an inflammatory process in the vessel wall with fibrous dysplasia. The disorder is of unknown cause, and there is no known therapy to arrest the problem although a number of drugs have been tried. Kalkarni and co-workers[23] reported the successful use of steroids in a patient with Takayasu's disease associated with abdominal aortic narrowing and renovascular hypertension. However, it is difficult to determine whether the steroids were really helpful or whether this was the natural course of the disease. We recently treated a similar patient with active aortitis and narrowing of the midaorta associated with renovascular hypertension and a high erythrocyte sedimentation rate. In this instance, steroids did not produce remission.

Midaortic Syndrome (Fig 151–4)

While patients in Japan and other Oriental countries tend to have Takayasu's disease with progressive occlusion of the branch vessels of the thoracic aorta, followed by abdominal and visceral arterial occlusion, Caucasian patients more commonly have occlusion of the abdominal aorta alone, also called subisthmic aortic coarctation.[31, 39] Undoubtedly, some cases are congenital, related to developmental arrest of vessel formation or possibly anomalous hypertrophy of the media.[51] In such instances, the subrenal aorta is ordinarily only a fibrous strand. Depending upon the degree of narrowing, ranging from partial narrowing to complete occlusion, symptoms may become evident any time during infancy or childhood. Hypertension is commonly associated whether or not the renal vessels are involved.

Much more commonly, however, the midaortic syndrome is acquired, as described by Wiest and co-workers,[50] Inada,[20] Sen et al.,[40] and Ben-Shoshan et al.[2] We have treated six such patients with an arteritis involving varying lengths of the midabdominal aorta, usually from the region of the renal vessels downward, but occasionally extending upward to involve the superior mesenteric or celiac axis origins. The disorder would appear to be inflammatory, possibly of immunologic or allergic origin. While other disorders such as neurofibromatosis have been associated with similar clinical pictures, no definite cause is evident in most cases.[3] Symptoms related to hypertension are ordinarily noted first; and, when the aortitis is in an active phase, the erythrocyte sedimentation rate is quite elevated. The active stage of aortitis lasted for a year or so in the majority of our patients. In one of our patients, progressive narrowing was observed over a 5-year period. Ben-Shoshan et al.,[2] Nennhaus and colleagues,[32] and Graham[16] have described various surgical approaches to the midaortic syndrome. In our hands, the most successful approach has been placement of a synthetic bypass graft

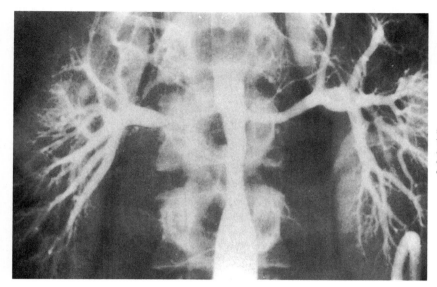

Fig 151–4.—Midaortic syndrome in a 13-year-old girl with severe hypertension. The aortogram is typical. She was treated by synthetic graft bypass from the upper abdominal aorta to the bifurcation and bilateral saphenous vein bypass to each renal artery, with complete relief of symptoms of claudication and hypertension.

from the upper abdominal or thoracic aorta to the level of the aortic bifurcation, followed by bypass grafting with saphenous vein from normal portions of the aorta, or from the synthetic bypass graft, to one or both critically narrowed renal arteries. If operation is performed when the disease is no longer acute, long-term relief of the occlusive manifestations of the disorder may be achieved. Patients must be followed for a lifetime, because reactivation can occur, as it did in one of the patients in our series.

Small Artery Disease

Hardy and co-workers[19] have summarized a large number of nonatherosclerotic occlusive lesions of small arteries, and many of these occur in childhood. Scleroderma, disseminated lupus erythematosus, dermatomyositis, and juvenile rheumatoid arthritis have all been reported associated with progressive occlusion of small arteries, particularly those of the distal fingers and toes.[51] Initially, the symptoms are primarily those of a vasoactive disorder typical of Reynaud's phenomenon. Later, an occlusive arteritis becomes evident, which produces atrophy of the tufts of the fingers and toes. If the disease burns out or can be arrested with anti-inflammatory drugs during the vasoactive phase of the arteritis, loss of the fingers and toes may be avoided. In selected instances, vasodilator drugs and sympathectomy as described by Dale and Lewis may be helpful.[9] Juvenile diabetics may present with a similar clinical picture, with occlusion of distal small arteries, but these patients do not often obtain relief from sympathectomy and in our experience usually must undergo amputation.

REFERENCES

1. Bell D.M., Morens D.M., Holman R.C., et al.: Kawasaki syndrome in the United States. *A.J.D.C.* 137:211, 1983.
2. Ben-Shoshan M., Rossi N.P., Karns M.E.: Coarctation of the abdominal aorta. *Arch. Pathol.* 95:221, 1978.
3. Bloor K., Williams R.T.: Neurofibromatosis and coarctation of the abdominal aorta with renal artery involvement. *Br. J. Surg.* 50:881, 1963.
4. Boijsen E., Efsing H.D.: Aneurysm of the splenic artery. *Acta Radiol. (Diagn.)* 8:29, 1969.
5. Braly B.D.: Neonatal arterial thrombosis and embolism. *J. Pediatr. Surg.* 58:869, 1965.
6. Campbell M.: Natural history of coarctation of the aorta. *Br. Heart J.* 32:633, 1970.
7. Colclough A.B., Barson A.J.: Infantile aortic aneurysm complicating umbilical arterial catheterization. *Arch. Dis. Child.* 56:795, 1981.
8. Coleman C.C.: Diagnosis and management of congenital arteriovenous fistulas of the head and neck. *Am. J. Surg.* 126:557, 1973.
9. Dale W.A., Lewis M.R.: Management of ischemia of the hand and fingers. *Surgery* 67:62, 1979.
10. Dean R.H.: Uncommon arteriopathies of childhood, in Dean R.H., O'Neill J.A.: *Vascular Disorders of Childhood.* Philadelphia, Lea Febiger, 1983, p. 98.
11. Fikar C.R., Armhein J.A., Harris J.P., et al.: Dissecting aortic aneurysm in childhood and adolescence: Case report and literature review. *Clin. Pediatr.* 20:578, 1981.
12. Fricker F.I., Park S.C., Neches W.H., et al.: Aneurysm of the aorta in children. *Chest* 76:305, 1979.
13. Frovig A.G., Loken A.C.: The syndrome of obliteration of the arterial branches of the aortic arch due to arteritis: Post-mortem angiographic and pathological study. *Acta Psychiatr. Neurol. Scand.* 26:313, 1951.
14. Galligioni F., Andrioli G.C., Marin G., et al.: Hypoplasia of the internal carotid artery associated with cerebral pseudoangiomatosis: Report of four cases. *Am. J. Roentgen. Rad. Ther. Nucl. Med.* 112:251, 1971.
15. Glovizcki P., Hollier L.H., Telander R.L., et al.: Surgical implications of Klippel-Trenaunay syndrome. *Ann. Surg.* 196:353, 1983.
16. Graham L.M.: Abdominal aortic coarctation and segmental hypoplasia. *Surgery* 86:519, 1979.
17. Gross R.E.: Arterial embolism and thrombosis in infancy. *A.J.D.C.* 70:61, 1945.
18. Harada K.: Acute febrile mucocutaneous lymph node syndrome with multiple aneurysms: Report of a case. *Pediatr. Cardiol.* 4:215, 1983.
19. Hardy J.D., Conn J.H., Fain W.R.: Nonatherosclerotic occlusive lesions of small arteries. *Surgery* 57:1, 1965.
20. Inada K.: Atypical coarctation of the aorta with special reference to its genesis. *Angiology* 16:608, 1965.
21. Ishikawa K.: Natural history and classification of occlusive thromboaortopathy (Takayasu's disease). *Circulation* 57:27, 1978.
22. Joyce P.F., Sundaran M., Riaz A., et al.: Embolization of extensive peripheral angiodysplasias. *Arch. Surg.* 115:665, 1980.
23. Kalkarni T.P., D'Cruz I.A., Gandhi M.J., et al.: Reversal of renovascular hypertension caused by nonspecific aortitis after corticosteroid therapy. *Br. Heart J.* 36:114, 1974.
24. Kitamura S.: Aortocoronary bypass grafting in a child with coronary artery obstruction due to mucocutaneous lymph node syndrome. *Circulation* 53:1035, 1976.
25. Knudsen R.P., Alden E.R.: Symptomatic arteriovenous malformations in infants less than 6 months of age. *Pediatrics* 64:238, 1979.
26. Malan E.: *Vascular Malformations.* Milan, Carlo Erba Foundation, 1974, p. 41.
27. Marfan B.A.J.: Un cas de déformation congénitale des quatre membres, plus prononcée aux extrémités, chactérisée par l'allongement des os avec un certain degré d'amincissement. *Bull. Mém. Soc. Méd. Hôp. Paris* 13:220, 1896.
28. Martorell F., Fabre J.: El sindrome de obliteracion de los troncos supra-aorticos. *Med. Clin.* 2:26, 1944.

29. McCullough C.J., Kenwright J.: The prognosis in congenital lower limb hypertrophy. *Acta Orthop. Scand.* 50:307, 1979.

30. McKusick V.A.: The Ehlers-Danlos syndrome, in *Hereditable Disorders of Connective Tissue*. St. Louis, C.V. Mosby Co., 1974, p. 292.

31. Milloy F., Gell E.H.: Elongate coarctation of the aorta. *Arch. Surg.* 78:759, 1959.

32. Nennhaus H.P., Havis H., Hunter J.A.: Surgical treatment of renovascular hypertension in children with a review of infradiaphragmatic arterial hypoplastic anomalies. *J. Thorac. Cardiovasc. Surg.* 54:246, 1967.

33. Numaguchi Y., Balsys R., Marc J.A., et al.: Some observations in progressive arterial occlusions in children and young adolescents: (moyamoya disease). *Surg. Neurol.* 6:293, 1976.

34. O'Neill J.A., Neblett W.W., Born M.L.: Management of major thromboembolic complications of umbilical artery catheters. *J. Pediatr. Surg.* 16:972, 1981.

35. Parkes-Weber F.: Angioma formation in connection with hypertrophy of limbs or hemi-hypertrophy. *Br. J. Dermatol.* 19:231, 1907.

36. Sako Y., Varco R.L.: Arteriovenous fistula: Results of management of congenital and acquired forms, blood flow measurements, and observations on proximal arterial degeneration. *Surgery* 67:40, 1970.

37. Schiller M., Gordon R., Shifrin E., et al.: Multiple arterial aneurysms. *J. Pediatr. Surg.* 18:27, 1983.

38. Schire V., Asherson R.H.: Arteritis of the aorta and its major branches. *Q. J. Med.* 33:439, 1964.

39. Schlessinger H.: Merkwurdige verschkiessung der aorta. *Wenscher Ges. Heilkund* 31:489, 1835.

40. Sen P.K., Kinare S.G., Engineer S.D., et al.: The middle aortic syndrome. *Br. Heart J.* 25:610, 1963.

41. Siegel M.J., McAlister W.H.: Aortic aneurysms in children. *Radiology* 132:615, 1979.

42. Spangler J.G., Kleinberg F., Fulton R.E., et al.: False aneurysm of the descending aorta. *A.J.D.C.* 131:1258, 1977.

43. Stockman J.A., Nigro M.A., Miskin M.M., et al.: Occlusion of large cerebral vessels in sickle-cell anemia. *N. Engl. J. Med.* 287:846, 1972.

44. Suzuki J., Takaku A.: Cerebrovascular "moyamoya" disease: Disease showing abnormal net-like vessels in base of brain. *Arch. Neurol.* 20:288, 1969.

45. Symbas P.N., Baldwin B.J., Silverman M.E., et al.: Marfan's syndrome with aneurysm of ascending aorta and aortic regurgitation. *Am. J. Cardiol.* 25:483, 1970.

46. Szilagyi D.E., Smith R.F., Elliott J.P., et al.: Congenital arteriovenous anomalies of the limbs. *Arch. Surg.* 111:423, 1976.

47. Takayasu M.: A case with peculiar changes of the central retinal vessels. *Acta Soc. Ophthal. Jap.* 12:554, 1908.

48. Thompson T.R., Tilleli J., Johnson D.E., et al.: Umbilical artery catheterization complicated by mycotic aortic aneurysm in neonates. *Adv. Pediatr.* 27:275, 1980.

49. Tice D.A., Clauss R.H., Keirle A.M., et al.: Congenital arteriovenous fistulae of the extremities. *Arch. Surg.* 86:460, 1963.

50. Wiest J.W., Traverso L.W., Dainko E.A., et al.: Atrophic coarctation of the abdominal aorta. *Ann. Surg.* 191:224, 1980.

51. Wood P.H.: *Diseases of the Heart and Circulation.* London, Eyre and Spottiswoode, 1956.

152
RICHARD H. DEAN

Renovascular Hypertension

ONE TO TWO PERCENT of children and up to 11% of adolescents have high blood pressure.[10] This frequency is similar to that of congenital heart disease; yet, although physicians routinely listen for murmurs and look for signs of congenital heart disease in children, they do not routinely measure blood pressure. Its recognition and management are important, because elevated pressures in vessels during the developmental years have deleterious effects on longevity. Unfortunately, because blood pressure is not routinely determined in early childhood, hypertension is usually severe by the time it is first detected; and it is a hypertensive crisis that leads to recognition of the condition. Because milder forms of hypertension are asymptomatic, the true incidence of hypertension during early childhood probably is underestimated. Nevertheless, even in instances of mild hypertension, a correctable cause must be sought.

Renovascular hypertension (RVH), second only to coarctation of the aorta as a cause of surgically correctable hypertension in children, has received sporadic attention in the literature over the past 30 years. Despite improved diagnostic methods and operative techniques, few medical centers are actively investigating the possibility of a renovascular origin of hypertension in children. Further, no universally accepted therapeutic guidelines are available to direct therapy once RVH is identified.

HISTORY.—A renovascular origin of hypertension was clearly demonstrated by Goldblatt[5] in 1934 in his classic experiment. He produced hypertension in the dog by creating renal artery stenosis with his ingenious clamp. After documenting that constriction of the renal artery caused hypertension, he enlightened the field of hypertension research further by showing that removal of the constricting clamp resulted in return of elevated pressures to normal. The first clinical recognition and treatment of this newly described form of correctable hypertension was probably the case reported by Leadbetter and Burkland[9] in 1938.

The first repair of renal artery stenosis in a child with subsequent cure of hypertension was performed in 1957 and reported in 1960 by Lambeth et al.[6] Their patient was evaluated for hypertension at the age of 33 months. Angiographic studies of this patient demonstrated severe stenosis of the superior branch of the right renal artery. Excision of the stenotic segment with reanastomosis of the branch resulted in prolonged cure of hypertension. Although nine children with renovascular hypertension had been reported prior to that report of successful revascularization, all had been treated by nephrectomy.

Although sporadic case reports of renovascular hypertension in children continued to appear during the late 1950s and early 1960s, this form of hypertension has been recognized with increasing frequency since the 1970s. Fry et al.[4] reported their cumulative experience with the operative management of 22 children at the University of Michigan in 1973. Finally, experience with the diagnostic evaluation of 107 hypertensive children and the operative management in 25 of 30 children with hypertension of renal origin at Vanderbilt University was reviewed by Lawson et al.[8] in 1977. Pertinent aspects of this review are detailed further in this chapter.

Etiology and Pathologic Anatomy

Hypertension may be due to a variety of underlying causes. Elevated blood pressure may be one of several manifestations of

Supported in part by National Institutes of Health Grant 5P17HL14192 to the Specialized Center for Research in Hypertension.

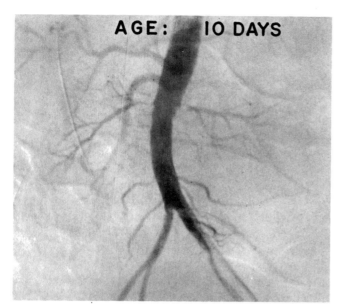

Fig 152–1.—Arteriogram of a hypertensive 10-day-old child showing severe bilateral orificial stenosis of the renal arteries. (From Dean R.H.: Renovascular hypertension during childhood, in Dean R.H., O'Neill J.A. Jr. (eds.): *Vascular Disorders of Childhood.* Philadelphia; Lea & Febiger, 1983. Used by permission.)

an illness, or it may be the single clue to an underlying disorder. Correctable forms of hypertension cover a spectrum of renal parenchymal, vascular, endocrine, neurologic, and metabolic disorders. Although each of these types can produce severe hypertension, the discussion here is directed only toward factors causing renal artery stenosis and renovascular hypertension.

Childhood renovascular lesions can be divided into two major categories: congenital and acquired. In many instances, however, the distinction is arbitrary, for lack of sufficient knowledge to classify the lesions precisely. Certainly, when renal hypoplasia is present, the renal arterial lesion is easily identified as congenital. In contrast, many isolated renal artery stenoses that are classified as fibromuscular dysplasia may be isolated coarctations involving only the renal artery. An example of such a case is seen in Fig 152–1. This child was admitted at the age of 1 week with congestive heart failure and pulmonary edema, with a blood pressure

of 210/130 mm Hg. Arteriography demonstrated severe bilateral orificial stenosis of the renal arteries. Seen later in childhood, such lesions would be classified as fibromuscular dysplasia. With identification at this early date, intrauterine developmental arrest of the renal artery segment is the most likely cause. Histologic examination is of little value in classifying such lesions, because fibromuscular dysplasia and coarctation may be indistinguishable. Both contain a mesenchymal cell component and a variable amount of collagen-rich fibrous tissue.

The majority of renal artery stenoses encountered in children are classified as fibromuscular dysplasia. Although classification of such lesions as fibromuscular dysplasia suggests that they have a common etiologic origin, the actual causes of such lesions are unknown; and they probably result from a variety of factors. Distinctly different from the "string-of-beads" appearance of medial dysplasia most frequently seen in adult females, fibrodysplastic lesions in children show no sex preference and are focal, discrete narrowings. Although the angiographic appearance of the lesions in childhood is consistent with intimal dysplasia, histologic correlation is rarely available. In contrast to the usual mid or distal location of fibrodysplastic lesions in adults, stenoses in children occur at any site along the length of the renal artery (Fig 152–2). Whether some of these represent congenital stenoses or acquired fibrodysplastic lesions is speculative. Bilateral involvement of the renal arteries with fibromuscular dysplasia has been recognized with increasing frequency in recent years. In the Vanderbilt University experience, of 16 children with fibromuscular dysplasia, 7 (44%) had bilateral involvement. Only three children had bilateral disease when initially examined. The other four developed contralateral stenosis 3 months to 10 years later (Fig 152–3).

Rarely, neurofibromatosis may be associated with renal artery stenosis and renovascular hypertension. Flynn and Buchanan[3] reviewed the literature and found 52 cases of renal vascular lesions in patients with neurofibromatosis; 32 of the individuals were male, and 70% were children. Characteristically, lesions involve the origin of the renal artery. Histologic study may show no difference from ordinary fibromuscular dysplasia. Abrams[1] has been quoted as stating that there does not appear to be any overgrowth of neural tissue within the arterial wall.

Renal artery stenosis can be secondary to previous trauma,[8] nonspecific arteritis (Takayasu's arteritis),[7] stenosis of the renal artery in a transplanted kidney, and as a late sequel of radiotherapy.[8] Finally, as a result of the use of umbilical artery catheter-

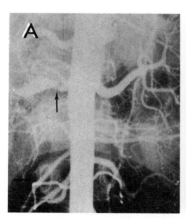
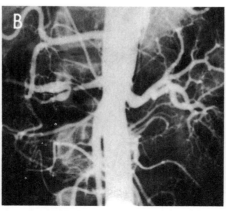
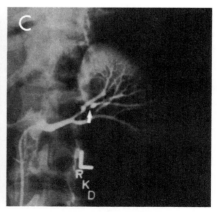

Fig 152–2.—Examples of locations and appearances of renal artery stenoses *(arrows)* found in children. (From Lawson J.D., Boerth R., Foster J.H., et al.: *Arch. Surg.* 112:1307, copyright 1977, American Medical Association. Used by permission.) **A,** orificial lesions frequently connote congenital coarctation variety lesions. **B,** mid-main renal artery lesions are seen more frequently in older children. **C,** branch renal artery lesions have been identified in children of all age groups.

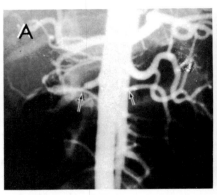
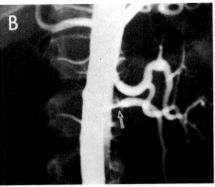
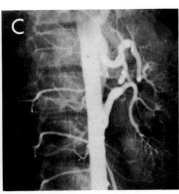

Fig 152–3.—Discovery of left renal artery stenosis after right nephrectomy. **A,** abdominal aortograms of a hypertensive 3-month-old boy showing severe stenosis *(arrows)* of the right renal artery. Note that the left renal artery looks normal. **B,** aortogram made because of recurrent hypertension 10 years after right nephrectomy showed severe left renal artery stenosis *(arrow).* **C,** this was successfully treated by saphenous vein bypass. (From Dean R.H.: Renovascular hypertension during childhood, in Dean R.H., O'Neill J.A. Jr. (eds.): *Vascular Disorders of Childhood.* Philadelphia, Lea & Febiger, 1983. Used by permission.)

ization in the newborn, the incidence of neonatal aortic thrombosis has increased. We have successfully managed a 15-month-old child who presented with RVH secondary to previous aortic and right renal artery thrombosis and recanalization.

Incidence

The incidence of renovascular hypertension in childhood is not known. However, the prevalence of hypertension in children must be grossly underestimated. Few screening programs for identification of hypertension in small children have been undertaken. Controversy over the definition of the upper limits of normal pressures in children remains unresolved. Mild hypertension is asymptomatic and, therefore, may go unrecognized for

years during early life. Pazdral et al.[11] emphasized the problem of lack of screening by showing that only 61 of 1,156 children (5.3%) evaluated in a Los Angeles screening program had their blood pressures recorded. Further, only six of 502 children (1.2%) seen who were under 3 years of age had blood pressures taken.

In 1977, we reported our experience with renovascular hypertension in children.[8] Although we saw 107 children during previous years, more uniform data have become available for classification purposes since the November 1971 institution of the Specialized Center for Research in Hypertension at Vanderbilt University Medical Center. Over the 5 years prior to 1977, 74 children were investigated. The causes of hypertension in these children are shown in Fig 152–4. Seven (78%) of the nine chil-

Fig 152–4.—Causes and frequency of surgically correctable hypertension during childhood. Data for this graph was gathered from 74 children evaluated for hypertension over 5 years. Note the frequency of correctable causes in first decade of life. *FMD* indicates fibromuscular dysplasia. (From Lawson J.D., Boerth R., Foster J.H., et al.: *Arch. Surg.* 112:1307, copyright 1977, American Medical Association. Used by permission.)

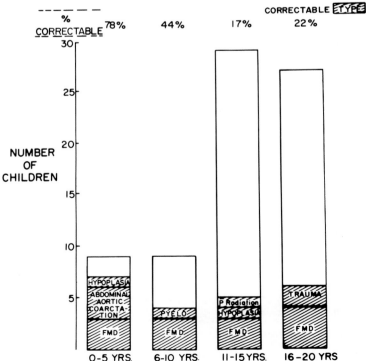
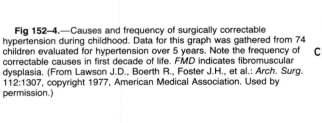

AGE AT TIME OF RECOGNITION

dren younger than six years of age had correctable forms of hypertension. Three had abdominal aortic coarctations; 3 had fibromuscular disease of the renal arteries; and 1 had a hypoplastic kidney. Four of the nine patients (42%) in the 6–10 year age group had correctable forms of hypertension, which included fibromuscular disease of the renal arteries in three patients and pyelonephritis in one. Similar causes of hypertension were less frequent in the 11–15-year and 16–20-year age groups, in which only 17% and 22% of the patients, respectively, had correctable forms of hypertension. Only patients referred for evaluation of hypertension are included in this analysis. Children with isthmic aortic coarctations, Wilms tumor, and other lesions in which hypertension was only an associated finding are excluded.

Clinical Presentation

The signs and symptoms of hypertension rarely are attributable to the elevated blood pressure per se, but rather are due to its effect on the target organs. In its early stages, the disease has few or no clinical manifestations. Little in the history, physical examination, or routine laboratory examination will help differentiate renovascular hypertension (RVH) from essential hypertension (EH) in children. A renovascular cause of hypertension is more likely than essential hypertension in children under 10 years of age. A history of abdominal or flank trauma may be related to the development of RVH. Recent onset and a family history of hypertension occur with equal frequency in RVH and EH. Cardiomegaly and retinopathy help gauge the severity of hypertension. In contrast to milder forms of hypertension, the vast majority of children with RVH are symptomatic, and markedly so, at the time of recognition of the hypertension. In our series, CNS signs and symptoms (headaches, extreme irritability, seizures, severe retinopathy), congestive heart failure, and cardiomegaly were the most common modes of presentation. Half of the children in this series had malignant hypertension by the time their blood pressure was recognized.

Diagnostic Evaluation

The general evaluation for all hypertensive patients can be summarized as follows:
1. History and physical examination
2. Hemogram, sequential multiple analysis-12, urinalysis, urine culture, serum potassium levels × 3
3. Electrocardiogram (ECG) and chest roentgenogram
4. Analysis of 24-hour urine collection for creatinine clearance, electrolytes, catecholamines, vanillylmandelic acid, and 17-OH steroids and ketosteroids
5. Rapid-sequence intravenous pyelogram (IVP)
6. Renal arteriography

Electrocardiography is important to gauge the extent of secondary myocardial hypertrophy. Serum electrolytes and serial serum potassium determinations can effectively exclude patients with primary aldosteronism if potassium levels are greater than 3.0 mg/dl. Evaluation of renal function is mandatory. Preexisting renal disease may reduce renal function and cause hypertension. Conversely, hypertension from any cause may produce intrarenal arteriolar nephrosclerosis and subsequent depression of renal function. Finally, assessment of the urinary 17-hydroxysteroid and 17-ketosteroid and vanillylmandelic acid levels will effectively identify the rare patient with a pheochromocytoma or functioning cortical tumor.

Rapid-Sequence IVP

This simple study is often employed as a screening test for RVH. The patient, having been dehydrated, receives a rapid infusion of contrast medium. Roentgenograms are obtained at 1, 2, 3, 4, 5, 10, 15, and 30 minutes. Findings suggestive of RVH include (1) unilateral delay in appearance of contrast medium; (2) decrease in renal length of greater than 1.5 cm, compared with the contralateral side; (3) ureteral notching from enlarged collateral arteries; (4) late unilateral hyperconcentration of the medium; and (5) defects in the renal outline suggesting infarction.

Although the rapid-sequence IVP might seem to have its greatest value as a relatively noninvasive screening study in this young age group, it has been particularly disappointing in children with renovascular hypertension. In our recent review, it was abnormal in only nine of 21 children (42%) with renovascular hypertension. In contrast, it is highly accurate in defining renal parenchymal disease. Therefore, although the rapid-sequence IVP gives valuable information relative to overall renal function and may suggest a renovascular origin of hypertension, the lack of any positive findings does not decrease the need for angiographic study of the renal vasculature in this age group.

Renal Arteriography

Aortography and renal arteriography should be performed in all children who are screened for correctable forms of hypertension. In all instances, to decrease the morbidity resulting from the procedure, severe hypertension is controlled with medication prior to performing the study. In infancy and early childhood, aortography alone is performed. Selective renal artery catheterization is reserved for evaluation of older children. In the younger group of children, general anesthesia is employed.

Anteroposterior and oblique views are especially important when examining children, in whom the normal vessels are smaller, and subtle lesions more easily missed. Figure 152–5 shows the anteroposterior and oblique views of the right renal artery in a 6-year-old child with a branch renal artery stenosis and secondary hypertension. Only on selective oblique views was the significant stenosis appreciated.

Although the potential risk of arteriography has limited its widespread acceptance as the screening test of choice in children, it is the only study that can identify all patients with potentially correctable renovascular hypertension. None of the other "screening studies" has the necessary sensitivity to guide the decision for further investigation. We have experienced no significant complications with the use of screening angiography in over 150 hypertensive children. Furthermore, the high probability of identifying a renovascular source of hypertension in very young patients argues even more strongly for an aggressive view of the diagnostic role of arteriography in them.

Renal Vein Renin Assays

Comparison of the renal venous renin activity from the two kidneys assesses the functional significance of anatomical lesions found with angiography. Several techniques have been employed over the past 20 years for obtaining renal vein renin assays (RVRA). If possible, all antihypertensive medications are discontinued 5 days prior to the study. Currently, patients undergoing RVRA receive furosemide 1 mg/kg of body weight, given orally the evening before the study for diuresis. Simultaneous bilateral renal venous catheterization is performed, the patient supine, and three paired samples are collected. The study is considered positive if at least two of the three paired samples show lateralization in activity with at least a 1.5–1.0 ratio between the involved side and uninvolved side. It is only recently that patients have had RVRA performed in this manner, but a 1.5–1.0 ratio has proved sufficient for a positive interpretation in all studies.

In 19 of 25 children who underwent operation (Table 152–1), RVRA was performed. The study was considered positive in 17 (89%) of these children. One of the two patients with nonlater-

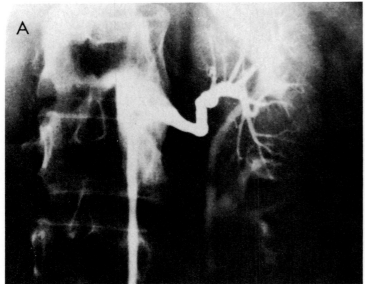

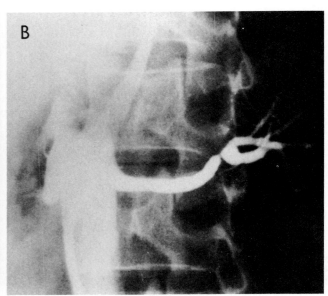

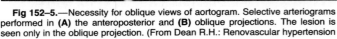

Fig 152–5.—Necessity for oblique views of aortogram. Selective arteriograms performed in **(A)** the anteroposterior and **(B)** oblique projections. The lesion is seen only in the oblique projection. (From Dean R.H.: Renovascular hypertension during childhood, in Dean R.H., O'Neill J.A. Jr. (eds.): *Vascular Disorders of Childhood.* Philadelphia, Lea & Febiger, 1983. Used by permission.)

alizing renin activity had equally severe bilateral fibromuscular dysplasia. Four of the six children not undergoing RVRA were treated early in our experience before the study was possible in smaller children. The final two patients had samples obtainable from only one kidney.

Split Renal Function Studies

Split renal function studies (SRFS) are employed only in older children of this group, the youngest in our experience being 9 years old. We believe the risk of the procedure to be prohibitive in younger children. The methods used to perform this test in our center have been previously described in detail.[2] Consistent lateralization of any magnitude in all three sample collection periods—decreased urine volume, increased para-aminohippuric acid concentration, and increased creatinine concentration—constitutes a positive study. Using these criteria, five of the seven patients (71%) undergoing the study had a positive test. One of two patients with a nonlateralizing study had bilateral fibromuscular disease, and the other had a shrunken kidney from chronic pyelonephritis. There were no complications of the study in any of the seven patients evaluated.

Operative Treatment

Preoperative Preparation

Patients with severe hypertension (diastolic pressures in excess of 120 mm Hg) should be controlled for several days prior to operation. We prefer the use of methyldopa as a diuretic for this

TABLE 152–1.—RESULTS OF
FUNCTIONAL STUDIES

TEST	NO. PERFORMED	NO. POSITIVE (%)
Renal vein renin assays	19	17 (89)
Split renal function studies	7	5 (71)

purpose, yet have supplemented this in children with intermittent use of intravenous diazoxide when necessary. In contrast to the recommended bolus technique of administration, we prefer to administer the diazoxide by intravenous infusion with constant monitoring of the blood pressure. Employing this method, one averts the distribution phase and has a more controlled stepwise and prolonged reduction in hypertension.

Operation is not undertaken until it is certain that aortography or SRFS have not caused an elevation in blood urea nitrogen or serum creatinine levels, in which case operation is delayed until renal function returns to its baseline.

Exposure

Exposure of the renal arteries is the most difficult aspect of renal artery surgery. A midline xiphoid-to-pubis incision provides excellent access to both renal arteries. To expose the left renal artery, the posterior peritoneum overlying the aorta is incised longitudinally, the duodenum is mobilized to the patient's right, and the left renal vein is dissected out and mobilized (Fig 152–6). By extending the posterior peritoneal incision to the left along the inferior border of the pancreas, an avascular plane behind the pancreas can be entered. The inferior mesenteric vein courses obliquely across the operative field and is often ligated and divided to facilitate the exposure. One must be certain that an ascending branch of the inferior mesenteric artery is not accompanying the vein. Division of the vein allows excellent exposure of the entire renal hilum on the left and is particularly helpful when distal lesions are to be managed. The left renal artery lies behind the left renal vein. In some cases, it is easier to retract the vein cephalad to expose the artery. In others, caudal retraction of the vein provides better access. Usually, the gonadal and adrenal veins, which enter the left renal vein, have to be ligated and divided to facilitate exposure of the renal artery. Another frequent tributary is a lumbar vein that enters the posterior wall of the left renal vein and is easily avulsed unless special care is taken in mobilizing the renal vein. The proximal portion of the right renal artery can be exposed through the base of the mesentery by ligating two or more pairs of lumbar veins,

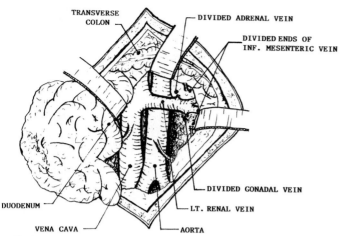

Fig 152–6.—Exposure of the left renal artery through the base of the mesentery. (From Dean R.H.: Renovascular hypertension during childhood, in Dean R.H., O'Neill J.A. Jr. (eds.): *Vascular Disorders of Childhood*. Philadelphia, Lea & Febiger, 1983. Used by permission.)

retracting the vena cava to the patient's right, and retracting the left renal vein cephalad (Fig 152–7). Usually, however, the right renal artery is best exposed by mobilizing the duodenum and right colon medially (Fig 152–8). The right renal vein is mobilized and usually retracted cephalad in order to expose the artery. In some patients, an accessory right renal artery arises from the anterior wall of the aorta about 1 inch above the origin of the inferior mesenteric artery. This artery is unusual in that its course is ordinarily anterior to the vena cava and then over to the lower pole of the right kidney, instead of the usual retrocaval course of the right renal artery. This artery can be easily injured if one is unaware of its presence.

Certain adjunctive measures are applicable in almost all renal arterial operations. Mannitol is administered intravenously early in the operation. Just prior to renal artery cross-clamping, 1.0

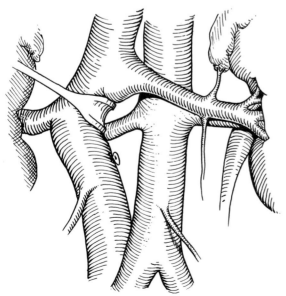

Fig 152–7.—Right renal artery lesion exposed, through the base of the mesentery, from the left by retracting the vena cava. (From Dean R.H.: Renovascular hypertension during childhood, in Dean R.H., O'Neill J.A. Jr. (eds.): *Vascular Disorders of Childhood*. Philadelphia, Lea & Febiger, 1983. Used by permission.)

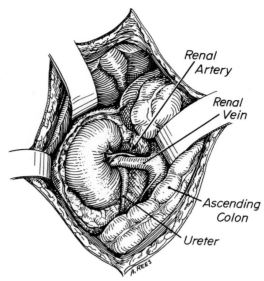

Fig 152–8.—Right renal artery lesions are usually exposed by reflecting the right colon and the duodenum to the left. (From Dean R.H.: Renovascular hypertension during childhood, in Dean R.H., O'Neill J.A. Jr. (eds.): *Vascular Disorders of Childhood*. Philadelphia, Lea & Febiger, 1983. Used by permission.)

mg/kg of heparin is given intravenously. Protamine is almost never required for reversal of the heparin at the end of the reconstruction.

Operative Techniques

A variety of operative techniques have been used to correct renal artery stenosis. Renal artery bypass is the preferred procedure, however, when managing renal artery lesions in children. Three graft materials are available for use: autogenous saphenous vein or hypogastric artery, and synthetic grafts. Saphenous vein is practical only in children over 10 years of age. Before that age, its relatively small size precludes its use as a substitute for the renal artery. Even in the second decade, its superiority is questioned because of its potential for aneurysmal degeneration during follow-up. In our follow-up angiography of saphenous vein aortorenal bypasses, we have found no grafts that became aneurysmally dilated when inserted in patients older than 25 years. In contrast, four of six (67%) saphenous veins used to bypass main renal artery lesions in patients younger than this developed aneurysmal dilatation.

Hypogastric artery is probably the superior graft for use during the first decade of life. Its comparative size, ease of procurement, and suturing characteristics are of increased practical value in this group. Wylie and associates[12] have extended the use of autogenous artery grafts in this group, recommending that a free bifurcation graft of common iliac, hypogastric, and external iliac arteries be procured for use when bilateral renal artery stenoses are to be corrected. In their scheme, leg perfusion is restored by interposing a synthetic graft to replace the excised iliac system. We do not share their enthusiasm for this method of management, but instead would stage the correction and use one hypogastric artery for each renal artery, leaving lower limb perfusion undisturbed.

Although the hypogastric artery appears to be the best choice for graft material in early childhood, the presence of fibromuscular disease in it must be excluded by frozen-section histologic study at operation prior to its use. We have rejected the hypogastric artery in one child on this basis. The single patient who

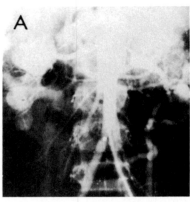
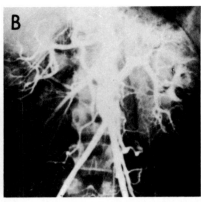
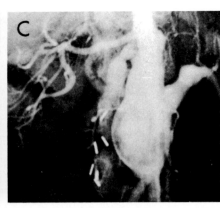

Fig 152–9.—Sequential arteriograms in child with multicentric arteriopathy. **A,** stenosis of left renal artery. **B,** early postoperative arteriogram showing some dilatation of the hypogastric artery used for aortorenal bypass and an external iliac vein used for aortosuperior mesenteric bypass. **C,** 3 years later, progressive aneurysmal dilatation had occurred. The grafts were subsequently replaced. (From Lawson J.D., Boerth R., Foster J.H., et al.: *Arch. Surg.* 112:1307, 1977, copyright 1977, American Medical Association. Used by permission.)

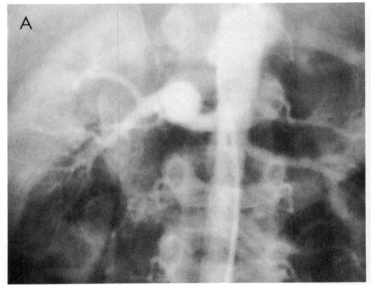

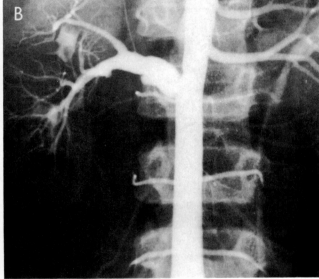

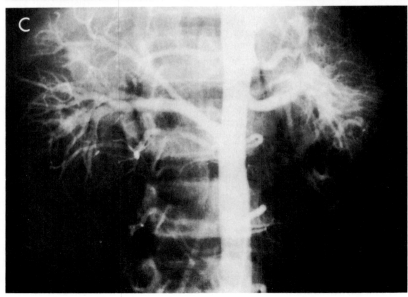

Fig 152–10.—Arteriograms of 7-year-old child with stenosis of the proximal right renal artery. **A,** stenosis and poststenotic dilatation. A 6-mm Dacron graft was inserted. **B,** early postoperative arteriogram shows the typical appearance of the Dacron graft in this position. **C,** 2 years later, arteriography shows excellent adaptation of Dacron graft without evidence of graft stenosis. (From Dean R.H.: Renovascular hypertension during childhood, in Dean R.H., O'Neill J.A. Jr.(eds.): *Vascular Disorders of Childhood.* Philadelphia, Lea & Febiger, 1983. Used by permission.)

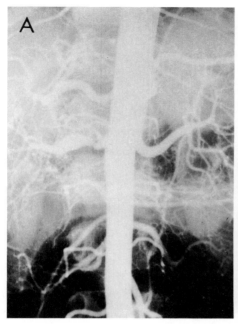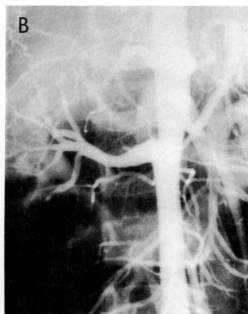

Fig 152–11.—Unilateral renal artery stenosis treated by reimplantation; **(A)** preoperative and **(B)** 1-week postoperative arteriograms in a 5-year-old child who underwent renal reimplantation of the right renal artery. (From Dean R.H.: Re- novascular hypertension during childhood, in Dean R.H., O'Neill J.A. Jr. (eds.): *Vascular Disorders of Childhood.* Philadelphia, Lea & Febiger, 1983. Used by permission.)

has required replacement of a renal artery bypass graft for aneurysmal degeneration is a child whose hypogastric artery was used to bypass a left renal artery stenosis (Fig 152–9). This child also required replacement of an iliac vein graft used to revascularize the superior mesenteric artery. Review of a specimen of the hypogastric artery used for bypass revealed fibromuscular dysplasia, which probably caused the aneurysmal degeneration. Unfortunately, follow-up angiography subsequent to the replacement of these grafts has shown the development of a branch renal artery aneurysm in the left kidney.

Synthetic material can be used successfully in selected children with renal artery stenosis. In many children with proximal renal artery stenosis and poststenotic dilatation, the distal renal artery is sufficiently large to accept a 6-mm Dacron graft. Serial follow-up studies of such grafts have shown excellent incorporation and long-term patency (Fig 152–10).

In selected children with orificial stenosis, the vessel beyond the stenosis may be redundant after it is freed from the surrounding retroperitoneal tissue. In such instances, transection of the vessel, spatulation, and reimplantation is the preferable method of revascularization (Fig 152–11). In these circumstances, the anastomotic orifice can be made large enough to ensure long-term patency and avoid any likelihood of late degeneration of the graft or stenosis.

Finally, nephrectomy may be required in the management of RVH in some children. This procedure should be considered as a secondary and ultimate alternative. Early in the history of the operative treatment of RVH, nephrectomy was employed frequently. In many of these children treated by nephrectomy, the subsequent appearance of contralateral disease threatened overall renal function and life. In our experience, fibromuscular disease ultimately proved to be bilateral in 44% of the children in whom nephrectomies were performed. Of the children who ultimately developed bilateral involvement, in 57% only unilateral disease was identified at the first evaluation and operation. Thus, the apparent absence of contralateral disease is insufficient reason to consider nephrectomy an acceptable method of treatment.

Nephrectomy should be reserved for children with unreconstructable vessels and uncontrollable hypertension. With advances in technology, even infants may be able to undergo revascularization. When growth of the child's vessels is required to permit revascularization, temporary control of hypertension by medication, if possible, is preferable to nephrectomy.

Results of Operative Treatment

Cure of hypertension by operative management should be expected in all children in whom all renovascular lesions are treated by bypass or replacement. In the report of Fry et al.,[4] 95% of children were cured by primary and secondary procedures. Table 152–2 shows the results of operative treatment in our center. Of the patients we treated operatively, 20 (72%) were cured. Six additional patients (21%) have had significant improvements in blood pressure control, but still require antihypertensive medications to remain normotensive. Two of these six patients have residual, uncorrected branch renal artery disease causing residual hypertension; and one patient has an uncorrected unilateral graft thrombosis after bilateral saphenous vein aortorenal bypasses. A fourth patient of these six had initially been cured of hypertension by nephrectomy at the age of 2 months. Ten years later, hypertension recurred secondary to contralateral renal artery stenosis. The two patients (7%) who did not improve after operation require special comment. The first child, 4 years old, had a nephrectomy for severe hypertension secondary to renal artery fibromuscular dysplasia. Hypertension

TABLE 152–2.—RESULTS OF
OPERATIVE TREATMENT

RESULT	NO. (%) OF PATIENTS
Cured	20 (72)
Improved	6 (21)
No change	2 (7)

soon recurred, and repeat arteriography showed severe contra-lateral branch renal artery fibromuscular dysplasia. The child died 6 months postoperatively in renal failure with severe hypertension. The second child had undergone a left nephrectomy and radiation 11 years previously for Wilms tumor. The hypertension, thought to be secondary to contralateral renal artery stenosis, was unimproved by renal artery reimplantation. Repeated arteriography at 5-month and 3-year postoperative intervals shows moderate stenoses in a lower pole branch of the renal artery bifurcation. Finally, 20 of the 23 patients (90%) without residual or untreated recurrent lesions have been cured. Amelioration of hypertension is highly predictable when all renovascular lesions can be corrected.

Follow-up studies of our 25 children have included 36 arteriograms made from 1 week to 11 years after operation. Four of the 13 children (32%), whose initial presenting symptom was unilateral fibromuscular dysplasia, displayed contralateral disease, recognized from 3 months to 10 years later. None of the saphenous vein grafts has undergone sufficient aneurysmal dilatation to require replacement. Furthermore, all grafts that were initially patent have remained open without developing any evidence of stenosis. The previously mentioned 10-year-old child, who had multicentric fibromuscular disease that probably caused aneurysmal dilatation of both a hypogastric artery used for renal artery bypass and an external iliac vein used to bypass a superior mesenteric artery occlusion, has had aneurysmal degeneration of his grafts, requiring replacement (see Fig 152–9).

Finally, the results of operative management of renovascular hypertension are quite acceptable and indicate that an aggressive diagnostic and therapeutic approach is appropriate for children with this problem. Many considerations peculiar to the pediatric age group, however, remain unanswered. Only through long-term intensive follow-up studies of these children will the natural history of their disease and the effects of operative management be more clearly defined.

REFERENCES

1. Abrams J.: Personal communication quoted by Fry W.J., Ernst C.B., Stanley J.C., et al.: Renovascular hypertension in the pediatric patient. *Arch. Surg.* 107:692, 1933.
2. Dean R.H., Foster J.H.: Criteria for the diagnosis of renovascular hypertension. *Surgery* 74:926, 1973.
3. Flynn M.P., Buchanan J.B.: Neurofibromatosis, hypertension and renal artery aneurysms. *South. Med. J.* 73:618, 1980.
4. Fry W.J., Ernst C.B., Stanley J.C., et al.: Renovascular hypertension in the pediatric patient. *Arch. Surg.* 107:692, 1973.
5. Goldblatt H.: Studies on experimental hypertension. *J. Exp. Med.* 59:347, 1934.
6. Lambeth C.B., Derrick J.R., Hansen A.E.: Stenosis of a branch of the renal artery causing hypertension in a child: Including a complication of translumbar renal arteriography. *Pediatrics* 26:822, 1960.
7. Lande A.: Takayasu's arteritis and congenital coarctation of the descending thoracic and abdominal aorta. *Am. J. Roentgenol.* 127:227, 1976.
8. Lawson J.D., Boerth R., Foster J.H., et al.: Diagnosis and management of renovascular hypertension in children. *Arch. Surg.* 112:1307, 1977.
9. Leadbetter W.F., Burkland C.E.: Hypertension in unilateral renal disease. *J. Urol.* 39:611, 1938.
10. Loggie J.M.H.: Hypertension in children and adolescents. *Hosp. Pract.* 10(6):81,1975.
11. Pazdral P.T., Lieberman H.M., Pazdral W.E.: Awareness of pediatric hypertension, measuring blood pressure. *JAMA* 235:2320, 1976.
12. Wylie E.J., Perloff D.L., Stoney R.J.: Autogenous tissue revascularization techniques in surgery for renovascular hypertension. *Ann. Surg.* 170:416, 1969.

153 William H. Weintraub

Peripheral Vascular Ischemia

Ischemia of the extremities in infants and children is a frequent diagnostic and management problem. The first report of vascular compromise leading to gangrene is ascribed to Martini in 1828.[74] In 1914, Von Khautz[135] presented a detailed list of the case reports in children up to age 15 years.[15] In 1945, Gross[43] added six additional cases to the world's literature and brought the total up to 41 cases.[72, 78, 111, 137] The number of cases has increased rapidly since.[128, 138, 140] Modern diagnostic modalities, aggressive monitoring techniques, and newer medications are partially responsible for this increase.

Incidence

Despite early reports suggesting an increased incidence in females, current literature details a more even distribution, with the exception of play-related trauma, where young boys predominate.[80, 82, 83, 87, 90, 113] Improved obstetric management, routine use of antibiotics in premature infants, and better management have reduced the risk of perinatal ischemic events. However, iatrogenic neonatal extremity ischemia is on the increase, because so many of the monitoring techniques and newer drugs have vascular implications or complications.

Etiologic Factors

Direct Vascular Insult

Arterial access for the purpose of monitoring blood gases or vital signs, or for cardiac catheterization, is being used with increasing frequency.[56, 66] Umbilical, radial, brachial, femoral, and axillary arteries are the most commonly chosen, and spasm and/or occlusion can result. Significant infusion of fluids or medications through the arterial line is not prudent, especially because arterial cannulation alone may result in ischemia. Inadvertent arterial injection of drugs can lead to frank gangrene.[73, 103, 131] This usually follows attempted intramuscular (IM) injections that accidentally become interarterial, and extreme care is needed for IM injections in infants and small children.[51, 131] Inadvertent pentobarbital injection into the brachial artery during induction of anesthesia can result in pain, numbness, blanching, and a reduced or absent pulse.[19,73,101] The ultimate consequence can be gangrene and amputation. Almost 10% of drug addicts in the United States are teenagers, and arterial injections in them are well documented.[19,70,123] Haller described gangrene in the upper extremities in five children after cardiac catheterization through the axillary artery.[34,45] Most centers now use the transfemoral approach for cardiac catheterization, which is safer because of the vessel's larger size and easier access.

Extremity gangrene after iatrogenic arterial manipulation is not caused by the transient "spasm" that is so often discussed.[106] Gangrene is usually the result of a correctable mechanical arterial injury or a thrombosis that can be appropriately diagnosed and acted upon promptly.[45]

Presentation of Vascular Compromise

Arterial injury or obstruction can occur anywhere in the body; occlusions of the axillary, brachial, ulnar, or radial artery obviously affect the flow to the arms, forearms, hands, and fingers, while problems in the aorta, iliac, femoral, or either tibial artery can create compromise to the legs, feet, or toes. If two or more extremities are involved, direct trauma is less likely to be the cause; and emboli, sepsis, drugs or systemic disease should be considered.

Arterial compromise presents with certain general patterns of signs and symptoms. However, infants and young children are often unable to communicate symptoms, and the clinician must rely on clinical signs. Arterial obstruction leads to reduced or absent pulses, coolness, pallor, decreased muscle function, diminished reflexes, and pain. This may be followed by significant color change and by swelling. Ultimately, a demarcation line develops representing decreased or absent viability. During the first 6 hours, it may be difficult to differentiate self-limiting arterial spasm from true correctable mechanical obstruction. Doppler pulses are often present in cases of spasm, while they are much less common in true obstruction.[138] The results are significantly better if the lesion is repaired in 6 hours or less. Repair is rarely effective after 18 hours.

The natural course of vascular ischemia depends on the site, duration, and degree of obstruction; the size of the vessel involved; and the adequacy of the collateral circulation in that area. If major peripheral vascular ischemia is not reversed within 12 to 24 hours, the ultimate fate of the extremity is almost surely sealed. The site of skin demarcation may change as collateral circulation takes effect, resulting in slightly *more* viable tissue remaining than was originally thought. The skin may not be an accurate indicator of the level of viability of the deeper tissues. The final result can vary from full recovery to dry gangrene and ultimate autoamputation. Between these two extremes, the child can end up with leg length discrepancy caused by impaired growth, survival of the extremity with reduced muscle function, decreased innervation, or just skin changes. The earlier the problem is defined and corrected, the more likely the results are to be favorable. Prior to the advent of modern vascular surgical techniques, these children were observed for 3–4 weeks for complete autoamputation in the belief that such conservative measures would preserve a maximal amount of tissue survival.[138] The newer forms of imaging techniques, early heparinization, and appropriate surgical reconstruction have led to a significant improvement in the survival of these extremities and in restoration of normal or near-normal function.[140]

Causes of Peripheral Ischemia

There are many and varied causes of peripheral vascular ischemia in children, as illustrated in the following outline:[77,85,121,138]

I. Direct vascular injury
  A. Intravascular cannulas
    1. Arterial catheters
    2. Venous catheters
  B. Inadvertent arterial injury
    1. Injections
    2. Addiction
    3. Iatrogenic causes
  C. Extremity trauma
    1. Compression
      a. Bandages
      b. Plaster cast and skeletal traction
    2. Direct arterial trauma (lacerations)
    3. Wringer injuries
II. Perinatal causes
  A. Prematurity
  B. Sepsis
  C. Difficult labor or delivery
  D. Disseminated intravascular coagulation (DIC)
III. Sepsis
  A. Bacterial
  B. Viral
IV. Medications
  A. Dopamine
  B. Epinephrine
  C. Norepinephrine
  D. Nitroprusside
  E. Metaraminol
V. Miscellaneous
  A. Congenital heart disease
  B. Diabetes
  C. Emboli and thrombi
  D. Vasculitis and collagen diseases
  E. Thermal insults
  F. Vascular anomalies
  G. Neoplasms
  H. Irradiation
  I. Sickle-cell disease

Intravascular Procedures

Most instances of extremity gangrene in children result from iatrogenic causes.[25,30,56,138] Although the original interarterial manipulation is usually justified, nonetheless an ischemic complication, when it does occur, can be a major disaster.

Extremity Gangrene Following Arterial Manipulation

The preferential use of the percutaneous technique for insertion of arterial catheters by the radiologist, cardiologist, and critical care specialist has led to a decrease in the risk of serious sequelae. Unfortunately, this ease of access has led to a concomitant increase in the number of procedures attempted, so that the actual number of complications continues to increase. Spasm is much less common with the percutaneous technique; but when spasm is present, it is almost always transient and spontaneously resolves in less than 6 hours.[68,70,71,113,138,141] However, because there is a 5–25% incidence of mechanical obstruction after the Seldinger (percutaneous) method,[84,96] patients with persistent signs and symptoms must be evaluated promptly and treated appropriately. Failure to recognize prolonged mechanical ischemia as opposed to spasm, and the resultant delay in instituting appropriate measures, can lead to limb loss, leg length discrepancy, or chronic vascular insufficiency. In the first hour or so after the ischemia is encountered, early institution of heparin therapy may reduce the likelihood of these late complica-

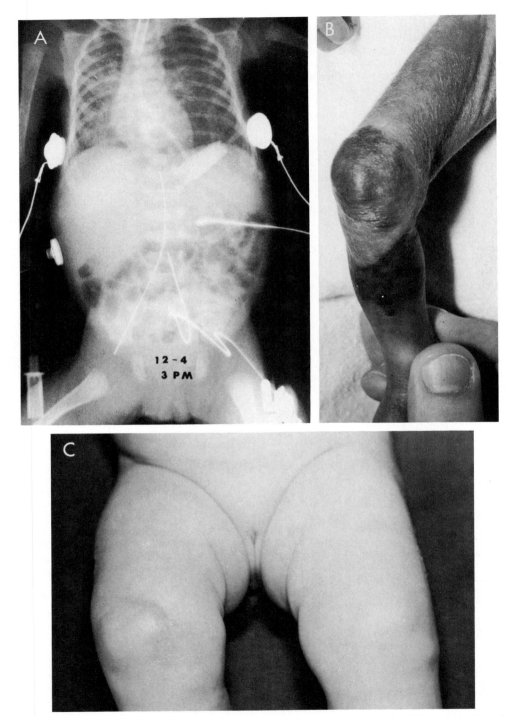

Fig 153–1.—Umbilical catheter embolism. **A,** second born of twins who, during attempted catheter removal, had accidental transection of right umbilical artery catheter demonstrated by x-ray to have embolized to the right iliac artery. The catheter was removed through an aortotomy. (There is a well-positioned left umbilical artery catheter in place.) **B,** postoperatively, the leg appeared nonviable. **C,** final result included only minor scarring near the knee, and no leg length discrepancy at 1 year of age.

tions, regardless of whether the child has arterial spasm or true injury.[6,120,140]

Umbilical artery catheters are frequently employed in neonatal critical care units. Catheter tip placement is important, as is the solution used to flush the line.[8] Many of these infants also have other risk factors for peripheral vascular ischemia (Fig 153–1). Color change in the toes is common and suggests the need for immediate evaluation.[19,31,40,61,86,94,102,105,109,118]

Arterial spasm arises from obvious causes like arterial sticks for monitoring or blood gas measurement, as well as less obvious causes such as skeletal traction or compression by plaster casts. Orthopedic manipulation has been shown in both laboratory experiments and in clinical situations to lead to spasm, ischemia, and even gangrene.[76,98,99] Dislocations or distractions of the elbow, knee, or ankle can lead to ischemic sequelae.[98,99,132] If the skeletal traction that precipitated the ischemia is deemed necessary, the extremity must be placed in more flexion to relieve the obstruction to the blood flow.[81,132]

Extremity Gangrene Following Venous Manipulation

Venipunctures are far more common than arterial sticks. Virtually every vein in the body has been used for an injection site, monitoring purposes, blood drawing, or infusions.[9,13,88,89] A skilled professional using the newer, sharper, smaller needles can use many different vessels in many and varied situations with excellent results. However, in the sickest of children, particularly fragile neonates or infants who are small and perhaps dehydrated, nearby arteries may occasionally be entered and injured.[3,13,88,100] If the injury to the artery is external to its muscular wall, then spasm is most likely and will result in a cool, pale extremity that gradually returns to normal. If the injury is deeper and includes the muscle wall, or in particular the intima, occlusion and thrombosis can result.[6] Even though the physician believes he was manipulating a vein, such an extremity must be treated as having an arterial injury and followed and treated accordingly.

There are several reports of extremity gangrene following

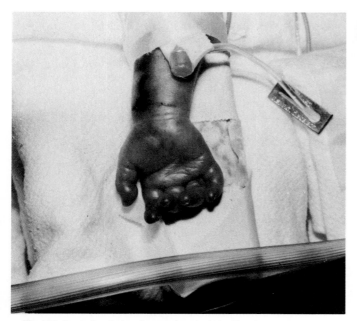

Fig 153–2.—Ischemic hand secondary to indwelling (1 week) intravenous catheter. The hand survived with no residua.

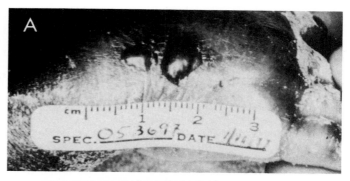

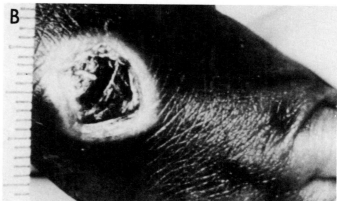

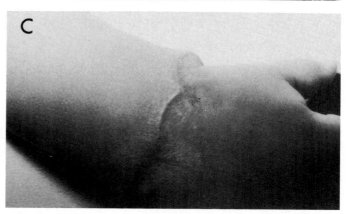

Fig 153–3.—Infiltration injury. **A,** dorsum of hand shortly after an infiltration of hyperalimentation solution. **B,** area of third-degree skin loss. **C,** final result after topical treatment only.

long-standing indwelling venous catheters.[13,59,92,112] The incidence is extremely small; but, considering the numbers of venous access procedures performed in pediatric centers, the risk is real. Peripheral venous locations are more likely to cause extremity gangrene than central venous lines, for obvious reasons (Fig 153–2).

Intravenous solutions are often hyperosmolar and chemically irritating. If the solution leaks out of the vein into the surrounding tissue, the skin and subcutaneous layers are at risk for ischemia or skin slough. Most clinicians deal daily with infiltrations, and fortunately most cases resolve spontaneously.[26] Skin grafting is rarely necessary. The area of the slough is treated like a small burn; and eventual healing follows, usually with minimal scarring (Fig 153–3).

Prematurity

Prematurely leaving the comforting environment of the uterus adversely alters most risks in infants. Alone or in combination with other etiologic factors, prematurity makes such infants more susceptible to arterial insult.[39] Some specific aspects of physiology in the premature directly increase susceptibility to vascular spasm, thrombi, emboli, or iatrogenic injury: (1) The abdominal organs have increased perfusion so that the peripheral circulation is relatively lower than in the full-term infant. (2) The resistance of capillaries to external compression improves with each intra-uterine week, so that the smaller premature infant is at increased risk for vascular compression from any cause. (3) Neurovascular control of capillary musculature is not well organized or developed in premature infants. (4) Premature infants are prone to sepsis.[1] All these phenomena make the premature patient and its peripheral vasculature more susceptible to spasm, thrombi, emboli, or iatrogenic injury.[37, 122]

Sepsis

Systemic sepsis is a frequent finding in patients of all ages with ischemic gangrene; however, a direct causal relationship is not usually evident.[17, 44, 63] Often in the younger patients and infants, dehydration also plays a supporting role. Viral or bacterial infections may either precede or coexist with ischemia.[2, 17, 18, 49] They can precede some vascular problems such as purpura fulminans, or in other circumstances occur simultaneously, as in gastroenteritis with dehydration and hyperosmolality.[21, 125] Such shifts in blood volume usually protect the central organs, exposing the extremities to increased risk. Some bacterial organisms like meningococcus produce exotoxins that cause consumption of coagulation factors and ultimately lead to vascular compromise.[26, 60]

Difficult or Prolonged Labor

An umbilical cord wrapped around an extremity is only one example of how labor or delivery can affect the peripheral vascular system of the newborn child.[46] Abnormal presentations such as footling, breech, face, as well as attempts at rotation during delivery, dystocia with generalized anoxia, or significant traction during delivery can all provoke mechanical factors with resultant peripheral vascular ischemia (Fig 153–4).[27, 41, 57]

Medications Affecting Peripheral Blood Flow

Many of the medications used to alter blood pressure or cardiac output place the peripheral vasculature at risk. Dopamine, a frequently used drug in the intensive care unit,[42] can and does reduce peripheral blood flow. In most circumstances, the reduced flow is transient and does not lead to serious distal ischemic insult. However, occasionally the fingers or toes appear mottled and cool. Careful evaluation of the patient's need for the particular vasoactive drug is necessary, and attempts should be made to change to another pressor agent. In selected circumstances, phentolamine (Regitine) can be administered to counteract the vasoconstrictive drug's effects on distal tissue.

In a newborn child with unexplained peripheral ischemia, the physician should obtain a careful medication history from the mother to rule out a transplacental origin of the child's vascular problem.

Congenital Heart Disease

Children with congenital heart disease can develop extremity gangrene spontaneously.[47] This is uncommon, but there are several proposed mechanisms. The ductus arteriosus normally undergoes obliteration by clotting within the duct when it is no longer in the mainstream of the vascular circuit. Thrombi within the ductus can break loose and cause pulmonary emboli, or with reversal of flow can cause systemic emboli and, rarely, extremity gangrene.[4] Prompt embolectomy is needed to prevent limb loss in these circumstances.[14, 43, 52, 63, 84]

The polycythemia of many patients with cyanotic congenital heart disease can predispose to extremity gangrene, as the blood flow is slowed by the increased viscosity.[67, 107] Clearly, these children are at greater risk when they become dehydrated from an intercurrent illness. Prevention is by careful monitoring, and correction of the child's state of hydration.[21, 138]

An occasional patient with congenital heart disease develops intracardiac thrombi near a septal defect.[138] This can become a source of emboli leading to extremity gangrene.

Diabetes

Infants of diabetic mothers are at risk of dehydration secondary to the osmotic load of the excess glucose in their blood. Renal vein thrombosis is a well-known manifestation of this problem in infants of diabetic mothers; extremity gangrene has been reported in these children as well.[66, 75] Careful observation of the status of such a child's hydration should be maintained to prevent a tragedy; however, thrombus formation with subsequent emboli can occur even in utero.[5, 27, 75, 134]

Vasculitis

Purpura Fulminans

First described in 1959,[92, 95, 108, 136, 137] this disease is usually preceded by an "uneventful and unremarkable" upper respiratory infection, which is then followed first by a small patch of purpura. Initially, all cultures (including throat) are reported as having normal flora, and blood coagulation factors may also be within normal limits. As the process continues, thrombocytopenia and hyperfibrinogenemia may be encountered.[57] The purpuric areas enlarge and begin to coalesce. Much of the area then becomes gangrenous. The vasculitis spreads to pressure points on the back, chest, and legs, and moves distally, affecting the fingers, toes, ears, and nose. As larger vessels become involved, an entire extremity can become gangrenous. There is a 50% mortality rate in this disease.[63] In the survivors, one or more of the extremities are severely and permanently damaged or lost, and scarring is usually seen in the other involved areas.

It is thought that purpura fulminans is a vasculitis secondary to a hypersensitivity following either a suspected or unsuspected process. Streptococcus or meningococcus have been implicated.[60] Steroids, heparin, and certain immunoactive drugs have some effect on the disease, but the course is often rapid, with complete evolution in only a few days (Fig 153–5).[17, 45]

Polyarteritis Nodosa

There have been many reports of polyarteritis nodosa in infants and children.[16, 38, 91, 114] This diffuse vasculitis affects children in many ways. First described in 1866, the pathogenesis remains elusive; and the initiating cause is unknown.[74] Signs and symptoms include fever, rash, conjunctivitis, abnormal cerebrospinal fluid, increased urinary sediment, cardiomegaly, and ECG changes. Somewhat more common in males, the onset is acute, resembling a viral illness; but the course is swift and frequently fatal.

Degenerative changes in the walls of medium and small arteries lead to thrombosis and aneurysm formation. This affects many organs, but changes in the coronary arteries and the CNS are

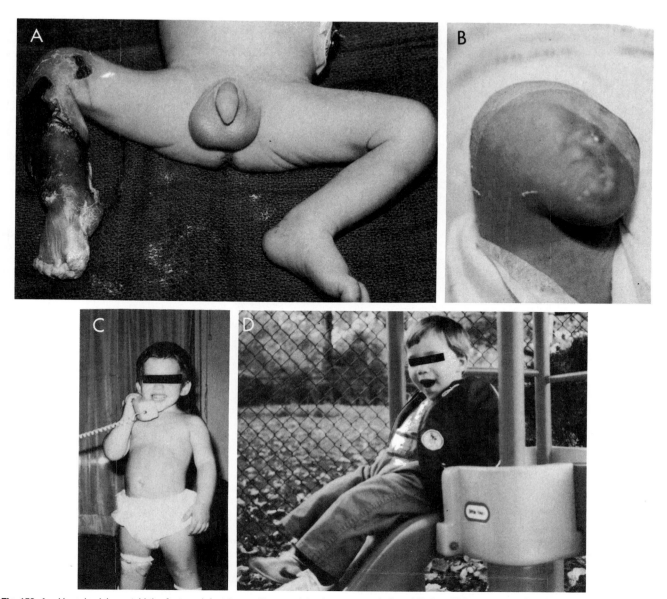

Fig 153–4.—Vascular injury at birth. **A,** term infant born with unexplained ischemia of the right leg that progressed to obvious gangrene despite aggressive therapy. It appeared that the knee might be nonviable. **B,** however, the knee was preserved. **C** and **D,** the child now runs well and is able to play freely with his friends.

the most life-threatening. Vaso-occlusive disease of the extremities is infrequent, but is highly suggestive of the diagnosis. Biopsy of a superficial artery is helpful.[16,93] We have experience with two patients, further suggested by peripheral ischemia, in whom we were able to confirm the diagnosis with rectal suction biopsies demonstrating the classic vascular changes. Treatment with azathioprine and prednisone has had some limited beneficial effect.[91]

Thermal Injury ((Burns and Frostbite)

Extremes of body temperature (low or high) can initiate ischemia or gangrene of the extremity, especially when there are wide swings in body temperature over a relatively short period of time. Frostbite is less common in children than in adults, but unfortunately flame burns and other forms of heat-induced injuries are all too common in the younger-age patient. Autoamputation may occur after thermal injury, or operative removal of the digit or extremity may be necessary during the care of the child with a thermal injury. Children with circumferential burns on an extremity are at risk of distal vascular compromise from the tourniquet effect of the encompassing 360-degree eschar. Early excision of the burn or at least escharotomy may be necessary to release the compression.

Treatment

The causes of extremity gangrene are numerous and varied. Treatment of an individual patient requires an understanding of the numerous clinical conditions that can lead to peripheral ischemia. Treatment is also dependent on the site and extent of the vascular compromise.

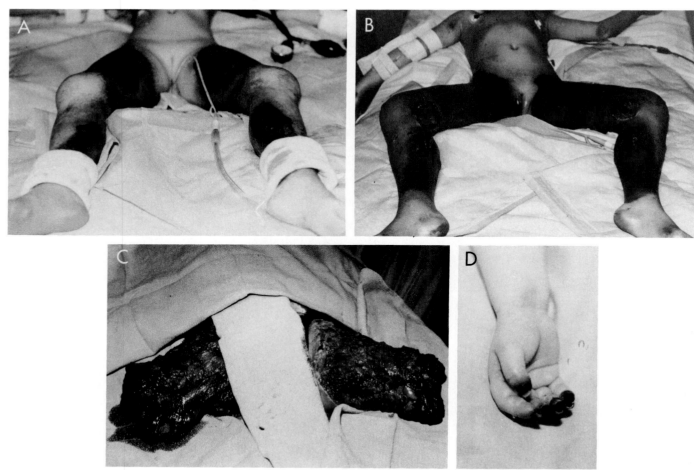

Fig 153–5.—Purpura fulminans. **A,** a child, followed for 24 hours with an erroneous diagnosis of mild idiopathic thrombocytopenic purpura, developed larger areas of purpura in the lower extremity. **B,** 48 hours later, she progressed to florid purpura fulminans and needed escharotomies. **C,** she required bilateral high thigh amputations. **D,** her hand developed distal gangrene. *(Continued.)*

General Considerations

If possible, all further pressure should be avoided on the extremity involved, by a soft surface that will provide gentle support and by a cradle cage placed over the extremity to protect it from pressure and from changes in temperature. Depending on the age of the patient and the extremity involved, the child should be allowed some active range-of-motion of the extremity. More commonly, the patient does not wish to move the extremity very much; and the limb is held in a neutral position. Room temperature should be maintained in the normal range of approximately 20 C. No attempt to raise or lower the temperature of the limb artificially should be considered (except in acute frostbite). Artificial thermal changes will most likely alter blood flow patterns in a disadvantageous way.

Tolazoline (Priscoline) may be given to provide distal arterial relaxation when it is believed that spasm plays a role. The dosage of tolazoline is 1 mg/kg/hr. Our most common indication for tolazoline occurs in the nursery in a child with an umbilical artery line who develops ischemic changes in the legs, feet, or toes. The tolazoline is infused just prior to the prompt removal of the catheter and then continued intravenously (IV) for 12–36 hours.

In older infants and children, heparin is used, at the dose of 3 mg/kg, particularly in those patients who have had known arterial injury. Heparin does not diminish the extent of injury, but may prevent progression of the thrombus.[36] If heparin is contraindicated, low molecular-weight dextran, in the dose of 1–3 ml/kg/hr IV, can partially diminish the blood viscosity.[6, 10, 11, 139, 140] We do not use paravertebral blocks, because, like others, we have not seen any benefit from them.[70]

Fortunately, most children, regardless of age, have return of their pulses within 6 hours; and treatment can be reduced and then discontinued. If resolution has not occurred, imaging techniques may be used in preparation for surgical repair. Digital venous angiography or nuclear flow studies are helpful and much safer in smaller children than arteriography, which itself can cause arterial injury. We have found that use of the Doppler, aided by the noninvasive imaging techniques, is almost always sufficient to follow and treat children with distal ischemia.

Gangrene will nonetheless develop in some children. In patients with evolving permanent damage, aseptic technique is used in caring for the gangrenous extremity. We prefer to treat these children with topical antimicrobial therapy. Silver sulfadiazine is applied gently every 12 hours. This cream has the advantage of crossing the barrier of any eschar, reducing the risk of infection beneath the necrotic tissue layer and preserving the maximal amount of viable deep tissue. Systemic antibiotics are used in a standard burn regimen. Tetanus prophylaxis is administered.

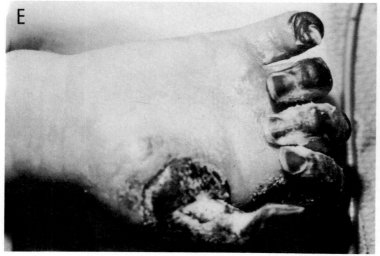

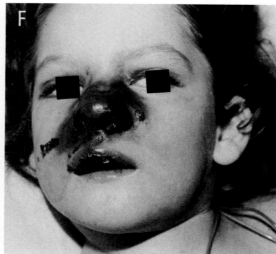

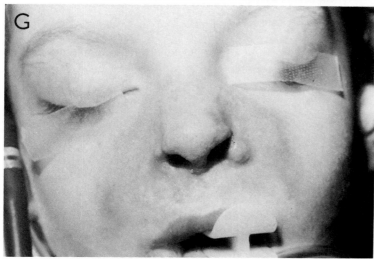

Fig 153–5 Cont.—E, the dry gangrene progressed, and she required amputation of several digits. **F,** the purpura appeared on her nose. **G,** final result of the scarring on her nose.

Patients suspected of polyarteritis nodosa have a superficial arterial or a rectal suction biopsy done to aid in the diagnosis and, if positive, are started on azathioprine at the dose of 5 mg/kg/day for 1 month, and then 2.5 mg/kg/day for 6 months.[23, 25] Routine immunosuppression precautions are instituted as well.

Steroids, in general, are not of significant benefit in extremity gangrene. However, in the few immunologically based phenomena such as purpura fulminans and Stevens-Johnson syndrome, steroids are reported to be somewhat helpful.[69, 95] The dose of prednisone is 1–5 mg/kg/day during the acute phase of the disease.[25, 104]

Disseminated Intravascular Coagulopathy (DIC)

When DIC is suggested by laboratory and clinical findings in a sick infant or child with extremity ischemia or gangrene, rapid treatment is necessary.[1, 22, 48] Fresh frozen plasma may be used to correct the coagulation factors, and platelets are administered as needed. Fresh whole blood has most of the coagulation factors present and may also help to correct the anemia that is almost routinely encountered. Occasionally, heparin may be used intravenously at the dose of 3 mg/kg until the coagulation factors stabilize or the patient has improved and the course of the DIC is corrected.[22] Not infrequently, this takes 2–3 days.

Sepsis is the most common precipitating factor in DIC and should be sought after and treated aggressively.[35] Prior to exact knowledge of the organism, ampicillin at the dose of 200 mg/kg/day, gentamicin at the dose of 5 mg/kg/day, and clindamycin at the dose of 10–15 mg/kg/day are begun. If shock is present, it is treated simultaneously. Anemia, acidosis, hyperpyrexia, and dehydration should be anticipated and rapidly reversed as encountered.[71]

Aggressive regimens may well save the child's life; however, some or all of the extremity may be lost. Hopefully, the extent is well defined and limited early, leaving the child with a minimally impaired extremity.[104]

Surgical Considerations

In most published series, between 50–100% of pediatric extremity ischemia or gangrene is related to iatrogenic intervention.[30, 58, 70, 104] When this type of direct arterial injury is the cause of extremity gangrene, the limb can be watched for only 6–8 hours at the maximum. The detailed methods for evaluation and treatment are in the chapter on arterial injury (see Chap. 25).

Figure 153–6 depicts our method of observation and intervention in children with extremity ischemia following arterial insult.

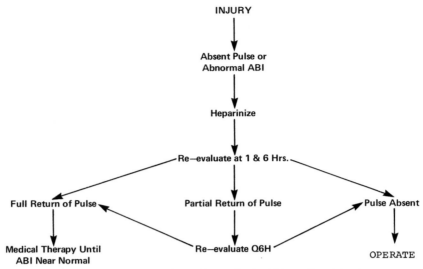

INJURY

↓

**Absent Pulse or
Abnormal ABI**

↓

Heparinize

↓

Re—evaluate at 1 & 6 Hrs.

Full Return of Pulse   **Partial Return of Pulse**   **Pulse Absent**

**Medical Therapy Until
ABI Near Normal**   **Re—evaluate Q6H**   **OPERATE**

Fig 153–6.—Algorithm for decision making in children with peripheral ischemia (*ABI* indicates ankle-brachial index; *Q6H,* every six hours.)

Its purpose is to differentiate spasm from mechanical injury. A patient whose pulse does not return after cardiac catheterization, or any arterial puncture, is immediately heparinized (1–3 mg/kg), unless there is some contraindication, like suspected bleeding. A careful search is then made for palpable or Doppler pulses.[142] The blood pressure in both the arm and leg is recorded. The Ankle-Brachial Index (ABI) is calculated by dividing the blood pressure in the ankle by the blood pressure in the arm. The index should be 1.0. If the leg is the affected limb, then an index of less than 0.9 suggests truly impaired flow. A ratio of greater than 1.1 is suggestive of upper-extremity arterial injury.[24, 119]

The pulses and pressures are measured again at 1 and 6 hours. If the pulses have not returned by 6 hours, operation is usually undertaken. If the pulses do reappear, then spasm is the likely diagnosis; and the heparin is continued for 2–4 days until the index is near normal. We have no experience with urokinase or

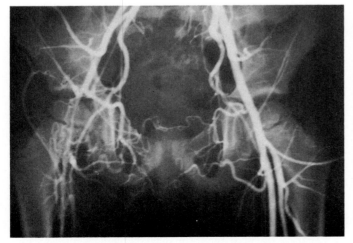

Fig 153–7.—Femoral artery occlusion after cardiac catheterization. Angiogram of right iliac artery several years after cutdown for cardiac catheterization. There is reconstitution of the femoral artery. Surgical reconstruction resulted in a minor increase in leg length.

streptokinase, but lytic therapy may play a role in selected patients.

Operative Technique

Although operation would seem the ideal treatment at this point, repair of very small vessels is not routinely successful. For this reason, we watch children under 5 kg longer than 6–8 hours. Fortunately, most peripheral ischemia in these small patients is self-limiting.[71, 84] We do have experience with two neonates who had plastic catheters break loose and pass into the leg. The aorta in these infants was successfully opened and the catheters removed (see Fig 153–1). This suggests that while arterial surgery below the inguinal crease may be difficult or impossible in the small neonate because of the tiny size of the involved vessel, one can consider aortotomy and thrombectomy in selected cases.[54, 55, 110, 116, 117, 128-130] In larger infants or children, surgical treatment may include resection with spatulated end-to-end anastomosis; local angioplasty, with or without a vein patch; or, if the site of the injury is near the elbow, groin, or knee, a reversed vein interposition. The details of these procedures are described in Chapter 25.

All patients are evaluated for compartment compression syndromes. Fasciotomy, with or without fibulectomy, should be performed early in those patients showing true compartment compression. Late fasciotomy has little positive effect.[29]

Children who have had peripheral ischemia must be followed for many years.[28, 32, 33] Signs of chronic vascular insufficiency may be manifest only as leg length discrepancies, slight muscle wasting, decreased pulses, or growth plate abnormalities on x-ray film.[79] Leg length discrepancies can be treated occasionally with further arterial reconstructions (Fig 153–7),[7, 65, 115, 140] or by orthopedic procedures to lengthen the involved extremity or reduce the length of the contralateral extremity.[64, 89]

Amputation is normally deferred as long as nondefinitive therapy does not threaten the patient's life or well-being.[30, 133] Because the skin loss is usually greater than the deep muscle and bone loss, the final level of amputation is distal to what might be first thought when looking at the involved skin. A most distal amputation can be done 2–6 weeks after resolution of the acute phase of the disease, and the end-result in such a child will often be a surprisingly useful extremity. Even in high thigh amputations, with early weight-bearing the results are usually quite gratifying (see Fig 153–4). [53, 124, 126, 127]

Results

Most arterial insults are iatrogenic, occur in a hospital, and usually are in the lower extremity. [30] The incidence of injury is higher in younger patients whose vessels are smaller. O'Neill[104] reports a 77% success rate in 92 children after arterial reconstruction, and Flanigan et al. [30] report a 91% success rate. Both authors believe early and aggressive therapy is responsible for their good results.

If, however, the ischemia is not reversed by medical or surgical therapy, the patient is at risk for significant leg length discrepancy. [12, 30] Even so, there is no direct relation of the duration of ischemia, the ABI, or the severity of ischemia, to the final presence or amount of length discrepancy. [7, 12] Although some investigators have achieved significant leg length improvement following late arterial reconstruction in an ischemic extremity, others have reported limited new growth. [50, 62, 71, 140]

Summary

Improvements in techniques have reduced the likelihood of peripheral ischemia in children undergoing invasive maneuvers, but an increase in the frequency of these various procedures has resulted in an increase in the absolute number of compromised extremities. Early recognition of possible ischemia is mandatory, and with well-planned observation, a decision as to the permanency of the insult can be made in less than 6 hours. Aggressive medical and surgical intervention can lead to a normal, or near normally functioning, extremity in almost every instance.

REFERENCES

1. Abrams C.A.: Hazards of overconcentrated milk formula: DIC and gangrene. *JAMA* 232:1136, 1975.
2. Adams J.M., Speer M.E., Rudolph A.M.: Bacterial colonization of radial artery catheters. *Pediatrics* 65:94, 1980.
3. Adams J.T., McEvoy R.K., DeWeese J.A.: Primary deep venous thrombosis of the upper extremity. *Arch. Surg.* 91:29, 1965.
4. Alstrup P., Anderson H.J., Schmidt K.G.: Neonatal aortic thromboembolism: Surgical treatment and coagulation studies. *Dan. Med. J.* 25:261, 1978.
5. Anabwani G.M.: Idiopathic gangrene in Nairobi children. *East Afr. Med. J.* 51:547, 1974.
6. Barnes J.M., Choata J.: Arterial spasm: An experimental study. *Br. J. Surg.* 30:74, 1942.
7. Bassett F.H. III, Lincoln C.R., King T.D., et al.: Inequality in the size of the lower extremity following cardiac catheterization. *South. Med. J.* 61:1013, 1968.
8. Bauer S.B., Feldman S.M., Gellis S.S., et al.: Neonatal hypertension: A complication of umbilical artery catheterization. *N. Engl. J. Med.* 293:1032, 1975.
9. Bauman F.G.: Gangrene of the arm in a newborn infant. *Ned. Tijdschr. Geneeskd.* 114:1077, 1970.
10. Bergan J.J., Trippel O.H., Kaupp H.A., et al.: Low molecular weight dextran in the treatment of severe ischemia. *Arch. Surg.* 91:338, 1965.
11. Bergentz S.E.: Indications of the use of low viscosity dextran in surgery. *Acta Chir. Scand.* 122:343, 1961.
12. Bloom J.D., Mozersky D.J., Buckley C.J., et al.: Defective limb growth as a complication of catheterization of the femoral artery. *Surg. Gynecol. Obstet.* 138:524, 1974.
13. Bosch D.T., Kengeter J.P., Beling C.A.: Femoral venipuncture. *Am. J. Surg.* 79:722, 1950.
14. Braly B.D.: Neonatal arterial thrombosis and embolism. *Surgery* 58:869, 1965.
15. Bronson E.B.: A case of gangrene in a newborn child. *Trans. Am. Dermatol. Assoc.* 158, 1902.
16. Chamberlain J.L. III, Perry L.W.: Infantile periarteritis nodosa with coronary and brachial aneurysms: A case diagnosed during life. *J. Pediatr.* 78:1039, 1971.
17. Charkes M.D.: Purpuric chickenpox: Report of a case. *Ann. Intern. Med.* 54:745, 1961.
18. Chaudhuri A.K.R., McKenzie P.: Peripheral gangrene after measles. *Br. Med. J.* 4:679, 1970.
19. Childi C.C., King D.R., Boles E.T. Jr.: An ultrastructural study of the intimal injury induced by an indwelling umbilical artery catheter. *J. Pediatr. Surg.* 18:109, 1983.
20. Cohen S.M.: Accidental arterial injection of drugs. *Lancet* 1:361, 1948.
21. Comay S.C., Karabus C.D.: Peripheral gangrene in hypernatremic dehydration of infancy. *Arch. Dis. Child.* 50:616, 1975.
22. Corrigan J.J. Jr., Jordan C.M.: Heparin therapy in septicemia with disseminated intravascular coagulation. *N. Engl. J. Med.* 283:778, 1970.
23. Crawford S.E., Riddler J.G.: Anaphylactoid purpura and gangrene of an extremity. *A.J.D.C.* 97:198, 1959.
24. Currarino G., Engle M.A.: The effects of ligation of the subclavian artery on the bones and soft tissues of the arms. *J. Pediatr.* 67:808, 1965.
25. Dameshek W., Schwartz R.: Treatment of certain "autoimmune diseases" with antimetabolites: A preliminary report. *Trans. Assoc. Am. Physicians* 73:113, 1960.
26. Dinguois R.O., Goabb W.C.: Postinfectious intramuscular thrombosis with gangrene. *Plast. Reconstr. Surg.* 31:58, 1963.
27. Dohan F.C.: Gangrene of an extremity in a newborn infant, with review of the literature. *J. Pediatr.* 5:756, 1934.
28. Drapanas T., Hewitt R.L., Weichert R.F., et al.: Civilian vascular injuries: A critical appraisal of three decades of management. *Ann. Surg.* 172:351, 1970.
29. Ernst C.B., Kaufer H.: Fibulectomy-fasciotomy: An important adjunct in the management of lower extremity arterial trauma. *J. Trauma* 11:365, 1971.
30. Flanigan D.P., Keifer T.J., Schuler J.J., et al.: Experience with iatrogenic pediatric vascular injuries. *Ann. Surg.* 198:430, 1983.
31. Flanigan D.P., Stolar C.J.H., Pringle K.C., et al.: Aortic thrombosis following umbilical artery catheterization. *Arch. Surg.* 117:371, 1982.
32. Fogarty T.J., Daily P.O., Shumway N.E., et al.: Experience with balloon catheter technique for arterial embolectomy. *Am. J. Surg.* 122:231, 1971.
33. Fogarty T.J., Krippaehne W.W.: Vascular occlusion following arterial catheterization. *Surg. Gynecol. Obstet.* 121:1295, 1965.
34. Formanek G., Frenc R.S., Amplatz K.: Arterial thrombus formation during clinical percutaneous catheterization. *Circulation* 41:833, 1970.
35. Fredlund P.E., Göransson G.: DIC with peripheral gangrene complicating appendicitis. *Br. J. Surg.* 61:903, 1974.
36. Freed M.D., Keane J.F., Rosenthal A.: The use of heparinization to prevent arterial thrombosis after percutaneous cardiac catheterization in children. *Circulation* 50:565, 1974.
37. Gilbert E.F.: Gangrene of an extremity in the newborn. *Pediatrics* 45:469, 1970.
38. Gillespie D.N., Burke E.C., Holley K.E.: Polyarteritis nodosa in infancy: A diagnostic enigma. *Mayo Clin. Proc.* 48:773, 1973.
39. Glaun B.P., Weinberg E.G., Malan A.F.: Peripheral gangrene in a newborn. *Arch. Dis. Child.* 46:105, 1971.
40. Goetzman B.W., Stadalnik R.C., Bogren H.G., et al.: Thrombotic complications of umbilical artery catheters: A clinical and radiographic study. *Pediatrics* 56:374, 1975.
41. Gottdiener J.S., Ellison R.C., Lorenzo R.L.: Arteriovenous fistula after fetal penetration at amniocentesis. *N. Engl. J. Med.* 293:1302, 1975.
42. Greene S.I., Smith J.W.: Dopamine gangrene. *N. Engl. J. Med.* 294:114, 1976.
43. Gross R.E.: Arterial embolism and thrombosis in infancy. *A.J.D.C.* 70:61, 1945.
44. Gyde O.H.: Gangrene of the digits after chickenpox. *Br. Med. J.* 4:284, 1970.
45. Haller A.J.: Extremity gangrene following brachial artery catheterization. Presented at the Annual Meeting, American Academy of Pediatrics, Washington, D.C., October 1976.
46. Hamamoto Y., Nomura S., Kudo E.: Congenital gangrene: An autopsy case of peripheral gangrene. *Bull. Osaka Med. Sch.* 17:73, 1971.
47. Hammerer I.: The risks involved in the heart catheter examination: A retrospective evaluation of the complications after 700 examinations. IV. Vascular complications. *Padiatr. Padol.* 14:405, 1979.
48. Hathaway W.E.: Care of the critically ill child: The problem of disseminated intravascular coagulation. *Pediatrics* 46:767, 1970.
49. Hawes W.J., Biehusen F.C.: Thrombocytopenia and massive gangrene following varicella. *Clin. Pediatr.* 5:161, 1966.

50. Hawker R.E., Palmer J., Bury R.G., et al.: Late results of percutaneous retrograde femoral arterial catheterization in children. *Br. Heart J.* 35:447, 1973.
51. Hawkins L.G.: The mainline accidental intra-arterial drug injection. *Clin. Orthop.* 94:268, 1974.
52. Heffelfinger M.J.: Neonatal gangrene with developmental abnormality of femoropopliteal artery. *Arch. Pathol.* 9:228, 1971.
53. Heller G., Alvari G.: Gangrene of the extremities in the newborn: Occurrence of functional recovery. *A.J.D.C.* 62:133, 1941.
54. Henry W., Johnson B.B., Peterson A.L.: Left common iliac arterial embolectomy in the newborn. *West J. Surg. Obstet. Gynecol.* 68:352, 1960.
55. Hensinger R.N.: Gangrene of the newborn. *J. Bone Joint Surg.* 57A:121, 1975.
56. Ho C.S., Krovetz L.J., Rowe R.D.: Major complications of cardiac catheterization and angiography in infants and children. *Johns Hopkins Med. J.* 131:247, 1972.
57. Hoffman S., Valderrama E., Gribetz I., et al.: Gangrene of the hand in a newborn infant. *Hand* 6:70, 1974.
58. Hohn A.R., Craenen J.: Arterial pulses following percutaneous catheterization in children. *Pediatrics* 43:617, 1969.
59. Hohn A.R., Lambert E.C.: Continuous venous catheterization in children. *JAMA* 197:140,1966.
60. Hoyne A.L., Smoller L.: Gangrene as a complication of scarlet fever. *J. Pediatr.* 18:242, 1941.
61. Huxtable R.F., Procor K.G., Beran A.V.: Effect of umbilical artery catheters on blood flow and oxygen supply to extremities. *Pediatr. Res.* 10:656, 1976.
62. Jacobsson B., Carlgren L.E., Hedvall G., et al.: A review of children after arterial catheterization of the leg. *Pediatr. Radiol.* 1:96, 1973.
63. Jager B.V.: Noninfectious thrombosis of a patent ductus arteriosus: Report of a case, with autopsy. *Am. Heart J.* 20:236, 1940.
64. Jahnke E.J., Howard J.M.: Primary repair of major arterial injuries. *Arch. Surg.* 66:646, 1953.
65. Jahnke E.J.: Late structural and functional results of arterial injuries primarily repaired: A study of 115 cases. *Surgery* 43:175, 1958.
66. Jaiyesemi F., Effiong C.E., Lawson E.A.L.: Congenital gangrene of an extremity in a Nigerian neonate. *Clin. Pediatr.* 15:283, 1976.
67. Jorgensen L., Packham M.A., Rowsell H.C., et al.: Deposition of formed elements of blood on the intima, and signs of intimal injury in the aorta of rabbit, pig, and man. *Lab Invest.* 27:341, 1972.
68. Katz A.M., Birnbaum M., Moylan J., et al.: Gangrene of the hand and forearm: A complication of radial artery cannulation. *Crit. Care Med.* 2:270, 1974.
69. Keat E.C.B., Shore J.H.: Gangrene of the legs in disseminated lupus erythematosus. *Br. Med. J.* 1:25, 1958.
70. Kinmonth J.B., Simeone F.A., Perlow V.: Factors affecting the diameter of large arteries: Particular reference to traumatic spasm. *Surgery* 26:452, 1949.
71. Klein M.D., Coran A.G., Whitehouse W.M. Jr., et al.: Management of iatrogenic arterial injuries in infants and children. *J. Pediatr. Surg.* 17:933, 1982.
72. Klob J.: Thrombose Ductus botalli. *Z. Gesellsch. Aerzt. Wien.* 15:4, 1859.
73. Knowles J.A.: Accidental intra-arterial injection. *A.J.D.C.* 111:552, 1966.
74. Lahner T.: Behçet's syndrome and auto-immunity. *Br. Med. J.* 1:465, 1967.
75. Lawrence R.D., McCance R.A.: Gangrene in infant associated with temporary diabetes. *Arch. Dis. Child.* 6:343, 1931.
76. Lebowitz M.H.: Gangrene of thumb following use of plethysmograph during anesthesia. *Anesthesiology* 32:164, 1970.
77. Lee D.H., Sapire D., Markowitz P., et al.: Radiation injury to abdominal aorta and iliac artery sustained in infancy. *S. Afr. Med. J.* 50:658, 1976.
78. Levy G.: Gangrene of the newborn. *A.J.D.C.* 62:381, 1941.
79. Lim L.T., Michuda M.S., Flanigan D.P., et al.: Popliteal artery trauma: 31 consecutive cases without amputation. *Arch. Surg.* 115:1307, 1980.
80. Lloyd A., Kemball M., Fraser G.: Peripheral gangrene in infants and in children. *Br. Med. J.* 1:468, 1967.
81. Louis D.S., Ricciardi J.E., Spengler D.M.: Arterial injury: A complication of posterior elbow dislocation. A clinical and anatomical study. *J. Bone Joint Surg.* 56A:1631. 1974.
82. Mackereth M., Lennihan R. Jr.: Gangrene of the extremities in infants and children. *Angiology* 23:688, 1972.
83. Magri P.: Gangrene of a lower limb in a newborn infant. *Clin. Ital.* 20:1666, 1968.
84. Mansfield P.B., Gazzania A.B., Litwin S.B.: Management of arterial injuries related to cardiac catheterization in children and young adults. *Circulation* 42:501, 1970.

85. Maragos G.D., Greene C.A., Lombardo A.J., et al.: Sickle cell anemia with thrombosis and gangrene of all four extremities. *Nebr. Med. J.* 56:3, 1971.
86. Marsh J.L., King W., Barrett C., et al.: Serious complications after umbilical artery catheterization for neonatal monitoring. *Arch. Surg.* 110:1203, 1975.
87. Martin W., Shore B.R.: Juvenile gangrene. *Ann. Surg.* 88:725, 1928.
88. McKay R.J.: Diagnosis and treatment: Risks of obtaining samples of venous blood in infants. *Pediatrics* 38:906, 1966.
89. Meagher D.P. Jr., Defore W.W., Mattox K.L., et al.: Vascular trauma in infants and children. *J. Trauma* 19:532, 1979.
90. Mehta M.G.: Peripheral gangrene in infancy: Report of three cases. *Indian J. Pediatr.* 40:154, 1973.
91. Melam H., Patterson R.: Periarteritis nodosa: A remission achieved with combined prednisone and azathioprine therapy. *A.J.D.C.* 121:424, 1971.
92. Millar D.S., Sebeck R.: Gangrene of the extremities in infants subsequent to intravenous therapy: Report of 5 cases. *A.J.D.C.* 90:153, 1955.
93. Miller J.J., Fries J.F.: Gangrene due to simultaneous vasculitis in a mother and newborn infant. *J. Pediatr.* 87:443, 1975.
94. Mokrohisky S.T., Levine R.L., Blumhagen J.D., et al.: Low positioning of umbilical artery catheters increases associated complications in newborn infants. *N. Engl. J. Med.* 299:561, 1978.
95. Morse T.S., Rowe M.I., Hartigan M.: Purpura fulminans. *Arch. Surg.* 93:268, 1966.
96. Mortensson W., Hallbrook T., Lundstrom N.R.: Percutaneous catheterization of the femoral vessels in children. II. Thrombotic occlusion of the catheterized artery: Frequency and causes. *Pediatr. Radiol.* 4:1, 1975.
97. Mortensson W.: Angiography of the femoral artery following percutaneous catheterization in infants and children. *Acta Radiol. (Diagn).* 17:581, 1976.
98. Mustard W.T., Simmons E.H.: Experimental arterial spasm of the lower extremities produced by traction. *J. Bone Joint Surg.* 35A:457, 1943.
99. Mustard W.T., Boles C.: A reliable method for relief of traumatic vascular spasm. *Ann. Surg.* 155, 339, 1962.
100. Nabseth D.C., Jones J.E.: Gangrene of the lower extremities after femoral venipuncture. *N. Engl. J. Med.* 268:1003, 1963.
101. Nathan P.: Gangrene of the hand following intra-arterial injection of barbiturate. *Hand* 7:175, 1975.
102. Neal W.A., Reynolds J.W., Jarvis C.W., et al.: Umbilical artery catheterization: Demonstration of arterial thrombus by aortography. *Pediatrics* 50:6. 1972.
103. Noles J.A.: Accidental intra-arterial injection of penicillin. *A.J.D.C.* 111:552, 1966.
104. O'Neill J.A. Jr.: Traumatic vascular lesions in infants and children, in Dean R.H., O'Neill J.A. Jr.: *Vascular Disorders of Childhood.* Philadelphia, Lea & Febiger, 1983, p. 181.
105. O'Neill J.A. Jr., Neblett W.W. III, Born M.L.: Management of major thromboembolic complications of umbilical artery catheters. *J. Pediatr. Surg.* 16:972, 1981.
106. Osborne A.H., Cobden R., Harvey J.P.: Gangrene of infant fingers. *JAMA* 221:1278, 1972.
107. Papageorgiou A., Stern L.: Polycythemia and gangrene of an extremity in an infant. *J. Pediatr.* 81:985, 1972.
108. Patterson J.H.: Dextran therapy of purpura fulminans. *N. Engl. J. Med.* 273:734, 1965.
109. Powers W.F., Swyer P.R.: Limb blood flow following umbilical arterial catheterization. *Pediatrics* 55:248, 1975.
110. Raffensperger J.G., D'Cruz I.A., Hastreiter A.R.: Thrombotic occlusion of the bifurcation of the aorta in infancy: A case with successful surgical therapy. *Pediatrics* 34:550, 1964.
111. Rauchfuss C.: Ueber Thrombose des Ductus arteriosus botalli. *Arch. Pathol. Anat.* 17:376, 1859.
112. Rich N.M., Hughes C.W., Baugh J.H.: Management of venous injuries. *Ann. Surg.* 171:724, 1970.
113. Richardson J.D., Fallat M., Nagaraj H.S., et al.: Arterial injuries in children. *Arch. Surg.* 116:685, 1980.
114. Roberts F.B., Fetterman G.H.: Polyarteritis nodosa in infancy. *J. Pediatr.* 63:519, 1963.
115. Rosenthal A., Anderson M., Thompson S.J., et al.: Superficial femoral artery catheterization: Effect on extremity length. *A.J.D.C.* 124:240, 1972.
116. Rothstein J.L.: Progress in pediatrics: Embolism and thrombosis of the abdominal aorta in infancy and in childhood. *A.J.D.C.* 49:1578, 1935.
117. Rubenson A., Jacobsson B., Sorensen S.E.: Treatment and sequelae of angiographic complications in children. *J. Pediatr. Surg.* 14:154, 1979.

118. Rudolph N., Wang H., Dragutsky D.: Gangrene of the buttock: a complication of umbilical artery catheterization. *Pediatrics* 53:106, 1974.
119. Sahn D.J., Goldberg S.J., Allen H.D., et al.: A new technique for noninvasive evaluation of femoral arterial and venous anatomy before and after percutaneous cardiac catheterization in children and infants. *Pediatr. Cardiol.* 49:349,1982.
120. Salerno F., Collins D.D., Redmond D.C.: External iliac artery occlusion in a newborn infant. *Surgery* 67:863, 1970.
121. Schenck R.R., Gilberti M.V.: Four cases of extremity gangrene and irradiation. *Arch. Surg.* 100:729, 1970.
122. Schenken J.R.: Gangrene of the extremities associated with hyaline membrane disease. *Clin. Pediatr.* 12:285, 1973.
123. Sengupta S.: Extremity gangrene following intra-arterial injection of procaine penicillin. *Aust. N.Z. J. Med.* 6:71, 1976.
124. Shaker I.J., White J.J., Signer R.D., et al.: Special problems of vascular injuries in children. *J. Trauma* 16:863, 1976.
125. Shehadi S.I., Slim M.S., Dabbons I.A.: Gangrene of lower extremities in infants following acute gastroenteritis. *Plast. Reconstr. Surg.* 42:530, 1968.
126. Skovanek J., Samamek A.: Chronic impairment of leg muscle blood flow following cardiac catheterization in childhood. *Am. J. Radiol.* 132:71, 1979.
127. Smith C., Green R.M.: Pediatric vascular injuries. *Surgery* 90:20, 1981.
128. Smith J.W., Currarino G., Goldberg H.P., et al.: Gangrene of the extremities in the newborn and infant. *Am. J. Surg.* 109:306, 1965.
129. Stout C., Koehl G.: Aortic embolism in a newborn infant. *A.J.D.C.* 120:74, 1970.
130. Strokes G.E., Shumacker H.B.: Spontaneous gangrene in infancy. *Angiology* 3:226, 1952.
131. Talbert J.L., Haslam R.H., Haller J.A.: Gangrene of the foot following intramuscular injection in the thigh. *J. Pediatr.* 70:110, 1967.
132. Thompson S.A., Mahoney L.J.: Volkmann's ischemic contracture. *J. Bone Joint Surg.* 33A:337, 1951.
133. Turin R.D., Mandel S., Hornstein L.: Fulminating purpura with gangrene of lower extremity necessitating amputation. *J. Pediatr.* 54:206, 1959.
134. Valderrawa E., Gribetz I., Strauss L.: Peripheral gangrene in a newborn infant of a diabetic mother. *J. Pediatr.* 80:101, 1972.
135. Von Khautz A.: Spontane Extremitätengangrän im Kindersalter. *Z. Kinderheikd.* 11:35, 1914.
136. Waddell W.B., Saltzman H.A., Fuson R.L., et al.: Purpuric gangrene treated with hyperbaric oxygenation. *JAMA* 191:971, 1965.
137. Wagener O.: Thrombenbildung am durchagangigen Ductus arteriosus (botalli). *Deutsch. Arch. Klin. Med.* 89:625, 1907.
138. Welch K.J.: Gangrene of the extremities, in Mustard W.T., et al. (eds.): *Pediatric Surgery*, ed. 2. Chicago, Year Book Medical Publishers, 1969.
139. White J.J., Talbert J.L., Haller J.A.: Peripheral arterial injuries in infants and children. *Ann. Surg.* 167:757, 1968.
140. Whitehouse W.M. Jr., Coran A.G., Stanley J.C., et al.: Pediatric vascular trauma: Manifestations, management, and sequelae of extremity arterial injury in patients undergoing surgical treatment. *Arch. Surg.* 111:1269, 1976.
141. Wigger H.J., Brainsilver B.R., Blanc W.A.: Thromboses due to catheterization in infants and children. *J. Pediatr.* 76:1, 1970.
142. Yao J.S.T.: Arterial survey with the Doppler ultrasonic velocity detector, in Rutherford R.B. (ed.): *Vascular Surgery*. Philadelphia, W.B. Saunders Co., 1977.

Index

in femoral focal deficiency, proximal, 1457, 1473
tibia, in neurofibromatosis, 1503
ulna, in neurofibromatosis, 1503
PSEUDOCYST
meconium, 929
meconium ileus and, 850, 851*, 853*
pancreas, 170, 1092–1095
ascites and, pancreatic, 927
diagnosis, 1093
differentiated from omental or mesenteric cysts, 922
etiology, 1093
etiology, by age, 1093*
imaging techniques, 160*
pancreatitis and, 1095*
pancreatitis causing, chronic recurring, 1094*
posttraumatic, 1093*
radiography, 1093*
spontaneous resolution, 170, 1094
treatment, 1093–1095
peritoneal, after ventriculoperitoneal shunt, 1435
PSEUDODIVERTICULUM: traumatic esophageal, 671
PSEUDOHERMAPHRODITISM
female, 1363, 1368, 1370–1372
masculinization of external genitalia in, 1371*
patients raised as females, 1371
male, 794, 1355, 1363, 1369–1370
dysgenetic, 1370
etiology, 1369*
hypospadias repair in, 1379*, 1380
patients raised as females, 1370
PSEUDOHYPERTELORISM, 427*
PSEUDOLEUKEMIA, 940
PSEUDOMEMBRANOUS
colitis due to antibiotics, 87
enterocolitis, 970
PSEUDOMONAS
aeruginosa, 78
burns and, 226
cellulitis and, 81
cephalosporin and, 86
agammaglobulinemia due to, X-linked, 89
in anorectal injuries, 1044
antigen after burns, 227
in appendicitis, 993
in enterocolitis, necrotizing, 951
in pancreatitis, 1088
PSEUDOMONAS
lung abscess due to, 658
sepsis, 84
with ecthyma gangrenosum, 84, 85*
PSEUDO-OBSTRUCTION, INTESTINAL, 987–988
home parenteral nutrition in, 107
PSEUDOPOLYPS: in colon, 942*
PSEUDOPRUNE, 1193
PSEUDOPUBERTY: isosexual precocious, and granulosa-theca cell tumors, 1345
PSEUDOSARCOMATOUS FASCIITIS: of jaw, 509
PSEUDOTUMOR, 1429
cerebri, 217, 1429–1430
lung, inflammatory, 664
PSOAS SHADOW: right, absence of, 168
PSYCHOGENIC CONSTIPATION, 1039, 1040
PSYCHOLOGICAL
considerations
after burns, 228
in kidney transplant, 369–370

factors
in ulcerative colitis, 970
in undescended testes, 798
responses to trauma, 133
PSYCHOMOTOR RETARDATION: and renal transplant, 360
PSYCHOSOCIAL
consequences of radiotherapy, 249
principles, 125–126
PSYCHOTHERAPY: in enuresis, 1214
PT, 113
PTC DEFICIENCY, 114
PTERYGIA: congenital, 1484
PTOSIS, 407–408, 410*
blepharophimosis and, 410*
levator muscle action in, 411*
levator resection for, 409–410, 412*–413*
operation
frontalis muscle in, 410
procedures, 408–410*
in pineal region tumors, 337
preoperative examination, 408, 410*
repair with fascia lata, 410, 413*, 414*
PUBERTAS PRAECOX, 337
PUBERTY
melanoma and, 1495
precocious, 560
in choriocarcinoma, 1349
isosexual pseudopuberty and granulosa-theca cell tumors, 1345
in ovarian tumors, 1341
teratoma and, intracranial, 266, 275
testicular torsion at, 1331
PUBIC BONES: in bladder closure, 1230
PUBIS APPROXIMATION: in cloacal exstrophy, 767
PUBOCOCCYGEAL LINE, 1024, 1025*, 1027
PUBORECTALIS MUSCLE, 1038
PUESTOW PROCEDURE
in pancreas divisum, 1090
in pancreatitis, chronic relapsing, 1088
PUGHE, J., 1022
PUJOL, A., 1336
PULMONARY
(See also Lung)
artery (see below)
aspiration and gastroesophageal reflux, 714
atresia (see Atresia, pulmonary)
blood flow
acidosis and, 591
in atrial septal defect, 1393
hypoxia and, 591
bronchopulmonary (see Bronchopulmonary)
capillary wedge pressure, 37, 38, 138
cardiopulmonary bypass (see Bypass, cardiopulmonary)
circulation, physiology of, 591–592
complications
of achalasia, 721
of meconium ileus, 856
embolism (see Embolism, pulmonary)
function, and burns, 221
hemorrhage, 641
hypertension (see Hypertension, pulmonary)
infarction (see Infarction, pulmonary)
interstitial emphysema (see Emphysema, pulmonary interstitial)
lymphangiectasia, 1508, 1509
tuberculosis (see Tuberculosis, pulmonary)
valve stenosis, pure, 1390
valvotomy (see Valvotomy, pulmonary)

vascular disease and atrioventricular canal defects, 1394
vascular resistance, 58, 59
in atrioventricular canal defects, 1394
in patent ductus arteriosus, 1399
in patent ductus arteriosus, in premature infant, 1399
after pulmonary atresia correction, 1391
after pulmonary stenosis correction, 1391
in ventricular septal defect, 1394
vasoconstriction, 31
vasodilators, and diaphragmatic hernia, 592
vein drainage, total anomalous, 1387, 1392–1393*
cardiac, 1392, 1393*
infracardiac, 1392, 1393*
supracardiac, 1392, 1393*
supracardiac, correction, 1393*
vein obstruction, 1392
after Mustard procedure, 1388
Pulmonary artery
anastomosis in heart transplant, 385
aneurysm, 615, 639
atretic, and heart-lung transplant, 386
banding
in aortic arch interruption, 1410
in coarctation of aorta, 1405
in truncus arteriosus, 1392
in ventricular septal defect, 1394
catheter, 37
pressure, 37, 38, 138
acidosis and, 591
hypoxia and, 591
wedge, 37, 38, 138
wedge, and crystalloids, 43
rupture, 38
shunt (see Shunt, systemic-to-pulmonary)
sling
anatomy, 1412–1413
angiogram, 1416*
esophagogram, 1416*
hyperinflation of right lung in, 1414
management, 1417
symptomatic, 1413
tracheal stenosis and, 636
tracheobronchial compression due to, 644
tracheomalacia and, 624
valved conduit from right ventricle to, in truncus arteriosus, 1392
PULMONIC
atresia and noncardiac operations, 1396
stenosis (see Stenosis, pulmonic)
PULSE
Doppler, in peripheral ischemia, 1537
oximetry, 71
PUNCTURE
arterial, 32
cervical, second lateral, 1423
cisternal, 1423
lumbar, 1423
subclavian vein, for parenteral nutrition, 103
subdural, 1420, 1423
ventricular, 1423
PUPIL SIZE: in brain herniation, 213
PURI, P., 690, 794
PURPURA
anaphylactoid (see Schönlein-Henoch below)
fulminans, 1540, 1542*–1543*
Henoch-Schönlein (see Schönlein-Henoch below)
nonthrombocytopenic, 112
Schönlein-Henoch, 112